Clinical Nuclear Medicine

Clinical Nuclear Medicine

Fourth edition

Edited by

Gary J.R. Cook
Consultant
Department of Nuclear Medicine
Royal Marsden Hospital
Surrey
UK

Michael N. Maisey
Emeritus Professor of Radiological Sciences
King's College
London
UK

Keith E. Britton
Emeritus Professor of Nuclear Medicine
Queen Mary, University of London and St Bartholomew's Hospital
London
UK

Vaseem Chengazi
Chief
Division of Nuclear Medicine
University of Rochester Medical Center
Rochester, NY
USA

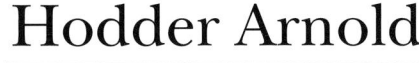

Hodder Arnold

A MEMBER OF THE HODDER HEADLINE GROUP

First published in Great Britain in 1983 by Chapman and Hall
Second edition 1991
Third edition 1998

This fourth edition published in 2006 by Hodder Arnold, an
imprint of Hodder Education and a member of the Hodder
Headline Group, 338 Euston Road, London NW1 3BH

http://www.hoddereducation.com

Distributed in the United States of America by
Oxford University Press Inc.,
198 Madison Avenue, New York, NY10016
Oxford is a registered trademark of Oxford University Press

*Hodder Headline's policy is to use papers that are natural, renewable and
recyclable products and made from wood grown in sustainable forests. The
logging and manufacturing processes are expected to conform to the
environmental regulations of the country of origin.*

Whilst the advice and information in this book are believed to be true and
accurate at the date of going to press, neither the author[s] nor the publisher
can accept any legal responsibility or liability for any errors or omissions that
may be made. In particular (but without limiting the generality of the preceding
disclaimer) every effort has been made to check drug dosages; however it is still
possible that errors have been missed. Furthermore, dosage schedules are
constantly being revised and new side-effects recognized. For these reasons the
reader is strongly urged to consult the drug companies' printed instructions
before administering any of the drugs recommended in this book.

British Library Cataloguing in Publication Data
A catalogue record for this book is available from the British Library

Library of Congress Cataloging-in-Publication Data
A catalog record for this book is available from the Library of Congress

ISBN-10   0 340 812397
ISBN-13   978 0 340 812396

1 2 3 4 5 6 7 8 9 10

Commissioning Editor: Sarah Burrows
Project Editor: Naomi Wilkinson
Production Controller: Joanna Walker
Cover Designer: Georgina Hewitt
Indexer: Laurence Errington

Typeset in 10/12 Minion by Charon Tec Ltd (A Macmillan Company), Chennai, India
www.charontec.com
Printed and bound in the UK by CPI Bath

What do you think about this book? Or any other Hodder Arnold
title? Please send your comments to www.hoddereducation.com

To all those around the world who have contributed and continue to contribute to educating the medical professionals and the public on the beneficial uses of radioactive materials in medicine and for society.

Contents

Colour plates appear between pages 168 and 169, and pages 488 and 489

Contributors	*xi*
Preface	*xvii*
Abbreviations	*xix*
Reference annotation	*xxiii*

SECTION A: CLINICAL TOPICS — 1

1. Molecular imaging — 3

    1A Molecular imaging — 5
    A.M. Scott, S.U. Berlangieri, and D.J. Macfarlane

    1B Peptide receptor imaging — 29
    D.J. Kwekkeboom and E.P. Krenning

    1C Radioimmunoscintigraphy — 39
    K.E. Britton and M. Granowska

    1D Monitoring treatment — 57
    R.P. Baum and V. Prasad

2. Principles of radionuclide therapy — 79
    K.E. Britton

3. The imaging of infection and inflammation — 93
    O.C. Boerman, C.P. Bleeker-Rovers, H.J. Rennen, W.J.G. Oyen, and F.H. Corstens

4. Pediatric imaging — 107
    I. Gordon

5. Sentinel lymph node imaging in clinical nuclear medicine — 121
    R. Allan, J. Rees, and R. Ganatra

SECTION B: CLINICAL SYSTEMS — 141

6. Functional imaging of cardiac disease — 145

    6A Functional imaging of coronary artery and congenital heart disease — 147
    S. Mahmood

    6B Left ventricular dysfunction — 183
    S.F. Barrington

7. Radionuclide imaging in thoracic disease — 195

    7A Ventilation perfusion imaging: a changing role for suspected pulmonary embolism — 197
    H.W. Gray

    7B Lung cancer — 223
    M.J. O'Doherty

    7C Other pulmonary applications — 239
    M.J. O'Doherty

8. Renal radionuclide studies   251

   8A Anatomy, physiology, and tracer handling   253
   K.E. Britton

   8B Non-imaging radionuclide assessment of renal function   269
   A.M. Peters

   8C Vesico-ureteric reflux and urinary tract infection   281
   L. Biassoni and I. Gordon

   8D Hypertension   297
   A. Hilson

   8E Obstruction of the outflow tract   305
   K.E. Britton

   8F Renal transplantation   315
   A. Hilson

   8G Renal tumors   321
   P. Shreve

9. Musculoskeletal radionuclide imaging   329

   9A Skeletal physiology and anatomy applied to nuclear medicine   331
   G.J.R. Cook

   9B Skeletal malignancy   337
   G.J.R. Cook and I. Fogelman

   9C Metabolic bone disease   355
   G.J.R. Cook and I. Fogelman

   9D Trauma and sports injuries   363
   H. van der Wall and S. Kannangara

   9E Radionuclide evaluation of the failed joint replacement   381
   C.J. Palestro

   9F Rheumatology and avascular necrosis   393
   P. Ryan

   9G Pediatric indications   403
   H.R. Nadel

10. Neuroimaging   413

   10A Dementia   415
   P.M. Kemp

   10B Functional imaging in cerebrovascular disease and neuropsychiatry   425
   R. Jayan and S. Vinjamuri

   10C Epilepsy   435
   S.F. Barrington

   10D Neuro-oncology   445
   R.B. Workman, T.Z. Wong, W. Young, and R.E. Coleman

   10E PET and SPECT imaging in movement disorders   457
   J. Booij, J. Zijlmans, and H.W. Berendse

11. Head and neck disease   465

   11A Head and neck cancer   467
   G.W. Goerres

   11B Salivary pathology   483
   G.W. Goerres

   11C Lachrymal studies   485
   G.W. Goerres

12. Endocrine disease   489

    12A Thyroid   491
    M.N. Maisey

    12B Parathyroid localization   511
    A.G. Kettle, C.P. Wells, and M.J. O'Doherty

    12C The adrenal gland   521
    R.T. Kloos, M.D. Gross, and B. Shapiro

13. The Breast and genital disease   541

    13A Breast cancer   543
    N. Avril, M. Bienert, and J.D. Schwarz

    13B Breast disease: Single photon and positron emission tomography   559
    J. Buscombe

    13C Testicular tumors   569
    S.F. Hain

    13D Impotence   575
    Q.H. Siraj

    13E Infertility   585
    M.P. Iturralde, Q.H. Siraj, and F. Hussain

    13F Testicular perfusion imaging   593
    Q.H. Siraj

    13G Gynecological cancer   601
    K.E. Britton and M. Granowska

    13H Prostate cancer   609
    K.E. Britton, M.J. Carroll, and V.U. Chengazi

14. The gastrointestinal tract   619

    14A Gastrointestinal bleeding   621
    P.J.A. Robinson

    14B Inflammatory bowel disease   629
    P.J.A. Robinson

    14C Functional studies of the gastrointestinal tract   637
    A. Notghi

    14D Positron emission tomography in gastrointestinal cancers   645
    G.J.R. Cook

    14E Gastrointestinal neuroendocrine tumors   653
    J. Buscombe and G. Gnanasegaran

15. Hepatobiliary disease: Primary and metastatic liver tumors   661
    R. Hustinx and O. Detry

16. Hematological, reticuloendothelial and lymphatic disorders   673

    16A Anemia and polycythemia   675
    R.W. Barber, N.G. Hartman, and A.M. Peters

    16B Imaging the spleen   685
    A.M. Peters

    16C Imaging of lymphomas   695
    L. Kostakoglu, M. Coleman, J.P. Leonard, and S.J. Goldsmith

    16D Lymphoscintigraphy   715
    A.M. Peters and P.S. Mortimer

17. Radionuclide therapy   725

    17A Thyroid disease   727
    S.E.M. Clarke

    17B Endocrine: Peptides   745
    M. de Jong, D. Kwekkeboom, R. Valkema, and E. Krenning

    17C Neuroblastoma   755
    C.A. Hoefnagel

    17D The skeleton   765
    V. Lewington

    17E The use of ^{32}P   773
    C. Parmentier

    17F The role of dosimetry   781
    G. Flux

SECTION C: TECHNICAL TOPICS   **789**

18. Pitfalls and artifacts in ^{18}F-FDG PET and PET/CT imaging   791
    G.J.R. Cook

19. Diagnostic accuracy and cost-effectiveness issues   799
    M.N. Maisey

20. Radiopharmaceuticals   813

    20A Introduction   815
    M. Frier

    20B Interactions and reactions   821
    M. Frier

    20C New single-photon radiopharmaceuticals   831
    S.J. Mather

    20D New radiopharmaceuticals for positron emission tomography   839
    E.M. Bednarczyk and A. Amer

21. Technology and instrumentation   847

    21A Solid state and other detectors   849
    R.J. Ott

    21B Image registration   861
    G. Flux and G.J.R. Cook

    21C Attenuation correction in positron emission tomography and single photon emission computed tomography 869
    D.L. Bailey

Index   881

Contributors

Rosemary Allan
St George's Healthcare NHS Trust
London
UK

Ahmed Amer
Drug Development Program
Department of Pharmacy Practice
University at Buffalo
Buffalo
USA

Norbert Avril
Department of Nuclear Medicine
St Bartholomew's Hospital
London
UK

Dale L. Bailey
Department of Nuclear Medicine
Royal North Shore Hospital
St Leonards
New South Wales
Australia

R.W. Barber
Department of Nuclear Medicine
Addenbrooke's Hospital
Cambridge
UK

Sally F. Barrington
Clinical PET Centre
St Thomas' Hospital
London
UK

Richard P. Baum
Department of Nuclear Medicine/Centre for PET
Zentralklinik Bad Berka
Bad Berka
Germany

Edward M. Bednarczyk
Departments of Nuclear Medicine, Pharmacy Practice
University at Buffalo, SUNY
Buffalo
USA

Henk W. Berendse
Department of Neurology
VU University Medical Center
Amsterdam
The Netherlands

Salvatore U. Berlangieri
Centre for PET
Austin Hospital
Melbourne
Australia

Lorenzo Biassoni
Department of Radiology
Great Ormond Street Hospital for Sick Children
London
UK

Maren Bienert
Department of Nuclear Medicine
Charité-University Medicine Berlin
Berlin
Germany

Chantal P. Bleeker-Rovers
Department of Nuclear Medicine
University Medical Center Nijmegen
Nijmegen
The Netherlands

Otto C. Boerman
Department of Nuclear Medicine
University Medical Center Nijmegen
Nijmegen
The Netherlands

Jan Booij
Department of Nuclear Medicine
University of Amsterdam
Academic Medical Center
Amsterdam
The Netherlands

Keith E. Britton
Cromwell Hospital
London
UK

John Buscombe
Department of Nuclear Medicine
Royal Free Hospital
London
UK

M.J. Carroll
Department of Nuclear Medicine
King's College Hospital
London
UK

V.U. Chengazi
Division of Nuclear Medicine
University of Rochester Medical Center
Rochester NY
USA

Susan E.M. Clarke
Nuclear Medicine Department
Guy's Hospital
London
UK

Morton Coleman
Department of Radiology, Division of Nuclear Medicine
The New York Presbyterian Hospital and
The Center for Lymphoma and Myeloma
Weill Medical College of Cornell University
New York
USA

R. Edward Coleman
Department of Radiology – Division of Nuclear Medicine
Duke University Medical Centre
Durham NC
USA

Gary J.R. Cook
Department of Nuclear Medicine
Royal Marsden Hospital
Sutton, Surrey
UK

F.H.M. Corstens
Nuclear Medicine Department
University Medical Center St Radboud
Nijmegen
The Netherlands

Olivier Detry
Department of Abdominal Surgery
University Hospital of Liège
Liège
Belgium

Glenn Flux
Physics Department
Royal Marsden Hospital
Sutton, Surrey
UK

Ignac Fogelman
Department of Nuclear Medicine
Guy's Hospital
London
UK

Malcolm Frier
Medical Physics Department
Diagnostics and Facilities Division
Queens Medical Centre
Nottingham University NHS Trust
Nottingham
UK

Rakesh Ganatra
Queen's Medical Centre
Nottingham University NHS Trust
Nottingham
UK

Gopinath Gnanasegaran
Guys and St Thomas' NHS Trust
London
UK

Stanley J. Goldsmith
Department of Radiology, Division of Nuclear Medicine
The New York Presbyterian Hospital and
The Center for Lymphoma and Myeloma
Weill Medical College of Cornell University
New York
USA

Isky Gordon
Department of Radiology
Great Ormond Street Hospital for Children
London
UK

Gerhard W. Goerres
Division of Nuclear Medicine
University Hospital Zurich
Zurich
Switzerland

M. Granowska
St Bartholomew's Hospital
London
UK

Henry W. Gray
Department Nuclear Medicine
Glasgow Royal Infirmary
Glasgow
UK

Milton D. Gross
Division of Nuclear Medicine
The University of Michigan
Ann Arbor, MI
USA

Sharon F. Hain
Clinical PET Centre
Guy's and St Thomas' Hospital and King's College
London
UK

N.G. Hartman
Department of Nuclear Medicine
Addenbrooke's Hospital
Cambridge
UK

Andrew Hilson
Department of Nuclear Medicine
Royal Free Hospital
London
UK

Cornelis A. Hoefnagel
Department of Nuclear Medicine
The Netherlands Cancer Institute
Amsterdam
The Netherlands

Fida Hussain
Nuclear Medical Centre, AFIP
Rawalpindi
Pakistan
and
Department of Nuclear Medicine
Royal Hospital Haslar
Gosport
Hants
UK

Roland Hustinx
Division of Nuclear Medicine
University Hospital of Liège
Liège
Belgium

M.P. Iturralde
Private Practice (retired)
Pretoria
South Africa

Radhakrishnan Jayan
Department of Nuclear Medicine
Royal Liverpool University Hospital
Liverpool
UK

Marion de Jong
Department of Nuclear Medicine, Erasmus MC
Rotterdam
The Netherlands

Siri Kannangara
Consultant Physician in Rheumatology
and Sports Medicine
Delmar Private Hospital
Dee Why
Australia

Paul M. Kemp
Department of Nuclear Medicine
Level D, Centre Block
Southampton University Hospitals Trust
Southampton
UK

Andrew Kettle
Nuclear Medicine Department
Kent & Canterbury Hospital
Canterbury
Kent
UK

R.T. Kloos
Departments of Medicine and Radiology
Divisions of Endocrinology, Diabetes and Metabolism and
Nuclear Medicine
The Ohio State University
Columbus, Ohio
USA

Lale Kostakoglu
Professor of Radiology
Mount Sinai Medical Center
New York, NY
USA

E.P. Krenning
Department of Nuclear Medicine
Erasmus MC
Rotterdam
The Netherlands

Dik J. Kwekkeboom
Department of Nuclear Medicine
Erasmus MC
Rotterdam
The Netherlands

John P. Leonard
Department of Radiology
Division of Nuclear Medicine
The New York Presbyterian Hospital and
The Center for Lymphoma and Myeloma
Weill Medical College of Cornell University
New York, NY
USA

Val Lewington
Royal Marsden Hospital
Department of Nuclear Medicine
Sutton, Surrey
UK

David J. Macfarlane
Queensland PET Service
Department of Nuclear Medicine
Royal Brisbane and Women's Hospital
Herston, Queensland
Brisbane
Australia

Shahid Mahmood
Nuclear Medicine and PET Centre
Mount Elizabeth Hospital
Singapore

Michael Maisey
King's College
London
UK

Stephen J. Mather
Department of Nuclear Medicine
St Bartholomew's Hospital
London
UK

Peter Mortimer
St George's Hospital
London
UK

Helen Nadel
BC Children's Hospital
Vancouver, BC
Canada

Alp Notghi
City Hospital
Birmingham
UK

Michael O'Doherty
Department of Nuclear Medicine
Kent & Canterbury Hospital
Canterbury
Kent
UK
and
Department of Nuclear Medicine
Guy's and St Thomas' Hospital
London
UK

Robert Ott
Physics Department
Royal Marsden Hospital
Sutton, Surrey
UK

Wim J.G. Oyen
Department of Nuclear Medicine
University Medical Center Nijmegen
Nijmegen
The Netherlands

Christopher J. Palestro
Albert Einstein College of Medicine of the Yeshiva University
Division of Nuclear Medicine
Long Island Jewish Medical Centre
New Hyde Park, NY
USA

Claude Parmentier
Nuclear Medicine Department
Institut Gustave Roussy
Villejuif
France

A. Michael Peters
Brighton Sussex Medical School
University of Sussex
Brighton
UK

Vikas Prasad
Department of Nuclear Medicine/Center for PET
Zentralklinik Bad Berka
Bad Berka
Germany

John Rees
Radiology Department
University Hospital Wales
Cardiff
South Glamorgan
UK

Huub J. Rennen,
Department of Nuclear Medicine
University Medical Center Nijmegen
Nijmegen
The Netherlands

Philip J.A. Robinson
Clinical Radiology Department
St James's University Hospital
Leeds
UK

Paul Ryan
Department of Nuclear Medicine
Medway Maritime Hospital
Gillingham, Kent
UK

Andrew Scott
Centre for PET and Ludwig Institute for Cancer Research
Austin Hospital
Melbourne
Australia

Joerg Dose Schwarz
Department of Gynecology
University Hospital Hamburg-Eppendorf
Germany

Brahm Shapiro
Division of Nuclear Medicine
The University of Michigan
Ann Arbor, MI
USA

Paul Shreve
Advanced Radiology Services
Grand Rapids, MI
USA

Qaisar H. Siraj
Department of Nuclear Medicine
Royal Hospital Haslar
Gosport
Hants
UK

Roelf Valkema
Department of Nuclear Medicine
Erasmus MC
Rotterdam
The Netherlands

Sobhan Vinjamuri
Department of Nuclear Medicine
Royal Liverpool University Hospital
Liverpool
UK

Hans van der Wall
Nuclear Medicine
Concord Hospital
Sydney, New South Wales
Australia

C.P. Wells
Department of Medical Physics
Kent & Canterbury Hospital
Canterbury
Kent
UK

Terence Wong
Department of Radiology – Division of Nuclear Medicine
Duke University Medical Center
Durham, NC
USA

Ronald B. Workman Jr
Department of Radiology – Division of Nuclear Medicine
Duke University Medical Center
Durham, NC
USA

Wen Young
Duke University Medical Center
Durham, NC
USA

Jan Zijlmans
Department of Neurology
VU University Medical Center
Amsterdam
The Netherlands

Preface

Clinical nuclear medicine continues to flourish as a result of the implementation of new techniques into the clinical evaluation of patients that impact on management and therapeutic decisions.

Since the previous edition, PET has become firmly established as a key clinical imaging modality and there is an emphasis on combined anatomical and functional imaging modality with PET/CT and SPECT/CT scannners as well as image registration techniques. These methods have become established in oncology, and cardiac, neurological and other applications are increasing. New SPECT and PET tracers continue to be developed to explore varied aspects of human physiology and biology and the discipline of targeted radionuclide therapy techniques continues to evolve and expand.

These new developments are of importance, not only for nuclear medicine, but also for a wide vareity of other disciplines, including the study of physiology and pathophysiology at a molecular level in both humans and animals. The ubiquity of these methods is a testament to the robustness of the radiotracer principle stimulating continuing advancement of radiotracers, techniques and instrumentation.

The text is structured in a similar manner to previous editions in an effort to describe relevant topics of current clinical importance rather than attempting to deal with all of the basic science. An initial section covers the broad principles and scope of important areas that are considered to impact more significantly on currrent and future clinical practice since the last edition. The second section covers the clinical systems where nuclear medicine influences clinical practice and a third section reviews a number of relevant technical topics.

In the drawning era of molecular medicine, establihsed and novel nuclear medicine techniques are firmly placed to ensure that this discipline remains at the heart of mainstream medical practice.

G.J.R.C., M.N.M., K.E.B. (London, UK)
V.C. (Rochester, USA)

Abbreviations

ACAT	acyl-CoA:cholesterol acyl transferase
ACD	annihilation coincidence detection
ACE	angiotensin-converting enzyme inhibitor
ACL	anterior cruciate ligament
ACS	acute coronary syndrome
ACTH	adrenocorticotrophic hormone
ADAM	2-((2-((dimethylamino)methyl) phenyl)thio)-5-iodophenylamine
AFP	alpha-fetoprotein
APA	aldosterone-producing adenoma
APC	activated protein C
APD	avalanche photodiode
ARPKD	autosomal recessive polycystic kidney disease
ATN	acute tubular necrosis
ATSM (^{62}Cu-ATSM)	^{62}Cu(II)-diacetyl-bis[$N(4)$-methylthiosemicarbazone]
BAH	bilateral adrenal hyperplasia
BBB	blood–brain barrier
BCPA	bidirectional cavo-pulmonary anastomosis
BGO	bismuth germanate
BMD	bone mineral density
BNP	B-type natriuretic peptide
BRASS	brain registration and analysis of SPECT studies
BSA	body surface area
C5a	complement factor 5a
CABBS	computer assisted blood background subtraction
CABG	coronary artery bypass graft
CAD	coronary artery disease
CAPD	chronic ambulatory peritoneal dialysis
CBF	cerebral blood flow
CCD	charged coupled device
CCK	cholecystokinin
CEA	carcino-embryonic antigen
CEA	cost-effectiveness analysis
CHD	congenital heart disease
CMR	complete metabolic response
CNH	cortical nodular hyperplasia
CNS	central nervous system
cps	counts per second
CRH	corticotropin-releasing hormone
CRMO	chronic recurrent multifocal osteomyelitis
CSF	colony stimulating factor
CT	computed tomography
CTPA	computed tomography pulmonary angiography
CVR	cerebrovascular reserve
CZT	cadmium zinc telluride
DCIS	ductal carcinoma *in situ*
DHEA	dehydroepiandrosterone
DIC	disseminated intravascular coagulation
DISIDA	diisopropylphenyl-carboxymethyl iminodiacetic acid
DLB	dementia of the Lewy body type
DLBCL	diffuse large B-cell NHL (q.v.)
DMSA	dimercaptosuccinic acid
DOTATOC	1,4,7,10-tetra-azacyclododecan-4,7,10-tricarboxy-methyl-1-yl-acetyl-D-Phe^1-Tyr^3-octreotide
DRF	differential renal function
DTBZ	dihydrotetrabenazine
DTPA	diethylenetriaminepentaacetic acid
DVT	deep vein thrombosis
DXA	dual-energy X-ray absorptiometry
ECD	L,L-ethyl cysteinate dimer
ECFV	extra-cellular fluid volume
Echo (or ECHO)	echocardiography
EDE	effective dose equivalent
EDTA	ethylenediaminetetraacetic acid
EDV	end diastolic volume
EECP	enhanced external counter pulsation
EF	ejection fraction
ELND	elective lymph node dissection
EORTC	European Organisation for Research and Treatment of Cancer
ERPF	effective renal plasma flow
f-Met-Leu-Phe	formyl-methionyl-leucyl-phenylalanine
FCH	fluorocholine (can have [^{18}F] fluorocholine, ^{18}F-FCH)

FDA	Food and Drug Administration (*in the USA*)
FDG	fluorodeoxyglucose
FHMA	ferric hydroxide macro-aggregates
FLT	fluorothymidine (can have [^{18}F] fluorothymidine, ^{18}F-FLT)
FMISO	fluoromisonidazole
FMRI	functional MRI
FNA	fine-needle aspiration (*in cytology*)
FoV	field of view
FRC	functional residual capacity
FTD	fronto-temporal dementia
5-FU	5-fluorouracil
FUO	fever of unknown origin
FUR	functional uptake rate
FvFTD	frontal varient of FTD
FWHM	full width at half maximum
GABA	gamma-aminobutyric acid
GADOX	gadolinium oxyorthosilicate, Gd$_2$O$_2$S (*also* GSO)
GAG	glycosaminoglycan
GBM	glioblastoma multiforme
GEP	gastro-entero-pancreatic
GFR	glomeruler filtration rate
GISTs	gastrointestinal stomach tumors
G-6-PD	glucose-6-phosphate dehydrogenase
GRD	gross residual disease
GRP	gastrin-releasing peptide
GSA	^{99m}Tc-DTPA-galactosyl-neoglyco-albumin
GSO	gadolinium oxyorthosilicate, Gd$_2$O$_2$S (*also* GADOX)
GTV	gross tumor volume
HAART	highly active antiretroviral therapy
HCG	human choriogonadotrophin
HD	Hodgkin's disease
HDL	high-density lipoprotein
HDP	hexamethylene diphosphonate
HDRBCs	heat-damaged red blood cells
HI	harmonics imaging
HIG	human immunoglobulin
HMFG	human milk fat globule
HMPAO	hexamethylpropylene amine oxime
HNP-1	human neutrophil peptide-1
HNSCC	head and neck squamous cell carcinomas
HPGe	high-purity germanium
HRT	hormone replacement therapy
HYNIC	hydrazinonicotinamide
^{123}I-β-CIT	2-β-carboxymethoxy-3-β-(4-[^{123}I]iodophenyl)-tropane
^{123}I-FP-CIT	N-ω-fluoropropyl-2-β-carboxymethoxy-3-β-(4-[^{123}I]iodophenyl)nortropane
IAEA	International Atomic Energy Agency (*in Vienna*)
IBZM	iodobenzamide
IDAs	iminodiacetates
IHD	ischemic heart disease
ITP	idiopathic thrombocytopenic purpura
IUDR	5-iodo-2′-deoxyuridine
IVC	inferior vena cava
IVU	intravenous urography
IVUS	intravascular ultrasound
JM	juxta-medullary
kcps	kilocounts per second (or thousands of counts per second)
LABC	locally advanced breast cancer
LAO	left anterior oblique
LBM	lean body mass
LDL	low-density lipoprotein
LOR	line of response
LS	lymphoscintigraphy
LSO	lutetium oxyorthosilicate
LTB$_4$	leukotriene B$_4$
LV	left ventricle
MAA	macro-aggregated albumin
MAG$_3$	mercaptoacetyl triglycine
MAO	monoamine oxidase
MBF	myocardial blood flow
MCE	myocardial contrast echocardiography
MCP-1	monocyte chemotactic protein-1
MDCT	multi-detector computed tomography
MDD	major depressive disorder
MDP	methylene diphosphonate
MIBG	*meta*-iodobenzylguanidine
MIBI	sestamibi; hexakis-2-methoxy-isobutylisonitrile
MIRD	Medical Internal Radiation Dose (committee)
MLPS	mean platelet life survival
MPTT	mean parenchymal transit time
MRD	minimal residual disease
MRG	metabolic rate of glucose
MRI	magnetic resonance imaging
MRS	magnetic resonance spectroscopy
MRSA	methicillin resistant *Staphylococus aureus*
MRTP	molecular radiation treatment planning
mRNA	messenger RNA
MTC	medullary thyroid carcinoma
MTD	mature teratoma differentiated; *also*, molecular (or metabolic) tumor diameter
MTI	molecular (or metabolic) tumor index

MTV	molecular (or metabolic) tumor volume		ROI	region of interest
MUGA	multiplanar gated angiography		RPF	renal plasma flow
MWPC	multiwire proportional chamber		RSD	reflex sympathetic dystrophy
			SAH	subarachnoid hemorrhage
NET	neuroendocrine tumor		SAP	serum amyloid P
NHL	non-Hodgkin's lymphoma		SCC	squamous cell carcinoma
NIS	sodium iodide symporter		SKM	simplified kinetic model
NMDA	N-methyl-D-aspartate		SLN	sentinel lymph node
NMR	nuclear magnetic resonance		SLNB	sentinel lymph node biopsy
NORA	normalized residual activity		SMC	6β-selenomethyl-19-norcholesterol
NSCLC	non-small cell lung carcinoma (cancer)		SMD	stable metabolic disease
			SNR	signal-to-noise ratio
OCD	obsessive–compulsive disorder		SPECT	single photon emission computed tomography
OIH	ortho-iodohippurate		SPM	statistical parametric mapping
OSEM	ordered-subsets estimation maximization		SPN	solitary pulmonary nodule
			SRI	strain rate imaging; also, somatostatin receptor imaging
PAF	platelet-activating factor		SRS	somatostatin receptor scintigraphy
PAP	placental alkaline phosphatase		SSTR	somatostatin receptor
PCI	percutaneous intervention		SUV	standardized uptake value
PDGF	platelet-derived growth factor			
PE	pulmonary embolism		T3	triiodothyronine
PEM	polymorphic epithelial mucin		T4	tetra-iodothyronine
PET	positron emission tomography		TBW	total body weight
PHA	phytohemaglutinin		TDI	tissue Doppler imaging
p.i.	post-injection		Tg	thyroglobulin
PMD	progressive metabolic disease		TLE	temporal lobe epilepsy
PMMA	polymethylmethacrylate		TMAE	tetrakis-dimethylamino ethylene
PMR	partial metabolic response		TNF-α	tumor necrosis factor alpha
PMT	photomultiplier tube		TRODAT	[2-[[2-[[[3-(4-chlorophenyl)-8-methyl-8-azabicyclo[3,2,1]oct-2-yl]methyl](2-mercaptoethyl)amino]ethyl]amino]ethanethiolato(3-)-N2,N,S2,S2'oxo-1R-(exo-exo)]
PNET	primary neuroectodermal tumors			
PNMT	phenylethanolamine-N-methyltransferase			
PRRT	peptide receptor radionuclide therapy			
PSA	prostate-specific antigen		TSH	thyroid-stimulating hormone
PSMA	prostate-specific membrane antigen		2-D	two-dimensional
PSPMT	position sensitive PMT		3-D	three-dimensional
PTCA	percutaneous transluminal coronary angioplasty		UHMW	ultra-high molecular weight
PTSM (64Cu-PTSM)	64Cu-pyruvaldehyde-bis(4N-methylthiosemicarbazone)		VEGF	vascular endothelial growth factor
PTTI	parenchymal transit time index		VLA	vertical long axis
PTV	planning target volume		VNA	vanillyl mandelic acid
PUO	Pyrexid of unknown origin		VOI	volume of interest
			VRI	visual response index
QALY	quality adjusted life years		VRS	visual response score
			VTE	venous thromboembolism
RBC	red blood cell		VTT	vascular transit time
rCBF	regional cerebral blood flow			
RF	relative function		WHO	World Health Organization
rhTSH	recombinant human TSH (q.v.)		WKTT	whole-kidney transit time
RNV	radionuclide ventriculography = MUGA (q.v.)		WLE	wide local excision

Reference annotation

The reference lists are annotated, where appropriate, to guide readers to primary articles, key review papers, and management guidelines, as follows:

- ● Seminal primary article
- ◆ Key review paper
- ✳ First formal publication of a management guideline

We hope that this feature will render extensive lists of references more useful to the reader and will help to encourage self-directed learning among both trainees and practicing physicians.

SECTION A

Clinical Topics

1. Molecular imaging   3

    1A Molecular imaging   5
    A.M. Scott, S.U. Berlangieri, and D.J. Macfarlane

    1B Peptide receptor imaging   29
    D.J. Kwekkeboom and E.P. Krenning

    1C Radioimmunoscintigraphy   39
    K.E. Britton and M. Granowska

    1D Monitoring treatment   57
    R.P. Baum and V. Prasad

2. Principles of radionuclide therapy   79
    K.E. Britton

3. The imaging of infection and inflammation   93
    O.C. Boerman, C.P. Bleeker-Rovers, H.J. Rennen, W.J.G. Oyen, and F.H. Corstens

4. Pediatric imaging   107
    I. Gordon

5. Sentinel lymph node imaging in clinical nuclear medicine   121
    R. Allan, J. Rees, and R. Ganatra

1

Molecular imaging

1A Molecular imaging

Overview	5	Molecular imaging in non-oncology applications	18
Molecular imaging methods and descriptions	8	Conclusions	24
Molecular imaging in oncology	12	References	24

1B Peptide receptor imaging

Introduction	29	Peptide receptor radionuclide therapy	34
Somatostatin receptors	29	Other radiolabeled peptides	34
Scintigraphy	29	Conclusions and perspective	35
Imaging results in neuroendocrine and other tumors	31	References	35
Imaging results in other diseases	34		

1C Radioimmunoscintigraphy

Introduction	39	Humanized monoclonal antibodies	44
Cancer radioimmunoscintigraphy	39	The radiolabel	44
The antigen	40	Clinical protocols and data analysis	47
The antibody	40	Clinical studies	48
The monoclonal antibody	41	Colorectal cancer	49
Biological factors affecting uptake	41	Recurrent colorectal cancer	51
Quality control	43	References	52

1D Monitoring treatment

Introduction	57	Apoptosis, gene expression and therapy monitoring	69
Basic principles of therapy monitoring	58	Dedication	71
Role of positron emission tomography and basic nuclear medicine in monitoring tumor response to therapy	62	References	71

Molecular imaging

A.M. SCOTT, S.U. BERLANGIERI, AND D.J. MACFARLANE

OVERVIEW

The radiotracer principle, used for both *in vitro* studies and clinical *in vivo* imaging, was first reported by George de Hevesy in the 1920s. His pioneering work laid the foundations for nuclear medicine imaging techniques, which have been successfully applied for decades in a broad range of human diseases. Radiolabeled tracers enable the imaging of physiologic events noninvasively, and the vast array of new targets and signaling pathways identified as playing key roles in disrupting normal cellular function can be potentially identified and quantified through these imaging techniques.

The term 'molecular imaging' initially appeared in the medical literature in the late 1990s. Despite a clear definition the term rapidly became widely incorporated within both the medical vocabulary and organizational titles. One conceptualization of the underlying construct of 'molecular targeting' is '… the specific concentration of a diagnostic tracer or therapeutic agent by virtue of its interaction with a molecular species which is distinctly present or absent in a disease state…'.[1] Although this appears to be a robust definition, it becomes problematic when classifying an agent such as 2-[^{18}F]-fluoro-2-deoxy-D-glucose (^{18}F-FDG), as glucose uptake is a feature of virtually all normal cells. Increased uptake is characteristic of many tumors due to the over-expression of the GLUT-1 glucose transporters. On the basis of the above definition, FDG would not constitute a molecular targeting (imaging) agent, although some authors have claimed that the over-expression of GLUT-1 qualifies it for the title.[2] Increasingly, however, molecular imaging is used to describe imaging technologies that provide unique information about the function of cellular processes, and this may extend to any aspect of cell

biology, molecular biology, cell signaling and genetics. While some uses of this term have extended to laboratory detection systems, including gene array and microscopy techniques used for identifying protein expression, and nontracer imaging methods including magnetic resonance imaging/magnetic resonance spectroscopy (MRI/MRS) and optical imaging, tracer-based imaging has a unique ability to quantify biological processes in living organisms.[3] There is also clear evidence that the development of new biomolecules requires sophisticated imaging techniques that are specifically designed for each new therapeutic.[4] Molecular imaging with tracers can therefore provide a link between disciplines and thus allow a cohesive pattern of normal and abnormal function to be identified.

When evaluating compounds for a molecular imaging strategy a variety of mechanistic factors need to be considered. These have been listed in Table 1A.1, broadly categorized as being relevant to ligand or target, although such a clear distinction is blurred by many of the factors being relevant to the ligand–target complex rather than its components. The pathophysiologic process involved in disease can also be identified and targeted, including blood flow, interstitial dynamics, trafficking within organs and cells, cell membrane kinetics, hypoxia and metabolic processes (ranging from glucose, to amino acids and proliferation, fatty acids and phosphoproteins).

The classic tracer approach to receptor targets involves the labeling of a tracer that simulates ligand that traverses the receptor cleft in a synapse (Fig. 1A.1). This is of tremendous importance in understanding the natural interactions of ligand and receptor in neurophysiology, as well as defining the role of altered binding kinetics in neurologic and psychiatric disorders. More recently it has become clear

Table 1A.1   *Characteristics of targets and ligands for molecular imaging*

Target	Ligand
Location	*Physical characteristics*
Within tissue	*Size*
Within cell	*Charge*
Membrane	*Lipophilicity/solubility*
Cytoplasm	*Radioisotope labeling*
Nucleus	*Delivery*
Accessibility	*Intravenous*
Perfusion	*Local administration*
Presence of barriers	*Vehicle, e.g. liposomes*
Capillary permeability	*Target binding*
Interstitial pressure	*Affinity*
Expression	*Specificity*
Density per cell	*Conformational changes*
Proportion of cells expressing	*Internalization of complex*
Conformation	*Biologic activity*
Biological modulation	*Toxicity*
Function	*Immunogenicity*
Physiologic	*Receptor activation/ blockade*
Kinetics	*Kinetics*
Metabolism	*Metabolism and catabolism*
Turnover rate relative to ligand	*Background clearance*
	Excretion

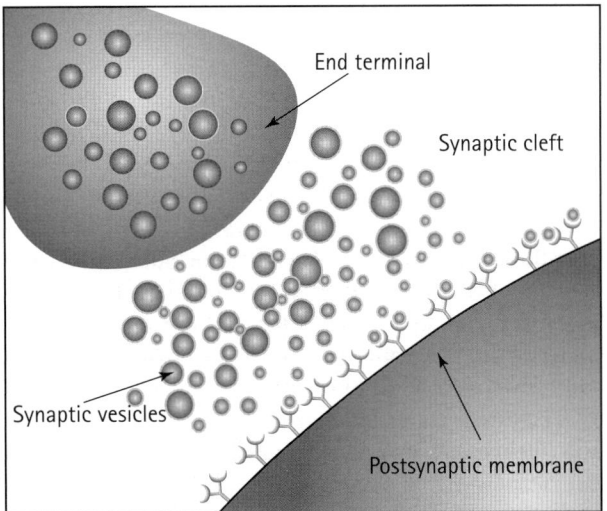

Figure 1A.1   *Diagram of a synapse. A neurotransmitter released from nerve endings traverses the synaptic cleft, and binds to post-synaptic membrane receptors.*

Labels on figure: End terminal; Synaptic cleft; Synaptic vesicles; Postsynaptic membrane.

that ligand–receptor interactions play a crucial role in many other disease states including diabetes and cancer, where receptor–receptor interactions and resistance to cognate ligand binding may have end-organ effects that promote disordered signaling, proliferation and cellular function. Receptor–ligand binding is, of course, only one facet of the possible molecular interactions that also extend to antigen–antibody, transporter–substrate and enzyme–substrate complexes. This may also extend to identification of altered conformation states of receptors which have implications in receptor activation and cellular signaling (including constitutive activation).[5] Although the classic definition of a receptor includes effector function upon ligand binding, with most imaging ligands biological effects are undesirable. For molecular imaging studies the quantity of imaging ligand is far below therapeutic levels, thus avoiding any adverse side events, and is specific for the target. Molecular imaging can allow identification of biochemical processes in normal and diseased cells and organs, and provide evidence of receptor expression that has implications in diagnosis and potential therapy, such as somatostatin receptor expression in carcinoid tumors (Fig. 1A.2).[6–8]

Trace-labeled peptides and proteins can be used for *in vivo* characterization of antigen expression suitable for targeted therapy approaches (Figs 1A.2 and 1A.3). In addition, trace-labeled infusions of antibodies can also provide dosimetry information that informs appropriate therapeutic doses required for radioimmunotherapy.[9,10] This has become an accepted methodology for confirmation of normal biodistribution of peptides/antibodies, and uptake in tumor, prior to therapy infusions. This is important for a number of reasons. Firstly, it identifies possible targeting of normal tissue which would lead to potential toxicity with a subsequent therapy infusion, therefore allowing patients to be stratified into modified dosing, or even not proceeding with therapy at all. Examples of this scenario include abnormal uptake in liver or spleen, or other tissues, that would impact on dose to those normal organs. Secondly, identification of uptake in tumor confirms antigen/receptor expression, which informs the potential for delivering adequate dose to tumor with subsequent therapy infusions. In view of the often heterogeneous nature of antigen/receptor expression in tumors, initial 'scout' imaging studies therefore provide confirmation of target antigen/receptor expression (*in vivo* immunohistochemistry) without requiring biopsy and pathology testing of samples. Thirdly, quantitative measurement of whole body clearance, and blood kinetics, as well as normal organ dose, can be performed from initial 'scout' infusions of radiolabeled peptide/antibody, and this dosimetry information may be used for actual dose calculation of the therapy dose. An example of this is the approved anti-CD20 mAb tositumomab (Bexxar™), where a 75 cGy whole-body dose (based on scout infusion) is used for therapy dosing in patients with non-Hodgkin's lymphoma.[9] These approaches are not confined to oncology, as the use of peptides/proteins to

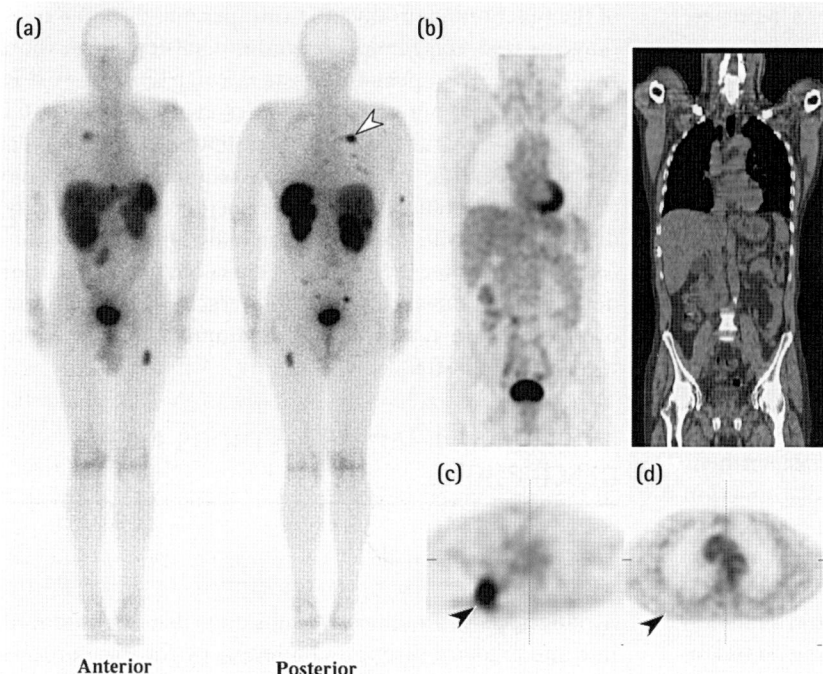

Figure 1A.2 *Receptor-based molecular imaging. A 56-year-old man with carcinoid presented with metastatic disease to liver, lung and bone which was somatostatin receptor positive on (a) planar and (c) SPECT ¹¹¹In-octreotide scan, but not metabolically active on ¹⁸F-FDG PET/CT (b, d).*

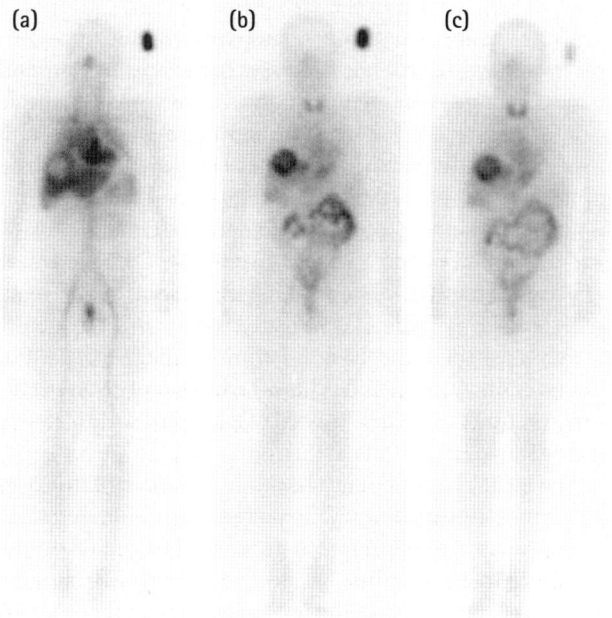

Figure 1A.3 *Biodistribution of ¹³¹I-labeled huA33 monoclonal antibody, which targets colorectal cancer. Anterior whole-body images are shown. (a) Initial blood pool image on day 1 of scout infusion of ¹³¹I-labeled huA33 in a patient with metastatic colorectal cancer, showing hypoperfusion of a large hepatic metastasis. (b) Day 6 following scout infusion, demonstrating specific uptake of ¹³¹I-huA33 in tumor. Central necrosis in tumor is evident. Some normal bowel activity is noted. (c) Biodistribution on day 6 following therapy dose of ¹³¹I-huA33, showing identical tumor uptake and organ distribution compared to the scout infusion.*

deliver therapeutic payloads can be used for many indications including cardiology (e.g. thrombosis and atheromatous plaque) and neurology (e.g. amyloid plaques).

Cellular signaling pathways have been shown to be key components of abnormal cellular function, and are often due to aberrant receptor activation. The identification of therapeutics based on specific signaling pathways checkpoints, or on active kinase domains of receptors, is one of the most active areas of drug development at present.[11] One approach has been to develop small molecules that bind to ATP pockets of intracellular kinase domains of cell surface receptors. These kinase domains act by phosphorylating key amino acid residues, which in turn lead to a downstream cascade of further activated molecules, and ultimately result in changes in cellular function such as proliferation, growth and apoptosis. Inhibitors of kinase domains of growth factor receptors have already shown clinical efficacy, and examples include gefitinib and erlotinib which inhibit the active kinase domain of the epidermal growth factor receptor.[12] Identification of kinase domains suited for small molecule inhibition, and particularly kinase mutations that may prevent efficacy, is a critical area where molecular imaging may play a role through trace labeling of substrate moieties, or downstream function activity (e.g. proliferation).

A further approach to imaging defined molecular events in living cells is through synthetic oligonucleotide constructs (aptimers and anti-sense fragments), which have been developed to bind target peptides and nucleic acid sequences. The expression of specific genes can be monitored by 'reporter genes'. In this construct the DNA sequence for the gene under investigation is spliced to that coding for a 'reporter', which may be a receptor or an enzyme.[3] Transcription of the target gene will be accompanied by transcription of the reporter, which can be detected by introduction of an appropriate ligand or radiolabeled substrate, which is potentially useful in monitoring gene therapy.[13]

The imaging of live cells has long been used in nuclear medicine for the diagnosis of infection, through labeling white blood cells with [111]In- or ^{99m}Tc-based oximes, as well as for blood pool studies in a range of conditions with ^{99m}Tc-labeled red blood cells. The advent of cell-based therapies for disease has expanded the use of molecular imaging to assisting with tracking cells to target organ sites, as well as monitoring pharmacodynamics of therapy *in situ*. Stem cells and progenitor cells have been used experimentally and in clinical trials to improve myocardial function after acute ischemia, and chronic heart failure.[14] The tracking of cells is an integral part of the assessment of successful delivery of cells to target areas and biodistribution. Cells can be labeled with tracers for single photon emission computed tomography (SPECT) and positron emission tomography (PET), as well as iron oxide particles for magnetic resonance imaging (MRI). Reporter genes have also been used for imaging (with PET) the successful transfer of genes to the myocardium.[14] Continuing challenges in this field include the optimization of cell selection and function, appropriate homing to myocardium, and effective myocardial functional improvement. In neurology, cell-based therapies are in clinical trials for the treatment of Parkinson's disease, and Huntington's disease, with some initial successes in symptomatic improvement.[15] PET has been used to monitor disease progression, and identify improvement in dopamine transport or glucose metabolism following stem cell treatment. Finally, the use of cell-based therapies in oncology is continuing to develop, particularly with blood-derived dendritic cells for vaccination strategies, as well as engineered T cells for direct tumor cell killing.[16,17] The tracking of cells with SPECT or PET tracers allows confirmation of functional trafficking to tumor or lymph nodes, and demonstrates the kinetics of retention in the target site, which can be used to evaluate the effectiveness of vaccination or cell homing. In addition, monitoring the metabolism of tumor can provide evidence of the functional outcome from cell-based therapy in oncology patients. Molecular imaging clearly has a major role to play in optimizing the development of cell-based therapies, and guiding future clinical trials.

Through an improved understanding of the fundamental basis of the human genetic code, combined with the relevance of transcription and protein expression (and post-translational changes), the mechanisms of normal cellular function can be studied. However, it has become clear that detection of a compound or compounds in an environment is insufficient, alone, as evidence of biological activity or interaction. This is exemplified by the genome, where the linkage between the presence of a gene and expression of the functioning product is a complex and dynamic relationship, and epigenetic changes and protein expression may be a more important link to cellular function.[18] It is through these approaches – genomics, transcriptomics and proteomics – that there is now the opportunity to develop new therapeutics, which in turn require more specific probes to detect and monitor cellular processes that typify disease, and may be modified by new 'designer' therapies.[19] As a consequence, the last decade has seen a rich vein of new potential imaging agents and targets, and the impact of molecular imaging in drug development continues to increase in importance.

MOLECULAR IMAGING METHODS AND DESCRIPTIONS

Tracers and ligands

A radiotracer is a radioactive substance that is introduced into and followed through a biological or chemical process by virtue of its radioactive signature, thus providing information on the course of the process or on the components or events involved. The introduction of this concept into modern scientific practice is identified as the seminal studies of ^{32}P disposition in the rat.[20]

Many nuclear medicine agents are physiologic radiotracers, following processes that are characteristic of normal tissues. Such processes represent the summation of multiple component steps involving both many gene products and often nonspecific physical processes such as diffusion. The input and output of the procedure can be quantified, but not the component steps within what is essentially a 'black box' (e.g. ^{99m}Tc-mercaptoacetyltriglycine (^{99m}Tc-MAG$_3$) renal scintigraphy).[1] However, the relationship between tracer uptake dynamics and organ function can be quantitatively measured and have a definitive diagnostic result, examples of which include characterization of renal perfusion and function (e.g. [99m]Tc MAG$_3$), biliary tract patency and dynamics (e.g. [99m]Tc DISIDA).

The term 'receptor' dates back to the work of Ehrlich in the early twentieth century. A modern definition describes a receptor as 'a molecular structure within a cell or on the surface characterized by (1) selective binding of a specific substance, and (2) a specific physiologic effect that accompanies the binding', and the partner 'ligand' as 'a molecule which binds to another, used especially to refer to a small molecule that binds specifically to a larger molecule' (Fig. 1A.1).[21] Although receptor–ligand studies have long been established in the neurosciences, it was only in the late 1970s that radiopharmaceuticals were being proposed to study changes in receptor concentration *in vivo*.[22] The first commercial agent in this class was ^{99m}Tc-diethylenetriaminepentaacetic acid-galactosyl-neoglycoalbumin (GSA), which is specific for the asialoglycoprotein receptor expressed solely on the surface of mammalian hepatocytes and used in assessment of hepatic functional reserve.[23,24] Commercial products such as ^{111}In-pentetreotide and ^{99m}Tc-depreotide (targeted to somatostatin tissue receptors), and ^{99m}Tc-apcitide (for the IIb/IIIa platelet receptor) soon followed, and a range of new diagnostic tracers are under development.

A variety of novel, complex techniques have been developed to accelerate the development of molecular imaging probes. In simple terms, these include:

- *Phage display libraries*, which involve mass expression of variable regions from antibody libraries using bacterial phage technologies. Fragments that react with the target are selected on the basis of affinity, and produced in quantity. They are then formed into low molecular weight constructs, usually either scFv or Fab.[25]
- *Aptimers* – artificially produced ≈10 kDa oligonucleotides with a three-dimensional (3-D) conformation allowing binding to target molecules, particularly proteins. This is a theoretically attractive technique, although the resulting molecules are relatively large, with limited stability and slow background clearance.[26]
- *Anti-sense fragments* – short oligonucleotide sequences can theoretically be produced with a very high specificity for a complementary sequence of DNA or mRNA. Disadvantages include a limited number of intranuclear targets, and tracer degradation by ribonucleases.[13,27]
- *High throughput screening of novel chemical libraries*, which although primarily used for identifying potential therapeutic molecules, can be used for defining imaging probes for precise intracellular signaling pathways.[28]

The development of new drugs is a complex process that takes tremendous resources and many years of effort. Molecular imaging is playing a major role in drug development through the identification and characterization of functional effects of drug activity, and trace labeling of the drugs to determine biodistribution *in vivo* can be a critical component of early drug development. While this approach has been successfully applied to monoclonal antibodies and peptides, the use of SPECT or PET tracers linked to new therapeutic molecules including signaling inhibitors and receptor-based drugs is being increasingly utilized.[8,29–31] The identification of biomarkers linked to disease is also an area of emerging importance, and may extend to novel imaging agents.[29,32,33]

It is clear that 'molecular imaging' is the focus of medical imaging research resources for the foreseeable future. When devising a 'molecular imaging' solution, the imaging paradigm and tracer selection should be selected on the basis of the biological question, rather than vice versa. The optimum imaging solution may require more than one component or modality. For use in drug development the relationships between the parameter being measured and the desired endpoint must also be clearly understood.[30]

Molecular imaging techniques

SPECT AND SPECT/CT

The detection of gamma rays emitted from radionuclides used for conventional nuclear medicine scans (e.g. [99m]Tc, ^{123}I, ^{111}In, ^{201}Tl) is performed using gamma cameras, which can acquire static (planar) images. When image data is acquired at multiple angles around the object of interest, a 3-D image is produced, and this technique is called single photon emission computed tomography (SPECT). SPECT imaging is an integral part of routine nuclear medicine practice, and provides the ability to identify and accurately locate physiologic processes.[34] The use of SPECT tracers that can identify receptor and antigen expression in tissue in neurology, cardiology and oncology patients is a key component of molecular imaging. Examples include detection of benzodiazepine and dopamine receptors, apoptosis, coagulation and infection (including cell-based trafficking), and peptides and antibodies directed against tumor associated antigens and receptors.

The introduction of SPECT/CT has had a significant impact on the interpretation of SPECT studies, by providing information relevant to the location of tracer uptake, as well as assisting in image registration (Figs 1A.4 and 1A.5). SPECT/CT has been shown to improve detection of disease and facilitate treatment planning particularly in oncology patients.[35,36] SPECT/CT can also be used for more accurate dosimetric measurement of uptake of tracers in organs and tumors, which can assist in treatment planning and assessment of therapeutic intent. In cardiology, the integration of blood flow information with CT provides improvements in attenuation correction and motion correction that assist with identifying viable myocardium.[37] Further studies are ongoing to explore the impact of SPECT/CT in patient management.

PET AND PET/CT

Positron emission tomography (PET) is an imaging technique that provides *in vivo* measurements in absolute units of a radioactive tracer. A scanner is used to detect coincident photons originating from an annhiliation event where a positron emitting isotope is located. One of the attractive aspects of PET is that the radioactive tracer can be labeled with short-lived radioisotopes of the natural elements of the biochemical constituents of the body. This provides PET with a unique ability to detect and quantify physiologic and receptor processes in the body, particularly in cancer cells, which is not possible by any other imaging technique.

The short-lived radionuclides (radioisotopes) required for PET are produced in cyclotrons. In PET clinical applications, the most commonly used positron-emitting tracer is ^{18}F-FDG.[38] The unique versatility of PET lies in the ability to study numerous physiologic and biochemical processes *in vivo*. For neuroreceptor studies, ^{11}C and ^{18}F compounds

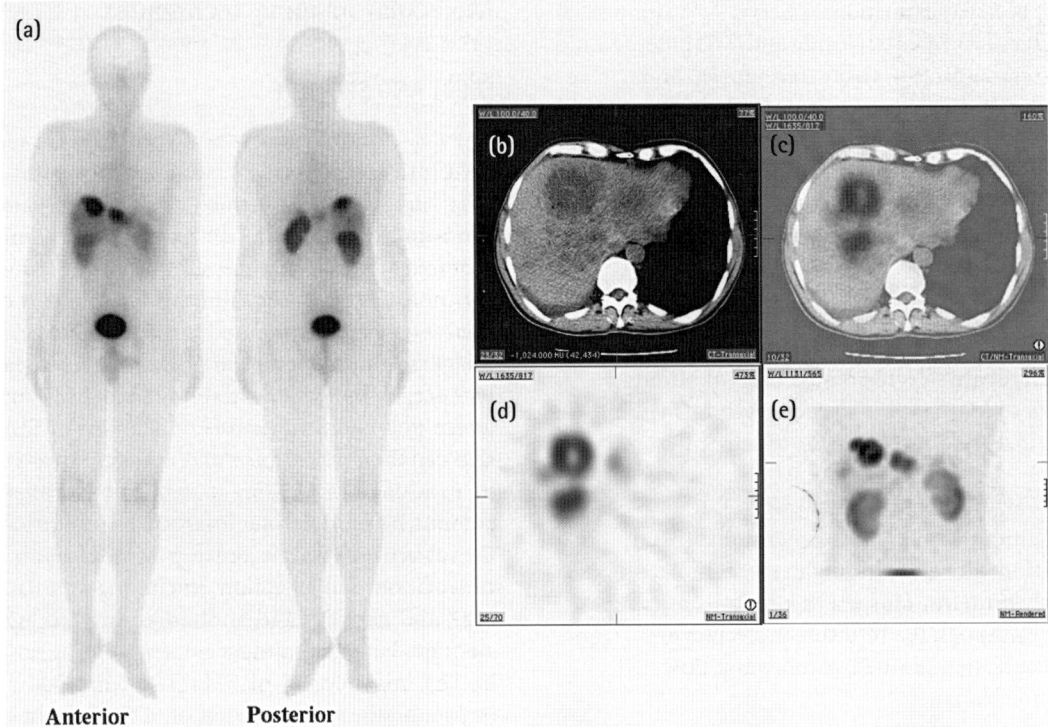

Anterior   Posterior

Figure 1A.4 *Receptor-based SPECT/CT molecular imaging. A 50-year-old man with metastatic carcinoid tumor underwent ^{111}In-octreotide SPECT/CT to determine the somatostatin positivity of liver metastases prior to consideration of therapy. Anterior and posterior whole body ^{111}In-octreotide scans (a) showed somatostatin receptor positive liver metastases, confirmed on (b) CT scan, (d) and (e) SPECT scan. Fused SPECT and CT images (c) confirm ^{111}In-octreotide uptake precisely corresponding to CT lesions.*

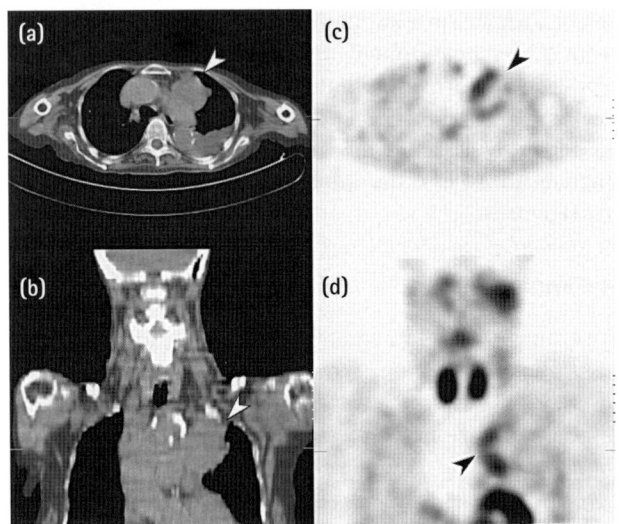

Figure 1A.5 *SPECT/CT imaging of a patient with hypercalcemia, who underwent a ^{99m}Tc-sestamibi scan (c) transaxial, and (d) coronal slices which showed incidental uptake in the left lung field (arrows, c, d). CT (a, transaxial; b, coronal) performed at the time as the SPECT, localized the activity to a left upper lobe pulmonary mass, suspected to be a pulmonary malignancy producing parathyroid hormone.*

Table 1A.2 *Commonly used positron-emitting radionuclides in clinical PET studies*

Radionuclide	Half-life
^{82}Rb	75 s
^{15}O	120 s
^{13}N	10 min
^{11}C	20.4 min
^{18}F	110 min
^{124}I	4.2 days
^{86}Y	13.6 h
^{64}Cu	12.8 h

are most commonly used (see Table 1A.4, page 21). The measurement of tissue blood flow, oxygen metabolism, glucose metabolism, amino acid and protein synthesis, nucleic acid metabolism, apoptosis and a broad array of neuroreceptor targets have all been demonstrated by PET. To exploit these physiologic and molecular targets, there are a number of positron emitting radioisotopes that have been used in clinical PET studies to date (Table1A.2).

The clinical role of PET has evolved considerably over the last decade. From its first applications principally in neurology and cardiology, the evaluation of oncology patients has become a pre-eminent clinical role for PET worldwide with oncology PET studies now representing almost 90% of clinical PET studies performed.[6,39,40] The dramatic rise in the number of PET oncology studies performed

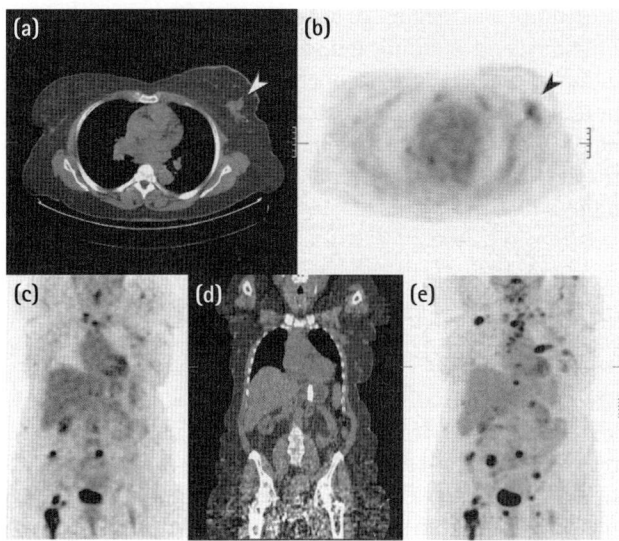

Figure 1A.6 *A 54-year-old woman with left breast carcinoma underwent a ^{18}F-FDG PET/CT scan. The breast tumor (arrow) is seen on (a) CT scan, and (b) ^{18}F-FDG PET scan. Whole-body PET/CT scans also demonstrate widespread metastatic disease (c, d, e).*

is related both to recent reimbursement approvals (particularly in the United States), as well as the increasing evidence for the role of PET in the staging, monitoring treatment response and biologic characterization of tumors. Cardiac PET remains an important imaging approach for the assessment of viable myocardium, and for perfusion assessment. The assessment of refractory epilepsy remains an important application of PET, and the evaluation of neurodegenerative disorders (particularly dementia) is an increasing area of clinical PET studies.

The development of combined PET/CT scanners has dramatically changed the approach to PET image interpretation, as the seamless integration of CT anatomic and PET images allows more accurate determination of abnormal sites of tracer uptake and potential clinical relevance (Fig. 1A.6).[41] The superior accuracy of PET/CT compared to PET alone has been reported in the assessment of many cancers including non-small cell lung cancer (NSCLC), colorectal cancer, lymphoma and melanoma.[42,43] Indeed, the area of PET/CT has emerged as one of the most prolific in prospective clinical trials and literature reports over the last 2 years.[40,44] PET/CT has impacted so significantly on the field that PET/CT scanners represented over 80% of all PET scanner sales in the US in 2005. One area of continuing debate regarding PET/CT is whether the CT should be used for attenuation correction and image registration (and thus a low mAs scan only is required), or whether a full contrast enhanced CT should be performed. Factors such as recent contrast enhanced CT availability, technical issues with performing routine contrast enhanced CT scans (and experience of operators), and cost-effectiveness of this approach are important issues that are guiding this debate. At the present time the vast majority of PET/CT

scans performed use CT only for attenuation correction and image registration. Further assessment of this technology, including the ability to integrate PET/CT data in radiotherapy treatment planning, is another area of significant importance for the management of oncology patients in the future.

In cardiology, the integration of blood flow and tissue metabolism with anatomic information of coronary artery position and blood flow are now possible with high resolution contrast CT and PET imaging. By acquiring dynamic, gated myocardial perfusion data, PET studies can provide insight into impairment of regional coronary blood flow reserve and microvascular endothelial dysfunction. Combining PET with multichannel CT angiography has the potential to provide information both on the presence and extent of anatomical luminal narrowing of coronary arteries, and the functional consequences of these changes, in one imaging session.[45] This technology is still at an early stage of development and implementation.

The use of PET/CT in neurology has some applications, although the principal anatomic modality remains MRI for the vast majority of neurological conditions. The early development of PET/MRI cameras is ongoing, and prototype systems for animal imaging have been reported.[46]

MRI, MRS, CT AND OPTICAL IMAGING

The analysis of cellular events and phenotype is an integral part of drug discovery, assessment of cellular trafficking, and response to drug exposure.[47] *In vivo* imaging of cellular and organ-based structure can be superbly evaluated with MRI, and recent advances in instrumentation and processing techniques permit additional assessment of physiology.[48] The development of a range of novel contrast agents, including nanoparticulate agents such as superparamagnetic agents, liposomes, perfluorocarbon nanoparticle emulsions, and dendrimers, permit the evaluation of lesion location and size, alterations in tissue structure, perfusion defects, cell migration and gene therapy.[49] MRI can also be integrated with MRS, which uses high magnetic fields and radio-frequency pulses to generate a nuclear magnetic resonance (NMR) spectrum which reflects the chemical environment within tissue. Nuclear magnetic resonance techniques are also opening new possibilities for imaging neurochemical events in the brain.[15] There are potential applications of MRI/MRS techniques in cardiology, neurology, oncology and infection for assessment of disease activity and metabolic characterization of cell function. The principal issues under development for functional imaging with MRI and MRS are the ability to quantify functional information, and the specificity for cellular processes.

The major recent advance in computed tomography (CT) scanning for molecular imaging is multi-slice 3-D image acquisition, which combined with contrast injection permits high resolution images of the anatomy and blood flow in major vessels (including coronary arteries).[50] High resolution images also allow unprecedented detail of organs such as CT colonography.

Optical imaging of fluorescence and bioluminescence in animal models allows the detection of luminescent probes induced in tissues through reporter genes or constitutive expression.[51] Cell-based therapies and xenograft experiments where cells have been transfected with luminescent probes (e.g. luciferase) can also be evaluated with this technique. This allows detection of cellular trafficking *in vivo*, and assessment of therapeutic interventions, without radiation exposure. Recent developments in instrumentation have resulted in improvements in depth of field and image resolution which have limited photonic detection techniques in the past. For optical imaging to fully realize its potential, further progress will be required in refining optical detection methods and data acquisition techniques.

Animal imaging

The ability to generate transgenic mice that have highly specific alterations in gene expression and phenotype creates enormous opportunities for understanding the pathophysiology of disease. Through molecular engineering techniques, genes can be removed (knock-out mice), added (knock-in mice), and there is also the ability to create conditional mutations and study gene dosage effects. The precise function of gene expression can therefore be evaluated, both for phenotypic effects as well as to study the implications of gene expression on the development of disease, and response to exogenous agents including therapeutics. More recently, this has extended to the use of gene silencing approaches using RNA interference which can prevent the in vivo expression of specific genes in transgenic mice, thus allowing confirmation of gene expression effects, and also potential therapeutic approaches in human diseases including cancer and infectious diseases.[52]

Molecular imaging has a major role to play in the characterization of transgenic mice through identification of the expression of receptors, and metabolism in organs. The use of bioluminescent markers expressed endogenously in mouse tissue can also be imaged and allow the pattern and temporal nature of gene/protein expression in live animals.[53] Immunodeficient mice can also be studied for assessment of organ/tumor metabolism, and therapeutic intervention (Plate 1A.1).[54,55] In addition, the response of animals to drug treatment can be directly imaged with SPECT/PET/CT/MRI and optical imaging techniques.[56] The biodistribution of novel compounds can also be accurately assessed using molecular imaging techniques allowing confirmation of stability and specificity of the compound in preclinical studies.[54]

The technology for imaging animals is similar to that required for humans, with the need for higher resolution being addressed through systems which combine functional and anatomic information (e.g. PET/CT, PET/MRI).[46,53,57]

The choice of imaging platform is based on the desired functional and anatomical information required. The evaluation of genetically manipulated animals or new designed biomolecules requires a thorough understanding of physiology, biochemistry and pharmacology, and molecular imaging has an important role in experimental approaches in these models.

MOLECULAR IMAGING IN ONCOLOGY

The role of molecular imaging in oncology traverses the breadth of cancer drug development, and patient management from initial diagnosis through to post-treatment monitoring. Tracer-based imaging techniques, principally involving SPECT and PET, permit the biologic characterization of tumors, and plays a key role in staging and restaging of disease, and monitoring therapy response. Through a greater understanding of the need for individual patient treatment planning based on tumor gene and protein expression profiles, and accurate staging information, molecular imaging plays an increasing role in treatment planning for patients. In addition, the introduction and success of new biologic therapies in oncology has created a need for accurate information on the precise biologic effects of therapy in individual patients, thus permitting alteration of treatment schedules and optimizing selection of drug therapy. Molecular imaging is perfectly suited to this requirement, and is increasingly being used to optimize treatment regimes in oncology patients.

Molecular characterization of tumors

Molecular imaging takes advantage of the phenotypic changes that occur in cancer cells to identify protein/receptor expression and metabolic changes that are specific for tumors or are over-expressed compared to normal tissue. The expression of specific receptors can be identified through imaging with SPECT and PET, allowing determination of appropriate treatment to be implemented. Examples of this include somatostatin receptor expression in neuroendocrine tumors, imaged with ^{111}In-pentetreotide and pheochromocytomas with *meta*-[^{123}I]iodobenzylguanidine (^{123}I-MIBG) (Figs 1A.2 and 1A.4).[58] Antigen expression in tumors can also be identified, and this information can be used to indicate the appropriateness of subsequent antibody-based therapy (Fig. 1A.3).[9,10] The grade of tumor can also be stratified with imaging, such as differentiation of low- and high-grade lymphoma with ^{18}F-FDG PET (Fig. 1A.7).[59]

The development of new biologic agents for tumors has also led to the need to characterize the receptor expression and signaling pathways in tumors, as well as metabolic changes, prior to therapy. As a result, molecular imaging of blood flow, proliferation, hypoxia and glucose metabolism

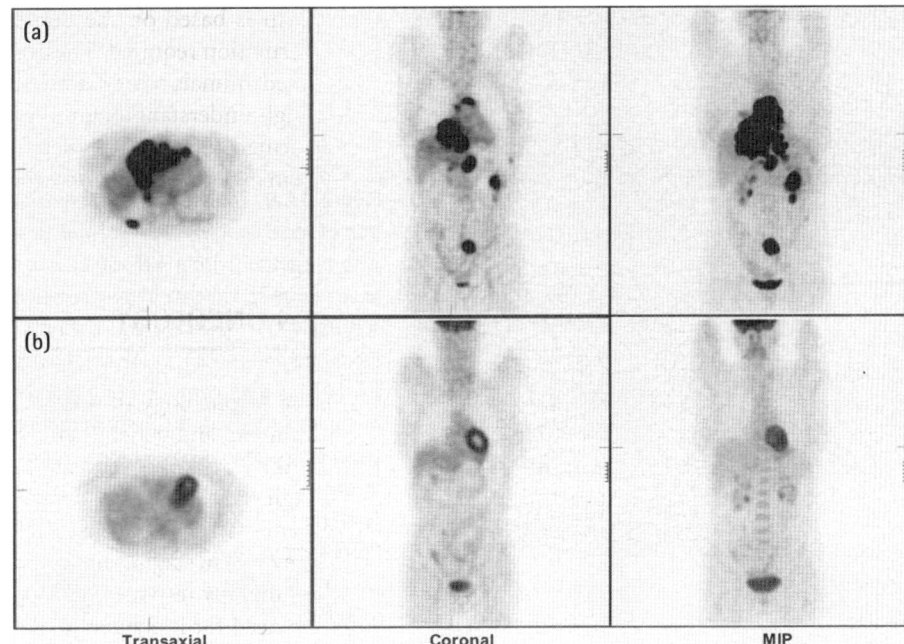

Figure 1A.7 *Staging and therapy response with PET. A 58-year-old woman with diffuse large B-cell lymphoma underwent ^{18}F-FDG PET at initial presentation (a) with ^{18}F-FDG-avid disease in the thorax and upper abdomen and following three cycles of chemotherapy (b) showing complete metabolic remission.*

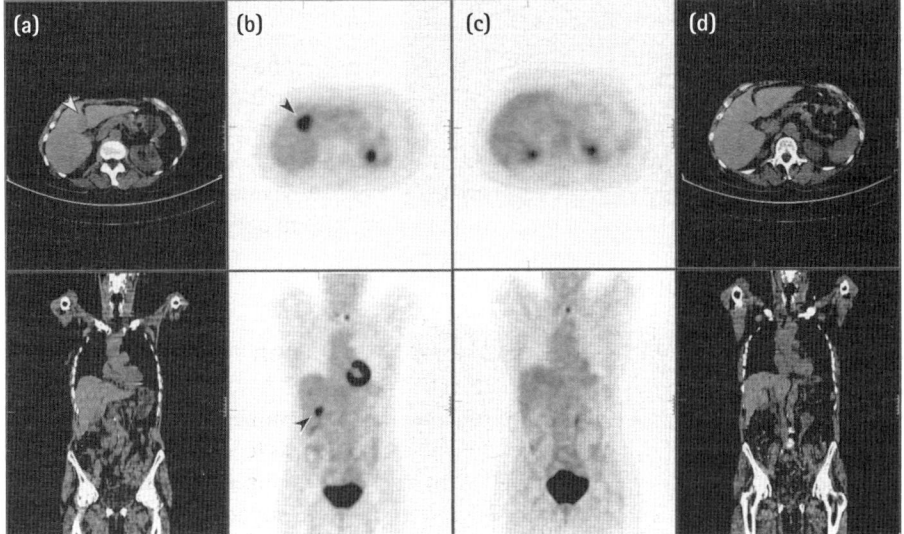

Figure 1A.8 *PET/CT assessment of therapy response. A 72-year-old woman with metastatic carcinoma of the colon to liver underwent ^{18}F-FDG PET/CT prior to (a, b) and following chemotherapy (c, d). The pre-therapy CT shows a low attenuation lesion in the liver (a, arrow) which is FDG-avid (arrow, b). On the post-therapy study (c, d), there has been anatomical and metabolic resolution of the hepatic metastasis.*

is increasingly required to facilitate optimal drug treatment (Figs 1A.8 to 1A.11). An example of this approach is the finding that tumoral hypoxia, assessed by ^{18}F-FMISO PET imaging, has been shown to be highly predictive of the efficacy of tirapazamine treatment in head and neck cancer.[60]

Prognostic information can also be obtained from molecular imaging, with the metabolic activity of tumors found to be a powerful independent predictor of prognosis and aggresive behavior of tumors in a range of malignancies including NSCLC, lymphoma, and esophageal cancer.[42,59,61,62] This application of molecular imaging is of considerable importance in being able to accurately stratify patients into high and low risk groups, and therefore assist in selecting treatment regimes that can produce optimal

outcomes of improved response and minimizing morbidity from futile and expensive therapies.

Staging and restaging

The accurate staging of tumors is dependent on both assessment of tumor, nodal spread and distant metastatic disease. The evaluation of tumor extent is of particular relevance to surgical resection, and both SPECT- and PET-based techniques may not be able to precisely identify the anatomical infiltration of surrounding tissues as accurately as anatomic imaging with CT, MRI or ultrasound (including endoscopic ultrasound). The principal role of SPECT- and PET-based

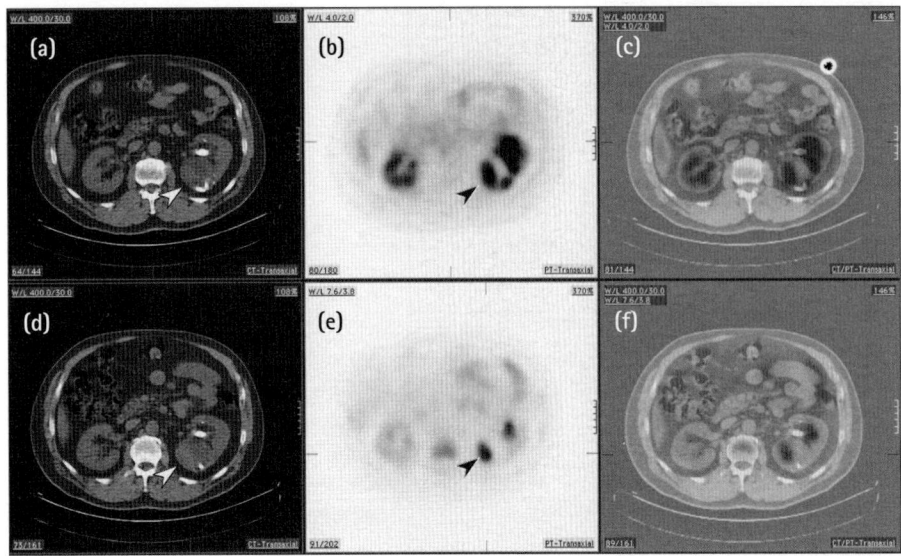

Figure 1A.9 *Molecular characterization of renal cancer. A 59-year-old man who presented with a left kidney mass (a, d, arrows) underwent preoperative staging with ^{18}F-FDG PET, which showed increased metabolism in the renal mass (b). PET imaging with ^{18}F-FLT, a marker of tumor proliferation, performed prior to surgery show increased proliferation in the tumor mass (e, arrow). Co-registered (c) ^{18}F-FDG PET/CT and (f) ^{18}F-FLT PET/CT images are also shown.*

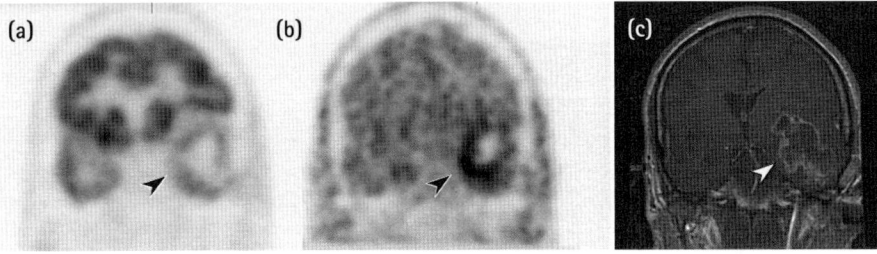

Figure 1A.10 *Molecular imaging of glioma. A 56-year-old man with glioblastoma multiforme in the left temporal lobe on MRI (c, arrow) underwent ^{18}F-FDG PET (a, arrow) which showed increased metabolic activity at the tumor margins. PET imaging with ^{18}F-FMISO, a hypoxic tissue marker (b, arrow) indicates significant tumor hypoxia along the medial temporal margin of the tumor.*

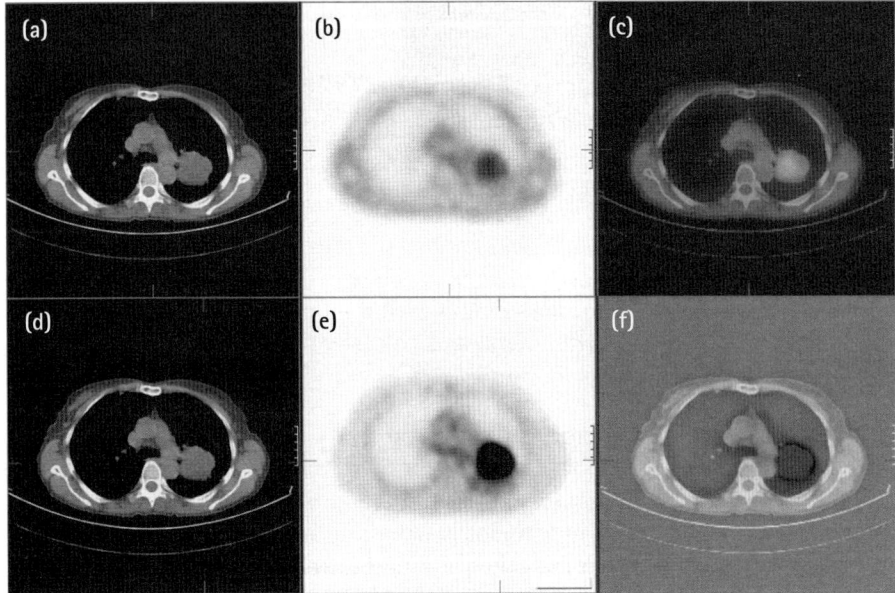

Figure 1A.11 *Hypoxia imaging of lung cancer. A 63-year-old woman with newly diagnosed left lung carcinoma on CT scan (a, d) underwent ^{18}F-FDG PET which showed intense uptake in the tumor mass (e). (f) Fused ^{18}F-FDG PET/CT image. (b) PET imaging with ^{18}F-FMISO shows moderate uptake indicating hypoxia in tumor. (c) Fused ^{18}F-FMISO/CT image.*

imaging is in defining the extent of nodal spread and distant metastases. The spread of tumor to locoregional lymph nodes may, however, be underestimated by anatomic and molecular imaging techniques due to the small size of metastatic disease – breast, melanoma, gastric and prostate cancer are examples of this. Sentinal node imaging has a pre-eminent role to play in assisting surgical identification of nodal spread, and preventing unnecessary

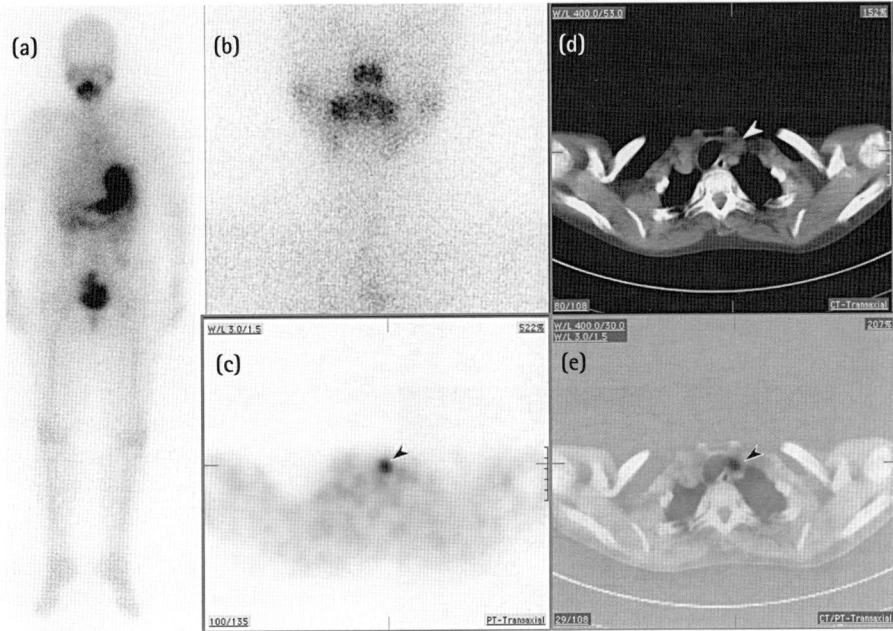

Figure 1A.12 *Molecular imaging of thyroid cancer. A 75-year-old woman with an initial diagnosis of papillary carcinoma of the thyroid with lymph node involvement, treated with surgery and radioiodine ablation, presents with a rising thyroglobulin and negative whole body* [131]*I scan (a, b). (c)* [18]*F-FDG PET shows a locally recurrent nodal metastasis (arrow), seen on (d) CT scan and (e) fused PET/CT scans, and subsequently confirmed at surgical resection.*

lymph node resection in a number of malignancies including breast cancer and melanoma.[63,64]

The staging of malignancies with planar and SPECT imaging has an established role in thyroid cancer, parathyroid tumors, neuroendocrine tumors, lymphoma and bone metastases (Figs 1A.2, 1A.4, 1A.5 and 1A.12). SPECT/CT has provided improved anatomic localization of lesions, and increased accuracy in diagnosis.[36] Although PET imaging with ^{18}F-FDG has shown advantages over gallium-67 citrate for lymphoma imaging, many centers still successfully utilize gallium-67 citrate scanning in the assessment of lymphoma patients. Conventional imaging may also be complemented by PET in some malignancies; in differentiated thyroid cancer lack of ^{123}I/^{131}I uptake in lesions showing positive ^{18}F-FDG PET often indicates a more agressive behavior of recurrent disase (Fig. 1A.12). In addition, while ^{18}F-FDG PET has a high sensitivity for bone metastases for a range of malignancies, conventional bone scans remain an important and sensitive test for screening for bony metastases in most cancer patients.

The principal role for clinical PET is in oncology. In most cancers, ^{18}F-FDG PET has been shown to be the most accurate noninvasive method to detect and stage tumors (Figs 1A.6, 1A.7 and 1A.8).[6,39,65–70] This has major implications in terms of improving the planning of treatment and avoiding unnecessary treatment and its associated morbidity and cost. High uptake of ^{18}F-FDG is not always seen in primary tumors, however, and many renal cell carcinomas, low-grade lymphomas, hepatocellular carcinomas and low-grade gliomas show low ^{18}F-FDG uptake. While a range of other PET tracers have been explored for the primary staging of malignancies, including ^{18}F-FLT, to date, virtually none have shown definitive improved sensitivity or accuracy compared to ^{18}F-FDG for primary tumor or spread of

disease. An exception to this is in glioma, where a range of tracers, including ^{11}C-methionine, has been shown to be accurate in defining extent of disease, and particularly characterizing low-grade gliomas.[71] In solitary pulmonary nodules, ^{18}F-FLT has been reported to have improved specificity for malignancy compared to ^{18}F-FDG, but the sensitivity is lower for primary and nodal spread, and histologic analysis of lesions is usually required.[72]

Evaluation of the evidence for PET in clinical oncology practice has, however, been complicated by the inherent diagnostic nature of this imaging technique. While standard evidence-based approaches to treatment require randomized controlled trials to establish the appropriate outcome or efficacy measures for assessment, imaging techniques provide information which is commonly used as only a part of the management paradigm of most patients. As such, the practical and ethical issues surrounding this make randomized controlled trials for PET extremely difficult to perform or inappropriate in the majority of clinical scenarios.[6,73] The establishment of diagnostic accuracy, and impact on patient management (including cost), are therefore the most appropriate levels of evidence that can be accurately obtained for PET in clinical practice.

Treatment planning

An emerging role of molecular imaging is in providing information that directly impacts on the mode of delivery of treatment to cancer patients. This can range from evaluation of the expression of receptors/antigens suited to biologic treatment, to the assessment of tumoral hypoxia prior to treatment with hypoxia-avid chemotherapy.[9,60,74] In addition, the ability of molecular imaging to accurately

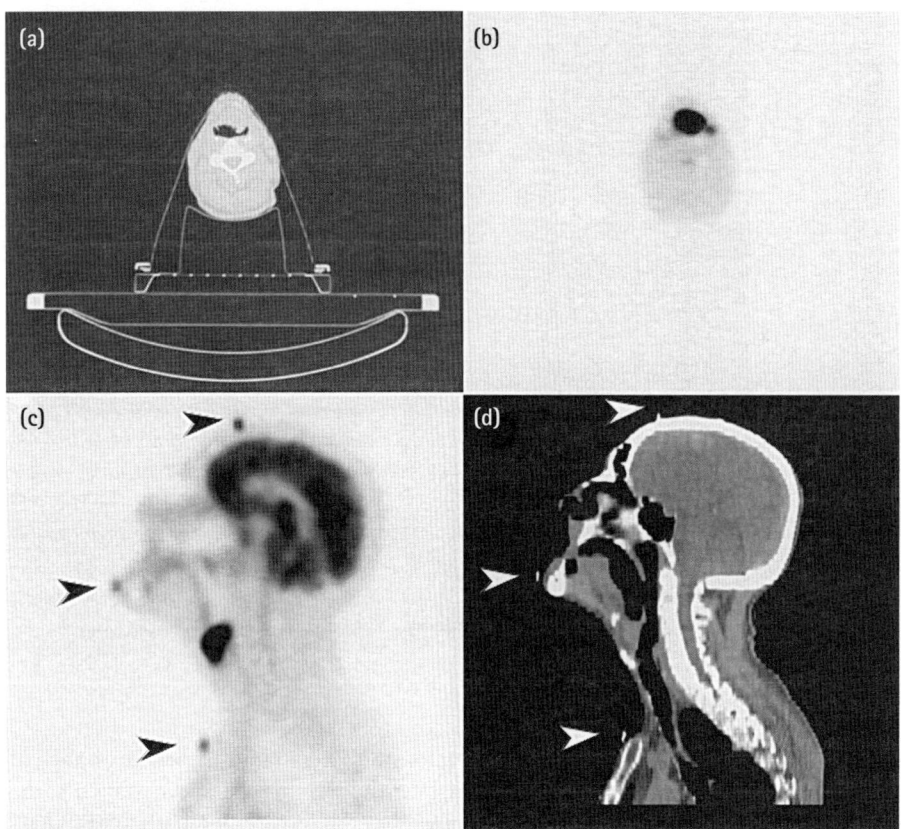

Figure 1A.13 *PET/CT in radiotherapy treatment planning. A 65-year-old man with squamous cell carcinoma of the epiglottis underwent ^{18}F-FDG PET/CT for radiotherapy planning. The patient was scanned using a flat radiotherapy palet and head restraint (a, b) with fiducial markers placed in the field of view (c, d) to assist in fusion of PET with CT.*

stage tumors can dramatically impact on management decision making including the appropriateness and type of surgery and radiotherapy that should be undertaken in individual patients.

The incorporation of molecular imaging techniques in the work-up of patients planned for radiotherapy has become an important new area of clinical investigation. The advent of 3-D conformal radiation therapy has resulted in a need to identify the optimal spatial regions for boosting radiation dose. PET has emerged as one of the most accurate methods to identify viable tumor in masses seen on CT/MRI, and the incorporation of PET data into treatment planning has been shown to markedly improve the accuracy of dose delivery and outcomes in treated patients.[40,75,76] ^{18}F-FDG PET has been shown to improve target volume, and assist in avoidance of relapse due to undiagnosed nodal or distant metastases, in a range of tumors including lung cancer and head and neck cancer.[40,75,76] In addition, the incorporation of PET/CT data directly into radiation treatment planning systems has been demonstrated to markedly improve the accuracy of radiation delivery to tumor (Fig. 1A.13). This is an area of continued development and it is likely that PET/CT will have an increasingly important role in radiotherapy of malignancy in the future.

A further application of imaging in treatment planning is in the confirmation of dose delivery for locoregional treatment of tumors with chemotherapy and radiolabeled compounds. For example, the treatment of hepatic tumors (primary hepatocellular carcinoma or metastatic disease usually from colorectal cancer primary) with infusion of chemotherapy or radiolabeled spheres directly into the hepatic artery requires the confirmation of the correct placement of vascular catheters prior to treatment (Fig. 1A.14). These techniques are invaluable whenever locoregional infusions are performed and catheter placement confirmation is required.[35]

Treatment response

The accurate and early assessment of response to therapy is a central theme in modern oncology practice. This is related in part to the emergence of biologic therapies (e.g. tyrosine kinase inhibitors, monoclonal antibodies, proteosome inhibitors) that target specific types of receptors or signaling/metabolic pathways that may or may not be relevant for each tumor type. The individualization of cancer therapies requires careful screening of tumors and patients for optimal treatment but, ultimately, response assessment early in treatment is the mainstay of patient care to ensure that optimal treatment is provided. Molecular imaging can clearly assist in identifying early response or nonresponse, across a broad range of tumor types with SPECT and PET imaging techniques.

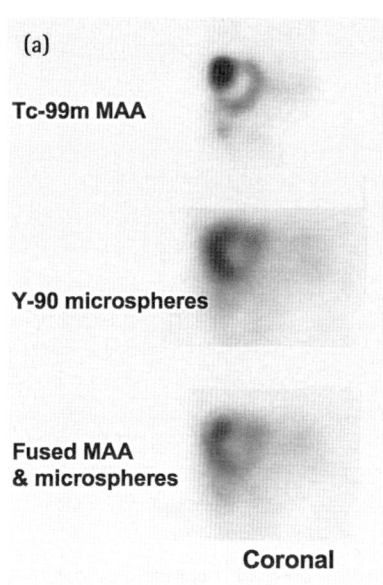

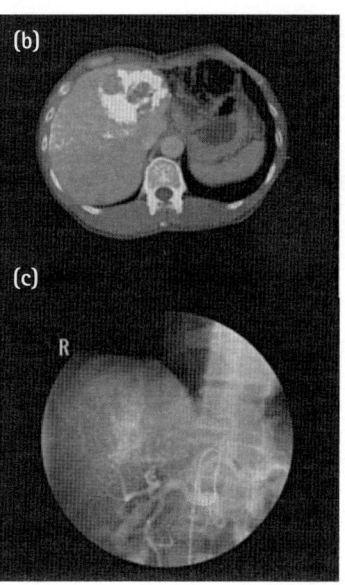

Figure 1A.14 *Locoregional therapy assessment with SPECT. (a) ^{99m}Tc-MAA injected into (c) hepatic artery catheter confirms perfusion to location of (b) metastatic disease in liver. ^{90}Y-microspheres were subsequently infused, and (a) SPECT imaging confirmed selective delivery to sites of metastatic disease.*

Planar and SPECT imaging can play a major role in the identification of early response, particularly in lymphoma treatment (^{67}Ga scans). A key component of assessment of tumor response following many types of cancer therapy is the 'flare' phenomenon, which can induce increased metabolic activity in tumors soon after treatment (particularly chemotherapy). This is particularly the case for bone scans soon after treatment when assessing extent of bony metastatic disease.

An emerging area of clinical utility of PET is in the monitoring of tumor response to therapy, principally with ^{18}F-FDG. Accurate evaluation of response to both chemotherapy and radiation therapy, often prior to CT scan changes, have been reported in glioma, colorectal, NSCLC, lymphoma, head and neck tumors, and soft tissue sarcomas (Figs 1A.7 and 1A.8, page 13).[39,67,75,77–82] PET is able to provide information on response to therapy earlier than most conventional imaging techniques, therefore providing confirmation of the efficacy of that treatment regime, or alternatively allowing an early change to alternate treatments that may have improved efficacy. The timing and reliability of ^{18}F-FDG PET studies in predicting tumor response is the subject of numerous prospective studies. The implications of this approach are significant in terms of optimizing treatments, minimizing unnecessary morbidity and reducing costs.

While ^{18}F-FDG is the principal tracer used for monitoring treatment response in oncology patients, a number of other tracers have been studied and are showing considerable promise. ^{18}F-FLT has been shown to accurately identify a range of tumors, and the assessment of proliferation response to therapy is being explored in a range of trials at present. Analysis of changes in blood flow or intratumoral hypoxia in response to anti-angiogenic therapy, and evaluation of reporter gene expression following gene therapy, are further examples of molecular imaging with PET impacting on assessment of novel therapeutics.[83]

Molecular imaging in oncology drug discovery

There has been a dramatic change in recent years in the techniques used to select new targets and new drugs for cancer. This has been driven by the information available following the sequencing of the human genome, and a greater understanding of the changes in gene expression and function that can be linked to oncogenesis. A key component of this process has been the identification of links between genes and epigenetic events, and the translation of proteins that play key roles on cellular function. In addition, the complexity of protein expression, with post-translational changes and multiple escape pathways in signaling pathways that are responsible for cell function, has meant that selection of targets for new anti-cancer drugs requires both insight into tumor biology and the ability to screen and test new drugs with high efficiency.

The use of molecular imaging is crucial in the development of these new generation compounds. An example of successful selection of target and drug, and the role of molecular imaging in development, is in gastrointestinal stromal tumors (GISTs). The majority of GIST tumors are characterized by an activating or gain-of-function mutation in the c-kit proto-oncogene.[84] This led to the development of a tyrosine kinase inhibitor that inhibits KIT phosphorylation (as well as Bcr-Abl and platelet derived growth factor receptor (PDGFR)), imatinib mesylate (Gleevec). Gleevec was shown to have marked efficacy for GIST tumors expressing this mutation, and has been approved for this indication. The role of molecular imaging in development of Gleevec was through the integral use of ^{18}F-FDG PET imaging in monitoring the profound effects of Gleevec on tumor metabolism within a short period of time following initiation of therapy, and even before tumor shrinkage occured on anatomic imaging (Fig. 1A.15).[85] This has led to ^{18}F-FDG PET being an integral part of the

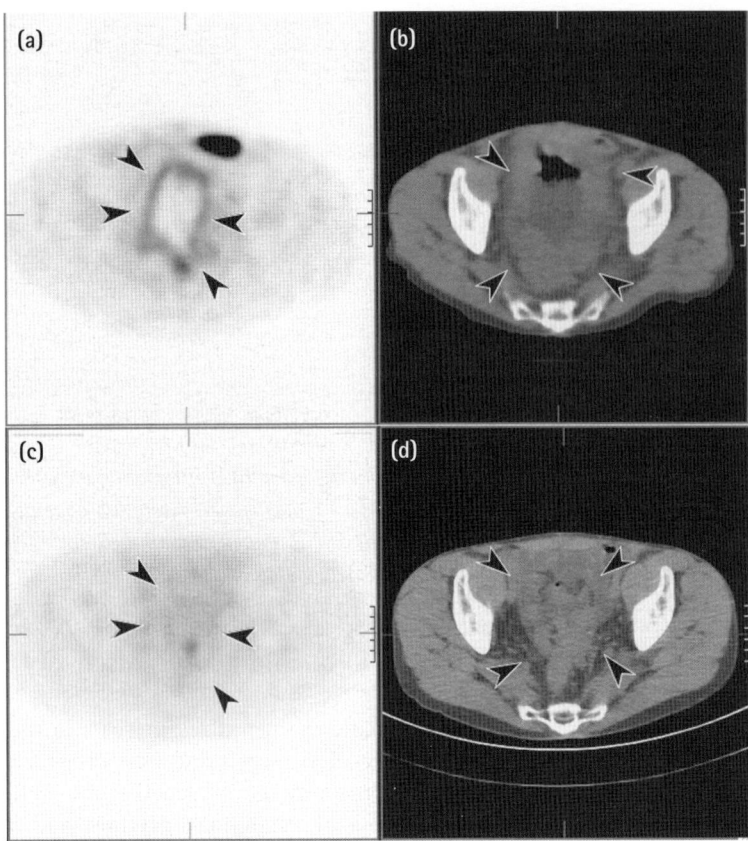

Figure 1A.15   *A 61-year-old man with a gastrointestinal stromal tumor of the rectum underwent ^{18}F-FDG PET/CT prior to treatment with Gleevec (a, arrows, b). The post-therapy ^{18}F-FDG PET/CT scan showed a residual mass on CT (d, arrows) but complete metabolic response on ^{18}F-FDG PET (c, arrows).*

routine assessment of patients being treated with Gleevec, both for response assessment and for detection of residual active disease. Interestingly, the development of KIT and PDGFR kinase mutations has been shown to occur in GIST tumors, and produce resistance to Gleevec therapy, and ^{18}F-FDG PET scans can demonstrate residual active tumor that express these mutations.

The specific trace labeling of new drugs can greatly facilitate drug development preclinically as well as in early phase clinical trials. Directly labeling drugs with SPECT or PET tracers allows the determination of interaction of the drug with its binding site. This is achieved through (1) radiolabeling the drug (or precursor) without change in function, and (2) validating uptake of the drug through competitive binding studies. The assessment of the biodistribution of the drug in *in vivo* preclinical models, as well as in human studies, provides essential information on the stability of the drug *in vivo*, pharmacokinetics, and the retention of binding specificity and affinity. This can be achieved with SPECT and PET tracers, and has been reported successfully for chemotherapy drugs, small molecules and both peptides and proteins (including monoclonal antibodies) (Fig. 1A.3, page 7).[6,9,54,55,86–90] The uptake of drug in tumor can also be assessed, which combined with pharmacokinetics and metabolite analysis allows validation of the targeting of drug to tumor, and can assist in selection of optimal formulation, and dosage and scheduling of treatment.

Pharmacodynamics is the evaluation of the effects of a drug on the physiology of a particular organ or system. Molecular imaging can impact on preclinical development of new drugs through the assessment of a broad array of physiologic changes in tumors, including changes in metabolism, proliferation, blood flow, and induction of events such as apoptosis *in vitro* and in animal models.[4,6,56] Pharmacodynamic changes in tumors can be assessed in early phase clinical trials, and this information can be used to inform the efficacy and optimal dosage schedule of novel anticancer biologics.

MOLECULAR IMAGING IN NON–ONCOLOGY APPLICATIONS

Cardiology

Routine cardiac nuclear medicine has centered on measures of myocardial perfusion and ventricular function. The utility of myocardial perfusion scans to identify areas of viable myocardium, and hence aid in risk stratification and treatment decisions, is well known and this is a common imaging test worldwide.[91] Quantification of ventricular function and ejection fraction is also widely used for assessment of cardiac patients and to assist in monitoring toxicity of chemotherapy. SPECT remains the principal nuclear medicine technique, and the introduction of SPECT/CT

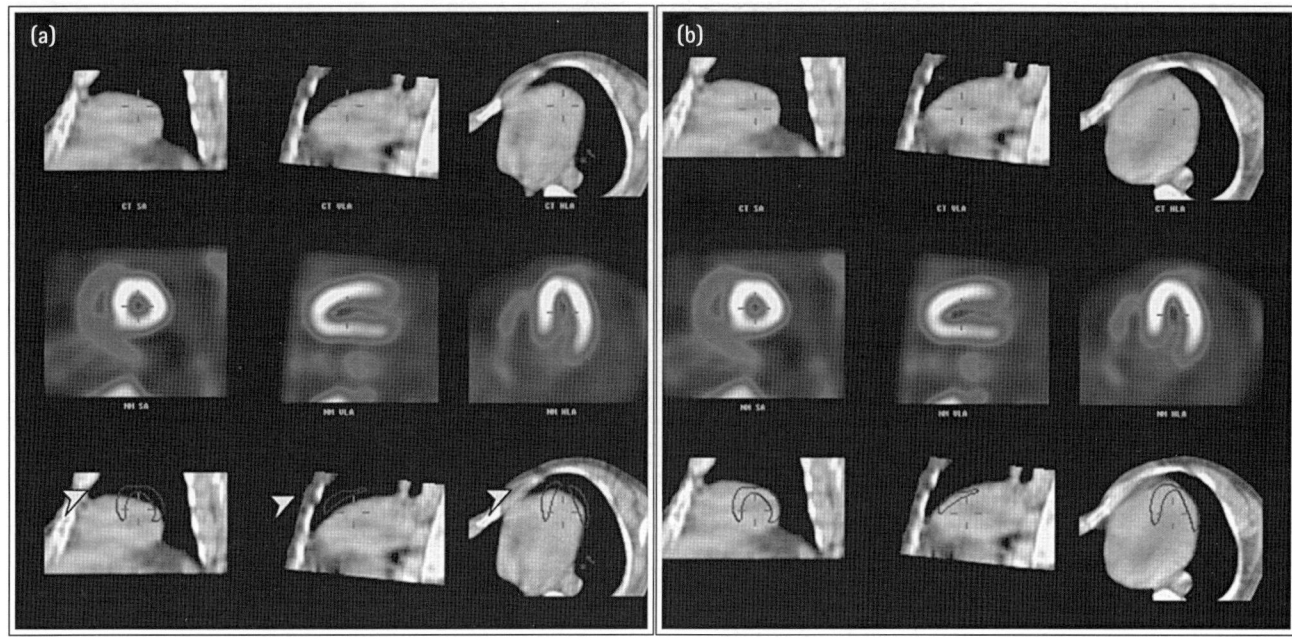

Figure 1A.16 *Myocardial SPECT/CT study. (a) SPECT and CT images show effects of respiratory motion on SPECT anatomic location (lower panel). (b) CT motion correction results in precise SPECT localization.*

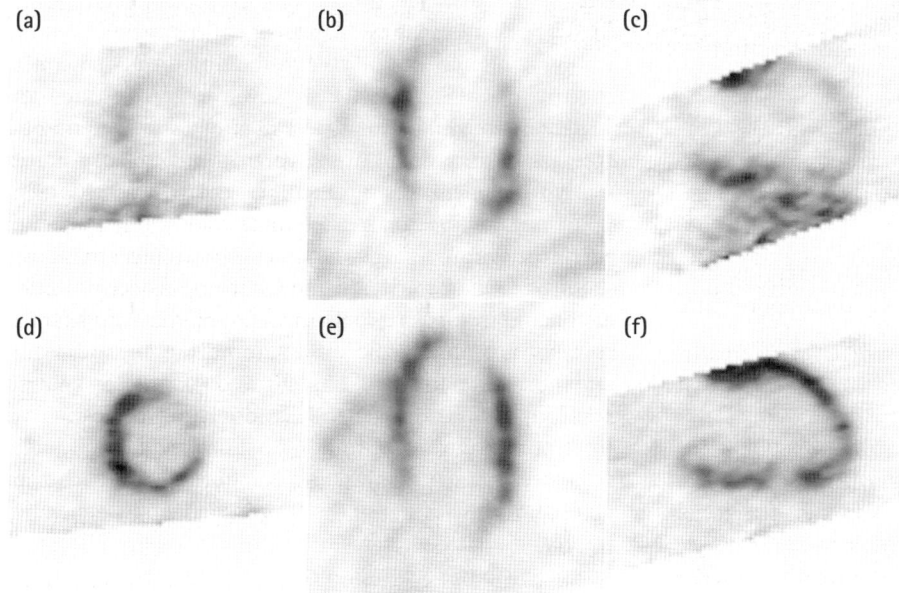

Figure 1A.17 *PET cardiac imaging. Perfusion imaging with $^{13}NH_3$ (a, b and c) shows a dilated left ventricle and impaired perfusion to extensive areas of the anterolateral and apical walls. ^{18}F-FDG imaging (d, e and f) shows viable myocardium in areas of reduced perfusion in the anteroapical walls.*

allows improvements in attenuation correction and motion correction (Fig. 1A.16). PET myocardial perfusion and metabolic imaging remains an important component of the work-up of many patients with ischemic heart disease and poor left ventricular function (Fig. 1A.17).

Molecular imaging of the myocardium has included assessment of sympathetic innervation, using ligands directed at specific components of the cardiac sympathetic nerve varicosities, including ^{123}I-MIBG (and PET derivatives), 6-[^{18}F]fluorometaraminol, ^{11}C-*meta*-hydroxyephedrine, ^{11}C-epinephrine, and ^{11}C-phenylephrine. These are all

analogs of norepinephrine, with substantial differences between agents in neuronal kinetics. Imaging of the parasympathetic system is more difficult due to its predominant location in the atria and nodes, and the much greater selectivity of the acetylcholine uptake carrier.[92] The heart and coronary blood vessels pose challenges to nuclear imaging, including small target volume, significant rapid motion, and adjacent blood pool activity.[93]

The realization that atherosclerotic plaque undergoes characteristic changes prior to rupture has led to considerable interest in detecting these 'vulnerable' or 'unstable'

Table 1A.3 *Pathological processes, targets, and ligands used in human subjects for imaging of vulnerable atherosclerotic plaque*

Process	Target	Example tracer
Lipid accumulation	LDL	^{123}I-LDL
	Oxidized LDL	^{99m}Tc-oxLDL
	Apolipoprotein B	
Activated macrophages	Labeled monocytes	^{111}In-monocytes
	Glucose	^{18}F-FDG
Endothelium	Endothelin	^{11}C-ABT-627, ^{18}F-SB209670
Apoptosis	Phosphatidylserine	^{99m}Tc-annexin V
Coagulation	Platelet IIb/IIIa	^{99m}Tc-P280
	Fibrin	^{131}I-fibrinogen

plaques. Key features include a large necrotic/lipid core, a fibrous cap with a marked infiltration of inflammatory cells, and few smooth muscle fibers.[94] Each of these features has provided impetus to develop a range of ligands, some of which are listed in Table 1A.3. It should be noted that none of these agents have been extensively studied in human subjects, with mixed results in trials to date.

Restoration of perfusion to ischemic myocardium by induction of angiogenesis has been an area of interest to cardiologists. Strategies to achieve this include direct intracoronary administration of autologous stem cells, vascular endothelial growth factor (VEGF), and DNA coding for VEGF.[91,95] Imaging of this process has predictably been required to monitor delivery and expression of the various agents. Probes include ^{111}In-VEGF12, $a_v\beta_3$ integrins, and reporter genes.[96,97] Unfortunately, none of these approaches have yielded encouraging responses in human trials.

Neurology

Until recently the role of nuclear medicine in clinical neuroimaging has largely comprised mapping of regional cerebral blood flow (e.g. [^{123}I]iodoamphetamine, ^{99m}Tc-ethylenecysteinediamine) and more recently glucose metabolism (^{18}F-FDG). This has only been augmented by the European availability of ^{123}I-ioflupane (DATScan, Amersham plc) since 2000. However, the receptor–ligand paradigm is most advanced in neurology, with the first *in vivo* studies dating to the early 1980s, and a very extensive array of research ligands and targets (Table 1A.4).[24,98]

Functional MRI (fMRI) has become ascendant in studies that require repeated examinations in a short period of time or high anatomical resolution. Magnetic resonance spectroscopy (MRS) is able to detect compounds at micromolar concentrations, whereas the threshold for scintigraphic techniques extends to 10^{-9} to 10^{-12} mol L^{-1}.[99] However, fMRS is able to characterize movement of some

compounds through chemical processes; for example, analysis of aerobic and anaerobic contributions to cerebral metabolism following administration of ^{13}C-glucose.[100] It is likely that optimum imaging solutions for some biological problems will involve a combination of modalities.

The specific applications of molecular imaging in neurology can be conceptualized in the following categories:

- Neurobiology and neuropathology
- Psychiatry
- Neuropharmacology
- Drug abuse and dependency
- Epilepsy
- Neurodegenerative conditions
- Dementing illnesses
- Movement disorders
- Brain ischemia
- Traumatic brain injury

Several characteristics of an imaging ligand are of particular interest when selecting agents for use in neurology, including potency, toxicity, plasma protein binding, penetration of the blood–brain barrier and the specific activity (and hence administered mass). This can be applied depending on the clinical situation and the pathophysiology of the disease process. For example, blood flow is highly relevant to the evaluation of epilepsy where anatomical imaging may not be able to identify the actual epileptogenic focus (Fig. 1A.18). However, receptor studies and metabolic imaging with ^{18}F-FDG may also have potential roles in the assessment of the patient with epilepsy, particularly when diagnosis is difficult (Figs 1A.18 and 1A.19).

As quantitative analysis of image datasets is frequently performed in neurological studies, meticulous attention is required to characterize the model of ligand–receptor interaction and factors that may impact upon this such as tracer metabolism, nonspecific binding, and presence of ligand and metabolites in blood. Model-based quantitative analyses relate input function (generally arterial time–activity curve) to response function through a defined model.[101] Kinetic, reference region, graphical and equilibrium approaches are all used, with selection of the appropriate model depending upon the system under study and available resources. As intimated above, quantitative analysis often requires arterial blood sampling and dynamic imaging. Examination of a neurotransmitter pathway in isolation is artificial and often not feasible *in vivo*, since every aspect of synthesis, release and metabolism of neurotransmitter is subject to complex feedback and modulation by both physiological and pathological processes.[102]

Amongst the wide variety of probes and targets, perhaps the two best established and characterized clinically are movement and dementing disorders, specifically Parkinson's disease and Alzheimer's disease.

Assessment of movement disorders, particularly differential diagnosis of Parkinson's disease, is a good example of a well-defined imaging paradigm applied to the dopaminergic

Table 1A.4 *Radiotracers available for studying neuropharmacology*

Biological application	Tracers
Blood flow	$H_2{}^{15}O$, ^{15}O-butanol ^{99m}Tc-HMPAO, ^{133}Xe, [^{123}I]iodoamphetamine (IMP)
Oxygen metabolism	$^{15}O_2$
Hypoxia	^{18}F-FMISO, ^{18}F-FAZA, ^{64}Cu-ATSM
Glucose metabolism	2-[^{18}F]fluoro-2-deoxy-D-glucose (FDG)
Dopamine storage/DDC activity	6-[^{18}F]fluorodopa (F-dopa), β-^{11}C-dopa
Monoamine vesicle transporters	^{11}C-dihydrotetrabenazine (DTBZ)
Dopamine transporters	^{11}C-CFT, ^{11}C-RTI 32, ^{18}F-CFT, ^{123}I-β-CIT
	^{123}I-FP-CIT, ^{123}I-IPT, ^{123}I-altropane
Dopamine D1 type sites	^{11}C-SCH 23390
Dopamine D2 type sites	^{11}C-raclopride, ^{11}C-FLB456, ^{11}C-methylspiperone, ^{18}F-spiperone, [^{18}F]fluorethylspiperone, [^{76}Br]bromospiperone, ^{123}I-epidepride, [^{123}I]iodobenzamide (IBZM)
Noradrenaline transporters	^{11}C-BATA
Noradrenaline $\alpha 2$	2-[^{18}F]fluorethoxyidazoxan
Serotonin storage	^{11}C-methyltryptophan
Serotonin transporters	^{11}C-DASB, ^{123}I-β-CIT
Serotonin HT_{1a}	^{11}C-WAY 100635
Serotonin HT_{2a}	^{11}C-MDL100907, ^{18}F-altanserin, ^{18}F-setoperone
Acetylcholinesterase activity	^{11}C-MP4A, ^{11}C-physostigmine
Cholinergic vesicle transporters	[^{18}F]fluoroethoxybenzovesamicol, ^{11}C-vesamicol, ^{123}I-benzovesamicol
Muscarinic M1 sites	^{11}C-tropanylbenzylate, ^{11}C-NMPB, ^{18}F-FP-TZTP, ^{123}I-QNB
Nicotinic sites	^{11}C-MPA, ^{11}C-A-85380, ^{18}F-A-85380, ^{123}I-A-85380
Histamine H1 sites	^{11}C-dothiepin
Opioid μ sites	^{11}C-carfentenil, ^{18}F-cyclofoxy
Opioid μ, κ, and δ sites	^{11}C-diprenorphine
Central benzodiazepine sites	^{11}C-flumazenil
Central benzodiazepine sites ($\alpha 5$ subunits)	^{11}C-RO15-4513
Peripheral benzodiazepine sites	^{11}C-PK11195, ^{18}F-PK11195, ^{123}I-PK11195
Substance P/NK1 sites	^{18}F-SPARQ, ^{11}C-GR205171
Adenosine A_{2A} sites	^{11}C-SCH 442416
NMDA voltage channels	^{11}C-CNS 5161
Amyloid	^{18}F-FDDNP, ^{11}C-PIB, ^{18}F-PIB, ^{11}C-SB13, ^{123}I-IMPY
Phosphoglycoprotein activity	^{11}C-carfentenil

Table modified from Brooks.[111]

system. Strategies to assess presynaptic dopaminergic function include:

- Amino acid decarboxylase activity through decarboxylation of [^{18}F]fluorodopa to [^{18}F]fluorodopamine
- Dopamine transporter density using variety of ligands, both SPECT and PET (e.g. tropanes)
- Activity of vesicular dopamine (monoamine) transporter type 2 (VMAT2) with ^{11}C-tetrahydrobenazine
- General metabolic activity using ^{18}F-FDG PET

Although all these approaches evaluate different aspects of disease biology, a recent review concluded that there was insufficient or contradictory evidence to support any of these approaches being used alone for diagnosis of Parkinson's disease, to assess disease progression, or effect of treatment.[103] However, it should be noted that ^{123}I-ioflupane (DATScan, Amersham plc) is approved in Europe to assist in distinguishing parkinsonian syndromes from essential tremor. A small series suggests that both visual interpretation and statistical parametric mapping of ^{18}F-FDG images using defined criteria can be employed to reliably distinguish classical from variant forms of parkinsonism.[104] As the study used a control group comprised of healthy normal subjects, validation in a larger population with co-morbidities is required before this can be considered for routine clinical practice.

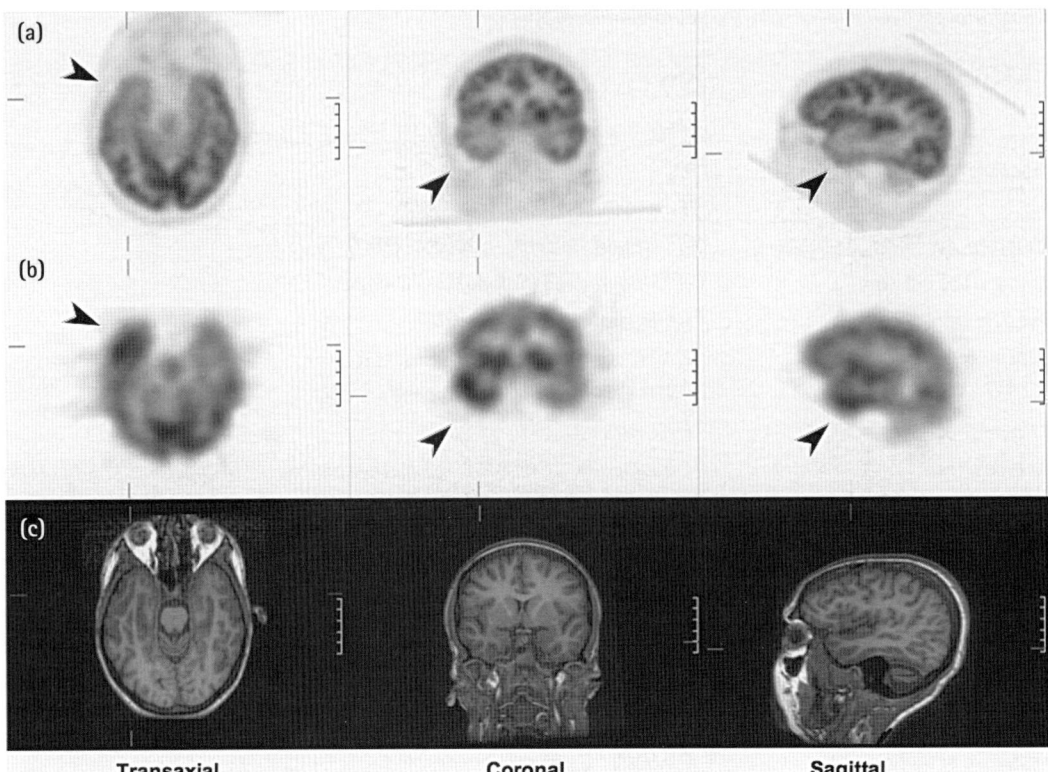

Transaxial   **Coronal**   **Sagittal**

Figure 1A.18 *SPECT and PET imaging of temporal lobe epilepsy. A 28-year-old woman with temporal lobe epilepsy, (c) lesion negative on MRI, showed (b) right temporal hyperperfusion on ictal SPECT (arrows), and (a) right temporal hypometabolism on* [18]*F-FDG PET (arrows).*

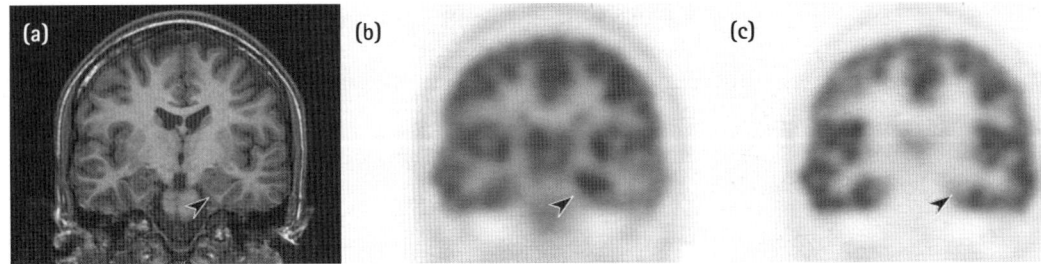

Figure 1A.19 *Molecular imaging of temporal lobe epilepsy. A 24-year-old woman with left temporal lobe epilepsy, (a) lesion negative on MRI (arrow), had a subclinical seizure during the uptake phase of the (b)* [18]*F-FDG PET study resulting in a focus of increased metabolism in the left mesial temporal cortex (arrow). (c) A* [11]*C-flumazenil study shows decreased density of benzodiazepine receptors in the left mesial temporal cortex (arrow).*

A key application of molecular imaging in neurology is Alzheimer's disease, which is estimated to affect approximately 2% of the population in developed countries, with approximately 50 compounds currently under investigation for treatment.[105] Imaging targets reflect the wide variety of potential therapeutic targets, and include cholinergic, dopaminergic and serotonergic systems; and benzodiazepine receptors, both central and peripheral. The hypothesis that Aβ has a causal role in Alzheimer's disease has led to a flurry of activity in developing an imaging agent. Given the putative role of Aβ plaques in neurotoxicity there has been considerable interest in imaging these. Most candidates are small molecules, derivatives of dyes and fluophores including thioflavin-T, Congo red, stilbene and acridine. The actual binding sites for these agents are still being elucidated.[106]

One of the more promising compounds to date is ^{11}C-PIB, which appears to exhibit selectivity for Aβ over other β-pleated sheets (Fig. 1A.20).[107] As cognitive impairment does not appear to clearly correlate with Aβ plaques, a variety of alternative hypotheses have been advanced, including neurotoxic effect being mediated by oligomeric Aβ rather than established plaques. Other proposals suggest that neurofibrillary tangles of hyperphosphorylated tau protein may be neurotoxic, but that this in turn lies downstream

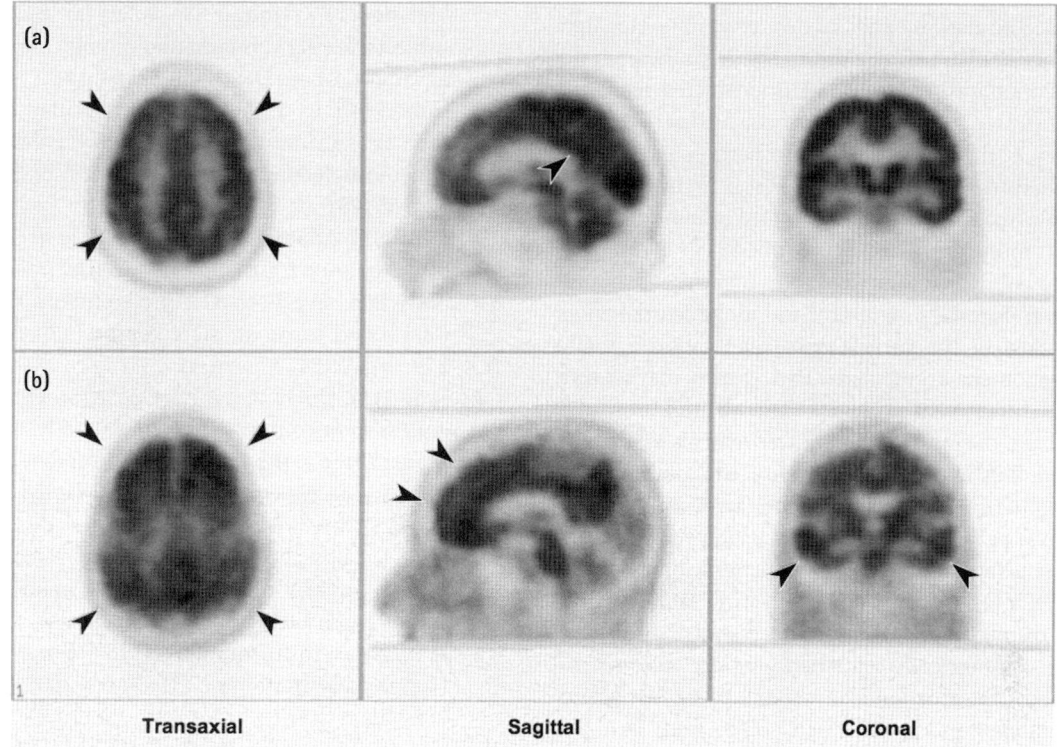

Transaxial	**Sagittal**	**Coronal**

Figure 1A.20 *Alzheimer's disease. A 90-year-old woman with cognitive impairment underwent (a) a ^{18}F-FDG PET scan which showed mild reduction in frontal, parietal and posterior cingulate metabolism (arrows). (b) A ^{11}C-PIB PET scan showed widespread cortical and subcortical amyloid deposition (arrows) typical of Alzheimer's disease.*

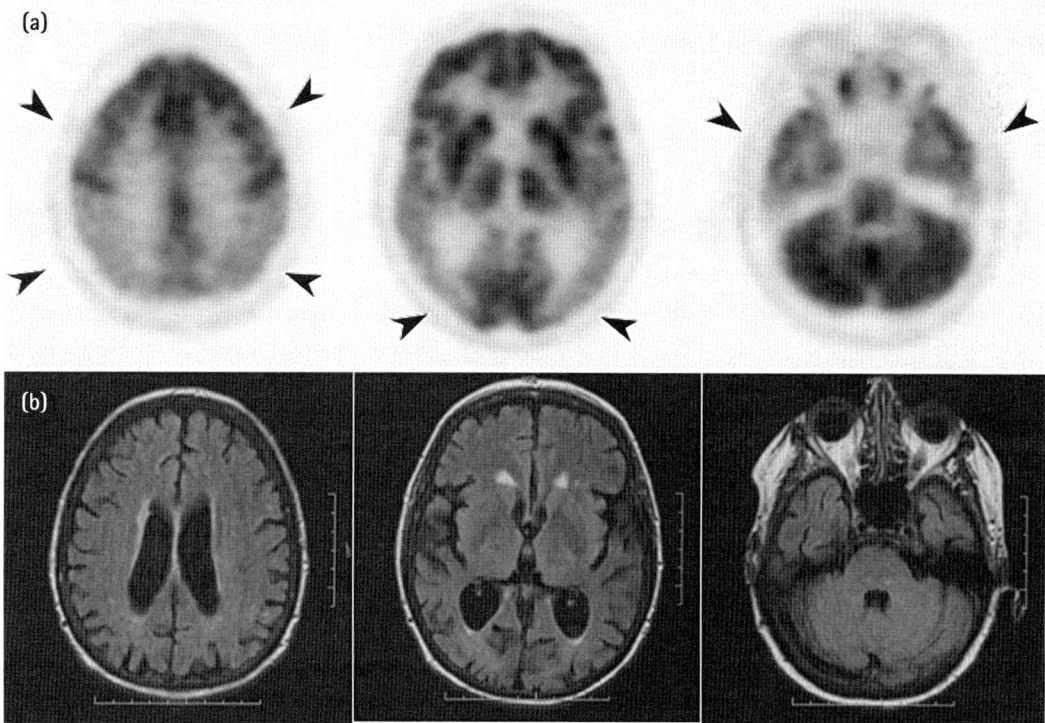

Figure 1A.21 *Alzheimer's disease variant. A 64-year-old woman with apraxia, neglect and Balint's syndrome, characterized by optic ataxia, optic apraxia and simultanagnosia, underwent (a) a ^{18}F-FDG PET scan, which showed bilateral hypometabolism in frontal, parietal and temporal cortex (arrows) extending posteriorly on the left consistent with the posterior cortical atrophy variant of Alzheimer's disease. (b) MRI shows enlarged ventricular spaces and ischemic white matter changes.*

from Aβ accumulation, and is not reversible through measures that deplete Aβ.[108] Alternative hypotheses hold aggregation of tau protein to be a neuroprotective response to oxidative stress.[109] Until the lack of concordance regarding aetiology, pathogenesis and clinicopathological correlates of Alzheimer's disease is resolved it is highly unlikely that a reliable imaging probe with clinical role in diagnosis or treatment monitoring can be identified.

This may be further complicated by Alzheimer's disease having several stages of progression and multifactorial etiology, with many of the current postulated causes actually being epiphenomena or responses. This, in turn, may require a multifaceted treatment process.[110] The identification of a single definitive diagnostic imaging test may also be problematic, and illustrates the importance of knowledge of the disease process to understand the target and process addressed by a particular molecular imaging probe. Indeed, ^{18}F-FDG is sensitive for detection of dementing illnesses even prior to development of symptoms, but may not be capable of reliably distinguishing the specific disease entity (Fig. 1A.21).[111,112] Sophisticated parametric image analysis, or combination of information from studies using two agents evaluating different processes (e.g. ^{11}C-DTBZ and ^{18}F-FDG) may help overcome this.[113] It should be realized that a diagnostic test is not necessarily the same as that which will be useful in determining prognosis or even treatment outcome. Validation of imaging paradigms in Alzheimer's disease is also complicated by lack of a 'gold standard' clinical diagnosis and in some cases, definite neuropathological criteria.[114] Many research studies use highly selected 'control' groups, raising the question as to applicability of imaging tests in an unselected population with co-existent diseases.[112]

CONCLUSIONS

Molecular imaging is a broad-based functional imaging approach that can characterize key components of normal cellular and organ function, and identify changes that occur in disease. Nuclear medicine studies can play a crucial role in drug discovery, assisting with patient diagnosis, defining extent of disease, monitoring and informing choices for optimal therapies, and improving patient management. The future will no doubt bring a vast array of new opportunities for tracer-based molecular imaging techniques.

REFERENCES

1   Britz-Cunningham SH, Adelstein SJ. Molecular targeting with radionuclides: state of the science. *J Nucl Med* 2003; **44**: 1945–61.

2   Sharma V, Luker GD, Piwnica-Worms D. Molecular imaging of gene expression and protein function *in vivo* with PET and SPECT. *J Magn Reson Imaging* 2002; **16**: 336–51.

3   Massoud TF, Gambhir SS. Molecular imaging in living subjects: seeing fundamental biological processes in a new light. *Genes Dev* 2003; **17**: 545–80.

4   Haberkorn U, Eisenhut M. Molecular imaging and therapy – a programme based on the development of new biomolecules. *Eur J Nucl Med Mol Imaging* 2005; **32**: 1354–9.

5   Johns TG, Adams TE, Wittrup KD, *et al.* Identification of the epitope for the EGFR-specific monoclonal antibody 806 reveals that it preferentially recognises an untethered form of the receptor. *J Biol Chem* 2004; **279**: 30375–84.

6   Scott AM. Current status of positron emission tomography in oncology. *Int Med J* 2001; **31**: 27–36.

7   Mansi L. From the magic bullet to an effective therapy; the peptide experience. *Eur J Nucl Med Mol Imaging* 2004; **31**: 1393–8.

8   Van Den Bossche B, Van de Wiele C. Receptor imaging in oncology by means of nuclear medicine: Current status. *J Clin Oncol* 2004; **22**: 3593–607.

9   Wahl RL. Tositumumab and ^{131}I therapy in non Hodgkins lymphoma. *J Nucl Med* 2005; **46(suppl 1)**: 28S–40.

10 Chong G, Lee F-T, Hopkins W, *et al.* Phase I trial of ^{131}I-huA33 in patients with advanced colorectal carcinoma. *Clin Cancer Res* 2005; **11**: 4818–26.

11 Bianco R, Melisi D, Ciardello F, Tortora G. Key cancer cell signal transduction pathways as therapeutic targets. *Eur J Cancer* 2006; **42**: 290–4.

12 Baselga J, Artega CL. Critical update and emerging trends in epidermal growth factor receptor targeting in cancer. *J Clin Oncol* 2005; **23**: 2445–59.

13 Blasberg R. PET imaging of gene expression. *Eur J Cancer* 2002; **38**: 2137–46.

14 Bengel FM, Schachinger V, Dimmeler S. Cell-based therapies and imaging in cardiology. *Eur J Nucl Med Mol Imaging* 2005; **32**: S404–16.

15 Kirik D, Breysse N, Björklund T, *et al.* Imaging in cell-based therapy for neurodegenerative disease. *Eur J Nucl Med Mol Imaging* 2005; **32**: S417–34.

16 Thompson M, Wall DM, Hicks RJ, Prince HM. *In vivo* tracking for cell therapies. *Q J Nucl Med Mol Imaging* 2005; **49**: 339–48.

17 Westwood JA, Smyth MJ, Teng MW, *et al.* Adoptive transfer of T cells modified with a humanized chimeric receptor gene inhibits growth of Lewis-Y-expressing tumors in mice. *Proc Natl Acad Sci USA* 2005; **102**: 19051–6.

18 Werner T. Promoters can contribute to the elucidation of protein function. *Trends Biotechnol* 2003; **21**: 9–13.

19 Simpson RJ, Dorow DS. Cancer proteomics from signaling networks to tumor markers. *Trends Biotechnol* 2001; **19**: S40–8.

20 Chievitz O, Hevesy G. Radioactive indicators in the study of phosphorus metabolism in rats. *Nature* 1935; **136**: 754–5.

21 Dorland WAN. *Dorland's Illustrated Medical Dictionary*, 30th edition. Philadelphia: W.B. Saunders; 2003.

22 Eckelman WC, Reba RC, Gibson RE, *et al.* Receptor-binding radiotracers: a class of potential radiopharmaceuticals. *J Nucl Med* 1979; **20**: 350–7.

23 Vera DR, Krohn KA, Stadalnik RC, Scheibe PO. Tc-99m-galactosyl-neoglycoalbumin: *in vivo* characterization of receptor-mediated binding to hepatocytes. *Radiology* 1984; **151**: 191–6.

24 Vera DR, Eckelman WC. Receptor 1980 and receptor 2000: twenty years of progress in receptor-binding radiotracers. *Nucl Med Biol* 2001; **28**: 475–6.

25 Winthrop MD, De Nardo GL, De Nardo SJ. Antibody phage display applications for nuclear medicine imaging and therapy. *Q J Nucl Med* 2000; **44**: 284–95.

26 Younes CK, Boisgard R, Tavitian B. Labelled oligonucleotides as radiopharmaceuticals: pitfalls, problems and perspectives. *Curr Pharm Des* 2002; **8**: 1451–66.

27 Tavitian B. *In vivo* antisense imaging. *Q J Nucl Med* 2000; **44**: 236–55.

28 Eckelman WC, Rohatagi S, Krohn KA, Vera DR. Are there lessons to be learned from drug development that will accelerate the use of molecular probes in the clinic? *Nucl Med Biol* 2005; **32**: 657–62.

29 Haberkorn U, Altman A. Radionuclide imaging in the post-genomic era. *J Cell Biochem* 2002; **39(suppl)**: 1–10.

30 Galbraith SM. Antivascular cancer treatments: imaging biomarkers in pharmaceutical drug development. *Br J Radiol* 2003; **76(Special issue no. 1)**: S83–6.

31 Yoshinaga K, Chow BJ, dekemp DA, *et al.* Application of cardiac molecular imaging using positron emission tomography in evaluation of drug and therapeutics for cardiovascular disorders. *Curr Pharm Res* 2005; **11**: 903–32.

32 Coon KD, Dunckley T, Stephan DA. Biomarker identification in neurologic diseases: improving diagnostics and therapeutics. *Expert Rev Mol Diagn* 2005; **4**: 361–75.

33 Maruvada P, Wang W, Wagner PD, Srivastava S. Biomarkers in molecular medicine: cancer detection and diagnosis. Biotechniques 2005; **Suppl**: 9–15.

34 Levin CS. Primer on molecular imaging technology. *Eur J Nucl Med Mol Imaging* 2005; **32**: S25–45.

35 Denecke T, Hildebrandt B, Lehmkuhl, L, *et al.* Fusion imaging using a hybrid SPECT–CT camera improves port perfusion scintigraphy for control of hepatic arterial infusion of chemotherapy in colorectal cancer patients. *Eur J Nucl Med Mol Imaging* 2005; **32**: 1003–10.

36 Palumbo B, Sivolella S, Palumbo I, *et al.* ^{67}Ga-SPECT/CT with a hybrid system in the clinical management of lymphoma. *Eur J Nucl Med Mol Imaging* 2005; **32**: 1011–7.

37 Berman DS, Hachamovitch R, Shaw LJ, *et al.* Roles of nuclear cardiology, cardiac computed tomography,

and cardiac magnetic resonance: assessment of patients with suspected coronary artery disease. *J Nucl Med* 2006; **47**: 74–82.

38 Som P, Atkins HL, Bandoypadhyay D, *et al.* A fluorinated glucose analog, 2-fluoro-2-deoxy-d-glucose (F-18): nontoxic tracer for rapid tumor detection. *J Nucl Med* 1980; **21**: 670–5.

39 Bar-Shalom R, Valdivia AY, Blaufox MD. PET imaging in oncology. *Semin Nucl Med* 2000; **30**: 150–85.

40 Ell PJ. The contribution of PET/CT to improved patient management. *Br J Radiol* 2006; **79**: 32–6.

41 Townsend DW, Carney JP, Yap JT, Hall NC. PET/CT today and tomorrow. *J Nucl Med* 2004; **45(suppl 1)**: 4S–14.

42 Schoder H, Larson SM, Yeung HW. PET/CT in oncology: integration into clinical management of lymphoma, melanoma, and gastrointestinal malignancies. *J Nucl Med* 2004; **45(suppl 1)**: 72S–81.

43 Lardinois D, Weder W, Hany TF, *et al.* Staging of non-small-cell lung cancer with integrated positron-emission tomography and computed tomography. *N Engl J Med* 2004; **348**: 2500–7.

44 von Schultess GK, Steinert HC, Hany TF. Integrated PET/CT: current applications and future directions. *Radiology* 2006; **238**: 405–22.

45 Lodge MA, Brasee H, Mahmoud F, *et al.* Developments in nuclear cardiology: transition from single photon computed tomography to positron emission tomography–computed tomography. *J Invasive Cardiol* 2005; **17**: 491–6.

46 Pichler BJ, Judenhofer MS, Catana C, *et al.* Performance test of an LSO-APD detector in a 7-T MRI scanner for simultaneous PET/MRI. *J Nucl Med* 2006; **47**: 639–47.

47 Lang P, Yeow K, Nichols A, Scheer A. Cellular imaging in drug discovery. *Nature Reviews Drug Discovery* 2005; **5**: 343–56.

48 Basilion JP, Yeon S, Botnar R. Magnetic resonance imaging: utility as a molecular imaging modality. *Curr Top Mol Biol* 2005; **70**: 1–33.

49 Caruthers SD, Winter PM, Wickline SA, Lanza GM. Targeted magnetic resonance imaging agents. *Methods Mol Med* 2006; **124**: 387–400.

50 Pache G, Saueressig U, Frydrychowicz A, *et al.* Initial experience with 64-slice cardiac CT: non-invasive visualization of coronary artery bypass grafts. *Eur Heart J* 2006; **27**: 976–80.

51 Ntziaxhristos V, Ripoll J, Wang LV, Weissleder R. Looking and listening to light: the evolution of whole-body photonic imaging. *Nat Biotechnol* 2005; **23**: 313–20.

52 Spankuch B, Strebhardt K. RNA interference-based gene silencing in mice: the development of a novel therapeutic strategy. *Curr Pharm Des* 2005; **11**: 3405–19.

53 Aboagye EO. Positron emission tomography imaging of small animals in anticancer drug development. *Mol Imaging Biol* 2005; **7**: 53–8.

54   Lee F-T, Rigopoulos A, Hall C, *et al.* Specific localization, gamma camera imaging, and intracellular trafficking of radiolabelled chimeric anti-G(D3) ganglioside monoclonal antibody KM871 in SK-MEL-28 melanoma xenografts. *Cancer Res* 2001; **61**: 4474–82.

55   Lee F-T, Hall C, Rigopoulos A, *et al.* Immuno-positron emission tomography (PET) of human colon xenograft bearing BALB/c nude mice using ^{124}I-CDR-grafted humanized A33 monoclonal antibody. *J Nucl Med* 2001; **42**: 764–9.

56   Dorow DS, Cullinane C, Conus N, *et al.* Multi-tracer small animal PET imaging of the tumour response to the novel pan-Erb-B inhibitor CI-1033. *Eur J Nucl Med Mol Imaging* 2006; **33**: 441–52.

57   Nieman BJ, Bock NA, Bishop J, *et al.* Magnetic resonance imaging for detection and analysis of mouse phenotype. *NMR Biomed* 2005; **18**: 447–68.

58   de Herder WW, Kwekkeboom DJ, Valkema R, *et al.* Neuroendocrine tumors and somatostatin: imaging techniques. *J Endocrinol Invest* 2005; **28**(**suppl 11**): 132–6.

59   Schoder H, Noy A, Gonen M, *et al.* Intensity of ^{18}fluorodeoxyglucose uptake in positron emission tomography distinguishes between indolent and aggressive non-Hodgkin's lymphoma. *J Clin Oncol* 2005; **23**: 4643–51.

60   Hicks RJ, Rischin D, Fisher R, *et al.* Utility of FMISO PET in advanced head and neck cancer treated with chemoradiation incorporating a hypoxia-targeting chemotherapy agent. *Eur J Nucl Med Mol Imaging* 2005; **32**: 1384–91.

61   Sasaki R, Komaki R, Macapinlac H, *et al.* [^{18}F]fluorodeoxyglucose uptake by positron emission tomography predicts outcome of non-small-cell lung cancer. *J Clin Oncol* 2005; **23**: 1136–43.

62   Rizk N, Downey RJ, Akhurst T, *et al.* Preoperative ^{18}[F]-fluorodeoxyglucose positron emission tomography standardized uptake values predict survival after esophageal adenocarcinoma resection. *Ann Thorac Surg* 2006; **81**: 1076–81.

63   Thompson JF, Uren RF. Lymphatic mapping in management of patients with primary cutaneous melanoma. *Lancet Oncol* 2005; **6**: 877–85.

64   James TA, Edge SB. Sentinel lymph node in breast cancer. *Curr Opin Obstet Gynecol* 2006; **18**: 53–8.

65   Damian DL, Fulham MJ, Thompson E, Thompson JF. Positron emission tomography in the detection and management of metastatic melanoma. *Melanoma Res* 1996; **6**: 325–9.

66   Lowe VJ, Boyd JH, Dunphy FR, *et al.* Surveillance for recurrent head and neck cancer using positron emission tomography. *J Clin Oncol* 2000; **18**: 651–8.

67   Shon IH, O'Doherty MJ, Maisey MN. Positron emission tomography in lung cancer. *Semin Nucl Med* 2002; **32**: 240–71.

68   van Tinteren H, Hoekstra OS, Smit EF, *et al.* Effectiveness of positron emission tomography in the preoperative assessment of patients with suspected non-small-cell lung cancer: the PLUS multicentre randomised trial. *Lancet* 2002; **359**: 1388–93.

69   Hain SF, Maisey MN. Positron emission tomography for urological tumours. *Br J Urol Int* 2003; **92**: 159–64.

70   Naumann R, Beuthien-Baumann B, Reiss A, *et al.* Substantial impact of FDG PET imaging on the therapy decision in patients with early-stage Hodgkin's lymphoma. *Br J Cancer* 2004; **90**: 620–5.

71   Scott AM, Poon A. PET Imaging of brain tumours. In: Ell PJ, Gambir S. (eds.) *Nuclear medicine in clinical diagnosis and treatment*, third edition. London: Churchill Livingstone, 2004: 345–59.

72   Buck AK, Hetzel M, Schirrmeister H, *et al.* Clinical relevance of imaging proliferative activity in lung nodules. *Eur J Nucl Med Mol Imaging* 2005; **32**: 525–33.

73   Valk PE. Randomized controlled trials are not appropriate for imaging technology evaluation. *J Nucl Med* 2000; **41**: 1125–6.

74   Scott AM, Lee F-T, Hopkins W, *et al.* Specific targeting, biodistribution and lack of immunogenicity of chimeric anti-GD3 monoclonal antibody KM871 in patients with metastatic melanoma – results of a phase I trial. *J Clin Oncol* 2001; **19**: 3976–87.

75   Kiffer JD, Berlangieri SU, Scott AM, *et al.* The contribution of ^{18}F-fluoro-2-deoxy-glucose positron emission tomographic imaging to radiotherapy planning in lung cancer. *Lung Cancer* 1998; **19**: 167–77.

76   Messa C, Di Muzio N, Picchio M, *et al.* PET/CT and radiotherapy. *Q J Nucl Med Mol Imaging* 2006; **50**: 4–14.

77   Findlay M, Young H, Cunningham D, *et al.* Noninvasive monitoring of tumor metabolism using fluorodeoxyglucose and positron emission tomography in colorectal cancer liver metastases: correlation with tumor response to fluorouracil. *J Clin Oncol* 1996; **14**: 700–8.

78   Berlangieri SU, Scott AM. Metabolic staging of lung cancer. *N Engl J Med* 2000; **343**: 290–2.

79   MacManus MP, Hicks RJ, Matthews JP, *et al.* Positron emission tomography is superior to computed tomography scanning for response-assessment after radical radiotherapy or chemoradiotherapy in patients with non-small-cell lung cancer. *J Clin Oncol* 2003; **21**: 1285–92.

80   Kostakoglu L, Goldsmith SJ. ^{18}F-FDG PET evaluation of the response to therapy for lymphoma and for breast, lung, and colorectal carcinoma. *J Nucl Med* 2003; **44**: 224–39.

81   Hawkins DS, Schuetze SM, Butrynski JE, *et al.* [^{18}F]Fluorodeoxyglucose positron emission tomography predicts outcome for Ewing sarcoma family of tumors. *J Clin Oncol* 2005; **23**: 8828–34.

82   Hoekstra CJ, Stroobants SG, Smit EF, *et al.* Prognostic relevance of response evaluation using [^{18}F]-2-fluoro-2-D-glucose positron emission tomography in patients with locally advanced non-small cell lung cancer. *J Clin Oncol* 2005; **23**: 8362–70.

83 Peñuelas I, Haberkorn U, Yaghoubi S, Gambhir SS. Gene therapy imaging in patients for oncology applications. *Eur J Nucl Med Mol Imaging* 2005; **32**: S384–403.

84 Demetri GD. Targting c-kit mutations in solid tumors: scientific rationale and novel therapeutic options. *Semin Oncol* 2001; **5(suppl 17)**: 19–26.

85 Blay JY, Bonvalot S, Casalia P, *et al.* Consensus meeting for the management of gastrointestinal stromal tumors. Report of the GIST Consensus Conference of 20–21 March 2004, under the auspices of ESMO. *Ann Oncol* 2005; **16**: 566–78.

86 Harte RJ, Matthews JC, O'Reilly SM, *et al.* Tumor, normal tissue, and plasma pharmacokinetic studies of fluorouracil biomodulation with *N*-phosphonacetyl-L-aspartate, folinic acid, and interferon alfa. *J Clin Oncol* 1999; **17**: 1580–8.

87 Saleem A, Harte RJ, Matthews JC, *et al.* Pharmacokinetic evaluation of *N*-[2-(dimethylamino) ethyl]acridine-4-carboxamide in patients by positron emission tomography. *J Clin Oncol* 2001; **19**: 1421–9.

88 Ackermann U, Tochon-Danguy H, Nerrie M, *et al.* Synthesis, ^{11}C labeling and biological properties of derivatives of the tyrphostin AG957. *Nucl Med Biol* 2005; **32**: 323–8.

89 Herbst RS, Mullani NA, Davis DW, *et al.* Development of biologic markers of response and assessment of antiangiogenic activity in a clinical trial of human recombinant endostatin. *J Clin Oncol* 2002; **20**: 3804–14.

90 Hutchinson OC, Collingridge DR, Barthel H, *et al.* Pharmacodynamics of radiolabeled anticancer drugs for positron emission tomography. *Curr Pharm* 2003; **9**: 931–44.

91 Strauss HW, Grewal RK, Pandit-Taskar N. Molecular imaging in nuclear cardiology. *Semin Nucl Med* 2004; **34**: 47–55.

92 Raffel DM, Wieland DM. Assessment of cardiac sympathetic nerve integrity with positron emission tomography. *Nucl Med Biol* 2001; **28**: 541–59.

93 Davies JR, Rudd JH, Weissberg PL. Molecular and metabolic imaging of atherosclerosis. *J Nucl Med* 2004; **45**: 1898–907.

94 Davies JR, Rudd JF, Fryer TD, Weissberg PL. Targeting the vulnerable plaque: the evolving role of nuclear imaging. *J Nucl Cardiol* 2005; **12**: 234–46.

95 Dobrucki LW, Sinusas AJ. Molecular imaging. A new approach to nuclear cardiology. *Q J Nucl Med Mol Imaging* 2005; **49**: 106–15.

96 Miyagawa M, Anton M, Haubner R, *et al.* PET of cardiac transgene expression: comparison of 2 approaches based on herpesviral thymidine kinase reporter gene. *J Nucl Med* 2004; **45**: 1917–23.

97 Wu AM, Yazaki PJ. Designer genes: recombinant antibody fragments for biological imaging. *Q J Nucl Med* 2000; **44**: 268–83.

98 Frost JJ. Molecular imaging of the brain: a historical perspective. *Neuroimaging Clin N Am* 2003; **13**: 653–8.

99 Talbot PS, Laruelle M. The role of *in vivo* molecular imaging with PET and SPECT in the elucidation of psychiatric drug action and new drug development. *Eur Neuropsychopharmacol* 2002; **12**: 503–11.

100 Morris PG. Synaptic and cellular events: the last frontier? *Eur Neuropsychopharmacol* 2002; **12**: 601–7.

101 Slifstein M, Laruelle M. Models and methods for derivation of *in vivo* neuroreceptor parameters with PET and SPECT reversible radiotracers. *Nucl Med Biol* 2001; **28**: 595–608.

102 Hartvig P, Bergstrom M, Antoni G, Langstrom B. Positron emission tomography and brain monoamine neurotransmission – entries for study of drug interactions. *Curr Pharm Des* 2002; **8**: 1417–34.

103 Ravina B, Eidelberg D, Ahlskog JE, *et al.* The role of radiotracer imaging in Parkinson disease. *Neurology* 2005; **64**: 208–15.

104 Eckert T, Barnes A, Dhawan V, *et al.* FDG PET in the differential diagnosis of parkinsonian disorders. *Neuroimage* 2005; **26**: 912–21.

105 Schmidt B, Braun HA, Narlawar R, *et al.* Drug development and PET-diagnostics for Alzheimer's disease. *Curr Med Chem* 2005; **12**: 1677–95.

106 Nordberg A. PET imaging of amyloid in Alzheimer's disease. *Lancet Neurol* 2004; **3**: 519–27.

107 Villemagne VL, Rowe CC, Macfarlane S, *et al.* Imaginem oblivionis: the prospects of neuroimaging for early detection of Alzheimer's disease. *J Clin Neurosci* 2005; **12**: 221–30.

108 LaFerla FM, Oddo S. Alzheimer's disease: A beta, tau and synaptic dysfunction. *Trends Mol Med* 2005; **11**: 170–6.

109 Lee HG, Perry G, Moreira PI, *et al.* Tau phosphorylation in Alzheimer's disease: pathogen or protector? *Trends Mol Med* 2005; **11**: 164–9.

110 Marlatt MW, Webber KM, Moreira PI, *et al.* Therapeutic opportunities in Alzheimer disease: one for all or all for one? *Curr Med Chem* 2005; **12**: 1137–47.

111 Brooks DJ. Positron emission tomography and single-photon emission computed tomography in central nervous system drug development. *NeuroRx* 2005; **2**: 226–36.

112 Jagust W. Molecular neuroimaging in Alzheimer's disease. *NeuroRx* 2004; **1**: 206–12.

113 Koeppe RA, Gilman S, Joshi A, *et al.* ^{11}C-DTBZ and ^{18}F-FDG PET measures in differentiating dementias. *J Nucl Med* 2005; **46**: 936–44.

114 Silverman DH, Small GW, Chang CY, *et al.* Positron emission tomography in evaluation of dementia: regional brain metabolism and long-term outcome. *JAMA* 2001; **286**: 2120–7.

Peptide receptor imaging

DIK J. KWEKKEBOOM AND ERIC P. KRENNING

INTRODUCTION

Peptide receptor scintigraphy in man started with the *in vivo* demonstration of somatostatin receptor positive tumors in patients using a radioiodinated somatostatin analog.[1] Later, other radiolabeled somatostatin analogs were developed, and two of these subsequently became commercially available. Because of the almost worldwide availability of radiopharmaceuticals for somatostatin receptor imaging, most of this chapter will focus on this type of receptor scintigraphy. At the end of the chapter other peptide receptor imaging agents will be briefly discussed.

SOMATOSTATIN RECEPTORS

Somatostatin is a regulatory peptide widely distributed in the human body, particularly in the endocrine glands, the nervous system, the gastrointestinal tract, as well as the immune system. In the nervous system, somatostatin acts as a neurotransmitter, whereas its hormonal activities include the inhibition of the physiologic and tumorous release of growth hormone, insulin, glucagon, gastrin, serotonin, and calcitonin.[2] Other actions are an antiproliferative effect on tumors, and also specific regulation of immune responses.[3]

The action of somatostatin is mediated through membrane-bound receptors, of which five have been cloned.[4] Only receptor subtype-2, subtype-5 and, to some extent, subtype-3 have a high affinity for the commercially available synthetic analogs octreotide, lanreotide or vapreotide.[5] Somatostatin receptors are expressed in several normal human tissues, including brain, pituitary, gastrointestinal tract, pancreas, thyroid, spleen, kidney, immune cells, vessels, and peripheral nervous system.[6–9]

Somatostatin receptors have also been identified in a large number of human neuroendocrine tumors, such as pituitary adenoma, pancreatic islet cell tumor, carcinoid, pheochromocytoma, paraganglioma, medullary thyroid cancer, and small-cell lung carcinoma. In addition, other tumors, such as meningioma, neuroblastoma, medulloblastoma, lymphoma, breast cancer, renal cell cancer, hepatocellular cancer, prostate cancer, sarcoma, and gastric cancer can express somatostatin receptors.[10] Non-tumoral lesions, like active granulomas and inflamed joints in active rheumatoid arthritis may also express somatostatin receptors.[11,12]

SCINTIGRAPHY

Radiolabeled somatostatin analogs

Because the radioiodinated somatostatin analog that was first used in patients, [^{123}I-Tyr^3]-octreotide, had several drawbacks, soon a chelated and ^{111}In-labeled somatostatin analog, [^{111}In-DTPA^0]-octreotide, was developed. [^{111}In-DTPA^0]-octreotide (Octreoscan®) is commercially available and is the most commonly used agent for somatostatin receptor imaging. The scanning protocol and scintigraphic results that are discussed below are therefore based on the use of [^{111}In-DTPA^0]-octreotide.

^{99m}Tc-depreotide (Neotect®) is another commercially available somatostatin analog that has been approved specifically for the detection of lung cancer in patients with pulmonary nodules.[13] Because of the relatively high abdominal background and the impossibility of performing delayed imaging due to the short half-life of the tracer, it is less suited for the detection of abdominal neuroendocrine tumors.[14]

[^{111}In-DOTA]-lanreotide is another somatostatin receptor imaging agent with a slightly different affinity profile than [^{111}In-DTPA[0]]-octreotide.[15] In comparison with Octreoscan, it has a lower sensitivity in demonstrating neuroendocrine tumor, but it may have advantages in other tumors, for instance in differentiated thyroid cancer.[16]

Scanning protocol

The preferred dose of [^{111}In-DTPA[0]]-octreotide (with at least 10 μg of the peptide) is about 200 MBq. With such a dose it is possible to perform single photon emission computed tomography (SPECT), which may increase the sensitivity.

Planar images are obtained with a double head or large field of view gamma camera, equipped with medium-energy parallel-hole collimators. The pulse height analyzer windows are centered over both ^{111}In photon peaks (172 keV and 245 keV) with a window width of 20%. The acquisition parameters for planar images (preferably spot views) are 300 000 preset counts or 15 min per view for the head and neck, and 500 000 counts or 15 min for the remainder of the body. If 'whole-body' acquisition is used, scan speed should not exceed 3 cm min^{-1}. Using higher scan speeds, like 8 cm min^{-1}, will result in failure to recognize small somatostatin receptor-positive lesions and lesions with a low density of these receptors.[17] For SPECT images with a triple-head camera the acquisition parameters are: 40 steps of 3° each, 128 × 128 matrix, and at least 30 s per step (45 s for SPECT of the head).

Planar and SPECT studies are preferably performed 24 h after injection of the radiopharmaceutical. A higher lesion detection rate by 24 h planar imaging over 4 h acquisition was reported by Jamar et al.,[18] as well as the additional value of SPECT imaging. Repeat scintigraphy after 48 h is especially indicated when 24 h scintigraphy shows accumulation in the abdomen, which may also represent radioactive bowel content.

Normal scintigraphic findings and artifacts

Normal scintigraphic features include visualization of the thyroid, spleen, liver, and kidneys, and in a portion of the patients of the pituitary and gallbladder (Fig. 1B.1). Recently, the visualization of one or both adrenal glands on SPECT images has also been reported in about 25% of patients without known adrenal pathology.[19] Also, the urinary bladder and the bowel are usually visualized. The visualization of the pituitary, thyroid, spleen, and adrenals is due to receptor binding. Uptake in the kidneys is for the most part

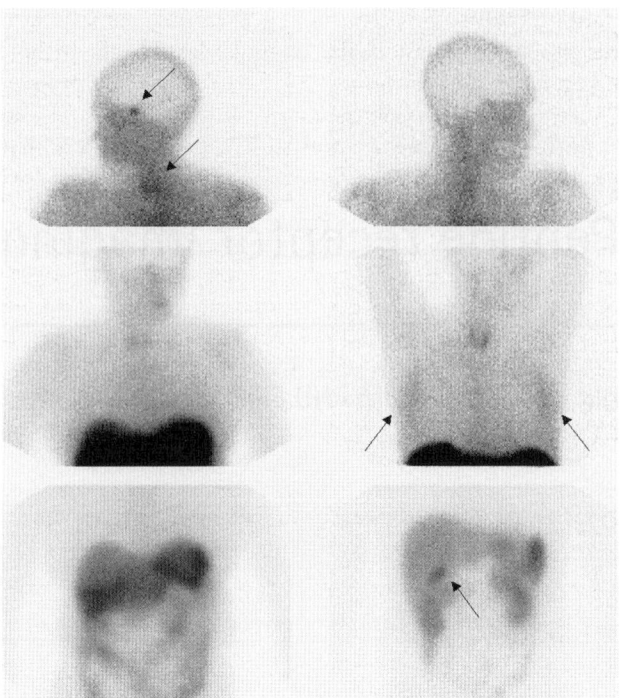

Figure 1B.1 *Normal distribution in somatostatin receptor imaging. Variable visualization of the pituitary and thyroid (arrows, upper panel). Faint breast uptake can sometimes be seen in women (right middle panel, arrows). Normal uptake in the liver, spleen, and the kidneys, and also some bowel activity in the lower panels. Gallbladder visualization in the lower right panel (arrow). Anterior views.*

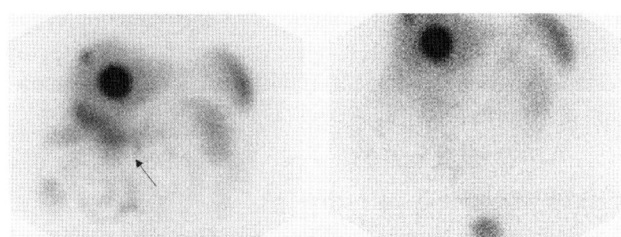

Figure 1B.2 *Anterior abdominal views in a patient with two liver metastases of a carcinoid tumor, 24 h (left) and 48 h post-injection (right). Intense uptake at the site of the tumors. Note that bowel radioactivity which is present in the abdomen at 24 h post-injection (arrow), has disappeared on the delayed images (right panel), due to the ongoing use of laxatives.*

due to re-absorption of the radiolabeled peptide in the renal tubular cells after glomerular filtration, although somatostatin receptors have been demonstrated in human renal tubular cells and vasa recta.[20] There is a predominant renal clearance of the somatostatin analog, although hepatobiliary clearance into the bowel also occurs, necessitating the use of laxatives in order to facilitate the interpretation of abdominal images (Fig. 1B.2).

False positive results of somatostatin receptor imaging (SRI) have been reported. In virtually all cases the term 'false positive' is a misnomer because somatostatin receptor-positive lesions that are not related to the pathology for which the investigation is performed, are present. Examples are the visualization of the gallbladder, thyroid abnormalities, accessory spleens, recent cerebrovascular accidents, activity at the site of a recent surgical incision, etc. Many of these have been reviewed by Gibril et al.[21] Also, chest uptake after irradiation and diffuse breast uptake in female patients can be mistaken for other pathology. In some patients, the co-existence of two different somatostatin receptor-positive diseases should be considered. During ongoing treatment with unlabeled octreotide, the uptake of [^{111}In-DTPA^0]-octreotide in somatostatin receptor-positive tumors and the spleen is diminished.

IMAGING RESULTS IN NEUROENDOCRINE AND OTHER TUMORS

Pituitary tumors

The majority of growth hormone-producing and clinically nonfunctioning pituitary adenomas can be visualized with SRI, but other pituitary tumors as well as pituitary metastases from somatostatin receptor-positive neoplasms, parasellar meningiomas, lymphomas or granulomatous diseases of the pituitary may be positive as well. Therefore the diagnostic value of SRI in pituitary tumors is limited.[22]

Endocrine pancreatic tumors

The majority of the endocrine pancreatic tumors can be visualized using SRI. Reported data on the sensitivity of SRI in patients with gastrinomas vary from about 60 to 90%,[23–26] and part of the discrepancy in results is likely due to insufficient scanning technique.

Using ultrasound, computed tomography (CT), magnetic resonance imaging (MRI), and/or angiography, endocrine pancreatic tumors can be localized in about 50% of cases.[27] Endoscopic ultrasound has been reported to be very sensitive in detecting endocrine pancreatic tumors, also when CT or transabdominal ultrasound fail to demonstrate the tumor.[28] Studies comparing the value of endoscopic ultrasonography with SRI in the same patients point to more favorable results for SRI.[24,26] In a prospective study in 80 patients with Zollinger – Ellison syndrome, Gibril et al.[25] found that SRI was as sensitive as all other imaging studies combined and advocated its use as the first imaging method to be used in these patients. Lebtahi et al.[29] reported that the results of SRI in 160 patients with gastro-entero-pancreatic (GEP) tumors modified patient classification and surgical therapeutic strategy in 25% of patients. Also, Termanini et al.[30] reported that SRI altered patient management in 47% of 122 patients with gastrinomas. However, results in patients with insulinomas are disappointing, possibly

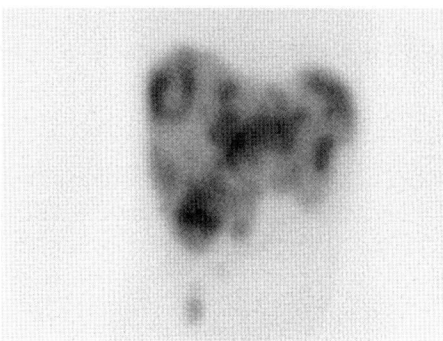

Figure 1B.3 *Anterior abdominal view in a patient with carcinoid syndrome. Irregular uptake in the liver with focal areas of increased uptake in carcinoid metastases. Also uptake in the presumed primary in the lower right abdomen.*

because part of these tumors may either be somatostatin receptor-negative or contain somatostatin receptors that do not bind octreotide.

Lebtahi et al.[14] compared ^{99m}Tc-depreotide (Neotect®) and [^{111}In-DTPA^0]-octreotide (Octreoscan®) in the same 43 patients with neuroendocrine tumors. With [^{111}In-DTPA^0]-octreotide 203 tumor sites in 39/43 (91%) patients were detected, whereas with ^{99m}Tc-depreotide, 77 sites in 28/43 (65%) patients were recognized. It can therefore be concluded that [^{111}In-DTPA^0]-octreotide scintigraphy is more sensitive for the detection of neuroendocrine tumors.

Carcinoids

Reported values for the detection of known carcinoid tumor localizations vary from 80 to nearly 100% (Figs 1B.2 and 1B.3).[31–33] Also, the detection of unexpected tumor sites, not suspected with conventional imaging, is reported by several investigators.[31,33]

Treatment with octreotide may cause a relief of symptoms and a decrease of urinary 5-HIAA levels in patients with carcinoid syndrome. In patients with carcinoid syndrome, SRI, in consequence of its ability to demonstrate somatostatin receptor-positive tumors, could therefore be used to select those patients who are likely to respond favourably to octreotide treatment. On the other hand, only for those patients who have somatostatin receptor-negative tumors, is chemotherapy effective.[34]

The impact on patient management is four-fold: SRI may detect resectable tumors that would be unrecognized with conventional imaging techniques; it may prevent surgery in patients whose tumors have metastasized to a greater extent than can be detected with conventional imaging; it may direct the choice of therapy in patients with inoperable tumors; and it may be used to select patients for peptide receptor radionuclide therapy (PRRT, see below).

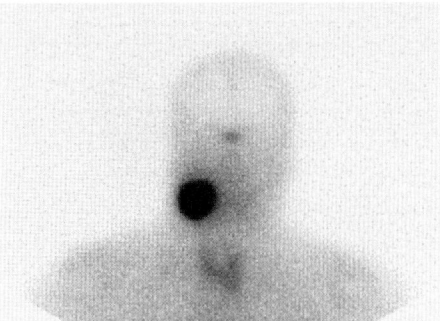

Figure 1B.4 *Anterior view of the head in a patient with a carotid body paraganglioma.*

Paragangliomas

In virtually all patients with paragangliomas, tumors are readily visualized (Fig. 1B.4).[35] Unexpected additional paraganglioma sites are frequently found. Multicentricity and distant metastases are each reported to occur in 10% of patients; in our study with SRI, we found multiple sites of pathology in nine of 25 patients (36%) with a known paraganglioma.[35] One of the major advantages of SRI is that it provides information on potential tumor sites in the whole body in patients with paraganglioma. It could thus be used as a screening test, to be followed by CT scanning, MRI or ultrasound of the sites at which abnormalities are found.

Medullary thyroid carcinoma and other thyroid cancers

In patients with medullary thyroid carcinoma (MTC) the sensitivity of SRI in detecting tumor localizations is 50–70% (Fig. 1B.5).[36,37] In a series of 17 patients with MTC whom we studied,[36] the ratio of serum calcitonin over carcino-embryonic antigen (CEA) levels was significantly higher in patients in whom SRI was successfully applied. This may imply that somatostatin receptors can be detected *in vivo* on the more differentiated forms of MTC. Also, SRI is more frequently positive in patients with high serum tumor markers and large tumors,[37] and seems therefore less suitable for demonstrating microscopic disease.

Although papillary, follicular, and anaplastic thyroid cancers, and also Hürthle cell carcinomas, do not belong to the group of classical neuro-endocrine tumors, the majority of patients with these cancers show uptake of radiolabeled octreotide during SRI.[38,39] Also, it is not necessary to withdraw patients from L-thyroxine suppression therapy in order to perform SRI.[40] Interestingly, differentiated thyroid cancers that do not take up radioactive iodine may also show radiolabeled octreotide accumulation.[38] In some patients, this could open new therapeutic options: surgery, if the number of observed lesions is limited, or, alternatively, PRRT if the uptake is sufficient.

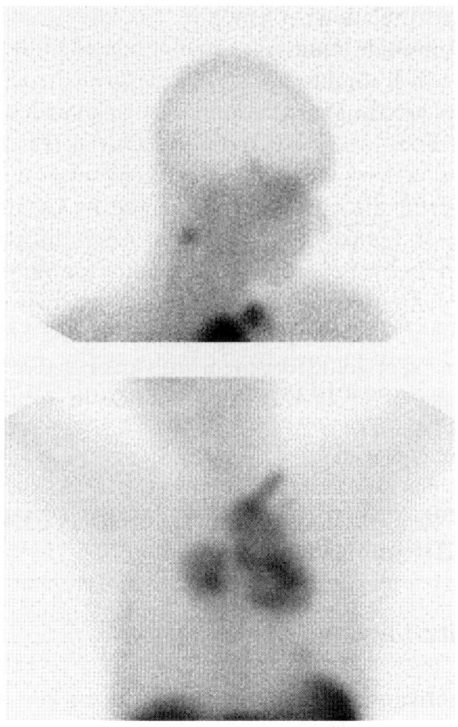

Figure 1B.5 *Lateral view of the head and anterior view of the chest in a patient with medullary thyroid carcinoma with bone metastases. There is visualization of a huge tumor mass in the chest with metastases in a rib and the cervical spine.*

Merkel cell tumors

Trabecular carcinomas of the skin or Merkel cell tumors, are aggressive neoplasms which tend to occur in skin exposed to the sun. Often these tumors metastasize and, despite therapy, disease-related death is high. In four out of the five patients studied with SRI in whom tumor had also been detected by CT and/or ultrasound, these sites were recognized on the scintigrams. In two patients SRI demonstrated more metastatic tumor localizations than previously recognized.[41]

Lung cancer

With SRI the primary tumors can be demonstrated in virtually all patients with small-cell lung cancer (SCLC).[42–44] A proportion of the known metastases may be missed, however. The unexpected finding of brain metastases, in particular, is reported by several authors.[42,43] Others, however, have reported the lack of any additional information with SRI.[45]

^{99m}Tc-depreotide was used in a multicenter trial comprising 114 patients who had indeterminate solitary pulmonary nodules (SPNs).[46] The sensitivity of ^{99m}Tc-depreotide scintigraphy for detecting malignancy was 97% and its specificity 73%. Six of seven false positive studies were caused by tracer accumulation in granulomas. The sensitivity of ^{99m}Tc-depreotide scintigraphy for detecting malignancy in SPN is comparable to that of [^{18}F]fluorodeoxyglucose (^{18}F-FDG) and might serve as an alternative for the latter.

Breast cancer

SRI localized 39 of 52 primary breast cancers (75%).[47] Imaging of the axillae showed nonpalpable cancer-containing lymph nodes in four of 13 patients with subsequently histologically proven metastases. In the follow-up after a mean of 2.5 years, SRI in 28 of the 37 patients with an originally somatostatin receptor-positive cancer, was positive in two patients with clinically recognized metastases, as well as in six of the remaining 26 patients who were symptom-free. SRI may be of value in selecting patients for clinical trials with somatostatin analogs or other medical treatments.

Malignant lymphomas

In vitro, somatostatin receptors can be detected in the majority of lymphomas. However, their density is often very low.[48] Although in many patients with non-Hodgkin's lymphoma (NHL) one or more lesions may be somatostatin receptor-positive; receptor-negative lesions also occur in a substantial number of patients.[49] Also, uptake of [^{111}In-DTPA^0]-octreotide in lymphomas is lower compared to the uptake in neuroendocrine tumors.[50] In a prospective study in 50 untreated patients with low-grade NHL, SRI was positive in 84% (42/50) of patients.[51] In 20% of patients, SRI revealed lesions that had not been demonstrated by conventional staging procedures. However, in 19 patients (38%), lesions were missed by SRI. Because of the limited sensitivity, SRI is recommended only in selected cases of low-grade NHL.

In 126 consecutive untreated patients with histologically proven Hodgkin's disease, the results of SRI were compared with physical and radiological examinations.[52] SRI was positive in all patients. The lesion-related sensitivity was 94% and varied from 98% for supradiaphragmatic lesions to 67% for infradiaphragmatic lesions. In comparison with CT scanning and ultrasonography, SRI provided superior results for the detection of Hodgkin's disease localizations above the diaphragm. In stages I and II supradiaphragmatic patients, SRI detected more advanced disease in 18% (15/83) of patients, resulting in an upstaging to stage III or IV, thus directly influencing patient management. These data support the validity of SRI as a powerful imaging technique for the staging of patients with Hodgkin's disease.

Melanoma

Positive results of SRI have been reported in 16 out of 19 patients with melanoma.[53] The exact impact of SRI on staging and patient management remains to be determined.

Neuroblastomas and pheochromocytomas

In about 90% of patients with neuroblastoma, SRI visualized tumor deposits.[54] Patients with neuroblastomas that are somatostatin receptor-positive *in vitro* have a longer survival compared with the receptor-negative ones.[55] A drawback of the use of SRI for localization of this tumor in the adrenal gland is the relatively high radioligand accumulation in the kidneys. Scintigraphy using *meta*-iodobenzylguanidine (MIBG) is preferred for its localization in this region.

In a large retrospective study in patients who underwent surgery for pheochromocytoma, the overall preoperative detection rate for tumors larger than 1 cm in diameter was 90% for ^{123}I-MIBG, and only 25% for SRI.[56] Most of the patients had primary benign pheochromocytomas. In patients with metastases, SRI detected lesions in seven of eight patients, including ^{123}I-MIBG negative cases. Therefore, it can be concluded that SRI should be tried in suspicious metastatic pheocromocytomas, especially if ^{123}I-MIBG is negative.

Cushing's syndrome

In a study of 19 patients with Cushing's syndrome, none of the pituitary adenomas of 8 patients with Cushing's disease or the adrenal adenoma of another patient could be visualized with SRI. In eight of the other 10 patients, the primary ectopic corticotropin or corticotropin-releasing hormone (CRH) secreting tumors were successfully identified with SRI.[57] Also, the successful localization of a 6 mm and a 10 mm diameter corticotropin-secreting bronchial carcinoid have been reported.[58,59] Therefore, SRI can be included as a diagnostic step in the work-up of Cushing's syndrome with a suspected ectopic corticotropin or CRH-secreting tumor. Others, however, conclude that although SRI may be helpful in selected cases, it is not a significant advance over conventional imaging.[60]

Brain tumors

SRI localizes meningiomas in virtually all patients.[61,62] Also astrocytomas have been visualized with SRI.[62] A prerequisite for their localization with this radioligand is a locally open blood–brain barrier. Especially in the lower graded astrocytomas this barrier may be unperturbed and the astrocytomas not visualized. It is presently not completely clear to what extent a positive octreoscan identifies somatostatin receptors located on glial tumor cells; recent studies have shown that many of these receptors may also be localized on tissues contaminating the tumor samples, such as neurofibres and vessels.[63] Therefore, the grading of glial-derived brain tumors with SRI should not be recommended.

IMAGING RESULTS IN OTHER DISEASES

In vivo SRI is also positive in a number of granulomatous and autoimmune diseases, like sarcoidosis, tuberculosis, Wegener's granulomatosis, DeQuervain's thyroiditis, aspergillosis, Graves' hyperthyroidism, and Graves' ophthalmopathy.[11,64,65] It is expected that SRI may contribute to a more precise staging and a better evaluation of several of these diseases.

Sarcoidosis

In a cross-sectional study in 46 patients with sarcoidosis, known mediastinal, hilar, and interstitial disease were recognized in 36 of 37 patients (Fig. 1B.6).[66] Also, such pathology was found in seven other patients who had normal chest X-rays. In five of these, SRI pointed to interstitial disease. SRI was repeated in 13 patients. In five of six patients in whom a chest X-ray monitored an improvement of disease activity, SRI also showed a decrease of pathologic uptake. In two of five patients in whom the chest X-ray was unchanged, although serum ACE concentrations decreased and lung function improved, a normalization was found with SRI. To determine the value of SRI in the follow-up of patients with sarcoidosis a prospective longitudinal study will have to be performed.

Uveitis may be the presenting symptom of sarcoidosis. In our experience, in patients with uveitis, SRI can not infrequently be of help because of the typical pattern of uptake in the mediastinum, lung hila, and parotid glands that can be seen in patients who eventually appear to have sarcoidosis, even when the chest X-ray or CT are normal. Thus, SRI can be used to reach a diagnosis, and also influence the decision of how to treat this type of patient.

Graves' disease

In Graves' hyperthyroidism, accumulation of radiolabeled octreotide in the thyroid gland is markedly increased and correlates with serum levels of free thyroxine and thyrotropin binding inhibiting immunoglobulins. *In vitro* studies showed that the follicular cells express somatostatin receptors in Graves' disease.[67] In clinically active Graves' ophthalmopathy the orbits show accumulation of radioactivity 4 h and 24 h after injection of [^{111}In-DTPA[0]]-octreotide.[64] SPECT is required for a proper interpretation of orbital scintigraphy. There is also a correlation between orbital [^{111}In-DTPA[0]]-octreotide uptake and clinical activity score and total eye score.[64,68] The clinical value of SRI in Graves' disease has yet to be established. Possibly this technique could select those patients with Graves' ophthalmopathy who might benefit from treatment with octreotide.[65,68]

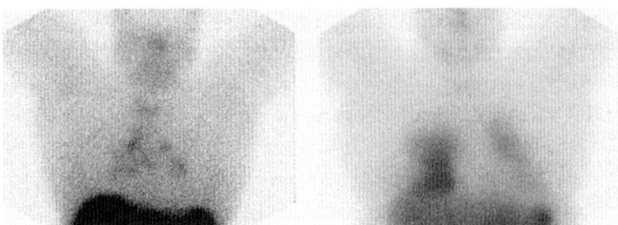

Figure 1B.6   *Bihilar (left image) and diffuse lung uptake (right image) in patients with sarcoidosis.*

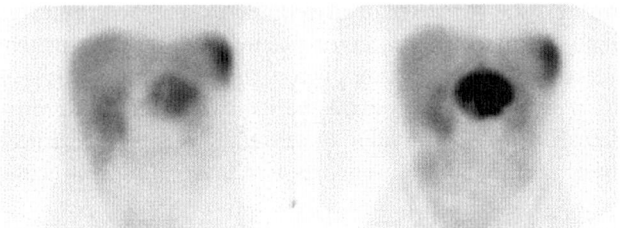

Figure 1B.7   *Images, 24 h post-injection, after [^{111}In-DTPA[0]]-octreotide (left panel) and after [^{177}Lu-DOTA[0],Tyr[3]]-octreotate (right panel) in a patient with an inoperable neuroendocrine pancreatic tumor. The uptake in the tumor sites is higher after [^{177}Lu-DOTA[0],Tyr[3]]-octreotate.*

PEPTIDE RECEPTOR RADIONUCLIDE THERAPY

In patients with somatostatin receptor-positive pathology, SRI is useful if it can localize otherwise undetectable disease, or if it can be used for treatment selection (usually the choice between symptomatic treatment with somatostatin analogs or other medical treatment). In patients with known metastatic disease, however, in whom little or no treatment alternatives are available, SRI has a limited role. This situation changes if imaging has a sequel in treatment. Recently, new somatostatin analogs such as [DOTA, Tyr[3]]-octreotide and [DOTA, Tyr[3]]-octreotate have been developed. This last compound has a considerably better binding affinity at subtype-2 receptors,[15] reflected by a three-fold to four-fold higher uptake than [^{111}In-DTPA[0]]-octreotide (Fig. 1B.7).[69] Because of the promising results in patients with neuroendocrine tumors of treatment with these somatostatin analogs coupled to yttrium-90[70–72] or the beta- and gamma-emitting radionuclide lutetium-177,[73] we expect that SRI will be increasingly used to select patients for such therapy (see Chapter 17B).

OTHER RADIOLABELED PEPTIDES

In vitro investigations have identified other peptide receptors expressed in high amounts by human tumors, opening new possibilities for peptide receptor scintigraphy. For instance, substance P receptors are expressed in high amounts in glioblastomas, MTC, and breast tumors.[74] This might be a basis for substance P receptor scintigraphy in these types of tumors. While such *in vivo* studies have not been performed in cancers, van Hagen *et al.*[75] reported the visualization of the thymus and disease-invaded sites in patients with autoimmune diseases, after the injection of an ^{111}In-labeled chelated substance P analog (^{111}In-DTPA-Arg[1]-substance P). It is speculated that this type of scintigraphy may be used to investigate the role of the thymus in immune-mediated diseases.

Virgolini *et al.*[76] reported the successful visualization of neuroendocrine tumors and adenocarcinomas with ^{123}I-vasoactive intestinal peptide (VIP). The cumbersome peptide labeling with ^{123}I is, amongst others, yet a limitation to the widespread use of this type of scintigraphy. However, the development of chelated VIP analogs, which can be labeled with ^{111}In, or of ^{99m}Tc-labeled compounds, might change this.[77]

Receptors for cholecystokinin (CCK) have been demonstrated *in vitro* in various tumors, especially MTC.[78] Depending on the analogs used, the reported results of scintigraphy with ^{111}In-labeled, DTPA-chelated CCK-B analogs in patients with MTC vary.[79,80] Interestingly, Béhé and Behr[80] reported the successful visualization of known lesions in all 43 studied patients, and also the targeting of at least one tumor site in 29 of 32 patients with negative conventional imaging studies.

One of the newer, promising peptide receptors to be targeted may possibly be the gastrin-releasing peptide (GRP) receptors which are expressed in high incidence and density in two frequently occurring cancers: breast and prostate carcinomas.[81,82] Van der Wiele *et al.*[83] were recently able to visualize with a ^{99m}Tc-labeled bombesin(7-14) analog both breast and prostate carcinomas, providing the proof of principle for GRP receptor scintigraphy *in vivo*.

CONCLUSIONS AND PERSPECTIVE

[^{111}In-DTPA[0]]-octreotide is a radiopharmaceutical with great potential for the visualization of somatostatin receptor-positive tumors. The overall sensitivity of SRI in localizing neuroendocrine tumors is high. In a number of neuroendocrine tumor types, as well as in Hodgkin's disease, inclusion of SRI in the localization or staging procedure may be very rewarding, in terms of cost-effectiveness, patient management, or quality of life. The value of SRI in patients with other tumors, such as breast cancer, or in patients with granulomatous diseases, has to be established.

Other radiolabeled peptide analogs hold great promise for the future, both for diagnosis and for therapy. Finally, the development of PRRT is expected to stimulate peptide receptor imaging.

REFERENCES

1 Krenning EP, Bakker WH, Breeman WAP, *et al.* Localization of endocrine related tumors with radio-iodinated analogue of somatostatin. *Lancet* 1989; **1**: 242–5.

2 Brazeau P. Somatostatin: a peptide with unexpected physiologic activities. *Am J Med* 1986; **81(Suppl 6B)**: 8–13.

3 Lamberts SWJ, Krenning EP, Reubi JC. The role of somatostatin and its analogs in the diagnosis and treatment of tumors. *Endocr Rev* 1991; **12**: 450–82.

4 Patel YC, Greenwood MT, Warszynska A, Panetta R, Srikant CB. All five cloned somatostatin receptors (hSSTR1-5) are functionally coupled to adenylyl cyclase. *Biochem Biophys Res Commun* 1994; **198**: 605–12.

5 Hoyer D, Epelbaum J, Feniuk W, *et al.* Somatostatin receptors. In: Girdlestrom D. (ed.) *The IUPHAR compendium of receptor characterization and classification.* London: IUPHAR Media, 2000: 354–64.

6 Sreedharan SP, Kodama KT, Peterson KE, Goetzl EJ. Distinct subsets of somatostatin receptors on cultured human lymphocytes. *J Biol Chem* 1989; **264**: 949–53.

7 Reubi JC, Horisberger U, Waser B, Gebbers JO, Laissue J. Preferential location of somatostatin receptors in germinal centers of human gut lymphoid tissue. *Gastroenterology* 1992; **103**: 1207–14.

8 Reubi JC, Schaer JC, Markwalder R, Waser B, Horisberger U, Laissue JA. Distribution of somatostatin receptors in normal and neoplastic human tissues: recent advances and potential relevance. *Yale J Biol Med* 1997; **70**: 471–9.

9 Csaba Z, Dournaud P. Cellular biology of somatostatin receptors. *Neuropeptides* 2001; **35**: 1–23.

10 Reubi JC. Regulatory peptide receptors as molecular targets for cancer diagnosis and therapy. *Q J Nucl Med* 1997; **41**: 63–70.

11 Vanhagen PM, Krenning EP, Reubi JC, *et al.* Somatostatin analogue scintigraphy in granulomatous diseases. *Eur J Nucl Med* 1994; **21**: 497–502.

12 Reubi JC, Waser B, Krenning EP, Markusse HM, Vanhagen M, Laissue JA. Vascular somatostatin receptors in synovium from patients with rheumatoid arthritis. *Eur J Pharmacol* 1994; **271**: 371–8.

13 Menda Y, Kahn D. Somatostatin receptor imaging of non-small lung cancer with ^{99m}Tc depreotide. *Semin Nucl Med* 2002; **32**: 92–6.

14 Lebtahi R, Le Cloirec J, Houzard C, *et al.* Detection of neuroendocrine tumors: (99m)Tc-P829 scintigraphy compared with (111)In-pentetreotide scintigraphy. *J Nucl Med* 2002; **43**: 889–95.

15 Reubi JC, Schaer JC, Waser B, *et al.* Affinity profiles for human somatostatin receptor sst1–sst5 of somatostatin radiotracers selected for scintigraphic and radiotherapeutic use. *Eur J Nucl Med* 2000; **27**: 273–82.

16 Virgolini I, Britton K, Buscombe J, Moncayo R, Paganelli G, Riva P. [111]In- and ^{90}Y-DOTA-lanreotide: results and implications of the MAURITIUS trial. *Semin Nucl Med* 2002; **32**: 148–55.

17 Van Uden A, Steinmeijer MVJ, De Swart J, *et al.* Imaging with octreoscan: haste makes waste. *Eur J Nucl Med* 1999; **26**: 1022P.

18 Jamar F, Fiasse R, Leners N, Pauwels S. Somatostatin receptor imaging with indium-111-pentetreotide in gastroenteropancreatic neuroendocrine tumors: safety, efficacy and impact on patient management. *J Nucl Med* 1995; **36**: 542–9.

19 Jacobsson H, Bremmer S, Larsson SA. Visualisation of the normal adrenals at SPET examination with ^{111}In-pentetreotide. *Eur J Nucl Med Mol Imag* 2003; **30**: 1169–72.

20 Reubi JC, Horisberger U, Studer UE, Waser B, Laissue JA. Human kidney as target for somatostatin: high affinity receptors in tubules and vasa recta. *J Clin Endocrinol Metab* 1993; **77**: 1323–8.

21 Gibril F, Reynolds JC, Chen CC, *et al.* Specificity of somatostatin receptor scintigraphy: a prospective study and effects of false-positive localizations on management in patients with gastrinomas. *J Nucl Med* 1999; **40**: 539–53.

22 Kwekkeboom DJ, de Herder WW, Krenning EP. Receptor imaging in the diagnosis and treatment of pituitary tumors. *J Endocrinol Invest* 1999; **22**: 80–8.

23 Kwekkeboom DJ, Krenning EP, Oei HY, van Eyck CHJ, Lamberts SWJ. Use of radiolabeled somatostatin to localize islet cell tumors. In: Mignon M, Jensen RT. (eds.) *Frontiers of gastro-intestinal research. Vol 23. Endocrine tumors of the pancreas.* New York: Karger, 1995: 298–308.

24 De Kerviler E, Cadiot G, Lebtahi R, Faraggi M, Le Guludec D, Mignon M. Somatostatin receptor scintigraphy in forty-eight patients with the Zollinger–Ellison syndrome. *Eur J Nucl Med* 1994; **21**: 1191–7.

25 Gibril F, Reynolds JC, Doppman JL, *et al.* Somatostatin receptor scintigraphy: its sensitivity compared with that of other imaging methods in detecting primary and metastatic gastrinomas. A prospective study. *Ann Intern Med* 1996; **125**: 26–34.

26 Zimmer T, Stolzel U, Bader M, *et al.* Endoscopic ultrasonography and somatostatin receptor scintigraphy in the preoperative localisation of insulinomas and gastrinomas. *Gut* 1996; **39**: 562–8.

27 Lunderquist A. Radiologic diagnosis of neuroendocrine tumors. *Acta Oncol* 1989; **28**: 371–2.

28 Rösch T, Lightdale CJ, Botet JF, *et al.* Localization of pancreatic endocrine tumors by endoscopic ultrasonography. *N Engl J Med* 1992; **326**: 1721–6.

29 Lebtahi R, Cadiot G, Sarda L, *et al.* Clinical impact of somatostatin receptor scintigraphy in the management of patients with neuroendocrine gastroenteropancreatic tumors. *J Nucl Med* 1997; **38**: 853–8.

30 Termanini B, Gibril F, Reynolds JC, *et al.* Value of somatostatin receptor scintigraphy: a prospective study in gastrinoma of its effect on clinical management. *Gastroenterology* 1997; **112**: 335–47.

31 Kwekkeboom DJ, Krenning EP, Bakker WH, *et al.* Somatostatin analogue scintigraphy in carcinoid tumors. *Eur J Nucl Med* 1993; **20**: 283–92.

32 Kalkner KM, Janson ET, Nilsson S, Carlsson S, Oberg K, Westlin JE. Somatostatin receptor scintigraphy in patients with carcinoid tumors: comparison between radioligand uptake and tumor markers. *Cancer Res* 1995; **55(Suppl 23)**: 5801–4.

33 Westlin JE, Janson ET, Arnberg H, Ahlstrom H, Oberg K, Nilsson S. Somatostatin receptor scintigraphy of carcinoid tumours using the [^{111}In-DTPA-D-Phe[1]]-octreotide. *Acta Oncol* 1993; **32**: 783–786.

34 Kvols LK. Medical oncology considerations in patients with metastatic neuroendocrine carcinomas. *Semin Oncol* 1994; **21(Suppl 13)**: 56–60.

35 Kwekkeboom DJ, Van Urk H, Pauw KH, *et al.* Octreotide scintigraphy for the detection of paragangliomas. *J Nucl Med* 1993; **34**: 873–878.

36 Kwekkeboom DJ, Reubi JC, Lamberts SWJ, *et al.* In vivo somatostatin receptor imaging in medullary thyroid carcinoma. *J Clin Endocrinol Metab* 1993; **76**: 1413–17.

37 Tisell LE, Ahlman H, Wängberg B, *et al.* Somatostatin receptor scintigraphy in medullary thyroid carcinoma. *Br J Surg* 1997; **84**: 543–7.

38 Postema PTE, De Herder WW, Reubi JC, *et al.* Somatostatin receptor scintigraphy in non-medullary thyroid cancer. *Digestion* 1996; **1(Suppl)**: 36–7.

39 Gulec SA, Serafini AN, Sridhar KS, *et al.* Somatostatin receptor expression in Hurthle cell cancer of the thyroid. *J Nucl Med* 1998; **39**: 243–5.

40 Haslinghuis LM, Krenning EP, de Herder WW, Reijs AEM, Kwekkeboom DJ. Somatostatin receptor scintigraphy in the follow-up of patients with differentiated thyroid cancer. *J Endocrinol Invest* 2001; **24**: 415–22.

41 Kwekkeboom DJ, Hoff AM, Lamberts SWJ, *et al.* Somatostatin analogue scintigraphy: a simple and sensitive method for the in vivo visualization of Merkel cell tumors and their metastases. *Arch Dermatol* 1992; **128**: 818–21.

42 Kwekkeboom DJ, Kho GS, Lamberts SW, Reubi JC, Laissue JA, Krenning EP. The value of octreotide scintigraphy in patients with lung cancer. *Eur J Nucl Med* 1994; **21**: 1106–13.

43 Bombardieri E, Crippa F, Cataldo I, *et al.* Somatostatin receptor imaging of small cell lung cancer (SCLC) by means of ^{111}In-DTPA octreotide scintigraphy. *Eur J Cancer* 1995; **31A**: 184–8.

44 Reisinger I, Bohuslavitzki KH, Brenner W, *et al.* Somatostatin receptor scintigraphy in small-cell lung cancer: results of a multicenter study. *J Nucl Med* 1998; **39**: 224–7.

45 Kirsch CM, von Pawel J, Grau I, Tatsch K. Indium-111 pentetreotide in the diagnostic work-up of patients with bronchogenic carcinoma. *Eur J Nucl Med* 1994; **21**: 1318–25.

46 Blum J, Handmaker H, Lister-James J, Rinne N. A multicenter trial with a somatostatin analog (99m)Tc depreotide in the evaluation of solitary pulmonary nodules. *Chest* 2000; **117**: 1232–8.

47 Van Eijck CH, Krenning EP, Bootsma A, *et al*. Somato-statin-receptor scintigraphy in primary breast cancer. *Lancet* 1994; **343**: 640–3.

48 Reubi JC, Waser B, Vanhagen M, *et al*. In vitro and in vivo detection of somatostatin receptors in human malignant lymphomas. *Int J Cancer* 1992; **50**: 895–900.

49 Van Hagen PM, Krenning EP, Reubi JC, *et al*. Somato-statin analogue scintigraphy of malignant lymphomas. *Br J Haemat* 1993; **83**: 75–9.

50 Leners N, Jamar F, Fiasse R, Ferrant A, Pauwels S. Indium-111-pentetreotide uptake in endocrine tumors and lymphoma. *J Nucl Med* 1996; **37**: 916–22.

51 Lugtenburg PJ, Lowenberg B, Valkema R, *et al*. Somatostatin receptor scintigraphy in the initial staging of low-grade non-Hodgkin's lymphomas. *J Nucl Med* 2001; **42**: 222–9.

52 Lugtenburg PJ, Krenning EP, Valkema R, *et al*. Somatostatin receptor scintigraphy useful in stage I–II Hodgkin's disease: more extended disease identified. *Br J Haematol* 2001; **112**: 936–44.

53 Hoefnagel CA, Rankin EM, Valdés Olmos, Israëls SP, Pavel S, Janssen AGM. Sensitivity versus specificity in melanoma imaging using iodine-123 iodobenzamide and indium-111 pentetreotide. *Eur J Nucl Med* 1994; **21**: 587–8.

54 Krenning EP, Kwekkeboom DJ, Bakker WH, *et al*. Somatostatin receptor scintigraphy with [^{111}In-DTPA-D-Phe^1]- and [^{123}I-Tyr^3]-octreotide: the Rotterdam experience with more than 1000 patients. *Eur J Nucl Med* 1993; **20**: 716–31.

55 Moertel CL, Reubi JC, Scheithauer BS, Schaid DJ, Kvols LK. Expression of somatostatin receptors in child-hood neuroblastoma. *Am J Clin Pathol* 1994; **102**: 752–6.

56 Van der Harst E, de Herder WW, Bruining HA, *et al*. [(123)I]metaiodobenzylguanidine and [(111)In] octreotide uptake in begnign and malignant pheochromocytomas. *J Clin Endocrinol Metab* 2001; **86**: 685–93.

57 De Herder WW, Krenning EP, Malchoff CD, *et al*. Somatostatin receptor scintigraphy: its value in tumor localization in patients with the Cushing syndrome caused by ectopic corticotropin and/or CRH secretion. *Am J Med* 1994; **96**: 305–12.

58 Philipponneau M, Nocaudie M, Epelbaum J, *et al*. Somatostatin analogs for the localization and preoperative treatment of an ACTH-secreting bronchial carcinoid tumor. *J Clin Endocrinol Metab* 1994; **78**: 20–4.

59 Weiss M, Yellin A, Husza'r M, Eisenstein Z, Bar-Zif J, Krausz Y. Localization of adrenocorticotropic hormone-secreting bronchial carcinoid tumor by somatostatin-receptor scintigraphy. *Ann Intern Med* 1994; **121**: 198–9.

60 Torpy DJ, Chen CC, Mullen N, *et al*. Lack of utility of (111)In-pentetreotide scintigraphy in localizing ectopic ACTH producing tumors: follow-up of 18 patients. *J Clin Endocrinol Metab* 1999; **84**: 1186–92.

61 Haldemann AR, Rosler H, Barth A, *et al*. Somatostatin receptor scintigraphy in central nervous system tumors: role of blood-brain barrier permeability. *J Nucl Med* 1995; **36**: 403–10.

62 Schmidt M, Scheidhauer K, Luyken C, *et al*. Somatostatin receptor imaging in intracranial tumours. *Eur J Nucl Med* 1998; **25**: 675–86.

63 Cervera P, Videau C, Viollet C, *et al*. Comparison of somatostatin receptor expression in human gliomas and medulloblastomas. *J Neuroendocrinol* 2002; **14**: 458–71.

64 Postema PTE, Krenning EP, Wijngaarde R, *et al*. [^{111}In-DTPA-D-Phe^1]-octreotide scintigraphy in thyroidal and orbital Graves' disease: a parameter for disease activity? *J Clin Endocrinol Metab* 1994; **79**: 1845–51.

65 Krassas GE, Dumas A, Pontikides N, Kaltsas T. Somatostatin receptor scintigraphy and octreotide treatment in patients with thyroid eye disease. *Clin Endocrinol (Oxford)* 1995; **42**: 571–80.

66 Kwekkeboom DJ, Krenning EP, Kho GS, Breeman WAP, Van Hagen PM. Octreotide scintigraphy in patients with sarcoidosis. *Eur J Nucl Med* 1998; **25**: 1284–92.

67 Reubi JC, Waser B, Friess H, Krenning EP, Büchler M, Laissue J. Regulatory peptide receptors in goiters of the human thyroid. *J Nucl Med* 1997; **38(Suppl)**: 266P.

68 Gerding MN, van der Zant FM, van Royen EA, *et al*. Octreotide-scintigraphy is a disease-activity parameter in Graves' ophthalmopathy. *Clin Endocrinol (Oxford)* 1999; **50**: 373–9.

69 Kwekkeboom DJ, Bakker WH, Kooij PP, *et al*. [^{177}Lu-DOTA^{0}Tyr^3]octreotate: comparison with [^{111}In-DTPA^0]octreotide in patients. *Eur J Nucl Med* 2001; **28**: 1319–25.

70 Waldherr C, Pless M, Maecke HR, *et al*. Tumor response and clinical benefit in neuroendocrine tumors after 7.4 GBq (90)Y-DOTATOC. *J Nucl Med* 2002; **43**: 617–20.

71 Paganelli G, Bodei L, Handkiewicz Junak D, *et al*. ^{90}Y-DOTA-D-Phe^1-Tyr^3-octreotide in therapy of neuroendocrine malignancies. *Biopolymers* 2002; **66**: 393–8.

72 Valkema R, Pauwels S, Kvols L, *et al*. Long-term follow-up of a phase 1 study of peptide receptor radionuclide therapy (PRRT) with [^{90}Y-DOTA^0,Tyr^3]octreotide in patients with somatostatin receptor positive tumours. *Eur J Nucl Med Mol Imaging* 2003; **30(Suppl 2)**: S232.

73 Kwekkeboom DJ, Bakker WH, Kam BL, *et al*. Treatment of patients with gastro-entero-pancreatic (GEP) tumours with the novel radiolabelled somatostatin analogue [^{177}Lu-DOTA(0),Tyr^3]octreotate. *Eur J Nucl Med Mol Imaging* 2003; **30**: 417–22.

74 Hennig IM, Laissue JA, Horisberger U, *et al.* Substance P receptors in human primary neoplasms. *Int J Cancer* 1995; **61**: 786–92.

75 Van Hagen PM, Breeman WAP, Reubi JC, *et al.* Visualization of the thymus by substance P receptor scintigraphy in man. *Eur J Nucl Med* 1996; **23**: 1508–13.

76 Virgolini I, Raderer M, Kurtaran A, *et al.* Vasoactive intestinal peptide-receptor imaging for the localization of intestinal adenocarcinomas and endocrine tumors. *N Engl J Med* 1994; **331**: 1116–21.

77 Thakur ML, Marcus CS, Saeed S, *et al.* ^{99m}Tc-labeled vasoactive intestinal peptide analog for rapid localization of tumors in humans. *J Nucl Med* 2000; **41**: 107–10.

78 Reubi JC, Schaer JC, Waser B. Cholecystokinin (CCK)-A and CCK-B/gastrin receptors in human tumors. *Cancer Res* 1997; **57**: 1377–86.

79 Kwekkeboom DJ, Bakker WH, Kooij PPM, *et al.* Cholecystokinin receptor imaging using an octapeptide DTPA-CCK analogue in patients with medullary thyroid carcinoma. *Eur J Nucl Med* 2000; **27**: 1312–17.

80 Béhé MP, Behr TM. Cholecystokinin (CCK)-B/gastrin receptor targeting peptides for staging and therapy of medullary thyroid cancer and other CCK-B receptor expressing malignancies. *Biopolymers* 2002; **66**: 399–418.

81 Markwalder R, Reubi JC. Gastrin-releasing peptide receptors in the human prostate: relation to neoplastic transformation. *Cancer Res* 1999; **59**: 1152–9.

82 Gugger M, Reubi JC. GRP receptors in non-neoplastic and neoplastic human breast. *Am J Pathol* 1999; **155**: 2067–76.

83 Van de Wiele C, Dumont F, Vanden Broecke R, *et al.* Technetium-99m RP527, a GRP analogue for visualisation of GRP receptor-expressing malignancies: a feasibility study. *Eur J Nucl Med* 2000; **27**: 1694–9.

Radioimmunoscintigraphy

K.E. BRITTON AND M. GRANOWSKA

INTRODUCTION

Nuclear medicine techniques are known for their sensitivity to changes of function induced by disease, but not for their specificity in determining the nature of the disease process. To address this problem, nuclear medicine has developed new procedures for tissue characterization additional to functional measurements, by receptor binding techniques and antigen–antibody interactions. The use of radiolabeled antibodies to image and characterize the nature of the disease process *in vivo* is called radioimmunoscintigraphy (RIS). In principle, the RIS technique is applicable to both benign (as in the identification of myocardial infarction by radiolabeled antimyosin) and malignant pathology.

CANCER RADIOIMMUNOSCINTIGRAPHY

Cancerous tissue differs from the normal tissue in a number of subtle ways that enables it to invade surrounding tissues. This ability appears to be determined mainly by the surface properties of the cancer cell. Differences have been found in the biochemistry, the adhesion properties, the receptor characteristics, the responses to cytokine and autocrine factors, and the antigenic determinants of the cancer cell surface, in comparison with an equivalent population of normal cells.

Thus, the modern approach to cancer detection attempts to exploit these features and to demonstrate the presence of a cancer not by relying on its physical attributes such as size, shape, position, space occupation, density, water content or reflectivity, for example, as for conventional radiology,

X-ray computed tomography (CT), magnetic resonance imaging (MRI) or ultrasound (US), but through the essential and specific 'cancerousness' of a cancer. This chapter is concerned with techniques designed to take advantage of the specific antigenic determinants of cancer tissue, in order to demonstrate the tumor, its local recurrence and its metastases. RIS is getting closer to achieving the goal of specific cancer detection.[1]

Five factors are required for RIS:

1. An antigen as specific as possible to the cancer and present in profusion at the cell surface
2. An antibody or antibody derivative capable of detecting and binding avidly to the cancer antigen
3. A radiolabel to give the best signal
4. A radiolabeling method with appropriate quality control to give a labeled antibody suitable for human use while maintaining full immunoreactivity
5. An imaging system optimized to the radionuclide that is used and the region under study, with single photon emission tomography (SPET) and/or serial image data analysis

The selective localization of cancer tissue by radiolabeled antibodies carries with it the hope of selective therapy and explains much of the motivation behind the development of RIS. However, for radioimmunotherapy (RIT) there are two additional requirements: the ratio of uptake of radiolabel by the target cancer compared with that in the most critical non-target organ should be a value of at least 10:1; and estimates of the absorbed radiation dose delivered to the tumor as compared to the critical non-target organ such as bone marrow and to the whole body pose severe limitations on the current techniques.

THE ANTIGEN

The key to RIS is the discovery of an antigen that is as specific as possible to the disease process under study. Four decades of saturation analysis techniques using antigen–antibody binding characteristics to measure hormones and other biological substances *in vitro* have shown the feasibility and specificity of this approach when the appropriate antigen or ligand is identified and purified. An avid and specific antibody is then raised against it. The part of an antigen with which an antibody reacts is called an 'epitope' or antigenic determinant.

The first problem for RIS is lack of specificity of the antigen for the disease process. There is no completely cancer-specific antigen, but a range of tumor-associated antigens may be used in the appropriate clinical context for the demonstration of cancer (Table 1C.1).

The expression of antigen by the cell is a dynamic process. It needs to be on the surface accessible to antibody. The higher the antigen density the greater the amount of antibody binding capacity. The possibility of binding is given by the binding constant K_B of the antigen–antibody reaction; current antibodies have K_B values of 10^{-9} to 10^{-10} $1\,mol^{-1}$. Antigen density can be increased by certain circumstances, such as exposure to gamma-interferon, but no practical clinical technique has been devised. Attachment to nuclear antigens would require the internalization of the antibody by endocytosis or other mechanisms that occur with certain antibodies.

The degree of antigen expression changes with time and the amount of the antigen on a cell surface can be reduced after exposure to a specific antibody and by other factors. This process is known as antigen modulation, which can lead to internalization and metabolism of the labeled antibody with either loss of the label or its fixation in the cell. Important for detection and crucial to radioimmunotherapy is the requirement that the antigen expression is not too heterogeneous. Ideally, all the cancer cells should express the chosen antigen. However, while this is usual in lymphoma, it is not so common in solid tumors. More usually some clumps of cells are antigen positive and others antigen negative. This does not affect RIS detection, but influences the success of RIT. Some cancers do not express a particular antigen at all. Thus, antibodies against placental alkaline phosphatase (PLAP) are excellent for RIS of ovarian cancer, but only 70% express this antigen.[2]

Current tumor-associated antigens are chosen in different ways (Table 1C.1). The de-differentiation antigens such as carcinoembryonic antigen (CEA), human choriogonadotrophin (HCG) and alpha-fetoprotein (AFP) are widely used. These are expressed in greater numbers on malignant cell surfaces than in normal tissues. They are secreted from such cells and are easily detectable in the blood and body fluids. Surprisingly, the injected antibody is not inactivated by, for example, circulating CEA and

Table 1C.1   *Examples of tumor-associated antigens*

Type of antigen	Monoclonal antibodies
Epithelial surface antigens	
These are separated from the blood by biological barriers and exposed by the architectural disruption of malignancy	*HMFG1, HMFG2, SM3, PR1A3*
Oncofetal antigens	*Anti-CEA, anti-alpha-fetoprotein*
Tumor-derived antigens	*B72.3, Mov 18*
Viral antigens	*Anti-hepatoma*
Synthetic antigens	*170 H82*
Receptor antigens	*Anti-EGF receptor*

immune-complex formation does not appear to be a problem unless serum CEA is over 500 ng ml^{-1}. However, these cancer antigens are not specific: CEA expression occurs in lung, bladder, breast, and gastric cancers and also in colorectal cancer. They can be increased in nonmalignant disease (e.g. Crohn's disease) and are present in the related normal tissues and colonic mucosa. The secretion of the antigen is essential for its use as a serum marker. It is not helpful for RIS, because the presence of the antigen, for example in a lymph node, does not mean the presence of a cancer cell. Virus-related antigens may be used, e.g. anti-hepatitis antibody for liver cancer. Idiotypic antigen may be used for the leukemias and lymphomas.

An alternative approach is to use normal epithelial tissue antigens lining ducts, which by their situation are not normally exposed to blood. Human milk fat globule (HMFG) is a glycoprotein (one of the polymorphic epithelial mucin (PEM) group) found in the lining epithelium of the lactiferous ducts of the breast, the internal lining of an ovarian follicle and in the crypts of the colon. The architectural disruption of the malignant process exposes these antigens in increased density directly to the bloodstream and antibodies against these, such as HMFG1, HMFG2 and SM3 (stripped mucin antigen) are used for RIS. The preferred antigen is membrane-fixed and specific to the cancer.

THE ANTIBODY

Antibodies are complex molecules: one part of the molecule is highly variable in terms of its structure (variable region, idiotype) and is associated with binding to antigen, while the other part varies little within different classes of antibodies (constant region, isotype). Biological functions of antibodies such as complement activation and binding to cell surface receptors are controlled by their constant 'Fc' regions. The basic structure of an IgG antibody molecule

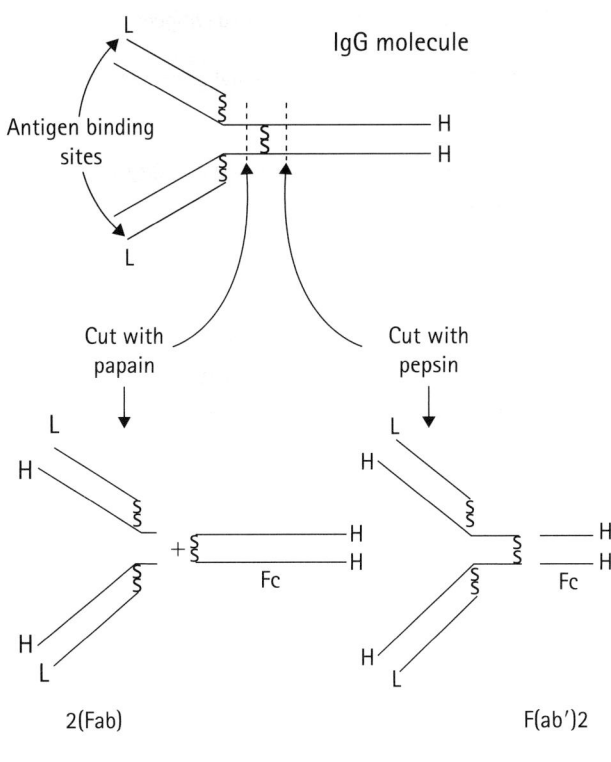

IgG molecule

Antigen binding sites

Cut with papain

Cut with pepsin

2(Fab)

F(ab')2

Fc

H = heavy chain
L = Light chain
S͢S = Disulphide bonds
Fab = fraction antigen binding – used as imaging reagents
Fc = fraction complement fixing

Figure 1C.1 *Structure of the IgG molecule.*

contains four polypeptide chains – two heavy and two light chains – held together by a variable number of disulfide bonds (Fig. 1C.1). It can be cleaved into smaller fragments that retain their ability to bind antigen by the two enzymes pepsin and papain. When radiolabeled, these fragments, because of their small size and loss of the biological Fc region, have markedly different pharmacokinetic and imaging properties compared with the whole antibody molecule. The specificity and accuracy of RIS depends on the production of a pure antibody against the selected antigen in a form acceptable for human use. This has been made possible through the development of monoclonal antibody technology.

THE MONOCLONAL ANTIBODY

A monoclonal antibody is the secreted product of a single B-lymphocyte clone. Since each B lymphocyte and its descendants are genetically destined to make a single antigen-combining site (idiotype), all the antibody molecules produced by a B-cell clone are homogeneous in terms of

their structure and antigen-binding specificity. In pathological terms, malignant transformation of a single B lymphocyte may give rise to a plasma cell tumor, a myeloma or plasmacytoma, that produces a homogeneous antibody product or myeloma protein. Tumors of this type produce monoclonal gammopathies that can be diagnosed serologically by detecting them as sharp narrow bands on serum electrophoretic scans. In the past, these monoclonal antibodies have been invaluable in elucidating the structure of antibodies. Kohler and Milstein[3] devised a way of making monoclonal antibodies in the laboratory by the technique of somatic cell hybridization. This involved the fusion of B lymphocytes with a myeloma cell line (adapted for growth *in vitro*) to make hybrid cells known as hybridomas. Essentially, these hybridomas retain the two important functions of their parental cells, namely the ability to produce specific antibodies and to grow indefinitely in tissue culture. To make a hybridoma secrete a single antibody, a non-antibody-secreting myeloma mutant is used.

In a normal antibody response to a foreign antigen, a large number of B lymphocytes are activated to secrete specific antibodies that bind to antigenic determinants expressed on the surface of the antigen. Added together, these antibodies constitute a polyclonal antibody response to a given antigen and they will have a range of antibody affinities. The term 'antibody affinity' refers to the summation of the attractive and repulsive forces existing between a single antibody-combining site, epitope and its antigenic determinant.

Each time a polyclonal antiserum is made to a given antigen it will contain a different mix of antibody affinities which collectively give a mean value (called avidity) for their binding to the antigen. This means polyclonal antisera are difficult to standardize from one batch to another. Also these antisera will contain only a small proportion (1%) of their total IgG antibody as the antigen-specific antibody and so further purification steps are required before they can be radiolabeled for RIS. Most of these problems can be avoided by using monoclonal antibodies. Unlike polyclonal antibodies, monoclonal antibodies bind to antigen with one specificity and one affinity and can be produced in large amounts in the laboratory under standard conditions. All these factors make them ideal standard reagents for a wide range of biological and clinical applications. The names of antibodies in clinical use have been systematized and have become largely unpronounceable (Table 1C.2).

BIOLOGICAL FACTORS AFFECTING UPTAKE

At present, only antibodies or their derivatives against tumor-associated antigens have been used for cancer RIS. Apart from specificity, the antibody must have access to the antigen, so that local factors are very important. The arrival of the antibody in the vicinity of the antigenic binding sites on the cells depends on physical factors: the flow to the

Table 1C.2 *Some monoclonal antibodies and derivatives in clinical use*

Official name	Common name	Nature
Capromab pendetide	Prostascint	^{111}In-DTPA CYT-356 anti-PSMA
–	Oncoscint	^{111}In-DTPA B72 3 anti-TAG
–	Hu-CC49	Humanized anti-TAG
Arcitumomab	CEA scan	^{99m}Tc-anti CEA-Fab'
Nofetumomab merpentan	Verluma	^{99m}Tc-NR-Lu-10-Fab'
Sulesomab	Leukoscan	^{99m}Tc-IMMO-MN3
Trastuzumab	Herceptin	Humanized IgG1 HER2
Rituximab	Mabthera	Murine IgG anti CD 20
Ibritumomab tiuxetan	Zevalin	^{90}Y-retuximab
Tositumomab	Bexxar	^{131}I-anti-B1 antibody
Epratuzumab	–	^{90}Y-DOTA anti-CD 22

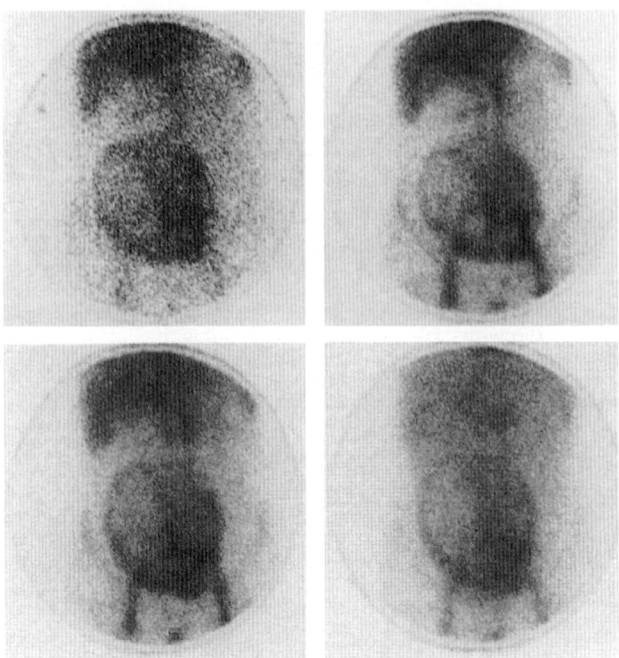

Figure 1C.2 *Radioimmunoscintigraphy with ^{123}I-labeled human milk fat globule 2 in patient with large fibroids in the uterus, anterior abdominal views at top left, 1 min; top right, 10 min; bottom left, 4 h; and bottom right, 22 h. Note the high early activity fading with time typical of non-specific uptake (compare with Fig. 1C.3).*

tumor, the capillary permeability and the effects of the cellular environment on the diffusion and convection of the antibody. The higher the avidity of the antibody for the antigen, the greater the probability of an interaction and binding on the cell membrane. The tumor blood supply is a major determinant of the kinetics of antibody uptake: the higher the flow, the more rapid the uptake, the earlier the imaging and the more short-lived the radionuclide label may be. Tumor blood supply is not under autonomic control, so attempts have been made to enhance tumor uptake by pharmacological vascular intervention. Tumor capillaries are abnormally leaky, allowing proteins to pass from the circulation to the tumor. This accounts for the nonspecific antibody uptake by tumors. Extracellular fluid-to-cell ratio of tumors is greater than normal tissues. The charge and composition of this fluid may affect the rate of uptake of antibody onto the tumor cell antigens. Intra-tumor pressure may be greater than its environment and reduce antibody penetration. Locally secreted antigens, such as the CEA from colorectal cancer may enhance the uptake in the environment of the tumor. Tumor growth leads to deprivation of central blood supply, with necrotic and cystic areas without specific antigen. In general, the larger the tumor, the smaller the fraction of cancer cells to tumor mass and the greater the degree of nonspecific uptake. An inverse relation between the uptake of anti-CEA by primary colorectal tumors and tumor mass has been shown.[4] Thus, the specific uptake of labeled antibody is designed best for demonstrating small tumors. Note also that each cancer cell should have over 5000 and preferably nearer 50 000 available epitopes to bind the monoclonal antibody. It is this biological magnification factor that helps RIS to compete with physical radiological techniques in tumor

detection. Other factors are also important in determining the uptake of antibody by cancer cell antigens. If the amount of antibody administered per study is increased, the amount taken up by both the tumor and its environment is greater, so the tumor-to-mucosa ratio does not show a corresponding increase. The more antibody that is given the greater the likelihood of side effects and formation of the human anti-mouse antibody, HAMA, particularly when over 2 mg of antibody is given.

The degree of tumor differentiation is important – poorly differentiated tumors taking up much less antibody per gram than the well-differentiated tumors; a four-fold difference in a study of colorectal cancer has been reported.[5] *In vivo* staging of cancer is not possible if normal lymph nodes draining the site of cancer take up a secreted antigen as frequently as the involved nodes, which occurs with CEA. Co-existing disease may compete for the antibody and large benign tumors may also take up the antibody. Another considerable influence on detection of small tumors is the degree and distribution of uptake in the blood and tissue background. Kinetic factors play an important part in the differentiation of specific and nonspecific antibody uptake and in the choice of radiolabel. Taking RIS of ovarian cancer as an example (see also Chapter 13G), whereas after an initial distribution period, nonspecific uptake decreases with time due to a falling blood and tissue fluid concentration and due to local metabolism by reticuloendothelial cells (Fig. 1C.2), specific uptake of antibody continues to increase

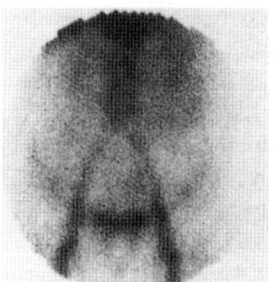 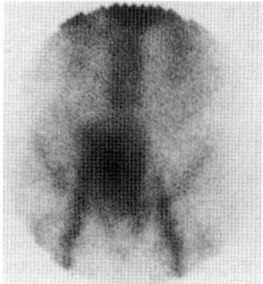 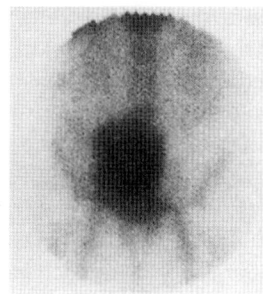

Figure 1C.3 *Radioimmunoscintigraphy with* ^{123}*I-labeled human milk fat globule 2 in a patient with a large ovarian adenocarcinoma, anterior abdominal views: left, 10 min; center, 4 h; right, 22 h. Note the increasing uptake with time typical of specific uptake (compare with Fig. 1C.2).*

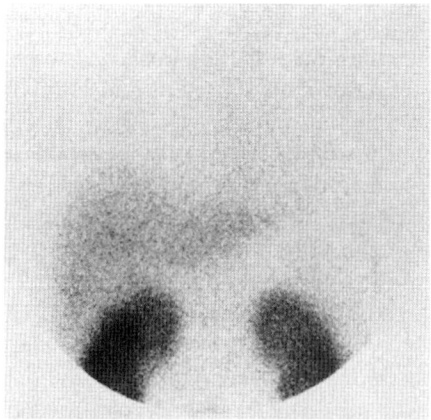 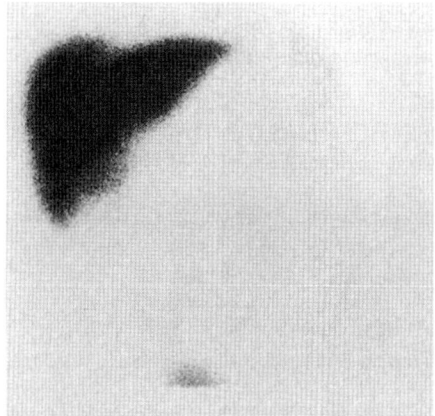

Figure 1C.4 *Radioimmunoscintigraphy with* ^{99m}*Tc-labeled F(ab')$_2$ fragment of 225.28S monoclonal antibody against high molecular weight melanoma antigen. Both images are at 20 min. Left: normal distribution with high renal uptake due to filtration, reabsorption, metabolism and deposition of* ^{99m}*Tc in the proximal tubules. Right: abnormal distribution due to allergic reaction (skin test negative, no previous exposure to antibody). There is very high liver uptake and low renal excretion due to immune complex formation which is too large to be filtered.*

with time over the first 24 h (Fig. 1C.3), although at a progressively slower rate as its concentration in the supplying blood falls.

The development of human anti-mouse antibodies, HAMA occurs in response to most injections of whole mouse monoclonal IgG gamma-globulin, particularly when intradermal skin testing was combined with intravenous injection. This was the main reason why skin testing was abandoned. There is usually no HAMA response to the first injection of F(ab')$_2$ fragments, but response to a second injection may occur in up to 50%. A strong HAMA response may significantly alter the biodistribution: its presence after the second injection of whole antibody may show a more rapid blood clearance to liver and other reticuloendothelial systems and slightly less tumor uptake.

Occasionally, a systemic reaction occurs (frequency about 1 per 1000 studies which is about the same as for a bone scan, provided that less than 2 mg antibody is used and patients with known allergy to foreign protein are excluded) and the liver uptake may be rapid. This is illustrated in Fig. 1C.4: on the left is the normal renal uptake of

^{99m}Tc-labeled F(ab')$_2$ 225.28S antimelanoma monoclonal antibody with low liver uptake at 20 min: on the right, the 20-min image in a patient with a negative skin test who had an episode of nausea and faintness shortly after injection of the same antibody shows high and rapid liver uptake.

QUALITY CONTROL

Since monoclonal antibodies are a biological product derived from cell culture, stringent quality control procedures are necessary to prevent undesirable products, particularly genetically active material and virus, from being present in the final product. A reasonable set of guidelines has been set out by a working party on the clinical use of antibodies,[6] but the regulations in Europe and USA are becoming increasingly demanding, including tests for numbers of unlikely mouse viruses at all stages of the production.

The European Directive on Clinical Trials which is being implemented requires much more detailed information and a formal sponsor who has to be willing to provide indemnity for any clinical trial including 'pilot' studies.

The rationale for the use of a monoclonal antibody or its derivative in RIS should include its demonstrated specificity and affinity for the chosen tumor and absence of reactivity with clinically relevant other tissues or tumors. It must be remembered that tissue sections have lost the biological barriers present in living tissues and may give a misleading apparent distribution of a monoclonal antibody in normal tissues. Human tumor xenograft uptake in an experimental animal such as the nude mouse may give misleadingly optimistic results since the human tumor antigens have no competition in the mouse, the ratio of tumor mass to mouse is inappropriately large and the tumor stroma is made up by mouse connective tissue. The findings may also be misleadingly pessimistic if antigenic modulation or cytochemical modification has occurred.

HUMANIZED MONOCLONAL ANTIBODIES

The limitations of monoclonal antibody production have been overcome by genetic engineering.[7,8] This requires the following:

1. The separation of the immunoglobulin gene sequences and their amplification by the polymerase chain reaction (PCR)
2. The use of an appropriate carrier to grow up or 'clone' the product, so that the amplified genes may be expressed
3. The selection of the 'antibody' for a particular antigen and for high affinity

In this way the frame or constant part (Fc portion) of the murine monoclonal antibody has been replaced by the equivalent Fc portion of a human monoclonal to give a 'chimeric antibody'.[9] The next approach was to replace all but the hypervariable region of the murine antibody by the human equivalent.[10] This is called a 'humanized', human reshaped or CDR (complementarity determinant region) grafted antibody. Usually the frame amino acids around the CDR may need to be altered also to improve stability and affinity.

The next advance was to develop phage antibodies.[11,12] Human B cells, of which there are millions, contain the genes for the heavy and light chains that make up an antibody. Foreign antigen exposure leads to its binding to the B cells causing their differentiation into memory cells and into plasma cells. These produce V (variable region) genes. These code for the particular antibody, which is released. The V (variable region) genes retained in the memory cells are subject to mutation, one result of which is to increase the binding affinity of the antibodies produced in response to a subsequent encounter with the antigen. It is possible to capture and insert these human V genes into bacteria and infect them with filamentous bacteriophages with the result that antibody components such as the variable region and

its frame may be expressed on the 'nose' of the bacteriophage. From immunized or even normal human B cells, all combinations of heavy and light chain V genes can be constructed each expressed on bacteriophages to form a 'combinatorial library' of such potential antibodies. To increase the number of heavy and light (V_H V_L) genes the polymerase chain reaction is used which is a method of amplifying DNA sequences (as in genetic fingerprinting). These genes can be combined to form gene products that are single chain fragments of one heavy and one light chain, called ScFv.[13] These can be grown up and expressed in the bacteriophage system.[11–15] Initially, the phage produced ScFv were of moderate affinity. The selection of the appropriate phage to grow up is done by an 'affinity' column in which the chosen antigen is fixed. Only phages with the appropriate antibody will bind when the mixture of phages is run through the column. The chosen phages are dissociated, grown up in bacteria and re-run through the column containing only a few of the chosen antigens. Only the phage with the highest affinity will then bind. This cloning and selection process gives ScFv of very high affinity which are produced into the culture medium by the phage-infected bacteria and harvested. In principle, antibodies can be made to any antigen, hapten or ligand without the bother of immunization. Success with an anti-CEA equivalent antibody MFE-23 is reported.[16] By genetic engineering two or more ScFv may be combined[17,18] and/or have linkers inserted with properties to enable easier labeling with radionuclides for RIS or RIT.[19–23] This combinatorial library approach circumvents the problems of obtaining human antibodies by immunizing humans which is clearly unethical for a range of toxic substances or malignant cells.

The immortalization of human peripheral B lymphocytes, e.g. from a patient who already has a cancer, is a problem which has been overcome in some situations.[24] The method of genetic engineering antibody-like molecules from combinatorial libraries with specific labeling sites is the way forward.

THE RADIOLABEL

What are the properties of an ideal radiolabel for radioimmunoscintigraphy and how do the available radionuclides match up? The key requirement for static imaging of a tumor through the distribution of a radiotracer is a high count rate delivered from the tissue-of-interest to the imaging system. The major determinants of the suitability of radionuclide for antibody labeling are the appropriateness of its energy for the modern gamma camera and its half-life. The shorter the half-life, the greater the activity that may be administered and the higher the count rate obtained, given an upper limit of the absorbed dose of radiation that is permitted for diagnostic nuclear medicine. Ideally, the half-life should be matched with kinetic information on the rate of antibody uptake by the target. If the uptake of antibody follows the Michaelis–Menten (enzyme–substrate) kinetics as expected, then the uptake rate is initially greatest, with a decrease in the fractional uptake of the amount administered as the blood concentration decreases with time. The temporal requirement concerns the rate of clearance of the injected antibody from the blood and tissues providing the environment for the target, in relation to its residence time on the target tissue. A typical biological clearance half-life of clearance of whole antibody from blood is 43 h, with a range of 24–64 h and an antibody fragment is cleared at approximately twice this rate, a biological half-life of 21.5 h, with a range of 15–30 h. For a typical whole antibody and a typical compact reasonable vascular tumor about 75% of the total uptake of labeled antibody occurs in the first 12 h, favoring the use of a radionuclide with a physical half-life ($T_{1/2}$) of about 12 h (e.g. for ^{123}I, $T_{1/2} = 13.2$ h). For some antibodies uptake will be more rapid, as Buraggi et al.[25] have shown for anti-melanoma antibody, giving an optimal time between 6 and 12 h, favoring a radiolabel such as ^{99m}Tc with a 6-h physical half-life. Other malignancies, such as prostate cancer and particularly relatively avascular tumors like scirrhous carcinoma of the breast, may show slower uptake requiring a longer-lived radionuclide such as ^{111}In (physical $T_{1/2} = 67.4$ h).

An appreciation of the need for higher sensitivity in order to detect small tumors requires an understanding of the sources of signal degradation. 'Noise' is a term used generally for anything that degrades the signal and has many sources, but the most important is the signal itself. Since one of the aims of RIS is to visualize recurrences or spread of cancer not detectable by conventional radiology, CT, MRI or US through the properties of a specifically targeted antibody, the optimization of a significant signal from a small target is essential. Most of the noise that prevents this objective is due to the weakness of the signal itself. This primary type of signal degradation severely reduces tumor detectability. Low count rates give 'noisy' images where the tumor is less separable from the background and the high variability of the background itself may produce 'noise blobs' that may be falsely interpreted as tumor signals.

This may be illustrated by consideration of RIS in a child with neuroblastoma using 40 MBq ^{131}I-labeled UJ13A (an antibody reacting with neuroblastoma) on one occasion (Fig. 1C.5(a)) and 40 MBq ^{123}I-labeled UJ13A 3 weeks later (Fig. 1C.5(b)). For the same activity and the same amount of antibody with ^{131}I as the radiolabel, the tumor is lost in the noisy background of liver, heart and spleen at 21 h, and can just be visualized at 70 h. In contrast, with ^{123}I as the

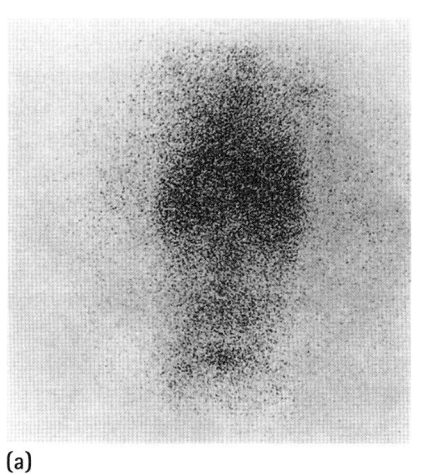

(a)

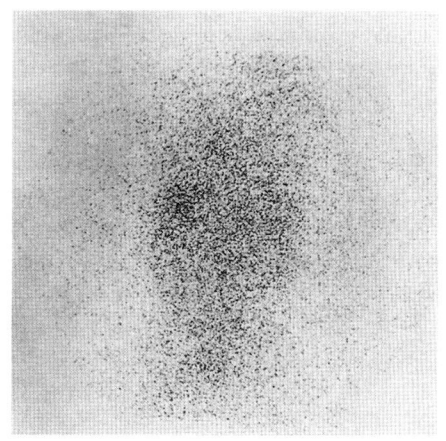

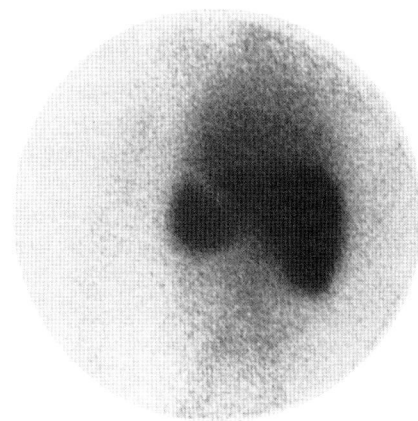

(b)

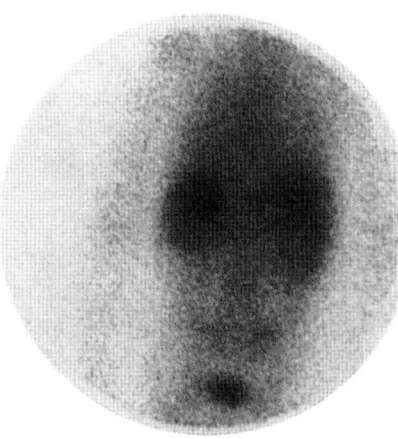

Figure 1C.5 *Radioimmunoscintigraphy of neuroblastoma using radioiodinated UJ13A in a 4-year-old child. (a) Posterior abdominal images 21 and 70 h after injection of 40 MBq ^{131}I-labeled UJ13A. General uptake is seen in the liver, spleen and blood pool at 21 h. Focal low-contrast uptake is seen at 70 h in the tumor. (b) Posterior abdominal images at 10 min and 21 h after injection of 40 MBq ^{123}I-labeled UJ13A in the same child. At 10 min the spleen and liver are identified with an area of reduced uptake superior to the spleen. At 21 h, a focal area of increased uptake is evident in the tumour superior to the spleen (see also Plate 1C.1).*

radiolabel, the spleen and liver are clearly outlined at 10 min and by 21 h the space seen superior to the spleen had been replaced by a focal area of high uptake in the tumor. With ^{131}I, the signal-to-noise ratio at 70 h was 25:1, but the signal was poor, whereas with ^{123}I, at 21 h the signal-to-noise ratio was 1.5:1, yet the tumor is evident. The tumor is evident at 4 h on a color-coded image (Plate 1C.1) when the tumor-to-background ratio was only 1.23:1. This example demonstrates the greater importance of the signal itself over the calculated signal-to-background ratio. For ^{123}I, the count content per pixel was 25 times that from ^{131}I, for the same administered activity. A good signal enables detection, however high the nonspecific background activity.[26] Thus, in principle, a pinhead-sized radiolabeled tumor will be visualized if it gives a good enough signal.

While the avidity, affinity and selectivity of the antibody are crucial to that signal, the choice of a radiolabel itself is very important. The requirements include the number of radiolabels allowable per antibody while retaining its immunoreactivity, the efficiency and abundance with which the gamma rays are emitted from the radiolabel, their gamma-ray energy, the total number of radioactive molecules that may be injected into the patient and the availability of the radiolabel. These all contribute to the choice of ideal radionuclide.

Even ignoring its excessive gamma-ray energy, ^{131}I with its half-life of 8 days and beta emission that gives 80% of the radiation due to this radionuclide *in vivo*, should no longer be used for modern RIS but limited to RIT. However, a beta-emitting radionuclide suitable for therapy which also emits a gamma ray whose energy is close to that of ^{99m}Tc such as ^{188}Re or ^{177}Lu has advantages for imaging and dosimetry. Pure beta emitters such as ^{90}Y and ^{32}P in therapeutic amounts are imageable through their Bremsstrahlung radiation using a wide window.

The immunoreactivity of the antibody must be preserved during the radiolabeling. This usually requires a radiolabel-to-antibody molar ratio of 1:1 or 2:1, since labeling of the antigen-combining site of the antibody must be avoided. Site-specific labeling of the Fc region of the antibody molecule away from the antigen-combining site is being developed to overcome this problem. Methods for labeling must therefore be 'gentle' so as not to denature the molecule by altering its three-dimensional conformation. Genetically engineered mouse antibodies which are 'humanized' to make them less immunogenic, may have a specific labeling site introduced. Improvements may be made to their antigen specificity. They may be produced by a continuous fermentation-like process. All these technological improvements should eventually overcome many of the present problems relating to quality control.

Radiolabeling

Radiolabeling with ^{131}I or ^{123}I is usually undertaken using the chloramine T or Iodogen techniques labeling the protein through the tyrosine radical. Radiolabeling with ^{111}In commonly uses the method described by Hnatowich *et al.*[27] in which the bicyclic anhydride of diethylenetriamine-pentaacetic acid (DTPA) is first coupled to the antibody with subsequent chelation of ^{111}In with this conjugate. To achieve good ^{111}In labeling, a balance has to be struck between the amount of DTPA attached to the antibody and the effects of this DTPA coupling on the physicochemical and biological properties of the antibody. Newer DTPA derivatives are more stable. A general finding with all ^{111}In-labeled antibodies given intravenously to patients is the high ^{111}In uptake in the liver. This occurs for a number of reasons: transchelation of ^{111}In onto plasma transferrin (6–10% per day), its binding to liver and sinusoid cells; the localization of antibodies in liver by virtue of its large blood supply; and antibody uptake by Kupffer cells of the reticuloendothelial system. New types of metal chelates and different methods of linking them to antibodies will help reduce this problem in the future.

Labeling antibodies with ^{99m}Tc

The *in vivo* stability of ^{99m}Tc-labeled monoclonal antibodies has been successfully improved by the development of new techniques. In a widely used method,[28] the S–S bonds holding the heavy chains are opened using 2-mercaptoethanol (2-ME). The antibody is concentrated by ultrafiltration to approximately 10 mg ml^{-1}. To a stirred solution of antibody, sufficient 2-ME is added to provide a 2-ME-to-antibody molar ratio of 1000:1. The mixture is incubated at room temperature for 30 min with continuous rotation. The reduced antibody is purified by gel filtration on Sephadex-G50 using phosphate-buffered saline as the mobile phase. The antibody fractions are collated and divided into 0.5-mg aliquots. These are frozen immediately at $-20°$C and stored ready for use. When imaging is required, the antibody aliquot is thawed and reconstituted (using a methylene disphosphonate (MDP) kit) with 5 ml 0.9% sterile saline. A 35 μl aliquot of MDP solution is added to the antibody aliquot and mixed. The required amount of ^{99m}Tc-pertechnetate (approximately 700 MBq) is added to the antibody/MDP mixture, which is gently shaken for 10 min. The labeling efficiency is assessed by thin-layer chromatography developed in 0.9% saline and should be over 95%; if below this, the labeled antibody can be further purified by gel filtration on Sephadex-G50. The ^{99m}Tc-labeled antibody is stable *in vivo* with an *in vitro* stability of a few hours. There is no thyroid uptake of ^{99m}Tc even after 24 h in patients who have received no thyroid-blocking medication. This technique has been used successfully for many different antibodies in clinical use in this department to date. An alternative method used a photoelectric system for labeling proteins with ^{99m}Tc.[29]

A new approach for labeling genetically engineered antibodies and peptides with ^{99m}Tc is to introduce a histidine tag for labeling via a ^{99m}Tc-carbonyl derivative.[21]

CLINICAL PROTOCOLS AND DATA ANALYSIS

A typical protocol is as follows:

1. Before injection of a labeled antibody, the patient must be asked about allergies. A history of severe allergic reactions or sensitivity to foreign protein is a contraindication to RIS. Skin testing is ineffective and sensitizes the patient.
2. The nature of the test is explained to the patient and informed consent is obtained.
3. Potassium iodide, 60 mg twice daily, is given the day before, during and for a day after the test for ^{123}I and for 2 weeks in the case of ^{131}I. No such preparation is required when ^{111}In or ^{99m}Tc is the label.
4. The patient is then positioned supine on the scanning couch under the gamma camera, which is fitted with an appropriate collimator and set up for the particular radionuclide.
5. The labeled antibody in an appropriate amount and activity is injected intravenously and for example, in the context of ovarian or colorectal cancer, anterior and posterior images of the lower and upper abdomen are obtained at 10 min, 6 h and 22 h for ^{123}I and ^{99m}Tc, and at 1, 48 and 72 h for ^{111}In. A minimum of 800 kcounts per view is recommended.

Evaluation of results

The series of transparent films or workstation displays are evaluated for the distribution of uptake in normal structures: vascular activity, bone marrow, liver, spleen, kidneys, gastrointestinal, and urinary activity; for sites of abnormal uptake; and for how the distribution of uptake varies with time. Thus, the activity in vascular structures, tissue background and at sites of nonspecific uptake after an initial increase in distribution seen on the 10-min images tends to decrease with time (Fig. 1C.2) whereas areas of specific uptake may show little or no uptake on the 10-min image, but show increasing uptake with time during the first 24 h (Fig. 1C.3). Gastrointestinal, liver, and marrow activity for ^{111}In and urinary activity for ^{123}I and ^{99m}Tc, may increase with time. Focal tumor uptake may be best seen at 6 h for ^{99m}Tc-labeled F(ab′)$_2$ RIS in ocular and cutaneous melanoma,[30,31] with ^{99m}Tc-labeled whole antibodies at 24 h for ovarian,[32,33] breast,[34–36] and colorectal cancer,[37] and for ovarian cancer with ^{123}I-labeled HMFG2.[38,39] In colorectal cancer, 24- or 48-h images may give the best contrast using ^{111}In-labeled anti-CEA (Plates 1C.2 and 1C.3) and 48- and 72-h images in prostate cancer. The key to identifying the tumor site are the changes occurring in the series of transparent films or workstation displays between the first early and the later images.

Image enhancement

The following additional techniques are used to improve the contrast between the target and its background:

- Background subtraction using a second radiopharmaceutical[40]
- Single photon emission tomography (SPET)[41]
- The use of F(ab′)$_2$ fragments[42]
- The use of a second antibody to speed the clearance of the radiopharmaceutical from the blood[43]
- Subtracting an early image from a later image[44]
- The use of a 'chase' in a two-or-three stage system[45,46]
- Kinetic analysis with probability mapping or statistical change detection[33–36,47] (see also Chapter 13H).

The Fab′ is a monovalent fragment and the F(ab′)$_2$ a bivalent fragment obtained by enzyme digestion of the whole antibody to remove the Fc portion, leaving the active antigen-binding site intact (Fig. 1C.1). The advantages of using an F(ab′)$_2$ fragment include: the absence of the Fc protein that binds specifically to the reticuloendothelial cells, tending to increase the liver, marrow, lymph node, and splenic uptake; a more rapid clearance (about two-fold) from blood; and a more rapid diffusion into the tumor tissue. The disadvantages include: usually lower avidity than the whole antibody; loss by glomerular filtration into the kidney followed by absorption and metabolism in the proximal tubules, depositing the metal ^{111}In and ^{99m}Tc there (but not ^{123}I, which is released by deiodinases); greater diffusibility into a wider volume of distribution than the whole antibody contributing to tissue background; and an additional preparative step. However, matched to a short-lived radionuclide such as ^{99m}Tc or ^{123}I, the advantages probably outweigh the disadvantages.

The main requirement for SPET is a high count rate from the target, so that the rotation can be completed in a time that is reasonable to expect a patient to remain still. This favors the use of the shorter-lived radionuclides for antibody labeling. It is the registration of sites of suspected abnormality in relation to anatomical landmarks that is the main problem for interpretation. Major vessel activity and incidental bone marrow uptake help, but the presence of activity in the bowel makes for difficulties. Co-location by SPET/CT systems or computer-assisted superimposition of separate SPET and CT images is helpful. The advantage of SPET is the increased contrast of the target in the plane of the section and particularly the ability to separate objects from in front of and behind the target, e.g. the bladder from a pelvic tumor, which may overlap on a conventional planar image. Another potential advantage is the ability to quantify the amount of activity in a region of the transverse section, for example, for dosimetry purposes. However, this is much more difficult than expected: errors occur due to less than perfect rotation and linearity of response of the camera, Poisson statistical noise, algorithm noise, artefacts due to overlapping tissue activities, the partial volume effect, patient and organ movement, and difficulties in correcting for scatter and for tissue attenuation. Accuracy is thereby considerably reduced and the anatomical relationships of tissues and target may be difficult to visualize and/or interpret. Once created, SPET sections cannot be repositioned. The SPET technique is a potentially useful adjunct to, but not a substitute for, planar imaging in RIS. Removal of unwanted objects, such as the bladder activity for prostate imaging, from the SPET data can be undertaken before reconstruction by 'image surgery'.[48] The advent of SPET/CT systems has given a great impetus to improving RIS, particularly in prostate cancer (see Chapter 13E).

It is clearly important to distinguish specific tumor uptake from nonspecific uptake and to reduce the effects to tissue and blood background. The concept of subtracting the early post-injection antibody images (showing distribution of activity in the blood and tissue) before significant tumor uptake has occurred, from the delayed images was introduced.[44] This approach overcomes the problem of subtracting the distribution of two radionuclides with differing energies and allows considerable enhancement of tumor uptake. However, it requires the repositioning and normalization of the two images. The repositioning must be reasonably accurate between the first and second visits of the patient and then the computer images must be completely superimposed. For each image of the patient, marker images are also obtained. For the latter the patient's bony landmarks (such as xiphisternum, costal margins, anterior superior iliac spines, and symphysis pubis) are marked with indelible ink and ^{57}Co radioactive markers are positioned over these. Transparent films of the marker positions on the persistence scope are made at the early visit. At each subsequent visit, the markers are replaced on the patient and the patient is repositioned until the image of the markers on the persistence scope fits that on the previously recorded films placed over the scope. The computer is also programmed so that the recorded images can be moved one pixel at a time, vertically, horizontally or by rotation so that an exact superimposition of the later image over the earlier image may be made in order that detailed analysis of the images may be performed, for example, by proportional subtraction of the early image from the later image.

A more sophisticated approach makes use of the kinetic information and also the count-rate distribution. As noted above, the specific tumor uptake increases with time whereas the nonspecific blood and tissue activity decreases with time. By analysing pairs of images separated in time, for example, the 10-min image with the 22-h image, for temporal changes in the count-rate distribution between the pairs of images, sites of specific uptake will be identified as positive derivations from a line of correspondence calculated from the count-rate frequency distribution of the two images for the areas where there has been no change between the two images. This technique of kinetic analysis with probability mapping satisfies the basic requirements of detectability of low contrast differences and insensitivity to statistical noise over the range encountered in a typical RIS study. Biopsy-proven 0.5-cm diameter deposits have been correctly identified using this approach.[47] Alternative change-detection algorithms based on statistical comparisons of multiple small regions in each image are being implemented, for example in the determination of axillary node involvement in primary breast cancer[34–36] and distinguishing benign from malignant adnexal masses[33] and Chapters 13D and 13E. Three-dimensional change detection analysis is being investigated in prostate cancer.[49]

CLINICAL STUDIES

When introducing any new imaging technique the crucial requirement is to define the principal circumstances under which it should be able to contribute to clinical management. Many diagnostic tests are undertaken in relation to a particular clinical problem and this strict criterion of a successful test is now being met by RIS. A number of generalizations about the technique in the management of malignant disease may be made:

- RIS has no role as a screening test for the presence of cancer in healthy people as it involves the injection of a foreign protein, a radioactive source and an antibody that is not completely cancer-specific.
- RIS is gaining a role in the evaluation of patients picked up on a preliminary investigation; e.g. the demonstration of an ultrasound abnormality in the pelvis may be supplemented using RIS to determine whether it contains ovarian cancer.[33]
- RIS is a natural counterpart to the increasing search for tumor markers in serum. However, the ideal antigen for detection in serum has to be released easily from the tumor as is CEA or AFP and most markers do not show a rise in serum until the tumor has reached a sufficient size to release enough antigen and/or some tumor necrosis has occurred. In contrast, for RIS an antigen well fixed to the tumor gives more specific results, localizes the site and is able to detect tumor before serum markers are elevated.
- RIS has a prime role in the re-evaluation of the patient after the management of the primary cancer by surgery, radiotherapy or chemotherapy, or combinations of these. It is of no clinical benefit to image by RIS, the large metastases already evident on ultrasound or CT. It is of particular benefit to show that a mass in the pelvis does not represent post-surgical fibrosis, but is a tumor recurrence; that a normal sized node does contain or that an enlarged lymph node does not contain metastases; and that a clinically or radiologically normal abdomen does, in fact, contain tumor, usually in the form of plaques, a few cells thick, which have no 'mass' for radiological detection. This role in demonstrating previously

unsuspected metastases has been confirmed in cutaneous melanoma,[31] in peritoneal plaques and pelvic recurrence of ovarian cancer[32,39] where ultrasound and CT are unreliable, in colorectal cancer recurrences,[37,50,51] in involved nodes that are clinically impalpable, in breast cancer,[34–36] and in recurrences of prostate cancer[49,52,53] and Chapters 13D and 13E.

- RIS is an essential precursor to RIT to demonstrate the *in vivo* uptake of the chosen antibody. Immunohistochemistry showing evidence of specific antibody binding by the patient's tumor cells is important but not sufficient evidence to justify RIT, particularly in solid tumors.

COLORECTAL CANCER

The detection of colorectal cancer depends on the clinical history and digital rectal examination, barium enema and/or endoscopy. Nuclear medicine techniques have no routine role in this phase of the patient's management. Their main applications were in the detection of para-aortic nodes and liver involvement, in the demonstration of recurrent cancer before serum markers were elevated, in the demonstration of the site of recurrent cancer when serum markers are elevated,[50] in the evaluation of the success of chemotherapy and/or radiotherapy, in the demonstration of the distribution of the recurrence for radiotherapy planning and surgery and in the demonstration of antibody uptake before consideration of RIT.

Radiolabeled monoclonal antibodies may be injected before surgery to enable the use of the per-operative probe.[24,54–59] This may aid in the detection of unsuspected disease, in the demonstration that a tumor bed is free of tumor after operation, in the demonstration that a piece of bowel for anastomosis is free from tumor and in showing that tissue removed at operation does or does not contain malignancy before being sent for frozen section.[54] The absorbed radiation dose to the operator is negligible.[60]

Tumor-associated antigens present in colorectal cancer are of several types. First, the epithelial surface antigens are separated from the blood by being in the inner surfaces of cells and by biological barriers, so do not react with a monoclonal antibody injected intravenously. However, with the architectural disruption that characterizes the malignant process, such antigens become exposed to blood and thus such colorectal tumors may be detected using radiolabeled monoclonal antibodies that react with these antigens. One such example is PR1A3 produced by the Imperial Cancer Research Fund, now Cancer Research-UK.[37,61] A well-used group are the oncofetal antigens such as the carcinoembryonic antigen, CEA.[35,40,62–65] Antibodies such as B-72.3 against the tumor-associated antigen TAG 72 are available.[66,67] Antigens may either be fixed to the tumor or released from the tumor. CEA is released from the tumor and therefore is available as a serum marker for cancer. However, a tumor must reach a certain size to release sufficient CEA to overcome uptake by the liver and reticulo-endothelial system and the normal biological variations in the blood to make it useful as a serum marker. Both CEA and B-72.3 are released by the tumor into lymphatics and therefore detection of the antigen in lymph nodes does not mean that tumor cells are present.[68] Conversely the PR1A3 antigen is fixed to the tumor. It is not found in lymph nodes draining a primary cancer and therefore detection of uptake in lymph nodes represents malignant involvement when PR1A3 is used.[37,69] When the cancer cell dies, the PR1A3 antigen is destroyed with it, whereas the CEA antigen may be still detectable in the environment of dead cancer cells.

It has now been shown that the CEA molecule is very complex. Its three-dimensional structure consists of a large extra-membrane portion with a tail buried in the surface membrane of the cell. The part known as CEA breaks off from this tail and thus is able to diffuse into the lymphatics and the blood vessels. This breaking off process causes a conformational change to conceal the antigen against which the monoclonal antibody PR1A3 is produced. Thus, PR1A3 only binds to the membrane fixed antigen. The sites of the two negative charges that bind to the antigen have been identified in the structure of the monoclonal antibody PR1A3. This information should help in the development of peptides derived from antibodies with even higher binding affinity to the cancer antigen.[70] Antibody fragments,[71,72] chimeric antibodies,[73] ScFv,[16,55,74–76] and human antibodies[77] have been studied. The principles remain the same although the timings differ.

Patient protocol

The test is explained in detail to the patient. Since these studies are usually performed under the control of an ethics committee, signed informed consent must be obtained from the patient. It is essential to ask the patient whether there is history of an allergy to foreign proteins and such patients should not be studied. The patient is then set on the imaging couch with the camera over the pelvis. The injection consists of 600 MBq of ^{99m}Tc monoclonal antibody or 120 MBq of ^{111}In monoclonal antibody of the chosen type. The amount of protein injected is normally <1 mg and this reduces the chance of side effects, sensitization or HAMA. Before and after the injection, the vital signs are observed.

^{111}IN–RADIOLABELED ANTIBODY

For ^{111}In-labeled antibody, the camera is set up with a medium-energy (up to 300 keV) general-purpose, parallel-hole collimator with windows of 15% around the 171 keV and 20% around the 247 keV photopeaks of ^{111}In. The camera is set so that the data are transferred automatically to the mini-computer for subsequent image analysis and presentation. The injection is given intravenously into an antecubital vein slowly over 10 s. Vital signs are recorded before and after the injection.

A series of images are made over the anterior and posterior lower abdomen, pelvis, upper abdomen and chest, starting about 10 min after the injection. Other images are taken at 24 and 72 h (Plates 1C.2 and 1C.3) with SPET at about 24 h. The camera undergoes a 360° rotation with 64 projections and takes about 32 min. It is essential the patient remains still during this period. Each planar image should contain at least 800 kcounts. To aid re-positioning, a similar image to each of the planar images maybe undertaken with radioactive markers over prominent bony landmarks.[5,78] The planar and SPECT images are analysed without clinical and radiological information and decisions are made as to whether a site of abnormal antibody uptake is seen.

Pre-targeted imaging of colorectal cancer undertaken using an ^{111}In bivalent hapten and a bispecific antibody conjugate has given satisfactory results.[79]

99MTC–RADIOLABELED MONOCLONAL ANTIBODY

For ^{99m}Tc, the gamma camera is set up with a low-energy, general-purpose or preferably a high-resolution, parallel-hole collimator. The photopeak is set at 140 keV with a 15% window and for data transfer on line to the mini-computer. The patient protocol is as above. A 600-MBq ^{99m}Tc-labeled dose of intact monoclonal antibody (either anti-CEA or PR1A3) is injected intravenously over 10 s. Images are taken of the upper and lower abdomen and pelvis, upper abdomen and chest anteriorly and posteriorly, at 10 min, 5–6 h, and 18–24 h (Fig. 1C.6). Each planar image should contain a minimum of 800 kcounts. Thyroid blockade is not required. The [99m]Tc Fab' fragment of anti-CEA has also been shown to be effective.[71]

Primary colorectal cancer

The identification of primary colorectal cancer is straightforward using ^{99m}Tc-anti-CEA or ^{99m}Tc-PR1A3. The 10-min image shows normal vascular, marrow, renal, urinary, and liver uptake. The 5-h and 22-h images show the focal area of increased uptake at the site of the cancer. Because of the release of CEA normal lymph nodes may be imaged (Plate 1C.3) and areas affected by inflammatory bowel disease. Through the series of images these areas of bowel show

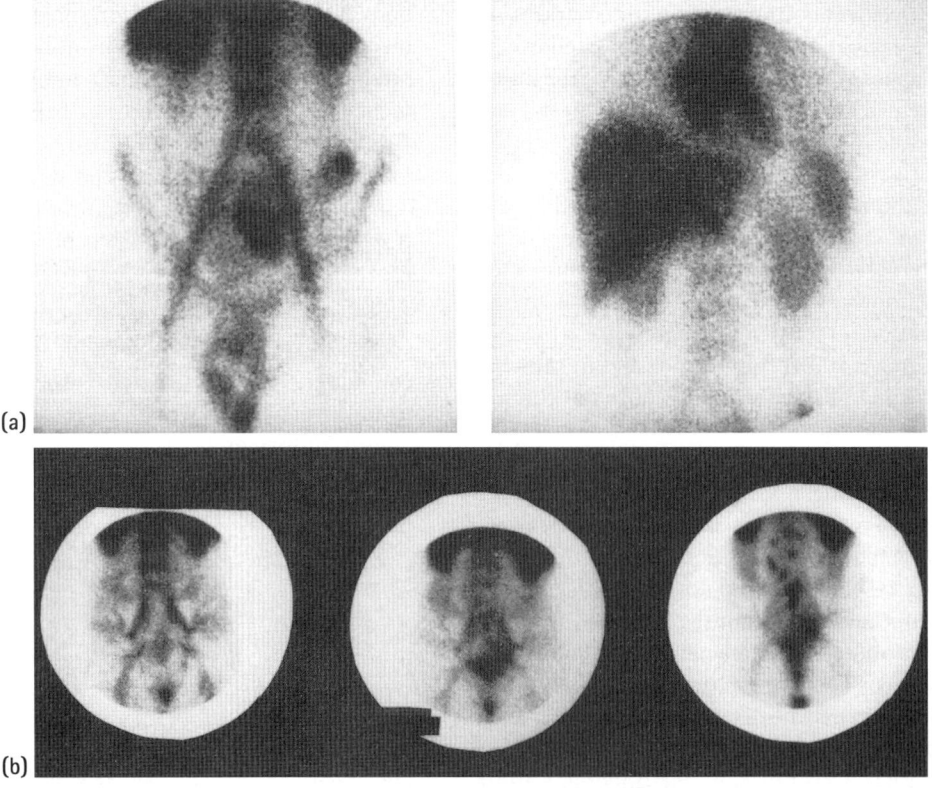

(a)

(b)

Figure 1C.6 *Colorectal cancer: radioimmunoscintigraphy with ^{99m}Tc-PR1A3. (a) Left: anterior view of the pelvis at 24 h. Focally increased uptake in the center of the pelvis due to primary sigmoid adenocarcinoma. In the left iliac fossa, a second unsuspected adenocarcinoma is seen. Right: liver metastasis in the same patient seen as a small focal area of increased uptake in the left lobe, not identified on ultrasound but confirmed at surgery. (b) Posterior view of the pelvis in a patient with recurrent rectal carcinoma. Left, 10 min; center, 5 h; right, 22 h. Increasing irregular uptake is seen in the pelvis confirming computed tomography findings, but further focal para-aortic uptake is seen which was unsuspected and made the patient inoperable.*

fixed uptake, whereas some secretion into normal bowel contents will show movement between the 5-h and the 24-h images. It is not unusual to see some diffuse uptake in the ascending colon, particularly if the patient has undergone bowel preparation before colonoscopy or surgery, where the slightly inflamed bowel becomes somewhat leaky to protein such as the gamma-globulin injected. Besides identifying the primary colorectal cancer, on occasion a second site of focal uptake may be seen; this may represent a second cancer, for example if the distal primary cancer has caused a stricture of the large bowel so that a colonoscope cannot pass (Fig. 1C.6(a)). Liver metastases may be detected. The injection of the ^{99m}Tc-labeled monoclonal antibody 24 h before surgery allows the imaging to be combined with the use of the pre-operative probe during surgery.

If rectal cancer is suspected, it is helpful to obtain a series of squat views at the three time points, since this may be the best indicator of the fact that a low-lying rectal cancer is posterior to the bladder. The planar anterior and posterior views may not define it due to superimposition with the bladder or genitalia, which usually appear vascular. Some genitalia activity persists with time and is thought to be due to binding of the Fc portion of the whole antibody to the gonadal tissue. SPET of the pelvis is always undertaken. This gives a good definition of the position of the bladder in relation to any abnormality in the pelvis. Note with excision of a rectal cancer, the bladder may lie more posteriorly than usual. The uterus may be seen as a vascular area on the early image but uptake fades with time.

Liver metastases

Liver metastases from colorectal cancer are mainly supplied by the hepatic artery, rather than the portal vein. Since the hepatic artery supply is less than the portal vein supply per unit volume of the liver, a liver metastasis will usually show as a defect in uptake on the 10-min image against the normal liver uptake, background and vascularity. Four patterns of liver metastases are seen on radioimmunoscintigraphy.

1. A defect in uptake seen on the 10-min image, which persists on the 5-h and 24-h images. This is usually large and may represent a space-occupying lesion due to a cause other than a liver metastasis.
2. A more typical pattern is a defect on the 10-min image that appears slightly smaller on the 5-h image and even smaller on the 24-h image, often with a halo of increased uptake around its periphery. This is typical of a moderate-sized liver metastasis.
3. A small metastasis in the liver may show as a defect on the 10-min image but appear undetectable on the 5-h and 24-h images since its uptake is balanced by the uptake in the normal liver. Without the 10-min image, this sort of liver metastasis, which is not uncommon, would not be detectable.

4. The last pattern is a normal 10-min image and a normal 5-h image, with a focal area of increased uptake seen on the 24-h image (Fig. 1C.6(a)). This is usually found in a very small metastasis (an accuracy of 92% can be achieved using ^{99m}Tc-PR1A3).[37]

Liver SPET may help to confirm the presence of a metastasis when interpreted in conjunction with the planar images. A very small focal metastasis with increased uptake may be detected on SPET when the planar scan is normal. It should be confirmed on all the orthogonal, coronal, transverse, and sagittal sections before being called a metastasis. SPET is not so helpful in large metastases where a defect may be difficult to distinguish from the normal variation of the liver lobes.

Focal areas of increased uptake in the para-aortic region should be interpreted with caution when anti-CEA is used, but indicates positive involvement when an antibody against a fixed antigen such as PR1A3 is used (Fig. 1C.6(b)). Rarely, lung metastases are identified but these usually occur only when the liver has been widely invaded. They are, however, not uncommon once liver metastases have been treated. Left supra-clavicular node metastases may be seen.

RECURRENT COLORECTAL CANCER

This is the main application of RIS.[80,81] Recurrences may be plaque-like, a few cells thick, over a wide area and not detectable by CT, MRI or ultrasound. They may be detectable on RIS, before any change in serum markers or symptoms. Dukes' C primary colorectal cancer has up to 50% chance of recurrence at 1 year. Imaging of such patients at a year after primary surgery, at a time when they may have no symptoms and a normal serum CEA, has shown evidence of recurrence in approximately 30% of cases. The RIS imaging technique is by its nature more sensitive than serum markers. With a good signal such as ^{99m}Tc, focal recurrences having the pattern of increasing uptake with time can be seen. Indeed, RIS may be the only modality capable of detecting such recurrences. As surgeons become confident with this technique, so surgery (with the help of the probe) or radiotherapy, may be undertaken on the basis of positive RIS alone. When serum markers are elevated, RIS can identify the site(s) of recurrence in the pelvis, abdomen or liver, even when other radiological modalities are negative. CT and MRI can demonstrate an abnormal mass in the pelvis or abdomen in a patient who has had surgery for primary colorectal cancer. However, these techniques are often unable to identify whether such a mass represents post-surgical, post-radiotherapy fibrosis, recurrent viable tumor, or indeed an inflammatory mass. The monoclonal antibody uptake will be absent if the mass is due to fibrosis; uptake will be early, and fade with time if the mass is due to an inflammatory process; and it will show no uptake on the early image with progressively increasing uptake with time, if the mass is due to a viable recurrent tumor. The greater extent of a recurrence in the abdomen may be seen by RIS due to the plaque-like spread of the tumor over the abdomen, whereas only the more mass-like part of the tumor recurrence may be appreciated on CT. Para-aortic lymph node involvement may be well visualized. There is no doubt now that FDG PET is a better detector of liver metastases than RIS in colorectal cancer.[82]

RIS in breast and ovarian cancer is considered in Chapter 13G and prostate cancer in Chapter 13H.

REFERENCES

● Seminal primary article
◆ Key review paper

● 1 Britton KE. Towards the goal of cancer-specific imaging and therapy. *Nucl Med Commun* 1997; **18**: 992–1007.

● 2 Epenetos AA, Carr D, Johnson PM, Bodmer WF, Lavender JP. Antibody guided radiolocalisation of tumours in patients with testicular or ovarian cancer using two radioiodinated monoclonal antibodies to placental alkaline phosphatase. *Br J Radiol* 1986; **59**: 117–25.

● 3 Kohler G, Milstein C. Continuous cultures of fused cells secreting antibody of proven defined specificity. *Nature* 1975; **256**: 495–7.

● 4 Williams LE, Barnes RB, Fass J, *et al.* Uptake of radiolabelled anti-CEA antibodies in human colorectal primary tumours as a function of tumour mass. *Eur J Nucl Med* 1993; **20**: 345–7.

● 5 Granowska M, Jass JR, Britton KE, Northover JMA. A prospective study of the use of ^{111}In-labelled monoclonal antibody against carcinoembryonic antigen in colorectal cancer and of some biological factors affecting its uptake. *Int J Colorect Dis* 1989; **4**: 97–108.

◆ 6 Begent, RHJ. Working party on clinical use of antibodies. *Br J Cancer* 1986; **54**: 557–68.

● 7 Winter G, Milstein C. Man-made antibodies. *Nature* 1991; **349**: 293–9.

◆ 8 Wu AM, Yazaki PJ. Designer genes: recombinant antibody fragments for biological imaging. *Q J Nucl Med* 2000; **44**: 268–83.

● 9 Morrison SL, Johnson JM, Herzenberg LA, *et al.* Chimeric antibody molecules: mouse antigen binding domains with human constant region domains. *Proc Natl Acad Sci USA* 1984; **81**: 6851–5.

● 10 Jones PT, Dear PH, Foote J, *et al.* Replacing the complementarity-determining regions in a human antibody with those from a mouse. *Nature* 1986; **321**: 522–5.

● 11 McCafferty J, Griffiths AD, Winter G, *et al.* Phage antibodies: filamentous phage displaying antibody variable domains. *Nature* 1990; **348**: 552–4.

● 12 Marks JD, Hoogenboom HR, Bonnert TP, *et al.* By-passing immunization: human antibodies from V-gene libraries displayed on phage. *J Mol Biol* 1991; **222**: 581–97.

● 13 Bird RE, Hardman KD, Jacobson JW, *et al.* Single-chain antigen-binding proteins. *Science* 1988; **242**: 423–6.

● 14 Clackson T, Hoogenboom HR, Griffiths AD, Winter G. Making antibody fragments using phage display libraries. *Nature* 1991; **352**: 624–8.

● 15 Chester KA, Begent RH, Robson L, *et al.* Phage libraries for generation of clinically useful antibodies. *Lancet* 1994; **343**: 455–6.

● 16 Begent RHJ, Verhaar MJ, Chester KA, *et al.* Clinical evidence of efficient tumor targeting based on single-chain Fv antibody selected from a combinatorial library. *Nature Med* 1996; **2**: 979–84.

● 17 Holliger P, Prospero T, Winter G. 'Diabodies': Small bivalent and bispecific antibody fragments. *Proc Natl Acad Sci USA* 1993; **90**: 6444–8.

● 18 Hu SZ, Shively L, Raubitschek A, *et al.* Minibody: A novel engineered anti carcinoembryonic antigen antibody fragment (single-chain Fv-CH3) which exhibits rapid, high-level targeting of xenografts. *Cancer Res* 1996; **56**: 3055–61.

● 19 George AJ, Jamar TF, Tai MS, *et al.* Radiometal labeling of recombinant proteins by a genetically engineered minimal chelation site: Technetium-99m coordination by single-chain Fv antibody fusion proteins through a C-terminal cysteinyl peptide. *Proc Natl Acad Sci USA* 1995; **92**: 8358–62.

● 20 Li L, Olafsen T, Anderson AL, *et al.* Reduction of kidney uptake in radiometal labeled peptide linkers conjugated to recombinant antibody fragments. Site-specific conjugation of DOTA-peptides to a Cys-diabody. *Bioconjug Chem* 2002; **13**: 985–95.

● 21 Waibel R, Alberto R, Willuda J, *et al.* Stable one-step technetium-99m labeling of His-tagged recombinant proteins with a novel Tc(I)-carbonyl complex. *Nat Biotechnol* 1999; **17**: 897–901.

● 22 Band HA, Creighton AM, Britton KE, *et al.* P-labelled antibodies for radioimmunotherapy: a review of recent developments and a preliminary report of the first phase I studies. *Tumor Targeting* 1995; **1**: 85–92.

● 23 Moffat FL, Vergas-Cuba RD, Serafini AN, *et al.* Preoperative scintigraphy and operative probe scintimetry of colorectal carcinoma using technetium-99m-88BV59. *J Nucl Med* 1995; **36**: 738–45.

● 24 Hanna MG, Haspel MV, McCabe R, *et al.* Development and application of human monoclonal antibodies. *Antibody Immunoconj Radiopharm* 1991; **4**: 67–75; and *J Nucl Med* 1995; **36**: 738–45.

◆ 25 Buraggi GL, Turrin A, Cascinelli N, *et al.* In: Donato L, Britton KE. (eds.) *Immunoscintigraphy*. London: Gordon and Breach, 1985: 215–53.

◆ 26 Britton KE, Granowska M. Radio-immunoscintigraphy in tumour identification. *Cancer Surveys* 1987; **6**: 247–67.

● 27 Hnatowich DJ, Childs RL, Lanteigne D, Najafi A. The preparation of DTPA-coupled antibodies radiolabelled with metallic radio-nuclides: an improved method. *J Immunol Methods* 1983; **65**: 147–57.

● 28 Mather SJ, Ellison D. Reduction-mediated Tc-99m labeling of monoclonal antibodies. *J Nucl Med* 1990; **31**: 692–7.

● 29 Stalteri M, Mather SJ. Technetium-99m labeling of an anti-tumour antibody PR1A3 by photoactivation. *Eur J Nucl Med* 1996; **23**: 42–4.

● 30 Bomanji J, Hungerford JL, Granowska M, Britton KE. Radioimmunoscintigraphy of ocular melanoma with 99-Tc-m labelled cutaneous melanoma antibody fragments. *Br J Ophthalmol* 1987; **71**: 651–8.

● 31 Siccardi AG, Buraggi GL, Callegaro L, *et al.* Multicentre study of immunoscintigraphy with radiolabelled monoclonal antibodies in patients with melanoma. *Cancer Res* 1986; **46**: 4817–22.

● 32 Granowska M, Britton KE, Mather SJ, *et al.* Radioimmunoscintigraphy with technetium-99m labelled monoclonal antibody, SM3, in gynaecological cancer. *Eur J Nucl Med* 1993; **20**: 483–9.

● 33 Ali N, Jan H, Van Trappen P, *et al.* Radioimmunoscintigraphy with Tc-99m labelled SM3 in differentiating malignant from benign adnexal masses. *Br J Obstet Gynaecol* 2003; **110**: 508–14.

34 Granowska M, Biassoni L, Carroll MJ, *et al.* Breast cancer Tc-99m SM3 radioimmunoscintigraphy. *Acta Oncol* 1996; **35**: 319–21.

● 35 Biassoni L, Granowska M, Carroll MJ, *et al.* Tc-99m labelled SM3 in the preoperative evaluation of axillary lymph nodes and primary breast cancer with change detection statistical processing as an aid to tumour detection. *Br J Cancer* 1998; **77**: 131–8.

● 36 Al Yasi AR, Carroll MJ, Granowska M, *et al.* Axillary node status in breast cancer patients prior to surgery by imaging with Tc-99m humanised anti PEM monoclonal antibody hHMFG1. *Br J Cancer* 2002; **86**: 870–8.

● 37 Granowska M, Britton KE, Mather SJ, *et al.* Radioimmunoscintigraphy with technetium-99m labelled monoclonal antibody, IA3, in colorectal cancer. *Eur J Nucl Med* 1993; **20**: 690–8.

● 38 Granowska M, Shepherd J, Britton KE, *et al.* Ovarian cancer: diagnosis using 123-I monoclonal antibody in comparison with surgical findings. *Nucl Med Commun* 1984; **5**: 485–99.

● 39 Granowska M, Britton KE, Shepherd JH. A prospective study of 123-I-labelled monoclonal antibody imaging in ovarian cancer. *J Clin Oncol* 1986; **4**: 730–6.

● 40 Goldenberg DM, Kim EE, Deland FH, *et al.* Radioimmunodetection of cancer with radioactive antibodies to carcinoembryonic antigen. *Cancer Res* 1980; **40**: 2984–92.

● 41 Berche C, Mach J-P, Lumbroso JD, *et al.* Tomoscintigraphy for detecting gastrointestinal and medullary thyroid cancers: first clinical results using radiolabelled monoclonal antibodies against carcinoembryonic antigen. *Br Med J* 1982; **285**: 1447–51.

● 42 Wahl RL, Parker CW, Philpott G. Improved radioimaging and tumour localisation with monoclonal (Fab′)$_2$. *J Nucl Med* 1983; **24**: 316–25.

● 43 Begent RHJ, Keep PA, Green AJ, *et al.* Liposomally entrapped second antibody improves tumour imaging with radiolabelled (first) anti-tumour antibody. *Lancet* 1983; **ii**: 739–41.

● 44 Granowska M, Britton KE, Shepherd J. The detection of ovarian cancer using 123-I monoclonal antibody. *Radiobiol Radiother (Berlin)* 1983; **25**: 153–60.

◆ 45 Paganelli G, Malcovati M, Fazio F. Monoclonal antibody pretargeting techniques for tumour localization: the avidin biotin system. *Nucl Med Commun* 1991; **12**: 211–34.

● 46 Paganelli G, Belloni C, Magnani P, *et al.* Two step targetting in ovarian cancer patients using biotinylated monoclonal antibodies and radioactive streptavidin. *Eur J Nucl Med* 1992; **19**: 322–9.

● 47 Granowska M, Nimmon CC, Britton KE, *et al.* Kinetic analysis and probability mapping applied to the detection of ovarian cancer by radioimmunoscintigraphy. *J Nucl Med* 1988; **29**: 599–607.

● 48 Chengazi VU, Nimmon CC, Britton KE. Forward projection analysis and image surgery: an approach to quantitative tomography. In: *Tomography in nuclear medicine, present status and future prospects.* Vienna: International Atomic Energy Agency, 1996: 31–44.

49 Carroll MJ, Britton KE. Fusing anatomical reference data to SPECT – application to 3D statistical change detection in prostate imaging. *Eur J Nucl Med* 2003; **30**: S330.

● 50 Chatal JF, Saccavini JC, Furnoleau P, *et al.* Immunoscintigraphy of colon carcinoma. *J Nucl Med* 1984; **25**: 307–14.

● 51 Corman ML, Galandiuk S, Block GE, *et al.* Immunoscintigraphy with 111-In-salumomoab pendetide in patients with colorectal adenocarcinoma: performance and impact on clinical management. *Dis Colon Rectum* 1994; **37**: 129–37.

● 52 Babaian RJ, Sayer J, Podoloff DA, *et al.* Radioimmunoscintigraphy of pelvis lymph nodes with [111]indium-labelled monoclonal antibody CYT-356. *J Urol* 1994; **152**: 1952–5.

53 Feneley MR, Chengazi VU, Kirby RS, *et al.* Prostate radioimmunoscintigraphy: preliminary results using technetium-labelled monoclonal antibody CYT-351. *Br J Urol* 1996; **77**: 373–81.

54 Howell R, Hawley PR, Granowska M, Morris G, Britton KE. Peroperative radio-immunodetection, PROD, of colorectal cancer using Tc-99m PR1A3 monoclonal antibody. *Tumori* 1995; **81(Suppl)**: 107–8.

● 55 Mayer A, Tsiompanou E, O'Malley D, *et al.* Radio-immunoguided sugery in colorectal cancer using a genetically engineered anti-CEA single-chain Fv antibody. *Clin Cancer Res* 2000; **6**: 1711–19.

● 56 Reuter M, Montz R, de Heer K, *et al.* Detection of colorectal carcinomas by investigative RIS in addition to preoperative RIS: surgical and immunohistochemical findings. *Eur J Nucl Med* 1992; **19**: 102–9.

● 57 Curtet C, Vuillez JP, Daniel G, *et al.* Feasibility study of radioimmunoguided surgery of colorectal carcinomas using indium-111 CEA specific monoclonal antibody. *Eur J Nucl Med* 1990; **17**: 299–304.

● 58 Aprile C, Prati U, Saponaro R, Roveda L, Carena M, Gastaldo L. Radioimmunolocalization of pelvic recurrences from rectosigmoid cancer employing ^{111}In-anti CEA F (ab')₂. *Nucl Med Biol* 1991; **18**: 51–2.

● 59 Muxi A, Pons F, Vidal-Sicart S, *et al.* Radio-immunoguided surgery of colorectal carcinoma with a In-111 labelled anti-TAG 72 monoclonal antibody. *Nucl Med Commun* 1999; **20**: 123–30.

● 60 Bares R, Muller B, Fass J, Buell V, Schumpelick V. The radiation dose to surgical personnel during intraoperative radioimmunoscintigraphy. *Eur J Nucl Med* 1992; **19**: 110–12.

● 61 Richman PI, Bodmer WF. Monoclonal antibodies to human colorectal epithelium: markers for differentiation and tumour characterisation. *Br J Cancer* 1987; **39**: 317–28.

● 62 Bischof Delaloye A, Delaloye B, Buchegger F, *et al.* Clinical value of immunoscintigraphy in colorectal carcinoma patients: a prospective study. *J Nucl Med* 1989; **30**: 1646–56.

◆ 63 Goldenberg DM, Larson SM. Radio-immunodetection in cancer identification. *J Nucl Med* 1992; **33**: 803–14.

● 64 Baum RP, Hertel A, Lorenz M, *et al.* Tc-99m anti-CEA monoclonal antibody for tumour immunoscintigraphy: first clinical results. *Nucl Med Commun* 1989; **10**: 345–8.

● 65 Lind P, Lechner P, Arian-Schad K, *et al.* Anti-carcinoembryonic antigen immunoscintigraphy (technetium-99m monoclonal antibody BW 431/26) and serum CEA levels in patients with suspected primary and recurrent colorectal carcinoma. *J Nucl Med* 1991; **32**: 1319–25.

● 66 Doerr RJ, Abdel-Nabi H, Krag D, Mitchell E. Radiolabelled antibody imaging in the management of colorectal cancer. *Arch Surg* 1991; **214**: 118–24.

● 67 Collier BD, Abdel Nabi G, Doerr RJ, *et al.* Immuno-scintigraphy performed with In-111-labelled CYT 103 in the management of colorectal cancer: comparisons with CT. *Radiology* 1992; **185**: 179–86.

● 68 Beatty JD, Duda RB, Williams LE, *et al.* Preoperative imaging of colorectal carcinoma with ^{111}In-labelled anticarcino-embryonic antigen monoclonal antibody. *Cancer Res* 1986; **46**: 6494–502.

● 69 Granowska M, Mather SJ, Britton KE. Diagnostic evaluation of ^{111}In and ^{99m}Tc radiolabelled monoclonal antibodies in ovarian and colorectal cancer: correlations with surgery. *Nucl Med Biol* 1991; **18**: 413–24.

● 70 Durbin H, Young S, Stewart LM, *et al.* An epitope on carcinoembryonic antigen defined by the clinically relevant antibody PR1A3. *Proc Natl Acad Sci USA* 1994; **91**: 4314–17.

● 71 Sirisriro R, Podoloff DA, Patt YZ, *et al.* [99]Tc[m]-IMMU4 imaging in recurrent colorectal cancer: efficacy and impact on surgical management. *Nucl Med Commun* 1996; **17**: 568–76.

● 72 Siccardi AG, Buraggi GL, Callegaro L, *et al.* Immuno-scintigraphy of adenocarcinomas by means of radio-labelled F (ab')₂ fragments of anti-carcinoembryonic antigen monoclonal antibody: a multicenter study. *Cancer Res* 1989; **49**: 3095–103.

● 73 LoBuglio AF, Wheeler RH, Trang J, *et al.* Mouse/human chimeric monoclonal antibody in man: kinetics and immune response. *Proc Natl Acad Sci USA* 1989; **86**: 4220–4.

● 74 Wu AM, Williams LE, Zieran L, *et al.* Anti-carcinoembryonic antigen (CEA) diabody for rapid tumor targeting and imaging. *Tumor Targeting* 1999; **4**: 47–58.

● 75 Pietersz GA, Patrick MR, Chester KA. Pre-clinical characterisation and in vivo imaging studies of an engineered recombinant technetium-99 labelled metallothionein-containing anti carcino embryonic antigen single-chain antibody. *J Nucl Med* 1998; **39**: 47–56.

● 76 Goel A, Baranowska-Kortylewicz J, Hinrichs SH. Tc 99m labelled divalent and tetravalent CC49 single chain Fv's. Normal imaging agents for rapid in vivo localisation of human: carcinoma. *J Nucl Med* 2001; **42**: 1519–27.

● 77 Krause BJ, Baum RP, Staib-Sebler E, Lorenz M, Niesen A, Hor G. Human monoclonal antibody [99m]Tc-88BV59 detection of colorectal cancer, recurrent or metastatic disease and immunogenicity assessment. *Eur J Nucl Med* 1997; **24**: 72–5.

◆ 78 Britton KE, Granowska M, Mather SJ. Radiolabelled monoclonal antibodies in oncology, I. Technical aspects. *Nucl Med Commun* 1991; **12**: 65–76.

● 79 Chetanneau A, Barbet J, Peltier P, *et al.* Pretargetted imaging of colorectal cancer recurrences using an ^{111}In-labelled bivalent hapten and a bispecific antibody conjugate. *Nucl Med Commun* 1994; **15**: 972–80.

◆ 80 Pinkas L, Robins PD, Forstrom LA, Mahoney DW, Mullan BP. Clinical experience with radiolabelled monoclonal antibodies in the detection of colorectal and ovarian carcinoma recurrence and review of the literature. *Nucl Med Commun* 1999; **20**: 689–96.

● 81 Baulieu S, Bourlier P, Scotto B, *et al.* The value of immunoscintigraphy in detection of recurrent colorectal cancer. *Nucl Med Commun* 2001; **22**: 1295–304.

● 82 Ruers TJ, Langenhoff BS, Neeleman N, *et al.* Value of positron emission tomography with (F-18)fluoro-deoxyglucose in patients with colorectal liver metastases: a prospective study. *J Clin Oncol* 2002; **20**: 388–95.

1D

Monitoring Treatment

RICHARD P. BAUM AND VIKAS PRASAD

INTRODUCTION

Medical science is constantly working towards understanding the basic cause of a disease and is no longer satisfied with morphological and gross cellular level pathology. The science has moved to the molecular level as the scientists have now realized that the cure to many devastating diseases lies in targeting molecular events. With the advent of new technologies like positron emission tomography (PET), magnetic resonance spectroscopy (MRS) and functional magnetic resonance imaging (fMRI), cumulatively mentioned as molecular imaging, it is now possible to not only image but also quantify the pathophysiology of a disease process at the molecular level. Most of the advances of these molecular imaging methodologies have been concentrated in the field of oncology. Demands from molecular imaging technologies have increased, keeping pace with the advances in treatment modalities to assess the response to therapy. Until now, conventional imaging tools like ultrasound (US), X-ray computed tomography (CT) and MRI have been assessing the response to therapy by measuring the change in anatomical size of a tumor. However, in the present era of advancing oncology, with the availability of so-called tailor-made drug therapy for individual patients, cytostatic drugs, cancer vaccines, immunotherapy and cytokines, it has become essential to gauge the therapy response of tumors at a very early stage, even prior to the changes in the anatomical size and clinical symptoms. Through molecular imaging, the ability to evaluate response to therapy at an early stage helps in reducing the toxicity and deciding whether the treatment protocol used is appropriate or an alternative therapy should be started.

Positron emission tomography (PET) has contributed considerably in properly assessing the response of tumors towards therapy by applying a whole armamentarium of radiopharmaceuticals. It has been used to monitor tumor metabolism, tissue perfusion, hypoxic tumor volume, cell proliferation, receptor status, uptake of therapeutic agents, shedding light on the mechanism of drug resistance, and many other tumor-specific interactions.[1] This chapter covers the role of PET in monitoring therapy response of the tumors listed in Table 1D.1. The different radiopharmaceuticals which have been mainly applied and the pathophysiological parameters underlying their use as well as the different tumor entities and the response predicted are mentioned in Table 1D.2.[2]

Table 1D.1 *Use of positron emission tomography to monitor the response of various tumors to therapy*

Malignancy	Molecular imaging method
Thyroid cancer	^{131}I, ^{18}F-FDG PET
Lung cancer	^{18}F-FDG PET
Breast cancer	^{18}F-FDG PET, ^{99m}Tc-sestamibi
Lymphoma	^{18}F-FDG PET
Colorectal cancer	^{18}F-FDG PET, ^{18}F-FU PET
Neuroendocrine tumor	SRS, ^{68}Ga-DOTA SMS analogs
Gastric carcinoma	^{18}F-FDG PET
Esophageal carcinoma	^{18}F-FDG PET
Gastrointestinal stromal tumor	^{18}F-FDG PET
Cervical carcinoma	^{18}F-FDG PET
Prostate cancer	^{11}C, ^{18}F-choline, ^{11}C-acetate PET
Brain tumor	^{18}F-FDG, ^{11}C-thymidine, ^{18}F-thymidine, ^{11}C-methionine, ^{18}F-tyrosine PET

Table 1D.2 *The response of tumors to various radiopharmaceuticals*

Radiopharmaceutical	Measured effect	Application in therapy response
^{18}F–FDG	Glycolysis, glucose consumption and metabolism	Staging, restaging, treatment response of different types of cancer
^{11}C-thymidine, ^{18}F-thymidine	DNA synthesis and tumor cell proliferation	Staging, restaging, treatment response of different types of cancer
^{11}C-methionine, [^{18}F]fluorothymidine	Protein synthesis and tumor cell proliferation	Staging, restaging, treatment response of different types of cancer
^{11}C-choline, ^{18}F-choline	Cell membrane metabolism and tumor cell proliferation	Staging, restaging, treatment response of different types of cancer
^{11}C-tyrosine, [^{18}F]fluorotyrosine and [^{18}F]fluoroethyltyrosine	Natural amino acid transport	Staging, restaging, treatment response of different types of cancer
^{11}C-acetate	Lipid synthesis	Staging, restaging, treatment response of different types of cancer
5-[^{18}F]fluorouracil	Accumulation of 5-FU in tumors	Prediction of tumor response to 5-FU (e.g. colorectal carcinoma)
[^{18}F]fluoro-17-β-estradiol	Estrogen receptor status	Monitoring response of estrogen receptor positive breast cancer
^{99m}Tc-annexin V, ^{18}F-annexin V	Apoptotic cell death	Monitoring treatment response of different types of cancer
[^{18}F]fluorodihydroxyphenylalanine	Dopamine synthesis and natural amino acid transport	Staging, restaging, treatment response of brain tumors and neuroendocrine tumors

Modified from the article by Juweid *et al.*[2]

Apart from PET, single photon emission computed tomography (SPECT) using sestamibi has been used in certain cancers for assessing multidrug resistance and in differentiating viable tumor tissue from scar or necrosis.[3–14] Thyroid cancer is one of the oldest examples, and probably the first cancer type, where nuclear medicine not only contributed significantly in therapy monitoring, but also in the treatment of disease, paving the way for future developments in the field (Fig. 1D.1).

BASIC PRINCIPLES OF THERAPY MONITORING

Therapy options available for treating cancer can be broadly classified into surgical and nonsurgical groups. Measuring the response in cancers belonging to the nonsurgical group is generally taken as therapy monitoring. The nonsurgical group comprises chemotherapy, radiation therapy, biological therapy and hormonal therapy. The stage at which a tumor is diagnosed and therapy instituted determines essentially the prognosis of the patient. The tumor volume, heterogeneity of the cell population in the tumor, growth cycle of cells at which the therapy is started, blood supply and oxygenation of tumor tissue affect significantly the outcome of therapy.[15] The principles of therapy monitoring, either by using anatomical or functional imaging, aim at having a

pre-treatment and post-treatment measurement of few or all of the above-mentioned parameters.

The World Health Organization (WHO) has defined criteria for assessing tumor response to therapy. According to these standardized criteria for the assessment of therapy response, the size of the tumor should be measured in two perpendicular diameters. Tumor response is defined as a therapy-induced reduction of the product of these two diameters by at least 50%. If no lesion remains visible after therapy, the response is classified as a complete response. Otherwise, the response is classified as a partial response. These criteria are based upon a study performed by Moertel and Hanley in 1976 using simple anatomical imaging by X-ray.[16–18] More recently, the RECIST (Response Evaluation Criteria in Solid Tumors) criteria (Table 1D.3) have been adopted, based upon longest measured diameter of the tumor, to classify therapy response into complete response, partial response, progressive disease and no response using CT, US and MRI.[19] Anatomical imaging has only limited success in predicting/monitoring the response of therapy because it primarily aims at measuring the anatomical change in size (volume and diameter), which is not a very reliable and specific marker for therapy response.[1,15] For solid tumors, reduction in tumor size may take considerable time.[20] Tumor response can also be analyzed histopathologically. Histopathological response is defined as the percentage of viable tumor cells as compared to the fibrosed tissue. It is generally expressed

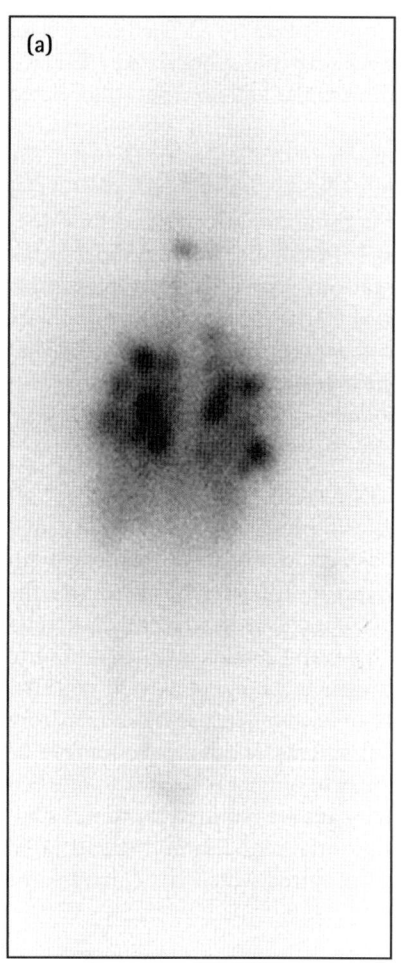

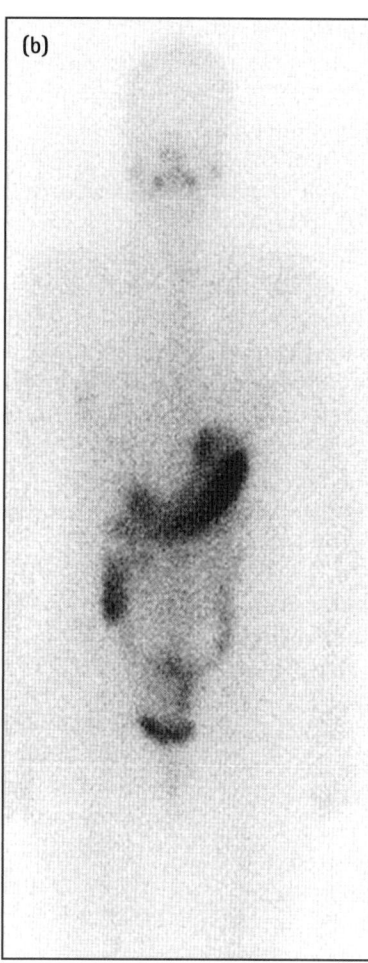

Figure 1D.1 *Iodine-131 scanning, the very first example of molecular imaging for monitoring therapy response in clinical practice: whole-body scans in a patient with disseminated lung metastases of differentiated thyroid cancer (papillary carcinoma, stage pT4b pN1a cM1) revealing strong iodine-131 uptake (a) after the first therapeutic dose (5.15 GBq). (b) Complete remission after the second dose (5.2 GBq) lasting now for 7 years. The 26 year-old female delivered 3 healthy children after therapy.*

Table 1D.3 *Criteria for tumor response based on anatomical and metabolic tumor imaging methods*

Report	Complete response	Partial response	Progressive disease	Stable disease
WHO	Complete disappearance of all disease manifestations in two observations at an interval of at least 4 weeks	Greater than or equal to 50% decrease in tumor size	Greater than 25% increase in tumor lesions and/or appearance of new foci of tumor	Increase or decrease in tumor size of less than 25%
RECIST	Disappearance of all tumor lesions	At least 30% decrease in the sum of longest diameter of tumor lesion	At least 20% increase in sum of the longest diameter of tumor lesion	Neither partial response nor progressive disease
EORTC (^{18}F-FDG PET)	No uptake of ^{18}F-FDG uptake in the target lesion	Reduction in SUV 15–25% after one cycle and greater than 25% afterwards	Increase in SUV greater than 25%, visible increase in extent of tumor uptake by 20%, appearance of new ^{18}F-FDG uptake in metastatic lesions	Increase in SUV less than 25% or decrease in SUV less than 15%, no visible change in extent of tumor

WHO, World Health Organization.
RECIST, Response Evaluation Criteria in Solid Tumors.
EORTC, European Organization for Research and Treatment of Cancer.

as a regression score. Histopathological response is currently the 'gold standard' for the evaluation of imaging modalities because these data have shown a very close correlation with patient survival. Patients with no or less than 10% residual tumor after therapy have been found to have an excellent prognosis. However, because of tumor heterogeneity, a biopsy specimen does not always provide reliable results.[20–25]

EORTC criteria for assessment of response to therapy using ^{18}F–FDG PET

Based on the guidelines[26] of the European Organization for Research and Treatment of Cancer (EORTC) on measurement of clinical and subclinical response of tumor using 2-[^{18}F]fluoro-2-deoxy-D-glucose (^{18}F-FDG) PET, progressive metabolic disease is defined as an increase in standardized uptake value (SUV) $> 25\%$, visible increase in the extent of tumor uptake $> 20\%$, and appearance of new hypermetabolic metastatic lesions. Stable disease is defined as an increase in SUV of $< 25\%$ or a decrease of $< 15\%$, no visible changes in extent, and partial metabolic response as reduction in SUV of 15–25% after 1 cycle and $> 25\%$ afterwards. Complete metabolic response is defined as complete resolution of ^{18}F-FDG uptake within tumor volume (Table 1D.3). Apart from defining general criteria for assessment of therapy response using ^{18}F-FDG PET, EORTC has also given patient-specific guidelines to be used while using ^{18}F-FDG PET. Patients must be fasted to achieve circulating glucose levels of 4–7 mmol L^{-1}. Patients with type I diabetes should be fasted overnight and scanned in the morning. The timing of scans is also critical. The pre-treatment scan should be acquired close to the start of treatment (not earlier than 2 weeks) and the post-treatment scan should be scheduled for assessment of the end point of therapy. There should be a gap of approximately 1–2 weeks between completion of chemotherapy cycle and PET scan. The recommendations also suggest normalization for body surface area (SUV$_{bsa}$) for SUV measurements. However, according to EORTC, kinetic analysis with calculation of metabolic rate of tracers (MR$_{glu}$) may be a better discriminator of subclinical response. For kinetic quantification, the Patlak approach is recommended, with dynamic image acquisition of at least 60 min duration with direct sampling of the arterial activity concentration.

Parameters used for monitoring response to therapy using PET

There are various methods available for assessing response to therapy using PET, which can be broadly classified into quantitative and visual parameters. The visual interpretation of pre-treatment and post-treatment scan suffers from a high degree of intra- and inter-observer variation. A more objective method of measuring response to therapy is the use of quantitative parameters.

QUANTITATIVE PARAMETERS USED TO MONITOR THERAPY RESPONSE

^{18}F-FDG is the only radiopharmaceutical that has been approved by the Food and Drug Administration in the United States for therapy monitoring.[2] The concentration of ^{18}F-FDG in tissue, as measured by PET, is the sum of three components: intracellular phosphorylated ^{18}F-FDG, non-phosphorylated intracellular and non-phosphorylated intravascular ^{18}F-FDG. The amount of phosphorylated ^{18}F-FDG is the only component that is directly related to the metabolic activity of tumor. Static measurement of ^{18}F-FDG takes into account all the three components and thus does not represent exact glucose metabolic rates in tumor.[20] Krak et al. reviewed in detail various approaches to overcome this problem of static imaging.[27] The two main approaches are the simplified tracer kinetic approach, e.g. Patlak–Gjedde analysis and the nonlinear regression analysis with a two-tissue compartment model.

NONLINEAR REGRESSION ANALYSIS

The net rate of ^{18}F-FDG phosphorylation can be calculated from a dynamic PET study using a two-compartment model and nonlinear regression analysis. It measures the time course of ^{18}F-FDG uptake by the tumor tissue and clearance of ^{18}F-FDG from the plasma over a minimum period of 1 h. However, despite its potential to provide the most accurate estimate of tumor glucose, it suffers from two major limitations: first, only one tumor lesion can be assessed at a time (as the field of view is limited to one bed position) and additional scans are required for tumor staging. Secondly, repeated arterial blood sampling and rapid dynamic acquisition are required which is a cumbersome procedure.

PATLAK–GJEDDE ANALYSIS

This technique uses simple linear regression analysis to determine the net rate of ^{18}F-FDG phosphorylation (K_i), as a measure of glucose metabolic rate of tumor. Patlak–Gjedde analysis in comparison with nonlinear regression analysis is significantly less sensitive to image noise and is easy to use. However, just as in nonlinear regression analysis, the field of view is limited to one bed position.

STATIC MEASUREMENT OF ^{18}F-FDG UPTAKE

The most commonly used parameter for assessment of therapy response is the SUV.[20] It is based upon a basic concept that the activity concentration after a sufficient time post-injection is correlated linearly with net ^{18}F-FDG phosphorylation rates provided the activity concentration is appropriately standardized.[28] Although there are a number of limitations and drawbacks in the assumption used for deduction of SUV, a strong correlation has been found between K_i determined by Patlak–Gjedde analysis and the SUV in follow-up of patients post-chemotherapy in non-small cell lung carcinoma (NSCLC). Both had almost similar diagnostic accuracy for the prediction of subsequent reduction of tumor size. A strong correlation was also observed between these two parameters and the overall survival post-chemotherapy.[29]

Basic principles of therapy monitoring

Table 1D.4 *Sources of error in tumor SUV measurements*

Error	Effect on SUV
Extravasation of ^{18}F-FDG injection, residual radioactivity in syringe	Smaller area under plasma time-activity curve leads to incorrectly low SUV
Variable time gap between injection and imaging	Measurement at longer uptake period leads to higher SUV
Inappropriate cross-calibration of dose calibration and scanner	Incorrect SUV reading
Failure to apply decay correction to injected activity	Incorrectly low SUV

Modified from the article by Weber.[20]

CHANGE IN TOTAL LESION GLYCOLYSIS: THE LARSON–GINSBERG INDEX

Based on the rationale that change in total glycolysis should correlate best with the change in the surviving fractions of tumor cells present in the whole tumor mass, Larson *et al.* have shown that the Larson–Ginsberg index correlates well with other therapy response parameters for locally advanced lung, gastric, esophageal and rectal cancer.[30] The volume of the lesion was determined using ^{18}F-FDG PET. For the calculation of the index, the difference in the pre-treatment and post-treatment glycolysis is taken into account according to the following formula:

$$\delta \text{TLG} = \frac{(\text{SUV}_{av,1} \times V_1) - (\text{SUV}_{av,2} \times V_2)}{\text{SUV}_{av,1} \times V_1} \times 100$$

where δTLG is the change in total lesion glycolysis (according to the Larson–Ginsberg index); V_1 and V_2 are the pre-treatment and post-treatment tumor volumes, respectively; and $\text{SUV}_{av,1}$ and $\text{SUV}_{av,2}$ are the average standardized uptake values for tumor volumes V_1 and V_2, respectively. Although ^{18}F-FDG has been used extensively to monitor therapy response, tumor uptake of glucose, as measured by PET, is influenced by many factors, as listed in Tables 1D.4 and 1D.5. In order to use ^{18}F-FDG PET for therapy monitoring, these factors have to be taken into account.

MOLECULAR (METABOLIC) TUMOR INDEX, MOLECULAR (METABOLIC) TUMOR DIAMETER AND MOLECULAR (METABOLIC) TUMOR VOLUME

These are relatively new parameters introduced by Baum *et al.* for quantifying therapy response by PET. By using routinely established software algorithms, it is now possible to quantify the molecular volume of a tumor by considering

Table 1D.5 *Factors affecting tumor uptake of ^{18}F-FDG measured by PET*

Factor	Effect
Size of lesion	Lesions with diameter <2 times resolution of PET scanner result in marked underestimation of radiotracer uptake in lesion
Heterogeneity of tumor	Underestimation of radiotracer uptake in necrotic center of tumor, for example
ROI definition	Small regions of interest have larger random errors, larger regions of interest have lower mean radiotracer uptake
Parameters for image reconstruction	Smoother reconstruction parameters result in lower radiotracer uptake values
Time interval between image acquisition and injection	Higher ^{18}F-FDG uptake with increasing time interval
Blood glucose level	Increasing blood glucose levels result in lower radiotracer uptake

Modified from the article by Weber.[20]

the three-dimensional PET image. The measured, maximum molecular diameter of the tumor is known as the MTD and the volume derived from it, because it represents the actual functional vital tumor tissue, is termed the molecular tumor volume (MTV). When FDG is utilized, the term metabolic tumor volume is used instead. By multiplying MTD and SUV, another index is derived, which represents the distribution of the radiopharmaceutical inside the tumor. The index is given a special name: molecular (or metabolic) tumor index (MTI) (Table 1D.6).

$$\text{MTI} = \text{SUV} \times \text{MTD}.$$

These parameters have also been used for the evaluation of radiation therapy response (Plates 1D.1 and 1D.2) and also in molecular radiation treatment planning (MRTP) and hold promise in therapy monitoring using alternative treatment options.[31]

Visual response parameters

Larson *et al.* have described a parameter for visual assessment of therapy response.[30] The visual response score (VRS) or visual response index (VRI) is based upon the visually estimated percentage change in the tumor volume and is recorded on a five-point response scale as shown in Table 1D.7.

Table 1D.6   *Quantitative parameters used for monitoring therapy response using* ^{18}*F-FDG PET*

	Method	Molecular event measured
1	*Nonlinear regression analysis*	*Dynamic PET using two-compartment model. Measures time course of ^{18}F-FDG uptake by tumor tissue and plasma clearance of ^{18}F-FDG over a minimum of 1 h*
2	*Patlak–Gjedde analysis*	*Determines the net rate of ^{18}F-FDG phosphorylation (K_i), as a measure of glucose metabolic rate of tumor*
3	*Standardized uptake value*	*Determines the concentration of ^{18}F-FDG in tumor tissue. The ^{18}F-FDG concentration in tumor tissue is the sum of three components: intracellular phosphorylated ^{18}F-FDG, non-phosphorylated intracellular ^{18}F-FDG and non-phosphorylated intravascular ^{18}F-FDG*
4	*Metabolic or molecular tumor index*	*Product of SUV and the maximum tumor diameter (metabolic tumor diameter), measured on ^{18}F-FDG PET or receptor density (e.g. measured on ^{68}Ga-DOTA-SMS PET/CT)*

Table 1D.7   *Five-point response scale to estimate change in tumor volume*

Score	Response
0	*No evidence of treatment effect, or tumor progression*
1+	*1–33% of tumor mass after treatment*
2+	*33–66% of tumor mass after treatment*
3+	*66–99% of tumor mass after treatment*
4+	*> 99% estimated response, complete remission*

ROLE OF POSITRON EMISSION TOMOGRAPHY AND BASIC NUCLEAR MEDICINE IN MONITORING TUMOR RESPONSE TO THERAPY

Lymphoma

Non-Hodgkin's lymphoma (NHL) and Hodgkin's disease (HD) comprise about 8% of all malignancies and are potentially curable. The prognosis of these malignancies depends upon stage and histology.[32,33] Early stage HD and NHL are treated with a combination of chemotherapy and radiotherapy or radiotherapy alone. Patients with stage III and stage IV disease require aggressive chemotherapy. Approximately 75–90% of early stage lymphoma patients respond to therapy. However, less than 50% of newly diagnosed advanced stage lymphoma patients are curable with standard treatment regimes.[34,35] The alternative treatment (bone marrow transplantation) then becomes the only option, thereby necessitating the need for evaluation of response to therapy early during therapy. Early recognition of resistance can lower the toxicity due to chemotherapy.

The International Workshop Criteria (IWC) are most commonly used for response assessment of NHL.[36] Although bone marrow biopsy and clinical and biochemical parameters are also taken into consideration, it is primarily based upon CT for measuring response to therapy.[36] CT cannot differentiate between viable tumor, necrosis or fibrosis in patients who have had complete clinical response, which occurs in approximately 40% of NHL patients treated with chemotherapy and/or radiotherapy.[36–50] ^{18}F-FDG PET has been shown to predict the presence or absence of tumor viability in residual masses with an accuracy of 80–90%.[41,42,44,45,50] These data clearly point towards the superiority of ^{18}F-FDG PET over CT for predicting the response to treatment in these patients. Juweid *et al.* tried to determine whether incorporation of ^{18}F-FDG PET in the already established IWC criteria has any added advantage over IWC criteria alone for assessment of response to therapy in patients with NHL[51] and concluded that IWC combined with ^{18}F-FDG PET provides a more accurate response classification in patients with aggressive NHL than IWC alone. Seeing the advancement in PET imaging, flow cytometry and immunohistochemistry in NHL and Hodgkin's lymphoma, Cheson *et al.* in their recommendations for revised response criteria for malignant lymphoma,

Table 1D.8 *Causes of false interpretation on ¹⁸F-FDG PET scans*

Tumor	False positive	False negative
Breast cancer	Inflammatory reactions in breast, immediately after surgery or biopsy, benign breast tumors (occasionally)	Tumor size < 1 cm, well differentiated tumor, e.g. tubular carcinoma, carcinoma in situ
NSCLC	Benign pulmonary lesions like sarcoidosis, tuberculosis, aspergillosis, coccidioidomycosis, Mycobacterium avium intracellulare infection, histoplasmosis, pneumonia and other infectious diseases	Bronchoalveolar carcinoma, carcinoid, well differentiated adenocarcinoma with tumor size < 1.0 cm
Lymphoma	Reactive lymph nodes, inflammatory/infectious processes like sarcoidosis, tuberculosis, fungal infection. Reactive bone marrow changes after therapy	Mucosa-associated lymphoma, tumor size < 1.0 cm, low grade lymphoma
Colorectal carcinoma	Immediately post-radiotherapy (radiation-induced mucositis)	Tumor size < 1.0 cm, especially in liver metastases, micrometastases in lymph nodes and proximity of the lymph nodes to the primary site
Brain tumor	Local inflammation post-radiotherapy, repair mechanism in necrotic tissue	Small volume of viable tissue, reversible decrease in metabolic activity immediately after radiation therapy, high radiation dose administered within short time interval

have concluded that PET is essential to monitor response in diffuse large B-cell NHL (DLBCL) and Hodgkin's lymphoma. In follicular lymphoma, mantle cell lymphoma and other indolent or aggressive histologies, PET is needed only if assessment of response is the major end point. Pre-treatment PET is strongly recommended (but not definitely required) to better define sites of disease which are likely to be PET positive (e.g. DLBCL, Hodgkin's lymphoma (HL), follicular lymphoma (FL) and mantle-cell lymphoma (MCL)). For those histological variants of lymphoma which are unlikely to be PET positive, a post-therapy scan should only be used if the scan prior to therapy was positive.[52]

Schoeder *et al.* determined the relationship between SUV of ¹⁸F-FDG and aggressiveness of NHL. They concluded that the SUV is lower in indolent than in aggressive NHL, that an SUV > 10 implies a high likelihood of aggressive NHL and that this information may provide insight in case there is discordance between biopsy and clinical behavior.[53]

¹⁸F-FDG PET can also be used for the determination of true extent of lymphoma recurrence if there is a clinical, biochemical or radiological suspicion.[54] However, the role of ¹⁸F-FDG PET scanning for routine post-therapy surveillance without clinical, biochemical or radiographic evidence of disease is controversial,[55] because of the false positive findings (Table 1D.8) due to increased ¹⁸F-FDG uptake e.g. in post-therapy inflammatory changes or rebound thymic hyperplasia.

There is also a potential role of ¹⁸F-FDG PET during the course of treatment to accurately assess early response to therapy (Fig. 1D.2). The primary aim of using ¹⁸F-FDG PET during the course of treatment is to tailor therapy based upon the information provided by the scan.[49,56,57] Spaepen

et al. have demonstrated that none of the NHL patients with a positive scan achieved a durable complete response, whereas around 90% of patients with a negative FDG PET scan remained in complete remission for 1107 days.[57]

Last but no means least, PET/CT has been shown to be superior to PET alone in staging and restaging of lymphoma patients with accuracies of 93% and 83%, respectively.[58] Although larger prospective studies will be needed, it already seems clear that PET/CT will be the main tool in lymphoma imaging and restaging in the future.

Lung cancer

Lung cancer is the leading cause of death in developed countries in both men and women. While there has been a decline in deaths from other cancers, that is not the case with lung cancer which is still increasing. The WHO has classified lung cancer into four subtypes: squamous cell carcinoma, adenocarcinoma, small-cell carcinoma and large-cell carcinoma. NSCLC accounts for 75–80% of all lung cancers, the remainder being small-cell carcinoma which has a poor prognosis because metastases are usually present at the time of diagnosis. TNM staging is at present the best tool for defining the prognosis and for choosing the optimal therapy from available treatment options (surgery, chemotherapy and radiotherapy).[59] It has been documented that TNM staging does not always give a correct explanation for differences in relapse and survival. For example, 35% of resected stage I NSCLC present with a relapse resulting in a 5-year survival rate of approximately 65%.[60] Therefore, it is of paramount importance to be able to predict and prevent these relapses either by using active chemotherapy or radiotherapy or both.

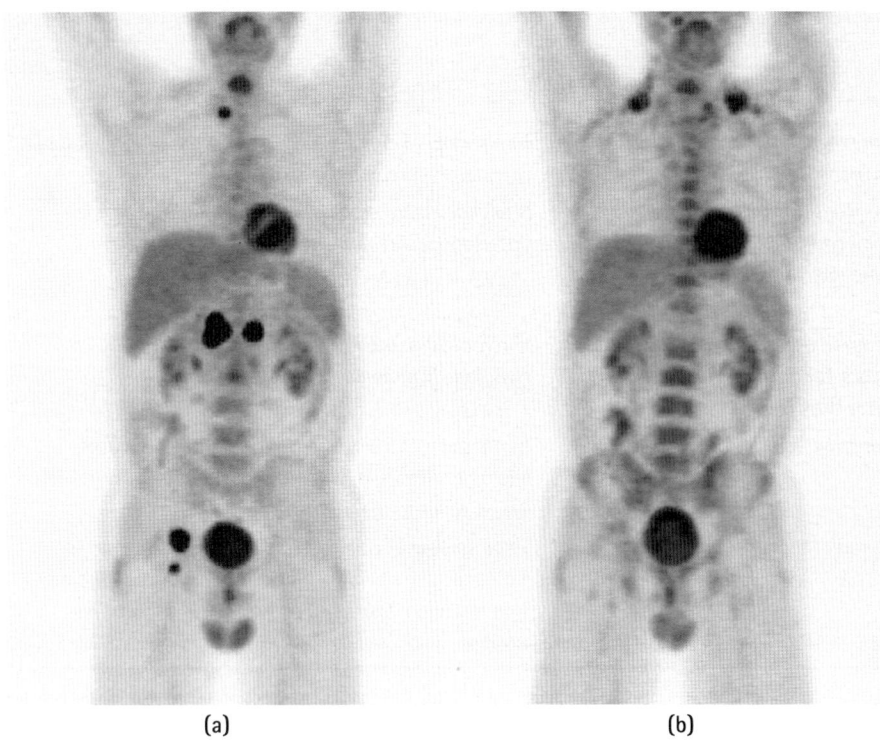

(a)   (b)

Figure 1D.2 *Early monitoring of therapy response in malignant lymphoma by F-18 FDG PET: Non-Hodgkin's lymphoma before chemotherapy (a) involving a cervical node, the spine, inguinal nodes and the right femur/acetabulum and after 2 cycles of CHOEP (b). Complete metabolic remission/cure (lasting now for 6 years) is demonstrated by FDG-PET whereas MRI and CT showed no significant change in anatomic size of the lesions and residual bulk tumor at the spine level after completion of 4 cycles of chemotherapy.*

Measures in tumor proliferation as estimated by *Ki*67 expression, a proliferating cell nuclear antigen, have prognostic value for survival and recurrence in resected NSCLC.[61,62] However, reduction in tumor size measured by conventional imaging is not a good predictor of response to treatment because there are resistant clones of cancerous cells which are present even in significantly shrunken tumor masses.[15] It has been documented that there is an upregulation of glucose transporter proteins (specifically GLUT-1) and an increase in hexokinase activity in NSCLC.[63] Using these perturbations in glucose metabolism, ^{18}F-FDG PET has been used extensively to monitor the response to therapy in patients with lung cancer.[64–66]

^{18}F-FDG PET is most useful in assessment of chemotherapy and radiotherapy in patients with locally advanced, bulky, inoperable NSCLC.[15] There is a chance of improving the survival rate in patients with advanced NSCLC, if induction therapy is used prior to surgery.[67] Patients with progressive disease after platinum-based therapy may have a survival benefit with the use of docetaxel as second-line chemotherapy.[68] It has been shown that patients with stage IIIA (N2) disease with no residual disease after induction therapy and surgery have a significantly higher 5-year survival rate (54%) as compared to patients with induction therapy (5-year survival rate of 17%) regardless of the response status.[67]

Patz *et al.* have assessed the prognostic value of ^{18}F-FDG PET in patients with NSCLC who received either chemotherapy, radiotherapy or surgery[69] and reported a statistically significant difference in the survival between patients with positive and negative ^{18}F-FDG PET findings. The median survival for patients with positive post-therapy ^{18}F-FDG PET study was 12.1 months as compared to 34.2 months in 85% of patients with negative ^{18}F-FDG PET results. Most early stage patients had negative results for the ^{18}F-FDG PET study. Weber *et al.* demonstrated that effective chemotherapy causes a rapid reduction in tumor glucose uptake:[29] 1-year survival rate was found to be 44% in patients with metabolic response as compared to only 10% in patients with no metabolic response. They concluded that ^{18}F-FDG PET can be used for predicting clinical outcome in patients receiving chemotherapy at a very early stage. The quantitative parameters used by Weber *et al.* were SUV, K_i and tumor-to-muscle ratio. They found a very close correlation between changes in SUV and K_i for prediction of therapy response with almost similar diagnostic accuracy. A similar correlation was observed between K_i and SUV in prediction of survival.

In comparison with CT, ^{18}F-FDG PET has been shown by Bury *et al.* to have higher sensitivity, specificity and negative predictive value in the detection of residual or recurrent disease.[70]

Cerfolio *et al.* performed a retrospective study to evaluate the role of maximum SUV in prediction of stage, recurrence and survival in NSCLC patients. The study clearly demonstrated that the maximum SUV of a pulmonary nodule on ^{18}F-FDG PET is an independent predictor of NSCLCs aggressiveness. Maximum SUV was also found to predict more accurately the recurrence rates for stages IB and II NSCLC and survival for patients with stage IB, II or IIIA as compared to TNM staging.[71]

Schmücking and Baum *et al.* found a strong correlation between the histologic regression rates and metabolic remission as detected by FDG PET.[72] This study clearly proved that ^{18}F-FDG PET precedes CT in measuring tumor

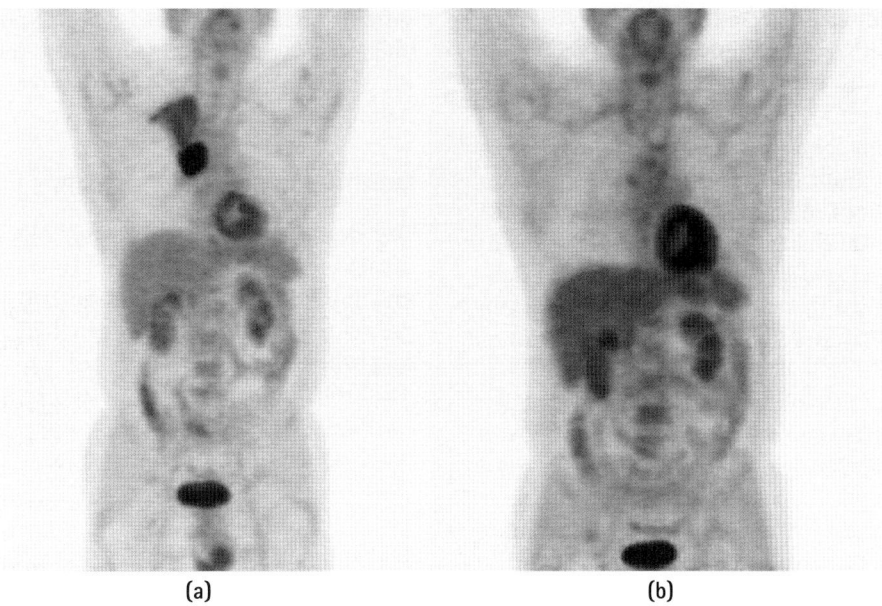

(a)   (b)

Figure 1D.3   *Molecular staging and follow-up of non-small cell lung cancer after therapy using F-18 FDG PET as compared to morphological imaging (CT scan): High glucose metabolism of primary lung cancer (molecular PET state mT3 mN0 mM0, SUVmax. 10.0, MTI 45.0) and faint uptake in retention pneumonia (a). CT stage was cT4 cN2 cM0. Complete metabolic remission (b) after chemotherapy (mT0 mN0 mM0, SUV 1.6) whereas CT showed persistent disease (no change). Surgical histology confirmed complete histomorphologic tumor regression without any vital tumor cells.*

response and predicting long-term therapeutic outcome in stage III NSCLC (Fig. 1D.3).

Yamamoto *et al.* have demonstrated the ability of FDG PET to predict response of primary tumor and nodal disease to preoperative induction chemoradiotherapy in patients with NSCLC. The study showed that the percentage change in SUV post-therapy was higher in pathological responders as compared to nonresponders.[73]

^{18}F-FDG PET has not only been used in radiotherapy for assessment of volumetric changes in the tumor post-therapy, but also to plan the therapy as such. This approach has been described by Baum *et al.* as metabolic or molecular radiation treatment planning (MRTP).[31] ^{18}F-FDG PET is used in conjunction with CT for calculating the planning target volume (PTV) and gross tumor volume (GTV) so that higher radiation dose can be used with minimum toxicity to the surrounding tissue. The rationale in using higher radiation dose is well documented in the Radiation Therapy Oncology Group (RTOG) study where it was clearly shown that the risk of intrathoracic first recurrence in cases with inoperable NSCLC declines with increasing radiation dose.[74] MTD, MTV and MTI are used for defining tumor volumes.

Apart from ^{18}F-FDG, ^{11}C-thymidine, which can be used for measuring tumor DNA synthesis, has been shown to be closely related to the effectiveness of cytotoxic therapy.[75,76] In a small group of small-cell lung cancer and sarcoma patients, ^{11}C-thymidine PET was superior to ^{18}F-FDG PET for measuring response to chemotherapy early after the institution of treatment.[77] However, larger, prospective randomized trials are needed to confirm this finding.

Breast cancer

Breast cancer is one of the leading causes of cancer death in women. The treatment options available depend upon the stage at which the cancer is diagnosed (Plate 1D.3). Approximately 25% of patients with breast cancer have tumors larger than 3 cm in size, or locally advanced disease at first presentation, defined as locally advanced breast cancer (LABC).[78] Neoadjuvant chemotherapy given prior to surgery and radiotherapy is the currently accepted treatment plan in such patients.[79–83] Early administration of systemic chemotherapy prior to local treatment is intended in such patients to downstage the primary tumor so that subsequent local treatment (surgery or radiotherapy) becomes more effective with less morbidity. It is also useful in elimination of occult distant metastases.[84] Complete pathological response to neoadjuvant chemotherapy is an important prognostic indicator of overall survival and of disease-free survival.[85] It is essential to monitor therapy in LABC patients as a significant number of patients do not respond to primary therapy and require an alternative or more prolonged chemotherapy.[86] Apart from this subgroup of patients, therapy monitoring is also useful in patients who have inoperable locally advanced disease as they generally receive chemotherapy and/or radiation therapy.[15]

MONITORING RESPONSE TO CHEMOTHERAPY

The prognostic relevance of a complete histopathologic response in patients receiving primary chemotherapy has been established. Patients having minimal residual disease

(MRD) have higher disease-free and survival rates as compared to patients with gross residual disease (GRD).[87,88] As the clinical response does not correlate well with the histopathological response, and because the side effects of primary chemotherapy are plenty, there is a definite need to segregate responders from nonresponders.[89] The conventional imaging methods, mammography, USG and MRI measure the anatomical change in tumor size. The advantage of ^{18}F-FDG PET over histopathology, the already established 'gold standard' for therapy monitoring, is that it can also assess distant metastases along with the primary tumor in the same session.

An overview of the literature suggests that among all the quantitative parameters used for therapy monitoring (e.g. the Patlak method and simple kinetic method) the SUV (corrected for plasma glucose) compares well with nonlinear regression analysis (NLR).[90] Static protocols are much more practical in a busy PET department.[27] The simplified kinetic model (SKM) was introduced by Hunter *et al.* in order to reduce the sensitivity of tumor uptake value to plasma clearance:[91] the ^{18}F-FDG uptake is normalized to the plasma integral, i.e. to the total amount of ^{18}F-FDG delivered to the tumor, by taking one or few venous blood samples during the course of the static scan. Although EORTC does not recommend correcting SUV for plasma glucose, a better correlation between SUV and NLR has been observed if plasma glucose is also taken into consideration.[92–94]

In order to make calculations of ^{18}F-FDG uptake and other quantitative parameters, the region of interest (ROI) plays a major role. The ROI technique used should be automated, user independent and insensitive to partial volume effects due to therapy-induced changes in tumor dimensions.[27] The data from simulation studies suggest that isocount contour tumor ROI, corrected for background activity, is the preferred ROI method for assessing response to therapy.[95]

^{18}F-FDG PET can be used for prediction of response to therapy after its completion and for early prediction of response to therapy. In a study performed by Vranjesevic *et al.*, ^{18}F-FDG PET was shown to be superior to the conventional imaging (CI) methods for predicting outcomes after the completion of chemotherapy, with positive and negative predictive values of 93% and 84% for ^{18}F-FDG PET, versus 85% and 59%, respectively for CI. In contrast to CI, ^{18}F-FDG PET can detect metabolic changes in breast cancer as early as 8 days after initiation of therapy.[96] Several studies also indicated that responders can be differentiated from nonresponders using ^{18}F-FDG PET after the first course of chemotherapy.[89,97,98]

MONITORING RESPONSE TO RADIOTHERAPY

MRTP, a new and novel approach to radiation therapy planning using ^{18}F-FDG PET helps in having more precise and more effective dose delivery to the tumor tissue. However, depending on the region where radiation is delivered, ^{18}F-FDG PET during and shortly after radiotherapy may suffer from lack of specificity because of radiation induced inflammatory changes in the tissue (especially mucosa of the head and neck or in the rectum) surrounding the tumor leading to higher than normal uptake of ^{18}F-FDG.[99]

MONITORING HORMONE THERAPY

The degree of estrogen receptor blockade and increased uptake of ^{18}F-FDG in the tumor (metabolic flare) early after initiation of tamoxifen are important single parameters to predict response to anti-estrogen therapy in estrogen receptor positive metastases. It is possible to differentiate responders from nonresponders to anti-estrogen therapy using ^{18}F-FDG PET and 16α-[^{18}F]fluoro-17β-estradiol (FES) or the Z-isomer of 11β-methoxy-17α-[^{123}I]iodovinylestradiol (Z-^{123}I-MIVE) SPECT alone.[100,101]

SESTAMIBI IN MULTIDRUG–RESISTANT BREAST CANCER

In spite of advances in cancer therapy, multidrug resistance, primarily due to expression of P glycoprotein (Pgp), specifically after chemotherapy, remains the major cause of treatment failure. ^{99m}Tc-sestamibi has been shown to be a substrate of Pgp. Using this principle, it has been documented that ^{99m}Tc-sestamibi is an important predictor of MDR in breast carcinoma. ^{99m}Tc-sestamibi imaging has also been used to monitor therapy response in locally advanced breast cancer and has been claimed to be as sensitive as ^{18}F-FDG PET in detecting treatment response.[3–12]

Colorectal carcinoma

Colorectal cancer is one of the most lethal cancers in western countries. Surgical treatment is curative in only 70–80% of patients at disease presentation, and the overall survival at 5 years is less than 60%. Improvement in adjuvant therapies, surgery and screening programs has led to significant improvement in quality of life and improvement in symptoms in advanced stage colorectal cancer.[102] Systemic chemotherapy has been shown to double the survival of patients with advanced stage colorectal cancer as compared to untreated control patients.[15]

5-Fluorouracil (5-FU) combined with radiotherapy has also demonstrated significant improvement in survival in primary unresectable colorectal cancer. With the availability of newer cytotoxic drugs for treatment (e.g. oxaliplatin and oral fluoropyrimidines), optimization of therapy has become essential.[15] ^{18}F-FDG PET has been shown to be very promising to solve this issue.

Guillem *et al.* assessed response to 5-FU and preoperative radiotherapy in a pilot study in patients with rectal cancer using ^{18}F-FDG PET (determining SUV, metabolic tumor volume, visual response score and changes in total lesion glycolysis as response parameters) and compared it with CT findings. They demonstrated that ^{18}F-FDG PET provides

Table 1D.9 *Response criteria for computed tomography, magnetic resonance imaging and ^{18}F-FDG positron emission tomography (based upon standardized uptake values) in colorectal carcinoma*

Technique	Response		No response	
	Complete response	Partial response	Stable disease	Progressive disease
CT, MRI	Absence of any evidence of tumor tissue	>65% decrease in estimated volume in case of unchanged T, down-staging of T category	No change in estimated volume (increase <40%, or decrease <65%), no change in T category	Increase in infiltration depth (>40%) in case there is no change in T or increase in T category
^{18}F-FDG PET	No glucose metabolism within the tumor volume, estimated by visual analysis	Decrease in SUV (requires determination of cut-off value)	No change in SUV (requires determination of upper and lower limit)	Increase in SUV (requires determination of cut-off value)

Modified from the article by Denecke et al.[108]

incremental information to the preoperative assessment of patients with rectal cancer. Response to 5-FU and radiotherapy could be assessed in 100% of the cases with PET as compared to only 78% with CT.[103] Victor et al. demonstrated that visual assessment of ^{18}F-FDG uptake could provide good medium term prognostic information in patients with advanced rectal cancer undergoing curative radical surgery.[104]

Early on, ^{18}F-FDG PET has also been used to monitor the response to radiotherapy. Haberkorn et al. demonstrated that ^{18}F-FDG PET, performed 6 weeks after completion of radiation therapy, revealed a statistically significant reduction in tumor uptake in only 50% of patients in spite of having obtained a satisfactory palliative effect. The discrepancy can be explained by the inflammatory reaction caused by radiation injury ('mucositis') immediately after radiotherapy. The recommended time interval for such a study therefore is 3–6 months. The same study has shown that serum carcinoembryonic antigen is less sensitive than ^{18}F-FDG PET in predicting tumor recurrence.[105]

Neoadjuvant radiotherapy is potentially useful in improving the results of surgery in patients with primary rectal cancer.[106,107] Multimodal preoperative approaches have necessitated monitoring of therapy to accurately assess response to therapy and appropriate restaging prior to surgery, especially for locally advanced tumors. Denecke et al. performed a study to analyze the role of MRI and CT (the currently accepted 'gold standard' for therapy) and ^{18}F-FDG PET in prediction of response to neoadjuvant radiochemotherapy in patients with locally advanced rectal cancer. The study clearly depicts the superiority of ^{18}F-FDG PET over CT and MRI (Table 1D.9) in predicting the outcome to preoperative multimodal treatment of locally advanced primary rectal cancer.[108]

Guillem et al. have demonstrated the usefulness of FDG PET in the assessment of response to pre-operative chemo-radiation in patients with locally advanced rectal cancer. Using the parameters SUV$_{max}$, δTLG and VRS it was shown that patients with a ΔSUV$_{max}$ = 62.5% and a

δTLG ⩾ 69.5% had significantly improved recurrence-free and disease-specific survival.[109]

It is clinically very important to know at an early stage whether neoadjuvant chemotherapy and/or radiotherapy is having an effect on the tumor or not. Findlay et al. performed sequential ^{18}F-FDG PET studies in colorectal cancer patients with liver metastases before and during the first 5 months of 5-FU chemotherapy. A strong correlation was found between the observed reduction in tumor metabolism at 5 weeks after the start of 5-FU and therapy outcome. It was also possible to distinguish between responders and nonresponders. However, there was no correlation between the changes in tumor metabolism at 1–2 weeks and therapy outcome, probably due to flare reaction.[110]

^{18}F-FDG PET has been shown to be superior to CT in predicting response to novel therapies like cryotherapy, hepatic embolization and radio-frequency ablation.[111]

^{18}F-FU has been used to assess the response to 5-FU chemotherapy. Dimitrakopoulou-Strauss et al., using ^{18}F-FU for assessing therapy response in colorectal cancer patients with liver metastases, have demonstrated that only those metastases which have ^{18}F-FU SUV > 3 at 120 min postinjection demonstrated a response to therapy.[112] Several studies have shown that those patients who have ^{18}F-FU SUV > 2.5, have higher chances of achieving stabilization of disease and have increased chances of survival.[112,113]

Thyroid cancer

The role of nuclear medicine in thyroid cancer started in 1942 when Keston et al. first described the accumulation of ^{131}I in thyroid metastases.[114] The underlying mechanism which permits usage of ^{131}I for imaging is the presence of the Na–I symporter which results in uptake of the tracer.[115,116] With the development of cyclotrons, two other isotopes of iodine, ^{123}I and ^{124}I, have found application in the management of patients with thyroid cancer. However, only ^{131}I is used for therapy because it emits beta particles along with gamma rays.

FOLLOW–UP AFTER SURGERY AND RADIOIODINE ABLATION

The information to be derived in the follow-up period post-surgery and radioiodine ablation is to know the extent of remnant thyroid, diagnose recurrence of carcinoma, detect distant metastases, and to define the presence of radioiodine uptake as a prerequisite for radioiodine therapy. Although US, multislice CT and MRI have some role in evaluation of patients after therapy, the conventional approach is to measure the thyroglobulin (Tg) level and to perform a whole-body iodine scan (^{131}I WBS) after ablative therapy and in the case of rising Tg levels.[117] In case there is remnant thyroid tissue and/or metastatic tissue, ablative dose/high dose of radioiodine therapy is given and a post-treatment scan is performed after therapy which may reveal an even higher number of metastatic lesions.[118]

^{18}F-FDG PET has also obtained a significant role in the management of patients with metastatic/recurrent differentiated thyroid cancer and negative ^{131}I WBS.[119] The exact localization of the thyroid metastases is essential in this subgroup of patients as there may be a change in therapeutic planning. The alternative treatments available for these patients are surgery, external radiation therapy, chemotherapy and redifferentiation therapy.[120–123] Contraindication to a planned surgery may be deduced from the results of ^{18}F-FDG PET. The usefulness of further radioiodine therapy comes under scrutiny if WBS negative sites exist (at more important sites) along with WBS positive tumor sites.[119]

^{18}F–FDG PET IN ANAPLASTIC THYROID CANCER

The role of ^{18}F-FDG PET in anaplastic thyroid cancer has not been extensively studied, but based upon preliminary studies, it can be concluded that ^{18}F-FDG PET may have a positive impact in the follow-up of patients after initial resection for the detection of metastatic or residual disease and also in patients with advanced disease who received chemotherapy for assessing therapeutic response.[124–126]

Brain tumors

Conventional imaging such as CT and MRI cannot differentiate accurately enough between recurrence and radiation injury.[127] Early detection of recurrence is essential because it leads to alteration in therapy which in turn may result in a better prognosis. Biopsy is also not useful because of sampling errors within large masses. ^{18}F-FDG PET has been used to differentiate between necrotic tissue post-radiation injury and recurrence with high sensitivity (approximately 80%) and specificity (ranging from 40 to 94%).[128,129] However, there are some conditions (enumerated in Table 1D.5) in which ^{18}F-FDG PET gives false positive and false negative

results.[130–132] Fusion imaging has been used with great success in patients with brain tumors. In patients treated with stereotactic surgery, Chao et al. have demonstrated an improvement in sensitivity from 65 to 80% with the use of MRI/^{18}F-FDG PET co-registration.[133]

Increase in ^{18}F-FDG uptake (as early as 4 h after radiotherapy) is significantly correlated with a decrease in tumor size.[134] Other radiotracers, such as [11]C- or ^{18}F-labeled tyrosine or ^{11}C-methionine or ^{11}C-thymidine, have been used with good results.[135–137] These PET tracers have higher tumor-to-background ratios and higher specificity as compared to ^{18}F-FDG as they are not significantly taken up by the normal brain. Several studies have demonstrated the utility of these PET tracers in radiotherapy monitoring of glioma patients.

Esophageal and gastric carcinoma

Preoperative chemotherapy has been used in both esophageal and gastric carcinoma although survival benefit in patients treated with preoperative chemotherapy and surgery in esophageal carcinoma or gastric carcinoma is limited.[138–142] However, a better prognosis for patients who respond to preoperative therapy as compared to nonresponders has been shown.[140,141,143–146] Weber et al. proved that a decrease in tumor uptake of ^{18}F-FDG by >35% as compared to the baseline value allowed accurate prediction of response in patients with locally advanced esophageal cancer as early as 14 days after initiation of chemotherapy.[147] Another study demonstrated that response to preoperative chemotherapy can be predicted early during the course of chemotherapy in patients with locally advanced gastric cancer by keeping a 35% fall in ^{18}F-FDG uptake as the baseline for differentiating between responders and nonresponders.[148] It has also been shown that the prognosis for patients who have nonresponding tumors (to preoperative chemotherapy) is even worse than for patients treated with surgery alone, which is probably related to the toxicity associated with chemotherapy, the selection of chemotherapy resistant clones and unnecessary delay in surgical treatment.[140,141,149]

Wieder et al. have demonstrated that the changes in the tumor metabolism on FDG PET is a more sensitive parameter for assessment of response to chemotherapy in patients with adenocarcinoma of esophagogastric junction as compared to the tumor size on CT scan.[150]

Prostate cancer

Prostate cancer is one of the most common cancers affecting men. Accurate imaging tools are essential for detection of residual, recurrent and metastatic prostate cancer. There are few PET radiotracers which have been used for therapy evaluation in prostate cancer. ^{11}C-acetate has been shown to be useful in detection of tumor recurrence in patients who had been treated previously with radiation therapy or prostatectomy.[151–156] Kishi *et al.* have used ^{11}C-choline for the determination of outcome of hormone therapy in prostate cancer patients. The tracer uptake was found to decrease in the primary tumor as well as in the metastases after androgen deprivation therapy.[157]

Cervical cancer

Cervical cancer is the leading cause of cancer-related death in women (especially in developing countries). The treatment options available to these patients are either surgery and/or radiation therapy or chemo-radiation therapy. Grisby *et al.* have demonstrated the usefulness of ^{18}F-FDG PET in evaluation of response and outcome post-therapy in a retrospective study. They concluded that persistent or new post-therapy abnormal ^{18}F-FDG uptake measures tumor response and might have predictive value in tumor recurrence and death due to cervical cancer.[158] ^{18}F-FDG PET may be particularly useful by selecting the most efficient therapy in patients with good prognosis and avoiding unnecessary expenses in those patients with poor prognosis. In a prospective study on the impact of ^{18}F-FDG PET on the management of disease and patient survival, Yen *et al.* demonstrated that ^{18}F-FDG PET modified the initial treatment plan in nearly 66% of all women.[159]

Gastrointestinal stromal tumor

Gastrointestinal stromal tumors (GISTs) constitute about 0.1–3.0% of all gastrointestinal tract neoplasms and 6% of all sarcomas.[160] The median time of survival of patients with metastatic GISTs from the time of diagnosis ranges between 12 and 19 months.[161,162] Imatinib mesylate has a proven role in the management of patients with recurrent or metastatic GIST after resection.[163] Gayed *et al.* retrospectively analyzed the role of ^{18}F-FDG PET and CT in staging and evaluating response to therapy in patients with recurrent or metastatic GIST after resection. The study demonstrated no significant difference between CT and ^{18}F-FDG PET in the initial staging of malignant GIST. However, ^{18}F-FDG PET was able to predict response to imatinib mesylate therapy 2 months earlier than CT in 22.5% of patients. A > 25% decrease and > 25% increase in SUV of ^{18}F-FDG on a post-therapy scan was taken as response to therapy and progression of disease, respectively. ^{18}F-FDG SUV < 25% was considered to denote stable disease.[164]

Neuroendocrine tumors

Neuroendocrine tumors (NETs) are a heterogeneous group of neoplasms which are characterized by their endocrine metabolism and histologic pattern. There are several imaging modalities available for diagnosis and staging of NETs. CT, MRI, USG and endosonography play a significant role in the initial diagnosis and staging.[165–167] As there is a high expression of somatostatin receptors on many NETs, somatostatin receptor scintigraphy (SRS) is increasingly used for diagnosis, staging, restaging and for assisting therapeutic decision making between surgery, somatostatin analogs and embolization therapy.[168] There has been growing evidence that SRS can be used for determining the prognosis of patients as somatostatin receptor positivity indicates good response to treatment with somatostatin analogs.[169] The two main radiopharmaceuticals that have been used most commonly up until now for diagnosis and staging of NETs are ^{111}In-pentetreotide and *meta*-[^{123}I]iodo-benzylguanidine (^{123}I-MIBG) or ^{131}I-MIBG.

^{131}I-MIBG therapy is one of the options available in MIBG-avid NETs. Menzel *et al.* have shown in a small group of patients that those tumors that have simultaneous uptake of MIBG and ^{18}F-FDG, showed a better response to therapy.[170]

With the advent of peptide receptor radionuclide therapy (PRRT) using [90]Y- and ^{177}Lu-labeled somatostatin analogs, it has become essential to predict and follow-up patients with NETs using SRS in order to evaluate the response to therapy as well as to choose the patients who will respond to PRRT (Plate 1D.4). Krenning *et al.* have proposed the prospective role of peptide receptor scintigraphy in combination with CT in the follow-up of therapy of gastroenteropancreatic neuroendocrine tumors.[171] New PET radiopharmaceuticals such as ^{68}Ga-DOTA-TOC or ^{68}Ga-DOTA-NOC have shown very promising results in therapy evaluation and diagnosis of NET patients. PET/CT using ^{68}Ga-labeled somatostatin analogs is increasingly used by some centers for treatment planning of patients with advanced NET (Figs 1D.4 and 1D.5). In a preliminary study, Hoffmann *et al.* have shown that ^{68}Ga-DOTA-TOC was superior to III In-octreotide SPECT (CT was taken as the reference for comparison) in detecting upper abdominal metastases.[172] Baum *et al.*, in a large series of patients (over 800 studies) have clearly demonstrated that receptor PET/CT using ^{68}Ga-labeled pansomatostatin analogs like DOTA-NOC has to be considered as the new 'gold standard' in imaging neuroendocrine tumors (initial staging, follow-up and therapy response evaluation) (Fig. 1D.6).

APOPTOSIS, GENE EXPRESSION AND THERAPY MONITORING

Apoptosis, programmed cell death, has been one of the most extensively studied biologic topics in the last decade. Annexin V is a calcium-dependent binding protein with high specificity for phophatidylserine. It binds to the surface of apoptotic cells. *In vivo* imaging of phosphatidylserine expression in apoptotic cells has been possible with ^{99m}Tc-recombinant human annexin V.[173] Many studies have demonstrated the potential role of imaging cell death in acute myocardial infarction, in tumors having high apoptotic index, and in

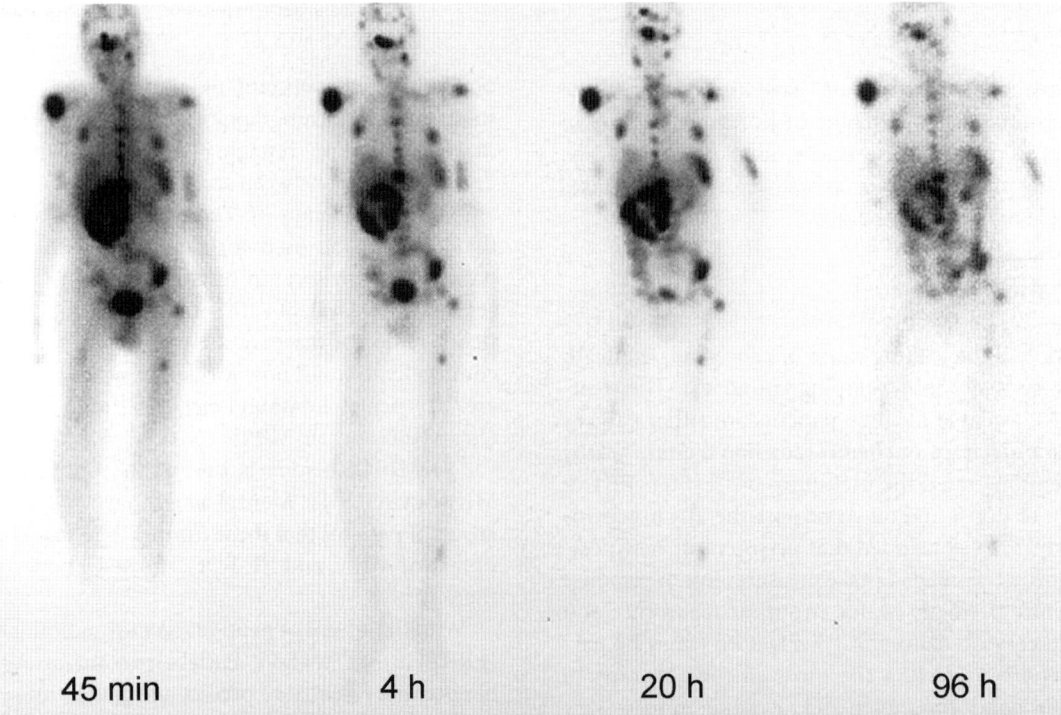

Figure 1D.4 *Monitoring therapy response depends also on the time of acquisition of the scans. Therefore, calculation of the tumor dose by dosimetry (e.g. using the MIRD algorithm) is a more objective method than only visual examination of scans. Serial whole-body scans (anterior views 45 min until 96 hrs after administration of In-111 DOTA-TOC) in a 19 year-old paraganglioma patient: dosimetry under peptide receptor radionuclide therapy (PRRT) with Y-90 DOTA-TOC (1.85 GBq), injected intra-arterially at the level of TH11/12 for treatment of an inoperable spine metastasis which caused paralysis of the legs. Intense uptake in the primary tumor (arising from the right adrenal) and in multiple bone metastases, with persistent accumulation over time (long tumor half-life).*

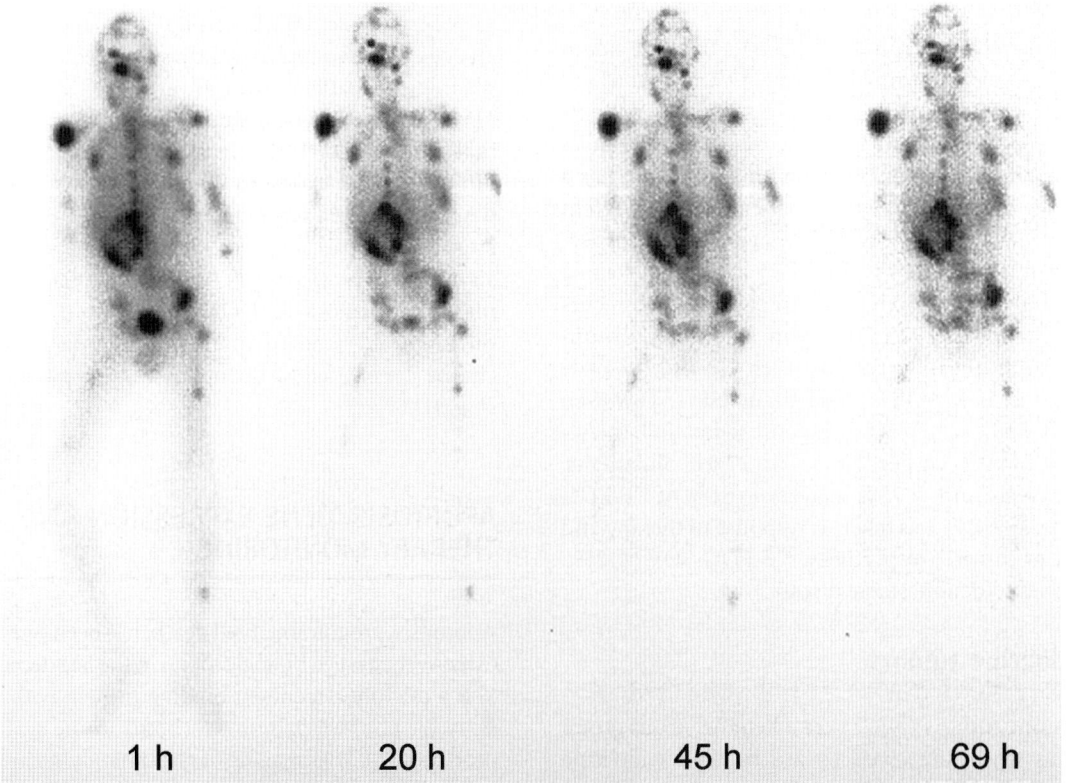

Figure 1D.5 *Post-therapy scans after administration of In-111 DOTA-TOC (co-injected intravenously with Y-90 DOTA-TOC, 1.85 GBq) 3 months later (same patient as described in Fig. 1D.4). There is still high, but significantly diminished uptake in the primary tumor and the metastases (molecular therapy response). Several months after the treatment, the patient started walking again and later on fully recovered from the paralysis (without any other form of therapy).*

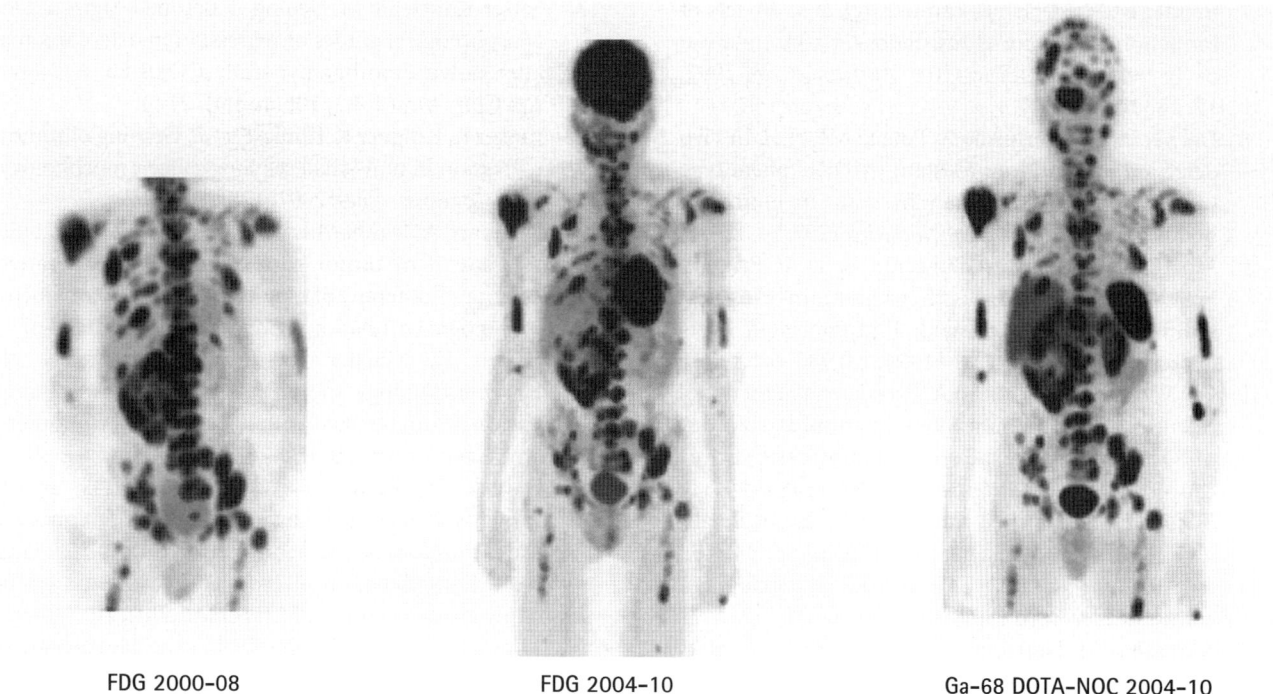

FDG 2000-08   FDG 2004-10   Ga-68 DOTA-NOC 2004-10

Figure 1D.6 *Monitoring therapy response depends also on the tracer used for displaying different molecular features of a cancer cell, e.g. glucose (F-18 FDG) metabolism vs. somatostatin receptor expression. Comparison between F-18 FDG PET scans (in August 2000 and in October 2004) and receptor PET (in October 2004) using Ga-68 labeled DOTA-NOC (same patient as described in Figs 1D.4 and 1D.5). High glucose metabolism and intense SMS-receptor expression in the same lesions is obvious ("match" between FDG-uptake and SMS-receptor expression).*

response to chemotherapy of lung and breast cancer, lymphoma and sarcoma.[174] [99mTc]-ethylenedicysteine–annexin V has been tested for *in vivo* and *in vitro* measurements of apoptosis in breast cancer with the purpose of evaluating response to radiation and chemotherapy. The study showed significantly increased uptake after paclitaxel treatment and radiation therapy *in vitro*.[175] Prognosis and early prediction of response to chemotherapy (after one course) has been shown in lung cancer, lymphoma and breast cancer using [99mTc]-annexin V.[176]

The future to treatment of many genetic disorders and deadly diseases lies in targeting and understanding gene expression. PET has been used for studying gene expression *in vivo* using translated enzymes or a receptor labeled with positron emitting ligands (reporter gene) which are specific for gene expression. The future holds good promise for PET reporter gene imaging which will help in quantification of gene expression and monitoring gene therapy.

DEDICATION

This chapter is dedicated to Prof. Dr. Gustav Hör, Professor Emeritus and former Director, Department of Nuclear Medicine, University Medical Center Frankfurt/Main, on the occasion of his 75th birthday. His continuous inspiration and support of molecular diagnosis and therapy in the field of Nuclear Medicine is greatly appreciated.

REFERENCES

● Seminal primary article
◆ Key review paper
✻ First formal publication of a management guideline

1 Giannopoulou C. The role of SPET and PET in monitoring tumor response to therapy. *Eur J Nucl Med* 2003; **30**: 1173–200.

◆ 2 Juweid ME, Cheson BD. Positron-emission tomography and assessment of cancer therapy. *N Engl J Med* 2006; **354**: 496–507.

3 Bae KT, Piwnica-Worms D. Pharmacokinetic modeling of multidrug resistance P-glycoprotein transport of gamma-emitting substrates. *Q J Nucl Med* 1997; **41**: 101–10.

4 Duran Cordobes M, Starzec A, Delmon-Moingeon L, *et al.* Technetium-99m-sestamibi uptake by human benign and malignant breast tumor cells: correlation with MDR gene expression. *J Nucl Med* 1996; **37**: 286–9.

5 Piwnica-Worms D, Rao VV, Kronauge JF, Croop JM. Characterization of multidrug resistance P-glycoprotein transport function with an organotechnetium cation. *Biochemistry* 1995; **34**: 12210–20.

6 Ballinger JR, Sheldon KM, Boxen I, *et al.* Differences between accumulation of [99mTc]-MIBI and [201Tl]-thallous chloride in tumor cells: role of P-glycoprotein. *Q J Nucl Med* 1995; **39**: 122–8.

7 Bender H, Friederich E, Zamora PO, *et al.* Effects of induction of multidrug resistance on accumulation of Tc-99m sestamibi in vitro. *Anticancer Res* 1997; **17**: 1833–9.

8 Del Vecchio S, Ciarmiello A, Potena MI, *et al.* In vivo detection of multidrug-resistant (MDR1) phenotype by technetium-99m sestamibi scan in untreated breast cancer patients. *Eur J Nucl Med* 1997; **24**: 150–9.

9 Moretti JL, Azaloux H, Boisseron D, *et al.* Primary breast cancer imaging with technetium-99m sestamibi and its relation with P-glycoprotein overexpression. *Eur J Nucl Med* 1996; **23**: 980–6.

10 Del Vecchio S, Ciarmiello A, Pace L, *et al.* Fractional retention of technetium-99m-sestamibi as an index of glycoprotein P-expression in untreated breast cancer patients. *J Nucl Med* 1997; **38**: 1348–51.

11 Kostakoglu L, Elahi N, Kiratli P, *et al.* Clinical validation of the influence of P-glycoprotein on technetium-99m-sestamibi uptake in malignant tumors. *J Nucl Med* 1997; **38**: 1003–8.

12 Mubashar M, Harrington KJ, Chaudhary KS, *et al.* ^{99m}Tc-sestamibi imaging in the assessment of toremifene as a modulator of multidrug resistance in patients with breast cancer. *J Nucl Med* 2002; **43**: 519–25.

13 Soler C, Beauchesne P, Maatougui K, *et al.* Technetium-99m sestamibi brain single-photon emission tomography for detection of recurrent gliomas after radiation therapy. *Eur J Nucl Med* 1998; **25**: 1649–57.

14 Yamamoto Y, Nishiyama Y, Toyama Y, *et al.* ^{99m}Tc-MIBI and ^{201}Tl SPET in the detection of recurrent brain tumours after radiation therapy. *Nucl Med Commun* 2002; **23**: 1183–90.

15 Kostakoglu L, Goldsmith SJ. ^{18}F-FDG PET evaluation of the response to therapy for lymphoma and for breast, lung, and colorectal carcinoma. *J Nucl Med* 2003; **44**: 224–39.

16 Miller AB, Hoogstraten B, Staquet M, Winkler A. Reporting results of cancer treatment. *Cancer* 1981; **47**: 207–14.

17 World Health Organization. *Handbook for Reporting Results of Cancer Treatment.* Offset publication No. 48. Geneva: WHO, 1979.

18 Moertel CG, Hanley JA. The effect of measuring error on the results of therapeutic trials in advanced cancer. *Cancer* 1976; **38**: 388–94.

* 19 Therasse P, Arbuck SG, Eisenhauer EA, *et al.* New guidelines to evaluate the response to treatment in solid tumors. European Organization for Research and Treatment of Cancer, National Cancer Institute of the United States, National Cancer Institute of Canada. *J Natl Cancer Inst* 2000; **92**: 205–16.

♦ 20 Weber WA. Use of PET for monitoring cancer therapy and for predicting outcome. *J Nucl Med* 2005; **46**: 983–95.

21 Salzer-Kuntschik M, Delling G, Beron G, Sigmund R. Morphological grades of regression in osteosarcoma after polychemotherapy: study COSS 80. *J Cancer Res Clin Oncol* 1983; **106(suppl)**: 21–4.

22 Junker K, Langner K, Klinke F, *et al.* Grading of tumor regression in non-small cell lung cancer: morphology and prognosis. *Chest* 2001; **120**: 1584–91.

23 Mandard A, Dalibard F, Mandard J, *et al.* Pathologic assessment of tumor regression after preoperative chemoradiotherapy of esophageal carcinoma: clinicopathologic correlations. *Cancer* 1994; **73**: 2680–6.

24 Becker K, Mueller JD, Schulmacher C, *et al.* Histomorphology and grading of regression in gastric carcinoma treated with neoadjuvant chemotherapy. *Cancer* 2003; **98**: 1521–30.

25 Bielack SS, Kempf-Bielack B, Delling G, *et al.* Prognostic factors in high-grade osteosarcoma of the extremities or trunk: an analysis of 1,702 patients treated on neoadjuvant cooperative osteosarcoma study group protocols. *J Clin Oncol* 2002; **20**: 776–90.

* 26 Young H, Baum R, Cremerius U, *et al.* Measurement of clinical and subclinical tumor response using F-18 FDG-PET: review and EORTC recommendations. *Eur J Cancer* 1999; **13**: 1773–82.

27 Krak NC, Hoekstra OS, Lammertsma AA. Measuring response to chemotherapy in locally advanced breast cancer: methodological considerations. *Eur J Nucl Med Mol Imaging* 2004; **31(suppl 1)**: S103–11.

28 Huang SC. Anatomy of SUV: standardized uptake value. *Nucl Med Biol* 2000; **27**: 643–6.

29 Weber WA, Petersen V, Schmidt B, *et al.* Positron emission tomography in non-small-cell lung cancer: prediction of response to chemotherapy by quantitative assessment of glucose use. *J Clin Oncol* 2003; **21**: 2651–7.

● 30 Larson SM, Erdi Y, Akhurst T, *et al.* Tumor treatment response based on visual and quantitative changes in global tumor glycolysis using PET-FDG imaging: The visual response score and the change in total lesion glycolysis. *Clin Positron Imag* 1999; **2**: 159–71.

31 Schmuecking M, Baum RP, Griesinger F, *et al.* Molecular whole body cancer imaging using positron emission tomography: consequences for therapeutic management and metabolic radiation treatment planning. *Recent Results Cancer Res* 2003; **162**: 195–202.

32 Armitage JO. Drug therapy: treatment of non Hodgkin's lymphoma. *N Engl J Med* 1993; **328**: 1023–30.

33 Jotti G, Bonandonna G. Prognostic factors in Hodgkin's disease: implications for modern treatment. *Anti-Cancer Res* 1998; **8**: 749–60.

34 Brandt L, Kimby E, Nygren P, Glimelius B. A systematic overview of chemotherapy effects in Hodgkin's disease. *Acta Oncol* 2001; **40**: 185–97.

35 Coiffier B, Gisselbrecht C, Vose JM, et al. Prognostic factors in aggressive malignant lymphomas: description and validation of prognostic index that could identify patients requiring a more intensive therapy. J Clin Oncol 1991; 9: 211–19.

36 Cheson BD, Horning SJ, Coiffier B, et al. Report of an international workshop to standardise response criteria for non-Hodgkin's lymphoma. J Clin Oncol 1999; 17: 1244–53.

37 Brodeur GM, Pritchard J, Berthold F, et al. Revisions of the international criteria for neuroblastoma diagnosis, staging, and response to treatment. J Clin Oncol 1993; 11: 1466–77.

38 Fuks JZ, Aisner J, Wiernik PH. Restaging laparotomy in the management of the non-Hodgkin's lymphomas. Med Pediatr Oncol 1982; 10: 429–38.

39 Stewart FM, Williamson BR, Innes DJ, et al. Residual tumor masses following treatment for advanced histiocytic lymphoma. Cancer 1985; 55: 620–3.

40 Surbone A, Longo DL, DeVita VT Jr, et al. Residual abdominal masses in aggressive non-Hodgkin's lymphoma after combination chemotherapy: significance and management. J Clin Oncol 1988; 6: 1832–7.

41 Coiffier B, Gisselbrecht C, Herbrecht R, et al. LNH-84 regimen: a multicenter study of intensive chemotherapy in 737 patients with aggressive malignant lymphoma. J Clin Oncol 1989; 7: 1018–26.

42 Canellos GP. Residual mass in lymphoma may not be residual disease. J Clin Oncol 1988; 6: 931–3.

43 Kaplan WD, Jochelson MS, Herman TS, et al. Gallium-67 imaging: a predictor of residual tumor viability and clinical outcome in patients with diffuse large-cell lymphoma. J Clin Oncol 1990; 8: 1966–70.

44 Front D, Bar-Shalom R, Mor M, et al. Aggressive non-Hodgkin lymphoma: early prediction of outcome with Ga-67 scintigraphy. Radiology 2000; 214: 253–7.

45 Vose JM, Bierman PJ, Anderson JR, et al. Single-photon emission computed tomography gallium imaging versus computed tomography: predictive value in patients undergoing high-dose chemotherapy and autologous stem-cell transplantation for non-Hodgkin's lymphoma. J Clin Oncol 1996; 14: 2473–9.

• 46 Jerusalem G, Beguin Y, Fassotte MF, et al. Whole-body positron emission tomography using ^{18}F-fluorodeoxyglucose for post-treatment evaluation in Hodgkin's disease and non-Hodgkin's lymphoma has higher diagnostic and prognostic value than classical computed tomography scan imaging. Blood 1999; 94: 429–33.

47 Spaepen K, Stroobants S, Dupont P, et al. Prognostic value of positron emission tomography (PET) with fluorine-18 fluorodeoxyglucose ([^{18}F]-FDG) after first-line chemotherapy in non-Hodgkin's lymphoma: is [^{18}F]-FDG-PET a valid alternative to conventional diagnostic methods? J Clin Oncol 2001; 19: 414–9.

48 Cremerius U, Fabry U, Neuerburg J, et al. Positron emission tomography with ^{18}F-FDG to detect residual disease after therapy for malignant lymphoma. Nucl Med Commun 1998; 19: 1055–63.

49 Römer W, Hanauske-Abel R, Ziegler S, et al. Positron emission tomography in non-Hodgkin's lymphoma: Assessment of chemotherapy with fluorodeoxyglucose. Blood 1998; 91: 4464–71.

50 Kostakoglu L, Goldsmith SJ. Fluorine-18 fluorodeoxyglucose positron emission tomography in the staging and follow-up of lymphoma: is it time to shift gears? Eur J Nucl Med 2000; 27: 1564–78.

* 51 Juweid ME, Wiseman GA, et al. Response assessment of aggressive non-Hodgkin's lymphoma by integrated international workshop criteria and fluorine-18-fluorodeoxyglucose positron emission tomography. J Clin Oncol 2005; 23: 4652–61.

52 Cheson BD, Pfistner B, Juweid ME. Recommendations for revised response criteria for malignant lymphoma. Blood 2005; 11: Abstract No. 18.

53 Schoder H, Noy A, Gonen M, et al. Intensity of ^{18}fluorodeoxyglucose uptake in PET distinguishes between indolent and aggressive non-Hodgkin's lymphomas. J Clin Oncol 2005; 23: 4643–51.

54 Juweid ME. Role of positron emission tomography in lymphoma. J Clin Oncol 2005; 23: 4577–80.

55 Jerusalem G, Beguin Y, Fassote MF, et al. Early detection of relapse by whole body emission tomography in the follow-up of patients with Hodgkin's disease. Ann Oncol 2003; 12: 123–30.

56 Kostakoglu L, Coleman M, Leonard JP, et al. PET predicts prognosis after 1 cycle of chemotherapy in aggressive lymphoma and Hodgkin's disease. J Nucl Med 2002; 43: 1018–27.

57 Spaepen K, Stroobants S, Dupont P, et al. Early staging positron emission tomography (PET) with fluorine-18 fluorodeoxyglucose ([^{18}F]-FDG) predicts outcome in patients with aggressive non-Hodgkin's lymphoma. Ann Oncol 2002; 13: 1356–63.

58 Allen-Auerbach M, Quon A, Weber WA, et al. Comparison between 2-deoxy-2-[(18)F] fluoro-D-glucose positron-emission tomography and positron-emission tomography/computed tomography hardware fusion for staging of patients with lymphoma. Mol Imaging Biol 2004; 6: 411–6.

59 van Rens MTM, de la Riviere AB, Elbers HRJ, van den Bosch JMM. Prognostic assessment of 2,361 patients who underwent pulmonary resection for non-small cell lung cancer, stage I, II, and IIIA. Chest 2000; 117: 374–9.

60 Naruke T, Goya T, Tsuchiya R, Suemasu K. Prognosis and survival in resected lung carcinoma

based on the new international staging system. *J Thorc Cardiovasc Surg* 1988; **96**: 440–7.

61 Lavezzi AM, Santambrogio L, Bellaviti N, *et al.* Prognostic significance of different biomarkers in non-small cell lung cancer. *Oncol Rep* 1999; **6**: 819–25.

62 Pence JC, Kerns BM, Dodge RK, Iglehart JD. Prognostic significance of the proliferation index in surgically resected non-small-cell lung cancer. *Arch Surg* 1993; **128**: 1382–90.

63 Nelson CA, Wang JQ, Leav I, *et al.* The interaction among glucose transport, hexokinase, and glucose-6-phosphatase with respect to ^{3}H-2-deoxyglucose retention in murine tumor models. *Nucl Med Biol* 1996; **23**: 533–41.

64 Hoekstra CJ, Stroobants SG, Smit EF, *et al.* Prognostic relevance of response evaluation using [^{18}F]-2-fluoro-2-deoxy-D-glucose positron emission tomography in patients with locally advanced non-small-cell lung cancer. *J Clin Oncol* 2005; **23**: 8362–70.

65 Hazelton TR, Coppage L. Imaging for lung cancer restaging. *Semin Roentgenol* 2005; **40**: 182–92.

66 Mavi A, Lakhani P, Zhuang H, *et al.* Fluorodeoxyglucose-PET in characterizing solitary pulmonary nodules, assessing pleural diseases, and the initial staging, restaging, therapy planning, and monitoring response of lung cancer. *Radiol Clin North Am* 2005; **43**: 1–21.

67 Martini N, Kris MG, Flehinger BJ, *et al.* Preoperative chemotherapy for stage IIIa (N2) lung cancer: the Sloan–Kettering experience with 136 patients. *Ann Thorac Surg* 1993; **55**: 1365–73.

68 Sorenson S, Glimelius B, Nygren P. A systematic overview of chemotherapy effects in non-small cell lung cancer. *Acta Oncol* 2001; **40**: 327–39.

69 Patz EF, Connolly J, Herndon J. Prognostic value of thoracic ^{18}F-FDG PET imaging after treatment for non-small cell lung cancer. *Am J Roentgenol* 2000; **174**: 769–74.

70 Bury T, Corhay JL, Duysinx B, *et al.* Value of ^{18}F-FDG PET in detecting residual or recurrent non-small cell lung cancer. *Eur Respir J* 1999; **14**: 1376–80.

● 71 Cerfolio RJ, Bryant A, Ohja Buddhiwardhan, *et al.* The maximum standardized uptake values on positron emission tomography of non-small cell lung cancer predict stage, recurrence and survival. *J Thoracic Cardiovasc Surg* 2005; **130**: 151–9.

● 72 Schmuecking M, Baum RP, Bonnet R, *et al.* Correlation of histologic results with PET findings for tumor regression and survival in locally advanced non-small cell lung cancer after neoadjuvant treatment. *Pathologe* 2005; **26**: 178–90.

73 Yamamoto Y, Nishiyama Y, Monden T, *et al.* Correlation of FDG-PET findings with histopathology in the assessment of response to induction

chemoradiotherapy in non-small cell lung cancer. *Eur J Nucl Med Mol Imaging* 2006; **33**: 140–7.

74 Perez CA, Stanley K, Rubin P, *et al.* Radiation Therapy Oncology Group. Patterns of tumor recurrence after definitive irradiation for inoperable non-oat cell carcinoma of the lung. *Int J Radiat Oncol Biol Phys* 1980; **6**: 987–94.

75 Vander Borght T, Labar D, Pauwels S, Lambotte L. Production of 2-[^{11}C]thymidine for quantification of cellular proliferation with PET. *Appl Radiat Isotopes* 1991; **42**: 103–4.

76 Shields A, Lim K, Grierson J, *et al.* Utilization of labeled thymidine in DNA synthesis: studies for PET. *J Nucl Med* 1990; **31**: 337–42.

77 Shields AF, Mankoff DA, Link JM, *et al.* Carbon-11-thymidine and ^{18}F-FDG to measure therapy response. *J Nucl Med* 1998; **39**: 1757–62.

78 Carter CL, Allen C, Henson DE. Relation of tumor size, lymph node status, and survival in 24,740 breast cancer cases. *Cancer* 1989; **63**: 181–7.

79 Eltahir A, Heys SD, Hutcheon AW, *et al.* Treatment of large and locally advanced breast cancers using neo-adjuvant chemotherapy. *Am J Surg* 1998; **175**: 127–32.

80 Formenti SC, Volm M, Skinner KA, *et al.* Preoperative twice-weekly paclitaxel with concurrent radiation therapy followed by surgery and postoperative doxorubicin-based chemotherapy in locally advanced breast cancer: a phase I/II trial. *J Clin Oncol* 2003; **21**: 864–70.

81 Hutcheon AW, Heys SD, Sarkar TK. Neoadjuvant docetaxel in locally advanced breast cancer. *Breast Cancer Res Treat* 2003; **79(suppl 1)**: S19–24.

82 Dixon JM, Jackson J, Renshaw L, *et al.* Neoadjuvant tamoxifen and aromatase inhibitors: comparisons and clinical outcomes. *J Steroid Biochem Mol Biol* 2003; **86**: 295–9.

83 Bonadonna G, Valagussa P, Zucali R, Salvadori B. Primary chemotherapy in surgically resectable breast cancer. *CA Cancer J Clin* 1995; **45**: 227–43.

84 Fisher B, Bryant J, Wolmark N, *et al.* Effect of preoperative chemotherapy on the outcome of women with operable breast cancer. *J Clin Oncol* 1998; **16**: 2672–85.

85 Wang HC, Lo SS. Future prospects of neoadjuvant chemotherapy in treatment of primary breast cancer. *Semin Surg Oncol* 1996; **12**: 59–66.

86 Heys SD, Eremin JM, Sarkar TK, *et al.* Role of multimodality therapy in the management of locally advanced carcinoma of the breast. *J Am Coll Surg* 1994; **179**: 493–504.

87 Machiavelli MR, Romero AO, Perez JE, *et al.* Prognostic significance of pathological response of primary tumor and metastatic axillary lymph nodes after neoadjuvant chemotherapy for locally advanced breast carcinoma. *Cancer J Sci Am* 1998; **4**: 125–31.

88 Honkoop AH, van Diest PJ, de Jong JS, *et al.* Prognostic role of clinical, pathological and biological characteristics in patients with locally advanced breast cancer. *Br J Cancer* 1998; **77**: 621–6.

89 Schelling M, Avril N, Nahrig J, et al. Positron emission tomography using [(18)F]fluorodeoxyglucose for monitoring primary chemotherapy in breast cancer. J Clin Oncol 2000; **18**: 1689–95.

90 Wu HM, Bergsneider M, Glenn TC, et al. Measurement of the global lumped constant for 2-deoxy-2-[^{18}F]fluoro-D-glucose in normal human brain using [^{15}O]water and 2-deoxy-2-[^{18}F]fluoro-D-glucose positron emission tomography imaging. A method with validation based on multiple methodologies. Mol Imaging Biol 2003; **5**: 32–41.

91 Hunter GJ, Hamberg LM, Alpert NM, et al. Simplified measurement of deoxyglucose utilization rate. J Nucl Med 1996; **37**: 950–5.

92 Krak NC, van der Hoeven JJ, Hoekstra OS, et al. Measuring [^{18}F]-FDG uptake in breast cancer during chemotherapy: comparison of analytical methods. Eur J Nucl Med Mol Imaging 2003; **30**: 674–81.

93 Hoekstra CJ, Hoekstra OS, Stroobants SG, et al. Methods to monitor response to chemotherapy in non-small cell lung cancer with^{18}F-FDG PET. J Nucl Med 2002; **43**: 1304–9.

94 Kroep JR, Van Groeningen CJ, Cuesta MA, et al. Positron emission tomography using 2-deoxy-2-[^{18}F]-fluoro-D-glucose for response monitoring in locally advanced gastroesophageal cancer: a comparison of different analytical methods. Mol Imaging Biol 2003; **5**: 337–46.

95 Boellaard R, Krak NC, Hoekstra OS, et al. Effects of noise, image resolution, and ROI definition on the accuracy of standard uptake values: a simulation study. J Nucl Med 2004; **45**: 1519–27.

96 Vranjesevic D, Filmont JE, Meta J, et al. Whole-body ^{18}F-FDG PET and conventional imaging for predicting outcome in previously treated breast cancer patients. J Nucl Med 2002; **43**: 325–9.

97 Jansson T, Westlin JE, Ahlstrom H, et al. Positron emission tomography studies in patients with locally advanced and/or metastatic breast cancer: a method for early therapy evaluation? J Clin Oncol 1995; **13**: 1470–7.

98 Bassa P, Kim E, Inoue T, et al. Evaluation of preoperative chemotherapy using PET with fluorine-18-fluorodeoxyglucose in breast cancer. J Nucl Med 1996; **37**: 931–8.

99 Lowe VJ. PET in radiotherapy. In: Oehr P, Biersack HJ, Coleman RE. (eds.) PET and PET-CT in oncology. New York, Berlin, Heidelberg: Springer, 2003: 303–8.

100 Mortimer JE, Dehdashti F, Siegel BA, et al. Metabolic flare: indicator of hormone responsiveness in advanced breast cancer. J Clin Oncol 2001; **19**: 2797–803.

101 Bennink RJ, van Tienhoven van G, Rijks LJ, et al. In vivo prediction of response to antiestrogen treatment in estrogen receptor-positive breast cancer. J Nucl Med 2004; **45**: 1–7.

102 Chu KC, Tarone RE, Chow WH, et al. Temporal patterns in colorectal cancer incidence, survival and mortality from 1950 through 1960. J Natl Cancer Inst 1994; **86**: 997–1006.

103 Guillem JG, Puig-La Calle Jr J, Akhurst T, et al. Prospective assessment of primary rectal cancer response to preoperative radiation and chemotherapy using 18-fluorodeoxyglucose positron emission tomography. Dis Colon Rectum 2000; **43**: 18–24.

104 Victor K, Cuong D, Drummond GE, et al. Findings on ^{18}F-FDG PET scans after neoadjuvant chemoradiation provides prognostic stratification in patients with locally advanced rectal carcinoma subsequently treated by radical surgery. J Nucl Med 2006; **47**: 14–22.

105 Haberkorn U, Strauss LG, Dimitrakopoulou A, et al. PET studies for fluorodeoxyglucose metabolism in patients with recurrent colorectal tumors receiving radiotherapy. J Nucl Med 1991; **32**: 1485–90.

106 Sauer R, Fietkau R, Wittekind C, et al. Adjuvant vs. neoadjuvant radiochemotherapy for locally advanced rectal cancer: the German trial CAO/ARO/AIO-94. Colorectal Dis 2003; **5**: 406–15.

107 Minsky BD. Primary treatment of rectal cancer: present and future. Crit Rev Oncol/Hematol 1999; **32**: 19–30.

108 Denecke T, Rau B, Hoffmann KT, et al. Comparison of CT, MRI and ^{18}F-FDG-PET in response prediction of patients with locally advanced rectal cancer after multimodal preoperative therapy: is there a benefit using functional imaging? Eur Radiol 2005; **15**: 1658–66.

109 Guillem JG, Moore HG, Akhurst T, et al. Sequential preoperative fluorodeoxyglucose-positron emission tomography assessment of response to preoperative chemoradiation: A means for determining longterm outcomes of rectal cancer. J Am Coll Surg 2004; **199**: 1–7.

110 Findlay M, Young H, Cunningham D, et al. Noninvasive monitoring of tumor metabolism using fluorodeoxyglucose and positron emission tomography in colorectal cancer liver metastases: correlation with tumor response to fluorouracil. J Clin Oncol 1996; **14**: 700–8.

111 Akhurst T, Larson S, Macapinlac H, et al. Fluorodeoxyglucose (^{18}F-FDG) positron emission tomography (PET) immediately post hepatic cryotherapy predicts recurrence of tumor in the liver. Proc Am Soc Clin Oncol 1999; **625a**: 2415 (abstract).

112 Dimitrakopoulou-Strauss A, Strauss LG, Schlag P, et al. Fluorine-18-fluorouracil to predict therapy response in liver metastases from colorectal carcinoma. J Nucl Med 1998; **39**: 1197–202.

113 Moehler M, Dimitrakopoulou-Strauss A, Gutzler F, et al. ^{18}F-labeled fluorouracil positron emission tomography and the prognoses of colorectal carcinoma patients with metastases to the liver treated with 5-fluorouracil. Cancer 1998; **83**: 245–53.

114 Keston AS, Ball RP, Frantz VK, et al. Storage of radioactive iodine metastasis from thyroid carcinoma. Science 1942; **95**: 362–3.

115 Filleti S, Bidart JM, Arturi F, *et al.* Sodium/iodide symporter: a key transport system in thyroid cancer cell metabolism. *Eur J Endocrinol* 1999; **141**: 443–57.

116 Levy O, De la Vieja A, Carrasco N, *et al.* The Na+/I− symporter (NIS): recent advances. *J Bioenerg Biomembr* 1998; **30**: 195–206.

117 Nusynowitz ML, Tauxe WN. Thyroid cancer. In: Aktolun C, Tauxe WN. (eds.) *Nuclear oncology.* Berlin Heidelberg: Springer-Verlag, 1999: 137.

118 Grünwald F, Kälicke T, Feine U, *et al.* Fluorine-18 fluorodeoxyglucose positron emission tomography in thyroid cancer: results of a multicentre study. *Eur J Nucl Med* 1999; **12**: 1547–52.

119 Lerch H, Schober O, Kuwert T, *et al.* Survival of differentiated thyroid carcinoma studied in 500 patients. *J Clin Oncol* 1997; **15**: 2067–75.

120 Fleine U. Fluor-18-deoxyglucose positron emission tomography in differentiated thyroid cancer. *Eur J Endocrinol* 1998; **138**: 492–6.

121 Farhati J, Reiners C, Stuschke M, *et al.* Differentiated thyroid cancer: impact of adjuvant external radiotherapy in patients with perithyroidal tumor infiltration (stage pT4). *Cancer* 1996; **77**: 172–80.

122 Grünwald F, Menzel C, Bender H, *et al.* Redifferentiation therapy induced radioiodine uptake in thyroid cancer. *J Nucl Med* 1998; **39**: 1903–6.

123 Schmid DT, Stoeckli SJ, Bandhauer F, *et al.* Impact of positron emission tomography on the initial staging and therapy in locoregional advanced squamous cell carcinoma of the head and neck. *Laryngoscope* 2003; **113**: 888–91.

124 Jadvar H, Fischman AJ. Evaluation of rare tumors with [F-18]fluorodeoxyglucose positron emission tomography. *Clin Positron Imaging* 1999; **2**: 153–8.

125 Conti PS, Durski JM, Bacqai F, *et al.* Imaging of locally recurrent and metastatic thyroid cancer with positron emission tomography. *Thyroid* 1999; **9**: 797–804.

126 Khan N, Oriuchi N, Higuchi T, *et al.* Review of fluorine-18-2-fluoro-2-deoxy-D-glucose positron emission tomography (18F-FDG-PET) in the follow-up of medullary and anaplastic thyroid carcinomas. *Cancer Control* 2005; **12**: 254–60.

127 Nelson SJ, Huhn S, Vigneron DB, *et al.* Volume MRI and MRSI techniques for the quantitation of treatment response in brain tumors: presentation of a detailed case study. *J Magn Reson Imaging* 1997; **7**: 1146–52.

128 Kahn D, Follett KA, Bushnell DL, *et al.* Diagnosis of recurrent brain tumor: value of 201Tl-SPECT vs 18F-fluorodeoxyglucose PET. *Am J Roentgenol* 1994; **163**: 1459–65.

129 Kim EE, Chung SK, Haynie TP, *et al.* Differentiation of residual or recurrent tumors from post-treatment changes with 18F-FDG PET. *Radiographics* 1992; **12**: 269–79.

130 Ricci PE, Karis JP, Heiserman JE, *et al.* Differentiating recurrent tumor from radiation necrosis: time for re-evaluation of positron emission tomography? *Am J Neuroradiol* 1998; **19**: 407–13.

131 Fischman AJ, Thornton AF, Frosch MP, *et al.* 18F-FDG hypermetabolism associated with inflammatory necrotic changes following radiation of meningioma. *J Nucl Med* 1997; **38**: 1027–9.

132 Janus TJ, Kim EE, Tilbury R, *et al.* Use of [18F]fluorodeoxyglucose positron emission tomography in patients with primary malignant brain tumors. *Ann Neurol* 1993; **33**: 540–8.

133 Chao ST, Suh JH, Raja S, *et al.* The sensitivity and specificity of 18F-FDG PET in distinguishing recurrent brain tumor from radionecrosis in patients treated with stereotactic radiosurgery. *Int J Cancer* 2001; **96**: 191–7.

134 Maruyama I, Sadato N, Waki A, *et al.* Hyperacute changes in glucose metabolism of brain tumors after stereotactic radiosurgery: a PET study. *J Nucl Med* 1999; **40**: 1085–90.

135 Chung JK, Kim YK, Kim SK, *et al.* Usefulness of 11C-methionine PET in the evaluation of brain lesions that are hypo- or isometabolic on 18F-FDG PET. *Eur J Nucl Med Mol Imaging* 2002; **29**: 176–82.

136 Voges J, Herholz K, Holzer T, *et al.* 11C-methionine and 18F-2-fluorodeoxyglucose positron emission tomography: a tool for diagnosis of cerebral glioma and monitoring after brachytherapy with 125I seeds. *Stereotact Funct Neurosurg* 1997; **69**: 129–35.

137 Nuutinen J, Sonninen P, Lehikoinen P, *et al.* Radiotherapy treatment planning and long-term follow-up with [(11)C]methionine PET in patients with low-grade astrocytoma. *Int J Radiat Oncol Biol Phys* 2000; **48**: 43–52.

138 Kelsen DP, Ginsberg R, Pajak TF, *et al.* Chemotherapy followed by surgery compared with surgery alone for localized esophageal cancer. *N Engl J Med* 1998; **339**: 1979–84.

139 Law S, Fok M, Chow S, *et al.* Preoperative chemotherapy versus surgical therapy alone for squamous cell carcinoma of the esophagus: a prospective randomized trial. *J Thorac Cardiovasc Surg* 1997; **114**: 210–7.

140 Kang YK, Choi DW, Im YH, *et al.* A phase III randomized comparison of neoadjuvant chemotherapy followed by surgery versus surgery for locally advanced stomach cancer. *Proc Am Soc Clin Oncol* 1996; **15**: 215 (abstract).

141 Songun I, Keizer HJ, Hermans J, *et al.* Chemotherapy for operable gastric cancer: results of the Dutch randomized FAMTX trial. *Eur J Cancer* 1999; **25**: 558–62.

142 Fujii M, Kosaki G, Tsuchiya S, *et al.* Randomized trial of preoperative adjuvant chemotherapy using oral 5-FU in operable gastric cancer. *Proc Am Soc Clin Oncol* 1999; **18**: 272a (abstract).

143 Roth JA, Pass HI, Flanagan MM, *et al.* Randomized clinical trial of preoperative and postoperative adjuvant chemotherapy with cisplatin, vindesine, and bleomycin for carcinoma of the esophagus. *J Thorac Cardiovasc Surg* 1988; **96**: 242–8.

144 Ajani JA, Mansfield PF, Lynch PM, *et al.* Enhanced staging and all chemotherapy preoperatively in patients with potentially resectable gastric carcinoma. *J Clin Oncol* 1999; **17**: 2403–11.

145 Lowy AM, Mansfield PF, Leach SD, *et al.* Response to neoadjuvant chemotherapy best predicts survival after curative resection of gastric cancer. *Ann Surg* 1999; **229**: 303–8.

146 Chak A, Canto MI, Cooper GS, *et al.* Endosonographic assessment of multimodality therapy predicts survival of esophageal carcinoma patients. *Cancer* 2000; **88**: 1788–95.

147 Weber WA, Ott K, Becker K, *et al.* Prediction of response to pre-operative chemotherapy in adenocarcinomas of the esophagogastric junction by metabolic imaging. *J Clin Oncol* 2001; **19**: 3058–65.

148 Ott K, Fink U, Becker K, *et al.* Prediction of response to pre-operative chemotherapy in gastric carcinoma by metabolic imaging: results of a prospective trial. *J Clin Oncol* 2003; **24**: 4604–10.

149 Nooter K, Kok T, Bosman FT, *et al.* Expression of the multidrug resistance protein (MRP) in squamous cell carcinoma of the oesophagus and response to pre-operative chemotherapy. *Eur J Cancer* 1998; **34**: 81–6.

150 Wieder HA, Beer AJ, Lordick F, *et al.* Comparison of changes in tumor metabolic activity and tumor size during chemotherapy of adenocarcinomas of the esophagogastric junction. *J Nucl Med* 2005; **46**: 2029–34.

151 Shreve PD, Iannone O, Weinhold P, *et al.* Cellular metabolism of (1-C14)-acetate in prostate cancer cells in vitro. *J Nucl Med* 2002; **43(suppl 5)**: 272P.

152 Seltzer MA, Jahan S, Dahlbom M, *et al.* C-11 acetate PET imaging of primary and locally recurrent prostate cancer: comparison to normal controls. *J Nucl Med* 2002; **43(suppl 5)**: 117P.

153 Kotzerke J, Volkmer BG, *et al.* Carbon-11 acetate positron emission tomography can detect local recurrence of prostate cancer. *Eur J Nucl Med Mol Imaging* 2002; **29**: 1380–4.

154 Oyama N, Akino H, *et al.* ¹¹C-acetate PET imaging of prostate cancer. *J Nucl Med* 2002; **43**: 181–6.

155 Oyama N, Miller TR, *et al.* ¹¹C-acetate PET imaging of prostate cancer: detection of recurrent disease at PSA relapse. *J Nucl Med* 2003; **44**: 549–55.

156 Dimitrakopoulou-Strauss A, Strauss LG. PET imaging of prostate cancer with ¹¹C-acetate. *J Nucl Med* 2003; **44**: 556–8.

157 Kishi H, Minowada S, Kosada N, *et al.* C-11 choline PET helps determine the outcome of hormonal therapy of prostate cancer. *J Nucl Med* 2002; **43(suppl 5)**: 117P.

158 Grigsby PW, Barry SA, Dehdashti F, *et al.* Post-therapy fluorodeoxyglucose positron emission tomography in carcinoma of the cervix: response and outcome. *J Clin Oncol* 2004; **22**: 2167–71.

159 Yen TC, See LC, Chang TC, *et al.* Defining the priority of using ¹⁸F-FDG PET for recurrent cervical cancer. *J Nucl Med* 2004; **45**: 1632–9.

160 Burkill GJ, Badran M, Al-Muderis O, *et al.* Malignant gastrointestinal stromal tumor: distribution, imaging features, and pattern of metastatic spread. *Radiology* 2003; **226**: 527–32.

161 Casper ES. Gastrointestinal stromal tumors. *Curr Treat Options Oncol* 2000; **1**: 267–73.

162 Dematteo RP, Maki RG, Antonescu C, Brennan MF. Targeted molecular therapy for cancer: the application of STI571 to gastrointestinal stromal tumor. *Curr Probl Surg* 2003; **40**: 144–93.

163 Van den Abbeele AD, Badawi RD. Use of positron emission tomography in oncology and its potential role to assess response to imatinib mesylate therapy in gastrointestinal stromal tumors (GISTs). *Eur J Cancer* 2002; **38(suppl 5)**: S60–5.

164 Gayed I, Vu T, Iyer R, *et al.* The role of ¹⁸F-FDG PET in staging and early prediction of response to therapy of recurrent gastrointestinal stromal tumors. *J Nucl Med* 2004; **45**: 17–21.

165 Becherer A, Szabo M, *et al.* Imaging of advanced neuroendocrine tumors with ¹⁸F-DOPA PET. *J Nucl Med* 2004; **45**: 1161–7.

166 Zimmer T, Ziegler K, Liehr RM, *et al.* Endosonography of neuroendocrine tumors of the stomach, duodenum, and pancreas. *Ann NY Acad Sci* 1994; **733**: 425–36.

167 De Angelis C, Carucci P, Repici A, Rizzetto M. Endosonography in decision making and management of gastrointestinal endocrine tumors. *Eur J Ultrasound* 1999; **10**: 139–50.

168 Slooter GD, Mearadji A, Breeman WA, *et al.* Somatostatin receptor imaging, therapy and new strategies in patients with neuroendocrine tumors. *Br J Surg* 2001; **88**: 31–40.

169 Kvols LK, Reubi JC, Horisberger U, *et al.* The presence of somatostatin receptors in malignant neuroendocrine tumor tissue predicts responsiveness to octreotide. *Yale J Biol Med* 1992; **65**: 505–18.

170 Menzel C, Graichen S, *et al.* Monitoring the efficacy of iodine-131 MIBG therapy using ¹⁸F-FDG PET. *Acta Med Austriaca* 2003; **30**: 37–40.

◆ 171   Krenning EP, Valkerma R, *et al.* Molecular imaging as in-vivo molecular pathology for gastro-enteropancreatin neuroendocrine tumors: implications for follow-up after therapy. *J Nucl Med* 2005; **46**: 76S–82S.

● 172   Hofmann M, Maecke H, Borner R, *et al.* Biokinetics and imaging with the somatostatin receptor PET radioligand ^{68}Ga-DOTATOC: preliminary data. *Eur J Nucl Med* 2001; **28**: 1751–7.

173   Blankenberg FG, Katsikis PD, Tait JF, *et al.* In vivo detection and imaging of phosphatidylserine expression during programmed cell death. *Proc Natl Acad Sci USA* 1998; **95**: 6349–54.

174   Blankenberg FG, Strauss HW. Will imaging of apoptosis play a role in clinical care? A tale of mice and men. *Apoptosis* 2001; **6**: 117–23.

175   Yang DJ, Azhdarinia A, Wu P. *In vivo* and *in vitro* measurement of apoptosis in breast cancer cells using ^{99m}Tc-EC-annexin V. *Cancer Biother Radiopharm* 2001; **16**: 73–83.

176   Green AM, Steinmetz ND. Monitoring apoptosis in real time. *Cancer J* 2002; **8**: 82–92.

2

Principles of radionuclide therapy

K.E. BRITTON

Introduction	79	The role of radionuclide therapy in cancer management	83
Imaging for therapy	79	References	86
Principles of localization	80	Appendix: Guidelines for systemic radionuclide therapy	
Intracellular localization	81	for cancer	89
Follow-up	82		

INTRODUCTION

Radionuclide therapy in oncology is dependent on using a radiolabeled agent designed to be as specific as possible to target just the disease process. Receptor-binding peptides and other chemicals, antigen binding monoclonal antibodies, their derivatives and genetically engineered analogs have these properties.

Nuclear medicine exploits the subtle differences between the cancer cell and the normal cell for the identification of cancer cells.[1] For peptides, receptor expression per cell may be increased to between 500 and 10 000 and antigen expression per cell for monoclonal antibodies to between 5000 and 50 000 as compared to their normal counterparts. This amplification factor allows cancer to be detected down to of the order of 2 mm in size, for example in normal sized lymph nodes and to be treated by internally targeted radionuclide therapy down to the level of micrometastases. Size, however, is not the main determinant of uptake, but the number of uptake or binding sites for the radiolabeled agent. Imaging gives confidence that therapeutic uptake will occur. Nuclear medicine imaging techniques also utilize the ability to visualize alterations in metabolism. These alterations in metabolism may occur in the tissues surrounding the tumor site or may occur in the tumor itself and either aid or reduce the effectiveness of therapy. As well as the uptake, the residence time of the radiopharmaceutical is important so that what is taken up stays a sufficient length of time for imaging and/or for therapy.

Most cancer surgery and radiotherapy is based on the physical extent of the disease and not the biological extent. Radiology requires a mass in tissue, displacing tissue, or infiltrating tissue for contrast. Nuclear medicine does not require a mass, since this identification technique is able to detect receptors or epitopes on ribbons, fingers or plaques of cancer cells as well as on the surfaces of cells in a mass.

IMAGING FOR THERAPY

Most cancer chemotherapy is based on clinical trials involving many patients and may or may not work in the individual. Nuclear medicine treats the individual in whom it has provided evidence for uptake of the agent before therapy. The imaging radionuclide (gamma emitting) is substituted with a therapy radionuclide (beta or alpha emitting) on the same agent so that only those patients in whom there has been demonstrated by imaging significant and specific tumor uptake (Table 2.1) are exposed to radiation therapy. More importantly all those patients without sufficient uptake of a good equivalent imaging agent are extremely unlikely to benefit from radionuclide therapy, a saving of time, effort, cost, and unnecessary radiation exposure. There are no data showing any outcome benefit for radionuclide therapy in image negative patients.

Iodine-123 is now used to detect recurrence during follow-up imaging of differentiated thyroid cancer instead of ^{131}I.[2] This is because it has over 20 times greater ability than an equal activity of ^{131}I to detect iodine-avid tissue.[3] meta-[^{123}I]iodobenzylguanidine (^{123}I-MIBG) is used for imaging to prove uptake to determine whether ^{131}I-MIBG therapy is appropriate.[4] A positive bone scan with ^{99m}Tc-methylene diphosphonate (^{99m}Tc-MDP) is used to see if therapy with ^{153}Sm-EHMDP would be appropriate for palliation of bone metastases.[5] Neuro-endocrine tumors (NETs) are imaged

Table 2.1 *Gamma imaging for beta therapy*

Disease/disorder	Imaging	Therapy
Recurrent thyroid cancer	^{123}I, ^{131}I	^{131}I
Neuroendocrine tumor	^{123}I-MIBG	^{131}I-MIBG
	^{111}In-octreotide	^{90}Y-DOTATOC
		^{90}Y-Octreother
		^{177}Lu-octreotide
	^{111}In-lanreotide	^{90}Y-lanreotide
Bone metastases	^{99m}Tc-MDP	^{153}Sm-EDTMP
		^{186}Re-HEDP
Non-Hodgkin's lymphoma	^{131}I-B1 Anti CD20*	^{131}I-B1 Anti CD20
	^{111}In-retuximab*	^{90}Y-retuximab

*For dosimetry also.

with indium-111[6] or ^{99m}Tc-octreotide derivatives[7] to see if yttrium-90[8,9] or ^{177}Lu-DOTATOC[10] therapy is appropriate. Alternatively, NETs may be imaged with ^{111}In-lanreotide to see if ^{90}Y-lanreotide therapy is appropriate.[11] The use of ^{90}Y-lanreotide, ^{90}Y-octreotide or ^{177}Lu-octreotate therapy is indicated in those NETs that are image positive on the respective octreotide analog imaging but are ^{123}I-MIBG negative. In non-Hodgkin's lymphoma ^{131}I-B1 anti-CD 20 antibody is used not only for imaging but also for dosimetry before therapy[12,13] and ^{111}In-retuximab should be regularly used for imaging and dosimetry before ^{90}Y-retuximab (Zevalin) therapy.[14,15] In prostate cancer ^{99m}Tc or ^{111}In-anti-PSMA may be used to see whether ^{90}Y anti-PSMA would be appropriate therapy in the future.[16]

Interleukin-2 binds with activated T cells and in melanoma it may be used therapeutically. Studies with ^{99m}Tc-labeled interleukin-2 have shown a relationship between the amount of uptake in melanoma and the degree of lymphocytic infiltration. The demonstration of uptake of ^{99m}Tc interleukin-2 may indicate whether or not interleukin-2 therapy would be appropriate in patients with melanoma.[17] Infusions of cytokines for cancer therapy are used increasingly. Some patients respond and some do not. It may be appropriate that evidence of uptake by the tumor environment is obtained by using radiolabeled cytokines to predict efficacy before expensive and maybe ineffective cytokine therapy with known side effects is undertaken. The same approach is applicable to chemotherapy agents.

PRINCIPLES OF LOCALIZATION

Biological factors affect uptake. The radionuclide therapy must have access to the tumor cells that are its target, so local factors are very important and are considered in Chapter 1F. These include metabolism, vascularity, cell membrane structure and function, and intracellular localization.

Metabolism: Bone metastases

While the most obvious target site for tumor imaging is the tumor itself, many radiopharmaceuticals used for tumor imaging have localized in the normal tissues surrounding the tumor. In the case of ^{99m}Tc-MDP bone scans, the tissue surrounding the tumor site reacts with increased osteoblastic activity. An increase in tracer uptake is observed adjacent to the tumor. As diphosphonate uptake is proportional to osteoblastic activity and since the changes in osteoblastic activity occur at an extremely early stage in the development of a bone metastasis, the radionuclide bone scan provides a sensitive tool for the detection of bone metastases.

This uptake of diphosphonates by active osteoblasts has been utilized to develop a palliative therapy for pain due to bone metastases. Samarium-153-labeled ethylenediamine-tetramethylenephosphonate (^{153}Sm-EDTMP)[5,18] and ^{186}Re-labeled etidronate (^{186}Re-HEDP) (diphosphonates labeled with beta-emitting radionuclides)[19,20] are currently under evaluation as therapy agents. Strontium-89, which behaves like calcium, is taken up both into normal bone and sites of increased osteoblastic activity, but clears much more slowly from the abnormal sites. It has been shown to have a clear-cut role in palliating bone pain and in reducing the likelihood of developing new painful bone metastatic sites (see Chapter 17D). Phosphorus-32 is incorporated into the DNA and RNA of rapidly dividing cells and so is used in the treatment of thrombocythemia and polycythemia (Chapter 17F). This property and the uptake of phosphate by bone have lead to the re-introduction of ^{32}P for the treatment of bone metastases, for which it is the cheapest option.[21]

The question remains as to which of these and other radionuclides should one choose for palliation of bone metastases? Bone pain is related to the intimate interaction of the surface of the tumor cell and the adjacent bone and inflammatory cells through the actions of cytokines including tumor necrosis factor and chemokines. If the only requirement is reduction of pain, then the radionuclide with the shortest range in the highest dose acceptable, that is with the shortest half-life is used. A 'short soft' agent, such as ^{153}Sm, would be the best (Table 2.2).[22] There is also the advantage of minimal marrow suppression due to its short range (2.5 mm). An even softer (range 0.27 mm) but long half-life agent such as ^{117}Sn might be selected to allow cancer cells time to enter their most radiosensitive part of the cell cycle just before division. Alternatively, many consider that the cancer cells in the marrow need treatment, so in spite of the effect on normal marrow at least reduction of the cancer cell burden might be achieved as well as pain relief. Thus a 'long hard' such as ^{89}Sr or a 'short hard' such as ^{188}Re, with the advantage of its generator production

Table 2.2   *Some radionuclides used for therapy*

Type of radiation	Radionuclide	Half–life (T$_{1/2}$)	Beta energy (MeV)	Range in tissue (mm)
Short soft	^{153}Sm	47 h	0.81*	2.5
Medium soft	^{177}Lu	6.7 days	0.50*	2.0
Long soft	^{117}Sn	13.6 days	0.16*	0.27
Short hard	^{188}Re	17 h	2.2*	11.0
	^{166}Ho	27 h	1.84*	8.4
Medium hard	^{90}Y	2.7 days	2.3	11.1
	^{186}Re	3.7 days	1.07*	4.5
Long hard	^{32}P	14.3 days	1.7	7.9
	^{89}Sr	50.5 days	1.49	7.0

*Also has a gamma ray suitable for imaging.

might be recommended. In an ideal world probably a combination of 'short soft' and 'long hard' would be chosen, with one of these having a low abundance of gamma-ray emission for imaging and dosimetry. The same principles apply to the choice of radionuclide therapy in other situations.

Vascularity: Liver metastases

Angiogenesis is a phenomenon frequently observed in tumors and this increased vascularization may be demonstrated as increased blood pool if a dynamic study is performed or a radiolabeled red cell study undertaken, which may have diagnostic utility. The uptake of all tumor agents depends on the tumor blood supply. As the clonogenic cancer cells are those inducing the blood supply and dividing most rapidly, so their treatment by internal radionuclide targeting is potentially more direct and effective than by external-beam radiotherapy, which gives a uniform dose to the cancer cells and stroma. Anti-angiogenic drugs might be given in combination with or after the administration of radionuclide therapy to prevent regeneration of tumor blood supply.

Use may be made of tumor blood supply in therapy, particularly for liver metastases. ^{131}I-labeled lipiodol[23] and ^{188}Re-labeled lipiodol[24] have been injected into the hepatic artery with successful reduction in the size of hepatic metastases. Blockage of the tumor capillary bed and delivery of a therapy radiation dose has also been achieved using ^{32}P- or ^{90}Y-labeled ceramic, resin or glass microspheres.[25–27]

Cell membranes: Monoclonal antibodies and receptor binding

Radiopharmaceutical localization may be achieved by binding to the tumor cell membrane, the bindee–binder

interaction. This may be through using an antigen–antibody reaction or by developing radiopharmaceuticals which bind to the receptors or transport proteins expressed on certain tumor cell membranes.

Over the past decade, research has been undertaken to identify tumor-specific antigens expressed on the membranes of tumor cells. The identification of these antigens has allowed the development of monoclonal antibodies and genetically engineered derivatives, which may be radiolabeled without losing their immunogenicity. Radioimmunoscintigraphy is described in Chapters 13G and 13H and radioimmunotherapy in Chapter 17F.

A targeting technique using two or more steps has been successfully developed using the biotin–avidin reaction. Unlabeled antibody is attached to either avidin or biotin and administered intravenously. After a suitable time interval, during which time the antibody has localized at tumor site(s), the radionuclide label attached to the reciprocal biotin or avidin is injected and attaches to the antibody localized on the cell membrane. This technique reduces the amount of nonspecific binding of antibody and increases target-to-background ratios. It has been applied in imaging and radionuclide therapy of solid tumors:[28–30] glioma,[31,32] colorectal cancer,[33] and lung cancer.[34]

Further measures to increase the specificity of monoclonal antibodies include the developments of chimeric antibodies, which have a murine variable region and a human constant region, humanized antibodies where only the complimentarity determinant regions (CDRs) are murine and genetically engineered fragments. The aim of these modified antibodies is to reduce nonspecific uptake caused by the immunogenicity of the murine element of the antibody, when used for radionuclide therapy. Human antimurine antibody (HAMA) develops in approximately 50% of patients studied using more than 2 mg of monoclonal antibodies and these antibodies may affect the biodistribution of subsequent radionuclide therapy doses of antibody, with the liver becoming the main site of uptake.

The presence of receptors on the cell membranes of certain tumor cells has led to the development of radiopharmaceuticals for therapy that bind to these membrane receptors. Yttrium-90-octreotide and ^{177}Lu-octreotate are examples (Chapter 17B).

INTRACELLULAR LOCALIZATION

Specific uptake: Chemical tumor agents

IODINE–123/131

Differentiated thyroid tumor cells of follicular and papillary cancer usually retain the ability to trap and organify iodine. This accessible metabolic pathway, combined with the availability of radioactive forms of iodine, has been fundamental to the development of radionuclide tumor imaging and therapy over the past 50 years. The radiopharmaceutical is specific to thyroid cancer, although nonspecific uptake in the salivary glands and stomach and excretion into the bowel and bladder may reduce the sensitivity of lesion detection in the abdomen and pelvis. Therapy with ^{131}I is successful in treating recurrent thyroid cancer and high tumor radiation doses may be achieved with sparing of surrounding normal tissues (Chapter 17A).

META-[[123/131]I]IODOBENZYLGUANIDINE

This is a guanethidine analog that is taken up into the chromaffin granules of neuroendocrine cells. Over the past 18 years, the role of this radiopharmaceutical has been evaluated in both the diagnosis and therapy of certain neuroendocrine tumors, particularly pheochromocytomas, neuroblastomas, carcinoid tumors, medullary thyroid tumors, and paragangliomas[35] Therapy with ^{131}I-MIBG has proved successful, particularly in 'carcinoid' tumors and neuroblastomas (Chapters 17B and 17C). Unlike ^{111}In-octreotide, radiolabeled MIBG is not so often taken up into gastroendocrine pancreatic (GEP) tumors. The reason for this lack of uptake in certain neuroendocrine tumors is related to the absence of chromaffin granules.[36] Interfering medication must always be excluded.[37]

Auger electrons and alpha particles

Although having reputedly a high linear energy transfer, Auger electrons have been disappointing as therapy agents for nuclear medicine. Iodine-125 and ^{125}I-MIBG have not been successful in thyroid cancer or NETs, respectively. Indium-111-octreotide has been disappointing in neuroendocrine tumors and less effective than either ^{90}Y-octreotide or ^{177}Lu-octreotate.[38]

Alpha particle emitters have very high linear energy transfer and the track of one or two particles in a cell is sufficient to kill it and equivalent to 400 cell traverses of beta particles. Its disadvantages include the requirement for internalization of the agent, limited supply, usually short half lives, difficult chemistry with the high recoil energy tending to cause radiolysis, radiation protection, and handling problems. Nevertheless, it is being used successfully in myeloid leukemia[39,40] and should be successful in metastatic melanoma.[41]

FOLLOW-UP

At present, nuclear medicine tests play an important role in the follow-up of patients with proven malignancy. It is helpful to study the patient before and after the initial intervention to determine the outcome. Radionuclide studies may be used to determine the completeness of surgery or other primary intervention, the presence of recurrence, the response to second-line treatment, the appropriateness of certain therapies, and organ function following therapy.

When radiotherapy or chemotherapy is the first-line treatment, radionuclide imaging, particularly [^{18}F]fluorodeoxyglucose (^{18}F-FDG) positron emission tomography (PET), may be used to determine the response of the primary tumor to therapy. Gallium-67 has been shown to be useful in assessing the presence of residual active tumor in patients treated with radiotherapy and/or chemotherapy for lymphoma. Computed tomography (CT) and magnetic resonance imaging (MRI) are unable to determine whether a post-treatment residual mediastinal mass contains active tumor or not and ^{67}Ga has been shown to be superior to these two anatomical techniques in this situation. It has been replaced by the use of ^{18}F-FDG PET, which is proving a sensitive method of detecting early local recurrence in patients with carcinoma, sarcoma and melanoma (Chapter 1C).

The presence of recurrence may be initially detected biochemically if an adequately specific biochemical marker exists. However, even a sensitive biochemical marker is unable to localize the recurrence or determine its suitability for further treatment.

A rising prostate-specific antigen (PSA) level in a patient with prostate cancer indicates recurrent disease. ^{99m}Tc-MDP bone scan or ^{111}In-labeled antibody against a prostate specific membrane antigen (PSMA) will determine whether the recurrence is in the skeleton or in the soft-tissue (Chapter13H).

An ^{111}In-octreotide scan will show the site of recurrent neuroendocrine tumor in a patient whose biochemical markers in blood and/or urine become elevated. The presence of whole-body information will also accurately identify whether the recurrence is single and suitable for surgery or multiple requiring a more palliative approach.

Tumor response

Tumor response to second-line treatment may be monitored using whole-body nuclear medicine imaging. ^{99m}Tc-MDP bone imaging remains the best method of monitoring the effects of chemotherapy in patients with breast cancer on bone metastases or in following patients undergoing hormone manipulation with bone metastases in prostate cancer.

^{18}F-FDG imaging and other PET agents are being assessed as a means of obtaining early information on the response of a tumor to second-line treatment such as chemotherapy since a reduction of uptake will precede the actual reduction in tumor mass (Chapter 1C). Loss of uptake of radiolabeled monoclonal antibodies or receptor-binding peptides is also providing evidence of response.

This often predates a change in tumor size seen by cross-sectional radiology response evaluation.

For solid tumors and lymphomas, complete remission (CR) is defined as complete resolution of all disease-related radiological abnormalities and the disappearance of all signs and symptoms related to the disease. Complete remission unconfirmed (CR(u)) is defined as complete resolution of all disease-related symptoms but with residual focal abnormalities. Generally, these comprise an unchanging lesion of ≤2 cm diameter by radiological evaluation. Partial remission (PR) is defined as a greater than 50% reduction in the sum of the products of the longest perpendicular diameter of all measurable lesions with no new lesions. Overall response rate (ORR) is the sum of CR and PR. Stable disease (SD) is defined as a less than 25% increase or less than 50% decrease in the sum of the products of the longest perpendicular diameters of all measurable lesions and progressive disease (PD) as a greater than or equal to 25% increase from the nadir value. At progression, marker lesions are usually required to be >2 × 2 cm diameter by radiographic evaluation, or >1 cm diameter by physical examination. Alternatively, the appearance of any new lesion (>2 × 2 cm in diameter by radiographic evaluation or >1 cm diameter by physical examination) also defines PD. Duration of response is defined as the length of time from the day of first evaluation with a response to the first day of documented progression and progression free survival as the time from start of treatment to first documented progression or death. Overall survival is defined from the date of start of therapy to death. For solid tumors the RECIST definitions are being promoted.[42,43]

Organ function post-therapy

As many oncology therapies are toxic to normal tissues, the function of normal organs may require monitoring during certain therapies. Certain chemotherapy agents are nephrotoxic and monitoring of the glomerular filtration rate is required to guide the dose of chemotherapy that may be used. Chromium-51-ethylenediaminetetraacetic acid (^{51}Cr-EDTA) is a well-established non-imaging technique for monitoring renal function in this situation. Some chemotherapeutic agents such as adriamycin and herceptin are cardiotoxic. Gated blood pool imaging is a reliable and reproducible technique for monitoring left ventricular ejection fraction in patients undergoing courses of chemotherapy.

THE ROLE OF RADIONUCLIDE THERAPY IN CANCER MANAGEMENT

Evaluating the appropriateness of radionuclide therapy as an option in the treatment of malignancy may be determined using a tracer study. Unlike other second-line treatments such as chemotherapy, the tracer study can be used to select those patients for whom radionuclide therapy is likely to be helpful. This selection not only spares patients who show no uptake on the tracer study from unnecessary treatment, but also saves valuable resources.[44] The requirement for a positive ^{123}I-MIBG tracer study is a prerequisite of treatment with therapy doses of ^{131}I-MIBG in patients with neuroendocrine tumors. The tracer dose will confirm both the presence and degree of MIBG uptake and also enables dosimetry calculations to be performed as appropriate. An ^{111}In-octreotide scan should be performed before undertaking therapy with somatostatin to confirm uptake, since the therapy is both expensive and has side effects, which may be avoided in scan-negative patients.

Thyroid cancer

Once the histological diagnosis of differentiated thyroid cancer is established by biopsy or incidentally following thyroid surgery, total thyroidectomy or completion thyroidectomy is undertaken. This usually leaves a little residual thyroid tissue so as to preserve the parathyroid glands and the recurrent laryngeal nerve. This residual thyroid tissue is then removed using an ablation dose of ^{131}I radionuclide therapy, typically 3 GBq (80 mCi), given to the patient who stays in a designated side ward. Four days after the ablation therapy, the patient is imaged with the gamma camera set up for ^{131}I with a high-energy collimator. This shows the amount of thyroid remnant. Occasionally it may show iodine-avid functioning metastases, but these are not usually seen until all normal thyroid tissue has been ablated. The ablation therapy is undertaken so that ^{131}I can be used to concentrate in and treat any subsequent thyroid metastases that are iodine avid. Removal of all normal thyroid tissue also allows the measurement for serum thyroglobulin (Tg) as another means of monitoring the patient with thyroid cancer during follow-up. Serial ^{131}I tracer imaging studies of the patient using 74–185 MBq (2–5 mCi) ^{131}I are performed then follow typically for a period of several years (Chapter 17A).

This approach using ^{131}I tracer for imaging has two main disadvantages. Iodine-131 is a poor imaging agent for the modern gamma camera. Therefore the desire was to increase the administered 'tracer' dose of ^{131}I to 370 MBq (10 mCi) for better imaging. Unfortunately, this creates stunning; that is, a small amount of radionuclide uptake prevents the benefit of a large amount of therapeutic administered activity. It has been shown that below 185 MBq, stunning is less likely to occur. Thus a typical administered dose for ^{131}I follow-up is 74–185 MBq (2–5 mCi) ^{131}I which is too low for good imaging. It was sometimes observed that the post-^{131}I therapy scan showed more iodine avid metastases than the tracer ^{131}I imaging study. Clearly, the detection of small or weakly iodine-avid metastases is likely to be better if undertaken after 5.5 GBq (150 mCi) ^{131}I as compared with 74 MBq (2 mCi). This type of finding has even led to patients receiving ^{131}I therapy with a negative ^{131}I tracer study and a raised Tg. But there is no outcome data for any benefit of ^{131}I therapy for weakly or non-iodine-avid thyroid cancer treated with [131]I. The alternative approach therefore is to use a radionuclide of iodine with better imaging properties so that the 'tracer' imaging has equivalent detectability for iodine avid metastases to that of imaging after ^{131}I therapy.

[123]I high dose tracer

Iodine-123 is a pure gamma emitter with an energy of 159 keV, close to that of [99m]Tc (140 keV). The combination of the modern gamma camera with a low energy collimator and ^{123}I imaging gives up to 20-fold greater detectability compared with an equivalent activity of [131]I.[3] A dose of 185 MBq (5 mCi) [123]I is equivalent to nearly 2 GBq (100 mCi) of [131]I. Yet the radiation dose to the thyroid from this activity of ^{123}I is less than a fifth of that due to 74 MBq (2 mCi) [131]I, so stunning does not occur using high dose ^{123}I and the quality of imaging is comparable with that following an ^{131}I therapy dose. Ideally, from this formula, 278 MBq (7.5 mCi) [123]I would be equivalent to 5.5 GBq (150 mCi) [131]I. A dose of 7.4 MBq (2 mCi) [123]I is too low, as results from Cohen et al.[45] showed a number of false negatives as compared to post- [131]I therapy imaging. Leger et al.[46] used less than 40 MBq (1 mCi) [123]I which is clearly too little. For SPET or SPET/CT studies, which are beneficial for detecting and localizing small remnants or disease and for distinguishing esophageal activity, 370 MBq ^{123}I is recommended.

We were one of the first groups to substitute ^{123}I for ^{131}I tracer imaging in the follow-up of thyroid cancer.[2,47,48] This approach is supported by Shankar et al.[49] and Park et al.[50] We have evaluated this technique in a pilot study and have now adopted a protocol where no ^{131}I tracer study is done in patients with differentiated thyroid cancer, through a protocol which uses a combination ^{123}I and Tg. The ^{123}I protocol is briefly as follows. Low risk patients after ^{131}I ablation therapy are followed only clinically and with Tg serially (off T3 for 8 days). If Tg rises an ^{123}I study is performed with imaging at 2 and 24 h after confirming that the TSH is greater than 30 mU L^{-1}.

High risk patients after ^{131}I ablation therapy all have imaging with ^{123}I at 6 months and Tg measurement (off T3 for 8 days, TSH >30 mU L^{-1}). If imaging and Tg are normal, follow-up is with Tg (off T3 8 days). If Tg subsequently rises a further ^{123}I study is performed. Any positive ^{123}I study leads to ^{131}I therapy which is repeated every 6 months until the post-^{131}I therapy scan is normal or until 45 GBq (1.2 Ci) is reached. When the post-^{131}I therapy scan becomes negative, follow-up is with Tg (off T3 for 8 days). If ^{123}I imaging is negative and Tg rises, then ^{123}I is repeated and if still negative, a conventional search for non-iodine-avid disease is made leading to surgery, radiotherapy or medical treatment as appropriate. Localization of non-iodine-avid thyroid disease used to be with ^{201}Tl but is now undertaken by either ^{99m}Tc-MIBI or ^{18}F-FDG PET in combination with radiological techniques, particularly MRI. These agents help to localize the site of the recurrence but are not specific for thyroid cancer and do not lead to specific radionuclide therapy.

Iodine-123 imaging avoids giving ^{131}I therapy in the absence of evidence of iodine-avid disease. To give therapy to a patient in whom the post-^{131}I therapy scan at 4 days shows no iodine uptake is a disaster. It is a waste of patient's time, unnecessary isolation and ward usage, and expense. It contravenes the basic principle of radionuclide therapy: that of requiring evidence of uptake by a cancer by imaging the gamma emission of an appropriate compound before using a substituted beta emitter on the same compound for therapy. No ^{131}I-MIBG therapy is given unless ^{123}I-MIBG imaging is positive, no ^{90}Y-octreother unless ^{111}In-octreotide imaging is positive, no [186]Re-HEDP therapy unless a ^{99m}Tc-MDP bone scan is positive etc. It contravenes the principle that unnecessary radiation should not be given. In the UK on the basis of the Ionising Radiation (Medical Exposure) Regulations 2000, ^{131}I therapy cannot be justified in the absence of evidence that there would be any benefit. This requirement for justification is met through the demonstration that the patient's thyroid carcinoma is iodine avid. Cyclotron-produced ^{123}I is becoming more widely available as the number of cyclotrons for producing FDG increases. A preliminary review of ^{123}I studies in 102 patients gave 37 concordant ^{123}I/pre-^{131}I post-therapy positive scans, seven concordant ^{123}I/pre-^{131}I post-therapy negative scans and three discordant results: one ^{123}I positive/^{131}I negative and one ^{131}I positive 3 months after an ^{123}I negative scan and one related to the use of retinoic acid (P < 0.001).[51]

Iodine-123 imaging does require attention to detail: it is used in a lesser chemical amount than ^{131}I and appears more sensitive to iodine interference and a careful history is required. Esophageal activity from saliva may affect interpretation; swallowing plenty of water before imaging and a 48 h image may help. It may be sensitive to lack of TSH stimulation, so it is important to check TSH is over 30 mU L^{-1}. If thyroglobulin continues to rise and ^{123}I imaging is persistently negative, which is quite a rare situation in our hands in differentiated thyroid carcinoma and may be due to interference by unsuspected iodine-containing agents or medication, we would evaluate each case on its merits. Is there ever an argument for ^{131}I therapy in non-iodine-avid disease?[48,52,53] Any uptake of ^{131}I is likely to be too trivial to be of benefit. Outcome data on the benefit of ^{131}I therapy is only for iodine-avid disease.

In conclusion, high dose ^{123}I imaging is an excellent predictor of the post-^{131}I therapy scan and when strategically combined with thyroglobulin has replaced ^{131}I tracer studies in our follow-up of differentiated thyroid cancer. If the trials of this approach are successful elsewhere, then in the future ^{123}I imaging is likely to replace ^{131}I tracer imaging in the follow-up of patients with differentiated thyroid cancer.

This combination of the best imaging and the best therapy to identify the individual who will benefit meets the guiding principle of radionuclide therapy. It will have an impact on the management of differentiated thyroid cancer.

Radionuclide therapy of neuroendocrine tumors

Neuroendocrine tumors have many different types of receptor and their assessment for radionuclide therapy follows the principles outlined above. ^{123}I-MIBG is used for imaging first, before deciding on ^{131}I-MIBG therapy (Chapter 17B). Indium-111 or ^{99m}Tc-octreotide derivative imaging is used before deciding on therapy using ^{90}Y or ^{177}Lu labeled to the same derivatives (Chapter 17B).

Radioimmunotherapy

The contrast between the protocols for ^{131}I-tositumomab therapy and ^{90}Y-ibritumomab tiuxetan is quite striking.[54] For ^{131}I-tositumomab therapy prior imaging and dosimetry is standard following the principles set out above,[55] whereas for ^{90}Y-ibitrumomab tiuxetan therapy, neither the appropriateness of therapy nor the tumor uptake is assessed at all, but the dose is given on a body weight basis.[56] This is justified on the basis of minimizing the bone marrow radiation but at the same time may result in undertreating the tumor burden. Bone marrow depression is likely to be more related to the degree of free ^{90}Y than the weight of the patient. Failure to demonstrate the uptake of the potential therapy agent by imaging a gamma emitting analog helps to exclude those patients whose tumors are without avidity for the therapy agent from unnecessary radiation treatment.

Assessing the likely therapy dose to the tumor is a basic principle of radionuclide therapy. This requires prior imaging and the assessment may be visual (for example tumor uptake more than liver uptake or equal to liver uptake for therapy or less than liver uptake for no therapy) or by detailed dosimetry.[55] In no nuclear medicine practice except for ^{90}Y-ibitrumomab tiuxetan therapy is the therapy dose calculated using body weight and in no way can body weight determine the dose to a tumor. The fact that on the basis of a whole-body calculation it can be argued that the bone marrow dose can be minimized, does not justify giving therapy to a tumor that has not been demonstrated to take up the agent. In our first case of non-Hodgkin's lymphoma treated with ^{90}Y-ibritumomab, in which we undertook dose calculation by the body weight as stipulated by the manufacturer's protocol, this gave in fact approximately one third of the dose limit of the bone marrow as assessed by prior imaging and dosimetry. In other words, three times the amount of activity could have been given to treat this patient's tumor from our dose calculation than that assessed on a body weight basis. Whereas there may be

an upper limit above which a further increase in therapy dose has no benefit to the patient with a tumor, there is clearly a lower limit at which insufficient therapy has no benefit for the patient. Wahl[13] argues convincingly for a tracer dose before therapy to optimize the dose.

The dilemma has to be faced. Should one insist on the nuclear medicine approach to cancer therapy, where potential nonresponders are excluded by negative imaging results or should one follow an approach whereby as long as the marrow is safe, it does not matter whether the tumor receives an adequate or inadequate amount of therapy or whether the patient receives unnecessary radionuclide therapy? The basic principles of nuclear medicine and radiation protection for radionuclide therapy should be followed without exception.[54]

Non-Hodgkin's lymphoma is now being treated using ^{131}I-anti-CD20 B1 antibody, tositumomab (Corixa) or ^{90}Y-anti-CD20 (Schering). Low-grade non-Hodgkin's lymphoma that has relapsed and remitted once or several times after chemotherapy finally relapsing is treated in a two-stage process. First, a small amount of ^{131}I-anti-CD20 B1 (185 MBq, 5 mCi) is infused after an infusion of 450 mg of the 'cold' antibody. Images are taken serially and the whole-body dose equivalent is calculated from this imaging study. Then a calculation is performed to obtain the administered activity for therapy to give a whole-body dose of 75 cGy. This therapy is then infused 1 week later after a further infusion of 450 mg of the unlabeled antibody. Remarkable response rates (ORR 95%) to ^{131}I-tositumomab have been reported in previously untreated advanced stage patients with follicular lymphoma.[57] Seventy-four percent of patients achieved a confirmed CR, and importantly, responses appeared to be durable, with a 5-year progression-free survival of 63%. Patients treated with transformation to large B-cell lymphoma had a similar response rate and duration of remission to therapy to those that had no evidence of transformation. A similarity in response rates (transformed 60% vs. indolent 57%) was also reported by Vose et al.[58] However, in the pivotal study of 23 patients with transformation,[59] the response rate was lower at 39%. Nevertheless, the results are encouraging, as transformation to large B-cell lymphoma presents a difficult clinical challenge with a typically poor outcome.[60] The ability of ^{131}I-tositumomab to achieve a high CR rate is in contrast to that observed with the unconjugated chimeric anti-CD20, rituximab.[61] The relative contribution of ^{131}I linked to tositumomab has been demonstrated in a randomized study comparing unconjugated tositumomab to the ^{131}I-tositumomab treatment schedule. Response rates for the unconjugated antibody were 28% (confirmed CR 8%) compared to 67% (confirmed CR 33%) for the radioiodide conjugate. The best response rates were observed in patients with follicular lymphoma (ORR 79% and CR/CR(u) 59%) representing the largest histological subgroup in our study.[62] This has similarly been observed with rituximab[61] and ^{90}Y-labeled ibritumomab tiuxetan.[63] In small lymphocytic lymphoma, a 62% response rate to ^{131}I-tositumomab has been documented when the data from a number of studies are collated. There is a poor response of this disease to rituximab.[61–66] Yttrium-90-Lym 1 is an alternative approach.[67]

Detection of human anti-mouse antibodies (HAMAs) on serum samples prior to therapy is a contraindication to further therapy as it diverts the antibody bound as an immune complex to the liver, so reducing any direct therapeutic effect. The frequency of HAMA development appears to be less than 5%. This appears to be related to previous exposure to chemotherapy and probably reflects the patient's inability to mount an immunological response.[59] When ^{131}I-tositumomab has been used as a front line therapy, HAMA developed in 63% of patients.[57] The appearance of HAMA had no influence upon response rate or duration or remission. The low seroconversion rate permits consideration of re-treatment in the majority of patients. A response rate of 56% has been reported with ^{131}I-tositumomab used in this context.[68] The presence of HAMA also does not appear to affect the later administration of rituximab. The HAMA response may lead to the development of an idiotype 2 human anti-tumor response, however, which may be beneficial.

An advantage of internal targeting and specific uptake by the targeted cell is the prolonged residence of the radioactivity in the tumor and a crossfire bystander effect for energetic beta-emitting particles so that cells not expressing the antigen may be treated. A disadvantage is that there is a need to handle high amounts of radioactivity so that the patient has to be confined to a special side ward with radiation protection precautions, particularly when ^{131}I is used, with the psychological problems of isolation. Only a few percent of the injected activity is taken up by the tumor. There is a high radiation dose to critical organs, e.g. the marrow especially in heavily chemotherapy pre-treated patients. The main problems are the regulatory delays and expenses of bringing such products to the market.

These problems may be overcome in the following ways. Confinement of the patient can be avoided by using a pure beta emitter such as ^{90}Y or ^{32}P. The high radiation dose to critical organs can be overcome by using a two- or three-stage approach.[28–34] The penetration of tumors can be helped by using small molecules. The regulatory problems can be overcome by using genetically engineered or synthetic mimic molecules, which can undergo better quality control than biological molecules. So, synthesized peptides or genetically engineered monoclonal antibody derivatives with specific receptor or epitope binding of high avidity will begin to replace monoclonal antibodies.

Individualization of therapy

Linking cancer radionuclide imaging with cancer therapy to identify the individual patient who should benefit is not a guarantee of successful treatment but indicates one way forward for individualizing chemotherapy by imaging its radiolabeled analog.[44] Should not medical oncology adopt and develop the same individualization of chemotherapy using, for example, ^{99m}Tc and ^{18}F-estrodial receptor agents and 5-[^{18}F]fluorouracil, as radionuclide therapy by only treating those patients in whom imaging shows that tumor localization of chemotherapy takes place?

In conclusion, radionuclide internal targeted therapy is beginning to prove itself where other therapy has failed or is not available. It should now be given earlier in the course of the disease. Nuclear medicine finds cancer in the individual and treats cancer in the individual by substituting a therapy radionuclide for a gamma-emitting imaging radionuclide when the image confirms potential therapeutic uptake.

REFERENCES

- ● Seminal primary article
- ◆ Key review paper
- ✳ First formal publication of a management guideline

● 1 Britton KE. Towards the goal of cancer specific imaging and therapy. *Nucl Med Commun* 1997; **18**: 992–1007.

● 2 Siddiqi A, Foley RR, Britton KE, *et al.* The role of I-123 diagnostic imaging in the follow up of patients with differentiated thyroid carcinoma as compared to I-131-scanning: avoidance of negative therapeutic uptake due to stunning. *Clin Endocrinol* 2001; **55**: 515–21.

● 3 Britton KE, Granowska M. Radioimmunoscintigraphy in tumour identification. *Cancer Surveys* 1987; **6**: 247–67.

● 4 Bomanji J, Levison DA, Flatman WD, *et al.* Uptake of I-123 metaiodobenzylguanadine by phaeochromocytomas, other paragangliomas and neuroblastomas: a histopathological comparison. *J Nucl Med* 1987; **23**: 973–8.

5 Serafini AN. Systemic metabolic radiotherapy with samarium-153 EDTMP for the treatment of painful bone metastasis. *Q J Nucl Med* 2000; **45**: 91–9.

● 6 Krenning EP, Kwekkeboom DJ, Bakkar WH, *et al.* Somatostatin receptor scintigraphy with [^{111}In-DTPA-D-Phe] and [^{123}I-tyr]-octreotide: the Rotterdam experience with more than 1000 patients. *Eur J Nucl Med* 1993; **20**: 716–31.

● 7 Decristoforo C, Melendez-Alafort L, Sosabowski J, Mather SJ. Tc-99m-HYNIC-[Tyr^3]-octreotide for imaging somatostatin receptor positive tumours: preclinical evaluation and comparison with In-111 octreotide. *J Nucl Med* 2000; **41**: 1114–19.

● 8 Otte A, Mueller-Brand J, Dellas S, *et al.* Yttrium-90-labelled somatostatin analogue for cancer treatment. *Lancet* 1998; **351**: 417–18.

● 9 Paganelli G, Zoboli S, Cremonesi M, *et al.* Receptor-mediated radiotherapy with Y-90-Dota-D-Phe^1-Tyr^3-octreotide. *Eur J Nucl Med* 2001; **28**: 426–34.

10 Kwekkeboom DJ, Bakker WH, Kam BL, *et al.* Treatment of patients with gastro-entero-pancreatic (GEP) tumours with the novel radiolabelled somatostatin analogue [(177)Lu- DOTA(0),Tyr(3)]octreotate. *Eur J Nucl Med Mol Imaging* 2003; **30**: 417–22.

11 Virgolini I, Szilvasi I, Kurtaran A, *et al.* Indium-111-DOTA lanreotide: biodistribution, safety and radiation absorbed dose in tumour patients evaluated by somatostatin receptor mediated radiotherapy. *J Nucl Med* 1998; **39**: 1928–36.

12 Kaminski MS, Zasadny KR, Francis IR, *et al.* Iodine-131 anti-B1 radioimmunotherapy for B cell lymphoma. *J Clin Oncol* 1996; **14**: 1974–81.

13 Wahl RL. The clinical importance of dosimetry in radioimmunotherapy with tositumomab and I-131 tositumomab. *Semin Oncol* 2003; **30(2 Suppl 4)**: 31–8.

14 Witzig T, White C, Wiseman G, *et al.* Phase 1–2 trial of IDEC-Y2B8 radioimmunotherapy for the treatment of relapsed or refractory CD20+ B-cell non-Hodgkin's lymphoma. *J Clin Oncol* 1999; **17**: 3793–803.

15 Wiseman GA, White CA, Stabin M, *et al.* Phase 1/11 Y-90-Zevalin (yttrium-90 ibrutumomab tiuxetan; IDEC-Y2B8) radioimmunotherapy dosimetry results in relapsed or refractory non-Hodgkin's lymphoma. *Eur J Nucl Med* 2000; **27**: 766–70.

16 Smith-Jones PM, Vallabhajosula S, Novarro V, *et al.* Y-90 huJ-591Mab specific to PSMA: radioimmunotherapy studies in nude mice with prostate cancer LN CaP tumour [Abstract]. *Eur J Nucl Med* 2000; **27**: 951.

17 Barone R, Chianelli M, Bottoni U, *et al.* In vivo detection of lymphocytic infiltration in melanoma using ^{99m}Tc-IL2 [Abstract]. *Eur J Nucl Med* 1996; **23**: 1217.

18 Olea E, Zhongyun P, parma EP, *et al.* Efficacy and toxicity of Sm-153 EDTMP in the palliative treatment of painful bone metastases. *World J Nucl Med* 2002; **1**: 21–8.

19 Maxon III HR, Thomas SR, Hertzberg VS, *et al.* Rhenium-186 hydroxyethylidene diphosphonate for the treatment of painful osseous metastases. *Semin Nucl Med* 1992; **22**: 33–40.

20 Liepe K, Kropp J, Runge R, Kotzerke J. Therapeutic efficacy of rhenium-188-HEDP in human prostate cancer skeletal metastases. *Br J Cancer* 2003; **89**: 625–9.

21 Fettich J, Padhy A, Nair N, *et al.* Comparative clinical efficacy and safety of phosphorus-32 and strontium-89 in the palliative treatment of metastatic bone pain: results of an IAEA coordinated research project. *World J Nucl Med* 2003; **2**: 226–31.

22 Britton KE. Highlights lecture of the European Association of Nuclear Medicine and the World Federation of Nuclear Medicine and Biology Congress, Berlin 1998. Where next and how? *Eur J Nucl Med* 1998; **25**: 1671–84.

23 Brans B, Bacher K, Vandevyver V, *et al.* Intra-arterial radionuclide therapy for liver tumours: effect of selectivity of catheterization and ^{131}I-lipiodol delivery on tumour uptake and response. *Nucl Med Commun* 2003; **24**: 391–6.

24 Sundram FX, Jeong J-M, Zanzonico P, *et al.* Transarterial rhenium-188 lipiodol in the treatment of inoperable hepatocellular carcinoma – an IAEA sponsored multicentre phase 1 study. *World J Nucl Med* 2002; **1**: 5–11.

25 Gray B, Van Hazel G, Hope M, *et al.* Randomised trial of SIR-spheres plus chemotherapy vs. chemotherapy alone for treating patients with liver metastases from primary large bowel cancer. *Ann Oncol* 2001; **12**: 1711–20.

26 Goin JE, Dancey JE, Hermann GA, *et al.* Treatment of unresectable colorectal carcinoma to the liver with intrahepatic Y-90 microspheres: dose ranging study. *World J Nucl Med* 2003; **2**: 216–25.

27 Wong CY, Salem R, Raman S, *et al.* Evaluating ^{90}Y-glass microsphere treatment response of unresectable colorectal liver metastases by [^{18}F]FDG PET: a comparison with CT or MRI. *Eur J Nucl Med Mol Imaging* 2002; **29**: 815–20.

28 Cremonesi M, Ferrari M, Chinol M, *et al.* Three step radioimmunotherapy with yttrium-90 biotin: dosimetry and pharmacokinetics in cancer. *Eur J Nucl Med* 1999; **26**: 110–18.

29 Stoldt HS, Aftab F, Chinol M, *et al.* Pretargeting strategies for radio-immunoguided tumour localisation and therapy. *Eur J Cancer* 1997; **33**: 186–92.

30 Breitz H, Weiden PL, Beaumier PL, *et al.* Clinical optimization of pretargeted radioimmunotherapy with antibody streptavidin conjugate and Y-90-DOTA biotin. *J Nucl Med* 2000; **41**: 131–40.

31 Paganelli G, Grana C, Chinol M, *et al.* Antibody guided three-step therapy for high grade glioma with yttrium-90 biotin. *Eur J Nucl Med* 1999; **26**: 348–57.

32 Paganelli G, Bartolomei M, Ferrari M, *et al.* Pretargeted locoregional radioimmunotherapy with ^{90}Y-biotin in glioma patients: phase I study and preliminary therapeutic results. *Cancer Biother Radiopharm* 2001; **16**: 227–35.

33 Paganelli G, Magnani P, Zito F, *et al.* Three-step monoclonal antibody tumor targeting in carcinoembryonic antigen-positive patients. *Cancer Res* 1991; **51**: 5960–6.

34 Dosio F, Magnani P, Paganelli G, *et al.* Three-step tumor pre-targeting in lung cancer immunoscintigraphy. *J Nucl Biol Med* 1993; **37**: 228–32.

35 Mukherjee JJ, Kaltsas GA, Islam N, *et al.* Treatment of metastatic carcinoid tumours, phaeochromocytoma, paraganglioma and medullary carcinoma of the thyroid with (131)I-meta-iodobenzylguanidine [(131)I-mIBG]. *Clin Endocrinol* 2001; **55**: 47–60.

• 36 Bomanji J, Levison DA, Flatman WD, *et al.* Uptake of I-123 metaiodobenzylguanidine by phaeochromo-cytomas, other parangangliomas and neuroblas-tomas. A histopathological comparison. *J Nucl Med* 1987; **23**: 973–8.

♦ 37 Solanki KK, Bomanji J, Mayes J, *et al.* A pharmaco-logical guide to medicines which interfere with the biodistribution of radiolabelled meta-iodobenzyl-guanidine. *Nucl Med Commun* 1992; **13**: 513–21.

• 38 De Jong M, Kwekkeboom D, Valkema R, Krenning EP. Radiolabelled peptides for tumour therapy: current status and future directions. Plenary lecture at the EANM 2002. *Eur J Nucl Med Mol Imaging* 2003; **30**: 463–9.

• 39 Jurcic JG, Larson SM, Sgouros G, *et al.* Targeted alpha particle immunotherapy for myeloid leukemia. *Blood* 2002; **100**: 1233–9.

• 40 Sgouros G, Ballangrud AM, Jurcic JG, *et al.* Pharmacokinetics and dosimetry of an alpha-parti-cle emitter labeled antibody: ^{213}Bi-HuM195 (anti-CD33) in patients with leukemia. *J Nucl Med* 1999; **40**: 1935–46.

• 41 Link EM. Targeting melanoma with ^{211}At/^{131}I-methylene blue: preclinical and clinical experience. *Hybridoma* 1999; **18**: 77–82.

✳ 42 Therasse P, Arbuck SG, Eisenhauer EA, *et al.* New guidelines to evaluate the response to treatment in solid tumours. *J Natl Cancer Inst* 2000; **92**: 205–16.

✳ 43 Therasse P. Measuring clinical response. What does it mean? *Eur J Cancer* 2002; **38**: 1817–23.

♦ 44 Britton KE, Granowska M. Cancer: find and treat the individual, the nuclear medicine approach. *World J Nucl Med* 2002; **1**: 75–9.

• 45 Cohen J, Kalinyak J, McDougall IR. Is 74 MBq ^{123}I useful for whole-body diagnostic scan in patients with differentiated thyroid cancer? *Nucl Med Commun* 2003; **24**: 453.

46 Leger FA, Izembart M, Dagousset F, *et al.* Decreased uptake of therapeutic doses of I-131 after 185 MBq I-131 diagnostic imaging for thyroid remnants in differentiated thyroid cancer. *Eur J Nucl Med* 1998; **25**: 242–6.

• 47 Britton KE, Foley RR, Siddiqi A, *et al.* I-123 imaging for the prediction of I-131 Therapy for recurrent differentiated thyroid cancer, RDTC, when I-131 tracer is negative but raised thyroglobulin [Abstract]. *Eur J Nucl Med* 1999; **26**: 1013.

48 Britton KE, Foley RR, Chew SL. Should hTG levels in the absence of iodine uptake be treated? *Eur J Nucl Med Mol Imaging* 2003; **30**: 794–5.

• 49 Shankar LK, Yamamoto AJ, Alavi A, Mandel SJ. Comparison of I-123 scintigraphy at 5 and 24 hours in patients with differentiated thyroid cancer. *J Nucl Med* 2002; **43**: 72–6.

50 Park HM. Invited commentary: I-123 almost a designer radioiodine for thyroid scanning. *J Nucl Med* 2002; **43**: 77–8.

51 Britton KE, Foley RR. Differentiated thyroid cancer, monitoring with high dose I-123 imaging [Abstract]. *J Nucl Med* 2004; **45(Suppl)**: 288p–9p.

52 Lind P. Should high hTg levels in the absence of iodine uptake be treated? For. *Eur J Med Mol Imaging* 2003; **30**: 157–60.

53 Biermann M, Schober O. Should high hTg levels in the absence of iodine uptake be treated? Against. *Eur J Med Mol Imaging* 2003; **30**: 160–3.

54 Britton KE. Radioimmunotherapy of non-Hodgkin's lymphoma. *J Nucl Med* 2004; **45**: 924–5.

• 55 Koral KF, Dewaraja R, Li J, *et al.* Update on hybrid conjugate-view SPECT tumour dosimetry and response in I-131 tositumomab therapy of previ-ously untreated lymphoma patients. *J Nucl Med* 2003; **44**: 457–64.

• 56 Wiseman GA, Kornmehl E, Leigh B, *et al.* Radiation dosimetry results and safety correlations from ^{90}Y-ibritumomab tiuxetan radioimmunotherapy for relapsed or refractory non-Hodgkin's lym-phoma: combined data from four clinical trials. *J Nucl Med* 2003; **44**: 465–74.

• 57 Kaminski MS, Tuck M, Regan D, *et al.* High response rates and durable remissions in patients previously untreated, advanced stage, follicular lymphoma treated with tositumomab and iodine I-131 tositumomab (Bexxar™) [Abstract]. *Blood* 2002; **100**: 1384.

• 58 Vose JM, Wahl RL, Saleh M, *et al.* Multicenter phase II study of iodine-131 tositumomab for chemotherapy-relapsed/refractory low-grade and transformed low-grade B-cell non-Hodgkin's lymphomas. *J Clin Oncol* 2000; **18**: 1316–23.

• 59 Kaminski MS, Zelenetz AD, Press OW, *et al.* Pivotal study of iodine I-131 tositumomab for chemotherapy-refractory low-grade or transformed low-grade B-cell non-Hodgkin's lymphomas. *J Clin Oncol* 2001; **19**: 3918–28.

• 60 Bastion Y, Sebban C, Berger F, *et al.* Incidence, pre-dictive factors, and outcome of lymphoma transfor-mation in follicular lymphoma patients. *J Clin Oncol* 1997; **15**: 1587–94.

• 61 McLaughlin P, Grillo-Lopez AJ, Link BK, *et al.* Rituximab chimeric anti-CD20 monoclonal anti-body therapy for relapsed indolent lymphoma: half of patients respond to a four-dose treatment pro-gram. *J Clin Oncol* 1998; **16**: 2825–33.

62 Davis T, Kaminski MS, Leonard J, *et al.* Results of a randomised study of Bexxar™ (tositumomab and I-131 tositumomab) vs unlabelled tositumomab in patients with relapsed or refractory low-grade or transformed non-Hodgkin's lymphoma (NHL) [Abstract]. *Blood* 2001; **98**: 843.

• 63 Witzig TE, Gordon LI, Cabanillas F, *et al.* Randomized controlled trial of yttrium-90-labeled ibritumomab tiuxetan radioimmunotherapy versus rituximab immunotherapy for patients with relapsed or refractory low-grade, follicular, or transformed B-cell non-Hodgkin's lymphoma. *J Clin Oncol* 2002; **20**: 2453–63.

● 64   Foran JM, Gupta RK, Cunningham D, *et al.* A UK multicentre phase II study of rituximab (chimaeric anti-CD20 monoclonal antibody) in patients with follicular lymphoma, with PCR monitoring of molecular response. *Br J Haematol* 2000; **109**: 81–8.

● 65   Wiseman GA, Gordon LI, Multani PS, *et al.* Ibritumomab tiuxetan radioimmunotherapy for patients with relapsed or refractory non-Hodgkin lymphoma and mild thrombocytopenia: a phase II multicenter trial. *Blood* 2002; **99**: 4336–42.

● 66   Witzig TE, Flinn IW, Gordon LI, *et al.* Treatment with ibritumomab tiuxetan radioimmunotherapy in patients with rituximab-refractory follicular non-Hodgkin's lymphoma. *J Clin Oncol* 2002; **20**: 3262–9.

● 67   De Nardo GL, O'Donnell RT, Shen S, *et al.* Radiation dosimetry for ^{90}Y-21T-BAD-Lym-1 extrapolated from pharmacokinetics using ^{111}In-2IT BAD-Lym-1 in patients with non-Hodgkin's lymphoma. *J Nucl Med* 2000; **41**: 952–8.

● 68   Kaminski MS, Estes J, Zasadny KR, *et al.* Radioimmunotherapy with iodine (131)I tositumomab for relapsed or refractory B-cell non-Hodgkin lymphoma: updated results and long-term follow-up of the University of Michigan experience. *Blood* 2000; **96**: 1259–66.

APPENDIX: GUIDELINES FOR SYSTEMIC RADIONUCLIDE THERAPY FOR CANCER

Introduction

Each patient must be considered on an individual basis, but there are common elements to all radionuclide therapy, as indicated in the following check list.

Indications

Patients referred for systemic radionuclide therapy for cancer must have had an imaging 'tracer' scan showing positive uptake by the tumor. This is an essential part of the justification of therapy procedure.

The imaging report should indicate that therapy with a beta-emitting equivalent of the imaging agent would be beneficial.

Contraindications

Pregnancy or breast-feeding
Negative 'tracer' scan or insufficient uptake to justify therapy
Over the safety limit from previous radionuclide therapies
Open discharging wounds, incontinence, severe systemic disease
Need for excessive close-contact nursing, terminality
Moderately to severely impaired renal or liver function
Moderate to severely impaired blood, leukocyte and or platelet count
Surgery contemplated in the near future

Referrers

The list of or criteria for competent referrers should be documented under local or national rules.

Referrers should indicate on the request card that the patient had a positive imaging 'tracer' scan before the first therapy, or else indicate the number and timing of previous radionuclide therapy.

They should confirm nonpregnancy (although a pregnancy test MUST be performed immediately prior to therapy if appropriate).

They should state the level of liver and renal function and the blood count or that these are satisfactory.

Booking method

These patients must be treated under an established protocol.

The patient or guardian must have spoken to the physicist/physician responsible for the therapy to arrange a date to discuss the procedure and radiation protection issues.

The patient information leaflet is to be given to patient by the clinician/nuclear medicine staff with confirmation of therapy date.

A radionuclide therapy side room must be booked for an appropriate number of nights following the day of administration, if it is not an outpatient procedure.

Waiting time and medication

The waiting time is generally dependent on the availability of the therapy ward side room.

Interfering drugs must be stopped for the appropriate period of time. Other sources of interference must be considered, for example iodine in skin preparations or hair dye.

Dietary recommendations may be advised.

All blood and urine investigations should be completed before the therapy is given.

The fitness, both mental and physical health, of the patient for isolation and self-caring must be assessed.

Ordering of radiopharmaceutical

Once the therapy date has been arranged, a request card signed by an authorized documented license holder for radionuclide therapy should be given to the radio-pharmacist or physicist responsible for nuclear medicine therapy, with the date of the therapy clearly written on the card.

The radiopharmaceutical and the dose required should be written on the card clearly by the prescriber and signed and dated. Deviations from the 'standard' dose should be explained and recorded.

Preparation and measurement of dose

The radionuclide therapy dose will usually arrive on the day of administration coordinated with the admission of the patient. The activity may not be sufficient to allow administration the following day. The packing notes should be given to the radiopharmacy technician to enter in the delivery book. Ensure the radionuclide therapy dose has defrosted, if appropriate. It is recommended to wear a white coat, film badge, and thermoluminescence finger badges. An instantaneous dosemeter is also useful. Gloves must be worn.

Check the request card and enter the patient details into the therapy administration book together with the relevant details from the lead pot containing the radionuclide therapy. Set the calibrator for the particular radionuclide and change the normal cylindrical holder for the one for therapy.

Measure the activity and have the reading witnessed. Confirm that the amount agrees to that on the manufacturer's lead pot, using the reference date, as well as the prescribed dose. Enter the amount in each vial into the therapy book.

Return the vials to their protective pots and put them on the administration trolley behind the lead shield. Set a radiation sign so that it is visible.

Personnel able to administer therapy

Designated nuclear medicine staff must be listed in the local rules.

A nuclear medicine physicist, physician or principal radio-pharmacist should oversee the administration.

Patient preparation

On the day of admission, the ward doctors and nurses should be requested to admit the patient within a reasonable time.

All necessary blood tests should be done prior to therapy; it is generally necessary to obtain the results of some of these before administering the dose.

If appropriate, nonpregnancy must be confirmed.

Prior to dose administration, explain the procedure to the patient and counsel them about the radiation risks and precautions necessary. Discuss the patient's home circumstances with them as this will affect their discharge date (a preliminary discussion will have been made at the initial contact).

Familiarize them with the therapy suite and advise how to minimize the waste produced. Discuss the procedure for receiving food etc.

A 'consent form' must be signed by the patient agreeing to remain in the therapy suite during treatment and to abide by any radiation protection advice given. It should be witnessed and signed by the operator.

Just before therapy administration, ensure that all relevant admission checks have been completed and that the patient has everything they require.

If intravenous therapy is to be given, the patient will have had an antecubital vein canulated by the appropriate nurse or physician administering the infusion of the therapy with appropriate precautions and shielding.

Therapy administration

Take the trolley to the ward and positively identify the patient using their name, address, and date of birth.

Switch on the radiation warning light outside the therapy suite or attach a 'Controlled Area' radiation sign to the door.

Flush the patient's cannula using a syringe of saline and then attach the giving set.

Spray the top of the radionuclide therapy vial with alcohol and then insert the infusion set arm. Insert the air vent needle with filter.

It is helpful to also insert a needle with a three-way tap on an extension tube at this time since the access to the vial top is very restricted.

Set the infusion rate to the rate indicated in the protocol, for example $300 \, \text{mL} \, \text{h}^{-1}$ and start the infusion. Once the vial has emptied, it may be flushed by injecting approximately 15 mL of saline

If the infusion is through a Hickman line, extra flushing is necessary to ensure that the radionuclide therapy does not remain in the tubing.

After the infusion has finished, the cannula may be removed unless the patient is likely to require intravenous antiemetics. Cannulas left *in situ* must be subsequently retrieved by nuclear medicine staff.

Collect all potential radioactive waste for return to nuclear medicine.

Ensure that the emergency telephone numbers and the digital dosemeter are outside the room together with plastic aprons, gloves, and overshoes.

Inform the nurses that the patient is 'loaded' or 'active' and write in the patient's notes that the therapy has been carried out and its details.

On returning to the department, measure the residual activity in the vials and using a dose rate meter, estimate the waste in the sharps bin containing the tubing.

Calculate the amount administered and write this in the therapy book, on the request card, and on the dose administration card.

Dispose of the empty vials in the sharps bin, label it with the date and activity, and take it to the main radioactive waste store at the first convenient moment. Enter the amount into the 'waste spreadsheet'.

Carry out full personal contamination monitoring using a radiation monitor and record the results. Monitor the therapy trolley also for contamination.

Post-therapy scan

Depending on the nature of the therapy agent a post-therapy scan is undertaken 1–5 days after the therapy. For pure beta emitters, the patient may be imaged with the gamma camera set for Bremsstrahlung. The nuclear medicine physicist should estimate the residual activity.

Decontamination of the therapy suite

After the patient has left the room, it must be decontaminated prior to the domestic cleaners entering. Follow the authorized procedure. Switch off the radiation sign or remove the 'Controlled Area' card. Once the room has been checked, inform either the domestic cleaner or the senior ward nurse that the room can be cleaned.

Follow-up

Clinical follow-up must be arranged with appropriate monitoring by clinical response, blood tests, nuclear medicine, and radiological imaging.

ACKNOWLEDGMENT

The help of Ms Rosemary R. Foley, clinical physicist, is gratefully acknowledged.

3

The imaging of infection and inflammation

OTTO C. BOERMAN, CHANTAL P. BLEEKER-ROVERS, HUUB J. RENNEN, WIM J.G. OYEN, AND FRANS H. CORSTENS

Introduction	93	Receptor binding ligands for imaging infection and inflammation	97
Radiopharmaceuticals available for imaging infection and inflammation	93	Tracers for visualizing infiltrating neutrophils	98
Imaging infection in patients with infectious or inflammatory disorders	95	Tracers for visualizing infiltrating mononuclear cells	100
		References	102

INTRODUCTION

Scintigraphic visualization of the localization of infection and inflammation is a challenging problem in clinical practice because it may have important implications for the management of patients with infectious or inflammatory disorders. In order to enable clinicians to rapidly commence the most appropriate treatment, adequate delineation and diagnosis of inflammatory foci in these patients is of critical importance. If the clinical history and physical examination are indecisive, the clinician can choose from several diagnostic modalities to determine the localization, extent, and severity of the disease. New, highly sensitive, radiological investigations like magnetic resonance imaging (MRI) and spiral computerized tomography (CT) are able to locate relatively small focal abnormalities. However, these radiological methods rely on morphological changes, and as a result they are less accurate in the early stages of infection or inflammation and are unable to discriminate active processes from anatomical changes due to a cured infection or after surgery (scar tissue).

In contrast, radiopharmaceuticals used for imaging infection and inflammation accumulate in the infectious/inflammatory lesion due to the locally changed physiological condition, such as enhanced blood flow, enhanced vascular permeability, or influx of leukocytes. Thus, scintigraphic imaging does not depend on morphological changes, but is based on physiochemical processes in tissues. Therefore, scintigraphic techniques can also visualize infectious foci in their early phases, when morphological changes are not yet apparent. In addition, scintigraphic imaging is an excellent noninvasive method of whole-body scanning that can determine the extent of the infectious or inflammatory disease throughout the body. Here the characteristics of the radiopharmaceuticals that are currently used for imaging infection and inflammation are reviewed. In addition, the status and potential of the agents that are currently under development are discussed.

RADIOPHARMACEUTICALS AVAILABLE FOR IMAGING INFECTION AND INFLAMMATION

To date there are at least four classes of radiopharmaceuticals that are commercially available for imaging infection or inflammation: (1) gallium-67 citrate, (2) radiolabeled leukocytes, (3) radiolabeled anti-granulocyte antibody preparations, and (4) 2-[^{18}F]fluoro-2-deoxy-D-glucose (^{18}F-FDG).

Gallium-67 citrate

The use of gallium-67 citrate for infection and inflammation imaging was described for the first time in 1971.[1,2] Upon intravenous injection ^{67}Ga binds to transferrin, and the ^{67}Ga–transferrin complex extravasates at the site of inflammation due to the locally enhanced vascular permeability.[3] In the inflammatory lesion ^{67}Ga may transchelate to lactoferrin as present in leukocytes.[4] Gallium-67 is excreted partly via the kidneys, and at later time points also via the gastrointestinal tract. Physiological uptake of ^{67}Ga is observed in the liver, bone, bone marrow, and bowel.

Radiolabeled leukocytes

Because it was known that leukocytes actively migrate from the circulation into the inflamed tissue, in the 1970s the *in vivo* localization of radiolabeled leukocyte preparations was studied. McAfee and Thakur[5] labeled leukocytes with ^{111}In complexed as ^{111}In-oxinate. After intravenous administration, the labeled cells home into the lungs with subsequent rapid clearance from them. The radiolabeled leukocytes rapidly clear from the blood and some of the cells accumulate in the infected/inflamed tissue, while a substantial portion of the leukocytes (presumably the damaged cells) accumulate in the spleen. Three phases can be distinguished in the migration of the radiolabeled leukocytes from the circulation into inflamed tissue: (1) adherence to the vascular endothelium due to locally enhanced expression of adhesion molecules; (2) diapedesis: active migration through the endothelial lining and the basal membrane; and (3) chemotaxis: active migration up the chemotactic gradient into the affected tissue. Ten years later, the labeling of leukocytes with ^{99m}Tc was developed using the lipophilic chelator hexamethylpropylene amine oxime (HMPAO).[6] Due to the more optimal radiation characteristics of ^{99m}Tc for scintigraphic application ^{99m}Tc-labeled leukocytes have replaced ^{111}In-labeled leukocytes for most indications.

Radiolabeled anti–granulocyte antibodies

The main limitation of the use of radiolabeled leukocytes is their cumbersome preparation. Therefore investigators have tried to develop a method that allows the *in vivo* labeling of leukocytes (as opposed to their labeling *ex vivo*). The use of radiolabeled monoclonal antibodies against surface antigens of granulocytes was one of the first approaches tested to accomplish *in vivo* labeling of leukocytes. Two of these preparations are now available as radiopharmaceuticals for infection/inflammation imaging: anti-CD67 IgG (anti-NCA-95, BW250/183),[7] and anti-CD66 Fab′ (Leukoscan®)[8–10] (Fig. 3.1), and a third preparation, the anti-CD15 IgM (Neutrospec®, anti-CD15)[11,12] was recalled from the market in December 2005, after two fatalities attributed to cardiopulmonary failure within 30 minutes of injection. With each of these ^{99m}Tc-labeled anti-granulocyte antibody preparations infectious and inflammatory foci can be delineated. The actual mechanism by which these antibody preparations accumulate in infectious or inflammatory lesions has been a matter of debate. Initially, it was thought that the antibodies would bind to circulating granulocytes and subsequently migrate to the lesion. Alternatively, the antibodies could also target cells that have already migrated into the interstitial space of an inflammatory lesion. For the anti-CD67 antibody it was shown that only 5–10% of the ^{99m}Tc activity in the blood was associated with circulating granulocytes.[13] Skehan *et al.* carefully compared the kinetics of ^{99m}Tc-labeled anti-CD66 Fab′ and

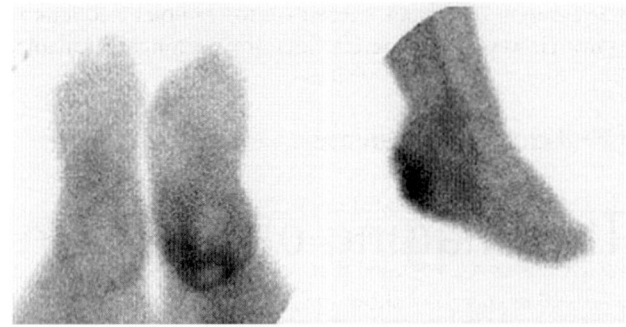

Figure 3.1 *Images of the feet of a 64-year-old female with diabetes 5 h after injection of ^{99m}Tc-anti-CD66 (Leukoscan®). Note the increased uptake in posterior aspect of left calcaneus with central photopenic area (left panel). The osteomyelitic lesion is also visualized on the left lateral view (right panel).*

^{99m}Tc-HSA in the blood, the inflammatory focus and in the control tissue.[14] This analysis confirmed that the ^{99m}Tc-anti-CD66 Fab′ fragments did not localize in inflammation as a result of binding to circulating granulocytes.

Apart from antibodies directed against surface antigens expressed on granulocytes, investigators have tried to use antibodies directed against bacteria which, theoretically, would allow specific detection of the micro-organism causing the infection.[15] However, these studies have shown that IgG molecules show enhanced extravasation in any inflamed tissue, due to the locally enhanced vascular permeability.[16] This finding was exploited by using human nonspecific polyclonal immunoglobulin (HIG) for infection and inflammation imaging. HIG was labeled with ^{111}In and ^{99m}Tc and extensively characterized clinically. Both ^{111}In and ^{99m}Tc-labeled HIG have a long circulatory half-life and physiological uptake in the liver and spleen. A general limitation is the long time span of at least 24 h between injection and diagnosis. In a comparative study, it was shown that ^{99m}Tc-HIG labeled via the chelator hydrazinonicotinamide (HYNIC) has *in vivo* characteristics highly similar to those of ^{111}In-HIG and in most cases is suitable for replacing the ^{111}In-labeled compound.[17] ^{99m}Tc-HIG imaging, however, has more limited sensitivity in chest disease and in chronic inflammatory processes than ^{111}In-HIG scintigraphy.[18] Direct comparison of ^{111}In-HIG and ^{111}In-leukocytes in 35 patients with various subacute infections showed a slightly, but significantly better overall accuracy of ^{111}In-HIG scintigraphy.[19] The major indication for imaging with radiolabeled HIG is localization of acute infection or inflammation of the musculoskeletal system.[20–22] In addition, ^{111}In-HIG scintigraphy is clinically useful in pulmonary infection, particularly in immunocompromised patients.[23–25] In conclusion, [111]In- or ^{99m}Tc-HIG scintigraphy can be successfully used in various infectious and inflammatory diseases with a diagnostic accuracy comparable to that of radiolabeled leukocytes. When facilities for labeling leukocytes are not available or severely granulocytic patients require imaging, HIG scintigraphy can be an alternative for radiolabeled leukocytes. However, commercial kits are no longer available, impeding its general clinical use.

[¹⁸F]fluorodeoxyglucose

The widespread successful use of 2-[¹⁸F]fluoro-2-deoxy-D-glucose (¹⁸F-FDG) for the detection of a wide range of malignancies has revealed that not only neoplastic cells but also leukocytes may show enhanced uptake of ¹⁸F-FDG. In fact, all activated leukocytes (granulocytes, monocytes, and lymphocytes) have enhanced uptake of ¹⁸F-FDG, and thus acute and chronic inflammatory processes can be imaged with FDG PET.[26] There have been many reports of ¹⁸F-FDG accumulation in different infections and inflammatory lesions,[27,28] and with the growing availability of PET scanners it is expected that the imaging of infection by using ¹⁸F-FDG PET will acquire its place in clinical practice in the near future. Obviously, FDG PET is not specific for infection because tumor lesions, inflammatory lesions, and granuloma will also be detected by this technique.

IMAGING INFECTION IN PATIENTS WITH INFECTIOUS OR INFLAMMATORY DISORDERS

Infected joint prostheses

An important group of patients referred to nuclear medicine physicians for the imaging of infection is patients with suspected infection of a joint prosthesis. In most patients the complications of prosthetic joint surgery are readily diagnosed. A significant number of patients with joint prostheses presents with aseptic loosening of the prosthesis (50% within 10 years after implantation) as can be determined radiographically.[29,30] However, 1–3% of the patients with joint prostheses present with infected implants[31] and the differentiation between aseptic loosening from infection can be difficult. In cases where there is a suspicion of any type of postoperative complication, a negative bone scintigraphy effectively rules out any complication.[32] However, the majority of the infections occur within 1 year after implantation, and at that time enhanced periprosthetic uptake is observed on the bone scan in most patients.[33] Therefore, an abnormal bone scan will require additional studies to determine the cause of the abnormality. Although not the ideal agent in these patients gallium-67 citrate can be used to delineate infected prostheses, with a moderate overall accuracy of 70–80%.[33,34] Radiolabeled leukocytes can very accurately delineate infections in this patient population. However, in many cases the physiological uptake of the labeled leukocytes in the bone marrow complicates the interpretation of the images. In combination with sulfur colloid, which accumulates in active marrow but not in infection, the diagnostic accuracy for diagnosing painful prosthesis exceeds 90% (Fig. 3.2).[35]

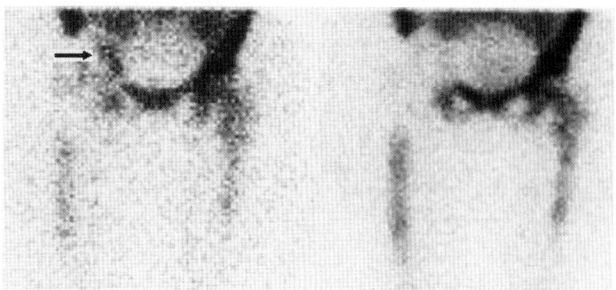

Figure 3.2 *Patient with a 2-year-old cementless right total hip replacement. Scintigraphic images after injection of ¹¹¹In-labeled leukocytes (left panel) and ⁹⁹ᵐTc-colloid bone marrow scan (right panel). Note the leukocyte uptake adjacent to the prosthesis (arrow) in an area without normal bone marrow activity. The prosthesis was infected with MRSA. (Images were kindly provided by Dr C.J. Palestro, Long Island Jewish Medical Center, Division of Nuclear Medicine, New Hyde Park, NY, USA.)*

Furthermore, infected prostheses can be diagnosed very accurately using radiolabeled anti-granulocyte antibody preparations. In a study of 53 patients with infected joint prostheses Leukoscan® (⁹⁹ᵐTc-labeled anti-CD66 Fab′) had a diagnostic accuracy of 88%, as compared to 81% for radiolabeled leukocytes.[8] Finally, the first PET studies indicate that ¹⁸F-FDG is exquisitely sensitive for delineating infected prostheses. However, ¹⁸F-FDG PET does not allow differentiation between aseptic loosening of prostheses and infected prostheses.[36,37]

Osteomyelitis

A three-phase bone scan in otherwise normal bone is able to diagnose osteomyelitis with high sensitivity and specificity. Obviously, in patients with other osseous abnormalities, the specificity of the bone scan is much lower. In those patients gallium-67 citrate or radiolabeled leukocytes can be applied to increase the specificity. Radiolabeled leukocytes are less suitable for diagnosing chronic low-grade osteomyelitis, however. In patients suspected of vertebral osteomyelitis radiolabeled leukocytes can not be used because these images will show a photopenic defect in the spine. The preferred technique for patients with disease localized in the vertebrae is a ⁹⁹ᵐTc-methylene diphosphonate (⁹⁹ᵐTc-MDP) scan and gallium-67 citrate scanning. In the case of spinal osteomyelitis, the ⁹⁹ᵐTc-MDP scan will show intense uptake in the affected vertebrae with a reduction of the space between the disks.

In several studies, ¹⁸F-FDG PET enabled correct visualization of spondylodiscitis.[28–40] ¹⁸F-FDG PET proved to be superior to MRI, gallium-67 citrate scintigraphy, and a three-phase bone scan in these patients.[39,41] ¹⁸F-FDG PET was also able to differentiate between mild infection and degenerative changes.[41,42] PET images are not disturbed by the presence of metallic implants, which is a major advantage when compared to CT and MRI. In addition, ¹⁸F-FDG

PET is a very sensitive tool even for chronic and low-grade infections. Thus, ^{18}F-FDG PET is very useful in cases of suspected osteomyelitis of the central skeleton[43] or chronic low-grade infections of the peripheral skeleton.[44,45]

Pulmonary infections

Gallium-67 citrate can be used for imaging of suspected pulmonary infections. In these patients the physiological uptake of ^{67}Ga in the gastrointestinal tract will not deteriorate the images. The sensitivity of gallium-67 citrate for imaging infections in the chest region is good, but the specificity is relatively low. Furthermore, due to the relatively high radiation burden and the delay of 1–3 days between injection and imaging time, nowadays gallium-67 citrate scanning is replaced by high-resolution chest computed tomography. Radiolabeled white blood cells can very effectively visualize sarcoidosis, interstitial pneumonia, tuberculosis, and other pulmonary infections. In many cases radiolabeled leukocytes or gallium-67 citrate can also be used to assess the location and extent of disease, differentiating active disease from scar tissue, guiding potential biopsy, and determining recurrence and response to therapy. More recent studies indicate that pulmonary infections can be imaged effectively with ^{18}F-FDG PET. Although the differentiation between neoplasm and infection with ^{18}F-FDG PET may be difficult, ^{18}F-FDG PET has a high sensitivity for imaging a variety of benign pulmonary disorders.[46]

Abdominal infections

Early treatment following rapid and accurate diagnosis of intra-abdominal infections has shown to improve outcome.[47–49] For this purpose, ultrasonography, CT, and MRI are currently considered the modalities of choice.[50] However, in early stages of infections without anatomical changes, or in postoperative patients with equivocal anatomical changes, scintigraphic imaging can be very useful.[51,52] Although gallium-67 citrate has a reasonable diagnostic accuracy for diagnosing abdominal infection, the physiological gastrointestinal uptake of this tracer limits the interpretation of the images.[53] Therefore gallium-67 citrate is not the agent of choice for diagnosing abdominal infections. Radiolabeled white blood cells are the most suitable radiopharmaceutical in these patients. Because ^{111}In-labeled leukocytes normally do not localize in the gastrointestinal tract, they have an advantage over ^{99m}Tc-labeled leukocytes. In a study of 170 patients suspected of abdominal infections the use of ultrasound, CT, and ^{111}In-leukocytes, the leukocyte scanning had a sensitivity of 86% for detecting abdominal abscesses.[54] Based on these data the authors recommended that patients who are not critically ill and/or who have no localizing signs should be studied first with ^{111}In-labeled leukocytes.

Fever of unknown origin

In patients with fever of unknown origin (FUO), imaging with radiolabeled leukocytes is not very helpful because in this patient population only 25–35% of the patients actually have an infection.[55] Patients with FUO can be classified into four categories: infections, tumors, noninfectious inflammatory diseases, and miscellaneous, and in this subgroup of patients an imaging agent that also gives diagnostic information in the patients without infection is more valuable. Because ^{18}F-FDG accumulates in inflammatory foci and in a wide range of neoplastic lesions it appears to be a very suitable agent in patients with FUO. The percentage of ^{18}F-FDG PET scans helpful in the diagnostic process in patients with FUO varied from 37 to 69%.[56–59] In a retrospective study of 16 patients with FUO in whom conventional diagnostics had not been conclusive, Lorenzen et al.[59] found that ^{18}F-FDG PET was helpful in 69%. Meller et al.[58] prospectively studied the utility of ^{18}F-FDG coincidence imaging in 20 patients with FUO. In 55% of these patients ^{18}F-FDG PET was helpful in establishing a final diagnosis. The positive predictive value was 90% and the negative predictive value was 75%, compared to a positive predictive value of 75% for ^{67}Ga scintigraphy in the same patients and a negative predictive value of 70%. In a prospective study of 58 patients with FUO, Blockmans et al.[60] demonstrated that ^{18}F-FDG PET was helpful in 41% of the patients. Gallium-67 scintigraphy was only helpful in 25% of a subgroup of 40 patients in the same study. In 35 patients with FUO, Bleeker-Rovers et al.[56] found that ^{18}F-FDG PET was helpful in the diagnostic process of 13 patients (37%), while the probability of a diagnosis was only 54% (Fig. 3.3).

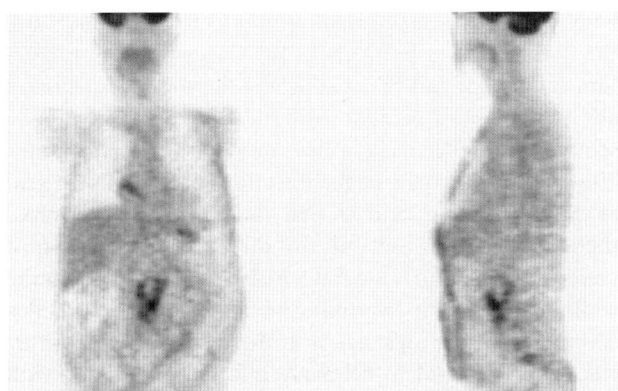

Figure 3.3 ^{18}F-FDG PET scan of a 59-year-old man with an infected aorta. The patient was admitted with fever, chills and pain in the lower abdomen. He had an aneurysm of the abdominal aorta. Blood cultures repeatedly showed Salmonella. Note the increased FDG uptake in the abdominal aorta. Surgical excision of the aneurysm confirmed the presence of a Salmonella infection of the aortic aneurysm.

Vascular graft infections

In general, to visualize infectious vascular lesions it is preferable that a radiopharmaceutical with a relatively short residence time in the circulation is used. The background activity of the images obtained with ^{67}Ga and radiolabeled IgGs in many cases is too high for accurate visualization of vascular lesions. Vascular infections can be very accurately detected with radiolabeled white blood cells. In a study in 162 patients with vascular graft infection, the overall sensitivity, specificity, and accuracy of ^{111}In-labeled leukocytes was 100%, 92.5%, and 97.5%, respectively.[61]

Although, so far, there is only limited clinical experience ^{18}F-FDG PET also appears to be a useful tool for detecting vascular infections. Stumpe et al.[41] studied 10 patients with suspected blood vessel graft infection with ^{18}F-FDG PET. In five patients with infection, the lesions were successfully identified while the scans in the patients without infection were negative. Similarly, Chacko et al.[44] reported the correct identification of vascular graft infection in three patients with ^{18}F-FDG PET.

Vasculitis

Vasculitis is a collective noun for a wide range of inflammatory vascular diseases characterized by the interaction of immune cells with cells of the vessel wall, such as giant cell arteritis, polymyalgia rheumatica, polyarteritis nodosa, Takayasu, Churge–Strauss, Wegener's granulomatosis, and vasculitis skin. The detection of vascular inflammation and monitoring of the activity of the disease is still a challenging clinical problem. Various radiopharmaceuticals have been tested for the diagnosis of vasculitis. Gallium-67 citrate scintigraphy had a 94% specificity and a 90% positive predictive value in patients with temporal arteritis.[62] Reuter et al.[63] showed that radiolabeled leukocyte scintigraphy was superior to conventional angiography and CT for detecting and monitoring vasculitis of the respiratory tract. In contrast, ^{111}In-leukocyte scintigraphy had a low sensitivity in patients with Takayasu arteritis.[64] More recent reports suggest that ^{18}F-FDG PET is a useful imaging technique for diagnosing and determining the extent of various forms of vasculitis. In 25 patients with biopsy-proven temporal arteritis or polymyalgia rheumatica Blockmans et al.[57] found a sensitivity of ^{18}F-FDG PET of 56%, a specificity of 98%, a positive predictive value of 93%, and a negative predictive value of 80%. Bleeker-Rovers studied the use of ^{18}F-FDG PET in 27 patients suspected of vasculitis. ^{18}F-FDG PET results were true positive in 10 patients, true negative in 14 patients and false negative in three patients, resulting in a positive predictive value of 100% and a negative predictive value of 82%.[65] These recent studies also suggest that ^{18}F-FDG PET may become a useful tool for evaluating the effect of treatment of vasculitis.

Each of the radiopharmaceuticals that are currently available for infection imaging has its limitations. The applicability of gallium-67 citrate is limited due to the physiological bowel uptake, the high radiation dose and the long time interval between injection and imaging. Despite the high diagnostic accuracy of radiolabeled leukocytes, the cumbersome and time-consuming preparation is an important limitation of this radiopharmaceutical. Furthermore, the diagnostic accuracy of radiolabeled anti-granulocyte antibody preparations in various patient populations is insufficient, while ^{18}F-FDG can only be applied in PET centers. Therefore, there is still a need for a better agent to image infection or inflammation. Currently this search focuses on agents that avidly bind to receptors expressed on cells involved in the inflammatory response.

RECEPTOR BINDING LIGANDS FOR IMAGING INFECTION AND INFLAMMATION

Inflammation is the response of tissues to injury in order to bring plasma proteins and peptides and immune cells to the site of damage. This tissue damage can be caused by contamination with a foreign species (bacteria, viruses, asbestos and others), neoplasm or trauma. If the inflammation is due to contamination with micro-organisms, the inflammation is referred to as an infection. In the first century, Cornelius Celsus wrote that there are four cardinal signs of inflammation: redness and swelling with heat and pain ('rubor et tumor cum calore et dolore'). In fact, up to now these characteristics are still used to recognize acute inflammation. In the first half of the twentieth century it was recognized that the inflammatory response consists of three components: (1) increased blood flow in the region, (2) increased permeability of the blood vessels in the inflamed tissue, and (3) influx of leukocytes. Due to these processes leukocytes and plasma are recruited in order to repair the injured tissue. The plasma contains defensive proteins such as antibodies, complement factors, and opsonins.

As indicated above, the currently used radiopharmaceuticals for infection imaging, gallium-67 citrate and radiolabeled leukocytes, exploit the enhanced vascular permeability and the influx of leukocytes in inflamed tissue, respectively. During the past two decades various analogs of receptor-binding ligands for receptors expressed on leukocyte subsets have been tested for imaging infection and inflammation. Apart from the defensive proteins in plasma, a large variety of chemical mediators (e.g. interleukins, chemotactic factors, vascular mediators) appear in the affected region which regulate the activity of the immune cells in the region. The immune cells involved (granulocytes, monocytes, and lymphocytes) have specific receptors on their cell surface for these chemical mediators. In general, these chemical mediators have a high affinity ($K_d = 10^{-8}$ to 10^{-10} M) for the receptors on the leukocyte plasma membrane. Their high affinity makes these mediators suitable vehicles for the scintigraphic visualization of the homing of leukocytes in infectious and inflammatory foci. An overview of the receptor-binding ligands involved and their role in the inflammatory response will be given here.

The inflammatory response

As mentioned above, the inflammatory response is triggered by tissue injury. Due to the injury mast cells and basophils release histamine, while platelets may release serotonin. Histamine and serotonin act on the blood vessels, enhancing vasodilatation, vascular permeability, and the expression of P-selectin and platelet activating factor (PAF). The enhanced P-selectin expression causes adhesion of neutrophils to the endothelial lining (rolling), helping PAF to interact with the PAF receptor. As a result, the expression of E-selectin is enhanced and the neutrophils are more avidly bound to the endothelial lining (arrest). Under the influence of chemotactic factors (complement factor 5a (C5a) and leukotriene B_4 (LTB$_4$)) the activated neutrophils migrate through the gaps between the endothelial cells, across the basement membrane (diapedesis) and up the chemotactic gradient. Due to the diapedesis the Hageman factor is activated, triggering the kinin and plasmin systems. This results in release of bradykinin and fibrinopeptides that further increase the blood supply and the vascular permeability in the region. The inflammatory response can also be initiated by bacterial products like endotoxin and formyl-methionyl-leucyl-phenylalanine (f-Met-Leu-Phe) that may act on monocytes and granulocytes, respectively.

The inflammatory response continues because locally produced prostaglandins increase vasodilation and permeability. Macrophages secrete the proinflammatory cytokines interleukin-1 (IL-1) and tumor necrosis factor-α (TNF-α), and these cytokines stimulate neutrophils and endothelial cells to release various chemokines (e.g. IL-8, NAP-2, PF-4, GCP-2, ENA-78, and IP-10) regulating the influx of neutrophils. In a later stage, chemotactic factors like monocyte chemotactic protein-1 (MCP-1) will also attract monocytes to the inflamed region. In this phase the invaded micro-organisms coated with opsonins (e.g. IgG, C3b) are phagocytosed by neutrophils and macrophages.

After the agent or micro-organism that caused the local tissue injury has been removed the inflammatory response is downregulated by a dedicated set of regulatory factors (PGE$_2$, TGF-β, IL-1ra, IL-10). These cytokines deactivate inflammatory cells and inhibit further production of proinflammatory cytokines and thus the region returns to a normal noninflamed state.

TRACERS FOR VISUALIZING INFILTRATING NEUTROPHILS

Bacterial chemotactic peptides

One of the first receptor-binding peptides that was tested for its ability to image infectious foci was the chemotactic peptide f-Met-Leu-Phe. This N-terminally formylated tripeptide is a chemotactic factor produced by bacteria. It binds to the formyl-peptide receptor that is expressed on granulocytes and monocytes. This G-protein coupled receptor (MW 62–85 kDa glycoprotein) is expressed on human neutrophils (6×10^4 receptors/cell).[66] f-Met-Leu-Phe has a high affinity ($K_d = 3$–4 nM) for this receptor.[67] The first work on this radiolabeled chemotactic peptide was reported by Zoghbi et al.[68] and McAfee et al.[69] They found that even low doses of peptide induced transient granulocytopenia. In 1991, Fischman et al.[70] described the synthesis of four DTPA-derivatized chemotactic peptide analogs and their labeling with ^{111}In. The receptor binding affinity and the biological activity of the peptides was preserved. The peptides were tested in rats with Escherichia coli infections. These analogs showed preferential localization in the focal infection within 1 h after injection. In rabbits with E. coli infections, ^{99m}Tc-labeled f-Met-Leu-Phe localized preferentially in the infected thigh muscle.[71] In a study in rabbits with E. coli infection, ^{123}I-labeled f-Met-Leu-Phe had a relatively low uptake in the abscess and relatively low abscess-to-background ratio.[72] Furthermore, a peptide dose as low as 10 ng kg^{-1} still had a pronounced effect on the leukocyte counts[73] and therefore several groups have developed antagonists to circumvent this side effect. However, these antagonists had lower uptake in infected tissue, most likely due to reduced affinity for the receptor.[74,75] Thus, preclinical studies have shown that infection imaging is feasible with radiolabeled chemotactic peptides, although their uptake in infectious foci is relatively low and the effects of these peptides on leukocyte counts seem to impede further clinical development.

Interleukin-1

Interleukin-1 (IL-1) binds with high affinity ($K_d = 10^{-9}$ to 10^{-11} M) to IL-1 receptors expressed on granulocytes, monocytes, and lymphocytes. Studies in mice with focal Staphylococcus aureus infections showed specific uptake of radioiodinated IL-1 at the site of infection.[76] Using IL-1 receptor blocking antibodies, it could be demonstrated that accumulation of the agent in the infectious foci was due to binding to the IL-1 type II receptor.[77] However, the biologic effects (e.g. hypotension, headache) of IL-1 even at very low doses (10 ng kg^{-1}) preclude clinical application of radiolabeled IL-1. Therefore, the naturally occurring IL-1 receptor antagonist (IL-1ra) was tested as an imaging agent. This equally sized (17 kDa) protein binds to both IL-1 receptor subtypes with similar high affinity as IL-1, but does not trigger the signal transduction pathway. In a comparative study in rabbits with E. coli infection, the abscess uptake of radioiodinated IL-1ra was similar to that of radioiodinated IL-1.[72] Based on these results in rabbits, ^{123}I-IL-1ra was tested in patients with rheumatoid arthritis. In these patients, inflamed joints were visualized. However, in patients the agent cleared mainly via the hepatobiliary route. Therefore this agent was unsuitable for visualizing infectious and inflammatory lesions in the abdomen, and therefore was not further characterized in patients.[78]

Interleukin-8

Interleukin-8 (IL-8) is a small protein (72 amino acids, 8.5 kDa) and belongs to the CXC subfamily of the chemokines. IL-8 binds to both types of CXC receptors (CXCR1 and CXCR2) that are expressed at high levels on human neutrophils.[79] The affinity of IL-8 for both receptor types is relatively high ($K_d = 0.3 \times 10^{-9}$ to 4×10^{-9} M). The potential of radiolabeled IL-8 to image inflammation was reported for the first time by Hay and colleagues.[80] The uptake of IL-8, radioiodinated via the chloramine-T method, in inflamed thigh muscle in rats, peaked at 1–3 h after injection. In a pilot study in eight diabetic patients these investigators showed that ^{123}I-IL-8 could visualize active foot infections.[81] The labeling method appeared to have major effects on the *in vivo* biodistribution of radioiodinated IL-8. The imaging characteristics of IL-8 labeled via the Bolton–Hunter method were clearly superior to those of IL-8 labeled via the iodogen method.[82] The specific activity of the radioiodinated IL-8 preparations was relatively low; in rabbits an imaging dose of ^{123}I-IL-8 (25 µg kg^{-1}) caused a transient drop of peripheral leukocyte counts to 45%, followed by a leukocytosis (170% of preinjection level) over several hours. Recently, we developed a ^{99m}Tc-labeled IL-8 preparation using HYNIC as a chelator.[83,84] This preparation was characterized in rabbits with focal infection and uptake in the abscess was extremely high (0.3–0.4%ID/g). As a result more than 15% of the injected activity accumulated in the abscess and abscess-to-muscle ratios exceeded 100.[83,85] ^{99m}Tc-IL-8 clearly delineated inflammatory foci in rabbits with colitis (Fig. 3.4). In neutropenic rabbits, the uptake of ^{99m}Tc-IL-8 in the inflamed muscle was less than 10% of the uptake obtained in rabbits with normal neutrophil counts, indicating that the uptake was dependent on the presence of IL-8 receptor-positive cells.[85]

The high specific activity of the preparation (50 MBq µg^{-1}) allows injection of very low doses of IL-8 for imaging (<0.1 µg kg^{-1}), and therefore even temporary cytopenia is not anticipated. Detailed analysis of serial images of rabbits that received ^{99m}Tc-IL-8 revealed that a substantial part of the ^{99m}Tc-IL-8 is trapped in the lungs immediately after i.v. injection. Concomitant with the clearance of the activity from the lungs (between 1 and 6 h p.i.) the accumulation of the activity in the abscess occurs, suggesting that the neutrophil-bound ^{99m}Tc-IL-8 that is initially trapped in the lungs migrates to the inflammatory focus.[85] Studies with ^{99m}Tc-IL-8 in patients with infectious and inflammatory disorders were initiated in November 2003.

Platelet factor 4

Platelet factor 4 (PF4), like IL-8, is a member of the CXC chemokines, but has no relevant affinity for either of the two CXC receptor types. In fact, the PF4 receptor has not been identified yet. PF4 is also called the 'body's heparin neutralizing agent'. At Diatide Research Laboratories (since 1999 part of the Berlex Laboratories, Seattle, USA) the peptide P483, with 23 amino acids, was synthesized. This peptide contains the heparin-binding region of PF4, a lysine-rich sequence to facilitate renal clearance and a CGCG sequence to allow labeling with [99m]Tc. When P483 was complexed with heparin its affinity for leukocytes increased and this complex (P483H) was studied in a rabbit model of infection. ^{99m}Tc-P483H clearly delineated the infectious foci as early as 4 h after injection. Upon intravenous injection high pulmonary uptake is observed.[86] ^{99m}Tc-P483H has been studied in 30 patients to test its applicability as an imaging agent for scintigraphic detection of infection and inflammation, and the results have been good (86% sensitivity, 81% specificity, 83% accuracy).[87] Due to the high physiological uptake in the lungs, the agent is not suited for detection of pulmonary infections. In addition, in some patients, excessive thyroid uptake was observed, which correlated with the peptide:heparin ratio.

Complement factor 5a

Complement factor 5a (C5a) and its natural metabolite C5a-des-Arg are involved in several stages of the inflammatory process. C5a-des-Arg only differs from C5a by the absence of the C-terminal Arg residue of C5a. Both act on a common receptor on different cell types, including neutrophils and monocytes. The receptor binding affinity of C5a is one order of magnitude higher than the affinity of C5a-des-Arg. The biologic activity of C5a-des Arg is considerably lower than that of C5a. In rabbits with intramuscular *E. coli* infection, ^{99m}Tc-C5a rapidly visualized the infection with high uptake of the radiolabel in the affected muscle while uptake of ^{99m}Tc-C5a-des-Arg in the abscess

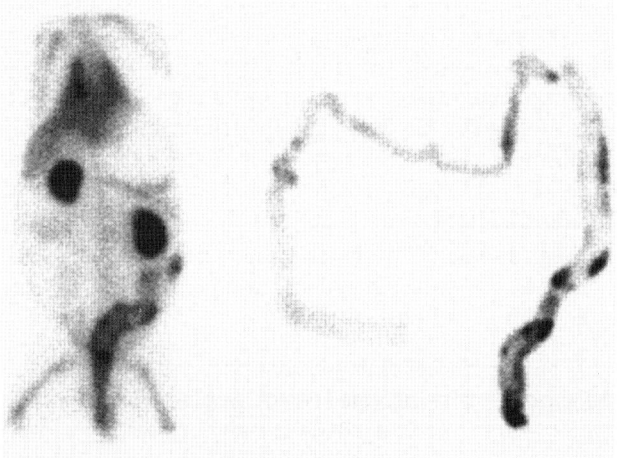

Figure 3.4 *Scintigraphic image of a rabbit with experimental colitis. Images were acquired 4 h after injection of ^{99m}Tc-IL-8 (left panel). Image of the dissected colon of the animal (right panel).*

was low.[88] Thus, none of the compounds in this study combined good imaging characteristics with reduced biologic activity.

Leukotriene B$_4$

Leukotriene B$_4$ (LTB$_4$) is a potent chemoattractant that activates granulocytes and macrophages and it is an important mediator in both acute and chronic inflammatory diseases. Two distinct types of leukotriene receptors have been identified (BLT1 and BLT2). LTB$_4$ has a high affinity for the BLT1 receptor ($K_d = 10^{-9}$M) that is mainly expressed on human neutrophils, while the recently characterized BLT2 receptor is a low-affinity receptor ($K_a = 23 \times 10^{-9}$M) expressed more ubiquitously. Binding of LTB$_4$ to BLT1 and BLT2 promotes chemotaxis and chemokinesis. In search for an effective infection-imaging agent, the LTB$_4$ receptor antagonist RP517 was synthesized. RP517 (MW 830 Da) has a quinolone function as a receptor binding moiety linked via a spacer arm to HYNIC to allow labeling with ^{99m}Tc (IC$_{50}$ = 2×10^{-9}M). In rabbits with E. coli infections, ^{99m}Tc-RP517 rapidly visualized the abscess with high abscess-to-background ratios.[89] RP517 labeled with ^{99m}Tc could also visualize experimental endocarditis in dogs.[90] However, ^{99m}Tc-RP517 is a highly lipophilic compound that is cleared mainly via the hepatobiliary route, resulting in high uptake in the digestive tract relatively early after injection. The high physiologic uptake in the intestines limits the applicability of ^{99m}Tc-RP517 as an infection-imaging agent.[89]

In order to produce a hydrophilic variant of RP517, a new compound, designated as DPC11870-11, was synthesized. DPC11870-11 (MW = 3127 Da) consists of two quinolone moieties for receptor binding linked via a cysteic acid-based hydrophilic backbone and a DTPA moiety to allow labeling with ^{111}In. In rabbits with intramuscular E. coli infection, ^{111}In-DPC11870-11 rapidly delineated the infection with high abscess-to-background ratios. The agent cleared exclusively via the kidneys and no accumulation of radioactivity was observed in the gastrointestinal tract. Blocking experiments with an excess of the nonradiolabeled agent indicated that the localization of ^{111}In-DPC11870-11 was dependent on the specific interaction with LTB$_4$ receptors expressed in the infected tissue.[91] Recently, ^{111}In-DPC11870-11 was tested for its ability to visualize abdominal inflammation. Chemically induced colonic inflammation could clearly be delineated in rabbits. The ^{111}In-DPC11870-11 rapidly accumulated in the inflamed colon and in the images the affected colon-to-nonaffected colon uptake ratios exceeded 10. The images obtained with ^{111}In-DPC11870-11 were superior to those obtained with ^{111}In-labeled leukocytes and to the PET images obtained after injection with ^{18}F-FDG.[92] The mechanism of accumulation of this tracer was studied in rabbits with soft tissue E. coli infection. Detailed analysis of serial images and biodistribution data of the rabbits revealed that 40–45% of the tracer localizes in the bone marrow within 1 h after injection, whereas the accumulation in the infected tissue occurred during the next few hours concomitant with clearance of the tracer from the bone marrow, suggesting that the targeted cells in the bone marrow migrate to the infectious focus. This hypothesis was confirmed by demonstrating that the tracer also localized in an abscess that was induced 4 h after injection of ^{111}In-DPC11870-11.[93] We now aim to synthesize a DPC11870-11 analog that can be labeled with ^{99m}Tc.

TRACERS FOR VISUALIZING INFILTRATING MONONUCLEAR CELLS

Interleukin-2

Chronic inflammation is characterized by infiltration of monocytes and lymphocytes. Thus to visualize chronic inflammatory processes, ligands of receptors on these mononuclear cells should be applied. Radiolabeled IL-2 (MW = 15 kDa) can target IL-2 receptors expressed on activated T lymphocytes. In a mouse model of autoimmune diabetes and in rats with renal allografts, ^{123}I-IL-2 adequately detected areas of lymphocytic infiltration. Specific accumulation of ^{123}I-IL-2 has been confirmed by ex vivo autoradiography.[94–96] IL-2 labeled with ^{123}I has been used successfully in patients with type 1 diabetes.[97] A method was developed that allowed the preparation of a ^{99m}Tc-IL-2 preparation with a high specific activity.[98] IL-2 labeled with ^{99m}Tc was able to identify a subgroup of patients with type 1 diabetes with persistent inflammation at the time of diagnosis that might benefit from the use of immunomodulating drugs to preserve beta-cell function.[99] Studies in patients with autoimmune disorders, such as Hashimoto thyroiditis, Graves' disease, Crohn's disease, and coeliac disease, demonstrated localization of ^{123}I- or ^{99m}Tc-labeled IL-2 at the site of lymphocytic infiltration.[100,101] In patients with active Crohn's disease, the focal uptake of ^{123}I-IL-2 in the intestinal wall decreased after corticosteroid therapy, and potentially this technique can be used to monitor the effect of therapy.[102] Scintigraphic results using ^{123}I-IL-2 in patients with coeliac disease were consistent with the histologically determined number of infiltrating IL-2 receptor-positive cells in the jejunal mucosa.[103] IL-2 labeled with ^{99m}Tc also accumulated in the thyroid glands of patients with Hashimoto's thyroiditis and Graves' disease.[104,105] These results suggest that radiolabeled IL-2 may be a useful tool to visualize T-cell infiltration in several autoimmune diseases.

Monocyte chemoattractant protein 1

The chemotactic cytokine monocyte chemoattractant protein 1 (MCP-1) is a monomeric polypeptide (MW = 6–7 kDa). MCP-1 is a chemotactic factor for monocytes but not neutrophils, because only monocytes express MCP-1 receptors. Two MCP-1-specific receptors have been cloned which signal in response to nanomolar concentrations of MCP-1. The two receptors differ in their carboxyl tails as a result of alternative splicing. MCP-1 labeled with ^{125}I showed rapid blood clearance in normal mice and in rabbits with experimental arterial lesions. The uptake of ^{125}I-MCP-1 in damaged artery walls was higher than in normal vessels and correlated with the histologically determined number of macrophages.[106] The uptake of ^{99m}Tc-labeled MCP-1 localized only in subacute inflammation in a rat model of sterile subacute and chronic turpentine-induced inflammation, reflecting the density of macrophages.[107] These preclinical data indicate that radiolabeled MCP-1 may be used to visualize infiltrates of monocytes and macrophages.

Tuftsin

Tuftsin is a chemotactic tetrapeptide derived from the Fc portion of IgG, which promotes chemotaxis and phagocytosis of neutrophils, monocytes and macrophages by binding to the tuftsin receptor. RP128 is a peptide that can be labeled with ^{99m}Tc designed to target this receptor. The ability of ^{99m}Tc-RP128 to detect central nervous system (CNS) inflammation was shown in experimental allergic encephalomyelitis, an animal model of multiple sclerosis. In addition, ^{99m}Tc-RP128 successfully monitored glucocorticoid suppression of inflammation, recording a typical dose–response to increasing steroid concentration.[108] In 10 patients with long-standing rheumatoid arthritis, ^{99m}Tc-RP128 was able to visualize clinically affected joints, although studies in healthy volunteers also showed physiological uptake in large joints.[109]

Antimicrobial agents

The agents described above have a specific affinity for receptors expressed on cells that are recruited during the inflammatory response, and these agents target the cells infiltrating the inflamed tissue. As these agents accumulate in the focus due to a common feature of infection and inflammation, they can not be used to differentiate between infection and inflammation. Agents that specifically target the infectious organism (e.g. bacteria, fungi or viruses) have the potential to distinguish microbial from non-microbial inflammation. During the last decade a few agents have been presented that aim to specifically visualize infectious foci by targeting the infectious organism.

CIPROFLOXACIN

The most intensively studied agent in this category is ^{99m}Tc-ciprofloxacin, also referred to as Infecton™ (Draximage, Kirkland, Canada), which is ciprofloxacin labeled with ^{99m}Tc. Ciprofloxacin is a fluoroquinolone antimicrobial agent that binds to prokaryotic topoisomerase IV and DNA gyrase

as expressed in proliferating bacteria.[110,111] It has been hypothesized that ^{99m}Tc-labeled ciprofloxacin could specifically target living bacteria *in vivo* and thus that ^{99m}Tc-ciprofloxacin is able to specifically visualize bacterial infection. In clinical practice, such an agent would be extremely useful, as it would allow discrimination between infection and inflammation due to other causes. The radiochemical characterization of ^{99m}Tc-ciprofloxacin has not been described yet and, so far, the coordination of the ^{99m}Tc species is unknown. The labeling procedure and the method to determine the radiochemical purity of the preparation have been described in detail.[112] The first results obtained with ^{99m}Tc-ciprofloxacin in 56 patients with known or suspected sites of infection were published in the *Lancet* in 1996, and suggested that ^{99m}Tc-ciprofloxacin had a high sensitivity (84%) for visualizing infection.[113] The efficacy of ^{99m}Tc-ciprofloxacin for imaging infections was evaluated in 879 patients in a large multicenter study coordinated by the International Atomic Energy Agency (IAEA). The overall sensitivity and specificity for infection were 85.5% and 81.6%, respectively.[114] The sensitivity and specificity varied according to the type of infection imaged, e.g. the sensitivity and specificity in prosthetic joint infections were 96% and 91%, respectively. Despite these impressive figures from this large multinational study, several reports dispute the claim that ^{99m}Tc-ciprofloxacin only visualizes bacterial infection. In rabbits with infected and uninfected knee prosthesis and in patients with osteomyelitis or with septic arthritis, the specificity of ^{99m}Tc-ciprofloxacin for bacterial infection was not found.[115,116] Recently, a series of factors were described that could explain these conflicting data.[117] It has been pointed out that proper preparation and careful assessment of the radiochemical purity of the ^{99m}Tc-labeled ciprofloxacin preparation is essential. A slight increase of reducing agent during the labeling of ciprofloxacin with ^{99m}Tc could lead to the formation of ^{99m}Tc-colloid.[112] Contamination of the ^{99m}Tc-ciprofloxacin preparation with colloid could explain the contradictory results. Similarly overdilution of the preparation could be detrimental. ^{99m}Tc-ciprofloxacin (Infecton™) is now being produced commercially in a new and standard kit form by Draximage Inc. (Kirkland, Canada) and is undergoing phase II clinical trials.

According to a similar approach, recently new tracers have been proposed for the specific visualization of fungal infections. ^{99m}Tc-labeled fluconazole was developed by Lupetti *et al.*[118] for the specific detection of *Candida albicans* and *Aspergillus fumigatus* infections in mice. Technetium-99m-fluconazole preferentially accumulated in infections induced *in vivo* by *C. albicans*, while accumulation in bacterial infections, *A. fumigatus* infections and sterile inflammation was significantly lower.

ANTIMICROBIAL PEPTIDES

Antimicrobial peptides (MW = 5–7 kDa) are produced by phagocytes, endothelial cells, and many other cell types and are an important component of the innate immune system. The basis of their antimicrobial activity is their direct interaction with the bacterial plasma membrane by electrostatic and hydrophobic interaction. The preferential binding of various antimicrobial peptides to bacteria was demonstrated *in vitro*.[119] Due to this preferential binding these peptides potentially can be used to discriminate bacterial infections from nonbacterial infections and sterile inflammations. The group in Leiden has labeled several (fragments of) antimicrobial peptides with ^{99m}Tc and characterized these labeled peptides *in vitro* and in mice and rabbits with experimental infection/inflammation.[119–121] A fragment of the antimicrobial peptide ubiquicidin (UBI 29-41) labeled with ^{99m}Tc showed some uptake (1–2%ID) in the infected thigh muscle at 30 min p.i. This enhanced uptake was specific because co-injection of an excess of unlabeled UBI 29-41 peptide resulted in a significantly lower uptake of ^{99m}Tc-UBI 29-41. In addition, uptake in muscle tissue with inflammation induced by inoculation of dead bacteria was also significantly lower. Recently, this peptide was studied in six children with suspected bone infection.[122] The agent cleared rapidly from the body (85% in 24 h), but uptake in the infectious lesions was low and target-to-background ratios were 2.18 ± 0.74.

Another antimicrobial peptide, human neutrophil peptide-1 (HNP-1) labeled with ^{99m}Tc, was characterized in mice with inflamed thigh muscles. The abscess-to-background ratios obtained with this tracer were low (3–5) and decreased with time.[123,124] In the peritoneal cavity of the infected mice, ^{99m}Tc-HNP-1 bound preferentially to bacteria rather than to leukocytes. The investigators propose that these peptides can be used to monitor the efficacy of antimicrobial therapy regimens and to distinguish between bacterial infection and sterile inflammation.

REFERENCES

- Seminal primary article
- Key review paper

- 1 Lavender JP, Lowe J, Barker JR, *et al.* Gallium 67 citrate scanning in neoplastic and inflammatory lesions. *Br J Radiol* 1971; **44**: 361–366.
- 2 Ito Y, Okuyama S, Awano T, *et al.* Diagnostic evaluation of Ga-67 scanning of lung cancer and other diseases. *Radiology* 1971; **101**: 355–362.
- 3 Tsan MF. Mechanism of gallium-67 accumulation in inflammatory lesions. *J Nucl Med* 1985; **26**: 88–92.
- 4 Weiner R. The role of transferrin and other receptors in the mechanism of ^{67}Ga localization. *Int J Rad Appl Instrum B* 1990; **17**: 141–149.
- 5 McAfee JG, Thakur ML. Survey of radioactive agents for the in vitro labeling of phagocytic leucocytes. I Soluble agents. II Particles. *J Nucl Med* 1976; **17**: 480–492.

- 6 Peters AM, Danpure HJ, Osman S, *et al.* Clinical experience with ^{99m}Tc-hexamethylpropyleneamineoxime for labelling leucocytes and imaging inflammation. *Lancet* 1986; **8513**: 946–949.
- 7 Becker W, Saptogino A, Wolf F. The single late Tc-99m granulocyte antibody scan in inflammatory diseases. *Nucl Med Commun* 1992; **13**: 186–192.
- 8 Becker W, Palestro CJ, Winship J, *et al.* Rapid imaging of infections with a monoclonal antibody fragment (Leukoscan®). *Clin Orthopaedics* 1996; **329**: 263–272.
- 9 Barron B, Hanna C, Passalaqua AM, *et al.* Rapid diagnostic imaging of acute, nonclassic appendicitis by leukoscintigraphy with sulesomab, a technetium 99m labeled antigranulocyte antibody Fab′ fragment. *Surgery* 1999; **125**: 288–296.
- 10 Harwood SJ, Valdivia S, Hung GL, Quenzer RW. Use of sulesomab, a radiolabeled antibody fragment, to detect osteomyelitis in diabetic patients with foot ulcers by leukoscintigraphy. *Clin Infect Dis* 1999; **28**: 1200–1205.
- 11 Thakur ML, Marcus CS, Henneman P, *et al.* Imaging inflammatory diseases with neutrophil-specific technetium-99m-labeled monoclonal antibody anti-SSEA-1. *J Nucl Med* 1996; **37**: 1789–1795.
- 12 Kipper SL, Rypins EB, Evans DG, *et al.* Neutrophil-specific ^{99m}Tc-labeled anti-CD15 monoclonal antibody imaging for diagnosis of equivocal appendicitis. *J Nucl Med* 2000; **41**: 449–455.
- 13 Becker W, Borst U, Fischbach W, *et al.* Kinetic data of in vivo labeled granulocytes in humans with a murine Tc-99m-labelled monoclonal antibody. *Eur J Nucl Med* 1989; **15**: 361–366.
- 14 Skehan SJ, White JF, Evans JW, *et al.* Mechanism of accumulation of ^{99m}Tc-sulesomab in inflammation. *J Nucl Med* 2003; **44**: 11–18.
- 15 Rubin RH, Young LS, Hansen WP, Nedelman M, Wilkinson R, Nelles MJ, *et al.* Specific and non-specific imaging of localized Fisher immunotype 1 Pseudomonas aeruginosa infection with radiolabeled monoclonal antibody. *J Nucl Med* 1988; **29**: 651–656.
- 16 Fischman AJ, Fucello AJ, Pellegrino-Gensey JL, Geltofsky J, Yarmush ML, Rubin RH, Strauss HW. Effect of carbohydrate modification on the localization of human polyclonal IgG at focal sites of bacterial infection. *J Nucl Med* 1992; **33**: 1378–1382.
- 17 Dams ET, Oyen WJ, Boerman OC, Claessens RA, Wymenga AB, van der Meer JW, Corstens FH. Technetium-99m labeled to human immunoglobulin G through the nicotinyl hydrazine derivative: a clinical study. *J Nucl Med* 1998; **39**: 119–124.
- 18 Chianelli M, Mather SJ, Martin-Comin J, Signore A. Radiopharmaceuticals for the study of inflammatory processes: a review. *Nucl Med Commun* 1997; **18**: 437–55.

● 19 Oyen WJ, Claessens RA, van der Meer JW, Corstens FH. Detection of subacute infectious foci with indium-111-labeled autologous leukocytes and indium-111-labeled human nonspecific immunoglobulin G: a prospective comparative study. *J Nucl Med* 1991; **32**: 1854–1860.

● 20 Oyen WJ, Claessens RA, van Horn JR, *et al.* Scintigraphic detection of bone and joint infections with indium-111-labeled nonspecific polyclonal human immunoglobulin G. *J Nucl Med* 1990; **31**: 403–412.

● 21 Nijhof MW, Oyen WJ, van Kampen A, *et al.* Evaluation of infections of the locomotor system with indium-111-labeled human IgG scintigraphy. *J Nucl Med* 1997; **38**: 1300–1305.

● 22 Oyen WJ, Claessens RA, Raemaekers JM, *et al.* Diagnosing infection in febrile granulocytopenic patients with indium-111-labeled human immunoglobulin G. *J Clin Oncol* 1992; **10**: 61–68.

● 23 Buscombe JR, Oyen WJ, Grant A, *et al.* Indium-111-labeled polyclonal human immunoglobulin: identifying focal infection in patients positive for human immunodeficiency virus. *J Nucl Med* 1993; **34**: 1621–1625.

● 24 Buscombe JR, Oyen WJ, Corstens FH, *et al.* A comparison of ^{111}In-HIG scintigraphy and chest radiology in the identification of pulmonary infection in patients with HIV infection. *Nucl Med Commun* 1995; **16**: 327–335.

● 25 Buscombe JR, Oyen WJ, Corstens FH. Use of polyclonal IgG in HIV infection and AIDS. *Q J Nucl Med* 1995; **39**: 212–220.

● 26 Kubota R, Yamada S, Kubota K, *et al.* Intratumoral distribution of fluorine-18-fluorodeoxyglucose in vivo: high accumulation in macrophages and granulation tissues studied by microautoradiography. *J Nucl Med* 1992; **33**: 1972–1980.

◆ 27 de Winter F, Vogelaers D, Gemmel F, Dierckx RA. Promising role of 18-F-fluoro-D-deoxyglucose positron emission tomography in clinical infectious diseases. *Eur J Clin Microbiol Infect Dis* 2002; **21**: 247–257.

● 28 Zhuang H, Alavi A. 18-Fluorodeoxyglucose positron emission tomographic imaging in the detection and monitoring of infection and inflammation. *Semin Nucl Med* 2002; **32**: 47–59.

● 29 Harris WH, Sledge CB. Total hip and total knee replacement (1). *N Engl J Med* 1990; **323**: 725–731.

● 30 Harris WH, Sledge CB. Total hip and total knee replacement (2). *N Engl J Med* 1990; **323**: 801–807.

● 31 Hanssen AD, Rand JA. Evaluation and treatment of infection at the site of a total hip or knee arthroplasty. *J Bone Joint Surg Am* 1998; **80**: 910–922.

● 32 Love C, Tomas MB, Marwin SE, *et al.* Role of nuclear medicine in diagnosis of the infected joint replacement. *Radiographics* 2001; **21**: 1229–1238.

◆ 33 Palestro CJ, Torres MA. Radionuclide imaging in orthopedic infections. *Semin Nucl Med* 1997; **27**: 334–345.

● 34 Spangehl MJ, Younger AS, Masri BA, Duncan CP. Diagnosis of infection following total hip arthroplasty. *Instr Course Lect* 1998; **47**: 285–295.

● 35 Palestro CJ, Swyer AJ, Kim CK, Goldsmith SJ. Infected knee prostheses: diagnosis with In-111 leukocyte, Tc-99m sulfur colloid, and Tc-99m MDP imaging. *Radiology* 1991; **179**: 645–648.

● 36 Zhuang H, Duarte PS, Pourdehnad M, *et al.* The promising role of ^{18}F-FDG PET in detecting infected lower limb prosthesis implants. *J Nucl Med* 2001; **42**: 44–48.

● 37 Love C, Pugliese PV, Afriyie MO, *et al.* Utility of F-18 FDG imaging for diagnosing the infected joint replacement. *Clin Positron Imaging* 2000; **3**: 159.

● 38 Schmitz A, Risse JH, Grunwald F, *et al.* Fluorine-18 fluorodeoxyglucose positron emission tomography findings in spondylodiscitis: preliminary results. *Eur Spine J* 2001; **10**: 534–539.

● 39 Gratz S, Dorner J, Fischer U, *et al.* ^{18}F-FDG hybrid PET in patients with suspected spondylitis. *Eur J Nucl Med Mol Imaging* 2002; **29**: 516–524.

● 40 Stumpe KD, Zanetti M, Weishaupt D, *et al.* FDG positron emission tomography for differentiation of degenerative and infectious endplate abnormalities in the lumbar spine detected on MR imaging. *Am J Roentgenol* 2002; **179**: 1151–1157.

● 41 Stumpe KD, Dazzi H, Schaffner A, von Schulthess GK. Infection imaging using whole-body FDG-PET. *Eur J Nucl Med* 2000; **27**: 822–832.

● 42 Stumpe KD, Notzli HP, Zanetti M, Kamel EM, Hany TF, Gorres GW, *et al.* FDG PET for differentiation of infection and aseptic loosening in total hip replacements: comparison with conventional radiography and three-phase bone scintigraphy. *Radiology* 2004; **231**: 333–41.

● 43 Guhlmann A, Brecht-Krauss D, Suger G, *et al.* Fluorine-18-FDG PET and technetium-99m antigranulocyte antibody scintigraphy in chronic osteomyelitis. *J Nucl Med* 1998; **39**: 2145–2152.

● 44 Chacko TK, Zhuang H, Nakhoda KZ, *et al.* Applications of fluorodeoxyglucose positron emission tomography in the diagnosis of infection. *Nucl Med Commun* 2003; **24**: 615–624.

● 45 de Winter F, Van de Wiele C, Vandenberghe S, *et al.* Coincidence camera FDG imaging for the diagnosis of chronic orthopedic infections: a feasibility study. *J Comput Assist Tomogr* 2001; **25**: 184–189.

◆ 46 Alavi A, Gupta N, Alberini JL, *et al.* Positron emission tomography imaging in nonmalignant thoracic disorders. *Semin Nucl Med* 2002; **32**: 293–321.

● 47 Fry DE, Garrison RN, Heitsch RD, *et al.* Determinants of death in patients with intra-abdominal abscess. *Surgery* 1980; **88**: 517–523.

● 48   Bohnen J, Boulanger M, Meakins JL, McLean AP. Prognosis in generalized peritonitis: relation to cause and risk factors. *Arch Surg* 1983; **118**: 285–290.

● 49   McLauchlan GJ, Anderson ID, Grant IS, Fearon KCH. Outcome of patients with abdominal sepsis treated in an intensive care unit. *Br J Surg* 1995; **82**: 524–529.

● 50   Montgomery RS, Wilson SE. Intraabdominal abscesses: image-guided diagnosis and therapy. *Clin Inf Dis* 1996; **23**: 28–36.

◆ 51   Gagliardi PD, Hoffer PB, Rosenfield AT. Correlative imaging in abdominal infection: an algorithmic approach using nuclear medicine, ultrasound, and computed tomography. *Semin Nucl Med* 1988; **18**: 320–334.

● 52   Lantto E. Investigation of suspected intra-abdominal sepsis: the contribution of nuclear medicine. *Scan J Gastroenterol* 1994; **29(Suppl 203)**: 11–14.

● 53   Staab EV, McCartney WH. Role of gallium 67 in inflammatory disease. *Semin Nucl Med* 1978; **8**: 219–234.

● 54   Knochel JQ, Koehler PR, Lee TG, Welch DM. Diagnosis of abdominal abscesses with computed tomography, ultrasound, and ^{111}In leukocyte scans. *Radiology* 1980; **137**: 425–432.

● 55   Knockaert DC, Vanderschueren S, Blockmans D. Fever of unknown origin in adults: 40 years on. *J Intern Med* 2003; **253**: 263–275.

● 56   Bleeker-Rovers CP, De Kleijn EM, Corstens FH, *et al.* Clinical value of FDG PET in patients with fever of unknown origin and patients suspected of focal infection or inflammation. *Eur J Nucl Med Mol Imaging* 2004; **31**: 29–37.

● 57   Blockmans D, Stroobants S, Maes A, Mortelmans L. Positron emission tomography in giant cell arteritis and polymyalgia rheumatica: evidence for inflammation of the aortic arch. *Am J Med* 2000; **108**: 246–249.

● 58   Meller J, Altenvoerde G, Munzel U, *et al.* Fever of unknown origin: prospective comparison of [^{18}F]FDG imaging with a double-head coincidence camera and gallium-67 citrate SPET. *Eur J Nucl Med* 2000; **27**: 1617–1625.

● 59   Lorenzen J, Buchert R, Bohuslavizki KH. Value of FDG PET in patients with fever of unknown origin. *Nucl Med Commun* 2001; **22**: 779–783.

● 60   Blockmans D, Knockaert D, Maes A, *et al.* Clinical value of [18F]fluoro-deoxyglucose positron emission tomography for patients with fever of unknown origin. *Clin Infect Dis* 2001; **32**: 191–196.

● 61   Liberatore M, Iurilli AP, Ponzo F, *et al.* Clinical usefulness of technetium-99m-HMPAO-labeled leukocyte scan in prosthetic vascular graft infection. *J Nucl Med* 1998; **39**: 875–879.

● 62   Genereau T, Lortholary O, Guillevin L, *et al.* Temporal [67]gallium uptake is increased in temporal arteritis. *Rheumatology (Oxford)* 1999; **38**: 709–713.

● 63   Reuter H, Wraight EP, Qasim FJ, Lockwood CM. Management of systemic vasculitis: contribution of scintigraphic imaging to evaluation of disease activity and classification. *QJM* 1995; **88**: 509–516.

● 64   Chen CC, Kerr GS, Carter CS, *et al.* Lack of sensitivity of indium-111 mixed leukocyte scans for active disease in Takayasu's arteritis. *J Rheumatol* 1995; **22**: 478–481.

● 65   Bleeker-Rovers CP, Bredie SJH, van der Meer JWM, *et al.* F-18-fluorodeoxyglucose positron emission tomography in diagnosis and follow-up of patients with different types of vasculitis. *Neth J Med* 2003; **61**: 323–329.

● 66   Niedel J, Davis J, Cuatrecasas P. Covalent affinity labeling of the formyl peptide chemotactic receptor. *J Biol Chem* 1980; **255**: 7063–7066.

● 67   Heiman DF, Gardner JP, Apfeldorf WJ, Malech HL. Effects of tunicamycin on the expression and function of formyl peptide chemotactic receptors of differentiated HL-60 cells. *J Immunol* 1986; **136**: 4623–4630.

● 68   Zoghbi S, Thakur M, Gottschalk A. Selective cell labelling: a potential radioactive agent for labeling of human neutrophils. *J Nucl Med* 1981; **22**: 32P.

◆ 69   McAfee JG, Subramanian G, Gagne G. Technique of leukocyte harvesting and labeling: problems and perspectives. *Semin Nucl Med* 1984; **14**: 83–106.

● 70   Fischman AJ, Pike MC, Kroon D, *et al.* Imaging focal sites of bacterial infection in rats with indium-111-labeled chemotactic peptide analogs. *J Nucl Med* 1991; **32**: 483–491.

● 71   Babich JW, Graham W, Barrow SA, *et al.* Technetium-99m-labeled chemotactic peptides: comparison with indium-111-labeled white blood cells for localizing acute bacterial infection in the rabbit. *J Nucl Med* 1993; **34**: 2176–2181.

● 72   Van der Laken CJ, Boerman OC, Oyen WJG, *et al.* Imaging of infection in rabbits with radioiodinated interleukin-1 (α and β), its receptor antagonist and a chemotactic peptide: a comparative study. *Eur J Nucl Med* 1998; **25**: 347–352.

● 73   Fischman AJ, Rauh D, Solomon H, *et al.* In vivo bioactivity and biodistribution of chemotactic peptide analogs in nonhuman primates. *J Nucl Med* 1993; **34**: 2130–2134.

● 74   Pollak A, Goodbody AE, Ballinger JR, *et al.* Imaging inflammation with Tc-99m labelled chemotactic peptides: analogues with reduced neutropenia. *Nucl Med Commun* 1996; **17**: 132–139.

● 75   Babich JW, Dong Q, Graham W, *et al.* A novel high affinity chemotactic peptide antagonist for infection imaging. *J Nucl Med* 1997; **38**: 268P.

● 76   Van der Laken CJ, Boerman OC, Oyen WJ, *et al.* Specific targeting of infectious foci with radioiodinated human recombinant interleukin-1 in an experimental model. *Eur J Nucl Med* 1995; **22**: 1249–1255.

● 77   Van der Laken CJ, Boerman OC, Oyen WJ, *et al.* Preferential localization of systemically administered radiolabeled interleukin-1α in experimental inflammation in mice by binding to the type II receptor. *J Clin Invest* 1997; **100**: 2970–2976.

78 Barrera P, van der Laken CJ, Boerman OC, *et al.* Localization of ^{123}I-IL-ra in affected joints in patients with rheumatic arthritis. *Rheumatology* 2000; **39**: 870–874.

79 Patel L, Charlton SJ, Chambers JK, Macphee CH. Expression and functional analysis of chemokine receptors in human peripheral blood leukocyte populations. *Cytokine* 2001; **14**: 27–36.

80 Hay RV, Skinner RS, Newman OC, *et al.* Scintigraphy of acute inflammatory lesions in rats with radiolabelled recombinant human interleukin-8. *Nucl Med Commun* 1997; **18**: 367–378.

81 Gross MD, Shapiro B, Fig LM, *et al.* Imaging of human infection with ^{131}I-labeled recombinant human interleukin-8. *J Nucl Med* 2001; **42**: 1656–1659.

82 Van der Laken CJ, Boerman OC, Oyen WJ, et al. Radiolabeled interleukin-8: scintigraphic detection of infection within a few hours. *J Nucl Med* 2000; **41**: 463–469.

83 Rennen HJ, Boerman OC, Oyen WJG, *et al.* Specific and rapid scintigraphic detection of infection with Tc-99m-labeled interleukin-8. *J Nucl Med* 2001; **42**: 117–123.

84 Rennen HJ, van Eerd JE, Oyen WJ, *et al.* Effects of coligand variation on the in vivo characteristics of Tc-99m-labeled interleukin-8 in detection of infection. *Bioconjug Chem* 2002; **13**: 370–377.

85 Rennen HJ, Boerman OC, Oyen WJ, Corstens FH. Kinetics of ^{99m}Tc-labeled interleukin-8 in experimental inflammation and infection. *J Nucl Med* 2003; **44**: 1502–1509.

86 Moyer BR, Vallabhajosula S, Lister-James J, *et al.* Technetium-99m-white blood cell-specific imaging agent developed from platelet factor 4 to detect infection. *J Nucl Med* 1996; **37**: 673–679.

87 Palestro CJ, Weiland FL, Seabold JE, *et al.* Localizing infection with a technetium-99m-labeled peptide: initial results. *Nucl Med Commun* 2001; **22**: 695–701.

88 Rennen HJ, Oyen WJ, Cain SA, *et al.* Tc-99m-labeled C5a and C5a-des-Arg74 for infection imaging. *Nucl Med Biol* 2003; **30**: 267–272.

89 Brouwers AH, Laverman P, Boerman OC, *et al.* A ^{99m}Tc-labelled leukotriene B4 receptor antagonist for scintigraphic detection of infection in rabbits. *Nucl Med Commun* 2000; **21**: 1043–1050.

90 Riou LM, Ruiz M, Sullivan GW, *et al.* Assessment of myocardial inflammation produced by experimental coronary occlusion and reperfusion with ^{99m}Tc-RP517, a new leukotriene B4 receptor antagonist that preferentially labels neutrophils in vivo. *Circulation* 2002; **106**: 592–598.

91 Van Eerd JE, Oyen WJ, Harris TD, *et al.* A bivalent leukotriene B4 antagonist for scintigraphic imaging of infectious foci. *J Nucl Med* 2003; **44**: 1087–1091.

92 Van Eerd JE, Laverman P, Oyen WJ, *et al.* Imaging of experimental colitis with a radiolabeled leukotriene B4 antagonist. *J Nucl Med* 2004; **45**: 89–93.

93 van Eerd JE, Oyen WJ, Harris TD, *et al.* Scintigraphic imaging of infectious foci with an ^{111}In-LTB4 antagonist is based on in vivo labeling of granulocytes. *J Nucl Med* 2005; **46**: 786–93.

94 Signore A, Parman A, Pozzilli P, *et al.* Detection of activated lymphocytes in endocrine pancreas of BB/W rats by injection of ^{123}I-interleukin-2: an early sign of type 1 diabetes. *Lancet* 1987; **8558**: 537–540.

95 Signore A, Chianelli M, Toscano A, *et al.* A radiopharmaceutical for imaging areas of lymphocytic infiltration: ^{123}I-interleukin-2. Labelling procedure and animal studies. *Nucl Med Commun* 1992; **13**: 713–722.

96 Abbs IC, Pratt JR, Dallman MJ, Sacks SH. Analysis of activated T cell infiltrates in rat renal allografts by gamma camera imaging after injection of 123-iodine-interleukin 2. *Transpl Immunol* 1993; **1**: 45–51.

97 Signore A, Picarelli A, Chianelli M, *et al.* I-interleukin-2 scintigraphy: a new approach to assess disease activity in autoimmunity. *J Pediatr Endocrinol Metab* 1996; **9(Suppl 1)**: 139–144.

98 Chianelli M, Signore A, Fritzberg AR, Mather SJ. The development of technetium-99m-labelled interleukin-2: a new radiopharmaceutical for the in vivo detection of mononuclear cell infiltrates in immune-mediated diseases. *Nucl Med Biol* 1997; **24**: 579–586.

99 Signore A, Chianelli M, Parisella MG, Capriotti G, Giacalone P, Di Leve G, Barone R. In vivo imaging of insulitis in autoimmune diabetes. *J Endocrinol Invest* 1999; **22**: 151–158.

100 Signore A. Interleukin-2 scintigraphy: an overview. *Nucl Med Commun* 1999; **20**: 938.

101 Signore A, Picarelli A, Annovazzi A, *et al.* ^{123}I-interleukin-2: biochemical characterization and in vivo use for imaging autoimmune diseases. *Nucl Med Commun* 2003; **24**: 305–316.

102 Signore A, Chianelli M, Annovazzi A, *et al.* ^{123}I-interleukin-2 scintigraphy for in vivo assessment of intestinal mononuclear cell infiltration in Crohn's disease. *J Nucl Med* 2000; **41**: 242–249.

103 Signore A, Chianelli M, Annovazzi A, *et al.* Imaging active lymphocytic infiltration in coeliac disease with iodine-123-interleukin-2 and the response to diet. *Eur J Nucl Med* 2000; **27**: 18–24.

104 Procaccini E, Chianelli M, Pantano P, Signore A. Imaging of autoimmune diseases. *Q J Nucl Med* 1999; **43**: 100–112.

● 105   Signore A, Chianelli M, Parisella MG, *et al.* In vivo imaging of insulitis in autoimmune diabetes. *J Endocrinol Invest* 1991; **22**: 151–158.

● 106   Ohtsuki K, Hayase M, Akashi K, *et al.* Detection of monocyte chemoattractant protein-1 receptor expression in experimental atherosclerotic lesions: an autoradiographic study. *Circulation* 2001; **104**: 203–208.

● 107   Blankenberg FG, Tait JF, Blankenberg TA, *et al.* Imaging macrophages and the apoptosis of granulocytes in a rodent model of subacute and chronic abscesses with radiolabeled monocyte chemotactic peptide-1 and annexin V. *Eur J Nucl Med* 2001; **28**: 1384–1393.

● 108   Paul C, Peers SH, Woodhouse LE, *et al.* The detection and quantitation of inflammation in the central nervous system during experimental allergic encephalomyelitis using the radiopharmaceutical ^{99m}Tc-RP128. *J Neurosci Methods* 2000; **98**: 83–90.

● 109   Caveliers V, Goodbody AE, Tran LL, *et al.* Evaluation of ^{99m}Tc-RP128 as a potential inflammation imaging agent: human dosimetry and first clinical results. *J Nucl Med* 2001; **42**: 154–161.

● 110   Anderson VE, Osheroff N. Type II topoisomerases as targets for quinolone antibacterials: turning Dr. Jekyll into Mr. Hyde. *Curr Pharm Des* 2001; **7**: 337–353.

● 111   Pan XS, Yague G, Fisher LM. Quinolone resistance mutations in *Streptococcus pneumoniae* GyrA and ParC proteins: mechanistic insights into quinolone action from enzymatic analysis, intracellular levels, and phenotypes of wild-type and mutant proteins. *Antimicrob Agents Chemother* 2001; **45**: 3140–3147.

● 112   Oh SJ, Ryu JS, Shin JW, Yoon EJ, Ha HJ, Cheon JH, Lee HK. Synthesis of ^{99m}Tc-ciprofloxacin by different methods and its biodistribution. *Appl Radiat Isot* 2002; **57**: 193–200.

● 113   Vinjamuri S, Hall AV, Solanki KK, Bomanji J, Siraj Q, O'Shaughnessy E, Das SS, Britton KE. Comparison of ^{99m}Tc-Infecton imaging with radio-labelled white-cell imaging in the evaluation of bacterial infection. *Lancet* 1996; **347**: 233–235.

◆ 114   Britton KE, Wareham DW, Das SS, *et al.* Imaging bacterial infection with ^{99m}Tc-ciprofloxacin (Infecton). *J Clin Pathol* 2002; **55**: 817–823.

● 115   Sarda L, Saleh-Mghir A, Peker C, Meulemans A, Cremieux AC, Le Guludec D. Evaluation of ^{99m}Tc-ciprofloxacin scintigraphy in a rabbit model of *Staphylococcus aureus* prosthetic joint infection. *J Nucl Med* 2002; **43**: 239–245.

● 116   Dumarey N, Blocklet D, Appelboom T, Tant L, Schoutens A. Infecton is not specific for bacterial osteo-articular infective pathology. *Eur J Nucl Med Mol Imaging* 2002; **2**: 530–535.

● 117   Das SS, Britton KE. Bacterial infection imaging. *World J Nucl Med* 2003; **2**: 173–179.

● 118   Lupetti A, Welling MM, Mazz U, Nibbering PH, Pauwels EKJ. Technetium-99m labelled fluconazole and antimicrobial peptides for imaging of *Candida albicans* and *Aspergillus fumigatus* infections. *Eur J Nucl Med* 2002; **29**: 674–679.

● 119   Welling MM, Mongera S, Lupetti A, *et al.* Radiochemical and biological characteristics of ^{99m}Tc-UBI 29-41 for imaging of bacterial infections. *Nucl Med Biol* 2002; **29**: 413–422.

● 120   Welling MM, Lupetti A, Balter HS, *et al.* ^{99m}Tc-labeled antimicrobial peptides for detection of bacterial and *Candida albicans* infections. *J Nucl Med* 2001; **42**: 788–794.

● 121   Lupetti A, Welling MM, Pauwels EK, Nibbering PH. Radiolabelled antimicrobial peptides for infection detection. *Lancet Infect Dis* 2003; **3**: 223–229.

● 122   Melendez-Alafort L, Rodriguez-Cortes J, Ferro-Flores G, *et al.* Biokinetics of ^{99m}Tc-UBI 29-41 in humans. *Nucl Med Biol* 2004; **31**: 373–379.

● 123   Welling MM, Hiemstra PS, van den Barselaar MT, Paulusma-Annema A, Nibbering PH, Pauwels EK, Calame W. Antibacterial activity of human neutrophil defensins in experimental infections in mice is accompanied by increased leukocyte accumulation. *J Clin Invest* 1998; **102**: 1583–1590.

● 124   Welling MM, Nibbering PH, Paulusma-Annema A, Hiemstra PS, Pauwels EK, Calame W. Imaging of bacterial infections with ^{99m}Tc-labeled human neutrophil peptide-1. *J Nucl Med* 1999; **40**: 2073–2080.

4

Pediatric imaging

ISKY GORDON

Introduction	107	Indications for functional imaging in children	113
Handling the child	107	References	119
Maturation of the infant as it affects functional imaging	111		

INTRODUCTION

Undertaking examinations on children can be an exciting and rewarding experience for all concerned when the department is tuned to the needs and requirements of children and their parents. Every nuclear medicine department has a significant capital investment, yet that which is required for the understanding and successful handling of children has no significant capital or revenue consequence. A successful examination can be defined as one in which a high quality study has been achieved, together with the child and parent feeling well content and with a feeling of achievement. This does not mean that the child can not or may not cry; in fact, a few tears may be totally appropriate and the family may still feel well content despite the tears. In order to achieve this, all members of the department must be in tune with the need to establish the correct atmosphere from the first moment the child and parent enter the department, including making the appointment, until they leave when the examination is complete. There are departments where the thought of undertaking a pediatric examination instils fear and trepidation among the staff. In such an environment, the child, parent, and staff may be traumatized by the examination which further adds to the feeling that children are 'difficult'. Some professionals believe that children can be treated like adults and simply told to lie still: the lack of awareness of the 'child's world' leads to inappropriate handling of the pediatric patient. Some institutions feel that sedation is the only way to ensure that the child fits into the paradigm of adult examinations, but sedation could be seen as a sign of a department inadequately prepared for the handling of children.[1-3]

HANDLING THE CHILD

There are many ways to prepare the department for children; this institution finds that use of the word 'pediatrics' as a mnemonic is well suited to covering all aspects that are specific and particular to children.

P: Preparation and parent

PREPARATION

Preparation is the key to success. To have the best chance of a high-quality nuclear medicine examination there must be adequate preparation of the child and his/her parents. To achieve this the staff in the department require training as well as an adequate awareness of the handling of the child and parent. Staff training and preparation should include the appointments staff, receptionists, nurses, and technicians, while much of the training is based on good practice. Nevertheless, it is easy to forget the basic principles of using simple language, ensuring that what has been said has been understood and not assuming that because the child/parent has been told that they have necessarily understood. The reception and appointment areas should not pose an architectural barrier; rather, there should be an open area where the staff are on the same level as the parent, with space for the family to sit.

Preparation of the child begins when the appointment is made: the attitude of the receptionist/appointments clerk must be positive and encouraging. Specific information sheets have been prepared for all types of examination so that the parent receives full details of what to expect and how long the procedure will take. This reinforces the attitude of the department, which is to be open and completely truthful at all times, including information about aspects of the examination which are considered unpleasant; for example, the intravenous injection of an isotope. The information sheet also suggests that the parent should bring the child's favorite book or cassette tape to the department so that the child can enjoy it during the examination. If the department has a video tape recorder and TV monitor in the gamma camera room, then the child's favorite video could also prove useful during the examination. This is not, however, an excuse not to prepare properly.

THE PARENT

The *parent* offers the best form of comfort and security for a child. For this reason it is essential that the parent has a very good understanding of what will happen and also knows why the specific examination needs to be undertaken. If possible, the entire procedure should be explained to the parent and it should be stressed that the child will reflect the attitude of the parent. At times the parent needs a great deal of help so that the proposed examination can be faced positively and can be a support to the child.

E: Explain

There is a need for a full and truthful *explanation* of the entire procedure, without exception. This should be given to the parent and child both when the appointment is made and also when they return for the actual examination. The referring clinician should give a full explanation to the family of the test that has been requested although, in truth, the clinician does not always know the full details. For this reason, staff in the nuclear medicine department should assume that the parent/child has either not been informed or has been misinformed about the details of the investigation requested. The explanation must be open and done in such a way as to allow the parent and/or child to ask questions. Every family will be apprehensive and a good explanation means that the one or other member of the family will ask questions or express anxiety over either the examination or how their child may perform. Many parents feel that their child will not behave properly and this further raises anxiety levels.

D: Dose

The *dose* of the radiopharmaceutical should be scaled down; this scaling should be best done based on body surface area, and conversion charts are available whereby the weight may be used to represent body surface area. The use of age is not recommended because this results in considerable variation in radiation burden to the child. There is also a minimum dose schedule below which the injected activity is too low to obtain adequate information (Tables 4.1 and 4.2).[4]

Table 4.1 *Dosage card. Fraction of adult administered activity*

3 kg = 0.1	22 kg = 0.50	42 kg = 0.78
4 kg = 0.14	24 kg = 0.53	44 kg = 0.80
6 kg = 0.19	26 kg = 0.56	46 kg = 0.82
8 kg = 0.23	28 kg = 0.58	48 kg = 0.85
10 kg = 0.27	30 kg = 0.62	50 kg = 0.88
12 kg = 0.32	32 kg = 0.65	52–54 kg = 0.90
14 kg = 0.36	34 kg = 0.68	56–58 kg = 0.92
16 kg = 0.40	36 kg = 0.71	60–62 kg = 0.96
18 kg = 0.44	38 kg = 0.73	64–66 kg = 0.98
20 kg = 0.46	40 kg = 0.76	68 kg = 0.99

(Information is from a chart produced by the Paediatric Committee of the European Association of Nuclear Medicine, reproduced with permission from the EANM.)

I: Injection and information

INJECTION

The *injection* should be undertaken preferably with a butterfly needle connected to a three-way tap. This allows the needle to be positioned and flushed with saline with the minimum possibility of dislodging it in a small vein. In the UK many healthcare professionals have been retrained and job descriptions have been altered so that in numerous institutions, well-trained technologists and/or nurses are now undertaking the injections. If one or two persons in a department undertake the majority of the examinations, these individuals become very experienced in the procedure and have a high success rate. In many departments the responsibility for i.v. injection is no longer that of the medical staff.

INFORMATION

In the UK almost all departments are now faced with a population of families who have different home languages. It is essential for the *information sheet* to be translated into the languages that are commonly used in different geographic areas.

Every specific nuclear medicine examination requires its own information sheet with the full details explained, including waiting times. Directions for finding both the hospital and the department should also be included with every information pack.[1]

A: Amuse, anesthetic cream, assess, and attitude

AMUSE

The child should be *amused* – never ignored – and should remain the central focus throughout the entire procedure. Staff should be actively discouraged from chatting to each

Table 4.2 *Recommended adult and minimum amounts, in megabecquerels*

Radiopharmaceutical	Adult	Minimum
^{99m}Tc-diethylene triaminepentaacetic acid (DTPA) (kidney)	200	20
^{99m}Tc-dimercaptosuccinic acid (DMSA)	100	15
^{99m}Tc-mercaptoacetyltriglycine (MAG$_3$)	70	15
^{99m}Tc-pertechnetate (cystography)	20	20
^{99m}Tc-methylene diphosphonate (MD)	500	40
^{99m}Tc-colloid (liver/spleen)	80	15
^{99m}Tc-colloid (marrow)	300	20
^{99m}Tc-spleen (denatured RBCs)	40	20
^{99m}Tc-RBC (blood pool)	800	80
^{99m}Tc-albumin (cardiac)	800	80
^{99m}Tc-pertechnetate (first pass)	500	80
^{99m}Tc-macro-aggregated albumin (MAA)/microspheres	80	10
^{99m}Tc-pertechnetate (ectopic gastric)	150	20
^{99m}Tc-colloid (gastric reflux)	40	10
^{99m}Tc-iminodiacetic acid (IDA) (biliary)	150	20
^{99m}Tc-pertechnetate (thyroid)	80	10
^{99m}Tc-hexamethylpropylene amine oxime (HMPAO) (brain)	740	100
^{99m}Tc-HMPAO (WBCs)	500	40
^{123}I-hippuran	75	10
^{123}I (thyroid)	20	3
^{123}I-amphetamine (brain)	185	18
meta-[^{123}I]iodobenzylguanidine (^{123}I-MIBG)	400	80
^{67}Ga	80	10

RBCs: red blood cells. WBCs: white blood cells.

(The information is from a chart produced by the Paediatric Committee of the European Association of Nuclear Medicine, reproduced with permission from the EANM.)

other during the examination. The parent should be informed and encouraged to communicate actively with the child. The use of books or a cassette tape recorder and/or a VTR also helps in ensuring that the child does not become bored. This helps in achieving high quality images.

ANESTHETIC CREAM

The application of a *local anesthetic agent* to all children approximately 45 min before the intravenous injection ensures that almost all injections are undertaken through anesthetized skin and are therefore pain free. Although the injection is pain free, the local anesthetic cream will not prevent all sensation, so the child will feel skin being cleaned and the pressure of the injection but not the pain. This must be explained to the family. It is interesting to note that although children are told that this will be a pain-free injection, they are still anxious beforehand and are only fully convinced that the injection is indeed pain free when it has been completed. This is an example of how many children hear what you say but are unable to incorporate this knowledge. Staff must understand that this is

normal behavior and not insist that the child 'behave properly' or 'stop crying'. Only after the examination is completed can the child integrate all the information. The parent also must be informed that this is 'acceptable behavior' and not shout at the child because he/she does not live up to the parent's expectation. The 45 min wait period was originally perceived by many members of this department as a negative aspect, but it is now used advantageously by both patients and staff. It provides a good opportunity for the staff to sit and talk to the child and parent and also allows time to encourage oral fluid intake which is valuable in many different examinations (mainly dynamic renal, bone and brain (Bicisate) scintigraphy). The use of a local anesthetic agent with the added time in the department and pain-free injection builds up a significant degree of confidence between the child, the parent, and the staff and adds to the patient's trust.

ASSESS

The child and parent should be *assessed*, especially when the appointment is being made, and also when the EMLA cream is being applied, as to the cooperation that can be expected from the child and parent. The sensitive receptionist/booking clerk may well detect the parent who needs additional reassurance and so spend a little longer explaining the procedure or calling one of the technicians to talk to the parents and child. At times, showing the parent and child the equipment at this stage is very useful. At this stage, certain children, such as those who are mentally retarded and require regional cerebral blood flow studies, may be assessed as requiring sedation or even general anesthesia.

ATTITUDE

Every member of the department who comes into contact with a parent or child must have a *child-centred attitude*. This may require special times set aside in adult departments when only children are examined in a gamma camera room for that session, or in smaller departments, where the entire department is dedicated to children for specific hours per week. The time invested by the staff in the department in ensuring that the parent has a positive attitude towards the examination, and knows the importance of his/her role in supporting the child reaps its reward when a successful examination has been completed. If a technologist who enjoys working with children can undertake all the pediatric examinations, then the attitude in the department becomes more positive since those technologists who are anxious when dealing with children know they will be spared that anxiety.

T: Technique and team

TECHNIQUE

For the best *technique*, wherever possible, the camera should be rotated so that it is face upwards with the child lying on top and as close to the camera face as possible. This ensures that the child does not feel 'sandwiched' between the table and the camera and so does not have his/her world excluded. The highest quality images are obtained when the child is in contact with the gamma camera face; this is possible for smaller children, who may lie on top of the camera. When a bed is used, the camera should be in contact with the bed.

TEAM

A *team* attitude for all staff, parent and child is very helpful. A successful examination is more frequently obtained when the child and parent feel that they have made a major contribution to the examination. Every nuclear medicine examination requires cooperation from the child and parent. If this is acknowledged and encouraged then a team atmosphere is built up. In addition, the technical staff receive positive feedback, which enhances staff morale. Thus a positive cycle is created where each successful examination builds confidence in all members of the team and

goes a long way to create the positive, open, constructive approach required.

R: Radiation burden

The principle is to keep the *radiation burden* as low as possible, but at the same time obtain a high-quality result, particularly if a nuclear medicine examination is required. A significant part of the radiation burden may come from the bladder when undertaking examinations of other organs. Frequent voiding will reduce the radiation but is not easy to obtain in children. If they are frequently offered their favorite drinks, however, this adds to the possibility that they will be happy and feel that the department is interested in their welfare: there may be no need to mention voiding because a child will empty his/her bladder frequently.

Occasionally, a particular organ may be studied with one or more different radiopharmaceuticals that are considered similar. Whenever this happens, the biodistribution of the radiopharmaceutical should be understood and usually the one with the shortest biological half-life used as this will give the lowest radiation burden. This applies currently to regional cerebral blood flow studies.

I: Immobilize and images

IMMOBILIZE

The vast majority of children can be *immobilized* using very simple techniques such as sand bags placed on either side of the child with or without Velcro straps. Certain institutions prefer using a vacuum pillow which is wrapped around the child, the air extracted and the child then immobilized by the extraction bag. Sedation is not the answer to immobilization. There are times when the child moves during an examination but computer programs are available to correct for this movement. This is often adequate for dynamic renography although for static scans there is inevitably a loss of image quality. In this institution we use list mode acquisition for static dimercaptosuccinic acid (DMSA) scans when the image requires repeating because of movement.

IMAGES

High-quality *images* are essential. This requires a priori knowledge of what is an adequate image. Static examinations, e.g. bone or DMSA scans, are examples of where a department must set standards. There is now an atlas of normal bone scans in children of different ages (see bone section below). There is a difference between an image which is diagnostic and a high-quality image. At times an image which is not ideal may be accepted because it gives the required clinical information and the child is too ill to repeat the procedure or an over-invasive approach would be needed in order to obtain a higher-quality image.

C: Camera, cooperation, and crying

CAMERA

High-quality images are required, and this demands the use of high-resolution collimators for all static images. The *camera* should be used face up, wherever possible. The child should always be as close to the camera face as is reasonably practicable; often this may be with the child in contact with the collimator face.

COOPERATION

The best *cooperation* is achieved by allowing the child and parent to feel part of the team and that they have actively participated in the entire procedure. This requires truthfulness and openness together with a degree of confidence on behalf of the staff. The more the child feels part of the team, the more cooperative he/she will be. There is little value in shouting at a child or parent because this quickly leads to an escalating confrontational situation. There are times when an examination should be abandoned in order to maintain the cooperation and confidence of the parent. A full explanation should be given of why the examination has not been completed and it should be re-booked at a time which is convenient to both the department and the parent. Such openness frequently results in the parent insisting that the examination is tried one last time and does not then have to be abandoned.

CRYING

Crying may be a sign of anxiety. A child may cry frequently before the examination begins and even before the i.v. injection is given. Staff need to be prepared to tolerate this crying and reassure the parent and child that nothing untoward is happening without trying to stop the crying. Allow children to cry but acknowledge their fear: talk to them and their parents.

S: Sedation

Sedation is not routinely carried out in pediatric nuclear medicine examinations in this institution or many others. This institution undertakes over 1300 dynamic renograms per year – 700 DMSA scans as well as both direct and indirect radionuclide cystography – and yet, during the past 10 years, sedation has been used for only two patients undergoing renal studies. A recent survey of examinations carried out in this department over two consecutive months showed that sedation was used in 4.3% of children who, mainly, were undergoing brain scans and in young children undergoing lung or bone scans. This group had a median age of 27 months with a range of 3–54 months. These findings are in keeping with those of Pintelon *et al.*[2] who suggested that sedation was infrequently required for pediatric nuclear medicine examinations if there was adequate preparation and trained, skilled staff.

In the small group of children who do require sedation, there is considerable debate as to what is the 'best' sedation. At the pediatric pre-congress meeting of the European Association of Nuclear Medicine in Brussels in 1995, a seminar was held where it became clear that there is no such thing as 'safe' sedation. There is a cost–benefit analysis between the different drugs, but the use of Medazolan with adequate monitoring and appropriately trained staff for resuscitation came out as the possible first choice technique. This small group of children do require a great deal of gamma camera time, disproportionate to their numbers. Children with intractable epilepsy who are undergoing rCBF studies as part of a work-up for surgery form the largest single group who require sedation and, at times, general anesthesia. This is especially true in those children who are also mentally retarded where preparation is not possible. When using sedation for bone scans, the child usually can not void and the bladder fills with isotope. This may well require a bladder catheter, but placing it in a sedated child may well wake him/her and so spoil the sedation. It is not possible, however, to simply catheterize all children who require sedation while bone scans are carried out. This department tries hard to prepare the parent and child as a means of keeping sedation to as small a group as possible.

MATURATION OF THE INFANT AS IT AFFECTS FUNCTIONAL IMAGING

It is often stated that the child is not a small adult. Nowhere is this more obvious than in the very young. Maturation affects every organ in the body and because nuclear medicine is based on organ function, so the appearances of each organ system vary with the degree of both maturation and growth.

The brain

The appearances of regional cerebral blood flow (rCBF) begin to resemble those of an adult by the age of 2 years (Plate 4.1). Little work has been done on the changes in blood flow in normal subjects between 2 years of age and adulthood, yet clearly there is psychological maturation even if brain growth is almost complete by 2 years of age.[5]

Stomach and salivary glands

There is failure of salivary gland uptake of [^{99m}Tc]pertechnetate in the newborn and during early infancy, while gastric uptake is either absent or severely limited during this period. This observation is important if there is gut bleeding in the very young and a suspicion of a Meckel's diverticulum is raised. The other practical aspect of this biodistribution

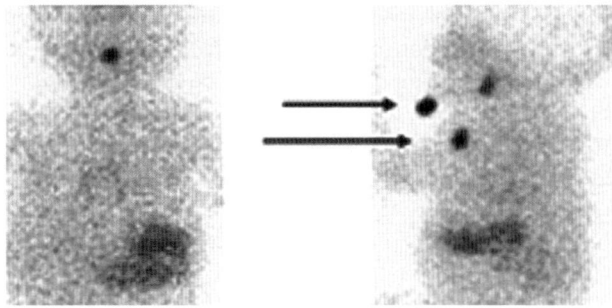

Figure 4.1 *A 1-week-old neonate with congenital hypothyroidism. On the anterior view of the $^{99m}TcO_4$ scan there is a single focus of uptake of tracer. This is midline and represents the hypoplastic thyroid gland. Note the lack of activity in the salivary glands and poor uptake by the stomach. The lateral view has markers on the chin and sternal notch, thus allowing the diagnosis of an ectopic gland situated at the base of the tongue.*

is that there is no need to undertake an anterior view of the neck in neonates with hypothyroidism because if activity is seen on the lateral view it can be assumed that it is thyroid and not salivary gland (Fig. 4.1).[6]

Lungs

While perfusion in children follows the same principles as that seen in adults, the effect of gravity has the opposite effect. In the dependent position in adults the dependent lung is both better perfused and ventilated while in childhood, the dependent lung is better perfused but has reduced ventilation. Thus in unilateral lung disease, placing the pathological lung dependent may result in better ventilation to the normal/better lung and will have beneficial effects on oxygen saturation.[7]

Kidneys: dynamic renography

Glomerular filtration reaches adult values (if factored to body surface area) by ± 2 years of age. However, the kidneys are not of adult size by this age and so growth will continue into the postpubertal phase with little or no further maturation. The early years of life are also characterized by a relatively large body surface area. The importance of this lies in the biodistribution of dynamic renal agents. Diethylenetriaminepentaacetic acid (DTPA), a small molecule, freely filtered, will cross the capillary membrane and so enter the extracellular space freely, thus lowering the blood concentration due to its biodistribution and not renal function. Mercaptoacetyltriglycine (MAG_3) on the other hand with a high protein binding will remain in the intravascular space and thus a higher concentration of tracer will be available to the kidney for uptake compared to DTPA especially in the first years of life.[8]

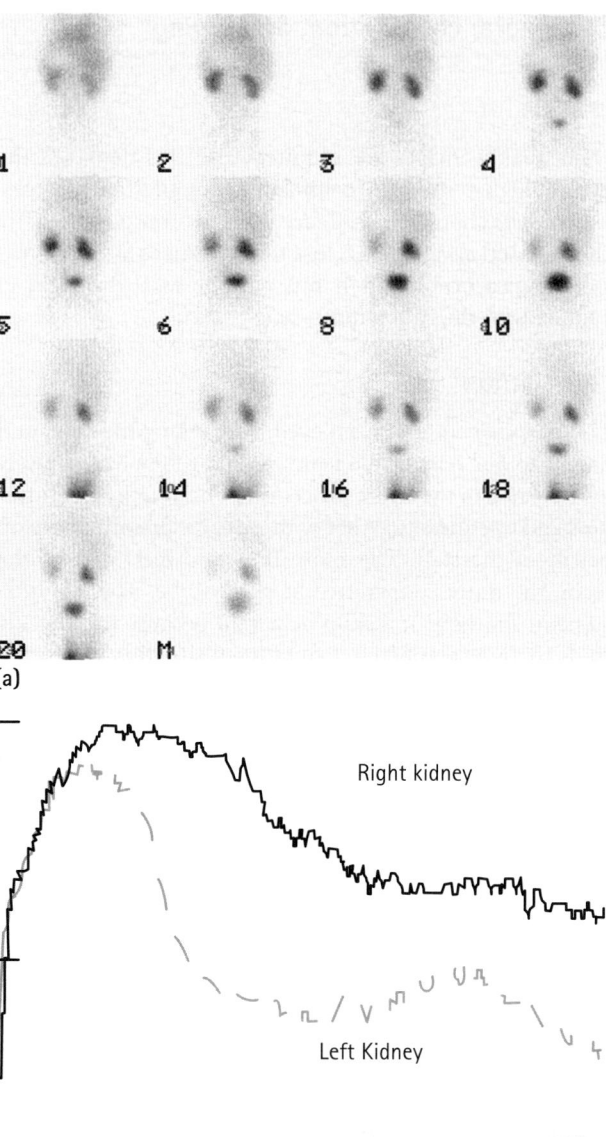

(a)

(b)

Figure 4.2 *Dynamic renal diuretic MAG_3 renogram in a 2-month-old neonate with prenatal diagnosis of unilateral right hydronephrosis. (a) The left kidney handles the tracer normally with tracer in the bladder by 4 min. The right kidney shows prompt uptake in the early images with moderate drainage by 20 min and further drainage by the end of the study. The image labelled 'M' is following a change in posture and micturition. (b) The renogram curves have steep upslope but following the peak there is a slow downslope even of the nonhydronephrotic kidney, typical of the normal neonate. The differential function showed that the right kidney contributed 46% to overall function.*

The dynamic MAG_3 renogram in early life is characterized by a high background with relatively poor visualization of the kidneys. Using DTPA the renogram curve is flat. However, the normal kidney has a short transit time and rapid transit into the bladder (Fig. 4.2(a) and (b)).

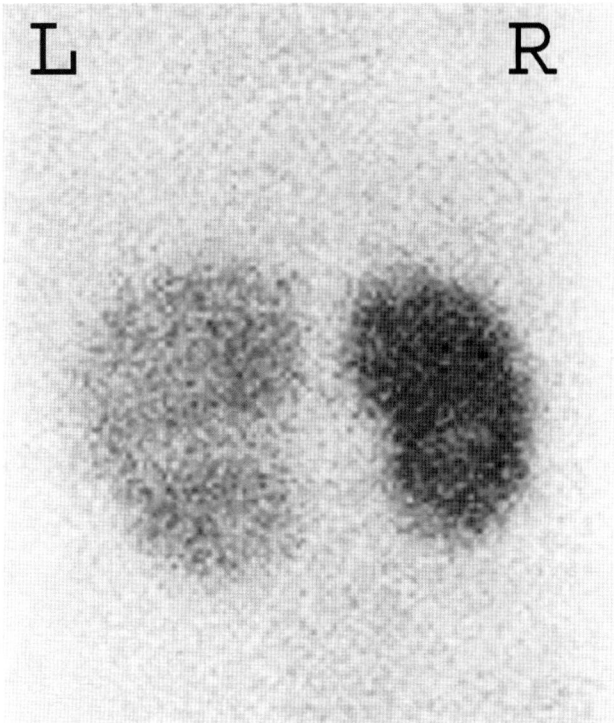

Figure 4.3 *A 10-week-old girl in renal failure secondary to severe neonatal hypoxia. Plasma creatinine elevated at 107 μmol L⁻¹. The ⁹⁹ᵐTc-DMSA shows a high background activity with poor uptake seen in both kidneys, worse on the left than the right. Differential function: left kidney 59% and right kidney 41%.*

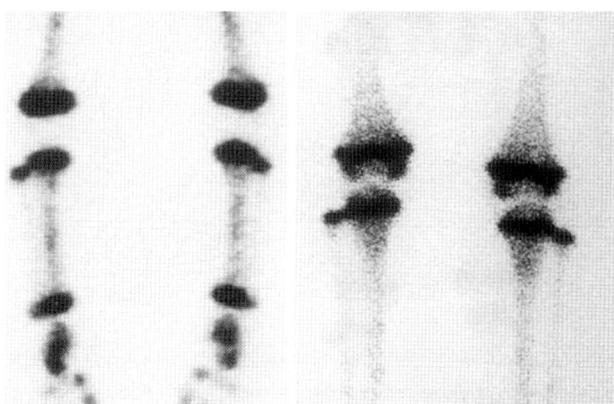

Figure 4.4 *Normal ⁹⁹ᵐTc-MDP bone scan at different ages. On the left is a normal posterior image of the knees of a 5-month-old child while on the right are the normal knees of a 4.6-year-old child. Note the marked difference in the appearances of the growth plates.*

Kidneys: static DMSA scan

Renal immaturity results in a high background in the first months of life as the tubules fail to take up the same amount of DMSA as the mature kidney. This does not preclude using DMSA but simply means that the detection of

focal parenchymal defects are more difficult because of the combination of small kidneys plus high background (Fig. 4.3).[9]

Bone scans

The growth plates of the skeleton concentrate the tracer to a greater degree than the remainder of the skeleton. This demands high-quality images of the growth plates as the common pathology seen in children often affects the growth plates. As the skeleton matures so the activity in the growth plates decreases and the normal appearances of the plates change with age (Fig. 4.4).[10]

INDICATIONS FOR FUNCTIONAL IMAGING IN CHILDREN

Brain

BRAIN DEATH

A dynamic technique with ⁹⁹ᵐTc-DTPA can be used to acquire images during the blood flow phase as well as a static image at ±3 min. On the latter image, an indication of activity in the venous sinuses is sought. Alternatively one of the lipophilic compounds (e.g. hexamethylpropylene amine oxime (HMPAO), ethyl cysteinate dimer (ECD)) can be injected and then single photon emission computed tomography (SPECT) or planar imaging can be undertaken (Plate 4.2).

BRAIN INJURY

Following brain injury the determination of rCBF using a lipophilic compound with SPECT will allow an assessment that many physicians in an intensive care unit find is valuable added information for completing a complex picture of injury (Plate 4.3).

EPILEPSY

The aim of rCBF imaging is to localize the epileptogenic focus that may be amenable to surgery. For this purpose both an ictal as well as an inter-ictal study is essential. Finding a hypoperfused region on an inter-ictal scan does not allow the conclusion that the region is the focus of the epilepsy. It is the difference between the ictal and inter-ictal rCBF study that enables the identification of the focus. The results of these studies need to be taken in conjunction with the full clinical, electrical and MRI findings in every case (Plate 4.4).[11]

PSYCHIATRIC DISTURBANCES

In pediatric psychiatry, the major use of rCBF is in research.[12]

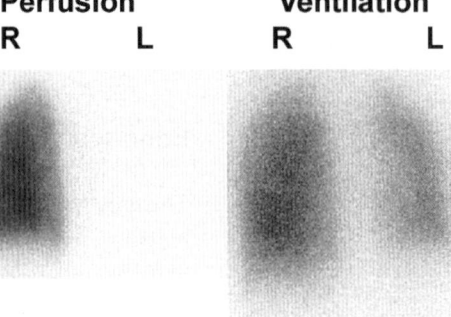

Perfusion
R L

Ventilation
R L

Figure 4.5 *A 1-year-old child with a hypoplastic left lung and associated interrupted pulmonary artery. The chest radiograph shows the mediastinum shifted to the left with a clear left hemi-diaphram. The left main bronchus is normally located. The anterior view of the ventilation scan (*^{81m}*Kr) reveals overall reduced ventilation, while the perfusion scan (*^{99m}*Tc-macroaggregates) shows only right lung perfusion.*

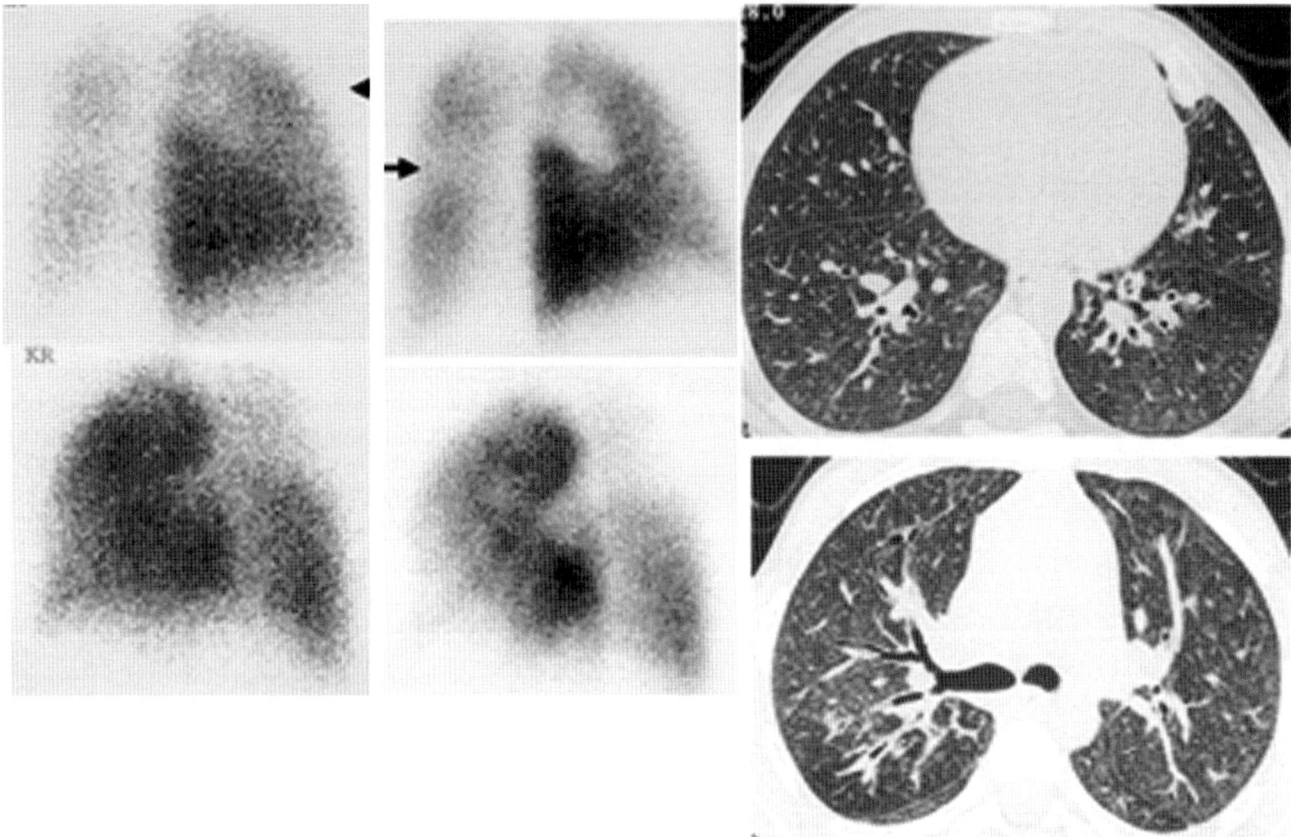

Figure 4.6 *A 12-year-old child with known immunodeficiency who was being followed-up. The high resolution CT scan shows diffuse disease throughout both lungs. The right and left posterior oblique images V/Q show multiple segmental defects that are mainly matched defects. This explained the increasing dyspnea that the child was suffering.*

The thyroid gland

NEONATAL HYPOTHYROIDISM

With the routine assessment of thyroid hormone levels in the early neonatal period, hypothyroidism is detected at a very young age. If this is confirmed on a second blood test with elevated thyroid-stimulating hormone (TSH), then an urgent thyroid scan is required. Using a dose of 10 MBq [^{99m}Tc]pertechnetate, lateral images of the neck are obtained

20 min later. One image is with markers on the chin and the top of sternum (Fig. 4.1).[6]

THYROID MASS/NODULE

This is an uncommon problem in childhood and the protocol is the same as for adults.

MASS IN NECK/UPPER MEDIASTINUM

As ectopic thyroid tissue is more common in children than adults, many surgeons wish to know if the mass in the

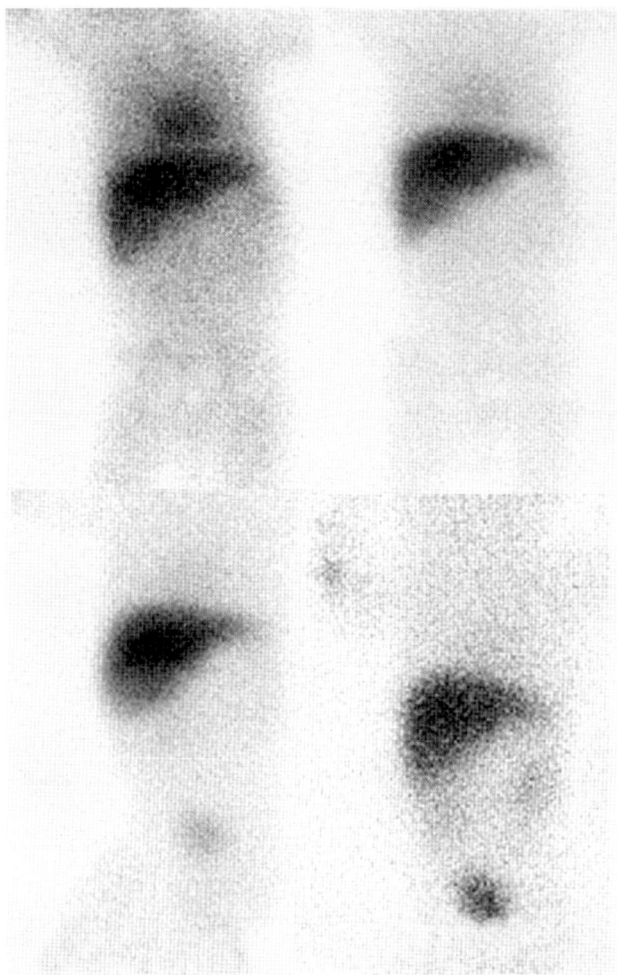

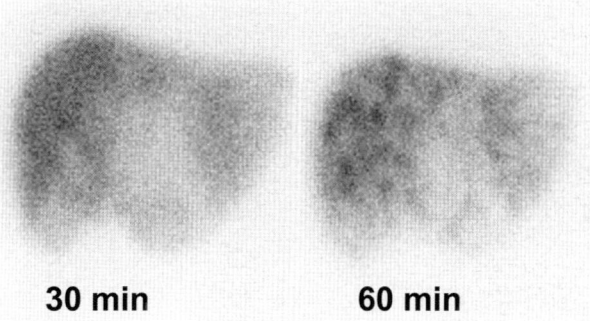

30 min   **60 min**

Figure 4.8 *99mTc-DISIDA scan in a child with autosomal recessive polycystic kidney disease (ARPKD). The 30 min image shows an enlarged left lobe of the liver. The 60 min image shows patchy tracer in the liver due to stasis in the bile ducts. These are typical features of ARPKD but not seen in 100% of cases. (See Fig. 4.10 also.)*

In the follow-up of children with chronic lung parenchymal damage (e.g. cystic fibrosis, immunodeficiency with recurrent respiratory tract infection), the V/Q scan can be used to assess regional lung function (Fig. 4.6).

The scan can also be useful for assessing pulmonary blood flow in congenital heart disease, including following interventions.

Gut

Indications for a radionuclide scan include swallowing disturbances, gastroesophageal reflux, and gastric emptying (esophagus and stomach). It may also be useful for studying intestinal bleeding, mainly for ectopic gastric mucosa (Meckel's). Inflammatory bowel disease (suspected or established) can be investigated by using 99mTc-HMPAO labeled white blood cells.[14]

Liver

Jaundice in the infant requires separation between biliary atresia and neonatal hepatitis. Biliary atresia requires surgery and is not associated with dilated biliary ducts, thus making it very difficult to use ultrasound to distinguish between these two conditions (Fig. 4.7).

In children with suspected autosomal recessive polycystic kidney disease the differential diagnosis may be wide in the neonatal period, further the typical radiological features seen in the early infancy may change with age so that by 5 years of age the appearances can mimic autosomal dominant polycystic disease. For this reason the changes seen in the liver add weight to the diagnosis. After 1 year of age the left lobe is enlarged and this may or may not be associated with dilatation of the biliary ducts. The latter signs are similar to those seen in Caroli's syndrome (Fig. 4.8).[15]

Figure 4.7 *99mTc-DISIDA in an infant with biliary atresia. The infant had progressive jaundice. The ultrasound examination was unremarkable. Phenobarbitone was given for 3 days prior to the 99mTc-DISIDA scan. Images over 24 h are displayed. The 5 min and 30 min images show high cardiac activity despite good uptake by the liver in the 1 min images. No gut activity is seen at any stage of the examination. The absence of gut activity means that biliary artresia can not be excluded but with such good liver uptake there is a very high probability that this is biliary atresia.*

upper mediastinum/neck is thyroid, so a [99mTc]pertechnetate scan is useful. The imaging protocol is the same as for a suspected thyroid mass plus including views of the upper mediastinum.

Lungs

Indications for a V/Q lung scan include the small/hypertranslucent lung on chest radiograph.[13] The V/Q scan readily detects the hypoplastic lung from the lung damaged by infection or foreign body. In the hypoplastic lung the associated anomalies of either interrupted pulmonary artery and sequestered segment can be readily detected on V/Q scans (Fig. 4.5).

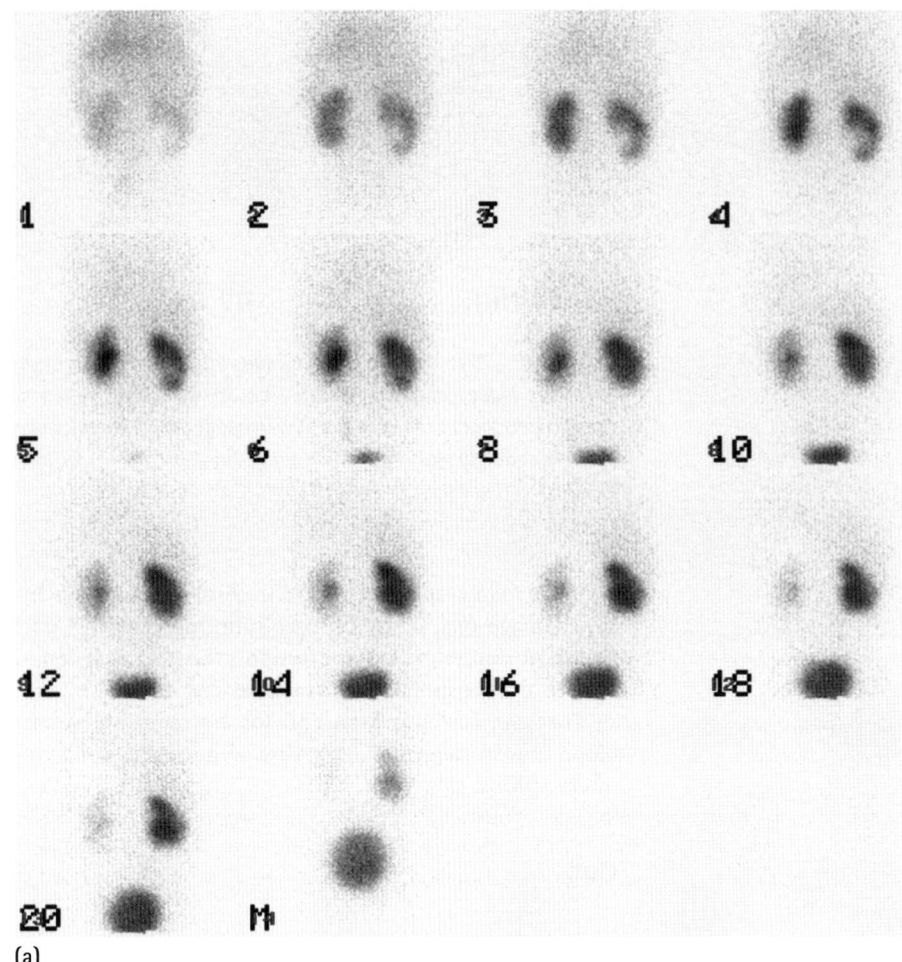

(a)

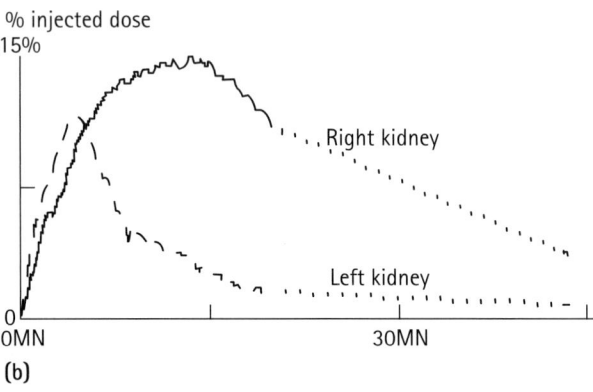

(b)

Figure 4.9 *Diuretic ^{99m}Tc-MAG$_3$ renogram in a 15-month-old infant with unilateral pelvic dilatation of the right kidney. Ultrasound showed a 22 mm AP diameter of the renal pelvis. The differential function of the right kidney was 42% (stable over the past 12 months) with good drainage only following a change in posture (pelvic excretion efficiency of 89% on the late image at 45 min). (a) Images over the first 20 min with an image at 45 min following a change in posture. Furosemide was given 2 min after the start of the study. (b) Background subtracted renal curves over the 45 min. The curves are discontinuous between 20 and 45 min as the infant is placed upright on the mother's shoulder after the 20 min acquisition and then replaced on the gamma camera at 45 min.*

Kidney

ASSESSMENT OF DIFFERENTIAL RENAL FUNCTION

If only differential renal function (DRF) is required, then a dynamic MAG$_3$ study will provide reliable results using the guidelines from the consensus report of International Radionuclides in Nephrology. The only exception is in the young infant with severe hydronephrosis.

DILATATION OF THE COLLECTING SYSTEM: DYNAMIC DIURETIC RENOGRAM

Assessment of hydronephrosis, especially in infants with the diagnosis of prenatal renal pelvic dilatation, requires specific attention to the acquisition, processing, and interpretation of the study. The protocol should follow the guidelines of the European Association of Nuclear Medicine. The estimation of differential function as well as assessment of drainage is difficult and has caused controversy.

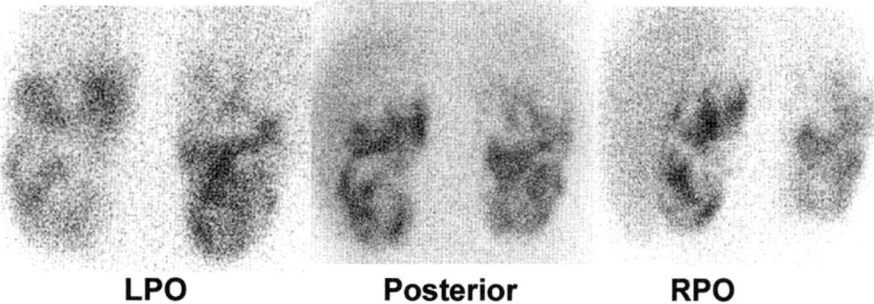

LPO   **Posterior**   **RPO**

Figure 4.10   *⁹⁹ᵐTc-DMSA scan in a child with ARPKD. The ultrasound showed symmetrically enlarged homogeneously bright kidneys. The ⁹⁹ᵐTc-DMSA scan shows bilateral defects with high background activity including activity in the liver. The combination of large symmetrical kidneys on ultrasound and a DMSA scan with multiple defects makes the diagnosis of ARPKD easy.*

Impaired drainage is not an indication for surgery, rather the long term function and degree of dilatation on ultrasound should guide management (Fig. 4.9(a) and (b)).[16–18]

SUSTAINED SYSTEMIC HYPERTENSION

This is similar to that done in adults with the knowledge that intrarenal pathology may exist on its own as a cause of the hypertension. This is found in fibro-muscular hyperplasia.

STATIC SCAN OF THE KIDNEYS

This type of scan can be used for assessment of parenchymal abnormalities, as follows:

- Urinary tract infection (see Chapter 8C).
- Suspected autosomal recessive polycystic kidney disease. The ultrasound and MRI findings show that the kidneys are uniformly enlarged with very small 'cysts' (dilated collecting ducts) seen evenly throughout the kidney. However, the ⁹⁹ᵐTc-DMSA scans reveal patchy uptake with large defects in both kidneys. This combination of enlarged homogenous kidneys on ultrasound in infancy and patchy uptake on DMSA confirms the diagnosis of autosomal recessive polycystic disease (Fig. 4.10).[15]
- In children with bilateral Wilms' tumors, there is a need to undertake kidney sparing surgery; this requires identification of the extent of the functioning renal tissue around each tumour in each kidney.
- Whenever an ectopic kidney is suspected, then function of this kidney should be undertaken using ⁹⁹ᵐTc-DMSA. This should include an anterior view.[19]
- If only one kidney is found on ultrasound and there is a suspicion of another kidney, e.g. in a child who is constantly wet or in a child with hypertension, then a ⁹⁹ᵐTc-DMSA scan is the most sensitive technique to find the very small kidney.

Bone scans[20]

INFECTION

In suspected osteomyelitis the ⁹⁹ᵐTc-methylene diphosphonate (⁹⁹ᵐTc-MDP) scan is a sensitive test for abnormal osteoblastic activity. If the pyrexia has been present for >24 h the bone scan is highly likely to be positive.

In suspected septic arthritis, the bone scan could be normal, hot or cold. When the clinical suspicion is septic arthritis of the hip, then a bone scan may rule out adjacent osteomyelitis, but has no role in the diagnosis of the arthritis.

BACK ACHE

Back ache is unusual in children. We have found that this must be taken seriously. If there are no neurological signs and the plain radiographs are normal, then a bone scan is indicated with SPECT of the spine. This should be undertaken prior to cross-sectional imaging, as this will then focus on the abnormal area seen on bone scan.

SUSPECTED HIP PATHOLOGY (INCLUDING PERTHES' DISEASE)

Adequate examination of the hip demands pinhole views to ensure that femoral head pathology is not overlooked (Fig. 4.11).

TRAUMA

When there is a suspicion of non-accidental injury and the radiographs are normal, then a bone scan is indicated. This should include spot views of the entire skeleton including oblique views of the ribs, a whole-body scan is not adequate.

After an episode of minor trauma, when there is persisting pain and negative radiographs, then a bone scan is very useful in proving that a fracture is present. A negative bone scan excludes significant bone pathology as a cause of the pain.

Pin hole collimator

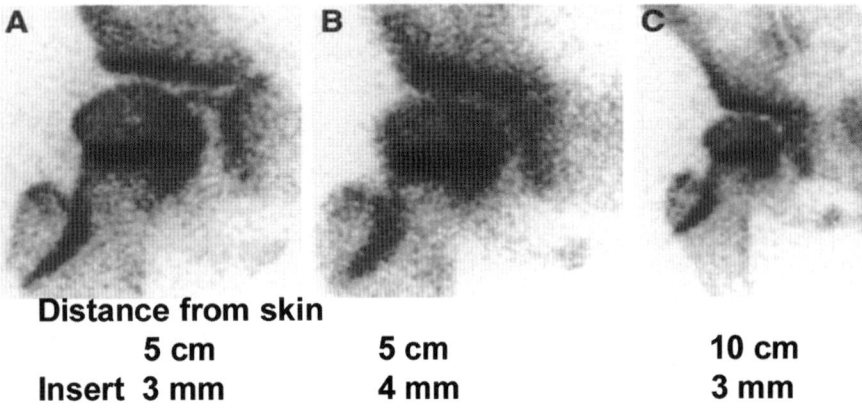

A **B** **C**

Distance from skin

5 cm	5 cm	10 cm
Insert 3 mm	4 mm	3 mm

Figure 4.11 *Bone scan with pinhole collimator, showing hips that are normal. The differences between the size of pinhole insert and the distance from the skin are important in the final quality of the image obtained. No department doing pediatric bone scans should be without a pinhole collimator.*

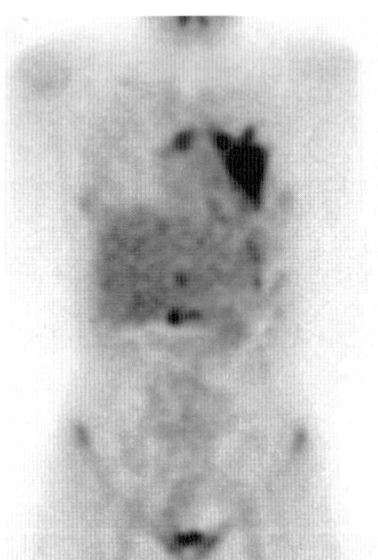
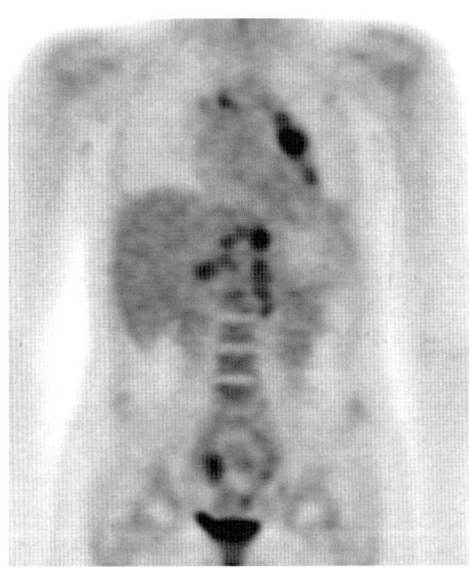

Figure 4.12 *A 6-year-old girl with Hodgkin's disease. Thoracic relapse treated with radiotherapy, Follow-up chest radiography showed persistent calcified lesion, but nil else. The PET scan shows active disease both above and below the diaphragm.*

DETECTION OF TUMORS

Primary tumors (both benign and malignant) can be detected. In children with known or suspected neuroblastoma, the use of *meta*-[^{123}I]iodo-benzylguanidine (^{123}I-MIBG) is essential for staging. This does not replace the need for a bone scan if the MIBG scan is normal.

Oncology – indications for PET–CT

BONE

PET–CT has a rapidly evolving role in the management of primary bone tumors including both osteosarcoma and Ewing's sarcome.[21] There is also a place for PET–CT in soft tissue sarcomas. The main indications include:

- Predicting outcome
- Monitor tumor response to neoadjuvant chemotherapy

- Differentiating post-operative changes from residual tumour or relapse
- Whole body imaging for detection of hematogenous spread

LYMPHOMA

Combined PET–CT imaging is becoming the new standard imaging modality for staging and re-staging of pediatric patients with lymphoma.[22] Indications:

- Staging
- Assessing response to therapy/prognostic value
- Monitoring status after the completion of therapy (Fig. 4.12)
- Evaluating for relapse

PET–CT has replaced PET, Ga-67 and in some cases CT.

REFERENCES

1 Harding LK, Harding NJ, Tulley NJ, *et al.* Improving information for nuclear medicine department outpatients. *Nucl Med Commun* 1994; **15**: 392–8.

2 Pintelon H, Jonckheer MH, Piepsz A. Paediatric nuclear medicine procedures: routine sedation or management of anxiety? *Nucl Med Commun* 1994; **15**: 664–6.

3 Gordon I. Issues surrounding preparation, information and handling the child and parent in nuclear medicine. *J Nucl Med* 1998; **39**: 490–4.

4 Piepsz A, Hahn K, Roca I, *et al.* A radiopharmaceutical schedule for imaging in paediatrics. Paediatric Task Group of the European Association of Nuclear Medicine. *Eur J Nucl Med* 1990; **17**: 127–9.

5 Rubinstein M, Denays R, Ham HR, *et al.* Functional imaging of brain maturation in humans using iodine-123 iodoamphetamine and SPECT. *J Nucl Med* 1989; **30**: 1982–5.

6 Kiratli PO, Gordon I, Nagaraj N. Neonatal hypothyroid disease: absent salivary gland evident on technetium-99m pertechnetate scan. *Clin Nucl Med* 2001; **26**: 310–13.

7 Davies H, Kitchman R, Gordon I, Helms P. Regional ventilation in infancy. *N Engl J Med* 1985; **313**: 1626–8.

8 Gordon I. Effect of normal infant maturation on nuclear medicine studies. *Nucl Med Commun* 1993; **4**: 827–9.

9 Smith T, Evans K, Lythgoe MF, *et al.* Tc-99m DMSA in children: Biodistribution, dosimetry, radiopharmaceutical schedule and age dependency. In: *Proceedings of the Sixth International Radiopharmaceutical Dosimetry Symposium.* Oak Ridge Associated Universities, Gatlinburg, Tennessee, 7–10 May 1997, pp. 665–78.

10 Hahn K, Fischer S, Gordon I. *Atlas of bone scintigraphy in the developing paediatric skeleton.* Heidelberg: Springer, 1993.

11 Cross JH, Boyd SG, Gordon I, *et al.* Ictal cerebral perfusion related to EEG in drug resistant focal epilepsy of childhood. *J Neurol Neurosurg Psychiat* 1997; **62**: 377–84.

12 Chowdhury U, Gordon I, Lask B, *et al.* Early-onset anorexia nervosa: is there evidence of limbic system imbalance? *Int J Eat Disord* 2003; **33**: 388–96.

13 Gordon I. Lung scanning in paediatrics. In: Peters AM. (ed.) *Nuclear medicine in radiological diagnosis.* London: Martin Dunitz, 2003: 641–50.

14 Jobling JC, Lindley KJ, Yousef Y, *et al.* Investigating inflammatory bowel disease – white cell scanning, radiology and colonoscopy. *Arch Dis Child* 1996; **74**: 22–6.

15 Zagar I, Anderson PJ, Gordon I. The value of radionuclide studies in children with autosomal recessive polycystic kidney disease. *Clin Nucl Med* 2002; **27**: 339–44.

16 Gordon I, Colarinha P, Fettich J, *et al.* Guidelines for standard and diuretic renography in children. *Eur J Nucl Med* 2001; **28**: BP21–30.

17 Eskild-Jensen A, Gordon I, Piepsz A, Frokiaer J. Interpretation of the renogram: problems and pitfalls in hydronephrosis in children. *BJU Intern* 2004; **94**: 887–92.

18 Eskild-Jensen A, Gordon I, Piepsz A, Frokiaer J. Clinical approach to the PUJ renogram: problems and pitfalls in hydronephrosis in children. *Urology* 2005; **94**: 887–92.

19 Gordon I. Indications for ^{99m}Tc-DMSA scans in paediatrics. *J Urol* 1987; **137**: 464–7.

20 Gordon I, Fischer S, Hahn K. *Atlas of bone scintigraphy in the pathological paediatric skeleton.* Heidelberg: Springer, 1996.

21 Brenner W, Bohuslavizki KH, Eary JF. PET imaging of osteosarcoma. *J Nucl Med* 2003; **44**: 930–42.

22 Hudson MM, Krasin MJ, Kaste SC. PET imaging in pediatric Hodgkin's lymphoma. *Pediatr Radiol* 2004; **34**: 190–8.

5

Sentinel lymph node imaging in clinical nuclear medicine

ROSEMARY ALLAN, JOHN REES, AND RAKESH GANATRA

Introduction	121	Breast carcinoma	127
Development of sentinel lymph node biopsy	121	Head and neck carcinoma	133
Definitions	122	Other cancers	133
Demonstrating the sentinel lymph node: lymphoscintigraphy	122	Standards	134
Malignant melanoma	123	Future developments	134
Surgical considerations	125	References	135

INTRODUCTION

Metastasis to regional lymph nodes is the main prognostic factor for many solid tumors, but this occurs in the minority of patients with clinical stage I and II disease. Unfortunately, both clinical examination and conventional cross-sectional radiological techniques understage nodal involvement because they can only detect metastases bulky enough to deform or enlarge lymph nodes. Changes in nodal shape (oval to circular), increase in size, enhancement with intravenous contrast, and loss of a fatty hilum are radiological indicators of malignant involvement. However, these characteristics are not specific because inflammatory nodes can display similar features. Until recently, the only reliable way to detect nodal involvement was to remove all regional lymph nodes and analyse them histologically. The treatment dilemma for early stage solid tumors without clinically involved regional lymph nodes is therefore: should all patients undergo elective lymph node dissection (ELND) when only the minority with occult nodal metastases will benefit, or should patients have clinical surveillance of their lymph nodes, knowing that this will be adequate treatment for most patients, but in some disease will progress? Sentinel lymph node biopsy (SLNB) aims to resolve this dilemma and marks a major advance in our ability to stage tumor spread. SLNB is essentially 'targeted' lymph node biopsy, where mapping the functional lymphatic drainage of a tumor locates the best lymph nodes for assessing disease spread.

Cabanas[1] first proposed the term 'sentinel lymph node' (SLN) in 1977. He hypothesized that lymphatic drainage from a tumor occurs in a stepwise and orderly manner, first to the SLN before passing on to other nodes in that lymphatic basin. Other nodes in the same drainage basin should therefore only contain metastases if there are metastases in the SLN. Cabanas used contrast lymphography to demonstrate the dorsal lymphatics of the penis and drainage to the SLN adjacent to the superficial epigastric vein in 100 patients with penile carcinoma. He then biopsied the SLN and patients underwent inguinofemoroiliac node dissection only if their SLN contained metastases. This was the first outcome study for SLNB; those patients whose SLN was clear of metastases had a much better 5 year survival (90%) than those in whom metastasis had occurred (70% if the SLN was the only node involved and 50% if others were too).

Other researchers were attempting to map lymphatic drainage of whole organs, skin, and tumors, using a variety of radiopharmaceuticals or blue dye. These studies challenged existing rules about lymphatic drainage, as laid down by Sappey in 1874, which were the basis of then current clinical practice.[2]

DEVELOPMENT OF SENTINEL LYMPH NODE BIOPSY

Further studies in the early 1990s refined the technique for identifying the SLN. Wong et al.[3] developed the use of

Table 5.1 *Complete procedure for a sentinel lymph node biopsy (SLNB)*

Procedure	Notes
1. Diagnosis, staging and counselling as appropriate for SLNB	*1. Tumor stages I and II, biopsy-proven, patient should understand the potential need to go on to ELND*
2. Sentinel lymph node imaging	*2. Day before or same day as surgery*
3. Surgery to remove SLNs	*3. Assisted by hand-held intra-operative gamma probe*
4. Histological analysis of SLNs	*4. Multisectioning, hematoxylin and eosin staining, immunohistochemistry ± polymerase chain reaction analysis*
5. ELND only if a patient's SLN(s) contains metastases	

ELND, elective lymph node dissection.

blue dye injected intradermally as an intra-operative aid to identify lymphatic tracks to one or more SLNs, first in a feline model and then in patients with malignant melanoma.[4] All patients then went on to have ELND. SLNs were identified in 194/237 (82%) of lymph node basins, with metastases in 40/237 specimens (17%) and only two non-sentinel nodes (of 3079 nodes) contained metastases, giving a false negative rate of <1%.

The disadvantage of using blue dye alone is that the surgeon cannot predict the location of SLNs prior to surgical incision, important in melanoma, as unexpected drainage pathways occur in 41%.[5] Pre-operative lymphoscintigraphy (LS) was introduced to solve this; by mapping tumor drainage, the skin overlying SLNs can be marked. Norman *et al.* had previously demonstrated that LS redirected surgical management in up to 59% of patients with head and neck or truncal melanoma[6] and Uren *et al.* found that LS improved detection of those drainage sites that contained metastases.[7]

The final step was the introduction of a hand-held gamma probe to aid surgical localization of radiolabeled lymph nodes.[8] SLN localization now reached 98%; all of the blue-stained nodes in this study were radiolabeled, but 10% of the SLNs would not have been found by LS alone.

Since then, multiple other studies both in melanoma and breast carcinoma have confirmed high success rates at retrieving SLNs in patients by this 'triple method' of pre-operative mapping with LS and intra-operative mapping with blue dye plus a hand-held gamma probe and this now represents the 'gold standard' technique.

The complete SLNB procedure is listed in Table 5.1 and is a multidisciplinary team procedure. The role of imaging is to provide the surgeon with a pre-operative route-map that localizes the SLNs, to identify all potentially involved lymph node draining basins that might require subsequent ELND, and to demonstrate any aberrant drainage pathways.[9] Following resection, SLNs are then sent for histological analysis which is much more detailed than previously performed on nodes from ELND.

SLNB has been most widely applied to malignant melanoma and to breast carcinoma, but is likely to be relevant to most solid tumors. If SLN theory really is valid, 'skip' metastases to non-sentinel nodes should not occur and this is virtually true in malignant melanoma (<2%).[4,9]

DEFINITIONS

The most concise definition of an SLN is 'any lymph node which receives drainage directly from the tumor site'[10] and, anatomically, SLNs should be connected to the tumor by their own individual lymphatic tracks. As there may be several lymphatic drainage tracks leading from a tumor site, each with different rates of lymphatic flow, there is frequently more than one SLN; moreover SLNs are not necessarily either the first draining node or the ones closest to the tumor. Second-tier nodes receive lymphatic drainage from SLNs before draining to other nodes in the lymph node basin. Aberrant nodes are SLNs outside a named lymphatic drainage basin, usually in the superficial tissues and interval nodes lie along a lymphatic track leading from a tumor to a named lymphatic drainage basin; both may contain metastases.[11]

DEMONSTRATING THE SENTINEL LYMPH NODE: LYMPHOSCINTIGRAPHY

Particles pass from the interstitium into the lymphatic capillaries via gaps in the endothelial cells, which are usually 10–25 nm in diameter, but are widened during exercise or massage. The capillaries then join into larger collecting vessels which eventually lead to lymph nodes. Flow rates within the lymphatic vessels are reduced by low temperature and external pressure and vary according to which part of the body is being drained, being fastest from the leg and foot and slowest from the head and neck.[12] Once within the lymphatic system, foreign particles are phagocytosed by macrophages and tissue histocytes situated predominantly in the subcapsular sinuses of lymph nodes.

The ideal radiocolloid is one which passes easily into the lymphatics and the optimum particle size for this is

5–50 nm.[13] Smaller particles may pass preferentially into the intravascular space and very large ones (>200 nm) cannot pass easily through the interstitium to enter the lymphatic system, so tend to remain at the injection site. ^{99m}Tc-nanocolloid (an albumin derivative, particle size 3–80 nm, 80% <30 nm) and ^{99m}Tc antimony sulfide colloid (particle size 10–15 nm) usually allow good visualization of lymphatic tracks, SLNs and aberrant drainage and are the preferred agents. However, because they migrate rapidly, they tend to demonstrate more second and third echelon nodes than larger radiocolloids, which may lead to more extensive surgery. Although ^{99m}Tc sulfur colloid has particle sizes up to 300 nm, it may be filtered to produce particles <200 nm, but then has to be used quickly. The choice of colloid is usually dictated by regional/national availability, with ^{99m}Tc nano- and antimony sulfide colloids being used in Europe and Australasia, whereas in the United States, ^{99m}Tc sulfur colloid is the only agent approved for use.

SLNs retain most of the blue dye and radiolabeled colloid that reaches them, but some may pass through SLNs to second-tier nodes, especially where lymphatic flow rates are high, as in the lower limb.[12,13] A small percentage of SLNs accumulate only either blue dye or colloid, but an SLN should take up one or other agent.

MALIGNANT MELANOMA

The likelihood of lymph node metastases in melanoma depends largely on staging of the primary tumor, which is determined histologically from a biopsy. The criteria for tumor (T) classification are tumor thickness in millimeters (Breslow thickness) and the presence or absence of ulceration; ulcerated melanomas are upstaged to the next level T substage compared with thicker non-ulcerated melanomas. Clark's level of invasion is an independent prognostic feature only for T1 melanomas <1 mm.[14]

Five-year survival of patients with nodal metastases at presentation is 40%, compared with 90% of those without such metastases. Five-year survival rates for thin (<1 mm Breslow thickness) melanomas are 95–100%, falling to 50% for thick (>4 mm) melanomas. Overall 5-year survival rates for intermediate thickness (Breslow 1–4 mm) range from 60% to 96%, although patients with melanomas 1–2 mm have 5-year survival rates much better than those with lesions 2.1–4 mm (80–96% vs 60–75%).[15] Approximately 20% of patients with intermediate thickness melanoma have occult lymph node metastases at presentation and the role of ELND in this group is controversial. Two randomized trials comparing immediate ELND with nodal observation failed to demonstrate an overall survival advantage from either option.[16,17] However, two other multicenter trials identified subgroups of patients who did benefit from ELND (those with tumors 1–2 mm thick and/or aged <60 years[18] and those with truncal melanoma and nodal metastases at ELND).[19] Some countries therefore proposed ELND plus wide local excision (WLE) of the tumor as the standard of care, whilst others adopted WLE plus nodal observation. SLNB was thus introduced into the management of early malignant melanoma[4] to select those patients likely to benefit from ELND.

Patient selection

The Society of Nuclear Medicine guidelines endorse SLNB in patients with melanomas 0.76–4 mm thick and with no clinical evidence of nodal or distal involvement.[20] Melanomas <0.75 mm have a 1% incidence of nodal metastases, but SLNB may be considered if adverse histological features such as ulceration, regression or Clark level >3 are present.[21] Patients with thick (>4 mm) non-ulcerated melanomas have a 50% better overall 3-year survival advantage if their SLNs are clear compared with those with ulcerated tumors and positive SLNs (85.9% vs 57.3%)[22] and SLNB may be also used in this group. At the time of writing, UK guidelines do not support SLNB as routine practice outside of clinical trials in specialist centers, but this may change when longer follow-up data are published.[15]

Lymphatic mapping is unlikely to be accurate in patients who have had previous extensive surgery, ELND[20] or trauma. Patients who do not consent to ELND should not undergo SLNB.

Sentinel lymph node lymphoscintigraphy

SLNB is performed ideally 2–3 weeks following diagnosis and staging, to allow any lymphatic disruption from biopsy to abate. The technique for lymphoscintigraphy is summarized in Table 5.2.

INJECTION TECHNIQUE

In order to mimic tumor lymphatic drainage, injections should be made into the intra- or subdermal space, because melanomas arise from transformed melanocytes situated at the junction of the dermis and epidermis. The average administered dose of radiocolloid is approximately 40 MBq, in divided aliquots of 10 MBq in 0.2–0.5 ml, tailored to the size of the excision biopsy site and administered via a 25–27G needle.[13,23] Larger volumes of injectate may force fluid down nonphysiological pathways. Inadvertent contamination is minimized by covering the patient's surrounding skin and the gamma camera face and covering the injection site with a gauze as the needle is being withdrawn.

IMAGE ACQUISITION

Imaging should begin immediately following injection and continue for at least 1 h, depending on the speed of lymphatic drainage. The dynamic series provides information

Table 5.2 *Technique for sentinel lymph node (SLN) lymphoscintigraphy*

Procedure	Notes
Preparation	• *Cover surrounding skin and gamma camera face with waterproof drape (e.g. incontinence pad)*
	• *LFOV gamma camera, LEAP collimator, 10% energy window centred on 140 keV energy peak*
Injection	• *40 MBq radiocolloid divided into small volume (0.05–0.2 ml) aliquots*
	• *Average of four injections placed intradermally around excision, concentrating on center of scar: more may be required with larger scars*
Image acquisition	• *Immediate dynamic acquisition for 15–20 min (128 × 128 matrix, 10 s frames)*
	• *Orthogonal static images (256 × 256 matrix for 300 s)*
	• *Continue for approximately 2 h*
	• *Delayed imaging may occasionally be required*
	• *Body outline view ([57]Co flood or point source)*
	• *Depth estimation of SLNs*
SLN marking	• *Surface locations of all SLNs located with [57]Co point source and marked indelibly at the shortest skin-node point*
	• *Patient in same position as surgery as far as possible*
	• *Match nodal classification with histologist*
Reporting lymphoscintigraphy	• *Review all imaging*
	• *Anatomical locations of SLNs ascertained*
	• *Written tabulation in patient's clinical record prior to operation*

LFOV, large field of view; LEAP, low-energy, all-purpose.

about lymphatic tracks and helps discriminate SLN from second-tier nodes, whilst the static high count images are necessary for SLN localization. All potential drainage basins should be imaged (e.g. axillae/inguinal regions plus popliteal/antecubital fossae for limb melanomas, axillae and inguinal regions for truncal melanomas, cervical regions and axillae for head and neck melanomas) and orthogonal views of all SLN acquired. Most centers use [57]Co point or flood sources for body outline views, although transmission images using the [153]Gd line source available on many gamma cameras for attenuation correction are described as being superior.[24]

DEPTH ESTIMATION

An estimation of the depth of any marked SLNs provides useful information in addition to that provided by lymphoscintigraphy and may help surgeons decide how aggressive they should be in pursuing marked SLNs at sites that are difficult to access, bearing in mind that SLNB is just a staging procedure. The easiest way of estimating the depth of an SLN is to place a radioactive marker on the skin site of the node and obtain an orthogonal image; the distance between the skin marker and the SLN can then be estimated.

Combined SPECT/CT systems should provide the most accurate depth estimation, particularly in the head and neck, where anatomy is complex and packed into subcentimeter distances that are below the resolution of the

gamma camera.[25] Ultrasonography may also prove useful in selected cases, although it can only visualize nodes corresponding with the sites marked, rather than deciding whether these nodes are sentinel or not.

Sentinel lymph node lymphoscintigraphy: interpretation

Anyone undertaking lymphoscintigraphy should familiarize themselves with potential drainage patterns and the reader is referred to the comprehensive review by Uren *et al.*[12] It is essential that images are reviewed on the computer console where windowing of low count areas can be performed.

Reviewing the dynamic series in cine-mode demonstrates the time-sequence of lymphatic flow and allows SLNs to be distinguished from non-SLN areas of focal activity. These include second-tier nodes and physiological sites of hold-up under the edges of muscles and at lymphatic confluences. One or more lymphatic tracks are usually identified converging on a SLN and second-tier nodes may appear slightly later (Fig. 5.1). Second-tier nodes are usually more central than SLNs, but may be hotter at the time of imaging. However, if there are multiple tracks apparently converging on one SLN and activity appears simultaneously in a more central node, that should also be considered as a SLN as one of the tracks may have bypassed the first SLN.[13]

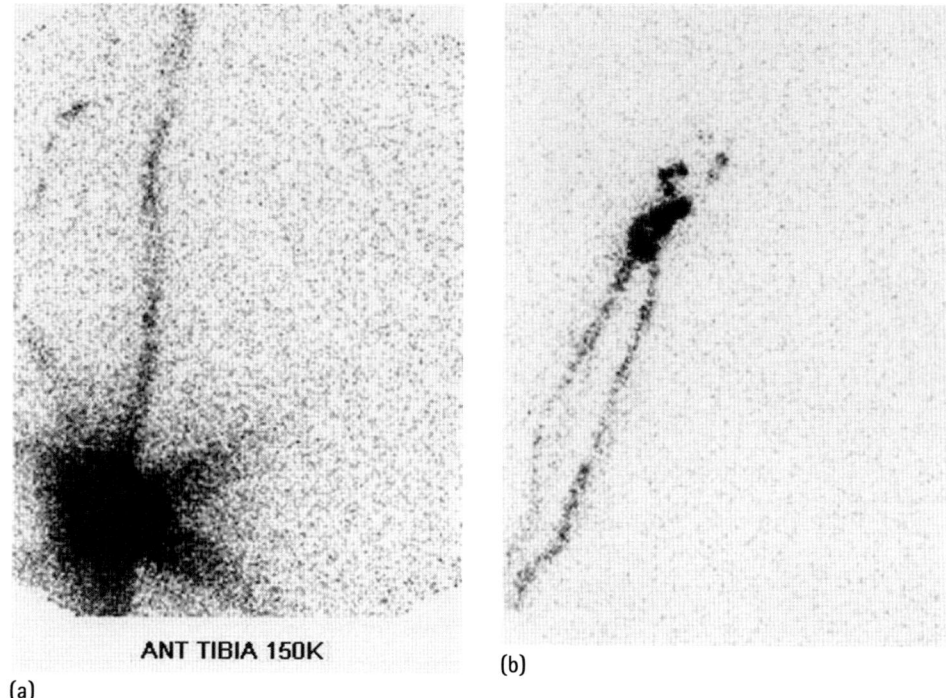

(a)

ANT TIBIA 150K

(b)

Figure 5.1 *(a and b) Melanoma in the right calf. Lymphatic drainage of the melanoma is via several lymphatic tracks leading from the injection site, which converge firstly on several closely adjacent sentinel lymph nodes in the right inguinal region and, subsequently, in second-tier nodes that are placed more centrally.*

Static images obtained in at least two projections and the body outline views identify the number and anatomical location of SLNs and the drainage basins they are situated in. Aberrant drainage should be anticipated; 12% of melanomas on the back drain to the triangular intermuscular space (Fig. 5.2) and 4% to para-aortic nodes, whilst 8% of lower limb melanomas drain to the popliteal fossa (Fig. 5.3).[7,11,22] One or more SLNs may overlie in one projection and appear as a single site, or may move with patient positioning (Fig. 5.2).

Slow drainage and non-drainage are encountered infrequently; slow drainage may be influenced by an individual's lymphatic clearance and requires delayed imaging if this can be coordinated with the patient's surgery. Theoretically, nodes that are replaced completely by tumor should not take up colloid and this appears to be true in breast carcinoma, where 73% patients in whom no SLN was found had extensive axillary nodal disease compared with 23% in whom a SLN was found.[26]

Marking the sentinel lymph node

SLNs are located by using a ^{57}Co point source during an image acquisition and the shortest skin-node distance marked. The patient should be in the same position as far as possible as for surgery, as the relationship of the overlying skin with the node can vary by up to 3–4 cm with patient movement. SLNs should be marked on the skin indelibly.

Some centers find it helpful to confirm the position with a gamma probe. When marking a SLN, it is advisable to use the same nodal tabulation as the histologist.

SURGICAL CONSIDERATIONS

Technique

Surgery is guided by intra-operative gamma probe counting and vital blue dye. Blue dye travels faster through the lymphatics than radiocolloid and is injected around the skin lesion at the time of surgery.[3] Before making an incision, the probe is used to verify the position of the node relative to the skin mark. Hot nodes are identified by comparison with background activity, with ratios of 2:1 to 20:1 being acceptable.[23,27] The probe is used to direct dissection; visualization being aided by blue dye. Hot nodes are removed, along with blue nodes that are not hot.

Intra-operative gamma probes

The intra-operative probe consists of the hand-held detector (the probe) which is linked to an electronic processing unit. Several types of probes are commercially available. The main differences are related to sensitivity, collimation

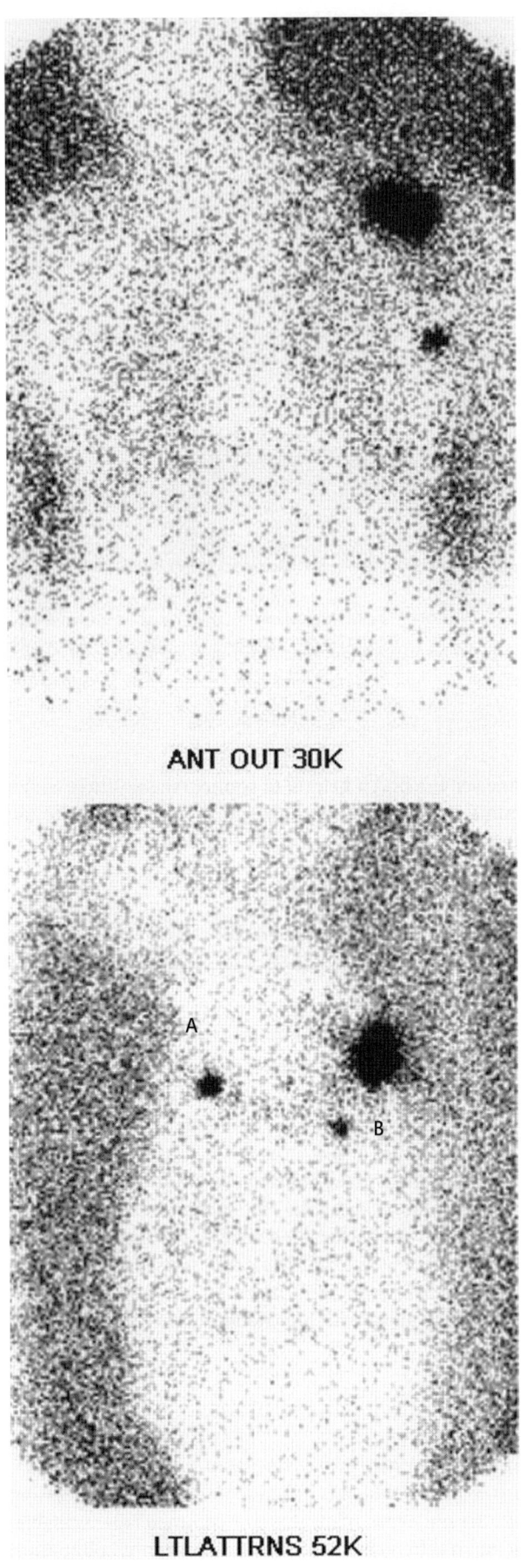

ANT OUT 30K

LTLATTRNS 52K

spatial resolution and count rate linearity. Studies have compared these probes and although there are variations in performance, most are suitable for SLN localization.[28,29]

Most of the activity injected is retained at the injection site and only about 5% is taken up by the SLN. Therefore, the probe should be directed away from the injection site when locating the SLN. For statistical significance, positive uptake should be taken as a minimum of three standard deviations above the background level.[28]

Histology

Each SLN that is removed is multisectioned and examined by conventional hematoxylin and eosin staining and immunohistochemistry with S-100 protein and HMB-45 (which detects an additional 12% of positive nodes).[27] The role of reverse transcriptase polymerase chain reaction is controversial[30] as it is extremely sensitive but can lead to false positive results.

Results

SLNB is now a recognized staging procedure and was included in the latest American Joint Committee for Cancer staging system for melanoma.[14] SLN status is a strong independent prognostic survival factor, with 3-year disease-specific survival being 69.9% and 96.8%, respectively, depending on whether the SLN contains metastases or not.[31] Many patients want this prognostic information in order to plan their lives, whether or not long-term survival is prolonged.[32]

The World Health Organization (WHO) declared SLNB as the standard of care in melanoma[33] after its trial (trial 14) of men with truncal melanomas 1.5–4 mm thick found 5-year survival rates in patients with occult nodal metastases were better (48.2%) in patients who had WLE and immediate ELND than in those who had WLE alone.[19] However, it is still not known if SLNB improves 5-year survival in all eligible patients and although individual centers are beginning to present their results,[34] the outcome of large randomized trials such as the Multicenter Selective Lymphadenectomy Trial are needed to resolve this.

Figure 5.2 *Melanoma in the left scapula region. Lymphatic drainage is to two sentinel lymph nodes (SLNs), although this is only appreciable on the lateral view. One SLN is in the left axilla and the second is situated too posteriorly to be in the axilla and was in the posterior triangular space. It is important to appreciate this because the surgical approach to the latter is through the back rather than via the axilla. This example also demonstrates how the position of SLNs may change with arm positioning; for the AP view the patient's arms are by their side and for the lateral view they are elevated.*

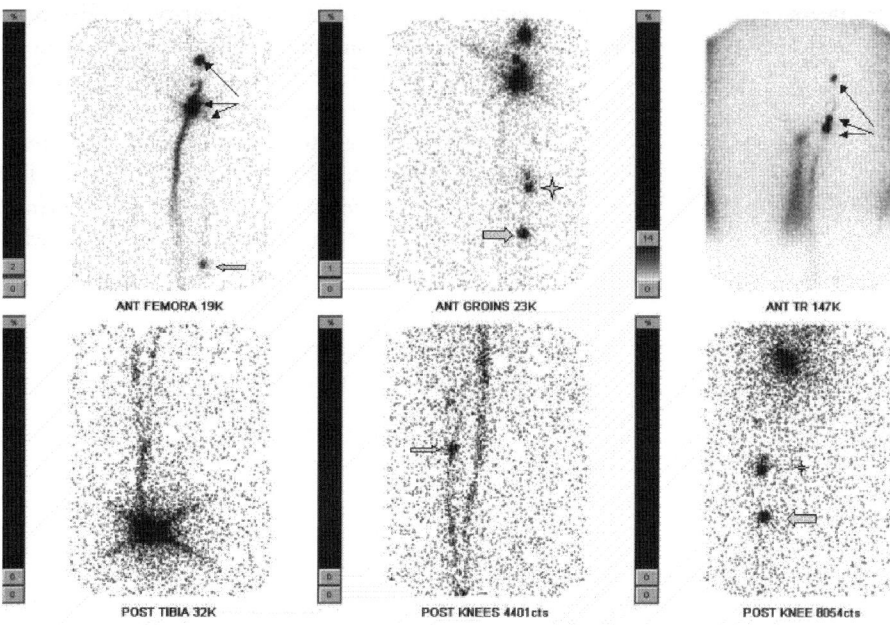

ANT FEMORA 19K

ANT GROINS 23K

ANT TR 147K

POST TIBIA 32K

POST KNEES 4401cts

POST KNEE 8054cts

Figure 5.3 *Melanoma in the left ankle. Early dynamic and delayed views demonstrate separate tracks leading to the left inguinal region and left popliteal fossa. There are two sentinel lymph nodes (SLNs) in the left inguinal region, but a track is visualized immediately leading to another node which fills almost synchronously with the first and should be considered another SLN. As well as the popliteal SLN, a further SLN was identified in the mid thigh, along the deep veins and lymphatics. All of these SLNs were stained blue at surgery. (Thin arrows, left inguinal SLN; block arrows, popliteal SLN; star, mid thigh SLN.)*

BREAST CARCINOMA

Introduction

Breast cancer is the commonest cancer in women in the UK, accounting for 27% of all cancer diagnoses.[35] The incidence in the UK is 92.7 per 100 000 and the overall incidence in Europe is 76.0.[36–38] Breast cancer shows the highest incidence and death rate of all cancers in women in the USA accounting for 135 cases per 100 000 of the population.[39]

Regional axillary lymph node status is one of the most important predictors of survival in breast cancer and the most important factor when deciding to use adjuvant treatment.[40,41] Other prognostic factors include tumor size, grade of tumor, lymphovascular invasion (causing hematogenous spread from the primary tumor) and receptor status.[42]

Conventionally, most women with invasive breast cancer have undergone operative axillary sampling or axillary clearance, both of which have associated morbidity.[43] The introduction of a breast cancer screening program has meant that very small tumors are detected.[44] Although this has resulted in an axillary positivity rate of as low as 3–7%, the average overall axillary positivity is still about 25%.[45] Therefore, at least 75% of women have 'unnecessary' axillary node sampling or axillary clearance. The morbidity associated with an axillary procedure include arm swelling, sensory disturbance, infection, shoulder stiffness and impaired shoulder movement. This is particularly troublesome in axillary clearance[46] but is also seen in axillary node sampling. The ideal situation, therefore, would be to stage the axilla with no or minimal intervention.

When nodes are palpable, percutaneous biopsy can be performed for histological staging. Ultrasound imaging can also be used to locate and sample impalpable nodes using fine needle aspiration. However, neither clinical nor conventional radiological evaluation of nodes is accurate. Up to 40% of patients with clinically negative axillae have lymph node metastases.[47] Therefore, alternative methods of evaluating the axillary nodal status have been sought.

The application of the sentinel node concept to breast cancer by Giuliano *et al.*[48] has revolutionized the management of patients with breast cancer. SLNB offers not only an accurate method of local staging but has also been shown to reduce morbidity from arm lymphedema. SLNB can be performed under local anesthesia in an attempt to reduce the risks of general anesthetics and allow the surgeon to preoperatively select the treatment given to the patient.[49,50]

The sensitivity of SLNB ranges from 80 to 96% but the method of calculating the false negative rate varies between studies and is not always equated to node positive patients.[51] Despite this lack of standardization and lack of long-term outcome data, the SLNB technique is becoming accepted internationally as a routine method of managing breast cancer. However, there are a number of variations in SLNB technique as practised by major centers which routinely use SLNB in the management of breast cancer. These include variation in the methods of localization, differences in injection technique, imaging differences and variation in the histopathological methods used to identify tumor cells (Table 5.3). Despite many of these variations, most centers achieve high success rates at localizing SLNs and most studies now aim only to optimize the technique in order to achieve small improvements in the rate of detection of the SLN.

Current indications

SLNB is indicated in stage T1 and 2 invasive breast carcinomas for staging the axilla. The concept can be applied to both

Table 5.3 *Technical variations in the sentinel lymph node biopsy technique in breast cancer*

Part of the procedure	Possible variations
Method of localization	Patent blue dye
	Lymphoscintigraphy
	Combination of these two methods
Colloid particle size used	Small (50 nm)
	Large (1000 nm)
	Mixed
Injection site	Intra-tumoral
	Peri-tumoral
	Sub-areolar
	Intra-dermal
	Subdermal
	Single/multiple injection sites
Use of breast massage following injection	
Single/dual isotope injection	
Radiopharmaceutical	
Administered activity	7–370 MBq
Volume	0.2–4 ml
Labelling method	In air or in a vacuum
Imaging technique	Intra-operative gamma probe only
	Pre-operative lymphoscintigraphy (± marking) and intra-operative gamma probe
	Use of two or several view lymphoscintigraphy
	Timing of lymphoscintigraphy
	Use of dynamic lymphoscintigraphy
Gamma detection probe	A variety available for SLNB
Sampling region	Axillary only
	Axillary plus internal mammary chain
Use of intra-operative histopathology	

palpable and impalpable primary tumors.[52] The technique has also been applied to, and shown to be useful in, men with breast cancer.[53] The use of SLNB in ductal carcinoma *in situ* (DCIS) and in patients undergoing prophylactic mastectomy remains controversial. However, a small proportion of patients who are thought to have DCIS are upstaged at surgery.[54] Therefore it seems logical to include this group of patients in surgery with SLNB.

With the introduction of a breast cancer screening program in many countries, including the UK and the USA, the number of screen-detected cancers is increasing. In a study of 110 women with unilateral breast cancer, Fernandez *et al.* showed that the concept of SLNB can be applied to screen-detected tumors using ultrasonographically guided tracer injection followed by scintigraphy.[55]

SLNB is obsolete in patients with proven distant spread of tumors. It appears less accurate at staging axillary disease in patients who have been treated with neoadjuvant chemotherapy[56] and will not be accurate in patients who have already had axillary surgery or radiotherapy.

Technical considerations and methods of locating the SLN in breast cancer

BLUE DYE

Giuliano *et al.* were the first to apply the blue dye technique for localizing the SLN to breast cancer.[57] The SLN is seen 3–10 min after injection of blue dye. However, due to the rapidity of transport of the dye, more than one node may stain blue in the same basin making the SLN (the first draining node) difficult to identify. In addition, the sentinel node is not always the nearest staining node to the primary tumor. Therefore, the localization of the SLN is more difficult using blue dye alone than LS alone or with the use of a combined technique. However, the technique has been shown to produce satisfactory localization of the SLN.[58] The main advantages of the blue dye technique are that it avoids radiation exposure to the patient and staff and reduces the cost and length of the procedure.

LYMPHOSCINTIGRAPHY

LS involves the injection of radiocolloid into the tumor, overlying skin or breast parenchyma followed by acquisition of images of the axilla with a gamma camera. Imaging is usually performed several hours after injection of the radiocolloid but early images may be obtained to identify the lymphatic pathways. An intra-operative hand-held gamma detector probe can later be utilized to locate the SLN.

Theoretically, preoperative LS should improve SLN localization by using this technique to identify and mark the node prior to surgery. However, as yet, no study has proved a significant advantage in localization over the use of an intra-operative gamma probe alone. The surgery, however, is more straightforward, and the technique may aid the identification of non-axillary SLNs. In addition, it has been shown that when the SN is not identified at preoperative LS, it is unlikely that it will be located at surgery.[59]

One of the factors which contributes to the nonlocalization of the SLN at preoperative LS is the number and orientation of the views acquired. Figures 5.4 and 5.5 demonstrate that the SLN is sometimes seen on certain views and not others, therefore, acquiring multiple views is likely to improve the detection rate of the SLN. Although not routinely performed, the lateral view is often a useful additional view.

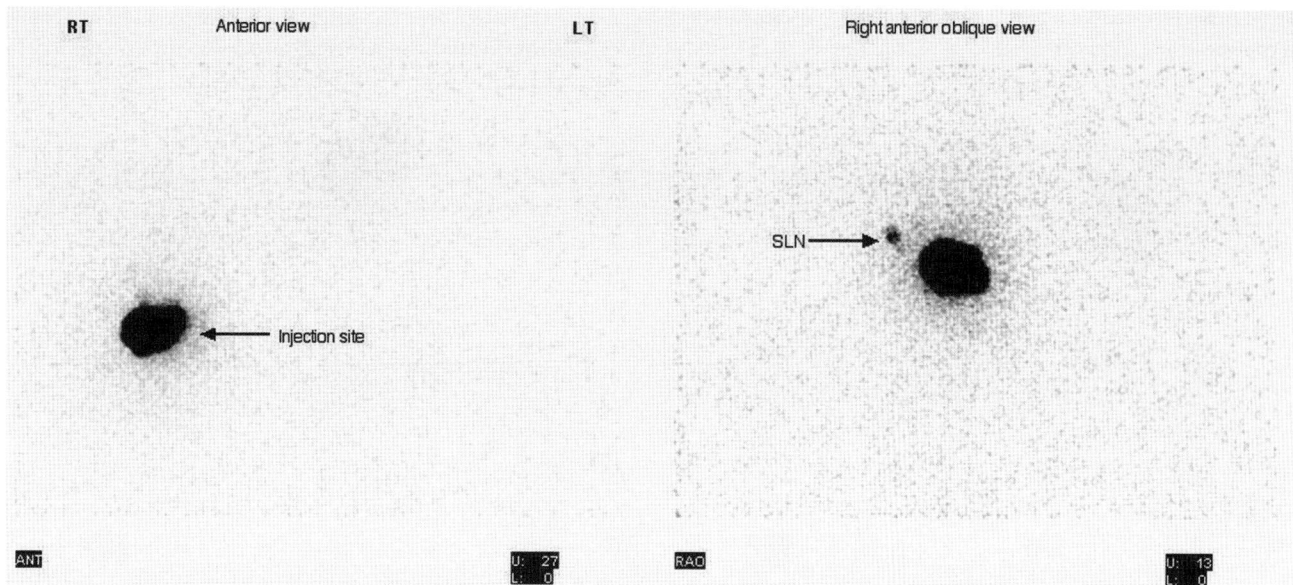

Figure 5.4   *Breast lymphoscintigraphy. The sentinel lymph node is only seen on right anterior oblique view, not on the anterior view.*

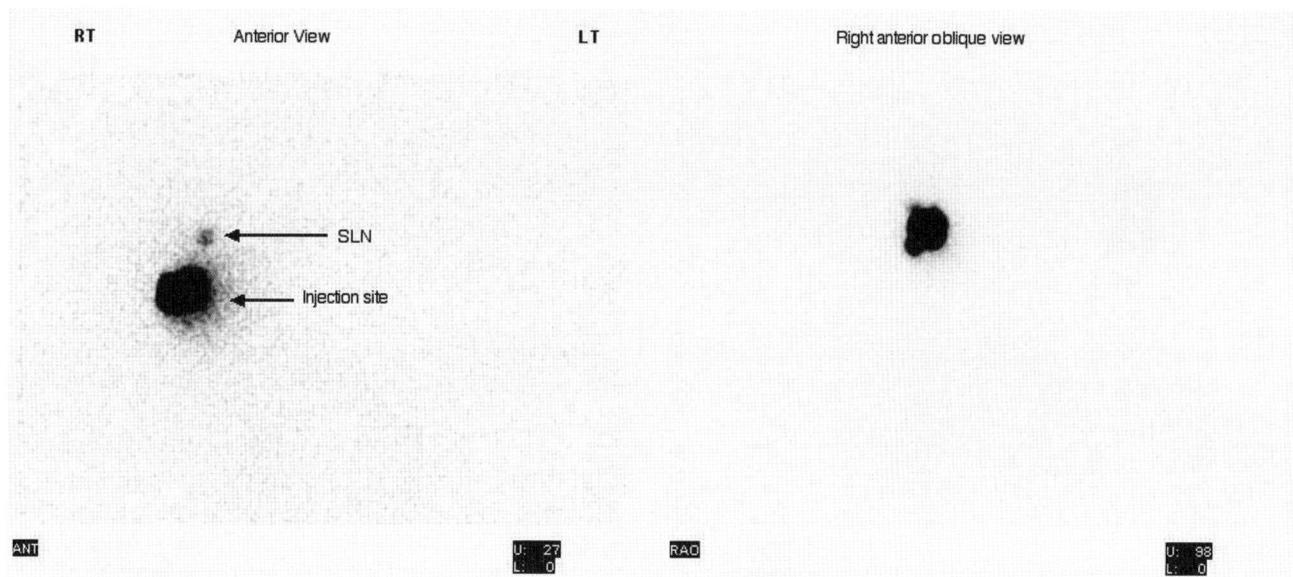

Figure 5.5   *Breast lymphoscintigraphy. The sentinel lymph node is only seen on anterior view, not on the right anterior oblique view.*

Dynamic preoperative LS has been used to identify the SLN. Although it improves the interpretation of preoperative SLN imaging for breast cancer, it does not contribute significantly to the successful detection of SLN.[60] Dynamic imaging increases the camera time and hence the cost of the procedure and is not used routinely, but can be helpful when first learning the technique.[61] Scatter from the injection site is another factor which can reduce the localization of the sentinel lymph node. It has been suggested that shielding of the injection site may improve the accuracy of LS in melanoma [62] and theoretically, this could also apply to breast cancer.

The timing of preoperative LS is also important because activity within the SLN decays with time and may make the SLN more difficult to identify. Figure 5.6 compares LS at 3 and 18 h, showing that low count SLNs are harder to identify with increasing intervals between injection and imaging. The same applies to longer intervals between injection and surgery and Koizumi *et al.* advocate increasing the administered activity of radiocolloid with increasing times to surgery.[63]

It should be remembered that the SLN is not necessarily the hottest node but is the first draining node in that nodal

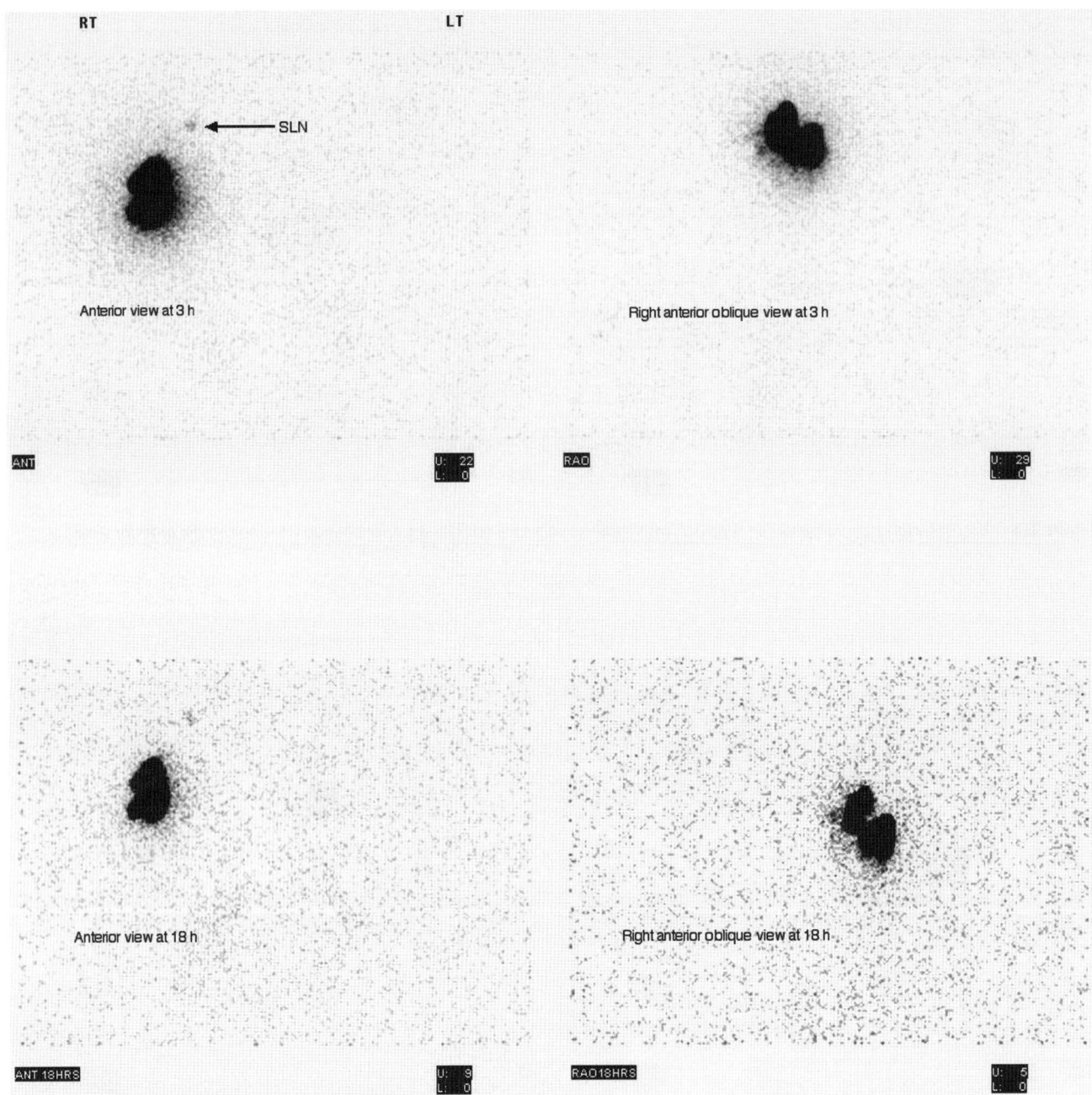

Figure 5.6 *Breast lymphoscintigraphy. Anterior and right anterior oblique views at 3 and 18 h. The sentinel lymph node, which is low-count, is seen at 3 h but is harder to see at 18 h because much of its activity has decayed.*

basin. It may be a relatively low count node compared with the others demonstrated at LS (Fig. 5.7). This can lead to confusion and false negatives, particularly when early images are not acquired.

As already discussed, the main advantage of preoperative lymphoscintigraphy is that once the SLN is located, the skin overlying it can be marked to simplify the surgical procedure. Transmission images obtained with a ^{57}Co flood source aid localization (Fig. 5.8).

COMBINED USE OF LYMPHOSCINTIGRAPHY AND BLUE DYE

Individually, both blue dye and LS produce satisfactory results, but the majority of studies using the combined technique of LS and blue dye have concluded that the combination increases the accuracy of identifying the SLN.[64,65] Most studies have shown that lymphoscintigraphy alone identifies more SLNs than the blue dye technique alone but a combined approach further improves the accuracy of detection.

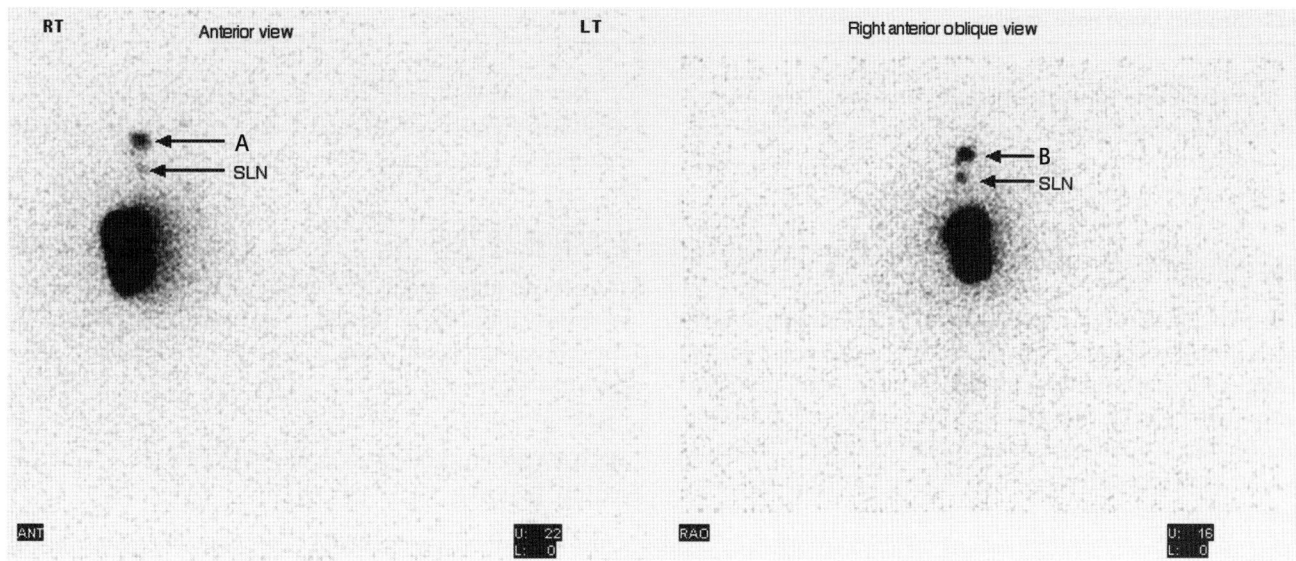

Figure 5.7 *Breast lymphoscintigraphy. Anterior and right anterior oblique views. The sentinel lymph node is the first draining node and is not necessarily the hottest node (a).*

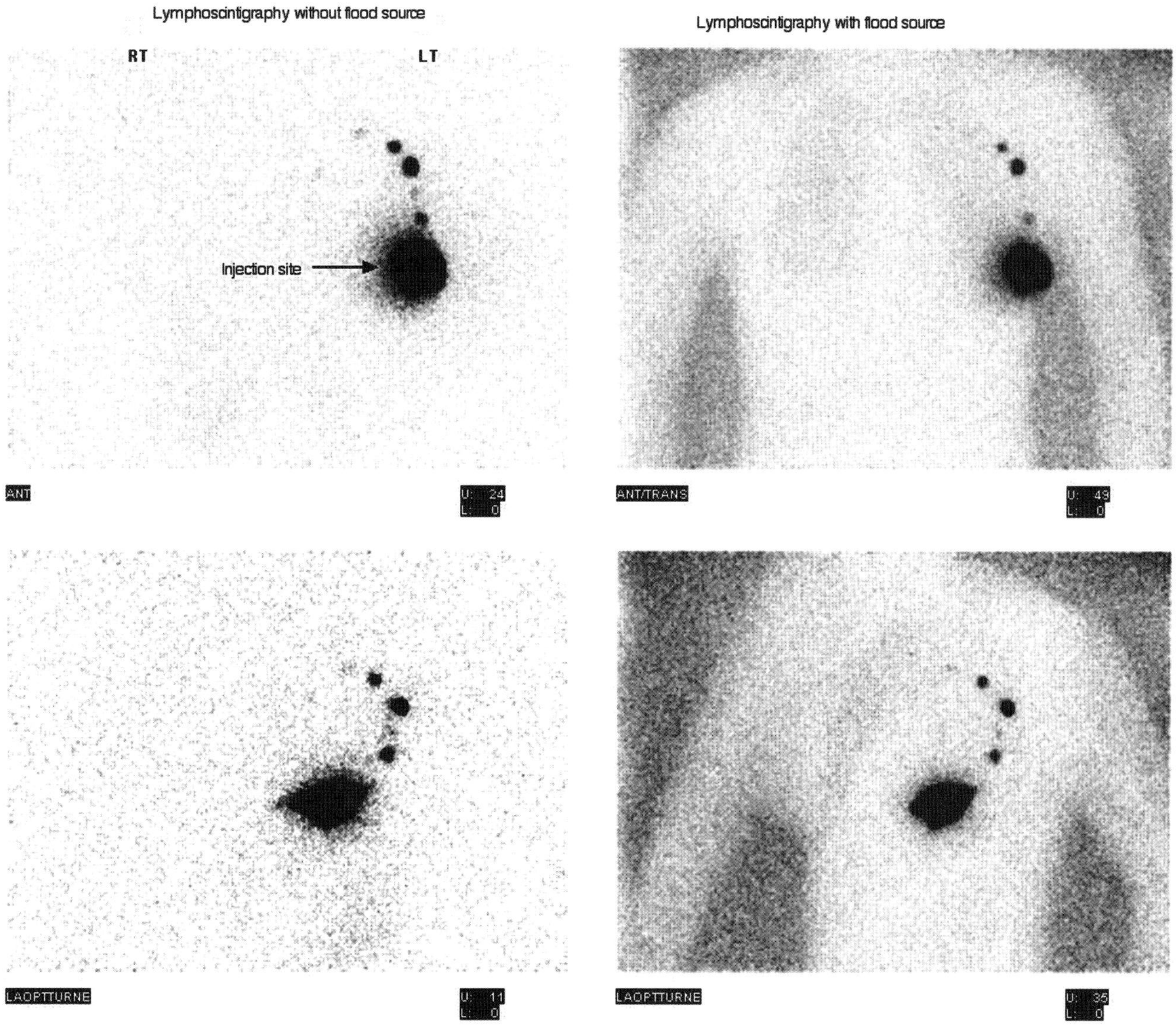

Lymphoscintigraphy without flood source

Lymphoscintigraphy with flood source

Injection site

Figure 5.8 *Breast lymphoscintigraphy. Anterior and left anterior oblique views with and without a* ^{57}*Co flood source. Images with a flood source can be useful in locating the sentinel lymph node at surgery.*

However, due to additional cost and time constraints, the combined technique is not used in every center; there is no international consensus as to which to use and local resources are usually the determining factors.

INJECTION SITE

The SLNB concept has been used to locate simultaneously both impalpable breast lesions and the SLN using a single preoperative intratumoral injection of radiotracer and the intra-operative use of a gamma probe detector.[66] A variety of injection sites have been used in SLNB (Table 5.3, page 8) and in experienced hands, all have been shown to be accurate at SLN localization.

RADIOPHARMACEUTICAL: ADMINISTERED ACTIVITY AND VOLUME

The administered dose of radiopharmaceutical has two effects. Firstly, it influences the rate of localization of the SLN and secondly, it raises issues of radiation exposure to both the patient and medical personnel involved in SLNB. The radiopharmaceutical dose injected varies from 7 to 370 MBq ($\approx$0.2 to 10 mCi). Van der Ent et al.[67] used the higher dose of 370 MBq ^{99m}Tc-nanocolloid to locate the SLN and concluded that it was more accurate for this purpose. Tanis et al.[68] reached the same conclusion using 370 MBq but also added that delayed imaging and re-injection of the radioactive tracer increases the visualization rate in a study of 495 clinically node negative patients. Most UK centers administer activities of 20–40 MBq, but as Valdes-Olmos et al.[69] found, it is important to have a high specific activity of tracer in the injectate to optimize SLN localization.

The volume of radiopharmaceutical varies from 0.2 to 4 ml but there is no consensus over the optimal volume suitable for locating the SLN in breast cancer.

LABELING METHOD

It has been suggested that labeling in a vacuum rather than in air may improve the detection rate of the SLN.[70] However, this adds complexity, time and cost and is not routinely performed.

HISTOPATHOLOGY AND MICROMETASTATIC NODAL DISEASE

One of the disadvantages of SLNB is that, where the node is positive, the patient requires a further operation for axillary clearance. Intra-operative histopathological analysis has been used in an attempt to avoid a two-stage procedure. However, an intra-operative frozen section has a higher false negative rate than conventional histology.[71] Intra-operative imprint cytology has shown encouraging results[72] but its role in routine SLNB has not been determined.

Standard histopathological techniques are based on the use of hematoxylin and eosin techniques. Newer methods including immunohistochemistry and polymerase chain reaction (PCR) techniques have led to the identification of micrometastases. As a result, the identification of micrometastases has improved.[73] SLNB and a focused pathological approach have resulted in upstaging 10–20% of breast cancers.[74] However, the significance of micrometastases is still under debate and it is uncertain whether the presence of micrometastases significantly alters prognosis. Evidence is emerging that their presence does reduce disease free

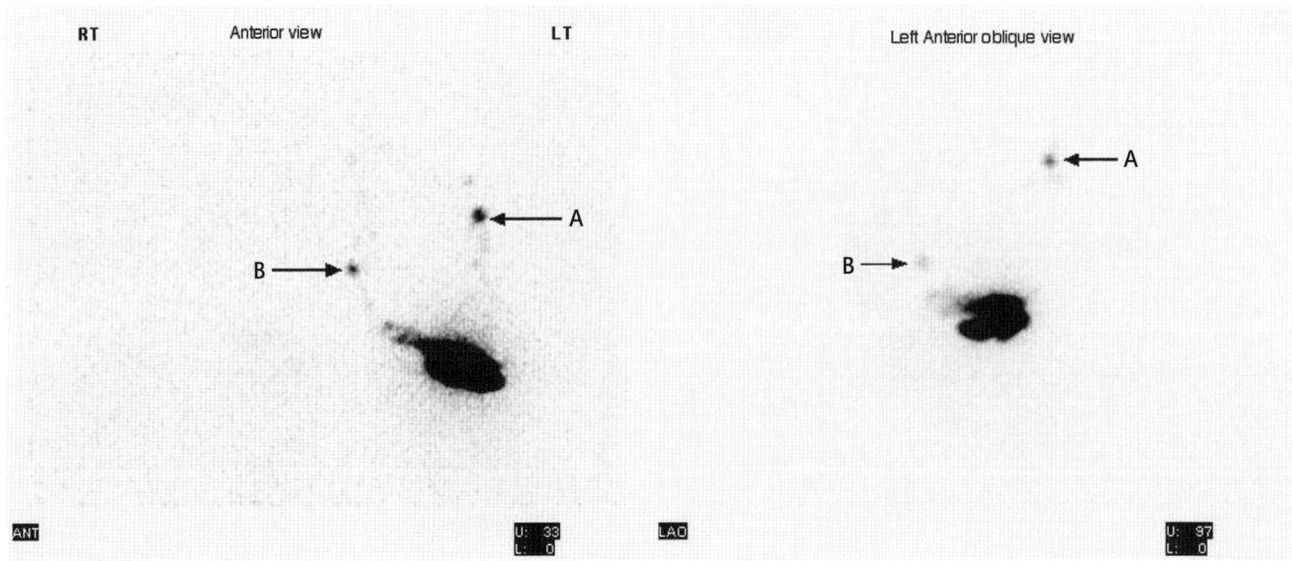

Figure 5.9   *Breast lymphoscintigraphy. Anterior and left anterior oblique views showing two nodes (A and B). A lies in the axilla and B lies in the internal mammary chain. Both should be regarded as sentinel lymph nodes.*

survival.[75–77] However, larger studies are needed to determine their impact on adjuvant therapy.

INTERNAL MAMMARY NODES

Although nodal spread to the axilla is the commonest lymphatic route,[75,78] metastasis to the internal mammary nodes is also seen, particularly from tumors located on the medial side of the breast.[79] Figure 5.9 shows an example of an internal mammary SLN from a primary in the medial half of breast.

It has been shown that all regions of the breast can drain to the internal mammary nodes.[80] Carcoforo showed that lymphoscintigraphy with SLNB was an accurate method to detect internal mammary chain metastases in patients with breast cancer.[81] Whether or not internal mammary nodes are detected during SLNB seems to depend on the technique used to inject the radiotracer. The use of peri-tumoral injection appears optimal to locate internal mammary sentinel nodes.[82]

However, it is still unclear whether internal mammary nodes metastases change prognosis. Studies by Veronesi *et al.* have found that removal of internal mammary nodes did not improve survival.[83,84] This has been substantiated by studies which have shown that overall survival does not appear to be affected by radiotherapy to this site.[85] However, some authors have suggested that localization of involved nodes in the internal mammary chain is important so that they can be included in the radiotherapy field.[86] Also, the presence of internal mammary nodes has been shown to put the patient into a poorer prognostic category[87] and it has been suggested that the presence of both positive axillary and internal mammary nodes confers an even worse prognosis. Tanis *et al.*[88] showed that SLNB was useful not only in identifying axillary and internal mammary sentinel nodes, but also other non-axillary sentinel nodes. In a separate study, Tanis *et al.* showed a remarkably high percentage of extra-axillary drainage (43%) in a study of 60 patients with impalpable breast cancer.[89] Dissection of internal mammary nodes does not have the same morbidity as axillary node dissection and although it is a relatively simple technique,[89,90] sampling of these nodes is not performed routinely.

Results

A number of studies have shown that SLNB is an accurate technique for staging the axilla.[57,58,91–94] However, a variety of methodologies have been employed and some technical aspects must be standardized.[95] A large randomized UK trial, the Axillary Lymphatic Mapping Against Nodal Axillary Clearance (ALMANAC) trial has now been completed, having recruited 1031 patients. Although not formally published at the time of writing, SLNB is associated with decreased arm morbidity, better quality of life, and cost-effectiveness compared to standard axillary treatment.[96]

There is a steep learning curve to the SLNB technique and it has been shown that results improve rapidly with experience in the technique.[97–99] The ALMANAC study required surgeons to perform 40 SLNBs under supervision before being deemed suitably trained.

Not all studies agree that negative SLNB correlates with negative axillary status.[100] Whether staging the axilla by SLNB confers any advantage over axillary clearance is not known and large multicenter randomized trials comparing differences in long-term patient outcome are needed.

Conclusion

Sentinel lymph node biopsy is being widely accepted as the standard of care in patients with early breast cancer despite lack of data on its impact on overall survival. Wide variations in the technique still exist and the lack of standardization is a major contributor to the differences in accuracy reported in the literature.

The major advantage of SLNB is the reduction of axillary morbidity. However, the significance of nodal micrometastases detected in SLNB is undetermined. The impact on cost to health services is also uncertain and further research is necessary before the technique replaces axillary lymph node dissection.

HEAD AND NECK CARCINOMA

The rationale for deploying SLNB in squamous cell head and neck carcinoma is that 15–20% of clinically N0 patients have occult nodal metastases and lymphatic drainage may be unpredictable. Elective lymph node dissection is used as a staging procedure to decide which patients should have the usual treatment of N+ disease, neck irradiation, but carries considerable morbidity. Special considerations are the close proximity of the injection site to potential SLNs and more technically demanding surgery. Shoaib *et al.* recommend the triple technique of blue dye + preoperative LS + intra-operative gamma probe guidance, as blue dye alone was unable to either localize SLNs reliably or to identify infiltrated nodes.[101]

OTHER CANCERS

Sentinel lymph node biopsy has also been performed in numerous other tumors including lung,[102] gastrointestinal,[103–105] bladder,[106] testicular,[107] vulval,[108] and cervical cancers,[109] but at present these are only feasibility studies.

STANDARDS

Any institution wishing to offer SLNB should ensure that its standards match those of larger centers. There is a surgical learning curve of 30 supervised cases for melanoma, after which SLNs can be located in 97–99% of patients, with an accuracy of >90%.[31] Accuracy is assessed by the incidence of SLN's that contain metastases (15–26% in melanoma and 30–35% in breast cancer) and of same-basin recurrence in SLNs reported to be negative;[27] the suggested standard is <5%.[110]

Complications of sentinel lymph node biopsy

Complications from surgery include those associated with blue dye, such as transient urine staining, skin tattooing and occasional anaphylaxis and those from the dissection itself. Sentinel lymph node biopsy is intended to avoid some of the morbidity of ELND; wound infection, lymphoceles or lymphedema occur in approximately 35%[111] of patients following ELND and these are also seen following 5% of SLNBs.[112] Radiocolloid is associated with anaphylactoid reactions very rarely.

Radiation protection

The majority of injected radiocolloid stays at the injection site, with approximately 1% passing into the lymphatic system; although the local dose rate at the injection site is high, virtually all of this is resected and overall does not represent a significant radiation dose to the patient. There have been relatively few studies addressing the issues of radiation safety of SLNB in breast cancer. Motta *et al.* monitored the radiation consequences of the SLNB procedure and concluded that it was a safe procedure and that the radiation dose to theater staff during SLN surgery was small.[113] Most of the studies investigating radiation exposure to patients and staff have concluded that levels of risk to either group are negligible.[114–116] Cumulative doses to personnel are low, with the surgeon receiving the highest dose of approximately 1% of annual dose limits per 100 operations.[23]

Tissue specimens should be stored for some hours so that radioactive decay minimizes the dose to pathology personnel; similarly, materials and equipment contaminated during the procedure should be stored before disposal or sterilization.

Resources

In the UK, from 1996 to 2000 the incidence of malignant melanoma increased by 25% to 7000 per annum, of which approximately 90% would be eligible for SLNB. The incidence of breast cancer increased by 12% over the same time period to 40 700 per annum, 80% of which would be

suitable for SLNB (Cancer Research UK). In countries where ELND is the current standard of care, the introduction of SLNB should reduce the number of operations and result in healthcare savings: in the USA the projected healthcare savings for melanoma are $172 million per year.[112] Similar economic advantages should result if SLNB replaces routine axillary dissection in breast cancer.[117] However, where ELND is not the standard of care (such as melanoma in Europe), introducing SLNB would add estimated UK costs of approximately £1300 per SLNB plus the additional costs of ELND in 20%.[118] These figures do not take into account the cost of additional equipment or staff recruitment and training costs which would be required for most countries to roll out an SLNB program.

FUTURE DEVELOPMENTS

Alternative methods of imaging the sentinel lymph node

No imaging investigation is likely to be sensitive enough for surgeons to be able to rely on a negative result (i.e. no uptake = no SLN metastases), given the intensive histological techniques necessary to demonstrate micrometastases. Even demonstration of uptake at one site would only be of limited value, as other potential drainage sites would not be demonstrated. The most sensitive radiopharmaceutical currently available, [^{18}F]fluorodeoxyglucose, failed to identify any of the positive SLNs in a series of melanoma patients where 14 (28%) had SLN metastases.[119] Others have looked at ultrasound-guided fine-needle aspiration in primary cancers that have a limited range of drainage pathways to lymph node basins accessible to ultrasonography. Nodal metastases were predicted correctly in 92% of patients with vulvar carcinoma.[120] However, even when guided by LS, this technique only detected 1 of 7 patients with SN metastases, and 1 in 14 patients with squamous carcinoma of the head and neck.[121] A strategy for imaging with a humanized Tc-99m monoclonal antibody has been presented to determine axillary node status prior to breast cancer surgery. A positive image leads to ELND without SLNB, a negative image indicates the need for SLNB. A specificity of 93% and a positive predictive value of 93% were obtained for impalpable nodes.[122]

Preliminary SLN lymphography using alternative contrast agents and imaging modalities (microbubbles/power Doppler ultrasonography[123]), iopamidol/computed tomography[124] and gadolinium/magnetic resonance imaging[125,126] cite potential advantages over lymphoscintigraphy. Ultrasonography may be better at detecting SLN close to the injection site, CT and MRI have much superior anatomical resolution and all techniques may visualize nodal metastases directly. However, it needs to be demonstrated whether these techniques are truly comparable with lymphoscintigraphy, particularly given the different particle sizes involved.

Scanning probes

Several manufacturers have developed hand-held gamma cameras, which allow real-time intra-operative imaging and preliminary clinical experience with these is beginning to be published.[127] Against the advantages of better intra-operative visualization and quicker imaging times than for lymphoscintigraphy, are the large size of the imaging head for entering the incision and poorer directional sensitivity, meaning that imaging probes cannot replace non-imaging probes and both will still be required.

Newer radiopharmaceuticals

Where injection usually has to be made endoscopically for tumors that are relatively inaccessible, neither radiocolloid nor blue dye are ideal sentinel lymph node localizing agents. Radiocolloid travels relatively slowly through the lymphatics, so has to be injected preoperatively. Blue dye travels quickly, so can only be injected intra-operatively, but may be difficult to see where fat is abundant; subsequent surgical mobilization may alter lymphatic flow.

^{99m}Tc-DTPA-mannosyl-dextran ('Lymphoseek') is a new nonparticulate lymph node-specific radiopharmaceutical which binds to macrophage surface receptors and accumulates in SLNs, with very little passing to second-tier nodes. It demonstrates faster clearance from injection sites than radiocolloids. Studies in breast cancer[128] and pig models of gastrointestinal cancer[129] have shown some concordance with existing agents.

REFERENCES

● Seminal primary article
◆ Key review paper

● 1   Cabanas RM. An approach for the treatment of penile carcinoma. *Cancer* 1977; **39**: 456–66.

2   Lock-Andersen J, Partoft S, Jensen MG. Patterns of the first lymph node metastases in patients with cutaneous malignant melanoma of axial location. *Cancer* 1988; **62**: 2073–7.

3   Wong JH, Cagle LA, Morton DL. Lymphatic drainage of skin to a sentinel lymph node in a feline model. *Ann Surg* 1991; **214**: 637–41.

● 4   Morton DL, Wen DR, Wong JH, Economou JS, Cagle LA, Storm K, *et al.* Technical details of intraoperative lymphatic mapping for early stage melanoma. *Arch Surg* 1992; **127**: 392–9.

5   Berman C, Norman J, Cruse CW. Lymphoscintigraphy in malignant melanoma. *Ann Plast Surg* 1992; **28**: 29–32.

6   Norman J, Cruse W, Espinosa C, Cox C, Berman C, Clark R, *et al.* Redefinition of cutaneous lymphatic drainage with the use of lymphoscintigraphy for malignant melanoma. *Am J Surg* 1991; **162**: 432–7.

7   Uren RF, Howman-Giles RB, Shaw HM, Thompson JF, McCarthy WH. Lymphoscintigraphy in high-risk melanoma of the trunk: predicting draining node groups, defining lymphatic channels and locating the sentinel node. *J Nucl Med* 1993; **34**: 1435–40.

8   Alex JC, Krag DN. Gamma-probe guided localisation of lymph nodes. *Surg Oncol* 1993; **2**: 137–43.

◆ 9   Reintgen D, Cruse CW, Wells K, *et al.* The orderly progression of melanoma nodal metastases. *Ann Surg* 1994; **220**: 759–67.

10   Morton D, Wen DR, Wong JH, *et al.* Technical details of intraoperative lymphatic mapping for early stage melanoma. *Arch Surg* 1992; **127**: 392–9.

11   Uren RF, Howman-Giles RB, Thompson JF, *et al.* Interval nodes. The forgotten sentinel nodes in patients with melanoma. *Arch Surg* 2000; **135**: 1168–72.

◆ 12   Uren RF, Howman-Giles RB, Thompson JF. Patterns of lymphatic drainage from the skin in patients with melanoma. *J Nucl Med* 2003; **44**: 570–82.

13   Uren RF, Thompson JF, Howman-Giles RB. *Lymphatic drainage of the skin and breast: locating the sentinel nodes.* The Netherlands: Harwood Academic Publishers, 1999.

14   Balch CM, Buzaid AC, Soon S-J, *et al.* Final version of the report of the America Joint Committee on Cancer Staging System for Cutaneous Melanoma. *J Clin Oncol* 2001; **19**: 3635–84.

15   Roberts DLL, Anstery AV, Barlow RJ, Cox NH, Corrie PG. UK guidelines for the management of cutaneous melanoma. *Br J Dermatol* 2002; **146**: 7–17.

16   Sim FH, Taylor WF, Ivins JC, Pritchard DJ, Soule EH. A propspective randomized study of the efficacy of routine elective lymphadenectomy in management of malignant melanoma: preliminary results. *Cancer* 1978; **41**: 948–56.

17   Veronesi U, Adamus J, Bandiera DC, Brennhovd IO, Cascinelli N, Claudio F. Inefficacy of immediate node dissection in stage 1 melanoma of the limbs. *N Engl J Med* 1977; **297**: 627–30.

18   Balch CM, Soon S-J, Bartolucci AA, Urist MM, Karakousis CP, Smith TJ. Efficacy of an elective regional lymph node dissection of 1 to 4 mm thick melanomas for patients 60 years of age and younger. *Ann Surg* 1996; **224**: 255–66.

19   Cascinelli N, Morabito A, Santinami M, MacKie RM, Belli F. Immediate or delayed dissection of regional nodes in patients with melanoma of the trunk: a randomised trial. *Lancet* 1998; **351**: 793–6.

20   Alazraki N, Glass EC, Castronovo F, Valdés Olmos RA, Podoloff D. Procedure guideline for lymphoscintigraphy and the use of intraoperative gamma probe for sentinel lymph node localization

in melanoma of intermediate thickness. *J Nucl Med* 2002; **43**: 1414–18.

21 Lens MB, Dawes JA, Newton-Bishop JA, Goodacre T. Tumour thickness as a predictor of occult lymph node metastases in patients with stage I and II melanoma undergoing sentinel lymph node biopsy. *Br J Surg* 2002; **89**: 1223–7.

22 Gershenwald JE, Mansfield PF, Lee JL, Ross MI. Role for lymphatic mapping and sentinel lymph node biopsy in patients with thick (≥4 mm) primary melanoma. *Ann Surg Oncol* 2000; **7**: 160–5.

23 Mariani G, Gipponi M, Moresco L, Villa G, Bartolomei M, Mazzarol G. Radioguided sentinel lymph node biopsy. *J Nucl Med* 2002; **43**: 811–27.

24 Clarke E, Notghi A, Harding K. Improved body-outline imaging technique for localisation of sentinel lymph nodes in breast surgery. *J Nucl Med* 2002; **43**: 1181–3.

25 Even-Sapir E, Lerman HL, Lievshitz G, Khafif A, Fliss DM, Schwartz A. Lymphoscintigraphy for sentinel node mapping using a hybrid SPECT/CT system. *J Nucl Med* 2003; **44**: 1413–20.

26 Vargas HI, Vargas MP, Venegas R, *et al.* Lymphatic tumour burden negatively impacts the ability to detect the sentinel lymph node in breast cancer. *Am Surg* 2003; **69**: 886–90.

27 Morton DL, Thompson JF, Essner R, Elashoff R, Stern S, Nieweg O. Validation of the accuracy of intra-operative lymphatic mapping and sentinel lymphadenectomy for early-stage melanoma: a multicenter trial. *Ann Surg* 1999; **230**: 453–63.

28 Perkins AC, Britten AJ. Specification and performance of the intra-operative gamma probe for sentinel node detection. *Nucl Med Commun* 1999; **20**: 309–15.

29 Tiorina T, Arends B, Huysmans D, *et al.* Evaluation of surgical gamma probes for radioguided sentinel node localisation. *Eur J Nucl Med* 1998; **25**: 1224–31.

30 Diest PJV. Histopathological workup of sentinel lymph nodes: how much is enough? *J Clin Pathol* 1999; **52**: 871–3.

31 Gershenwald JE, Thompson W, Mansfield PF, Lee JL, Colome MI, Tseng C. Multi-institutional melanoma lymphatic mapping experience: the prognostic value of sentinel lymph node status in 612 stage I or II melanoma patients. *J Clin Oncol* 1999; **3**: 967–83.

32 Wookey S. What is a prognosis worth? *BMJ* 2000; **321**: 1285.

33 Cascinelli N. WHO declares lymphatic mapping to be the standard of care for melanoma. *Oncology* 1999; **13**: 288.

34 Estourgie SH, Nieweg OE, Kroon BBR, Hoefnagel CA. Lymphatic mapping in melanoma? 250 patients with a median follow-up of six years. *Eur J Nucl Med* 2003; **20(Suppl. 2)**: S154.

35 UK Cancer Research Campaign. *CRC CancerStats: incidence.* London: Cancer Research Campaign, 1998.

36 Bray F, Sankila R, Ferlay J, Parkin DM. Estimates of cancer incidence and mortality in Europe in 1995. *Eur J Cancer* 2004; **38**: 99–166.

37 European Network of Cancer Registries, EUROCIM Version 4.0. European Incidence Database V2.3. ICD-10 Dictionary (2001). Lyon: International Association for Research on Cancer, 2001.

38 European Network of Cancer Registries, EUROCIM Version 4.0. European Mortality Database V2.3 (2001). Lyon: International Association for Research on Cancer, 2001.

39 Ries LA, Eisner MP, Kosary CL, *et al. SEER cancer statistics review, 1975–2000.* Bethesda: National Cancer Institute, 2003.

40 Bonadonna G, Brusamolino E, Valagussa P, *et al.* Combined chemotherapy as an adjuvant treatment in operable breast cancer. *N Engl J Med* 1976; **294**: 405–10.

41 Fisher ER, Constantino J, Fisher B, *et al.* Pathologic findings from the National Surgical Adjuvant Breast Project (Protocol 4). Discriminants for 15-year survival. *Cancer* 1993; **71**: 2141–50.

42 Nemoto T, Vana J, Bedwani RN, *et al.* Management and survival of female breast cancer: results of a national survey by the American College of Surgeons. *Cancer* 1980; **45**: 2917–24.

43 Ivens D, Hoe AL, Podd TJ, *et al.* Assessment of morbidity from complete axillary dissection. *Br J Cancer* 1992; **66**: 136–8.

44 Cady B, Stone MD, Schuler JG, *et al.* The new era in breast cancer: invasion, size and nodal involvement dramatically decreasing as a result of mammographic screening. *Arch Surg* 1996; **131**: 301–8.

45 Ranaboldo CJ, Mitchel A, *et al.* Axillary nodal status in women with screen-detected breast cancer. *Eur J Surg Oncol* 1993; **19**: 130–3.

46 Lin PP, Allison DC, Wainstock J, *et al.* Impact of axillary lymph node dissection on the therapy of breast cancer patients. *J Clin Oncol* 1993; **11**: 1536–44.

47 de Mascarel I, Bonichon F, Coindre JM, *et al.* Prognostic significance of breast cancer axillary lymph node micrometastases assessed by two special techniques: re-evaluation with longer follow-up. *Br J Cancer* 1992; **66**: 523–7.

● 48 Guiliano AE, Kirgan DM, Guenther JM, *et al.* Lymphatic mapping and sentinel lymphadenectomy for breast cancer. *Ann Surg* 1994; **220**: 391–401.

49 Mariotti S, Buonomo O, Guadagni F, *et al.* Minimal sentinel node procedure for staging early breast cancer. *Tumori* 2002; **88**: S45–S47.

50 Van-Berlo CLH, Hess DA, Nijhuis PAH, *et al.* Ambulatory sentinel node biopsy under local anaesthesia for patients with early breast cancer. *Eur J Surg Oncol* 2003; **29**: 383–5.

◆ 51 Strickland AH, Beechey-Newman N, Steer CC, *et al.* Sentinel node biopsy: an indepth appraisal. *Crit Rev Oncol/Haematol* 2002; **44**: 45–70.

52 McIntosh SA, Ravichandran D, Balan KK, *et al.* Sentinel lymph node biopsy in impalpable breast cancer. *Breast* 2001; **10**: 82–3.

53 De Ciccio C, Baio SM, Veronesi P, *et al.* Sentinel node biopsy in male breast cancer. *Nucl Med Commun* 2004; **25**: 139–43.

54 Morrow M. Axillary dissection: when and how radical? *Semin Surg Oncol* 1996; **12**: 321–7.

55 Fernandez A, Escobedo A, Benito E, *et al.* Sentinel node localization in patients with non-palpable breast cancer. *Nucl Med Commun* 2002; **23**: 1165–9.

56 Fernandez A, Cortes M, Benito E, *et al.* Gamma probe sentinel node localization and biopsy in breast cancer patients treated with a neoadjuvant chemotherapy scheme. *Nucl Med Commun* 2001; **22**: 361–6.

● 57 Giuliano AE, Kirgan DM, Guenther JM, *et al.* Lymphatic mapping and sentinel lymphadenectomy for breast cancer. *Ann Surg* 1994; **220**: 391–401.

● 58 Giuliano AE, Jones RC, Brennan M, *et al.* Sentinel lymphadenectomy in breast cancer. *J Clin Oncol* 1997; **15**: 2345–50.

59 Kollias J, Gill PG, Coventry BJ, *et al.* Clinical and histological factors associated with sentinel node identification in breast cancer. *Aust NZ J Surg* 2000; **70**: 485–9.

60 Lee AC, Keshtgar MRS, Waddington WA, Ell PJ. The role of dynamic imaging in sentinel lymph node biopsy in breast cancer. *Eur J Cancer* 2002; **38**: 784–7.

◆ 61 Mariani G, Moresco L, Viale G, *et al.* Radioguided sentinel lymph node biopsy in breast cancer surgery. *J Nucl Med* 2001; **42**: 1198–215.

62 Maza S, Valencia R, Geworski L, *et al.* Temporary shielding of hot spots in the drainage areas of cutaneous melanoma improves accuracy of lymphoscintigraphic sentinel lymph node diagnostics. *Eur J Nucl Med* 2002; **29**: 1399–402.

63 Koizumi M, Nomura E, Yamad Y, *et al.* Sentinel node detection using ^{99m}Tc-rhenium sulphide colloid in breast cancer patients: evaluation of 1 day and 2 day protocols and a dose-finding study. *Nucl Med Commun* 2003; **24**: 663–70.

64 Mariani G, Villa G, Gipponi M, *et al.* Mapping sentinel lymph node in breast cancer by combined lymphoscintigraphy, blue-dye, and intra-operative gamma-probe. *Cancer Biother Radiopharm* 2000; **15**: 245–52.

65 Villa G, Gipponi M, Buffoni F, *et al.* Localization of the sentinel lymph node in breast cancer by combined lymphoscintigraphy, blue dye and intra-operative gamma probe. *Tumori* 2000; **86**: 297–9.

66 Feggi L, Basagila E, Corcione S, *et al.* An original approach in the diagnosis of early breast cancer: use of the same radiopharmaceutical for both non-palpable lesions and sentinel node localisation. *Eur J Nucl Med* 2001; **28**: 1589–96.

67 Van der Ent FW, Kenger RA, Van der Pol HA. Sentinel node biopsy in 70 unselected patients with breast cancer: increased feasibility by using 10 mCi radiocolloid in combination with a blue dye tracer. *Eur J Surg Oncol* 1999; **25**: 24–9.

68 Tanis PJ, Van-Sandick JW, Nieweg OE, *et al.* The hidden sentinel node in breast cancer. *Eur J Nucl Med* 2002; **29**: 305–11.

69 Valdes-Olmos RA, Tanis PJ, Hoefnagel CA, *et al.* Improved sentinel node visualization in breast cancer by optimizing the colloid particle concentration and tracer dosage. *Nucl Med Commun* 2001; **22**: 579–86.

70 Gommans GMM, Van-Dongen A, Van-der-Schors TG, *et al.* Further optimisation of (99m)Tc-nanocoll sentinel node localisation in carcinoma of the breast by improved labelling. *Eur J Nucl Med Mol Imag* 2001; **28**: 1450–5.

71 Dixon JM, Mamman U, Thomas J. Accuracy of intra-operative frozen-section analysis of axillary nodes. Edinburgh Breast Unit team. *Br J Surg* 1999; **86**: 392–5.

72 Ratanawichitrasin A, Biscotti CV, Levy L, *et al.* Touch imprint cytological analysis of sentinel lymph nodes for detecting axillary metastases in patients with breast cancer. *Br J Surg* 1999; **86**: 1346–8.

73 Dowlatshahi K, Fan M, Snider HC, *et al.* Lymph node micrometastases from breast carcinoma: reviewing the dilemma. *Cancer* 1997; **80**: 1188–97.

74 Turner RR, Guiliano AE, Hoon DS, *et al.* Pathological examination of sentinel lymph node for breast carcinoma. *World J Surg* 2001; **25**: 798–805.

75 de Mascarel I, Bonichon F, Coindre JM, *et al.* Prognostic significance of breast cancer axillary lymph node micrometastases assessed by two special techniques: re-evaluation with longer follow-up. *Br J Cancer* 1992; **66**: 523–7.

76 Hainsworth PJ, Tjandra JJ, Stillwell RG, *et al.* Detection and significance of occult metastases in node-negative breast cancer. *Br J Surg* 1993; **80**: 459–63.

77 International (Ludwig) Breast Cancer Study Group. Prognostic importance of occult axillary lymph node micrometastases from breast cancers. *Lancet* 1990; **335**: 1565–8.

78 Tassenoy A, Van-der-Veen P, Bossuyt A, *et al.* Lymphatic pathways of the upper medial quadrant of the breast in healthy women: radiotracer study of the sentinel lymph node. *Lymphology* 2002; **35**: 153–60.

79 Handley RS. Carcinoma of the breast. *J R Coll Surg* 1975; **57**: 59–66.

80 Veronesi U, Cascinelli N, Greco M, *et al.* Prognosis of breast cancer patients after mastectomy and dissection of the internal mammary nodes. *Ann Surg* 1985; **202**: 702–7.

81 Carcoforo P, Basaglia E, Soliani G, Bergossi L, *et al.* Sentinel node biopsy in the evaluation of the internal

mammary node chain in patients with breast cancer. *Tumori* 2002; **88**: S5–S7.

82 Rouman RM, Geuskens LM, Valkenberg JG. In search of the true sentinel node by different injection techniques in breast cancer patients. *Eur J Surg Oncol* 1999; **25**: 347–51.

83 Veronesi U, Cascinelli N, Bafalino R, *et al.* Risk of internal mammary lymph node metastases and its relevance on prognosis of breast cancer patients. *Ann Surg* 1983; **198**: 681–4.

84 Veronesi U, Marubini E, Mariani L, *et al.* The dissection of internal mammary nodes does not improve the survival of breast cancer patients. 30-year results of a randomised trial. *Eur J Cancer* 1999; **35**: 1320–5.

85 Obedian E, Haffty BG. Internal mammary nodal irradiation in conservatively managed breast cancer patients: is there a benefit? *Intern J Radiat Oncol Biol Phys* 1999; **44**: 997–1003.

86 Struikmans H, Van Rijk PP. Optimizing radiotherapy of the internal mammary chain in breast cancer by scintigraphy. *Radiother Oncol* 1996; **41**: 15–20.

87 Cody HS, Urban JA. Internal mammary node status: a major prognosticator in axillary node-negative breast cancer. *Ann Surg Oncol* 1995; **2**: 32–7.

88 Tanis PJ, Nieweg OE, Valdes-Olmos RA, *et al.* Impact of non-axillary sentinel node biopsy on staging and treatment of breast cancer patients. *Br J Cancer* 2002; **23**: 705–10.

89 Tanis PJ, Deurloo EE, Valdes-Olmos RA, *et al.* Single intralesional tracer dose for radio-guided excision of clinically occult breast cancer and sentinel node. *Ann Surg Oncol* 2001; **8**: 850–5.

90 Van-der-Ent FWC, Kengen RAM, Van-der-Pol HAG, *et al.* Halsted revisited: internal mammary sentinel lymph node biopsy in breast cancer. *Ann Surg* 2001; **234**: 79–84.

● 91 Krag D, Weaver D, Ashikaga T, *et al.* The sentinel node in breast cancer – a multicenter validation study. *N Engl J Med* 1998; **339**: 941–6.

● 92 McMasters KM, Tuttle TM, Carlson DJ, *et al.* Sentinel lymph node biopsy for breast cancer: a suitable alternative to routine axillary dissection in multi-institutional practice when optimal technique is used. *J Clin Oncol* 2000; **18**: 2560–6.

● 93 Borgstein PJ, Pijpers R, Comans EF, *et al.* Sentinel lymph node biopsy in breast cancer: guidelines and pitfalls of lymphoscintigraphy and gamma probe detection. *J Am Coll Surg* 1998; **186**: 275–83.

● 94 Haigh PI, Hansen NM, Qi K, *et al.* Biopsy method and excision volume do not affect success rate of subsequent sentinel lymph node dissection in breast cancer. *Ann Surg Oncol* 2000; **7**: 21–7.

95 Zavagno G, Busolin R, Bozza F, *et al.* Sentinel node biopsy in breast cancer. *Breast* 2000; **9**: 139–43.

96 Clarke D, Khonji NI, Mansel RE. Sentinel node biopsy in breast cancer: the ALMANAC trial. *World J Surg* 2001; **25**: 819–22.

97 Castalegno PS, Sandrucci S, Bello M, *et al.* Sentinel lymph node and breast cancer staging: Final results of the Turin multicenter study. *Tumori* 2000; **86**: 300–3.

98 McMasters KM, Wong SL, Chao C, *et al.* Defining the optimal surgeon experience for breast cancer sentinel lymph node biopsy: a model for implementation of new surgical techniques. *Ann Surg* 2001; **234**: 292–9.

99 Mechella M, De-Cesare A, Di-Luzio E, *et al.* A study of sentinel node biopsy in T1 breast cancer treatment: Experience of 48 cases. *Tumori* 2000; **86**: 320–1.

100 Pelosi E, Arena V, Baudino B, *et al.* Sentinel node detection in breast carcinoma. *Tumori* 2002; **88**: S10–S11.

101 Shoaib T, Soutar DS, Prosser JE, *et al.* A suggested method for sentinel node biospy in squamous cell carcinoma of the head and neck. *Head & Neck* 1999; **21**: 728–33.

102 Melfi FM, Chella A, Menconi GF, *et al.* Intraoperative radioguided sentinel lymph node biopsy in non-small cell lung cancer. *Eur J Cardio-Thoracic Surg* 2003; **23**: 214–20.

103 Peley G, Farkas E, Sinkovics I, *et al.* Inguinal sentinel lymph node biopsy for staging anal cancer. *Scand J Surg* 2002; **91**: 336–8.

104 Hundley JC, Shen P, Shiver SA, Geisinger KR, Levine EA. Lymphatic mapping for gastric adenocarcinoma. *Am Surg* 2002; **68**: 931–5.

105 Nastro P, Sodo M, Dodaro CA, Acampa W, Bracale U, Renda A. Intraoperative radiochromoguided mapping of sentinel lymph node in colon cancer. *Tumori* 2002; **88**: 352–3.

106 Malmstrom PU, Ren ZP, Sherif A, de la Torre M, Wester K, Thorn M. Early metastatic progression of bladder carcinoma: molecular profile of primary tumour and sentinel lymph node. *J Urol* 2002; **168**: 2240–4.

107 Tanis PJ, Horenblas S, Valdés Olmos RA, Hoefnagel CA, Nieweg OE. Feasibility of sentinel node lymphoscintigraphy in stage I testicular cancer. *Eur J Nucl Med Mol Imag* 2004; **29**: 670–3.

108 Hulla JAD, Doting E, Piers DA, Hollema H, Aalders JG, Koops HS. Sentinel lymph node identification with technetium-99m-labeled nanocolloid in squamous cell carcinoma of the vulva. *J Nucl Med* 1998; **39**: 1381–5.

109 Levenback C, Coleman RL, Burke TW, Lin WN, Erdman W, Deavers M, *et al.* Lymphatic mapping and sentinel node identification in patients with cervix cancer undergoing radical hysterectomy and pelvic lymphadenopathy. *J Clin Oncol* 2002; **20**: 688–93.

110 Nieweg OE, Tanis PJ, Rutgers EJT. Summary of the Second International Sentinel Node Conference. *Eur J Nucl Med* 2001; **28**: 646–9.

111 Swan MC, Furniss D, Cassell OC. Surgical management of metastatic inguinal lymphadenopathy. *BMJ* 2004; **329**: 1272–6.

112 Reintgen D, Albertini J, Milliotes G, Marshburn J, Cruse W, Rapaport D. Investment in new technology research can save future health care dollars. *J Florida Med Assn* 1997; **84**: 175–9.

113 Motta C, Turra A, Farina B, *et al*. Radioguided surgery of breast cancer: Radiation protection survey. *Tumori* 2000; **86**: 372–4.

114 Cremonesi M, Ferrari M, Sacco E, *et al*. Radiation protection in radioguided surgery of breast cancer. *Nucl Med Commun* 2004; **25**: 919–24.

115 Eshima D, Fauconnier T, Eshima L, *et al*. Radiopharmaceuticals for lymphoscintigraphy: including dosimetry and radiation considerations. *Semin Nucl Med* 2000; **30**: 25–32.

116 Waddington WA, Keshtgar MRS, Taylor I, *et al*. Radiation safety of the sentinel lymph node technique in breast cancer. *Eur J Nucl Med Mol Imag* 2000; **27**: 377–91.

117 Howard-Jones E. A Preliminary study of cost. In: Keshtgar MRS, Wassington WA, Lakhani SR, Ell PJ. (eds) *The sentinel node in surgical oncology*. Springer-Verlag: Berlin, 1999; pp. 183–6.

118 Hettiaratchy SP, Kang N, Kirkpatrick N, Allan R, Cook M, Powell WBEM. Sentinel lymph node biospy in malignant melanoma:a series of 100 consecutive patients. *Br J Plastic Surg* 2000; **53**: 559–62.

119 Acland KM, Healy C, Calonje E, O'Doherty M, Nunan T, Page C. Comparison of positron emission tomography scanning and sentinel node biopsy in the detection of micrometastases of primary cutaneous malignant melanoma. *J Clin Oncol* 2001; **19**: 2674–8.

120 Hall TB, Barton DP, Trott PA, *et al*. The role of ultrasound-guided cytology of groin lymph nodes in the management of squamous cell carcinoma of the vulva: 5-year experience in 44 patients. *Clin Radiol* 2003; **58**: 367–71.

121 Höft S, Muhle C, Brenner W, Sprenger E, Maune S. Fine-needle aspiration cytology of the sentinel lymph node in head and neck cancer. *J Nucl Med* 2002; **43**: 1585–90.

122 Al-Yasi AR, Carroll MJ, Ellison D, *et al*. Axillary node status in breast cancer patients prior to surgery by imaging with Tc-99m humanised anti-PEM monoclonal antibody, HMFG1. *Br J Cancer* 2002; **86**: 870–8.

123 Wisner ER, Ferrara KW, Short RE, Ottoboni TB, Gabe JD, Patel D. Sentinel node detection using contrast-enhanced power doppler ultrasound lymphography. *Invest Radiol* 2003; **38**: 358–65.

124 Suga K, Yuan Y, Okada M, *et al*. Breast sentinel lymph node mapping at CT lymphography with iopamidol: preliminary experience. *Radiology* 2004; **230**: 543–52.

125 Suga K, Yuan Y, Ogasawara N, Okada M, Matsunaga N. Localisation of breast sentinel lymph nodes by MR lymphography with a conventional gadolinium contrast agent. Preliminary observations in dogs and humans. *Acta Radiologica* 2003; **44**: 35–42.

126 Torchia MG, Misselwitz B. Combined MR lymphangiography and MR imaging-guided needle localisation of sentinel nodes using Gadomer-17. *Am J Roentgenol* 2002; **179**: 1561–5.

127 Pitre S, Ménard L, Ricard M, Solal M, Garbay J-R, Charont Y. A hand-held imaging probe for radioguided surgery: physical performance and preliminary clinical experience. *Eur J Nucl Med* 2003; **30**: 339–43.

128 Wallace AM, Hoh CK, Vera DR, Darrah DD, Schulteis G. Lymphoseek: a molecular radiopharmaceutical for sentinel node detection. *Ann Surg Oncol* 2003; **10**: 531–8.

129 Méndez J, Wallace AM, Hoh CK, Vera DR. Detection of gastric and colonic sentinel nodes through endoscopic administration of ^{99m}Tc-DTPA-mannosyl-dextran in pigs. *J Nucl Med* 2003; **44**: 1677–81.

SECTION B

Clinical Systems

6. Functional imaging of cardiac disease   145

  6A Functional imaging of coronary artery and congenital heart disease   147
  S. Mahmood

  6B Left ventricular dysfunction   183
  S.F. Barrington

7. Radionuclide imaging in thoracic disease   195

  7A Ventilation perfusion imaging: a changing role for suspected pulmonary embolism   197
  H.W. Gray

  7B Lung cancer   223
  M.J. O'Doherty

  7C Other pulmonary applications   239
  M.J. O'Doherty

8. Renal radionuclide studies   251

  8A Anatomy, physiology, and tracer handling   253
  K.E. Britton

  8B Non-imaging radionuclide assessment of renal function   269
  A.M. Peters

  8C Vesico-ureteric reflux and urinary tract infection   281
  L. Biassoni and I. Gordon

  8D Hypertension   297
  A. Hilson

  8E Obstruction of the outflow tract   305
  K.E. Britton

  8F Renal transplantation   315
  A. Hilson

  8G Renal tumors   321
  P. Shreve

9. Musculoskeletal radionuclide imaging   329

  9A Skeletal physiology and anatomy applied to nuclear medicine   331
  G.J.R. Cook

  9B Skeletal malignancy   337
  G.J.R. Cook and I. Fogelman

  9C Metabolic bone disease   355
  G.J.R. Cook and I. Fogelman

  9D Trauma and sports injuries   363
  H. van der Wall and S. Kannangara

  9E Radionuclide evaluation of the failed joint replacement   381
  C.J. Palestro

9F Rheumatology and avascular necrosis　　　393
P. Ryan

9G Pediatric indications　　　403
H.R. Nadel

10. Neuroimaging　　　413

10A Dementia　　　415
P.M. Kemp

10B Functional imaging in cerebrovascular disease and neuropsychiatry　　　425
R. Jayan and S. Vinjamuri

10C Epilepsy　　　435
S.F. Barrington

10D Neuro-oncology　　　445
R.B. Workman, T.Z. Wong, W. Young, and R.E. Coleman

10E PET and SPECT imaging in movement disorders　　　457
J. Booij, J. Zijlmans, and H.W. Berendse

11. Head and neck disease　　　465

11A Head and neck cancer　　　467
G.W. Goerres

11B Salivary pathology　　　483
G.W. Goerres

11C Lachrymal studies　　　485
G.W. Goerres

12. Endocrine disease　　　489

12A Thyroid　　　491
M.N. Maisey

12B Parathyroid localization　　　511
A.G. Kettle, C.P. Wells, and M.J. O'Doherty

12C The adrenal gland　　　521
R.T. Kloos, M.D. Gross, and B. Shapiro

13. The Breast and genital disease　　　541

13A Breast cancer　　　543
N. Avril, M. Bienert, and J.D. Schwarz

13B Breast disease: Single photon and positron emission tomography　　　559
J. Buscombe

13C Testicular tumors　　　569
S.F. Hain

13D Impotence　　　575
Q.H. Siraj

13E Infertility　　　585
M.P. Iturralde, Q.H. Siraj, and F. Hussain

13F Testicular perfusion imaging　　　593
Q.H. Siraj

13G Gynecological cancer　　　601
K.E. Britton and M. Granowska

13H Prostate cancer　　　609
K.E. Britton, M.J. Carroll, and V.U. Chengazi

14. The gastrointestinal tract　　　619

14A Gastrointestinal bleeding　　　621
P.J.A. Robinson

14B Inflammatory bowel disease   629
P.J.A. Robinson

14C Functional studies of the gastrointestinal tract   637
A. Notghi

14D Positron emission tomography in gastrointestinal cancers   645
G.J.R. Cook

14E Gastrointestinal neuroendocrine tumors   653
J. Buscombe and G. Gnanasegaran

15. Hepatobiliary disease: Primary and metastatic liver tumors   661
R. Hustinx and O. Detry

16. Hematological, reticuloendothelial and lymphatic disorders   673

16A Anemia and polycythemia   675
R.W. Barber, N.G. Hartman, and A.M. Peters

16B Imaging the spleen   685
A.M. Peters

16C Imaging of lymphomas   695
L. Kostakoglu, M. Coleman, J.P. Leonard, and S.J. Goldsmith

16D Lymphoscintigraphy   715
A.M. Peters and P.S. Mortimer

17. Radionuclide therapy   725

17A Thyroid disease   727
S.E.M. Clarke

17B Endocrine: Peptides   745
M. de Jong, D. Kwekkeboom, R. Valkema, and E. Krenning

17C Neuroblastoma   755
C.A. Hoefnagel

17D The skeleton   765
V. Lewington

17E The use of ^{32}P   773
C. Parmentier

17F The role of dosimetry   781
G. Flux

6

Functional imaging of cardiac disease

6A Functional imaging of coronary artery and congenital heart disease

Coronary artery disease	147	The future of radionuclide imaging	169
Imaging techniques	148	Congenital heart diseases	169
Clinical applications of radionuclide imaging	156	References	172

6B Left ventricular dysfunction

Measuring left ventricular function: equilibrium radionuclide ventriculography	183	Definitions of ischemic syndromes	185
		Techniques to image viable myocardium	185
Reversing left ventricular dysfunction: the rationale for imaging myocardial viability	184	Cardiac sympathetic innervation imaging	189
		References	189

Functional imaging of coronary artery and congenital heart disease

SHAHID MAHMOOD

CORONARY ARTERY DISEASE

Coronary artery disease (CAD) has become a global epidemic, responsible for almost 30% of deaths worldwide.[1–3] Cardiovascular diseases were responsible for nearly 16.7 million fatalities globally in 2002, with the majority in developing countries.[1,4]

In the developed countries, there has been an encouraging decrease in mortality due to CAD, with a persistent rise in the developing countries like China and eastern European countries.[4] Similarly, there has been a six-fold increase in the incidence of CAD in the Indian urban population.[4,5] Collectively, all such developing countries account for more than 70% of the world population.

The variations in culture, ethnicity, race, socioeconomic status and lifestyle are responsible for differences in the prevalence and incidence of CAD.[4,6–8] Many studies have demonstrated a higher incidence of cardiovascular morbidity in non-Caucasians, compared with Caucasians.[6–8] The classical risk factors, such as a higher amount of saturated fat in the diet, elevated serum cholesterol, hypertension and diabetes are the main factors that contribute to CAD in western Europeans. In contrast, in eastern European countries, a higher incidence of smoking, excessive alcohol intake along with diets rich in saturated fat and poorer social conditions play a major contributory role. In the rapidly developing economies like China, it is further compounded by sedentary lifestyles, rapid industrialization, urbanization and increased stress in daily life. In the Indian population, higher levels of lipoprotein-a and insulin resistance play additional crucial roles in disease development.[8,9]

A family history of heart disease is associated with two- to seven-fold higher risk of CAD.[10] The control of modifiable risk factors is the best option to prevent premature CAD, regardless of cultural, social, ethnic and economic variations.[11]

Pathogenesis of coronary atherosclerosis

Coronary artery disease depicts the presence of coronary atherosclerosis, which is initiated during adolescence and increases throughout life with progressive narrowing of the vessel lumen and impaired myocardial blood flow (Fig. 6A.1). The process of atherosclerosis can be considered as 'a healing attempt of endothelial injury, caused by the risk factors'. Lipid and cholesterol metabolism is the primary known genetic factor in atherosclerosis, with already more than 150 types of mutation discovered. A multitude of complex factors, such as CD-40L signaling, *Chlamydia* antigens, oxidized low-density lipoprotein (LDL), macrophage apoptosis and macrophage–lymphocyte interactions contribute in the process of atherogenesis. There are also inter-relationships between endothelial injury, and risk factors, such as family history, smoking, diabetes mellitus, hypertension, obesity, hyperlipidemia, and a sedentary lifestyle. In older age, the endothelial dysfunction becomes more pronounced, causing reduced arterial compliance and increased vessel stiffness representing 'vascular aging'. This leads to a higher incidence of hypertension and atherosclerotic disease.

Atherosclerotic plaques characteristically occur in vascular regions where blood undergoes sudden changes in velocity and direction of flow, causing shear stress on the endothelial surface. Such segments are mostly present at the bifurcations, origin of smaller branches and areas of marked curvature and geometric irregularities. The development of fatty streaks between the endothelium and the internal elastic lamina secondary to oxidation of LDLs is the first critical step in the initiation and pathogenesis of atherosclerotic lesions. Over time, an extracellular lipid core, layers of smooth muscle and a connective tissue matrix with a fibrous cap constitutes an intermediate lesion. Endothelium secretes various chemicals to preserve the vascular tone. The risk factors speed up endothelial dysfunction and vascular inflammation, causing impaired endothelium-dependent dilation and paradoxical vasoconstriction. Endothelial dysfunction leads to inactivation of nitric oxide by the excess production of free radicals and reduced transcription of nitric oxide synthase messenger RNA (mRNA). Reduced nitric oxide results in increased platelet adhesion, increased plasminogen activator inhibitor, decreased plasminogen activator and increased tissue factor, enhancing platelet thrombus formation. Simultaneously, oxidized LDL activates inflammatory processes at the level of gene transcription, with recruitment of monocytes/macrophages. The circulating monocytes infiltrate the intima of the vessel wall, and these tissue macrophages act as scavenger cells, taking up LDL cholesterol and forming the characteristic 'foam cell', which is a hallmark of early atherosclerosis. These activated macrophages also release additional factors aggravating endothelial dysfunction. The soft atherosclerotic plaques may either organize over time with a fibrous cap and some calcification or may rupture, exposing the underlying thrombogenic core of lipid and necrotic material to circulating blood, resulting in platelet adhesion, aggregation, and progressive luminal narrowing, responsible for acute coronary syndromes.

There is an increasing body of evidence suggesting that atherosclerotic progression could be result of micro inflammation mediated by pro-inflammatory cytokines. A relationship between total infectious burden and extent of atherosclerosis has been proposed, whereby multiple infectious pathogens may act synergistically to cause vascular damage.[12] Biochemical markers such as elevated levels of C-reactive protein and interleukin-6 signal more rapidly advancing coronary artery disease and unstable plaques, requiring aggressive preventive measures.[13] The statins lower circulating levels of C-reactive protein,[14] either due to an anti-inflammatory effect or secondary to their effect on hepatic lipid homeostasis. Therefore, multitude and complexity of pathogenesis of CAD calls for individualization of treatment decisions for each patient, considering clinical symptoms, risk factors, the type and location of the lesions involving coronary arteries, extent and severity of ischemia, cardiac function and prognosis.

IMAGING TECHNIQUES

Knowledge of functional parameters such as flow, perfusion, function and metabolism is crucial for diagnosis, prognosis and management decisions. Echocardiography and Doppler, magnetic resonance imaging and radionuclide imaging are the commonly used modalities for functional imaging. Echocardiography and Doppler is the method of choice for most of the congenital and valvular heart diseases. MRI is being increasingly used for both complex congenital heart, as well as coronary artery diseases. There is a large amount of clinical data supporting the use of radionuclide imaging for evaluation of extent, severity and prognosis of coronary artery disease.

Radionuclide imaging in coronary artery disease

The quest to understand cardiac physiology in health and disease paved the way for the development of radionuclide imaging techniques. Hermann Blumgart pioneered the first human use of radioactivity in cardiovascular medicine using radon gas to measure human pulmonary circulation time.[15] Later, Geiger tubes and scintillators were used in the development of 'radiocardiography' for assessment of cardiac and pulmonary hemodynamics. With the invention of the Anger camera, true noninvasive cardiac imaging became a reality. Initially, left ventricular function was assessed by serial sequential imaging of the heart, establishing the first-pass technique for assessment of function and shunting.[16,17] Potassium-43 and ^{83}Rb were the first tracers

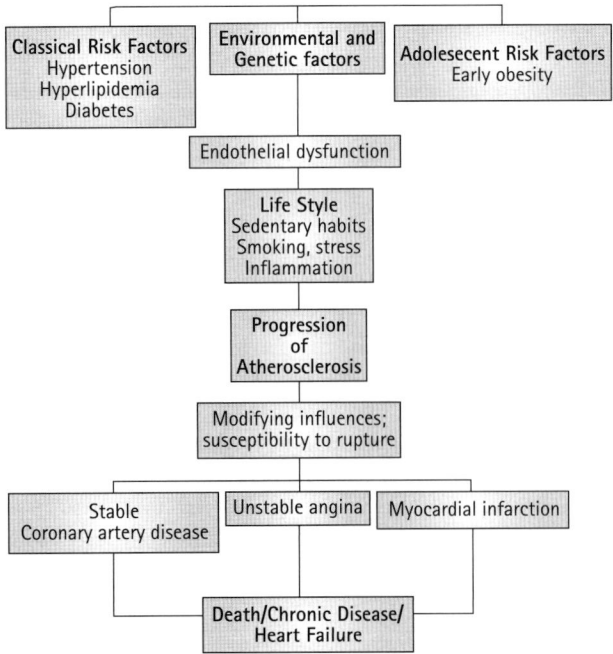

Figure 6A.1 *Flow diagram demonstrating key steps in initiation and gradual progression of coronary artery atherosclerosis. The initial event in the pathogenesis is endothelial dysfunction, which with other contributory factors progresses to atherosclerosis.*

used for myocardial imaging, but were not suitable for gamma camera imaging. With the introduction of ^{201}Tl, assessment of myocardial perfusion in conjunction with dynamic and pharmacological stress became the 'gold standard'.[18–20] Introduction of single photon emission computerized tomography (SPECT) revolutionized the scope of clinical nuclear medicine, with its biggest impact on the radionuclide cardiac imaging.[21,22] It is often not recognized that nuclear medicine was the one of the first medical specialties to incorporate computers into clinical practice.

Tracers for myocardial perfusion imaging using gamma camera

Currently, various SPECT and PET tracers are available, each depicting a unique functional aspect of cardiovascular imaging. There is still continuing research for the development of an ideal tracer for myocardial perfusion imaging, as none of the currently available tracers fulfils all the properties of an ideal radiopharmaceutical for gamma camera imaging (Table 6A.1).

THALLIUM-201

Thallium (Greek: 'thallous' meaning a green shoot) is a soft metal. Of its various isotopes, ^{201}Tl has been the principal tracer used for assessment of myocardial perfusion for more than three decades.[18,22,23] It has low gamma emissions and therefore relatively abundant X-ray emissions of ^{201}Hg are used for imaging. Thallium-201 is administered intravenously as thallous chloride, with a first-pass extraction efficiency of approximately 85%. It is a potassium analog and the uptake is not only dependent on the Na$^+$/K$^+$ pump,

but partially on a separate non-energy dependent facilitated diffusion (Fig. 6A.2). Myocardial uptake is approximately 3.5–4.3% of the administered dose.

The myocardial segments with reduced flow rates have relatively low uptake and a slower clearance rate, compared to the well-perfused segments. This generates a gradient between these hypoperfused segments and the vascular space, leading to an influx of ^{201}Tl from the vascular into the intracellular space. This appears as relatively increased uptake on the delayed images 'reversible defects' and clinically termed 'myocardial ischemia'.

TECHNETIUM-99m BASED-TRACERS

Many ^{99m}Tc-based radiopharmaceuticals with different characteristics have been introduced (Table 6A.2).[24] However, of all these, currently only sestamibi and tetrofosmin are available for clinical use. Other tracers such as teboroxime,[25,26] furifosmin[27,28] and NoET[29] have either been withdrawn or have not been approved for clinical use due to various shortcomings.

SESTAMIBI

Sestamibi (hexakis-2-methoxy-2-isobutyl isonitrile) was the first approved ^{99m}Tc-based tracer for myocardial perfusion imaging. The uptake is strongly dependent on plasma membrane and mitochondrial membrane potentials[30] (Fig. 6A.3). Its relatively low first-pass extraction fraction compared to ^{201}Tl is partially compensated by higher counts, yielding diagnostic and prognostic information similar to that of ^{201}Tl.[31–33]

Table 6A.1 *Properties of an ideal tracer*

- *Higher extraction fraction*
- *High contrast ratio (myocardium:blood pool ratio)*
- *Sufficient retention time for image acquisition*
- *No immediate redistribution*
- *Lowest possible radiation burden to the patient*
- *Low energy, with stable half-life*

None of the currently available tracers has extraction fraction of 100%.

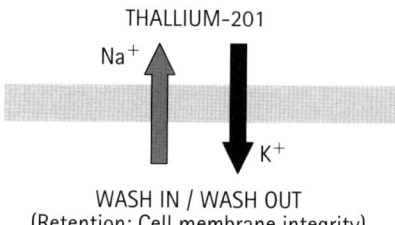

THALLIUM-201

Na$^+$

K$^+$

WASH IN / WASH OUT
(Retention: Cell membrane integrity)

Figure 6A.2 *Mechanism of uptake for ^{201}Tl, which is a potassium analog and uptake is mostly dependent upon the Na$^+$/K$^+$ pump. Thallium-201 redistributes and intracellular retention suggests integrity of cell wall (myocardial viability).*

Table 6A.2 *Comparison between properties of different tracers for myocardial perfusion*

Property	Thallium	Teboroxime	Sestamibi	Tetrofosmin	Furifosmin	NOET
Extraction (max)	0.80	0.89	0.39	0.30	0.26	0.48
Extraction (5 min)	0.60	0.71	0.41	0.30	0.12	0.24
Cell injury reduces uptake	++++	±	++++	++++	++	++
Myocardial clearance	Moderate	Rapid	Slow	Slow	Slow	Moderate
Redistribution	Yes	No	Not significant	Not significant	No	Yes

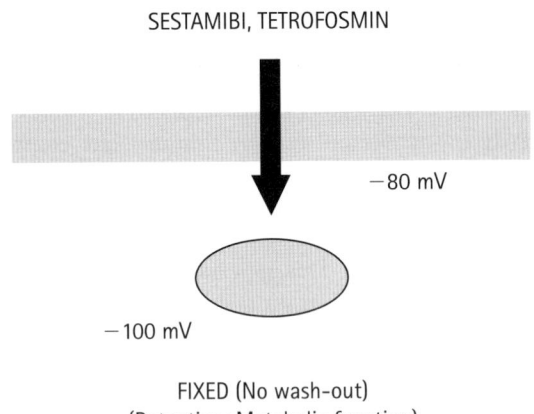

SESTAMIBI, TETROFOSMIN

−80 mV

−100 mV

FIXED (No wash-out)
(Retention: Metabolic function)

Figure 6A.3 *Mechanism of uptake for* ^{99m}Tc-*based available tracers. The uptake of* ^{99m}Tc-*sestamibi and* ^{99m}Tc-*tetrofosmin is dependent on plasma membrane and mitochondrial membrane potentials. They do not redistribute like* ^{201}Tl.

TETROFOSMIN

Technetium-99 m tetrofosmin is a cationic diphosphine compound, with rapid clearance from background organs. It has slightly lower extraction fraction than sestamibi at high flow rates,[34] which may underestimate the severity and extent of true ischemic burden in certain patients.[35] However, many studies have shown good comparison with other agents, without loss of significant diagnostic accuracy.[35,36] Due to its rapid rate of liver clearance, dedicated fast protocols can be employed that also increase patient throughput in busy centers.[37]

A NEW TRACER: N-DBODC5

Many other new agents are still under development in various laboratories. One of these is ^{99m}Tc-N-DBODC5 (bis (dimethoxypropylphosphinoethyl)-ethoxyethylamine (PNP5))-(bis (N-ethoxyethyl)-dithiocarbamato (DBODC)) nitride (N-PNP5-DBODC). This new agent appears to be promising with rapid clearance from the blood pool, and better heart-to-liver ratios in the initial animal studies.[38] The results of clinical trials are still awaited.

PET tracers for myocardial perfusion

PET offers several advantages over SPECT imaging, including less complex attenuation correction, superior resolution and, *in vivo*, noninvasive measurement of coronary flow in mL min^{-1} g^{-1}.

RUBIDIUM-82

Rubidium-82 has a very short half-life (75 s), and therefore multiple serial studies can be performed on the same day.[39] It concentrates in the myocardium in a manner similar to potassium and thallium, depending upon the Na$^+$/K$^+$ ATP pump. The quality of images depends on the tracer infusion

duration and necessitates appropriate infusion and imaging protocols.

[^{13}N]AMMONIA

[^{13}N]Ammonia is probably the best PET tracer for imaging and quantification of myocardial blood flow (70–80% myocardial extraction fraction).[40] After passively diffusing into the myocardium, it is converted into glutamine and is retained in the myocardial cells. Most studies have demonstrated sensitivity and specificity of more than 95% for detection of coronary artery disease.[41,42] Moreover, ECG-gated [^{13}N]ammonia permits simultaneous assessment of myocardial perfusion, ventricular geometry, and contractile function.[43]

[^{15}O]WATER

[^{15}O]Water is a freely diffusible tracer (half-life of 2.1 min), quantitatively correlating closely with perfusion assessed by means of microspheres. However, the simultaneous presence of water in the vascular space and myocardium poses difficulties in visual interpretation and requires quantification models.[44]

Non-perfusion tracers

TRACERS FOR ASSESSMENT OF METABOLISM

Glucose, fatty acids, and acetate are the predominant contributors of myocardial metabolism and can be evaluated using various physiological tracers.[45]

GLUCOSE METABOLISM: [^{18}F]FLUORODEOXYGLUCOSE

Fluorodeoxyglucose (FDG) is a glucose analog and is labeled with ^{18}F. FDG competes with glucose for uptake with conversion into FDG-6-phosphatase, without any further significant metabolism.[46] ^{18}F-FDG is considered the 'gold standard' for detection of viable myocardium.[47,48] FDG cardiac studies should ideally performed following glucose loading, using a hyperinsulinemic–euglycemic clamping technique. However, the technique is time consuming and therefore many centers adopt simpler methods.

FATTY ACID METABOLISM

Fatty acid oxidation is readily affected in a variety of cardiac pathologies.

Carbon-11 palmitate washout rates are associated with the oxidative metabolism of fatty acids. However, the quantitative assessment of ^{11}C-palmitic acid is complicated, as it also requires simultaneous assessment of myocardial blood flow.[49]

Carbon-11 acetate has been used for evaluation of fatty acid metabolism in recent myocardial infarction.[50] It demonstrates reduced clearance in the central area, with gradual normalization of the clearance rates towards the periphery.

Fluorine-18 6-thia-hepta-decanoic acid (^{18}*F-FTHA)* is a false long-chain fatty acid substrate and inhibitor of fatty acid metabolism and has been used for assessment of myocardial fatty acid metabolism.[51]

A variety of iodinated fatty acid compounds is also available for assessment of fatty acid metabolism with conventional gamma cameras. These include straight chains, such as iodopheyl pentadecanoic acid (IPPA), and branch-chain fatty acid compounds, such as beta-methyl iodophenyl pentadecanoic acid (BMIPP).[52] The BMIPP uptake is relatively increased compared to perfusion (reverse mismatch) in cases of acute myocardial infarction and chronic coronary artery disease. Due to its unique 'ischemic memory property', ^{123}I-BMIPP offers potential advantage to image ischemia without a stress test, up to 30 h after an anginal episode.

TRACERS FOR CARDIAC NEUROTRANSMISSION

The cardiac sympathetic stimulation affects the contractile and electrophysiological status of the heart and results in increased heart rate and contractility (chronotropic and inotropic effects) as well as atrioventricular conduction (dromotropic effect). With aging, there is decrease in cardiac function, primarily due to reduced responsiveness to the beta-adrenergic stimulation. The cardiac sympathetic activity is also affected in patients with myocardial infarction, life threatening ventricular arrhythmias, heart failure, cardiomyopathies and diabetes. Radionuclide imaging is currently the only imaging modality capable of investigating the integrity of neuronal status. PET imaging is more accurate than SPECT, due to advantages of superior resolution, attenuation correction and better quantitation.

[^{18}F]fluorodopamine reflects norepinephrine synthesis, while ^{11}C-hydroxyephedrine, ^{11}C-ephedrine, and *meta*-[^{123}I] iodobenzylguanidine (^{123}I-MIBG) are helpful in assessing pre-synaptic reuptake and storage.[53,54] Beta antagonists such as ^{11}C-CGP, ^{11}C-carazolol and [^{18}F]fluorocarazolol can be used to evaluate beta-adrenoceptor expression and density at the post-synaptic level.[53,55]

^{123}I-MIBG is a norepinephrine analog, with uptake by the sympathetic nerve terminals.[54] Even a mild degree of ischemia could be detrimental to the myocardial sympathetic neuronal activity. Increased washout rates are correlated with sympathetic denervation.[56,57] Myocardial infarction destroys not only the myocardium but also results in destruction of neurons that were destined to supply innervations in areas in which myocardial tissue is still viable. Therefore, MIBG imaging demonstrates a relatively larger defect than the associated perfusion deficit.[56,58] However, the denervation is not absolute and partial residual sympathetic innervation permits perception of anginal pain. MIBG has also been used to evaluate autonomic neuropathy in diabetics, heart failure and cardiomyopathies.[54]

TRACERS FOR IMAGING APOPTOSIS

Apoptosis is an evolutionary genetically controlled mechanism of 'programmed cell death'.[59,60] In comparison with necrosis, apoptosis occur in isolated cells, without inflammation. Annexin-V, an endogenous human protein, has been used as a new agent for apoptosis imaging in a variety of diseases.[61–63] It binds to a cell membrane-associated enzyme, phosphatidylserine, which is released during the early stages of apoptosis. It can be labeled by ^{99m}Tc for SPECT or ^{18}F for PET and fluorescein or rhodamine for optical imaging.[62,64]

TRACERS FOR IMAGING NECROSIS

In the past, myocardial necrosis could be detected by ^{99m}Tc-pyrophosphate or by ^{111}In-antimyosin antibody imaging, but both of these were unable to detect necrosis in the very early stages.[62] Indium-111 DTPA-antimyosin-Fab is a Fab monoclonal antibody fragment which has been used in past for imaging myocarditis and transplant rejection.[62,65,66]

Technetium-99 m D-glucarate is a myocardial infarct-avid imaging agent, concentrating only in severely injured myocardial segments within a few minutes of cardiac insult. It yields negative images in unstable angina, with a reported specificity of 100%.[62,67,68] It can also be taken up by ischemic but viable myocardium.

TRACERS FOR IMAGING HYPOXIA

Over the past several years, a vast effort has been put into the development of radiopharmaceuticals capable of defining hypoxic tissue in neurological, cardiovascular and oncological pathologies. The first series of radiopharmaceuticals were fluorinated analogs of the hypoxic cell sensitizer, misonidazole. Low oxygen, but not low flow per se, is responsible for retention of such tracers in the myocardium. [^{18}F]-Fluoromisonidazole (^{18}F-FMISO) demonstrated increased retention in hypoxic myocardium, but not in infarcted myocardium on PET imaging.[69] Another PET radiotracer, ^{62}Cu-diacetyl-bis-N^4-methylthiosemicarbazone (^{62}Cu-ATSM) has also been used for hypoxic imaging.

Technetium-99 m-labeled hypoxia-imaging tracers such as nitroimidazole and HL91 have also been developed for gamma camera imaging.[70,71]

In clinical routine, there has not been great interest for using new tracers such as these, particularly in the acute setting. This is primarily because myocardial perfusion imaging provides important clinical, management and additional prognostic information. Recent advances in noninvasive cardiac imaging methodologies may have a further impact on the development and use of such new tracers.

Exercise stress testing

The exercise ECG stress test is the most widely noninvasive method used for clinical evaluation of CAD. There are two major methods of exercise stress testing, (i.e. dynamic

Table 6A.3   *Types of stress test*

1. Exercise treadmill test
   - *Treadmill exercise*
   - *Bicycle (ergometer) exercise*
2. *Pharmacological stress test*
   - *Vasodilators*
     - *Adenosine (ATP)*
     - *A2 adenosine agonists*
     - *Dipyridamole (Persantine)*
   - *Inotropes*
     - *Dobutamine*
     - *Arbutamine*
3. *Combination: adenosine/dipyridamole with dynamic exercise*

A pharmacological vasodilator stress test can also be combined with a dynamic stress test.

exercise and pharmacological stress), used in combination with myocardial perfusion imaging (Table 6A.3). Other methodologies including isometric handgrip exercise stress test, atrial pacing simulation, cold pressor and mental stress tests are less feasible in clinical routine.

DYNAMIC (PHYSICAL) STRESS TEST

Physical exercise is a physiological stress test. It not only provokes perfusion and ventricular function abnormalities, but also provides crucial clinical information regarding symptoms, exercise capacity, and hemodynamic parameters, helping diagnostic and prognostic assessment.[72,73] The bicycle (ergometer) or treadmill exercise are two standard techniques, involving either symptom-limited exercise testing to elicit symptoms and/or hemodynamic/electrocardiographic changes. During the stress test, the double product (HR × systolic BP) reflects myocardial oxygen demand and ideally should be greater than 20 000 or at least double the patient's resting value. An adequate stress test is imperative for reliable results. A heart rate less than 85% of the maximal target heart rate in asymptomatic patients leads to suboptimal perfusion imaging results.[74] The indications for immediate cessation and contraindication of the stress test are listed in Tables 6A.4 and 6A.5.

STRESS TEST PROTOCOLS

Many stress test protocols have been devised, with the Bruce protocol being the test of choice in most laboratories. The standard Bruce exercise protocol begins walking at 1.7 mph with a 10% incline, with subsequent gradual increase in speed and grade every 3 min. In cases of unstable symptoms or deconditioned patients, the modified Bruce protocol is favored. The modified Bruce protocol starts at a lower workload. Nine minutes of the modified Bruce protocol are equal to the workload achieved at 3 min of the standard Bruce protocol.

Table 6A.4   *Indication for termination of a stress test*

- *Attainment of predicted target heart rate or double product*
- *Classic angina*
- *More than 3 mm of flat/downsloping ST segment depression or ST elevation*
- *Drop in systolic BP ≥ 20 mmHg*
- *Ventricular arrhythmia*

ST segment depression may not actually correspond to the ischemic region, while ST segment elevation typically relates to the site of ischemia. Patients with reduced BP during stress test have high likelihood of severe CAD.

Table 6A.5   *Contraindications of a stress test*

Absolute contraindications
- *Uncontrolled unstable angina*
- *Uncontrolled heart failure*
- *BP ≥ 200/115 mmHg*
- *Severe pulmonary hypertension*

Relative contraindications
- *Severe aortic stenosis*
- *Hypertrophic obstructive cardiomyopathy*
- *Recent MI*

Recent MI used to be an absolute contraindication but, currently, the pharmacological stress test appears to be safe.

Table 6A.6   *Indications of a pharmacological stress test*

- *Bundle branch block (right/left, bifascicular, pacing)*
- *Poor physical conditioning*
  Back pain
  Amputations
  Severe arthritis
  Other diseases, e.g. cancer, stroke, on dialysis
- *Peripheral arterial disease*
- *Poor patient motivation to exercise*
- *Lung disease (in COPD adenosine/dipyridamole are contraindicated)*
- *Medications (e.g. beta-blocking drugs)*

PHARMACOLOGICAL STRESS TEST

A pharmacological stress test is carried normally out in patients unable to exercise (Table 6A.6). The pharmacological stress agents are categorized into two sub-groups:

- Vasodilators: adenosine and dipyridamole
- Inotropes: dobutamine and arbutamine

VASODILATORS

The degree of coronary hyperemia attained with coronary vasodilators, exceeds that achieved by dynamic exercise,

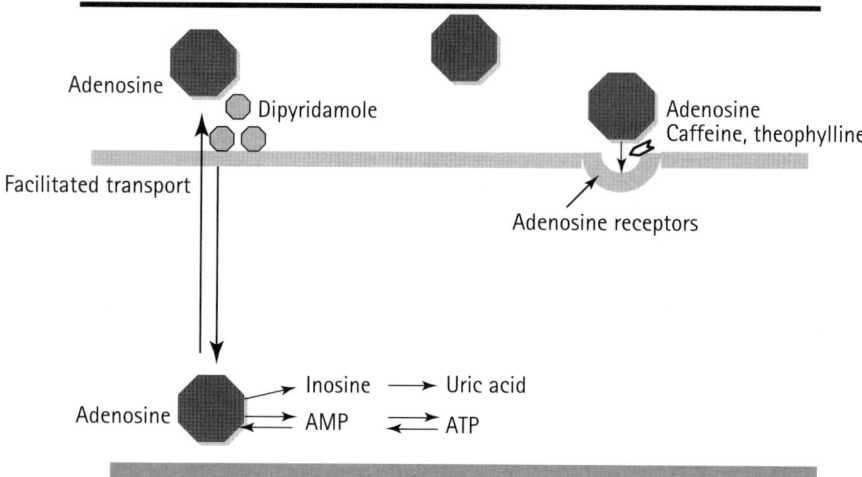

Figure 6A.4 *Mechanism of action of dipyridamole and adenosine. Dipyridamole inhibits intracellular uptake of adenosine, elevating levels of circulating adenosine. Adenosine binds to adenosine receptors leading to vasodilatation. The effect of adenosine is blocked by caffeine and theophylline derivatives.*

achieving a similar diagnostic accuracy to that of dynamic exercise.[75–78]

Adenosine, a physiological vasodilator, is a naturally occurring purine, present in the body as a result of dephosphorylation of adenosine monophosphate (AMP) and intracellular degradation of *S*-adenosyl-homocysteine (SAH). Adenosine is rapidly taken up into erythrocytes and vascular endothelium from blood and is either converted into adenosine triphosphate or metabolized into uric acid (Fig. 6A.4). The effect of adenosine is primarily through its effect on adenosine receptors, causing vascular smooth muscle cell relaxation with coronary (increased flow) and systemic vasodilatation (decreased BP).[79] The effect on coronary vasodilatation is required for perfusion imaging.

The most common side effects are flushing, shortness of breath, gastrointestinal discomfort and mild nonspecific chest pressure, with occasional (2–5%) AV block.[80] Due to a short half-life, discontinuation of the infusion immediately resolves most side effects. It should not be used if there is evidence or suspicion of SA node disease.[81]

Dipyridamole blocks cellular uptake of endogenous adenosine, causing an indirect but variable degree of coronary vasodilatation.[82] An adequate pharmacological effect can be judged by an increase in HR by more than 10 beats per minute (bpm), a decrease in diastolic blood pressure and symptomatology.

Dipyridamole and adenosine are contraindicated in patients with a second or higher degree atrioventricular block (Table 6A.7). They should be used with caution in cases of first-degree block, which may progress to a higher degree of block,[83] particularly with dipyridamole due to its longer half-life.

It should be recognized that the chest pain associated with vasodilators is not specific for myocardial ischemia. Normally, the patients with angina-like pain and normal

Table 6A.7 *Contraindications to the use of adenosine and dipyridamole*

- *COPD*
- *Second or third degree AV block*
- *Sick sinus syndrome*
- *<90 mmHg systolic blood pressure*
- *Use of dipyridamole during the previous 24 h*
- *Use of xanthine derivatives in the previous 12 h*

Xanthine derivatives like aminophylline, theophylline and caffeine act as an antagonist for A2A receptors and block adenosine. Therefore, no caffeine should be consumed within 12 h before the test with adenosine and dipyridamole.

coronary angiograms have a low pain threshold and reduced tolerance to pain induced by adenosine.[84]

The coupling of dipyridamole or adenosine infusions with dynamic stress is safe.[85–89] Most of the initial studies implemented a low level of dynamic exercise,[89] while only a few later studies used higher levels of exercise. The main advantages of adding physical stress to vasodilator pharmacological stress are reduction in adverse effects and improved image quality.[89–91] Adenosine combined with exercise also predicts a higher number of coronary events than adenosine infusion alone (3.91% vs. 3.20%).[91]

INOTROPES

The two inotropes dobutamine and arbutamine are synthetic catecholamines. *Dobutamine* is a sympathomimetic agent and has been widely used as a stress agent not only in myocardial perfusion imaging, but also for echocardiography and MRI. Through its effect on the beta-1 receptors, dobutamine increases heart rate and myocardial contractility; it augments cardiac output, while its direct effect on coronary arterioles causes mild coronary dilation. Dobutamine stress myocardial perfusion imaging has overall sensitivity, specificity and accuracy of 88%, 74% and 84%, respectively, for CAD.[92–94]

The use of dobutamine in myocardial perfusion imaging is usually selective, being limited to patients with contraindications to dipyridamole and adenosine. It should not be used in cases of bundle branch block, significant hypertension or hypotension, other types of significant arrhythmias, and aortic stenosis (Table 6A.8).

Dobutamine infusion is commonly started at a rate of $10\,\mu g\,kg^{-1}\,min^{-1}$, increasing in increments of $10\,\mu g\,kg^{-1}\,min^{-1}$, at 3-min intervals (Fig. 6A.5). The perfusion tracer is injected at peak stress. The commonest reported side effects of dobutamine are chest pain, palpitations, headache, flushing and dyspnea.[95,96]

Arbutamine is a short-acting potent nonselective beta-adrenergic agonist with mild alpha-1 sympathomimetic activity. It has 10 times greater affinity for beta receptors than that of dobutamine and is safe and effective.[97] Arbutamine is no longer available commercially, however, due to its infrequent use, higher cost, and the complexity of the closed-loop drug delivery system.

CHOICE OF STRESS TEST

In any given clinical situation, the choice of the appropriate stress test is extremely important for diagnostic accuracy. The standard paradigms in patients for the evaluation of CAD is to use dynamic exercise testing, provided they are estimated to be able achieve a good level of exercise. Pharmacological stress with adenosine or dipyridamole is used in patients with early post-MI, aortic stenosis, left bundle branch block, cerebral vascular accident and with exercise limitations due to peripheral vascular disease, hip/knee prosthesis and arthritis.[98,99] Pharmacological stress with dual-isotope imaging could also be helpful in very busy departments, to increase throughput.[37] Dobutamine is normally reserved for patients with bronchospasm or asthma. As mentioned earlier, simultaneous coupling of dynamic exercise with dipyridamole or adenosine infusion could be a more useful standardized approach, except where contraindicated.[100]

Gated SPECT

Electrocardiographic (ECG) gating of blood pool images has been well established for more than three decades. With advances in technology, it has also been possible to gate myocardial perfusion SPECT data, permitting simultaneous evaluation of myocardial perfusion, left ventricular (LV) volumes, ejection fraction (EF), regional wall motion and thickening in a single study.[101,102] In a gated study, the cardiac cycle is divided into multiple phases (frames) and counts from each phase of the cardiac cycle are associated with a temporal frame within the computer.[103]

The LV function obtained from the post-stress test gated dataset is not a true representative of resting LV function in patients with stress-induced ischemia.[104,105] In many patients with post-stress test perfusion abnormalities, a relative drop in ejection fraction is also present, compared with resting data (Plate 6A.1a,b). This information is crucial in defining prognosis. Therefore, we prefer to gate both stress and rest studies, regardless of 1-day and 2-day protocols.

Acquisition and processing of myocardial perfusion SPECT

High-quality images are not only important for the confidence of the reporting physician, but also to gain the trust of referring physicians. Different acquisitions and processing variables affect the ultimate quality of SPECT images. Myocardial perfusion scintigraphy can be performed with either single isotopes e.g. ^{201}Tl or ^{99m}Tc tracers, or using a

Table 6A.8   *Contraindications of the dobutamine stress test*

- *Uncontrolled unstable angina*
- *Hemodynamically significant LVOT obstruction*
- *Uncontrolled hypertension or BP > 200/115 mmHg*
- *Recent MI*
- *Prior history of ventricular tachycardia*
- *Atrial tachyarrhythmias*

The dobutamine stress test should not be performed in LVOT obstruction like aortic stenosis or hypertrophic obstructive cardiomyopathy, recent MI and severe arrhythmias. LVOT: left ventricular outflow tract.

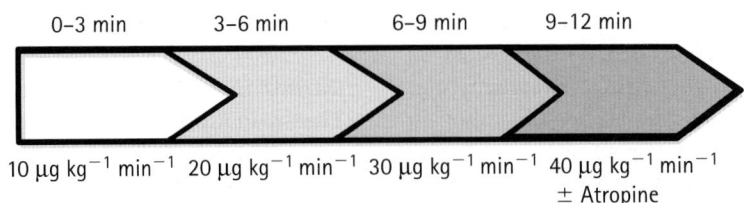

Figure 6A.5   *Protocol for a dobutamine stress test. Dobutamine, a sympathomimetic agent, is infused at a rate of $10\,\mu g\,kg^{-1}\,min^{-1}$ up to 40–$50\,\mu g\,kg^{-1}\,min^{-1}$. If an adequate heart rate is not achieved by that time and there are no clinical contraindications, 0.25–0.5 mg of atropine can be administered slowly, intravenously, to achieve an optimal target heart rate.*

dual-isotope protocol, with variable acquisition and processing parameters. Although different guidelines are available for imaging from various societies and institutions, there is still variability between individual users.

In gated SPECT studies, data are gated with the peak of the R wave on ECG and data for different phases (frames) of the cardiac cycle are acquired.[106] Currently, most manufacturers allow the acquisition of up to 32 frames per RR interval. In practice, eight frames is often a reasonable compromise. Inconsistent and rapid alterations of heart rate during acquisition may reject too many beats, resulting in variable numbers of frames and counts in each projection. On the cine loop, this appears as a 'flickering' artifact. Therefore, an acceptance window for bad-beat rejection must be specified. If the window is too wide, arrhythmic beats may be included and therefore results may be downgraded.[106,107] Despite the advantages of the functional information provided by gated SPECT, the perfusion data should not be compromised due to arrthymias. Therefore, in patients with severe arrhythmia, such as atrial fibrillation, frequent ventricular ectopics, and high degree heart block, gated SPECT should be performed with caution. While the ungated-SPECT data are checked for any motion or external attenuation artifacts, the ECG-gated raw images must additionally be evaluated for presence of arrthymia-generated artifacts, as mentioned earlier.

The newer generation of SPECT system offers choice of attenuation. If available, both attenuation and scatter correction should be applied. Attenuation correction has the benefit of improved diagnostic accuracy and confidence (Plate 6A.2), but requires a modified approach to image interpretation.[108] With the recent introduction of SPECT–CT systems, fast and more accurate attenuation correction should be possible. This would likely reduce quality control procedures required for attenuation correction hardware and problems with the transmission line sources.

Image display must include comparative slices (approximately 6 mm width) of stress and rest studies presented in three planes. For perfusion assessment from gated cardiac SPECT, it is standard practice to ungate the gated datasets, and process as non-gated SPECT studies (Plate 6A.3). Appropriate reconstruction algorithms and filtering, with appropriate definition of oblique angles of the LV are crucial for incomparable quality of SPECT slices. Filtered back-projection is the most commonly used technique to reconstruct SPECT images. It has to be ensured that the images are neither over-smoothed nor too noisy but still preserve all the detail.[109] Two-dimensional semi-quantitative analysis of myocardial perfusion can be achieved through bull's eye display or polar maps to document the extent and severity scores of the defects (Plate 6A.4).

The gated raw data sets are processed separately, to generate reconstructed slices for functional assessment. The use of appropriate filters in processing is crucial, as pre-filtering tends to result in higher value of ejection fraction, than post-processing filters.[110] Automatic software is then used to determine functional parameters like ejection fraction, volumes and wall thickening and motion abnormalities. The three most common software packages are 4D-MSPECT (University of Michigan), Emory Cardiac Toolbox or ECTb (Emory University) and QGS (Cedars-Sinai) (Plate 6A.5). Direct comparative analysis has demonstrated good correlation between all three packages.[111,112] The QGS uses an edge detection method using endocardial and epicardial surface points and makes geometric assumptions (Gaussian fit) to calculate LV end-systolic and end-diastolic volumes. The Emory Toolbox uses a count-based technique to define the same points. In clinical routine, we recognize that QGS provides relatively lower volumes and ejection fraction than ECTb. Similar observations have been made by others.[113,114] However, the QGS tends to overestimate LVEF and LV volumes in smaller hearts, most likely due to limited spatial resolution of SPECT. In such cases, a count-based technique like Emory Cardiac Toolbox may be an appropriate choice.

Interpretation of myocardial perfusion SPECT images

It is necessary to standardize reporting criteria to ensure consistency and reliability. In the UK, one audit documented a lack of good quality reports.[115]

The stress test is an important component of the procedure and therefore, ECG, hemodynamic response, typical angina, exercise capacity, and ST-segment changes during exercise must be described in the final report.

The raw data must be examined before reporting reconstructed SPECT slices, to visualize patient motion, soft tissue or external attenuation or non-cardiac uptake (Plate 6A.6), preferably using a gray scale. Increased lung uptake of ^{201}Tl in post-stress test images indicates poor LV function and carries a poor prognosis.[116] It is important to comment on LV configuration prior to describing perfusion defects.[117] A small or contracted LV is unlikely to be associated with any significant ischemia, whereas a post-stress transiently dilated LV or drop in ejection fraction would be related with significant ischemic burden (Plates 6A.7 and 6A.8). The perfusion defects can be either reversible or fixed and are best reported using a 9- or 20-segment model, as also suggested in many guidelines[118] (Plate 6A.9). The description of extent and severity of the defects is subjective and may be a source of inter-observer variability. It is therefore useful to standardize criteria for each laboratory by consensus among the reporting physicians. The easiest way is to use percentage uptake of the tracer in the myocardium as a guide for severity (Plate 6A.10 and Table 6A.9). Quantitative methods of the sum score can also be used. With improvement in SPECT systems, it is frequent to visualize the right ventricle. In 30–40% of patients with inferior wall infarction or merely disease in RCA, RV free wall abnormalities can be seen and are a bad prognostic sign (Plate 6A.11).

The pattern of reverse redistribution is seen particularly with ^{201}Tl imaging (Plate 6A.12). However, ^{99m}Tc compounds may also show similar characterization. Although, at times, it may be a normal variable in patients with known CAD, it most likely represents sub-endocardial scarring distal to the patent proximal coronary artery.[119] The post-stress images appear normal due to increased coronary hyperemia masking a sub-endocardial scar. Absence of hyperemia in the overlying myocardium during resting images reveals the defect as reduced uptake in the scar. We have frequently noted this pattern in patients undergoing thrombolytic therapy post-PTCA and post-coronary artery bypass graft (CABG).

LBBB, LVH, long membranous/short muscular septum, apical thinning, and myocardial bridges, coronary artery spasm and anomalous origins of coronary arteries are a source of false-positive myocardial perfusion studies in absence of obstructive CAD. The diaphragm and breast are major causes of attenuation artifacts (Table 6A.10). Gated

Table 6A.9 *Visual assessment of defect severity*

Extent

- *Severe: Less than approx. 35% maximal myocardial counts*
- *Moderate: 45–60% of maximal counts*
- *Mild: Approx. 60–80% of maximal counts*
- *Minimal: 70–85%*

Degree of reversibility

- *Complete: More than approx. 85% reversible*
- *Partial: 30–85% reversible*
- *Primarily/partially fixed: 15–30% reversible*
- *Fixed: Less than 15% reversible*

The percentage of maximal counts on the color/gray scales are used for the visual interpretation of the defect severity. Although in most cases counts of more than 80% are considered normal, it is also common to observe minimal change between stress and rest images. The counts could be between 70 and 85% on stress images. This is a narrow range and could be difficult to detect. However, such changes could reflect either minor microvascular or mild early disease. This is also found in many patients with very high calcium scores. Despite a relatively lower risk in such patients, more careful clinical assessment is required, as such patients could also be candidates for medical management, such as statins and risk modification.

Table 6A.10 *Identification of attenuation artifacts and other types of pathophysiological diagnoses identifiable on a gated SPECT study*

- *Fixed defect + wall thickening (no evidence of MI) = Attenuation*
- *Fixed defect + wall thickening (history of previous MI) = Viable tissue*
- *Fixed defect + no wall thickening = Infarction*
- *Normal perfusion + no wall thickening = Stunning*

SPECT is helpful in differentiating between true perfusion defects and artifacts.[101,102] Gating may increase the confidence level, but appears to have little impact in interpretation with experienced physicians.[120] Small sub-endocardial infarcts with perfusion abnormalities may demonstrate normal wall motion and good thickening on the gated SPECT, underestimating the true extent of underlying disease. However, a good prognosis is still expected in such patients.

CLINICAL APPLICATIONS OF RADIONUCLIDE IMAGING

Radionuclide imaging is a clinically helpful methodology for various diagnostic and management challenges and providing necessary prognostic information in patients with CAD (Table 6A.11).

Diagnosis of coronary artery disease

In the past, rest–stress gated blood pool and first-pass imaging were the commonly used radionuclide techniques for establishing diagnosis, estimating severity and predicting prognosis of coronary artery disease. LV functional parameters are excellent indicators of prognosis and risk stratification, but have lower specificity.[121] Over recent years, myocardial perfusion imaging with [201]Tl- and ^{99m}Tc-labeled agents has gradually substituted these methodologies, with diagnostic accuracies ranging from 84 to 94%.[33,35,122,123] In a meta-analysis of 3425 patient studies, organized by the National Institute for Clinical Excellence (NICE) in the UK, myocardial perfusion imaging has established diagnostic sensitivity of 87%.[124] Myocardial perfusion imaging may underestimate true ischemic burden due to balanced hypoperfusion, in certain patients with multi-vessel disease.[125] Gated myocardial perfusion SPECT could be of help in such

Table 6A.11 *Main indications and uses of myocardial perfusion scintigraphy*

- *Detection of CAD (diagnosis)*
- *Assessment of extent and severity of CAD (ischemic burden)*
- *Prognostication and risk stratification*
- *Management decision and monitoring of therapies (interventional and medical)*
- *Acute coronary syndrome*
- *Myocardial viability*
- *Future: Gene/stem cell therapy?*

It is likely that, in near future, coronary CT angiography will become routine for the noninvasive diagnosis and screening of CAD. MPI would still have a role in hemodynamic assessment of lesion risk stratification, and in various management decisions and the detection of hibernating myocardium.

cases, by demonstrating reduced ejection fraction and wall motion abnormalities.[118]

PET has approximately 10% higher diagnostic accuracy than SPECT. Attenuation correction, with high spatial and temporal resolutions, and absolute measurements of coronary flow reserve in mL min^{-1} g^{-1} are the added advantages.[126]

Recently, a newer generation of SPECT–CT devices has been launched. CT provides faster attenuation–scatter correction for the SPECT data, improving diagnostic accuracy.[127] The American Society of Nuclear Cardiology and the Society of Nuclear Medicine have also recommended implementation of attenuation and scatter correction even for gated SPECT, preferably using sequential transmission–emission imaging protocols, like the one used in SPECT–CT systems.[128] Myocardial perfusion SPECT imaging is capable of identifying hemodynamically significant ischemia, thus aiding management decisions, but does not detect atherosclerosis and may underestimate early disease. On the other hand, CT has the capability of detecting coronary calcifications and atherosclerotic changes. Therefore, SPECT–CT may permit better delineation of the extent and severity of underlying coronary artery stenosis, enhancing the clinical information, particularly in equivocal and minor lesions, in conduit or stent re-stenosis and disease progression in the native coronary arteries, with an impact on management decisions (Plate 6A.13 (a) and (b)). This could only be achieved if a multi-slice CT (minimum of 16 slices) is incorporated into the SPECT–CT.

SCREENING FOR CORONARY ARTERY DISEASE

The higher incidence of CAD with escalating costs of treatment emphasizes the need of early screening and prevention.[129] Therefore, the objective for the future would be not only to identify high-risk individuals for CAD but also to identify disease in the asymptomatic, low- and intermediate-risk groups. This would allow management strategies to be defined with the expectation of reducing future coronary ischemic events.

The assessment of risk factors is helpful for defining the pre-test likelihood of CAD. An ideal screening methodology should be capable of not only detecting early obstruction or abnormal coronary flow but also predicting future cardiac events. The use of coronary angiography has demonstrated improved outcomes.[130] However, due to its invasive nature and higher costs, it cannot be used as a screening or early diagnostic tool.

Stress ECG is the most commonly used screening test but it has the lowest predictive accuracy. Radionuclide imaging, particularly myocardial perfusion scintigraphy, is a well-established, cost-effective, noninvasive methodology with high predictive accuracy.[131,132] A positive SPECT study would be consistent with hemodyamically significant disease, regardless of the degree of anatomical luminal obstruction.

Myocardial contrast echocardiography (MCE) has also revealed comparable results with myocardial perfusion SPECT imaging,[133] but such studies are limited. Coronary calcium scoring using electron-beam and multi-slice CT, and, recently, noninvasive coronary CT angiography have also been employed as screening methodologies.[134,135] Calcium scores of less than 100 indicate a low risk to patients. However, myocardial perfusion abnormalities have been observed in approximately 9% patients with coronary calcium scores of ranging between 1 and 10, and 20% with scores of 11–100.[136] Abnormal scans have also been detected in 12% of the middle-aged asymptomatic population, with absent coronary calcium.[136] Therefore, myocardial perfusion SPECT imaging provides important diagnostic information, even in cases of low or absent coronary calcium scores. Myocardial perfusion scans are normal in approximately 17.5% patients with coronary calcium score of more than 100.[137] Conversely, perfusion abnormalities can also be detected in apparently 'normal' coronary angiogram, representing earliest changes in coronary flow reserve, secondary to endothelial and microcirculatory dysfunctions, and precede anatomical and morphological transformations.[138]

Newer generation multi-slice CT scanners are gradually being widely adopted for noninvasive angiography.[135,139] With recent 64 slice CT scanners, sensitivities and specificities of 94% and 97%, respectively, and a negative predictive value of 99% has been reported for hemodynamically significant lesions.[140] Multi-slice CT coronary angiography appears also to be capable of identifying both soft and hard plaque, supplementing the information gleaned from risk factors and myocardial perfusion imaging.[141] However, data on the plaque recognition is still preliminary.

Cardiovascular magnetic resonance imaging can evaluate the presence of CAD by direct visualization of coronary stenosis and measurement of flow, assessment of myocardial perfusion, metabolism, wall motion abnormalities and infarcted (nonviable) myocardium.[141–143] Compared to CT angiography, it is unlikely, however, that it would attain wide clinical acceptance for screening in the near future.

The Association for Eradication of Heart Attack (AEHA), in developing SHAPE (Screening for Heart Attack Prevention and Education), has advocated that traditional risk factors alone should not be used for screening beyond the age of 45 years in men and 55 years in women, and everyone beyond that age should undergo a comprehensive assessment. However, as mentioned above, absence of coronary calcification does not preclude myocardial ischemia. If myocardial perfusion imaging is included in such an approach, it would greatly enhance incremental risk stratification and early detection of coronary disease (Fig. 6A.6).

Positron emission tomography has the capability of quantifying the functional abnormalities in perfusion and coronary flow reserve.[41,43,44] The recent emergence of a combination of PET with multi-slice CT could provide information of both modalities.[141] The functional information such as reduced coronary flow reserve in pre-clinical

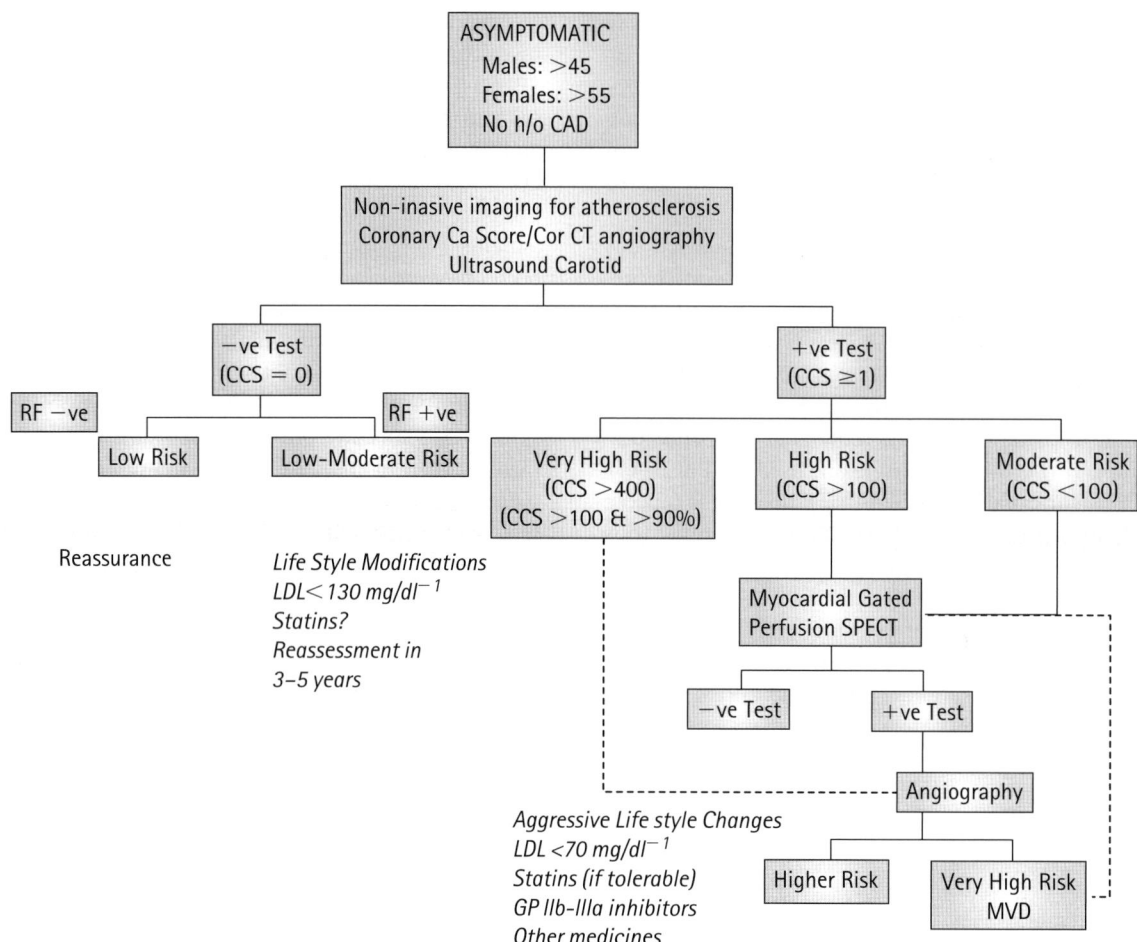

Figure 6A.6 *With coronary calcium scoring and wider use of multi-slice CT for coronary angiography, the role of myocardial perfusion SPECT may change and it play a more important role in coronary artery disease. While traditional risk factors and calcium score could define the likelihood of coronary atherosclerosis, the moderate- and high-risk patients would benefit from further sub-categorization into moderate-, high- and extremely high-risk groups. Even high-risk patients with MVD also benefit from myocardial perfusion SPECT imaging to define the culprit lesion. (Modified from Association for Eradication of Heart Attack (AEHA) and Screening for Heart Attack Prevention and Education (SHAPE).)*

non-obstructive disease, can precisely be correlated with affected anatomical segments of coronary vessels. Such information would be crucial for development, use and follow-up of targeted drug delivery systems. Evidence is still lacking to show that such high-cost screening methodology or early treatment would reduce the incidence of MI or sudden cardiac death.

SYNDROME X

Patients with classic angina-like chest pain often associated with ST segment changes, positive stress test, normal coronary angiograms, with no evidence of coronary spasm on provocation testing are termed 'syndrome X' or 'microvascular angina'[144] and this is more common in women than in men.

Cardiac syndrome X is a different entity from metabolic syndrome X (Reaven syndrome or insulin resistance syndrome), which is a major risk factor in the development of coronary disease. Cardiac syndrome X has relatively low mortality, compared to very high mortality in metabolic syndrome X.

Several possible mechanisms like endothelial dysfunction, increased thromboxane A2 from platelet aggregation and increased sympathetic activity have been attributed, as causes of abnormal coronary microvascular tone in syndrome X patients (Fig. 6A.7).

Myocardial perfusion SPECT imaging can elicit heterogeneous perfusion abnormalities and reverse redistribution on ^{201}Tl SPECT imaging in patients with syndrome X.[145] Therefore, reverse redistribution on ^{201}Tl SPECT imaging should be considered as diagnostically helpful in cases of suspected syndrome X, representing sub-endocardial ischemia due to microvascular changes. Echocardiography, PET and MRI, can also measure coronary blood flow at baseline and post-adenosine-induced hyperemia, depicting a varied distribution of regional myocardial blood indicative of focal myocardial ischemia.

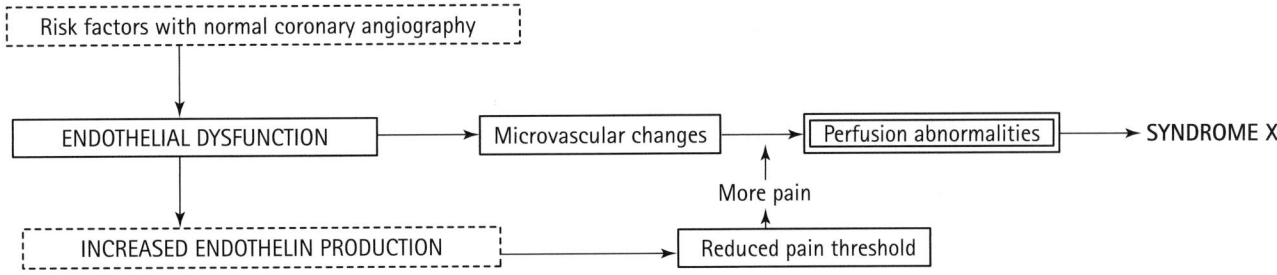

Figure 6A.7 *Possible mechanism of perfusion abnormalities in syndrome X. Endothelial dysfunction increases endothelin production, a vaso-constrictor by the vascular endothelium, reducing the pain threshold and aggravating the microvascular changes. This leads to more perfusion abnormalities, despite normal angiography.*

VARIANT OR PRINZMETAL'S ANGINA

This is characterized by recurrent, transient attacks of coronary vasospasm, causing chest pain and ST-segment elevation on ECG. The patients with variant angina have a higher risk of MI (20–30%) and also life-threatening cardiac arrhythmias. The exact cause of spasm has not been established yet. A variety of processes like autonomic dysfunction, platelet-derived vasoactive substances and hypersensitivity to endothelial-derived factors play a part towards probable mechanisms for spasm.

The diagnosis of coronary spasm is difficult, as mostly the symptoms occur out of hospital. Gated myocardial perfusion SPECT can exhibit wall motion abnormalities (stunning), even hours after an episode has occurred. Pharmacological activated PET studies can also induce spasm and quantify coronary flow and perfusion, but are not feasible in clinical routine.

Abnormalities in fatty acid metabolism persist long after an ischemic episode or even reperfusion.[146] Iodine-123 BMIPP has unique 'memory' of an ischemic event by demonstrating fatty acid metabolism abnormalities several hours after an episode of angina that occurs outside hospital.

ACUTE CORONARY SYNDROME

Acute coronary syndrome (ACS) is a common manifestation of CAD and represents a continuum of pathophysiological conditions like unstable angina, non-S-T elevation MI and acute S-T elevation MI.[147,148]

The diagnosis, evaluation and management of acute coronary syndrome (ACS) continue to be a clinical challenge. In unstable angina, the cardiac enzymes such as troponin and CK-MB are within normal limits in most of the patients. Myocardial perfusion imaging is of great help and can elicit perfusion abnormalities suggesting hemodynamically abnormal flow in such cases. The high sensitivity and negative predictive value of myocardial perfusion imaging provides discriminatory power.[149–151]

The cardiac markers like troponin are positive in approximately 30% patients with unstable angina, indicating a

higher-risk group.[152,153] Such patients are likely to benefit most with platelet GPIIa/IIIb inhibitors. Failures to stabilize on medical treatment, high risk on myocardial perfusion imaging, or multiple repeated episodes of unstable angina are indications for priority cardiac catheterization (Fig. 6A.8).

Myocardial perfusion scintigraphy is the most appropriate and cost-effective choice, to evaluate acute chest pain with a nondiagnostic ECG, and is likely to affect patient management decisions.[154] Patients with negative imaging results have smaller infarcts and less extensive coronary disease. In one multi-center trial (ERASE) of 2475 patients with chest pain or symptoms of acute myocardial ischemia, with normal or nondiagnostic initial ECG results, use of myocardial perfusion imaging improved the management decisions for patients without initial ECG abnormalities and also reduced unnecessary hospitalization.[155] Gated myocardial perfusion SPECT is even more helpful in refining initial clinical prognosis of such patients into low, intermediate, or high risk.

It is estimated that 2–8% of patients with acute MI are discharged inappropriately.[156] Addition of gated myocardial perfusion SPECT to the clinical information and cardiac troponin levels provides complementary incremental information in difficult cases of myocardial infarction.

Echocardiography is also often used for evaluation of chest pain due to ease of availability and capability of bedside imaging. Echocardiography has excellent negative predictive value, comparable with myocardial perfusion SPECT.[157] Besides wall motion abnormalities, it helps in the evaluation of left ventricular function and other complications of CAD, like papillary muscle involvement and acute mitral valve regurgitation. Newer imaging options like harmonic imaging and contrast echocardiography further improve the diagnostic accuracy. However, in a small subset of patients, echocardiography may have poor image quality. Multi-slice/multi-detector CT (MSCT/MDCT) and cardiac MR have also been used to identify patients with acute coronary syndromes. With wall motion analysis, first pass and delayed contrast enhanced imaging has demonstrated a sensitivity of 84% and specificity of 85% for detection of acute coronary

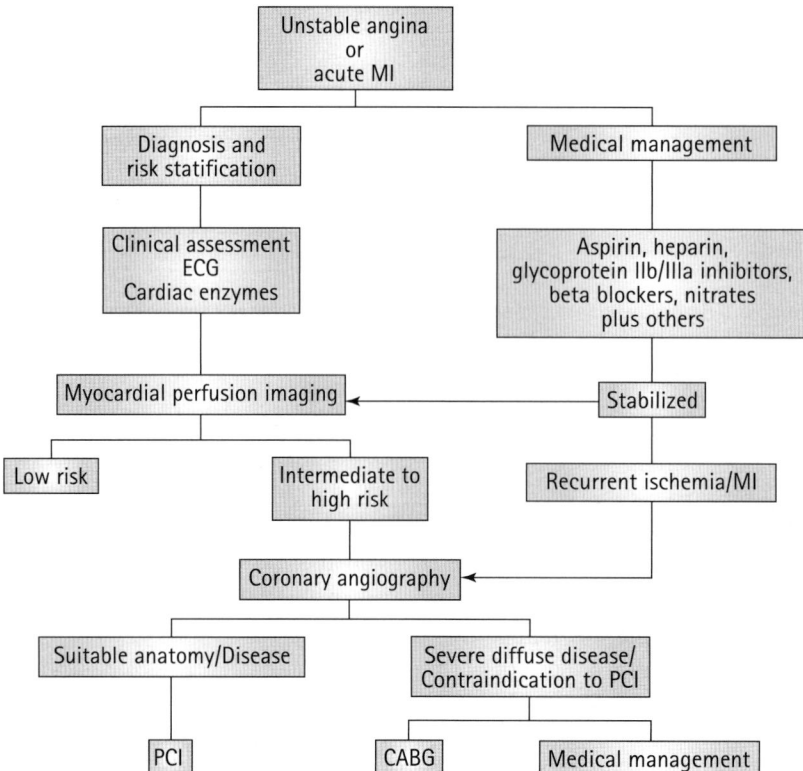

Figure 6A.8   *Role of myocardial perfusion imaging in management of acute coronary syndromes.*

syndromes.[158] There have been also some initial encouraging reports regarding the use of MDCT in acute chest pain and recognition of soft plaques.[159] So far, radionuclide imaging appears to be a most promising technique, due to the added advantage of risk stratification.[160]

DIABETES AND CORONARY ARTERY DISEASE

The Framingham study revealed increased risk of coronary disease in diabetic patients.[161–163] Diabetes causes more extensive coronary artery disease, debilitating many patients with congestive heart failure or angina. In type I diabetes mellitus, there is 35% cardiovascular mortality by the age of 55 years.[164] Women with diabetes have five to seven times higher risk of cardiovascular mortality than in those without diabetes.[163,165]

Hyperglycemia not only leads to impaired endothelial function, preceding clinically overt CAD, but it also contributes to the worsening of major coronary risk factors like obesity, dyslipidemia and hypertension. Therefore, even the presence of diabetes alone must be considered as CAD-equivalent.

Silent ischemia is a common finding in diabetics, making diagnosis difficult on routine exercise stress testing. Interestingly, angina or silent ischemia appears to be more frequent in diabetics with normal angiographic coronary arteries. Early diagnosis and intervention in diabetic patients with silent ischemia could be beneficial. In the

Coronary Artery Surgery Study (CASS), diabetic patients with silent ischemia had a higher mortality than did nondiabetic patients with silent ischemia and revascularization offered a better outcome than pharmacological therapy in such a group.[166] Smoking, low high-density lipoprotein (HDL) and micro-albuminuria are considered as predictors of silent ischemia in diabetes. However, such prediction cannot be translated into the severity of disease or prognosis, which can be achieved only by radionuclide imaging.

Due to a low probability of significant obstructive CAD in uncomplicated diabetics, most physicians tend to screen diabetic patients only in the presence of complications or ECG abnormalities. However, due to high risk of cardiac and non-cardiac complications, assessment of myocardial perfusion in all patients with type 2 diabetes, at the time of diagnosis and thereafter would be apposite. Sequential radionuclide imaging with PET or SPECT would be helpful in follow-up of the disease development and progression in such a higher-risk population group.

There has been no well-designed prospective study available concerning the early diagnostic and prognostic implication of myocardial perfusion imaging in truly asymptomatic diabetics. The Detection of Ischemia in Asymptomatic Diabetes (DIAD) trial intends to assess prevalence and severity of myocardial ischemia in asymptomatic diabetic population. Initial results have revealed 22% of asymptomatic diabetic patients with abnormalities suggestive of silent ischemia, with 5% having major perfusion abnormalities.[167] It is therefore plausible that improved diagnostic accuracy of myocardial perfusion imaging in diabetics, would translate into improved clinical outcomes.

Prognosis and risk stratification

Traditionally, the ECG stress test is still being used not only for diagnosis but also for prognostic assessment. Nevertheless, pre-defined low-risk patients on an ECG stress test, with abnormal myocardial perfusion scintigrams, have a higher incidence of major coronary events (up to 6.2%).[168] Use of myocardial perfusion SPECT and, particularly gated SPECT are standardized and tested methodologies applicable to all groups and classes of patients for identification of high-risk subset of patients, and aid rational and targeted treatment decisions.[169–171]

The patients with a normal stress perfusion scan have a favorable prognosis even in the presence of CAD.[168–172] In an analysis of 21 studies comprising 53 762 patients, myocardial perfusion imaging successfully identified a subset of low-risk patients in whom further invasive procedures might be avoided.[173]

The lower incidence of major coronary events in low-risk groups has also been demonstrated in other studies.[170,174] The overall survival rate in the low risk groups ranges from 99.3 to 99.7%.[169,170,172–174] In a meta-analysis of 39 studies (69 655 patients), moderate to severe abnormal scans, multi-vessel perfusion abnormalities, or a summed stress score of more than 8, the perceived high-risk patient population had an approximate annual incidence rate of 5.9%, while the low-risk group had an annual rate of 0.6% for major coronary events.[171]

Various parameters, such as extent of perfusion defects and degree of reversibility, and left ventricular function on myocardial perfusion scintigraphy, have been attributed for risk assessment (Tables 6A.12 and 6A.13).[175] Moderate to severe reversible perfusion defects (ischemia) suggest a relatively higher risk compared to fixed defects for any major coronary events in future, whereas mildly abnormal scans suggest an intermediate risk (approximately 2.7%), but a high likelihood of presence of CAD (Plate 6A.14 (a) and (b). Patients with mild perfusion abnormalities are likely candidates for medical therapy, provided their functional status and quality of life are not compromised. Conversely, severe and extensive reversible defects predict an adverse prognosis and provide incremental information, requiring early revascularization (Plate 6A.7).

Transient left ventricular dilatation in the post-stress test images represents ventricular impairment secondary to ischemic burden and is associated with high risk.[176] The relative risk increases 3.3 times for patients with moderate-to-severe transient LV dilatation and 1.6 times for mild dilatation.[91] An increased lung/heart ratio on a ^{201}Tl study is also a useful prognostic indicator of clinical

Table 6A.12 *Various parameters of risk stratification on myocardial perfusion SPECT imaging*

1. *Number of reversible defects (extent of ischemia)*
2. *Degree of perfusion abnormality (severity of ischemia)*
3. *Involvement of multiple vascular territories*
4. *Left ventricular dilation*
5. *Increased lung thallium uptake*
6. *Left ventricular ejection fraction*

Table 6A.13 *The number of segments in relation to risk*

Number of segments involved	Risk	Expectation of an event per year
0	Very low	< 1%
1–2	Low	1–5%
3–4	Moderate	5–15%
5–6	High	15–25%
> 7	Extremely high	> 25%

A higher number of reversible defects indicates a higher risk.

outcome, as it accurately mimics the degree of left ventricular dysfunction.[116]

LV systolic function has a powerful impact on the future outcome of patients with and without CAD. Every 1% drop of ejection fraction (post-stress) leads to a 3% increase in the risk.[91] In the past, gated equilibrium blood pool radionuclide angiocardiography with planar and SPECT approaches and first-pass studies have been used to assess LV functional parameters (Plates 6A.15 and 6A.16). These have been replaced with gated myocardial perfusion SPECT, permitting combined assessment of perfusion and function to predict adverse cardiac events more accurately.[177] On post-stress test images, abnormal left ventricular ejection fraction has been associated with a rate of 7.4% for major cardiac events, compared with 1.8% for normal ejection fraction.[178] Similarly, the presence of segmental wall motion abnormalities are also a predictor of a high annual event rate of 6.1%, compared to 1.6% for a normal wall motion.[178] Myocardial infarction is predicted by perfusion defects only, whereas cardiac death is associated with the number of vascular territories involved, detected by abnormal LVEF and perfusion abnormalities. This means that patients with normal or near-normal LV function have a better prognosis, even in the presence of coronary artery disease, whereas patients with poor ventricular function and ischemia are at higher risk of death.

Gated SPECT also permits measurement of LV end diastolic volumes, imparting decisive clinical information regarding LV remodeling and therapeutic decision-making in patients with LV dysfunction and viable myocardium. An end diastolic volume (EDV) of greater than 70 mL is also a prognostic indicator and is normally associated with worsening of survival over years.[179]

Older patients with CAD also have a poor prognosis. The poor prognosis in the elderly population could also be related to the aging vessels and reduced collateral formation. One study has confirmed reduced collaterals from 47.5% below the age of 50 years, to 43.4% between 60 and 69 years and 34.5% above 70 years of age.[180] Like other population groups, transient LV dilatation and the presence of myocardial ischemia are also applicable predictors of cardiac death and MI in elderly patients.[181]

The gender difference has a major impact in not only the clinical presentation and diagnosis, but also prognosis. Women with CAD usually have more unstable disease.[163,182] Approximately 63% of women die suddenly from CAD without any prior symptoms. The 1-year mortality rate for women is estimated at 42%, compared to 24% for men. In 26 years of follow-up of the Framingham Heart Study, chest pain was the most frequent presenting symptom in women (47% vs. 26% in men).[163] The incidence of myocardial infarction was higher in men, while the women had higher in-hospital (36% vs. 31% for men) and 1-year mortality rates (45% vs. 10% for men). The diabetic females with abnormal perfusion studies also have a relatively higher risk for future coronary events than males (5.2 vs. 2.7).[91] Myocardial perfusion imaging provides crucial incremental prognostic information in females and helps in management decisions, prioritizing high-risk females for invasive strategies.[183,184] Clinically, high-risk females with abnormal scans have a higher incidence of unstable angina and congestive heart failure, whereas high-risk males are more likely to be victims of cardiac deaths and myocardial infarctions. The treatment strategies for prevention of myocardial infarction and cardiac death differ. Therefore, prognostic stratification with gated SPECT would be able to differentiate between these two end-points, with selection of appropriate management.

Clinical parameters, including extent and severity of disease, left ventricular function, gender, hypertension, left ventricular hypertrophy, diabetes mellitus, hyperlipidemia, smoking, stress, race and plaque stability are important determinants of future cardiac events in patients with CAD. All of these impact individually on the 'event-free interval' in subjects with normal myocardial perfusion scans[185] and therefore, must always be kept in mind when managing patients with normal scans. A quantitative method of prognostic score has been devised and validated in 5873 patients for risk assessment using myocardial perfusion scintigraphy and some of the risk factors (Table 6A.14).[186] A score of <49 distinguishes low risk, while 49–57 is related to intermediate risk and >57 confers a higher risk group for future coronary events (0.9%, 3.3% and 9.5% cardiac deaths per year, respectively). However, further evaluation of such a quantitative score would be necessary before adopting it into clinical routine.

POST-MYOCARDIAL INFARCTION RISK STRATIFICATION

Acute MI results in a number of clinical complications and poor outcome. In acute chest pain, a combination of the

Table 6A.14 *Quantitative prognostic score*

Score	Parameter
1.	*Evidence of atherosclerosis on non-invasive imaging, i.e. an age- and sex-adjusted calcium score of the coronary arteries above the 75th percentile or an increased intima-media thickness ratio of the carotid on ultrasound.*
2.	*Lipoprotein (a) $\geqslant 30\,mg\,dL^{-1}$*
3.	*C-reactive peptide $>3\,mg\,L^{-1}$ (in absence of any obvious inflammation)*
4.	*Homocysteine $\geqslant 12\,\mu mol\,L^{-1}$*
5.	*$\geqslant 4$ risk factors (particularly in positive family history of CAD)*

The above formula has been validated to evaluate prognosis quantitatively in 5873 patients. A score of more than 57 identifies high-risk patients.[186]

Table 6A.15 *Advantages of pre-discharge myocardial perfusion SPECT imaging in post-MI patients*

- *Detection, and localization of ischemia*
- *Assessment of viable myocardial tissue*
- *Assessment of LV function by gated SPECT*
- *Early risk stratification*

troponin T assay and myocardial perfusion SPECT imaging would be ideal for risk stratification (Table 6A.15). Normally patients with MI undergo a pre-discharge sub-maximal stress test, which is a suboptimal approach for risk assessment. However, a myocardial perfusion SPECT study with a pharmacologically induced stress test can easily be performed within a few days following an acute insult, with superior risk stratification and direction for appropriate management selection.[187–189] A 40% incidence of future coronary events in patients with severe ischemia, 18% in cases of mild ischemia and 11% without ischemia has been documented on the pre-discharge dobutamine stress gated myocardial perfusion SPECT study.[190] Adenosine stress myocardial perfusion SPECT imaging has also demonstrated its advantages and safety for risk stratification in the INSPIRE (AdenosINe ^{99m}Tc-Sestamibi SPECT Post-InfaRction Evaluation) trial.[191] The low-risk group (perfusion defect size <20%) was treated medically. The high-risk group (perfusion defect size >20% with an ischemic defect size >10%), was further subdivided into two subgroups on the basis of LVEF >35% or LVEF <35%. Two hundred and five patients with LVEF of >35% were randomized and subjected either to intensive medical therapy only or intensive medical therapy with coronary revascularization, with follow-up myocardial perfusion SPECT imaging. The increased extent of perfusion defects was associated with higher cardiac event rate of approximately 7% per year. In

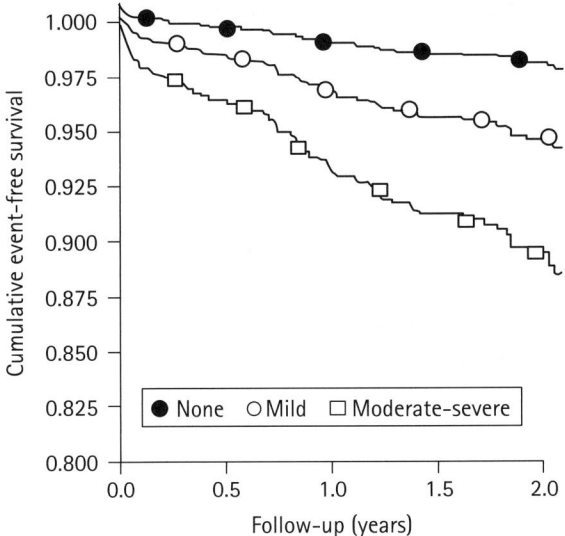

Figure 6A.9 *Effect of post-stress transient LV dilatation on the cumulative survival of patients. The degree of LV dilatation is directly related to the survival. Patients without LV dilatation had better survival than those with LV dilatation. (From: Thomas GS et al. J Am Coll Cardiol 2004; 43: 213–23.)*

the high-risk group, both management strategies resulted in similar reduction in ischemic burden and major coronary events.

A normal myocardial perfusion scan post-MI is associated with an annual cardiac death rate of 0.5% during the first 3 years and 1.3% in the subsequent 3 years.[192] Myocardial perfusion imaging is also superior to echocardiography in risk stratification of acute uncomplicated MI.[193]

In the early post-thrombolytic era, the prognostic value of radionuclide imaging was disputed because of biased studies, including low-risk patients only, as high-risk patients already had interventional or thrombolytic therapy.[194] The benefits of myocardial perfusion imaging in post-thrombolytic cases have been documented in many studies.[195]

Gated myocardial perfusion SPECT studies in post-MI patients are not only helpful in initial risk stratification, but also in follow-up, as they may alter treatment decisions and ultimately improve outcomes[91] (Figs 6A.9 and 6A.10).

Therapy management

Despite new advances in pharmacological therapies and improvement in revascularization procedures, the ultimate course is still a relentless progression of CAD. Therefore, selection and monitoring of the appropriate management strategy and the ability to identify further disease progression are crucial for good clinical outcome. The selection of any chosen therapy is primarily dictated by clinical symptoms, risk factors and severity of disease. Radionuclide

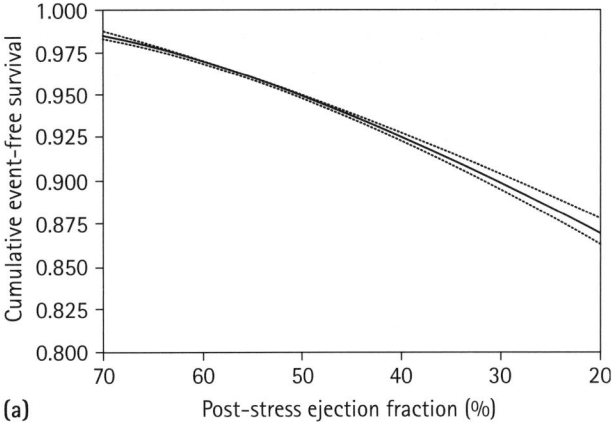

(a)

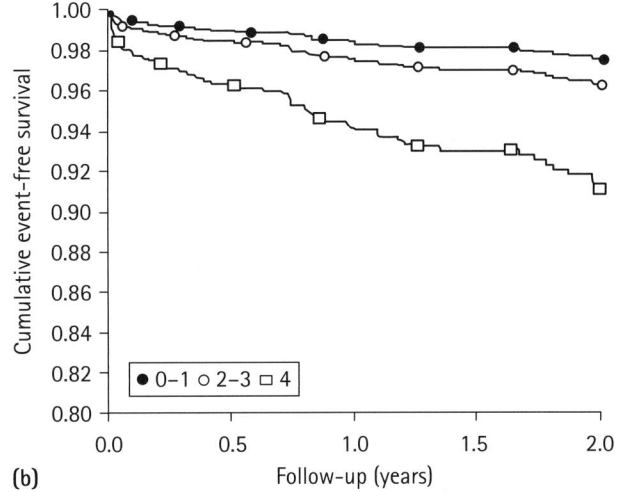

(b)

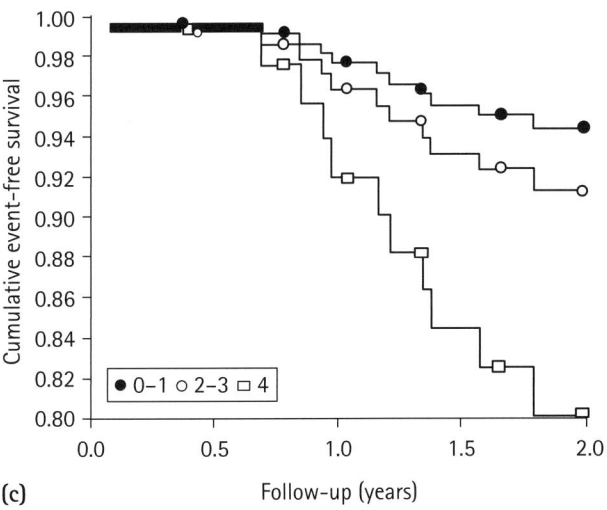

(c)

Figure 6A.10 *Effect of post-stress test ejection fraction on the survival rate. (a) Lower ejection fraction is related with poor survival, suggesting LV as predictor of death. (b) Cumulative survival stratified by reversibility score in patients with LVEF of ⩾40% and (c) LVEF <40% is associated with reduced event free interval. (From: Thomas GS et al. J Am Coll Cardiol 2004; 43: 213–23.)*

imaging, particularly myocardial perfusion, is helpful not only in appropriate management selection, but also in the follow-up of patients with CAD (Plates 6A.7 and 6A.8).

REVASCULARIZATION THERAPY

Percutaneous intervention (PCI) and CABG surgery are two well-established methodologies of coronary revascularization.

PERCUTANEOUS INTERVENTIONS

The presence of moderate to severe ischemia is a prerequisite for optimal patient selection for an interventional procedure. Cardiac catheterization documents the extent of coronary disease, but is unable to assess the hemodynamic significance of a coronary lesion. Incorporation of intravascular ultrasound (IVUS) for vessel wall imaging, assessment of the plaque morphology and post-stenotic flow leads to an approximately 20% alteration in the management strategy.[196] The newer generation of IVUS probes are built on the interventional balloons providing ability to image beyond proximal segments.[197] Despite certain benefits of IVUS-guided coronary stent implantation regarding target–lumen revascularization, the routine use of IVUS has not gained wide clinical acceptance.[197] There is also insufficient published data to support its benefit in prognostic categorization or reduction of major future coronary events. Myocardial perfusion SPECT imaging, on the other hand, is an established and validated technique to document the hemodynamic significance of stenosis, guiding appropriate selection for interventional procedures with important prognostic information.[198]

Post-intervention re-stenosis is still a major clinical challenge, requiring close follow-up of these patients. The use of stents, aspirin, clopidogrel and glycoprotein IIb/IIIa inhibitors all have contributed to lower the rate of restenosis to less than 10% in optimal conditions.[199] The newer generation of coated stents with antiproliferative drugs like sirolimus and paclitaxel appeared to further reduce the restenosis rate.[200,201] However, the incidences of restenosis and complications still occur.[202] Radionuclide imaging is useful in post-intervention follow-up of patients[203–205] (Plates 6A.17a,b). In cases of post-PCI incomplete revascularization, follow-up myocardial perfusion imaging determines the extent of remodeling or restenosis. Sensitivities ranging from 76 to 94% and specificities of 46 to 84% have been documented to predict restenosis.[203–206] Myocardial perfusion abnormalities are also detected in many patients following primary or rescue PCI in AMI, despite brisk restoration of coronary flow.[207] It is common to observe a partially reversible or persistent perfusion defect soon after a successful interventional procedure, even in patients without recent MI.[208] This is probably due to post-intervention stunning, distal embolization and vascular trauma. Such defects resolve subsequently over time (Plates 6A.18 (a) to (c)). For the best accuracy and higher predictive value, myocardial perfusion imaging should be delayed 2–4 weeks after an interventional procedure (Plates 6A.19a,b).

CORONARY ARTERY BYPASS GRAFT SURGERY

Complete revascularization with coronary artery bypass graft surgery is expected to lower the incidence of coronary events and improve functional capacity by alleviating symptoms. During recent years, more surgical procedures are being performed without cardiopulmonary bypass (off-pump CABG). Although off-pump surgery appears to be safer, it may lower the graft-patency rate compared to on-pump.[209] The minimally invasive coronary artery bypass (MIDCAB) approach is also being used in suitable cases. There is a 10–15% re-occlusion rate of the grafts after 5 years. The long-term patency rate of internal mammary artery grafts is superior to that of venous grafts.[210] Diabetes mellitus, hyperlipidemia, hypertension and smoking accelerate disease progression not only in the bypass grafts but also in the native arteries. The recurrence of symptoms post-CABG is indicative of either graft closure or disease progression in the native vessels.[211] However, myocardial ischemia and occlusion may still occur in asymptomatic patients. Post-CABG, malperfusion syndrome or silent residual ischemia can be present in patients without obstructive coronary disease.[212] The presence of myocardial ischemia in the absence of any significant obstructive disease, due to mismatch between LAD and LIMA diameters at the anastomotic site, has a similar clinical impact on the prognosis for major coronary events in future, as with obstructive disease.[213] Myocardial perfusion imaging is useful in such a group of patients. A high-risk scan is indicative of incomplete revascularization, and requires aggressive management strategies including repeat intervention by PCI or surgical means, if necessary.

Due to the increased number of percutaneous interventions over recent years, most patients undergoing surgical revascularization have LV dysfunction, extensive disease, multiple risk factors or prior failed interventions. Radionuclide imaging is very helpful, not only in appropriate selection of patients with viable myocardium for surgical revascularization, but also to demonstrate procedural success.

The development of high resolution CT and MR has made it possible to study grafts with very high sensitivity.[214] However, anatomically obstructive vessels are not always the best predictors of prognosis of future cardiac events. Myocardial perfusion imaging has the strength to predict progression or graft occlusion, but more importantly in risk stratification with implications on the long-term outcome of such patients.[215,216]

Many patients with diffuse coronary artery disease cannot be amenable to revascularization procedures and their management remains a difficult task. A variety of alternative treatments like laser revascularization with transmyocardial or percutaneous approach and enhanced external counter pulsation (EECP) have been attempted to relieve symptoms in such patients.[217,218] Introduction of robotics and endoscopes may make surgical revascularization less invasive and more precise in future.[219] However, the effectiveness of such therapies cannot be assessed by anatomical imaging modalities like CT, and currently myocardial perfusion imaging appears to be most useful in evaluating success of such treatment options.[218,220]

MEDICAL MANAGEMENT AND RISK MODIFICATION

Pharmacological therapy is part of the long-term management of coronary artery disease. Nitrates, calcium antagonists, beta-blockers and ACE inhibitors used alone or in combination effectively improve symptoms and reduce the extent of myocardial ischemia. ACE inhibitors increase the bioavailability of bradykinin and nitric oxide (NO), leading to improvement in myocardial perfusion. Clopidogrel blocks adenosine diphosphate-activated platelets. In combination with aspirin, it lowers the future risk of coronary events by 20%.[221] The HMG-CoA reductase inhibitors or 'statins' significantly lower future cardiac events by improving cholesterol profile and stabilize the plaque, with improvement of myocardial perfusion and coronary flow reserve.

Sequential radionuclide imaging allows measurement of efficacy of most of the anti-ischemic drugs and the effect of risk factor modifications in terms of reduction in extent and severity of perfusion deficits or improved coronary flow reserve by SPET and PET imaging.[222–224]

Medical treatment appears to be as efficient as interventional procedures.[224,225] However, further direct head-to-head comparisons are indispensable between these two strategies. The COURAGE (Clinical Outcomes Utilizing Percutaneous Coronary Revascularization and Aggressive Drug Evaluation) trial is an ongoing study comparing efficacies of pharmacological and interventional approaches using myocardial perfusion SPECT.[226] The trial is due for completion in 2006 and may bring new insights into current management strategies.

Assessment of myocardial viability

Recurrent episodes of coronary ischemia and reperfusion may result in necrosis, stunning, hibernation or preconditioning (Table 6A.16). While preconditioning is a cardioprotective phenomenon, necrosis, stunning and hibernation are pathological events, contributing to left ventricular dysfunction.

Myocardial stunning is characterized by reversible left ventricular dysfunction, with relatively preserved resting myocardial blood flow secondary to an acute brief ischemic episode including post-thrombolysis, during PCIs, cardiac surgery and coronary artery spasm. Persistent (chronic) underperfusion of the myocardium leads to sustained abnormal contractile function, and recovers only after restoration of oxygen supply with interventions such as revascularization. During the early phase, despite reduction

Table 6A.16 *Types of viable myocardium*

Type of myocardium	Features
Normal	Adequate oxygen supply under stress (normal perfusion)
Ischemic	Reduced flow at stress (reversible perfusion defects)
Myocardial infarct	Damaged (necrotic) myocardium
Hibernating	Viable myocardium due to reduced perfusion causing impairment of function
	There is decoupling of metabolism–function, with improvement in function, after revascularization
Stunned	Normally perfused myocardium with regional wall motion abnormalities. It recovers on its own, without any intervention

The hibernating myocardium is chronic mechanically impaired tissue secondary to hypo-perfusion or repetitive stunning, whereas stunning represents transient depression of function, due to an acute transient episode of reduced coronary flow. In stunning, there are disproportionate abnormalities of wall motion and perfusion. The perfusion could be normal or mildly reduced compared with larger area of wall motion abnormalities.

in the myocardial flow reserve, resting perfusion remains normal. However, in due course, the hemodynamic progression of the underlying disease leads to a state of dysfunction with reduced resting flow, consistent with the initial definition of 'hibernation'.[227,228] The diminished coronary flow downgrades function, thereby decreasing oxygen demand and preventing cell death. This 'flow–function' match was expressed 'smart heart', signifying hibernating myocardium as an 'exquisitely regulated tissue, successfully adapting its functionality to the prevailing circumstances'. However, later studies have demonstrated that regional blood flow is not reduced in hibernating myocardium.[229,230] Under coronary vasodilatation using adenosine the coronary flow reserve appears to be severely blunted.[230] This strengthens the concept that hibernating myocardium is most likely due to repetitive episodes of stunning. The presence of blunted coronary flow reserve post-vasodilatation and histological changes in the hibernating myocytes suggests that hibernation is an 'ischemic suffering with capability of restoring normal function', and does not stand for the successful adaptation of 'smart heart' as contemplated earlier.

CLINICAL IMPLICATIONS

Clinically, in a patient with known CAD, symptoms of dyspnea rather than angina would be more pertinent to detection of viable myocardium. Myocardial hibernation represents an unstable state from which patients can have either further deterioration of cardiovascular condition,

Table 6A.17 *Different available techniques for the detection of viable myocardium*

Myocardial metabolism on PET
- ^{18}F-FDG

Cell membrane integrity
- Rb
- ^{201}Tl

Cellular metabolism
- ^{99m}Tc-sestamibi
- ^{99m}Tc-tetrofosmin

  (Nitrates/trimetazadine enhanced)

Contractility
- LDD echocardiography
- LDD MRI

Microvascular damage
- Delayed enhancement on MRI

LDD: low dose dobutamine.

Table 6A.18 *Criteria for viable myocardium on ^{201}Tl images*

- *Normal uptake*
- *Evidence of ischemia on stress–redistribution images*
- *> 10% increase in activity in fixed defects on re-injection or delayed resting images*
- *Uptake of >50% on redistribution–re-injection images*

causing worsening of clinical condition and death or recuperate to a better status and improved clinical outcome, with coronary revascularization.[231] Coronary revascularization is expected to prevent further episodes of stunning, re-infarction, fibrosis and electrophysiological instability. Approximately 55–60% of the hibernating myocardium is expected to demonstrate functional improvement. The ventricular functional recovery is expected to occur, only if ≥25% of the LV is viable.[232–234] Revascularization of non-viable tissue does not offer any prognostic advantage, whereas revascularization of viable myocardium may lead to 80% reduction in the annual mortality rate, compared with medical treatment alone.[235]

DIFFERENT TECHNIQUES FOR DETECTING HIBERNATING MYOCARDIUM

Post-revascularization improvement of ventricular function is still a singular 'gold standard' determinant of viable myocardium. Most of the imaging techniques exploit various characteristics of myocytes based upon either a 'perfusion–contraction match' or 'perfusion–metabolism mismatch' for identification of hibernating myocardium[232–234] (Table 6A.17).

POSITRON EMISSION TOMOGRAPHY

Fatty acids are the major source of energy in a normal heart. However, in hibernating myocardium, normal free fatty acid metabolism switches to glucose as the main energy source reflected as increased ^{18}F-FDG avidity in hypoperfused segments. Additionally, the rich glycogen content and increased number of glucose membrane transporters (GLUT1, GLUT4) in hibernating myocardium also contribute towards enhanced FDG uptake. Increased ^{18}F-FDG uptake is therefore considered a marker of viability. A perfusion–metabolism mismatch on ^{18}F-FDG PET is highly predictive of hibernating myocardial viability, with a high likelihood of partial/complete functional recovery, post-revascularization. ^{18}F-FDG PET is therefore considered the 'gold standard' for the detection of viable myocardium, with a sensitivity of 93% and specificity of 58%.[48,54,232,233,235] The lower specificity of ^{18}F-FDG can probably be improved further, with dobutamine-gated PET, with information regarding contractile reserve.[236]

Simultaneous flow assessment with [^{13}N]ammonia, or [^{15}O]water, with ^{18}F-FDG PET is useful to differentiate between stunned and hibernating myocardium. Stunning can be identified if dysfunctional segments have normal myocardial blood flow (MBF) (≥0.6 mL min^{-1}g^{-1}); while dysfunctional segments with reduced MBF (<0.6 mL min^{-1}g^{-1}) and metabolic rate of glucose (MRG) of ≥0.25 μmol g^{-1} min^{-1} represent hibernating myocardium.[237]

SINGLE PHOTON EMISSION TOMOGRAPHY

Cell membrane integrity: ^{201}Tl Rubidium-82 and ^{201}Tl are potassium analogs, and their retention therefore reflects cellular membrane integrity (viable myocardium). Thallium-201 has an advantage of being cheaper and more easily available. The most accurate suggested ^{201}Tl protocols are either stress–redistribution–re-injection or rest–redistribution.[233,235,238–240] The stress–redistribution–re-injection protocol provides information about both ischemia and viability, while the rest–redistribution protocol assesses viability only. Re-injection of ^{201}Tl leads to a higher blood concentration of ^{201}Tl required for redistribution to severe perfusion defects. The criteria for the diagnosis of hibernating myocardium on ^{201}Tl imaging are listed in Table 6A.18. The ^{201}Tl stress–redistribution–re-injection protocol has a concordance in 88% of the segments, with FDG PET for the presence or absence of viable myocardium. The sensitivity and specificity of thallium imaging is approximately 90% and 54% for detecting and accurately predicting improvement of the regional LV dysfunction.[233,235,238,239]

Cellular metabolism: ^{99m}Tc tracers Technetium-99 m-labeled compounds such as sestamibi and tetrofosmin are retained by the myocardium as a result of cell membrane integrity and mitochondrial function and metabolism, reflecting myocyte viability.[233] Dual-isotope SPECT/PET studies are also feasible for the detection of hibernating myocardium.[241] Nitrates (oral, sublingual or intravenous) enhance tracer uptake in severely hypoperfused regions, improving the accuracy of ^{99m}Tc tracers and ^{201}Tl for identification of viable myocardium.[242–245]

Administration of another anti-ischemic drug, trimetazidine, also improves sestamibi uptake in the myocardium, with results similar to that of nitrate administration[246,247] (Plate 6A.20). Most likely, trimetazidine stimulates carbohydrate oxidation during ischemia, with further increase in glucose metabolism, and thus enhances sestamibi uptake. Dobutamine-gated SPECT can also be used to evaluate contractile reserve, for the detection of myocardial viability.[245]

ECHOCARDIOGRAPHY

Myocardial infarction results in thinning of ventricular wall and wall motion abnormalities. Improvement in function or wall motion of such a segment would be consistent with presence of viable myocardium. Reduced regional end diastolic wall thickness, with hyper-echoic texture is diagnostic of scar tissue (nonviable myocardium) on echocardiography. Low-dose dobutamine infusion ($5–10\,\mu g\,kg^{-1}\,min^{-1}$) enhances systolic contraction in dyskinetic segments and reflects viable myocardium on echocardiographic examination.[234,248] A high dose infusion of dobutamine ($30–40\,\mu g\,kg^{-1}\,min^{-1}$) induces ischemia, resulting in reversal of the initial improvement in wall thickening. This 'biphasic' response (i.e. improvement at low dose and deterioration at high doses) is predictive of the improvement in the contractile function, post-revascularization. A dobutamine challenge requires a minimum of 5 g or 6% of total myocardium, for genesis of wall motion abnormality. Similarly, myocardial damage of <25% of the ventricular wall thickness or <3% of left ventricular mass is unlikely to produce any segmental motion abnormality. This means that dobutamine echocardiography may fail to spot apparently viable myocardium in such cases.

Contrast echocardiogram, with micro-bubbles, also appears to be a promising technique. Harmonics imaging (HI) combined with two-dimensional echocardiography enhances the sensitivity of echocardiographic techniques for detection of viable myocardium. A velocity of less than $5\,cm\,s^{-1}$ at the epicardial and of $11\,cm\,s^{-1}$ at the endocardial layers on tissue Doppler imaging (TDI), identifies hibernating myocardium. Strain rate imaging (SRI) demonstrates decreased systolic lengthening with increased post-systolic shortening in viable myocardial segments.[249] SRI appears to be superior to dobutamine stress echocardiography and TDI, for such use.

CARDIAC MAGNETIC RESONANCE IMAGING

Magnetic resonance imaging (MRI) provides high-quality images with a spatial resolution of 1–2 mm and temporal resolution of 25–50 ms. In the past, detection of wall motion abnormalities by low-dose dobutamine was the only way for assessing myocardial viability on MRI, with a relatively lower sensitivity of 50%, compared with radionuclide imaging, but higher specificity of 81%.[250,251]

During recent years the development of high-performance gradient hardware, and ultra-fast pulse sequences have stimulated interest in cardiac MRI, with new imaging protocols being established. Of these, delayed contrast-enhanced MRI appears to be sensitive for detection of nonviable myocardial tissue and feasible in a clinical routine. After intravenous bolus administration of Gd-DTPA, normal myocardium demonstrates initial increased signal intensity, followed by rapid washout. During the early images (first-pass), the damaged myocardium does not enhance, ('hypo-enhanced' or 'no refold' segments), signifying complete obstruction of blood flow (myocardial infarction). These areas demonstrate 'delayed hyper-enhancement' (up to 10 min after contrast administration). In fact, this is not really 'hyper-enhancement', rather retention of the Gd molecule, due to leakage into the interstitial space, associated with cell necrosis and capillary plugging, resulting in impaired washout.[252] The delayed enhancement reflects non-viable myocardium (scar), due to any cause like necrosis not necessarily only due to CAD. Due to its inherent high resolution, MRI has the capability of detecting tiny infarcts secondary to microvascular disease as a potential cause of unexplained LV dysfunction. The delayed contrast enhancement on MRI appears to be superior to low-dose dobutamine echocardiography and ^{201}Tl SPECT, with similar accuracy to ^{18}F-FDG PET.[253,254] However, cardiac MRI appears to be superior to radionuclide imaging for the identification of segments that are unlikely to recover function with better spatial resolution, permitting simultaneous assessment of morphology and function and is less expensive than ^{18}F-FDG PET.

With the newer generation of multi-detector CT equipment, contrast-enhanced computed tomography has also been used to assess perfusion and viable myocardium.[255] However, data are still preliminary.

ELECTRICAL CHANGES

The diminished perfusion and function of hibernating myocardium results in reduced electrical potentials. On ECG, low ST dispersion (<70 ms) post-MI is indicative of viable myocardium, and has a sensitivity of 83% and specificity of 71% for predicting functional recovery, post-revascularization.[256] Direct epicardial electrophysiological mapping has also been reported to predict functional recovery. A cut-off value of 8.75 mV has been recommended to differentiate between hibernating and scarred myocardial tissue, with a sensitivity of 94% and specificity of 83%.[257] This is a safe noninvasive technique. However, no large prospective studies are yet available.

CHOICE OF TECHNIQUE

In the current era of cost containment in healthcare, it is crucial to identify and detect hibernating myocardial segments prior to revascularization. The presence of at least 20% of viable myocardium is essential for improvement in left ventricular function, post-coronary revascularization. Myocardial perfusion SPECT imaging using ^{201}Tl or ^{99m}Tc tracers is a more sensitive, widely available technique and should be the first-line approach for detection of hibernating myocardium.[251,258] Dobutamine echocardiography is superior to dobutamine-gated SPECT and enhances specificity by complementing information gathered from the radionuclide studies. Metabolic imaging with ^{18}F-FDG PET is relatively expensive and is not widely available. In future, with more MRI installations, we may see increased use of MRI for detection of nonviable myocardium.

Heart failure

The improved clinical outcomes and better survival rates in CAD have resulted in a higher incidence of heart failure. Patients with heart failure normally require repeated hospital admissions with an ever-increasing burden on the existing healthcare systems. In addition, patients become debilitated. In the UK, in 2000 alone, heart failure costs approximated £625 million to the National Health Service.

The management goals in heart failure therapy are to improve quality of life, reduce unnecessary hospital admissions and improve prognosis. B-type natriuretic peptide (BNP) levels correlate with the severity and prognosis of heart failure,[259] and currently are being used for assessment and management of heart failure.

Most patients with heart failure have a significant amount of viable myocardium. Therefore, revascularization, by any means in such cases, will not only potentially decrease the cost, but also improve the ultimate clinical outcome.[260,261] The quantity of viable myocardium is an important factor not only for post-revascularization improvement but also for medical management and many of the alternative devices like synchronization. Several available techniques to detect hibernating myocardium have already been discussed in preceding sections. The perceptible survival benefit of revascularization or other therapies may not be associated with improvement in symptoms in patients with residual viability but advanced cardiac remodeling.

Various drugs, including beta-blockers and angiotensin-converting enzyme inhibitors, are being used to impede progression and improve symptoms with expectations to reduce mortality in patients with heart failure.[262,263] Serial gated equilibrium blood pool radionuclide angiocardiography or gated SPECT studies can effectively monitor the success of different therapeutic options. Gated myocardial perfusion SPECT is an excellent and cheaper way for not only obtaining reproducible measurements of ventricular volumes and ejection fractions but also for assessing perfusion, with the advantage of more accurate prediction of prognosis in patients with heart failure. The Surgical Treatment of Ischemic Congestive Heart Failure (STICH) trial is an ongoing multicenter randomized trial comparing treatment options of medical therapy alone to medical plus surgical therapy. The trial is due for completion by 2008 and additionally is expected to further strengthen the role of gated myocardial perfusion SPECT in the management decisions in patients with heart failure.

In the future, a variety of newer therapeutic options, including assist devices, artificial hearts and transplantation of progenitor cells, may be available routinely for patients with advanced heart failure.[264–268] Additionally, there are also several other surgical therapies under clinical investigation in the effort to reverse or restore the remodeled left ventricle. Radionuclide imaging has the ability to play an important role in the appraisal of such new techniques.[269]

The progression of heart failure is related to sympathetic nervous system dysfunction. Increased sympathetic activity leads to increased norepinephrine levels, with a higher incidence of arrhythmias and sudden cardiac death. The heart-to-mediastinal count ratio obtained using ^{123}I-MIBG has been utilized as an indicator of prognosis in heart failure,[53,270,271] but the normal range of heart-to-mediastinum ratio varies between different gamma camera systems. Autonomic failure on ^{123}I-MIBG cardiac imaging may also be indicative of early Parkinson's disease (Fig. 6A.11).

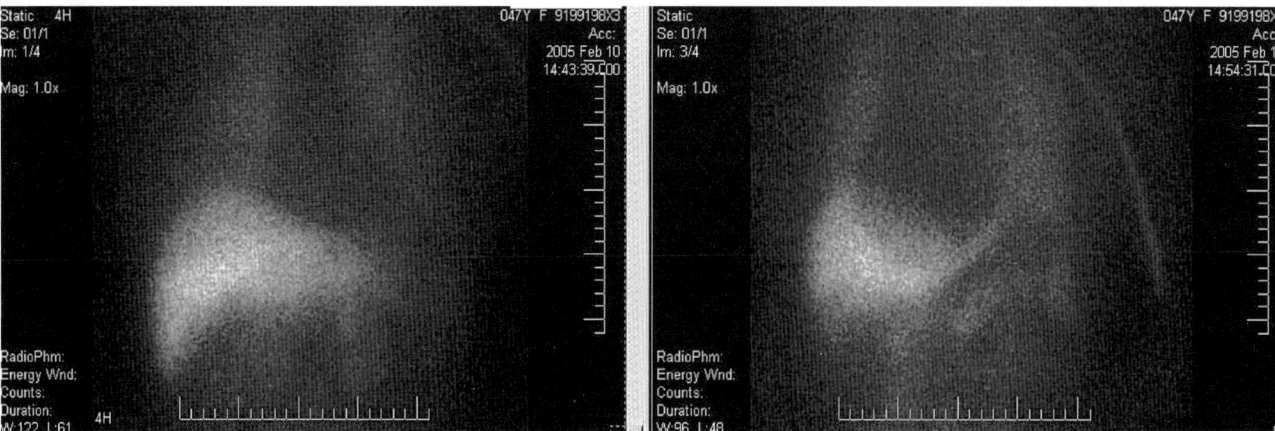

Figure 6A.11 ^{123}I-MIBG imaging for cardiac innervation. The 4-h p.i. planar images in anterior and LAO projection demonstrate no significant uptake of MIBG in the myocardium, suggesting pure autonomic failure in case of early Parkinson's disease. (Image courtesy of Dr Constantin Dragoiescu, Leiden University Medical Centre, the Netherlands.)

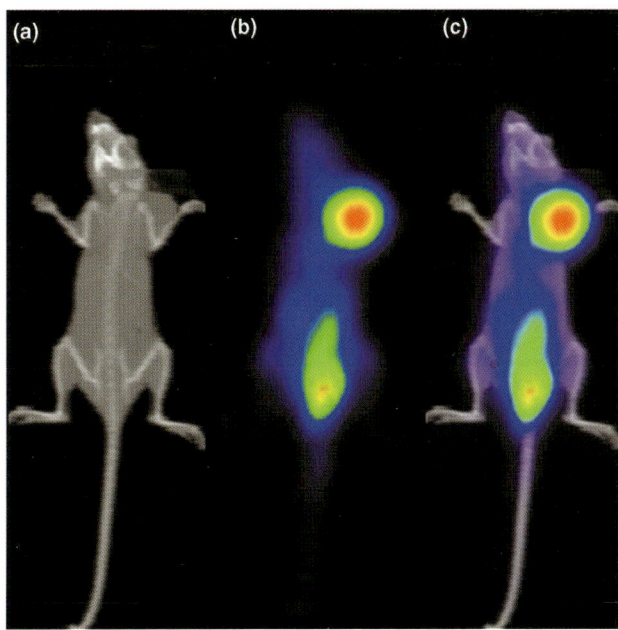

Plate 1A.1 *Animal PET/CT study of tumor proliferation in vivo. (a) Surface-rendered CT scan of BALB/c nude mouse; (b) coronal ^{18}F-FLT PET image, showing high uptake in the renal cell cancer xenograft; (c) PET/CT fused images of tumor proliferation. See page 12.*

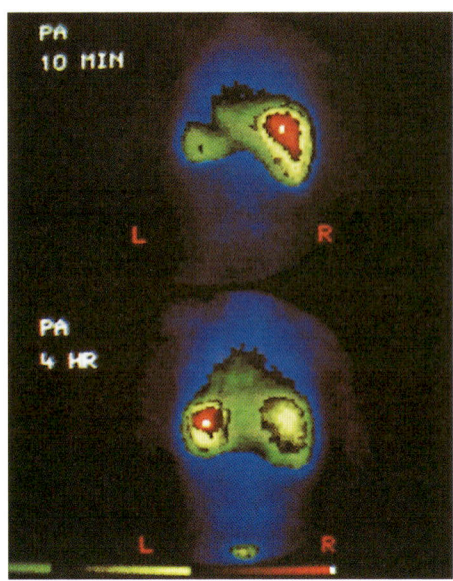

Plate 1C.1 *Radioimmunoscintigraphy of neuroblastoma using radioiodinated UJ13A in a 4-year-old child. Posterior abdominal images at 10 min and 4 h with* ^{123}*I-UJ13A. At 4 h the tumor is evident as a focal area of high uptake (red) in contrast to the spleen and liver (green). See page 46.*

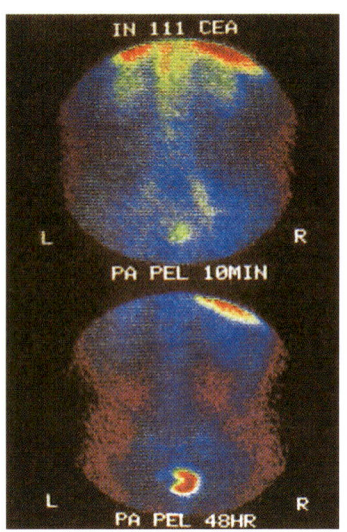

Plate 1C.2 *Radioimmunoscintigraphy with* ^{111}*In-labelled anti-carcinoembryonic antigen monoclonal antibody in a rectal carcinoma. Posterior abdominal views: top, 10 min and bottom, 48 h. Slight vascularity is seen at 10 min in the pelvis while the 48 h image shows uptake in a reverse 'C' in the pelvis with a small focal area of uptake to its left in a lymph node. Renal but not urinary activity is seen at 10 min. High liver, spleen, and marrow uptake is seen on both views. See page 47.*

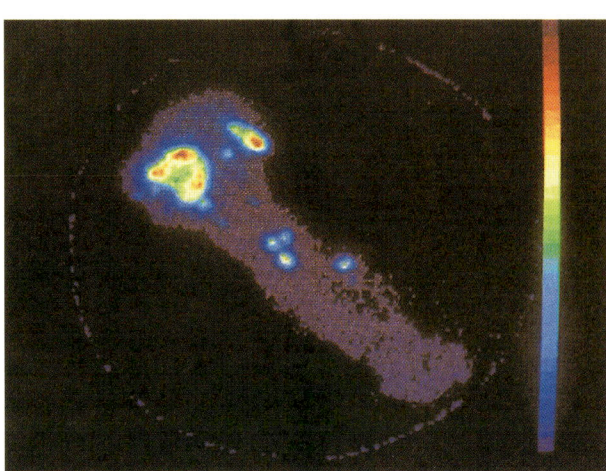

Plate 1C.3 *Radioimmunoscintigraphy with* ^{111}*In-labelled anti-carcinoembryonic antigen (CEA) monoclonal antibody in a rectal carcinoma tumor specimen. Image of the surgical specimen was taken at 72 h after injection showing the tumor uptake in red and yellow (the cut is made opposite to the mesentry to display the bowel lumen so the tumor has been divided) and uptake in lymph nodes. Note that none of the lymph nodes contained tumor cells on histology. These images are of unbound CEA antigen falsely implying tumor presence in the nodes (Duke's B, see text). See page 47.*

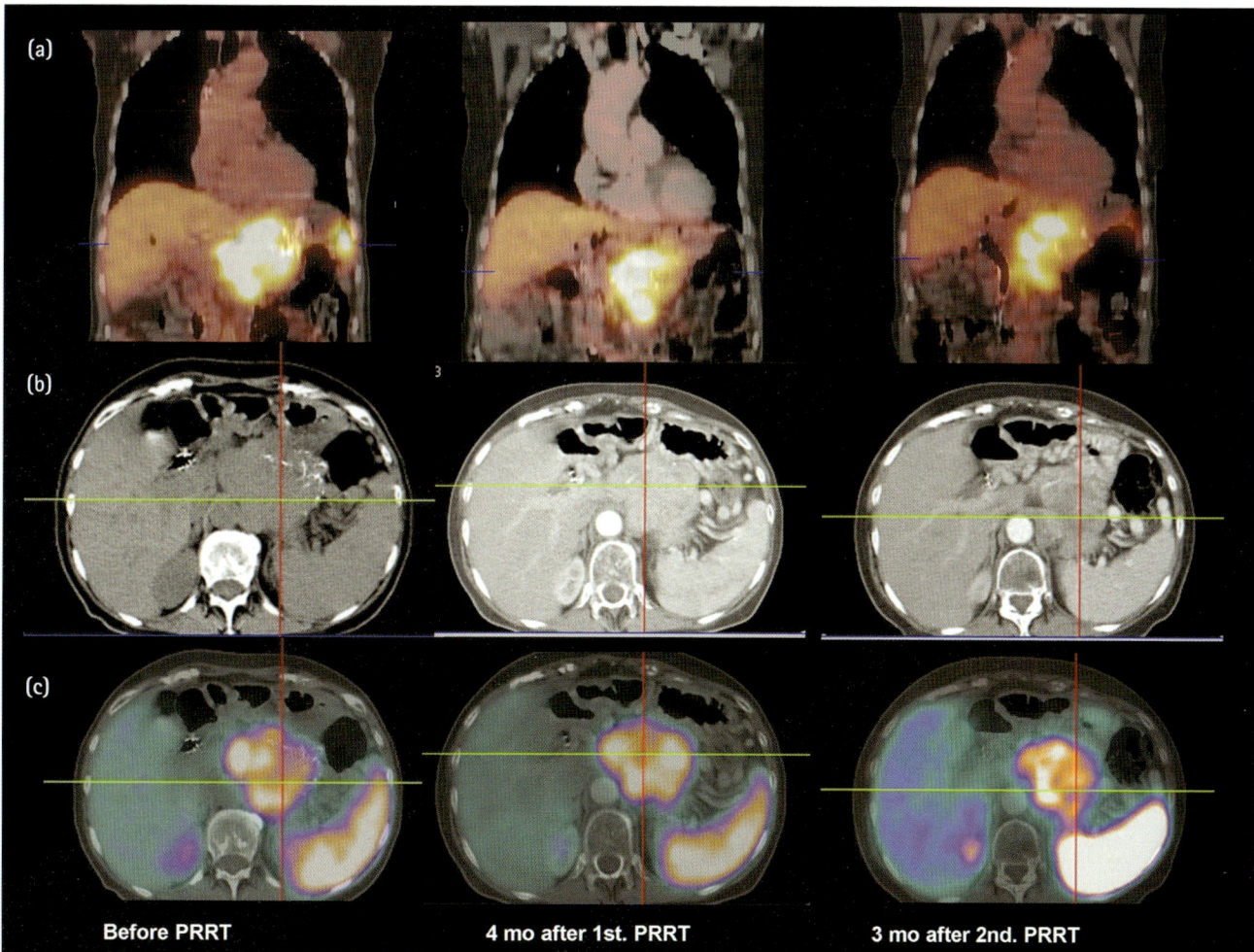

(a)

(b)

(c)

| Before PRRT | 4 mo after 1st. PRRT | 3 mo after 2nd. PRRT |

Plate 1D.1 *Large, inoperable neuroendocrine carcinoma of the pancreatic tail with infiltration of the stomach. Ga-68 DOTA-NOC receptor PET/CT (a: coronal PET slices, b: transversal CT slices, and fused images (c) before intra-arterial PRRT using Y-90 DOTA-TATE, 4 months after the first treatment, and 3 months after the second intra-arterial therapy) show high, but heterogeneous SMS-receptor expression. Before treatment, the 66 year-old patient needed multiple blood transfusions despite intense conventional treatment, including chemotherapy and octreotide. After the second PRRT the bleedings stopped completely. See page 61.*

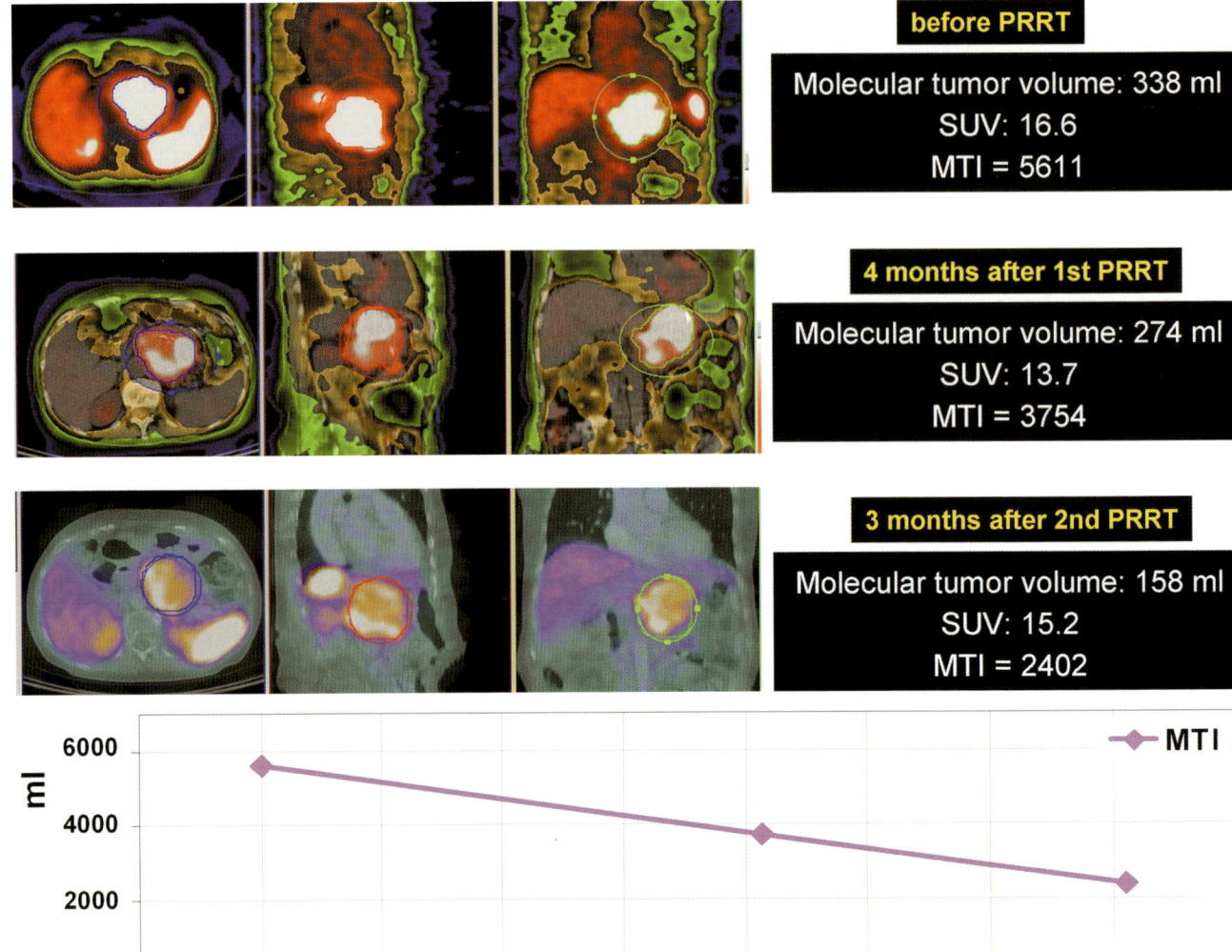

Plate 1D.2 *Measuring therapy response by calculating the molecular tumor index using ROI technique and Ga-68 DOTA-NOC receptor PET/CT (MTI = molecular tumor volume (MTV) multiplied by standardized uptake value (SUV). The significant decrease of MTI over time correlated with the improvement of the clinical symptoms of the patient. See page 61.*

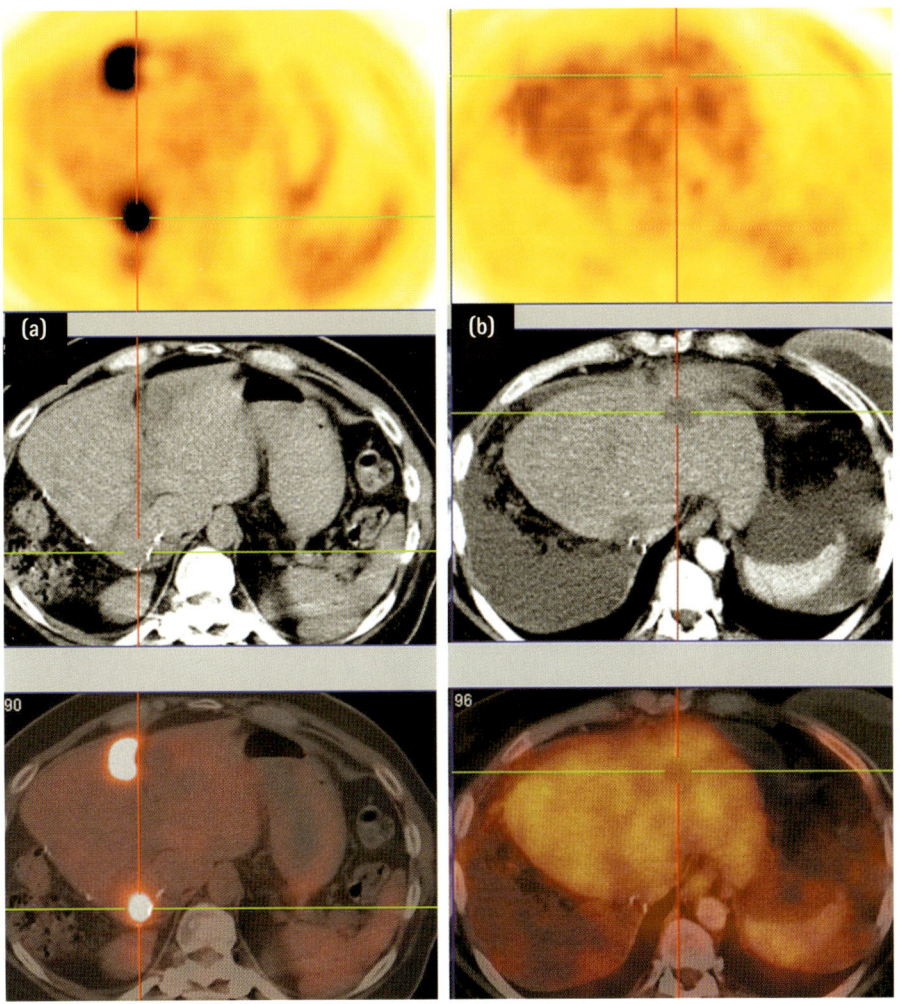

Plate 1D.3 *Monitoring therapy response by F-18 FDG PET/CT before (a) and after (b) selective internal radiation therapy (SIRT) of breast cancer metastases to the liver using Yttrium-90-SIR-Spheres. After intra-arterial radioembolization, FDG-PET demonstrates complete metabolic regression whereas CT scan shows still hypodense hepatic lesions ("metabolism precedes morphology"). See page 65.*

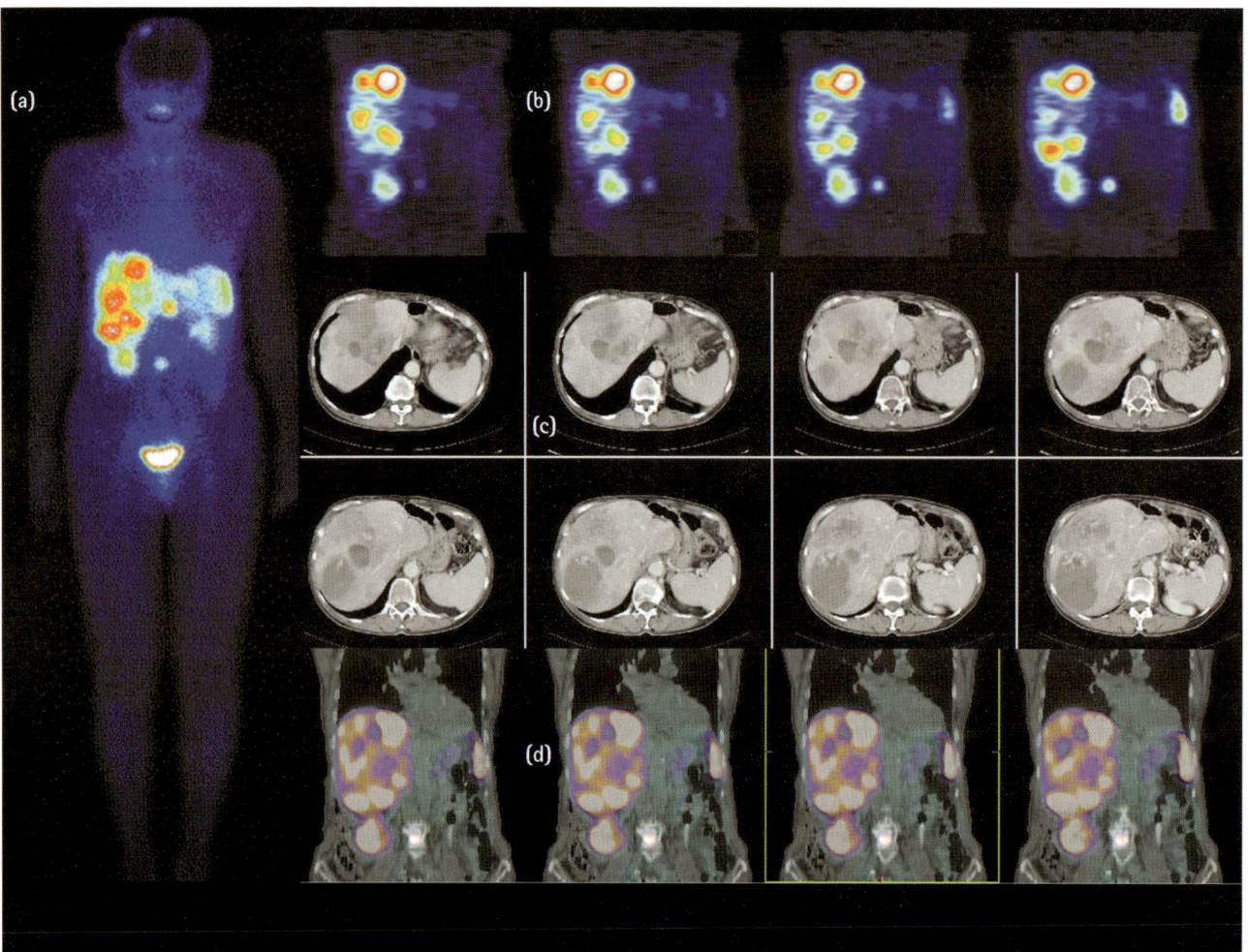

Plate 1D.4 *Measuring therapy response by imaging depends heavily on the modalities used for monitoring, e.g. whole-body vs. regional scans, planar vs. SPECT vs. PET, molecular properties of the tumor cells (i.e. expression of somatostatin receptors) vs. anatomic size (as displayed by CT scan): Tc-99m EDDA Hynic TOC whole-body scan (anterior view (a): 1 hr p.i.) and SPECT slices (coronal view (b) 2 hrs p.i.) demonstrating multiple liver metastases of a well-differentiated neuroendocrine lung cancer (bronchus carcinoid) operated 17(!) years before. In addition, bone metastases in the lumbar spine and in the skull can be seen. (c) and (d) show the transaxial CT and the coronal PET slices of the same patient using Ga-68 DOTA-NOC PET/CT with intense accumulation of the somatostatin analogue in the liver metastases. See page 69.*

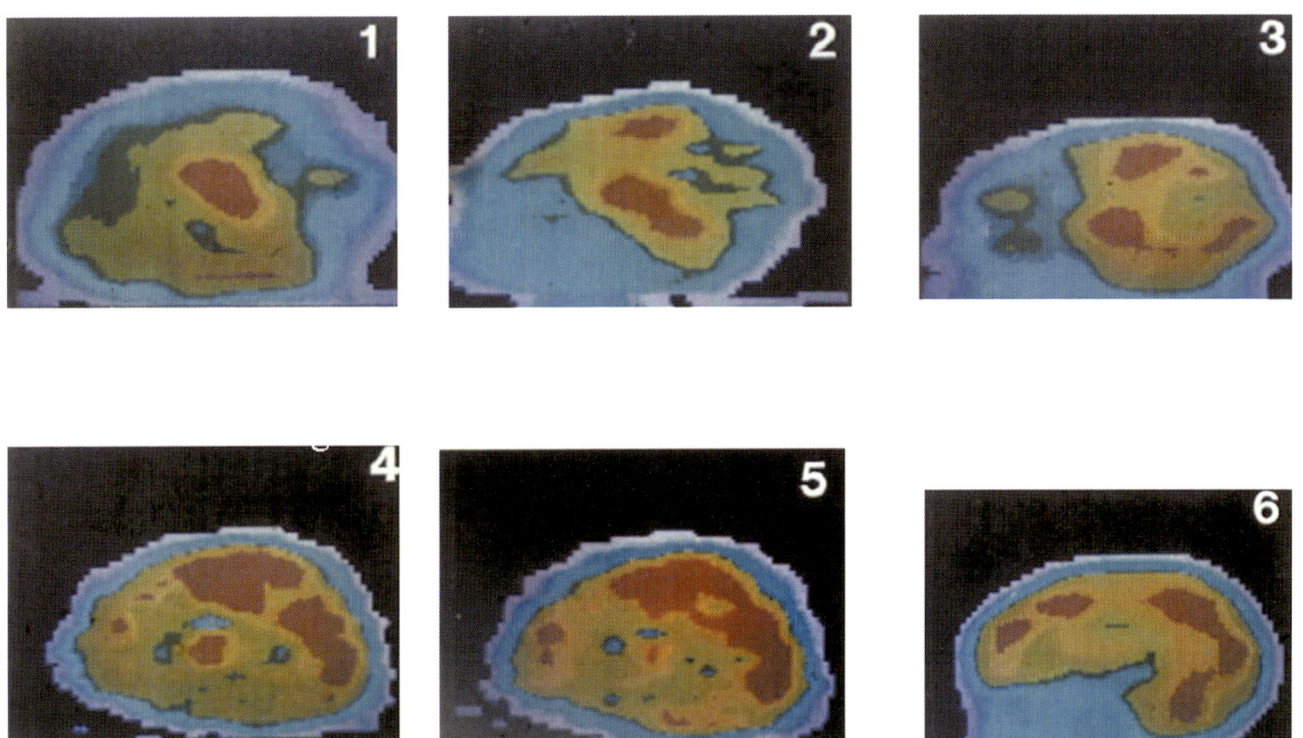

Plate 4.1 *Sequential sagittal midline images of rCBF scans in normal infants showing the distribution of tracer with age. Number 1 corresponds to a 36 week gestation neonate; number 2 to a neonate at term; and number 3 is a neonate at 4 weeks of age. Number 4 is at 3 months of age, while number 5 is at 6 months of age. In a 2 year-old child the distribution resembles that of the adult (number 6). See page 111.*

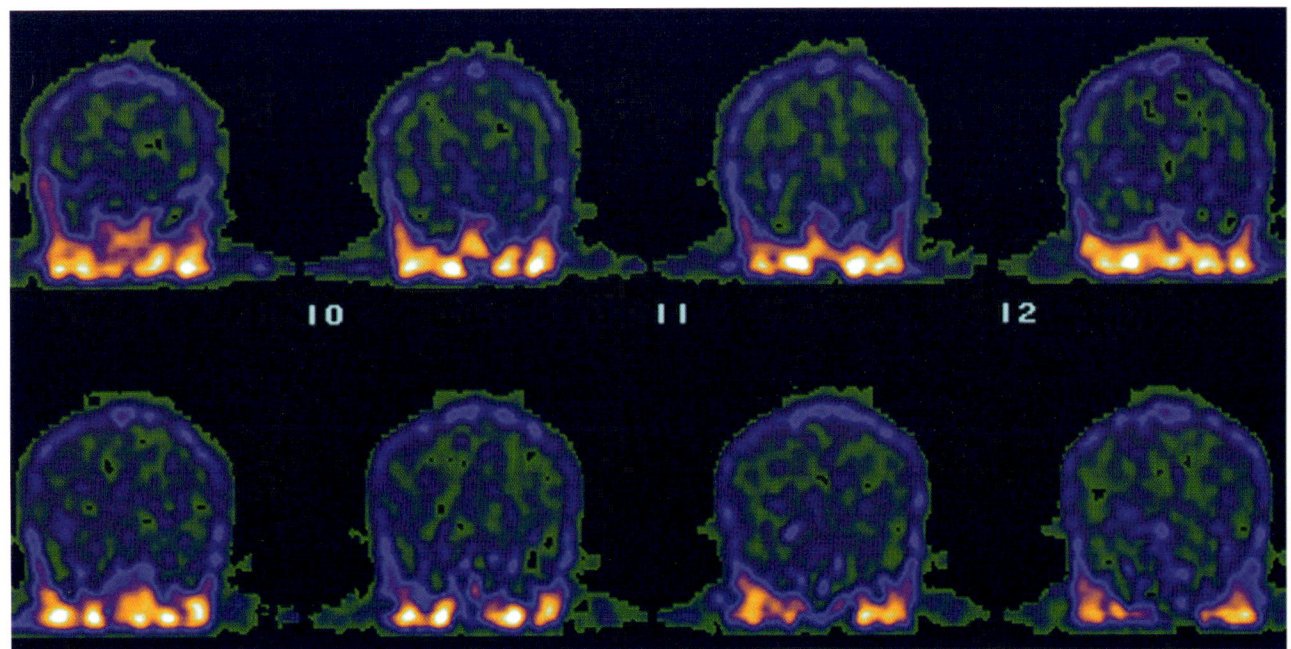

Plate 4.2 *Brain death in a 4-year-old following trauma. The coronal SPECT views of the ^{99m}Tc-HMPAO rCBF study fail to show any accumulation in the anterior, posterior or middle cranial fossa. See page 113.*

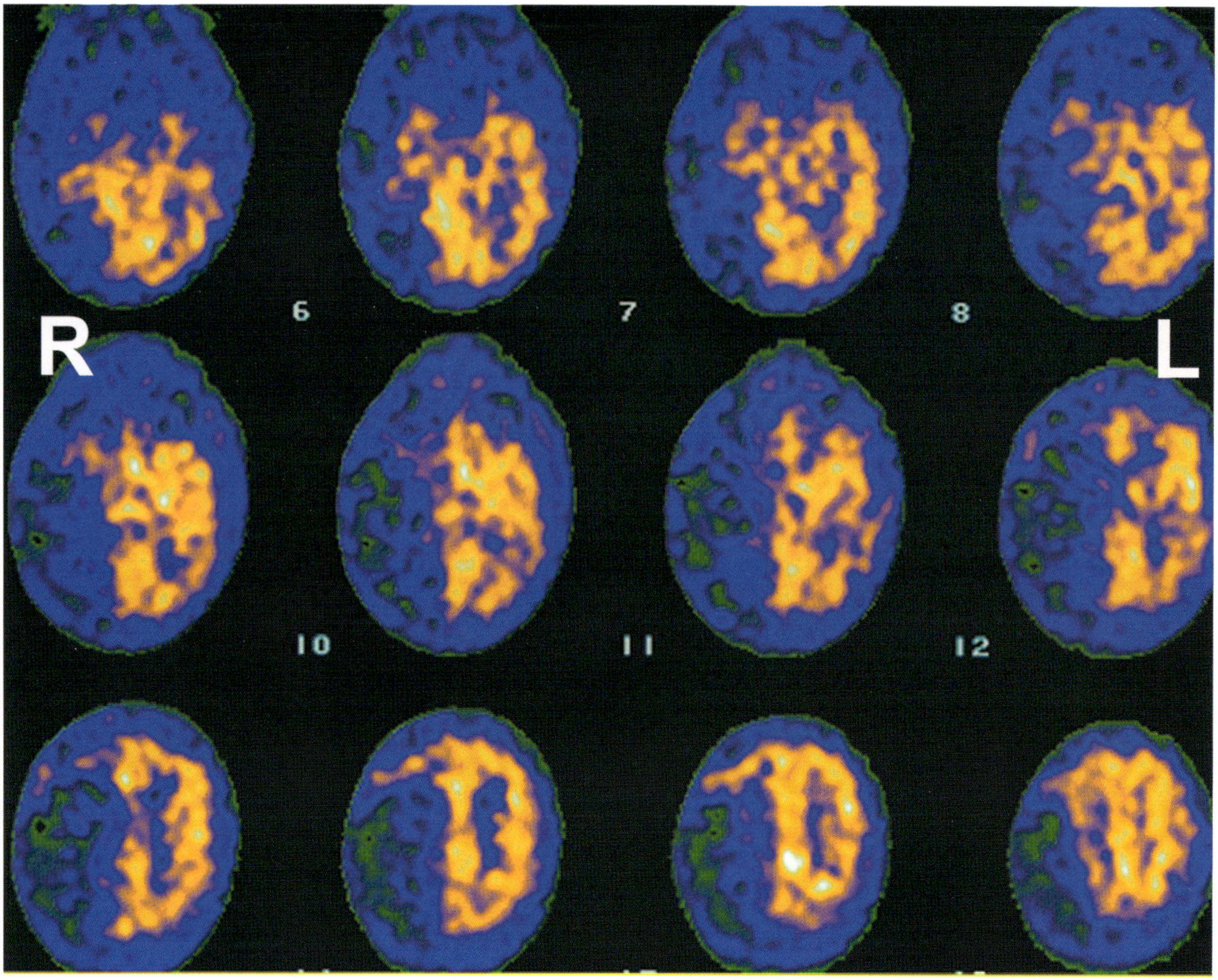

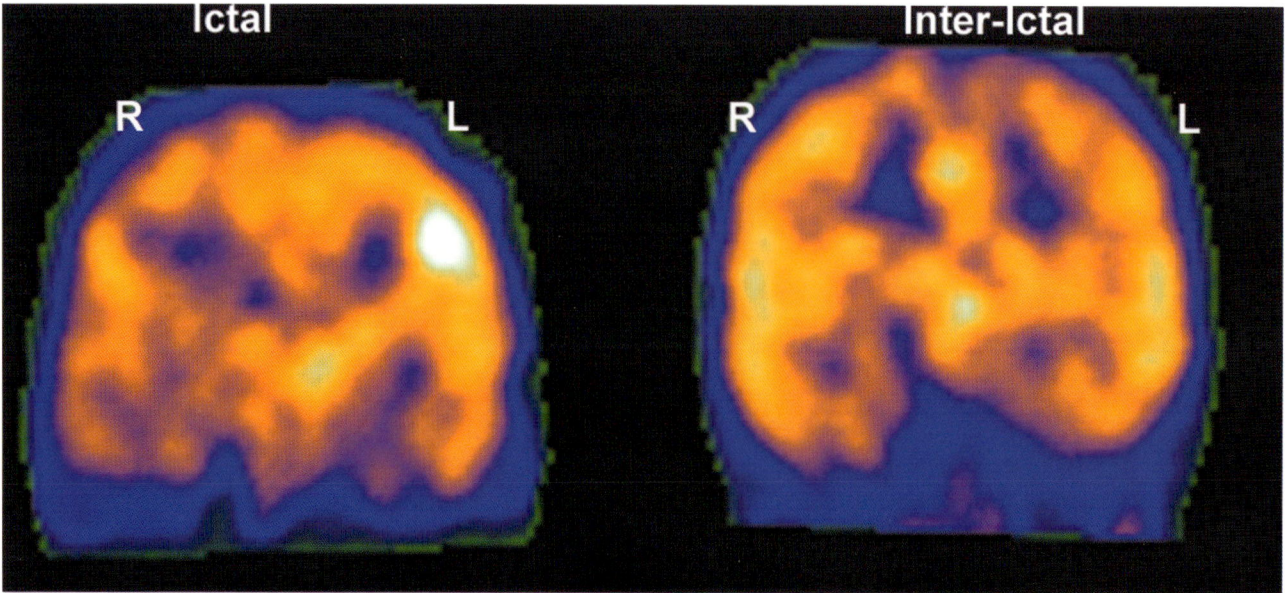

Plate 4.3 *Following a subarachnoid hemorrhage, this 13-year-old girl was in intensive care and required artificial ventilation. The intensive team were discussing the possible outcome with the parents. The transaxial SPECT views of the ^{99m}Tc-HMPAO rCBF study shows patchy uptake by the left cerebral cortex with virtually no uptake on the right. When the child started having cardiac arrests, the rCBF abnormalities plus the clinical state helped the team and parents come to a mutually agreed decision about resuscitation. See page 113.*

Plate 4.4 *Intractable epilepsy in a 5-year-old child. The coronal slice of the ^{99m}Tc-ECD ictal rCBF shows focal increased activity in left pari-etal lobe with generalized increase in the remainder of the left hemisphere. The inter-ictal ^{99m}Tc-ECD rCBF scan shows slight asymmetry with left hemisphere being reduced compared to the right. Crossed cerebellar diaschisis was also seen (not illustrated). This is both a lateralizing and localizing study of the epileptogenic focus in the left parietal lobe. See page 113.*

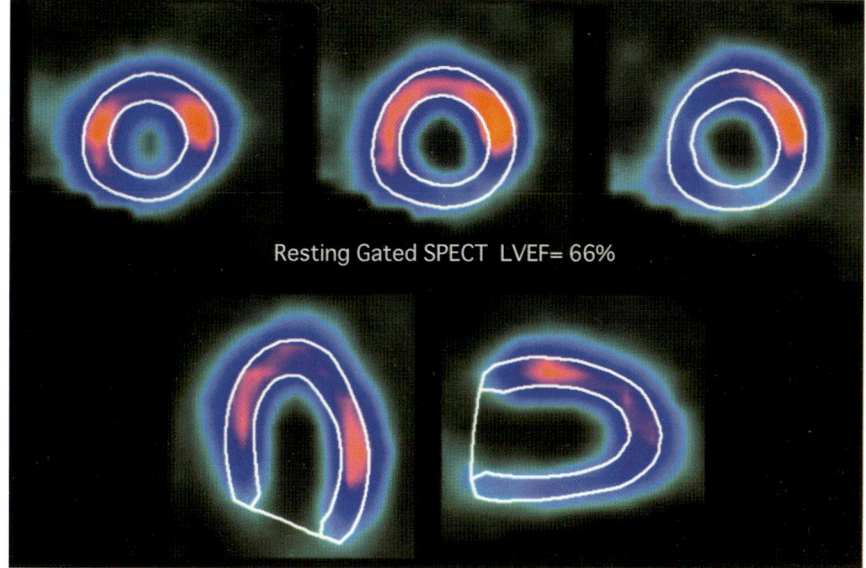

Resting Gated SPECT LVEF= 66%

(a)

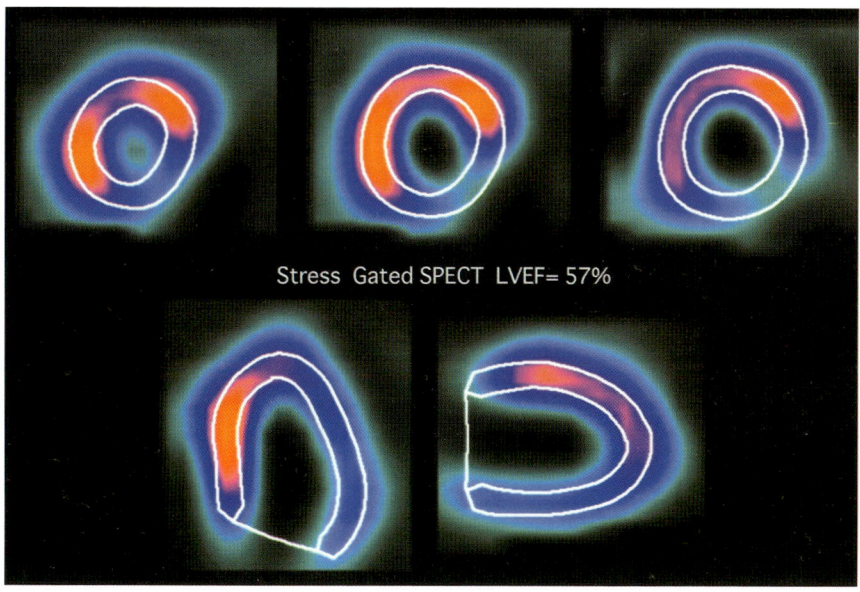

Stress Gated SPECT LVEF= 57%

(b)

Plate 6A.1 *Left ventricular (LV) functional parameters at rest and stress. Resting left ventricular ejection fraction of (a) 66%, and (b) reduced to 57% in post-stress test images. See page 154.*

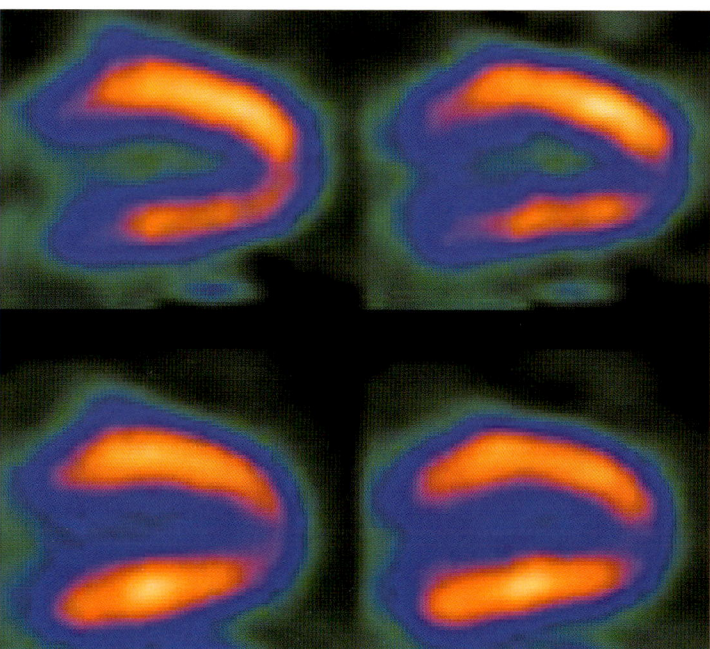

Plate 6A.2 *Effect of attenuation correction. The upper row images demonstrate conventional vertical long axis slices, without attenuation correction and demonstrate relatively low uptake in the inferior wall. Attenuation corrected images in the second row demonstrate markedly increased uptake in the inferior wall, after attenuation correction is applied, changing the ratio of uptake between anterior and inferior walls. (Image courtesy of Dr J. Bomanji, UCL Hospitals, London, UK.) See page 155.*

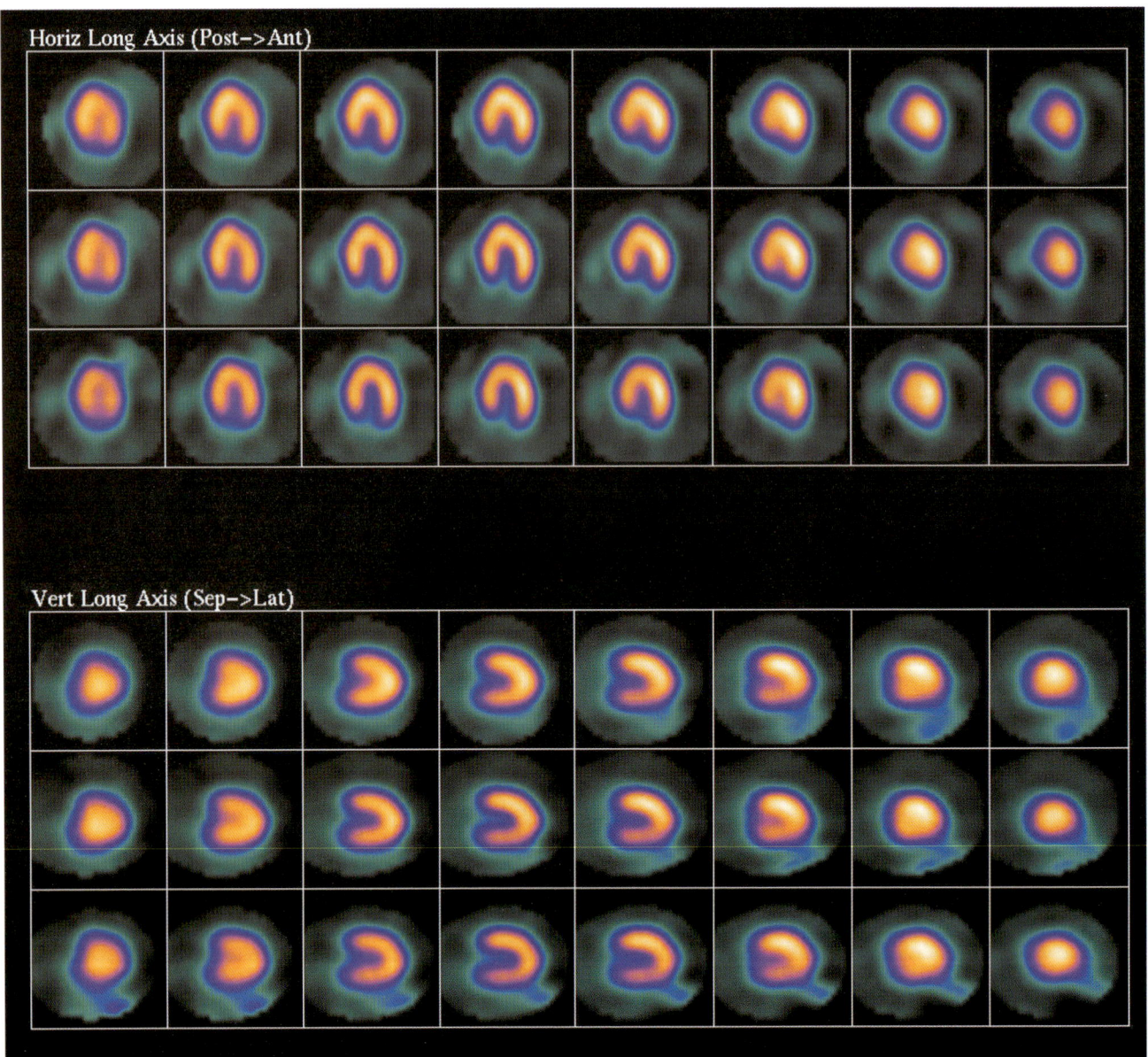

Horiz Long Axis (Post->Ant)

Vert Long Axis (Sep->Lat)

Plate 6A.3 *Simultaneous display of the reconstructed ^{99m}Tc sestamibi gated stress and ungated stress–rest vertical long and horizontal long axes slices, with no evidence of ischemia. See page 155.*

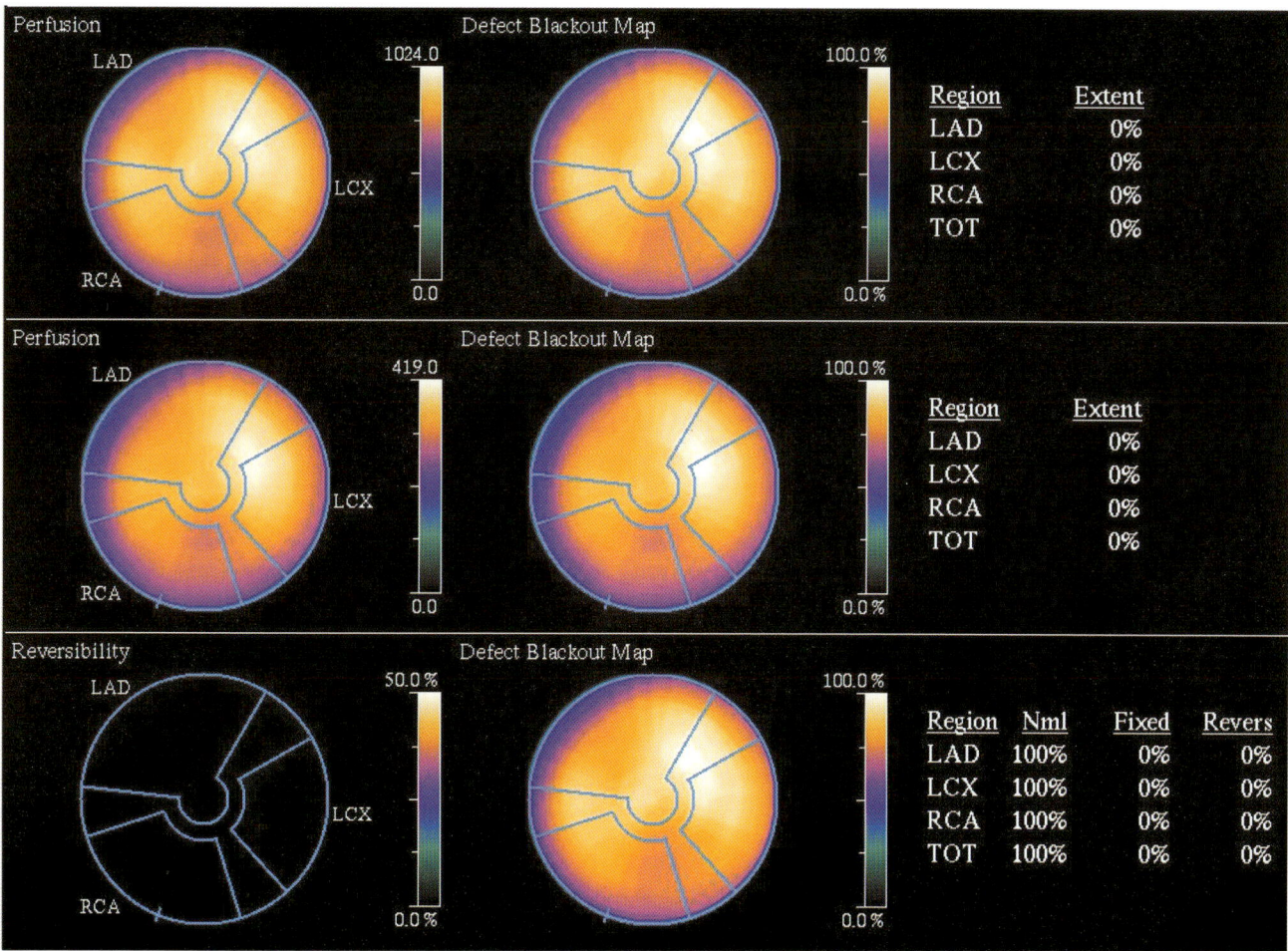

Plate 6A.4 *Quantitative assessment of myocardial perfusion (polar maps) in a study with no evidence of ischemia. See page 155.*

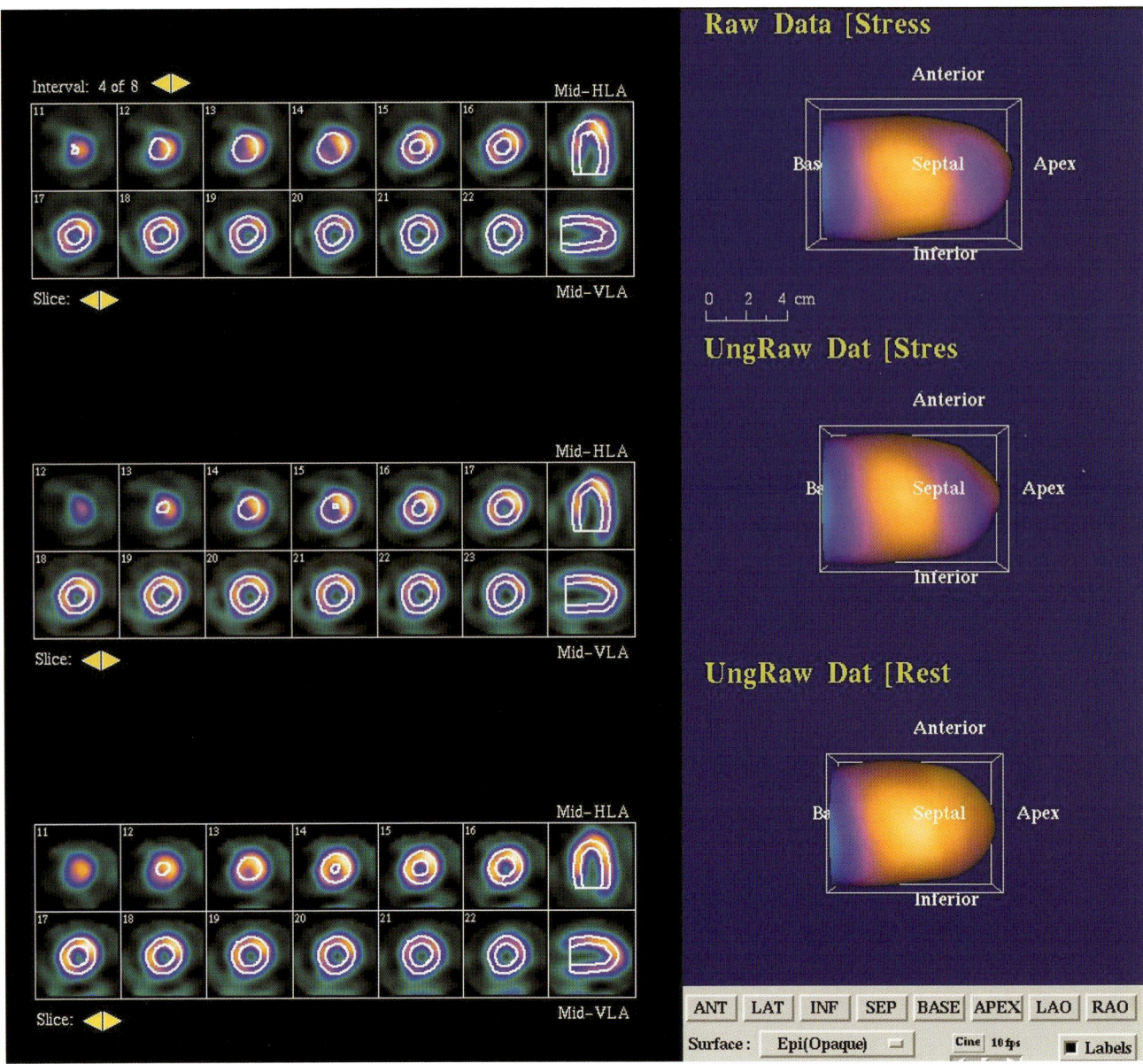

Plate 6A.5 *Assessment of perfusion and function using 4DMSPECT. The left-side panel shows gated and ungated short-axis slices demonstrating severe reversible ischemia of the antero-septal region. The right-side panel displays a three-dimensional map of the left ventricle. See page 155.*

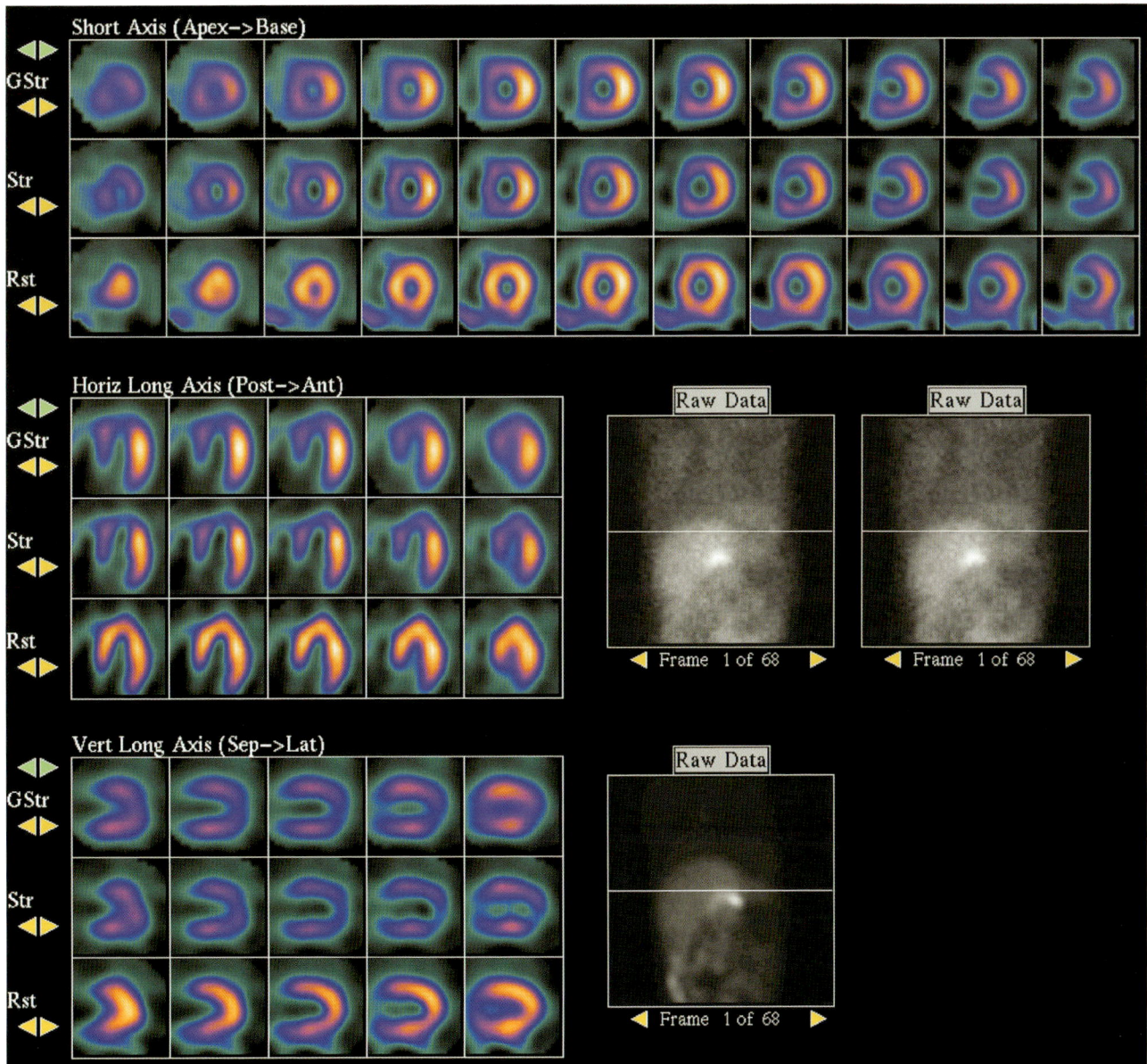

Plate 6A.6 *Simultaneous display of the reconstructed gated stress and ungated stress–rest slices with raw data sets. The evaluation of the gated and ungated raw data sets constitutes an important step for quality control of the study. The above study demonstrates severe reversible ischemia of the anterior and inferior walls, apex and septum. Coronary angiogram confirmed multi-vessel disease. See page 155.*

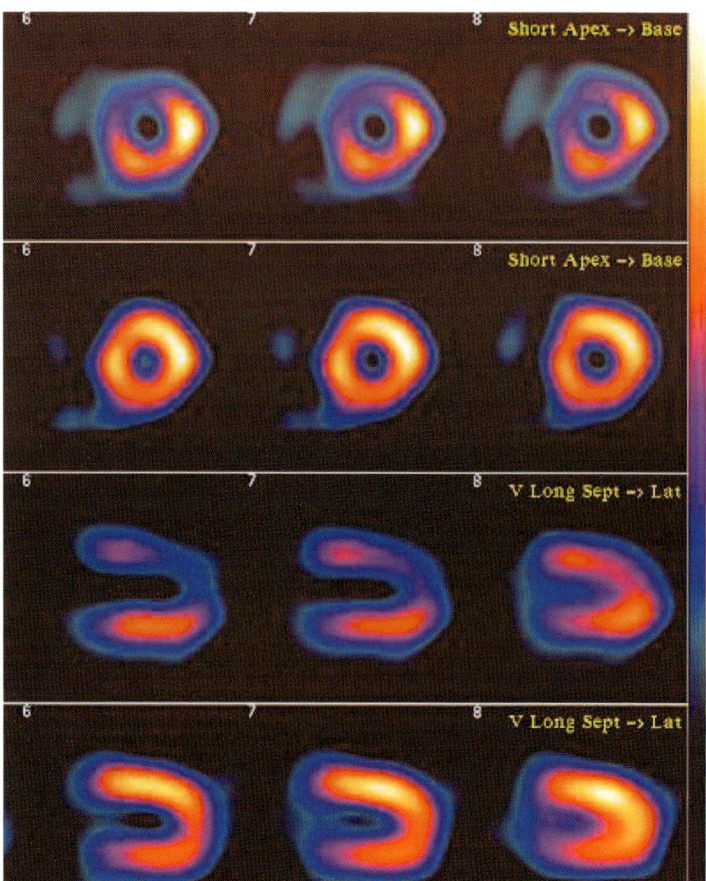

Plate 6A.7 *Thallium-201 stress–redistribution images in a patient with single vessel disease. The figure demonstrates transient LV dilatation in the post-stress test images, with severe reversible ischemia. The coronary angiogram demonstrated a critical LAD lesion, with minor disease in the distal RCA. The patient was treated with percutaneous intervention and medical therapy. See page 155.*

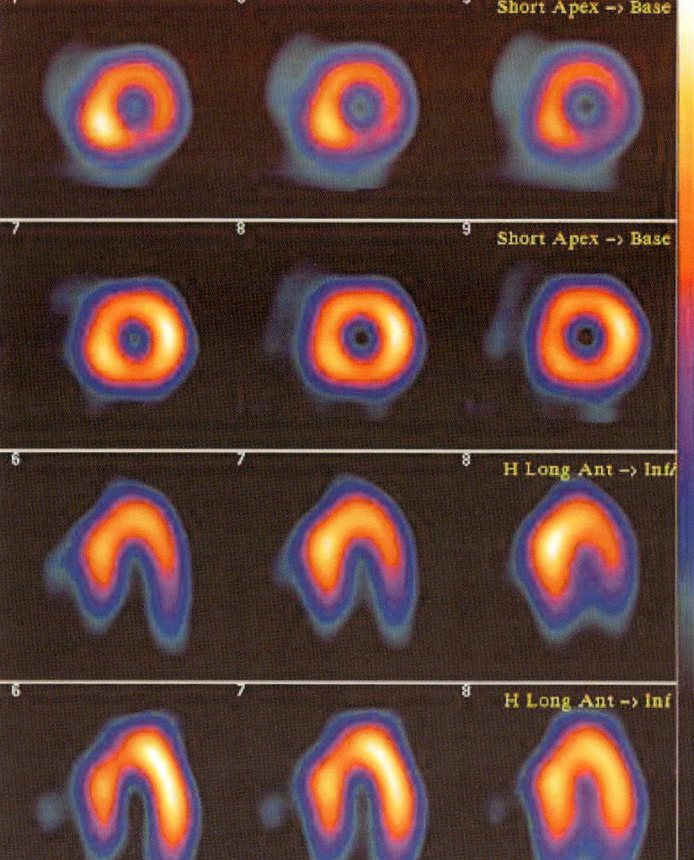

Plate 6A.8 *Comparison of ^{201}Tl stress–redistribution images in a second patient with single-vessel disease. The figure reveals moderate ischemia of the lateral wall, without transient LV dilatation in the post-stress images. The angiogram of this patient had approximately 60% lesion with diffuse involvement of the OM1, with mild diffuse disease (<40%) in RCA and some minor irregularities in LAD. The patient was asymptomatic but diabetic. Medical management was initiated, with the intention for subsequent close follow-up. See page 155.*

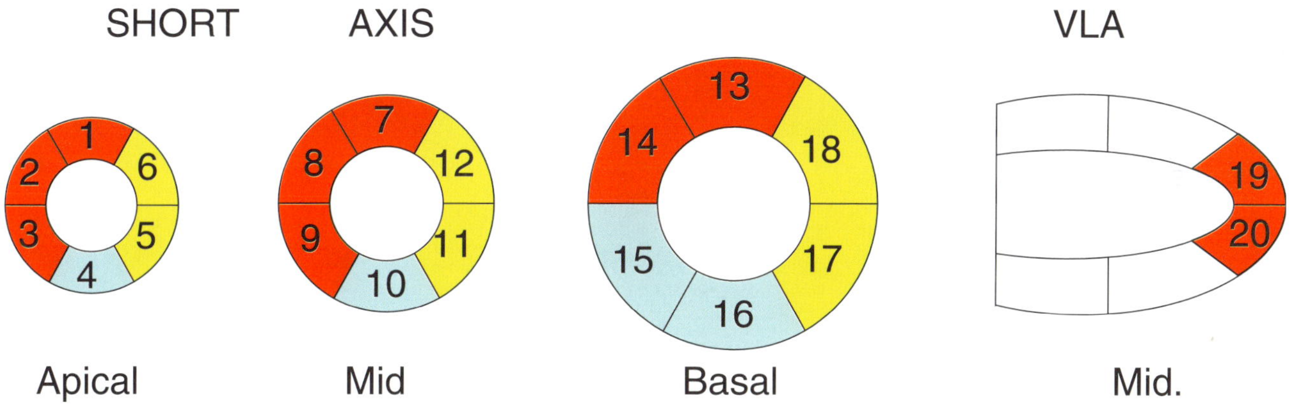

SHORT AXIS   VLA

Apical   **Mid**   **Basal**   **Mid.**

	Apical	Mid.	Basal
Anterior	1	7	13
Antero-septal	2	8	14
Infero-septal	3	9	15
Inferior	4	10	16
Antero-lateral	6	12	18
Infero-lateral	5	11	17
Antero-apical	19		
Apico-inferior	20		

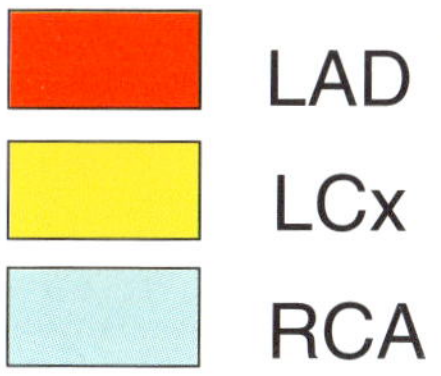

- ■ LAD
- ■ LCx
- ■ RCA

Plate 6A.9 *Twenty–segment model for reporting of myocardial perfusion SPECT images. Three short-axis cuts at the apex, mid and basal levels of LV are used. It should be remembered that one segment of apical inferior wall is supplied by LAD (VLA, vertical long axis).[118] See page 155.*

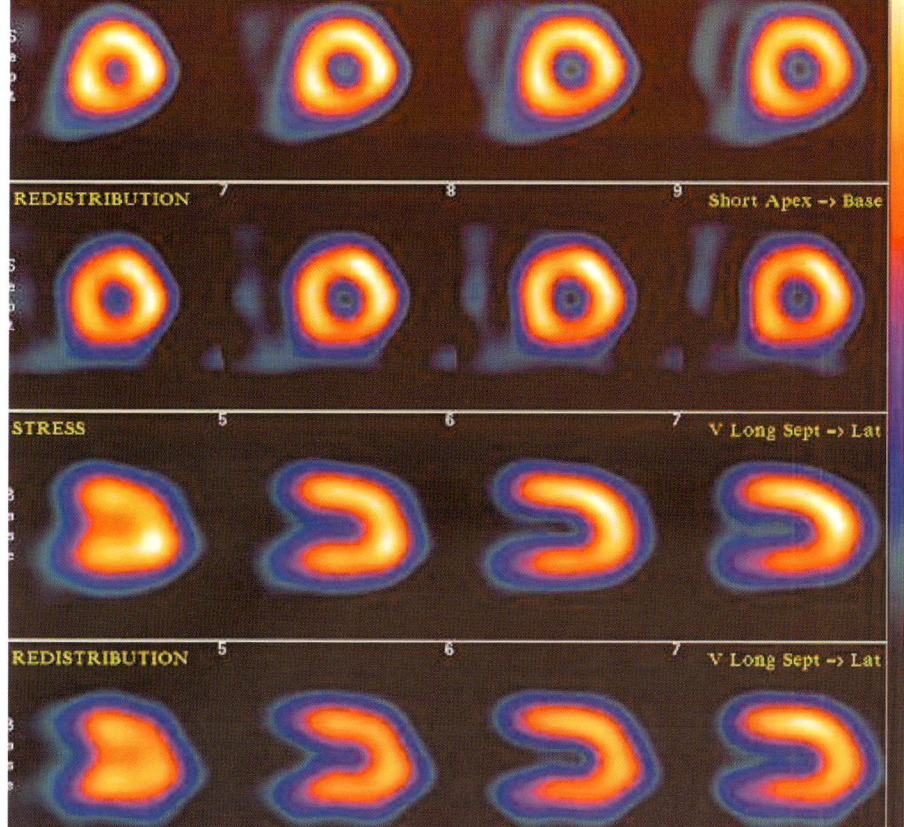

Plate 6A.10 *Stress–redistribution ^{201}Tl slices, revealing normal tracer uptake in the myocardium. See page 155.*

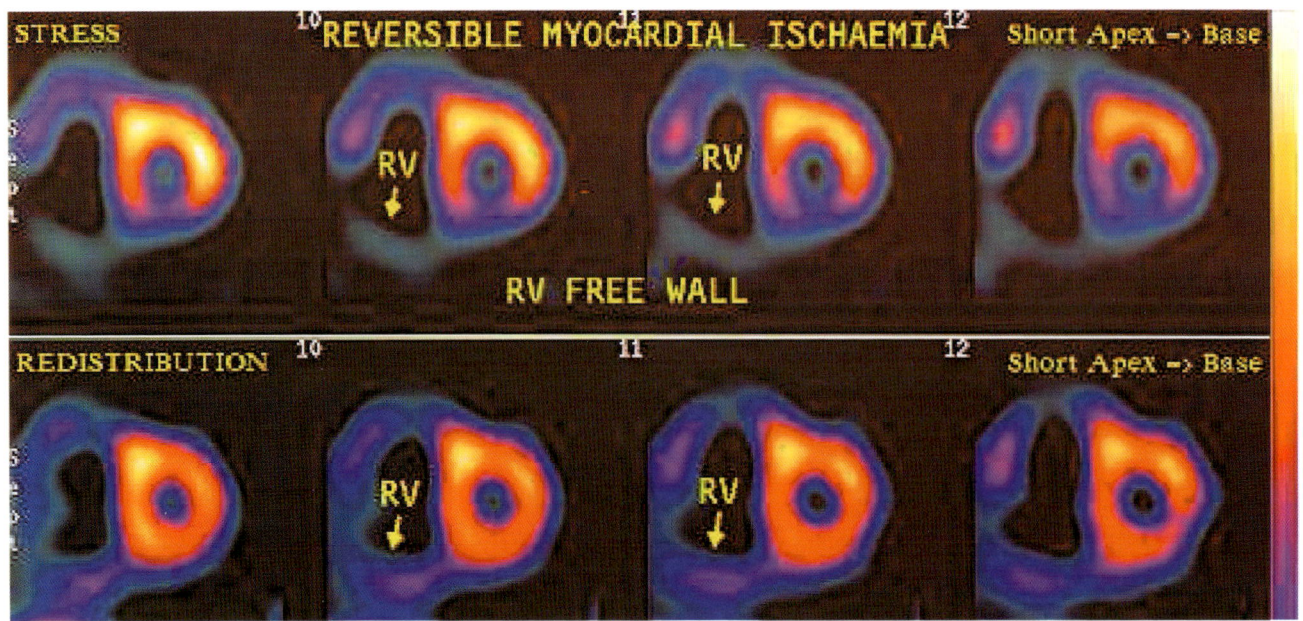

Plate 6A.11 *Dilated RV is obvious, with reduced uptake in the RV wall on the stress images. The redistribution images demonstrate improvement in uptake, consistent with RV ischemia. See page 155.*

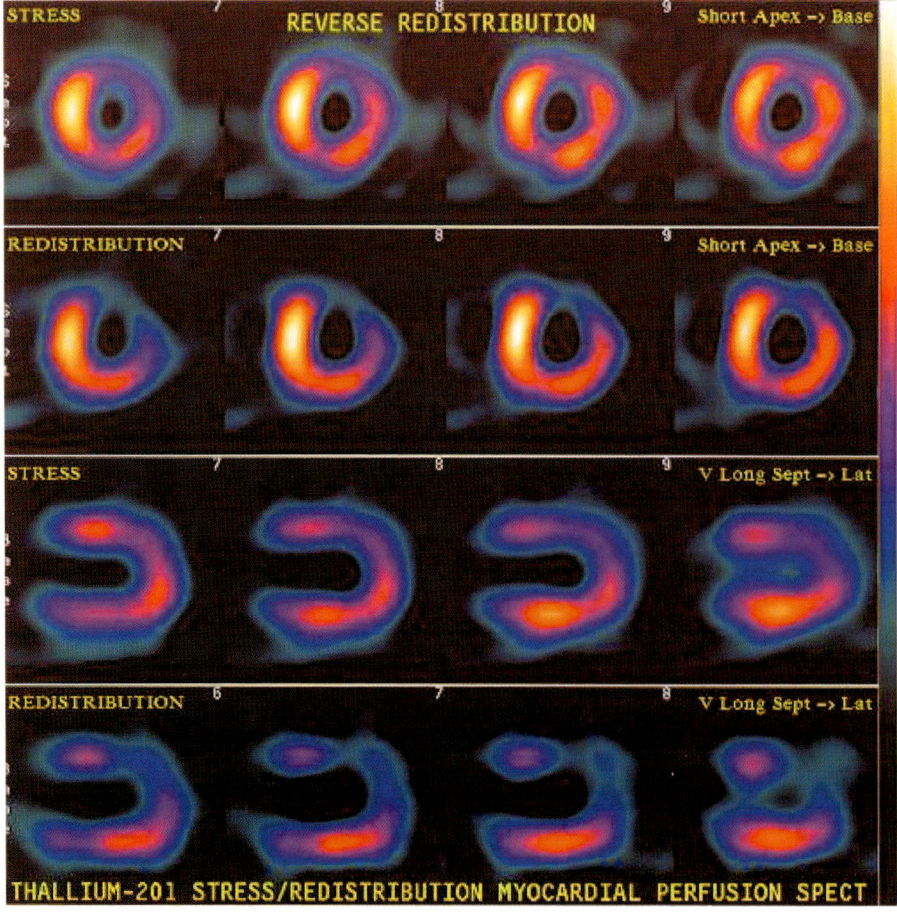

Plate 6A.12 *Thallium-201 SPECT demonstrating reduced uptake in the anterior and small segment of antero-lateral walls on the stress slices, with further reduction in the uptake in the anterior wall in the redistribution slices, demonstrating reverse redistribution. This 43-year-old male patient was admitted in emergency with acute chest pain and was given tissue plasminogen activator. A coronary angiogram demonstrated re-canalized proximal LAD, post-thrombolysis. See page 156.*

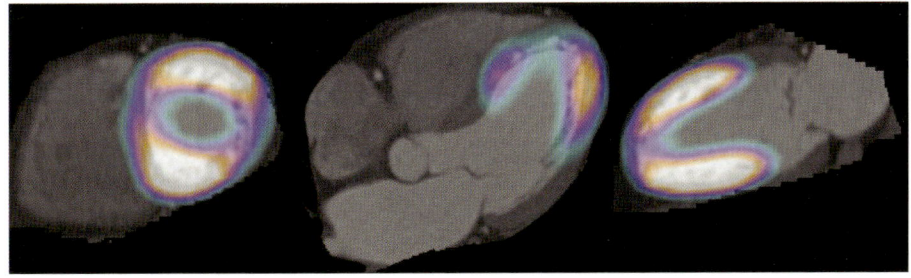

(a)

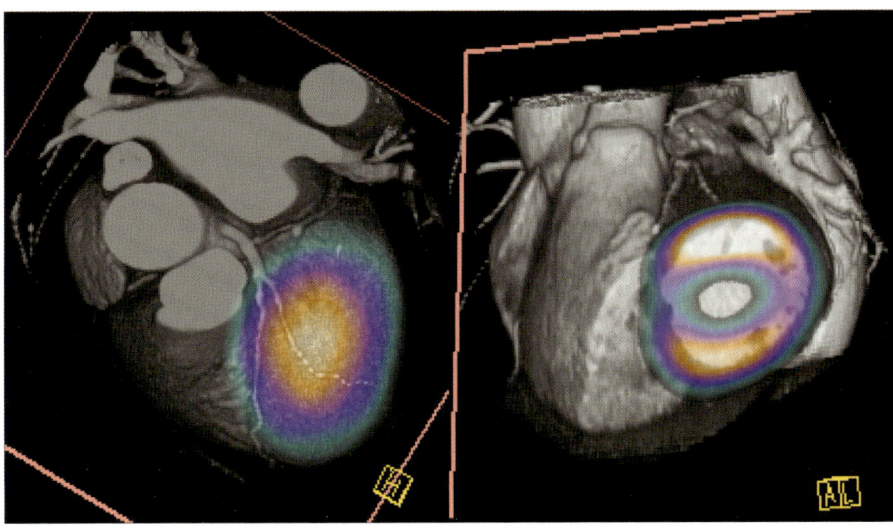

(b)

Plate 6A.13 *(a) Fused SPECT–CT short axis, HLA and VLA slices. (b) The SPECT–CT data fused with 64-slice CT coronary angiography. There is diffuse disease involving LAD, Dx and LCx. Stress myocardial perfusion demonstrates small areas of reduced perfusion septum and lateral wall. Perfusion is well preserved to most of the anterior and inferior walls. Medical management was initiated. SPECT–CT not only provides fast accurate attenuation and scatter correction for the SPECT studies, but is also capable of correlating it to the anatomical lesion or calcium scoring seen on the coronary CT images. See page 157.*

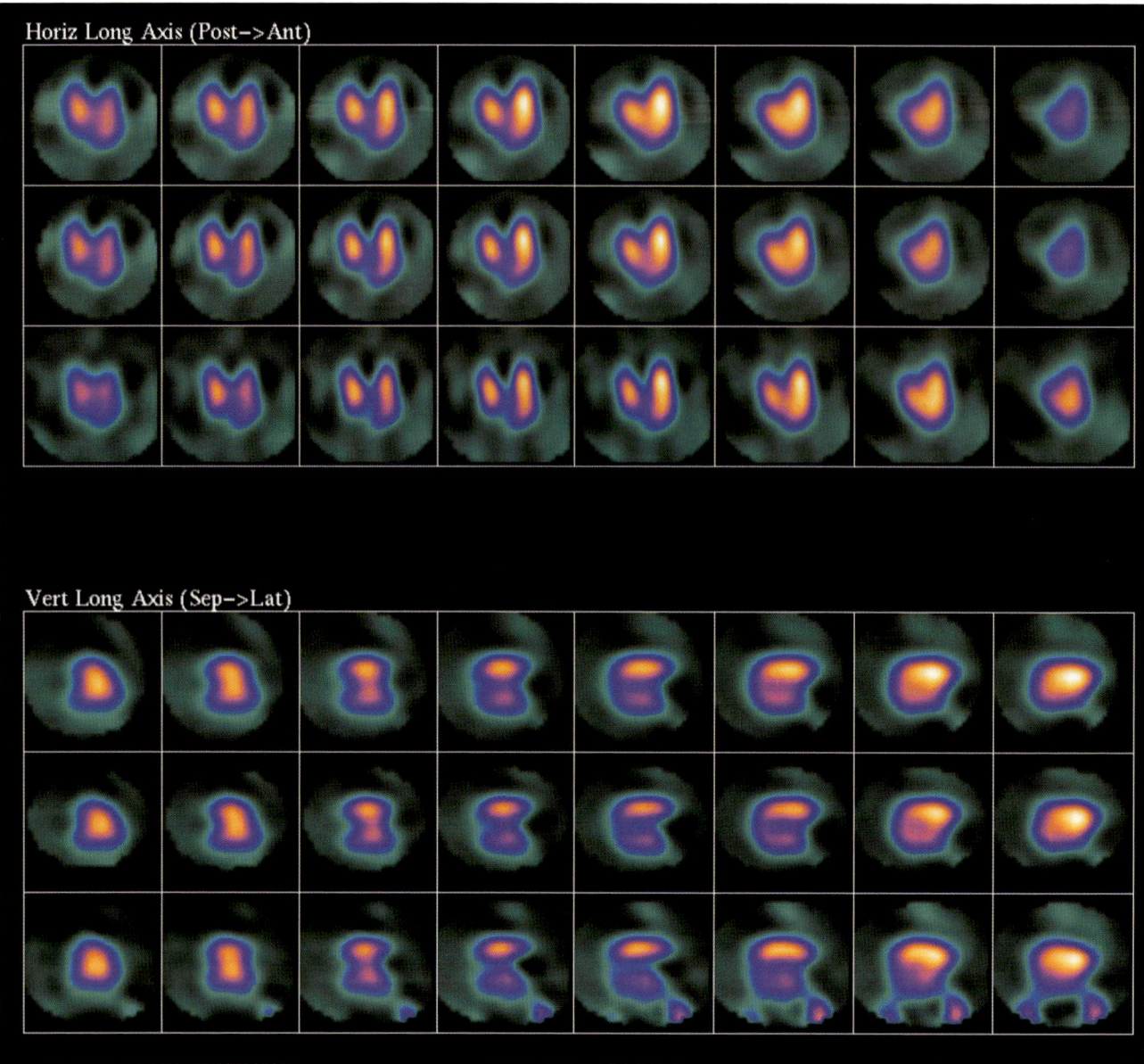

Horiz Long Axis (Post->Ant)

Vert Long Axis (Sep->Lat)

(a)

Plate 6A.14 *(a) Gated myocardial perfusion SPECT slices demonstrating a fixed defect in the apex, due to apical infarct. This young patient complained of chest pain but a coronary calcium scoring did not reveal any significant pathology. Ultimately, a few days later the patient was re-admitted with another episode of chest pain and elevated troponin. A gated myocardial perfusion SPECT study did not reveal any significant residual ischemia. In the absence of any significant coronary calcium burden, it is likely that the episode occurred because of unstable soft plaque. See page 161.*

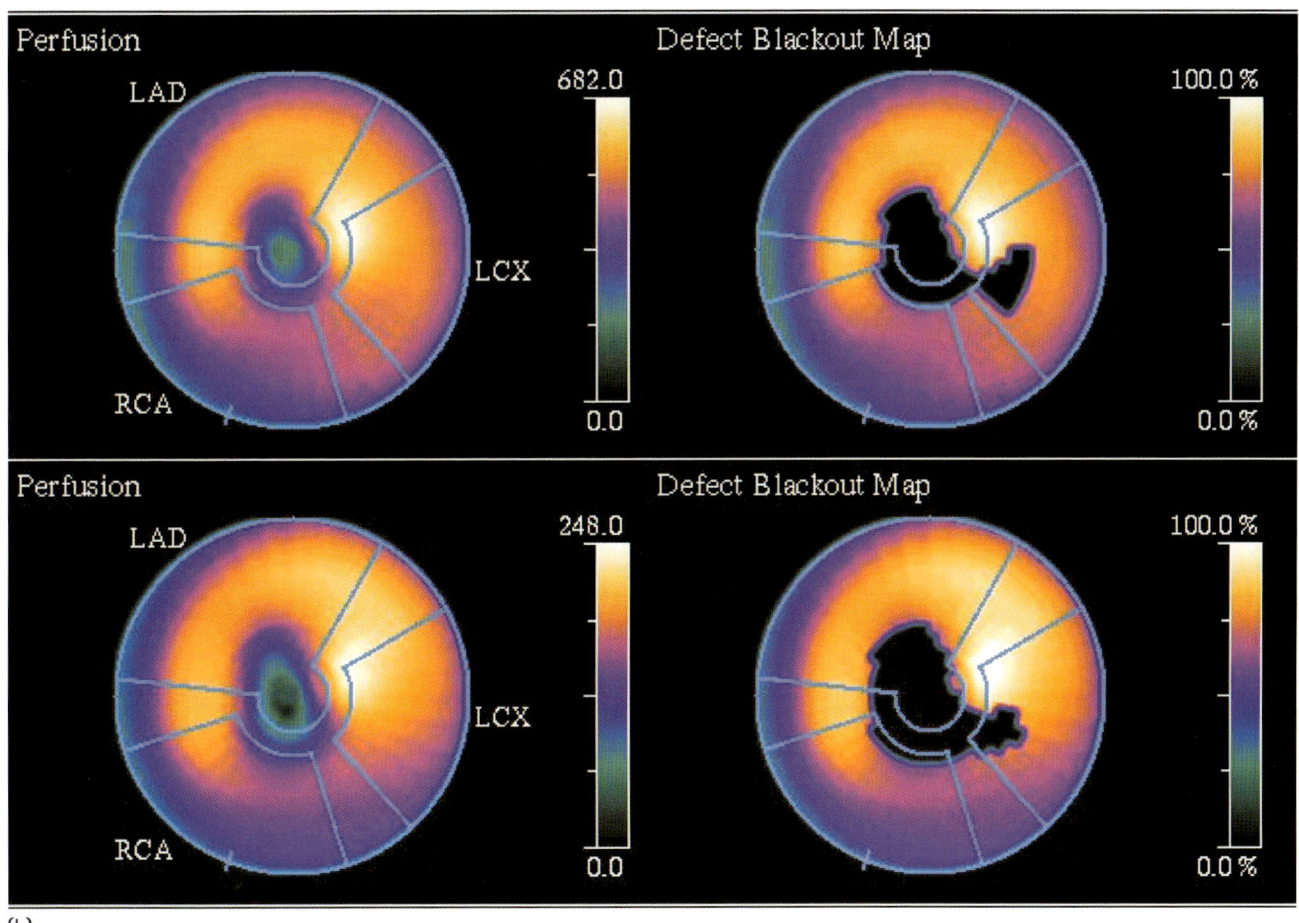

(b)

Plate 6A.14 *(Continued)* *(b) The quantitative polar maps also confirmed an apical infarct, with no residual ischemia. See page 161.*

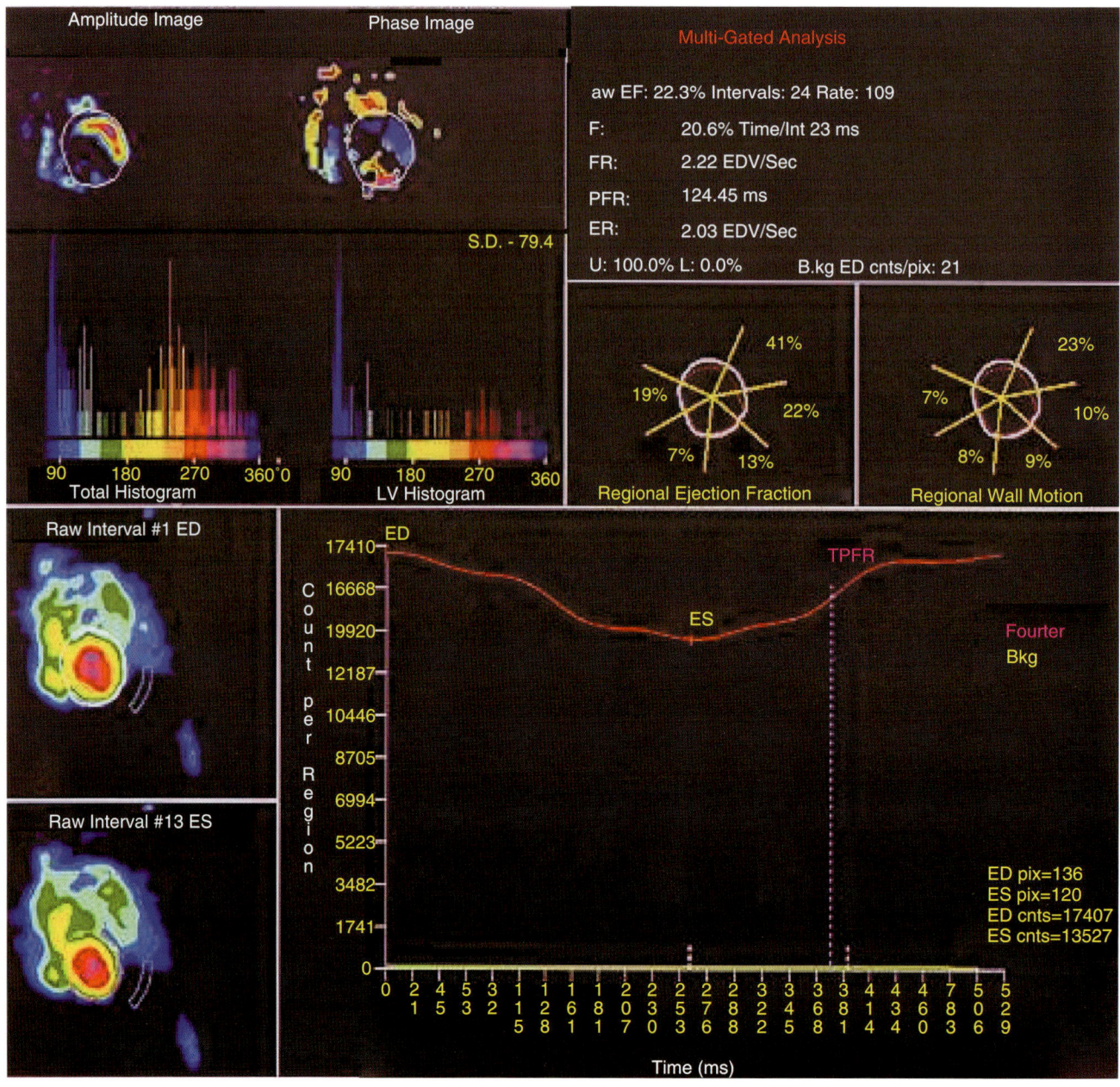

Plate 6A.15 *Gated blood pool radionuclide angiocardiography. A typical scan display demonstrating poor LVEF of 22%, with changes in amplitude and phase images. See page 161.*

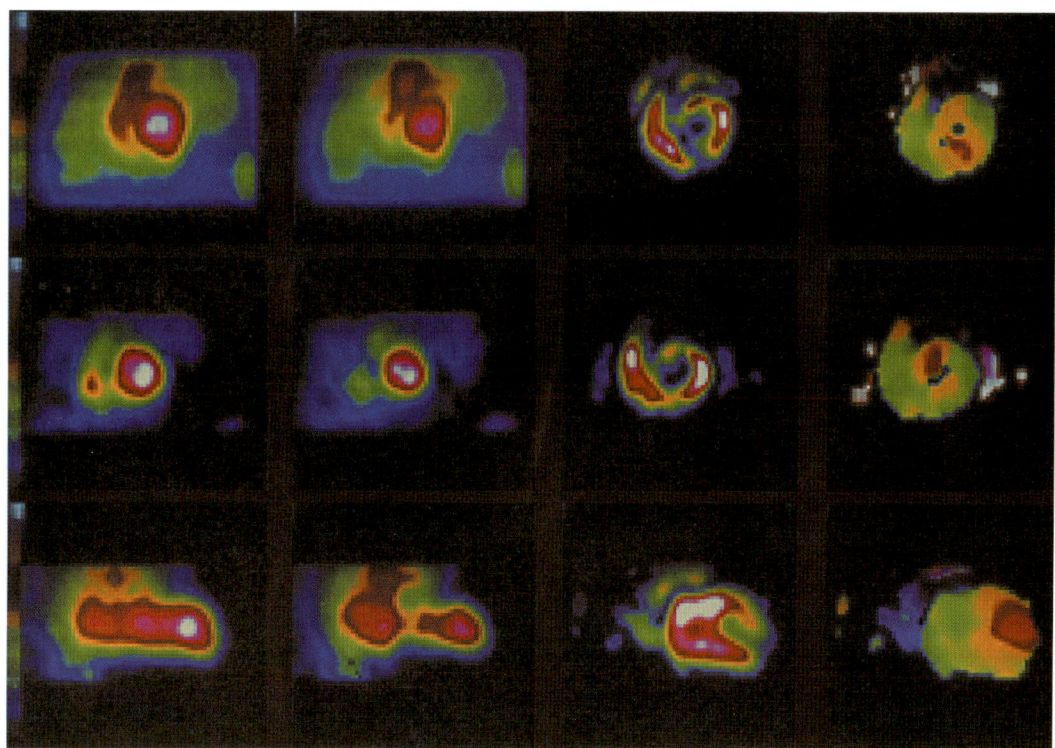

Plate 6A.16   *MUGA SPECT study. Reconstructed horizontal and short and vertical long axis slices in which amplitude and phase images are demonstrated. There is evidence of poor LV function, with marked changes in the apex on the phase images, consistent with dyskinetic region (apical aneurysm). See page 161.*

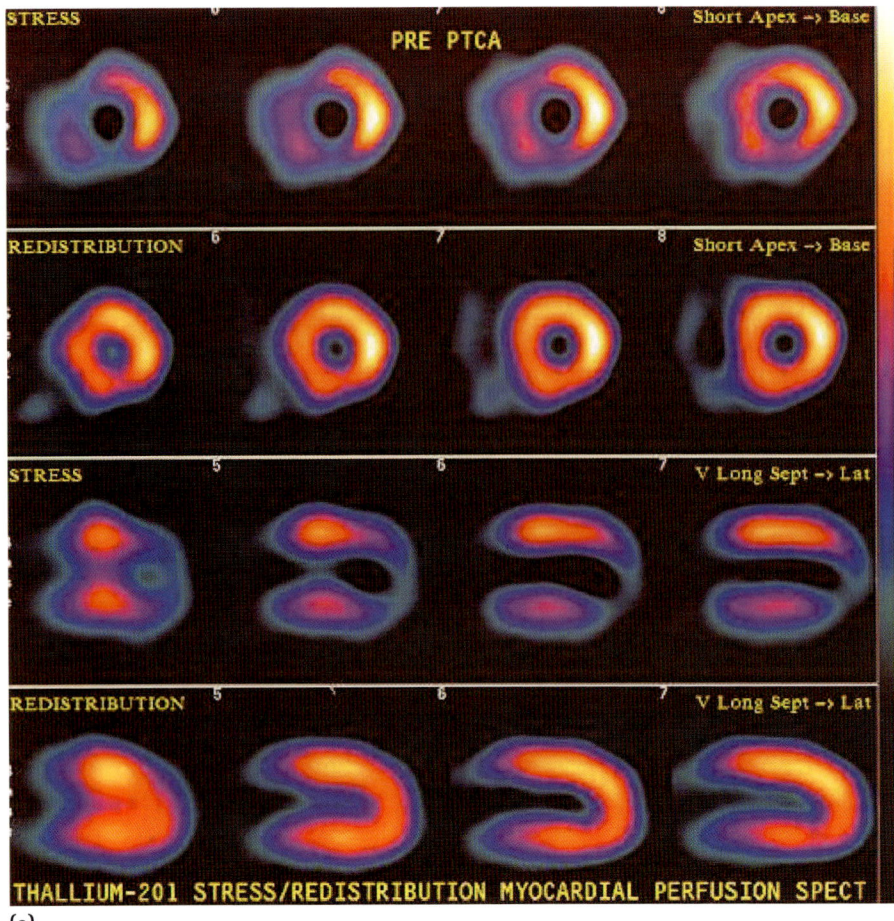

(a)

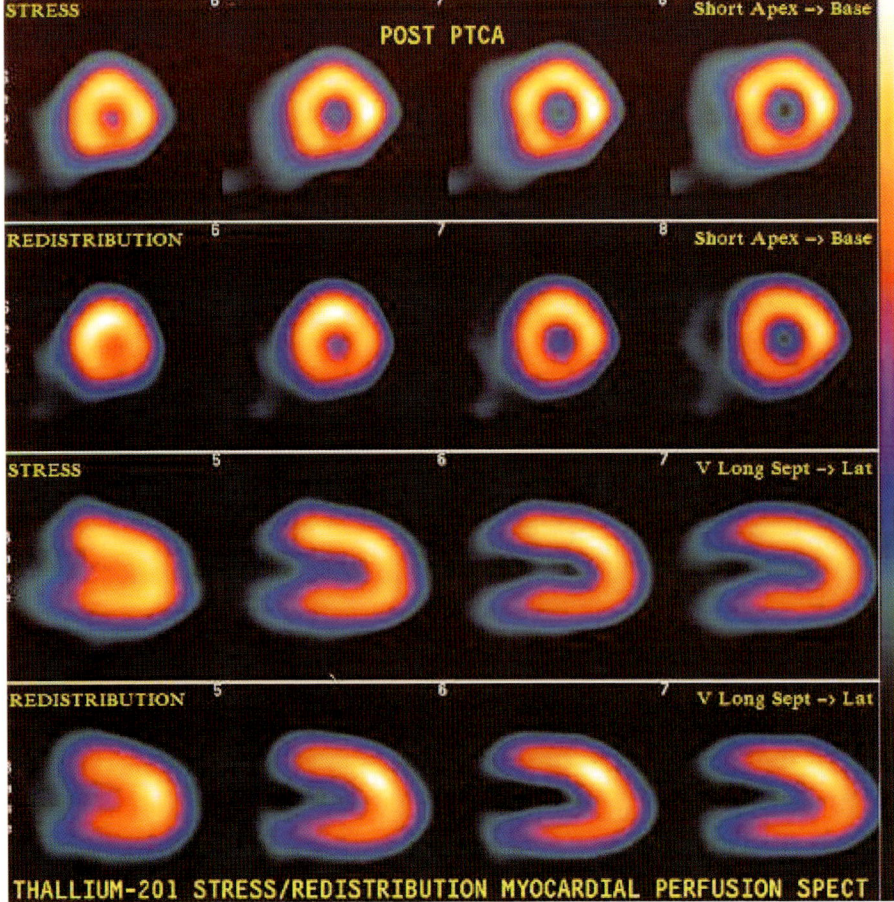

(b)

Plate 6A.17 *Pre-PCI and post-PCI ^{201}Tl myocardial perfusion SPECT images in a case of successful complete revascularization. (a) The pre-PTCA images demonstrate extensive ischemia involving apex, anteroseptal region and inferior wall. (b) Post-PCI images demonstrate normal uptake, with no evidence of any residual ischemia. See page 164.*

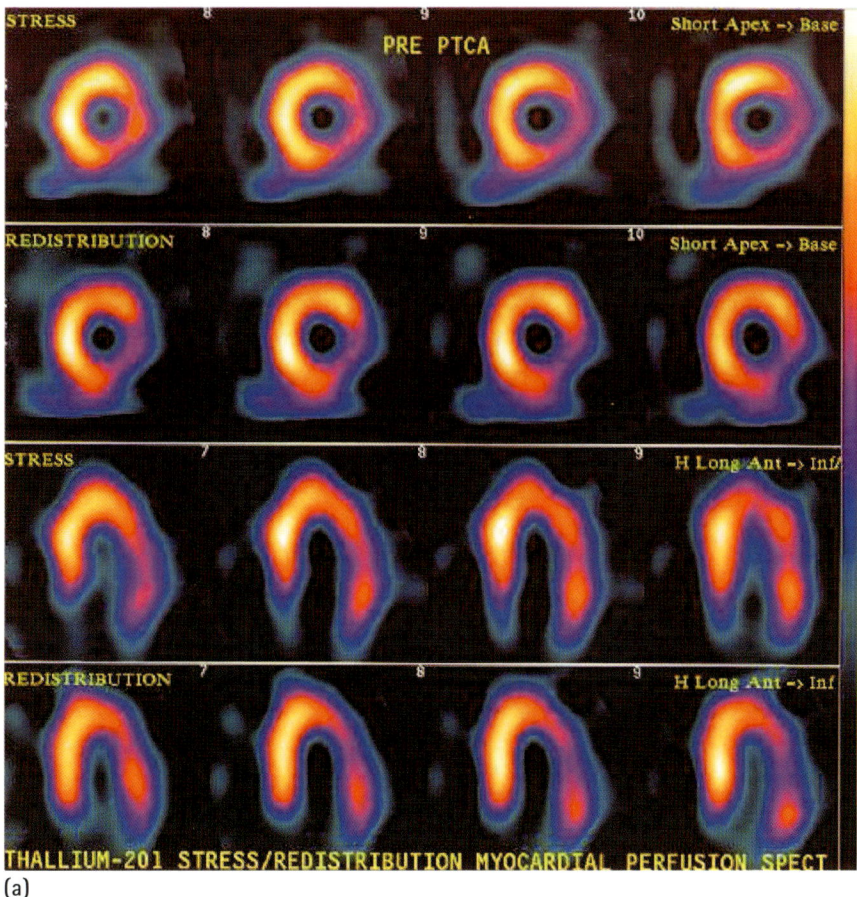

(a)

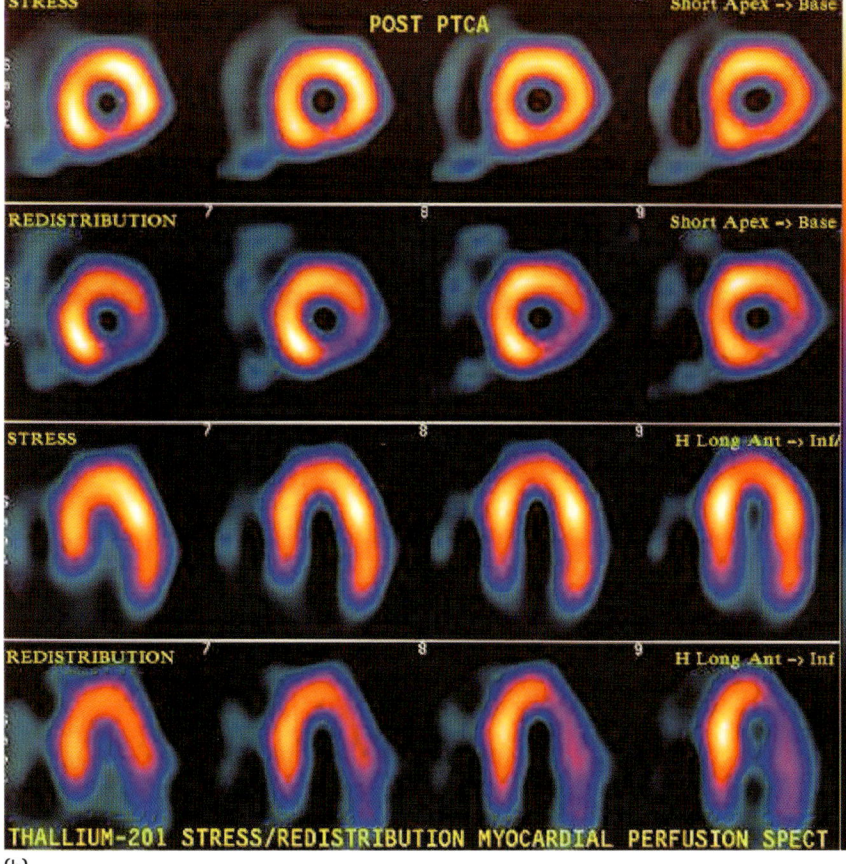

(b)

Plate 6A.18 *Post-intervention changes in myocardial perfusion. (a) The pre-PTCA images demonstrate severely reduced uptake in the lateral wall, on the stress–redistribution images. (b) Post-PCI images 1 month later reveal marked improvement in the perfusion status at stress, with reverse redistribution; most likely representing associated sub-endocardial ischemia. See page 164.*

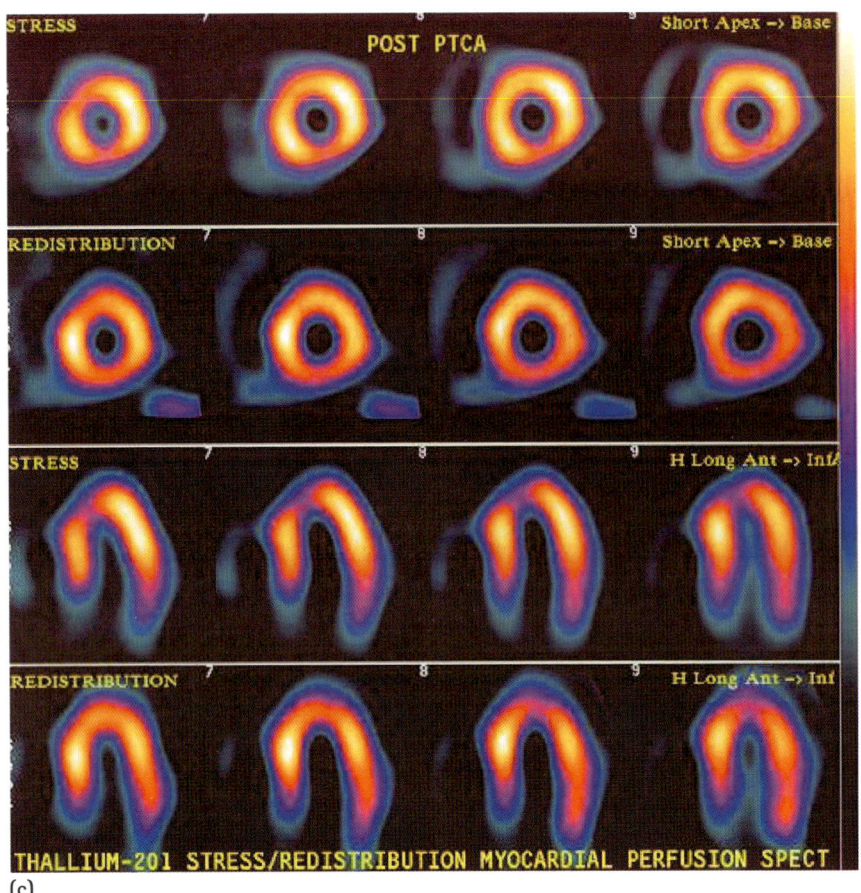

STRESS
POST PTCA
Short Apex –> Base

REDISTRIBUTION
Short Apex –> Base

STRESS
H Long Ant –> Inf

REDISTRIBUTION
H Long Ant –> Inf

THALLIUM-201 STRESS/REDISTRIBUTION MYOCARDIAL PERFUSION SPECT

(c)

Plate 6A.18 *(Continued)* (c) Subsequent, ^{201}Tl myocardial perfusion SPECT images 6 months later do not demonstrate reverse redistribution, suggesting improvement in the infero-lateral wall. However, a small segment of reversible ischemia is noted in the apex, most likely due to disease progression in the native artery. Coronary angiogram demonstrates mild progression of disease in the distal LAD, with no evidence of re-stenosis in the LCx. See page 164.

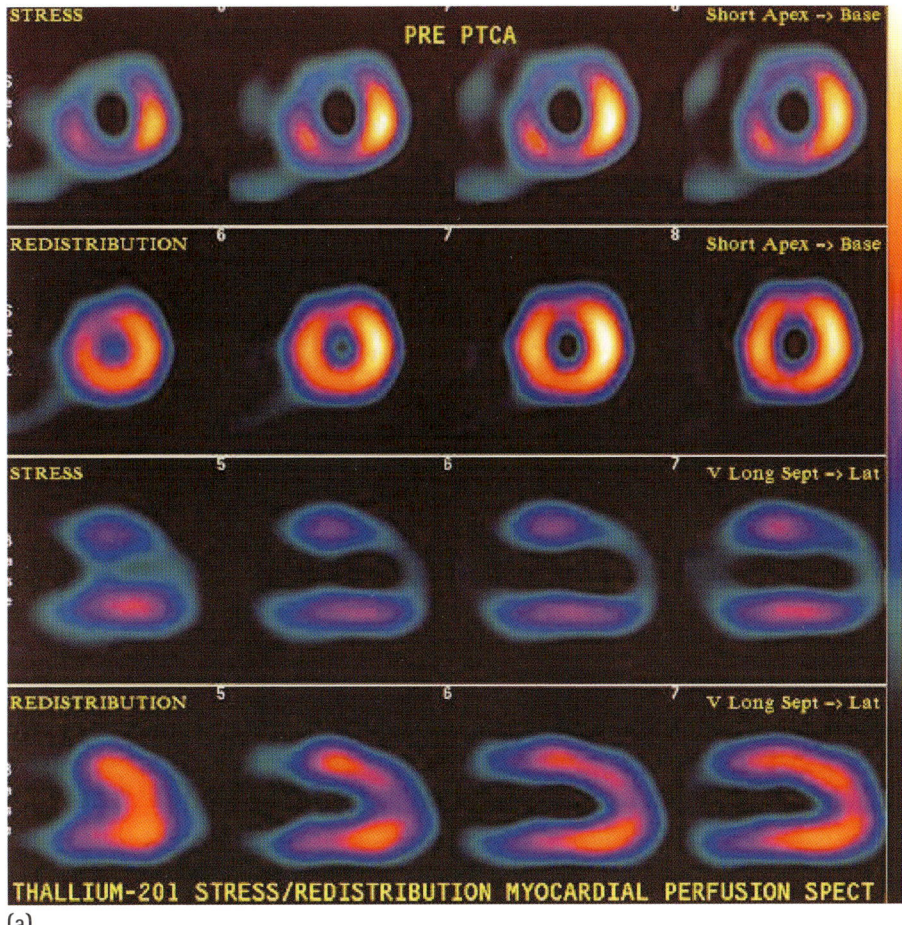

(a)

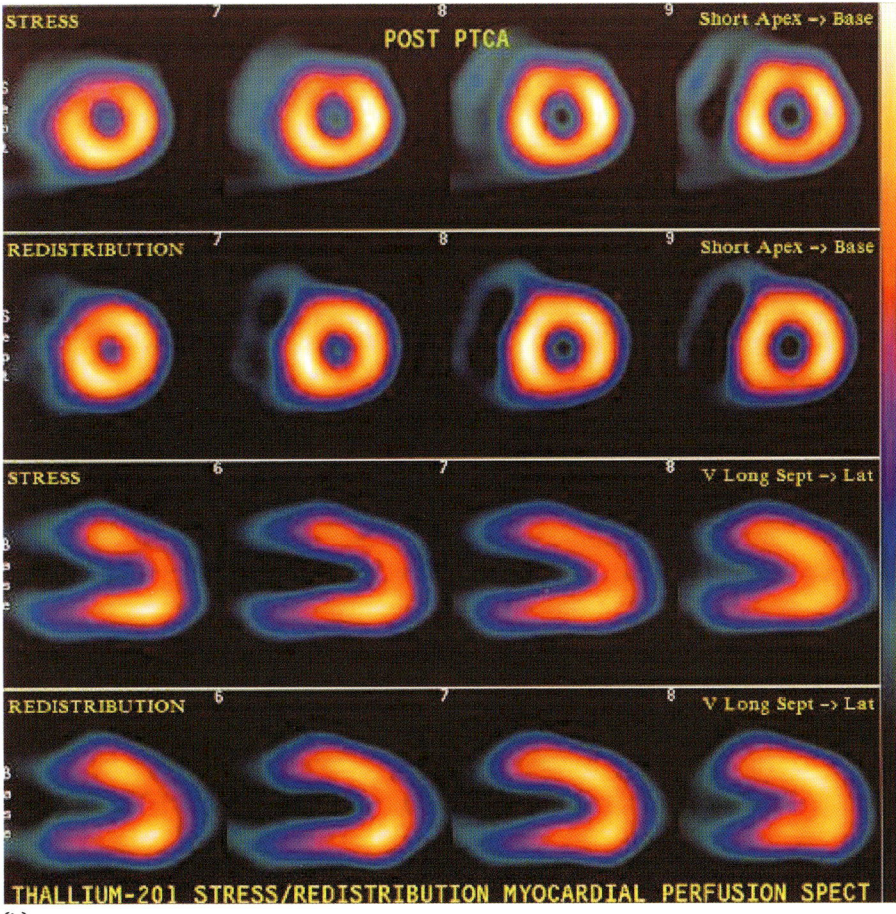

(b)

Plate 6A.19 *Pre- and post-PCI ^{201}Tl myocardial perfusion SPECT images in a case of re-stenosis. (a) The pre-PTCA images demonstrate severe ischemia of the apex and anteroseptal region, with moderate changes in the inferior wall. (b) Post-PCI images demonstrate mild ischemia of anterior wall, 4 weeks post-intervention, without symptoms. A repeat angiogram confirmed approximately 50% in-stent re-stenosis in LAD. See page 164.*

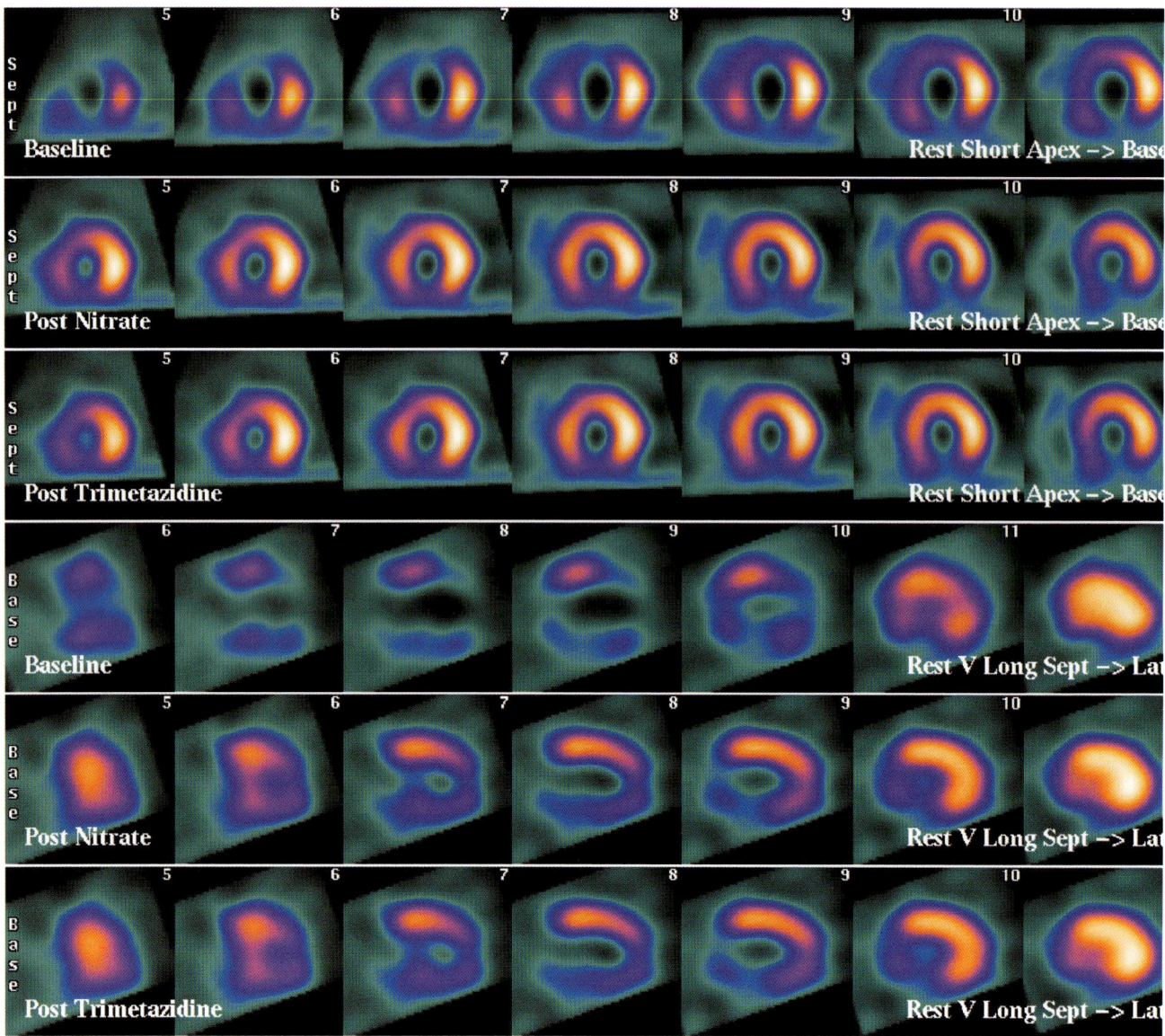

Plate 6A.20 *Technetium-99 m sestamibi myocardial perfusion SPECT for hibernating myocardium. Patient had baseline scan on day 1. On day 2 a SPECT scan after 10 mg of oral nitrate was performed. On day 3, the third acquisition after trimetazidine administration was performed. The reconstructed images demonstrate an absence of uptake in the apex, with severely reduced uptake in the anterior wall, septum and inferior wall. Both post-nitrate and trimetazidine SPECT images reveal improvements, with no significant difference between two interventions. See page 167.*

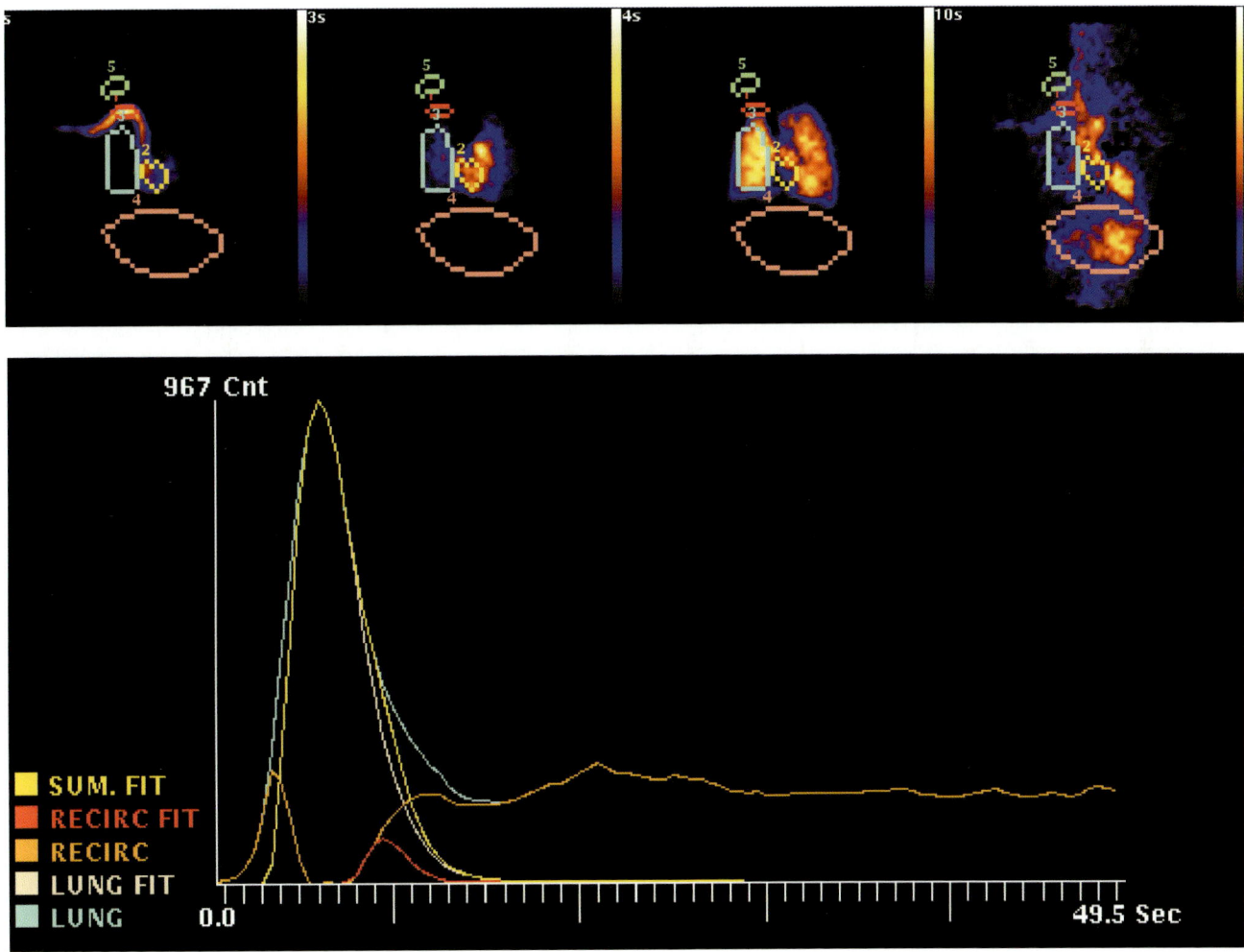

Plate 6A.21   *Normal first-pass study. (a–d) Different regions of interest are placed for analysis on SVC, RV, lungs and LV. (e) The time–activity curves are generated from these ROIs. (Image courtesy of Dr Gary Cook, London, UK.) See page 171.*

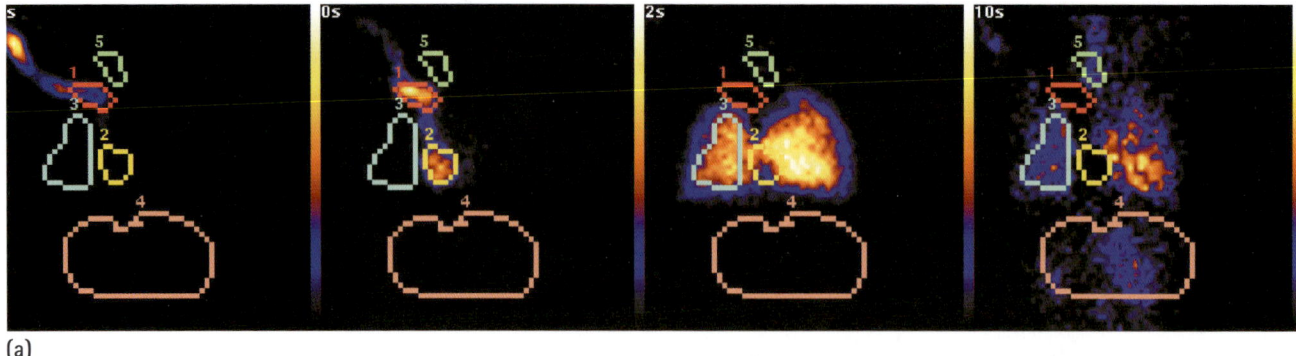

(a)

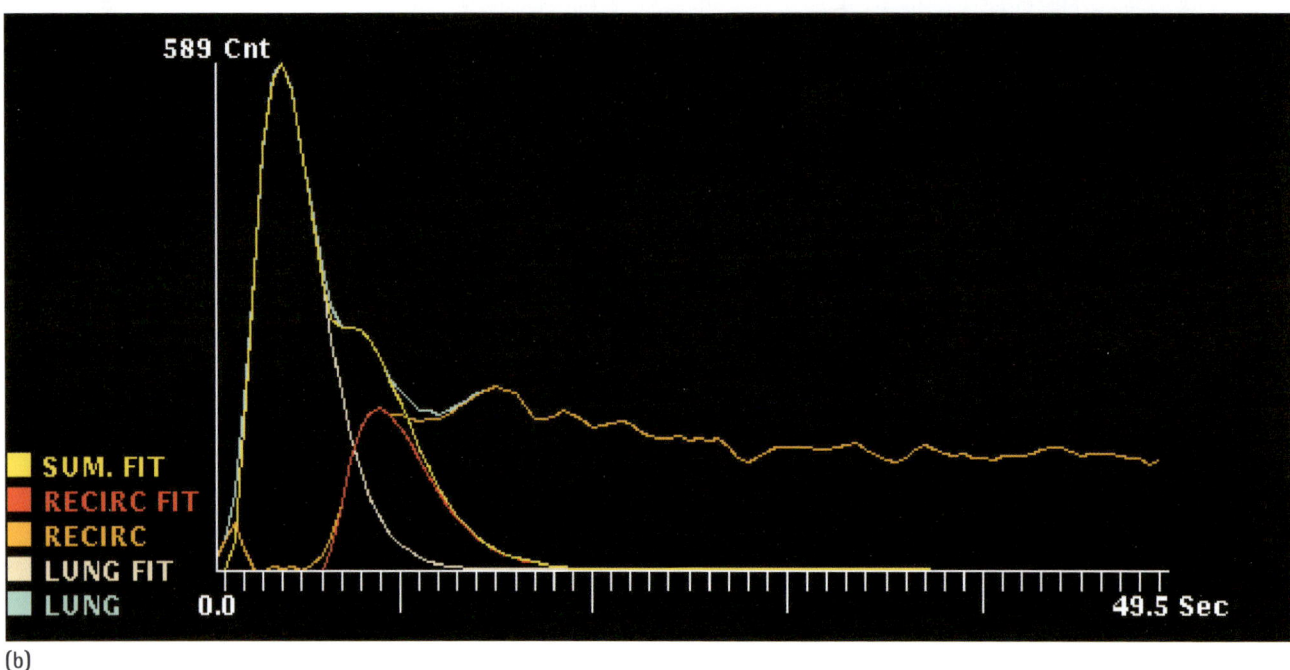

(b)

Plate 6A.22 *Shunt quantification from a first-pass study. (a) Different regions of interest. (b) Time–activity curves demonstrating delayed lung clearance with L–R shunt with a Qp:Qs ratio of 1.65:1 (Image courtesy of Dr Gary Cook, London, UK.) See page 171.*

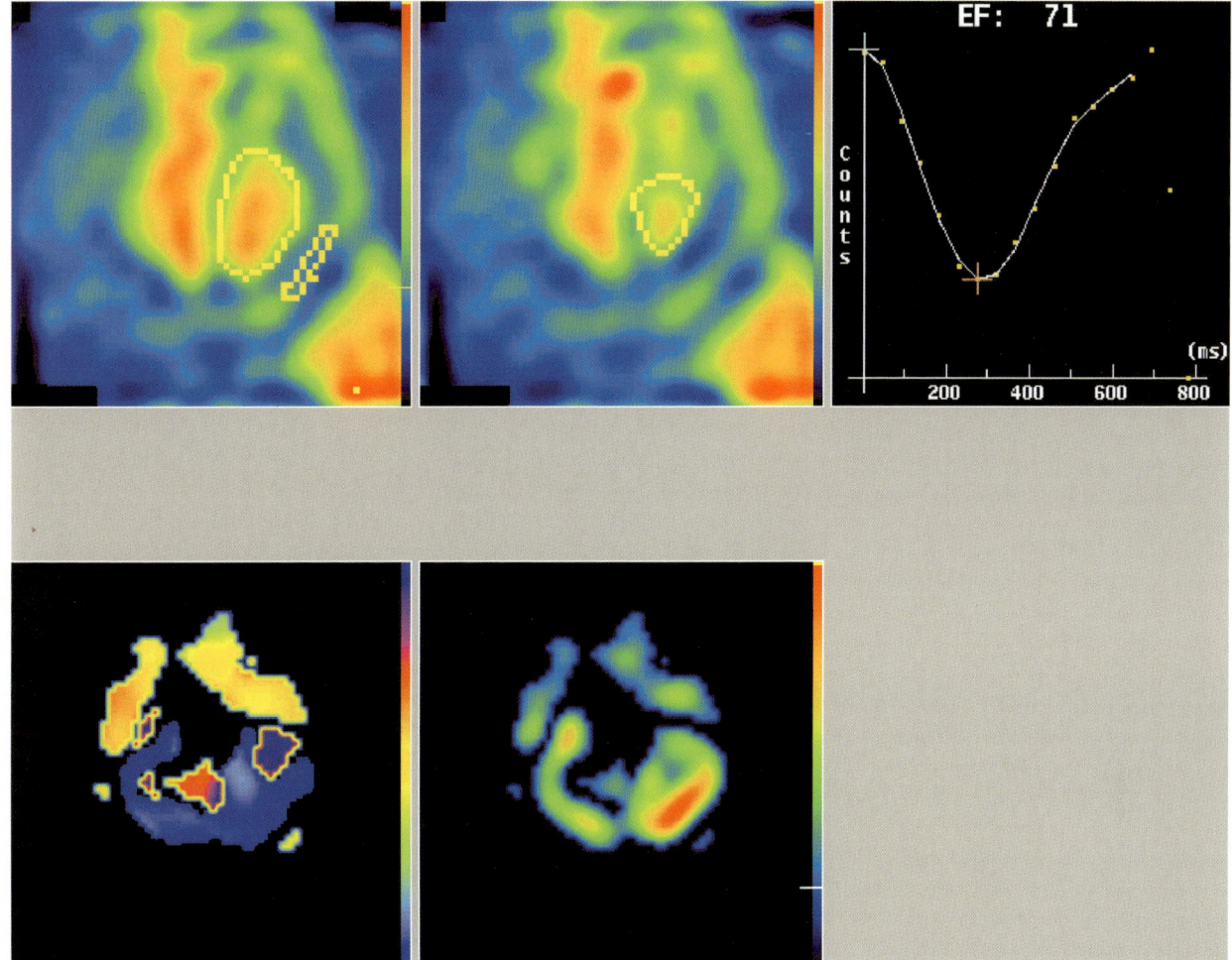

Plate 6B.1 *A normal radionuclide ventriculogram. The end diastolic (top left) and end systolic images are shown (top middle) with the regions of interest defined around the left ventricle and the background region. The phase (bottom left) and amplitude (bottom right) images are also shown. Note that the atria contract 180° out of phase with the ventricles and that there is relatively uniform contraction of the left ventricle. The count profile through the cardiac cycle is shown (top right) and the ejection fraction is 71% with the end diastolic and end systolic counts indicated by the cross-hairs. See page 184.*

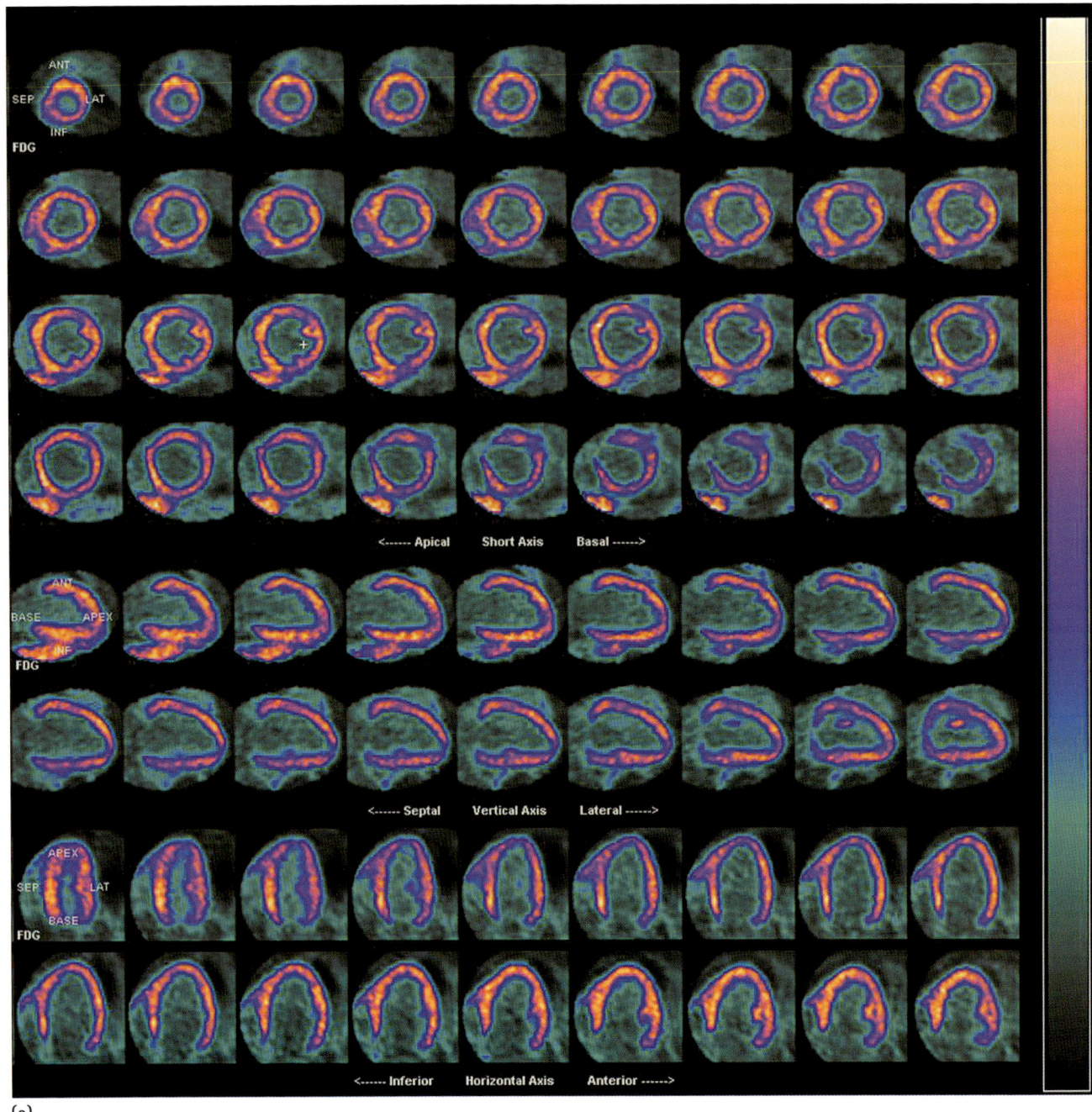

(a)

Plate 6B.2 *(a) [^13N]Anmonia (perfusion). See page 189.*

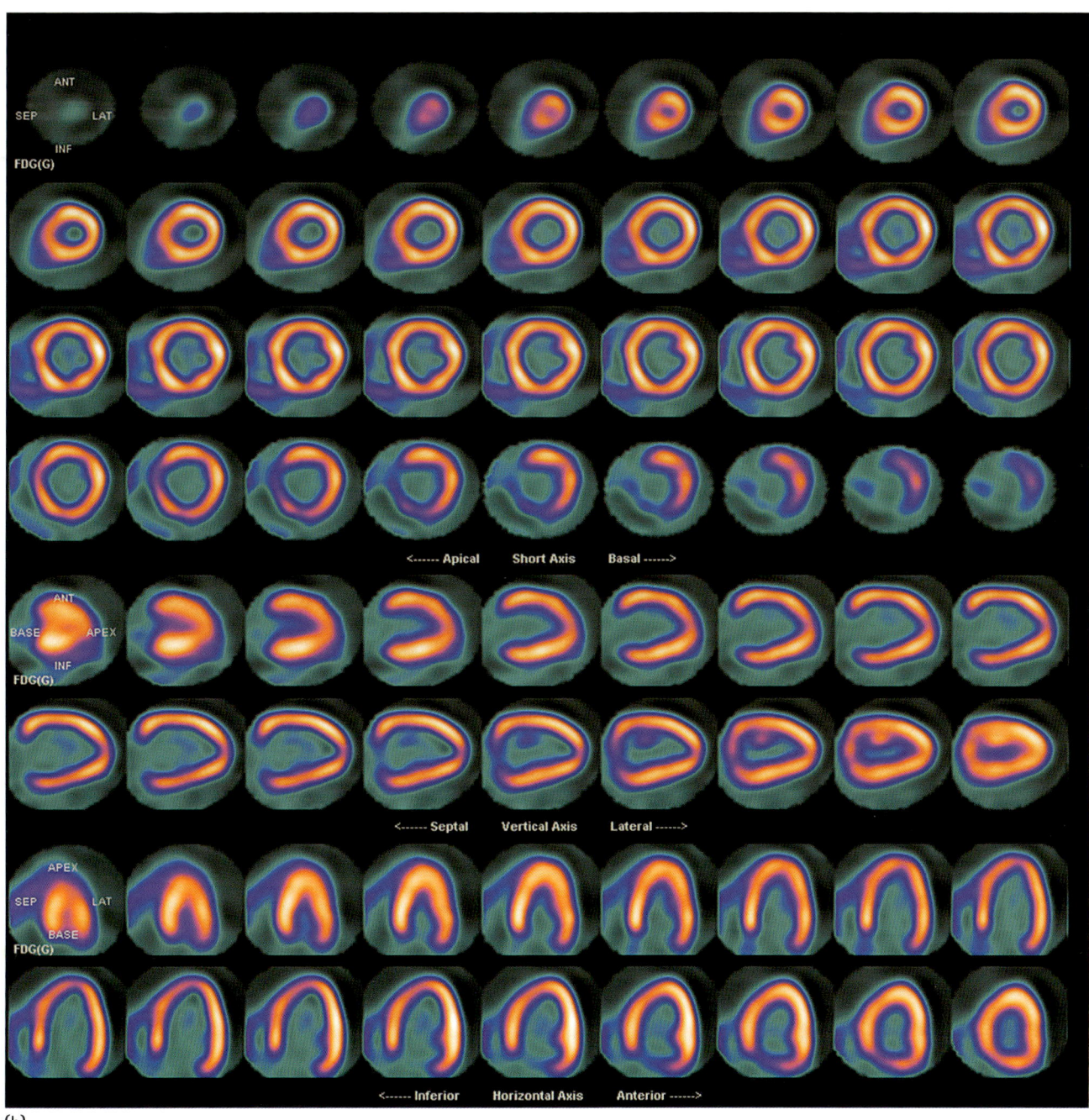

(b)

Plate 6B.2 *(Continued)* *(b)* ^{18}*FDG (metabolism). See page 189.*

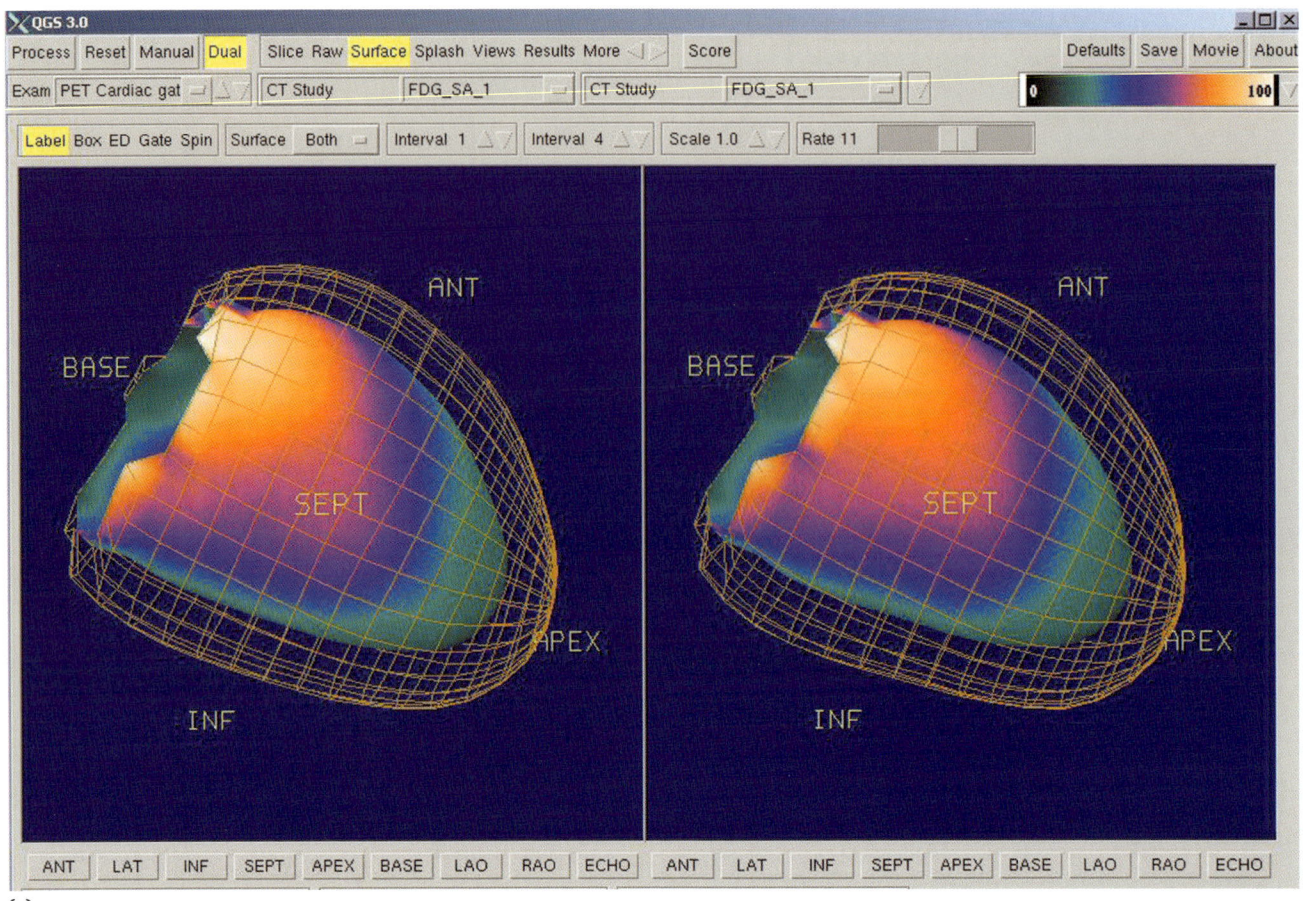

(c)

Plate 6B.2 *(Continued)* *(c) Surface views: end diastole and end systole. Endocardial (inner) and epicardial (outer) surfaces are shown. INF, inferior; ANT, anterior; SEPT, septum. See page 189.*

Apoptosis is one of the underlying pathological processes not only in heart failure, but also in acute myocardial infarction, myocarditis and acute transplant rejection.[59,60,272,273] Annexin-V can be used for noninvasive detection of apoptosis, with labeling either by ^{99m}Tc for SPECT or ^{18}F for PET imaging.[61,64]

The prevention of apoptosis (anti-apoptotis) is one potentially new and attractive future therapeutic option for treating cardiac diseases. However, it is unlikely that the prevention of apoptosis will be of benefit to full functional recovery.

THE FUTURE OF RADIONUCLIDE IMAGING

There is a substantial body of evidence in support of the clinical role of radionuclide imaging in the management of CAD, as cited in the preceding sections. Despite enthusiasm for echocardiography and MRI for the assessment of myocardial perfusion, none of these has been able to substitute radionuclide methodology completely, particularly in CAD. With the recent development of multi-slice/multi-detector CT technology, it is likely that CT coronary angiography will be integrated into clinical routine for screening intermediate- and high-risk asymptomatic patients. However, with more disease detection by coronary CT angiography, it is expected that more patients would require functional assessment of the obstructive lesions and risk stratification prior to interventional procedures and the established role of myocardial perfusion scintigraphy as 'gatekeeper' to interventional procedures would be even more imperative. Coronary CT angiography is also of limited use in very high coronary calcium scores. This particularly applies to elderly patients with expected high coronary calcium scores. In such cases, radionuclide myocardial perfusion SPECT should be the first test of choice. Therefore, if such approaches are adopted into clinical routines, the number of radionuclide procedures would increase in near future.

The myocardial perfusion and left ventricular function can also be assessed with the newer generation of multi-detector CT. However, it is unlikely that such an approach would gain wide clinical acceptance in the near future, due to lack of clinical validity. Rather, with more MR installations and experience, we may observe that part of the work of viability detection by radionuclide imaging is shared by MR imaging.

The advent of hybrid imaging techniques like PET–CT and SPECT–CT permits straightforward fusion of the two datasets. In the next few years, we will be seeing more information being gathered by such hybrid imaging techniques, redefining the clinical applications of radionuclide imaging.

The current areas of research for radionuclide imaging are assessment of endothelial dysfunction, imaging plaques, apoptosis, necrosis, hypoxia, receptor imaging and metabolic transduction pathways, each one with different clinical implications. During the last few years, there has been progress in angiogenesis and cell transplantation biology, with the ambition of making cardiac repair an achievable therapeutic option.[266–268] It is possible that in the future, stem cell transplants could become a clinical reality for regeneration of the damaged myocytes. Radionuclide imaging is the most promising methodology for evaluating the effectiveness of such therapeutic options: there is huge potential for future growth and for exploring the key mechanisms for molecular and genetic therapies.[274]

CONGENITAL HEART DISEASES

The developmental malformations and congenital heart diseases (CHDs) are the leading noninfectious cause of infant mortality (Table 6A.19). Approximately 10% of first trimester miscarriages are estimated to be due to congenital cardiac anomalies.[275] Early surgical correction of congenital heart defects reduces the future impact due to ventricular dysfunction, endocarditis, and complications secondary to cyanosis.

There is a steady rise in the number of survivors of congenital heart diseases into adult life, with or without treatment. Many of these adults, particularly from developing and under-developed countries, have not had any previous surgical correction procedure performed. Aortic valve disease, coarctation, pulmonary stenosis, atrial septal

Table 6A.19 *Major congenital heart diseases*

- *Patent ductus arteriosus: left-to-right shunt, except in Eisenmenger's syndrome*
- *Coarctation of the aorta*
- *Ventricular septal defect: most common congenital heart disease*
  - *Membranous septum: commonest*
  - *Muscular septum*
  - *Supracristal: involving outflow tracts (normally in tetralogy of Fallot)*
  - *Posterior: involving the inflow portion of the septum (AV canal)*
- *Atrial septal defects*
  - *Secundum type*
  - *Ostium primum*
  - *Sinus venosus*
- *Tetralogy of Fallot: most common cyanotic heart disease*
- *Transposition of the great vessels*
- *Ebstein's anomaly*
- *Single ventricle*
- *Persistent truncus arteriosus (with hypothyroidism and thymic aplasia)*
- *Cardiomyopathies*
- *Coronary abnormalities*

defect, and patent ductus arteriosus are the most common lesions in this group of patients.

Non-invasive imaging in congenital heart diseases

CHD requires thorough evaluation and assessment prior to any surgical repair. In long-standing cases there could be shunt reversal (Eisenmenger's syndrome) or cyanosis or volume overload leading to ventricular dysfunction. Cyanosis and under-perfusion of the lungs initiates the development of aorto-pulmonary collaterals, while long-standing increased pulmonary flow may increase pulmonary vascular resistance.

ECHOCARDIOGRAPHY AND MAGNETIC RESONANCE IMAGING

Trans-thoracic echocardiography, in general, and in a few selected cases trans-esophageal echocardiography remains the first-line imaging technique in CHD, as it mostly eliminates the need for cardiac catheterization in children. Three-dimensional reconstruction of the echocardiographic data further enhances detection of structural abnormalities. The magnitude of the shunts can also be determined quantitatively by the Qp:Qs ratio, where Qp is the pulmonary flow and Qs is the systemic flow. Color flow Doppler is not only useful for estimating septal defects, but also for valvular areas and regurgitation. Doppler is also helpful in estimation

of the Qp:Qs ratio in left-to-right shunts and residual septal defects, post-operatively.[276] Fetal cardiac imaging has opened new doors for the management of CHD.[277]

Developments in multi-sclice CT and MRI permit high-resolution noninvasive detection of anomalous coronary arteries and CHDs of complicated anatomy.[278] MR provides better functional information than CT, without any ionizing radiation, and overcomes issues of acoustic window that occur in echocardiography. Furthermore, the larger field of view of CT and MR helps to cover a wider body area in one scan, compared to echocardiography, with the ability to diagnose incidental extra-cardiac abnormalities.

RADIONUCLIDE IMAGING

The main indications/uses of radionuclide imaging in CHD are:

- Detection and quantitation of shunts
- Determination of ventricular function
- Assessment of lung ventilation and perfusion
- Assessment of myocardial perfusion

DETECTION AND QUANTITATION OF SHUNTS

First-pass radionuclide angiocardiography is a simple and rapid method for detection and quantification of shunts[279] (Table 6A.20). After the first peak of radioactivity in the lungs, a small second recirculation peak is seen, by approximately 8 s, after the tracer has passed through the systemic

Table 6A.20   *First-pass radionuclide angiography for shunt quantification*

Left-to-right shunt

Tracer	*[^{99m}Tc]pertechnetate*
Volume/activity	*Smallest possible volume (0.1 mL), with high specific activity*
Administration	*Intravenous bolus, and flush with normal saline*

Image acquisition

- *Serial images at intervals of 20–25 ms*
- *Position: anterior/RAO*
- *Total counts: 800 000 counts s^{-1} for 30–60 s*

Image analysis

- *The bolus passes from the right ventricle to the lungs and then to the left ventricle, before entering systemic circulation*
- *ROIs are drawn over bolus, RV, lungs and LV as well as background and time–activity curves are generated and pulmonary-to-systemic circulation is calculated*

Calculation of the left-to-right shunt

The pulmonary/systemic ratio (Qp/Qs) is given by A/(A − B), where A is the area under the first peak, and B is the area under the second peak

Right-to-left shunt

Tracer	*^{99m}Tc-MAA*

Calculation of the right-to-left shunt

The right-to-left shunt is given by (C$_{body}$ − C$_{lung}$)/C$_{body}$, where C$_{body}$ is the total body counts and C$_{lung}$ is the total lung counts

For left-to-right shunts, [^{99m}Tc]pertechnetate (with or without stannous chloride) is used. For right-to-left shunts ^{99m}Tc-MAA is preferred.

circulation and returned to the heart. The shunting is expressed as pulmonary-to-systemic flow ratios (Qp:Qs) (Plate 6A.21a–e).

A *left-to-right ventricular shunt* would demonstrate an early recirculation to the right heart, with early reappearance or persistence of activity in the lungs. Regions of interest drawn over the lungs, excluding the heart provide the most accurate quantification of shunt flow. Due to the shunt, the expected exponential decline in the lung counts in the curve is not seen and counts may actually increase sufficiently to cause a second curve peak. The size of the early re-circulation peak in the pulmonary time–activity curve is directly proportional to the size of the shunt. A high background activity is also demonstrated. Gamma variate function approximations over the initial and re-circulation segments of the pulmonary transit curve help in the accurate quantification of left-to-right shunts between 1.2 and 3.5:1 (Plate 6A.22 (a) and (b)).

In cases of atrial septal defects, first-pass radionuclide evaluation of left-to-right shunts is comparable to the oximetric technique.[280] The first-pass radionuclide technique is also a useful and reliable method for post-surgical follow-up in cases of ASD.

The presence of activity in the left ventricle or aorta, prior to normal lung activity is highly suggestive of the presence of a *right-to-left shunt*. Technetium-99 m MAA is preferably used. There is, however, some minimal bypass from the pulmonary vasculature (approximately 3–6%). Technetium-99 m MAA has the ability to quantify the intrapulmonary right to left shunt even after bidirectional cavopulmonary anastomosis (BCPA), occurring most likely due to sustained and inappropriate vasodilatation.

Knowledge of the degree of intrapulmonary shunting is crucial for future management. The diversion of systemic venous return to the pulmonary arteries, without a sub-pulmonary ventricle (Fontan operation) is palliative management for the most of the patients with single ventricle. The Fontan procedure may be done as a single or staged procedure and has various variations. The presence of more than a 25% shunt requires subsequent completion of the modified Fontan procedure due to increased cyanosis.[281]

DETERMINATION OF VENTRICULAR FUNCTION

Left ventricular dysfunction complicates the management of long-standing congenital heart defects and is associated with biventricular volume overload. Gated blood pool equilibrium radionuclide angiocardiography is a reproducible method for assessment of function.

In patients with ASD, gated equilibrium blood pool radionuclide angiocardiography is not only helpful in assessment of function but also in diagnosing left to right shunts. Unlike assessing pulmonary-to-systemic flow ratios (Qp:Qs) as in first pass studies, the ratio of right to left end diastolic ventricular volumes is used, demonstrating RV diastolic overload. This is assuming that LV volume and function are normal. In secundum type ASDs, the diastolic

count and stroke volume ratios show a good correlation with the oximetric technique.[282,283]

In atrial shunts, the Qp:Qs ratio is related to SCRV/SCLV (right ventricular stroke counts/left ventricular stroke counts), while in ventricular and ductal shunts it is correlated with SCLV/SCRV.[284]

Exercise-gated blood pool equilibrium radionuclide angiocardiography provides more accurate assessments of the surgical results and prognosis in children above the age of 15 years. Biventricular dysfunction is frequently present after intra-atrial repair of transposition of the great arteries.[285] Radionuclide angiography also has a high specificity in patients without severely impaired left ventricular function and a left-to-right shunt through an atrial septal defect.

Evaluation of right ventricular function is still best performed by radionuclide imaging techniques (first pass/radionuclide angiography) or MRI rather than echocardiography.

ASSESSMENT OF MYOCARDIAL PERFUSION

Anomalous origin of coronary arteries is rare, seen in 1% of patients undergoing cardiac catheterization.[286] Coronary anomalies have been implicated in chest pain, sudden death, cardiomyopathy, syncope, dyspnea, ventricular fibrillation, and myocardial infarction. Multi-slice CT and MR are capable of detecting such anatomical anomalies with ease. However, the presence of ischemia can be detected with myocardial perfusion SPECT.[287–290] Early diagnosis and surgical repair should result in a better prognosis. Gated myocardial perfusion SPECT is excellent not only for assessment of ischemic burden, but also in the evaluation of treatment response.

POSITRON EMISSION TOMOGRAPHY

The prerequisite of molecular imaging is to assess cellular and biochemical functions and PET is likely to remain a key technique. Molecular imaging with radionuclide techniques is expected to contribute substantially to basic science and research.

The Fontan procedure is one of the surgical procedures performed in many complex congenital heart diseases. After surgical repair, the coronary flow reserve and right ventricular function could still be impaired requiring further surgical interventions.[281,287,290,291] PET imaging is capable of not only detecting abnormalities of cardiac perfusion in such cases, but also various dystrophies, cardiomypathies and related arrhythmogenesis.[292,293]

Despite its unique potential, radionuclide imaging is still under-utilized in the clinical research of CHDs. With the strength of molecular imaging with PET, it is hoped that radionuclide imaging will be able to play an important role in better understanding the underlying pathogenesis of congenital disorders. However, it is unlikely that it will have any significant impact on the current clinical management options.

REFERENCES

1 Chockalingam A, Balaguer-Vintro I. (eds.) *Impending global pandemic of cardiovascular diseases: Challenges and opportunities for the prevention and control of cardiovascular diseases in developing countries and economies in transition*. World Heart Federation White Book. Barcelona, Spain: Prous Science, 1999.

2 UK Department of Health. Indicators of the nation's health: male death rates by selected causes. Available at http://www.performance.doh.gov.uk/hpsss/tbl_a3.htm.

3 Kochanek KD, Smith BL. *Deaths: Preliminary data for 2002*. National vital statistics reports number 52(13). Hyattsville, Maryland: National Center for Health Statistics, 2004. Available at http://www.cdc.gov/nchs/data/nvsr/nvsr52/nvsr52_13.pdf

4 Yusuf S, Reddy S, Ounpuu S, *et al.* Global burden of cardiovascular diseases part II: Variations in cardiovascular disease by specific ethnic groups and geographic regions and prevention strategies. *Circulation* 2001; **104**: 2855.

5 Reddy KS. Cardiovascular disease in the non-western countries. *N Engl J Med* 2004; **350**: 2438–40.

6 Galasko GIW, Senior R, Lahiri A. Ethnic differences in the prevalence and aetiology of left ventricular systolic dysfunction in the community: the Harrow heart failure watch. *Heart* 2005; **91**: 595–600.

7 Maynard C, Fosher LD, Passamani ER, *et al.* Blacks in the Coronary Artery Surgery Study: risk factors and coronary artery disease. *Circulation* 1986; **74**: 64–71.

8 Enas EA. Lipoprotein (a) is an important genetic risk factor for premature coronary artery disease in Asian Indians. *Am J Cardiol* 2001; **88**: 201–20.

9 Manolio T. Novel risk markers and clinical practice. *N Engl J Med* 2003; **349**: 1587–9.

10 Myers RH, Kiely DK, Cupples LA, Kannel WB. Parental history is an independent risk factor for coronary artery disease: the Framingham Study. *Am Heart J* 1990; **120**: 963–9.

11 Yusuf S, Hawken S, Ounpuu S, *et al.* (The INTERHEART Study investigators). Effect of potentially modifiable risk factors associated with myocardial infarction in 52 countries (the INTERHEART study): case–control study. *Lancet* 2004; **364**: 937–52.

12 Danesh J, Whincup P, Walker M, *et al.* Low grade inflammation and coronary heart disease: prospective study and updated meta-analyses. *Br Med J* 2000; **321**: 199–204.

13 Danesh J, Wheeler JG, Hirschfield GM, *et al.* C-reactive protein and other circulating markers of inflammation in the prediction of coronary heart disease. *N Engl J Med* 2004; **350**: 1387–97.

14 Nissen SE, Tuzcu EM, Schoenhagen P, *et al.* Statin therapy, LDL cholesterol, C-reactive protein, and coronary artery disease. *N Engl J Med* 2005; **352**: 29–38.

15 Blumgart HC, Weiss S. Studies on the velocity of blood flow, VII: the pulmonary circulation times in normal resting individuals. *Clin Inv* 1927; **4**: 399–425.

16 Mason DT, Ashburn WL, Harbert JC, *et al.* Rapid sequential visualization of the heart and great vessels in man using the wide-field Anger scintillation camera. Radioisotope angiography following the injection of technetium-99 m. *Circulation* 1969; **39**: 19–28.

17 Gibbons RJ, Lee KL, Pryor D, *et al.* The use of radionuclide angiography in the diagnosis of coronary artery disease. *Circulation* 1983; **68**: 740–6.

18 Lebowitz E, Greene MW, Fairchild R, *et al.* Thallium-201 for medical use. I. *J Nucl Med* 1975; **16**: 151–5.

19 Phost GM. Differentiation of transiently ichaemic from infracted myocardium by serial imaging after a single dose of thallium-201. *Circulation* 1977; **55**: 294–302.

20 Verani MS, Marcus ML, Razzak MA, *et al.* Sensitivity and specificity of thallium-201 perfusion scintigram under exercise in the diagnosis of coronary artery disease. *J Nucl Med* 1978; **19**: 773–82.

21 Tamaki N, Yonekura Y, Mukai T, *et al.* Stress thallium-201 transaxial emission computed tomography: quantitative versus qualitative analysis for evaluation of coronary artery disease. *J Am Coll Cardiol* 1984; **4**: 1213–21.

22 Fintel DJ, Links JM, Brinker JA, *et al.* Improved diagnostic performance of exercise thallium-201 single photon emission tomography over planar imaging in the diagnosis of coronary artery disease: a receiver operating characteristic analysis. *J Am Coll Cardiol* 1989; **13**: 600–12.

23 Beller GA. Myocardial perfusion imaging with thallium-201. *J Nucl Med* 1994; **35**: 674–80.

24 Beller GA, Watson DD. Physiological basis of myocardial perfusion imaging with the technetium-99 m agents. *Semin Nucl Med* 1991; **21**: 173–81.

25 Leppo JA, DePuey EG, Johnson LL. A review of cardiac imaging with sestamibi and teboroxime. *J Nucl Med* 1991; **32**: 2012–22.

26 Chua T, Kiat H, Germano G, *et al.* Rapid back to back adenosine stress–rest Tc-99 m teboroxime myocardial perfusion SPECT using a triple-detector camera. *J Nucl Med* 1993; **34**: 1485–93.

27 Gerson MC, Lukes J, Deutsch E, *et al.* Comparison of technetium 99 m Q12 and thallium for detection of angiographically documented coronary artery disease in humans. *J Nucl Cardiol* 1994; **1**: 499 (Abstract).

28 Mahmood S, Bomanji J, Ayub M, *et al.* Tc-99 m furifosmin (Q12) myocardial perfusion SPECT in the detection of coronary artery disease. *J Nucl Cardiol* 1997; **4(suppl 2)**: S45 (Abstract).

29 Vanzetto G, Fagret D, Ghezzi C. Tc-99 m N-NOET: chronicle of a unique perfusion imaging agent and a missed opportunity? *J Nucl Cardiol* 2004; **11**: 647–50.

30 Wackers FJTh, Berman DS, Maddahi J, *et al.* Technetium 99 m hexakis 2-methoxyisobutyl isonitrile: human biodistribution, dosimetry, safety and preliminary comparison to thallium-201 for myocardial perfusion imaging. *J Nucl Med* 1989; **30**: 301–11.

31 Berman DS, Kiat H, Van Train KF, *et al.* Comparison of SPECT using technetium-99 m agents and thallium-201 and PET for the assessment of myocardial perfusion and viability. *Am J Cardiol* 1990; **66**: 72E–9E.

32 Maddahi J, Kiat H, Van Train KF, *et al.* Myocardial perfusion imaging with technetium-99 m sestamibi SPECT in the evaluation of coronary artery disease. *Am J Cardiol* 1990; **66**: 55E–62E .

33 Sochor H. Technetium-99 m sestamibi in chronic coronary artery disease: the European experience. *Am J Cardiol* 1990; **66**: 91E–6E.

34 Kelly JD, Forster AM, Higley B, *et al.* Technetium-99 m tetrofosmin as a new radiopharmaceutical for myocardial perfusion imaging. *J Nucl Med* 1993; **34**: 222–7.

35 Shanoudy H, Raggi P, Beller GA, *et al.* Comparison of technetium-99 m tetrofosmin and thallium-201 single-photon emission computed tomographic imaging for detection of myocardial perfusion defects in patients with coronary artery disease. *J Am Coll Cardiol* 1998; **32**: 331–7.

36 Kapur A, Latus KA, Davies G, *et al.* A comparison of three radionuclide myocardial perfusion tracers in clinical practice: the ROBUST study. *Eur J Nucl Med Mol Imaging* 2002; **29**: 1608–16.

37 Mahmood S, Gunning M, Bomanji JB, *et al.* Combined rest thallium201/stress techneium-99 m tetrofosmin SPECT: feasibility and diagnostic accuracy of a 90-minute protocol. *J Nucl Med* 1995; **36**: 932–5.

38 Hatada K, Riou LM, Ruiz M, *et al.* Tc-99 m N-DBODC5, a new myocardial perfusion imaging agent with rapid liver clearance: comparison with Tc-99 m sestamibi and Tc-99 m tetrofosmin in rats. *J Nucl Med* 2004; **45**: 2095–101.

39 Selwyn AP, Allan RM, L'Abbate A, *et al.* Relation between regional myocardial uptake of rubidium-82 and perfusion: absolute reduction of cation uptake in ischemia. *Am J Cardiol* 1982; **50**: 112–21.

40 Schelbert HR, Phelps ME, Huang SC, *et al.* N-13 ammonia as an indicator of myocardial blood flow. *Circulation* 1981; **63**: 1259–72.

41 Yonekura Y, Tamaki N, Senda M, *et al.* Detection of coronary artery disease with ^{13}N-ammonia and high-resolution positron emission tomography. *Am Heart J* 1987; **113**: 645–54.

42 Tamaki N, Yonekura Y, Senda M, *et al.* Value and limitation of stress thallium-201 single photon emission computed tomography: comparison with nitrogen-13 ammonia positron tomography. *J Nucl Med* 1988; **29**: 1181–8.

43 Khorsand A, Graf S, Eidherr H, *et al.* Gated cardiac N-13 NH$_3$ PET for assessment of left ventricular volumes, mass, and ejection fraction: comparison with electrocardiography gated ^{18}F-FDG PET. *J Nucl Med* 2005; **46**: 2009–13.

44 Bergmann SR, Fox KAA, Rand AL, *et al.* Quantification of regional myocardial blood flow in vivo with O-15 water. *Circulation* 1984; **70**: 724–33.

45 Opie LH. Fuels: aerobic and anaerobic metabolism. In: Opie LH. (ed.) *The heart. Physiology, from cell to circulation.* Philadelphia, PA: Lippincott-Raven, 1998: 295.

46 Gambhir SS, Schwaiger M, Huang SC, *et al.* Simple noninvasive quantification method for measuring myocardial glucose utilization in humans employing positron emission tomography and fluorine-18 deoxyglucose. *J Nucl Med* 1989; **30**: 359–66.

47 Mäki M, Luotolahti M, Nuutila P, *et al.* Glucose uptake in the chronically dysfunctioning but viable myocardium. *Circulation* 1996; **93**: 1658–66.

48 Ghesani M, Depuey EG, Rozanski A. Role of F-18 FDG positron emission tomography (PET) in the assessment of myocardial viability. *Echocardiography* 2005; **22**: 165–77.

49 Bergmann SR, Weinheimer CJ, Markham J, *et al.* Quantitation of myocardial fatty acid metabolism using PET. *J Nucl Med* 1996; **37**: 1723–30.

50 Brown M, Marshall DR, Sobel BE, *et al.* Delineation of myocardial oxygen utilization with carbon-11-labeled acetate. *Circulation* 1987; **3**: 687–96.

51 Schulz G, von Dahl J, Kaiser HJ, *et al.* Imaging of beta-oxidation by static PET with 14(R,S)-[^{18}F]fluoro-6-thiaheptadecanoic acid (FTHA) in patients with advanced coronary heart disease: a comparison with [18]FDG-PET and [99]Tc[m]-MIBI SPET. *Nucl Med Commun* 1996; **17**: 1057–64.

52 Yazaki Y, Isobe M, Takahashi W, *et al.* Assessment of myocardial fatty acid metabolic abnormalities in patients with idiopathic dilated cardiomyopathy using I-123 BMIPP SPECT: correlation with clinicopathological findings and clinical course. *Heart* 1999; **81**: 153–9.

53 Carrió I. Cardiac neurotransmission imaging. *J Nucl Med* 2001; **42**: 1062–76.

54 Gamici PG. Positron emission tomography and myocardial imaging. *Heart* 2000; **83**: 473–80.

55 Berridge MS, Nelson AD, Zheng L, *et al.* Specific beta-adrenergic receptor binding of carazolol measured with PET. *J Nucl Med* 1994; **35**: 1665–76.

56 McGhie AI, Corbett JR, Akers MS, *et al.* Regional cardiac adrenergic function using I-123 meta-iodobenzylguanidine tomographic imaging after acute myocardial infarction. *Am J Cardiol* 1991; **67**: 236–42.

57 Nakata T, Nagao K, Tsuchihashi K, *et al.* Regional cardiac sympathetic nerve dysfunction and the diagnostic efficacy of metaiodobenzylguanidine tomography in stable coronary artery disease. *Am J Cardiol* 1996; **78**: 292–7.

58 Hartikainen J, Mä ntysaari M, Kuikka J, *et al.* Extent of cardiac autonomic denervation in relation to angina

on exercise test in patients with recent acute myocardial infarction. *Am J Cardiol* 1994; **74**: 760–3.

59 Fisher SA, Langille BL, Srivastava D. Apoptosis during cardiovascular development. *Circ Res* 2000; **87**: 856–64.

60 Colucci WS. Apoptosis in heart. *N Engl J Med* 1996; **335**: 1224–6.

61 Kolodgie FD, Petrov A, Virmani R, *et al.* Targeting of apoptotic macrophages and experimental atheroma with radiolabeled annexin V: a technique with potential for noninvasive imaging of vulnerable plaque. *Circulation* 2003; **108**: 3134–9.

62 Flotats A, Carrió I. Non-invasive in vivo imaging of myocardial apoptosis and necrosis. *Eur J Nucl Med Mol Imaging* 2003; **30**: 615–30.

63 Narula J, Kietselaer B, Hofstra L. Role of molecular imaging in defining and denying death. *J Nucl Cardiol* 2004; **11**: 349–57.

64 Murakami Y, Takamatsu H, Taki J, *et al.* ^{18}F-labelled annexin V: a PET tracer for apoptosis imaging. *Eur J Nucl Med Mol Imaging* 2004; **31**: 469–74.

65 Yasuda T, Palacios IF, Dec GW, *et al.* Indium 111-monoclonal antimyosin antibody imaging in the diagnosis of acute myocarditis. *Circulation* 1987; **76**: 306–11.

66 Hesse B, Mortensen SA, Folke M, *et al.* Ability of antimyosin scintigraphy monitoring to exclude acute rejection during the first year after heart transplantation. *J Heart Lung Transplant* 1995; **14**: 23–31.

67 Beanlanders RSB, Ruddy TD, Bielawski L, *et al.* Differentiation of myocardial ischemia and necrosis by technetium-99 m-glucaric acid kinetics. *J Nucl Cardiol* 1997; **4**: 274–82.

68 Mariani G, Villa B, Bossettin PF, *et al.* Detection of acute myocardial infarction by ^{99m}Tc-labeled D-glucaric acid imaging in patients with acute chest pain. *J Nucl Med* 1999; **40**: 1832–9.

69 Martin GV, Caldwell JH, Graham MM, *et al.* Noninvasive detection of hypoxic myocardium using fluorine-18-fluoromisonidazole and positron emission tomography. *J Nucl Med* 1992; **33**: 2202–8.

70 Ng CK, Sinusas AJ, Zaret B, *et al.* Kinetic analysis of technetium-99 m-labeled nitroimidazole (BMS181321) as a tracer of myocardial hypoxia. *Circulation* 1995; **92**: 1261–8.

71 Okada RD, Johnson G, Nguyen KN, *et al.* Tc-99 m HL91 'hot spot' detection of ischemic myocardium *in vivo* by gamma camera imaging. *Circulation* 1998; **97**: 2557–66.

72 Froelicher VF, Fearon WF, Ferguson CM, *et al.* Lessons learned from studies of the standard exercise ECG test. *Chest* 1999; **116**: 1442–51.

73 Miranda CP, Lehmann KG, Froelicher VF. Correlation between resting ST segment depression, exercise testing, coronary angiography, and long-term prognosis. *Am Heart J* 1991; **122**: 1617–28.

74 Iskandrian AS, Heo J, Kong B, *et al.* Effects of exercise level on the ability of thallium-201 tomographic imaging in detecting coronary artery disease: analysis of 461 patients. *J Am Coll Cardiol* 1989; **14**: 1477–86.

75 Nguyen T, Heo J, Ogilby JD, *et al.* Single-photon emission computed tomography with thallium-201 during adenosine-induced coronary hyperemia: correlation with coronary arteriography, exercise thallium imaging, and two-dimensional echocardiography. *J Am Coll Cardiol* 1990; **16**: 1375–83.

76 Verani MS, Mahmarian JJ, Hixson JB, *et al.* Diagnosis of coronary artery disease by controlled coronary vasodilation with adenosine and thallium-201 scintigraphy in patients unable to exercise. *Circulation* 1990; **82**: 80–7.

77 Miyagawa M, Kumano S, Sekiya M, *et al.* Thallium-201 myocardial tomography with intravenous infusion of adenosine triphosphate in diagnosis of coronary artery disease. *J Am Coll Cardiol* 1995; **26**: 1196–201.

78 Pearlman JD, Boucher CA. Diagnostic value for coronary artery disease of chest pain during dipyridamole–thallium stress testing. *Am J Cardiol* 1988; **61**: 43–5.

79 Wilson RF, Wyche K, Christensen BV, *et al.* Effects of adenosine on human coronary arterial circulation. *Circulation* 1990; **82**: 1595–606.

80 Cerqueira MD, Verani MS, Schwaiger M, *et al.* Safety profile of adenosine stress perfusion imaging: results from the Adenoscan Multicenter Trial Registry. *J Am Coll Cardiol* 1994; **23**: 384–9.

81 Pennell DJ, Mahmood S, Ell PJ, *et al.* Bradycardia progressing to cardiac arrest during adenosine thallium myocardial perfusion imaging in occult sino-atrial disease. *Eur J Nucl Med* 1994; **21**: 170–2.

82 Knabb RM, Gidday JM, Ely SW, *et al.* Effects of dipyridamole on myocardial adenosine and active hyperemia. *Am J Physiol* 1984; **247**: H804–10.

83 Lette J, Tatum JL, Fraser S, *et al.* Safety of dipyridamole testing in 73,806 patients: the Multicenter Dipyridamole Safety Study. *J Nucl Cardiol* 1995; **2**: 3–17.

84 Lagerqvist B, Sylven C, Waldenstrom A. Lower threshold for adenosine-induced chest pain in patients with angina and normal coronary angiograms. *Br Heart J* 1992; **68**: 282–5.

85 Walker PR, James MA, Wilde R, *et al.* Dipyridamole combined with exercise for thallium-201 myocardial imaging. *Br Heart J* 1986; **55**: 321–9.

86 Hall ML, Mahmood S, Ell PJ. Safety of combined dipyridamole–exercise thallium-201 myocardial perfusion scintigraphy. *Nucl Med Commun* 1992; **13**: 217 (Abstract).

87 Thomas G, Prill N, Majumdar H, *et al.* Treadmill exercise during the adenosine infusion is safe, results in fewer adverse reactions and improves myocardial image quality. *J Nucl Cardiol* 2000; **7**: 439–46.

88 Holly TA, Satran A, Bromet DS, *et al.* The impact of adjunctive adenosine infusion duiring exercise myocardial perfusion imaging: results of the Both Exercise and Adenosine Stress Test (BEAST) trial. *J Nucl Cardiol* 2003; **10**: 291–6.

89 Mahmood S, Gupta NK, Gunning M, *et al.* Tl-201 myocardial perfusion SPET: adenosine alone or combined with dynamic exercise. *Nucl Med Commun* 1994; **15**: 586–92.

90 Vitola JV, Brambatti JC, Caligaris F, *et al.* Exercise supplementation to dipyridamole prevents hypotension, improves electrocardiogram sensitivity and increases heart to liver activity ratio on Tc-99 m sestamibi imaging. *J Nucl Cardiol* 2001; **8**: 652–9.

91 Thomas GS, Miyamoto MI, Morello AP, *et al.* Technetium-99 m based myocardial perfusion imaging predicts clinical outcome in the community outpatient setting: the Nuclear Utility in the Community (NUC) study. *J Am Coll Cardiol* 2004; **43**: 213–23.

92 Mason JR, Palac RT, Freeman ML, *et al.* Thallium scintigraphy during dobutamine infusion: nonexercise-dependent screening test for coronary disease. *Am Heart J* 1984; **107**: 481–5.

93 Pennell DJ, Underwood SR, Swanton RH, *et al.* Dobutamine thallium myocardial perfusion tomography. *J Am Coll Cardiol* 1991; **18**: 1471–9.

94 Geleijnse ML, Elhendy A, Fioretti PM, *et al.* Dobutamine stress myocardial perfusion imaging. *J Am Coll Cardiol* 2000; **36**: 2017–27.

95 Pennell DJ, Underwood SR, Ell PJ. Safety of dobutamine stress for thallium-201 myocardial perfusion tomography in patients with asthma. *Am J Cardiol* 1993; **71**: 1346–50.

96 Dakik HA, Vempathy H, Verani MS. Tolerance, hemodynamic changes, and safety of dobutamine stress perfusion imaging. *J Nucl Cardiol* 1996; **3**: 410–4.

97 Kiat H, Iskandrian AS, Villegas BJ, *et al.* Arbutamine stress thallium-201 single-photon emission computed tomography using a computerized closed-loop delivery system. Multicenter trial for evaluation of safety and diagnostic accuracy. The International Arbutamine Study Group. *J Am Coll Cardiol* 1995; **26**: 1159–67.

98 Pennell DJ. Pharmacological cardiac stress: when and how? *Nucl Med Commun* 1994; **15**: 578–85 (Review).

99 Tak T, Gutierrez R. Comparing stress testing methods: available techniques and their use in CAD evaluation. *Postgrad Med* 2004; **115**: 61–70.

100 Thomas GS, Miyamoto MI. Should simultaneous exercise become the standard for adenosine myocardial perfusion imaging? *Am J Cardiol* 2004; **94**: 3D–10D.

101 Abidov A, Germano G, Hachamovith R, Berman DS. Gated SPECT in assessment of regional and global left ventricular function: a major tool of modern nuclear imaging. *J Nucl Cardiol* 2006; **13**: 261–79.

102 Heller GV. Gated SPECT imaging: increasing the armamentarium of nuclear cardiology. *J Nucl Cardiol* 1998; **5**: 442–4.

103 Germano G, Nichols K, Cullom SJ. Gated perfusion SPECT: technical considerations. In: DePuey EG, Garcia EV, Berman DS. (eds.) *Cardiac SPECT imaging*, second edition. Philadelphia, PA: Lippincott Williams and Wilkins, 2001: 103–15.

104 Johnson LL, Verdesca SA, Aude WY, *et al.* Postischemic stunning can affect left ventricular ejection fraction and regional wall motion on post-stress gated sestamibi tomograms. *J Am Coll Cardiol* 1997; **30**: 1641–8.

105 Mut F, Beretta M, Núñez M, *et al.* Does post-stress gated perfusion SPECT reflect stunned myocardium in patients undergoing ischemic stress test? *J Nucl Cardiol* 1999; **6**: S68.

106 Paul KA, Nabi HA. Gated myocardial perfusion SPECT: basic principles, technical aspects, and clinical applications. *J Nucl Med Technol* 2004; **32**: 179–87.

107 Nichols K, Yao SS, Kamran M, *et al.* Clinical impact of arrhythmias on gated SPECT cardiac myocardial perfusion and function assessment. *J Nucl Cardiol* 2001; **8**: 19–30.

108 Hendel RC, Corbett JR, Cullom SJ, *et al.* The value and practice of attenuation correction for myocardial perfusion SPECT imaging: a joint position statement from the American Society of Nuclear Cardiology and the Society of Nuclear Medicine. *J Nucl Cardiol* 2002; **9**: 135–43.

109 Ohnishi H, Ota T, Takada M, *et al.* Two optimal prefilter cutoff frequencies needed for SPECT images of myocardial perfusion in a one-day protocol. *J Nucl Med Technol* 1997; **25**: 256.

110 Wheat JM, Currie GM. QGS ejection fraction reproducibility in gated SPECT comparing pre-filtered and post-filtered reconstruction. *Nucl Med Commun* 2006; **27**: 57–9.

111 Lum DP, Coel MN. Comparison of automatic quantification software for the measurement of ventricular volume and ejection fraction in gated myocardial perfusion SPECT. *Nucl Med Commun* 2003; **24**: 259–66.

112 Nakajima K, Higuchi T, Taki J, *et al.* Accuracy of ventricular volume and ejection fraction measured by gated myocardial SPECT: comparison of 4 software programs. *J Nucl Med* 2001; **42**: 1571–8.

113 Santana CA, Garcia EV, Folks R, *et al.* Comparison of left ventricular function between two programs: QGS and Emory Cardiac Toolbox (ECTb). *J Nucl Med* 2001; **42**: 166P.

114 Nichols K, Santana CA, Folks R, *et al.* Comparison between ECTb and QGS for assessment of left

ventricular function from gated myocardial perfusion SPECT. *J Nucl Cardiol* 2002; **9**: 285–93.

115   Prvulovich EM, Jarritt PH, Vivian GC, *et al.* Quality assurance in myocardial perfusion tomography: a collaborative BNCS/BNMS audit programme. British Nuclear Cardiology Society/British Nuclear Medicine Society. *Nucl Med Commun* 1998; **19**: 831–8.

116   Mahmood S, Buscombe JR, Ell PJ. The use of thallium-201 lung/heart ratios. *Eur J Nucl Med* 1992; **19**: 807–14.

117   Morton KA, Alzaraki NP, Taylor AT, *et al.* SPECT thallium-201 scintigraphy for the detection of left-ventricular aneurysm. *J Nucl Med* 1987 **28**: 168–72.

118   Cerqueira MD, Weisaman NJ, Dilsizian V, *et al.* Standardized myocardial segmentation and nomenclature for tomographic imaging of the heart: a statement for healthcare professionals from the Cardiac Imaging Committee of the Council on Clinical Cardiology of the American Heart Association. *Circulation* 2002; **105**: 539–42.

119   Pace L, Cuocolo A, Maurea S, *et al.* Reverse redistribution in resting thallium-201 myocardial scintigraphy in patients with coronary artery disease: relation to coronary anatomy and ventricular function. *J Nucl Med* 1993; **34**: 1688–94.

120   Chatziioannou SN, Moore WH, Dhekne RD, *et al.* Gating of myocardial perfusion imaging for the identification of artifacts: is it useful for experienced physicians? *Texas Heart Inst J* 2000; **27**: 14–18.

121   Lee KL, Pryor DB, Pieper KS, *et al.* Prognostic value of radionuclide angiography in medically treated patients with coronary artery disease. *Circulation* 1990; **82**: 1705–17.

122   Beller GA, Zaret BL. Contributions of nuclear cardiology to diagnosis and prognosis of patients with CAD. *Circulation* 2000: **101**: 1465–78.

123   Beller GA. First Annual Mario S Verani Memorial Lecture: Clinical value of myocardial perfusion imaging in coronary artery disease. *J Nucl Cardiol* 2003; **10**: 529–42.

124   Underwood SR, Anagnostopoulos C, Cerqueira M, *et al.* Myocardial perfusion scintigraphy: the evidence consensus conference organised by the British Cardiac Society, the British Nuclear Cardiology Society and the British Nuclear Medicine Society, endorsed by the Royal College of Physicians of London and the Royal College of Radiologists. *Eur J Nucl Med Mol Imaging* 2003; **31**: 261–91.

125   Rehn T, Griffith LS, Achuff SC, *et al.* Exercise thallium-201 myocardial imaging in left main coronary artery disease: sensitive but not specific. *Am J Cardiol* 1981; **48**: 217–23.

126   Gould KL. PET perfusion imaging and nuclear cardiology. *J Nucl Med* 1991; **32**: 579–606.

127   Masood Y, Liu YH, Depuey G, *et al.* Clinical validation of SPECT attenuation correction using x-ray computed tomography-derived attenuation maps: multicenter clinical trial with angiographic correlation. *J Nucl Cardiol* 2005; **12**: 676–86.

128   Hendel RC, Corbett JR, Cullom SJ, *et al.* The value and practice of attenuation correction for myocardial perfusion SPECT imaging: a joint position statement from the American Society of Nuclear Cardiology and Society of Nuclear Medicine. *J Nucl Cardiol* 2002; **9**: 135–43.

129   Epstein SE, Quyumi A, Bonow RO. Sudden cardiac death without warning: possible mechanisms and implications for screening asymptomatic populations. *N Engl J Med* 1989; **321**: 320–3.

130   Bhatt DL, Roe MT, Peterson ED, *et al.* Utilization of early invasive management strategies for high-risk patients with non-ST-segment elevation acute coronary syndromes: results from the CRUSADE Quality Improvement Initiative. *JAMA* 2004; **292**: 2096–104.

131   Hachamovitch R, Hayes SW, Friedman JD, *et al.* Stress myocardial perfusion SPECT is clinically effective and cost-effective in risk-stratification of patients with a high likelihood of CAD but no known CAD. *J Am Coll Cardiol* 2004; **43**: 200–8.

132   Poornima IG, Miller TD, Christian TF. Utility of myocardial perfusion imaging in patients with low-risk treadmill scores. *J Am Coll Cardiol* 2004; **43**: 194–9.

133   Jeetley P, Hickman M, Kamp O, *et al.* Myocardial contrast echocardiography for the detection of coronary artery stenosis: a prospective multicenter study in comparison with single-photon emission computed tomography. *J Am Coll Cardiol* 2006; **47**: 141–5.

134   Kondos GT, Hoff JA, Sevrukov A. Electron-beam tomography coronary artery calcium and cardiac events: a 37-month follow-up of 5635 initially asymptomatic low- to intermediate-risk adults. *Circulation* 2003; **107**: 2571–6.

135   Hoffmann MHK, Shi H, Schmitz BL, *et al.* Non-inasive coronary angiography with multislice computed tomography. *JAMA* 2005; **293**: 2471–8.

136   Blumenthal RS, Becker DM, Yanek LR, *et al.* Comparison of coronary calcium and stress myocardial perfusion imaging in apparently healthy siblings of individuals with premature coronary artery disease. *Am J Cardiol* 2006; **97**: 328–33.

137   Thompson RC, McGhie AI, Moser KW, *et al.* Clinical utility of coronary calcium scoring after non-ischemic myocardial perfusion imaging. *J Nucl Cardiol* 2005; **12**: 392–400.

138   Rodes-Cabau J, Candell-Riera J, Angel J, *et al.* Relation of myocardial perfusion defects and non-significant coronary lesions by angiography with insights from intravascular ultrasound and coronary pressure measurements. *Am J Cardiol* 2005; **96**: 1621–6.

139   Gracia M J. Non-invasive coronary angiography. Hype or new paradigm? *JAMA* 2005; **293**: 75–8, 2531–3.

140 Leschka S, Alkadhi H, Plass A, *et al*. Accuracy of MSCT coronary angiography with 64-slice technology: first experience. *Eur Heart J* 2005; **6**: 1482–7.

141 Berman DS, Hachamovitch R, Shaw LJ, *et al*. Roles of nuclear cardiology, cardiac computed tomography, and cardiac magnetic resonance: assessment of patients with suspected coronary artery disease. *J Nucl Med* 2006; **47**: 74–82.

142 Sommer T, Hackenbroch M, Hofer U, *et al*. Coronary MR angiography at 3.0 T versus that at 1.5 T: initial results in patients suspected of having coronary artery disease. *Radiology* 2005; **234**: 718–25.

143 Prasad SK, Assomull RG, Pennell DJ. Recent developments in non-invasive cardiology. *Br Med J* 2004; **329**: 1386–9.

144 Beltrame JF. Advances in understanding the mechanisms of angina pectoris in cardiac syndrome X. *Eur Heart J* 2005; **26**; 946–8.

145 Fragasso G, Rossetti E, Dosio F, *et al*. High prevalence of the thallium-201 reverse redistribution phenomenon in patients with syndrome X. *Eur Heart J* 1996; **17**: 1482–7.

146 Kawai Y, Tsukamoto E, Nzaki Y, *et al*. Significance of reduced uptake of iodinated fatty acid analogues for the evaluation of patients with acute chest pain. *J Am Coll Cardiol* 2001; **38**: 1888–94.

147 Libby P. Current concepts of the pathogenesis of the acute coronary syndromes. *Circulation* 2001; **104**: 365–72.

148 Rosamond TL. Initial appraisal of acute coronary syndrome: understanding the mechanisms, identifying patient risk. *Postgrad Med* 2002; **112**: 29–42.

149 Christian TF, Clements IP, Gibbons RJ. Non-invasive identification of myocardium at risk in patients with acute myocardial infarction and non-diagnostic electrocardiogram with technetium-99 m sestamibi. *Circulation* 1991; **83**: 1615–20.

150 Allman KC, Freedman SB. Emergency department assessment of patients with acute chest pain: myocardial perfusion imaging, blood tests, or both? *J Nucl Cardiol* 2004; **11**: 87–89.

151 Duca MD, Giri S, Wu AH, *et al*. Comparison of acute rest myocardial perfusion imaging and serum markers of myocardial injury in patients with chest pain syndromes. *J Nucl Cardiol* 1999; **6**: 570–6.

152 Kontos MC, Fratkin MJ, Jesse RL, *et al*. Sensitivity of acute rest myocardial perfusion imaging for identifying patients with myocardial infarction based on a troponin definition. *J Nucl Cardiol* 2004; **11**: 12–19.

153 Anand DV, Lahiri A. Myocardial perfusion imaging versus biochemical markers in acute coronary syndromes. *Nucl Med Commun* 2003; **10**: 1049–54.

154 Weissman IA, Dickinson CZ, Dworkin HJ, *et al*. Cost-effectiveness of myocardial perfusion imaging with SPECT in the emergency department evaluation of patients with unexplained chest pain. *Radiology* 1996; **199**: 353–7.

155 Kapetanopoulos A, Heller GV, Selker HP, *et al*. Acute resting myocardial perfusion imaging in patients with diabetes mellitus: results from the Emergency Room Assessment of Sestamibi for Evaluation of Chest Pain (ERASE Chest Pain) trial. *J Nucl Cardiol* 2004; **11**: 570–7.

156 Pope JH, Aufderheide TP, Ruthazer R, *et al*. Missed diagnoses of acute cardiac ischemia in the emergency department. *N Engl J Med* 2000; **342**: 1163–70.

157 Kontos MC, Hinchman D, Cunningham M, *et al*. Comparison of contrast echocardiography with single-photon emission computed tomographic myocardial perfusion imaging in the evaluation of patients with possible acute coronary syndromes in the emergency department. *Am J Cardiol* 2003; **91**: 1099–2102.

158 Kwong RY, Schussheim AE, Rekhraj S, *et al*. Detecting acute coronary syndrome in the emergency department with cardiac magnetic resonance imaging. *Circulation* 2003; **107**: 531–7.

159 White CS, Kuo D, Kelemen M, *et al*. Chest Pain evaluation in the emergency department: can MDCT provide a comprehensive evaluation? *Am J Roentgenol* 2005; **185**: 533–40.

160 Barnett K, Feldman JA. Noninvasive imaging techniques to aid in the triage of patients with suspected acute coronary syndrome: a review. *Emerg Med Clin North Am* 2005; **23**: 977–98.

161 Garcia MJ, McNamara PM, Gordon T, *et al*. Morbidity and mortality in diabetics in the Framingham population: sixteen year follow-up study. *Diabetes* 1974; **23**: 105–111.

162 Stamler J, Vaccaro O, Neaton JD, *et al*. Diabetes, other risk factors, and 12-year cardiovascular mortality for men screened in the Multiple Risk Factor Intervention Trial. *Diabetes Care* 1993; **16**: 434–44.

163 Lerner DJ, Kannel WB. Patterns of coronary heart disease morbidity and mortality in the sexes: a 26-year follow-up of the Framingham population. *Am Heart J* 1986; **111**: 383–90.

164 Asia Pacific Cohort Studies Collaboration. The effects of diabetes on the risks of major cardiovascular diseases and death in the Asia-Pacific region. The Asia Pacific Cohort Studies Collaboration. *Diabetes Care* 2003; **26**: 360–6.

165 Huxley R, Barzi F, Woodward M. Excess risk of fatal coronary heart disease associated with diabetes in men and women: meta-analysis of 37 prospective cohort studies. *Br Med J* 2006; **332**: 73–8.

166 Weiner DA, Ryan TJ, Parsons L, *et al*. Significance of silent myocardial ischemia during exercise testing in patients with diabetes mellitus: a report from the Coronary Artery Surgery Study (CASS) registry. *Am J Cardiol* 1991; **68**: 729–34.

167 Wackers FJTh, Young LY, Inzucchi SE, *et al.*, for the Detection of Ischemia in Asymptomatic Diabetics (DIAD) Investigators. Detection of silent myocardial ischemia in asymptomatic diabetic subjects. *Diabetes Care* 2004; **27**: 1954–61.

168 Gibbons RJ, Hodge DO, Berman DS, *et al.* Long-term outcome of patients with intermediate-risk exercise electrocardiograms who do not have myocardial perfusion defects on radionuclide imaging. *Circulation* 1999; **100**: 2140–5.

169 Schuijf JD, Poldermans D, Shaw LJ, *et al.* Diagnostic and prognostic value of non-invasive imaging in known or suspected coronary artery disease. *Eur J Nucl Med Mol Imaging* 2006; **33**: 93–104.

170 Bateman TM, Prvulovich E. Assessment of prognosis in chronic coronary artery disease. *Heart* 2004; **90**: 10–15.

171 Shaw LJ, Iskandrian AE. Prognostic value of gated myocardial perfusion SPECT. *J Nucl Cardiol* 2004; **11**: 171–85.

172 Shaw LJ, Hachamovitch R, Heller GV, *et al.* Noninvasive strategies for the estimation of cardiac risk in stable chest pain patients. The Economics of Noninvasive Diagnosis (END) Study Group. *Am J Cardiol* 2000; **86**: 1–7.

173 Mowatt G, Brazzelli M, Gemmell H, *et al.* Systematic review of the prognostic effectiveness of SPECT myocardial perfusion scintigraphy in patients with suspected or known coronary artery disease and following myocardial infarction. *Nucl Med Commun* 2005; **26**: 217–29.

174 Shaw LJ, Hendel R, Borges-Neto S, *et al.* for the Myoview Multicenter Registry. Prognostic value of normal exercise and adenosine ^{99m}Tc-tetrofosmin SPECT imaging: results from the multicenter registry of 4,728 patients. *J Nucl Med* 2003; **44**: 1–6.

175 Borges-Neto S, Shaw LK, Tuttle RH, *et al.* Incremental prognostic power of single-photon emission computed tomographic myocardial perfusion imaging in patients with known or suspected coronary artery disease. *Am J Cardiol* 2005; **95**: 182–8.

176 Abidov A, Bax JJ, Hayes SW, *et al.* Transient ischemic dilation ratio of the left ventricle is a significant predictor of future cardiac events in patients with otherwise normal myocardial perfusion SPECT. *J Am Coll Cardiol* 2003; **42**: 1818–25.

177 Petix NR, Sestini S, Coppola A, *et al.* Prognostic value of combined perfusion and function by stress technetium-99 m sestamibi gated SPECT myocardial perfusion imaging in patients with suspected or known coronary artery disease. *Am J Cardiol* 2005; **95**: 1351–7.

178 Travin MI, Heller GV, Johnson LL, *et al.* The prognostic value of ECG-gated SPECT imaging in patients undergoing stress Tc-99 m sestamibi myocardial perfusion imaging. *J Nucl Cardiol* 2004; **11**: 252–63.

179 Sharir T, Germano G, Kavanagh PB, *et al.* Incremental prognostic value of post-stress left ventricular ejection fraction and volume by gated myocardial perfusion single photon emission computed tomography. *Circulation* 1999; **100**: 1035–42.

180 Kurotobi T, Sato H, Kinjo K, *et al.* Reduced collateral circulation to the infarct related artery in elderly patients with acute myocardial infaction. *J Am Coll Cardiol* 2004; **44**: 28–34.

181 Zafrir N, Mats I, Solodky A, *et al.* Prognostic value of stress myocardial perfusion imaging in octogenarian population. *J Nucl Cardiol* 2005; **12**: 671–5.

182 Johnson BD, Kelsey SF, Bairey Merz CN. Clinical risk assessment in women: chest discomfort. Report from the WISE study. In: Shaw LJ, Redberg RF. (eds.) *Coronary disease in women: evidence-based diagnosis and treatment.* Totowa, NJ: Humana Press, 2003: 129–41.

183 Mieres JH, Rosman DR, Shaw LJ. The role of myocardial perfusion imaging in special populations: women, diabetics, and heart failure. *Semin Nucl Med* 2005; **35**: 52–61.

184 Milan E. Coronary artery disease. The other half of the heaven. *Q J Nucl Med Mol Imaging* 2005; **49**: 72–80.

185 Hachamovitch R, Hayes S, Friedman JD, *et al.* Determinants of risk and its temporal variation in patients with normal stress myocardial perfusion scans: what is the warranty period of a normal scan? *J Am Coll Cardiol* 2003; **41**: 1329–40.

186 Hachamovitch R, Hayes SW, Friedman JD, *et al.* A prognostic score for prediction of cardiac mortality risk after adenosine stress myocardial perfusion scintigraphy. *J Am Coll Cardiol* 2005; **45**: 722–9.

187 Heller GV, Brown KA, Landin RJ, *et al.* Safety of early intravenous dipyridamole technetium 99 m sestamibi SPECT myocardial perfusion imaging after uncomplicated first myocardial infarction. Early Post MI IV Dipyridamole Study (EPIDS). *Am Heart J* 1997; **134**: 105–11.

188 Mahmarian JJ, Mahmarian AC, Marks GF, *et al.* Role of adenosine thallium-201 tomography for defining long-term risk in patients after acute myocardial infarction. *J Am Coll Cardiol* 1995; **25**: 1333–40.

189 Dakik H, Wendt JA, Kimball K, *et al.* Prognostic value of adenosine Tl-201 myocardial perfusion imaging after acute myocardial infarction: results of a prospective clinical trial. *J Nucl Cardiol* 2005; **12**: 276–83.

190 Spinelli L, Petretta M, Acampa W, *et al.* Prognostic value of combined assessment of regional left ventricular function and myocardial perfusion by dobutamine and rest gated SPECT in patients with uncomplicated acute myocardial infarction. *J Nucl Med* 2003; **44**: 1023–9.

191 Mahmarian JJ, Shaw LJ, Olszewski GH, *et al.* Adenosine sestamibi SPECT post-infarction evaluation (INSPIRE)

trial: a randomized, prospective multicenter trial evaluating the role of adenosine Tc-99 m sestamibi SPECT for assessing risk and therapeutic outcomes in survivors of acute myocardial infarction. *J Nucl Cardiol* 2004; **11**: 458–69.

192 Schinkel AF, Elhendy A, Bax JJ, *et al.* Prognostic implications of a normal stress technetium-99 m-tetrofosmin myocardial perfusion study in patients with a healed myocardial infarct and/or previous coronary revascularization. *Am J Cardiol* 2006; **97**: 1–6.

193 Acampa W, Spinelli L, Petretta M, *et al.* Prognostic value of myocardial ischemia in patients with uncomplicated acute myocardial infarction: direct comparison of stress echocardiography and myocardial perfusion imaging. *J Nucl Med* 2005; **46**: 417–23.

194 Verani MS. Risk assessment after myocardial infarction: have the rules changed with thrombolytic therapy? *J Nucl Cardiol* 1996; **3**: S50–9.

195 Burns RJ, Gibbons RJ, Yi Q, *et al.* CORE Study Investigators. The relationships of left ventricular ejection fraction, end-systolic volume index and infarct size to six-month mortality after hospital discharge following myocardial infarction treated by thrombolysis. *J Am Coll Cardiol* 2002; **39**: 30–6.

196 Nissen SE, Yock P. Intravascular ultrasound: novel pathophysiological insights and current applications. *Circulation* 2001; **103**: 604–16.

197 Orford JL, Lerman A, Holmes DR. Utility of routine intravascular ultrasound guidance of percutaneous coronary intervention: a critical reappraisal. *Overview J Am Coll Cardiol* 2004; **43**: 1335–42.

198 Francis JK, Michael GB Beverly HL, *et al.* ACC/AHA/ASNC guidelines for the clinical use of cardiac radionuclide imaging. Executive summary: a report of the American College of Cardiology/ American Heart Association Task Force on Practice Guidelines (ACC/AHA/ASNC committee to revise the 1995 guidelines for the clinical use of cardiac radionuclide imaging). *J Am Coll Cardiol* 2003; **42**: 1318–33.

199 The EPISTENT Investigators (Evaluation of Platelet IIb/IIIa Inhibitor for Stenting). Randomised placebo-controlled and balloon-angioplasty-controlled trial to assess safety of coronary stenting with use of platelet glycoprotein-IIb/IIIa blockade. *Lancet* 1998; **352**: 87–92.

200 Schluter M, Schofer J, Gershlick AH, *et al.* Direct stenting of native de novo coronary artery lesions with the sirolimus-eluting stent: a post hoc subanalysis of the pooled E- and C-SIRIUS trials. An overview. *J Am Coll Cardiol* 2005; **45**: 10–13.

201 Werner GS, Krack A, Schwarz G, *et al.* Prevention of lesion recurrence in chronic total coronary occlusions by paclitaxel-eluting stents. *J Am Coll Cardiol* 2004; **44**: 2301–6.

202 Price MJ, Cristea E, Sawhney N, *et al.* Serial angiographic follow-up of sirolimus-eluting stents for unprotected left main coronary artery revascularization. *J Am Coll Cardiol* 2006; **47**: 871–7.

203 Alazraki NP, Krawczynska EG, Kosinski AS, *et al.* Prognostic value of thallium-201 SPECT for patients with multivessel coronary disease post-revascularization: results from the Emory angioplasty-surgery trial. *Am J Cardiol* 1999; **84**: 1369–74.

204 Galassi AR, Foti R, Azzarelli S, *et al.* Usefulness of exercise tomographic myocardial perfusion imaging for detection of restenosis after coronary stent implantation. *Am J Cardiol* 2000; **85**: 1362–4.

205 Rajagopal V, Gurm HS, Brunken RC, *et al.* Prediction of death or myocardial infarction by exercise single photon emission computed tomography perfusion scintigraphy in patients who have had recent coronary artery stenting. *Am Heart J* 2005; **149**: 534–40.

206 Stone GW, Peterson MA, Lansky AJ, *et al.* Impact of normalized myocardial perfusion after successful angioplasty in acute myocardial infarction. *J Am Coll Cardiol* 2002; **39**: 591–7.

207 Jaffea R, Haimb S Ben, Karkabi B, *et al.* Myocardial perfusion abnormalities early (12–24 h) after coronary stenting or balloon angioplasty: implications regarding pathophysiology and late clinical outcome. *Cardiology* 2002; **98**: 60–6.

208 Rodés J, Domingo E, Candell J, *et al.* Specificity of exercise–dipyridamole Tc-99 m-tetrofosmin myocardial tomography early after successful coronary stent implantation. *Eur Heart J* 1999; **20**: 617 (Abstract).

209 Khan NE, De Souza A, Mister R, *et al.* A randomized comparison of off-pump and on-pump multivessel coronary-artery bypass surgery. *N Engl J Med* 2004; **350**: 21–8.

210 Goldman S, Zadina K, Moritz T, *et al.* Long-term patency of saphenous vein and left internal mammary artery grafts after coronary artery bypass surgery: results from a Department of Veterans Affairs Cooperative Study. *J Am Coll Cardiol* 2004; **44**: 2149–56.

211 Alderman EL, Kip KE, Whitlow PL, *et al.* Native coronary disease progression exceeds failed revascularization as cause of angina after five years in the Bypass Angioplasty Revascularization Investigation (BARI). *J Am Coll Cardiol* 2004; **44**: 766–74.

212 Gaudino M, Trani C, Luciani N, *et al.* The internal mammary artery malperfusion syndrome: late angiographic verification. *Ann Thorac Surg* 1997; **63**: 1257–61.

213 Zafrir N, Madduri J, Mats I, *et al.* Discrepancy between myocardial ischemia and luminal stenosis in patients with left internal mammary artery grafting to left anterior descending coronary artery. *J Nucl Cardiol* 2003; **10**: 663–8.

214 Schlosser T, Konorza T, Hunold P, *et al.* Noninvasive visualization of coronary artery bypass grafts using

16-detector row computed tomography. *J Am Coll Cardiol* 2004; **44**: 1224–9.

215 Nallamothu N, Johnson JH, Bagheri B, *et al.* Utility of stress single-photon emission computed tomography (SPECT) perfusion imaging in predicting outcome after coronary artery bypass grafting. *Am J Cardiol* 1997; **80**: 1517–21.

216 Iskandrian AE, Heo J, Mehta D, *et al.* Gated SPECT perfusion imaging for the simultaneous assessment of myocardial perfusion and ventricular function in the BARI 2D trial: an initial report from the Nuclear Core Laboratory. *J Nucl Cardiol* 2006; **13**: 83–90.

217 Horvath KA, Aranki SF, Cohn LH, *et al.* Sustained angina relief 5 years after transmyocardial revascularization with a CO_2 laser. *Circulation* 2001; **104(suppl I)**: 81–4.

218 Lam L, Mahmood S. Enhanced external counterpulsation. *Asian Cardiovasc Thorac Ann* 2003; **11**: 92–4.

219 Yuh DD, Simon BA, Fernandez-Bustamante A, *et al.* Totally endoscopic robot-assisted transmyocardial revascularization. *J Thorac Cardiovasc Surg* 2005; **130**: 120–4.

220 Burns SM, Brown S, White CA, *et al.* Quantitative analysis of myocardial perfusion changes with transmyocardial laser revascularization. *Am J Cardiol* 2001; **87**: 861–7.

221 Yusuf S, Zhao F, Mehta SR, *et al.* Effects of clopidogrel in addition to aspirin in patients with acute coronary syndromes without ST-segment elevation. *N Engl J Med* 2001; **345**: 494–502.

222 Schwartz RG, Pearson TA, Kalaria VG, *et al.* Prospective serial evaluation of myocardial perfusion and lipids during the first six months of pravastatin therapy: coronary artery disease regression single photon emission computed tomography monitoring trial. *J Am Coll Cardiol* 2003; **42**: 600–10.

223 Gould KL, Ornish D, Scherwitz L, *et al.* Changes in myocardial perfusion abnormalities by PET after long-term intense risk factor modification. *JAMA* 1995; **274**: 894–901.

224 Berman DS, Kang X, Schistermana EF, *et al.* Serial changes on quantitative myocardial perfusion SPECT in patients undergoing revascularization or conservative therapy. *J Nucl Cardiol* 2001; **8**: 428–37.

225 Blumenthal RS, Cohn G, Schulman SP. Medical therapy versus coronary angioplasty in stable coronary artery disease: a critical review of the literature. *J Am Coll Cardiol* 2000; **36**: 668–73.

226 Boden WE, O'Rourke RA, Teo KK, *et al.* Design and rationale of the Clinical Outcomes Utilizing Percutaneous Coronary Revascularization and Aggressive Drug Evaluation (COURAGE) trial. Veterans affairs Cooperative Studies Program no. 424. *Am Heart J* 2006; **151**: 1173–9.

227 Knight C, Fox KM. The vicious circle of ischemic left ventricular dysfunction. *Am J Cardiol* 1995; **75(suppl)**: 10E–15E.

228 Vanoverschelde JLJ, Wijns W, Borgers M, *et al.* Chronic myocardial hibernation in humans: from bedside to bench. *Circulation* 1997; **95**: 1961–71.

229 Hearse DJ. Myocardial ischemia: can we agree on a definition for the 21st century? *Cardiovasc Res* 1994; **28**: 1737–44.

230 Vanoverschelde J, Melin JA. The pathophysiology of myocardial hibernation: current controversies and future directions. *Prog Cardiovasc Dis* 2001; **43**: 387–98.

231 Rahimtoola SH. Clinical aspects of hibernating myocardium. *J Mol Cell Cardiol* 1996; **28**: 2397–401.

232 Bax JJ, van der Wall E, Harbinson M. Radionuclide techniques for the assessment of myocardial viability and hibernation. *Heart* 2004; **90**: 26–33.

233 Underwood SR, Bax JJ, vom Dahl J, *et al.* Imaging techniques for the assessment of myocardial hibernation. Report of a Study Group of the European Society of Cardiology. *Eur Heart J* 2004; **25**: 815–36.

234 Bax JJ, Poldermans D, Elhendy A, *et al.* Improvement of left ventricular ejection fraction, heart failure symptoms and prognosis after revascularization in patients with chronic coronary artery disease and viable myocardium detected by dobutamine stress echocardiography. *J Am Coll Cardiol* 1999; **34**: 163–9.

235 Allman KC, Shaw LJ, Hachamovitch R, *et al.* Myocardial viability testing and impact of revascularization on prognosis in patients with coronary artery disease and left ventricular dysfunction: a metaanalysis. *J Am Coll Cardiol* 2002; **39**: 1151–8.

236 Santana CA, Shaw LJ, Garcia EV, *et al.* Incremental prognostic value of left ventricular function by myocardial ECG-gated FDG PET imaging in patients with ischemic cardiomyopathy. *J Nucl Cardiol* 2004; **11**: 542–50.

237 Hernandez-Pampaloni M, Bax JJ, Morita K, *et al.* Incidence of stunned, hibernating and scarred myocardium in ischaemic cardiomyopathy. *Eur J Nucl Med Mol Imaging* 2005; **32**: 314–21.

238 Dilsizian V, Rocco TP, Freedman M, *et al.* Thallium reinjection after stress–redistribution imaging: enhanced detection of ischaemic and viable myocardium. *N Engl J Med* 1990; **323**: 141–6.

239 Bonow RO, Dilsizian V, Cuocolo A, *et al.* Identification of viable myocardium in patients with chronic coronary artery disease and left ventricular dysfunction. Comparison of thallium scintigraphy with reinjection and PET imaging with 18-F-fluorodeoxyglucose. *Circulation* 1991; **83**: 26–37.

240 Mahmood S, Buscombe, JR, Hall ML, *et al.* Assessment of myocardial viability with ^{201}Tl SPET and reinjection technique: a quantitative approach *Nucl Med Commun* 1992; **13**: 783–9.

241 Slart RH, Bax JJ, de Boer J, *et al.* Comparison of ^{99m}Tc-sestamibi/^{18}FDG DISA SPECT with PET for the detection of viability in patients with coronary artery disease and left ventricular dysfunction. *Eur J Nucl Med Mol Imaging* 2005; **32**: 972–9.

242 Giorgetti A, Marzullo P, Sambuceti G, *et al.* Baseline/post-nitrate Tc-99 m tetrofosmin mismatch for the assessment of myocardial viability in patients with severe left ventricular dysfunction: comparison with baseline Tc-99 m tetrofosmin scintigraphy/FDG PET imaging. *J Nucl Cardiol* 2004; **11**: 142–51.

243 Bisi G, Sciagra R, Santoro GM, *et al.* Rest Tc-99 m sestamibi tomography in combination with short term administration of nitrates: feasibility and reliability for prediction of post revascularization outcome of asynergic territories. *J Am Coll Cardiol* 1994; **24**: 1282–9.

244 Basu S, Senior R, Raval U, *et al.* Superiority of nitrate-enhanced thallium-201 over conventional redistribution thallium-201 imaging for prognostic evaluation after MI and thrombolysis. *Circulation* 1997; **96**: 2932–7.

245 Leoncini M , Marcucci G, Sciagra R, *et al.* Nitrate-enhanced gated technetium 99 m sestamibi SPECT for evaluating regional wall motion at baseline and during low-dose dobutamine infusion in patients with chronic coronary artery disease and left ventricular dysfunction: comparison with two-dimensional echocardiography. *J Nucl Cardiol* 2000; **7**: 426–31.

246 Ciavolella M, Greco C, Tavolaro R, *et al.* Acute oral trimetazidine administration increases resting technetium 99 m sestamibi uptake in hibernating myocardium. *J Nucl Cardiol* 1998; **5**: 128–33.

247 Mahmood S, Javaid A, Ayub M, *et al.* Effect of pharmacological intervention on detection of viable myocardium: nitrates vs. trimetazidine. *Eur J Nucl Med* 2000; **42**: 922 (Abstract).

248 Yao SS, Chaudhry FA. Assessment of myocardial viability with dobutamine stress echocardiography in patients with ischemic left ventricular dysfunction. *Echocardiography* 2005; **22**: 71–83.

249 Sutherland GR, Di Salvo G, Claus P, *et al.* Strain and strain rate imaging: a new clinical approach to quantifying regional myocardial function. *J Am Soc Echocardiogr* 2004; **17**: 788–802.

250 Waiterb D, Hillisa GS, McKiddie FI, *et al.* Dobutamine magnetic resonance imaging as a predictor of myocardial functional recovery after revascularisation. *Heart* 2000; **83**: 40–6.

251 Gunning MG, Anagnostopoulos C, Knight CJ, *et al.* Comparison of Tl-201, technetium-99 m tetrofosmin and dobutamine magnetic resonance imaging in identifying hibernating myocardium. *Circulation* 1998; **98**: 1869–74.

252 Kim RJ, Wu E, Rafael A, *et al.* The use of contrast enhanced magnetic resonance imaging to identify reversible myocardial dysfunction. *N Engl J Med* 2000; **343**; 1488–90.

253 Kuhl HP, Beek AM, van der Weerdt AP, *et al.* Myocardial viability in chronic ischaemic heart disease: comparison of contrast-enhanced magnetic resonance imaging with F-18 FDG PET. *J Am Coll Cardiol* 2003; **16**: 1341–8.

254 Klein C, Nekolla SG, Bengel FM, *et al.* Assessment of myocardial viability with contrast-enhanced magnetic resonance imaging: comparison with positron emission tomography. *Circulation* 2002; **105**: 162–7.

255 Nikolaou K, Javier Sanz J, Poon M, *et al.* Assessment of myocardial perfusion and viability from routine contrast-enhanced 16-detector-row computed tomography of the heart: preliminary results. *Eur Radiol* 2005; **15**: 864–71.

256 Schneider CA, Voth E, Baer FM, *et al.* QT dispersion is determined by the extent of viable myocardium in patients with chronic Q-wave myocardial infarction. *Circulation* 1997; **96**: 3913–20.

257 Vahlhaus C, Bruns HJ, Stypmann J, *et al.* Direct epicardial mapping predicts the recovery of left ventricular dysfunction in chronic ischaemic myocardium. *Eur Heart J* 2004; **25**: 154–7.

258 Sloof GW, Knapp Jr FF, van Lingen A, *et al.* Nuclear imaging is more sensitive for the detection of viable myocardium than dobutamine echocardiography. *Nucl Med Commun* 2002; **24**: 375–81.

259 Berger R, Huelsman M, Stecker K, *et al.* B-type natriuretic peptide predicts sudden death in patients with chronic heart failure. *Circulation* 2002; **105**: 2391–6.

260 Rizzello V, Poldermans D, Biagini E, *et al.* Benefits of coronary revascularisation in diabetic and non-diabetic patients with ischaemic cardiomyopathy: role of myocardial viability. *Eur J Heart Fail* 2005; **8**: 314–20.

261 Tomaselli GF, Zipes DP. What causes sudden death in heart failure? *Circ Res* 2004; **95**: 754–63.

262 Braunwald E. Expanding indications for beta-blockers in heart failure. *N Engl J Med* 2001; **344**: 1711–2.

263 Cleland JG, Pennell DJ, Ray SG, *et al.* Myocardial viability as a determinant of the ejection fraction response to carvedilol in patients with heart failure (CHRISTMAS trial): randomised controlled trial. *Lancet* 2003; **362**: 14–21.

264 Abraham WT, Fisher WG, Smith AL, *et al.* for the MIRACLE Study Group. Cardiac resynchronization in chronic heart failure. *N Engl J Med* 2002; **346**: 1845–53.

265 Rose EA, Gelijns AC, Moskowitz AJ, *et al.* Long-term mechanical left ventricular assistance for end-stage heart failure. *N Engl J Med* 2001; **345**: 1435–43.

266 Benjamin IJ, Schneider MD. Learning from failure: congestive heart failure in the postgenomic age. *J Clin Invest* 2005; **115**: 495–9.

267 Schumacher B, Pecher P, von Specht B, *et al.* Induction of neoangiogenesis in ischemic myocardium by human growth factors. *Circulation* 1998; **97**: 645–50.

268 Janssens S, Dubois C, Bogaert J, *et al.* Autologous bone marrow-derived stem-cell transfer in patients with ST-segment elevation myocardial infarction: double-blind, randomised controlled trial. *Lancet* 2006; **367**: 113–21.

269 Sciagra R, Giaccardi M, Porciani MC, *et al.* Myocardial perfusion imaging using gated SPECT in heart failure patients undergoing cardiac resynchronization therapy. *J Nucl Med* 2004; **45**: 164–8.

270 Merlet P, Valette H, Dubois RJ, *et al.* Prognostic value of cardiac metaiodobenzylguanidine imaging in patients with heart failure. *J Nucl Med* 1992; **33**: 471–7.

271 Shinichiro F, Aritomo I, Shinji H, *et al.* Usefulness of meta-[^{123}I]iodobenzylguanidine myocardial scintigraphy for predicting cardiac events in patients with dilated cardiomyopathy who receive long-term beta blocker treatment. *Nucl Med Commun* 2005; **26**: 97–102.

272 Rossig L, Fichtlscherer S, Heeschen C, *et al.* The proapoptotic serum activity is an independent mortality predictor of patients with heart failure. *Eur Heart J* 2004; **25**: 1620–5.

273 Wencker D, Chandra M, Nguyen K, *et al.* A mechanistic role for cardiac myocyte apopotosis in heart failure. *J Clin Invest* 2003; **111**: 1497–504.

274 Strauss HW, Grewal RK, Pandit-Taskar N. Molecular imaging in nuclear cardiology. *Semin Nucl Med* 2004; **34**: 47–55.

275 Hoffman JIE, Kaplan S. The incidence of congenital heart disease. *J Am Coll Cardiol* 2002; **39**: 1890–900.

276 Ueda Y, Hozumi T, Yoshida K, *et al.* Non-invasive automated assessment of the ratio of pulmonary to systemic flow in patients with atrial septal defects by the colour Doppler velocity profile integration method. *Heart* 2002; **88**: 278–82.

277 Devore GR, Polanko B. Tomographic ultrasound imaging of the fetal heart: a new technique for identifying normal and abnormal cardiac anatomy. *J Ultrasound Med* 2005; **24**: 1685–96.

278 Boxt LM. Magnetic resonance and computed tomographic evaluation of congenital heart disease. *J Magn Reson Imaging* 2004; **19**: 827–47.

279 Hurwitz RA, Treves S, Keane JF. Current value of radionuclide angiocardiography for shunt quantification and management in patients with secundum atrial septal defect. *Am Heart J* 1982; **103**: 421–5.

280 Kelbaek H, Aldershvile J, Svendsen JH, *et al.* Evaluation of left-to-right shunts in adults with atrial septal defect using first-pass radionuclide cardiography. *Eur Heart J* 1992; **13**: 491–5.

281 Vettukattil JJ, Slavik Z, Lamb RK, *et al.* Intrapulmonary arteriovenous shunting may be a universal phenomenon in patients with the superior cavopulmonary anastomosis: a radionuclide study. *Heart* 2000; **83**: 425–8.

282 Brunotte F, Laurens MH, Cloez JL, *et al.* Sensitivity and specificity of radionuclide equilibrium angiocardiography for detection of haemodynamically significant secundum atrial septal defect. *Eur J Nucl Med* 1986; **12**: 468–70.

283 Kress P, Bitter F, Stauch M, *et al.* Radionuclide ventriculography: a noninvasive method for the detection and quantification of left-to-right shunts in atrial septal defect. *Clin Cardiol* 1982; **5**: 192–200.

284 Eterovic D, Dujic Z, Popovic S, *et al.* Gated versus first-pass radioangiography in the evaluation of left-to-right shunts. *Clin Nucl Med* 1995; **20**: 534–7.

285 Parrish MD, Graham Jr TP, Bender HW, *et al.* Radionuclide angiographic evaluation of right and left ventricular function during exercise after repair of transposition of the great arteries. Comparison with normal subjects and patients with congenitally corrected transposition. *Circulation* 1983; **67**: 178–83.

286 Angelini P, Velasco JA, Flamm S. Coronary anomalies: incidence, pathophysiology, and clinical relevance. *Circulation* 2002; **105**: 2449.

287 Kondo C. Myocardial perfusion imaging in paediatric cardiology. *Ann Nucl Med* 2004; **18**: 551–61.

288 Finlay JP, Howman-Giles R, Gilday DL, *et al.* Thallium-201 myocardial imaging in anomalous left coronary artery arising from the pulmonary artery. Applications before and after medical and surgical treatment. *Am J Cardiol* 1978; **42**: 675–80.

289 Cowie MR, Mahmood S, Ell PJ. The diagnosis and assessment of an adult with anomalous origin of the left coronary artery from the pulmonary artery. *Eur J Nuc Med* 1994; **21**: 1017–9.

290 Hauser M, Bengel FM, Hager A, *et al.* Impaired myocardial blood flow and coronary flow reserve of the anatomical right systemic ventricle in patients with congenitally corrected transposition of the great arteries. *Heart* 2003; **89**: 1231–5.

291 Senzaki, H, Masutani S, Kobayashi J, *et al.* Ventricular afterload and ventricular work in fontan circulation: comparison with normal two-ventricle circulation and single-ventricle circulation with Blalock–Taussig shunts. *Circulation* 2002; **105**: 2885–92.

292 Quinlivan RM, Lewis P, Marsden P, *et al.* Cardiac function, metabolism and perfusion in Duchenne and Becker muscular dystrophy. *Neuromusc Disord* 1996; **6**: 237–46.

293 Quinlivan RM, Robinson RO, Maisey MN. Positron emission tomography in paediatric cardiology. *Arch Dis Child* 1998; **79**: 520–2.

Left ventricular dysfunction

S.F. BARRINGTON

MEASURING LEFT VENTRICULAR FUNCTION: EQUILIBRIUM RADIONUCLIDE VENTRICULOGRAPHY

Clinical indications and comparison with other techniques

Left ventricular ejection fraction (EF) is an important prognostic indicator in heart disease and may be used to guide treatment. It is also an important measure used to monitor unwanted effects of cardiotoxic chemotherapeutic agents such as adriamycin. These are the main clinical indications for equilibrium radionuclide ventriculography (RNV) also referred to as multiplanar gated angiography (MUGA). Regional wall motion can also be evaluated including the assessment of left ventricular aneurysm. First-pass radionuclide angiography allows for accurate assessment of LV function but is mainly used for the assessment of intracardiac shunting. Perfusion imaging has largely replaced rest and stress RNV for the assessment of ischemic heart disease.

Echocardiography offers an alternative method to measure EF without the need to expose the patient to ionizing radiation. Developments including the use of contrast agents and tissue harmonic imaging have improved endocardial border detection so that the precision and accuracy of echocardiographic measurements now approach those of RNV[1,2] and most cardiologists favor the use of echocardiography to assess ventricular function. Echocardiography does rely on geometric assumptions to calculate ventricular volumes, however, which may be less valid in severely impaired ventricles. In one study comparing echocardiography with RNV after myocardial infarction, calculation of EF was not possible in 27% of patients using echocardiography.[3]

The technique is also very operator dependent and it may be difficult to obtain good quality images in patients with lung disease. Gated SPECT can be used to assess LV function but edge detection is more difficult in patients who have significant perfusion defects. It is, of course, these patients in whom accurate estimation of EF is most important. RNV therefore still has a role to play in the assessment of LV function and is often preferred for monitoring chemotherapy agents because it has better precision than echocardiography and gated SPECT. RNV is still used as the 'gold standard' technique in studies evaluating other techniques to measure EF.[1,4]

Equilibrium RNV: imaging technique

The basis for equilibrium RNV is to image the blood pool within the cardiac chambers using a tracer, which labels red cells. There are three techniques used. All rely on the fact that [^{99m}Tc]pertechnetate diffuses passively into red cells and in the presence of a reducing agent such as stannous ions binds to hemoglobin. In the *in vitro* method, a blood sample is taken and the red cells are separated from whole blood and incubated with stannous ions then [^{99m}Tc] pertechnetate. In the *in vivo* method stannous ions, usually 10–20 μg kg^{-1}, are injected 20 min prior to the tracer. The best labeling efficiency is achieved with the *in vitro* method but the *in vivo* method is much easier to perform. The modified *in vitro* method is a compromise, which enables high labeling efficiencies of 90–95% to be achieved without the need for complex blood-handling procedures. The stannous agent is given first intravenously. After 15–30 min a blood sample of 5–10 mL is withdrawn into a syringe prefilled with anticoagulant and [^{99m}Tc]pertechnetate. The blood is mixed and incubated with the tracer in the syringe for 10 min and re-injected.

Gated acquisitions are performed. Images are usually acquired in anterior and left anterior oblique (LAO) projections. An additional left lateral or left posterior oblique projection gives better images of the inferior wall. The LAO view with caudal tilt gives the best separation of the right and left ventricles. The R wave on the ECG is used as a trigger to collect data from multiple cardiac cycles. The cardiac cycle is divided into intervals or 'frames' of set times typically 16 or more per cycle. The time duration of the frames is chosen according to the patient's mean R–R interval, which is sampled prior to the acquisition. The data from frame 1 of each cycle is summed, the data from frame 2 of each cycle is summed and so on until adequate counts are acquired, typically 200 000–400 000 counts per frame. Alternatively, data may be acquired for a set number of beats (usually 500–1000 beats). A composite image is thus built up of the chambers of the heart during an 'average' cardiac cycle. The method relies on a regular heart rhythm so that the R–R interval is reasonably constant. Beats that are shorter or longer than the mean R–R interval recorded during the sampling period by >10% are rejected by the computer. Images may also be acquired in list mode where the computer instead of 'binning' the data collected into separate frames collects all the data as a 'list'. The coordinates of each scintillation event are stored in the memory alongside the ECG gating and time markers. List mode allows the data to be processed after acquisition and a suitable R–R interval chosen and beats longer than this to be rejected. Whilst this allows for more flexible handling of the data, list mode also requires larger amounts of computer memory and more processing time than frame mode acquisition which generally gives adequate images and satisfactory quantification.

Equilibrium RNV: imaging analysis

Images are displayed scaled to the hottest pixel and usually a temporal and spatial smooth is applied. Visual inspection of a cine loop gives an impression of the wall motion and contractility and chamber size. Regional wall motion abnormalities can be assessed. Regional shortening of a radius from the centre of the ventricle to the endocardial edge of the chamber between diastole and systole should be at least 25%.

For quantification purposes, regions of interest (ROIs) are drawn around the left and right ventricle using the unsmoothed LAO image, either manually or using an automatic edge detection algorithm. A background region is drawn inferolateral to the heart over several pixels avoiding the spleen and great vessels (Plate 6B.1). This is to correct for the counts recorded in the image that arise from structures in front of the heart and may contribute 30–60% of the total counts. Accurate background correction is vital

for accurate calculation of EF. The background counts are subtracted from each pixel in the ventricular ROIs. A time–activity curve is generated for each frame in the cardiac cycle. The LVEF is calculated as follows:

$$\frac{\text{end diastolic counts} - \text{end systolic counts}}{\text{end disastolic counts}}.$$

The normal value for resting LVEF is in the range of 50–70%. The RVEF can be calculated in a similar fashion but is more difficult to quantify because there is significant overlap of the right ventricle by the right atrium. Regional EF may be calculated by dividing the ventricle into radii from the geometric center and analyzing the count rate during the cardiac cycle for multiple segments.

The data can be used to generate functional images using Fourier analysis. This is a mathematical technique which fits the left ventricular time–activity curve for each individual pixel to the first harmonic Fourier transform, equivalent to a symmetrical cosine curve with a period equal to the period of the cardiac cycle. The phase and amplitude of the fitted curve is displayed for each pixel in the 'phase' and 'amplitude' images. The phase image reflects when in the cardiac cycle (from 0 to 360°) each pixel is contracting maximally. The amplitude image reflects the greatest magnitude of contraction for each pixel. Inspection of the phase image should show that the ventricles contract simultaneously and that the atria contract approximately 180° later (Plate 6B.1). The data may also be displayed as a histogram, which has two peaks for atrial and ventricular contraction. Aneurysms with paradoxical movement and contraction will be out of phase with the remainder of the ventricle. The amplitude image should be relatively homogeneous although amplitude is usually larger at the base of the left ventricle than the apex. Difference in amplitude within the left ventricle occurs with regional reductions in contractility. More complex analysis can be performed to generate ventricular volumes, filling and emptying rates but these are rarely used clinically.[5]

REVERSING LEFT VENTRICULAR DYSFUNCTION: THE RATIONALE FOR IMAGING MYOCARDIAL VIABILITY

Patients with ischemic heart disease (IHD) may develop left ventricular (LV) dysfunction following ischemia or infarction. If there is sufficient viable myocardium within areas subtended by coronary artery stenoses then revascularization of these regions may improve function. Rahimtoola[6] first described this concept and used the term 'hibernation' to describe the 'smart heart' that could adapt to the harsh conditions of low flow by downgrading function and be restored to full function with revascularization.[7–16] Revascularization also results in improved survival.[17–19] In a recent meta-analysis which included results from 24 studies involving 3088 patients, the annual mortality of patients with 'viability' was 16% with medical treatment compared to 3.2% for those who underwent revascularization ($P < 0.0001$).[20] Revascularization may also attenuate the deleterious effects of ongoing LV remodeling.[21]

Most data suggest that there is no survival benefit conferred on patients with 'nonviable' dysfunctional myocardium by revascularization.[17,19,22–24] One study only suggested that patients with severe coronary artery disease (three-vessel disease and/or left main stem stenosis) did better with revascularization than medical treatment even without evidence of viability, although the reduction in relative risk was much higher for those patients with viability.[24] Two studies indicated a relatively benign course for patients without viability over 18 months with survival $\geqslant 80\%$,[17,25] but others with longer follow-up have reported survival rates around 50–65%.[24,26–29] One of the problems with interpretation of these data is that patients with nonviable myocardium tend not to be offered revascularization and the number of patients in this category is small. For this reason a randomized trial of medical treatment versus revascularization is under way: the Surgical Treatment for Ischaemic Heart Failure (STICH) trial, which is expected to report in 2008.

In the meantime, patients with IHD and significant viability, probably between 25–50% of the myocardium,[26,30–34] who have LV dysfunction should be offered revascularization. Viability assessment should be undertaken prior to revascularization.[35] Angina appears to improve regardless of the presence of viability[22,26] and therefore viability testing may be more important in patients with predominant symptoms of heart failure. Patients with angina and no viability still represent a high-risk group for revascularization, however.[35]

DEFINITIONS OF ISCHEMIC SYNDROMES

Acute ischemia is accompanied by abnormal contractile function, which is restored to normal immediately after restoration of blood flow. It involves anaerobic glycolysis with the production of lactate. *Infarction* is accompanied by persistent irreversible contractile dysfunction, the degree of which will depend upon the extent of injury and the time course of events, which determines whether there has been sufficient time for a collateral circulation to develop. Between these two extremes lie two further ischemic syndromes characterized by persistent yet reversible dysfunction. These are referred to as *stunning* and *hibernation*.

Stunned myocardium has abnormal contraction, which persists for a time beyond the restoration of normal blood flow.[36,37] Contractile function eventually recovers spontaneously. Impairment in function is thus temporary but reversible. Stunning is accompanied by normal resting blood flow and aerobic metabolism. Clinical manifestations include the temporary impairment of function that occurs in the peri-infarct region after myocardial infarction and following extracorporeal circulation during coronary artery bypass

surgery.[38] Function can be transiently restored to normal with positive inotropic agents, such as dobutamine.[39,40]

Hibernation was initially described as myocardium showing abnormal contraction in the presence of chronic reduction in blood flow which was reversible with restoration of normal blood flow.[6,41,42] It was considered to be an adaptation of the myocardium to resting hypoperfusion with downgrading of function to match the reduction in blood flow.[43] The prerequisite that abnormal function must be accompanied by chronic resting hypoperfusion was subsequently challenged.[44] Recovery of function was demonstrated in myocardium with impaired resting blood flow[45] and myocardium with normal and near normal resting flow[10,46–48] but impaired coronary flow reserve.

This led to the hypothesis that recurrent episodes of ischemia with insufficient time between episodes for cardiac function to recover may lead to chronic impairment of function.[46] This is called 'repetitive stunning'. Impaired resting blood flow is also accompanied by impaired coronary flow reserve which is more profound than that which accompanies normal resting flow[49] and it may be that 'repetitive stunning' leads on to 'hibernation' and that the two entities co-exist, often accompanied by areas of infarction.

Whatever the mechanism underlying the development of chronic 'reversible' left ventricular dysfunction, function is restored only by revascularization and a looser use of the term 'hibernation' than the original description is now often used. *Hibernation* is taken to mean dysfunctional areas of the myocardium subtended by coronary artery stenoses where function is improved by revascularization.[35] It is this use of the term hibernation that will generally be used in this chapter.

TECHNIQUES TO IMAGE VIABLE MYOCARDIUM

Several different functional imaging techniques are available for the detection of hibernation clinically:

- Single photon emission computed tomography (SPECT) uses tracers such as ^{99m}Tc-sestamibi and ^{201}Tl which rely on active cellular transport mechanisms for retention in viable tissue.
- Positron emission tomography (PET) detects preserved or increased metabolic activity using fluorodeoxyglucose (FDG) in dysfunctional myocardium.
- Echocardiography detects contractile reserve in dysfunctional myocardium with dobutamine. Cine magnetic resonance imaging (MRI) has also been used with dobutamine analogous to the use of echocardiography.

Contrast-enhanced MRI has been used in viability assessment[50] with increased permeability and leakage of gadolinium occurring into scar tissue. The technique is not currently in widespread clinical use but the improved

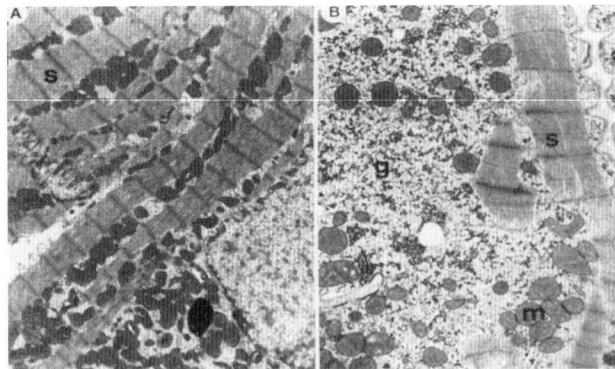

Figure 6B.1 *This figure shows electron microscopic samples of normal myocardium (left) and hibernating myocardium (right). Note there are fewer sarcomeres (S) and increased accumulation of glycogen (g) in the section from hibernating myocardium. (Reproduced with permission from the* Am J Physiol *1995; **268(3, pt 2)**: H1272.)*

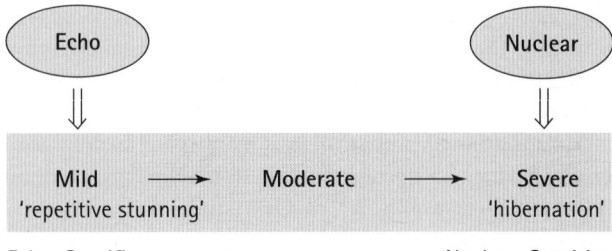

Figure 6B.2 *This illustrates the spectrum of structural changes that underlie the development of ischemic left ventricular dysfunction. Echo may be best at detecting myocardium with mild structural changes and nuclear techniques at detecting myocardium with more severe structural changes. This explains why echo is a test with higher specificity whilst nuclear techniques tend to have higher sensitivity.*

resolution of MRI compared with nuclear and echocardiographic techniques may prove to be a substantial advantage.

Structural changes accompany the development of ischemic LV dysfunction. Loss of contractile material with replacement by glycogen and fibrosis has been reported in biopsy specimens of patients undergoing surgery[46,51] (Fig. 6B.1). The changes may vary from mild to severe and this has implications for imaging. At the mild end of the spectrum, resting perfusion is normal but there is reduced coronary flow reserve. The myocytes probably remain intact with little fibrosis and minimal loss of contractile material. These myocytes are likely to exhibit contractile reserve upon stimulation of beta-adrenoreceptors with dobutamine. They will also accumulate tracers such as sestamibi and thallium that rely on the integrity of the cell membrane for their uptake and display either normal or enhanced glucose metabolism, which can be monitored with FDG. Inducible ischemia may be present on stress testing with perfusion tracers. The time course of recovery for these myocytes would be expected to be rapid and complete. Indeed, myocardium, which responds to dobutamine stimulation on echocardiography, has been demonstrated to improve in the operating theater.[15,52]

Towards the severe end of the spectrum, LV dysfunction may be accompanied by reduced resting perfusion. The myocytes may have significant loss of contractile material with increased fibrosis. The time course of recovery of function postoperatively, which is likely to depend on the re-synthesis of intracellular contractile material may be protracted.[48,52–54] Cells may no longer respond to dobutamine but will continue to accumulate tracers such as thallium and sestamibi which rely only on cellular membrane integrity for their uptake.[55] Glucose metabolism also is preserved and the cells take up FDG.[56] Gunning *et al.* demonstrated that the fraction of the biopsy thickness occupied by myocytes was higher in patients showing contractile reserve

using dobutamine magnetic resonance imaging preoperatively than those without contractile reserve but with evidence of viability using technetium or thallium SPECT.[57] Of course, myocardium with small 'islands' of viable cells may appear viable on nuclear imaging but the viable cells may be too few in number for functional recovery to occur.

This may explain why nuclear techniques relying on cell membrane integrity or metabolism are more sensitive in the detection of hibernating myocardium whilst echocardiographic techniques relying on inotropic reserve are more specific (Fig. 6B.2).

SPECT imaging

The tracers currently in use are ^{201}Tl (as thallous chloride) and lipophilic ^{99m}Tc compounds such as ^{99m}Tc-sestamibi and newer agents such as ^{99m}Tc-tetrofosmin. The easier availability, lower radiation dose and better image quality are good reasons to prefer technetium agents to thallium and they are probably at least[8,58] if not more accurate in the detection of viability.[55,59,60] Thallium was used, however, in preference to technetium agents for many years owing to its ability to redistribute in the myocardium, which was thought to be a theoretical advantage, allowing uptake of the tracer in areas of very low flow.

For viability imaging, technetium tracers are injected at rest, when delivery of the tracer is likely to be highest in areas of low flow. Sestamibi is the agent about which there is the most published data, but it is likely that other agents such as ^{99m}Tc-tetrofosmin have similar utility. These agents diffuse passively across the cell membrane and are then sequestered within mitochondria. Retention depends upon the integrity of the cell membrane and mitochondrial function[61,62] which can only be maintained if there is active metabolism.[62] Sestamibi is therefore a marker of viability not a simple perfusion agent (although the presence of 'reversible ischemia'

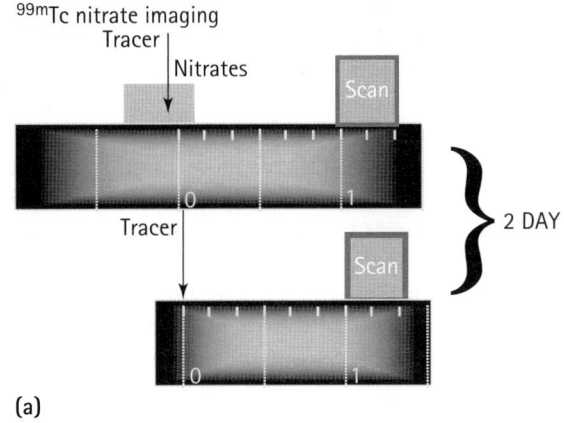

(a)

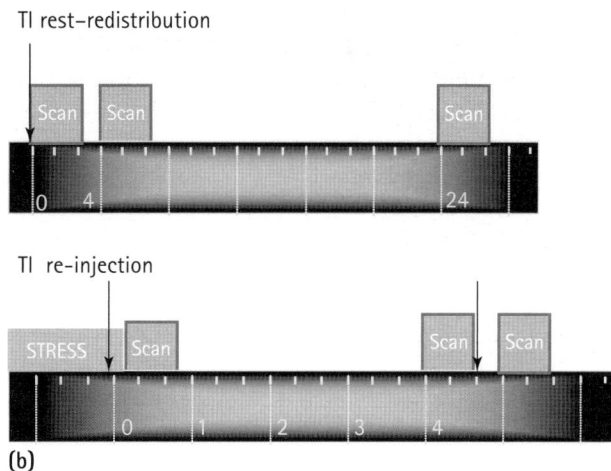

(b)

Ammonia and FDG PET Scan

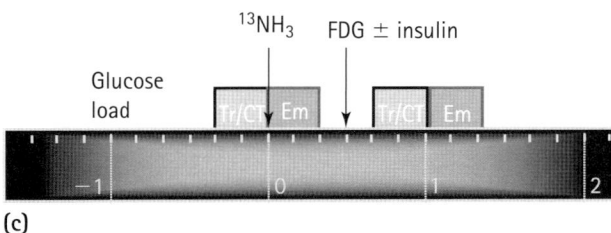

(c)

Figure 6B.3 *Scan protocols are shown for viability imaging with technetium tracers and nitrates (a), thallium redistribution and re-injection imaging (b), and ammonia and FDG PET scanning (c).*

may in itself be predictive of hibernation).[63] The uptake of sestamibi is inversely correlated with the amount of fibrosis in biopsy specimens of patients undergoing revascularization and the ability of sestamibi to detect hibernating myocardium is superior to using a perfusion tracer such as [13N]ammonia.[64,65] The sensitivity of sestamibi injected at rest for the detection of hibernating myocardium is approximately 80% with a specificity of approximately 60–70%.[59,66]

Nitrates have been used to augment the uptake of technetium tracers. Nitrates dilate epicardial vessels and increase flow through collateral channels.[67] The change in size of a perfusion defect before and after the administration of intravenous isosorbide dinitrate is a good predictor of functional recovery with revascularization[68–70] (Fig. 6B.3 (a)). The best parameters to use are reduction in the size of the perfusion defect by at least 10% on the nitrate image compared to a resting image acquired without administration of nitrates or resting uptake of tracer $\geqslant$65% relative to the maximum uptake on the nitrate image.[70] The sensitivity and specificity has been reported as 77–95% and 69–88% respectively using sestamibi with nitrates in small groups of patients.[68,70–72]

Thallium is a metallic element which is transported into cells both via the sodium–potassium adenosine triphosphate pump and by passive diffusion. The coronary circulation extracts 88% of the tracer in one pass and the uptake of thallium into normal myocardium is rapid.[73] Conversely, in ischemic areas, where perfusion is diminished either during stress or at rest, uptake is lower than in normal tissue.

However, thallium also washes out of the cell in proportion to blood flow, so that clearance from ischemic areas is slower than normal tissue, leading to an apparent increase in counts in areas of initially low uptake. This change in the distribution of the tracer with time is referred to as 'redistribution'. Thallium has similar sensitivity to sestamibi for viability assessment but lower specificity of around 47–54% depending on the technique used.[59,66] There are two types of technique used referred to as 'redistribution' and 're-injection' imaging.

In redistribution imaging, thallium is injected at rest and imaged immediately followed by a second redistribution image acquired at 4–24 h after injection. Delaying imaging allows maximal uptake to occur in areas of low flow but this has to be weighed against the loss of counts that occurs with time. 'Re-injection' imaging was introduced to enable combined assessment of stress-induced ischemia and viability. Using this approach, an image is taken following stress then a further image is taken at 4 h. A second injection of thallium is given if defects have failed to fill in to boost the concentration of thallium in severely ischemic areas.[74] However, re-injection imaging does appear to be less accurate than redistribution imaging[59] (Fig. 6B.3 (b)).

The accuracy of these agents is probably lower than FDG PET[60,64,75] although this may not necessarily affect patient management. In one study where referring doctors were blinded as to which method was used to assess viability, there was no difference in outcome between patients scanned using SPECT and those scanned using PET.[76] The lower accuracy of SPECT may be partly due to the properties of FDG as a tracer and also to the problems associated with attenuation[65,77] which may be circumvented in time with attenuation correction algorithms, but these are unlikely to correct the problem completely.[78]

It should be noted though that the negative predictive value for SPECT is very high, however, and a patient with no evidence of viability within dysfunctional myocardium on SPECT is unlikely to benefit from revascularization.

In reporting, a threshold value below which the myocardium is deemed to be nonviable is often used. Different thresholds have been applied mostly ranging between 50 and 65% of the maximum uptake in the heart for SPECT agents. This semi-quantitative approach is more reliable than just visual assessment[8] but it should be remembered that a threshold represents an arbitrary value and viability is not an 'all or none' phenomenon. The likelihood of recovery increases with increasing uptake of tracer and in an individual patient this has to be weighed against the other factors important in the clinical decision of whether to proceed to revascularization.

PET imaging

The tracer most commonly used is $[^{18}F]$fluorodeoxyglucose (^{18}F-FDG) which is an analog of glucose. Glucose metabolism is preserved or increased in hibernating myocardium due to increased expression of glucose transporters[79] or to increased glycogen synthesis secondary to other mechanisms such as translocation of GADPH.[80] In dysfunctional myocardium, the presence of FDG uptake in sites of normal or impaired flow, most commonly assessed with the perfusion tracer $[^{13}N]$ammonia, has been used to distinguish viable myocardium from infarcted myocardium where both flow and glucose metabolism are impaired. These are the so-called 'normal', 'mismatch' and 'matched' patterns of uptake on PET scanning.[81] It has been suggested that the correlates of the 'normal', 'mismatch' and 'match' patterns on PET are 'stunned', 'hibernating' and 'infarcted' myocardium, respectively. Mild matched reduction probably represents nontransmural scar and severe matched reduction represents transmural scar.[82] The sensitivity of FDG PET is approximately 85–90% and the specificity is 70–75%.[59]

FDG can be imaged using a dedicated PET camera which is usually referred to as FDG PET or with a gamma camera operating in coincidence mode in FDG SPECT. The gamma camera is not well suited to detecting high-energy emissions and this leads to a loss in sensitivity and count rate performance. Whether this is of importance clinically in cardiac imaging where it is usually the visualization of large areas of FDG uptake which is important, remains to be seen and some comparative studies of FDG imaging using PET and SPECT technology have already been published.[83,84]

FDG imaging may be performed alone or in combination with perfusion imaging, which may give added predictive value.[85] However, the fact that FDG alone is a powerful predictor of recovery is important because of the development of commercially run cyclotrons situated centrally which supply increasing numbers of peripherally located scanners. Such scanners can perform FDG imaging (half-life 110 min) but not perfusion imaging using PET tracers because of their short half-life (<10 min). FDG imaging may also be performed using cardiac gating which enables function and metabolism to be assessed simultaneously (Fig. 6B.3c). Patients are usually scanned after an oral glucose load because in the fasting state there is variable myocardial uptake and poor quality images are obtained in 40–50% of cases.[86] Additional doses of insulin may be given to enhance uptake in the myocardium, especially in diabetic patients. The use of a hyperinsulinemic–euglycemic clamp gives better image quality than more simple approaches but does not alter the ratio of uptake in normal versus hibernating versus infarcted myocardium and is generally used in clinical studies only where more simple approaches have failed.[87] The threshold used for FDG for viability in earlier studies was around 50–55% although data from studies using discriminant analysis suggest that a higher threshold of 60–65% may be more appropriate.[33,60]

The advent of PET/CT may have a significant impact on cardiac imaging. The situation of a multislice (16–64 slice) CT scanner in the same gantry as the PET scanner allows for combined assessment of anatomy, function and wall motion. CT coronary angiography, perfusion, metabolism and contractility can be performed in a single scanning session. The clinical utility of this combined approach compared to 'standard' methods remains to be seen.

Echocardiography

In echocardiography the contractility of the myocardium can be visualized using ultrasound in response to dobutamine. In viable but dysfunctional myocardium, dobutamine stimulates beta-receptors at low dose with improvement in wall motion and contractility. Myocardial perfusion also increases due to autoregulation where blood flow increases to keep up with the increased oxygen demand associated with improved contractility to generate sufficient ATP. There is probably also a direct effect on coronary arteries causing vasodilatation. Improved contractility may be seen using 'low dose' dobutamine (up to $20\,\mu g\,kg^{-1}\,min^{-1}$).[9] At higher doses ($20$–$40\,\mu g\,kg^{-1}\,min^{-1}$), however, the chronotrophic effects of dobutamine on heart rate and systolic blood pressure outweigh the inotropic effects and cardiac workload outstrips myocardial oxygen supply. Ischemia ensues with production of lactate and the development of acidosis associated with worsening wall motion. This biphasic response of dobutamine is the best predictor of hibernation.[16]

The sensitivity of echocardiography is around 80% overall but is lower in patients with large areas of akinesis where nuclear techniques, particularly PET perform better.[13,32]

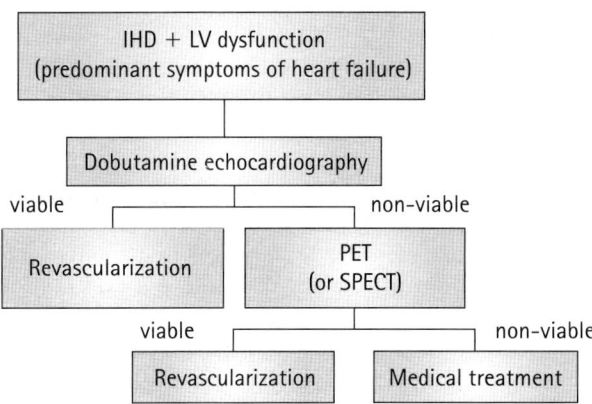

Figure 6B.4 *Suggested algorithm for investigating a patient with ischemic heart disease and left ventricular dysfunction.*

Echocardiography has higher specificity of 79–84% than the nuclear techniques for the reasons discussed above. It has been suggested therefore that the most appropriate investigative algorithm may be one that employs echocardiography as a first-line test.[60,88] It is easy to perform, relatively cheap and does not use ionizing radiation. If echo demonstrates the presence of viable myocardium, the patient should be considered for revascularization. However, because it is less sensitive than nuclear techniques, patients who do not appear to have viable myocardium on echo should undergo a second-line test, either FDG or technetium imaging (Fig. 6B.4).

Myocardial contrast echocardiography (MCE) using intracoronary injection of microbubbles has also been used to evaluate viability.[89,90] This reflects perfusion and appears to be sensitive but much less specific than dobutamine echocardiography. Unsurprisingly, there is a high degree of concordance between thallium and MCE in the assessment of viability.[90]

CARDIAC SYMPATHETIC INNERVATION IMAGING

meta-Iodobenzylguanidine (MIBG) is an analog of guanethidine, which is taken up into sympathetic nerve terminals like noradrenaline. The distribution of ^{123}I-MIBG in the heart reflects adrenergic receptor density. MIBG uptake is diminished in infarcted myocardium and may also be reduced in the peri-infarct region.[91] The presence of sympathetic denervation in the peri-infarct region using MIBG and thallium imaging is associated with an increased incidence of ventricular arrhythmias in patients following myocardial infarction.[91,92] Patients with right ventricular outflow tract and idiopathic ventricular tachycardia also have reduced MIBG uptake suggesting sympathetic denervation and increased sympathetic sensitivity as a possible mechanism for the development of malignant arrhythmias.[93] Merlet *et al.* demonstrated a reduced incidence of sudden death in patients with dilated cardiomyopathies with ischemic and non-ischemic etiologies when cardiac MIBG uptake was normal.[94]

Increased sympathetic activity is cardioprotective in the early stages of heart failure but prolonged sympathetic activity results in sympathetic denervation which has been implicated in the development of heart failure. Adrenergic neurotransmitters may mediate the development of the fibrogenic changes, which result in LV remodeling. Reduced uptake and increased washout of MIBG correlates with worsening ejection fraction, increased circulating levels of noradrenaline and progressive heart failure symptoms.[95,96] Drugs that alter the prognosis of patients with heart failure, such as angiotensin converting enzyme inhibitors, increase the uptake of MIBG within the heart.[97] MIBG imaging may also be able to predict those patients who are likely to benefit from treatment with beta-blockers.

Possible future roles for MIBG cardiac imaging are therefore:

- To identify patients at increased risk of malignant arrhythmias and direct placement of intracardiac defibrillator devices[98]
- As an index of LV remodelling and to monitor the efficacy of medical treatment.[98]

The assessment of patients with LV dysfunction represents a challenge which nuclear medicine in combination with other techniques such as echocardiography and MRI is well placed to meet.

Case history

The patient had three-vessel coronary artery disease with impaired left ventricular function (ejection fraction 25%) (Plate 6B.2). He had symptoms of heart failure without angina. PET/CT was requested to determine whether there was significant hibernating myocardium.

REFERENCES

- Seminal primary article
- Key review paper

1 Mele D, Campana M, Sciavo M, *et al.* Impact of tissue harmonic imaging in patients with distorted left ventricles: improvement in accuracy and reproducibility of visual, manual and automated echocardiographic assessment of left ventricular ejection fraction. *Eur J Echocardiogr* 2003; **4**: 59–67.
2 Senior R, Sridhara BS, Basu S, *et al.* Comparison of radionuclide ventriculography and 2D echocardiography for the measurement of left ventricular ejection fraction following acute myocardial infarction. *Eur Heart J* 1994; **15**: 1235–9.

3   Jensen-Urstad K, Bouvier F, Hojer J, *et al.* Comparison of different echocardiographic methods with radionuclide imaging for measuring left ventricular ejection fraction during acute myocardial infarction treated by thrombolytic therapy. *Am J Cardiol* 1998; **81**: 538–44.

4   Nahar T, Croft L, Shapiro R, *et al.* Comparison of four echocardiographic techniques for measuring left ventricular ejection fraction. *Am J Cardiol* 2000; **86**: 1353–62.

5   Nousiainen T, Vanninen E, Jantunen E, *et al.* Concomitant impairment of left ventricular systolic and diastolic function during doxorubicin therapy: a prospective radionuclide ventriculographic and echocardiographic study. *Leuk Lymphoma* 2002; **43**: 1807–11.

● 6   Rahimtoola SH. A perspective on the three large multicenter randomized clinical trials of coronary bypass surgery for chronic stable angina. *Circulation* 1985; **72(6 Pt 2)**: V123–V135.

7   Perrone-Filardi P, Pace L, Prastaro M, *et al.* Assessment of myocardial viability in patients with chronic coronary artery disease. Rest–4-hour–24-hour ^{201}Tl tomography versus dobutamine echocardiography. *Circulation* 1996; **94**: 2712–9.

8   Udelson JE, Coleman PS, Metherall J, *et al.* Predicting recovery of severe regional ventricular dysfunction. Comparison of resting scintigraphy with ^{201}Tl and ^{99m}Tc-sestamibi. *Circulation* 1994; **89**: 2552–61.

● 9   Vanoverschelde JL, D'Hondt AM, Marwick T, *et al.* Head-to-head comparison of exercise–redistribution–reinjection thallium single-photon emission computed tomography and low dose dobutamine echocardiography for prediction of reversibility of chronic left ventricular ischemic dysfunction. *J Am Coll Cardiol* 1996; **28**: 432–42.

10   Gerber BL, Vanoverschelde JL, Bol A, *et al.* Myocardial blood flow, glucose uptake, and recruitment of inotropic reserve in chronic left ventricular ischemic dysfunction. Implications for the pathophysiology of chronic myocardial hibernation. *Circulation* 1996; **94**: 651–9.

● 11   Tillisch J, Brunken RC, Schwaiger MD, *et al.* Reversibility of cardiac wall-motion abnormalities predicted by positron tomography. *N Engl J Med* 1986; **314**: 884–8.

12   Tamaki N, Yonekura Y, Yamashita K, *et al.* Positron emission tomography using fluorine-18 deoxyglucose in evaluation of coronary artery bypass grafting. *Am J Cardiol* 1989; **64**: 860–5.

13   Baer FM, Voth E, Deutsch HJ, *et al.* Predictive value of low dose dobutamine transesophageal echocardiography and fluorine-18 fluorodeoxyglucose positron emission tomography for recovery of regional left ventricular function after successful revascularization. *J Am Coll Cardiol* 1996; **28**: 60–9.

14   Cigarroa CG, deFilippi CR, Brickner ME, *et al.* Dobutamine stress echocardiography identifies hibernating myocardium and predicts recovery of left ventricular function after coronary revascularization. *Circulation* 1993; **88**: 430–6.

15   La Canna G, Alfieri O, Giubbini R, *et al.* Echocardiography during infusion of dobutamine for identification of reversible dysfunction in patients with chronic coronary artery disease. *J Am Coll Cardiol* 1994; **23**: 617–26.

16   Afridi I, Kleiman NS, Raizner AE, Zoghbi WA. Dobutamine echocardiography in myocardial hibernation. Optimal dose and accuracy in predicting recovery of ventricular function after coronary angioplasty. *Circulation* 1995; **91**: 663–70.

17   Afridi I, Grayburn P, Panza JA, *et al.* Myocardial viability during dobutamine echocardiography predicts survival in patients with coronary artery disease and severe left ventricular systolic dysfunction. *J Am Coll Cardiol* 1998; **32**: 921–6.

18   Meluzìn J, Cigarroa CG, Brickner ME, *et al.* Dobutamine echocardiography in predicting improvement in global left ventricular systolic function after coronary bypass or angioplasty in patients with healed myocardial infarcts. *Am J Cardiol* 1995; **76**: 877–80.

19   DiCarli MF, Davidson M, Little R, *et al.* Value of metabolic imaging with positron emission tomography for evaluating prognosis in patients with coronary artery disease and left ventricular dysfunction. *Am J Cardiol* 1994; **73**: 527–33.

● 20   Allman KC, Shaw L, Hachamovitch R, Udelson JE. Myocardial viability testing and impact of revascularization on prognosis in patients with coronary artery disease and left ventricular dysfunction: a meta-analysis. *J Am Coll Cardiol* 2002; **39**: 1151–8.

21   Narula J, Dawson M, Singh B, *et al.* Noninvasive characterisation of stunned, hibernating, remodeled and nonviable myocardium in ischemic cardiomyopathy. *J Am Coll Cardiol* 2000; **36**: 1913–9.

22   Chaudhry F, Tauke J, Alessandrini R, *et al.* Prognostic implications of myocardial contractile reserve in patients with coronary artery disease and left ventricular dysfunction. *J Am Coll Cardiol* 1999; **34**: 738.

23   DiCarli MF, Maddahi J, Rokhsar S, *et al.* Long-term survival of patients with coronary artery disease and left ventricular dysfunction: implications for the role of myocardial viability assessment in management decisions. *J Thorac Cardiovasc Surg* 1998; **116**: 997–1004.

24   Pasquet A, Robert A, D'Hondt AM, *et al.* Prognostic value of myocardial ischaemia and viability in patients with chronic left ventricular ischaemic dysfunction. *Circulation* 1999; **100**: 141–8.

25   Lee KS, Marwick TH, Cook SA, *et al.* Prognosis of patients with left ventricular dysfunction, with and without viable myocardium after myocardial

infarction. Relative efficacy of medical therapy and revascularization. *Circulation* 1994; **90**: 2687–94.

26 Bax JJ, Poldermans D, Elhendy A, *et al*. Improvement of left ventricular ejection fraction, heart failure symptoms and prognosis after revascularisation in patients with chronic coronary artery disease and viable myocardium detected by dobutamine stress echocardiography. *J Am Coll Cardiol* 1999; **34**: 163–9.

27 Meluzìn J, Cerny J, Frélich M, *et al*. Prognostic value of the amount of dysfunctional but viable myocardium in revascularized patients with coronary artery disease and left ventricular dysfunction. *J Am Coll Cardiol* 1998; **32**: 912–20.

28 Pagley PR, Beller GA, Watson DD, *et al*. Improved outcome after coronary bypass surgery in patients with ischemic cardiomyopathy and residual myocardial viability. *Circulation* 1997; **96**: 793–800.

29 Senior R, Kaul S, Lahiri A. Myocardial viability on echocardiography predicts long-term survival after revascularization in patients with ischemic congestive heart failure. *J Am Coll Cardiol* 1999; **33**: 1848–54.

30 DiCarli MF, Asgarzadie F, Schelbert HR, *et al*. Quantitative relation between myocardial viability and improvement in heart failure symptoms after revascularization in patients with ischemic cardiomyopathy. *Circulation* 1995; **92**: 3436–44.

31 Flameng WJ, Shivalkar B, Spiessens B, *et al*. PET scan predicts recovery of left ventricular function after coronary artery bypass operation. *Ann Thorac Surg* 1997; **64**: 1694–701.

32 Pagano D, Townend JN, Littler WA, *et al*. Coronary artery bypass surgery as treatment for ischemic heart failure: the predictive value of viability assessment with quantitative positron emission tomography for symptomatic and functional outcome. *J Thorac Cardiovasc* Surg 1998; **115**: 791–9.

33 Bax JJ, Fath-Ordoubadi F, Boersma E, *et al*. Accuracy of PET in predicting functional recovery after revascularisation in patients with chronic ischaemic dysfunction: head-to-head comparison between blood flow, glucose utilisation and water-perfusable tissue fraction. *Eur J Nucl Med* 2002; **29**: 721–7.

34 Bax JJ, Visser FC, Poldermans D, *et al*. Relationship between preoperative viability and postoperative improvement in LVEF and heart failure symptoms. *J Nucl Med* 2001; **42**: 79–86.

35 Pitt M, Lewis M, Bonser RS. Coronary artery surgery for ischemic heart failure: risks, benefits, and the importance of assessment of myocardial viability. *Prog Cardiovasc Dis* 2001; **43**: 373–86.

● 36 Braunwald E, Kloner RA. The stunned myocardium: prolonged, postischemic ventricular dysfunction. *Circulation* 1982; **66**: 1146–9.

37 Braunwald E, Rutherford JD. Reversible ischemic left ventricular dysfunction: evidence for the 'hibernating myocardium'. *J Am Coll Cardiol* 1986; **8**: 1467–70.

38 Maseri A, Lanza G, Sanna T, *et al*. Coronary blood flow and myocardial ischaemia. In: Fuster V, Alexander R, O'Rourke R, Roberts R, King S, Wellens H. (eds.) *The heart*, 10th edition. New York: McGraw-Hill, 2001: 1109–30.

39 Pierard L, De Landsheere C, Berthe C, *et al*. Identification of viable myocardium by echocardiography during dobutamine infusion in patients with myocardial infarction after thrombolytic therapy: comparison with positron emission tomography. *J Am Coll Cardiol* 1990; **15**: 1031.

40 Smart S, Sawada SG, Ryan T. Low-dose dobutamine echocardiography detects reversible dysfunction after thrombolytic therapy of acute myocardial infarction. *Circulation* 1993; **88**: 405–15.

41 Rahimtoola SH. Coronary bypass surgery for chronic angina – 1981. A perspective. *Circulation* 2000; **65**: 225–41.

42 Diamond GA, Forrester JS, deLuz PL, *et al*. Post-extrasystolic potentiation of ischemic myocardium by atrial stimulation. *Am Heart J* 1978; **95**: 204–9.

● 43 Rahimtoola SH. The hibernating myocardium. *Am Heart J* 1989; **117**: 211–21.

◆ 44 Vanoverschelde JL, Melin JA. The pathophysiology of myocardial hibernation: current controversies and future directions. *Prog Cardiovasc Dis* 2001; **43**: 387–98.

45 Maes A, Flameng W, Nuyts J, *et al*. Histological alterations in chronically hypoperfused myocardium. *Circulation* 1994; **90**: 735–45.

● 46 Vanoverschelde JL, Wijns W, Depre C, *et al*. Mechanisms of chronic regional postischemic dysfunction in humans. New insights from the study of noninfarcted collateral-dependent myocardium. *Circulation* 1993; **87**: 1513–23.

47 Marinho NV, Keogh BE, Costa DC, *et al*. Pathophysiology of chronic left ventricular dysfunction. New insights from the measurement of absolute myocardial blood flow and glucose utilization. *Circulation* 1996; **93**: 737–44.

48 Shivalkar B, Maes A, Borgers M, *et al*. Only hibernating myocardium invariably shows early recovery after coronary revascularization. *Circulation* 1996; **94**: 308–15.

49 Marzullo P, Parodi O, Sambuceti G, *et al*. Residual coronary reserve identifies segmental viability in patients with wall motion abnormalities. *J Am Coll Cardiol* 1995; **26**: 342–50.

50 Kim R, Wu E, Rafael A, *et al*. The use of contrast-enhanced magnetic resonance imaging to identify reversible myocardial dysfunction. *N Engl J Med* 2000; **343**: 1445–53.

51 Ausma J, Thone F, Dispersyn GD, *et al*. Dedifferentiated cardiomyocytes from chronic hibernating myocardium are ischemia-tolerant. *Mol Cell Biochem* 1998; **186**: 159–68.

52 Alfieri O, La Canna G, Giubbini R, *et al*. Recovery of myocardial function. The ultimate target of coronary revascularization. *Eur J Cardiothorac Surg* 1993; **7**: 325–30.

53 Bax JJ, Visser FC, Poldermans D, *et al*. Time course of functional recovery of stunned and hibernating segments after surgical revascularization. *Circulation* 2001; **104(12, suppl 1)**: I314–I318.

54 Haas F, Augustin N, Holper K, *et al*. Time course and extent of improvement of dysfunctioning myocardium in patients with coronary artery disease and severely depressed left ventricular function after revascularisation: correlation with positron emission tomographic findings. *J Am Coll Cardiol* 2000; **36**: 1927–34.

◆ 55 Udelson JE. Steps forward in the assessment of myocardial viability in left ventricular dysfunction. *Circulation* 1998; **97**: 833–8.

56 Pagano D, Townend JN, Parums DV, *et al*. Hibernating myocardium: morphological correlates of inotropic stimulation and glucose uptake. *Heart* 2000; **83**: 456–61.

57 Gunning MG, Kaprielian R, Pepper J, *et al*. The histology of viable and hibernating myocardium in relation to imaging characteristics. *J Am Coll Cardiol* 2002; **39**: 428–35.

58 Gunning MG, Anagnostopoulos C, Knight CJ, *et al*. Comparison of ^{201}Tl, ^{99m}Tc-tetrofosmin, and dobutamine magnetic resonance imaging for identifying hibernating myocardium. *Circulation* 1998; **98**: 1869–74.

● 59 Bax JJ, Wijns W, Cornel JH, *et al*. Accuracy of currently available techniques for prediction of functional recovery after revascularization in patients with left ventricular dysfunction due to chronic coronary artery disease: comparison of pooled data. *J Am Coll Cardiol* 1997; **30**: 1451–60.

60 Barrington S, Chambers J, Hallett W, *et al*. Comparison of sestamibi, thallium, echocardiography and PET for the detection of hibernating myocardium. *Eur J Nucl Med* 2004; published online 6 November 2003 Springer-Verlag, Heidelberg.

61 Beanlands RS, Dawood F, Wen WH, *et al*. Are the kinetics of technetium-99m methoxyisobutyl isonitrile affected by cell metabolism and viability? *Circulation* 1990; **82**: 1802–14.

62 Piwnica-Worms D, Kronauge JF, Chiu ML. Uptake and retention of hexakis (2-methoxyisobutyl isonitrile) technetium(I) in cultured chick myocardial cells. Mitochondrial and plasma membrane potential dependence. *Circulation* 1990; **82**: 1826–38.

63 Gonzalez P, Massardo T, Munoz A, *et al*. Is the addition of ECG gating to technetium-99m sestamibi SPET of value in the assessment of myocardial viability? An evaluation based on two-dimensional echocardiography following revascularization. *Eur J Nucl Med* 1996; **23**: 1315–22.

64 Maes A, Borgers M, Flameng W, *et al*. Assessment of myocardial viability in chronic coronary artery disease using technetium-99m sestamibi SPECT. *J Am Coll Cardiol* 1997; **29**: 62–8.

65 Dakik H, Howell J, Lawrie G, *et al*. Assessment of myocardial viability with ^{99m}Tc-sestamibi tomography before coronary artery bypass surgery. *Circulation* 1997; **96**: 2892–8.

66 Wijns W, Vatner SF, Camici PG. Hibernating myocardium. *N Engl J Med* 1998; **339**: 173–81.

67 He Z, Verani MS. Evaluation of myocardial viability by myocardial perfusion imaging: should nitrates be used? *J Nucl Cardiol* 1998; **5**: 527–32.

68 Bisi G, Sciagra R, Santoro GM, Fazzini PF. Rest technetium-99m sestamibi tomography in combination with short-term administration of nitrates: feasibility and reliability for prediction of postrevascularization outcome of asynergic territories. *J Am Coll Cardiol* 1994; **24**: 1282–9.

69 Sciagra R, Bisi G, Santoro GM, *et al*. Comparison of baseline-nitrate technetium-99m sestamibi with rest–redistribution thallium-201 tomography in detecting viable hibernating myocardium and predicting post revascularization recovery. *J Am Coll Cardiol* 1997; **30**: 384–91.

70 Sciagra R, Leoncini M, Marcucci G, *et al*. Technetium-99m sestamibi imaging to predict left ventricular ejection fraction outcome after revascularisation in patients with chronic coronary artery disease and left ventricular dysfunction: comparison between baseline and nitrate-enhanced imaging. *Eur J Nucl Med* 2001; **28**: 680–7.

71 Maurea S, Cuocolo A, Soricelli A, *et al*. Enhanced detection of viable myocardium by technetium-99m-MIBI imaging after nitrate administration in chronic coronary artery disease. *J Nucl Med* 1995; **36**: 1945–52.

72 Li ST, Liu XJ, Lu ZL, *et al*. Quantitative analysis of technetium-99m 2-methoxyisobutyl isonitrile single-photon emission computed tomography and isosorbide dinitrate infusion in assessment of myocardial viability before and after revascularization. *J Nucl Cardiol* 1996; **3(6 Pt 1)**: 457–63.

73 Weich H, Strauss HW, Pitt B. The extraction of thallium-201 by the myocardium. *Circulation* 1977; **56**: 188–91.

74 Dilsizian V, Rocco TP, Freedman NM, *et al*. Enhanced detection of ischemic but viable myocardium by the reinjection of thallium after stress–redistribution imaging. *N Engl J Med* 1990; **323**: 141–6.

75 Bax JJ, Cornel JH, Visser FC, *et al*. Prediction of recovery of myocardial dysfunction after revascularization. Comparison of fluorine-18 fluorodeoxyglucose/thallium-201 SPECT, thallium-201 stress–reinjection SPECT and

dobutamine echocardiography. *J Am Coll Cardiol* 1996; **28**: 558–64.

76 Siebelink H, Blanksma P, Crijns H, *et al.* No difference in cardiac event-free survival between positron emission tomography-guided and single-photon emission computed tomography-guided patient management. *J Am Coll Cardiol* 2001; **37**: 81–8.

77 Soufer R, Dey HM, Ng CK, Zaret BL. Comparison of sestamibi single-photon emission computed tomography with positron emission tomography for estimating left ventricular myocardial viability. *Am J Cardiol* 1995; **75**: 1214–9.

78 Matsunari I, Boning G, Ziegler SI, *et al.* Attenuation-corrected ^{99m}Tc-tetrofosmin single-photon emission computed tomography in the detection of viable myocardium: comparison with positron emission tomography using ^{18}F-fluorodeoxyglucose. *J Am Coll Cardiol* 1998; **32**: 927–35.

● 79 Depre C, Vanoverschelde JL, Melin JA, *et al.* Structural and metabolic correlates of the reversibility of chronic left ventricular ischemic dysfunction in humans. *Am J Physiol* 1995; **268(3 Pt 2)**: H1265–H1275.

● 80 Elsasser A, Schlepper M, Klovekorn W, *et al.* Hibernating myocardium: an incomplete adaptation to ischaemia. *Circulation* 1997; **96**: 2920–31.

81 Marshall R, Tillisch JH, Phelps ME, *et al.* Identification and differentiation of resting myocardial ischemia and infarction in man with positron computed tomography, ^{18}F-labeled fluorodeoxyglucose and N-13 ammonia. *Circulation* 1983; **67**: 766–78.

◆ 82 Schelbert HR. Measurements of myocardial metabolism in patients with ischaemic heart disease. *Am J Cardiol* 1998; **82**: 61K–7K.

83 Srinivasan G, Kitsiou AN, Bacharach SL, *et al.* [^{18}F]fluorodeoxyglucose single photon emission computed tomography: can it replace PET and thallium SPECT for the assessment of myocardial viability? *Circulation* 1998; **97**: 843–50.

84 Matsunari I, Yoneyama T, Kanayama S, *et al.* Phantom studies for estimation of defect size on cardiac (18)F SPECT and PET: implications for myocardial viability assessment. *J Nucl Med* 2001; **42**: 1579–85.

85 Knuuti MJ, Saraste M, Nuutila P, *et al.* Myocardial viability: fluorine-18-deoxyglucose positron emission tomography in prediction of wall motion recovery after revascularisation. *Am Heart J* 1994; **127**: 785–96.

86 Schelbert HR. Euglycemic hyperinsulinemic clamp and oral glucose load in stimulating myocardial glucose utilisation during positron emission tomography. *J Nucl Med* 1992; **33**: 1263–6.

87 Knuuti MJ, Nuutila P, Ruotsalainen U, *et al.* Euglycemic hyperinsulinemic clamp and oral glucose load in stimulating myocardial glucose utilization during positron emission tomography. *J Nucl Med* 1992; **33**: 1255–62.

88 Pagano D, Bonser RS, Townend JN, *et al.* Predictive value of dobutamine echocardiography and positron emission tomography in identifying hibernating myocardium in patients with postischaemic heart failure. *Heart* 1998; **79**: 281–8.

89 deFilippi CR, Willett DL, Irani WN, *et al.* Comparison of myocardial contrast echocardiography and low-dose dobutamine stress echocardiography in predicting recovery of left ventricular function after coronary revascularization in chronic ischemic heart disease. *Circulation* 1995; **92**: 2863–8.

90 Nagueh SF, Vaduganathan P, Ali N, *et al.* Identification of hibernating myocardium: comparative accuracy of myocardial contrast echocardiography, rest-redistribution thallium-201 tomography and dobutamine echocardiography. *J Am Coll Cardiol* 1997; **29**: 985–93.

91 McGhie AI, Corbett JR, Akers MS, *et al.* Regional cardiac adrenergic function using I-123 meta-iodobenzylguanidine tomographic imaging after acute myocardial infarction. *Am J Cardiol* 1991; **67**: 236–42.

92 Stanton MS, Tuli MM, Radtke NL, *et al.* Regional sympathetic denervation after myocardial infarction in humans detected noninvasively using I-123-metaiodobenzylguanidine. *J Am Coll Cardiol* 1989; **14**: 1519–26.

93 Wichter T, Hindricks G, Lerch H, *et al.* Regional myocardial sympathetic dysinnervation in arrhythmogenic right ventricular cardiomyopathy. An analysis using ^{123}I-meta-iodobenzylguanidine scintigraphy. *Circulation* 1994; **89**: 667–83.

94 Merlet P, Benvenuti C, Moyse D, *et al.* Prognostic value of MIBG imaging in idiopathic dilated cardiomyopathy. *J Nucl Med* 1999; **40**: 917–23.

95 Merlet P, Pouillart F, Dubois-Rande JL, *et al.* Sympathetic nerve alterations assessed with ^{123}I-MIBG in the failing human heart. *J Nucl Med* 1999; **40**: 224–31.

96 Schofer J, Spielmann R, Schuchert A, *et al.* Iodine-123 meta-iodobenzylguanidine scintigraphy: a noninvasive method to demonstrate myocardial adrenergic nervous system disintegrity in patients with idiopathic dilated cardiomyopathy. *J Am Coll Cardiol* 1988; **12**: 1252–8.

97 Somsen GA, van Vlies B, de Milliano PA, *et al.* Increased myocardial [^{123}I]-metaiodobenzylguanidine uptake after enalapril treatment in patients with chronic heart failure. *Heart* 1996; **76**: 218–22.

◆ 98 Udelson JE, Shafer CD, Carrio I. Radionuclide imaging in heart failure: assessing etiology and outcomes and implications for management. *J Nucl Cardiol* 2002; **9(5, suppl)**: 40S–52S.

7

Radionuclide imaging in thoracic disease

7A Ventilation perfusion imaging: a changing role for suspected pulmonary embolism

Introduction	197	Diagnosis of venous thromboembolism	206
Anatomy and physiology	197	Conclusion	220
Ventilation perfusion imaging	199	References	220

7B Lung cancer

Introduction	223	Detection of recurrent non-small cell lung cancer	230
Solitary pulmonary nodules	224	Chemotherapy/radiotherapy	230
Staging of non-small cell lung cancer	226	Positron emission tomography–computed tomography	232
Assessment of distant metastases	227	Small-cell lung cancer	233
Management change and cost-effectiveness of		Mesothelioma	233
fluorodeoxyglucose positron emission tomography		Conclusion	234
in non-small cell lung cancer	227	References	235
Fluorodeoxyglucose positron emission tomography	230		

7C Other pulmonary applications

Introduction	239	Granulomatous diseases of the lung	243
Inflammation and infection	239	Sarcoidosis	243
Lung permeability measurements	240	HIV positive patients	245
Method of measuring DTPA transfer	242	Other immunosuppressed conditions	247
Idiopathic interstitial lung diseases	242	Conclusion	248
Adult respiratory distress syndrome	243	References	248

Ventilation perfusion imaging: a changing role for suspected pulmonary embolism

H.W. GRAY

INTRODUCTION

Venous thromboembolism (VTE), otherwise known as pulmonary embolism (PE), can behave like a dangerous predator gnawing at the very strands of life itself. It can develop slowly, usually unseen, and often bursts into full clinical view with frightening rapidity and a potentially life-threatening cardio-pulmonary illness. Most experts believe from the evidence that up to 25% of sufferers will die within the first 4 weeks with a significant number succumbing within the first hour.[1,2]

Diagnosis of PE can be difficult for clinical staff because it shares early symptoms and signs with so many more benign cardio-pulmonary conditions[3]. While we in nuclear medicine have rarely been involved in treatment or prevention, we have had an important role in diagnosis of PE and in its exclusion for those cases where the clinical pre-test probability of PE was low to medium. The important task of eliminating PE from the clinical equation has always been helped by the speed at which VQ imaging can be performed and interpreted. This particular role is increasing in frequency at present and is permitting physicians, surgeons, obstetricians and family doctors to safely redirect their diagnostic energies to alternate diagnoses for those patients with suspicious symptoms but normal chest X-rays.

In the last 10 years, the most exciting development in PE diagnosis for specialists in internal medicine has been the development, refining and deployment of computed tomography pulmonary angiography (CTPA). Most clinicians and radiologists are now confident that with modern multidetector row machines (MDCT) and 1–2 mm chest slices,

the majority of major vessel and segmental emboli can be detected.[4] Negative MDCT appears to correlate well with a low risk of subsequent PE.[5]

It seems reasonable therefore to ask whether there is a need to continue the provision of VQ imaging now that CTPA is more widely available than nuclear medicine services throughout our smaller hospitals in the UK. This chapter therefore will explore the rationale for VQ imaging in the age of CT scanning, its strengths, weaknesses and indications particularly as they each relate to MDCT pulmonary angiography.

ANATOMY AND PHYSIOLOGY

Lung structure

The lungs are essentially two thin-walled elastic sponges within the chest that communicate with the atmosphere via the naso-pharynx and trachea and are really receptacles for the environment. Gas is transported to the alveoli by a system of branching airways of decreasing caliber and length. The number of airways increases from 1 at the level of trachea to 130 000 at the level of the terminal bronchioles while the internal diameter falls to about 0.4 mm at the level of the respiratory and alveolar ducts. Airflow is maximal in the trachea (200 cm s^{-1}) and slows towards the periphery such that gas flow occurs solely by diffusion in the terminal bronchioles and beyond. The volume of the conducting airways is 150 mL whereas the volume of gas within the lungs at functional residual capacity (FRC) is 2.3 L.

Alveoli, minute sacks of diameter 200 μm, are grouped into acini each supplied by a terminal bronchiole and acinar arteriole. Their walls are made up of a thin layer of alveolar cells surrounded by a confluent mesh of fine-walled capillaries supported by interstitial tissue. There are 300 million alveoli in each lung and the total surface area of alveolar wall for gas exchange is around $80\,m^2$ in the adult lung.

The distribution of ventilation is not uniform and is influenced by gravity and the rate and depth of breathing. Alveoli at the lung apices are more distended at FRC because of the greater trans-pulmonary pressures therefore ventilation per unit lung volume is greater at the lung bases.

The pulmonary circulation is distinctive as it accommodates the entire circulating blood volume ($6\,L\,m^{-1}$) and provides a huge surface area for gas exchange at low pressure. From the right or left pulmonary artery, venous blood is transported to the gas-exchanging areas by successive arterial divisions numbering 17 resulting in a vast number of vessels (200–300 million). The internal diameter of the pulmonary vessels diminishes from 1.86 cm in the main pulmonary artery to 8.3 μm in the alveolar capillaries.

Regional blood flow is non-uniform because of gravity. Because of this, perfusion per unit volume is lower at the lung apex than at the lung base in the upright position. Acinar venules drain oxygenated blood into segmental, lobar then main pulmonary veins and thence to the left atrium and ventricle for distribution to body organs. A separate bronchial circulation supplies arterial blood to lung tissues down to the level of the smallest bronchiole.

The lungs are organized into lobes with an upper, middle and lower on the right and an upper and lower on the left. The lobes are further subdivided into segments each supplied by a specific segmental bronchus and pulmonary artery and drained by a pulmonary vein. The branching structure of the bronchi (Fig. 7A.1) is similar to that for pulmonary vessels.

Lung function

Breathing is essentially an involuntary mechanical process controlled by the respiratory center in the medulla oblongata through nervous and chemical feedback mechanisms. Inspiration occurs when efferent nerve impulses from the respiratory center contract the diaphragmatic and intercostal muscles. As air enters the lungs, stretch receptors in the airways start firing. The more the lungs inflate, the faster the stretch receptors feedback impulses. When the lungs are inflated sufficiently, signals from the respiratory center stop for a short time and exhalation follows automatically.

The respiratory center in the medulla oblongata contains central chemoreceptors sensitive to the CO_2 concentration in the arterial blood. The carotid bodies in the wall of the carotid arteries and the aortic bodies on the aortic arch represent the peripheral chemoreceptors that sense both changes in CO_2 concentration and pH levels and to a

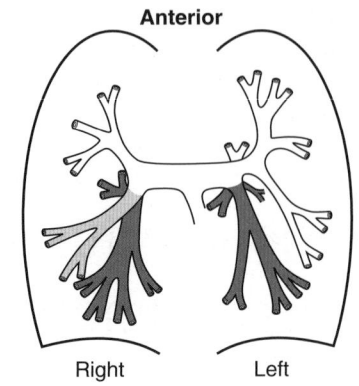

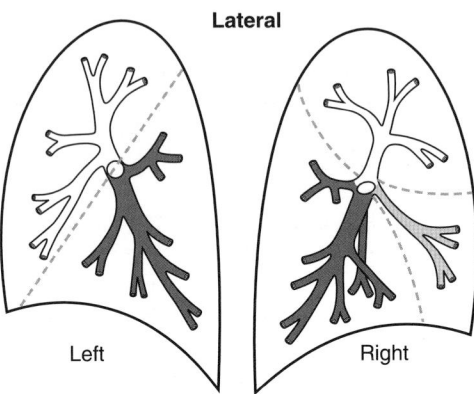

Figure 7A.1 *Branching structure of the larger pulmonary vessels. Segmental arteries include 1-apical, 2-posterior, 1,2-apicoposterior, 3-anterior, 4-lateral (r) or superior lingular (l), 5-medial (r) or inferior lingular (l), 6-apical, 7-medial basal, 8-anterior basal, 9-lateral basal, 10-posterior basal.*

lesser extent, changes in O_2 concentration. By these means, a normal pressure of O_2 in arterial blood (P_aO_2) between 11 and 13 kPa (83–98 mmHg) and CO_2 (P_aCO_2) at 4.8–6 kPa (36–45 mmHg) are maintained. A resting blood flow through the lungs of $5\,L\,min^{-1}$ carries $11\,mmol\,min^{-1}$ of O_2 from lungs to body tissues. A resting ventilation of $6\,L\,min^{-1}$ carries $9\,mmol\,min^{-1}$ ($200\,mL\,min^{-1}$) of CO_2 out of the body. The normal lung has a great reserve capacity for increasing both the lung blood flow and the ventilation during exercise.

Ventilation perfusion matching

There is usually an efficient matching between ventilation and perfusion in the normal lung. This match can be adversely affected by primary disorders of the heart, pulmonary vasculature or lung parenchyma. A lung sector ventilated but unperfused increases the physiological deadspace. A sector perfused but unventilated causes physiological shunting which leads to desaturation of the arterial blood. Pulmonary vessels, however, compensate by displaying the phenomenon of hypoxic vasoconstriction. When alveolar P_{O_2} falls below 70 mmHg, regional perfusion diminishes to prevent or reduce physiological shunting. This reflex serves to preserve the balance (matching) of ventilation and perfusion as close to normal as possible.

In an erect individual, perfusion will tend to be inadequate at the lung apices (mismatched) while the reverse occurs at the bases. This results from gravitational forces acting upon a low pressure pulmonary circulation (2 kPa or 15 mmHg) and will therefore change on recumbancy. In that position, perfusion will be greatest posteriorly and least anteriorly. Ventilation is abbreviated to 'V' in pulmonary physiology while 'Q' represents perfusion from '*quellen*' in German for springing or gushing forth.

VENTILATION PERFUSION IMAGING

Perfusion imaging

When a thoroughly mixed tracer in arterial blood is completely removed in a single passage through an organ, the final distribution of the tracer within that organ is proportional to the relative blood flow in different areas within that organ. The unique properties of the pulmonary circulation permit regional pulmonary perfusion to be imaged following the intravenous injection of ^{99m}Tc-labeled human macro-aggregated albumin (MAA). These particles, which measure 10–40 μm in diameter, impact in the terminal arterioles and other pre-capillary vessels and have a lung residence time long enough for imaging. All commercial MAA is manufactured from plasma known to be virus free and the safety record of MAA over 35 years has been exemplary. Early on, however, a number of deaths did occur in patients with severe pulmonary hypertension which indicated that particle numbers were important in cases where disease had reduced the number of pulmonary vessels. It is now recognized that 60 000 particles is the minimum required to avoid spurious non-uniformity in the acquired image. Conversely, increasing the number of particles above 200 000 has little effect on image quality. Most now agree that the ideal number of particles for injection to provide an acceptable perfusion scan lies between 100 000 and 200 000 and that the ideal particle size is between 10 and 40 μm. In patients with pulmonary hypertension, particle numbers should be between 60 000 and 80 000. For children less than 1 year, between 10 000 and 20 000 particles is advised while for those under 3 years, between 30 000 and 50 000 is the recognized standard.

If 200 000 particles are administered to a normal adult subject, fewer than 0.1% of the total number of arterioles will be blocked giving a safety margin of around 1000:1.

Side effects from MAA are very uncommon, the majority being allergic in nature. Initial concerns about cerebral toxicity have been assuaged and ^{99m}Tc-MAA has been used for over 30 years to assess right-to-left intra-cardiac shunts in children and adults though the dose of albumin should be limited to 0.2 mg or 100 000 particles (Fig. 7A.2).

Prior to intravenous injection, the vial or syringe containing the ^{99m}Tc-MAA should be shaken gently to resuspend particles that have settled. A normal MAA dose for VQ imaging in the UK is 80 MBq ($\approx$2 mCi) while 240 MBq ($\approx$6 mCi) is used in the USA. A slow intravenous bolus injection over 30 s is best while the patient breathes normally. This ensures a uniform distribution within the pulmonary circulation. MAA adheres to plastic so giving sets should be avoided. Withdrawal of blood into the syringe prior to injection should also be avoided as blood can cause particle aggregation. The resulting clump of MAA impacts in lung to provide a highly radioactive perfusion artefact (Fig. 7A.3).

There is no correct position for the patient at the time of MAA injection. The author favors the supine position for injection to permit adequate visualization of the apices. Clearly, one has to accept a relative sparing of the anterior lung.

^{99m}Tc-MAA is eliminated from the lung microvasculature by dissociation of the ^{99m}Tc label and mechanical dispersion of the protein particle. The dissociation of ^{99m}Tc begins within the hour (t_{fi} = 50 min) while the mechanical dispersion of the albumin particle is slower with a $t_{1/2}$ of nearer 5 h.

The radiation absorbed dose (effective dose equivalent) following a standard ^{99m}Tc-MAA perfusion scan is approximately 1 mSv (100 mrem). In pregnancy, where the dose of MAA is 50% of normal, the dose to the uterus is low at 0.14 mGy (14 mrad). Breast feeding must be interrupted for 24 h after a perfusion scan but the milk can be refrigerated and used the following day. Staff-absorbed dose from a standard 80 MBq is 1.5 μSv (150 μrem).

Perfusion imaging continues to be performed routinely using multiple view planar imaging. Images are acquired using a low energy, all-purpose collimator, a large-field-of-view camera centered upon a 140 keV peak and a 20% window. Images of between 200 000 and 1 000 000 counts are acquired in six projections: anterior, posterior, left and right posterior oblique and either right and left lateral or right and left anterior oblique projections.

In a normal study (Fig. 7A.4, page 202), the lung margins are concave and uninterrupted reflecting the diaphragm, chest wall and lung apical contours. On the anterior and posterior projections, the medial borders are indented by the hilar structures, the heart and the spine, respectively. The hilar apparatus is observed centrally on the oblique and lateral views, as is the scapula in the posterior oblique. The cardiac impression is seen anteriorly, and on the left anterior oblique and lateral projections.

Pulmonary emboli characteristically appear as lobar, segmental or subsegmental pleural-based perfusion defects. Planar perfusion scintigraphy may underestimate the size of the defects[6] and there is some evidence that single photon emission tomography improves the detection of segmental defects (Fig. 7A.5, page 203) in PE.[7] Single photon

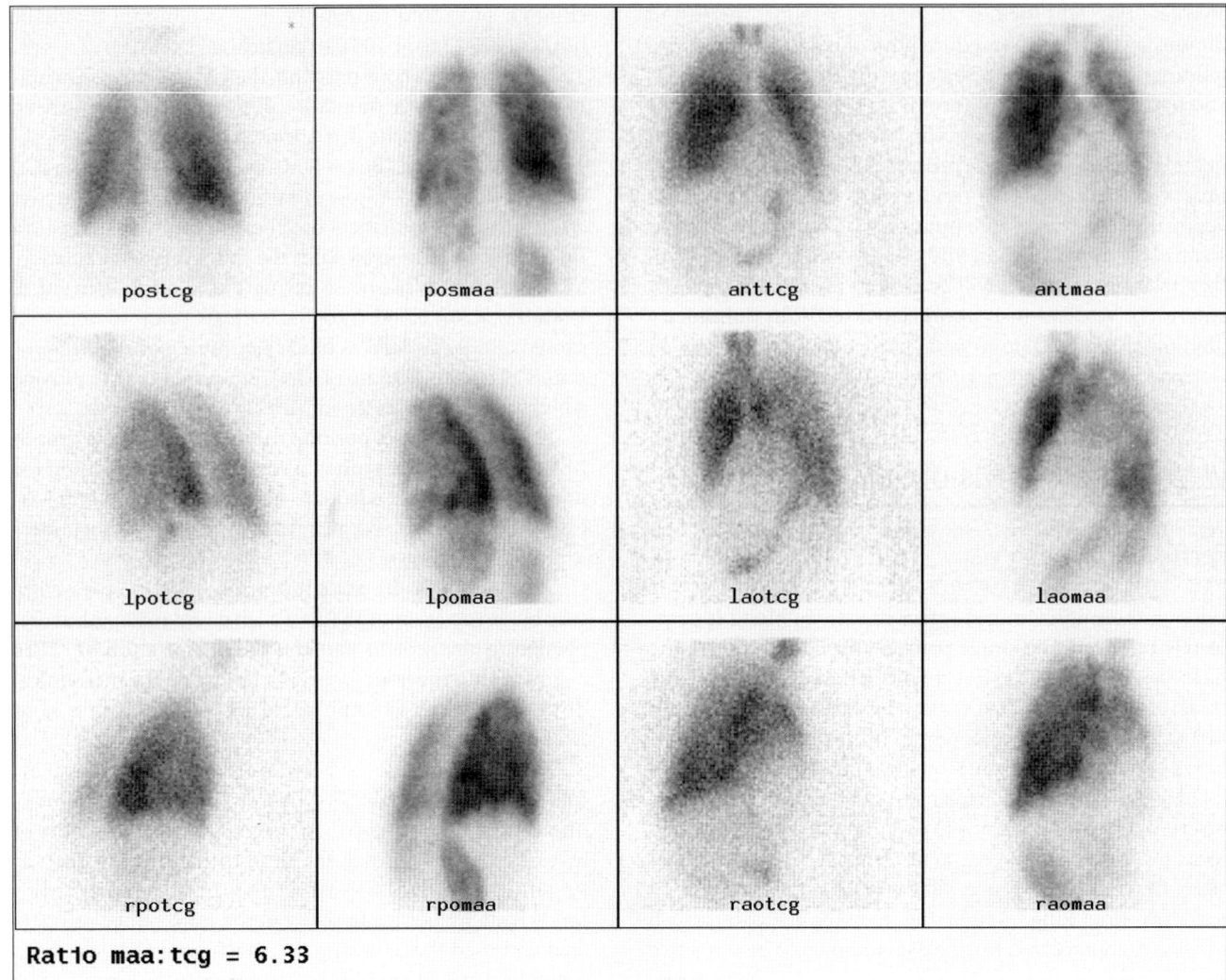

Figure 7A.2   *Ventilation and perfusion lung scan showing renal macro-aggregated albumin (MAA) activity from right-to-left shunt. Brain images with equivalent activity are not shown.*

emission computerized tomography (SPECT), however, is more taxing for the breathless patient because of longer data acquisition in the supine position so it has been used infrequently in the UK up until now.

Resolution of pulmonary emboli can occur at different rates in different patients. Thrombus dissolution occurs mainly by thrombolysis or mechanical dispersion. Most authorities therefore advise scanning within 24 h of the presenting symptom. One other advantage of early scanning is the ability to image while the chest X-ray is clear of parenchymal density. When lung consolidation or infiltration appears, VQ imaging is often of little value for diagnosis of PE and cannot exclude it either.

Ventilation imaging

Ventilation imaging complements perfusion imaging by revealing those perfusion defects likely to be related to PE and those to chronic airways disease. Perfusion defects are present in regions of acute or chronic airways obstruction because regional hypoxia results in compensation by reflex arteriolar vasoconstriction in the same area. Perfusion abnormalities can therefore be classified as matched to ventilation (i.e. likely to be due to airways obstruction) or mismatched to ventilation (i.e. unlikely to be the result of airways obstruction).

Four techniques for ventilation imaging can be performed in most departments, namely ^{133}Xe, ^{81m}Kr, ^{99m}Tc-labeled aerosols or ^{99m}Tc-labeled Technegas.

RADIOACTIVE XENON

Xenon-133 has, until recently, formed the basis for ventilation assessment for 30 years and is still widely used in North America. An inert gas, it decays by beta emission with a half-life of 5.3 days and produces 81-keV photons at 37% abundance. Xenon is best inhaled prior to imaging with

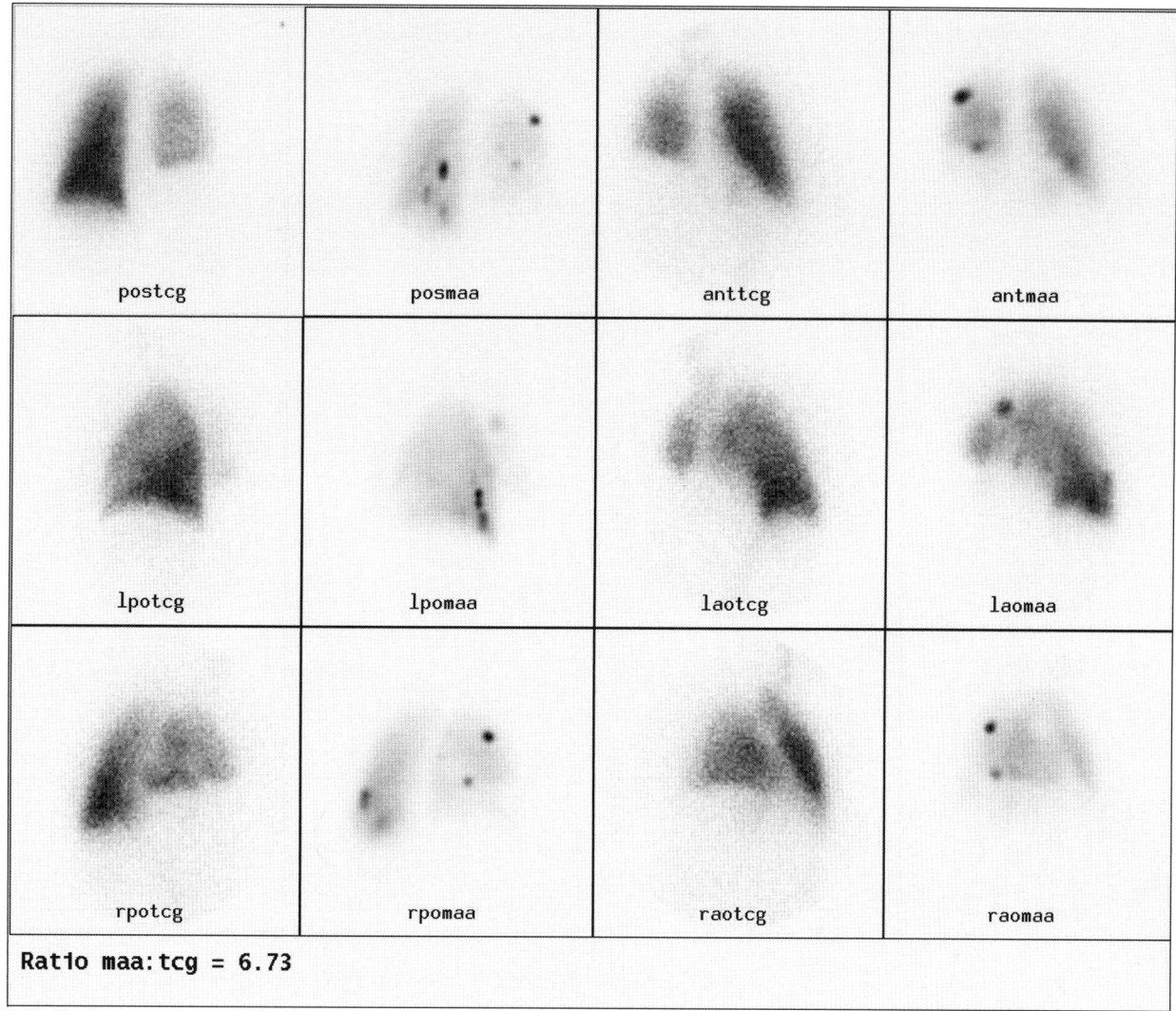

Figure 7A.3 *Ventilation and perfusion lung scan showing multiple clumps of macro-aggregated albumin (MAA) producing highly radioactive perfusion artifacts.*

^{99m}Tc-MAA and requires a fair degree of cooperation from the patient. The two principal methods of acquiring meaningful data are the single breath and the multiple breath steady state techniques (equilibrium and washout).

The single breath and breath hold after inhalation of ^{133}Xe provides a useful image of regional ventilation. In the UK a dose of 37 MBq (1 mCi) is used, while in the USA 370 MBq (10 mCi) is used. The posterior projection has been standard in the UK, while in the USA anterior and posterior projections are obtained using dual-headed cameras. The ^{133}Xe gas is best injected directly into the inhalation circuit as close as possible to the patient's mouth and at the start of the deep inspiration. Unfortunately, ill patients with dyspnea find the breath hold particularly difficult to perform.

The multiple breath steady state technique consists of three phases: namely wash-in, equilibrium and washout following introduction of ^{133}Xe into the spirometer circuit. During re-breathing (wash-in period), most of the aerated

portions of lung will achieve a uniform and an equilibrium concentration of ^{133}Xe. The equilibrium images reflect the regional lung volume but no information whatever on regional ventilation rate. In the USA, anterior, posterior, left anterior oblique and right anterior oblique views are obtained.

During the washout phase, the patient breathes room air and sequential dynamic imaging reflects the rate of clearance of the radioactive gas from the lungs. Well-ventilated areas of lung clear the ^{133}Xe fairly rapidly.

In obstructive lung disease, there will be delay in the wash-in of areas that are poorly ventilated but the equilibration views may be relatively normal. The washout views show delayed clearance of gas from areas of poor ventilation and appear as areas of persisting radioactivity. The washout images are more sensitive for airways obstruction than the single-breath images (Fig. 7A.6, page 204). Dual-camera technology permits imaging in anterior, posterior,

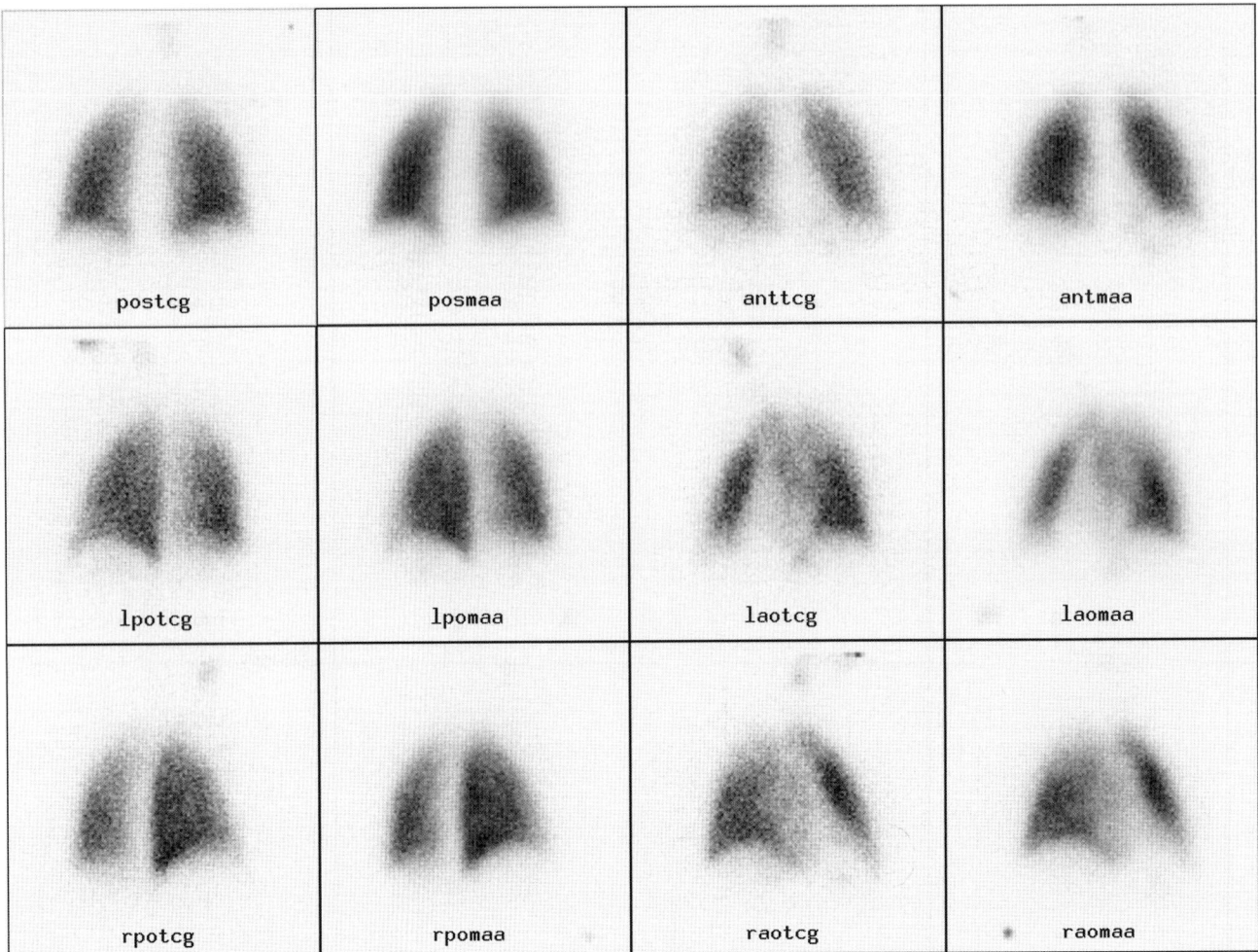

Figure 7A.4 *Normal category six-view* ^{99m}*Tc-Technegas ventilation (left) and* ^{99m}*Tc-macro-aggregated albumin (MAA) perfusion (right) scan performed sequentially. Count rate of perfusion was more than five times that of ventilation images.*

and even posterior oblique can be obtained to image the lateral segments of the lower lobes.

The long half-life of ^{133}Xe and its weight mean that contamination of the atmosphere from a careless patient can lead to ^{133}Xe at floor level for many days. Accordingly, radiation safety demands that expiration is closely supervised and that expired breath is passed through a charcoal trap or vented to atmosphere.

The effective dose equivalent for each 37 MBq of ^{133}Xe administration is approximately 0.3 mSv and the staff dose is estimated to be 0.1 μSv from each patient.

KRYPTON-81m

Krypton-81m, produced from an ^{81}Rb generator, is the ideal inert gas for ventilation studies. The patient is injected with ^{99m}Tc-MAA and the first perfusion image acquired. Next, the patient breathes a mixture of ^{81m}Kr in air or oxygen produced by passing a stream of water-humidified air or oxygen through the generator. This permits the ventilation image to be acquired in the same position after altering the

energy window of the gamma camera. The procedure is then repeated following the acquisition of each subsequent perfusion image. The half-life of 13 s means that ^{81m}Kr decays very quickly within the lungs with none of the xenon tendency to build up in underventilated areas. The image signal is therefore equivalent to a 'single breath' with xenon and opposite to the xenon washout. It also results in a tiny radiation dose (effective dose equivalent (EDE) 0.1 mSv) to the patient and a minute dose for staff (0.1 μSv).

The relatively high photon energy of 190 keV from ^{81m}Kr is ideal for dual imaging with ^{99m}Tc and permits acquisition of separate perfusion and ventilation signals with excellent positional match and comparability (Fig. 7A.7). High-quality perfusion images with ^{99m}Tc-MAA can also be obtained because the krypton in the lungs disappears rapidly due to its short half-life when the gas is eliminated from the inspired air.

The short half-life of the generator results from the short parental half-life (^{81}Rb: $t_{1/2}$ 4.5 h) and means that a new generator is required each day. In the UK, the twice weekly cyclotron production of ^{81}Rb and considerable expense rather limits its availability and application except in some larger

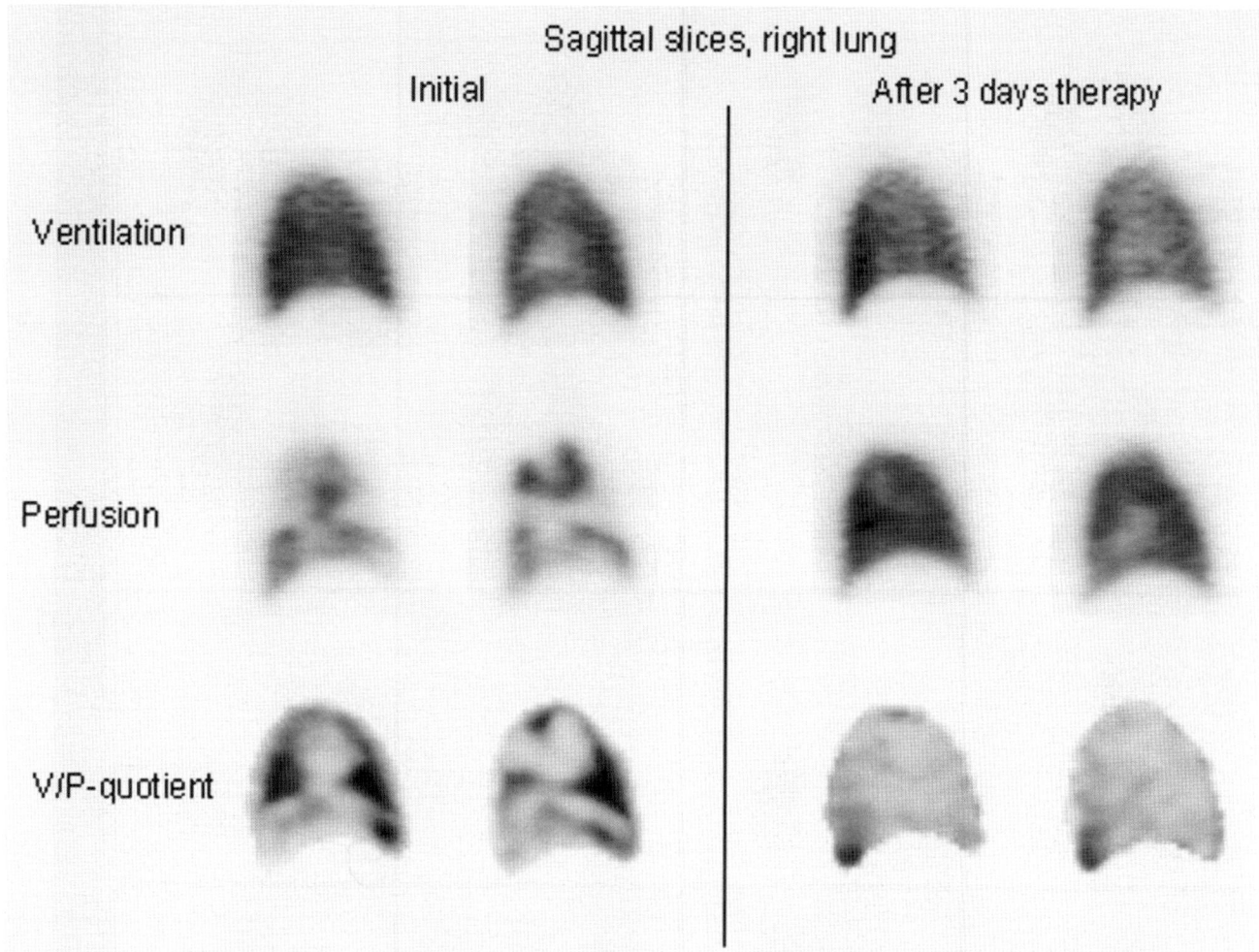

Figure 7A.5 *Sagittal slices of right lung from a patient on presentation with pulmonary embolism and 3 days after heparin therapy. Clear-cut mismatched segmental abnormalities of perfusion were seen which largely resolve following treatment. (Image kindly provided by Dr Bajc.)*

centers. Several patients (eight at least) need to be studied with each generator for the costs to mirror other ventilation agents.

The final problem with the technique relates to the many high-energy photons from the ^{81m}Rb. They mandate considerable lead shielding for the generator making it heavy and awkward to handle and maneuver within the department.

AEROSOL VENTILATION

When ^{81m}Kr is unavailable or impractical, ^{99m}Tc aerosols provide a ventilation signal that not only has an ideal energy but also is provided in six views, independently acquired, to position match with perfusion. An aerosol is basically a mixture of liquid droplets or solid particles that are stable as a suspension in air. Aerosols are usually defined by the size of their particles.

Following inhalation, aerosol particles are removed from the inhaled air by inertial and gravitational forces. Impaction on mucosal surfaces at the bifurcation of large airways occurs due to the changes in airflow direction at high

speed. Impaction also occurs at any air velocity when an aerosol particle makes a chance contact with the bronchial wall. Sedimentation of particles or settlement occurs due to gravity in the smaller airways and alveolar spaces. Finally, diffusion of particles is the natural tendency for suspended particles to drift randomly with the alveolar air resulting in chance contact with the respiratory membranes. The probability of particle contact with respiratory membrane is enhanced by hygroscopic growth of the particle, coalescence of several particles within the airways or by slow tidal breathing and breath holding. Particles of mean diameter 1–5 μm are deposited in the lower respiratory tract whereas particles < 1 μm penetrate the alveolar compartment. While 10% only of these ultrafine particles are retained in the alveoli, they provide the optimum image for assessing regional ventilation.

AEROSOL DROPLET PARTICLES

These are produced by either a jet or ultrasonic device primed with ^{99m}Tc-DTPA which should produce a majority

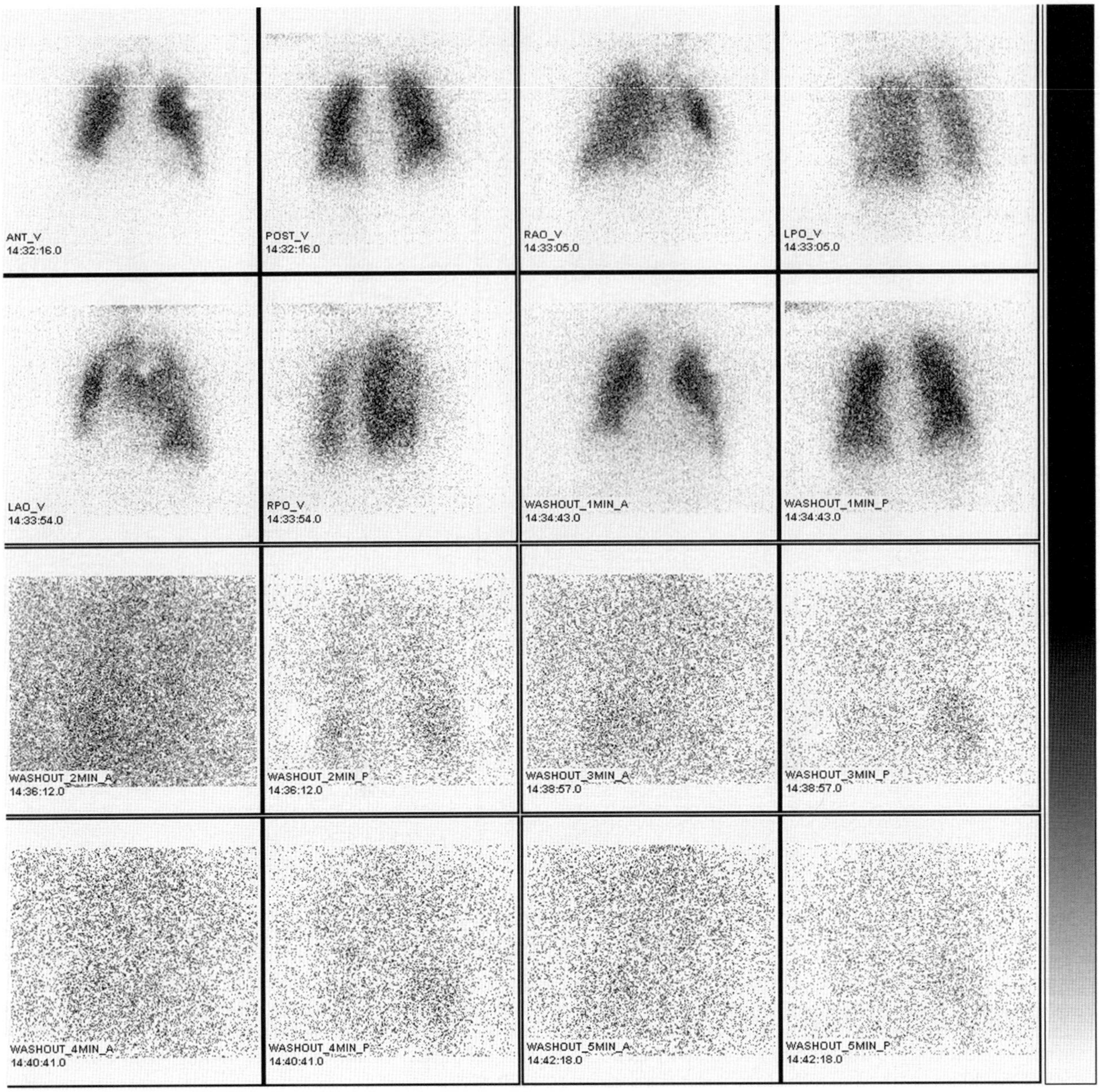

ANT_V
14:32:16.0

POST_V
14:32:16.0

RAO_V
14:33:05.0

LPO_V
14:33:05.0

LAO_V
14:33:54.0

RPO_V
14:33:54.0

WASHOUT_1MIN_A
14:34:43.0

WASHOUT_1MIN_P
14:34:43.0

WASHOUT_2MIN_A
14:36:12.0

WASHOUT_2MIN_P
14:36:12.0

WASHOUT_3MIN_A
14:38:57.0

WASHOUT_3MIN_P
14:38:57.0

WASHOUT_4MIN_A
14:40:41.0

WASHOUT_4MIN_P
14:40:41.0

WASHOUT_5MIN_A
14:42:18.0

WASHOUT_5MIN_P
14:42:18.0

Figure 7A.6 *Equilibration images for ^{133}Xe (upper two rows) and washout (lower two rows) in a patient with obstructive airways disease showing retention particularly at the right base. (Image kindly provided by Dr Holmes.)*

of particles less than 1 μm in size. The jet nebulizer is frequently used to provide ultrafine particles and it functions on the Bernoulli principle. Oxygen at a standard flow rate of 8 L min^{-1} is passed through a small hole known as a Venturi. The resulting fall in surrounding air pressure produces atomization of the liquid in the feeding bowl. Such nebulizers reliably produce aerosols with 90–95% of the particles less than 1 μm in diameter. The ultrasonic technology used in such equipment varies. The most recent advance uses an electronic micropump. At the heart of the generator is an aperture plate that contains 1000 precision-tapered holes surrounded by a vibrational element. Vibration at $> 100\,000$ s^{-1} causes each micro-aperture to act as a

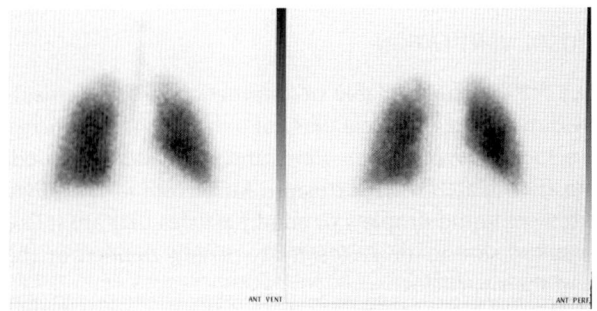

ANT VENT   ANT PERF

Figure 7A.7 *An anterior ^{81m}Kr ventilation image (left) and matched perfusion image with ^{99m}Tc-MAA (right) showing normal ventilation and perfusion. (Image kindly provided by Dr Hilson.)*

micropump, drawing the radiopharmaceutical through the holes to form consistently sized droplets.

The most commonly used solute in the UK has been ^{99m}Tc-DTPA (diethylene triaminepentaacetic acid). Patients normally inhale aerosols of DTPA in a room separate from the gamma camera and preferably fitted with negative pressure or venting facilities to prevent camera contamination. Breathing for 1–2 min is required to provide appropriate images. The jet nebulizer unit for single use is housed in a lead-lined container and charged with 740–1110 MBq of ^{99m}Tc-DTPA in 2 mL saline. The patient uses a nose clip to prevent contamination of the surrounding air and the exhaled aerosol is trapped in an appropriate filter.

The high activity required in the nebulizer bowl necessitates adequate shielding to protect patient and technologist. Most devices rely on the patient re-breathing through a mouthpiece so that the undeposited or unretained aerosol is collected on an exhalation circuit filter. Contamination of the atmosphere is possible. Ventilation studies performed under a ceiling extraction hood is much the safest method of preventing contamination of staff.

The quality of images obtained with ^{99m}Tc-DTPA aerosols is usually excellent but in patients with major acute or chronic airways disease with airway narrowing, central deposition of the tracer can make image interpretation problematic. The other disadvantage of aerosols is the potential radioactive contamination of the surrounding air which occurs when patients whose breathing is laborious relax their facial muscles too much during exhalation and the seal between mouthpiece and lips is broken.

Since ^{99m}Tc will be used for both ventilation and perfusion, activity from the ventilation study will be indistinguishable from activity resulting from the perfusion. The simplest way to minimize this problem is to ensure that the ventilation activity is only 20% of the perfusion activity. Normally, the ventilation study is performed with the gamma camera in the posterior position to ensure that no more than 20% of the perfusion count rate is administered. Clearly this is important because PE may not be appreciated if ventilation in the region of the perfusion abnormality is normal and neatly fills up the defect.

The effective dose equivalent for each 20 MBq administered is 0.6 mSv (60 mrem) and the staff dose is estimated to be 0.3–0.5 μSv (30–50 μrem).

TECHNEGAS GENERATOR PARTICLES

This radiopharmaceutical is an ultrafine dispersal of ^{99m}Tc-labeled carbon particles in the inert gas argon produced in a compact commercial generator. Technically, ^{99m}Tc is evaporated onto a carbon crucible. The crucible is then heated to 2500°C instantaneously in an atmosphere of 100% argon producing the Buckminsterfullerine molecule of carbon within which ^{99m}Tc atoms are trapped. Technegas particles are probably < 200 nm in diameter and around 20% deposit in the alveolar compartments with only 5% in the upper airways.

The patient is positioned in front of the gamma camera and during slow inhalation through the disposable delivery set, the count rate is monitored until 1600 counts s^{-1} is reached. This often occurs after three to five breathing cycles and results in a deposition activity of 20 MBq with a ventilation-to-perfusion ratio of 1:5 following the 100 MBq of ^{99m}Tc-MAA.

The ventilation images in multiple projections are usually of excellent technical quality (Fig. 7A.4). Excess particulate deposition in the proximal airways is much less than with aerosols but does occur in moderate to severe chronic obstructive airways disease.

Four to six breaths of argon may produce a transient fall in oxygen saturation and symptoms of dizziness in patients with significant cardio-respiratory disease. Pre-scan administration of supplemental oxygen for 2–3 min is recommended for all patients who fall into this category.

TECHNICAL ASPECTS OF AEROSOL VENTILATION

Particle size is of critical importance for efficient aerosol imaging. Larger particles of 5 μm are respirable with comfort but deposit in the large airways. Only those of 2 μm and less will reach peripheral respiratory bronchioles and alveoli and provide the images of alveolar ventilation that are required. The very large and large particles suffer inertial impaction on large central air passages and sediment under gravity in the larger bronchi. Smaller particles will diffuse further downstream into alveoli and impact by turbulent diffusion. While 0.5 μm particles are most likely to reach the periphery, alveolar deposition is best between 0.05 and 0.2 μm. Even at that particle size, deposition mechanisms are very inefficient so most of the inhaled particles are exhaled to be safely collected for disposal by a filter on the exhalation circuit.

Lung deposition of an aerosol increases with time and is inversely proportional to the airways diameter. Unfortunately, chronic obstructive airways disease with airway narrowing and distortion leads to high localized central deposition of the particles resulting in central hot spots. This will occur even with the smallest of particles (Fig. 7A.8). High inhalation flow rates will increase central airways deposition so pre-test training and ongoing encouragement to inhale in a calm and unhurried manner is most important.

^{99m}Tc is the radionuclide for both aerosol ventilation and MAA perfusion studies and therefore simultaneous studies are not possible. Since aerosol droplet particles are cleared quite rapidly from the lung, a delay between ventilation and perfusion of 1 h usually suffices to reduce the ^{99m}Tc lung background to acceptable levels. The alternative that permits better time management is to use a lower activity of ^{99m}Tc for the ventilation study and image for a longer time to compensate. The perfusion dose should be increased to swamp the residual ventilation activity by least four-fold. This four-fold preponderance of perfusion over ventilation is ideal and should be checked for during each

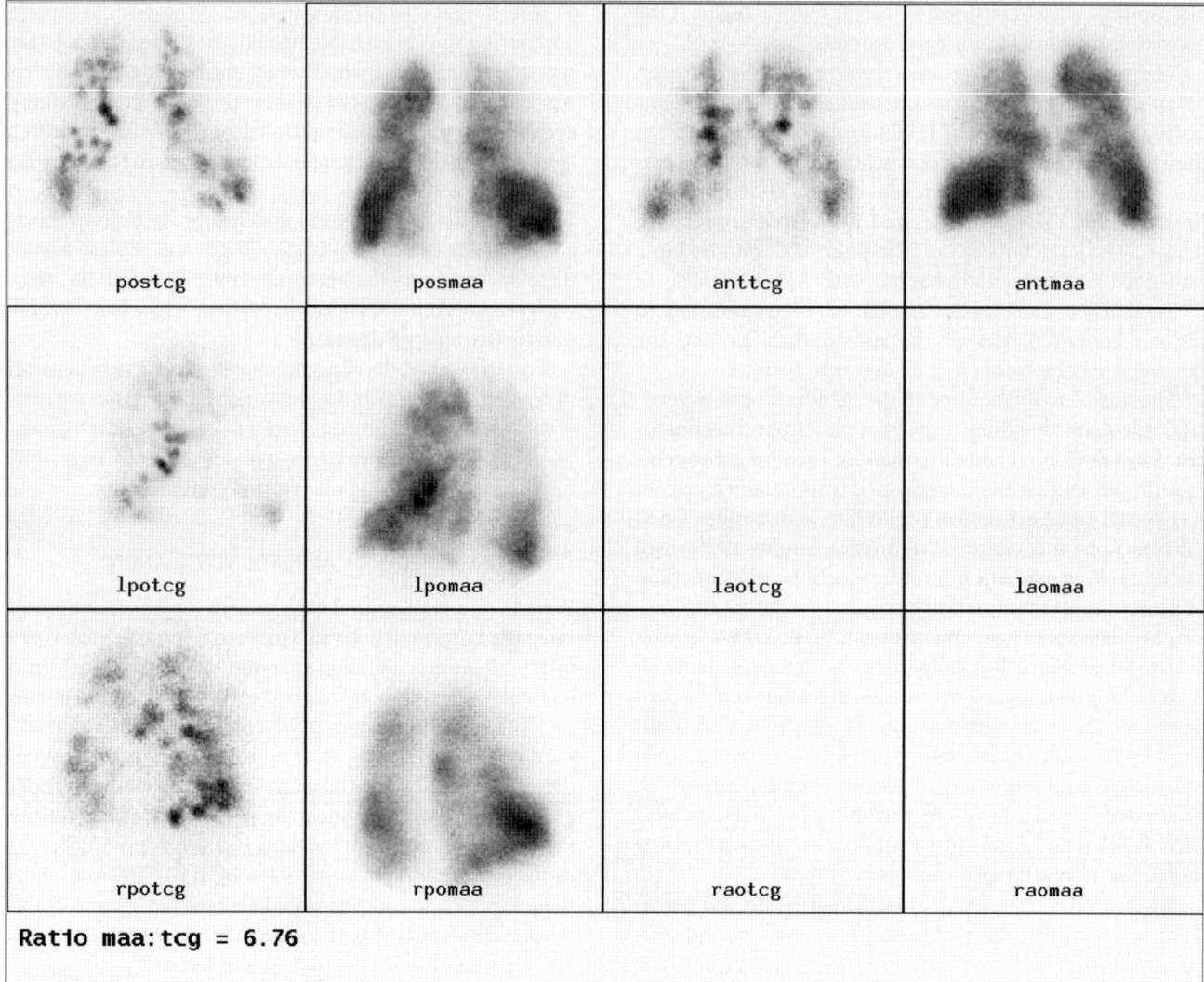

Figure 7A.8 *Technegas ventilation image with a central deposition of tracer and poor peripheral penetration with focal deposition peripherally. Patchy perfusion (right) confirms chronic parenchymal lung disease.*

study. Too low a ratio could result in the ventilation signal filling-in mismatched perfusion defects thereby confusing a diagnosis of PE.

DIAGNOSIS OF VENOUS THROMBOEMBOLISM

Origins of venous thromboembolism

The origin of deep vein thrombosis (DVT) is usually in the venous sinusoids of the calf muscles or within the valves of the ilio-femoral channel.[8] Often seeded as a platelet cluster on endothelium, the thrombus grows with the laying down of alternate layers of red cells enmeshed in fibrin and more platelets. The thrombus may enlarge further and propagate proximally into larger veins bringing with it an increased risk

of dislodgement from the endothelial tether.[9] If it dislodges, the thrombus may drift passively with the venous return towards the heart like a guided missile, eventually resulting in pulmonary embolism. The increase in pulmonary vascular resistance resulting from degrees of obstruction of the pulmonary arteries may result in acute right ventricular failure, hypotension and death.[10]

DVT and PE are separate but related aspects of the same dynamic process, VTE, which not only shares risk factors and treatment but also requires a coordinated approach to diagnosis. VTE continues to be a clinical problem because it is common – our population is aging – and also because of our continuing difficulties in the clinical diagnosis of this perplexing malady. Only 50% of cases with clinical signs of DVT have the disease on objective testing[11] whereas approximately 40% of apparently uncomplicated cases of DVT have PE shown by perfusion imaging.[12] It is known from autopsy that most patients with fatal PE have demonstrable DVT[8] but only 20% have symptoms of that DVT before death.

Risk factors for venous thromboembolism

Risk factors are conditions associated with an increased incidence of disease and include vascular injury, hemostatic and environmental factors.[13] Vascular injury and endothelial damage that increase the risk of platelet adherence and aggregation are least common and include central venous catheters in children and intravenous drug abuse.

GENETIC HEMOSTATIC RISK FACTORS

In 1993, the first description of activated protein C resistance appeared. APC resistance is a frequent prothrombotic marker associated with a single point mutation in the factor V gene and has been called factor V Leiden.[14] The mutation eliminates the protein C cleavage site making the factor V resistant to inactivation by activated protein C normally found within the blood on endothelium. Other genetic risk factors include antithrombin deficiency, protein C or S deficiency, prothrombin 20210A, high plasma concentrations of factor VIII and hyperhomocysteinemia.

ACQUIRED HEMOSTATIC RISK FACTORS

In the UK, VTE is the leading cause of maternal death and there is evidence that much of the pregnancy-related thrombosis is related to genetic abnormalities of hemostasis.

First-generation oral contraceptives increased the risk of VTE by a direct estrogen effect. The risk fell with second-generation drugs but increased again in third-generation pills containing the new progestogens desogestrel and gestodene, possibly due to production of APC resistance similar to factor V Leiden. Even the low dose of estrogen for hormone replacement therapy (HRT) appears to double the risk of VTE.

Cancer confers a four-fold increase in the risk of VTE and such patients receiving immunosuppressive or cytotoxic chemotherapy are at even higher risk. Finally, autoantibodies specific for negatively charged phospholipids (lupus anticoagulant or anticardiolipin antibody) can be associated with arterial and venous thrombosis, miscarriage and PE.

ENVIRONMENTAL RISK FACTORS

Environmental risk factors are usually associated with decreased blood flow through the venous channels. Multiple factors such as immobilization, paralysis after stroke or paraplegia, hospitalization following surgery, and plaster casts are well recognized. Recent studies have shown that even confinement in a care facility such as a hospital or nursing home is an independent risk factor for VTE. Travelers' thrombosis has become prominent over the last few years and increases with the length of the journey.

Clinical presentation of venous thromboembolism

Theoretically, there should be no problem with the clinical diagnosis of VTE. Clot in the legs is the most common preliminary for PE in 65–95% of cases so presentation of leg symptoms should assist the clinical diagnosis of PE. Unfortunately, the majority of patients with proven PE have no leg symptoms whatever on presentation and diagnosis.[15,16] Conversely, patients with clear-cut DVT may have totally asymptomatic PE. In a group of 350 cases with proven DVT, PE was clearly present by VQ imaging or pulmonary angiography in 56% but symptoms of PE were absent in 26% of cases.[17]

PE poses a considerable diagnostic challenge for our clinical colleagues. Younger patients may present few of the classical symptoms and signs while many older patients present with PE masquerading as an acute coronary syndrome, an acute exacerbation of chronic obstructive airways disease or heart failure.

For clinicians, clearly, the important first step is to consider VTE as a diagnostic possibility – the clinical suspicion. Regrettably, the symptoms and signs are inadequate for assessing the clinical risk of PE. In PIOPED (*vide supra*), patients with PE presented with dyspnea (73%), pleuritic pain (66%), cough (37%), and hemoptysis (13%). Signs of PE included tachypnea (70%), crackles (51%), tachycardia (30%), a fourth heart sound (24%) and a loud pulmonary second sound (23%).[15,16] Unfortunately, the frequency of such symptoms and signs in patients without PE were similar making the distinction of PE from no-PE impossible on clinical grounds alone. Use of risk factors (*vide infra*) was found to be more helpful in practice.

Clinical diagnosis of venous thromboembolism

Most experienced physicians will admit that mental alertness, knight's-move thinking, a low threshold of suspicion and luck are each required at one time or another to pick up the many cases of VTE presenting in the clinical setting either as inpatients or outpatients. Senior physicians who have been caught out in the past to the detriment of their patients are probably the most effective at bedside diagnosis.[18] It cannot be reiterated too often that those in nuclear medicine, physicians or radiologists, need an accurate assessment of this clinical risk of VTE for their VQ report to ensure an accurate final diagnosis. This clinical information permits the VQ reporter to change the relative risk of PE from the lung scan category alone to the absolute risk obtained when the VQ category analysis is combined with an accurate clinical assessment. It also helps to clarify which imaging test is most appropriate for diagnosis in any particular case. Realistically, nuclear medicine physicians and radiologists cannot retain such clinical skills indefinitely so

Table 7A.1   *Clinical risk of pulmonary embolism*

High (70–80%)	Medium (20–70%)	Low (5–20%)	Very unlikely (<5%)
≥3 risk factors	1 or 2 risk factors	No risk factors	d-dimer < 500 ng ml^{-1}
Documented deep vein thrombosis		Other symptoms/signs	(Vidas)

Important risk factors include: past history of pulmonary embolism/deep vein thrombosis, immobilization, surgery in last 3 months, age > 65 years, cancer ± chemotherapy, thrombophilia.

communication with the referring clinician will often provide the relevant clinical appraisal.[19]

If a clinical opinion on level of PE risk is not immediately available, the alternative for the nuclear medicine physician is the use of in-house diagnostic tools or checklists that can stratify cases into the likely clinical prevalence of PE. Specifically, 5–10% prevalence is a low pre-test probability/risk of PE, 10–70% is a medium pre-test and 70–80% prevalence is a high pre-test clinical probability/risk.

While user-friendly diagnostic tools have been published[20,21] the author prefers a more simple in-house assessment of the clinical pre-test probability of PE and finds it just as useful as the more complicated algorithms (Table 7A.1).[13,22] Firstly, patients with a proven DVT by Doppler ultrasound have a high clinical pre-test risk of PE and included in this group are those with three or more risk factors. Secondly, patients with one or two risk factors are given a medium clinical pre-test risk. The important risk factors in this simplified algorithm include a history of previous PE or DVT, surgery within the last 3 months, immobility for whatever reason (plaster cast, stroke, long journey etc), age older than 65 years, cancer particularly if prescribed chemotherapy and thrombophilia indicated by VTE within members of the close family.[23]

Clearly, patients over 65 years require only two other risk factors to be in the high risk group. Thirdly, those younger than 65 years without risk factors and with a clear chest radiograph but symptoms in relation to the cardio-respiratory system such as sudden dyspnea or pleuritic chest pain have a low clinical pre-test probability/risk of VTE. VTE is not excluded but is clearly much less likely.

Investigations for venous thromboembolism

Until recently, arterial blood gases for hypoxemia and measurement of the alveolar–arterial oxygen gradient were standard investigations in suspected PE. These tests could be helpful but in a significant number with PE, the P_aO_2 and alveolar–arterial oxygen gradient were normal. Today, the laboratory tests and imaging for thrombus are much more sensitive and specific.[24,25]

D-DIMER MEASUREMENT

The first screening test for VTE in the emergency department is the rapid quantitative ELISA (Vidas) d-dimer measurement

for cross-linked fibrin derivatives produced when fibrin is degraded by plasmin.[26,27]

Raised levels of d-dimer > 500 ng mL^{-1} do not infer the presence of VTE because of general nonspecificity. Raised d-dimer levels are commonly found in hospitalized patients, after myocardial infarction, pneumonia, sepsis and cancer, in obstetric practice and after surgery. By contrast, a normal d-dimer concentration (500 ng mL^{-1}) has a high negative predictive value for excluding VTE in up to 98% of cases. No further investigation for VTE is required in the majority after this result. At the Emergency Department of Brigham and Women's Hospital, they found that approximately 50% of individuals with a history consistent with VTE had normal d-dimer results. Only two cases out of 547 with a normal d-dimer concentration had VTE giving sensitivity for acute PE of 96.4% and a negative predictive value of 99.6%.[28]

MULTIDETECTOR ROW SPIRAL COMPUTED TOMOGRAPHY

Advanced computed tomographic pulmonary angiography is an excellent imaging investigation for PE down to subsegmental levels and is more sensitive for peripheral thrombus than conventional CTPA.[4]

Four CT slices can be acquired simultaneously during each rotation of the X-ray source and the total examination time is eight times faster than with conventional single row detector systems. The resolution is an amazing 1.25 mm and subsegmental thrombus can often be seen. The sensitivity for PE is up to 90%.[29] Another advantage of chest CT is that alternative diagnoses can be revealed in the lung parenchyma that cannot be recognized on conventional chest X-ray. Clearly, cases with a history of allergy to contrast or with renal failure require another test. Emergency CT is the investigation of choice for those with life-threatening PE since it reliably demonstrates central clot and acute RV dilatation.[30]

LEG ULTRASOUND

Leg ultrasound is currently used to prove a clinical DVT or after an indeterminate VQ scan since identification of venous thrombosis obviates the need for further testing. Regrettably, it is a poor test since peripheral thrombus is only detected in one third to one half of all those with PE[31,32] unless serial tests are used.[33]

ECHOCARDIOGRAPHY

This is only really helpful in massive PE. The transesophageal route improves sensitivity but availability is limited.[34,35]

MAGNETIC RESONANCE ANGIOGRAPHY

This appears promising but it has reduced sensitivity compared with CT and there is limited access.[36,37]

Current role for VQ imaging

The recent improvements in CT technology are most welcome. For sick patients, CT is often quicker to perform than VQ in smaller hospitals, rarely needs further testing, may provide another diagnosis when PE has been excluded, is available now in most hospitals and is easier to arrange urgently out of hours. Nuclear medicine can now concentrate its involvement on its strengths, namely the exclusion or diagnosis of PE in cases with a normal chest X-ray. Firstly, VQ imaging with a normal chest X-ray can exclude PE in the majority of patients with a low or medium clinical pre-test probability at less than 7% of the radiation dose to the breast from MDCT. Breast dose from VQ imaging is 0.6 mSv from IRCP publications while MDCT is 8–10 mSv (www.impactscan.org). Secondly, VQ imaging with a normal chest X-ray can correctly pick out PE with a high probability scan category in four out of five cases with proven disease. This probably accounts for 30–35% of all those presenting with PE. It is clear that the crucial factor for successful VQ imaging is often the chest X-ray. If it is normal, a diagnostic VQ scan is likely. If abnormal with consolidation or pleural fluid, a nondiagnostic study is likely though on occasion, mismatched abnormalities in the clear lung or a perfusion defect greater in size than the effusion do strongly point to PE. Clearly, however, CTPA is more sensitive and specific than VQ imaging with abnormal chest X-rays.

Regrettably, VQ imaging has all the weaknesses of a functional test. The diagnosis of acute PE in the presence of multiple mismatches can be strongly inferred but only confirmed absolutely with contrast studies of lung or lower limb. Secondly, it is usually nondiagnostic when there is consolidation on chest X-ray unless, of course, there are also mismatched perfusion abnormalities of the contralateral lung with a clear lung field on X-ray. Thirdly, it is very difficult to interpret consistently in chronic heart and lung disease. These groups and those with consolidation can represent up to 40–50% of inpatients previously sent for VQ imaging in the UK. Finally, and quite unlike CTPA, VQ imaging never provides the interpreter with a credible alternative diagnosis in cases without PE unless COPD is clearly seen on the ventilation images.

Since CTPA has become routinely available in our teaching and district hospitals, the indications for VQ imaging have become clearer. Current wisdom suggests that VQ imaging is the screening test of choice for suspected PE when the d-dimer is abnormal, the chest X-ray is normal and when the clinical pre-test probability for PE is low or medium. It is likely that young women will preferentially have VQ imaging given the higher breast dose from MDCT. The nuclear medicine service should perform the VQ scan as soon as practical after the clinical suspicion is raised to permit its completion before the development of pulmonary infarction which complicates VQ scan interpretation. Delay of more than 48 h is considered unwise by most since diagnostic perfusion abnormalities can resolve within days.

It is likely that VQ imaging in patients with normal chest X-rays and raised d-dimer will provide a post-test PE risk of 5% or less in more than two thirds of that category presenting to the department. Equally, a post-test PE risk of 90% or more can be expected in at least one third of those with PE (with a normal chest X-ray). If the post-test risk is >10% or <85% (i.e. diagnostic doubt), CTPA should be used to clarify and refine the diagnosis further.

Ventilation perfusion scan interpretation

Ventilation/perfusion lung scanning can reveal a normal physiological pattern, physiological abnormalities of perfusion secondary to positional changes during the injection of MAA, or the effects of diverse disease processes including VTE and COPD on pulmonary physiology. The downside is that every perfusion defect is nonspecific. The pathological basis for the abnormality is most likely to be proven by contrast studies. The upside is that a normal VQ scan completely excludes PE and perfusion defects that conform to segmental or lobar boundaries are highly correlated with acute or previous PE particularly when multiple and bilateral and with normal accompanying ventilation. Recognizing this basic nonspecificity, most experienced reporters use probability terms in their report to reflect and communicate their understanding of the level of certainty or uncertainty that prevails. A very low probability term indicates the least likely to harbor PE while the high probability category is most likely. Many patterns of ventilation and perfusion are undecipherable and are quite unhelpful for diagnosis. Such images can be called indeterminate to reflect the difficulties in interpretation or intermediate to reflect the median probability of PE (neither high nor low). CTPA is always required for accurate diagnosis under these circumstances. It is fortunate that abnormalities on the chest X-ray often indicate when the VQ imaging will be indeterminate and allow us to move smartly to CTPA if available.

Now that CTPA often takes the difficult and the emergency cases, consistent and accurate interpretation of VQ scans when the chest X-ray is normal is simpler than before but remains a challenging cognitive task with three steps: firstly, the integration of the perfusion and ventilation signal with the X-ray to provide the VQ category of scan, secondly, the assessment of the pre-test clinical probability of PE either by the VQ reporter or from the referring clinical staff and thirdly, the integration of the scan category with the pre-test clinical probability of PE to provide the final post-test diagnosis. The author favors a 'neoclassical' approach to VQ scan analysis that recognizes that the nearer to normal the perfusion, the less the PE risk but at the end of the day, it is the pre-test clinical probability of PE that determines the post-test risk. For example, while the risk of PE after a low probability category scan is 3% with a low probability pre-test clinical probability, the risk is up to 10% with a medium pre-test risk where there are =2 risk factors. The risk is up to 35% in the presence of a DVT where the clinical risk is high.[38]

Several solid and reliable principles of lung scan interpretation can be recognized. They permit a more accurate and reproducible categorization of these scans and their associated PE risk and guide those who currently provide a VQ scanning service for clinical and radiological colleagues. They also provide a rational basis for educating clinical colleagues and teaching juniors.

The *first principle* states that a normal perfusion scan (Fig. 7A.4) excludes PE for clinical purposes no matter the clinical presentation. Twenty to 25% of those without PE will present with a normal scan and it is by far the most valuable diagnostic finding in VQ scanning. In pregnancy it is particularly helpful where there is a need to limit the use of ionizing radiation. A near-normal perfusion scan with a widened mediastinum or raised hemi-diaphragm with clear fields on X-ray is just as valuable and can be followed immediately by a search for another cause for the symptoms.

The *second principle* states that PE can present with any perfusion abnormality but the risk of acute PE will depend upon the site of abnormality as well as upon the pattern of the VQ abnormality or abnormalities. For example, the smaller the perfusion abnormality or abnormalities (Fig. 7A.9), the more matched they are to concordant abnormal ventilation (Fig. 7A.10) and the more numerous, the lower the risk of PE. Most matched abnormalities in chronic pulmonary disease are clearly nonsegmental but rarely, it is possible for PE to produce matching defects by release of active mediators that cause local bronchoconstriction. It is the segmental appearance of abnormalities that raises suspicion and risk of PE, and clearly not the matching of V and Q. Under these unusual circumstances, CTPA should be seriously considered as the next most appropriate investigation.

Of course, some patterns of V and Q abnormality can never be interpreted with sufficient accuracy and will always attract a 'don't know' label. Such patterns include extensive parenchymal lung disease with multiple and widespread V and Q abnormalities throughout both lung fields, multiple matched and mismatched perfusion abnormalities (Fig. 7A.11), a single mismatched perfusion abnormality of whatever size (Fig. 7A.12), and, in certain circumstances of high clinical risk, a single segmental match. The single segmental mismatch is thought to have the highest risk of PE in the group at about 30–60%.

Clearly, the larger the abnormalities, the more segmental and more mismatched in appearance, the higher the risk of PE. A high probability lung scan category is usually clear cut (Fig. 7A.13) with multiple mismatched segmental

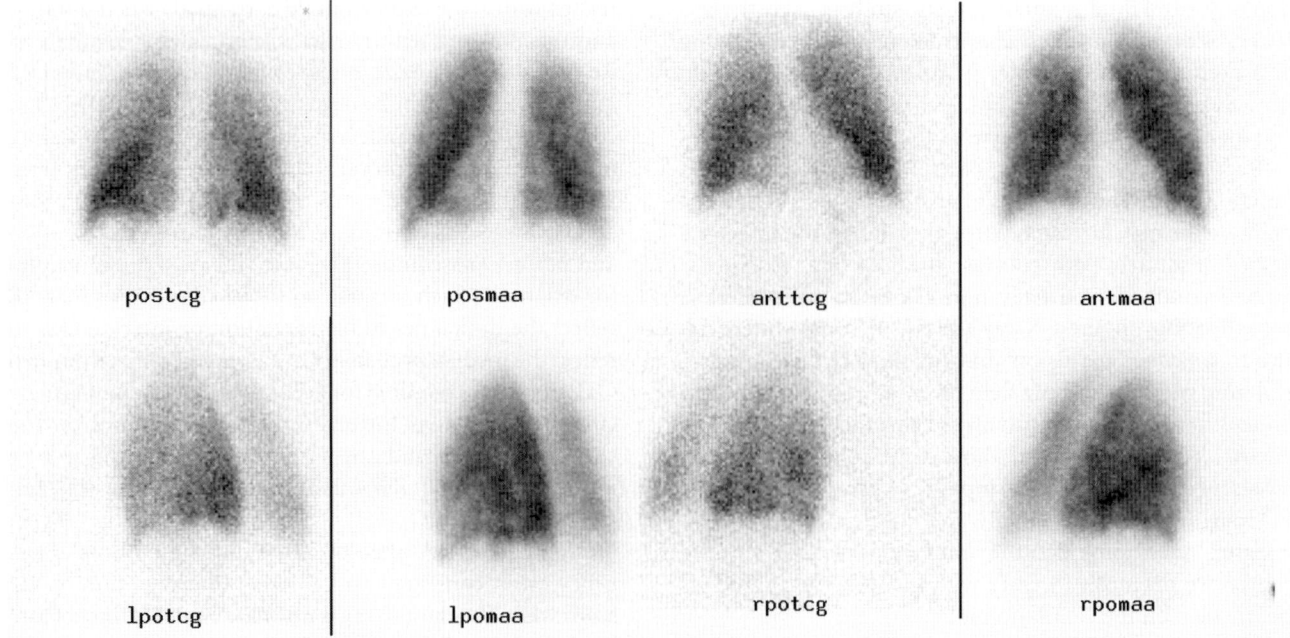

Figure 7A.9   *Almost normal Technegas ventilation (left) with minor matched perfusion abnormalities (<25% seg) on the perfusion image (right). Very low probability category scan for pulmonary embolism.*

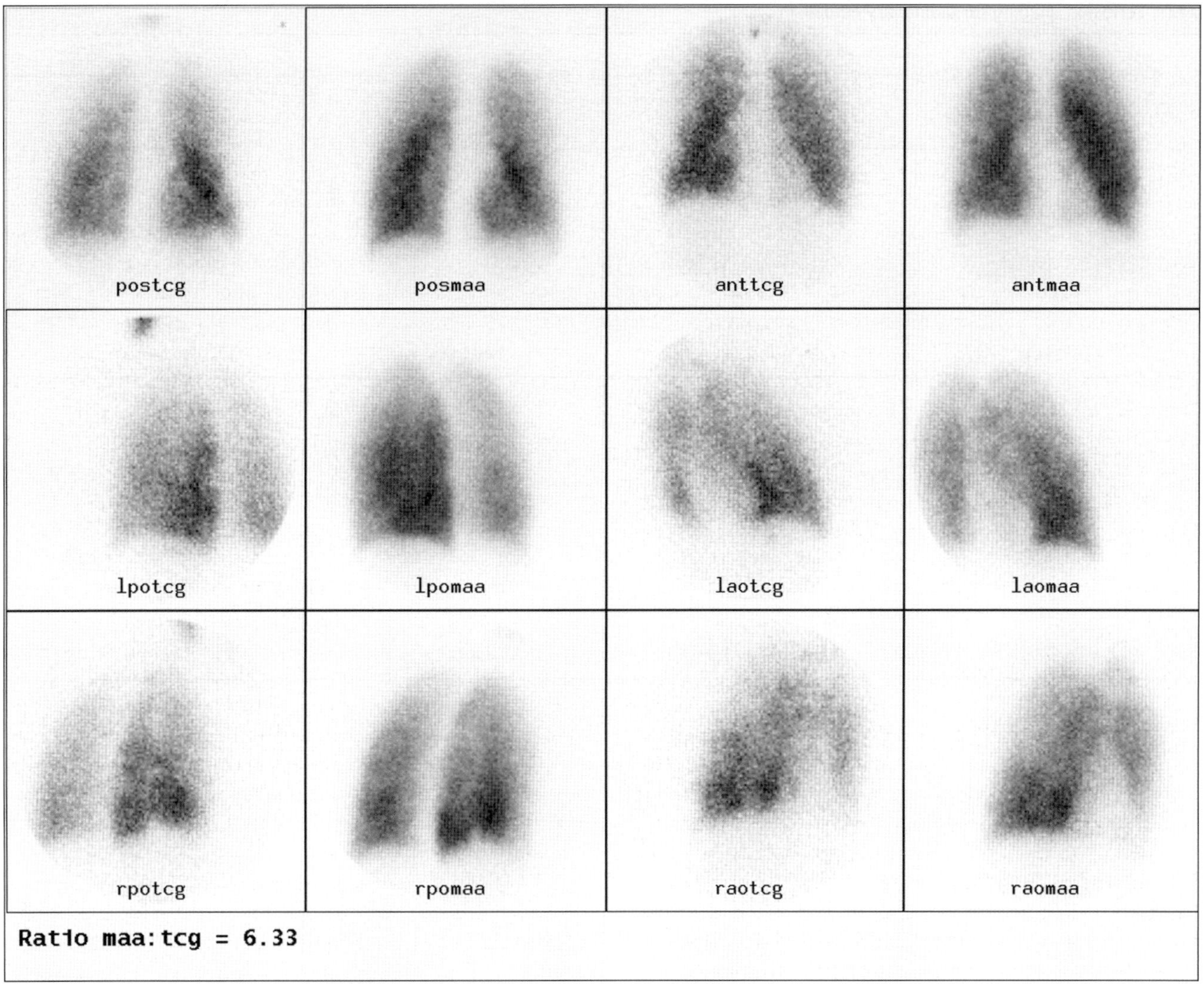

postcg
posmaa
anttcg
antmaa
lpotcg
lpomaa
laotcg
laomaa
rpotcg
rpomaa
raotcg
raomaa
Ratio maa:tcg = 6.33

Figure 7A.10 *Matched right apical defect and a focal match at the right base in a patient with a normal chest X-ray. Low probability category lung scan.*

postcg
posmaa
lpotcg
lpomaa
anttcg
antmaa
rpotcg
rpomaa

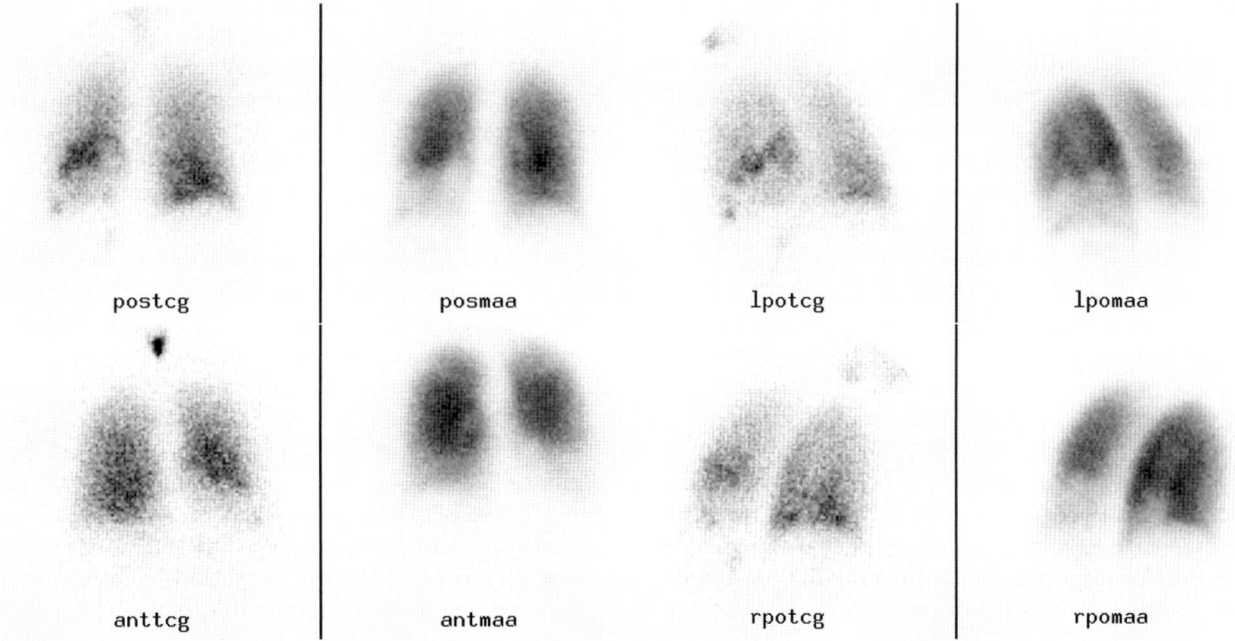

Figure 7A.11 *Left basal match and right posterior segment mismatch in a patient with a normal chest X-ray following delivery. Intermediate or indeterminate lung scan category but CTPA was negative for pulmonary embolism.*

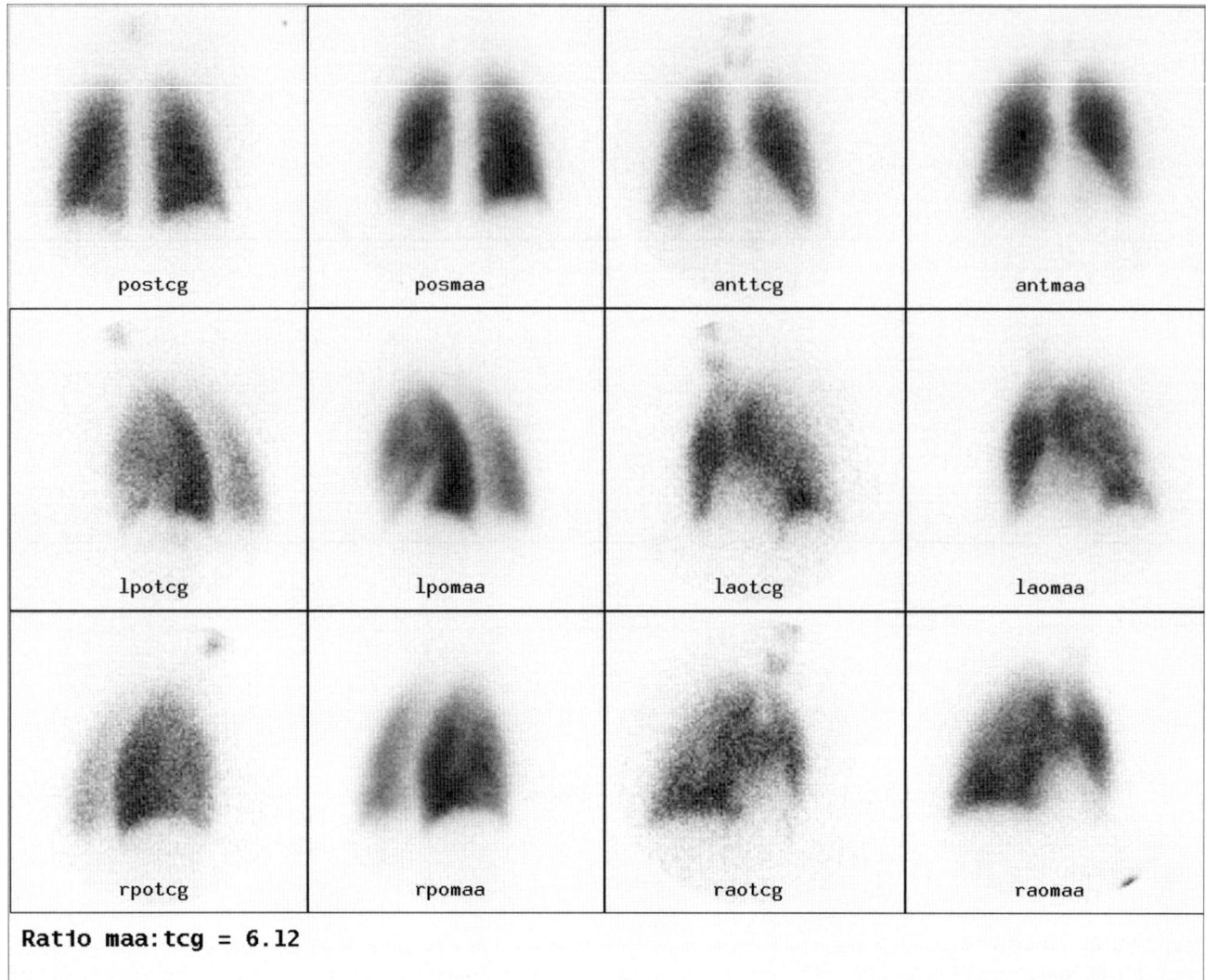

postcg   posmaa   anttcg   antmaa

lpotcg   lpomaa   laotcg   laomaa

rpotcg   rpomaa   raotcg   raomaa

Ratio maa:tcg = 6.12

Figure 7A.12   *Single mismatch of the inferior lingular segment with a normal chest X-ray. Indeterminate or intermediate category lung scan.*

and/or lobar abnormalities but this pattern can be seen in patients with previous PE but with unresolved changes and negative CTPA (Fig. 7A.14). While whole lung mismatching is unusual (Fig. 7A.15) and often secondary to a central lung cancer, PE is possible and therefore CTPA is essential for differential diagnosis. CTPA may also be wise if the mismatches are small (Fig. 7A.16).

The *third principle* states that a good quality erect and contemporaneous chest X-ray is essential for accurate VQ scan interpretation and must be available to assist the decision about proceeding to VQ imaging or CTPA. It is clear that any parenchymal abnormality on the chest X-ray increases the risk of PE in an unquantifiable manner and can degrade the diagnostic potential of most VQ imaging preformed in this scenario (Fig. 7A.17 (a) to (c)). PE can be present in up to 60% with a single triple matched perfusion defect but VQ imaging cannot distinguish PE from no PE.

VQ imaging can be diagnostic of PE in cases presenting with a single area of consolidation on X-ray but only when the triple match on the abnormal lung field is accompanied by mismatched perfusion abnormalities on the other clear lung field (Fig. 7A.18, page 216). This happens in only 10% of cases with PE. Since CTPA provides the full diagnosis in >90% of cases with a chest X-ray abnormality, VQ scanning is usually only indicated when CTPA cannot be performed.

Occasionally, reverse mismatching can be found in an area of radiological consolidation caused by pneumonia (Fig. 7A.19, page 217). This unusual appearance with relative preservation of some perfusion does not exclude PE but makes it unlikely. CTPA would again be wise under these circumstances.

The *fourth principle* states that the pre-test clinical probability of PE, that is the PE risk as determined by the clinical presentation, is itself an independent risk factor for PE along with the lung scan category and the d-dimer level (if normal). Bayes' theorem provides the mathematical expression for combining the pre-test clinical probability of PE and the PE probability from the lung scan category to provide a more closely defined post-test probability of PE. This

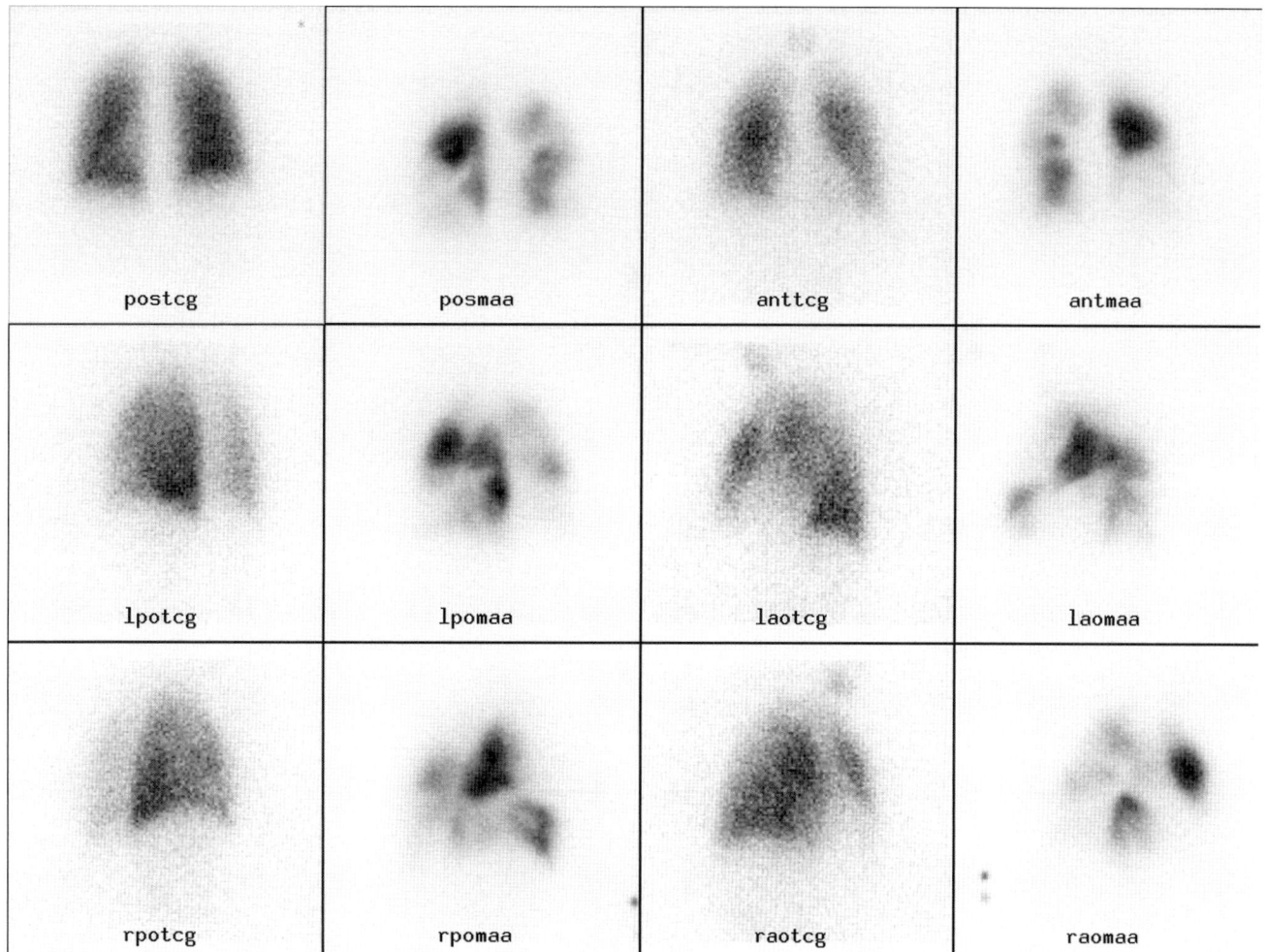

Figure 7A.13   *Six-view Technegas ventilation (left) and perfusion (right) images in a patient with a high pre-clinical risk of pulmonary embolism (PE). Multiple segmental and lobar mismatched perfusion abnormalities with normal ventilation confirm a high probability category of lung scan for PE.*

post-test value is more accurate than either of the above variables taken singly (Fig. 7A.20, page 218). Bayes' theorem is only annulled by the presence of a normal perfusion scan where PE is excluded for clinical purposes whatever the history (Tables 7A.2, 7A.3 and 7A.4, page 218). A normal d-dimer is almost as good at excluding PE at 96% of cases.

The *fifth principle* states that the VQ scan and chest X-ray should be interpreted and its category determined whenever possible before becoming appraised of the clinical details of the patient's presentation. This can ensure that the two independent variables, VQ scan category assessment and pre-test probability of PE, remain independent during the analysis of the VQ study. Clearly, this can be difficult in practice if the VQ scan reader has to assess the patient's suitability for VQ scanning in the first place but it is an important standard to be kept if possible. The British Thoracic Society Guidelines[30] agree and state 'that knowledge of the clinical probability should not influence description of the VQ scan category, but is essential for interpreting the report's meaning' (i.e. for the derivation of the post-test risk of PE).

The *sixth principle* states that a Vidas d-dimer level below the upper limit of normal (i.e. <500 units) is an accurate method of excluding VTE and eliminating the need for VQ or CTPA. However, the false negative rate is likely to lie between 2 and 4%. Accordingly, one should consider further imaging with VQ scanning or CTPA after a negative d-dimer if the clinical history is highly suggestive of PE.

A basic algorithm for the analysis of lung scans is given in Figure 7A.21, page 219.

Formation of a post-test diagnosis

Modification of the PIOPED dataset[38] permits the development of neoclassical criteria for lung scan categorization (Table 7A.5, page 219) which increases the accuracy of the post-test probability estimate. For example, Figure 7A.20 illustrates how low and very-low probability scans reduce the presenting clinical probability of PE (indicated by the line of identity) to provide for the clinical staff the more accurate lower post-test probability of PE. When the

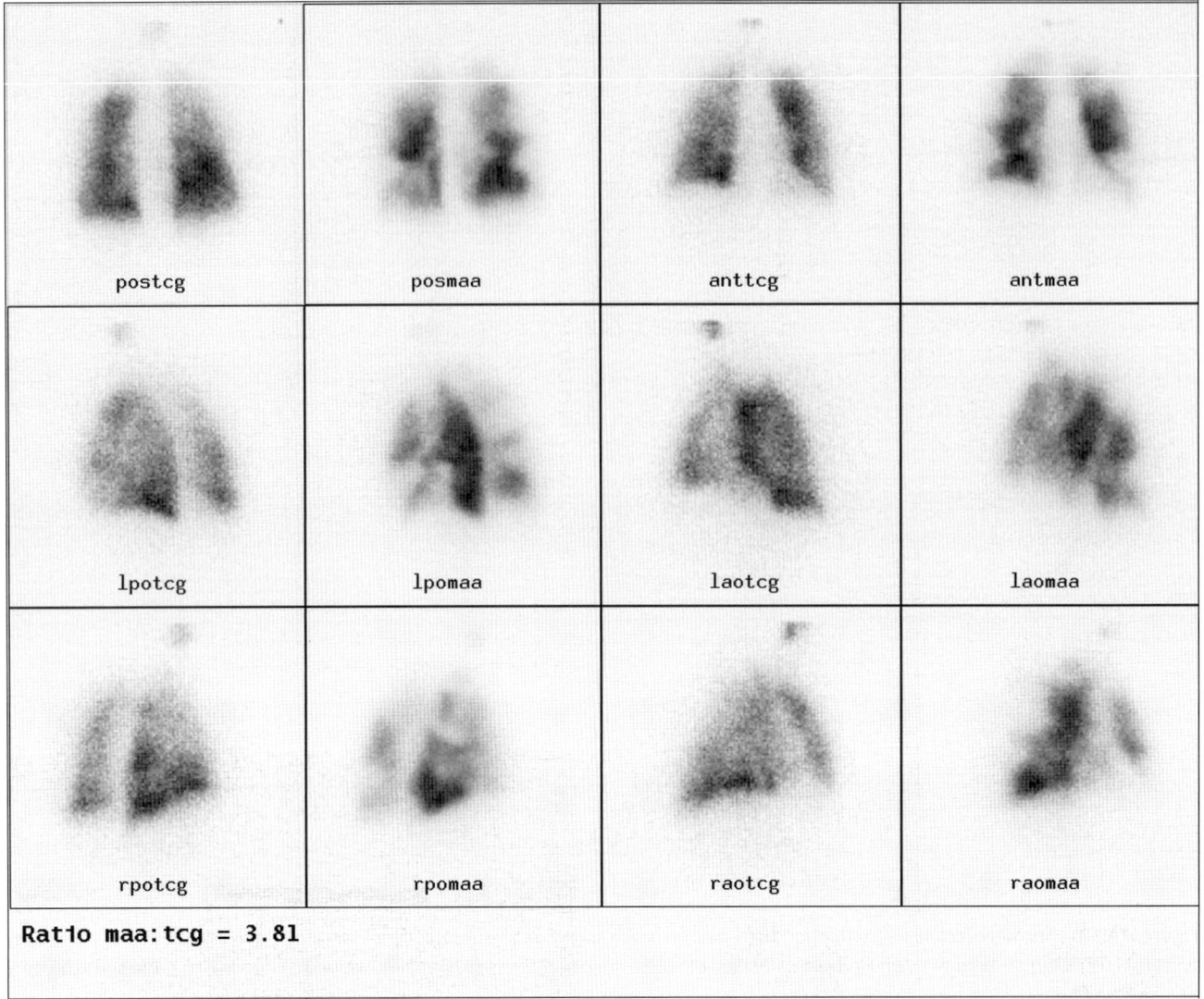

Figure 7A.14 *Multiple segmental and multi-segmental mismatched perfusion abnormalities 2 years after documented pulmonary embolism. CTPA was negative and ECHO revealed minor pulmonary hypertension.*

clinical pre-test probability is low (i.e. 10%), a LP category scan reduces that risk to 4% while a VLP scan category reduces it to 2% post-test. The most valuable results for clinical staff and patients therefore are a normal scan which eliminates PE absolutely and a LP and VLP scan category without risk factors (low clinical pre-test) that excludes PE to a significant degree. When there are up to two risk factors present (medium pre-test) a LP scan reduces the 30% risk to 10% and the VLP scan to 5–8% post-test. It is more than likely that the VLP scan category with matched subsegmental perfusion defects and up to two risk factors (medium risk) will be an acceptable endpoint to investigation not only because the probability of PE is very low but also because CTPA would struggle to resolve vessels in the peripheral lung fields.

When the pre-test clinical probability is high in the presence of a DVT or three risk factors (70% risk), a LP category scan reduces that risk to 20–40% and a VLP category scan to 10–20% post-test. The actual risk of PE after a LP

category scan may not be low at all since the risk clearly varies between 4 and 40% depending upon the clinical presentation. One could say that it was a 'lower than clinical' probability. The HP category scan is also a 'higher than clinical' probability.

Using strict criteria for VQ scan interpretation and a careful selection of cases with low or medium clinical pre-test risk, an accurate post-test diagnosis can be provided for each clinical presentation and VQ scan category combination (Tables 7A.2, 7A.3 and 7A.4, page 218). For example, no further investigation is required when a patient presents with a low clinical pre-test probability of PE (i.e. no risk factors with elevated d-dimer) and a normal, very low or low probability category scan with matching defects since the ongoing risk of PE is so small. If up to two risk factors for VTE are noted in the clinical history (medium pre-test), a normal scan eliminates PE, a VLP category makes it highly unlikely (around 5%), while a HP scan is virtually diagnostic

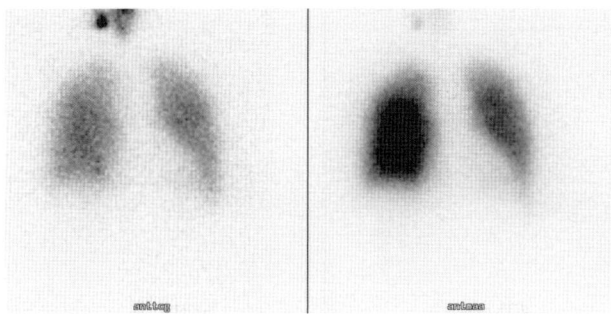

Figure 7A.15 *Relative hypoperfusion of whole left lung compared to ventilation with a normal chest X-ray which in this case was shown to be pulmonary embolism by CTPA. Lung cancer is a more usual cause of this abnormality.*

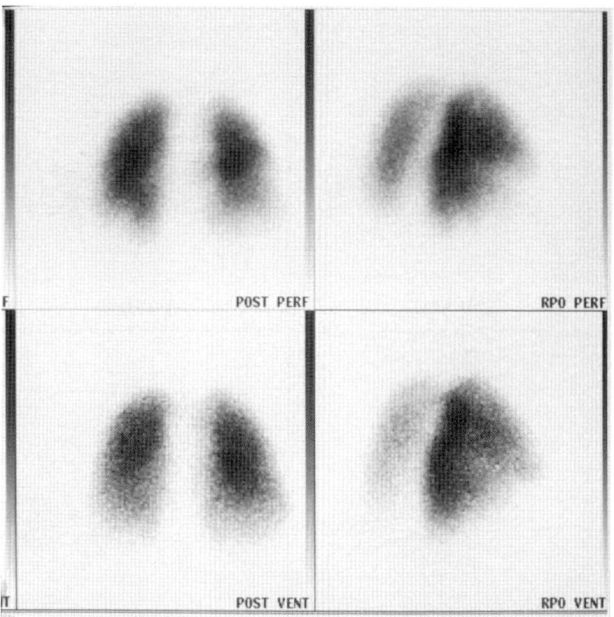

Figure 7A.16 *Small mismatches mainly of right lung with a normal chest X-ray. Pulmonary embolism was confirmed at pulmonary angiography. (Image kindly provided by Dr Hilson.)*

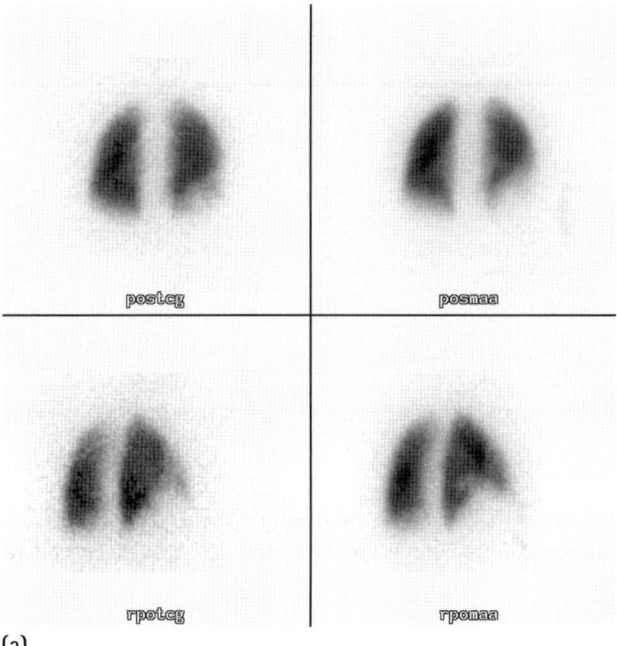

(a)

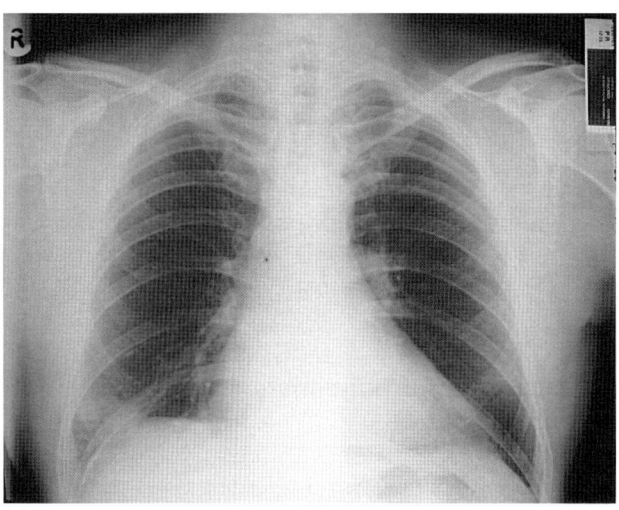

(b)

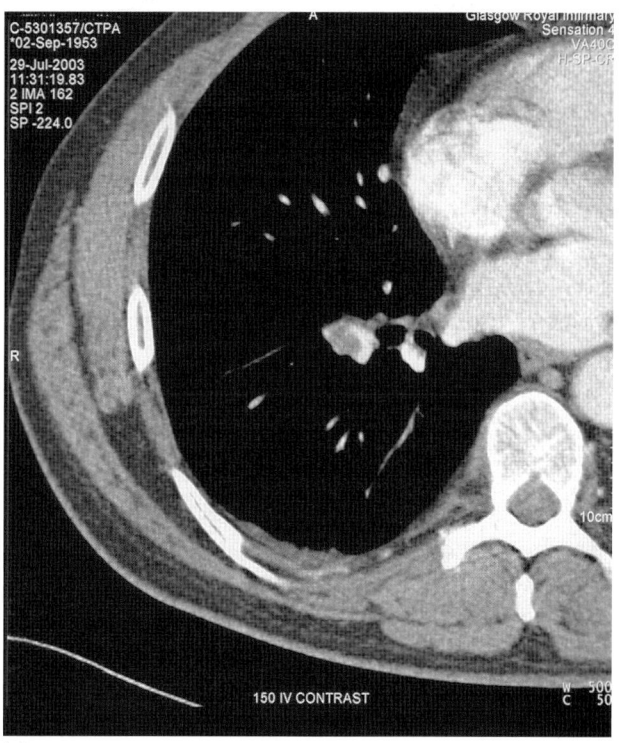

(c)

Figure 7A.17 *(a) Posterior and right posterior oblique Technegas and perfusion images showing a triple-matched defect of the right anterior and lateral segments confirming an indeterminate VQ scan category. (b) Chest X-ray showing right lower lobe consolidation matching the VQ abnormality. (c) PE confirmed by CTPA on the right.*

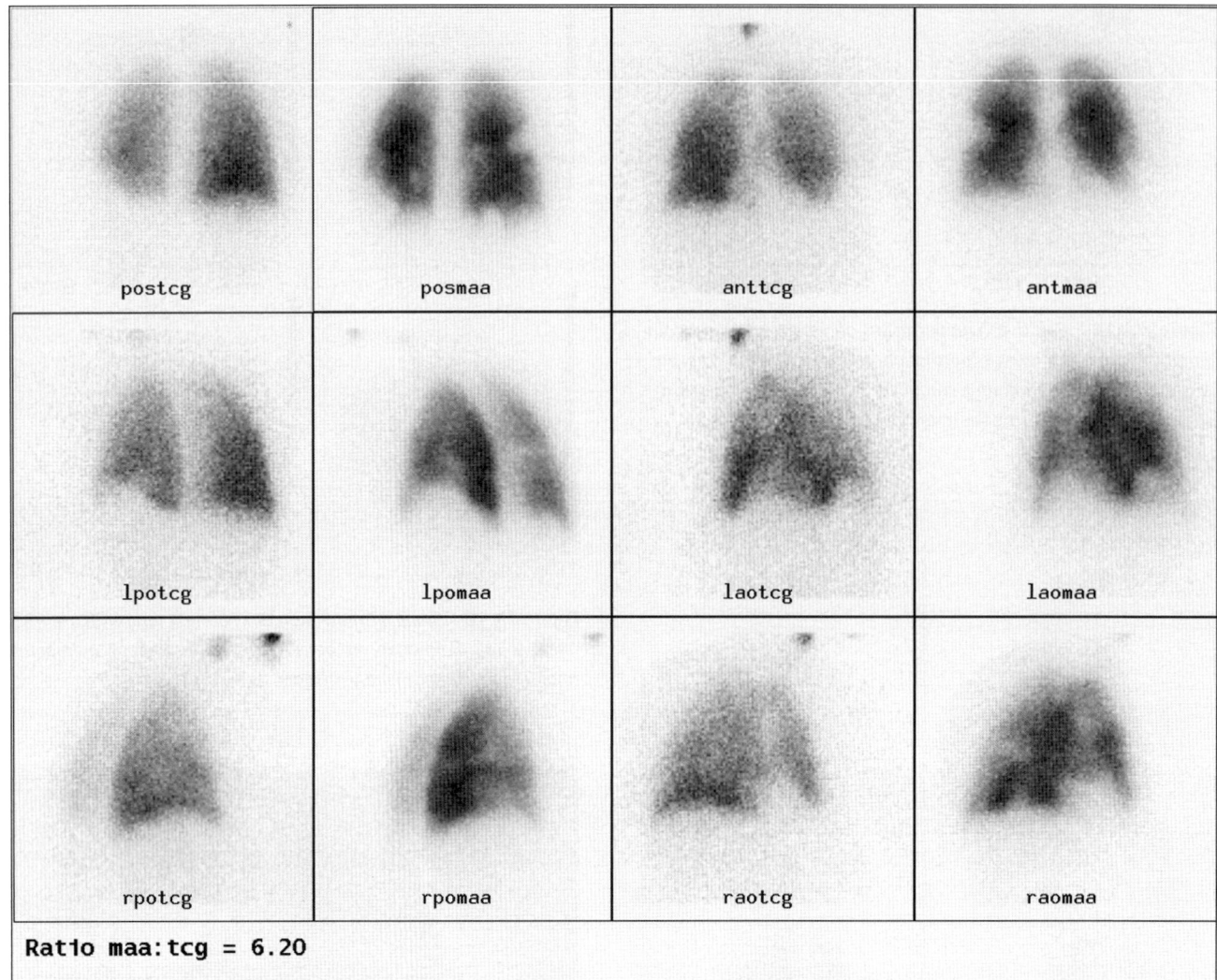

Figure 7A.18 *Ventilation perfusion abnormality at left base matching consolidation on chest X-ray. Multiple mismatched segmental abnormalities in upper left and right lung where the lung fields are clear indicating a high probability category lung scan. CTPA confirmed bilateral pulmonary embolism.*

of PE. In cases with a DVT or three or more risk factors, a normal scan eliminates PE and a HP scan is diagnostic of PE. Clearly, all the other combinations of clinical and VQ scan category are nondiagnostic or unhelpful to varying degrees. VQ imaging with a normal chest X-ray will exclude PE in over two thirds of cases.

Communication of the risk of pulmonary embolism after lung scanning

Communication of the results of VQ scanning is crucial yet experience has shown that our probability jargon causes a modicum of confusion among junior clinicians. It is certainly possible that the addition of a numerical estimate of risk along with the verbal report clarifies that risk.[39] Accordingly, it is belt-and-braces to communicate the post-test diagnosis providing both a verbal report and a percentage risk of PE on completion of the procedure. The

percentage risk can be obtained from an analysis of the original PIOPED data (Fig. 7A.20).[38] A discussion with the clinical staff immediately following the VQ study may permit the nuclear medicine physician to clarify the impact of the post-test result on the provisional diagnosis. At this point, the need for further investigation with CTPA or Doppler of legs can be explored. Tables 7A.2, 7A.3 and 7A.4 provide the data on categorical analysis, clinical presentation and post-test risk with verbal and numerical report responses outlined. We eagerly await the new data from the PIOPED 2 clinical study using VQ imaging and CTPA.

Consideration of pulmonary embolism risk in pregnancy

Venous thromboembolism is a leading cause of maternal morbidity and mortality in pregnancy and can occur in up

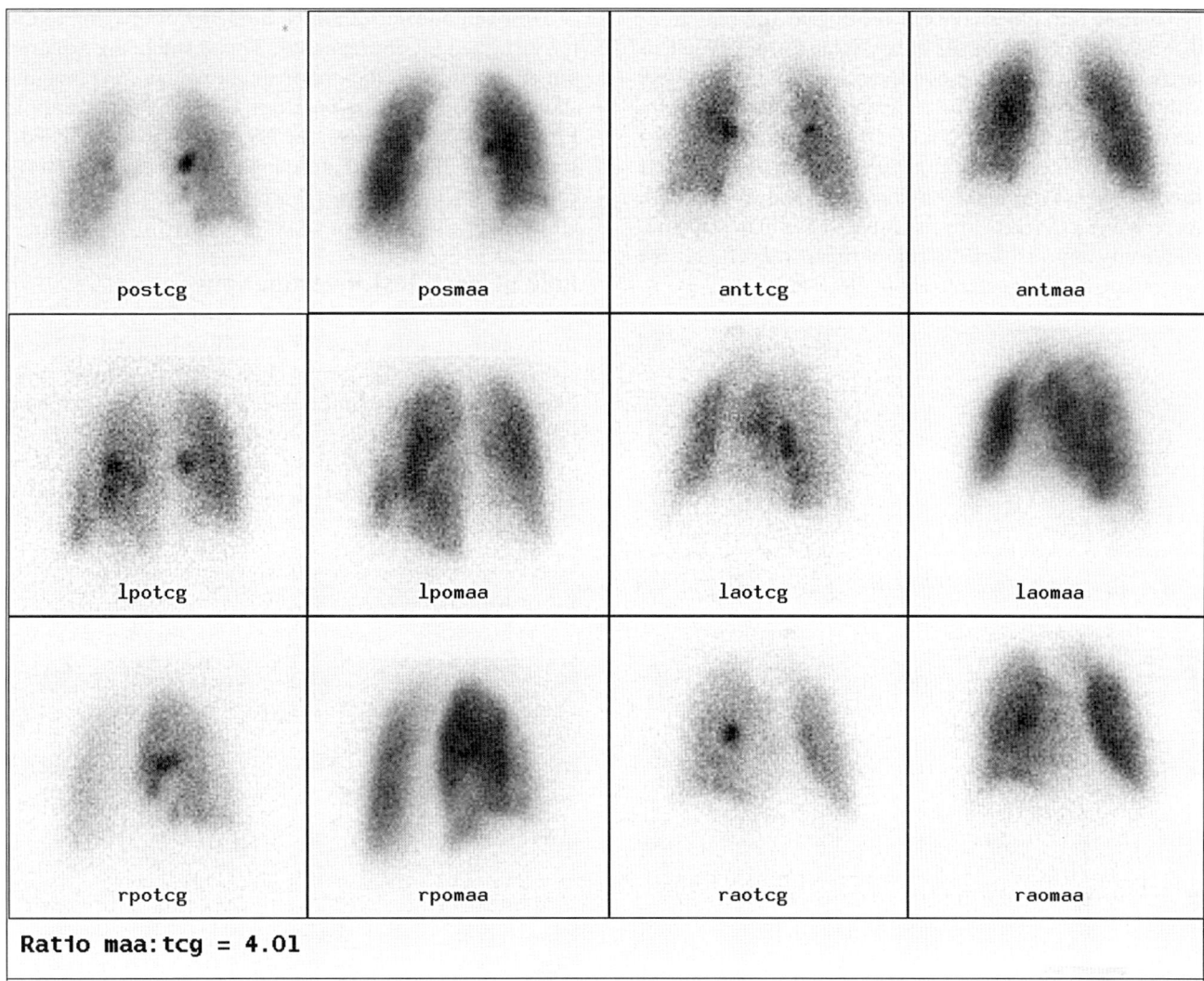

Figure 7A.19   *Pneumonic consolidation of the left lower lobe on chest X-ray with matched ventilation defect. Reversed mismatch of perfusion seen here is often seen in pneumonia but CTPA is essential to exclude pulmonary embolism. CTPA negative in this case.*

to 0.3% of all pregnancies.[40] Pregnancy increases the risk of VTE astonishingly five times over a nonpregnant woman of similar age[41] and there is some evidence that the risk of VTE is increased equally throughout each of the three trimesters and early postpartum period.[42]

VTE diagnosis in pregnancy is clearly crucial. Several groups have suggested guidelines that maximize the efficacy of diagnosis and minimize the fetal exposure to ionizing radiation.[43,44] Prior to the widespread deployment of CTPA, VQ imaging was the primary diagnostic modality in pregnancy.[45] VQ imaging was always recognized to have limited specificity particularly in patients with abnormal chest X-rays but in the subgroup of young and healthy individuals with normal X-rays, it has been shown to produce clinically useful results in the majority of women imaged.[46]

Since the deployment of CTPA, a reassessment of indications for VQ imaging and CTPA is continuing.

There is little doubt (Table 7A.6) that the theoretical risk following a linear hypothesis of inducing a cancer is double for the mother after CTPA given the effective dose of 1.7 mSv compared with 0.8 mSv for half-dose VQ imaging.[47] Conversely, the fetus is exposed to more radiation dose after half-dose VQ imaging compared to CTPA because of the systemic administration of tracers against the tight collimation of the CT beam on the upper torso. These doses from both modalities are low and are considered to result in an acceptable exposure. Clearly, in view of the risk to the fetus of maternal death, the most important consideration is the actual diagnosis of potential VTE since it is preventable and treatable. There is a theoretical risk from the use of non-ionic contrast media of which the commonly used are iohexol and ioversol. A small number of case reports highlight transient neonatal hypothyroidism as a potential end-result of the iodine load. Biochemical screening postpartum may therefore be appropriate after CTPA. There is a small risk of idiosyncratic contrast reaction following intravenous exposure but this is rarely seen with modern non-ionic media.

There is one other concern relating to the radiation-absorbed dose to the female breast tissue from CTPA. This can be up to 8 mGy with modern machines but even higher with older equipment. The comparative breast dose from half-dose VQ imaging is 0.3 mGy. In addition, and contrary to intuition, the theoretical lifetime risk of breast cancer after CTPA or VQ is highest in the young and reduces with age.[48] While a concern, this risk must be put in perspective. The reality appears that the risk of breast cancer after the contraceptive pill equates to about 38 CTPAs.

How can one decide which modality of imaging to use for suspected PE of pregnancy? This is still being explored but currently, as in the nonpregnant women, VQ imaging should be chosen when the chest X-ray is normal and the PE risk is low to moderate. (i.e. PE requires to be excluded). If the risk of PE is moderate to high with cardio-respiratory complications and particularly with an abnormal chest X-ray, CTPA is the modality of choice.

Role of post-test investigations

In the author's experience of a teaching hospital, VQ scan analysis in cases with normal chest X-rays and subsequent integration with the clinical data excludes PE in up to two thirds of cases and picks up one third of cases of PE. Some other cases have a 'PE unlikely' report (LP category with up to two risk factors) resulting in a less useful risk of 10%.

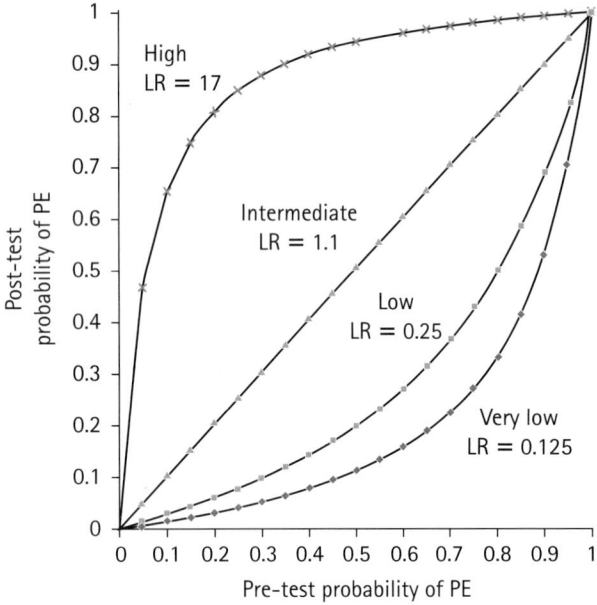

Figure 7A.20 *The conditional probability graph for PE diagnosis is constructed using the likelihood ratios (LRs) calculated from the re-aligned PIOPED 1 data. The graph combines the clinical pre-test probability and the VQ categories into the post-test probability of PE.*

Table 7A.2 *Diagnosis of venous thromboembolism: the low clinical pre-test probability*

Scan category	Risk of pulmonary embolism (VQ + clinical) (%)	Post-test result
Normal	0	PE excluded
Near normal	0	PE excluded
Very low probability	2	PE highly unlikely
Low probability	3	PE highly unlikely*
Indeterminate probability	10–15	Diagnosis uncertain
High probability	50–60	Diagnosis uncertain

PE, pulmonary embolism.

*Risk due to a LP single match is unknown but probably approximately 5% or more.

Table 7A.3 *Diagnosis of venous thromboembolism: the medium clinical pre-test probability*

Scan category	Risk of pulmonary embolism (VQ + clinical) (%)	Post-test result
Normal	0	PE excluded
Near normal	0	PE excluded
Very low probability	5	PE highly unlikely
Low probability	10	PE unlikely*
Indeterminate probability	20–30	Diagnosis uncertain
High probability	80–90	PE likely

PE, pulmonary embolism.

*Risk due to a LP single match is unknown but probably approximately 15%.

Table 7A.4 *Diagnosis of venous thromboembolism: the high clinical pre-test probability*

Scan category	Risk of pulmonary embolism (VQ + clinical) (%)	Post-test result
Normal	0	PE excluded
Near normal	5	PE unlikely
Very low probability	10–20	Diagnosis uncertain
Low probability	20–40	Diagnosis uncertain
Indeterminate probability	40–70	Diagnosis uncertain
High probability	95	PE highly likely

PE, pulmonary embolism.

Clearly those cases require a further test to lower the PE risk into a more useful diagnostic range. A negative well-performed Doppler ultrasound of both legs would reduce this risk by half to 5% that is clinically useful.[49,50]

Patients with abnormal chest X-rays, significant cardio-respiratory disease or with VQ imaging providing a report 'diagnosis uncertain' all have a PE risk between 10 and 60%. CTPA is the only investigation that can clarify the diagnosis in these groups that may represent up to 35% of all cases of suspected PE.

Each hospital or institution will need to formulate its individual imaging strategy for suspected PE in cases with an abnormal d-dimer but it is likely that an abnormal chest X-ray and/or a > 10% risk of PE following VQ imaging will

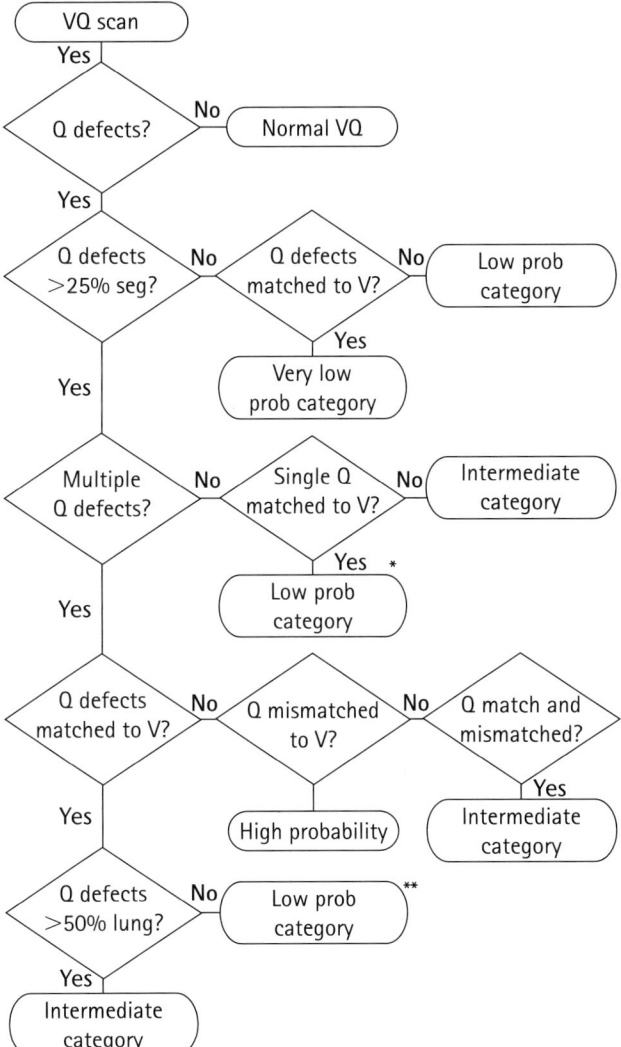

Figure 7A.21 *A basic algorithm for VQ scan interpretation. The flow chart starts with a normal chest X-ray. *Likelihood of pulmonary embolism is higher than with multiple matches. **Multiple matched segmental abnormalities should raise a suspicion of pulmonary embolism.*

Table 7A.5 *Neoclassical criteria for VQ scan interpretation: modified PIOPED*

High probability

*Two or more moderate/large mismatched perfusion defects**

Prior heart and lung disease probably requires more abnormalities (i.e. four or more)

Triple match in one lung with one or more mismatch in the other with clear lung field on X-ray

Intermediate probability

Difficult to categorize or not described as very low, low or high, including all cases with a chest X-ray opacity, pleural fluid or collapse

Single moderate VQ match or mismatch without corresponding radiograph abnormality

Low probability

Large or moderate focal VQ matches involving no more than 50% of the combined lung fields with no corresponding radiograph abnormalities

Small VQ mismatches with a normal chest X-ray

Very-low probability

Small VQ matches with a normal chest X-ray

Near-normal

Perfusion defects due to raised hemi-diaphragm, cardiomegaly, enlarged hila or aorta

Normal

No perfusion abnormalities

Large defects are >75% segment, moderate defects are 25–75% segment and small defects are <25% segment.

Table 7A.6 *Theoretical risk of inducing cancer after VQ imaging or CTPA*

Modality	Total effective dose (mSv)	Additional lifetime risk of fatal cancer	Fetal dose (mGy)	Additional risk of fatal cancer to age 15
VQ imaging	0.8	1 in 21 000	0.18	1 in 194 000
CTPA	1.7	1 in 10 000	0.015	1 in 2.2 million
Comparative baseline risk		1 in 4.5 for whole life		1 in 1300 to age 15

Information from Brennan.[47]

be automatic triggers for immediate CTPA. Either Doppler ultrasound or immediate CTPA could be used for the 10% risk cases (i.e. LP scan category and medium clinical risk).

There is also an argument for performing a perfusion lung scan at the completion of anticoagulant therapy for PE to provide a baseline image for use should the patient represent with chest symptoms.[51] This is a sensible precaution. The perfusion abnormalities secondary to PE can be long-lasting and can result in diagnostic confusion should the patient require re-imaging.

CONCLUSION

It appears highly likely that VQ imaging will remain a pivotal screening test for patients suspected of possible PE but with normal chest X-rays. It is likely that CTPA will become routine for cases with an abnormality of chest X-ray or those with intermediate or indeterminate VQ scan categories secondary to cardio-respiratory disease. Most departments of nuclear medicine will experience an increase in the proportion of scans that are diagnostic as the clinical risk of their referred population falls.

REFERENCES

1 Dalen JE, Alpert JS. Natural history of pulmonary embolism. *Prog Cardiovasc Dis* 1975; **17**: 259–70.

2 Goldhaber SZ. Pulmonary embolism. *Lancet* 2004; **363**: 1295–305.

3 Benotti JR, Ockene IS, Alperts S, *et al.* The clinical profile of unresolved pulmonary embolism. *Chest* 1983; **84**: 669–78.

4 Coche E, Verschuren F, Keyeux A, *et al.* Diagnosis of acute pulmonary embolism in outpatients: comparison of thin-collimation multi-detector row spiral CT and planar ventilation perfusion scintigraphy. *Radiology* 2003; **229**: 757–65.

5 Kavanagh EC, O'Hare A, Hargaden G, *et al.* Risk of pulmonary embolism after negative MDCT pulmonary angiography findings. *Am J Roentgenol* 2004; **182**: 499–504.

6 Morrell NW, Nijran KS, Jones BE, *et al.* The understanding of segmental defects in radionuclide lung scanning. *J Nucl Med* 1993; **34**: 370–4.

7 Bajc M, Olsson CG, Olsson B, *et al.* Diagnostic evaluation of planar and tomographic ventilation/perfusion lung images in patients with suspected pulmonary emboli. *Clin Physiol Funct Imaging* 2004; **24**: 249–56.

8 Sevitt S, Gallagher N. Venous thrombosis and pulmonary embolism. A clinico-pathological study in injured and burned patients. *Br J Surg* 1961; **48**: 475–89.

9 Line BR. Pathophysiology and diagnosis of deep vein thrombus. *Semin Nucl Med* 2002; **31**: 90–101.

10 Elliot G. Pulmonary physiology during pulmonary embolism. *Chest* 1992; **101**: 163S–71.

11 Hull RD, Hirsh J, Carter CJ, *et al.* Pulmonary angiography, ventilation lung scanning and venography for clinically suspected pulmonary embolism with abnormal perfusion scan. *Ann Intern Med* 1983; **98**: 891–9.

12 Moser KM, Fedulla PF, Littlejohn JK, *et al.* Frequent asymptomatic pulmonary embolism in patients with deep vein thrombosis. *J Am Med Assoc* 1994; **271**: 223–5.

13 Gray HW. The natural history of venous thromboembolism: impact on ventilation/perfusion scan reporting. *Semin Nucl Med* 2002; **32**: 159–72.

14 Dahlback B, Carlsson M, Svensson PJ. Familial thrombophilia due to a previously unrecognised mechanism characterised by poor anticoagulant response to activated protein C: prediction of a co-factor to activated protein C. *Proc Natl Acad Sci USA* 1993; **90**: 1004–8.

15 Stein PD, Henry JW, Gottschalk A. Reassessment of pulmonary angiography for the diagnosis of pulmonary embolism: relation of interpreter agreement to the order of the involved pulmonary arterial branch. *Radiology* 1999; **210**: 689.

16 The PIOPED Investigators. Value of the ventilation/perfusion scan in acute pulmonary embolism. Results of the prospective investigation of pulmonary embolism diagnosis (PIOPED). *J Am Med Assoc* 1990; **263**: 2753.

17 Stein PD, Athanasoulis C, Alavi A *et al.* Complications and validity of pulmonary angiography in acute pulmonary embolism. *Circulation* 1992; **85**: 462.

18 Gray HW. The languages of lung scan interpretation. In: Freeman LM. (ed.) *Nuclear medicine annual.* Philadelphia PA: Lippincott Williams and Wilkins, 2001: 23–47.

19 Perrier A, Miron MJ, Desmarais S, *et al.* Using clinical evaluation and lung scan to rule out suspected pulmonary embolism. *Arch Intern Med* 2000; **160**: 512–6.

20 Wicki J, Perneger TV, Junod A, *et al.* Assessing clinical probability of pulmonary embolism in the emergency ward: a simple score. *Arch Intern Med* 2001; **161**: 92–7.

21 Wells PS, Ginsberg JS, Anderson DR, *et al.* Use of a clinical model for safe management of patients with suspected pulmonary embolism. *Ann Intern Med* 1998; **129**: 997–1005.

22 Neilly JB, Davidson J, McCarter D, *et al.* CT pulmonary angiography in patients with suspected pulmonary embolism [abstract]. *Nucl Med Commun* 2000; **21**: 392.

23 Heit JA, Silverstein MD, Mohr DW, *et al.* The epidemiology of venous thromboembolism in the community. *Thromb Haemost* 2001; **86**: 452–63.

24 Stein PD, Goldhaber SZ, Henry JW, *et al.* Arterial blood gas analysis in the assessment of suspected acute pulmonary embolism. *Chest* 1996; **109**: 78–81.

25 Stein PD, Goldhaber SZ, Henry JW. Alveolar-arterial oxygen gradient in the assessment of acute pulmonary embolism. *Chest* 1995; **107**: 139–43.

26 Bounameaux H, De Moerloose P, Perrier A, *et al.* D-dimer testing in suspected venous thromboembolism: an update. *Q J Med* 1997; **90**: 437–42.

27 Kelly J, Hunt BJ. Role of d-dimers in diagnosis of venous thromboembolism. *Lancet* 2002; **359**: 456–8.

28 Dunn KL, Wolf JP, Dorfman DM, *et al.* Normal d-dimer levels in emergency department patients suspected of acute pulmonary embolism. *J Am Coll Cardiol* 2002; **40**: 1475–8.

29 Revel MP, Petrover D, Hernigova A, *et al.* Diagnosing pulmonary embolism with four-detector row helical CT: prospective evaluation of 216 outpatients and inpatients. *Radiology* 2005; **234**: 265–73.

30 British Thoracic Society Standards of Care Committee Pulmonary Embolism Guideline Development Group. British Thoracic Society Guidelines for the management of suspected acute pulmonary embolism. *Thorax* 2003; **58**: 470–84.

31 Turkstra F, Kuijer PM, vanBeek EJ, *et al.* Diagnostic utility of ultrasonography of leg veins in patients suspected of having pulmonary embolism. *Ann Int Med* 1997; **126**: 775–81.

32 MacGillavry M, Sanson M, Buller H, *et al.* Compression ultrasonography of the leg veins in patients with clinically suspected pulmonary embolism: is a more extensive assessment of compressibility useful? *Thromb Haemost* 2000; **84**: 973–6.

33 Wells PS, Ginsberg JS, Anderson DR, *et al.* Use of a clinical model for safe management of patients with suspected pulmonary embolism. *Ann Int Med* 1998; **129**: 997–1005.

34 Miniati M, Monti S, Pratali L, *et al.* Value of transthoracic echocardiography in the diagnosis of pulmonary embolism: results of a prospective study in unselected patients. *Am J Med* 2001; **110**: 528–35.

35 Steiner P, Lund GK, Debatin JF, *et al.* Acute pulmonary embolism: value of transthoracic and transesophageal echocardiography in comparison with helical CT. *Am J Roentgenol* 1996; **167**: 931–6.

36 Oudkerk M, van Beek EJR, Wielopolski P, *et al.* Comparison of contrast enhanced magnetic resonance angiography and conventional pulmonary angiography for the diagnosis of pulmonary embolism: a prospective study. *Lancet* 2002; **359**: 1643–7.

37 Stein PD, Woodard PK, Hull RD, *et al.* Gadolinium enhanced magnetic resonance angiography for detection of acute pulmonary embolism. An in-depth review. *Chest* 2003; **124**: 2324–8.

38 Gray HW, Bessent RG. Pulmonary exclusion: a practical approach to low probability using the PIOPED data. *Eur J Nucl Med* 1998; **25**: 271–6.

39 Gray HW, McKillop JH, Bessent RG. Lung scan reporting language: what does it mean? *Nucl Med Commun* 1993; **14**: 1084–97.

40 Barbour LA, Pickard J. Controversies in thromboembolic disease during pregnancy: a critical review. *Obstet Gynecol* 1995; **86**: 621–33.

41 Prevention of venous thrombosis and pulmonary embolism. NIH Consensus Development. *J Am Med Assoc* 1986; **256**: 744–9.

42 Toglia MR, Weg JG. Venous thromboembolism during pregnancy. *N Engl J Med* 1996; **335**: 108–14.

43 Demers C, Ginsberg JS. Deep vein thrombosis and pulmonary embolism in pregnancy. *Clin Chest Med* 1992; **13**: 645–56.

44 Russell JR, Stabin MG, Sparks RB, *et al.* Radiation absorbed dose to the embryo/fetus from radiopharmaceuticals. *Health Phys* 1997; **73**: 756–69.

45 Bouselle PM, Reddy SS, Villas PA, *et al.* Pulmonary embolism in pregnant patients: survey of ventilation–perfusion imaging policies and practices. *Radiology* 1998; **207**: 201–6.

46 Chan WS, Ray JG, Murray S, *et al.* Suspected pulmonary embolism in pregnancy. *Arch Int Med* 2002; **162**: 1170–5.

47 Brennan A. Personal communication, 2004.

48 NHSBSP. *Review of radiation risk in breast screening.* Publication 54, Table 4. February 2003.

49 Hull RD, Rascob G, Ginsberg J, *et al.* A non-invasive strategy for the treatment of patients with suspected pulmonary embolism. *Arch Int Med* 1994; **154**: 289–97.

50 Huisman MV, Buller HR, ten Cate JW, *et al.* Serial impedance plethysmography for suspected deep vein thrombosis in outpatients: the Amsterdam General Practitioners Study. *N Engl J Med* 1986; **314**: 823–8.

51 Bomanji J, Alawadhi H, Beale A, *et al.* Clinical outcomes of patients with suspected pulmonary embolism using ^{99m}Tc-Technegas as a ventilatory agent for lung scanning. *Nucl Med Commun* 1992; **13**: 467–77.

Lung cancer

M.J. O'DOHERTY

INTRODUCTION

The management of patients with disease often poses a variety of questions and differing requirements for the patients, clinicians, and the healthcare providers:

1. The patient needs to know the diagnosis, the extent of the disease, the best management of the disease, and the likely prognosis when the best management option has been decided.
2. The clinician needs to know all the patient's requirements and the most appropriate way of satisfying them.
3. The government or the funding body needs to know the cost of achieving the patient's and the clinician's requirements and the benefits to the patient.

Patients with pulmonary nodules, masses or pleural disease may have benign or malignant disease. The clinician managing the patient requires the establishment of a diagnosis, staging, and a means of evaluating response to treatment. After the appropriate treatment has been adopted there may also be a requirement to identify disease recurrence. The health provider(s) (those groups holding the purse strings) often have a notional sum of money that is attached to the value of investigative techniques and their benefits to patient care and quality of life. This notional sum varies with country but is often quoted as under approximately €50 000 or $50 000 or between £30 000 and £35 000.

Nodules found in the lung are described as pulmonary nodules if less than 3–4 cm in diameter whereas lesions larger than this are described as pulmonary masses and are frequently malignant.[1] The causes of a solitary primary nodule (SPN) are highly variable and dependent on the part of the world the individual is from or resident in. They are extremely common affecting up to 0.2% of adults[2] with 20–50% of cases being malignant.[1] This prevalence of pulmonary nodules may well change dramatically if computed tomography (CT) screening for lung cancer in a population who are at risk is introduced.

Carcinoma of the lung may be divided histologically into non-small cell lung cancer (NSCLC), small cell lung cancer (SCLC) and other less common causes of lung cancer. NSCLC represents approximately 82% of all lung cancers. There are approximately 35 000 deaths from lung cancer in the UK and 158 000 in the USA each year.[1] NSCLC can be subdivided into squamous cell carcinoma, adenocarcinoma, and large cell carcinoma. The prevalence of adenocarcinoma is increasing compared with squamous carcinoma. The International System for Staging Lung Cancer (Table 7B.1)[3] identifies the extent of disease and is related to the survival of such patients with NSCLC. SCLC patients normally have extensive disease at presentation but staging is no less important and is usually expressed as limited or extensive disease. Patients with very limited disease may have a better prognosis. The overall mortality from NSCLC remains high with 5-year survival figures in Europe between 8 and 11% and in the USA as high as 14%. The prognosis for disseminated disease is poor with 5-year survival figures of less than 5% and as good as 60–80% for nonmetastatic disease. The high mortality for disseminated disease requires a method to identify these patients at an early stage such that their management can be directed appropriately.

There are multiple diagnostic tests available for use in carcinoma of the lung including computerized tomography, magnetic resonance imaging, ultrasound imaging,

Table 7B.1   *Revisions of the International System for Staging Lung Cancer: Pathological stage classification and 5-year survival data*

Stage	TNM classification	Survival (%)
IA	T1N0M0	67
IB	T2N0M0	57
IIA	T1N1M0	55
IIB	T2N1M0	39
	T3N0M0	38
IIIA	T3N1M0	25
	T3N2M0	23
IIIB	T4N0–2M0	7
	T1–4N3M0	3
IV	Any T, Any N, M1	1

Adapted from Mountain CF. Revisions in the International System for Staging Lung Cancer. *Chest* 1997; **111**: 1710–17.

single photon imaging, and positron imaging. These latter functional imaging techniques have grown rapidly with a particular emphasis on positron emission tomography (PET) including tracers such as [^{18}F]fluorodeoxyglucose, ^{11}C-methionine, ^{11}C-choline, ^{11}C-acetate, [^{18}F]fluorothymidine, and hypoxia tracers such as ^{18}F-misonidazole and ^{64}Cu-ATSM.[1,4–8] There has also been the development of single photon imaging with the introduction of ^{99m}Tc-depreotide.[9–11]

This chapter will explore the role that PET and SPECT have in the investigation of SPNs and lung cancer.

SOLITARY PULMONARY NODULES

There are a number of problems associated with SPNs for functional imaging, these are predominantly related to the size of the lesion as well as metabolic activity/antigen expression. Prevalence of benign causes of SPNs in a given population will also affect the sensitivity and specificity of the test. Furthermore, lesion size may become a dominant factor if a screening program is introduced using CT, since smaller lesions will be detected and these may be beyond the resolution of existing equipment. If the prevalence of SPNs less than 1 cm in size rises, the sensitivity of functional imaging in this group will fall.

Single photon emission computerized tomography

A variety of radiotracers have been used to assess lung nodules including ^{67}Ga, ^{201}Tl, ^{99m}Tc-sestamibi, ^{99m}Tc-tetrofosmin, and ^{99m}Tc-depreotide. As with PET imaging pulmonary nodules less than 1 cm and in some instances less than

1.5 cm in size are not visualized with ^{67}Ga, ^{201}Tl, ^{99m}Tc-sestamibi, and ^{99m}Tc-tetrofosmin. Gallium-67 is poor at differentiating mediastinal disease and has been reported to be falsely negative in up to 22% of pulmonary nodules.[12] Thallium-201 has variable sensitivity and specificity and is therefore not used to assess SPNs.[1,13] Technetium-99m-sestamibi and ^{99m}Tc-tetrofosmin have had differing success. The sensitivity of ^{99m}Tc-sestamibi is reportedly between 86 and 89%[14] for the detection of malignancy in pulmonary nodules. This compares favorably with other methods of assessing the primary nodule, unfortunately in the assessment of the mediastinum this is less effective than fluorodeoxyglucose (FDG) PET.[4] Technetium-99m-sestamibi does have a potential advantage in that rapid washout or nonvisualization of a known tumor may indicate the presence of P-glycoprotein and provide a method of assessing chemoresistance. Technetium-99m-tetrofosmin has reported sensitivities between 61 and 94%,[1] but FDG PET was found to be superior in detecting the primary lesion and mediastinal metastases.

Technetium-99m-depreotide, which has high affinity binding to somatostatin receptors 2, 3, and 5, is a relatively new tracer. There are few studies on this product to know how useful it will be in the assessment of pulmonary nodules. There are three published studies using depreotide alone, two by Blum *et al.*[9,10] and one by Grewal *et al.*[11] The studies by Blum were initially of a group of 30 patients and the subsequent study of 114 patients 77% of whom subsequently had a malignancy.[9,10] The mean lesion size in this latter group was 2.8 ± 1.6 cm. The sensitivity was 96% and specificity 73% in this group, similar to reports using ^{99m}Tc-sestamibi. The surprising number of malignancies in this group may reflect selection bias or larger lesions that are inherently more likely to be malignant. A study with a larger number of benign lesions would be needed to assess true sensitivity. Grewal *et al.* with a smaller number of patients (*n* 39) found a sensitivity of 100% but a specificity of 43% indicating a worrying number of false positives but no false negatives.[11] At present the staging value of depreotide is not known. The concern is that when larger numbers of patients are studied the specificity may not be sufficient to justify further investigation since the false positive rate will be too high. Kahn *et al.*[15] have compared prospectively ^{99m}Tc-depreotide and FDG PET in the same patients using a full ring PET scanner. This prospective study of 166 patients had 157 evaluable subjects and the sensitivity and specificity for PET were 96% and 71% for the primary solitary pulmonary nodule and for depreotide 94% and 51%, respectively. An assessment was also made of mediastinal and hilar nodal disease such that the sensitivity and specificity for FDG was 81% and 77%, respectively, and for depreotide 68% and 70%. The specificity for FDG PET was statistically better than depreotide for the primary lesion, but there was no difference for the nodal staging. In this series there were 122 malignancies and 35 benign lesions. This paper is unusual in that the sensitivity and specificity for nodal staging is very different to the PET literature in known malignancy and emphasizes this difficulty especially if there is granulomatous disease. At present it would appear the sensitivity is such that any positive study needs further investigation and then if proven to be lung cancer will require a FDG PET study to assess the mediastinum. This duplication could be prevented if there were adequate provision of PET. However, a negative study would appear to allow clinical follow-up, although the data is sparse at the present time.

A comparison of ^{99m}Tc-sestamibi and ^{99m}Tc-tetrofosmin with ^{99m}Tc-depreotide is required to examine what test is suitable for smaller hospitals to perform as cost-effectively as possible to assess patients with SPN.

Positron emission tomography

Over 2000 patients with histological or long-term follow-up confirmation have been published in peer-reviewed English language publications. The interpretation of the uptake of FDG has used both visual and semiquantitative measures with some using a cut-off value for the SUV of 2.5 to delineate malignancy. The sensitivity for FDG PET ranges from 83 to 100% with an overall sensitivity calculated from the pooled data of 95.9% and the specificity calculated from pooled data of 78.1%.[1] There is a variety of false positive and false negative results with FDG PET, the former predominantly caused by inflammation and are summarized in Table 7B.2.

False negative results are normally due to the small size of lesions or their degree of differentiation with the more differentiated slow growing tumors potentially negative.[1] Although bronchiolo-alveolar cell carcinomas are a recognized cause for false negative results this appears to depend on the histological type[16] and in our experience it is often positive on FDG PET with a lobar pattern of uptake. Lesions smaller than 1 cm may be falsely negative, especially at the bases where respiratory motion degrades the resolution of the scanner. It remains to be seen whether the combination of PET–CT will improve this size limit. Ultimately, however, it is the metabolic activity of the tumor that is the determinant, with a number of reports demonstrating that SPNs of less than 1 cm can be detected.[1]

A number of cost–benefit analyses have been performed to evaluate the role of FDG PET in SPNs. Gambhir et al.[17] and Dietlein et al.[18] compared differing strategies for FDG PET in the evaluation of SPNs. These evaluations used differing starting points. Gambhir et al. demonstrated that those patients with an intermediate pre-test probability of malignancy (12–69%) had the greatest cost-effectiveness whereas above this probability a CT only probability was more cost-effective and below this probability a watch and wait policy was most cost-effective. Dietlein et al. also found that for an intermediate pre-test probability of malignancy a strategy employing FDG PET yielded an increase in life

Table 7B.2 *Causes of false positive findings with fluorodeoxyglucose positron emission tomography for characterization of solitary primary nodules*

- *Granulomas*
  Tuberculosis
  Sarcoidosis
  Wegeners granulomatosis
- *Histoplasmosis*
- *Coccidioidomycosis*
- *Acute blastomycosis*
- *Cryptococcus neoformans*
- *Chronic inflammation (including histiocytic and in association with an anthracosilicotic nodule)*
- *Aspergillus infection (including invasive aspergillosis and aspergilloma)*
- *Abscess*
- *Schwannoma*
- *Chrondrohamartomas*
- *Neurofibroma*

expectancy at an increased cost of 3218 euros per life year gained.[18] Gould et al. evaluated a larger number of possible strategies but reached a similar conclusion that intermediate probability patients were best assessed using CT and PET.[19]

FDG PET is accurate in characterizing SPNs but there is controversy as to when it should be used. I suspect this will vary with the health system of a particular country, the availability of CT (and an experienced person to perform fine-needle aspirations), and the availability and cost of PET. In most countries the access to CT is likely to be high and at a relatively low cost and therefore the strategies that do not assess CT as an entry criterion to the use of PET are of little value. It is also unlikely in the current climate that every SPN of intermediate probability will be investigated with PET since in most cases an attempt to obtain a tissue diagnosis will be performed. Therefore PET should be reserved for those who have had a failed biopsy, or those in whom an attempt at a biopsy would be too great a risk or indeed those who do not wish to have a biopsy. Figure 7B.1 shows an algorithm for the role of FDG PET in the detection of SPNs. In these cases a 'metabolic biopsy' can be performed with PET to delineate those who could have a wait-and-watch policy or those who need a more invasive attempt at obtaining tissue.[20] Most of the cost-effectiveness strategies regard high probability SPNs as not cost-effective for PET. There is evidence that a significant proportion of patients (18%; 4/23) with T1N0 had N2 mediastinal lymph node metastases[21] and therefore this group should perhaps be viewed in terms of staging for known NSCLC described below.

Carbon-11-methionine and ^{11}C-tyrosine have been used to evaluate SPNs and appear to have equivalent findings to

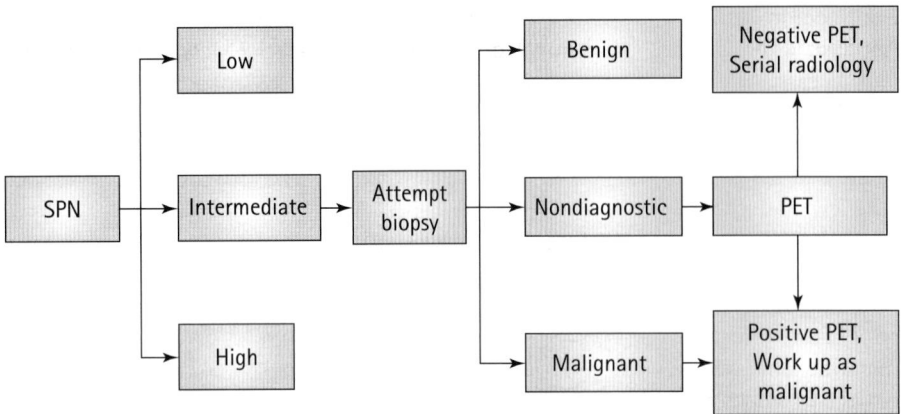

Figure 7B.1 *Algorithm for the role of fluorodeoxyglucose positron emission tomography (FDG PET) in the detection of solitary pulmonary nodules.*

FDG[22–24] but because of the short half-life it is unlikely that this route of investigation will take off. [^{18}F]Fluoromethyl-tyrosine may have a higher positive predictive value than FDG with the potential to separate nonmalignant from malignant causes of SPNs.[25]

STAGING OF NON–SMALL CELL LUNG CANCER

It is essential to accurately stage patients with NSCLC to enable the most appropriate management decisions. This is equally important to identify those patients who may be treated with curative intent – either by surgery or radical radiotherapy – as those who need palliative care instituted e.g. appropriate chemotherapy or pain control. It should be self-evident that the avoidance of inappropriate management should improve the quality of a patient's life by avoiding unnecessary surgery, instituting appropriate supportive care – psychological as well as drug related therapy. Disease stage is also the major predictor of prognosis (Table 7B.1). The International System for Staging Lung Cancer employs the TNM staging system.[3,26]

The most successful outcome for NSCLC is obtained by surgical intervention in those with disease limited to the hemithorax and involving resectable tissue, that is not extending beyond N1 lymph nodes and T3 disease. N2 disease (ipsilateral mediastinal or subcarinal nodes or both) is not normally resectable since the prognosis is much poorer regardless of what treatment is offered.[3] Although some argue that limited or minimal N2 disease (defined by CT) can be resected and the small improvement in survival is worth the procedure. Perhaps minimal 'N2P' disease should be defined and evaluated – that is minimal N2 disease defined by FDG PET. It is also possible that FDG uptake in the primary tumor may also indicate a group of patients with poorer prognosis (see below).

Currently, two techniques, CT and mediastinoscopy, are the most common tests performed to determine operability although with the advances in magnetic resonance imaging (MRI) whether this continues to be the case remains to be seen. CT is the most useful technique for T staging tumors and is the most available technique for the assessment of the mediastinum – some argue that CT should be performed prior to bronchoscopy to determine the extent of disease. Nodal staging has to use standard criteria to assess the involvement of lymph nodes by tumor. This normally assesses lymph nodes >1 cm in the short axis and the transverse plane as containing tumor.[27] However, this assumption is unreliable since reactive nodes will enlarge or lymph nodes containing tumor may not enlarge. McLoud *et al.* showed that 13% of normal sized lymph nodes (<1 cm in diameter) contained tumor, 25% of lymph nodes between 1 and 1.9 cm in diameter had tumor and only 37% of lymph nodes >2 cm contained tumor.[28] If the above criteria for nodal involvement with tumor are used then CT has a sensitivity of 79%, a specificity of 78% and an accuracy of 79%.[29] Other studies have suggested sensitivity and specificity of 60–65% and 60–77% for CT.[30,31]

The T stage

The T stage is dependent on the size and anatomic location of the primary tumor (whether the tumor is invading neighboring structures). FDG PET is not suited to the determination of size or invasion nor are any of the single photon tracers. This stage is best left to imaging that has high resolution and therefore good anatomic detail, for example CT.

Staging the mediastinum

Single photon emission tracers have not been found to have high enough sensitivity[32] or specificity to be useful in mediastinal assessment of disease.[1]

The role of FDG PET in lung cancer was one of the first clinical PET uses agreed by the health insurers for reimbursement in the USA. The majority of the studies performed since 1994 are retrospective studies performed in centers dedicated to the use of PET. Ho Shon *et al.* reviewed the literature up to 2002 and demonstrated that over 2000 patients were studied and meta-analyses performed by a variety of groups have demonstrated the potential role of

Table 7B.3 *Causes of false positive findings in fluorodeoxyglucose positron emission tomography in thoracic lymph node staging*

* Hyperplastic lymph node/reactive hyperplasia/active inflammation/nonspecific inflammation

    Bronchiectasis

    Upper respiratory tract infection

    Pneumonia of any cause

    Vaccinations

    Other infections e.g. aspergillosis, tuberculosis
* Active granulomatous disease e.g. sarcoid
* Wegener's granulomatosis
* Rheumatoid disease
* Proximity of tumor to mediastinum
* Pneumoconiosis
* Anthracosis/silicoanthracosis

FDG PET.[1,30,33,34] Since this literature review there have been a number of important contributions including prospective evaluations of the role of FDG PET compared to the standard work-up of patients with lung cancer considered for surgery.[35,36] This study was followed by a cost-effectiveness evaluation.[37] These studies have really substantiated the observational studies and the cost-effectiveness papers using pooled data. The only cautionary note relates to the number of thoracotomies performed on patients with benign lesions in this prospective study.

Over 2000 patients with histologically proven bronchogenic carcinoma have been studied, of whom over 1700 histological confirmations of thoracic lymph node status is available.[1] In this group of patients the median sensitivity and specificity were 83.3% and 92.2%, respectively. The most important role of FDG PET is to detect the presence or absence of N2 and N3 mediastinal lymph node metastases. The high negative predictive value means that if FDG PET is negative and there are no other contra-indications to surgery then the patient may proceed directly to surgery without the need for invasive surgical staging.[38,39] This is primarily because the invasive staging, mediastinoscopy, has a similar false negative rate to PET and in most countries has a similar cost to a PET scan but a higher morbidity.

False positive FDG PET findings in the mediastinal staging of lung carcinoma may occur, predominantly due to inflammatory pathologies. The reported causes for false positive findings are listed in Table 7B.3 but these are relatively infrequent. Since false positive results may deny a patient potentially curative surgery further investigation with mediastinoscopy should be performed to avoid denying a patient curative surgery.[38,39]

Ho Shon et al. reported that of 894 patients in 16 studies, 292 patients (32.7%) had N2/N3 mediastinal nodal metastases.[1] Compared to CT, FDG PET correctly altered nodal disease stage for the presence or absence of mediastinal nodal disease in 149 patients (16.7%). Interestingly, marginally more patients were downstaged ($n = 83$) than upstaged ($n = 66$) with FDG PET. Valk et al. reported a 24% nodal stage alteration for all nodal stages.[40]

Although N2/N3 lymph nodes that are positive should have further investigation, it is possible to identify some individuals where the degree of uptake on visual inspection is high and the nodal involvement is sequential through the mediastinum (Fig. 7B.2). It is unlikely therefore that this involvement is anything other than metastatic disease such that further investigation need not be pursued. The uptake of FDG in mediastinal lymph nodes has generally been observed after 1–1.5 h. These times may be suboptimal given information in the literature suggesting that delayed imaging of 2 h after FDG injection gives an increased likelihood of identifying distant metastases.[41] The development of new scanning technology may inadvertently result in earlier scanning times and reduce the sensitivity of FDG PET and therefore this needs careful consideration with PET–CT systems where the pressure on throughput may cause scanning to be performed after an uptake of 1 h.

ASSESSMENT OF DISTANT METASTASES

FDG PET can stage disease both within the thorax and in the rest of the body, with the exception of the brain. The studies that have looked at the detection of metastatic disease are small and predominantly retrospective observational studies. Ho Shon et al. reviewed nine studies, a total of 837 patients with 190 found to have metastatic disease. PET detected 94% of metastases and was the only imaging modality to detect distant metastases in 48% of patients. PET also excluded metastatic disease in 53 patients with presumed metastatic disease on other imaging. FDG PET has been shown to be both sensitive and specific for the detection of osseous metastases (Fig. 7B.3). Two recent studies comparing FDG PET and bone scintigraphy demonstrated that FDG PET was more specific and had a higher negative predictive value than bone scintigraphy; one study showed a specificity 98% vs. 66% and the other 88% vs. 78%.[42,43] FDG PET has been compared with various conventional imaging techniques including chest CT (from lung apex to liver), brain CT or MRI, and bone scintigraphy with FDG PET finding 6–9% more patients with metastatic disease.[42,44]

MANAGEMENT CHANGE AND COST-EFFECTIVENESS OF FLUORODEOXYGLUCOSE POSITRON EMISSION TOMOGRAPHY IN NON–SMALL CELL LUNG CANCER

While it may be evident that FDG PET has an impact on the management of patients there are few prospective studies

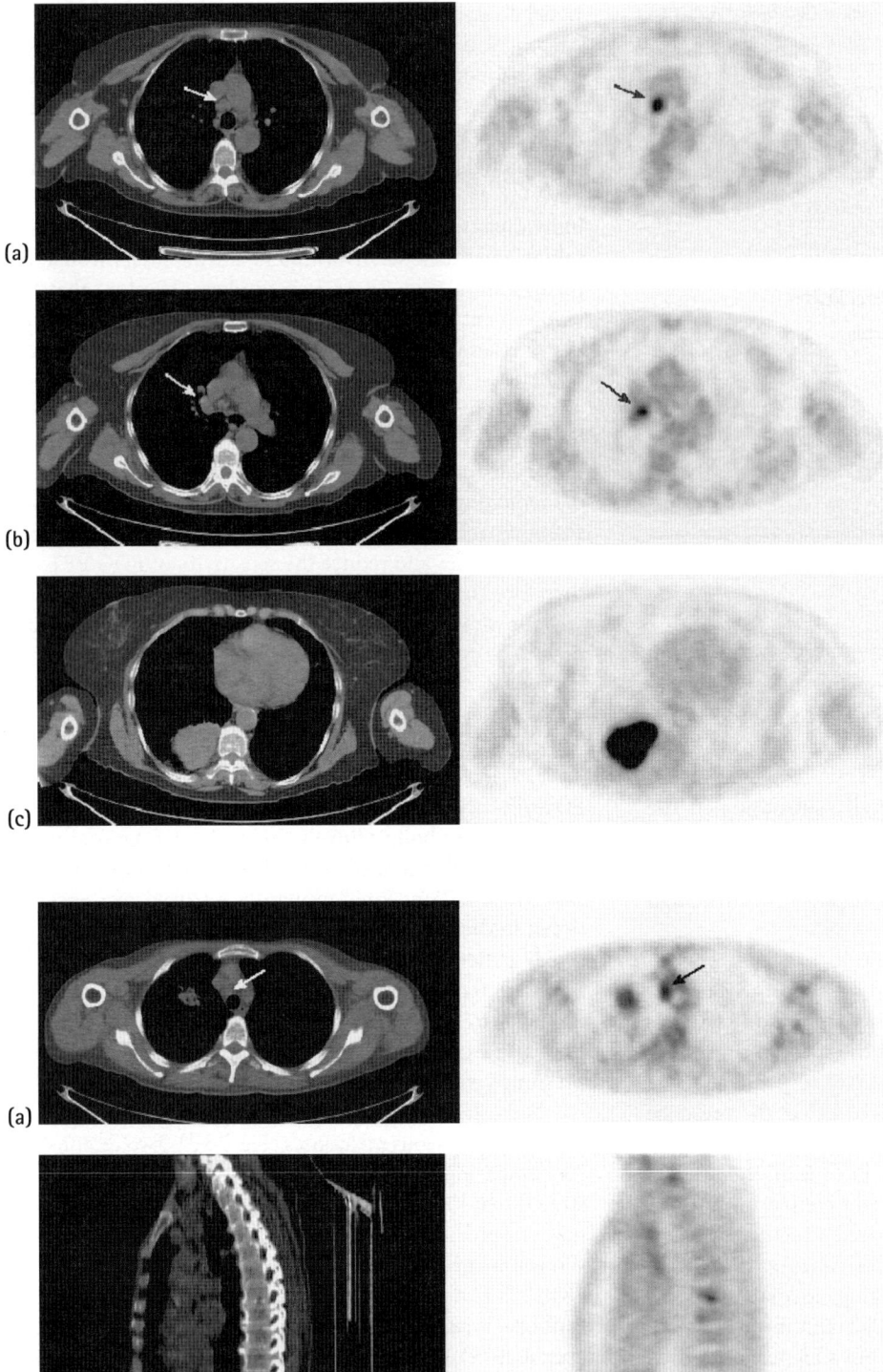

Figure 7B.2 *FDG PET–CT acquired images of a patient referred for staging prior to surgery. The patient was considered operable on conventional staging with computed tomography (CT) scans from the neck to the lower border of the liver. The scan demonstrates the sequential CT and PET images. The PET scan demonstrates the abnormal uptake in (a) the pre- and paratracheal nodes (nodal disease arrowed), (b) right hilum (arrowed), and (c) uptake in the primary tumor. (Abbreviations as in the legend to Fig. 7B.1.)*

Figure 7B.3 *FDG PET–CT acquired images of a patient referred for staging prior to surgery. The patient was considered operable on conventional staging with CT scans from the neck to the lower border of the liver. The primary tumor and a paratracheal node (arrowed) are shown in (a). The scan (b) demonstrates metastatic disease in the vertebrae (D1,7,8), the increased uptake in D7 correlated with a lytic abnormality seen on the CT scan. (Abbreviations as in the legends to Figs 7B.1 and 7B.2.)*

demonstrating an effect on outcome or indeed on quality of life. Alterations in management have been suggested to lie between 20 and 40%.[45,46] Van Tinteren *et al.* performed a prospective study evaluating a conventional work-up for operability and a conventional work-up with PET and showed a 50% reduction in futile thoracotomies with the use of PET.[36] It has to be noted that some of these changes were because of a finding of a benign lung lesion rather than malignancy. If this is allowed for there are still 20% of patients who were saved futile thoracotomies. It is perhaps of interest that most of the observational studies in the literature would point to the same outcome as this randomized controlled trial (RCT). An effect on overall outcome is unlikely to be apparent in any future prospective studies

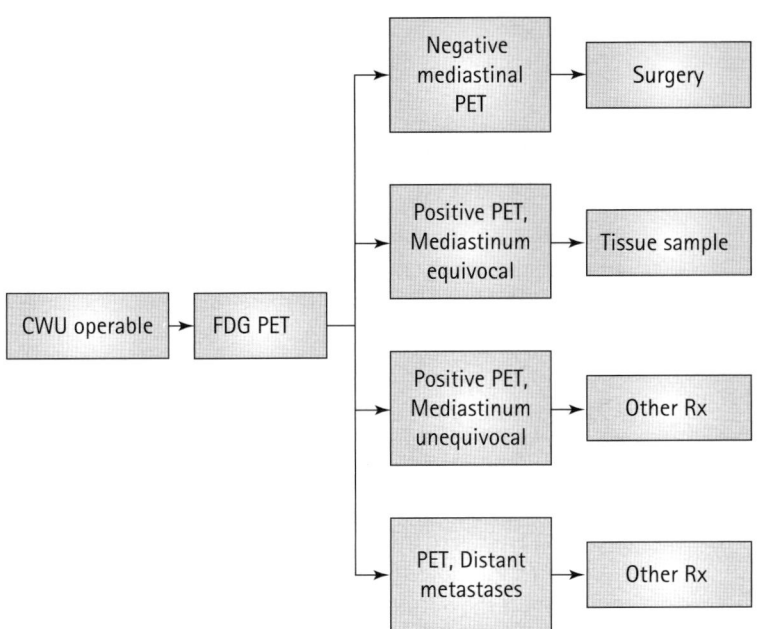

Figure 7B.4 *An algorithm for the use of FDG PET in staging patients with non-small cell lung cancer prior to surgery. (CWU = conventional work-up; other abbreviations as in the legend to Fig. 7B.1.)*

because the overall prognosis is poor from lung cancer. On the whole, RCTs are not designed to test the most appropriate diagnostic test; this is best achieved by direct comparison of the best test available and the new test. This assessment can be best achieved using the individual patient as their own control for imaging investigations. The use of RCTs in outcome assessment will be primarily influenced by the treatment methods and if these are poor then the overall result will remain poor.

The difficulty with assessments of cost-effectiveness of PET is that although the patients may be managed more appropriately by transferring to a palliative course of action the downstream costs of such a switch may be more expensive. Therefore an earlier switch may not be cost saving and yet would be more appropriate management. The areas for reduction of cost are in the reduction of use of mediastinoscopic procedures and of futile thoracotomy in those with metastatic disease. PET is not 100% accurate and therefore no patient should be denied surgery if there is any possibility that the PET result could be wrong and therefore confirmation of distant disease with other imaging or with biopsy needs to be undertaken.

Cost-effectiveness studies have been performed using modelling strategies and on the whole these have arrived at similar conclusions and agree with the one RCT performed.[37] Scott et al.[33] and later Dietlein et al.[34] found that FDG PET was most cost-effective when done on those patients where the CT was negative for nodal metastases with biopsy to confirm PET positive results. The difference was in the incremental cost-effectiveness ratio (ICER) where Scott et al. predicted US$25 286,[33] whereas Dietlein et al. measured an ICER of 143 euros.[34] In the UK, the National Institute for Clinical Excellence (NICE) has also reviewed cost-effectiveness of PET in lung cancer using UK costs and has come to the conclusion that PET is cost-effective in the

presurgical assessment of patients with no evidence of mediastinal or distant metastases on conventional imaging. The analysis also suggests that PET has a cost-effective role in the assessment of patients for radical radiotherapy.[47]

Verboom et al.[37] have recently analysed the cost data from the PLUS study.[36] This study is the first prospective analysis of cost-effectiveness of PET in NSCLC. In this study 188 patients with suspected NSCLC were randomized into a conventional work-up (CWU) group and a conventional work-up (CWU + PET) group with the addition of PET. One of the drawbacks of this study was that in the CWU and the CWU + PET groups there was a large number of patients with benign disease. Despite this the absolute reduction of patients undergoing futile thoracotomy was 20% and the overall cost for a CWU patient was 9573 euros and for the CWU + PET group 8284 euros. The sensitivity analysis performed showed that these results were robust for the CWU + PET. These results really confirm the modeling results performed on the observational data in the literature by Dietlein et al.[34]

The clinical use of FDG PET can be explained by the diagram shown in Fig. 7B.4. FDG PET should be used in those patients with normal-sized lymph nodes on CT. Those patients who are FDG PET negative should proceed directly to surgery. Those patients who have positive FDG PET in mediastinal lymph nodes should have a mediastinoscopy. The one caveat to this would be those patients where there is abnormal uptake in a chain of nodes illustrating sequential spread can be regarded as having metastatic disease. Those patients who have increased uptake in single nodes need further investigation and biopsy of the mediastinum prior to curative surgery.

Although the cost-effectiveness analysis shows only borderline benefit in patients with enlarged lymph nodes,[34] I believe patients with a small number of enlarged nodes who would otherwise be operable should have a FDG PET scan. If there is no evidence of metastases the patient could go on to have curative surgery.

FLUORODEOXYGLUCOSE POSITRON EMISSION TOMOGRAPHY

A number of studies have examined uptake of FDG in the primary tumor to see if this is an independent prognostic indicator. Our own group retrospectively reviewed 77 patients with NSCLC considered for resection and found that an SUV > 20 was of significant prognostic value with a median survival of just 6 months in this group of patients compared with those with an SUV less than 20.[48] Other studies[49,50] found an SUV > 10 or SUV > 7 were correlated with significantly poorer survivals. Ahuja *et al.* additionally found that if the SUV > 10 was combined with a tumor size of less than 3 cm the median survival was just 5.7 months.[49] The variation in SUV measurements needs to be examined more closely and standardized between different departments such that the uptake measurements can be used to act as a prognostic marker wherever the patient is seen.

The value of quantitative measurements needs to be recognized. The poor prognosis associated with high SUV despite the lack of identification of metastatic spread by PET suggests that the patients already have micrometastatic disease with these high values. The evidence is not yet strong enough to suggest that this is the case, but if this is the case then alternative treatments such as chemotherapy may need to be offered to this patient group early and not be put forward for surgical intervention. Further work needs to be done in this area and also clarification as to whether SUV measurements are sufficient or whether alternative methods of quantification are required. This also opens the debate as to whether three-dimensional or two-dimensional acquisition is better to perform quantitative measurement and issues related to CT attenuation correction.

DETECTION OF RECURRENT NON–SMALL CELL LUNG CANCER

Following therapy for previous carcinoma of the lung, interpretation of anatomical imaging owing to treatment induced distortions can be difficult. CT appearances are often thought of as nonspecific, whereas FDG PET has been found to be sensitive in the detection of residual/recurrent disease (97–100%) (Fig. 7B.5). Specificities ranged from 61.5 to 100%.[51–56] There are a number of causes of false positive results following therapy including recent surgery, radiation pneumonitis, and tumor necrosis. These are due to FDG uptake into macrophage infiltration.[55] Uptake may remain within 3–6 months of radiotherapy

and if there is doubt a repeat study may be helpful as false positive uptake has been shown to decline with time.[55]

CHEMOTHERAPY/RADIOTHERAPY

Radiotherapy, chemotherapy, and the best supportive care provide the mainstay of treatment of patients with lung cancer. PET can contribute to these therapies in a variety of ways.

Chemotherapy

One of the biggest growth areas in PET will be the monitoring of treatment response. Almost all other aspects of oncology have embraced the molecular definition of tumors: now is the time for molecular imaging to contribute to oncology and cast off the outmoded measurement of volume change as the measure of treatment response. These volume changes normally follow cell death, but only after a significant period of time has elapsed. FDG response after chemotherapy has been described more fully in patients with lymphoma although observations have been made in NSCLC following chemotherapy.[57–61] These studies showed that complete reduction of FDG uptake correlated with a complete response but even in those with a >50% reduction the prognosis was improved compared to those with no change in uptake. Two more recent publications appear to contradict these studies, suggesting a poor sensitivity with regard to the assessment of mediastinal nodes and their response to chemoradiotherapy but the specificity was high.[62,63] The response of the primary lesion showed a sensitivity and specificity of 75% and 90.5%, respectively.[62] These papers illustrate the requirement to confirm the optimum timing after chemo-radiotherapy especially in view of the large number of false positive results in the mediastinal lymph nodes (Fig. 7B.6).

The timing after chemotherapy is also a matter of debate. A recent article by Spaepen *et al.* demonstrated the time course of FDG uptake in an animal model for lymphoma and the histopathological change in the implanted tumors with time. This study showed that the macrophage infiltration occurred at approximately 5 days and tumor regrowth started at approximately 10 days.[64] This is not necessarily how all tumors will behave but it emphasizes the importance of the timing of the scans after chemotherapy. FDG PET scans performed very soon after chemotherapy may have increased uptake due to a tumor 'flare'.[65] The exact timing of scans remains to be seen in lung cancer.

Radiotherapy

Any successful treatment of cancer should be reflected by metabolic changes prior to changes in size of the tumor.

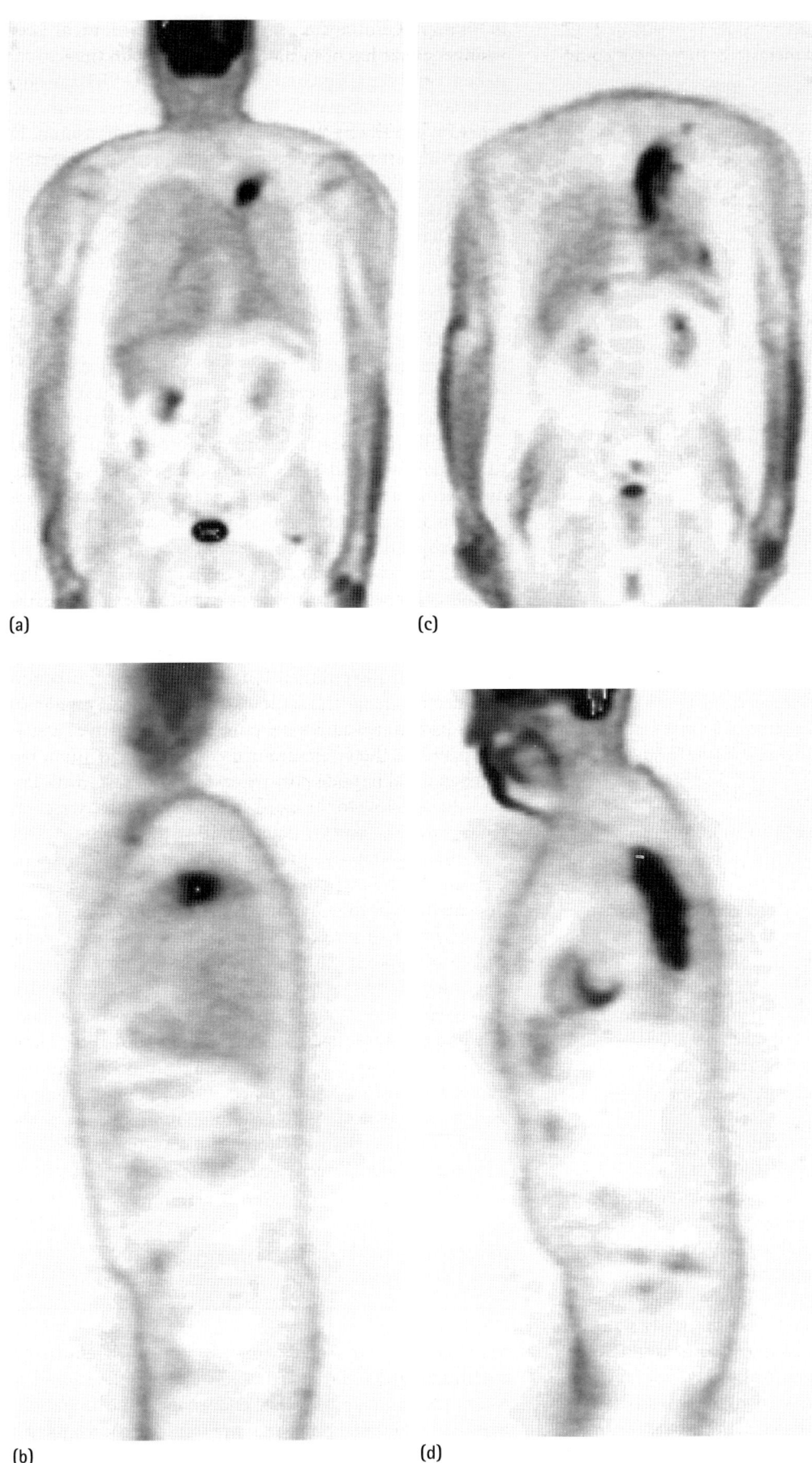

(a)

(c)

(b)

(d)

Figure 7B.5 *A non-attenuation corrected FDG PET study on a patient who had a scan prior to surgery demonstrates FDG uptake in the left upper lobe tumor on (a) the coronal and (b) the sagittal images. Following surgery the patient developed non-specific chest discomfort. The subsequent scan demonstrates high FDG uptake paravertebrally and extending over the left upper lobe on the (c) coronal and (d) the sagittal images consistent with recurrent malignancy. (Abbreviations as in the legend to Fig. 7B.1.)*

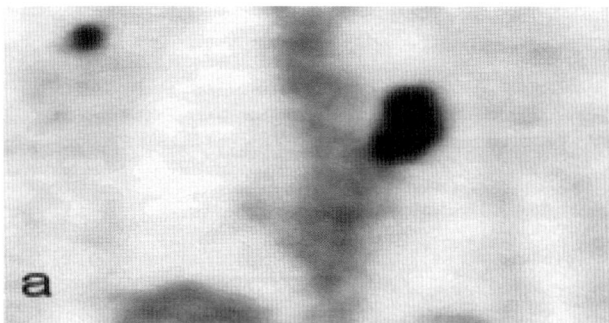

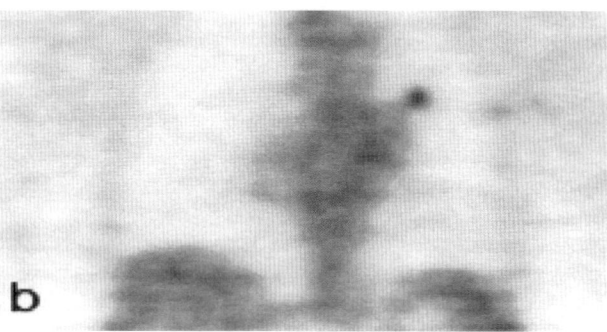

Figure 7B.6 *An attenuation corrected FDG PET study on a patient who had known malignant disease and associated metastatic disease in the right shoulder (a) and was given chemotherapy. The scan shows reduction of FDG uptake in the primary tumor, although there is still a small amount of residual disease, and marked reduction in the right shoulder. (Abbreviations as in the legend to Fig. 7B.1.)*

There are few data with regard to monitoring response following radiotherapy in patients with lung cancer and indeed whether such measurements are useful. There are even fewer data on when following radiotherapy these changes are maximal. The data that are available suggest that the tumors with high FDG uptake respond best to radiotherapy and that persisting FDG uptake reflects the likelihood of relapse.[54,66,67] Following radiotherapy radiation pneumonitis[55] can cause persistent uptake and a delay of 3 to 6 months is suggested following treatment to obtain a meaningful measure of response in those treated with radical radiotherapy.

The more basic question is can PET influence radiotherapy planning. The advent of the combined PET–CT systems suggests that PET usage can be incorporated more easily into radiotherapy planning. There are still issues related to data acquisition and transfer to radiotherapy planning systems. The introduction of respiratory gating approaches to delivery of radiotherapy also raises the issue related to PET data acquisition. FDG PET clearly alters the patient's stage and extent of disease and one would expect this therefore to alter radiotherapy planning.[68–72] However, most of these FDG PET studies are in those patients with normal-sized lymph nodes and the presence of enlarged nodes may alter the sensitivity and specificity of FDG PET

in these circumstances. It therefore remains to be seen whether alteration of radiotherapy field is beneficial to the patients and alters outcome. The use of FDG PET can alter treatment predominantly by changing the treatment volumes by identifying more disease in the mediastinum, by identifying areas of atelectasis rather than tumor extension, and by identifying distant disease in patients who are being considered for radical radiotherapy. A number of studies have demonstrated reduction of radiotherapy treatment volumes ranging from 26.7 to 35%; these studies, however, did not apply these plans to actual treatment and assess their effects. Another group identified the effect of FDG PET on radiotherapy planning of patients considered for radical radiotherapy with 25% of patients classed as stage III by conventional staging found to have distant metastases and therefore unsuitable for radical treatment.

Radiotherapy clearly has to account for the primary tumor and nodal disease. Traditional radiotherapy planning recommends the inclusion of large parts of the mediastinum that is macroscopically unaffected to allow for microscopic disease.[72] The question is whether FDG PET and CT used in combination can limit the extent of this radiotherapy without detriment to outcome. These issues remain unresolved. Grills *et al.*[73] have recently compared treatment planning using intensity modulated radiotherapy (IMRT), three-dimensional conformal radiotherapy and elective nodal irradiation. This group suggested that IMRT had limited additional value in node negative patients compared to three-dimensional conformal radiation, but was beneficial in node positive cases and in cases with target volumes close to the esophagus. It is clear that the combination of PET and CT could improve the selection of the radiotherapy, improve toxicity to the normal tissues, and increase the radiation dose to malignant sites. The value of PET needs to be tested in these treatment methods.

The other very relevant area is the assessment of the degree of hypoxia with tumors since this may influence response to radiotherapy. There are a variety of agents that can assess tissue hypoxia including [^{18}F]fluoromisonidazole and the thiosemicarbazone, labelled with ^{64}Cu. These agents are capable of demonstrating the distribution of hypoxia and also measure the response to interventions to change the oxygen tensions. A more interesting area is the use of ^{64}Cu-diacetyl-bis(N^4-methylsemicarbazone) as both a hypoxia localizing agent and a therapy agent.[8]

POSITRON EMISSION TOMOGRAPHY–COMPUTED TOMOGRAPHY

Manufacturers are already concentrating their efforts on combining metabolic and anatomic imaging. The question is how far this imaging will go and what are the limitations to its use. Combination of anatomic and functional images have taken place for a number of years either in the eye of the interpreter by routine visual comparison or by software fusion of images acquired on two separate devices or by fusion on in-line anatomical/functional devices. The routine use of such image fusion must provide additional information that is of value to the patient and to the clinician managing the patient. The simplest way in which the combination of PET and CT images may benefit the patient is that the metabolic site is more clearly demonstrated to the clinician who is normally used to looking at CT images but not PET images. Demonstration of the PET abnormality overlaid on the CT image can convince a sceptical clinician that the abnormality is real by demonstrating its location more clearly. The other role is perhaps in radiotherapy planning by defining the PET abnormalities on the anatomic image used for planning.

Although some have shown that simple visual comparison of the PET and CT or the use of image fusion has been shown to increase the certainty of calling abnormalities on PET but did not alter sensitivity or specificity compared to PET alone.[74] Others have reported that visual comparison of FDG PET with CT improved accuracy from 88% with PET alone (with the aid of the transmission image) to 96%.[1,75]

More recent studies have started to evaluate the use of combined PET–CT systems. The issues that have to be considered are many including the justification of the additional radiation dosimetry for which a definite benefit for the patient needs to be demonstrated. The value in different parts of the body needs to be shown and accurate registration also needs to be proven. Whether the image registration in the chest is accurate is clearly a problem due to the respiratory motion. This needs to be fully evaluated, in particular for radiotherapy planning, especially with the advent of radiotherapy devices also able to gate radiotherapy on respiratory motion.

PET–CT systems potentially have a number of advantages which include the availability of a CT at the time of the PET scan albeit at present without the range of contrast agents required for full assessment. This lessens the impact of not having the full diagnostic CT scans available when reporting PET studies and also ensures that there is a recent up to date study for comparison. The CT part of the scanners will also provide a whole-body attenuation map for the emission PET scan reducing the need for a dedicated transmission study through the chest for quantification, and therefore significantly enhance patient throughput. Furthermore, a low dose CT may be used to create the attenuation map, whilst minimizing patient dose, providing the means to register to a diagnostic CT. There have been early studies to assess these issues but on the whole they have been poorly performed.[76,77]

SMALL–CELL LUNG CANCER

The role of FDG PET in this group of patients remains to be evaluated. The tumors are FDG avid. The value of whole-body staging is not established. There is a potential difference in management of a small number of patients with limited disease and widespread disease and a potential role will be evaluating treatment response to chemotherapy. Little work has been performed in this field.[78]

MESOTHELIOMA

Mesothelioma is uncommon and has a poor prognosis. The problem confronting clinicians normally is to obtain a diagnosis, identify the extent of the disease within the thorax (Fig. 7B.7) and then identify extrathoracic disease (Fig. 7B.8). Gerbaudo has recently reviewed the use of FDG PET in mesothelioma.[79] This possible use has only been explored in small studies all of which appear to come to a similar conclusion, suggesting sensitivity values between 92 and 97% and specificities between 75 and 100% for the detection of the primary tumor. The specificity and sensitivity are said to be improved by using the SUV > 2.0 as a threshold for benign pleural disease compared to malignant disease. In our own experience and that of others the highest uptake normally is the place to biopsy to obtain a diagnosis. There is also a suggestion from published data that the higher the SUV values the poorer the prognosis. These data are from small studies, however, and need corroboration with larger prospective studies. FDG PET studies

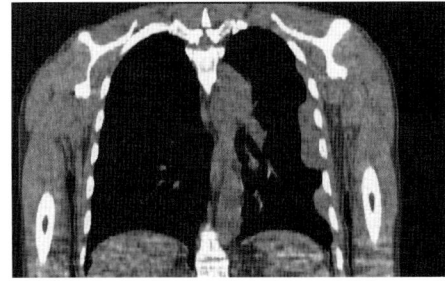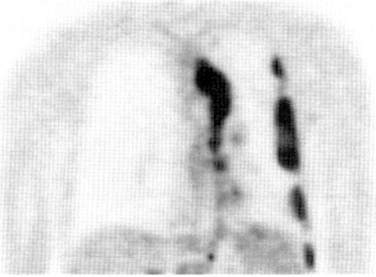

Figure 7B.7 *FDG PET–CT scan in a patient with known mesothelioma to determine the extent of disease. The FDG PET scan demonstrates extensive uptake in the pleura, correlating with the CT scan, and no mediastinal or distant spread. (Abbreviations as in the legends to Figs 7B.1 and 7B.2.)*

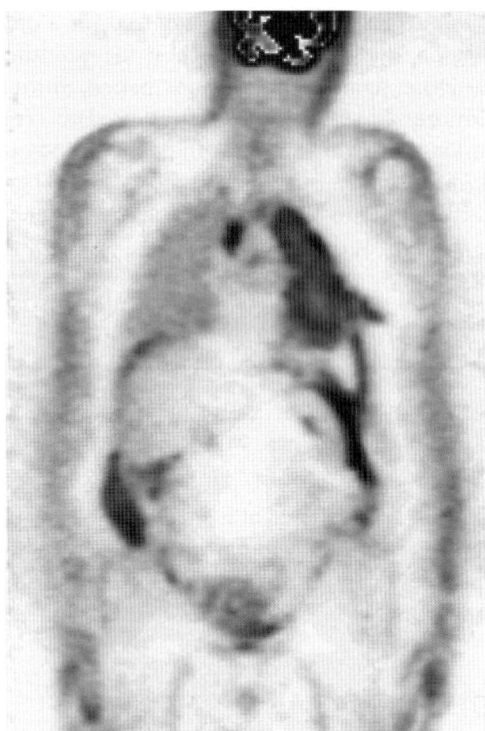

Figure 7B.8 *A non-attenuation corrected FDG PET study on a patient who had a known mesothelioma in the chest with no apparent disease elsewhere on CT examination. The PET scan demonstrates extensive disease in the chest and the abdomen. This was confirmed by biopsy. (Abbreviations as in the legends to Figs 7B.1 and 7B.2.)*

also identify metastatic disease more readily than conventional imaging both within the N1 and N2 nodes and distant metastatic disease. Although there is a suggestion in limited disease that trimodality therapy (extrapleural pneumonectomy, radiation therapy, and chemotherapy) may be the treatment of choice there is disagreement over this. There is evidence that if patients have N2 disease, large volume of disease or distant metastasis the prognosis is very poor and therefore heroic surgery would not be contemplated. A role for PET is therefore clearly apparent to try to identify the subgroups that might benefit from either more aggressive treatment or best supportive care. This is an area that does need further study since the peak incidence of mesothelioma in the UK is predicted to occur over the next 10 years.

CONCLUSION

Carcinoma of the lung is a genetic disease and, on the whole, oncologists have embraced the measurement of molecular changes in tumors from laboratory science to give insight into the development of cancers and demonstrate potential targets for treatment. It is only logical that

they should embrace molecular imaging in a similar way. The radiotracers available are expanding and will give direction to therapy and therapy response in the future. These areas will include the use of a variety of tracers to target cell processes. These tracers must include FDG but will extend into tracers that reflect protein metabolism, DNA turnover, and target specific cell markers, angiogenesis factors as well as cell surface markers and tumor hypoxia. The value also of the use of tracers to evaluate P-glycoprotein expression and the multidrug resistance gene expression will also come to the fore. This has been examined in lung cancer with ^{99m}Tc-sestamibi and predicting response to paclitaxel-based therapy.[80] The role of single photon tracers has recently been reviewed.[81] The use of radiotracers in drug development will also reduce the length of phase 1 studies by accurately reflecting biodistribution and the possible toxic effects of the drugs. These studies will not only reduce the cost of drug development but will also reduce the number of patients experiencing toxic effects and speed up the development and introduction of useful drugs to treat lung cancer.

Lung cancer is still a major cause of worldwide mortality and morbidity and at present the outcome is still poor. FDG PET has been extensively studied predominantly with observational studies and cost-effectiveness modelling studies in NSCLC and solitary pulmonary nodules. These retrospective studies have broadly agreed with the few prospective studies performed and the one randomized controlled trial of FDG PET compared with conventional work-up prior to surgery. This latter study demonstrates the utility and the cost-effectiveness of FDG PET. These findings have recently been supported by the American College of Surgeons Oncology Group study who found that PET avoided unnecessary surgery in 1 in 5 patients.[82] The American Cardiothoracic Society has recently suggested that: 'For patients who are candidates for surgery, where available, a whole body FDG PET scan is recommended to evaluate the mediastinum' and 'In patients with abnormal FDG PET scan findings, further evaluation of the mediastinum with sampling of the abnormal lymph node should be performed prior to surgical resection of the primary tumor'.[83] The American Society of Clinical Oncology has similar recommendations with regard to PET for locoregional disease. The Society goes further with regard to distant disease 'For the staging of distant metastatic disease, an FDG PET scan is recommended when there is no evidence of distant metastatic disease on CT scan of the chest' with further recommendations with regard to bone metastases, adrenal, and liver metastases.[84] Similar conclusions have been drawn by the National Institute for Clinical Excellence in the UK.[47] The current evidence-based indications are outlined in Table 7B.4.

Seventy to eighty percent of patients, however, are not suitable for surgery or radical radiotherapy and therefore undergo radiotherapy, chemotherapy or best supportive care. The challenge is to assess the role of PET in these

Table 7B.4 *Indications for positron emission tomography in lung cancer*

Current indications

- *FDG PET is a useful technique in patients with solitary pulmonary nodules of intermediate probability for lung cancer in whom a biopsy is not possible or biopsy attempts have failed*
- *FDG PET should be used to evaluate all patients with T(1,2,3) N (0,1) stage lung cancer on CT prior to surgical intervention*
- *FDG PET should be considered in patients with minimal N2 disease on CT that would otherwise be considered for surgery*
- *FDG PET should also be used in patients with equivocal distant metastases where other imaging or tissue biopsy has failed to exclude or confirm metastatic disease*
- *FDG PET should be used in all patients considered for radical radiotherapy treatment to exclude distant disease*

Future roles

- *Radiotherapy planning applications of FDG PET still need evidence related to its role*
- *The role of FDG PET in response monitoring in lung cancer has to be evaluated*
- *The determination of the value of other positron-emitting tracers for evaluating lung cancer is ongoing*

FDG, fluorodeoxyglucose; PET, positron emission tomography; CT, computed tomography.

areas. PET does not just use FDG and the exciting areas to be explored are to determine whether PET tracers can be used to individualize patient care by categorizing patients into groups that may benefit from particular types of therapy. Further exploration of the use of FDG PET in predicting prognosis, evaluating tissue hypoxia (either to direct therapy or to try to alter the hypoxia) and the optimum method of determining response to therapy is required. The days of using volume change as a measure of response are likely to be numbered and molecular response measures introduced to facilitate early therapy decisions.

REFERENCES

- Seminal primary article
- Key review paper
- First formal publication of a management guideline

◆ 1 Ho Shon I, O'Doherty MJ, Maisey MN. PET in lung cancer. *Semin Nucl Med* 2002; **32**: 240–71.

2 Shulkin AN. Management of the indeterminate solitary pulmonary nodule: a pulmonologist's view. *Ann Thorac Surg* 1993; **56**: 743–4.

● 3 Mountain CF. Revisions in the International System for Staging Lung Cancer. *Chest* 1997; **111**: 1710–17.

4 Higashi K, Ueda Y, Matsunari I, *et al.* ^{11}C-acetate PET imaging of lung cancer: comparison with (18)F-FDG PET and (99m)Tc-MIBI SPET. *Eur J Nucl Med Mol Imaging* 2004; **31**: 13–21.

5 Hara T. ^{11}C-choline and 2-deoxy-2-[^{18}F]fluoro-D-glucose in tumor imaging with positron emission tomography. *Mol Imaging Biol* 2002; **4**: 267–73.

6 Buck AK, Halter G, Schirrmeister H, *et al.* Imaging proliferation in lung tumors with PET: ^{18}F-FLT versus ^{18}F-FDG. *J Nucl Med* 2003; **44**: 1426–31.

7 Pieterman RM, Que TH, Elsinga PH, *et al.* Comparison of (11)C-choline and (18)F-FDG PET in primary diagnosis and staging of patients with thoracic cancer. *J Nucl Med* 2002; **43**: 167–72.

● 8 Lewis J, Sharp TL, Laforest R, *et al.* Tumour uptake of copper-diacetyl-bis(N(4)-methylsemicarbazone): effect of changes in tissue oxygenation. *J Nucl Med* 2001; **42**: 655–61.

9 Blum J, Handmaker H, Lister-James J, Rinne N. A multicenter trial with a somatostatin analog (99m)Tc depreotide in the evaluation of solitary pulmonary nodules. *Chest* 2000; **117**: 1232–8.

10 Blum JE, Handmaker H, Rinne NA. The utility of a somatostatin-type receptor binding peptide radiopharmaceutical (P829) in the evaluation of solitary pulmonary nodules. *Chest* 1999; **115**: 224–32.

11 Grewal RK, Dadparvar S, Yu JQ, *et al.* Efficacy of Tc-99m depreotide scintigraphy in the evaluation of solitary pulmonary nodules. *Cancer J* 2002; **8**: 400–4.

12 Abdel-Dayem HM, Scott A, Macapinlac H, *et al.* Tracer imaging in lung cancer. *Eur J Nucl Med* 1994; **21**: 57–81.

13 Kashitani N, Makihara S, Maeda T, *et al.* Thallium-201-chloride and technetium-99m-MIBI SPECT of primary and metastatic lung carcinoma. *Oncol Rep* 1999; **6**: 127–33.

14 Tanaka S, Asao T, Ubukata M, *et al.* Effectiveness of Tc-99m MIBI scintigraphy in diagnosing lung cancer. *Surg Today* 1997; **27**: 623–6.

● 15 Kahn D, Menda Y, Kernstine K, *et al.* The utility of ^{99m}Tc depreotide compared with F-18 fluorodeoxyglucose positron emission tomography and surgical staging in patients with suspected non-small cell lung cancer. *Chest* 2004; **125**: 494–501.

16 Yap C, Schiepers C, Fishbein M, *et al.* FDG-PET imaging in lung cancer: how sensitive is it for bronchioloalveolar carcinoma? *Eur J Nucl Med Mol Imag* 2002; **29**: 1166–73.

● 17 Gambhir SS, Shepherd JE, Shah BD, *et al.* Analytical decision model for the cost-effective management of solitary pulmonary nodules. *J Clin Oncol* 1998; **16**: 2113–25.

● 18 Dietlein M, Weber K, Gandjour A, *et al.* Cost-effectiveness of FDG-PET for the management of solitary pulmonary nodules: a decision analysis based on cost reimbursement in Germany. *Eur J Nucl Med* 2000; **27**: 1441–56.

● 19 Gould MK, Sanders GD, Barnett PG, *et al.* Cost-effectiveness of alternative management strategies for patients with solitary pulmonary nodules. *Ann Intern Med* 2003; **138**: 724–35.

20 Hain SF, Curran KM, Beggs AD, *et al.* FDG-PET as a 'metabolic biopsy' tool in thoracic lesions with indeterminate biopsy. *Eur J Nucl Med* 2001; **28**: 1336–40.

21 Tahara RW, Lackner RP, Graver LM. Is there a role for routine mediastinoscopy in patients with peripheral T1 lung cancers? *Am J Surg* 2000; **180**: 488–91.

22 Inoue T, Kim EE, Wong FC, *et al.* Comparison of fluorine-18-fluorodeoxyglucose and carbon-11-methionine PET in detection of malignant tumors. *J Nucl Med* 1996; **37**: 1472–6.

23 Nettelbladt OS, Sundin AE, Valind SO, *et al.* Combined fluorine-18-FDG and carbon-11-methionine PET for diagnosis of tumors in lung and mediastinum. *J Nucl Med* 1998; **39**: 640–7.

24 Pieterman R, Willemsen A, Appel M, *et al.* Visualisation and assessment of the protein synthesis rate of lung cancer using carbon-11 tyrosine and positron emission tomography. *Eur J Nucl Med Mol Imaging* 2002; **29**: 243–7.

25 Inoue T, Koyama K, Oriuchi N, *et al.* Detection of malignant tumors: whole body PET with fluorine 18 alpha-methyl tyrosine versus FDG – preliminary study. *Radiology* 2001; **220**: 54–62.

26 Maisey MN, Wahl RL, Barrington SF. *Atlas of clinical positron emission tomography.* London: Arnold, 1999.

27 Glazer GM, Gross BH, Quint LE, *et al.* Normal mediastinal lymph nodes: number and size according to American Thoracic Society mapping. *Am J Roentgenol* 1985; **144**: 261–5.

● 28 McLoud TC, Bourgouin PM, Greenberg RW, *et al.* Bronchogenic carcinoma: analysis of staging in the mediastinum with CT by correlative lymph node mapping and sampling. *Radiology* 1992; **182**: 319–23.

29 Dales RE, Stark RM, Raman S. Computed tomography to stage lung cancer. Approaching a controversy using meta-analysis. *Am Rev Respir Dis* 1990; **141**: 1096–101.

30 Dwamena BA, Sonnad SS, Angobaldo JO, *et al.* Metastases from non-small cell lung cancer: mediastinal staging in the 1990s – meta-analytic comparison of PET and CT. *Radiology* 1999; **213**: 530–6.

★ 31 British Thoracic Society. Guidelines on the selection of patients with lung cancer for surgery. *Thorax* 2001; **56**: 89–108.

32 Nosotti M, Santambrogio L, Gasparini M, *et al.* Role of (99m) Tc-hexakis-2-methoxy-isobutylisonitrile in the diagnosis and staging of lung cancer. *Chest* 2002; **122**: 1361–4.

● 33 Scott WJ, Shepherd J, Gambhir SS. Cost-effectiveness of FDG-PET for staging non-small cell lung cancer: a decision analysis. *Ann Thorac Surg* 1998; **66**: 1876–83.

● 34 Dietlein M, Weber K, Gandjour A, *et al.* Cost-effectiveness of FDG-PET for the management of potentially operable non-small cell lung cancer: priority for a PET-based strategy after nodal-negative CT results. *Eur J Nucl Med* 2000; **27**: 1598–609.

35 Pieterman RM, van Putten JW, Meuzelaar JJ, *et al.* Preoperative staging of non-small-cell lung cancer with positron-emission tomography. *N Engl J Med* 2000; **343**: 254–61.

● 36 Van Tinteren H, Hoekstra O, Smit E, *et al.* Effectiveness of positron emission tomography in the preoperative assessment of patients with suspected non-small cell lung cancer: the PLUS multicentre randomised trial. *Lancet* 2002; **359**: 1388–92.

● 37 Verboom P, Van Tinteren H, Hoekstra OS, *et al.* Cost-effectiveness of FDG-PET in staging non-small cell lung cancer: the PLUS study. *Eur J Nucl Med Mol Imaging* 2003; **30**: 1444–9.

38 Vansteenkiste JF, Stroobants SG, De Leyn PR, *et al.* Lymph node staging in non-small-cell lung cancer with FDG-PET scan: a prospective study on 690 lymph node stations from 68 patients. *J Clin Oncol* 1998; **16**: 2142–9.

39 Poncelet AJ, Lonneux M, Coche E, *et al.* PET-FDG scan enhances but does not replace preoperative surgical staging in non-small cell lung carcinoma. *Eur J Cardiothorac Surg* 2001; **20**: 468–74.

40 Valk PE, Pounds TR, Hopkins DM, *et al.* Staging non-small cell lung cancer by whole-body positron emission tomographic imaging. *Ann Thorac Surg* 1995; **60**: 1573–81.

41 Hustinx R, Smith RJ, Benard F, *et al.* Dual time point fluorine-18 fluorodeoxyglucose positron emission tomography: a potential method to differentiate malignancy from inflammation and normal tissue in the head and neck. *Eur J Nucl Med* 1999; **26**: 1345–8.

42 Marom EM, McAdams HP, Erasmus JJ, *et al.* Staging non-small cell lung cancer with whole-body PET. *Radiology* 1999; **212**: 803–9.

43 Gayed I, Vu T, Johnson M, *et al.* Comparison of bone and 2-deoxy-2-[^{18}F]fluoro-D-glucose positron emission tomography in the evaluation of bony metastases in lung cancer. *Mol Imag Biol* 2003; **5**: 26–31.

44 Bury T, Dowlati A, Paulus P, *et al.* Whole-body ^{18}FDG positron emission tomography in the staging of non-small cell lung cancer. *Eur Respir J* 1997; **10**: 2529–34.

45 Saunders CA, Dussek JE, O'Doherty MJ, *et al.* Evaluation of fluorine-18-fluorodeoxyglucose whole body positron emission tomography imaging in the

staging of lung cancer. *Ann Thorac Surg* 1999; **67**: 790–7.

46 Weng E, Tran L, Rege S, *et al.* Accuracy and clinical impact of mediastinal lymph node staging with FDG-PET imaging in potentially resectable lung cancer. *Am J Clin Oncol* 2000; **23**: 47–52.

* 47 National Collaborative Centre for Acute Care. Lung cancer: the diagnosis and treatment of lung cancer. 2005. www.nice.org.uk/CGO24NICEguideline.

48 Dhital K, Saunders CA, Seed PT, *et al.* [(18)F] Fluorodeoxyglucose positron emission tomography and its prognostic value in lung cancer. *Eur J Cardio-thorac Surg* 2000; **18**: 425–8.

49 Ahuja V, Coleman RE, Herndon J, *et al.* The prognostic significance of fluorodeoxyglucose positron emission tomography imaging for patients with non-small cell lung carcinoma. *Cancer* 1998; **83**: 918–24.

50 Vansteenkiste JF, Stroobants SG, Dupont PJ, *et al.* Prognostic importance of the standardized uptake value on (18)F-fluoro-2-deoxy-glucose-positron emission tomography scan in non-small-cell lung cancer: an analysis of 125 cases. Leuven Lung Cancer Group. *J Clin Oncol* 1999; **17**: 3201–6.

51 Inoue T, Kim EE, Komaki R, *et al.* Detecting recurrent or residual lung cancer with FDG-PET. *J Nucl Med* 1995; **36**: 788–93.

52 Kubota K, Yamada S, Ishiwata K, *et al.* Positron emission tomography for treatment evaluation and recurrence detection compared with CT in long-term follow-up cases of lung cancer. *Clin Nucl Med* 1992; **17**: 877–81.

53 Patz EF, Jr., Lowe VJ, Hoffman JM, *et al.* Persistent or recurrent bronchogenic carcinoma: detection with PET and 2-[F-18]-2-deoxy-D-glucose. *Radiology* 1994; **191**: 379–82.

54 Hebert ME, Lowe VJ, Hoffman JM, *et al.* Positron emission tomography in the pretreatment evaluation and follow-up of non-small cell lung cancer patients treated with radiotherapy: preliminary findings. *Am J Clin Oncol* 1996; **19**: 416–21.

55 Frank A, Lefkowitz D, Jaeger S, *et al.* Decision logic for retreatment of asymptomatic lung cancer recurrence based on positron emission tomography findings. *Int J Radiat Oncol Biol Phys* 1995; **32**: 1495–512.

56 Bury T, Corhay JL, Duysinx B, *et al.* Value of FDG-PET in detecting residual or recurrent nonsmall cell lung cancer. *Eur Respir J* 1999; **14**: 1376–80.

57 Minn H, Kangas L, Kellokumpu-Lehtinen P, *et al.* Uptake of 2-fluoro-2-deoxy-D-[U-^{14}C]-glucose during chemotherapy in murine Lewis lung tumor. *Int J Rad Appl Instrum B* 1992; **19**: 55–63.

58 Abe Y, Matsuzawa T, Fujiwara T, *et al.* Clinical assessment of therapeutic effects on cancer using ^{18}F-2-fluoro-2-deoxy-D-glucose and positron emission tomography: preliminary study of lung cancer. *Int J Radiat Oncol Biol Phys* 1990; **19**: 1005–10.

59 Vansteenkiste JF, Stroobants SG, De Leyn PR, *et al.* Potential use of FDG-PET scan after induction chemotherapy in surgically staged IIIa–N2 non-small-cell lung cancer: a prospective pilot study. The Leuven Lung Cancer Group. *Ann Oncol* 1998; **9**: 1193–8.

60 Weber WA, Petersen V, Schmidt B, *et al.* Positron emission tomography in non-small-cell lung cancer: prediction of response to chemotherapy by quantitative assessment of glucose use. *J Clin Oncol* 2003; **21**: 2651–7.

61 Cerfolio RJ, Ojha B, Mukherjee S, *et al.* Positron emission tomography scanning with 2-fluoro-2-deoxy-D-glucose as a predictor of response of neoadjuvant treatment for non-small cell carcinoma. *J Thorac Cardiovasc Surg* 2003; **125**: 938–44.

62 Ryu J-S, Choi NC, Fischmann AJ, *et al.* FDG-PET in staging and restaging non-small cell lung cancer after neoadjuvant chemoradiotherapy: correlation with histopathology. *Lung Cancer* 2002; **35**: 179–87.

63 Akhurst T, Downey RJ, Ginsberg MS, *et al.* An initial experience with FDG-PET in the imaging of residual disease after induction therapy for lung cancer. *Ann Thoracic Surg* 2002; **73**: 259–66.

64 Spaepen K, Stroobants S, Dupont P, *et al.* [^{18}F]FDG PET monitoring of tumour response to chemotherapy: does [^{18}F]FDG uptake correlate with the viable tumour cell fraction? *Eur J Nucl Med Mol Imag* 2003; **30**: 682–8.

65 Dehdashti F, Flanagan FL, Mortimer JE, *et al.* Positron emission tomographic assessment of 'metabolic flare' to predict response of metastatic breast cancer to antiestrogen therapy. *Eur J Nucl Med* 1999; **26**: 51–6.

66 O'Doherty MJ. PET in oncology, I – lung, breast, soft tissue sarcoma. *Nucl Med Commun* 2000; **21**: 224–9.

67 Vanuytsel LJ, Vansteenkiste JF, Stroobants SG, *et al.* The impact of (18)F-fluoro-2-deoxy-D-glucose positron emission tomography (FDG-PET) lymph node staging on the radiation treatment volumes in patients with non-small cell lung cancer. *Radiother Oncol* 2000; **55**: 317–24.

68 Kiffer JD, Berlangieri SU, Scott AM, *et al.* The contribution of ^{18}F-fluoro-2-deoxy-glucose positron emission tomographic imaging to radiotherapy planning in lung cancer. *Lung Cancer* 1998; **19**: 167–77.

69 Munley MT, Marks LB, Scarfone C, *et al.* Multimodality nuclear medicine imaging in three-dimensional radiation treatment planning for lung cancer: challenges and prospects. *Lung Cancer* 1999; **23**: 105–14.

70 Nestle U, Walter K, Schmidt S, *et al.* ^{18}F-deoxyglucose positron emission tomography (FDG-PET) for the planning of radiotherapy in lung cancer: high impact in patients with atelectasis. *Int J Radiat Oncol Biol Phys* 1999; **44**: 593–7.

71 Giraud P, Grahek D, Montravers F, *et al.* CT and (18)F-deoxyglucose (FDG) image fusion for optimization of conformal radiotherapy of lung cancers. *Int J Radiat Oncol Biol Phys* 2001; **49**: 1249–57.

72 Nestle U, Hellwig D, Schmidt S, *et al.* 2-Deoxy-2-[^{18}F]fluoro-D-glucose positron emission tomography in target volume definition for radiotherapy of patients with non-small-cell lung cancer. *Mol Imaging Biol* 2002; **4**: 257–263.

73 Grills IS, Yan D, Martinez AA, Vicini FA, Wong JW, Kestin LL. Potential for reduced toxicity and dose escalation in the treatment of inoperable non-small-cell lung cancer: a comparison of intensity-modulated radiation therapy (IMRT), 3D conformal radiation, and elective nodal irradiation. *Int J Radiat Oncol Biol Phys* 2003; **57**: 875–90.

74 Fischer B, Mortensen J, Hojgaard L. Positron emission tomography in the diagnosis and staging of lung cancer: a systematic quantitative review. *Lancet Oncology* 2001; **2**: 659–66.

75 Lowe VJ, Hoffman JM, DeLong DM, *et al.* Semiquantitative and visual analysis of FDG PET images in pulmonary abnormalities. *J Nucl Med* 1994; **35**: 1771–6.

76 Lardinois D, Weder W, Hany TF, *et al.* Staging of non-small-cell lung cancer with integrated positron-emission tomography and computed tomography. *N Engl J Med* 2003; **348**: 2500–7.

77 Antoch G, Stattaus J, Nemat AT, *et al.* Non-small cell lung cancer: dual-modality PET/CT in preoperative staging. *Radiology* 2003; Sept 25th [E-publication]

◆ 78 Zhao DS, Valdivia AY, Li Y, Blaufox MD. ^{18}F-fluorodeoxyglucose positron emission tomography in small cell lung cancer. *Semin Nucl Med* 2002; **32**: 272–5.

◆ 79 Gerbaudo VH. ^{18}F-FDG imaging of malignant pleural mesothelioma: *scientiam impendere vero. Nucl Med Commun* 2003; **24**: 609–14.

80 Hsu WH, Yen RF, Kao CH, *et al.* Predicting chemotherapy response to paclitaxel-based therapy in advanced non-small-cell lung cancer (stage IIIb or IV) with a higher T stage (>T2). Technetium-99m methoxyisobutylisonitrile chest single photon emission computed tomography and P-glycoprotein expression. *Oncology* 2002; **63**: 173–9.

81 Van de Wiele C, Rottey S, Goethals I, *et al.* ^{99m}Tc sestamibi and ^{99m}Tc tetrofosmin scintigraphy for predicting resistance to chemotherapy: a critical review of clinical data. *Nucl Med Commun* 2003; **24**: 945–50.

82 Reed CE, Harpole DH, Prosther KE, *et al.* Results of the American College of Surgeons Oncology Group Z0050 Trial: the utility of positron emission tomography in staging potentially operable non-small cell lung cancer. *J Thorac Cardiovasc Surg* 2003; **126**: 1943–51.

✳ 83 Silvestri GA, Tanoue LT, Margolis ML, *et al.* The noninvasive staging of non-small cell lung cancer: the guidelines. *Chest* 2003; **123**: S147–56.

✳ 84 Pfister DG, Johnson DH, Azzoli CG, *et al.* American Society of Clinical Oncology Treatment of Unresectable Non-Small Cell Lung Cancer Guideline: Update 2003. *JCO* 2004; **22**: 330–52.

FURTHER READING

Ho Shon I, O'Doherty MJ, Maisey MN. PET in lung cancer. *Semin Nucl Med* 2002; **32**: 240–71.

Zhao DS, Valdivia AY, Li Y, Blaufox MD. ^{18}F-fluorodeoxyglucose positron emission tomography in small-cell lung cancer. *Semin Nucl Med* 2002; **32**: 272–5.

Other pulmonary applications

M.J. O'DOHERTY

INTRODUCTION

Airway diseases are a major cause of morbidity and mortality in the UK, accounting for a large number of visits of patients to the primary care physicians. The variety of diseases includes pulmonary inflammation and infection as well as lung cancer. The lung presents a huge exposed surface to the air allowing the entrance of a variety of particulate matter onto the epithelial surfaces. These particulate substances encompass a range of pathogens (e.g. bacteria, viruses, fungi) as well as particulate matter, which may promote an antigenic response (e.g. pollens, house dust mite), particles that are potentially carcinogenic as in cigarette smoke, or fibers such as asbestos producing other responses in the pleura.

The exposed surface is, of course, important for gas exchange, but is also potentially available for the absorption of drugs across the epithelial/endothelial interface. The delivery of drugs to the lung to treat respiratory disease has been established using a variety of particle generators. The lung represents a body organ that may be studied with a variety of radionuclide techniques; areas of possible interest are outlined in Table 7C.1. The major use of pulmonary nuclear medicine is in the investigation of ventilation/perfusion inequality, particularly with reference to pulmonary emboli. However, there are a variety of other areas requiring the use of radionuclide techniques to explore pulmonary pathophysiology.

INFLAMMATION AND INFECTION

The initiation of an inflammatory response is linked to changes in the vascular supply to the affected part of the

Table 7C.1 *Radionuclides and imaging the lung*

Single photon imaging
- *Mucociliary clearance*
- *Aerosol deposition of drugs*
- *Lung permeability/transfer*
- *Ventilation/perfusion imaging*
  Pulmonary emboli
  Preoperative lung cancer assessment
  Congenital vascular/ventilation anomalies
- *Vascular/endothelial permeability*
- *Inflammation and infection*
- *Tumor imaging*

Positron emission imaging
- *Regional vascular volume*
- *Regional lung density*
- *Regional metabolism*
- *Drug deposition*
- *Receptor imaging*
- *Ventilation/perfusion imaging*
- *Vascular/endothelial permeability*
- *Inflammation and infection*
- *Tumor imaging*

lung. Such changes include hyperemia and increased vascular permeability, leading to swelling of local tissues due to interstitial edema. Damage to the endothelium and epithelial surface of the lung leads to leakage of fluid, proteins, and cells into the air spaces. The primary response may be to damage the epithelium, resulting in cell death and damage to the vascular endothelium. These inflammatory responses may be excessive, leading to alveolar flooding or consolidation, and affecting the aeration of the distal bronchioles and alveoli due to constriction of smooth muscle in the airways, and also by collapse and mucus plugging of airways. Airway diseases will affect the air supply to these regions, and the concomitant vasoconstriction will compromise the blood supply. Conversely, inflammation within the vascular supply due to arteritis may affect ventilation to a lesser extent. These abnormalities can be detected using conventional ventilation/perfusion imaging.

Severe widespread damage to the lung resulting in the syndrome of adult respiratory distress can be caused by a variety of disease processes. This condition results in the need to ventilate the patient, with few other therapeutic options available at the current time. A greater understanding of the physiology, and a marker for its severity – other than blood gases – would be potentially helpful in the assessment of new treatments. A number of nuclear medicine techniques, including lung epithelial transfer/permeability and endothelial permeability measurements, have been used to assess damage.

The other group of patients that may present particular problems for the imager are the immunosuppressed. An awareness of the cause(s) is the prime need and it is therefore essential to be informed of the immune competence of the individual when reporting scans. Immunosuppression as a result of T- or B-cell dysfunction may be associated with a variety of illnesses. These may be a direct result of the disease, the therapy given for the disease or the result of inadequate therapy. The problems in the immunosuppressed individual may be considered in relation to the underlying disease e.g. leukemia, lymphoma, human immunodeficiency virus (HIV) or congenital immune deficiency syndromes; the chemotherapy or drug treatment used, e.g. bleomycin lung, allergic alveolitis; the organ transplanted – heart or lung and the possibility of rejection. The important point is that patients with fevers do not necessarily have underlying infection or inflammation but may have a tumor or tumor recurrence. The pulmonary system is commonly affected in the immunocompromised host and is associated with a high mortality. Different reasons for immunosuppression are associated with different incidences of causes of a fever for example transplant patients on chemotherapy have a higher incidence of cytomegalovirus infection than HIV positive patients. The HIV positive patients have a spectrum of illness that perhaps deserves a special consideration.

Pneumocystis carinii pneumonia (PCP) is becoming a less common problem in HIV positive patients since the introduction of highly active antiretroviral therapies (HAARTs) but it still represents a major cause of respiratory problems. There is an increasing problem with bacterial infections including *Streptococcus pneumonia, Haemophilus influenzae, Pseudomonas* infections and mycobacterial infection. Some 10–15% of patients with PCP have a normal or atypical chest X-ray (CXR). A further diagnostic difficulty

with the so-called 'typical PCP CXR' is the differentiation of PCP from other causes of an abnormal CXR – such as mycobacterial infections, Kaposi's sarcoma (KS), lymphocytic interstitial pneumonitis or nonspecific interstitial pneumonitis. HRCT can be of help, although in one study, two observers made a confident diagnosis in only 48% of the cases, most of whom had PCP or KS.

Inflammation and infection in the lung are most commonly assessed using ^{67}Ga imaging, but other agents including somatostatin, labeled antibodies, labeled immunoglobulins, labeled peptides, fluorodeoxyglucose (FDG) and labeled leucocytes, are also used. Gallium-67 has been used in the assessment of granulomatous disease for many years; its role has been extended by the advent of HIV infection and by its application in a variety of other diseases that affect the thorax, and this will be discussed.

Finally, the use of aerosols in the lung, both as therapeutic and investigative agents, deserves a mention. A variety of devices have been used to deliver aerosols to patients' lungs, for pulmonary scanning and for medication in the form of bronchodilators, steroids, antibiotics, surfactants, etc. The use of radiolabels provides a rapid means of assessing the pulmonary delivery of drugs and allows comparison of patient response to the amount of drug delivered.[1] Drug delivery using radionuclides including positron emission tomography (PET) labeled tracers provides a rapid method of assessing delivery devices in normal respiring subjects or ventilated patients.[2,3]

LUNG PERMEABILITY MEASUREMENTS

An assessment of the integrity of the alveolar capillary interface has been performed using molecules delivered to the alveolar airspace to examine the epithelial integrity, and to the capillary bed to examine the endothelial permeability. Radiopharmaceuticals of various shapes, sizes, and charge, have been used for the assessment of permeability, ^{99m}Tc-diethylenetriaminepentaacetic acid (^{99m}Tc-DTPA) being the most common. The procedure for measuring ^{99m}Tc-DTPA transfer is simple, and the measure indicates the integrity of the alveolar–capillary interface.[4] The alveolar–capillary interface represents a large surface exposed to air, through which gas exchange occurs, but this barrier also allows soluble compounds to cross. The rate at which these molecules can cross the barrier is dependent on several factors, including membrane pore radii size, membrane charge, presence or absence of surfactant, the molecular gradient, etc. The transfer of molecules of different size and charge is used for elucidating disease processes.

Measurements made with the radionuclide techniques are not direct estimates of permeability, since this requires knowledge of the rate of flux of a molecule along a known concentration gradient across a known surface area. Therefore, all that these methods measure is the flux of the

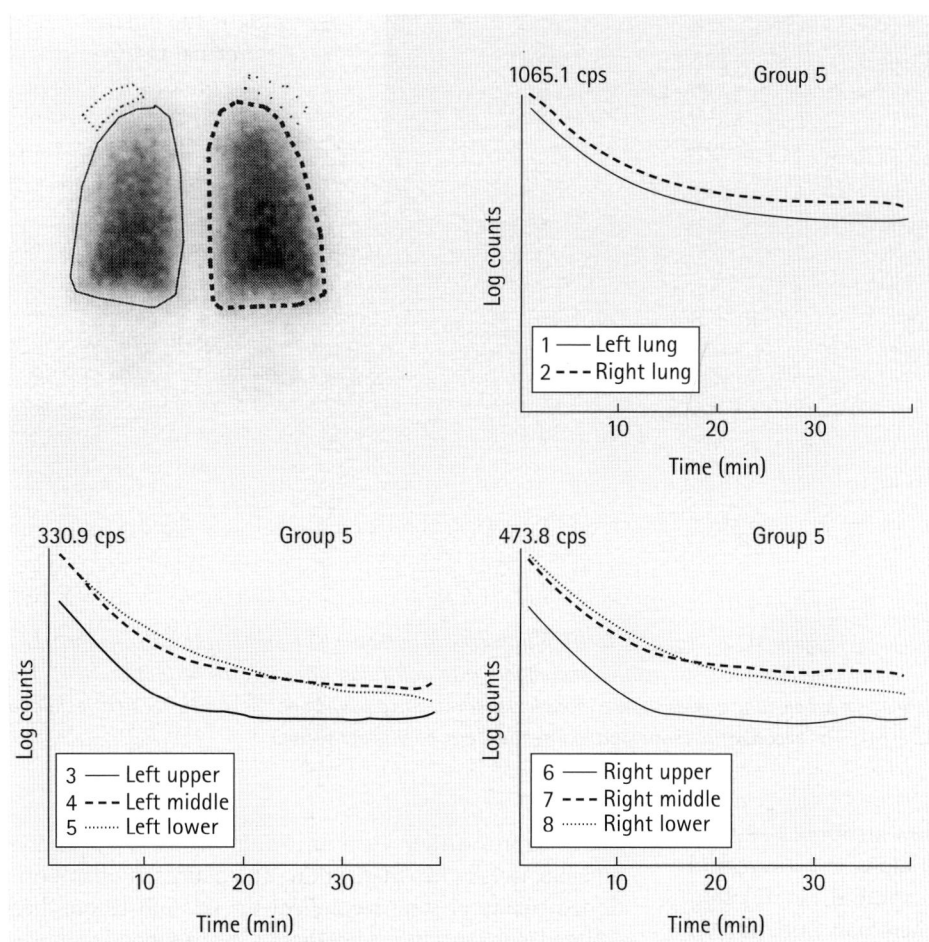

Figure 7C.1 *Lung ⁹⁹ᵐTc-DTPA transfer in a patient with* Pneumocystis carinii *pneumonia. Top left image demonstrates the even distribution of aerosol in both lungs and the regions of interest for background correction and the whole lung regions of interest. The top right shows the whole lung ⁹⁹ᵐTc-DTPA transfer curves for the right and left lungs.*

radionuclide that is at best an indirect measure of permeability. The recent study evaluating the transfer of ⁹⁹ᵐTc-DTPA and ¹¹¹In-DTPA (biotinylated) illustrates the problem whereby the transfer may be related to increase in pores or decrease in surfactant in smokers, the ratio between these agents however may give a better indication of damage to the epithelium in smokers.[5]

Initial studies by Taplin and colleagues[6] showed that [⁹⁹ᵐTc]pertechnetate clearance from the lung was very rapid, both in normal and abnormal subjects, whereas the higher molecular weight ⁹⁹ᵐTc-DTPA cleared more slowly; this has subsequently been confirmed by using molecules of even greater size. Other alterations to clearance have been found by changing the lipophilicity and the charge of the compound by using charged or neutral dextrans and using exametazamine, antipyrine, pertechnegas etc. Alterations in permeability have been found in a variety of conditions including smoking,[7] collagen diseases,[8] and fibrosing alveolitis.[9,10] Permeability may also be altered by the use of various drugs (both chemotherapeutic and recreational), and by administration of carbon monoxide and histamine. There are a variety of physiological factors that affect permeability, including exercise and the lung region (upper regions are more permeable than lower). The permeability measures are normally associated with a

monoexponential clearance, although biexponential clearance has been observed with respiratory distress syndrome and with alveolitis associated with *Pneumocystis carinii* pneumonia. Barrowcliffe and Jones[11] demonstrated fast clearance values with multi-exponential clearance in several patients. This phenomenon has been observed by other groups in severe lung injury.[11–15] Noncardiogenic pulmonary edema appears to result in accelerated clearance of ⁹⁹ᵐTc-DTPA as compared with cardiogenic pulmonary edema.[11,15]

The use of the technique in HIV-positive patients has been described and reviewed.[16] The half-time of DTPA transfer in HIV-positive patients is described normally by a single exponential curve with mean half-times of 20 min for smokers and 60 min for nonsmokers (k values 2.5% per min and 0.8% per min); approximately 10% of smokers may have a multi-exponential curve. In our studies, the appearance of a biphasic curve and a rapid first component (half-time of < 4 min (12.5% per min)) is the hallmark of alveolitis (Figs 7C.1 and 7C.2). In patients with HIV infection, PCP is still the most likely cause of alveolitis – hence the biphasic pattern – although this pattern may also be seen in patients with CMV infection, lymphocytic interstitial pneumonitis and nonspecific interstitial pneumonitis. In this patient population, the test has a high sensitivity and specificity for PCP, but there are false negative results.[17]

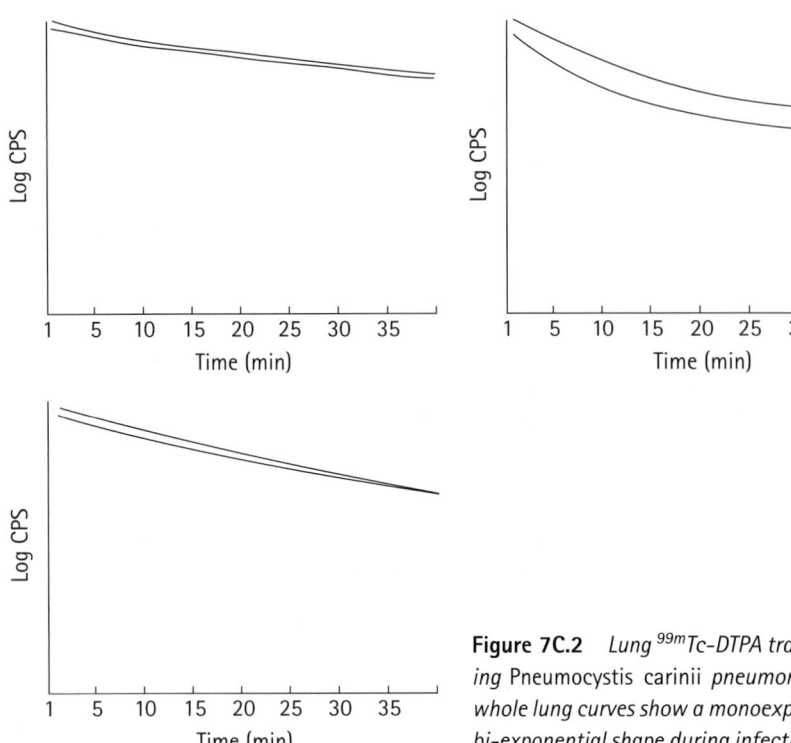

Figure 7C.2 *Lung* ^{99m}*Tc-DTPA transfer in a patient when normal (top left) and then during* Pneumocystis carinii *pneumonia (top right) and after treatment (bottom left). The whole lung curves show a monoexponential pattern when normal and after treatment and bi-exponential shape during infection. cps, counts per second.*

The false negative results usually show an abnormally fast transfer rate, but not with a typical biphasic pattern, and therefore further investigation (e.g. sputum examination or bronchoscopy) is suggested rather than initiation of treatment for PCP. In other bacterial infections, the transfer times are not biphasic (except for *Legionella pneumophila*).[17] Rosso *et al.*[18] have demonstrated by using only the first 7 min of the time–activity curve that the clearance rate for PCP is higher than for other pulmonary conditions. The biggest area of overlap was in patients who had a cytotoxic lymphocyte alveolitis. The most interesting comparison from this study was with ^{67}Ga scintigraphy, which was shown to have lower sensitivity than ^{99m}Tc-DTPA (72% vs. 92%) for infectious pulmonary complications. This was even more marked for patients who had a normal CXR and normal blood gases. A normal CXR with normal DTPA clearance virtually excluded pulmonary infection/inflammation that needed therapy.

Kula *et al.* have also recently demonstrated that patients infected with hepatitis C can have increased transfer of ^{99m}Tc-DTPA. This is a monoexponential increase and therefore even in patients with a mixed viral infection, HIV and hepatitis C, there should be no confusion over the presence of an alveolitis.[19]

METHOD OF MEASURING DTPA TRANSFER

Lung ^{99m}Tc-DTPA transfer (permeability, clearance) relies on the inhalation of an aerosol of ^{99m}Tc-DTPA (particle size of approximately 1 μm or less) for as short a period as possible, usually less than 1 min. The patient is often positioned supine or semi-recumbent for this inhalation, then scanned in that posture, since there is less likelihood of movement. The camera head is situated posteriorly, or occasionally anteriorly, and data can be acquired using a gamma camera equipped with a high-sensitivity collimator and linked to an on-line computer. Dynamic acquisition of 30-s or 1-min duration frames is obtained over a period of 20–60 min. The acquisition protocol varies from center to center. If background activity correction is used, then an intravenous injection of ^{99m}Tc-DTPA is given to allow the background region activity to be related to the lung regions. From the resultant time–activity curves, the half-time or clearance rate can be derived (with or without background correction).

A discussion on the need for background correction is beyond the scope of this chapter but the need for background subtraction will increase with the faster transit rates in the more diseased lungs.[12,20–26] The permeability is measured in terms of either a half-time ($T\frac{1}{2}$) of transfer (expressed in minutes) or a clearance rate, k (expressed as the percent per minute reduction in initial activity). The two values are easily related by the formula $T\frac{1}{2} = 0.693/k$.

IDIOPATHIC INTERSTITIAL LUNG DISEASES

This group of diseases affects predominantly the pulmonary interstitium and the etiology of a large proportion of these is known, e.g. noninfectious and infectious granulomatous disease, drug-induced lung disease, inhalation of toxic gases or allergic substances. In idiopathic pulmonary fibrosis the cause is unknown and tends to be relentlessly progressive. The histopathology reflects different stages of insult to the lungs with areas of fibrosis and other areas of acute disease activity. There is a predilection for the lower lobes of the lungs. Computed tomography is the mainstay of the early detection of the disease and provides the identification of the optimal site to biopsy. The difficulty with this disease process is the inexorable decline in respiratory function and death normally within 5 years of diagnosis and the paucity of therapeutic methods. High-resolution computed tomography (CT) has been studied as a possible prognostic tool and recently various ways of analyzing ^{99m}Tc-DTPA permeability/transfer have been evaluated to assess whether this measurement can identify patients with active alveolitis rather than stable fibrosing alveolitis.[27] Technetium-99m-DTPA clearance may discriminate those patients with a poor prognosis in those patients with a usual interstitial pneumonia.[9] It may also be used to identify patients who have an alveolitis from those with a vascular disease as found in patients with systemic sclerosis.[8]

ADULT RESPIRATORY DISTRESS SYNDROME

The American Thoracic Society and the European Society of Intensive Care Medicine define acute lung injury as 'a syndrome of inflammation and increasing permeability that is associated with a constellation of clinical, radiological and pathophysiological abnormalities that cannot be explained by, but may coexist with, left atrial or pulmonary capillary hypertension', and the adult respiratory distress syndrome (ARDS) as 'a more severe form of acute lung injury'. The link is therefore between structural change and pathophysiological changes resulting in the clinical syndrome. The ARDS has been evaluated with lung permeability measurements, both of the vascular endothelium and the epithelial surfaces. These techniques reflect the structural damage that can be done to the lung membranes. The movement of proteins from the vascular space into the interstitium and airspace through the endothelium and the epithelium is the most appropriate measurement to make. The measurements have included epithelial permeability measurements using ^{99m}Tc-DTPA, as well as inhaled charged dextrans or intravenously administered tracers including ^{113m}In-transferrin, ^{68}Ga-transferrin, ^{18}F and ^{99m}Tc-dextrans. Most assessments in ARDS would be performed using intravenously administered tracers although lung ^{99m}Tc-DTPA transfer has been shown to have a fast transfer rate.[14] The amount of damage to the endothelium has also been shown to be severe using ^{113m}In-transferrin accumulation within the lung.[28] Braude *et al.*[29] demonstrated a correlation between ^{99m}Tc-DTPA transfer and the ^{113m}In-transferrin measurement in patients with ARDS. The degree of structural damage has been assessed using PET techniques in humans[30,31] and dogs[32,33]

by measuring the changes in blood flow using $H_2^{15}O$, protein flux using ^{68}Ga-transferrin, and blood volume using $C^{15}O$ measurements. The measurements made include the transcapillary escape rate and the normalized slope index, which are mathematically equivalent. One may question the clinical role of these measurements, since blood gas measurements, right heart pressure measurements, and the chest X-ray evaluation can assess the damage to the lung. However, bedside permeability measurements can be used to define the severity of the disease and linked to the degree of lung injury. These measurements can then be used to monitor therapy, to help understand how the disease process progresses, and to provide requisite information for developing various therapeutic strategies.

GRANULOMATOUS DISEASES OF THE LUNG

There are a number of hypotheses as to the formation of granulomas within the lung – varying between the sensitization of lymphocytes by antigens producing lymphokines that attract monocytes and inhibit macrophages, to theories that propose agents that activate macrophages which then secrete factors that attract monocytes. Whatever the etiology, there are a variety of granulomatous diseases affecting the lung that may be infective in origin (e.g. mycobacterial infection), possibly immune complex (e.g. Wegener's granulomatosis, Churg–Strauss syndrome), foreign body-induced (e.g. talc granulomatosis) or undetermined cause (e.g. sarcoidosis).[34,35] Gallium-67 scanning has been demonstrated to have increased uptake in these conditions. The primary role of scanning is to define the disease activity as well as the extent of the disease. The most investigated disease is sarcoidosis.

SARCOIDOSIS

Sarcoidosis is a multisystem inflammatory granulomatous disease with an incidence varying between 2 and 18 per 100 000 of the world population. The disease predominantly affects the pulmonary system, but almost any organ can be affected. The conventional classification of the disease using the chest X-ray (CXR) is stage 0, normal CXR; stage I, bilateral hilar lymphadenopathy; stage II, bilateral hilar lymphadenopathy and lung changes; and stage III, lung changes alone. However, the CXR is highly insensitive, and up to 60% of patients with granulomas in the parenchyma may have a normal CXR. With a predominant hilar and mediastinal adenopathy, the differential diagnosis is essentially between lymphoma and sarcoidosis – unless the patient has underlying malignancy or immunosuppression. The differential diagnosis is weighted towards sarcoid if the patient is black Afro-Caribbean or of Irish descent. Computed tomography and high-resolution CT

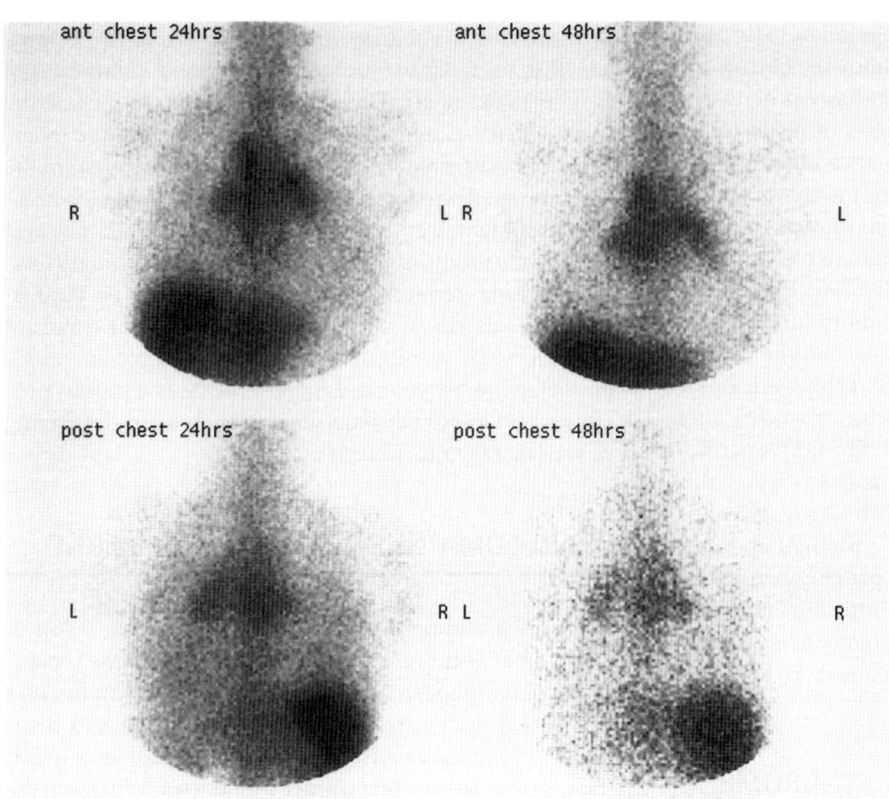

Figure 7C.3 *Gallium-67 scan in a patient with sarcoidosis, demonstrating increased gallium accumulation in the hilar and mediastinal lymph nodes at 24 and 48 h post-injection. There is no parenchymal lung involvement.*

show abnormalities not present on CXR, with reports that a first-choice diagnosis of sarcoid was provided with 57% of radiographic findings and 76% of CT scan readings. Computed tomography was superior to magnetic resonance imaging (MRI) in the assessment of parenchymal disease; although the correlation between the CT abnormality and the pulmonary function was good, there was no correspondence with the degree of alveolitis, and therefore prediction of disease response was poor (see Clarke *et al.* (1994) in the Further Reading section at the end of this chapter).

Using the ^{99m}Tc-DTPA technique (as discussed above), lung permeability has also been shown to be increased in pulmonary sarcoidosis. Increased ^{99m}Tc-DTPA flux across the epithelial membrane of the lung has been observed in types I, II, and III pulmonary sarcoidosis.[36–38] There is increased permeability associated with a deterioration in pulmonary function, which can be decreased by treating patients with steroids.[36] This increased permeability is likely to be related to the degree of inflammation associated with sarcoidosis. The rate of ^{99m}Tc-DTPA transfer has no definite relationship to the serum angiotensin converting enzyme levels, or to the lymphocyte amounts in bronchoalveolar lavage fluid.

Radionuclide assessment of sarcoidosis has normally involved the use of ^{67}Ga, but more recently the disease has been assessed using [^{18}F]fluorodeoxyglucose (FDG) and ^{111}In-octreotide. Gallium scanning at 24, 48, and 72 h has been performed nominally injecting 110 MBq ^{67}Ga and imaging over the thorax and the head. Diffuse uptake in the lung can be seen in sarcoid involving the lung parenchyma,

and this may be associated with intense uptake in the mediastinum and the hilum when these nodes are involved (Figs 7C.3 and 7C.4). The intensity of uptake in the lung relates to disease activity.[39] Uptake patterns have been described as the 'lambda' distribution (mediastinal and hilar uptake) and 'panda' pattern when there is increased uptake in the lachrymal, parotid and nasal areas. The combination is likely to be pathognomonic of sarcoidosis.[40,41] Gallium-67 imaging is seen as a method of following the activity of disease in response to therapy.[42,43] Quantification has been attempted using Ga to assess response of diffuse parenchymal uptake to therapy.[44] The combination of a negative gallium scan and biochemical markers is predictive of the absence of active sarcoidosis. Sarcoidosis in muscle or skin will only be detected by gallium if large areas are involved; gallium scanning should be reserved for atypical cases or to determine sites for biopsy.

Indium-111-octreotide has also been used to image granulomatous diseases (including sarcoidosis), but no direct comparison with gallium has been performed.[45] Abnormal uptake in the lung parenchyma as well as in lymph nodes has been observed. This was found to be more sensitive than radiological imaging. The uptake does fall with response to treatment, but this was only seen in two out of five patients who were followed-up; the other three remained positive with apparent failure of response to therapy by other parameters.

FDG PET imaging in sarcoidosis has been attempted, and owing to the nonspecific accumulation of FDG into

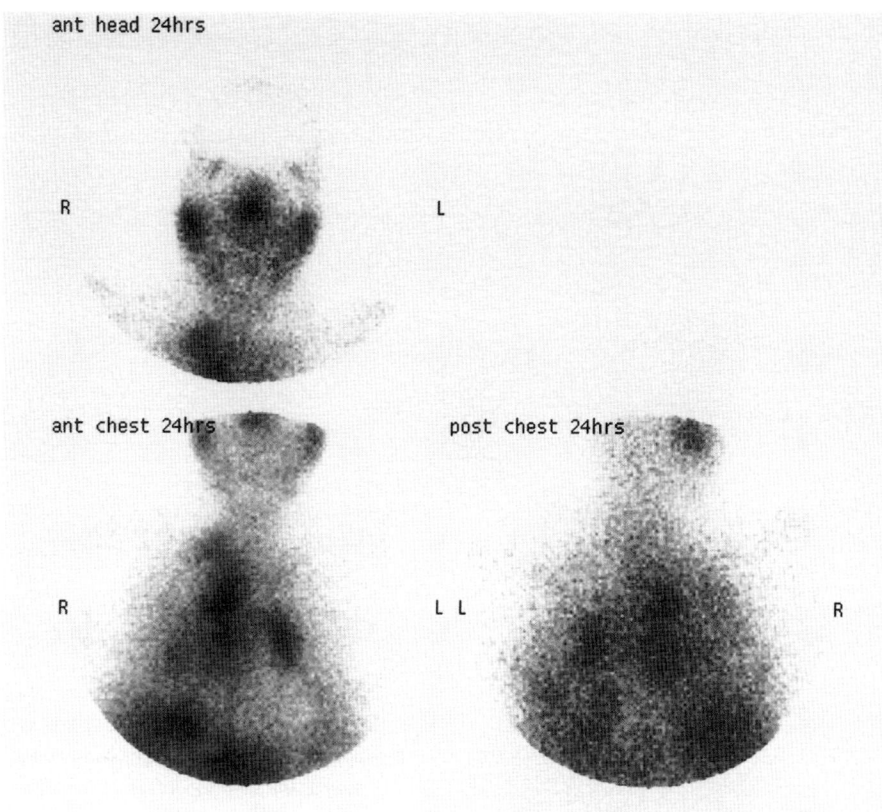

ant head 24hrs

R   L

ant chest 24hrs   post chest 24hrs

R   L L   R

Figure 7C.4 *Gallium-67 scan in a patient with sarcoidosis, demonstrating high uptake in the parotid glands, nasal area and lower uptake in the lachrymal glands. Increased uptake is seen in the hilar, medistinal and supraclavicular lymph nodes. There is also low-grade diffuse uptake in the lung parenchyma with a negative cardiac silhouette on the anterior view.*

inflammatory cells,[46] the disease can be visualized.[47] The uptake is high in both lymph nodes and lung parenchyma, as might be expected.[47,48] Regional glucose metabolism per gram of lung tissue can be calculated using FDG; this has been shown to be elevated in sarcoidosis with these abnormal levels returning to normal during treatment with steroids.[49] The improvement in glucose metabolism was reflected by an improvement in the level of serum angiotensin-converting enzyme and was thought to reflect 'disease activity'.

Positron emission tomography and the lung

The use of PET radiotracers in the lung presents the ability not only to assess tumors, but also inflammation and infection (see Alavi *et al.* (2002) in the Further Reading section). FDG is taken up by a variety of nonmalignant conditions (see Chapter 7B). These areas of uptake are normally seen as an incidental finding in patients with malignancy and tumor response is being assessed or tumor relapse is being reviewed. Uptake can be seen in a variety of infections and also in inflammation, e.g. esophagitis. A particular area of inflammation which is creating interest is pulmonary fibrosis with measures being developed to try and monitor the degree of reaction in the lungs using a fluoroproline.[50] Hara *et al.* have evaluated the role of ^{11}C-choline and FDG in the distinction of tuberculosis from lung cancer and found that choline had a low uptake in tuberculous infections

compared to lung cancer.[51] The separation was less distinct for lesions less than 2 cm in size and therefore further work needs to be performed before routine use. There is also a role in the assessment of FDG uptake in Takayasu's disease to assess disease activity. The variety of tracers allows the assessment of regional metabolism in disease, regional blood volume, and flow as well as permeability measurements. Interest is also advancing in the measurement of receptors in the lung, their site and distribution as well as their abundance, using labeled β-receptor agonists[52] and angiotensin-converting enzyme inhibitors.

HIV POSITIVE PATIENTS

Gallium scans

Scans are usually performed at 24, 48 and, occasionally, 72 h after injecting 74–185 MBq of [67]Ga. Patients with PCP normally show diffuse distribution throughout both lung fields, such that a negative cardiac silhouette is seen;[53,54] this diffuse uptake has been documented with cytomegalovirus (CMV). The uptake can be graded, and should be equal to, or higher than, that in the liver, to enable a confident diagnosis of diffuse lung disease, but the uptake is highly variable in PCP (Fig. 7C.5), and occasionally it is lower (above soft tissue activity, but less than the liver uptake).

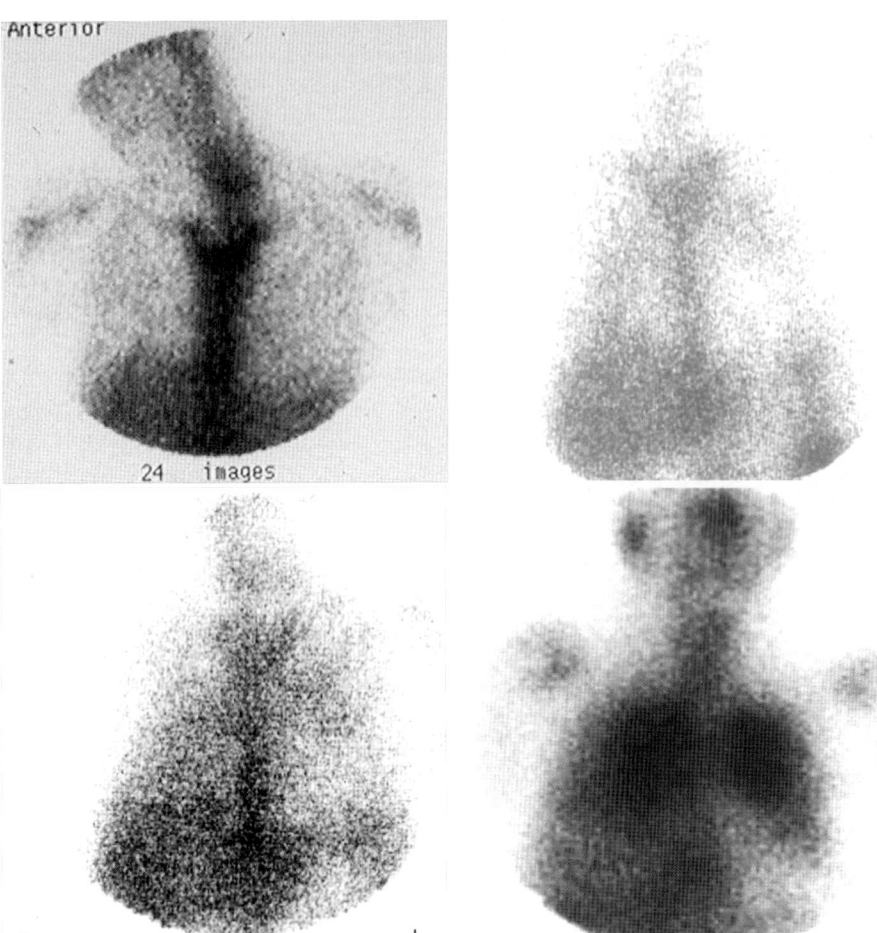

Figure 7C.5 *Gallium-67 scan in a patient with normal thoracic uptake and patients with* Pneumocystis carinii *pneumonia. The scan top left is normal distribution of* ^{67}*Ga, the scan top right shows low grade uptake (less than bone marrow), the scan bottom left shows uptake equivalent to bone marrow and liver and the bottom left high grade uptake.*

The sensitivity and specificity of ^{67}Ga are 80–90% and 50–74%, respectively,[55] rising to 100% in those patients with a normal CXR.[56] Early scanning at 4 h has been used, and the ratio between lung and liver uptake recorded to distinguish between a normal and an abnormal scan, although limitations with this approach would be expected in patients with liver disease. Atypical uptake confined to the upper lobes can be seen with PCP. One advantage of ^{67}Ga is that uptake throughout the body can be observed, and thus lung uptake with associated parotid uptake is suggestive of interstitial pneumonitis or sarcoidosis. Diffuse or patchy lung uptake with high lymph node uptake may be due to atypical mycobacterial infection, but may equally be due to lymphoma associated with an opportunistic lung infection. In patients with a lung infiltrate on the CXR, a gallium scan may show either lobar or multiple lobar focal defects, due to infection or tumor (Fig. 7C.6). If this uptake is associated with bone involvement, then atypical fungal infection or lymphoma should be considered in the differential diagnosis. In the presence of an abnormal CXR, the scan may be useful if it is entirely normal, since this would be consistent with KS (Fig. 7C.7); if the scan is abnormal then super-added infection patients with a wasting syndrome to exclude focal pathology should be considered.

Gallium undoubtedly has a role in the investigation of a persistent PUO in this patient group when there are no specific localizing features or in patients with a wasting syndrome to exclude focal pathology. Thallium-201 has been used in a small number of patients to localize KS. Following injection of approximately 90 MBq of ^{201}T1, images acquired immediately after the injection and up to 3 h later showed uptake in the skin lesions, lymph nodes, and the lung (lung uptake was confirmed as due to KS in one third of the patients). It is not known whether thallium is taken up in persistent generalized lymphadenopathy, which may present a source of confusion. Fluorodeoxyglucose and methionine PET studies have also not shown conclusive uptake.[57]

Gallium uptake in the myocardium has to be regarded as either inflammation in the myocardium or pericardium unless this is more focal when uptake in pericardial lymph nodes due to tumor may be the cause.

Antibody studies

The advantage of using antibodies available in the kit form over leukocyte imaging is a shorter preparation time and

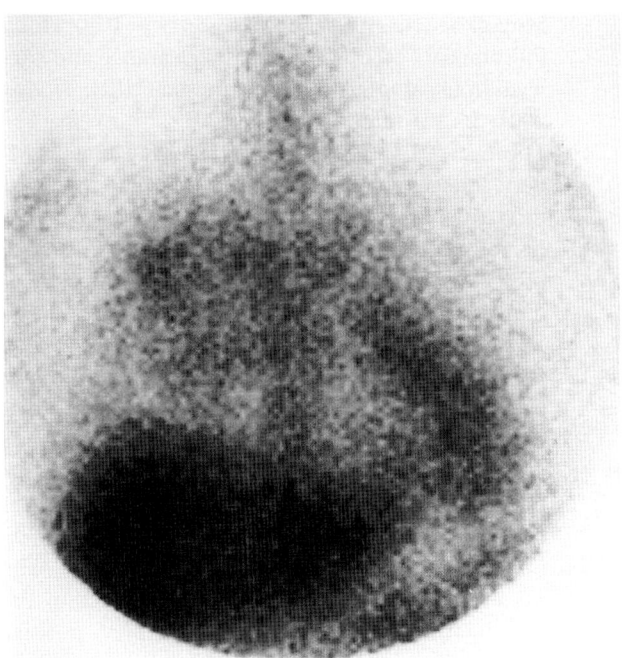

Figure 7C.6 *Gallium-67 scan in a patient with pneumococcal pneumonia. The scan shows increased uptake in the upper right lung and lower left lung. (Reprinted with permission from O'Doherty MJ, Nunan TO. Nuclear medicine and AIDS.* Nucl Med Commun *1993; 14: 830–48.)*

reduced blood handling. Currently, these products use ^{111}In as the radionuclide, and therefore there is potentially a time delay before the study can be performed. Localization of ^{111}In-polyclonal antibodies (^{111}In-HIgG) has been demonstrated in lungs infected with PCP in both animal and human studies. Imaging with ^{111}In-HIgG and ^{99m}Tc-HIgG has been performed, with the former having superior sensitivity and specificity than the latter. This was thought to be due to the later imaging with ^{111}In-HIgG. Diffuse uptake was seen with PCP and focal uptake with bacterial infections. Poor uptake of antigranulocyte antibody in HIV patients with infection has been demonstrated.[58]

Imaging of PCP has been performed in HIV-positive patients using ^{99m}Tc-labeled Fab' fragment raised in mice against *Pneumocystis carinii*. In this selected population, the 24-h images had a sensitivity of 86% and a specificity of 87%. The technique raises the interesting possibility of its use in the detection of extrapulmonary disease.

OTHER IMMUNOSUPPRESSED CONDITIONS

The problems are often associated with infection in the lung parenchyma which should be obvious using ^{67}Ga but more usually these would be assessed using a CXR. In heart

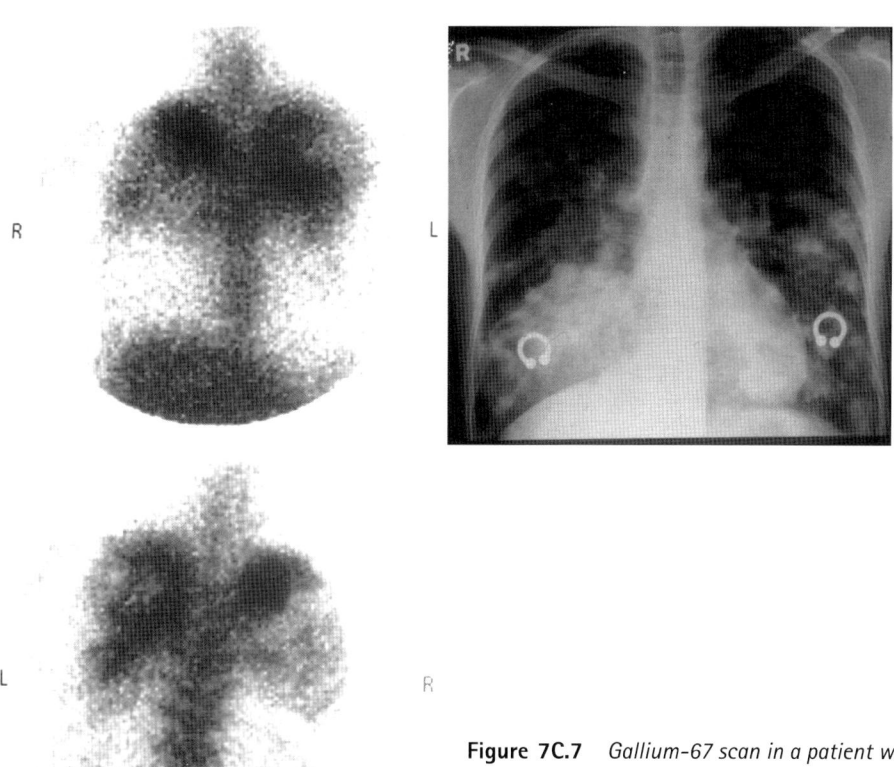

Figure 7C.7 *Gallium-67 scan in a patient with* Pneumocystis carinii *pneumonia in the upper lobes and Kaposi's sarcoma in the lower lobes. The chest X-ray demonstrates abnormal soft tissue densities in the lower lobes and clear upper lobes. The ^{67}Ga scan demonstrates no uptake in the Kaposi's sarcoma (the cause of the soft tissue density in the lower lobes) and marked uptake in the infected areas (upper zones) confirmed by bronchoscopy.*

lung transplantation there is a suggestion that quantitative ventilation/perfusion scans could detect early rejection with nonhomogeneity developing in the perfusion scan. Technetium-99m-DTPA clearance has been used with the finding of a very rapid clearance in those patients who are developing rejection; the data suggest this is a very simple way of monitoring patients and is more sensitive than FEV_1 measurements. Caution needs to be given to such measurements since CMV or PCP would give similar findings.

CONCLUSION

Radionuclide imaging techniques applied to the thorax are limited since a chest radiograph or CT can answer most questions. The tests that are available are outlined above and contribute when the CXR is normal or when there are abnormalities on the CT or CXR which are nondiagnostic. There is an increasing role for the quantitative aspects of radionuclide studies to explore changes in physiology, metabolic changes in disease, delivery and distribution of drugs in the lung.

REFERENCES

● Seminal primary article
◆ Key review paper

◆ 1   O'Doherty MJ, Miller RP. Aerosols for therapy and diagnosis. *Eur J Nucl Med* 1993; **20**: 1201–13.
◆ 2   Dolovich MB. Measuring total and regional lung deposition using inhaled radiotracers. *J Aerosol Med* 2001; **14(Suppl 1)**: S35–44.
3   Thomas SHL, O'Doherty MJ, Fidler HM, *et al.* Pulmonary deposition of a nebulised aerosol during mechanical ventilation. *Thorax* 1993; **48**: 154–9.
4   Staub NC, Hyde RW, Crandall E. Workshop on techniques to evaluate lung alveolar microvascular injury. *Am Rev Respir Dis* 1990; **141**: 1071–7.
5   Mason GR, Peters AM, Bagdades E, *et al.* Evaluation of pulmonary alveolar epithelial integrity by the detection of restriction to diffusion of hydrophilic solutes of different molecular sizes. *Clin Sci (London)* 2001; **100**: 231–6.
● 6   Taplin CV, Chopra SK, Uszler JM. Imaging experimental pulmonary ischaemic lesions after inhalation of a diffusible radioaerosol. Recent experience and further developments. *J Nucl Med* 1978; **19**: 567–8.
● 7   Jones JG, Minty BD, Lawler P, *et al.* Increased epithelial permeability in cigarette smokers. *Lancet* 1980; **I**: 66–8.
8   Kon OM, Danil Z, Black CM, du Bois RM. Clearance of inhaled technetium-99m-DTPA as a clinical index of pulmonary vascular disease in systemic sclerosis. *Eur Respir J* 1999; **13**: 133–6.

9   Mogulkoc N, Brutsche MH, Bishop PW, *et al.* Pulmonary ^{99m}Tc-DTPA aerosol clearance and survival in usual interstitial pneumonia (UIP). *Thorax* 2001; **56**: 916–23.
10   Thomeer MJ, Dehaes B, Mortelmans L, Demedts M. Pertechnegas lung clearance in different forms of interstitial lung disease. *Eur Respir J* 2002; **19**: 31–6.
● 11   Barrowcliffe MP, Jones JC. Pulmonary clearance of ^{99m}Tc-DTPA in the diagnosis and evolution of increased permeability pulmonary oedema. *Anaesth Intens Care* 1989; **17**: 422–32.
● 12   Jefferies AL, Coates C, O'Brodovich H. Pulmonary epithelial permeability in hyaline membrane disease. *N Engl J Med* 1984; **311**: 1075–80.
● 13   O'Doherty MJ, Page CJ, Bradbeer CS, *et al.* Alveolar permeability in HIV patients with *Pneumocystis carinii* pneumonia. *Genitourin Med* 1987; **63**: 268–70.
14   O'Doherty MJ, Page CJ, Bradbeer CS, *et al.* The place of lung ^{99m}Tc-DTPA aerosol transfer in the investigation of lung infections in HIV positive patients. *Respir Med* 1989; **83**: 395–401.
15   Mason CR, Effros RM, Uszler JM, *et al.* Small solute clearance from the lungs of patients with cardiogenic and noncardiogenic pulmonary edema. *Chest* 1985; **88**: 327–34.
16   O'Doherty MJ. ^{99m}Tc DTPA transfer/permeability in patients with HIV disease. *Eur J Nucl Med* 1995; **39**: 231–42.
17   Leach R, Davidson C, O'Doherty MJ, *et al.* Non-invasive management of fever and breathlessness in HIV positive patients. *Eur J Respir Med* 1991; **4**: 19–25.
18   Rosso S, Cuillon JM, Parrot A, *et al.* Technetium-99m-DTPA aerosol and gallium-67 scanning in pulmonary complications of human immunodeficiency virus infection. *J Nucl Med* 1992; **33**: 81–7.
19   Kula M, Gulmez I, Tutus A, *et al.* Impaired lung epithelial permeability in hepatitis C virus antibody positive patients detected by ^{99m}Tc-DTPA aerosol scintigraphy. *Nucl Med Commun* 2002; **23**: 441–6.
20   Oberdorster C, Utell MJ, Weber DA, *et al.* Lung clearance of inhaled 99m-Tc DTPA in the dog. *J Appl Physiol* **1984**; 57: 589–95.
21   Langford JA, Lewis CA, Cellert AR, *et al.* Pulmonary epithelial permeability: vascular background effects on whole lung and regional half-time values. *Nucl Med Commun* 1986; **7**: 183–90.
22   Kohn H, Kohn B, Klech H, *et al.* Urine excretion of inhaled technetium-99m-DTPA: an alternative method to assess lung epithelial transport. *J Nucl Med* 1990; **31**: 4419.
23   Groth S, Pedersen M. Pulmonary permeability in primary ciliary dyskinesia. *Eur Respir J* 1989; **2**: 64–70.
24   Barrowcliffe MP, Otto C, Jones JC. Pulmonary clearance of ^{99m}Tc-DTPA: influence of background activity. *J Appl Physiol* 1988; **64**: 1045–9.

25 O'Doherty MJ, Page CJ, Croft DN, Bateman NT. Lung ^{99m}Tc DTPA transfer: a method for background correction. *Nucl Med Commun* 1985; **6**: 209–15.

26 O'Doherty MJ, Page CJ, Croft DN, Bateman NT. Regional lung 'leakiness' in smokers and nonsmokers. *Nucl Med Commun* 1985; **6**: 353–7.

27 Wells AU, Hansell DH, Harrison DK, *et al.* Clearance of inhaled ^{99m}Tc DTPA predicts the clinical course of fibrosing alveolitis. *Eur Respir J* 1993; **6**: 797–802.

28 Basran CS, Byrne AJ, Hardy IC. A noninvasive technique for monitoring lung vascular permeability in man. *Nucl Med Commun* 1985; **3**: 3–10.

29 Braude S, Apperley J, Krausz T, *et al.* Adult respiratory distress syndrome after allogeneic bone marrow transplantation: evidence for a neutrophil independent mechanism. *Lancet* 1985; **i**: 1239–42.

30 Kaplan JD, Calandrino PS, Schuster DP. A positron emission tomographic comparison of pulmonary vascular permeability during the adult respiratory distress syndrome and pneumonia. *Am Rev Respir Dis* 1991; **143**: 150–4.

31 Velazquez M, Weibel ER, Kuhn C, *et al.* PET evaluation of pulmonary vascular permeability: a structure–function correlation. *J Appl Physiol* 1991; **70**: 2206–16.

32 Mintun MA, Dennis OR, Welch MJ, *et al.* Measurements of pulmonary vascular permeability with PET and gallium-68-transferrin. *J Nucl Med* 1987; **28**: 1704–16.

33 Mintun MA, Warfel TE, Schuster DP. Evaluating pulmonary vascular permeability with radiolabeled proteins: an error analysis. *J Appl Physiol* 1990; **68**: 1696–706.

34 Bekerman C, Hoffer PB, Bitran JD, Gupta RC. Gallium-67 citrate imaging studies of the lung. *Semin Nucl Med* 1980; **10**: 286–301.

35 Alavi A, Palevsky HI. Gallium-67-citrate scanning in the assessment of disease activity in sarcoidosis. *J Nucl Med* 1992; **33**: 751–55.

36 Chinet T, Jaubert P, Dusser D, *et al.* Effects of inflammation and fibrosis on pulmonary function in diffuse lung fibrosis. *Thorax* 1990; **45**: 675–8.

37 Dusser DJ, Collignon MA, Stanislas-Leguern C, *et al.* Respiratory clearance of ^{99m}Tc DTPA and pulmonary involvement in sarcoidosis. *Am Rev Respir Dis* 1986; **134**: 493–7.

38 Watanabe N, Inoue T, Oriuchi H, *et al.* Increased pulmonary clearance of aerosolised ^{99m}Tc-DTPA in patients with a subset of stage I sarcoidosis. *Nucl Med Commun* 1995; **16**: 464–7.

39 Line BR, Hunninghake GW, Keogh BA, *et al.* Gallium-67 scanning to stage the alveolitis of sarcoidosis: correlation with clinical studies, pulmonary function studies and bronchoalveolar lavage. *Am Rev Respir Dis* 1981; **123**: 440–6.

40 Sulavik SB, Spencer RP, Palestro CJ, *et al.* Specificity and sensitivity of distinctive chest radiographic and/or ^{67}Ga images in the noninvasive diagnosis of sarcoidosis. *Chest* 1993; **103**: 403–9.

41 Sulavik SB, Spencer RP, Weed DA, *et al.* Recognition of distinctive patterns of gallium-67 distribution in sarcoidosis. *J Nucl Med* 1990; **31**: 1909–14.

42 Baughman RP, Fernandez M, Bosken C. Comparison of gallium-67 scanning, bronchoalveolar lavage and serum angiotensin converting enzyme levels in pulmonary sarcoidosis: predicting response to therapy. *Am Rev Respir Dis* 1984; **129**: 676–81.

43 Lawrence EC, Teague RB, Cottlieb MS. Serial changes in markers of disease activity with corticosteroid treatment in sarcoidosis. *Am J Med* 1983; **74**: 747–56.

44 Alberts C, Van der Schoot JB. Standardized quantitative ^{67}Ga scintigraphy in pulmonary sarcoidosis. *Sarcoidosis* 1988; **5**: 111–18.

45 Vanhagen PM, Krenning EP, Reubi JC, *et al.* Somatostatin analogue scintigraphy in granulomatous disease. *Eur J Nucl Med* 1994; **21**: 497–502.

46 Kubota R, Yamada S, Kubota K, *et al.* Intratumoral distribution of fluorine-18-fluorodeoxyglucose in vivo: high accumulation in macrophages and granulocytes studied by microautoradiography. *J Nucl Med* 1992; **33**: 1972–80.

47 Lewis PJ, Salama A. Uptake of fluorine18-fluorodeoxyglucose in sarcoidosis. *J Nucl Med* 1994; **35**: 1647–9.

48 Pantin CF, Valind SO, Sweatman M, *et al.* Measures of the inflammatory response in cryptogenic fibrosing alveolitis. *Am Rev Respir Dis* 1988; **138**: 1234–41.

49 Brudin LH, Valind SO, Rhodes CG, *et al.* Fluorine-18 deoxyglucose uptake in sarcoidosis measured with positron emission tomography. *Eur J Nucl Med* 1994; **21**: 297–305.

50 Wallace WE, Gupta NC, Hubbs AF, *et al.* cis-4-[(18)F]fluoro-L-proline PET imaging of pulmonary fibrosis in a rabbit model. *J Nucl Med* 2002; **43**: 413–20.

51 Hara T, Kosaka N, Suzuki T, *et al.* Uptake rates of ^{18}F-fluorodeoxyglucose and ^{11}C-choline in lung cancer and pulmonary tuberculosis. *Chest* 2003; **124**: 893–901.

52 Qing F, Rahman SU, Rhodes CG, *et al.* Pulmonary and cardiac beta-adrenoceptor density in vivo in asthmatic subjects. *Am J Respir Crit Care Med* 1997; **155**: 1130–4.

53 Bitran J, Beckerman C, Weinstein R, *et al.* Patterns of gallium-67 scintigraphy in patients with acquired immunodeficiency syndrome and the AIDS related complex. *J Nucl Med* 1987; **28**: 1103–6.

54 Kramer EL, Sanger II, Caray SM, *et al.* Gallium-67 scans of the chest in patients with acquired immunodeficiency syndrome. *J Nucl Med* 1987; **28**: 1107–14.

55 Tumeh SS, Belville JS, Pugatch R, McNeil B. Ga-67 scintigraphy and computed tomography in the diagnosis of pneumocystis carinii pneumonia in patients with AIDS. A prospective comparison. *Clin Nuc Med* 1992; **17**: 387–94.

56 Tuazon CV, Delaney MD, Simon CL, *et al.* Utility of gallium-67 scintigraphy and bronchial washings in the diagnosis and treatment of *Pneumocystis carinii* pneumonia in patients with the acquired immunodeficiency syndrome. *Am Rev Respir Dis* 1985; **132**: 1087–92.

● 57 O'Doherty MJ, Barrington SF, Campbell M, *et al.* PET scanning and the human immunodeficiency virus positive patient. *J Nucl Med* 1997; **38**: 1575–83.

58 Prvulovich FM, Miller RF, Costa DC, *et al.* Immunoscintigraphy with a ^{99m}Tc labelled anti-granulocyte monoclonal antibody in patients with human immunodeficiency virus infection and AIDS. *Nucl Med Commun* 1995; **16**: 838–45.

FURTHER READING

Alavi A, Gupta N, Alberini J-L. Positron emission tomography imaging in nonmalignant thoracic disorders. *Semin Nucl Med* 2002; **32**: 293–321.

Clarke D, Mitchell AWM, Dick R, James CD. The radiology of sarcoidosis. *Sarcoidosis* 1994; **11**: 90–9.

O'Doherty MJ, Peters AM. Pulmonary technetium-99m diethylene triamine pentaacetic and aerosol clearance as an index of lung injury. *Eur J Nucl Med* 1997; **24**: 81–7.

8

Renal radionuclide studies

8A Anatomy, physiology, and tracer handling

Introduction	253	Renal radiopharmaceuticals	260
Anatomy	253	Renal functions	262
Physiology	253	Conclusion	264
Technique and interpretation	255	References	264
Renal models	256		

8B Non-imaging radionuclide assessment of renal function

Introduction	269	Transit (residence) time and distribution volume	273
Clearance	269	Indexing glomerular filtration rate to body size	275
Measurement of clearance	270	Conclusion	278
Measurement of glomerular filtration rate	270	References	278
Extraction fraction	273		

8C Vesico-ureteric reflux and urinary tract infection

Nuclear medicine techniques	281	Conclusion	292
Urinary tract infections: The clinical context and aim of imaging	287	References	294
The contribution of nuclear medicine to the management of urinary tract infections	289		

8D Hypertension

Introduction	297	The captopril renal radionuclide study	300
Renovascular hypertension	297	Technique of captopril intervention and interpretation	300
Mean parenchymal transit time	299	References	303

8E Obstruction of the outflow tract

Chronic outflow resistance	305	Pelvic dilation or obstructing uropathy	308
Obstructive nephropathy and obstructing uropathy	305	References	312
Output efficiency	306	Appendix: adult renal radionuclide study	313

8F Renal transplantation

Introduction   315
Clinical problems   315
Pharmaceuticals   316
The immediate postoperative period   316
The early postoperative period   316

The later postoperative period   317
The functioning graft and later complications   318
Infection   318
Technical methodology   319
References   319

8G Renal tumors

Scintigraphic evaluation of renal tumors using single   321
    photon tracers
Clinical management of renal tumors   321
Scintigraphic evaluation of renal tumors using positron 322
    tracers

Radionuclide treatment of renal tumors   324
References   326

Anatomy, physiology, and tracer handling

K.E. BRITTON

INTRODUCTION

The kidney is a conservative organ. In principle, it retains what the body needs and what is not needed is excreted. The fundamental purpose of nephro-urology is the preservation and improvement of renal function. The contribution that renal radionuclide studies make to this goal is increasing through the application of renal 'stress' tests: frusemide-induced diuresis is used for the evaluation of outflow disorder, while captopril enhances the determination of functionally significant renovascular disorder. These are in parallel with the developments in renal radiological techniques, which are usually complementary.

ANATOMY

The easiest way to locate the kidneys is to feel for the lumbar spine and the costal margins following the line of the ribs medially and cranially. A disk 10 cm in diameter may then be set with its medial edge towards the lumbar spine and the lowest rib overlying a quarter of its upper surface. The kidneys move with respiration and with change of posture, falling forward in the prone and sitting forward positions, so investigations are best performed with the patient reclining. In this position the two kidneys are at approximately equal depths, less than 1 cm difference in 75% of cases. The actual depth of the kidney in any individual varies from 4 to 11 cm; therefore, it is usual to calculate individual renal function as a fraction or percentage of the total and measure the total function separately to avoid the need to measure the absolute radiotracer content of each kidney. To correct for tissue attenuation, renal depth may be estimated

directly or indirectly, but is not necessary when the kidneys are in their normal position and a ^{99m}Tc agent is used.

In each kidney there are about one million nephrons, each composed of a glomerulus, proximal tubule, loop of Henle, and distal tubule connected to the about 20 collecting ducts. These connections between the distal tubules and the collecting duct are at the cortico-medullary junction, not in the medulla through which the collecting ducts run to join each other to form the 10–20 ducts of Bellini.

It is not known exactly how the kidneys work but it is clear that the physical arrangement of the filters, tubes, and loops made up of living cells is important; that the interaction of physical phenomena: forces, resistances, filtration, diffusion, osmosis, pressure gradients and flows with active transport mechanisms, enable the system to work; and that a hierarchy of control systems – the cell and intercellular channels, tubulo-glomerular balance, nephron autoregulation, the juxtaglomerular apparatus, intrarenal flow distribution and hormonal interactions – maintain not only the function of the kidney but also conserve and support the internal environment of the body. The maintenance of salt and water balance and the control of osmolality and acidity of the body and the levels of plasma potassium, calcium, and phosphate ions are essential functions. Important substrates such as glucose and amino acids are retained while unnecessary metabolites such as uric acid, urea, sulfate, creatinine, and guanidine derivatives are excreted. The kidney also produces and responds to a range of hormones.

PHYSIOLOGY

The kidney has a number of basic properties. It has the ability to take solutes up from the blood whether by filtration or secretion, which is best called its *uptake function.* In the special circumstance where the kidneys are the only exit for the solute from the body, then the rate of loss from the blood is equal to the rate of uptake by the kidney. This is the basis of the measurement of total kidney function. The kidney has the ability to move solutes along its nephrons, which is its *transit function.*[1] The solutes may be absorbed in whole or part and be retained or returned to the blood, its *reabsorption function.* In the special case where the solute is nonreabsorbable, which applies to several renal radiopharmaceuticals, then, if there is an increase in salt and water reabsorption as in functionally significant renovascular disease or obstructive nephropathy, the transit function is altered and the transit time through the renal parenchyma is prolonged. In renovascular disorder the transit time is prolonged through both cortical and juxtamedullary nephrons and collecting ducts. In obstructive nephropathy the transit time is prolonged through the cortical nephrons, but usually is shortened through the juxtamedullary nephrons and collecting ducts due to loss of medullary concentrating ability, which is a consequence of an increased resistance to outflow. After transit through the kidney, the solutes move through the pelvis and ureter, its *excretory function.* No more can come out of the kidney than went in previously. If less comes out in a given time than went in, then an increased resistance to outflow is predicted. The balance between excretory function and uptake function is measurable by the output (outflow) efficiency. The kidney also has receptors for hormones, which may modify its reabsorptive functions. For example, increased secretion and binding of the anti-diuretic hormone vasopressin increases the permeability of the collecting duct to water. The kidney also has the ability through enzymes to modify solutes, such as the activation of vitamin D.

Outcome analysis of therapeutic interventions or surgery is an increasingly important requirement for evidence-based medicine and essential to the individual. In nuclear medicine the term 'measurement-based medicine' may be more appropriate. Both encourage the growth of objective, physiologically based, noninvasive measurements with small and explicit errors. Renal radionuclide studies are well set for the future.

Considering the use of radiolabeled nonreabsorbable solutes as measurers of renal function, one can define the following functions.

- A '*washout*' *rate,* lambda, (λ), or alpha 3, (α_3) function such that the rate of loss from the blood is equal to a global kidney function for a particular compound whose exit from the body is only via the kidney.[2] The units are per second (s^{-1}) and the result is independent of gender, height, and weight.
- An *uptake function* by each kidney is their relative function in terms of the contribution of each kidney to total renal function as a percentage of total; or else as a rate of uptake of the solute by each kidney from the

blood, the fractional uptake rate (FUR)[3] in units of per second or per megasecond. FUR is independent of age, gender, height, and weight. An uptake function for cortical nephrons as a percentage of total kidney uptake may also be measured[4–6] and is relevant to understanding essential hypertension.[7–9]

- *Transit function* may be measured for the whole kidney (parenchyme and pelvis) as the whole kidney transit time; for the renal parenchyme alone, the mean parenchymal transit time (MPTT);[10,11] and for the outer cortex, the parenchymal transit time index (PTTI),[1,12,13] where PTTI plus the minimum transit time (min TT) equals MPTT.
- The balance between uptake function and *excretory function* may be measured by the output (outflow) efficiency (OE),[14–17] for a particular time period, usually 30 min, OE_{30}.

These measurements are physiological, have normal values, are reproducible, and are able to demonstrate pathophysiological processes when they are abnormal. Note that these measurements are either based only on the units of time or have no units (percentage). None involve the measurement or estimation of a volume or a volume of distribution so they are robust.

These measurements may be compared with some of the traditional measurements of renal function. Smith[18] encouraged the measurement of glomerular filtration rate (units of 'per time') whereas in fact it is glomerular filtration flow (units of volume/time, $mL\ min^{-1}$) that is measured. It is erroneously called the glomerular filtration rate. Van Slyke[19,20] introduced the concept of 'clearance', that a part of the blood volume can be considered to be free of a solute, which the kidneys have removed, whereas the rest of the blood contains it. A real leap of the imagination is needed to visualize such a situation given that the blood circulates and is not static.[21]

Single-shot measurements after the injection of a radiolabeled nonreabsorbable solute that undergoes compartmental analysis assume an instantaneous mixing of the injectate in its blood volume of distribution. They have to assume that the basic rule of compartmental analysis is valid: the rate of mixing in any one compartment is fast as compared with the rate of exchange between it and another compartment. They require a volume of the solute's distribution, usually related to the extracellular volume, to be obtained to give a result in $mL\ min^{-1}$. All the above traditional methods have in common the requirement to measure or estimate volume of distribution in some form, but from the single-shot measurement, the rate of washout measured as lambda or as alpha 3, the slope of the second exponential of the 'washout' curve is the key measurement. This is explained in the following.

When a solute is injected into the bloodstream, its volume of distribution increases with time. Its mixing in any compartment takes time. The measurement of the volume

Table 8A.1 *Comparison of pharmacokinetic parameters of ^{99m}Tc-mercaptoacetyltriglycine (^{99m}Tc-MAG$_3$) and radioiodine-labeled ortho-iodohippurate (OIH)*

Parameter	MAG$_3$	OIH	Ratio
Half-life, T_{fi} (min^{-1})	35	32	1.09
Volume (L)	16	25	0.65
Clearance (L min^{-1})	292	461	0.61

of distribution is the source of most errors in the traditional estimations of renal function. Two radiolabeled solutes such as hippuran and MAG$_3$ have almost the same values for lambda and alpha 3, but MAG$_3$ has a volume of distribution approximately 65% of that of hippuran.[22] Since the effective renal plasma flow (ERPF) is given by $V \times \lambda$, where V is the volume of distribution, the ERPF calculated for MAG$_3$ is approximately two thirds of that for hippuran, even though their rates of loss from the blood and rates of uptake by the kidneys are very similar (Table 8A.1). If the volumes of distribution are not measured but are estimated from height and weight, then the measurements of hippuran and MAG$_3$ have the same volume of distribution in an individual and therefore give similar answers. This is a typical paradox, which derives from the concept of clearance and its need for a volume of distribution.

The calculated volume of distribution from height and/or weight and the measured individual volumes of distribution give discordant answers: for the Gates method,[23] clearance of ^{99m}Tc-MAG$_3$ = 0.91 $\times$ c_{hip}; while for the direct measure, clearance of ^{99m}Tc-MAG$_3$ = 0.65 $\times$ c_{hip}, where c_{hip} is the concentration of radioiodinated hippuran.

TECHNIQUE AND INTERPRETATION

The patient requires hydration with about 500 mL fluid at least 30 min before the test so that the urine flow during the test is 1–4 mL min^{-1}. The patient should empty the bladder before the study and the time at the start of emptying is recorded. Time and volume may be measured after the study to obtain a urine flow in milliliters per minute. The patient should receive a reassuring explanation of the test before entering the gamma camera room. The patient may be studied reclining or supine. The supine position is generally recommended since the kidneys are less likely to descend but a postmicturition image is essential. The sitting position, particularly sitting forward, and the standing position are not advised as they allow the kidneys to drop and move anteriorly, making positioning and quantification less reliable. The reclining position is a suitable compromise. The gamma camera is positioned so that its face is set back about 20° off the vertical plane. The field of view must include the left ventricle and the kidneys. The bladder may

be imaged at the end of the study pre- and postmicturition, if it is not in the field of view together with the kidneys. The patient sits on a comfortable backless chair with side-arms and reclines back against the camera face. With the arm abducted, the injection of the chosen radiopharmaceutical is given preferably in less than 1 mL, rapidly into a deep antecubital vein. Alternatively, a 'butterfly' needle with a sterile extension tube and three-way tap may be used. The injectate is introduced into the extension tube and flushed in using 10–20 mL saline. This system also allows access for a subsequent injection of frusemide for the diuresis technique. Data are collected for 30 min, or longer if the pelvis is not visualized and for at least 10 min after an injection of frusemide if that technique is used. Frusemide (40 mg) should be injected at 18–20 min in the adult, but it may be necessary to wait for 30 min before injection for a child (0.5 mg kg^{-1} body weight administered).

Image data are transferred to the computer with a 10-s frame rate. This frame rate is optimal for further image data analysis. It is not necessary to record the first 30 s at 1-s intervals as the interpretation of the curves is generally unreliable due to the vascularity of peri-renal organs (except in renal transplants positioned in the iliac fossa, visualized anteriorly, for the perfusion index). Images on transparent film (analog images) are usually collected at 30-s intervals for the first 180 s; and then at 5-min intervals for the remainder of the study. The following features should be noted:

- The heart, the length of time the activity in the left ventricular cavity is visible; prolonged with renal impairment
- The patency and tortuosity of the aorta and possible aneurysm
- Whether the times of arrival and tracer distribution are equal in the two kidneys; prolongation on one side may occur with an inflow disorder
- The site and position of the kidneys relative to the liver and spleen; possible space-occupying lesion between
- Whether the cortical outline of each kidney is complete; possible scar due to infection or infarction
- Whether there are any defects in the parenchyme; possible tumor, cyst or parenchymal infection or scar
- The cortico-pelvic transfer time, that is the time from first appearance in the cortex to first appearance in the pelvis

A dilated calyx should fill at the pelvic retention stage, but not if it contains a stone. A cyst in the parenchyme will not show any tracer uptake, whereas a vascular tumor may show initial tracer vascular activity which may persist for longer than that in adjacent normal tissue and be followed by a focal defect in the distribution of activity due to the absence of normal nephrons.

Corticopelvic transfer will normally be seen to occur as the tracer moves from parenchyme to pelvis as the lateral edge of the kidney, noted on the 1-min to 2-min frames, appears to move medially as the test progresses. It is prolonged in renovascular disorder.[24] Pelvic, calyceal and/or ureteric retention of tracer occurs when the capacity of these structures has increased through dilation but cannot be used to distinguish whether obstruction is or is not present. The ureter should not be considered to have retained tracer unless its whole length or that down to a block can be seen to persist over several images. Blobs of activity in the ureter are of no significance and do not mean ureteric hold-up. The bladder is usually visualized at the end of the test. A ureterocele or a diverticulum of the bladder may be observed.

On visual inspection a normal pair of renal activity–time curves (renograms) are characterized by their symmetry. A normal renal activity–time curve has a steeply rising part usually lasting 20–30 s and ending with an apparent discontinuity of the slope. This is called the first phase and is an artefact compounded by a rising kidney curve and a falling blood clearance curve. It is absent in the renogram when it is corrected for tissue and blood background. The renogram then rises over the next few minutes towards the peak and this is called the second phase If there is no peak to the renograms, as is the case in certain diseases, it can be said that the second phase continues to rise. After the second phase is the peak which, if the chart specification is correct, should be sharp. The record descends after the peak in normal subjects and this is called the third phase. If there is no peak (in disease) then there is no third phase.

Abnormal renograms are characterized by a loss of sharpness of the peak and alteration of either the second or third phase, or both of these. Absence of the second phase does not necessarily mean total absence of renal function; absence of the third phase certainly does not necessarily mean obstruction to outflow. Differences in peak time between two renograms of over 1 min are of clinical significance only if either the second or third phase of the renogram with the delayed peak is impaired.

Small rapid fluctuations seen in the second or third phase are statistical in nature. When there are fluctuations in renal blood flow, for example due to anxiety, sudden noise or discomfort, an unsteady state occurs and larger irregularities may occur. These last over 2 min and generally return to the line of the third phase. Since ureteric peristalsis is about six contractions per minute and since increase in resistance to flow in the ureter leads to a rise in distending pressure and reduced force but increased frequency of peristalsis, these irregularities are not due to ureteric 'spasm', which does not occur in man.[1,25] Hydronephrosis or reflux of urine may be associated with large alterations of the third phase, with irregularities descending below the line of the third phase.

The report of an abnormal renogram should be in two parts, the description and the interpretation in the individual clinical context. After describing the images, the abnormal renogram is reported. The first phase should be ignored. The second phase may be called 'absent', 'impaired', 'normal' and/or 'continuing to rise' when no peak occurs. The third phase may be called 'absent', 'impaired' or normal. The time

to peak varies nonlinearly with the state of hydration and urine flow. It is indirectly related to the rate of salt and water reabsorption by the nephrons and to the state of the pelvis. It is a crude index of the tracer transit through the parenchyma and pelvis. Normal peak times vary from 2.0 to 4.5 min with a mean of 3.7 min at a urine flow of 1 mL min^{-1}.

If renograms without third phases are symmetrically abnormal, pre-renal or renal parenchymal disorder is the most likely explanation. If the renograms without third phase are asymmetrical, then, depending on context, bilateral renovascular or bilateral outflow disorder are likely. In the context of bilateral outflow obstruction, the kidney that should be operated upon first to relieve the outflow obstruction is that with the better uptake function.[26] A successful operation is followed by an improvement in the rate of rise of the second phase. However, the third phase may remain absent or impaired for weeks or even months after successful operation. Apparent retention in the pelvis may also be overcome by standing the patient up and then repositioning. A pre- and postmicturition image of the lower urinary tract is recommended, when there is evidence of pelvic retention of activity during the study.

RENAL MODELS

There are two types of measurement, 'descriptive' and 'physiological', that can be made from renal radionuclide studies. There at least 20 different points or times that have been taken empirically from the renograms, such as the time for the curve to fall from peak to half its height, the height of the curve at the end of the first phase, and so on. Such measurements are descriptive, and enable one to classify the shape of the curve and to compare one curve with another, which may be called 'curveology'. It should not be expected that such values have inherent physiological significance. This has to be demonstrated empirically by clinical observation and by correlation with other tests applied to the kidney. Denneberg[27] was the first to warn of dangers of comparing points on the curve and of taking ratios of points on the curve in the belief that these represented renal physiology. Secondly, there are those measurements that relate directly to the physiology and pathophysiology of the kidney through a 'physiological model'.

Nuclear medicine is a bridge between a particular clinical problem and a particular test using radionuclides. The physiological model comes first and defines the type of mathematics to be applied. This in turn gives the parameters and metameters that may be derived and then displayed. In order to develop a physiological model to use a physical measurement in a physiological situation, it is necessary to perceive how the measurement relates to a simplified version of reality. The truer the model is to reality (the more isomorphic), the more reliable the mathematical analysis.

The image is a window to an analysis program. Physiological measurements are those derived from image data analysis, which have a physiological basis. It is hoped that renal radionuclide studies will move forward with physiological renal function measurements that are time based or unitless: alpha 2 or lambda, FUR, MPTT, PTTI, OE. Changes in these measurements are directly related to pathophysiology and they avoid the conceptual and practical errors in volume of distribution measurement. The measurement of time is accurate, reproducible and understandable. It is appropriate in the evaluation of renal outflow disorders and renovascular disorders. The time dependency of biological processes is one of nuclear medicine's greatest strengths.

Keynes said that 'measurements ensure meaning'. However, measurements may not be meaningful. For every measurement there is a set of biological and physical assumptions, a set of biological and physical sources of error. There is a range only within which the measurement is applicable and this should be made explicit.

A descriptive parameter, NORA (normalized residual activity), compares the renal activity taking the slope of the kidney curve between 2 and 3 min with the value at 20 min.[28,29] Since a measurement of uptake function is used in the calculation of both NORA and the output efficiency it is reasonable to expect that both of these parameters will show some correlation. This is found in practice when renal function is near normal but with reduced renal function the error on OE remains small but that for NORA becomes large. This effect can be corrected by a special normalization method.[30]

It is important to understand that the application of mathematics or a mathematical model to the analysis of data depends on the physiological model that represents as simply and truly as possible the reality of the clinical situation. A crude example is the statement that blood is in a space (compartmental) and that the kidney is made up of tubes (linear). The more anatomically and physiologically acceptable (isomorphic) the physiological model is, the more possible it is to understand deviations from normal data obtained in pathological situations. Conversely, data analysis based on an incorrect physiological model, while appearing correct in the original test system, may well give uninterpretable or wrongly interpreted results in pathophysiological situations. Just as there are rules for mathematics so there are for physiology and each model has its own rules and assumptions. Thus, a conceptually isomorphic model gives both the physiological basis for choosing a particular form of mathematical analysis and for interpreting a particular measurement. It allows an appreciation of the biological assumptions and sources of error that are inherent in such an interpretation in the context of renal disorders. These are in addition to the more readily documented random and systematic measurement errors due to the physical basis of the external counting technique.

Two different models are typically used in assessing dynamic studies: the compartmental model and the linear system model.

The compartmental model

The compartmental model is most often isomorphic to fluid collections, for example, the interchange of tracer between blood and extracellular fluid. If a tracer that is only taken up by the organ under study is chosen, the rate of loss from, for example, blood plasma will equal the rate of uptake by the chosen organ, the uptake function of the organ.

The uptake function may also be determined relatively in paired organs, in parts of organs and in sites of suspected pathology. The popularity of compartmental models led to their attempted and incorrect use in the kidney, in which they are not isomorphic. As well as all the assumptions required by indicator dilution theory, an important feature of a compartmental model is that the rate of mixing in one compartment has to be rapid compared with the rate of exchange between the compartments. This situation is reasonable for a tracer introduced into the blood, but hardly likely to occur in a kidney made up of tubes of nephrons which show no cross-mixing of their contents.

Provided that a compartmental model is justified as for plasma clearance, then the results of compartmental analysis of the data may be applied to the compartments. Compartmental (exponential) analysis may be applied to curves obtained from many different sites. It is only when they are obtained from a site with which a compartmental model is isomorphic that the results of the compartmental analysis may be meaningfully related to the model and to the clinical problem.

Linear system

A linear system has and requires the assumptions of stationarity: if an input at a single time gives a particular response, then the same input at a later time will give the same response; and linearity that the sum of all the inputs will give a response which is the total of all of the individual responses to all the individual inputs. Looking at the kidneys from the point of view of these two models, it is evident that the compartmental model may be applied to the extracellular fluid, plasma and renal uptake, but it cannot realistically apply to the outer cortex, inner cortex and medulla because there is no mixing between the contents of the individual nephrons running through these regions. Because the nephrons are tubes there has to be a tube model and the model that deals best with tubes is the linear system. Compounds are taken up and move progressively forward along the tubes. Thus, the linear system is applicable to the nephrons of the kidney. There is a delay due to the tubular uptake of MAG_3 or hippuran and/or filtration of DTPA of less than 1 s. There is a longer delay in the cortical nephrons (about 3 min) and for the juxtamedullary nephrons (about 5.5 min). There is a short delay in the normal pelvis (about 20 s).

The appropriate mathematics for a linear system is called deconvolution analysis. This is conceptually quite simple.

A.A. Milne described the game of 'Pooh sticks' where you all stand on a bridge over a river and you all drop sticks in together. You all rush to the other side of the bridge to see which stick is the winner. To understand that simple game as a child is to understand deconvolution analysis. There was a spike input into the system, the simultaneous entry of sticks. The system has responded in some way so that there was an output response which is the distribution of path lengths, some long and some short, and thus a distribution of path times. If the input and output are known you can work out what has happened in that river, that is the distribution of path times, and so you have undertaken deconvolution analysis. If you know the input and output you can find the transit time distribution. Alternatively, if the bridge was made of glass and you had a helicopter flying above it you could actually watch the cumulative effect of all these sticks moving. That is in fact what happens with an activity–time curve from the kidney from a gamma camera over it. You are looking at all the sticks as packets of activity moving through the kidney. As there are multiple paths the input, which was a spike input, will be distributed in time at the output. In other words, if a bolus were injected into the renal artery you would get a distribution of output times. If you know input and total content curve, the renograms, or input and output, or total content and output, you can work out the transit times through the kidney by deconvolution and it is not that difficult.

How is it done in practice? The blood clearance curve obtained from the region of interest over the left ventricle is considered as a series of little spike inputs, decreasing in size over time. The renograms are considered to be the sum of all the responses to this complex input. Deconvolution analysis gives the single response that would have been obtained from a spike injection into the renal artery. Therefore, deconvolving the blood clearance curve and the renograms shows that the renograms are made up of all those similar impulse response functions, also called retention functions, resulting from that input. Thus, from this content curve (the renograms) deconvolution gives the response that would have been obtained from a direct injection of a spike of activity into the renal artery. The beauty of this technique for all of nuclear medicine is that although the injection is given to the patient through an easily accessible vein, it allows the determination noninvasively of what would have been obtained if the injection had been directly and invasively into an artery supplying the organ of interest.

This impulse retention function is quite complicated (Fig. 8A.1). After the input there are renal artery-to-vein transit times. After this short falling portion of the impulse response with time there is a plateau as the activity goes along all the nephrons. Then there is a shoulder to the impulse response and that point defines a minimum transit time, minTT that is common to all nephrons. This minimum transit time can be functionally related to the collecting ducts which are common to all nephrons. The

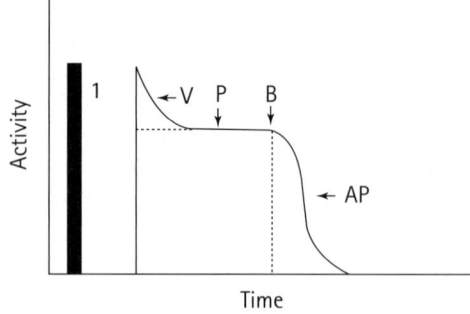

Figure 8A.1 *Parenchymal impulse retention function. The plateau P is extrapolated to the vertical axis to exclude the vascular component V. B gives the time of change from the plateau to a falling activity and delineates the minimum transit time. The mean parenchymal transit time is given by the area divided by the height of the plateau of the impulse retention function. The parenchymal transit time index is given by the area AP for transit times longer than the minimum divided by the height of the plateau of the impulse retention function. The transit times are measured in seconds.*

distribution of transit times just after the shoulder is called the parenchymal transit time index (PTTI).

Time is a fundamental biological variable which is determined by nuclear medicine techniques, which radiology conventionally does not consider. Time can be measured accurately, is easily understood and is universal. For deconvolution there should be a good bolus of high activity for good statistics because these impulse retention functions are rather noisy. A 10-s frame rate is optimal and must be used. The input is obtained from the left ventricle region of interest, and the content curve from the whole kidney or from a region of interest from the parenchyme excluding any pelvis or calyceal elements. Note that any part of the parenchyme is representative of the whole because it is time not counts that is the variable.

METHOD

Transit time analysis requires an adequate dose injected 100–150 MBq ^{99m}Tc-MAG$_3$ and a 10-s frame rate for 20 min: 128×128 matrix. A high quality bolus is required so that the first frame of the left ventricular activity–time curve includes its peak. The left ventricular activity–time curve is taken as the input which is divided into multiple decreasing delta input functions. The activity from the parenchyme after using a careful peripheral region of interest to avoid calyces and pelvis is deconvolved using the inverse matrix algorithm with the constraints of non-negativity and monotonicity and minimal smoothing. A 10-s frame rate gives better separation of the lung/heart from the kidneys. It gives a sharper input function, which is essential as compared to a 20-s frame rate and it allows the plateau of the impulse retention function to be seen which may not be detectable using a 20-s frame rate.

Deconvolution become straightforward only where a protocol is used to ensure stability and robustness of the solution given the statistical noise in the data obtained. The choice of pre-processing, filtering and the inclusion of prior knowledge in the form of mathematical constraints is important. These include monotonicity, which means curves that must have only one peak and be without major irregularities in them, so there is a need for a quiet and content patient; and non-negativity: if there are negative deviations these are removed.[31] The curves should not be smoothed because that will cause data loss. The first value should be the maximum which should be so if the patient has been given a bolus input and if the computer is started just prior to the moment of injection. If not so, then use the maximum input value and adjust the time base. For the impulse retention function, the shoulder is defined visually or with a gradient operator or by differentiation, and extrapolated back to give the plateau. That shoulder point separates the minimum transit time and the parenchymal transit times index. The main problems with deconvolution analysis are a poor bolus, an anxious patient (or doctor), human error since the program is interactive, too little parenchyme or too little left ventricle in the chosen regions of interest and computer failure. Nowadays the computers are stable and the main requirement is to obtain the data in a form that appropriately meets the constraints.

Transit times

The parts of a nephron can be related to its transit times (Fig. 8A.2). The mean whole kidney transit time is related to the peak of the renograms. It is nondiscriminatory, partly parenchyme, partly pelvis and related to the peak of the renograms. When the pelvis is separated out, the pelvic transit time and the mean parenchymal transit time (MPTT)

are obtained. MPTT is used to determine the presence of renovascular disorder. MPTT is divided into the minimum transit time and the residue of the impulse retention function, the parenchymal transit time index. This PTTI is the transit time representing activity mainly in the proximal nephron. It is most dependent on salt and water and is used to determine whether the patient has an obstructive nephropathy or not. The minimum transit time represents the time of transit through the collecting ducts and is dependent on urine flow rate. Hence its subtraction from the mean parenchymal transit time helps to compensate for differences in urine flow rate. The pelvic transit time is the time through the pelvis and is prolonged if the pelvis is enlarged, whatever the cause such as dilation without obstruction. This is because there will be eddying and mixing in an enlarged pelvis. The renal transit times can be summarized as follows. The very short time for ^{99m}Tc-labeled DTPA to pass the glomerular filter and the slight difference in timing between this and the secretion of ^{99m}Tc-labeled MAG$_3$ or ^{123}I-labeled *ortho*-iodohippuran (OIH) into the proximal tubular lumen are quite lost in consideration of the nephron transit times when the data sampling interval is 10 s. The whole kidney transit time (WKTT) is given by the total transit time through the renal parenchyme and pelvis. The mean parenchyme transit time (MPTT) is that through the whole of the parenchyme and added together with the pelvic transit time (PvTT) equals WKTT. The mean parenchymal transit time is made up of a minimum transit time (minTT) common to all nephrons, and parenchymal transit time index (PTTI). The whole kidney transit time corrected for the minimum transit time is called the whole kidney transit time index (WKTTI). Thus

$$WKTT = MPTT + PvTT,$$
$$MPTT = MinTT + PTTI,$$
$$WKTT = MinTT + WKTTI.$$

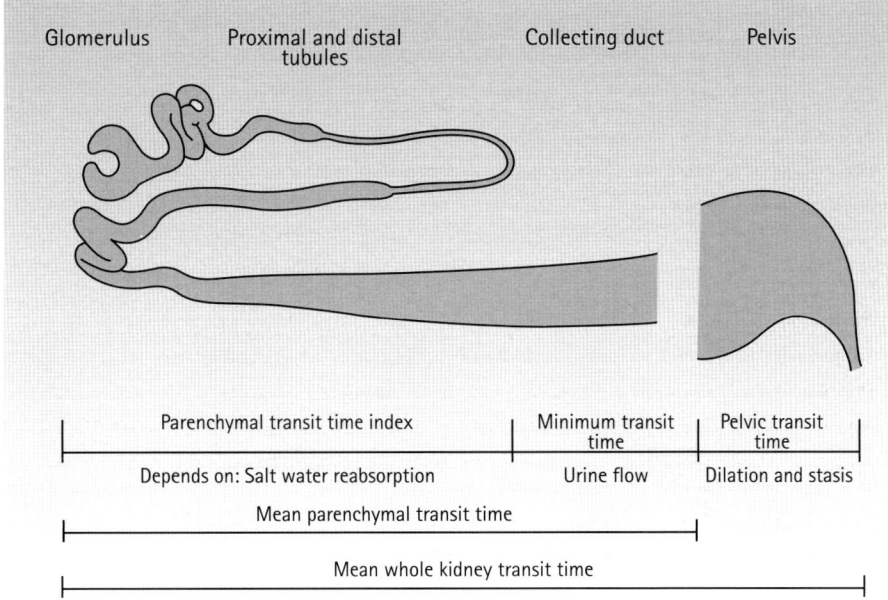

Figure 8A.2 *Renal functions from transit times. The mean parenchymal transit time excludes the pelvic transit time and is best for evaluating renovascular disorder. The minimum transit time common to all nephrons is related to flow in the collecting ducts common to all nephrons and is subtracted from the mean parenchymal transit time to give the parenchymal transit time index, which is best for evaluating obstructive nephropathy. (Redrawn with permission from the* British Journal of Urology.*)*

Normal ranges are PTTI = 10–156 s, MPTT = 100–240 s and WKTTI = 20–170 s.

When first published, the transit times were given in 2-s intervals and compared with the antegrade perfusion pressure measurements.[12] In those patients where there was outflow obstruction according to the criterion of a resistance increasing the pressure to over 20 cm of water pressure, then the parenchymal transit time index was over 160 s. However, in the patients with pelvic dilatation with no evidence of a positive pressure response to the antegrade perfusion measurements, the PTTI value was up to 142 s. The normal value was taken as 156 s and below.

It is necessary to separate the pelvis from the parenchyme. Often it is obvious and a region of interest can be drawn. A reliable way when the separation is not obvious is to make a mean time image. The 2-min image of the kidney has no pelvis or calyceal activity because nothing has reached there yet. This is the first template. At 15 min, if the border between pelvis or calyces and parenchyme cannot be drawn, then the matrix of pixels and the activity–time curve in each pixel is obtained. This is representative of a mean time by an area over height method for each pixel. If it is a parenchymal pixel it will have a short mean time. If it is a calyceal pixel it will have at least 2 min before activity appears and therefore it will have a longer mean time. If the mean time image is obtained and color-coded so that any pixel that has a short mean time has a low intensity and any pixel with a long mean time has a high intensity, a generous region of interest can be drawn around the pelvicalyceal system[12,13,32] or it can be automated.[33] The parenchymal region is thus defined, from which the parenchymal activity–time curve is obtained for deconvolution with the blood clearance curve. From the intact nephron hypothesis, a part of the kidney parenchyme is representative of the whole, unless there is a calyceal obstruction in one calyx, in which case the kidney divides into two regions and each is treated separately.

RENAL RADIOPHARMACEUTICALS

The main agents are shown in Table 8A.2.

^{99m}Tc-labeled mercaptoacetyltriglycine

The disadvantages of the current renal imaging agents ^{99m}Tc-labeled DTPA and radioiodinated OIH have led many workers to search for a better agent. The properties of an ideal substitute for radioiodinated OIH are as follows. It should be labeled with ^{99m}Tc. It should have an extraction efficiency at least three times greater than ^{99m}Tc-labeled DTPA, i.e. over 60%, and preferably better than radioiodinated OIH. It should be a stable compound easily prepared from a robust kit, cheap to purchase and easy to use. It should show weak or no protein binding to improve glomerular filtration and tubular secretion.

Compounds based on a linking of three nitrogen atoms and one sulfur atom with ^{99m}Tc, N_3–S, were developed by Fritzberg et al.,[34] leading to MAG$_3$, mercaptoacetyltriglycine, which was shown to be tubular secreted by probenecid inhibition studies and equivalent to radioiodinated OIH. The three nitrogen atoms and the sulfur atom of MAG$_3$ are in a ring structure which is able to bind reduced technetium in a stable way. It also contains the appropriate combination of polar and nonpolar groups that make it suitable for proximal tubular uptake, anionic transport and secretion, as a ^{99m}Tc-labeled replacement for OIH. The MAG$_3$ kit preparation contains a benzoyl group to protect the ring structure and this must be displaced by a boiling step to enable ^{99m}Tc to bind to the ring. MAG$_3$ is supplied

Table 8A.2 *Comparison of renal radiopharmaceuticals for gamma camera studies*

	^{99m}Tc–DTPA	^{99m}Tc–MAG$_3$	^{99m}Tc–EC	^{123}I–OIH
ERPF, fraction of	0.2	0.67	0.75	1
Dose (MBq)	300	100	80	60
Kidney count rate	Low	High	High	High
Background	High	Low	Low	Low
Extraction efficiency	20%	58%	65%	87%
Weak protein binding	<5%	90%	50%	70%
Fraction filtered	99%	2%	10%	6%
Volume of distribution	Large	Small	Moderate	Large
Availability	Routine	Routine	Not	Weekly
Boiling step	No	Yes	No	No
Impurities	Rare	Lipophilic	–	Free iodine, iodobenzoate
Cost	Low	Moderate	–	High

DTPA, diethylenetriaminepentaacetic acid; MAG$_3$, mercaptoacetyltriglycine; EC, ethylene dicysteine; OIH, *ortho*-iodohippurate; ERPF, effective renal plasma flow.

in the form of white powder in sealed glass vials. A lead-shielded water bath is prepared and brought to the boil. About 185 MBq (5 mCi) of [99mTc]pertechnetate is eluted in the standard way from a technetium generator. The volume dilution of the pertechnetate stock to give the required activity should be only with physiological 0.9% saline.

An amount should be calculated so that the volume to be added to the vial of MAG3 is not less than 4 mL and not more than 10 mL. The vial is then placed in the boiling water and left there for 10 min. It is then removed and cooled under running tap water or by immersion in cold water. Investigations of this method of preparation have shown that a number of modifications may be made to improve its convenience in routine use. First, the addition of 99mTc to the MAG3 powder may take place at a time convenient to the radiopharmacist at the time of elution of the generator for routine dispensing. Up to 4 h may be allowed to elapse before the boiling step. It is important, however, to avoid the entrance of air into the system and keep the product cold. After boiling for 10 min the kit is cooled and can be divided into four portions in four sterile syringes. Each is capped and frozen at 4°C – the 'cold' MAG3 method.[34] When the patient arrives, the syringe may be thawed under a table lamp and used. By spreading this arrangement through the day, eight renal studies can be prepared using two MAG3 vials. Radiochromatography shows that the impurities increase with time after the boiling step at room temperature. At 1 h, less than 5% of nontubularly secreted MAG3 is present, made up of three or more components, two of which are lipophilic and slowly taken up by the liver and excreted in the bile and intestine. The amount of this hepatic-excreted contaminant depends on the preparation conditions and the length of time between boiling and injection, and not on the level of renal function. The 'cold' MAG3 method reduces this liver contaminant a hundred-fold.[35] Delaying imaging in a patient with poor renal function will slow stomach, intestinal and colonic activity with time.

Accidental omission of the boiling step leaves benzoyl MAG3, which is a 99mTc-labeled DTPA-like renal agent. By 5 h without boiling, much of the benzoyl group has dissociated and 90% is in the form of 99mTc-labeled MAG3. No adverse effects, either clinical or biochemical, have been demonstrated using 99mTc-labeled MAG3. This compound shows between 78 and 93% of weak protein binding, which reduces its glomerular filtration to 2% in the same way and to greater extent than radioiodinated OIH (6%).

The clearance studies showed that 99mTc -MAG3 had a 65% smaller volume of distribution than 131I-labeled hippuran and a similar blood clearance half-life (slow component ratio 99mTc-labeled MAG3 to 123I-labeled hippuran is 1.09:1). The clearance relationship is

$$ERPF_{hip} = (1.5 \times ERPF_{Tc}) + c$$

where $ERPF_{hip}$ and $ERPF_{Tc}$ are the ERPF values for hippuran and 99mTc-labeled MAG3, respectively, and c is a constant that is equal to 40 mL min^{-1}. The SEM is 8%.

Although its clearance had a linear relationship with effective renal plasma flow, 99mTc-labeled MAG3 is not yet proposed as a substitute for the absolute measurement of glomerular filtration rate (GFR) or ERPF by the appropriate agents.[36,37] The reproducibility of 99mTc-MAG3 studies was assessed by Klingensmith et al.[38]

Clinical studies performed have shown it to be a successful radiopharmaceutical for routine renal work, combining the physiological advantages of OIH with the benefits of using 99mTc label.[22,39] An administered activity of 100 MBq of 99mTc-MAG3 is used for routine renal imaging, for relative function measurements, for renal transit time analysis and for frusemide diuresis studies. It is suitable for use for renal transplants and for the measurement of the intrarenal plasma flow distribution. Its use is preferred in children generally and for reflux studies.

99mTc–ethylene dicysteine

This agent, although not yet commercially available in western Europe and the USA may replace 99mTc-MAG3 because it does not require a boiling step and has a greater extraction efficiency: 75% of that of hippuran. It may be used for the full range of renal radionuclide studies.[40–43] It has a volume of distribution similar to that of hippuran, but lower protein binding (Table 8A.2).

99mTc–diaminocyclohexane

This agent is cationically transported through tubules, a property in common with thiamine, cyclosporin and cis-platinum, as well as being glomerular filtered. It may have a role in assessing cyclosporin toxicity.[44–46] It is not commercially available.

99mTc-labeled dimercaptosuccinic acid

99mTc-labeled dimercaptosuccinic acid (DMSA) is representative of a class of compounds that are taken up and fixed by the kidneys with less than 5% being excreted. In order to avoid urinary excretion and liver uptake attention to detail is required in its preparation. It is necessary to keep air (oxygen) out of the vials and use the compound preferably within 30 min of preparation otherwise it may show increased urinary loss which may interfere with the measurement of renal function. The compound binds weakly to plasma proteins and then is glomerular filtered[47] and taken up by the kidney tubules. If renal function is poor, uptake in the liver is seen. Acidosis also affects renal uptake.[48] A total of 100 MBq (2.7 mCi) is administered intravenously and static images may be taken at 1 h if renal function is good, or 3–6 h if renal function is poor. Single photon emission computed tomography (SPECT) studies with DMSA have indicated that they may have advantages over planar studies.[49]

^{51}Cr-ethylenediaminetetraacetic acid

^{51}Cr-EDTA is used for GFR measurement through serial blood samples (see Chapter 8B).

Although many other radiopharmaceuticals have been used to evaluate renal function, ^{99m}Tc-MAG$_3$, ^{99m}Tc-DMSA, and ^{51}Cr-EDTA will meet all routine clinical requirements.

RENAL FUNCTIONS

Relative renal function

The measurement of relative renal function is one of the major contributions of radionuclide renal studies to the practice of urology.[25] Kidneys that appear poorly functioning on intravenous urography were shown to have an important contribution to total renal function in patients with hydronephrosis and/or obstructing uropathy. The practice of removing 'bad' looking kidneys was replaced by conserving function as far as possible. In adults, a function of 5% or less was deemed irrecoverable and a level of 15% or more recoverable with a borderline range in between. The relative renal function improved after successful operation. The factors that influence the accuracy of the measurement include the level of total renal function, the variation in renal depth, the measurement technique, the correction for background activity and the radiopharmaceutical used.

Relative function was first measured with probe renography. A computer-assisted blood background subtraction (CABBS) method improved accuracy.[24] Secker-Walker and Coleman[50] showed relative function could be measured using the gamma camera approach which is now standard. The timing of the relative function measurement is best solved by recording the activities at 10-s intervals and plotting the ratio left/(left + right). The time interval over which this is constant gives the time to measure the relative function.[25] While, usually, 1.5 min (after unsteady state conditions are over) to 2.5 min (before any loss from the kidney), this may be delayed in obstructing uropathy or in renal impairment.[51]

Variation in renal depth has been addressed by Wujanto et al.[52] for ^{99m}Tc-DMSA where anterior and posterior geometric means are recommended for adults. Gruenewald et al.[53] recommend depth correction by measurement from skin to kidney of the uptake of ^{99m}Tc-DTPA not by a height–weight formula. Attenuation correction for DMSA makes no difference.[54] Prigent et al.[55] in the consensus and the BNMS quality guidelines[56] no longer recommend depth correction for ^{99m}Tc-radiolabeled pharmaceuticals. The correction for background regions has been addressed by Piepsz et al.[57] for ^{99m}Tc-MAG$_3$ studies in healthy volunteers using ^{99m}Tc-DMSA as the standard. They recommend the integral method with perirenal correction for background and the Patlak–Rutland plot. This region should avoid the renal hilum as recommended by the BNMS guidelines.[56] Moonen et al.[58] support the integral method with ^{99m}Tc-DTPA. Samal et al.[33] showed how fuzzy logic and factor analysis aid region of interest selection and the measurement of relative function.

The best choice of radiopharmaceutical is ^{99m}Tc-MAG$_3$.[55,56,59] ^{99m}Tc-MAG$_3$ and ^{99m}Tc-DTPA showed no difference in the measurement of relative function but MAG$_3$ is extracted from the blood 3.3 times more than DTPA.[60] Al-Nahhas et al.[39] found $r = 0.94$ for relative function for these two radiopharmaceuticals. ^{99m}Tc-DMSA is usually limited to children and measurement of relative renal function was audited by Fleming et al.[61] who found that 98% of the results were within 5%. They recommend that the technique be better standardized.

Fractional uptake rate

The main advance has been the direct measurement of the fractional uptake rate (FUR) using the Patlak–Rutland plot as described by Rutland et al.[3] This is a measure of the rate constant for the uptake by each kidney in per seconds (times a million as megaseconds for convenience). The fraction of tracer in the blood taken up by an organ in unit time:

$$\mathrm{FUR} = \frac{KB(0)}{D}$$

where K is the slope of the Rutland–Patlak plot and $B(0)$ is the blood curve value extrapolated back to time zero. D is the total dose administered, corrected for camera sensitivity, depth, and table attenuation.[3]

FUR is independent of volume of distribution, age, height, weight and gender. It is potentially the most reliable measure of relative renal function for the future. Its measurement relates to the recommendation to use lambda or alpha 2 for the slope of the blood clearance curve in per second for assessing overall renal function.

In conclusion, ^{99m}Tc-MAG$_3$ is recommended for the measurement of relative renal function using the integral method with background correction to give the percentage uptake left/(left + right), normal range 43–57%. The fractional uptake rate is the method for the future.

Transit function

The time it takes for a non-reabsorbable solute to move along a nephron depends mainly on the rate of proximal tubular salt and water reabsorption and the concentrating ability of the medulla to reabsorb water from the collecting ducts. This, in turn, depends in the proximal tubules on the intratubular pressure (increased with resistance to outflow) and the peritubular capillary pressure (decreased in renovascular disorder). Thus the MPTT is prolonged in renovascular disorders.[10] As the medullary concentration gradient is diminished in the presence of increased resistance to outflow, correction for this by subtraction of the minimum transit time gives a PTTI, a sensitive indicator of obstructive nephropathy.[12,13]

Deconvolution analysis is a method of obtaining the renal transit times.[25,59,62–66] The whole kidney transit time was found to be 3.6 ± 1.1 min.[67] This relates to the peak of the renal activity–time curve. Renovascular hypertension is associated with a prolonged MPTT.[10,68] This predicts the outcome of correcting renal artery stenoses by angioplasty or surgery as to whether or not hypertension will be improved.[69] The effect of the captopril stress enhancing the diagnosis of renovascular disorder was shown by Russell et al.,[70] who found MPTT was better than peak time in relation to arteriographic findings. Simpler indices may be used such as the cortico-pelvic transfer index, $r = 0.66$ with MPTT,[24] or R20/3, $r = 0.47$ with MPTT.[70]

In obstructive nephropathy, PTTI is successful in distinguishing its presence from a non-obstructed kidney with pelvic dilatation.[12,13,39,71] Measurements in extracorporeal shock wave lithotripsy (ESWL) for renal stone[72] showed a transient prolongation of MPTT. In chronic renal failure Prvulovich et al.[73] using ^{99m}Tc-ethylene dicysteine for MPTT measurements showed very similar results to those with ^{99m}Tc-MAG$_3$. In diabetic nephropathy MPTT helps to distinguish the benefit of angiotensin-converting enzyme inhibitors from detriment.[74]

In renal transplants the use of the vascular transit time (VTT) has been helpful.[75] Measurements in well functioning transplants are similar to those in normal kidneys.[76] Onset of complications may be assessed.[77–79]

Transit time analysis can also be used to separate the contribution of cortical nephron flow to total effective renal plasma flow. The reduction of cortical nephron flow in essential hypertension[80] is improved by angiotensin-converting enzyme inhibitor.[8] The effect of vasodilatation with indoramin in healthy subjects is not selective.[81]

In conclusion, measurements of renal transit times provide a physiological approach: MPTT in the diagnosis of renal vascular disorder, PTTI for obstructive nephropathy and VTT in the evaluation of renal transplant function.

Intra-renal flow distribution

Xenon washout was purported to represent inner cortical, outer cortical and medullary flow in the kidney, but, by using a compartmental model whose assumptions did not apply to a system of tubes, this empirical approach was eventually shown to be invalid. The physiological approach makes use of the fact that cortical nephrons have short loops, and juxta-medullary nephrons have long loops of Henle. Therefore a transit time distribution is likely to be bimodal. A bimodal distribution of nephrons was demonstrated by Chasis et al.[82] using the tubular maximum clearance of p-amino hippuric acid (PAH). A bimodal distribution was shown by probe renography[25] and a new technique using the gamma camera[4] has been improved by Nimmon et al.,[6] so that the percentage contribution of cortical nephrons to each kidney can be determined (Table 8A.3).

Cortical nephrons differ from juxta-medullary nephrons in that they show autoregulation due to the activity of the juxta-glomerular apparatus. Their afferent arterioles are muscular and are controlled by intra-renal angiotensin II. Efferent arterioles are not muscular. Juxta-medullary nephrons show no autoregulation, their afferent arterioles are not muscular but their efferent arterioles are muscular and under extra-renal and circulating angiotensin II control as well as vasopressin and prostaglandins. Thus the effect of angiotensin II inhibitors such as captopril differs on the two populations of nephrons. It causes an increase in afferent arteriolar flow in cortical nephrons due to inhibiting the intrarenal angiotensin II effect. It causes a decrease in glomerular filtration rate in juxta-medullary nephrons due to releasing their control due to circulating

Table 8A.3 *Cortical nephron flow as a percentage of total*

	Blood pressure		Cortical nephron flow		
	Mean	Range	Mean (%)	SEM	P value
Essential hypertension, 13 patients					
Combined	118	105–150	74.6	± 1.5	
Left kidney			74.8	± 2.3	
Right kidney			74.4	± 2.0	
Normotension, 21 patients	93	83–100			
Combined			83.9	± 0.7	<0.002*
Left kidney			84.2	± 0.85	
Right kidney			83.9	± 1.2	

*Combined essential hypertension versus normotension.

angiotensin, causing the efferent arterioles to become dilated. Thus in essential hypertension which has overconstriction of afferent arterioles of cortical nephrons,[7] the flow rate increases and transit time shortens, whereas in renal artery stenosis that is functionally significant or renovascular disorder due to small vessel disease, the glomerular filtration rate falls and the mean parenchymal transit times are prolonged. This forms part of the basis of the success of the captopril intervention study in the distinction between renovascular and essential hypertension.

The similarity of the right and left cortical nephron flow percentages in Table 8.1.3 indicates the robustness of the technique. The evidence that the cortical nephron flow is reduced in essential hypertension compared with normotensives is demonstrated. The action of captopril in improving percentage cortical nephron flow in essential hypertensives to greater than normal was also demonstrated.[7,9]

CONCLUSION

The demonstration that physiological methods are more reliable than empirical methods continues to be an important part of renal radionuclide studies progression for the future. The technology is sufficiently advanced for the replacement of empirical measures by physiological measurements. Abnormal or unusual results can then be interpreted upon a physiological frame of reference and the correct inferences drawn. In the future we should have alpha 3 or lambda for the measurement of overall renal function, FUR for the method of relative function, outflow efficiency for the assessment of obstructing uropathy, PTTI for the assessment of obstructive nephropathy and the measurements of MPTT, cortical nephron and juxta-medullary nephron flow in the assessment of essential hypertension and the response to captopril. Nuclear medicine physicians with an interest in nephrology should promote physiological measurements of kidney function in health and disease.[21]

REFERENCES

● Seminal primary article
◆ Key review paper
✳ First publication of a management guideline

◆ 1 Britton KE, Brown NJG, Nimmon CC. Clinical renography: 25 years on. *Eur J Nucl Med* 1996; **23**: 1541–6.

● 2 Peters AM, Henderson BL, Lui D. Comparison between terminal slope rate constant and 'slope/intercept' as measures of glomerular filtration rate using the single-compartment simplification. *Eur J Nucl Med* 2001; **28**: 320–6.

● 3 Rutland M, Que L, Hassan IM. FUR – one size suits all. *Eur J Nucl Med* 2000; **27**: 1708–13.

● 4 Gruenewald SM, Nimmon CC, Nawaz MK, Britton KE. A non invasive γ-camera technique for the measurement of intra renal flow distribution in man. *Clin Sci* 1981; **61**: 385–9.

5 Britton KE, Nawaz MK, Nimmon CC, *et al.* Total and intrarenal flow distribution in healthy subjects. *Nephron* 1986; **43**: 265–73.

6 Nimmon CC, Samal M, Backfrieder W, Britton KE. An improved method for the determination of the intrarenal transit time distribution. *Eur J Nucl Med* 2000; **27**: 994.

● 7 Britton KE. Essential hypertension: a disorder of cortical nephron control. *Lancet* 1981; **II**: 900–2.

● 8 Al-Nahhas A, Nimmon CC, Britton KE, *et al.* The effect of ramipril, a new angiotensin converting enzyme inhibitor on cortical nephron flow and effective renal plasma flow in patients with essential hypertension. *Nephron* 1990; **54**: 47–52.

◆ 9 Britton KE. The kidney and genital system. In: *Molecular nuclear medicine*. Feinendegen LE, Shreeve WW, Eckelman WC, Bahk Y-W, Wagner HW (eds). Berlin: Springer, 2003; pp. 574–82.

● 10 Al-Nahhas A, Marcus AJ, Bomanji J, *et al.* Validity of the mean parenchymal transit time as a screening test for the detection of functional renal artery stenoses in hypertensive patients. *Nucl Med Commun* 1989; **37**: 171–7.

● 11 Gruenewald SM, Stewart JH, Simmons KC, Crocker EF. Predictive value of quantitative renography for successful treatment of atherosclerotic renovascular hypertension. *Aus NZ J Med* 1985; **15**: 617–22.

● 12 Britton KE, Nimmon CC, Whitfield HK, *et al.* Obstructive nephropathy, successful evaluation with radionuclides. *Lancet* 1979; **I**: 905–7.

● 13 Britton KE, Nawaz MK, Whitfield HN, *et al.* Obstructive nephropathy: comparison between parenchymal transit time index and frusemide diuresis. *Br J Urol* 1987; **59**: 127–32.

● 14 Chaiwatanarat T, Padhy AK, Bomanji JB, *et al.* Validation of renal output efficiency as an objective quantitative parameter in the evaluation of upper urinary tract obstruction. *J Nucl Med* 1993; **34**: 845–8.

● 15 Saunders CAB, Choong KKL, Larcos G, Farlow D, Gruenewald SM. Assessment of pediatric hydronephrosis using output efficiency. *J Nucl Med* 1997; **38**: 1483–6.

16 Cosgriff PS, Morrish O. The value of output efficiency measurement in resolving equivocal frusemide responses. *Nucl Med Commun* 2000; **21**: 390–1.

● 17 Jain S, Cosgriff PS, Turner DTL, Aslam M, Morrish O. Calculating the renal output efficiency as a method for clarifying equivocal renograms in adults with suspected urinary tract obstruction. *Br J Urol Int* 2003; **92**: 485–7.

◆ 18 Smith HW. *The kidney, structure and function in health and disease.* New York: Oxford University Press, 1951.

19 Moller E, McIntosh JF, Van Slyke DD. Studies in urea excretion II. *J Clin Invest* 1928; **6**: 427–65.

20 Van Slyke DD, Rhoades CP, Hiller A, Alving AS. Relationships between urea excretion, renal blood flow, renal oxygen consumption and diuresis: the mechanism of urea excretion. *Am J Physiol* 1934; **109**: 336–74.

21 Britton KE. The mythology of renal function measurement. *World J Nucl Med* 2003; **2**: 263–4.

● 22 Jafri RA, Britton KE, Nimmon CC, *et al.* 99m-Tc MAG3: a comparison with I-123 and I-131 ortho-iodohippurate in patients with renal disorder. *J Nucl Med* 1988; **14**: 453–62.

● 23 Gates GF. Glomular filtration rate. Estimation from fractional renal accumulation of ^{99m}Tc-DTPA (stannous), *Am J Radiol* 1982; **138**: 565–70.

24 Makoba GI, Nimmon CC, Kouykin V, *et al.* Comparison of a corticopelvic transfer index with renal transit times. *Nucl Med Commun* 1996; **17**: 212–5.

◆ 25 Britton KE, Brown NJG. *Clinical renography.* London: Lloyd Luke, 1971.

26 Sreenevasan G. Bilateral renal calculi. *Ann R Coll Surg Engl* 1974; **55**: 3–12.

27 Denneberg T. Critical analysis of the renogram tracing in normal subjects and diseased states. In: *Radioisotopes in the diagnosis of diseases of the kidneys and urinary tract.* Timmermanns L, Merchie G (eds). International Congress Series, number 178. Amsterdam: Excerpta Medica, 1969; pp. 222–7.

● 28 Piepsz A, Tondeur M, Ham H. NORA: a simple and reliable parameter for estimating renal output with or without frusemide challenge. *Nucl Med Commun* 2000; **21**: 317–23.

29 Piepsz A, Kuyvenhoven JD, Tondeur M, Ham H. Normalized residual activity: usual values and robustness of method. *J Nucl Med* 2002; **43**: 33–8.

30 Nimmon CC, Samal M, Britton KE. Elimination of the influence of total renal function on renal output efficiency and normalised residual activity. *J Nucl Med* 2004; **45**: 587–93.

31 Nimmon CC, Lee TY, Britton KE, *et al.* Practical application of deconvolution techniques to dynamic studies. In: *Medical radionuclide imaging*, Vol. I. Vienna: International Atomic Energy Agency, 1981; pp. 367–88.

● 32 Whitfield HN, Britton KE, Hendry WF, Nimmon CC, Wickham JEA. The distinction between obstructive uropathy and nephropathy by radioisotope transit times. *Br J Urol* 1978; **50**: 433-6.

● 33 Samal M, Nimmon CC, Britton KE, Bergmann H. Relative renal uptake and transit time measurements using functional factor images and fuzzy regions of interest. *Eur J Nucl Med* 1998; **25**: 48–54.

● 34 Fritzberg AR, Sudhaker K, Eshima D, *et al.* Synthesis and biological evaluation of Tc-99m MAG3 as a hippuran replacement. *J Nucl Med* 1986; **17**: 111–16.

35 Solanki KK, Al Nahhas A, Britton KE. Cold Tc-99m MAG3. In: *Trends and possibilities in nuclear medicine.* Schmidt HAE, Buraggi GL (eds). Stuttgart: Schattauer Verlag, 1989; pp. 443–6.

36 Bubeck B, Brandau W, Weber E, *et al.* Pharmacokinetics of technetium-99m-MAG3 in humans. *J Nucl Med* 1990; **31**: 1285–93.

● 37 Rehling M, Nielsen BV, Pedersen EB, *et al.* Renal and extra renal clearance of ^{99m}Tc-MAG3: a comparison with ^{125}I-OIH and ^{51}Cr-EDTA in patients representing all levels of glomerular filtration rate. *Eur J Nucl Med* 1995; **22**: 1379–84.

● 38 Klingensmith WC, Briggs DE, Smith WI. Technetium-99m MAG3 renal studies; normal range and reproducibility of physiologic parameters as a function of age and sex. *J Nucl Med* 1994; **35**: 1612–17.

● 39 Al-Nahhas AA, Jafri RA, Britton KE, *et al.* Clinical experience with ^{99m}Tc-MAG3, mercaptoacetyltriglycine and a comparison with ^{99m}Tc-DTPA. *Eur J Nucl Med* 1988; **14**: 453–62.

● 40 Van Nerom C, Bormans C, Bauwens J, *et al.* Comparative evaluation of Tc-99m LL ethylene dicysteine and Tc-99m MAG3 in volunteers. *Eur J Nucl Med* 1992; **33**: 551–7.

41 Ozker R, Onsel C, Kabasakal L, *et al.* Technetium-99m-*N,N* ethylene dicysteine: a comparative study of renal scintigraphy with technetium-99m MAG3 and iodine-131-OIH in patients with obstructive renal disease. *J Nucl Med* 1994; **35**: 840–5.

● 42 Gupta NK, Bomanji JB, Waddington W, Lui D, Costa DC, Verbruggen AM. Technetium-99m-L-L ethylene dicysteine scintigraphy in patients with renal disorders. *Eur J Nucl Med* 1995; **22**: 617–24.

43 Kostadinova I, Simeonova A. The use of ^{99m}Tc-EC captopril test in patients with hypertension. *Nucl Med Commun* 1995; **16**: 128–31.

● 44 Padhy AK, Solanki KK, Bomanji JB, *et al.* Clinical evaluation of ^{99m}Tc diaminocyclohexane, a renal agent with cationic transport: results in healthy normal volunteers. *Nephron* 1993; **65**: 294–8.

45 Sonmezoglu K, Demir M, Erdil TY, *et al.* Evaluation of renal function in patients with psoriasis on low dose cyclosporin regimen by using Tc-99m diaminocyclohexane (DACH). *Eur J Nucl Med* 1998; **24**: 1630–6.

46 Taylor A, Hansen L, Marzilli LG. Biodistribution and renal excretion of isomers of the cationic tracer, (99m)Tc diaminocyclohexane (DACH): biodistribution of cationic renal tracers. *Nucl Med Biol* 2001; **28**: 299–302.

● 47 Peters AM, Jones DH, Evans K, Gordon I. Two routes for 99m-Tc-DMSA uptake into the renal cortical tubular cell. *Eur J Nucl Med* 1988; **14**: 555–61.

48 Yee CA, Lee HB, Blaufox MD. ^{99m}Tc DMSA renal uptake: influence of biochemical and physiological factors. *J Nucl Med* 1981; **22**: 1054–8.

49 Williams E, Parker D, Roy R. Multiple-section radionuclide tomography of the kidney: a clinical evaluation. *Br J Radiol* 1986; **59**: 975–83.

50 Secker-Walker RH, Coleman RE. Estimating relative renal function. *J Urol* 1976; **115**: 621–5.

51 Sennewald K, Taylor A. A pitfall in calculating differential renal function in patients with renal failure. *Clin Nucl Med* 1993; **18**: 377–81.

● 52 Wujanto R, Lawson RS, Prescott MC, Testa HJ. The importance of using anterior and posterior views in the calculation of differential renal function using ^{99}Tc^m-DMSA. *Br J Radiol* 1987; **60**: 869–72.

53 Gruenewald SM, Collins LT, Fawdry RM. Kidney depth measurement and its influence on quantitation of function from gamma camera renography. *Clin Nucl Med* 1985; **10**: 398–401.

54 Nimmo MJ, Merrick MV, Allen PL. Measurement of relative renal function. A comparison of methods and assessment of reproducibility. *Br J Radiol* 1987; **60**: 861–4.

✳ 55 Prigent A, Cosgriff P, Gates GF, *et al.* Consensus report on quality control of quantitative measurements of renal function obtained from the renogram: International Consensus Committee of Radionuclides in Nephrourology. *Semin Nucl Med* 1999; **29**: 146–59.

✳ 56 BNMS guidelines. Dynamic renal radionuclide studies. www.bnms.org.uk/bnms.htm 2003.

57 Piepsz A, Tondeur M, Ham H. Relative ^{99m}Tc-MAG3 renal uptake: reproducibility and accuracy. *J Nucl Med* 1999; **40**: 972–6.

58 Moonen M, Jacobsson L, Granerus G, Friberg P, Volkmann R. Determination of split renal function from gamma camera renography: a study of three methods. *Nucl Med Commun* 1994; **15**: 704–11.

59 Britton KE, Al Nahhas AA, Jafri RA, Bomanji J, Solanki K, Nimmon CC. ^{99m}Tc MAG3 - a renal radiopharmaceutical in routine use. In: *Proceedings of the 18th International Symposium on Radioactive Isotopes in Clinical Medicine and Research, Badgastein.* Höfer R, Bergmann H (editors). Stuttgart: Schattauer, 1988; pp. 321–2.

60 Rutland MD, Que L. A comparison of the renal handling of ^{99}Tc^m-DTPA and ^{99}Tc^m-MAG3 in hypertensive patients using an uptake technique. *Nucl Med Commun* 1999; **20**: 823–8.

● 61 Fleming JS, Cosgriff PS, Houston AS, *et al.* UK audit of relative renal function measurement using DMSA scintigraphy. *Nucl Med Commun* 1998; **19**: 989–97.

● 62 Brown NJG, Britton KE. The renogram and its quantitation. *Br J Urol* 1969; **41(Suppl)**: 15–25.

● 63 Kenny RW, Ackery DM, Fleming JS, Goddard BA, Grant RW. Deconvolution analysis of the scintillation camera renography *Br J Radiol* 1975; **48**: 481–6.

64 Reeve J, Crawley JC, Goldberg AD, *et al.* Abnormalities of renal transport of sodium *o*-[^{131}I]iodohippurate (hippuran) in essential hypertension. *Clin Sci Mol Med* 1978; **55**: 241–7.

65 Rutland MD. A comprehensive analysis of renal DTPA studies. I. Theory and normal values. *Nucl Med Commun* 1985; **6**: 11–20.

66 Russell CD, Japanwalla M, Khan S, Scott JW, Dubovsky EV. Techniques for measuring renal transit time. *Eur J Nucl Med* 1995; **22**: 1372–8.

67 Piepsz A, Ham HR, Erbsmann F, *et al.* A co-operative study on the clinical value of dynamic renal scanning with deconvolution analysis. *Br J Radiol* 1982; **55**: 419–33.

● 68 Gruenewald SM, Collins LT. Renovascular hypertension: quantitative renography as a screening test. *Radiology* 1983; **149**: 287–91.

● 69 Gruenewald SM, Stewart JH, Simmons KC, Crocker EF. Predictive value of quantitative renography for successful treatment of atherosclerotic renovascular hypertension. *Aust NZ J Med* 1985; **15**: 617–22.

70 Russell CD, Japanwalla M, Khan S, Scott JW, Dubovsky EV. Renal vascular transit times and tubular transit time dispersion for ^{99m}Tc-MAG3. *Nucl Med Commun* 1997; **18**: 832–8.

● 71 Lupton EW, Lawson RS, Shields RA, Testa HJ. Diuresis renography and parenchymal transit times in the assessment of renal pelvic dilatation. *Nucl Med Commun* 1984; **5**: 451–9.

72 Ilgin N, Iftehar SA, Vural G, Bozkirli I, Gokcora N. Evaluation of renal function following treatment with extra corporeal shock wave lithotripsy ESWL: the use of whole kidney parenchymal and pelvic transit times. *Nucl Med Commun* 1998; **19**: 155–9.

● 73 Prvulovich EM, Bomanji JB, Waddington WA, *et al.* Clinical evaluation of technetium-99m L,L-ethylenedicysteine in patients with chronic renal failure. *J Nucl Med* 1997; **38**: 809–14.

● 74 Datseris I, Bomanji JB, Brown EA, *et al.* Captopril renal scintigraphy in patients with hypertension and chronic renal failure. *J Nucl Med* 1994; **35**: 251–4.

● 75 Rutland MD. A comprehensive analysis of renal DTPA studies II. Renal transplant evaluation. *Nucl Med Commun* 1985; **6**: 21–30.

76 Gonzales A, Puchal R, Bajen MT, *et al.* ^{99}Tc^m-MAG3 renogram deconvolution in normal subjects in normal functioning kidney grafts. *Nucl Med Commun* 1994; **15**: 680–4.

77 Gemmell HG, Smith FW, Innes A, Edward N, Catto GR. The value of Tc-DTPA transit times and

NMRT1 measurements in monitoring the progress of renal transplants. *Nucl Med Commun* 1985; **6**: 67–74.

● 78 Chaiwatanarat T, Loarpatanaskul S, Poshyachinda M, *et al.* Deconvolution analysis of renal blood flow: evaluation of postrenal transplant complications. *J Nucl Med* 1994; **35**: 1792–6.

79 Mizuiri S, Hayashi I, Takano M, *et al.* Fractional mean transit time in transplanted kidneys studied by technetium-99m DTPA: comparison of clinical and biopsy findings. *J Nucl Med* 1994; **35**: 84–9.

● 80 Gruenewald SM, Nimmon CC, Nawaz MK, Britton KE. A non invasive γ-camera technique for the measurement of intra renal flow distribution in man. *Clin Science* 1981; **6**: 385–9.

81 Britton KE, Nawaz MK, Nimmon CC, *et al.* Total and intrarenal flow distribution in healthy subjects. Technique, acute effects of ibopamine and of indoramin. *Nephron* 1986; **43**: 265–73.

● 82 Chasis H, Redish J, Golding W, Ranges HA. The use of sodium *p*-aminohippurate for the functional evaluation of the human kidney. *J Clin Invest* 1945; **24**: 583–9.

Non-imaging radionuclide assessment of renal function

A. MICHAEL PETERS

INTRODUCTION

Radionuclide assessment of renal function without imaging is based on two general measurements: (1) clearance and (2) body fluid volumes. Compounds of interest with respect to clearance include (1) hippurates, for measuring so-called effective renal plasma flow, and (2) inulin, ^{99m}Tc-diethylenetriaminepentaacetic acid (^{99m}Tc-DTPA), ^{51}Cr-ethylenediaminetetraacetic acid (^{51}Cr-EDTA), and radiological contrast for measuring glomerular filtration rate (GFR). ^{99m}Tc-mercaptoacetyltriglycine (^{99m}Tc-MAG$_3$) clearance is also occasionally measured as a test of renal function. Body fluid volumes of interest in relation to renal function include plasma volume, extracellular fluid volume (ECFV) and total body water (TBW). Lean body mass (LBM), measured by dual photon X-ray absorptiometry, is closely related to TBW. With respect to fluid volumes, only ECFV will be considered in this chapter.

CLEARANCE

Clearance can be defined as a virtual volume of fluid from which an indicator or tracer (used interchangably in this chapter) is completely extracted in unit time, and, accordingly, has units of mL min^{-1} (or mL min^{-1} g^{-1} or mL min^{-1} mL^{-1} when normalized to tissue mass or volume); i.e. units of flow (or perfusion). It can be applied to 'moving' fluid (when indicator is extracted from flowing blood) or to 'static' fluid (when indicator, for example, moves from an organ or tissue compartment into blood or into an adjacent compartment). In the case of the former, clearance is equal to the product of blood flow and indicator extraction fraction. In the case of a fluid compartment, clearance from that compartment is equal to the removal rate of indicator (mg min^{-1}) divided by indicator concentration (mg mL^{-1}) in the compartment. So if the concentration is 100 mg L^{-1} and the flux 10 mg min^{-1}, then 10% of 1 L of compartmental fluid will have been cleared in 1 min, representing a clearance of 100 mL min^{-1}.

There are several forms of clearance: blood clearance, plasma clearance, free-water clearance, organ clearance, whole-body clearance and urinary clearance. Blood or plasma clearance is the volume of blood or plasma from which indicator is removed per unit of time. For indicators freely distributed between red cells and plasma (e.g. ^{133}Xe) blood and plasma clearances are identical, but for tracers confined to plasma (e.g. ^{51}Cr-EDTA), plasma clearance is lower than blood clearance and is equal to

$$C \times (1 - h)$$

where C is the blood clearance and h is the hematocrit (i.e. packed cell volume).

Organ blood or plasma clearance is the volume of blood or plasma cleared in unit time of tracer taken up by that organ. Whole-body blood or plasma clearance is the sum of blood or plasma clearances of all organs contributing to the removal of the indicator from blood or plasma, and is therefore identical to blood or plasma clearance, depending on the properties of the indicator. Urinary clearance is the volume of blood or plasma cleared of tracer that is excreted in urine. ^{99m}Tc-dimercaptosuccinic acid (^{99m}Tc-DMSA) is a good example to illustrate these clearances.[1] Thus, because it does not enter red cells, blood clearance ($\approx$100 mL min^{-1}) exceeds plasma clearance ($\approx$60 mL min^{-1}). Plasma clearance, in turn, is greater than renal (plasma) clearance ($\approx$35 mL min^{-1}) because other tissues also accumulate it, whilst its urinary (plasma) clearance is lower still ($\approx$7 mL min^{-1}) since about 80% of tracer taken up by the kidney is retained in the parenchyma. In contrast, for ^{51}Cr-EDTA, plasma, renal, and urinary clearances are all essentially identical because no other tissue takes it up and because all tracer taken up by the kidney ultimately appears in the urine. Just as blood clearance is higher than plasma clearance for a tracer unable to enter red cells, plasma clearance is higher than plasma water clearance because dissolved solutes, mainly macromolecules, make a small volumetric contribution to plasma volume.

MEASUREMENT OF CLEARANCE

Clearance may be measured under steady state or non-steady state conditions. In general, radionuclide techniques are used to measure clearance under non-steady state conditions; i.e. following bolus injection of tracer. Measurement of single organ clearance requires imaging, unless it is the only organ accumulating tracer in which case organ clearance is identical to plasma or blood clearance. Plasma clearance is measured by dividing the amount of tracer administered by the area under the plasma time–concentration curve between zero time and infinity. If the tracer freely distributes between red cells and plasma, then the concentration will be the same for whole blood and plasma and the clearances therefore the same; if confined to plasma, the whole-blood concentration will be less than plasma concentration, so the area under the clearance curve will be smaller and the quotient (and therefore clearance) larger.

MEASUREMENT OF GLOMERULAR FILTRATION RATE

Measurement of glomerular filtration rate (GFR) is based on clearance measurements of indicators that do not bind to plasma proteins, do not enter the intracellular compartment (including red cells) and are cleared from plasma exclusively by glomerular filtration. Such indicators include inulin, ^{51}Cr-EDTA, ^{99m}Tc-DTPA, ^{125}I-iothalamate and radiological contrast agents, such as iohexol, and can be called filtration markers. The requirements of an ideal filtration marker are:

- Free filtration at the glomerulus
- No binding to red cells or plasma proteins
- No extra-renal uptake (unless it is completely reversible, as in the interstitial fluid space)
- No tubular secretion (although provided the indicator is completely retained in the tubular epithelium, tubular re-absorption is theoretically allowed if plasma clearance is being measured)

- No diffusion across the tubular membrane following filtration; this occurs at its extreme in acute tubular necrosis, but also at lower rates in other clinically less obvious forms of tubular injury.[2]

GFR can be measured either under steady state or non-steady state conditions. The classical method involves the measurement of the urinary clearance of inulin at steady state. Under such circumstances, the product of urinary flow rate and urinary concentration is equal to the product of GFR and plasma concentration. The technique, however, is cumbersome, difficult to perform, and essentially obsolete for routine clinical use and has been replaced by the bolus injection technique with measurement of plasma clearance under non-steady state conditions.

The plasma clearance curve of a filtration marker following bolus intravenous injection is conventionally described as *bi*-exponential over 4 h. The first exponential, which lasts up to about 2 h, is taken to represent exchange of indicator between plasma and interstitial fluid of the whole body. This is a misrepresentation of the true kinetics because the clearance curve actually consists of three exponentials. Although this is obvious from arterial sampling[3–5] (Fig. 8B.1), the first exponential, which lasts only about 20 min, is attenuated on antecubital venous sampling because it is the result of tracer exchanging across capillary endothelium throughout the body, a large component of which is in muscle and skin, including the forearm. The first exponential has the largest zero-time intercept of the three exponentials. This is evident from a venous clearance curve when the sum of the intercepts of the second and third exponentials (conventionally the first and second) are summed and divided into the injected dose. When the

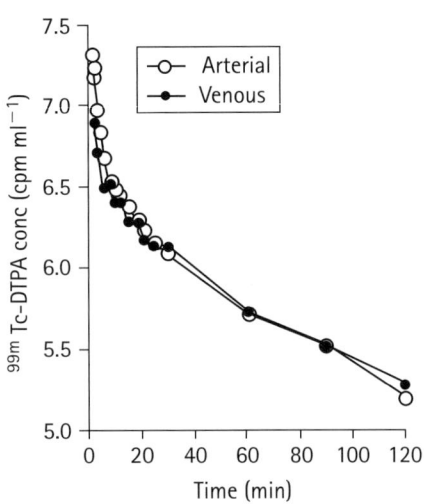

Figure 8B.1 *Arterial (unfilled circles) and venous (filled circles) concentrations up to 120 min following intravenous injection of ^{99m}Tc-DTPA in a subject with normal renal function. Note the logarithmic ordinate and presence of a fast early exponential up to about 30 min.*

indicator is ^{99m}Tc-DTPA (MW 500 Da), this generates a volume of about 10 L instead of plasma volume (3 L)[5,6] which would be generated if the first exponential did not exist. Interestingly, the volume so generated varies inversely with molecular size of the indicator, being about 7 L for inulin[6] (MW 6 kDa) and about 12 L for bromide anion.[5] The second exponential (conventionally the first) represents exchange of tracer between subcompartments in the interstitial space.[3,4,7,8] These subcompartments are in series[3,4] rather than in parallel[7,8] (i.e. the tracer moves between plasma and the first subcompartment before penetrating a deeper subcompartment) and presumably correspond to the so-called fluid and gel phases of the interstitial space.[9] The gel phase consists largely of a matrix of huge macromolecules called glycosaminoglycans (GAGs) that is penetrated by diffusible solutes at rates inversely dependent on molecular size. The third exponential, that the clearance curve approaches by about 2 h after injection, represents GFR; indeed, as discussed further below it is close to the fractional rate at which the extracellular fluid is filtered at the glomerulus.

Since plasma clearance is equal to the administered amount of tracer divided by the entire area under the plasma clearance curve, and since the area under an individual exponential is equal to its zero time intercept divided by its rate constant, the formal equation for GFR is

$$\text{GFR} = \frac{\text{administered activity}}{A/\alpha_1 + B/\alpha_2 + C/\alpha_3}. \tag{8B.1}$$

where A/α_1, B/α_2 and C/α_3 each correspond to one of the three exponentials.

Because the first exponential (A/α_1) is brief, its enclosed area is small and it can be ignored, giving the simplified equation

$$\text{GFR} = \frac{\text{administered activity}}{B/\alpha_2 + C/\alpha_3}. \tag{8B.2}$$

Because the terminal exponential reflects GFR, it is an acceptable approximation to base GFR on the curve recorded between 2 and 4 h. This gives the even more simplified equation

$$\text{GFR} = \frac{\text{administered activity}}{C/\alpha_3}. \tag{8B.3}$$

The area given by B/α_2 in Eqn 8B.2 is not negligible so this approach, widely known as the one compartment simplification, overestimates GFR by an amount which broadly depends on the area recorded under the third exponential. Because this latter area varies inversely with GFR, the error introduced by ignoring B/α_2 decreases with decreasing function but is about 15% at normal filtration function. Because of this relation, the recorded GFR can be corrected by a sliding factor that has a magnitude dependent on the

recorded value of GFR or α_3. Several formulae or 'algorithms', that are generally second order polynomials (i.e. have the form $y = a + bx + cx^2$), have been described for making this correction. Most are based on GFR[10–12] but one is based on α_3.[13] They all make the assumption that, from person to person, α_2 is invariable and that the intercept C is constant in relation to B. Because GFR obviously varies with body size, it must be scaled to body size, conventionally to a body surface area of 1.73 m^2 (see below), prior to the application of an algorithm based on GFR. It is more rational, however, to use α_3 since this is the variable which, in the presence of constant α_2 and B/C, is the primary determinant of the error arising from the erroneous assumption that the filtration marker distributes instantaneously throughout a single, well-mixed compartment.

The ratio, administered activity/C, is a volume. It is an approximation to and exceeds the volume of distribution of the filtration marker, V_d, and would be equal to V_d if the indicator *did* mix instantaneously throughout its volume of distribution immediately after injection. As such, Eqn 8B.3 can be rearranged to give GFR in terms of the product of α_3 and an approximate volume of distribution, V_d', i.e.

$$\text{GFR} \simeq V_d' \times \alpha_3. \tag{8B.4}$$

Simplified worked example

This is intended only as a summary of the technique; it is suggested that for more details on the practical aspects of GFR measurement, the recently published British Nuclear Medicine Guidelines be consulted.[14]

1. Make up indicator, e.g. ^{51}Cr-EDTA, in solution ready for injection.
2. Add x units of indicator to a flask containing 1 L of water. Mix completely and remove 1 mL (the standard) for counting in a well counter.
3. Administer the rest, y units, to the patient by intravenous injection. The exact amounts added to the flask and given to the patient (or at least their ratio, x/y) are best measured by weighing the syringes before and after each expulsion.
4. Take venous blood samples of 10 mL each from the arm opposite to the one injected with indicator at about 2, 3, and 4 h after injection, noting the exact time in each case.
5. Centrifuge the blood samples and remove 1 mL plasma from each for counting in a well counter along with the standard. Higher volumes may be counted but should then be matched by the volume of the standard counted and appropriate adjustments made to step 10 (below).
6. Measure the concentration of indicator in each plasma sample and in the standard (as counts per milliliter).
7. Plot the values for plasma on semi-logarithmic graph paper, or use a hand-held calculator, to calculate the half-life of the straight line fitted to the three points.

8. Calculate α_3 from the half-life ($T_{1/2}$), i.e.
   $\alpha_3 = 0.693/T_{1/2}$.
9. Extrapolate the line back to zero time to obtain the plasma counts per mL at zero time.
10. Compare the counts per mL in plasma at zero time (N_{plasma}) with the counts per milliliter in the standard (N_{std}); V'_d in liters is then equal to

$$\frac{N_{std}}{N_{plasma}} \times \frac{y}{x}.$$

11. Then the one-compartment GFR $= \alpha_3 \times V'_d$.
12. To correct for the one-compartment simplification and to scale for body size either
    (i) scale the GFR to $1.73\,m^2$ (having calculated the patient's body surface area from height and weight and a suitable formula – see below) and then correct the GFR/$1.73\,m^2$ using an algorithm based on GFR; or
    (ii) correct the GFR using an algorithm based on α_3 *before* scaling to $1.73\,m^2$

When GFR is measured in patients with severe renal decompensation, it needs to be measured accurately to be of any clinical use. Measurement, however, is difficult in such patients using the bolus injection, plasma clearance technique because it is not regarded as reliable when the GFR is less than about $20\,mL\,min^{-1}$ per $1.73\,m^2$, even though the one compartment assumption leads to almost no error at this level of filtration. Thus, bolus injection of ^{51}Cr-EDTA with sampling at 3–5 h overestimates GFR by almost 50% compared with steady state urinary inulin clearance,[15] suggesting delayed indicator mixing. Delayed mixing, even if only minimal, takes on greater importance in renal failure since in the presence of greatly impaired filtration, there is more time for indicator to diffuse into fluid spaces that are slowly penetrated, thereby overestimating clearance. Several groups have approached the problem of renal failure by taking very delayed samples (i.e. the day following injection) using iohexol[16] or ^{51}Cr-EDTA.[17] This approach, however, has been inadequately validated and, aside from the problems of delayed mixing, is subject to error through two possible further mechanisms: firstly, binding of indicator to plasma protein that increases as a function of time and, secondly, the diurnal variation in GFR. A further simplification of GFR measurement is to use a single sample. The rationale of this can be appreciated from Figure 8B.2, which shows that, everything else being equal (i.e. kinetics of distribution, time up to complete mixing of indicator throughout the ECFV, and relative volumes of various subcompartments), the concentration to which the indicator falls up to a specified time after injection is dependent only on α_3 and hence on GFR. The immediate result, i.e. the measured plasma concentration is compared with the administered activity to derive a virtual distribution volume (V_t), which is an inverse function of GFR. By plotting V_t against a

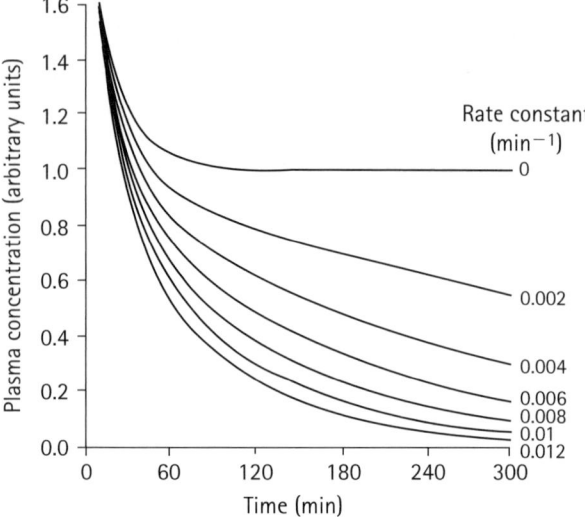

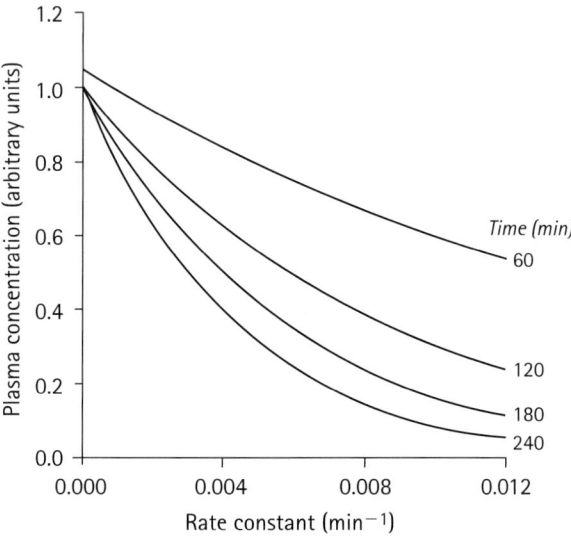

Figure 8B.2 *Basis of one-sample methods for measuring glomerular filtration rate (GFR) which generate a virtual volume of indicator distribution equal to the quotient, administered activity divided by sample concentration. The decrease in concentration (arbitrary units) between the time of injection and the time of sampling depends on (1) the actual volume of distribution of the indicator, (2) the rate of equilibration of the indicator throughout this volume of distribution, and (3) GFR. The illustrations are based on a bi-exponential plasma clearance in which the zero-time intercepts of the two exponentials are identical and the fast exponential has a rate constant of $0.05\,min^{-1}$. Upper panel: the relationship between plasma concentration and sampling time for different rate constants of the terminal exponential; lower panel: the relationship between plasma concentration and terminal rate constant for different sampling times.*

multi-sample measurement of GFR that can be regarded as a 'gold standard' in a large population of individuals, regression equations have been derived from which a single prospective measurement of V_t can be converted to a GFR value.[18,19] Whilst single-sample techniques are clearly less labor-intensive than multi-sample techniques and by and large appear to be reliable, any errors in an individual measurement remain silent, so quality assurance is a problem.

EXTRACTION FRACTION

The proportion of indicator entering an organ in arterial blood that is retained in the organ during a single pass is called the extraction faction, E, and

$$E = \frac{C_a(t) - C_v(t)}{C_a(t)} \qquad (8B.5)$$

where C_a and C_v, the arterial and organ venous indicator concentrations, respectively, are dependent on time in the non-steady state situation. If E is unity then blood flow, Q, is equal to clearance, Z, otherwise

$$E = \frac{Z}{Q}. \qquad (8B.6)$$

Invasive techniques, such as renal vein catheterization, are required to measure E.

The extraction fraction of a filtration marker is the quotient GFR/renal plasma flow (RPF), and is normally 0.2. Understanding E is important with respect to the use of hippurates or MAG_3 to measure renal plasma flow, since the assumption is made that the renal extraction fraction is unity, so that $Z = Q$, and renal plasma flow is equal to plasma clearance. For hippurates and even more so for MAG_3, extraction fraction is less than unity, especially in renal disease, and for hippurates may fall to values as low as 50%.[19,20] This fact is acknowledged by the use of the term effective renal plasma flow (ERPF) which may be significantly less than RPF, especially when it is based on MAG_3. Some drugs, such as angiotensin-converting enzyme inhibitors[20] and cyclosporin[21] have been shown to decrease hippurate extraction fraction even further so that ERPF is virtually uninterpretable without knowledge of renal venous concentration.

TRANSIT (RESIDENCE) TIME AND DISTRIBUTION VOLUME

After intravenous injection, an indicator mixes throughout its distribution volume (V_d). If the indicator is not cleared or cleared very slowly from that volume, then its concentration in plasma will obviously become essentially constant when mixing is completed. Moreover, it will remain in the volume for a long time and its mean transit time, T, through (or residence time in) the volume will be infinitely long. For substances that are not cleared slowly, mean transit time through the distribution volume can be measured

from the parameters of the plasma clearance curve following bolus injection using the equation

$$T = \frac{A/\alpha_1^2 + B/\alpha_2^2 + C/\alpha_3^2}{A/\alpha_1 + B/\alpha_2 + C/\alpha_3}. \qquad (8B.7)$$

On the basis of the same principles as for simplification of GFR measurement, this equation can be simplified:

$$T = \frac{B/\alpha_2^2 + C/\alpha_3^2}{B/\alpha_2 + C/\alpha_3}. \qquad (8B.8)$$

Further simplification leads to

$$T = \frac{C/\alpha_3^2}{C/\alpha_3} \qquad (8B.9)$$

which reduces to

$$T = \frac{1}{\alpha_3}.$$

Just as second-order polynomials have been derived that correct GFR for the one-compartment assumption, one has also been published that relates true T to $1/\alpha_3$.[22]

Residence time is directly proportional to the distribution volume and inversely proportional to clearance; i.e.

$$T = \frac{V_d}{Z} \qquad (8B.10)$$

or

$$V_d = T \times Z. \qquad (8B.11)$$

Filtration markers have a physiological distribution volume close to ECFV. The anatomical limits of this volume are difficult to define because, although the great majority of the ECFV is accessible to such indicators, small subcompartments are variably penetrated by them depending on indicator molecular size. Moreover, the accessible ECFV appears to be heterogeneous, consisting of two subcompartments, the gel and fluid phases, that have volumes that are functions of the molecular sizes of the indicators used to measure them, as discussed above. In general, however, once an indicator has penetrated and mixed throughout its distribution volume, its disappearance rate, both from plasma and interstitial fluid, expressed as the fractional rate constant α_3, is a positive function of GFR and a negative function of distribution volume. This rate constant is therefore an expression of GFR which is already indexed to ECFV[22,23] and has been used on its own as a measurement of GFR in what has become known as the slope only technique (in distinction to the conventional slope–intercept

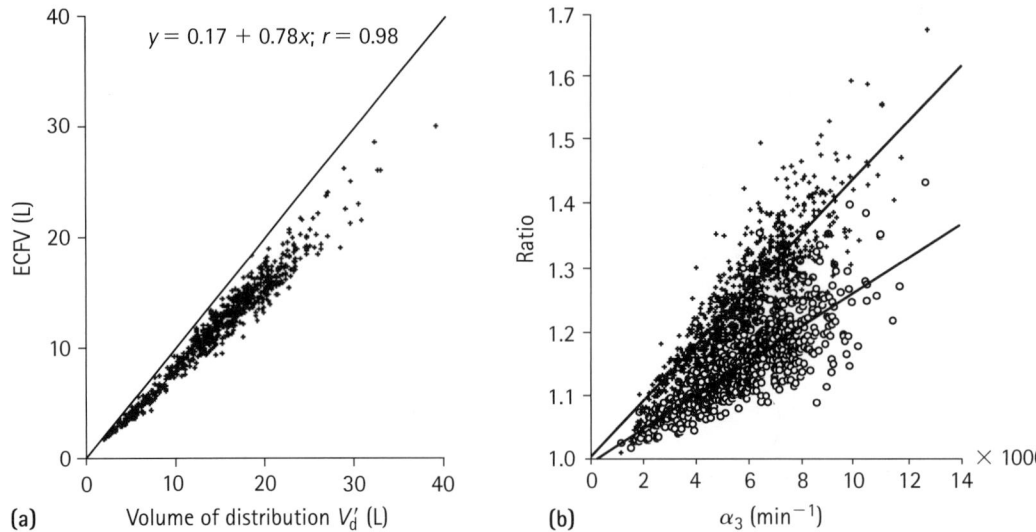

Figure 8B.3 *(a) The relationship between volume of distribution (V'_d), calculated as administered activity divided by intercept of terminal exponential and not indexed for body size, and ECFV (calculated as GFR divided by GFR/ECFV, both corrected for the one-compartment assumption[10,22]) in 753 routine clinical studies in which three accurately timed blood samples were taken at about 120, 180 and 240 min. The line is the regression line. Note that, across the entire range of renal function V'_d overestimates ECFV on average by 22%. (b) The overestimation of ECFV by V'_d (expressed as the ratio V'_d/ECFV; filled circles: y = 1.0 + 0.044; r = 0.89) is dependent on α_3, exceeding ECFV by more than 30% in the presence of normal filtration function. Raw GFR (uncorrected for the one-compartment assumption) also overestimates corrected GFR (expressed as their ratio; unfilled circles: r = 0.99 + 0.027; r = 0.8) but not as much as V'_d overestimates ECFV. The lines are regression lines.*

technique). Although α_3 approximates to GFR/ECFV (which, like α_3, has units of mL min^{-1} mL^{-1}), it slightly underestimates it because of the one-compartment assumption. Indeed, a concentration gradient becomes established between interstitial fluid and plasma throughout the body in which interstitial concentration is normally about 15% higher. This gradient, which can be quantified theoretically,[24] has been confirmed by direct measurement in the forearm[25] and must exist otherwise indicator would never be cleared from the interstitial fluid space. The greater α_3, the greater the concentration gradient and the more α_3 underestimates GFR/ECFV. The plasma–interstitial fluid concentration gradient is zero when α_3 is zero, i.e. when there is no filtration function. The extent to which α_3 underestimates GFR/ECFV is always smaller than the corresponding error in GFR arising from the one-compartment assumption[22] (Fig. 8B.3). For the body in general, but not the kidneys, the venous plasma concentration of a filtration marker soon exceeds the arterial concentration by an amount that is also a function of α_3. Early on in the plasma clearance curve, however, during the process of mixing, arterial concentration is higher than venous as tracer penetrates the extravascular space. This whole-body ateriovenous gradient reverses at about 20 min, and this is the time at which intravascular and extravascular concentrations are transiently equal. Although arterial and extra-renal venous time–concentration curves therefore have slightly different time courses, the total areas enclosed under them between time zero and infinity are identical.

For filtration markers, V_d is usually approximated (to V'_d) in routine clinical practice by dividing the intercept of the terminal exponential of the clearance curve into the injected dose (see Eqn 8B.4). V'_d overestimates true V_d because substantial amounts of indicator are lost through glomerular filtration between injection and the completion of mixing throughout the distribution volume, which takes about 2 h (Fig. 8B.3a). T and Z can both be measured from the parameters of a multisample clearance curve and used in Eqn 8B.11 to calculate 'true' V_d (i.e. ECFV), which, in standard man, is normally about 13 L.[24,26–28] It is worth noting that the overestimation of V_d by V'_d is greater than the overestimation of GFR resulting from the one-compartment assumption. Thus, re-arranging Eqn 8B.4 gives

$$V'_d = \frac{GFR}{\alpha_3}. \qquad (8B.12)$$

Now GFR in Eqn 8B.12 is already overestimated by the one-compartment assumption while α_3 is an underestimation of GFR/ECFV (as explained above), so V_d must be overestimated to an even greater extent than GFR (Fig. 8B.3b).

Extraction fraction (E), clearance ($Z = Q \times E$), transit time (T), and distribution volume ($T \times Z$) are all closely related and important variables in renal nuclear medicine and are summarized in Table 8B.1 for various commonly used renal radiopharmaceuticals.

Table 8B.1   *Kinetics of commonly used renal radiopharmaceuticals*

Tracer	Plasma clearance (renal clearance), Z (mL min^{-1})	Renal extraction fraction, E	whole body mean transit time, T (min)	Volume of distribution, V (mL)
DTPA/EDTA	120 (120)	0.2	104	12 500
MAG$_3$	350 (300)	0.5	15	5250
Hippuran	500 (500)	0.8	15	7500
DMSA	60 (35)	0.06	120	7200

DTPA, diethylenetriaminepentaacetic acid; EDTA, ethylenediaminetetraacetic acid; MAG$_3$, mercaptoacetyltriglycine; DMSA, dimercaptosuccinic acid. Data for MAG$_3$ are from Peters *et al.*[53] Data for DMSA are from Peters *et al.*[1] *Note:* $V = T \times Z$.

INDEXING GLOMERULAR FILTRATION RATE TO BODY SIZE

Routine clinical measurement of GFR is performed in three main patient groups:

- Nephro-urological disease, to quantify renal disease and monitor renal function
- Cancer, to predict the toxicity of renally excreted anti-cancer drugs which, although not nephrotoxic, are toxic to other organs, especially bone marrow
- Diseases that are effectively treated by drugs which, although not principally excreted through the kidneys, are nevertheless nephrotoxic, for example cyclosporin in the treatment of psoriasis and platinum-based drugs used in the treatment of cancer.

The interpretation of the derived value for GFR differs in the three circumstances. In nephro-urological disease, it is necessary to know GFR in relation to the body dimensions of the individual and therefore to scale it (or index it) to a whole-body variable. Body surface area (BSA) is the variable conventionally used as the reference for indexing and can be estimated from published relationships between height, weight and BSA[29,30] using the general equation

$$\mathrm{BSA} = aw^b \times h^c$$

where w is weight, in kilograms; h is height, in centimeters; and a, b, and c are all constants. In one such equation, described by Haycock *et al.*,[30] a, b, and c are 0.024265, 0.5378, and 0.3964, respectively.

In cancer, GFR is measured in order to maximize the therapeutic benefit of a drug whilst minimizing its toxicity, so it is desirable to know the unscaled GFR of the individual since this will determine the area under the plasma drug concentration–time curve.[31] For recipients of nephrotoxic drugs, it makes little difference whether an absolute or indexed value is used (unless the patient is still growing) since the main goal of GFR measurement is longitudinal assessment for the detection of drug-induced deterioration. Nevertheless, it is usually required to know the baseline renal status so an indexed value is preferable.

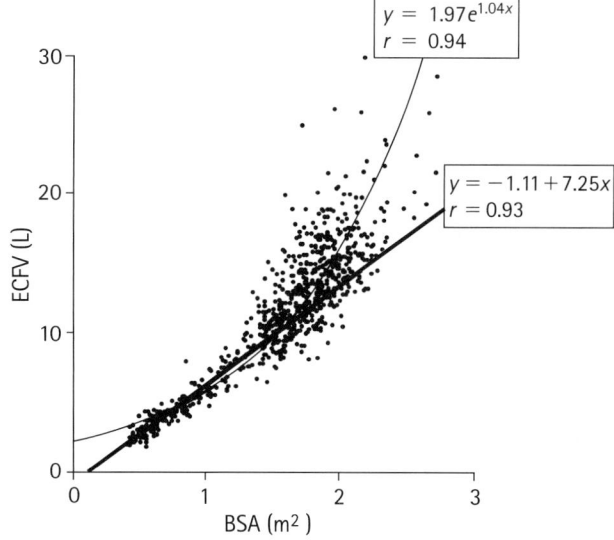

$$y = 1.97e^{1.04x}$$
$$r = 0.94$$

$$y = -1.11 + 7.25x$$
$$r = 0.93$$

Figure 8B.4   *Relationship between ECFV and body surface area (BSA) in the same 753 routine clinical studies shown in Fig. 8B.3 with blood sampling at 120, 180, and 240 min after injection. ECFV was calculated as GFR divided by GFR/ECFV, both corrected for the one-compartment assumption.*[10,22] *The curved line is the exponential fit to all points. The straight, bold line is the linear fit to patients with BSA $< 1.36\,m^2$ (i.e. children; n = 184).*

Several authors have questioned the value of BSA, not only as an index for GFR but also as an index for other physiological variables such as cardiac output.[32] Alternatives that have been suggested with respect to GFR include TBW,[33] LBM,[34,35] plasma volume,[36] the square of height,[37] and ECFV.[22,38–41] Recent attention has focussed on ECFV (Fig. 8B.4) and evidence has been presented to suggest that it is physiologically more appropriate than BSA for indexing GFR, especially in children.[27,38,40,41] This is not surprising as it is intuitive that GFR should be indexed to a volumetric variable rather than one based on area. Moreover, the prime function of glomerular filtration is to regulate the volume and composition of the ECF. α_3, by itself, is a close approximation to GFR/ECFV and can therefore be used as a convenient and attractive expression of GFR that is already indexed for the size of the individual. Injected activity, corrections for radionuclide decay and preparation of a standard are not required, avoiding several potential sources of error. GFR/ECFV, however, is always greater than α_3 by an amount that is a nonlinear function of α_3, but, as already mentioned, the relation between them can be defined by a second-order polynomial from which α_3 can be multiplied by a correction factor (greater than unity) based on itself to give 'true' GFR/ECFV.[21]

In infants and small children, GFR/ECFV is a closer reflection of true filtration function than GFR/BSA.[27,40,41] In general, GFR/ECFV shows a tendency to remain unchanged in circumstances in which ECFV may depart significantly from normal. Thus, GFR decreases reversibly as a result of hypovolemia[42] but GFR/ECFV changes less and more accurately reflects the fact that no renal decompensation exists. GFR is, however, closely defended so it does not necessarily follow changes in ECFV in a linear fashion. Moreover, whilst normal men have a slightly higher value of GFR/BSA (130 mL min^{-1} per 1.73 m^2) compared with normal women (120 mL min^{-1} per 1.73 m^2), the two genders have identical values of GFR/ECFV.[26] Indeed, α_3 seems to be a biological constant insofar as it varies little between several species in which it has been measured with values close to 0.01 min^{-1} in dogs of widely varying size, human children and adults, calves, and horses.[43] There are, moreover, several examples in clinical practice where GFR/BSA clearly increases or decreases but because of parallel changes in ECFV, GFR/ECFV changes less, e.g. diabetes mellitus,[44–46] pituitary dysfunction,[47,48] normal pregnancy,[49,50] and the short term physiological response to surgery.[51]

In clinical practice, GFR/ECFV, indexed to an ECFV of 12.9 L,[41] generally shows good agreement with GFR/BSA indexed to a BSA of 1.73 m^2 [22,40] (Fig. 8B.5), except in children in whom filtration function is apparently better when GFR is indexed to ECFV instead of BSA.[27,41] This arises from the fact that children have a high BSA in relation to their weight, just as a concrete sphere the size of a golf ball has a higher area to weight ratio than a concrete sphere the size of a football. Consequently, the difference between GFR/BSA and GFR/ECFV increases as a function of surface area (Fig. 8B.6). Interestingly, although for any shape – cylindrical, spherical or cuboid – the ratio of volume (or weight) to surface area increases as a nonlinear function of surface area, weight to surface area ratio in humans is a remarkably close linear function of surface area, indicating that humans change shape as they grow[41] (Fig. 8B.7), thereby further undermining the validity of BSA as an indexation variable.

The use of α_3 by itself in the 'slope only' approach is disadvantaged by a critical dependence on accurate measurement of α_3, and three or preferably four blood samples are recommended for its estimation. Accurate measurement of α_3 is less critical in the conventional slope–intercept technique because of the tendency for an error in α_3 to be offset by a resulting opposing error in the intercept.[23] Using a

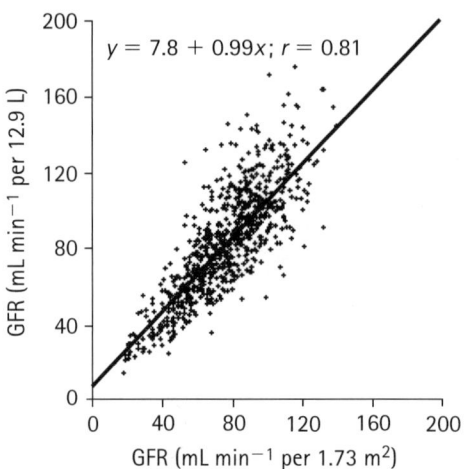

Figure 8B.5   *Correlation between GFR indexed to body surface area and GFR indexed to ECFV in the same 753 routine clinical studies shown in Figs 8B.3 and 8B.4 in which three blood samples were taken at 120, 180, and 240 min. GFR per 1.73 m^2 was corrected using the algorithm of Brochner-Mortensen.[10] GFR per liter ECFV was obtained from α_3 using the algorithm of Peters[22] and multiplied by 12.9 (taking ECFV to be 12.9 L in a standard man). The line is the regression line.*

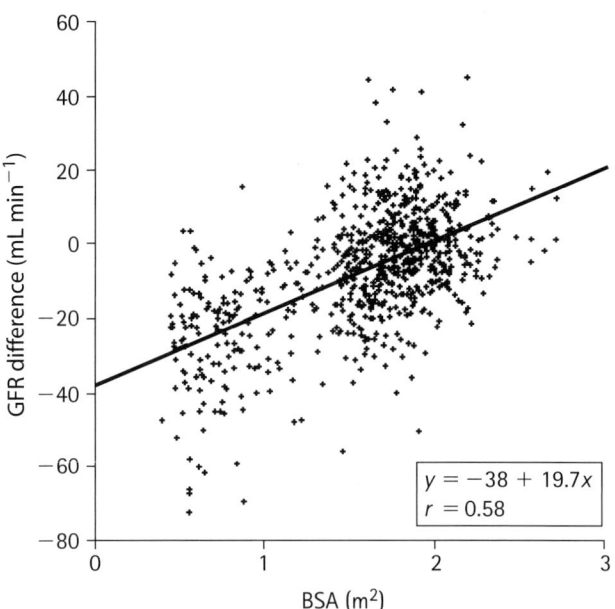

Figure 8B.6   *In children, GFR per 1.73 m^2 is less than GFR per 12.9 L ECFV. Overall, the difference between the two forms of expressing GFR correlates significantly with body surface area. The line is the regression line (n = 753).*

simple calculator, this can be confirmed from Eqn 8B.3. Nevertheless, other errors, such as in the measurement of administered activity and in the preparation of the standard, may adversely affect the accuracy of the slope–intercept technique and diminish its advantage over the slope-only technique[52,53] within which they do not arise. Further errors,

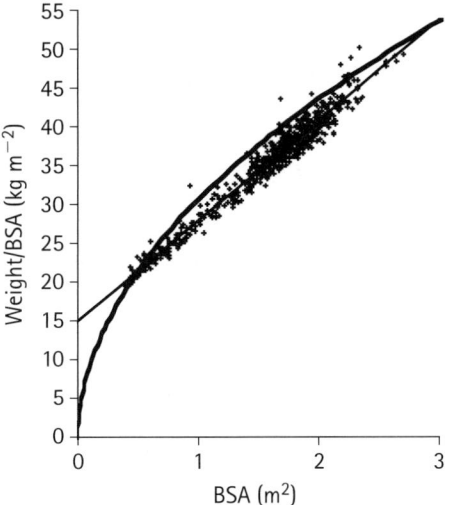

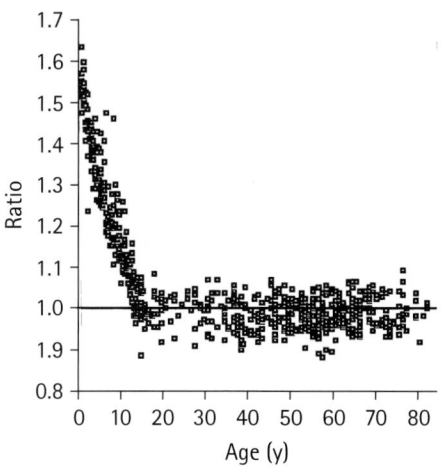

Figure 8B.7   *The volume to surface area ratio of a cylinder of any specific dimensions increases non-linearly with surface area (bold continuous line). In contrast, in humans, the weight per unit surface area increases linearly (fine line = regression line; n = 753), indicating that as they grow humans change shape from a relatively short fat shape to a long thin one and then back to short and fat.*

Figure 8B.8   *In children, GFR indexed to a new equation based on ECFV (see text) exceeds GFR indexed to the Haycock equation. The ratio of the two is expressed as a function of age (n = 753). In adults the ratio is essentially unity.*

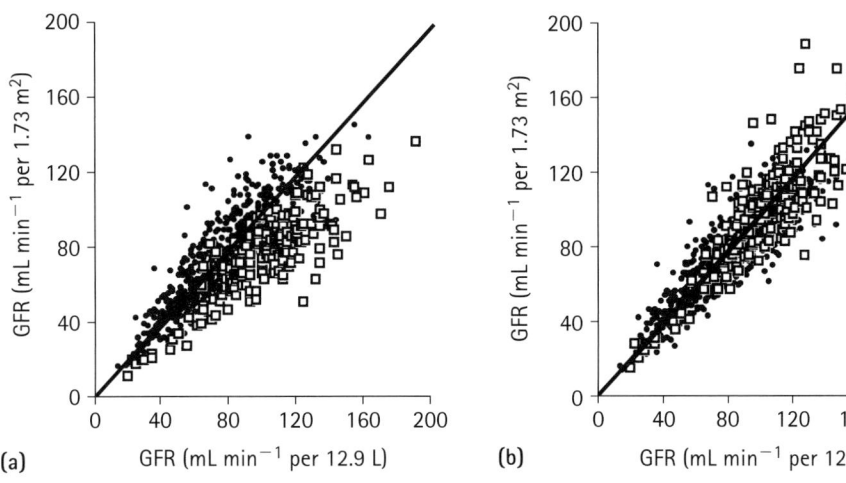

(a)

(b)

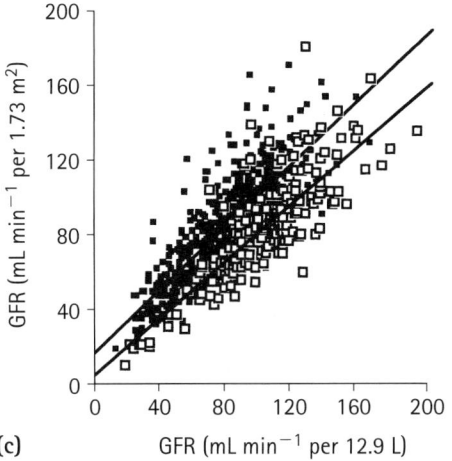

(c)

Figure 8B.9   *(a) In adults, GFR indexed to ECFV agrees reasonably well with GFR indexed to body surface area estimated using the Haycock equation (r = 0.86; n = 569), but in children, the Haycock equation underestimates GFR relative to adults (r = 0.85; n = 184). (b) Replacement of the Haycock equation with a new equation (weighted for ECFV, see text) brings children (r = 0.84) and adults (r = 0.87) 'into line'. (c) Use of the square of height (taking height squared of a standard man as 3 m²) in place of the new equation fails to do this; i.e. continues to underestimate GFR in children (r = 0.82) relative to adults (r = 0.82). The lines in (a) and (b) are the lines of identity and in (c) are the regression lines. Adults are shown as filled symbols and children as unfilled symbols.*

moreover, may arise in the estimation of BSA, especially in patients in whom BSA is difficult to measure, for instance paraplegics, amputees, and the bed-ridden.

An attractive approach to GFR indexation that continues to recognize the differences between children and adults is to use an equation for estimating body size that is weighted towards ECFV rather than BSA. One, analogous to the Haycock[30] and Du Bois[29] equations, i.e. of the form

$$ECFV = aw^b \times h^c$$

has recently been described in which the values of a, b, and c are 0.02154, 0.6469, and 0.7236, respectively, and weight (w) and height (h) are again in kilograms and centimeters.[41] In children, this equation gives higher values of indexed GFR than indexation with the Haycock equation but the two equations give similar values in adults (Fig. 8B.8). Using a reference[41] ECFV of 12.9 L (analogous to a reference BSA of 1.73 m^2) the new equation gives indexed GFR that correlates more closely with GFR/ECFV than does GFR indexed to BSA using the original Haycock equation. Moreover, it abolishes the discrepancy with GFR/ECFV in children that the original equation displays (Fig. 8B.9).

CONCLUSION

Clinical measurement of GFR is now almost exclusively performed in nuclear medicine departments so nuclear medicine physicians have a responsibility to understand the principles of the kinetics of filtration markers. There is a wide range of approaches to the determination of renal function in clinical practice, especially GFR, with the usual trade-off between clinical simplicity and accuracy. A major disadvantage of the single sample techniques is lack of quality control. A reasonable approach, which is not too labour intensive, is to obtain three or four blood samples and either express GFR in relation to ECFV by measuring only α_3 or perform the conventional slope–intercept technique, using α_3 as a means of quality control. Firstly, the correlation coefficient of the fit to the three or four points should exceed 0.99 and, secondly, the value of GFR, indexed either using the original Haycock equation or preferably one weighted towards ECFV, should broadly agree with GFR/13 L ECF. Thus, in a 10-year-old child, an absolute GFR measured by slope–intercept of 60 mL min^{-1} and an α_3 of 0.0075 min^{-1} would be compatible, but in say a large adult, an absolute GFR of 135 mL min^{-1} would not sit comfortably alongside an α_3 of 0.003 min^{-1}, and should prompt a search for a potential error.

REFERENCES

1 Peters AM, Jones DH, Evans K, Gordon I. Two routes for ^{99m}Tc-DMSA uptake into the renal cortical tubular cell. *Eur J Nucl Med* 1988; **14**: 555–61.

2 Peters AM, Heckmatt JZ, Hasson N, *et al*. Renal haemodynamics of cyclosporin nephrotoxicity in children with juvenile dermatomyositis. *Clin Sci* 1991; **8**: 153–9.

3 Cousins C, Gunasekera RD, Mubashar M, *et al*. Comparative kinetics of microvascular inulin and Tc-99m DTPA exchange. *Clin Sci* 1997; **93**: 411–17.

4 Cousins C, Mohammadtaghi S, Mubashar M, *et al*. Clearance kinetics of solutes used to measure glomerular filtration rate. *Nucl Med Commun* 1999; **20**: 1047–54.

5 Cousins C, Skehan SJ, Rolph S, *et al*. Comparative microvascular exchange kinetics of [^{77}Br]bromide and ^{99m}Tc-DTPA in humans. *Eur J Nucl Med* 2002; **29**: 655–62.

6 Gunasekera RD, Allison DJ, Peters AM. Glomerular filtration rate in relation to extracellular fluid volume: similarity between Tc-99m-DTPA and inulin. *Eur J Nucl Med* 1996; **23**: 49–54.

7 Henthorn TK, Avram MJ, Frederiksen MC, Atkinson AJ. Heterogeneity of interstitial fluid space demonstrated by simultaneous kinetic analysis of the distribution and elimination of inulin and gallamine. *J Pharmacol Exp Therap* 1982; **222**: 389–94.

8 Krejcie TC, Henthorn TK, Niemann CU, *et al*., Recirculatory pharmacokinetic models of markers of blood, extracellular fluid and total body water administered concomitantly. *J Pharmacol Exp Therap* 1996; **27**: 1050–7.

9 Katz MA. Interstitial space – the forgotten organ. *Med Hypotheses* 1980; **6**: 885–98.

10 Brochner-Mortensen J. A simple method for the determination of glomerular filtration rate. *Scand J Clin Lab Invest* 1972; **30**: 271–4.

11 Fleming JS, Wilkinson J, Oliver RM, *et al*. Comparison of radionuclide estimation of glomerular filtration rate using technetium-99m-DTPA and chromium-51-EDTA. *Eur J Nucl Med* 1991; **18**: 391–5.

12 Blake GM, Roe D, Holt S, *et al*. Measurement of GFR by ^{51}Cr-EDTA plasma clearance: the correction for the one-pool assumption [Abstract]. *Nucl Med Commun* 1993; **14**: 295.

13 Peters AM, Henderson BL, Lui D, *et al*. Appropriate corrections to glomerular filtration rate and volume of distribution based on the bolus injection and single compartment technique. *Physiol Measurement* 1999; **20**: 313–27.

14 Fleming JS, Zivanovic MA, Blake GM, *et al*. Guidelines for the measurement of glomerular filtration rate using plasma sampling. *Nucl Med Commun* 2004; **25**: 759–69.

15 Jagenburg R, Attman PO, Aurell M, Bucht H. Determination of glomerular filtration rate in advanced renal insufficiency. *Scand J Urol Nephrol* 1978; **12**: 133–7.

16 Frennby B, Sterner G, Almen T, *et al*. The use of iohexol clearance to determine GFR in patients with severe chronic renal failure – a comparison between different clearance techniques. *Clin Nephrol* 1995; **43**: 35–46.

17 Brochner-Mortensen J, Freund LG. Reliability of routine clearance methods for assessment of glomerular filtration rate in advanced renal insuffiency. *Scand J Clin Lab Invest* 1981; **41**: 91–7.

18 Martensson J, Groth S, Rehling M, Gref M. Chromium-51-EDTA clearance in adults with a single-plasma sample. *J Nucl Med* 1998; **39**: 2131–7.

19 Li Y, Lee HB, Blaufox MD. Single-sample methods to measure GFR with technetium-99m-DTPA. *J Nucl Med* 1997; **38**: 1290–5.

20 Wenting GJ, Tan-Tjiong HL, Derkx FH, *et al.* Split renal function after captopril in unilateral renal artery stenosis. *Br Med J* 1984; **288**: 886–90.

21 Battilana C, Zhang HP, Olshen RA, *et al.* PAH extraction and estimation of plasma flow in diseased human kidneys. *Am J Physiol* 1991; **261**: F726–F733.

22 Peters AM. Expressing glomerular filtration rate in terms of extracellular fluid volume. *Nephrol Dial Transplant* 1992; **7**: 205–10.

23 Waller DG, Keast CM, Fleming JS, Ackery DM. Measurement of glomerular filtration rate with technetium-99m-DTPA: comparison of plasma clearance techniques. *J Nucl Med* 1987; **28**: 372–7.

24 Ladegaard-Pedersen J. Measurement of extracellular fluid volume and renal clearance by a single injection of inulin. *Scand J Clin Lab Invest* 1972; **29**: 145–53.

25 Brun C, Hilden T, Raaschou F. The significance of the difference in systemic arterial and venous plasma concentrations in renal clearance methods. *J Clin Invest* 1949; **28**: 144–52.

26 Brochner-Mortensen J. A simple single injection method for the determination of the extracellular fluid volume. *Scand J Clin Lab Invest* 1980; **40**: 567–73.

27 Peters AM, Henderson BL, Lui D. Indexed glomerular filtration rate as a function of age and body size. *Clin Sci* 2000; **98**: 439–44.

28 Brochner-Mortensen J. The extracellular fluid volume of normal man determined as the distribution volume of Cr-51-EDTA. *Scand J Clin Lab Invest* 1982; **42**: 261–4.

29 Du Bois D, Du Bois EF. A formula to estimate the approximate surface area if height and weight are known. *Arch Intern Med* 1916; **17**: 863.

30 Haycock GB, Schwartz GJ, Wisotsky DH. Geometric method for measuring body surface area: a height–weight formula validated in infants, children and adults. *J Pediatrics* 1978; **93**: 62–6.

31 Calvert AH, Newell DR, Gumbrell LA, *et al.* Carboplatin dosage: prospective evaluation of a simple formula based on renal function. *J Clin Oncol* 1989; **7**: 1748–56.

32 Turner ST, Reilly SL. Fallacy of indexing renal and systemic hemodynamic measurements for body surface area. *Am J Physiol* 1995; **268**: R978–88.

33 McChance RA, Widdowson EM. The correct physiological basis on which to compare infant and adult renal function. *Lancet* 1952; **1**: 860–2.

34 Boer P. Estimated lean body mass as an index for normalization of body fluid volumes in man. *Am J Physiol* 1984; **247**: F632–5.

35 Kurtin PS. Standardization of renal function measurements in children: kidney size versus metabolic rate. *Child Nephrol Urol* 1989; **9**: 337–9.

36 Peters AM, Allison H, Ussov W Yu. Measurement of the ratio of glomerular filtration rate to plasma volume from the Tc-99m DTPA renogram. *Eur J Nucl Med* 1994; **21**: 322–7.

37 Mitch WE, Walser M. Nutritional therapy in renal disease. In: Brenner BM. (ed.) *The kidney*, 6th edition. Philadelphia: WB Saunders, 2000: 2298–340.

38 Peters AM, Gordon I, Sixt R. Normalisation of glomerular filtration rate in children: body surface area, body weight or extracellular fluid volume? *J Nucl Med* 1994; **35**: 438–44.

39 White AJ, Strydom WJ. Normalization of glomerular filtration rate measurements. *Eur J Nucl Med* 1991; **18**: 385–90.

40 Friis-Hansen B. Body water compartments in children: changes during growth and related changes in body composition. *Pediatrics* 1961; **28**: 169–75.

41 Bird NJ, Henderson BL, Lui D, Ballinger JR, Peters AM. Indexing glomerular filtration rate to suit children. *J Nucl Med* 2003; **44**: 1037–43.

42 Cervenka L, Mitchell KD, Navar LG. Renal function in mice: effects of volume expansion and angiotensin II. *J Am Soc Nephrol* 1999; **10**: 2631–6.

43 Gleadhill A. Quantitative assessment of renal function in domestic animals; measurement of glomerular filtration rate by the plasma clearance of technetium-diethylenetriaminepentaacetic acid. PhD thesis, University of London, 1996; 60–9.

44 Brochner-Mortensen J, Ditzel J. Glomerular filtration rate and extracellular fluid volume in insulin-dependent patients with diabetes mellitus. *Kidney Int* 1982; **21**: 696–8.

45 Hommel E, Mathiesen ER, Giese J, *et al.* On the pathogenesis of arterial blood pressure elevation early in the course of diabetic nephropathy. *Scand J Clin Lab Invest* 1989; **49**: 537–44.

46 Feldt-Rasmussen B, Matheisen ER, Deckert T, *et al.* Central role for sodium in the pathogenesis of blood pressure changes independent of angiotensin, aldosterone and catecholamines in type 1 (insulin-dependent) diabetes mellitus. *Diabetologia* 1987; **30**: 610–17.

47 Ikkos D, Ljunggren H, Luft R. Glomerular filtration rate and renal blood flow in acromegaly. *Acta Endocrinol* 1956; **21**: 226–36.

48 Falkheden T, Sjogren B. Extracellular fluid volume and renal function in pituitary insufficiency and acromegaly. *Acta Endocrinol* 1964; **46**: 80–6.

49 Sims EAH, Krantz KE. Serial studies of renal function during pregnancy and the puerperium in normal women. *J Clin Invest* 1958; **37**: 1764–74.

50 Brown A, Zammit VC, Lowe SA. Capillary permeability and extracellular fluid volumes in pregnancy-induced hypertension. *Clin Sci* 1989; **77**: 599–604.

51 Neilsen OM, Engell HC. Increased glomerular filtration rate in patients after reconstructive surgery on the abdominal aorta. *Br J Surg* 1986; **73**: 34–7.

52 Peters, AM, Henderson BL, Lui D. Comparison between terminal slope rate constant and 'slope/intercept' as measures of glomerular filtration rate using the single compartment simplification. *Eur J Nucl Med* 2001; **28**: 320–6.

53 Peters AM, Anderson P, Gordon I. The volume of distribution of MAG3. *J Nucl Med* 1991; **32**: 900–1.

Vesico–ureteric reflux and urinary tract infection

LORENZO BIASSONI AND ISKY GORDON

NUCLEAR MEDICINE TECHNIQUES

The pediatric nuclear medicine unit

A child is not a small adult. Pediatric pathology is different from that of an adult and a knowledge of embryology is required. Handling pediatric patients requires special techniques as a child should not move during the examination. This is achieved by winning the child's confidence and trust, amusing him or her and actively involving the parents in the examination. The technologists and radiographers should enjoy working with children. To achieve a satisfactory examination all pediatric nuclear medicine tests require a longer camera time than the equivalent tests in adults. A standard single-head gamma camera is adequate for the vast majority of pediatric examinations but a little attention to decoration, an audio/video tape player, a collection of illustrated children's books and tapes, are all extremely helpful. To ensure high-resolution images the child should be very close to the camera – on the camera face itself if possible.

The child's journey through the nuclear medicine department

JUSTIFICATION AND AUTHORIZATION OF A NUCLEAR MEDICINE TEST

The justification of a nuclear medicine procedure requires that information about the clinical status is available and previous examinations relevant to the procedure are reviewed. Information related to the structural renal abnormalities (hydronephrosis, duplex kidney, ectopic kidney, expansive lesions) may be of help in deciding on additional views and the appropriate time for imaging. The clinical question asked should be clear, so that the appropriate views are acquired to answer the question.

APPOINTMENT LETTER

A detailed clear full explanation of the particular test including duration of the scan and all the waiting times should be included. The parents should be told to bring the child's favorite book to be read or tape to be played during the acquisition of the images in order to keep the child entertained. Clear instructions on how to get to the nuclear medicine department (with maps and signs) is essential. This will reduce anxiety in both parents and child.

PRIOR TO INJECTION

Anesthetic cream should be applied for all intravenous injections 45–60 min before the injection. This waiting time can be useful in explaining again the entire procedure to the child and parents. The child should be encouraged to drink before and after every radiotracer injection. Dilution and more rapid excretion of the isotope eliminated via the kidneys and bladder is facilitated and the absorbed dose to these organs reduced. Drug sedation is almost never used for any renal radionuclide examination but can be critical for other examinations especially in a child with malignancy.

INJECTION OF THE RADIOPHARMACEUTICAL

Only members of staff trained in pediatric intravenous injections should undertake this procedure. A butterfly needle (caliber 25 or 27 gauge) connected to a three-way tap and a saline syringe flush or a small caliber cannula is strongly advised. Staff experienced in venopuncture reduces

Table 8C.1 *Dosage card. Fraction of adult administered activity*

3 kg = 0.1	22 kg = 0.50	42 kg = 0.78
4 kg = 0.14	24 kg = 0.53	44 kg = 0.80
6 kg = 0.19	26 kg = 0.56	46 kg = 0.82
8 kg = 0.23	28 kg = 0.58	48 kg = 0.85
10 kg = 0.27	30 kg = 0.62	50 kg = 0.88
12 kg = 0.32	32 kg = 0.65	52–54 kg = 0.90
14 kg = 0.36	34 kg = 0.68	56–58 kg = 0.92
16 kg = 0.40	36 kg = 0.71	60–62 kg = 0.96
18 kg = 0.44	38 kg = 0.73	64–66 kg = 0.98
20 kg = 0.46	40 kg = 0.76	68 kg = 0.99

(Information is from a chart produced by the Paediatric Committee of the European Association of Nuclear Medicine, reproduced with permission from the EANM.)

the tension for themselves as well as for the parents and child, and ensures a quiet environment. The administered amount of radioactivity in children is scaled on a body surface basis. The Paediatric Committee of the European Association of Nuclear Medicine (EANM) has produced a dosage card that can help in calculating the amount of radioactivity to be injected in a child (Tables 8C.1 and 8C.2). The amount of radioactivity to be injected in a child ranges from a minimum dose of 15 MBq for dimercaptosuccinic acid (DMSA) and mercaptoacetyltriglycine (MAG$_3$) and 20 MBq for diethylenetriaminepentaacetic acid (DTPA) to a maximum administered dose of 80 MBq for DMSA, 70 MBq for MAG$_3$ and 200 MBq for DTPA.

Static cortical scintigraphy

DMSA is extracted by the proximal renal tubules reaching a plateau of uptake in the kidneys 6 h after the injection with 40–65% of the injected dose taken up by the kidneys. With significant hydronephrosis part of the tracer may remain in the renal collecting system and thus lead to a falsely high estimation of the differential function; delayed images and the use of a diuretic may be helpful to avoid this artefact.

INDICATIONS

The DMSA scan provides information on focal parenchymal renal function. In particular, it can be used in the following clinical contexts:

- Urinary tract infection: detection of renal scarring (at least 6 months after the infection)
- Detection of acute pyelonephritis
- Detection of ectopic renal tissue
- In congenital abnormalities (e.g. duplex kidney, dysplastic renal tissue, small kidney), to assess the amount of functioning renal tissue

Table 8C.2 *Recommended adult and minimum amounts, in megabecquerels*

Radiopharmaceutical	Adult	Minimum
^{99m}Tc-DTPA (kidney)	200	20
^{99m}Tc-DMSA	100	15
^{99m}Tc-MAG$_3$	70	15
^{99m}Tc-pertechnetate (cystography)	20	20
^{99m}Tc-MDP	500	40
^{99m}Tc-colloid (liver/spleen)	80	15
^{99m}Tc-colloid (marrow)	300	20
^{99m}Tc-spleen (denatured RBCs)	40	20
^{99m}Tc-RBC (blood pool)	800	80
^{99m}Tc-albumin (cardiac)	800	80
^{99m}Tc-pertechnetate (first pass)	500	80
^{99m}Tc-MAA/microspheres	80	10
^{99m}Tc-pertechnetate (ectopic gastric)	150	20
^{99m}Tc-colloid (gastric reflux)	40	10
^{99m}Tc-IDA (biliary)	150	20
^{99m}Tc-pertechnetate (thyroid)	80	10
^{99m}Tc-HMPAO (brain)	740	100
^{99m}Tc-HMPAO (WBCs)	500	40
^{123}I-hippuran	75	10
^{123}I (thyroid)	20	3
^{123}I-amphetamine (brain)	185	18
^{123}I-MIBG	400	80
^{67}Ga	80	10

RBCs: red blood cells. WBCs: white blood cells.

(The information is from a chart produced by the Paediatric Committee of the European Association of Nuclear Medicine, reproduced with permission from the EANM.)

- Evaluation of relative renal function in severe hydronephrosis
- Evaluation of intra-renal functionally significant renal artery stenosis.

ACQUISITION AND ANALYSIS

Imaging should begin 2–4 h after the injection with the child lying supine either directly on the surface of a low-energy high-resolution collimator or as close as possible to it. Routine views include posterior plus right and left posterior oblique projections with magnification. Three hundred thousand to 500 000 counts are acquired (alternatively, the acquisition is carried out for a preset time of at least 5 min). An anterior view is required either when there is a suspicion of an ectopic kidney or when only one kidney has been visualized on the routine views. Some institutions prefer to use a pin-hole collimator; the acquisition time may then be longer. With an uncooperative child, a dynamic

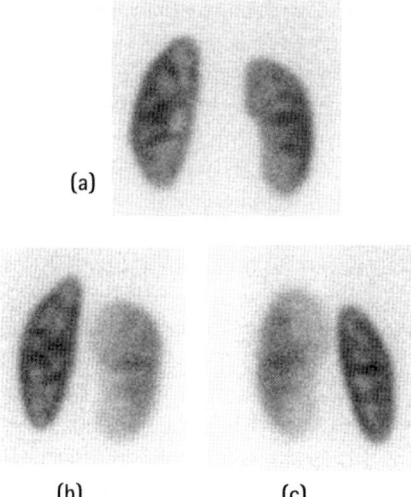

(a)

(b)   (c)

Figure 8C.1 *Normal dimercaptosuccininic acid (DMSA) scan. A high quality DMSA scan allows the observer to distinguish some features of renal internal architecture: the columns of Bertin should appear slightly hyperactive compared to the surrounding cooler medulla and the adjacent collecting system. The renal outline should be clearly defined. The use of the high resolution collimator, together with the acquisition of a sufficient number of counts and a child who does not move, allows a high quality study. In the figure, the posterior view (a), left posterior oblique (b) and right posterior oblique (c) views are shown.*

acquisition over a preset time with reframing to a single image after correcting for movement can help. During the dynamic acquisition one should try to keep the child as still as possible. The routine use of single photon emission computed tomography (SPECT) has not been shown to help clinical management and may be potentially misleading.

Differential renal function (DRF) is calculated after drawing regions of interest (ROIs) around each kidney as well as an ROI around each kidney for background subtraction. An estimate of background should include superior, lateral, and inferior tissue around the renal ROI. A DRF between 45 and 55% is considered normal, although some institutions consider values between 42 and 58% as normal. The contribution of an ectopic kidney to the total renal function is calculated using the geometric mean of the background subtracted counts from the renal ROIs in the posterior and anterior views (the square root of each kidney's background subtracted ROI counts in the anterior view multiplied for the same counts in the posterior view). The radiation burden of a DMSA scan is approximately 1 mSv per examination, regardless of the age of the child, as long as the dose injected is according the body surface area.

INTERPRETATION

In a high-quality DMSA the kidney outline should be clear and the internal architecture readily seen (Fig. 8C.1). The

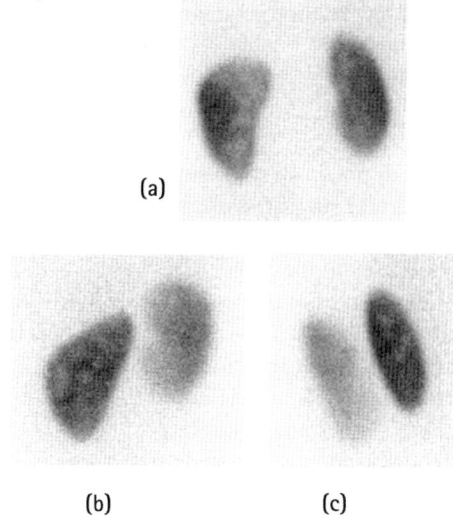

(a)

(b)   (c)

Figure 8C.2 *Dimercaptosuccinic acid (DMSA) scan: Normal variants. Two kidneys of different shape, both showing good uptake of DMSA and equal function. A prominent splenic impression (b) on the left kidney. The posterior view (a) with the left (b) and the right (c) oblique posterior views are shown.*

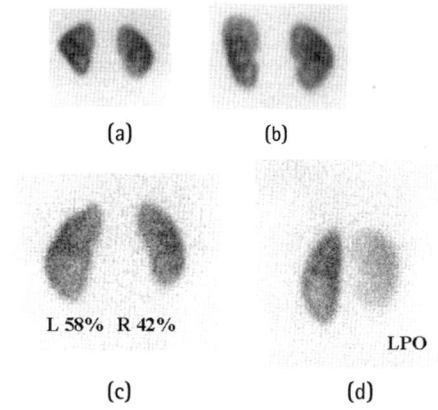

(a)   (b)

L 58% R 42%   LPO

(c)   (d)

Figure 8C.3 *Dimercapsuccinic acid (DMSA) scan: Normal variants. A triangular shape left kidney (a). Two kidneys of different shape but with equal differential function (b). An uncomplicated left duplex kidney (c) with a normal right kidney. The left kidney is larger than the right and contributes 58% to total function (right 42%). The features on the left, confirmed by the ultrasound examination, suggest a duplex system with very good uptake in both the upper and the lower moieties. An uncomplicated duplex is considered a normal variant as it functions as a single unit. Although the relative function of the left kidney is slightly higher (58%) than what is considered normal and consequently the right kidney only contributes 42% to total renal function, it is important to report the right kidney as normal as well.*

normal variants (Figs 8C.2 and 8C.3) of the renal outline on DMSA scan are well recorded:[1]

- The renal outline can be flat without suggesting a lesion
- The lateral aspect of the upper portion of the left kidney can be flattened (splenic impression)

- A kidney may have a triangular shape, with flattened external sides
- The transverse axis can sometimes be shorter at one pole than at the other thus giving the impression of a 'pear-shaped' kidney
- One or both poles can sometimes show relatively reduced uptake simply because of the contrast between the hyperactive columns of Bertin in the mid-portion of the kidney and the poles
- The number and size of the column of Bertin vary from patient to patient (variable thickness of the cortex), this may cause false interpretation of the images
- The presence of fetal lobulation in the lateral aspect of the kidney should not be interpreted as a scar
- The slender kidney, with a short transverse axis in the posterior view: this is often a rotated kidney.

An uncomplicated duplex kidney may look bigger than the contralateral kidney and its relative function as calculated by the computer can be higher than the accepted normal range (45–55%). It is important to remember that an uncomplicated duplex functions as a single unit and from a functional point of view is considered a normal variant. If the contralateral kidney does not show any abnormality, even if the number indicating its relative function is borderline low (Fig. 8C.3 (c) and (d)), it is important to describe both kidneys as functionally normal.

An abnormal DMSA scan is sensitive although not specific in the detection of a parenchymal lesion. A focal defect may be due to: cysts, scars, acute inflammatory infiltrate, tumours, vascular pathology or obstruction. In the context of urinary tract infection (UTI) several patterns of abnormality have been described on a DMSA scan[2] (Figs 8C.4 and 8C.5) performed either in the acute phase of the UTI or later on. The DMSA scan is a highly sensitive technique[3–6] and more sensitive than either ultrasound or intravenous urogram (IVU)[7,8] in the detection of focal cortical defects. While a MAG$_3$ scan gives comparable DRF results, at best it is only 80% sensitive in the detection of a focal parenchymal defect compared to a DMSA scan.[9]

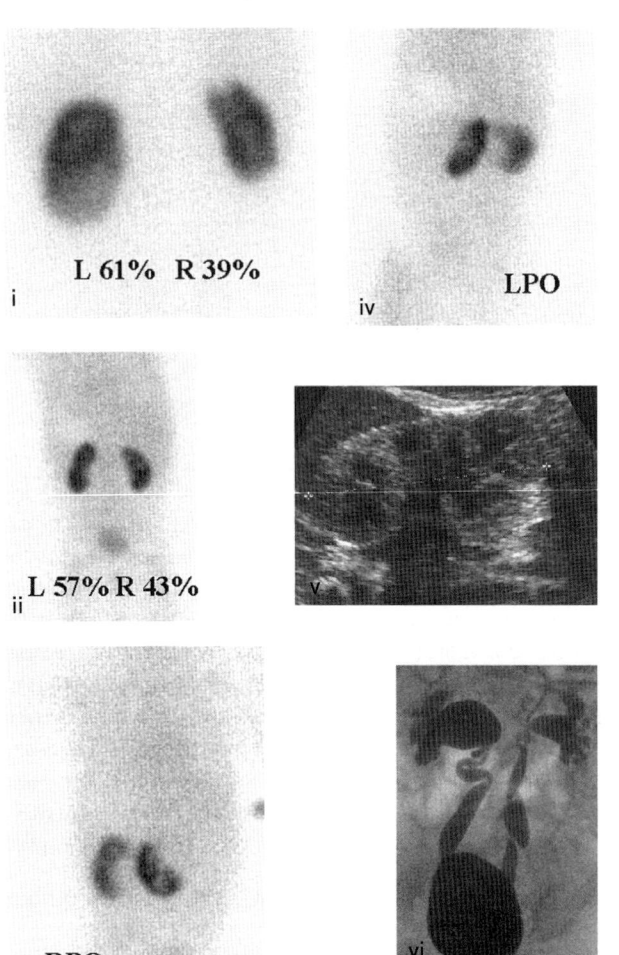

(a)

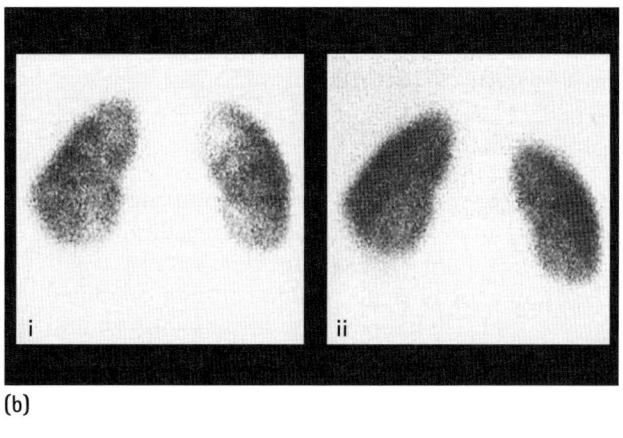

(b)

Figure 8C.4 *Acute dimercaptosuccinic acid (DMSA) scan. (a) A DMSA scan performed on a 1-year-old boy 4 weeks after the onset of symptoms suggestive of pyelonephritis (i). The left kidney shows reduced uptake at the lower pole with preserved outline. The right kidney shows focally reduced uptake at the upper pole, with a breached outline. Another example of acute DMSA in a 6-week-old infant admitted with a proven urinary tract infection (UTI) and systemic symptoms (ii, iii, iv). Several abnormalities in both kidneys are seen, best in the oblique views, with preservation of the cortical outline. Differential function left kidney 57%, right kidney 43%. The ultrasound (v) was done while the UTI was normal. The micturating cystogram (vi) shows bilateral reflux on filling. The urethra was normal. (b) A DMSA scan during an episode of acute pyelonephritis which shows two abnormalities at both poles (i), which resolve completely at follow-up DMSA 6 months later (ii).*

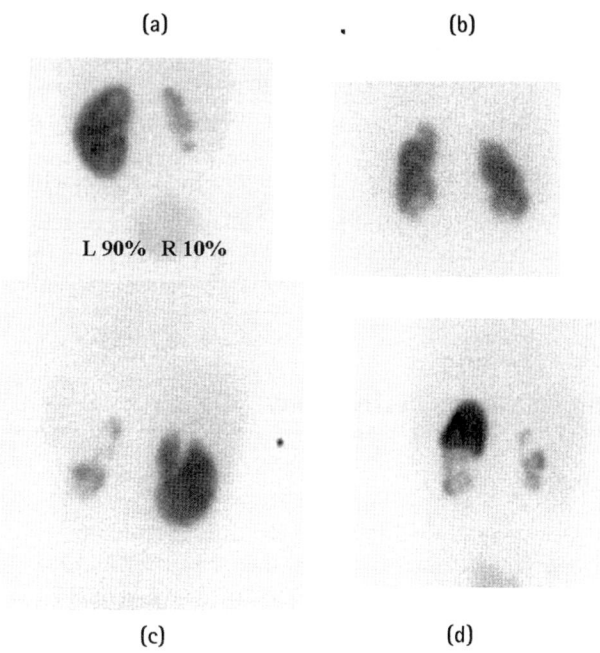

(a)   .   (b)

L 90%   R 10%

(c)   (d)

Figure 8C.5 *Renal scarring on a dimercaptosuccinic acid (DMSA) scan. (a) DMSA scan was done in a 13-month-old boy, a year after a severe urinary tract infection (UTI). This shows a globally contracted right kidney with several renal scars. The right kidney contributes 10% to total renal function (left 90%). This child had a first DMSA done 4 weeks after the onset of the symptoms, which showed very similar features. (b) Bilateral focal renal scars on a DMSA done in a 11-year-old boy with a history of recurrent UTI and bilateral vesico-uretic reflux. His glomerular filtration rate (GFR) was 67 ml min^{-1} at the time of the scan. (c) A 7-year-old boy with a recurrent UTI and poor compliance to treatment and prophylaxis. The DMSA scan shows a severely damaged left kidney which contributes only 12% to total renal function (right 88%). However, the right kidney is also abnormal and shows a typical wedge shaped renal scar in its upper pole. (d) A 4-year-old boy with a history of recurrent UTI, renal stones in the right kidney and a left duplex kidney. The DMSA scan shows a grossly abnormal right kidney with several scars. The left kidney shows poor function in the lower moiety and good function in the upper moiety.*

Indirect radionuclide cystography

Indirect radionuclide cystography (IRC) gives physiological information about bladder emptying and the presence of vesico-ureteric reflux. The major advantage of IRC is that no catheter is required and bladder emptying can be observed under normal circumstances. This is especially important in older girls with recurrent UTI, in whom a dysfunctional bladder can significantly increase the risk of focal renal damage. IRC should be considered as a continuation of the dynamic renal scintigraphy, which provides the DRF and information on drainage, while IRC informs on the upper tract status with a full and empty bladder and gives physiological information on bladder emptying

(Plate 8C.1). IRC is undertaken at the end of the dynamic radionuclide renal study, when the bladder is full of radioactive urine and the child wants to void. Children must be toilet trained so that voiding may occur on demand (usually children over 3 years of age). IRC does not entail bladder catheterization. As the child is actively encouraged to drink throughout the study period, there is usually frequent bladder emptying thus reducing the already low radiation burden from the MAG$_3$. With IRC performed over a 3-h period (from tracer injection to complete bladder emptying) the effective dose is 0.7 mSv;[10] in routine clinical practice the vast majority of IRC scans are completed in less than 3 h, thus significantly reducing the already low radiation burden.

INDICATIONS

- Detection and follow-up of vesico-ureteric reflux (VUR) in children who are toilet trained
- Assessment of the effect of the full and empty bladder on the drainage of the dilated upper tracts
- Evaluation of bladder function (completeness and promptness of bladder emptying).

ACQUISITION AND ANALYSIS OF THE INDIRECT RADIONUCLIDE CYSTOGRAPHY

This is conveniently divided into the two parts, the acquisition and analysis of the renal scintigraphy followed by IRC.

DYNAMIC RENAL SCINTIGRAPHY

The ideal tracer has a high extraction fraction and tubular agents are preferred to DTPA. With the child supine on the gamma camera, the tracer is injected and dynamic data (either 10 or 20 s per frame) are acquired for 20 min. Analysis requires reframing the data so that images over the entire period are displayed as well as curves from ROIs over both kidneys. Specific attention should be paid to the collecting system on the late images (see guidelines on European Association of Nuclear Medicine and Society of Nuclear Medicine websites: www.eanm.org and www.snm.org).

INDIRECT RADIONUCLIDE CYSTOGRAPHY

Once the dynamic renal scintigraphy is finished, the child returns to the waiting room and is encouraged to drink. When s/he is ready to micturate, the child is taken back to the gamma camera room where there is a quiet and peaceful atmosphere with as few people as possible. Boys stand while girls sit on the commode with their back to the camera, which is positioned vertically at a slight angle using a general purpose collimator. Imaging must include kidneys and bladder using magnification if possible. A frame rate of 5 s per frame maximum should be used. If compressed images are used, then a 1 s per frame acquisition is utilized. The length of the acquisition varies with the time the child takes to void. The dynamic acquisition should start before the child begins micturition and continue until after the end of micturition. Thirty seconds worth of data both before and after micturition is ideal. The voided urine volume should be measured. An IRC is considered finished when both the kidneys and the bladder are empty. If activity persists in the kidneys and bladder after the first micturition, the child is sent back to the waiting room, encouraged to drink, and a new IRC is acquired when the child wants to void again. If activity persists in a dilated collecting system, another IRC 15 min after oral frusemide administration is performed to exclude obstruction.

PROCESSING

ROIs are drawn over the bladder and kidneys and curves generated. A compressed image may be useful as this allows the entire study to be displayed in the form of two histograms, with time on the x-axis, anatomy and activity on the y-axis, representing the count rate in the region above the bladder. A cine of the raw data should be carefully reviewed with specific attention to both bladder emptying and changes in activity over each renal area. The diagnosis of renal reflux requires an increase in counts of at least two standard deviations from baseline activity before the start of micturition (Fig. 8C.6).

PITFALLS

Stasis of tracer in the renal collecting system at the end of the dynamic renal scintigraphy will make detection of VUR challenging. A large amount of refluxed urine can still be seen as an increase in counts over the kidney and ureter during and immediately after micturition. Smaller volumes of refluxed urine may be difficult to visualize. A low or ectopic kidney, especially if superimposed on the bladder, can make detection of reflux difficult. Reflux into a dilated lower ureter cannot be detected.

Direct isotope cystography

INDICATIONS

- Detection of VUR in non-toilet trained children (normally, children younger than 3 years of age)
- Detection of VUR in older girls with recurrent UTI with a normal IRC when the clinical suspicion of VUR is high.

PROCEDURE

There are three different techniques in use to undertake the direct isotope cystography (DIC), two using a catheter and the third using a supra-pubic approach.

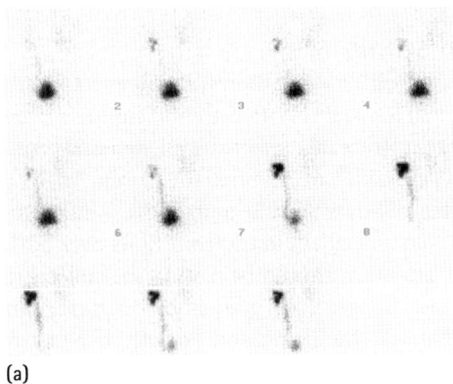

(a)

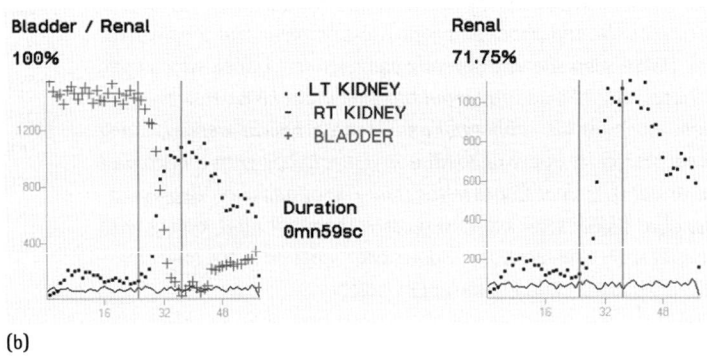

(b)

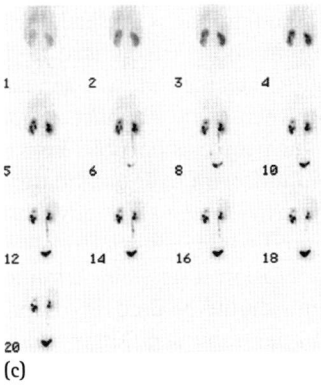

(c)

Figure 8C.6 *Indirect radionuclide cystography (IRC) showing vesico-ureteric reflux. A 9-year-old girl with a history of recurrent urinary tract infection and a left duplex kidney had IRC using mercaptoacetyltriglycine (MAG$_3$). The renal scintigraphy (c) shows two equally functioning kidneys. The left duplex kidney shows slightly better function in the upper than in the lower moiety. The IRC (a) shows good bladder emptying with clear evidence of reflux into the left lower moiety. This is confirmed by the time–activity curves (b).*

THE CATHETER TECHNIQUES

These require the passage of a small French feeding tube into the bladder and the urine drained off. Disposable nappies (usually three) are then placed with the catheter end outside the nappies. The child is placed supine on the gamma camera using a low-energy general-purpose collimator. A possible technique is the instillation of 20 MBq ^{99m}Tc-pertechnetate via a three-way tap followed by saline until the child micturates. The alternative technique involves good mixing of the tracer in the saline bag and then filling the bladder with the tracer and the saline mixture. The volume instilled is 30 ml per year of age, plus 60 ml. Dynamic data acquisition (5 s per frame) begins once the tracer is instilled and should continue throughout until micturition is complete, plus 30 s. If VUR is shown during the filling phase, data are collected for a further 30 s and then the bladder is drained. If the child has not micturated at the end of the filling phase then a new acquisition begins until the child micturates. The EANM guidelines recommend administration of antibiotics routinely after the test and this is the practice of the authors. There is debate over the timing of the first dose and the length of administration.

THE SUPRA-PUBIC TECHNIQUE

This requires a percutaneous injection of 10–20 MBq of ^{99m}Tc-pertechnetate or ^{99m}Tc-labeled MAG$_3$ into the full bladder after the application of anesthetic cream. Gamma-camera images of the bladder and renal areas are recorded during a 5 min resting period and during micturition.[11]

The DIC is very sensitive for renal reflux as it continually monitors the kidney area for the duration of the study (Fig. 8C.7). It does not give information on ureteric reflux nor can it provide a grading for reflux, as does radiological micturating cysto-urography (MCUG). Its main advantage is the very low radiation burden (0.012 mSv, i.e. one quarter of a chest X-ray) .

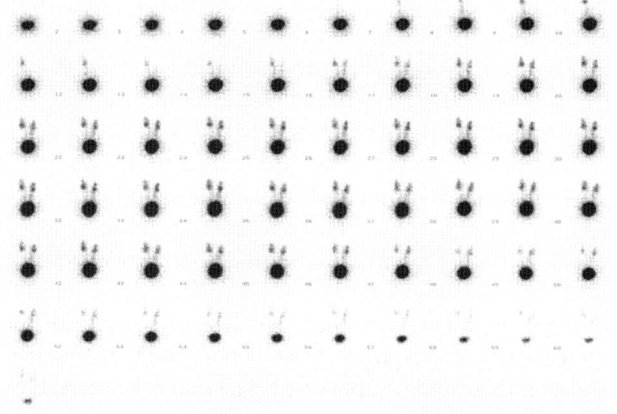

Figure 8C.7 *Direct isotope cystography. A 2-year-old girl with bilateral duplex kidneys and bilateral vesico-ureteric reflux.*

Comparison between direct isotope cystography and indirect radionuclide cystography

DIC allows monitoring of the kidneys during bladder filling and emptying, while IRC can only detect VUR during bladder emptying. With DIC the bladder fills in a non-physiological way, whereas in IRC the bladder is filled by the kidneys and this is a physiological study. Therefore IRC allows the pattern, completeness, and promptness of bladder emptying to be studied. Some institutions show poor correlation between direct and indirect cystography[12] while others show good correlation. All authors agree that if reflux is demonstrated by one of the techniques then it is true reflux, but if no reflux is demonstrated, then this means that reflux was not detected on that occasion and this differs from saying that the child did not have reflux.

URINARY TRACT INFECTIONS: THE CLINICAL CONTEXT AND AIM OF IMAGING

Introduction

Urinary tract infection (UTI) is a common pediatric condition. The inflammatory process may be limited to the bladder (cystitis), may involve the upper collecting system (pyelitis) or the renal parenchyma (pyelonephritis). Acute pyelonephritis may cause permanent renal damage. The goal in the management of children with UTI is to prevent or diminish renal damage as well as reduce the chances of a recurrent UTI. Conditions that require surgery must be identified. The presence and the extent of acute renal inflammatory involvement have been recognized as important risk factors for permanent renal damage. Several reports have suggested that renal scarring can be prevented or diminished by a prompt diagnosis and a rapid start of antibiotic therapy.

The rationale for investigation of a child with a urinary tract infection

A UTI may identify a group of children with an underlying structural abnormality that may require surgery. Acute pyelonephritis may cause permanent renal damage and the belief is that its long-term consequences inevitably include hypertension, complications of pregnancy, and chronic renal failure. These complications are now hotly debated.

HYPERTENSION

There is little long-term follow-up of blood pressure in children with renal damage secondary to UTI. To date, only one epidemiological study has been published and this

Table 8C.3 *Abnormalities of the urinary tract detected by imaging*

- *Congenital abnormalities (duplex kidneys, crossed fused kidneys, ectopic kidneys, posterior urethral valves)*
- *Hydronephrosis (especially with reduced function and poor drainage)*
- *Bladder dysfunction*
- *Extent of renal inflammatory involvement during acute pyelonephritis*
- *Presence of renal cortical scars*
- *High grade vesico-uretic reflux in a child with abnormal kidneys*

Table 8C.4 *Clinical risk factors for permanent renal damage in a child with urinary tract infection*

- *Systemic symptoms*
- *Fever and young age (<1 year)*
- *Recurrent urinary tract infection*
- *Bacteremia/septicemia*
- *Unusual microorganism (Proteus, Klebsiella, Pseudomonas)*
- *Nonresponders to treatment*

does not support the hypothesis that hypertension is more common in children with a damaged kidney.[13] However, other studies in small selected groups suggest an increased risk of hypertension of between 10 and 23%.[14,15]

COMPLICATIONS OF PREGNANCY

These are said to be more common in the presence of scarred kidneys, yet the literature does not support this.[16] Furthermore, most women who are pregnant attend antenatal clinics where blood pressure is routinely measured. In those countries with limited availability of antenatal clinics there are also inadequate facilities for the investigation of children with UTI.

CHRONIC RENAL FAILURE

There is little evidence to support the contention that renal scarring secondary to UTI will lead to chronic renal failure or transplant or dialysis.[17–19]

CONGENITAL ABNORMALITIES

The discovery of renal tract malformations that may require surgery or intervention in children with a UTI will reduce the morbidity of the UTI. These conditions include posterior urethral valves, complicated duplex kidneys, hydronephrosis, and calculi (Table 8C.3).

It may be concluded that the rationale for imaging children with a UTI is to discover an underlying malformation and/or reduce the morbidity (including renal damage).

Risk factors: Which children require imaging?

Not all children with UTI need imaging. Children with UTI at low risk, clinically, do not need imaging. Selection

of an appropriate group of children who warrant imaging requires the identification of the susceptible child. The most important group of children who should undergo imaging includes infants with a febrile UTI. The second most important group includes those children with recurrent UTI. Other groups include children with systemic symptoms, those who do not respond to treatment as expected, or have an unusual micro-organism as the cause of UTI (e.g. *Proteus, Pseudomonas*) (Table 8C.4).

Vesico-ureteric reflux and renal damage

The traditional view has been that VUR is a major risk factor for renal damage and therefore children with UTI should be tested for reflux. The Working Party of the Royal College of Physicians suggested that VUR should be excluded in children under 5 years of age,[20] and Hoberman *et al.*[21] recommended that a cystogram should be the first imaging test in children under 2 years of age with a UTI. In recent years, the role of VUR in the development of renal damage in children with UTI has been questioned. It has been found that not all children with reflux develop renal damage and children with UTI can have significant renal damage in absence of demonstrable reflux.[2,3,22–24] A study from Gothenburg[25] confirmed these findings when they investigated the first proven UTI in 162 boys and 142 girls aged in the range 5 days to 23.8 months. All children underwent ultrasound, MCUG and DMSA within 3 months of a UTI and had a follow-up DMSA scan between 1 and 2 years from the UTI. Results showed that 22% of boys and 31% of girls had VUR, and the first DMSA was abnormal in 51% of cases. Seven children had dilated VUR (grade III), all with normal US and DMSA. At follow-up five of them had no further VUR. The conclusion reached was that when both ultrasound and the early DMSA were normal then there was no benefit from MCUG and this could be omitted. If either ultrasound or DMSA were abnormal then MCUG was required. There are two meta-analyses[26,27] and neither of them supports the view that VUR, as such, is a risk factor. The conclusion of the meta-analysis by Wheeler *et al.* was: 'It is uncertain whether the identification and treatment of children with VUR confers a clinically important benefit.' The natural history of VUR is benign with 13% stopping spontaneously every year[28] and lower grade VUR stopping more quickly than higher grade VUR. Furthermore, VUR is an intermittent phenomenon with the same child showing a variation in VUR in the same day under the same physiological circumstances. The development of new scars is quite unusual and is more commonly seen in children with recurrent UTI and bladder dysfunction.[29–31]

The relevance of these data in children with UTI is that VUR is a sign elicited in a department of radiology/nuclear medicine and not a disease. The importance of VUR is in children with recurrent UTI and in young children with a UTI and an abnormal kidney.

In summary, aim of imaging in UTI is to discover malformations of the renal tract and find any renal damage (Table 8C.3). Children with documented renal damage and/or recurrent UTI need imaging to detect possible reflux. In children with recurrent UTI, imaging focused specifically on studying bladder function is important as bladder dysfunction is a major risk factor for recurrent UTI and renal damage.

THE CONTRIBUTION OF NUCLEAR MEDICINE TO THE MANAGEMENT OF URINARY TRACT INFECTIONS

The reference method for the detection of focal renal parenchymal damage is the ^{99m}Tc-DMSA scan, which can be done either during the acute episode to detect renal inflammatory involvement or several months after an infection, to assess if the kidney is scarred. Assessment of bladder function is especially important in children with recurrent UTI who may damage their kidneys significantly if their bladder is dysfunctional.

Acute urinary tract infection

The clinical/laboratory features of acute pyelonephritis and pyelitis are often non-specific. The latter may not damage the kidney, while the former may result in renal scarring. At times it is difficult clinically to distinguish between upper and lower tract infections. An accurate diagnosis of acute pyelonephritis requires a DMSA scan in the acute phase and a normal DMSA scan excludes this diagnosis. However, an abnormal DMSA scan in the acute phase does not imply that the kidney will be scarred. A late scan (at least 6 months after the UTI) is required in order to detect renal scarring (Fig. 8C.5(a)).

Animal experiments have shown the sensitivity and specificity of the DMSA scan in the setting of acute UTI. Pigs with acute pyelonephritis experimentally provoked by vesico-ureteric reflux of infected urine underwent DMSA scans in the acute and late phases. Histopathological correlation was obtained. DMSA had a sensitivity of 87–89% and a specificity of 100% in detecting and localizing lesions.[32] Missed lesions on DMSA were microscopic foci of inflammation not evident on gross examination and not associated with significant parenchymal damage.[3,22] These findings were also seen in the late DMSA scans in the pigs. In the context of acute DMSA scanning, Risdon et al.[4] described three types of abnormal kidney. When there was focally reduced uptake of DMSA and the renal outline was lost, all these kidneys went on to scarring. When the renal outline was intact, some of these kidneys returned to normal.

It has been suggested that an acute DMSA has prognostic significance. In their paper, Biggi et al.[33] stratified patients into high, intermediate and low risk of renal scarring according to the extent of parenchymal involvement and the presence or absence of VUR. The low risk group (normal acute DMSA with/without VUR) had a risk of scarring of 0%. In the intermediate risk group (small lesions – less than 25% parenchymal involvement – with/without VUR; extensive lesions without VUR) the risk of scarring ranged between 14 and 38%. In the high risk group (extensive lesions with VUR) the risk of scarring was 88%.

In the clinical setting of the sick child with high fever but a negative screen for infection, a DMSA scan may be useful if focal defects are seen suggesting renal inflammatory involvement due to kidney infection with a sterile urine.

Cortical scarring

The most common use of DMSA scanning is in diagnosing permanent cortical renal damage (Fig. 8C.5). While DMSA is very sensitive in detecting focal renal damage, it is not specific, as any cause of focal cortical damage can show up as a focal defect on a DMSA scan. In order to distinguish reversible from irreversible focal renal damage, a late DMSA scan is required. A recent study reported that only 15% of children with focal defects on DMSA scans performed in the acute phase of a UTI showed persistent focal defects six months later.[21] Furthermore, 47% of children with focal renal damage seen at DMSA scan done at 2–6 months after the UTI may still be reversible if the DMSA is repeated 2 years later.[34] Similar results has been obtained by other groups.[35]

Assessment of bladder function

In the older child with recurrent UTI, bladder dysfunction is an important risk factor for developing renal damage especially if VUR is present. A good history and the urinary flow chart are the first indispensable steps of a full assessment of bladder function. Dynamic renal scintigraphy with an IRC

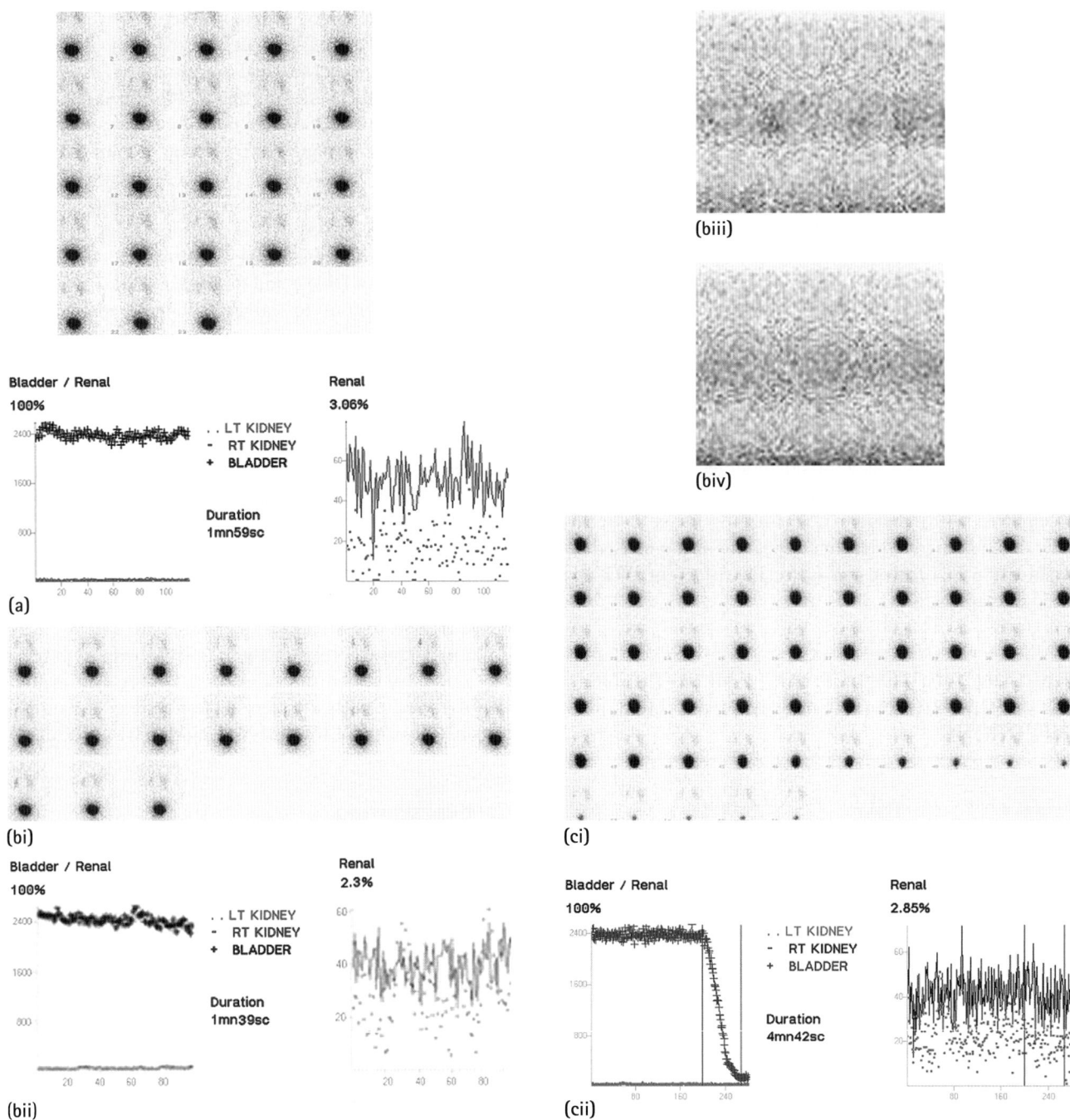

Figure 8C.8 *Indirect radionuclide cystography (IRC) showing bladder dysfunction. A 15-year-old boy had a recent episode of pyelonephritis. IRC using mercaptoacetyltriglycine (MAG₃) was utilized as part of the imaging tests. The renal scintigraphy showed reduced function in the left kidney (33%), which had not changed when compared to a previous MAG₃ scan in 1994. Repeat IRC was required as the boy did not void completely at the first attempt. (a) First IRC (done at 12:37 hours): no bladder emptying seen. No reflux demonstrated. (b) Second IRC (done at 12:47 hours): no bladder emptying, although there is reflux into the left kidney, confirmed by the compressed image (c). (c) Third IRC (done at 12:56 hours): good bladder emptying with no reflux during micturition. This case illustrates a particular case of bladder dysfunction called bladder instability (continuous but ineffective contractions of the detrusor with reflux while the child is not voiding). Also, the case shows the variability of reflux in the same patient and at different times (reflux with no void and no reflux during micturition).*

represents a complete physiological investigation of the entire nephro-urological system. The information gained includes renal function, drainage, bladder dynamics (especially during micturition) and the presence of VUR (Fig. 8C.6).

The IRC informs on both completeness of bladder emptying and rate of emptying. The main patterns of bladder

dysfunction detected with the IRC are the following (Figs 8C.8 and 8C.9):

- Incomplete bladder emptying
- Slow bladder emptying
- Stepwise void

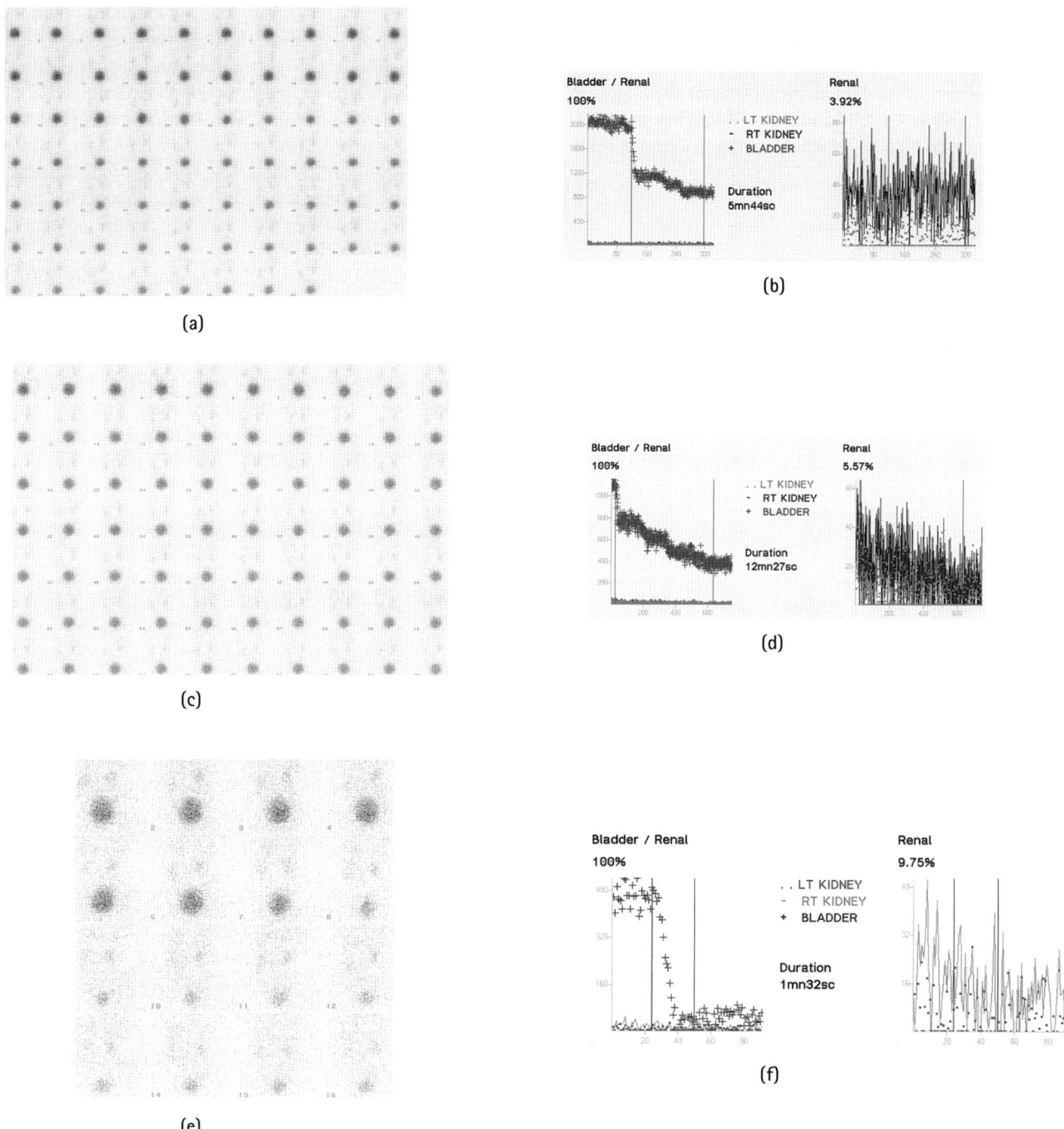

Figure 8C.9 *Indirect radionuclide cystography (IRC) showing bladder dysfunction. A 13-year-old girl with a history of recurrent urinary tract infection had this IRC scan using mercaptoacetyltriglycine (MAG$_3$) as part of her follow-up investigations. The renal scintigraphy (images not presented) showed reduced function in the right kidney (36% of total function). Drainage was good bilaterally. The girl had significant bladder dysfunction and required three attempts at IRC in order to empty her bladder completely. The first IRC (a and b) shows an initial brisk void followed by a partial, prolonged void, with no evidence of reflux. The second IRC (c and d) shows a very prolonged and partial void, again with no reflux. On the third IRC (e and f) she manages to void to completion but no reflux is demonstrated. This case shows another example of bladder dysfunction, compatible with dis-coordination of the detrusor sphincter: in this condition it is difficult to empty the bladder completely.*

Complete inability to void at the first attempt, followed by a subsequent good void to completion, does not necessarily mean that the bladder is dysfunctional; it could be due to psychological inhibition to void in an unusual environment.

In the presence of dilated upper tracts and recurrent UTI (e.g. in the follow-up of boys with posterior urethral valves) the dynamic renal scintigraphy and the IRC allow an assessment of renal function, drainage of the calyces and pelvis as well as the state of the ureters with the bladder full and empty. Voiding rate, completeness of voiding, and voided volume can also be assessed.

The detection of bladder dysfunction can shed light on the cause of a recurrent UTI and suggests that bladder voiding training is likely to be beneficial in that particular child.

CONCLUSION

Children with a UTI and risk factors for renal damage (Table 8C.4) require imaging. The DMSA scan is the reference examination to declare the renal parenchyma normal or abnormal. This scan will also detect all the major congenital abnormalities (duplex kidneys, ectopic kidneys, etc). Every susceptible child with an abnormal DMSA scan requires a cystogram. Boys under 3 years of age require a baseline radiological MCUG to assess the urethra. Follow-up scans can be done with a DIC until they are 3 years old and with dynamic renal scintigraphy and IRC thereafter. Girls should undergo a radionuclide cystogram (DIC if they are less than 3 years old, IRC if older) because of the low radiation burden. Recurrent urinary infection is associated with significantly increased risk of renal damage, especially if the bladder is dysfunctional. This occurs usually in the older child, often girls, and they require a dynamic renal scintigraphy with IRC.

In imaging children with UTI, the emphasis has shifted to the identification of the susceptible group and in this group the trend is moving away from detection of reflux as the major risk factor towards the identification of renal involvement using DMSA, either in the acute phase or late, as the main predictor of irreversible renal damage. The most susceptible groups are children under one year of age with fever and a UTI and older children with recurrent UTI.

Case history

PD is a girl who was born on 17 April 1997. In her first year of life she had a pyelonephritis followed by recurrent UTI. After commencing her on antibiotics, her general practitioner referred her to a children's hospital. The consultant pediatric nephrologist who took over her care, as part of her management, asked for some imaging. An ultrasound was performed on 13 October 1998 and showed a left kidney measuring 5.1 cm in length and a right kidney 6.6 cm. There was global cortical thinning on the left, particularly at the upper and lower poles, and dilatation of the left ureter down to the VUJ. The right kidney showed some small areas of cortical thinning. The bladder had a normal outline and normal bladder wall thickness. A DMSA scan done at the same time showed slightly reduced and irregular uptake in the left kidney and several focal defects. The right kidney showed a focal defect at the upper pole extending to the outer margin of the upper portion (Fig. 8C.10(a)). The left kidney contributed 39% to total renal function, right kidney 69%.

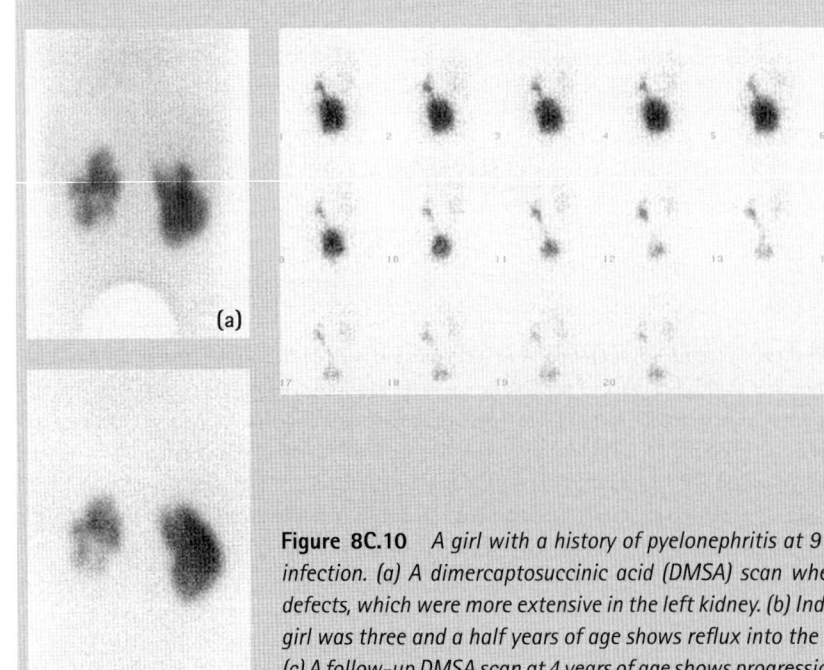

(a)

(b)

(c)

Figure 8C.10 *A girl with a history of pyelonephritis at 9 months of age followed by recurrent urinary tract infection. (a) A dimercaptosuccinic acid (DMSA) scan when the girl was 18 months showed bilateral focal defects, which were more extensive in the left kidney. (b) Indirect radionuclide cystography performed when the girl was three and a half years of age shows reflux into the left kidney and almost complete bladder emptying. (c) A follow-up DMSA scan at 4 years of age shows progression of scarring at the lower pole of the left kidney and some improvement in the right kidney.*

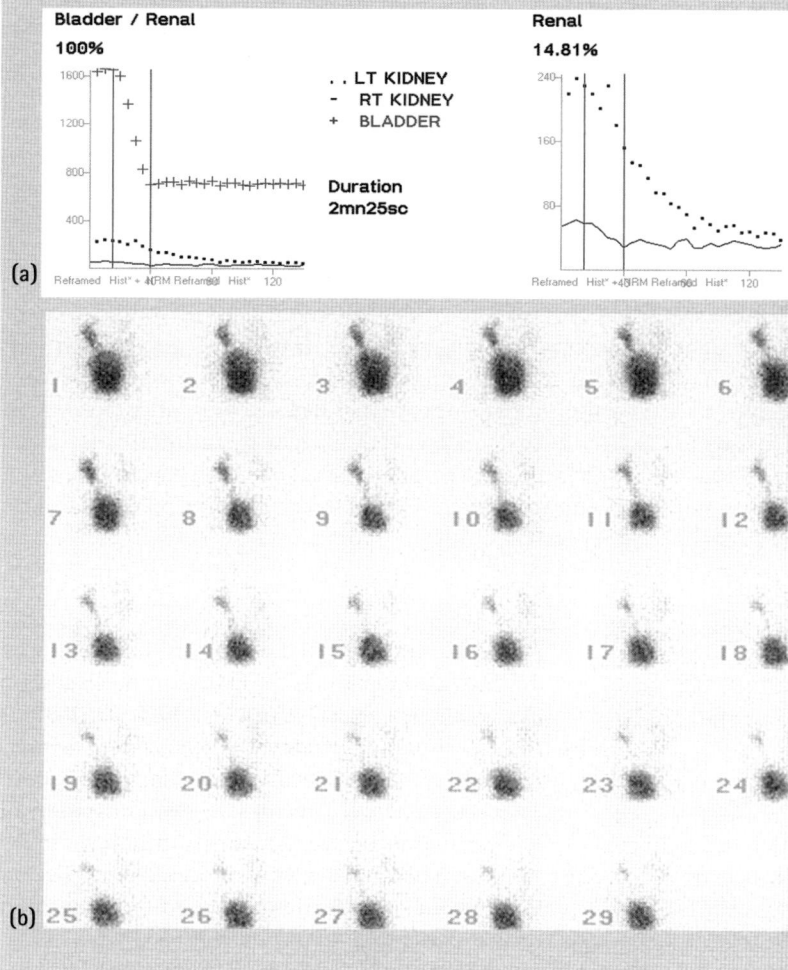

Figure 8C.11 *(a) Indirect radionuclide cystography done when the girl was five and a half years of age shows incomplete bladder emptying on the third attempt (the first two attempts were unsuccessful). (b) Time–activity curves confirming the incomplete bladder emptying.*

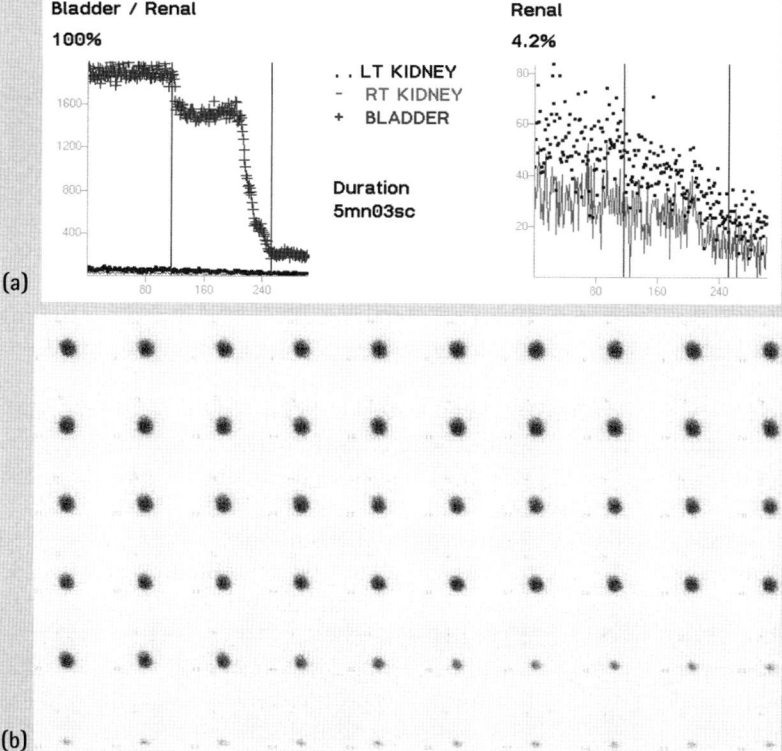

Figure 8C.12 *A follow-up indirect radionuclide cystography scan shows further evidence of bladder dysfunction (stepwise void) on both the scintigraphy (a) and the time–activity curves (b).*

A follow-up ultrasound a year later showed dilatation of the left pelvis and calyces and no dilatation on the right. Bilateral scars were confirmed. No calculi seen. Following recurrent UTI, a MAG$_3$ scan in October 2000 showed a fall in function in the left kidney (29%). Indirect radionuclide cystography confirmed the presence of a left sided vesico-ureteric reflux. The bladder emptied almost to completion with a voided volume of 189 ml (Fig. 8C.10(b)). A DMSA scan was performed a few months later to confirm the fall in function of the left kidney; this showed a scarred left kidney with more extensive focal defects than on previous DMSA of 1998 (especially at the lower pole) and a relative function of the left kidney of 28% (right kidney 72%) (Fig. 8C.10(c)).

The girl continued to have recurrent UTI and follow-up MAG$_3$/IRC in September 2002 showed relative renal function (left kidney 23%, right kidney 77%) that was not very different; the IRC demonstrated only one partially successful void with significant urinary retention in the bladder out of three attempts. No reflux was observed on that occasion (Fig. 8C.11 (a) and (b)).

Another MAG$_3$/IRC scan, performed a year later (November 2003) after three recurrent UTIs in a month, confirmed the impression of bladder dysfunction, with an incomplete stepwise void after a previous unsuccessful attempt (Fig. 8C.12 (a) and (b)). No significant change in the relative renal function was observed.

This case illustrates the importance of young age and systemic symptoms as risk factors for development of renal damage. It also illustrates that recurrent UTI can cause progression of renal damage even after 2 years of age. It finally shows that bladder dysfunction is a major risk factor for recurrent UTI and an appropriate bladder training programme can be beneficial in preventing further recurrent UTI.

REFERENCES

● Seminal primary article
◆ Key review paper
∗ First formal publication of a management guideline

● 1 Piepsz A, Blaufox MD, Gordon I, et al. Consensus on renal cortical scintigraphy in children with urinary tract infection. Scientific Committee of Radionuclides in Nephrourology. Semin Nucl Med 1999; 29: 160–74.

◆ 2 Rushton HG. The evaluation of acute pyelonephritis and renal scarring with technetium ^{99m}Tc-dimercaptosuccinic acid renal scintigraphy: evolving concepts and future directions. Pediatr Nephrol 1997; 11: 108–20.

3 Rosenberg AR, Rossleigh MA, Brydon MP, et al. Evaluation of acute urinary tract infections in children by dimercaptosuccinic acid scintigraphy: a prospective study. J Urol 1992; 148: 1746–9.

4 Risdon RA, Godley ML, Parkhouse HF, et al. Renal pathology and the Tc^{99m} DMSA image during the evolution of the early pyelonephritic scar: an experimental study. J Urol 1994; 151: 767–73.

5 Craig JC, Irwig L, Ford M, et al. Reliability of DMSA for the diagnosis of renal parenchymal abnormality in children. Eur J Nucl Med 2000; 27: 1610–16.

◆ 6 Goldraich NP, Goldraich IH. Update on dimercaptosuccinic acid renal scanning in children with urinary tract infection. Pediatr Nephrol 1995; 9: 221–6.

7 Goldraich NP, Ramos OL, Goldraich IH. Urography versus DMSA scan in children with vesicoureteric reflux. Pediatr Nephrol 1989; 3: 1–5.

8 Majd M, Nussbaum Blask AR, Markle BM, et al. Acute pyelonephritis: comparison of diagnosis with ^{99m}Tc-DMSA, SPECT, spiral CT, MR imaging, and power Doppler US in an experimental pig model. Radiology 2001; 218: 101–8.

9 Gordon I, Anderson PJ, Lythgoe MF, Orton M. Can Tc^{99m} MAG3 replace Tc^{99m} DMSA in the exclusion of a focal renal defect? J Nucl Med 1992; 33: 2090–3.

10 ARSAC. Notes for guidance on the clinical administration of radiopharmaceutical and use of sealed radioactive sources. Didcot, UK: Administration of Radioactive Substances Advisory Committee, 1998.

11 Wilkinson GA. Percutaneous direct radionuclide cystography in children: description of technique and early experience. Pediatr Radiol 2002; 32: 511–17.

12 Majd M, Kass EJ, Belman AB. Radionuclide cystography in children: comparison of direct (retrograde) and indirect (intravenous) techniques. Ann Radiol 1985; 28: 322–8.

∗ 13 Wennerstrom M, Hansson S, Hedner T, et al. Ambulatory blood pressure 16–26 years after the first urinary tract infection in childhood. J Hypertens 2000; 18: 485–91.

∗ 14 Goonasekera CDA, Shah V, Wade AM, et al. 15 year follow-up of renin and blood pressure in reflux nephropathy. Lancet 1996; 347: 640–3.

15 Patzer L, Seeman T, Luck C, et al. Day and night time blood pressure in children with higher grades of renal scarring. J Pediatr 2003; 142: 117–22.

16 Martinell J, Jodal U, Lidin-Janson G. Pregnancies in women with and without renal scarring after urinary tract infections in childhood. BMJ 1990; 300: 840–4.

∗ 17 Wennerström M, Hannson S, Jodal U, et al. Renal function 16 to 26 years after the first urinary tract infection in childhood. Arch Pediatr Adolesc Med 2000; 154: 339–45.

∗ 18 Craig JC, Irwig LM, Knight JF, Roy LP. Does treatment of vesicoureteric reflux in childhood prevent end-stage renal disease attributable to reflux nephropathy? Pediatrics 2000; 105: 1236–41.

* 19 American Academy of Pediatrics, Committee on Quality Improvement, Subcommittee on Urinary Tract Infection. The diagnosis, treatment and evaluation of the initial urinary tract infection in febrile infants and young children. *Pediatrics* 1999; **103**: 843–52.

* 20 Royal College of Physicians. Report of a working group of the research unit. Guidelines for the management of acute urinary tract infection in childhood. *JR Coll Phys Lond* 1991; **25**: 36–42.

* 21 Hoberman A, Charron M, Hickey RW, *et al.* Imaging studies after a first febrile urinary tract infection in young children. *N Engl J Med* 2003; **348**: 195–202.

22 Majd M, Rushton HG, Jantausch B, Wiedermann BL. Relationship among vesico-ureteral reflux, P-fimbriated *E. coli*, and acute pyelonephritis in children with febrile urinary tract infections. *J Pediatr* 1991; **119**: 578–85.

23 Jacobsson B, Soderlundh S, Berg U. Diagnostic significance of ^{99m}Tc dimercaptosuccinic acid (DMSA) scintigraphy in urinary tract infections. *Arch Dis Child* 1992; **67**: 1338–42.

24 Benador D, Benador N, Slosman DO, *et al.* Cortical scintigraphy in the evaluation of renal parenchymal changes in children with pyelonephritis. *J Pediatr* 1994; **124**: 17–20.

25 Stokland E, Hansson S, Jodal U, Sixt R. An alternative approach to investigation of children with urinary tract infection. *Ped Radiol* 2001; **31**: S32.

26 Wheeler D, Vimalachandra D, Hodson EM, *et al.* Antibiotics and surgery for vesicoureteric reflux: a meta-analysis of randomised controlled trials. *Arch Dis Child* 2003; **88**: 688–94.

27 Gordon I, Barkovics M, Pindoria S, *et al.* Primary vesico-ureteric reflux as a predictor of renal damage in children hospitalised with urinary tract infection: a systematic review and meta-analysis. *J Am Soc Nephrol* 2003; **14**: 739–44.

28 Schwab Jr CW, Wu HY, Selman GH, *et al.* Spontaneous resolution of vesico-ureteric reflux: a 15 year perspective. *J Urol* 2002; **168**: 2594–9.

29 Smellie JM, Ransley PG, Normand IC, *et al.* Development of new renal scars: a collaborative study. *Br Med J (Clin Res Edition)* 1985; **290**: 1957–60.

● 30 Olbing H, Smellie JM, Jodal U, Lax H. New renal scars in children with severe VUR: a 10 year study of a randomised treatment. *Pediatr Nephrol* 2003; **18**: 1128–31.

31 Vernon SJ, Coulthard MG, Lambert HJ, *et al.* New renal scarring in children who at age 3 and 4 years had had normal scans with dimercaptosuccinic acid: follow-up study. *Br Med J* 1997; **315**: 905–8.

32 Parkhouse HF, Godley ML, Cooper J, *et al.* Renal imaging with ^{99m}Tc-DMSA in the detection of acute pyelonephritis: an experimental study in the pig. *Nucl Med Commun* 1989; **10**: 63–70.

● 33 Biggi A, Dardanelli L, Cussino P, *et al.* Prognostic value of acute DMSA scan in children with first urinary tract infection. *Pediatr Nephrol* 2001; **16**: 800–4.

34 Ditchfield MR, Summerville D, Grimwood K, *et al.* Time course of transient cortical scintigraphy defects associated with acute pyelonephritis. *Pediatr Radiol* 2002; **32**: 849–52.

35 Jacobsson B, Svensson L. Transient pyelonephritic changes on 99^m-technetium-dimercaptosuccinic acid scan for at least five months after infection. *Acta Paediatr* 1997; **86**: 803–7.

Hypertension

A. HILSON

INTRODUCTION

For the patient, the taking of treatment for hypertension is essentially the paying of the premium of an insurance policy, in that long-term reduction of blood pressure reduces the incidence of the complications of heart failure, stroke and renal impairment. The incidence of myocardial infarction also falls if other risk factors are controlled at the same time. Depending on the selection of patients attending the general practitioner or the special clinic, and their age, the incidence of causes for hypertension varies between 1 in 20 and 1 in 8. The most common cause is bilateral renal disease. Depending on further selection, between 1 and 5% of hypertensives can be shown to have a renal or adrenal disorder for which correction by surgery will lead to amelioration of hypertension. Since virtually all hypertension responds to the right combination of drugs, the question is whether the pursuit of these few is worthwhile. This depends on whether the clinical tests demonstrating those likely to benefit from surgery are sufficiently simple, noninvasive, reliable and cost-effective; and whether the patient should be denied the right to choose a possibility of cure, whether by surgery or angioplasty as an alternative to a life-time of drug taking. For those who answer these questions affirmatively the search for these few may be considered as a five-stage process:

1. Identification of the hypertensives in the population
2. Selection of hypertensives who possibly have correctable lesions
3. Demonstration of those with the functional pattern of renovascular disorder
4. Definition of the surgical anatomy
5. Making the choice between angioplasty, a restorative operation and nephrectomy.

What is required is an evaluation of what each technique can and cannot do, and the scientific basis for its use; and for each hospital to outline a strategy of investigation and management. This will be different for different hospitals, partly because of the differing prevalence of renovascular hypertension, partly because of different availability of equipment, and partly because of differing expertise in the use and interpretation of results obtained with such equipment. Thus, as in most of medicine, there is no one right way of solving a diagnostic or patient management problem (Table 8D.1).

In essential hypertension, the renal images are of similar size, the renograms are symmetrical, and relative functions and peak times are also similar. The mean parenchymal transit times are normal. Cortical nephron flow is reduced equally in each kidney and may be improved by angiotensin-converting enzyme inhibitors.[1,2]

RENOVASCULAR HYPERTENSION

In renovascular hypertension the crucial clinical problem is whether successful correction of an arterial stenosis to one kidney is likely to relieve the hypertension. Renovascular hypertension may be defined as being present in those patients in whom an occlusive lesion (or lesions) of the large or small arteries or arterioles is associated with a particular pattern of renal function and in whom angioplasty, surgical repair of the lesion, or nephrectomy is likely to relieve the hypertension.

If no corrective procedure is undertaken to be followed by prolonged relief of hypertension, the diagnosis of renovascular hypertension remains in doubt, although the pattern of disordered renal function may be typical. Five statements

Table 8D.1 *Hypertension: assessment of renovascular hypertension*

1. *Renal radionuclide study*
   Baseline
   Captopril intervention
2. *Positive study: large-vessel or small-vessel disease?*
   Small vessel
       Clinical, urine: infection, casts, proteins, sugar, etc.
       Renal function, glomerulonephritis, diabetes, etc.
   Large vessel
       Doppler US, MRA
3. *Positive study: is control of blood pressure good?*
   Serial renal radionuclide studies
4. *Positive study: is control of blood pressure poor or deterioration in renal function?*
5. *Renal artery stenosis*
   Angioplasty, surgery or nephrectomy if relative function is less then 7% of total
6. *Improvement in hypertension*
   Serial renal radionuclide studies to demonstrate improvement in renal function and to detect return of renovascular disorder, e.g. due to restenosis

Hypertension: alternative approaches

1. *Small kidney or not?*
   US (IVU, CT, MRI)
2. *Reduced flow or not?*
   Doppler US (MRI)
3. *Renal artery stenosis, incidental on angiography, e.g. for peripheral vascular disease.*
4. *Proceed to assessment of presence of renovascular disorder*
   Renal radionuclide studies: baseline captopril or captopril intervention alone

may be made about renal radionuclide studies in renovascular hypertension:

1. Renovascular disorder is not renal artery stenosis.
2. Renovascular disorder is most commonly due to small-vessel disease, usually bilateral.
3. Renal radionuclide studies do not distinguish small-vessel from large-vessel disease as the cause of renovascular hypertension.
4. Angiographic renal artery narrowing is common, particularly in the elderly, where it is typically due to atherosclerotic disease of the aorta encroaching on the ostia of the renal arteries. The renographic demonstration of the characteristic functional abnormality suggests that there is renovascular disorder causing hypertension. Proof is only given when correction of the renovascular disorder (or nephrectomy) gives prolonged correction of the hypertension and returns the functional abnormality to normal.

5. It is not uncommon to find a small kidney on one side in hypertensive patients. Smith[3] stated if all small kidneys in this situation were excised, about 25% of patients would recover from hypertension. His challenge was how to tell which 25%.

The other kidney is important. It must not have renovascular disorder for relief of a contralateral renal artery stenosis to improve hypertension.

This functional pattern has three features relevant to radionuclide studies. First, there is an increased proximal tubular water and salt reabsorption related to the slight relative reduction in peritubular capillary pressure due to the occlusive arterial or arteriolar lesions. A nonreabsorbable solute such as ^{99m}Tc-mercaptoacetyltriglycine (^{99m}Tc-MAG$_3$) will therefore become relatively concentrated within a pool of fluid that travels more slowly along the nephron. The time to peak of the renogram which represents a crude measure of the mean transit time of MAG$_3$ entering and leaving the kidney will be prolonged as compared with a normal kidney. A reduction of the perfusion pressure is associated with a reduction of medullary blood flow whose consequence is an improvement in the concentration gradient in the medulla with increased reabsorption of water from the collecting duct, and a slowing of flow in it with further prolongation of the time of transit of a nonreabsorbable solute. Thus, the mean parenchymal transit time (MPTT) of a nonreabsorbable solute, whether it be *ortho*-iodohippurate (OIH), diethylenetriaminepentaacetic acid (DTPA), MAG$_3$, ethyl cysteinate dimer (ECD), or whatever, will be increased. In the absence of outflow system disorder and in a normally hydrated person this explains why a difference of over a minute between peak times in the two renograms is an indicator of prolonged MAG$_3$ transit.[4] Similarly, the corticopelvic transfer time is prolonged beyond 190 s.[5]

Second, the blood supply and therefore delivery of the radiopharmaceutical to the kidney with renovascular disorder is reduced below normal due to the occlusive arterial or arteriolar lesions. An uptake function less than 42% of total function is abnormal, and the second phase of the renogram of the affected (usually smaller) kidney is impaired. It should be noted, however, that renal artery stenosis is not an all-or-none phenomenon and in the early 'unstable' stage only a difference in peak time may be seen, without reduction in function.

The third requirement is that the 'non-affected' kidney has not itself undergone small vessel renovascular disorder as a consequence of hypertension. This may be demonstrated by the normality of the renogram from the unaffected kidney. A non-affected kidney should have an effective renal plasma flow (ERPF) of at least 300 mL min^{-1}.

The selection from amongst all hypertensive patients of those who might have a renovascular disorder used to be most simply undertaken by probe renography.[6,7] These authors showed that 99.4% of 980 essential hypertensives with normal renograms were correctly assumed to be free of significant unilateral renal parenchymal or renovascular disease. They found no benefit in pursuing further investigations for renovascular disorder in hypertensives with normal results of renography. Taking angiographic demonstration of renal artery stenosis as the 'gold standard', Britton and Brown[8] showed that 90% of patients with a 'false positive' probe renogram had elevated peripheral renins, indicating the likelihood of small-vessel disorder causing 'high-renin' essential hypertension. Renal radionuclide studies do not and cannot, in principle, distinguish small-vessel from large-vessel causes of renovascular disorder. Nordyke et al.[9] found that 15% of their hypertensive patients had abnormal findings from standard probe renography, and in one third of these after further tests, surgery for renovascular disorder was undertaken and ameliorated hypertension.

These findings may be contrasted with the use of rapid sequence intravenous urography (IVU). One in four patients with successfully corrected renovascular disorder have an undiagnostic rapid sequence IVU; hypertension per se is no longer an indication for an IVU. Ultrasound is used by some as a screen for unequal renal size and will also demonstrate pelvic dilatation, but it gives no functional information. Doppler ultrasound is an approach to demonstrating the presence of a renal artery stenosis causing an increased pressure gradient through change in the wave form and time characteristics of the response. It is cost effective when carried out by an expert, but there is a failure rate of up to 17%.[10]

Using a conventional gamma-camera technique, different authors place different emphases on the features that are extractable from the study. A conventional region of interest around each kidney and a C-shaped background for each kidney are used to obtain whole kidney background-corrected activity–time curves. Rapid recording of the initial arrival of activity at the kidney using 2-s frames and with a region of interest (ROI) over the left ventricle or aorta demonstrates the aortic to renal 'appearance time', which may be prolonged if renal plasma flow is reduced. However, the technique is not reliable in the diagnosis of renovascular disorders, because of the arrival of activity in vascular underlying and overlying tissue such as the gastrointestinal tract.

The distribution of uptake in the kidneys at 2 min is important and will be decreased in significant renovascular disorders. Reduction of size is typical of but not specific for renovascular disorder and a normal-sized kidney does not exclude it. Parenchymal defects such as infarct, small or large cystic disease and pyelonephritic scars may be noted. Functionally significant branch artery stenosis may be identified as delayed parenchymal uptake at one pole of a kidney. However, this is commoner in children, and is best demonstrated using dimercaposuccinic acid (DMSA). Such appearances are due to local prolongation of the tracer's mean parenchymal transit time. Duplex kidneys may be shown, one moiety of which is ischaemic.

Asymmetry of renal uptake function is the first step towards the demonstration of stable, unilateral, functionally significant renovascular disorder.

MEAN PARENCHYMAL TRANSIT TIME

The second requirement is the demonstration of an abnormally prolonged mean parenchymal transit time, which reflects the second disorder of renal function in the ischaemic kidney: that of increased salt and water reabsorption due to a tiny reduction of peritubular capillary pressure relative to the intratubular luminal pressure in the proximal tubules. Third, there is also an increase in medullary concentrating ability through the reduction in juxtamedullary (JM) nephron flow. JM nephrons cannot autoregulate in response to the fall in perfusion pressure and their efferent arteriolar tone is heightened by the increased circulating angiotensin II. The flow of fluid in the collecting ducts is thus reduced. In consequence, the MPTT is prolonged in renovascular disorder because of both the prolonged minimum transit time and a prolonged parenchymal transit time index (PTTI). The separation of the pelvis from the parenchyme for the calculation of MPTT is important since it obviates the effect of changes in pelvic transit time by which the specificity of the whole kidney transit time (WKTT) or peak time of activity–time curve is reduced. Thus, in renovascular hypertension, the MPTT of a nonreabsorbable solute, whether it be hippuran, DTPA, MAG$_3$ or ECD will be increased. This is usually reflected as a delayed peak to the renogram.

In a normal hydrated hypertensive patient, a mean parenchymal transit time over 240 s or, in a small kidney, over 1 min more than the contralateral kidney should lead to a captopril intervention study. Taken together with an uptake function of less than 42%, this is strongly suggestive of functionally significant renovascular disorder. Such a finding does not distinguish between large-vessel and small-vessel disease. Normals (kidney donors) showed equal percentage relative function (RF%) of 50 ± 8%, and MPTT of 171 ± 43 s. Hypertensive patients with radiologically significant unilateral renal artery stenosis showed RF% less than 30% and a prolonged MPTT of 344 ± 76 s. The contralateral unaffected kidney showed a normal MPTT of 186 ± 32 s, similar to that of hypertensive patients without renal artery stenosis (222 ± 87 s). The prolonged MPTT in unilateral renal artery stenosis was significantly different from the other groups.[11] Bilaterally prolonged MPTT was seen in patients with impaired renal function due to small-vessel disease. Bilateral functionally significant renal artery stenosis is rare and causes bilateral prolongation of MPTT. Renal activity–time curves and MPTT findings more usually demonstrate that one stenosis is significant at the time of the study when arteriography shows bilateral stenoses.

A congenitally small kidney or a small kidney due to pyelonephritis unilaterally will have a normal parenchymal transit time if it is an incidental occurrence in a hypertensive patient. The unilaterally small pyelonephritic kidney with a prolonged mean parenchymal transit time may be considered usually to have renovascular disorder contributing to hypertension. Smith[12] and Luke et al.[13] showed that only about one quarter of nephrectomies for unilaterally small kidneys in hypertensives would relieve hypertension.

It should also be noted that the demonstration of a renal artery stenosis incidentally in a hypertensive patient, for example undergoing aortography for peripheral vascular disease, does not mean it is necessarily contributing to hypertension, particularly in the elderly. Essential hypertension and atheroma are both common and less than 1% of all hypertension is due to renal artery stenosis. Fibromuscular hyperplasia is typically found in the artery of a tall or thin woman and is commoner in the USA than in Europe. It is a correctable cause of renovascular disorder.

The functional changes of renovascular disorder can be summarized as follows:

1. Loss of autoregulation of cortical nephrons, due to maximal arteriolar dilation in response to the fall in perfusion pressure
2. Increased passive reabsorption of salt and water in the proximal tubule due to a slight relative reduction of peritubular capillary pressure as compared with intraluminal pressure
3. Increased urinary concentration in the medulla due to reduced medullary blood flow
4. Prolonged parenchymal transit time of nonreabsorbable solutes such as DTPA, OIH and MAG$_3$ causing a prolongation of MPTT, typically giving rise to a delayed peak to the renogram
5. Renin production and release into the circulation
6. Increased efferent arteriolar tone of the JM nephrons due to the increased circulating angiotensin II

Significant renovascular disorder can occur with normal peripheral and renal vein renins. Renal size is not a reliable indication of relative renal function. The presence of renovascular disorder may be found in the presence of normal renal arteries on angiography in the situation of, for example, glomerulonephritis, pyelonephritis, diabetic or interstitial nephritis.

THE CAPTOPRIL RENAL RADIONUCLIDE STUDY

The difference between essential hypertension and renovascular disorder can be enhanced by the use of an angiotensin-converting enzyme (ACE) inhibitor such as captopril. The enhancement of the functional abnormality of renovascular disorder is through the following mechanisms.

Reduction of blood pressure

An ACE inhibitor will tend to reduce blood pressure and thus reduce the perfusion pressure to cortical and juxtamedullary nephrons. However, it is not the reduction of blood pressure that is the important stimulus. Reduction of blood pressure can be obtained by many other hypotensive agents that do not have the characteristics of ACE inhibitors in improving the diagnosis of renovascular disorder. So small, nonblood pressure-lowering doses of captopril (e.g. 25 mg) are to be preferred to larger doses.

Effect of ACEs on angiotensin II

Angiotensin II has a vasoconstrictor effect on efferent arterioles. In the human kidney the efferent arterioles of cortical nephrons have virtually no muscle in them, and therefore there is very little, if any, effect of circulating angiotensin II on the efferent arterioles of cortical nephrons (their control is through the afferent arterioles). However, the JM nephrons have thick muscular efferent arterioles which control their blood flow. Circulating angiotensin II is an important vasoconstrictor for these. ACE inhibition causes a fall in circulating angiotensin II and thus a loss of constriction of the efferent arterioles of the JM nephrons. This lack of resistance causes a dramatic fall in JM nephron glomerular filtration rate, which is one of the features of captopril intervention.

Inhibition of renal angiotensin II activity

Captopril will inhibit the intrarenal angiotensin II activity in the juxtaglomerular apparatus. Thus, if an afferent arteriole of a cortical nephron is not fully vasodilated in an autoregulatory response to the arterial or arteriolar narrowing, then it will dilate further, tending to increase the flow through a cortical nephron. In essential hypertension where afferent arterioles of cortical nephrons are vasoconstricted to a greater extent than normal, their vasodilation due to captopril[1] is the main reason for the improvement in MPTT.

Effect on tubular function

Angiotensin II has an activity on tubular function which will be affected by ACE inhibitors, prolonging further the transit time of nonreabsorbable solutes. In essential hypertension this effect will not be seen.

TECHNIQUE OF CAPTOPRIL INTERVENTION AND INTERPRETATION

^{99m}Tc-DTPA is only suitable for the test if renal function is good. Iodine-123-hippuran, ^{99m}Tc-MAG$_3$ or ^{99m}Tc-ECD are to be preferred if renal function is poor, or if there is a small kidney.

The data should be recorded from the start in 10-s frames from ROIs over the left ventricular cavity and over the two kidneys. The left ventricular cavity activity–time curve gives a good input function for subsequent deconvolution. The baseline curve normally has an impaired second phase, a delayed peak and sometimes an impaired third phase in functionally significant renovascular disorder. The delayed peak time is a crude reflection of the prolonged MPTT. After captopril, the second phase may or may not become more impaired. The peak time will be further delayed and the third phase may not be seen at all. There is a deterioration of the curve, depending on to what extent the blood flow and glomerular filtration rate have fallen. The MPTT should be obtained by deconvolution of the input function and the parenchymal activity–time curve to give the MPTT whose normal value is less than 240 s with a borderline range of 220–240 s. In functionally significantly renovascular disorder due to large- or small-vessel disease, this is typically prolonged greater than 240 s,[11] and with the captopril test it is prolonged even further.[14] Whether a baseline renal radionuclide study is required as well as the captopril intervention will depend on the referral pattern of patients to the department. Primary or secondary referral will require it, whereas tertiary referral may not.

If one kidney appears smaller than the other, but its activity–time curve is normal or MPTT is borderline, captopril intervention may be recommended.

For captopril intervention, the patient should be off diuretics for 3 days, off captopril for 2 days, and off other ACE inhibitors for 7 days. The patient should be normally hydrated and reclining against the gamma camera. Blood pressure should be monitored before and at intervals of 5–10 min after oral administration of captopril (25 mg). The renal radionuclide study should start if the diastolic pressure falls 10 mmHg or at 1 h. ^{99m}Tc-MAG$_3$ (100 MBq; up to 3 mCi) is given as a bolus and recordings made at a frame rate of 10 s for 30 min. A baseline study when renal function is fair may be followed 2 h later by captopril intervention on the same day, provided that the patient is properly prepared.

The interpretation of the response to captopril should be based on both visual and numerical criteria. The images may show an increased cortico-pelvic transfer time. The activity–time curve changes were classified by Oei et al.[15] Typically, a normal-shaped renogram shows change from a reduction in second phase and a further delay in peak time at least over 60 s to a rising curve without a peak. The poorer the initial renogram, the less the visual change with captopril intervention. The relative function typically shows a 5% reduction on the affected side. These criteria were used for the successful European multicenter trial of captopril intervention.[16] Using ^{99m}Tc-DTPA, angiography sensitivity for unilateral renal artery stenosis was 73% and for bilateral stenosis 91%. Taking the overall population, specificity was 84% for unilateral and 92% for bilateral stenosis, and prediction of reduction of hypertension was 93% for unilateral and 88% for bilateral stenosis. A 5% reduction in relative function may not be seen and this lack of change should not exclude a positive response, if other criteria are positive and the MPTT is prolonged. A greater than 10% reduction in relative function with ACE inhibitor is fairly specific.

Nally et al.[17] proposed probabilistic criteria for interpretation:

- *Low probability*: normal findings or improvement in abnormal baseline findings after ACE inhibition. (This is typical of essential hypertension.)
- *Indeterminate probability*: abnormal baseline unchanged by ACE inhibition. Specificity for renal artery stenosis is poor since such features may be due to small-vessel disease. MPTT helps to evaluate this population. Prolongation of MPTT from borderline to abnormal indicated renovascular disorder is present due to small- or large-vessel disease, but from abnormal to very prolonged is likely to be due to critical renal artery stenosis.[14] No change or improvement in MPTT makes renovascular disorder unlikely.
- *High probability*: marked deterioration of the renogram with ACE inhibition.

Taylor and Nally[18] have reviewed published studies and a consensus report on ACE inhibitor renography recommends good practice.[19] Once the combination of unilaterally reduced uptake, prolonged MPTT, a positive captopril test, and a contralateral normal kidney is found in a hypertensive patient – particularly if blood pressure is difficult to control – the next step, after considering that small-vessel disease is unlikely, is renal arteriography (Table 8D.1). The patient's blood pressure must be controlled as well as possible. This procedure should include a free aortic injection as well as selective catheterization to check the renal ostium and the number of renal arteries.

Selective renal vein sampling for plasma renin activity is still practised in a few centers, and may be helpful in difficult cases. As well as the renal vein samples, a low inferior vena cava (IVC) sample must be obtained. It should be noted that over three quarters of the renin that leaves by the renal vein entered by the renal artery, so the correct estimation of renin output is given by individual kidney plasma flow × the renin arteriovenous difference. However, a renal vein renin activity twice that from the non-affected kidney has been used as an indicator of renovascular disorder.[20]

The decision to intervene or not depends partly on the contribution that the affected kidney makes to total uptake function. It is often said that nephrectomy is indicated if this is less than 7% and a restorative operation if it is more than 16% of total function. Between these limits, the decision depends on other factors such as the complexity of the surgical anatomy, the overall renal function, and the clinical state of the patient. However, it is probably more sensible to think of single-kidney glomerular filtration rate (GFR). Many of these patients have a grossly reduced GFR, possibly as a result of small-vessel disease combined with cholesterol emboli, and even a doubling of GFR may make little difference to overall renal function, although there may be some improvement in blood-pressure control.[21] In bilateral renal artery stenosis it is usual that only one is functionally significant. The relative roles of surgery and angioplasty (with or without stenting) are still unclear, and the outcome of several major studies is awaited. The success of the captopril intervention and MPTT measurement in predicting the outcome of angioplasty of the renal artery stenosis and the importance of using MPTT in the follow-up to detect restenosis have been demonstrated.

Finally, to answer Smith's original question: if 100 hypertensive patients with a small kidney on one side and a normal kidney on the other side have all the small kidneys excised, about 25% of these patients will lose their hypertension. How to choose the 25%? The answer is by identifying the typical findings of a renovascular disorder on baseline and captopril renal radionuclide studies. If the shape of the renogram and/or the MPTT are normal on the side of the small kidney, it is not causing renovascular disorder.

In conclusion, the renal radionuclide study, with baseline and captopril intervention provide the appropriate cost-effective way of demonstrating renovascular disorder in hypertension.[10] The techniques of IVU, ultrasound, X-ray, computed tomography and magnetic resonance imaging may demonstrate that a kidney is small or has a reduced blood flow but are unable to demonstrate the particular functional disorder of renovascular hypertension. Demonstration of a narrowed renal artery and its anatomy is required before angioplasty and surgery, but does not show whether it is functionally significant. The renal radionuclide study shows the presence or absence of renovascular disorder both before and after correction of a renal artery stenosis.

A captopril intervention study enables the evaluation of whether ACE inhibition is of benefit or is detrimental to renal function in patients with renal impairment.[22,23] Recently, aspirin as an inhibitor of prostaglandin-mediated vasodilation in the kidney, has been proposed as an alternative to captopril for intervention.[24]

Case history

A 55-year-old man presented with recent onset of hypertension, accompanied by a rise in his serum creatinine. A ^{99m}Tc-MAG$_3$ renogram (Fig. 8D.1, upper row) was performed which showed impaired function in both kidneys, with marked reduction of uptake in the upper half of the right kidney. A repeat study following captopril was performed (Fig. 8D.1, lower row) which showed further deterioration in the upper right kidney. The function of the left kidney improved. Angiography confirmed stenosis of a segmental right renal artery, which was dilated with improvement in his blood pressure and renal function, confirming the diagnosis of renin/angiotensin-driven hypertension arising from this kidney, with secondary impairment in function of the left kidney.

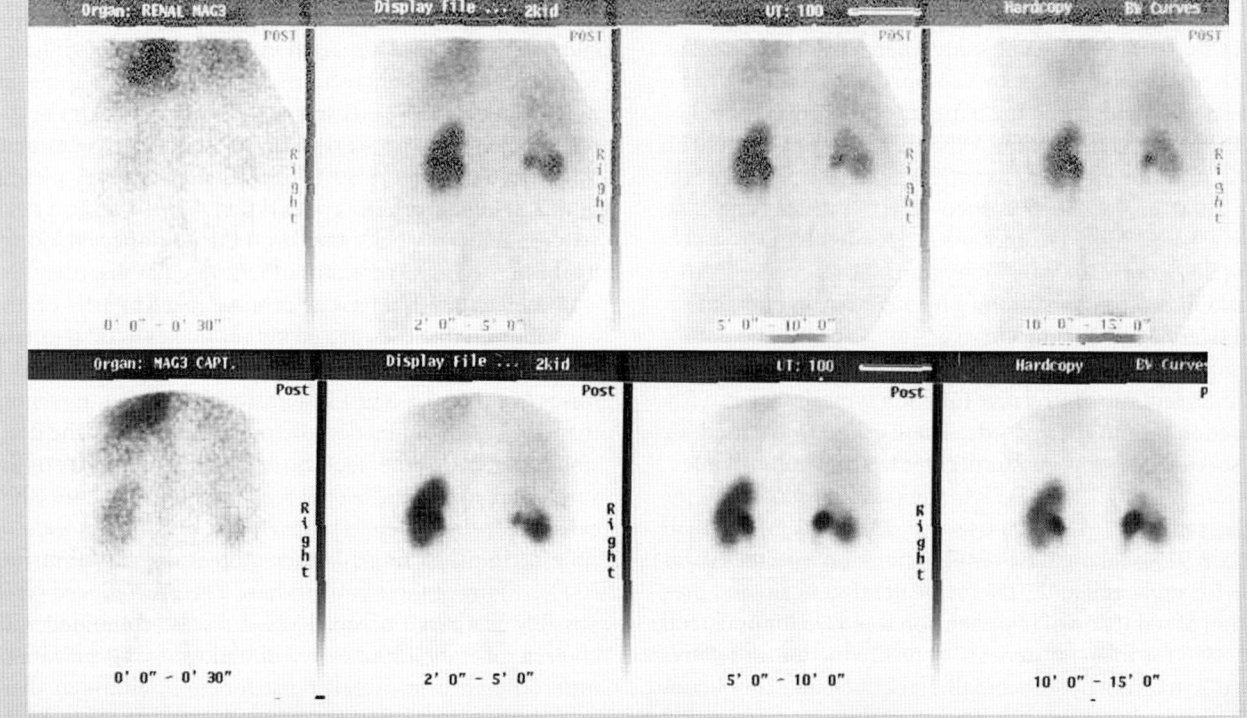

Figure 8D.1 *A 55-year-old man with recent onset hypertension.*

REFERENCES

1 Britton KE. Essential hypertension: a disorder of cortical nephron control? *Lancet* 1981; **ii**: 900–2.

2 Al-Nahhas A, Nimmon CC, Britton KE, *et al.* The effect of ramipril, a new angiotensin converting enzyme inhibitor on cortical nephron flow and effective renal plasma flow in patients with essential hypertension. *Nephron* 1990; **54**: 47–52.

3 Smith HW. *The kidney: structure and function in health and disease.* Oxford: Oxford University Press, 1951.

4 Russell CD, Japanwalla M, Khan S, *et al.* Techniques for measuring renal transit time. *Eur J Nucl Med* 1995; **22**: 1372–8.

5 Makoba GI, Nimmon CC, Kouykin V, *et al.* Comparison of a corticopelvic transfer index with renal transit times. *Nucl Med Commun* 1996; **17**: 212–5.

6 Mogensen P, Munck O, Giese J. ^{131}I-hippuran renography in normal subjects and patients with essential hypertension. *Scand J Clin Invest* 1995; **35**: 301–6.

7 Giese J, Mogensen P, Munck O. Diagnostic value of renography for detection of unilateral renal or renovascular disease in hypertensive patients. *Scand Clin Lab Invest* 1975; **35**: 307–10.

8 Britton KE, Brown NJG. *Clinical renography.* London: Lloyd Luke, 1971.

9 Nordyke RA, Gilbert FI, Simmons EC. Screening for kidney diseases with radioisotopes. *JAMA* 1969; **208**: 493–8.

10 Blaufox MD, Middleton ML, Bongiovanne J, Davis BR. Cost efficacy of the diagnosis and therapy of renovascular hypertension. *J Nucl Med* 1996; **37**: 171–7.

11 Al-Nahhas A, Marcus AJ, Bomanji J, *et al.* Validity of the mean parenchymal transit time as a screening test for the detection of functional renal artery stenosis in hypertensive patients. *Nucl Med Commun* 1989; **10**: 807–15.

12 Smith HW. Unilateral nephrectomy in hypertensive disease. *J Urol* 1956; **76**: 685–701.

13 Luke RG, Kennedy AC, Briggs JD, *et al.* Result of nephrectomy in hypertension associated with unilateral renal disease. *Br Med J* 1968; **3**: 764–8.

14 Datseris IE, Sonmezoglu K, Siraj QH, *et al.* Predictive value of captopril transit renography in essential hypertension and diabetic nephropathy. *Nucl Med Commun* 1995; **16**: 4–9.

15 Oei HY, Hoogeveen EK, Kooij PPM, *et al.* Sensitivity of captopril renography for detecting renal artery stenosis based on visual evaluation of sequential images performed with ^{99m}Tc-MAG$_3$. In: O'Reilly PH, Taylor A, Nally JV. (eds.) *Radionuclides in nephrourology.* Philadelphia: Field and Wood, 1994: 43–50.

16 Fommei E, Ghione S, Hilson AJW, *et al.* Captopril radionuclide test in renovascular hypertension: a European multicentre study. *Eur J Nucl Med* 1993; **20**: 635–44.

17 Nally JW, Chen C, Fine E, *et al.* Diagnostic criteria of renovascular hypertension with captopril renography. *Am J Hypertension* 1991; **4**: S749–52.

18 Taylor A, Nally JV. Clinical applications of renal scintigraphy. *Am J Radiol* 1995; **164**: 31–41.

19 Taylor A, Nally JV. Consensus report on ACE inhibitor renography for the detection of renovascular hypertension. *J Nucl Med* 1996; **37**: 1876–82.

20 Maxwell MH, Marks LS, Varady PD, *et al.* Renal vein renin in essential hypertension. *J Lab Clin Med* 1975; **86**: 901–9.

21 Scoble J, Mikhail A, Reidy J, Cook G. Individual kidney function in atherosclerotic renal-artery disease. *Nephrol Dial Transplant* 1998; **13**: 1049–50.

22 Datseris IE, Bomanji JB, Brown EA, *et al.* Captopril renal scintigraphy in patients with hypertension and chronic renal failure. *J Nucl Med* 1994; **35**: 251–4.

23 Blaufox MD. Should the role of captopril renography extend to the evaluation of chronic renal disease? *J Nucl Med* 1994; **35**: 254–6.

24 Maini A, Gambhir S, Singhal M, Kher V. Aspirin renography in the diagnosis of renovascular hypertension: a comparative study with captopril renography. *Nucl Med Commun* 2000; **21**: 325–31.

Obstruction of the outflow tract

K.E. BRITTON

CHRONIC OUTFLOW RESISTANCE

The physical factors are force, resistance, pressure, flow, and time. The force is that of cardiac output, the resistance is that of the nephron and urinary outflow tract. The combination of force and resistance leads to a pressure, which is a consequence, not a cause. Where there is flow in the system, flow will occur from the higher pressure to the lower pressure down the pressure gradient and for any particular compound a time can be measured from input to output. Thus time is able to be used as a measure of resistance. In chronic outflow resistance the force is unchanged. The cardiac output remains the same whether there is a renal stone or not, but the resistance increases. The change in the pressure gradient is from the source of the force to the site of the resistance that is from the glomerular filter to the site of the resistance not just the pelvis. Flow slows. Time, the transit time, is prolonged for nonreabsorbable solutes, such as ^{99m}Tc-mercapto-acetyltriglycine (^{99m}Tc-MAG$_3$). Therefore transit time can be used as a surrogate measure of outflow resistance. Transit time measurements are made by deconvolution analysis (see Chapter 8A).

OBSTRUCTIVE NEPHROPATHY AND OBSTRUCTING UROPATHY

In outflow disorders, definitions are important:

- *Obstructive uropathy* is a change in the outflow tract which is suggestive of an obstructing process being present, such as pelvic dilatation seen on ultrasound. Dilatation does not mean obstruction and absence of pelvic dilatation does not exclude obstruction.

- *Obstructing uropathy* is a change in the outflow tract due to an increased resistance to flow above normal. 'Obstructing' instead of 'obstructive' uropathy indicates confirmation of the presence of an obstructing process.
- *Obstructive nephropathy* is the effect of an obstructing process on the function of the kidney.
- *Diuresis renography* is the use of a pharmacologically active diuretic before, during or after injection of the radionuclide labeled agent excreted by the kidney. The convention is to use minus time, e.g. -15 min (F $-$ 15), at the time of injection (F0) or plus time, e.g. at $+18$ min (F $+$ 18) to indicate the timing of the injection of the diuretic to that of the radiopharmaceutical.[1]
- *Obstructing process* is an increase above normal of the resistance to outflow and this has a number of different consequences on the physical appearance and function of the kidney and outflow tract. Acute obstruction is the province of intravenous urography (IVU) and ultrasound. Chronic obstruction to outflow means chronically increased resistance to outflow. There is still fluid flowing down the ureter in the presence of a chronically increased resistance to outflow.

The causes of chronic obstruction include pelvi-ureretic junction disorder, stones, malignancies of various sorts, benign structures and other benign causes of narrowing of the outflow tract such as retroperitoneal fibrosis. After a clinical history and examination, a plain X-ray of the abdomen, intravenous urography and/or ultrasound is done to see if there is obstructive uropathy from evidence of dilatation of the outflow tract, stone or other pathology. A renal radionuclide study follows to show if there is an increased resistance to outflow, an obstructing uropathy causing an obstructive nephropathy. Antegrade perfusion pressure measurements, antegrade or retrograde contrast studies might follow, or computed tomography or magnetic resonance imaging for pathology.

Direct antegrade perfusion of the pelvis with pressure measurements is the technique of Whitaker.[2] He showed that, if under local anesthetic the cortex of the kidney is punctured in order to hold the needle steady into the pelvis, then the pelvis may be perfused with saline at different rates, typically $10\,mL\,min^{-1}$. A pressure transducer system records if there is a rising pressure due to this high flow. If there is no change in pressure, the flow rate is increased to $20\,mL\,min^{-1}$ and if there is still no pressure rise, then there is no abnormal resistance to outflow. In other words, although the pelvis is dilated there is no obstructing uropathy. On the other hand, if there is an increasing pressure that exceeds 15 cm of water or 13 mmHg, there is an abnormal resistance to outflow. This technique was used as a standard. The disadvantages are that it is invasive and if there is leakage around the needle, the pressure will fail to rise in the patient with an obstructing uropathy. Alternatively, the IVU can be used with an injection of frusemide at 20 min to cause a diuresis. If the dilated pelvis 15 min later increases in size by over 22% on planimetry, that would be an indication of an obstructing uropathy.[3] If it does not increase in size or increases by less than 10%, then it is taken as the normal response to frusemide. In the past, many patients underwent surgery because of loin pain and dilated pelvis on the urogram on the side of the pain, but with no evidence of resistance to outflow. The presence of a dilated pelvis on ultrasound or urography cannot by itself be used to distinguish an abnormally increased resistance to outflow from normal.

The renal radionuclide study gives a whole range of events: images, activity–time curves, relative function, the response to frusemide, the output efficiency, and measurements of transit times including the parenchymal transit time index (PTTI). It shows the responses of the kidney to the obstructing process, the obstructive nephropathy. A surgeon wants to operate on the outflow tract, not to make it look like normal, but actually to improve or prevent the deterioration of the renal function as well as relieving pain. A set of images with ^{99m}Tc-MAG$_3$ which show retention in the pelvis may or may not respond to frusemide given at 18–20 min. Either the diuretic caused no response and the response is considered 'obstructive', or there is a 'normal' response which is considered 'non-obstructive'. The problem is that there is an important indeterminate group which is often wrongly called 'partial obstruction' – wrongly, because partial obstruction is no answer to the problem. The surgeon cannot do half an operation. He or she must make the decision to operate or not and this depends on whether there is an increased resistance to outflow causing an obstructive nephropathy or not. The weakness of the frusemide response is that it is often indeterminate in the patients with the difficult problems,

particularly when renal function is impaired.[4] Whereas the use of F − 15 reduces the equivocal rate in well functioning kidneys, it has yet to be shown that F − 15 technique is of benefit when renal function is impaired.

In a patient with hydronephrosis, the activity–time curve is usually a rising curve, even when the relative function of the two kidneys is the same. Clearly, there is a function of the kidney which is different between the hydronephrotic and the normal kidney and this is the time required for the activity taken up by the kidney to move through the nephrons, the pelvis and out of the system. It is the transit time. The transit times and the uptake functions are two independent variables (see Chapter 8A) that can be used to evaluate an obstructive nephropathy.

OUTPUT EFFICIENCY

Uptake and output components

The activity–time curve recorded over a kidney using an externally placed detector or gamma camera represents the variation with time of the quantity of radiation arriving at the detector from radioactive material within its field of view. When the organ of interest is the kidney and a probe detector is used the activity–time curve has been called the 'renogram' and the technique 'renography'. When the gamma camera is used, the term 'renal radionuclide study' is preferred for the technique and 'renogram' is used loosely for the activity–time curve recorded from a region of interest taken to include the kidney.

This 'renal' activity–time curve is a complex composite curve, $R(t)$. One component is the curve representing the variation with time of the quantity of activity in nonrenal tissue in the chosen region of interest, mainly in front of and behind the kidney. Another component represents activity in the renal vasculature not taken up by the kidney. The important component of interest is how the amount of radiotracer activity taken up by the kidneys varies with time, which is called the kidney activity–time curve $K(t)$. This may be considered to have been derived or obtained theoretically in an idealized situation free of blood and tissue background activity. In practice, the kidney curve is obtained as the resultant activity–time curve after appropriate assumptions or corrections have been applied to the composite activity–time curve $R(t)$, obtained from the gamma camera, for tissue and blood background activity, depth, attenuation, and size of region of interest. The supply curve is the blood clearance curve, which is usually obtained from a region of interest posteriorly over the left ventricle in the field of view of the camera. After an initial peak, it decreases rapidly and then less rapidly with time as the radiopharmaceutical is taken up by the kidneys.

Since the nonrenal blood and tissue component of the composite externally recorded activity–time curve, is proportional to the blood clearance curve, the relationship between $R(t)$ and $K(t)$ is given by

$$R(t) = K(t) + F \int B(t)\mathrm{d}t \qquad (8E.1)$$

where F is a constant called the blood background subtraction factor. For probe renography the factor F was calculated using a prior injection of radiolabeled human serum albumin.[5,6] The kidney activity–time curve, $K(t)$ – also called the kidney content curve – is itself complex and it can be separated into uptake and removal components.[5,6] Such a separation not only aids an understanding of the underlying physiology but also leads to new ways of analysis for determining renal blood flow,[7–9] and for determining the radiotracer output curve and response to frusemide.[10,11]

Taking ^{99m}Tc-labeled MAG$_3$ as an example, it is evident that before any MAG$_3$ leaves the kidney parenchyme to enter the pelvis in urine, the amount of MAG$_3$ in the kidney depends on the amount which has been supplied to it in the blood and the renal extraction efficiency. The early part of the kidney activity–time curve during the minimum transit time of MAG$_3$ from its tubular uptake site along the nephron and before any urinary loss of MAG$_3$ activity occurs, represents the accumulation with time of MAG$_3$ in the kidney.

The kidney is in effect integrating the uptake of the supplied and extracted MAG$_3$. The MAG$_3$ supplied to the kidney in renal arterial blood can take one of two paths: either it remains in the intrarenal blood circulation returning via the renal vein, or it is taken up by the tubules (with 2% filtered at the glomerulus). The renal artery to renal vein transit time is of the order of 4 s with a range of 3–20 s. The renal uptake of MAG$_3$, the fraction of blood activity taken up per second, designated $U(t)$ (the uptake constant), will be proportional to the blood activity and the total uptake (during the period of the minimum parenchymal transit time, t) will be proportional to the integral of the blood curve $B(t)\mathrm{d}t$.[5]

This is the uptake component $Q(t)$ of $K(t)$:

$$Q(t) = U(t) \int B(t)\mathrm{d}t. \qquad (8E.2)$$

Then, combining Eqns 8E.1 and 8E.2, during the minimum transit time, t, when $K(t) = Q(t)$:

$$R(t) = U(t) \int B(t)\mathrm{d}t + FB(t). \qquad (8E.3)$$

Alternatively, dividing both sides of the equation by $B(t)$:

$$\frac{R(t)}{B(t)} = \frac{U(t) \int B(t)\mathrm{d}t}{B(t)} + F. \qquad (8E.4)$$

Equation 8E.4 is in the form $y = mx + c$, the equation of a straight line. The intercept F and the slope $U(t)$ can be obtained by plotting the externally detected renal activity–time curve $R(t)$ divided by the actual background $B(t)$ data against the integral of $B(t)$, $\int B(t)$ divided by $B(t)$. This approach to the measurement of the background component

and the individual kidney (IK) uptake constant (i.e. IKGFR for DTPA and IKERPF for radioiodinated OIH) has been developed by Rutland[7,8] and applied not only to renal events but also to the renal arterial inflow and outflow. The same logic has been applied to the separate determination of the extravascular and intravascular components of the nonrenal activity in the renal region of interest by Peters et al.[9,12,13] in selecting the most appropriate region for the background correction of $R(t)$ to give $K(t)$.

Since during the minimum transit time period, $K(t)$ is proportional to $\int B(t)\mathrm{d}t$, consider a situation where no activity appears in the urine for a long time, as with complete outflow obstruction; then the kidney continues to integrate the supply for as long as this period and $K(t)$ becomes the uptake component, $Q(t)$, a 'zero output' curve. Therefore the curve of the integral of the blood clearance curve, $\int B(t)\mathrm{d}t$, can be considered as a representation of the kidney curve that would have been obtained if no activity had left the kidney. Then, by fitting (using a least-squares technique) the integral of the blood clearance curve to the uptake phase of a particular normal or abnormal kidney curve that decreases with time after a delay period, the difference between the two curves (fitted $\int B(t)\mathrm{d}t$ and $K(t)$) gives the cumulative output, also called the removal or output component, $O(t)$ (Fig. 8E.1). Differentiation of the removal component gives the tracer output curve, which is the variation with time of the quantity of tracer leaving the kidney. This should act as a reminder that the falling phase (third phase) of a kidney activity–time curve is not an 'excretory' phase, but an 'amount of tracer left behind in the kidney' phase. Only by deriving the tracer output curve in this way can the true 'excretory' activity–time curve be obtained. The use of the integral of the blood clearance curve fitted to the second phase of the renogram was published in *Clinical Renography*.[5] This was the original 'Patlak/Rutland' plot. It was used to calculate what was then called the isotope removal factor. To obtain a reliable Patlak plot, a 10-s frame rate is advised as it gives six or so points for fitting the integral of the blood clearance curve to the second phase of the activity–time curve from the kidney, whereas a rate of 20 s per frame gives only three such points. Peters[13] described the graphical analysis of the Patlak–Rutland plot.

By comparing the removal component with the uptake component an estimate of the efficiency of the process of excretion can be made. An isotope removal factor can be calculated for a series of renal transit times in order to make this comparison. For example, a kidney recovering after operation for pelvi-uretic obstruction would show progressive improvement of the isotope removal factor with time.[5,6] This approach has been developed by Chaiwatanarat et al.[11] to determine the appropriateness of the renal response to frusemide, particularly when renal function is impaired. The output efficiency (OE(t)%), is obtained from the removal component $O(t)$ as a percentage of the uptake component $Q(t)$. This gives the OE$_{30}$% for a 30 min study.

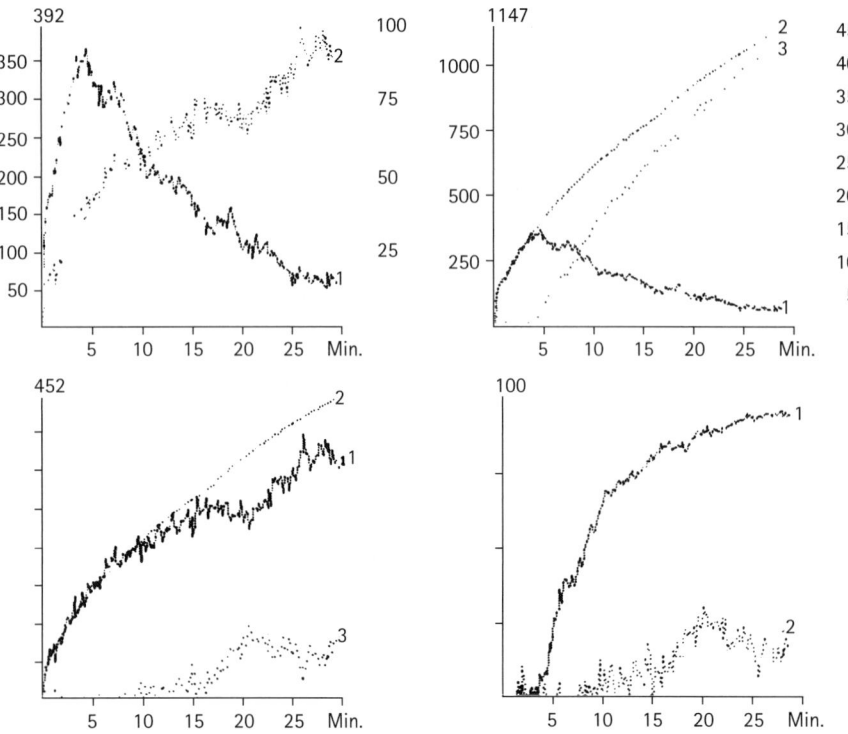

Figure 8E.1 *Outflow efficiency. Top left shows a normal renogram (1) and a renogram that continues to rise (2). Top right shows the production of the cumulative output curve (3) by subtracting the renogram curve (1) from the integral of the blood clearance curve (2) fitted to the second phase of the renogram. The cumulative output is similar to the cumulative input and the outflow efficiency is over 90%. Bottom left, the renogram with a rising curve has the integral of the blood clearance curve fitting to it (2). The difference between the two is the poor cumulative output (3). Bottom right shows the two cumulative outputs. For (1), the cumulative output is normal. For (2), the cumulative output has an outflow efficiency of less than 25% confirming an obstructing uropathy.*

$$OE(t)\% = \left[\frac{Q(t)}{O(t)}\right] \times 100. \qquad (8E.5)$$

The output efficiency may be calculated both before and after frusemide. The normal range of $OE_{30}\%$ post-frusemide in patients with a dilated pelvis is better than 78% and similar to the normal range in patients with no outflow disorder. This means that over 78% of that which entered the kidney has left it by 30 min. An inappropriately impaired response to frusemide gives a value below 78%. A general discussion of these analysis methods is given by Britton and Brown,[5,6,14] Peters,[12,13] and Rutland.[7,8,15]

The normal output (outflow) efficiency was established in healthy persons (22 kidneys) in whom the OE_{30} ranged from 82 to 98%, mean 92%, SD 4.5%. The mean $- 3\,SD =$ 78%, so a normal value of greater than 78% was chosen. In 11 patients with subsequently confirmed obstructing uropathy, the OE_{30} mean was 56%, range 30–76%, SD 20%. In 53/54 patients who were suspected of having outflow obstruction but which was not confirmed, the mean was 94%, range 79–99%, SD 6.3%. The patient with an obstructed value for OE_{30} passed a renal stone before outcome evaluation. In a comparison of output efficiency (OE_{30}) and the frusemide response (FR) assessed visually, the sensitivity for OE_{30} was 91% and for FR 9/11 82%. The specificity for OE_{30} was 94% and for FR 87%. The accuracy of OE_{30} was 94% and for FR 86% There were no equivocal results for OE_{30}, but seven equivocal results for FR.[11]

In a study of 100 patients Cosgriff and Morrish[16] showed that only two patients had an output efficiency between 70 and 78% and that the equivocal response to frusemide was reduced by 15% to 2%. Jain et al.[17] extended this work to 162 patients, 320 kidneys and showed that OE_{30} enabled a reduction in the equivocal, that is, the uninterpretable frusemide (F + 15) responses from 9% to 3.4%. This supports the validation of output efficiency in the determination of the presence of chronic resistance to outflow. Output efficiency is a useful way of evaluating the frusemide response. It allows the response to be related to the level of renal function and is physiologically based. It provides an objective numerical result and a normal range. It reduces the equivocal rate of the frusemide response to under 4%.

PELVIC DILATION OR OBSTRUCTING UROPATHY

Consider the question of outflow dilatation. Dilatation does not mean obstruction and this is the problem for an over-enthusiastic ultrasound reader. Lack of dilatation also does not mean lack of obstruction. In an oliguric renal transplant there may be no dilation of the pelvis associated with a low urine flow and yet there may be an obstructive nephropathy present because of increased resistance to flow.

Obstruction means an increased resistance to outflow above normal. Obstructing uropathy is the effect of this resistance on the outflow.

Frusemide diuresis (FD) is the commonest method of evaluating obstructing uropathy with a renal radionuclide study. The approach is to intervene usually 18–20 min into

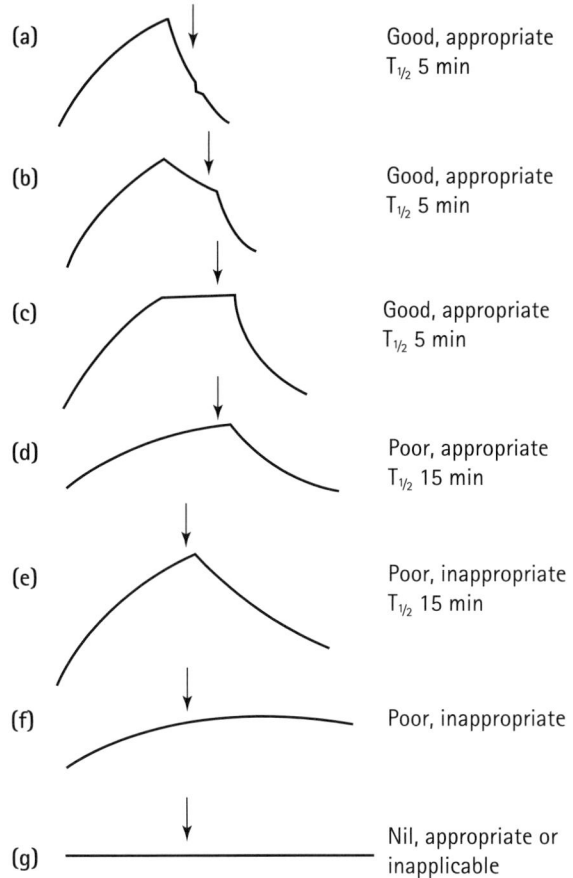

Figure 8E.2 *Responses to frusemide. Curves a, b, and c have good responses to frusemide (arrowed) with a half-life (T½) of the post-frusemide curve of 5 min. Curve d shows an impaired second phase and a poor response to frusemide, T½ = 15 min, but it can be seen that the response is appropriate to the second phase. Curve e shows a normal second phase and a poor response to frusemide (T½ = 15 min). Here the response is inappropriate to the second phase, indicating an obstructing uropathy. Curve f shows a very impaired second phase with an even more impaired third phase indicating an inappropriate response and an obstructing uropathy. Curve g shows that if nothing goes in it is appropriate that nothing comes out of the kidney.*

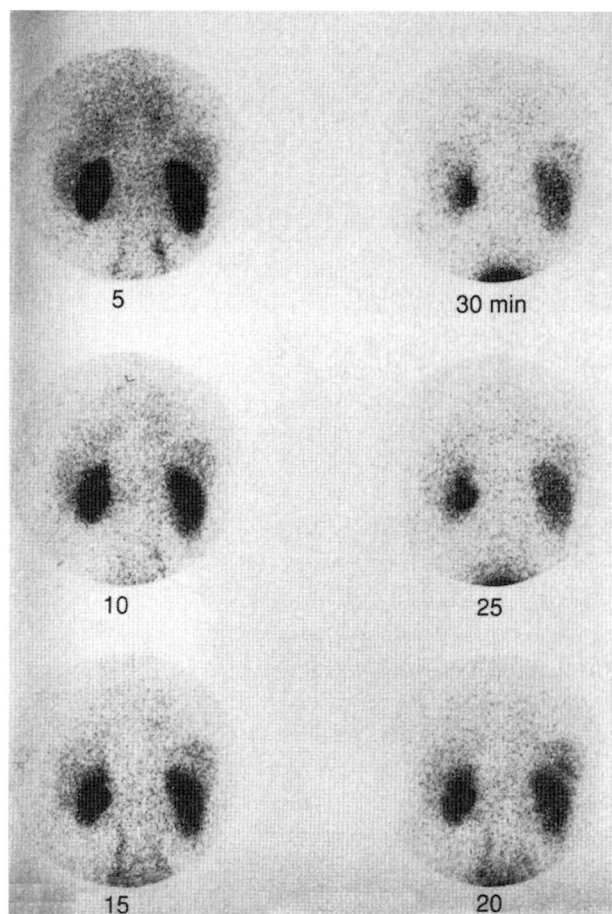

(a)

Figure 8E.3 *Pelvic dilatation. (a) A series of ^{99m}Tc-MAG_3 images. Frusemide was given at 18 min and there is some slight response visually.*

the study by giving an intravenous injection of frusemide, also called furosemide or Lasix (40 mg for an adult, $0.5\,mg\,kg^{-1}$ for a child, to a maximum of 20 mg) (see Appendix). It was introduced by Rado *et al.*[18] and evaluated and promoted by O'Reilly *et al.*[19] It is well recognized that a dilated pelvis, hydronephrosis, in the absence of an obstructive nephropathy is a relatively benign condition. The diuresis induced by frusemide helps to clear a dilated baggy unobstructed pelvis of active urine and causes a rapid fall in the activity–time curve.[1,4] O'Reilly *et al.*[20] using FD and gamma camera renography showed no obstruction occurred in 25 out of 28 patients with a negative FD over a 5-year follow-up. Kinn *et al.*[21] in 38 out of 83 patients with

hydronephrosis having no pyeloplasty showed it was a benign condition.

The frusemide response can be evaluated in a number of different ways and there are several visual classifications of the responses into various types; for example, empirically into F0 to F6 or into I, II, IIIa, IIIb (equivocal) and IV.[3,4,22–25] Visual criteria may be interpreted as normal or non-obstructive, obstructive, and indeterminate. Frusemide responses were categorized by a half-life after the injection of frusemide or some similar measurement made empirically from the activity–time curve. The post-frusemide half-life may be prolonged if renal function is good and there is a resistance of flow, or if renal function is poor and there is no resistance to flow. The output depends on the input.

Consider an alcoholic trying to get the last drop of alcohol out of the bottle. He has learned that if there is no alcohol in the bottle he cannot get any out of it. If the bottle was half full and there was an unextractable cork which had a very small hole in it, then he might know that he might be able to get something out of it but he cannot get it out quickly enough to satisfy him. What comes out depends on what is there. This is obvious, but when it is applied to the

Percentage Left Renal Uptake = 32.9%

Background_Subracted_Curves

```
1     +
1        +
1     +
1
1
1          +
1   +     +
1         +
1           +
1         + *******
1        ***+ +      *****
1     **       ++       ***   *
1     *            +       ** **
1  **         ++            *****
1             ++++++          ********
1 *              +++++ +   +++      *****
1                  + +++   +++++++++   **
1*                              +++++++++++++
1                                    *****+ +
+                                        *
*
```
- ·

L kidney (BBS) : * R kidney (BBS): +
L kidney OUTF%: * 94.% R kidney OUTF%: + 96. %
Kidney Transit Times in units of one second

	PTTI	WKTTI	MIN PTT	MEAN PTT	MEAN WTT
Left:	61	409	100	161	509
Right:	36	58	100	136	158
NORMAL RANGE					
	<156	<170		<270	

(b)

Figure 8E.3 *(Continued)* *(b) Activity–time curves: the left kidney (*) shows an impaired second phase and a somewhat more impaired third phase which is difficult to assess visually. The outflow efficiency, however, was 94% and the parenchymal transit time index 61 s – both normal – indicating no obstructive nephropathy or obstructing uropathy. The right kidney (+) is normal.*

kidney somehow this principle may be forgotten. Consider the frusemide response: if a little goes in then the correct response is only a little coming out. If a lot goes in then one must expect a lot to come out. If nothing goes in, nothing will come out, and that is not an abnormal response, it is normality. Thus, in evaluating the response from the activity–time curves, instead of saying that the responses are good or bad, what should be said is that the responses are appropriate or not appropriate. Take a normal curve which is rising and then falling after giving the frusemide, and the half-life is 5 min (Fig. 8E.2(a), (b) and (c)). Another curve showed good uptake and a poor output, with a half-life of 15 min (Fig. 8E.2(e)). A further curve (Fig. 8E.2(d)) shows a poorly rising curve, second phase, and a poor falling curve, third phase, also with a half-life of 15 min. In this case it is an appropriate response in that with only a little going in, there is only a little going out, whereas it is certainly inappropriate when there is a lot going into the kidney and only a little coming out (Fig. 8E.2(e)). Thus, one cannot distinguish frusemide response by looking only at the post-frusemide curve or a 20-min percent fall, or an excretion index post frusemide or by measuring a half-life.[26] What comes out of the kidney must be related to what went into it. Visually, the response to frusemide should be reported as appropriate or inappropriate to the second phase of the renogram or equivocal/indeterminate. Finally, a situation of 'nothing in' and 'nothing out' is totally appropriate (Fig. 8E.2(g)). Clinical examples are given in Figs 8E.3 and 8E.4.

When resistance to outflow is increased, the FD shows an obstructive pattern and pyeloplasty improves relative function.[27–29] Problems with FD are reduced renal function, particularly if one kidney has a GFR of less than $15 \, \text{mL} \, \text{min}^{-1}$.[30] There is less chance of recovery if the relative function is less than 35% due to fibrosis at the pelvi-ureteric junction.[31] Insufficient volume expansion was shown by Howman-Giles et al.[32] to be another cause of poor results. Equivocal visual results occur in about 15% of patients when frusemide is given about 20 min after the injection of the radiopharmaceutical, F + 20. Repeating the study by injecting the frusemide 15 min before (F − 15) was shown to improve equivocal results,[31,33–35] but this may not be seen when renal function is reduced. A consensus on the methodology of FD[1] was updated in 2003.[36] Conway[37] has reviewed the method in children (see pediatric section). Spencer et al.[38] have shown how FD correlates with magnetic resonance excretory urography in the hydronephrosis of pregnancy.

The radiopharmaceutical has changed from ^{131}I-OIH or ^{99m}Tc-DTPA to ^{99m}Tc-MAG$_3$ with FD. Hvid-Jacobson et al.[39] showed that ^{99m}Tc-MAG$_3$ was better than ^{131}I-OIH. Ozker et al.[40] showed that ^{99m}Tc-EC was also better than ^{131}I-OIH. Al-Nahhas et al.[41] evaluated ^{99m}Tc-MAG$_3$ which was preferred to ^{99m}Tc-DTPA.

The visual frusemide response has been compared with the other approaches to the assessment of outflow resistance. In chronic outflow resistance, transit time analysis particularly the PTTI has been validated against antegrade

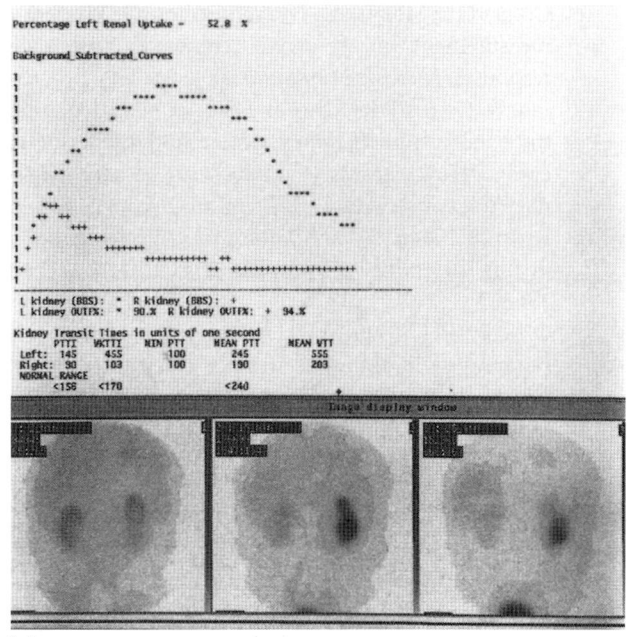

(a)

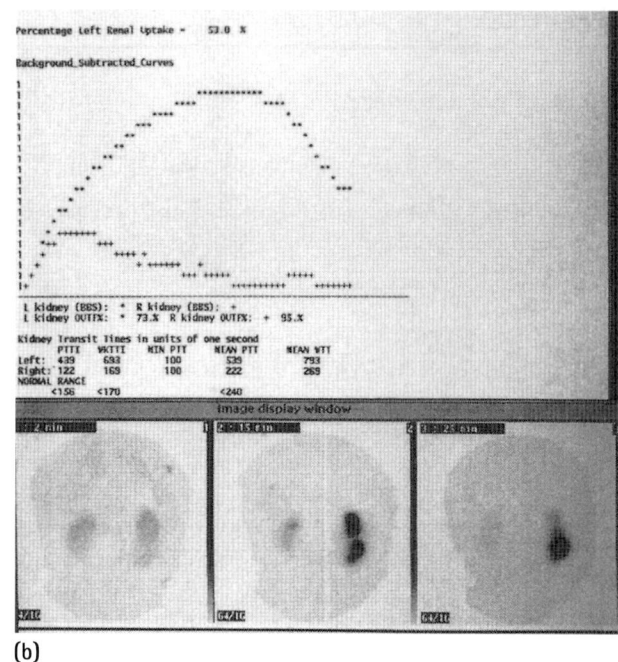

(b)

Figure 8E.4 *Progression of obstructive nephropathy. (a) ^{99m}Tc-MAG$_3$ study. The left kidney curve (*) rises to a delayed peak and falls. The third phase appears appropriate to the second phase. Outflow efficiency 90%, parenchymal transit time index (PTTI) 145 s close to the upper range of normal. (b) ^{99m}Tc-MAG$_3$ study, 1 year later. The left kidney curve looks similar to that of 1 year earlier with a rounded delayed peak and a third phase that appears appropriate to the second phase. There has been no change in relative function. However, the left kidney outflow efficiency has fallen to 73% and the PTTI has risen to 439 s, confirming the presence of obstructive nephropathy and obstructing uropathy. This diagnosis could not have been made on assessment of the curves and images alone.*

perfusion pressure measurements. Nine patients with pelvic outflow obstruction by this method had a range of PTTI from 160 to 306 s, mean 206 s. Four patients with dilated pelvis without obstruction had a PTTI range of 82–142 s with a mean of 104 s. From this the normal value of less than 156 s for PTTI was obtained.[42] In comparison of PTTI with frusemide, for the diagnosis of obstructive nephropathy, there was concordance in 116 normal patients. Those patients with proven outflow resistance PTTI found 59 out of 61 whereas frusemide was correct in 55 out of 61. Neil *et al.*[43] showed PTTI and FD correlated well, $P < 0.025$, but that dynamic computed tomography was poor in determining obstruction or not. The correlation between PTTI determined with ^{99m}Tc-DTPA and ^{99m}Tc-MAG$_3$ was $r = 0.83$.[41] Bahar *et al.*[44] showed PTTI was able to identify obstructive nephropathy as well as FD, sensitivity PTTI 96%, FD 92%. Extracorporeal shock wave lithotripsy (ESWL) may also be assessed using parenchymal and pelvic transit times.[45,46]

Output efficiency corrects the response to frusemide for the level of renal function as described above. Normal OE$_{30}$ is greater than 78% of what is taken up by the kidney is excreted within 30 min. A similar normal value of greater than 79% is seen in children.[47] The OE$_{30}$ value is becoming the standard method for measuring the response to frusemide in addition to the visual interpretation. Frusemide diuresis and output

efficiency are applicable to renal transplant studies[48,49] (see Chapter 8G).

Serial studies may be used to monitor the patient if no treatment is considered necessary or to monitor the response to treatment. The percentage contribution of each kidney to total renal function is measured directly after the first 1.5 min of the activity–time curve until a time before there is any loss from the renal parenchyma (see Chapters 8A and 8B). The measurement of relative renal function helps to determine which kidney to operate on first if there is bilateral obstructing uropathy. It is the one with the better relative uptake function.[50] In the context of chronic resistance to outflow a restorative operation or approach is recommended if one kidney contributes 15% or more of total function, whereas a contribution of less than 5% in an adult is unlikely to show recoverable function in response to treatment. The PTTI and OE provide complementary and often more sensitive means than the relative function for assessing response to surgery or other therapy for obstructing uropathy.

In conclusion, renal radionuclide studies clearly determine the presence of obstructive nephropathy and obstructing uropathy in patients with a dilated pelvis through frusemide diuresis, output efficiency and parenchymal transit time index measurements. They form an essential part of the evaluation of patients with suspected obstruction to the renal outflow tract.

REFERENCES

● Seminal primary article
◆ Key review paper
* First formal publication of a management guideline

* 1   O'Reilly P, Aurell M, Britton KE, *et al.* Consensus in diuresis renography. *J Nucl Med* 1996; **37**: 1872–6.

● 2   Whitaker RM. An evaluation of 170 diagnostic pressure flow studies of the upper urinary tract. *J Urol* 1979; **121**: 602–4.

● 3   Whitfield HN, Britton KE, Hendry WF, *et al.* Frusemide intravenous urography in the diagnosis of pelviureteric junction obstruction. *Br J Urol* 1979; **51**: 445–8.

● 4   Kletter K, Nurnberger N. Diagnostic potential of diuresis renography: limitations by the severity of hydronephrosis and by impairment of renal function. *Nucl Med Commun* 1989; **10**: 51–61.

◆ 5   Britton KE, Brown NJG. *Clinical renography.* London: Lloyd Luke, 1971.

6   Britton KE, Brown NJG. The value in obstructive nephropathy of the hippuran output curve derived by computer analysis of the renogram. In: *Proceedings of the International Symposium on Dynamic Renal Studies with Radioisotopes in Medicine.* Vienna: International Atomic Energy Agency, 1971; 263–75.

● 7   Rutland MD. A comprehensive analysis of renal DTPA studies. I. Theory and normal values. *Nucl Med Commun* 1985; **6**: 11–20.

8   Rutland MD, Stuart RA. A comprehensive analysis of renal DTPA studies II. Renal artery stenosis. *Nucl Med Commun* 1986; **7**: 879–85.

● 9   Peters AM, Gordon I, Evans K, *et al.* Background in the ^{99m}Tc-DTPA renogram: analysis of intravascular and extravascular components. *Am J Physiol Imaging* 1987; **2**: 66–71.

10   Nimmon CC, Britton KE, Bomanji JB, *et al.* In: Schmidt HAE, Csernay L. (eds.) *Proceedings of the European Nuclear Medicine Congress.* Stuttgart: Schattauer Verlag, 1988; 472–6.

● 11   Chaiwatanarat T, Padhy AK, Bomanji JB, *et al.* Validation of renal output efficiency as an objective quantitative parameter in the evaluation of upper urinary tract obstruction. *J Nucl Med* 1993; **34**: 845–8.

● 12   Peters AM. A unified approach to quantification by kinetic analysis in nuclear medicine. *J Nucl Med* 1993; **34**: 706–13.

● 13   Peters AM. Graphical analysis of dynamic data the Patlak–Rutland plot. *Nucl Med Commun* 1994; **15**: 669–72.

◆ 14   Britton KE, Brown NJG, Nimmon CC. Clinical renography 25 years on. *Eur J Nucl Med* 1996; **23**: 1541–6.

15   Rutland MD. Tracer flows and difficult organs. *Nucl Med Commun* 1994; **16**: 31–7.

16   Cosgriff PS, Morrish O. The value of output efficiency measurement in resolving equivocal frusemide responses. *Nucl Med Commun* 2000; **21**: 390–1.

● 17   Jain S, Cosgriff PS, Turner DTL, *et al.* Calculating the renal output efficiency as a method for clarifying equivocal renograms in adults with suspected urinary tract obstruction. *Br J Urol Int* 2003; **92**: 485–7.

● 18   Rado JP, Banos C, Tako J. Radioisotope renography during frusemide lasix diuresis. *Nucl Med (Stuttgart)* 1968; **7**: 212–21.

● 19   O'Reilly PH, Testa HJ, Lawson RS, *et al.* Diuresis renography in equivocal urinary tract obstruction. *Br J Urol* 1978; **50**: 76–80.

● 20   O'Reilly PH, Lupton EW, Testa HJ, *et al.* The dilated non-obstructed renal pelvis. *Br J Urol* 1981; **53**: 205–9.

● 21   Kinn AC. Ureteropelvic junction obstruction: long-term follow-up with and without surgical treatment. *J Urol* 2000; **164**: 652–6.

● 22   Britton KE, Nawaz MK, Whitfield HN, *et al.* Obstructive nephropathy: comparison between parenchymal transit time index and frusemide diuresis. *Br J Urol* 1987; **59**: 127–32.

● 23   O'Reilly PH, Testa HJ, Lawson RS, *et al.* Diuresis renography in equivocal urinary tract obstruction. *Br J Urol* 1978; **50**: 76–80.

◆ 24   O'Reilly PH. The diuresis renogram 8 years on: an update. *J Urol* 1986; **136**: 993–9.

25   Bahar TH. Chronic urinary schistosomiasis: patterns of abnormalities in radionuclide Tc-99m-DTPA diuretic renogram. *Acta Pathol Microbiol Immunol Scand* 1988; **Suppl**: 54–8.

26   Amarante J, Anderson PJ, Gordon I. Impaired drainage on diuretic renography using half-time of excretion efficiency is not a sign of obstruction in children with a prenatal diagnosis of unilateral renal pelvic dilatation. *J Urol* 2003; **119**: 1828–31.

27   Probst P, Ackermann D, Noelpp U, Roesler H. Obstructive uropathy: frusemide test and analysis of renographic curve patterns. *Nuklearmedizin* 1983; **22**: 128–35.

28   Muller-Schauenburg W, Hofmann U, Feine U, *et al.* Criteria for ureteral obstruction by functional imaging of upper urinary tract. *Contrib Nephrol* 1987; **56**: 225–31.

◆ 29   Sarkar SD. Diuretic renography: concepts and controversies. *Urol Radiol* 1992; **14**: 79–84.

● 30   Brown SC, Upsdell SM, O'Reilly PH. The importance of renal function in the interpretation of diuresis renography. *Br J Urol* 1992; **69**: 121–5.

● 31   Howman-Giles R, Uren R, Roy LP, Filmer RB. Volume expansion diuretic renal scan in urinary tract obstruction. *J Nucl Med* 1987; **28**: 824–8.

● 32   English PJ, Testa HJ, Lawson RS, *et al.* Modified method of diuresis renography for the assessment of equivocal pelvi-ureteric junction obstruction. *Br J Urol* 1987; **58**: 10–14.

● 33 Ahlawat R, Basarge N. Objective evaluation of the outcome of endopyelotomy using Whitaker's test and diuretic renography. *Br J Urol* 1995; **76**: 686–91.

34 Sultan S, Zaman M, Kamal S, *et al.* Evaluation of ureteropelvic junction obstruction (UPJO) by diuretic renography. *J Pak Med Assoc* 1996; **46**: 143–7.

35 Roarke MC, Sandler CM. Provocative imaging. Diuretic renography. *Urol Clin North Am* 1998; **25**: 227–49.

∗ 36 O'Reilly PH. Standardization of the renogram technique for investigating the dilated upper urinary tract and assessing the results of surgery. *Br J Urol Int* 2003; **91**: 239–43.

● 37 Conway JJ. 'Well-tempered' diuresis renography: its historical development, physiological and technical pitfalls, and standarized techniques protocol. *Semin Nucl Med* 1992; **22**: 74–84.

38 Spencer JA, Tomlinson AJ, Weston MJ, Lloyd SN. Early report: comparison of breath-hold MR excretory urography, Doppler ultrasound and isotope renography in evaluation of symptomatic hydronephrosis in pregnancy. *Clin Radiol* 2000; **55**: 446–53.

● 39 Hvid-Jacobson K, Thomsen HS, Nielsen SL. Diuresis renography, a simultaneous comparison of ^{131}I-hippuran and ^{99m}Tc-MAG3. *Acta Radiol* 1990; **31**: 83–6.

● 40 Ozker K, Onsel C, Kabasakal L, *et al.* Technetium-99m-*N*-*N*-ethylene dicysteine – a comparative study of renal scintigraphy with technetium-99m MAG3 and iodine-131-OIH in patients with obstructive renal disease. *J Nucl Med* 1994; **35**: 840–5.

● 41 Al-Nahhas AA, Jafri RA, Britton KE, *et al.* Clinical experience with ^{99m}Tc-MAG3 mercaptoacetyl triglycine, and a comparison with ^{99m}Tc-DTPA. *Eur J Nucl Med* 1988; **14**: 453–62.

● 42 Britton KE, Nimmon CC, Whitfield HK, *et al.* Obstructive nephropathy, successful evaluation with radionuclides. *Lancet* 1979; **I**: 905–7.

43 Neal DE, Simpson W, Bartholomew P, Keavey PM. Comparison of dynamic computed tomography, diuresis renography and DTPA parenchymal transit time in the asssessment of dilatation of the upper urinary tract. *Br J Urol* 1985; **57**: 515–19.

44 Bahar RH, Kouris K, Sabha M, *et al.* The value of parenchymal transit time index of Tc-99m DTPA diuretic renography in the evaluation of surgery in chronic bilharzial obstructive uropathy. *Am J Physiol Imaging* 1991; **6**: 121–8.

45 Bomanji J, Boddy SAM, Britton KE, *et al.* Radionuclide evaluation of pre- and post-extracorporeal shock wave lithotripsy for renal calculi. *J Nucl Med* 1987; **28**: 1284–9.

● 46 Ilgin N, Iftehar SA, Vural G, *et al.* Evaluation of renal function following treatment with extra corporeal shock wave lithotripsy ESWL: the use of whole kidney parenchymal and pelvic transit times. *Nucl Med Commun* 1998; **19**: 155–9.

● 47 Saunders CAB, Choong KKL, Larcos G, *et al.* Assessment of pediatric hydronephrosis using output efficiency. *J Nucl Med* 1997; **38**: 1483–6.

● 48 Nankivell BJ, Cohn DA, Spicer ST, *et al.* Diagnosis of kidney transplant obstruction using MAG3 diuresis renography. *Clin Transplant* 2001; **15**: 11–18.

● 49 Spicer ST, Chi KK, Nankivell BJ, *et al.* Mercaptoacetyltriglycine diuretic renography and output efficiency measurement in renal transplant patients. *Eur J Nucl Med* 1999; **26**: 152–4.

● 50 Sreenevasan G. Bilateral renal calculi. *Ann R Coll Surg Engl* 1974; **55**: 3–12.

APPENDIX: ADULT RENAL RADIONUCLIDE STUDY

Parameters

Radiopharmaceutical: ^{99m}Tc-mercaptoacetyltriglycine (^{99m}Tc-MAG$_3$)
Energy: 140 keV
Window: 20%
Activity: 100–150 MBq
Collimator: Low-energy, high-resolution

Procedure

The patient should be normally hydrated.
Give 500 mL water 30 min before commencing the procedure.
The patient should empty the bladder before the procedure starts.
A urine flow of 1–3 mL min^{-1} is optimal.
Set up a two-way tap infusion set for injection and saline flush.
Place the patient in a reclining position against the camera face which is tilted back 15–20° so the kidneys fall back against the muscles. Many practitioners prefer to image the patient supine, but this does not allow natural gravitational drainage and a post-micturition view is essential. Ensure that the left ventricle and kidneys are in the posterior field of view.

Dynamic aspects

The injection is given as a good bolus or a flush system.
Start the computer just before the moment of injection but not later. Obtain 180 × 10-s frames, at 128 × 128 resolution. Frames of 10 s each are optimal for the Patlak plot and deconvolution analysis for transit times.

For frusemide (furosemide, Lasix), inject 40 mg ($0.5 \, mg \, kg^{-1}$ in child aged 1–16 years to a maximum of 20 mg) after 100–110 frames of 10 s at 16–18 min. Warn the patient of the diuretic effects.

Do not interrupt the study for the injection of frusemide.

All patients should empty the bladder after the study.

A post-micturition standing posterior image of kidneys and bladder is required if there is evidence of pelvic retention at the end of the study.

Frusemide may also be given at the time of injection F0, or 15 min before the injection (F − 15), particularly if a previous F + 16–18 min response has been equivocal and output efficiency measurement is not available.

If a micturition study is requested to assess reflux (see Chapter 8G), start computer just before micturition starts: 180×1-s frames, at 128×128 resolution.

Renal transplantation

A. HILSON

INTRODUCTION

Renal transplantation has been in a routine procedure for over almost half a century, yet still continues to evolve. Its development has coincided with the period of major growth of nuclear medicine, and so it is not perhaps surprising that nuclear medicine has a significant role to play.

This starts with the *assessment of the potential donor*. Nowadays, with the shortage of cadaveric organs relative to the demand, there is an increasing trend of using organs from living donors. It is obviously necessary to ensure that the donor has two normal kidneys before one is removed. The protocol which is used in our center is to start with an ultrasound scan to ensure that there are two normally sited kidneys with no major abnormalities. If this is normal, we proceed to static scintigraphy with ^{99m}Tc-dimercaptosuccinic acid (^{99m}Tc-DMSA) to ensure that there is no major scarring, and that the divided function is normal. At the same visit, we also estimate the donor's glomerular filtration rate (GFR) with ^{51}Cr-ethylenediaminetetraacetic acid (^{51}Cr-EDTA), giving us the total GFR and the single-kidney GFR for each kidney. If these are satisfactory, the vascular and pelvi-ureteric anatomy are assessed using contrast-enhanced magnetic resonance angiography and urography. We then have a full set of data on the structural and functional state of the potential donor.

It must be remembered that the recipient will have been in renal failure, and this may exacerbate the complications this produces. In particular, there is a high incidence of (often undiagnosed) cardiac vascular disease,[1] which increases the operative risk.[2] For this reason, many centers require a myocardial perfusion study prior to surgery. In practice, this means regular (every 2–3 years) studies on all potential recipients.

CLINICAL PROBLEMS

Nuclear medicine has a significant role to play in the management of renal transplant recipients in the postoperative period. To understand this role, it is necessary to review briefly the clinical problems.

In the immediate postoperative period, there may be a worry about the vascular supply to the kidney. Over the 24–48 h following the operation, the kidney shows the effect of the (inevitable) ischemic injury it has undergone. This process is known as acute tubular necrosis (ATN). It may lead to total anuria by the end of 48 h. At the same time, the kidney is being exposed to the recipient's immune system, and this inevitably leads to an element of acute rejection. With modern immunosuppression, this is usually mild and occurs more slowly than was the case before the introduction of cyclosporin A as an immunosuppressant. Typically, a mild cell-mediated rejection develops at about 7–10 days (with modern tissue-typing, the full-blown accelerated or hyper-acute rejection of the past, developing in the first 48 h, is rarely seen). This rejection involves the parenchyma and especially the vasculature (which is, of course, of donor origin). It also involves the donor ureter, which may lose its peristalsis.

Over a longer time scale, the management depends on the use of maintenance therapy including cyclosporin A. This is not straightforward, as a low dosage may lead to rejection, while chronic higher dosage leads to renal damage. This is initially parenchymal, but if maintained or severe leads to vascular change. Over a period of years, the kidney may also undergo chronic rejection, which is poorly understood, but involves both vasculature and parenchyma. At any stage, but especially in the immediate postoperative period, there may be surgical complications.

PHARMACEUTICALS

Experience has shown that there is no significant advantage to either ^{99m}Tc-mercaptoacetyltriglycine (^{99m}Tc-MAG$_3$) or ^{99m}Tc-DTPA in the investigation of renal transplants, although it is often convenient to use one agent in any given patient until expertise has been gained.

THE IMMEDIATE POSTOPERATIVE PERIOD

If there is no suspicion of surgical complications, and patient is passing good volumes of urine with the serum creatinine level falling satisfactorily, then it is preferable to leave the baseline study until about 48 h after surgery, when the effect of ATN is likely to be maximal.

If the patient is passing satisfactory volumes of urine (30 mL h^{-1} above any previous urine output), but the serum creatinine is not falling, this most likely represents moderate-to-severe ATN. Occasionally, patients who have been maintained on regular hemodialysis may develop a 'hypovolemic circulatory failure' without fluid loss. Treatment consists of fluid replacement, but occasionally a nuclear medicine study may be requested to confirm renal perfusion.

Complete anuria postoperatively is always a cause of alarm. If there is a suspicion of a vascular complication, this represents an emergency, and the kidney must be studied immediately with whatever pharmaceutical is to hand. The study should always be reviewed with either the surgeon concerned or his operation note, to be sure what the vascular supply to the kidney was: it is not uncommon for the graft to have two or more arteries, and it may be necessary to look for evidence of a polar or posterior surface infarct.

The image should also be examined for evidence of a photon-deficient area above or around the kidney, representing a collection. If one is seen, a delayed image must be obtained to see whether it fills in with the ^{99m}Tc-DTPA or ^{99m}Tc-MAG$_3$, representing a urine collection. This may happen even if the graft is apparently producing no urine, as the ureter may have become detached from the bladder and there may be a total leak. It is important to remember that all renal transplant recipients have had an incision in the bladder for the re-implantation of the ureter. For this reason, the bladder is always drained with a urethral or supra-pubic catheter. This must *never* be clamped, as this may produce a leak, especially if the patient is in the polyuric phase of recovery from renal failure.

If the collection does not fill in, but urine is being produced, it may be a hematoma. Ultrasound may be helpful here, as fluid collections such as urine are well shown by ultrasound. If no separate collection is shown ultrasonographically, then a hematoma is more likely, as fresh hematomas in the transplant bed are often not identified on ultrasound, as they consist of a solid echogenic clot that cannot be clearly separated from the retroperitoneal muscle on which the graft is lying.

The worst situation that may be seen is that of the dreaded 'black hole', so named from the early days when images were recorded on Polaroid instant film, and a non-perfused kidney was seen as a black hole surrounded by a rim of inflammatory activity. This is generally considered an indication for instant intervention: the surgeon should be contacted as soon as this is seen on the screen, even before the study is finished, as the only hope is for urgent vascular surgery.[3]

THE EARLY POSTOPERATIVE PERIOD

On the baseline study performed at about 48 h, it is usual to see some evidence of ATN. This is shown on a ^{99m}Tc-DTPA study as a mild-to-moderate impairment of perfusion, with the presence of a blood pool within the kidney at 2 min, but little or no excretion. With ^{99m}Tc-MAG$_3$ the perfusion changes are similar, but the parenchyma shows progressive accumulation of tracer, with varying excretion. Indeed, if no excretion is seen, it may not be possible to exclude obstruction (although this is extremely uncommon in renal transplants). This is one of the very unusual times when a dual-pharmaceutical study may be necessary: if a ^{99m}Tc-DTPA study shows gross impairment, a ^{99m}Tc-MAG$_3$ study may be reassuring to show that there is uptake of tracer by tubular cells, which is probably a good prognostic sign. Conversely, if a ^{99m}Tc-MAG$_3$ study shows progressive uptake, a ^{99m}Tc-DTPA study showing that there is no functional peak, but rather a blood pool, may be taken as proof of ATN.

The impairment of perfusion typical of ATN may be assessed more accurately by use of numerical methods. The most widely used compares the upslope of the curve from a region of interest (ROI) drawn over the transplanted kidney with the upslope of a curve from an ROI over the iliac artery. This gives a perfusion index, which reflects renal transplant perfusion (Fig. 8F.1). In simple ATN there is mild-to-moderate impairment of perfusion, but this improves steadily with time.[4] It used to be necessary to carry this out on alternate days because of the lack of other methods of investigation and the fear of rejection, but now it is more usual to carry it out once or twice per week in the oliguric period.

Some centers use a measurement of ^{99m}Tc-MAG$_3$ clearance as a measurement of renal blood flow.[5] Whilst there is no doubt that this measurement changes with pathology, this is more complicated, as the clearance reflects not only blood flow, but also extraction fraction, which may change with pathology.

Regardless of the agent used, it is essential to record the presence or absence of excretion, and imaging of the bladder

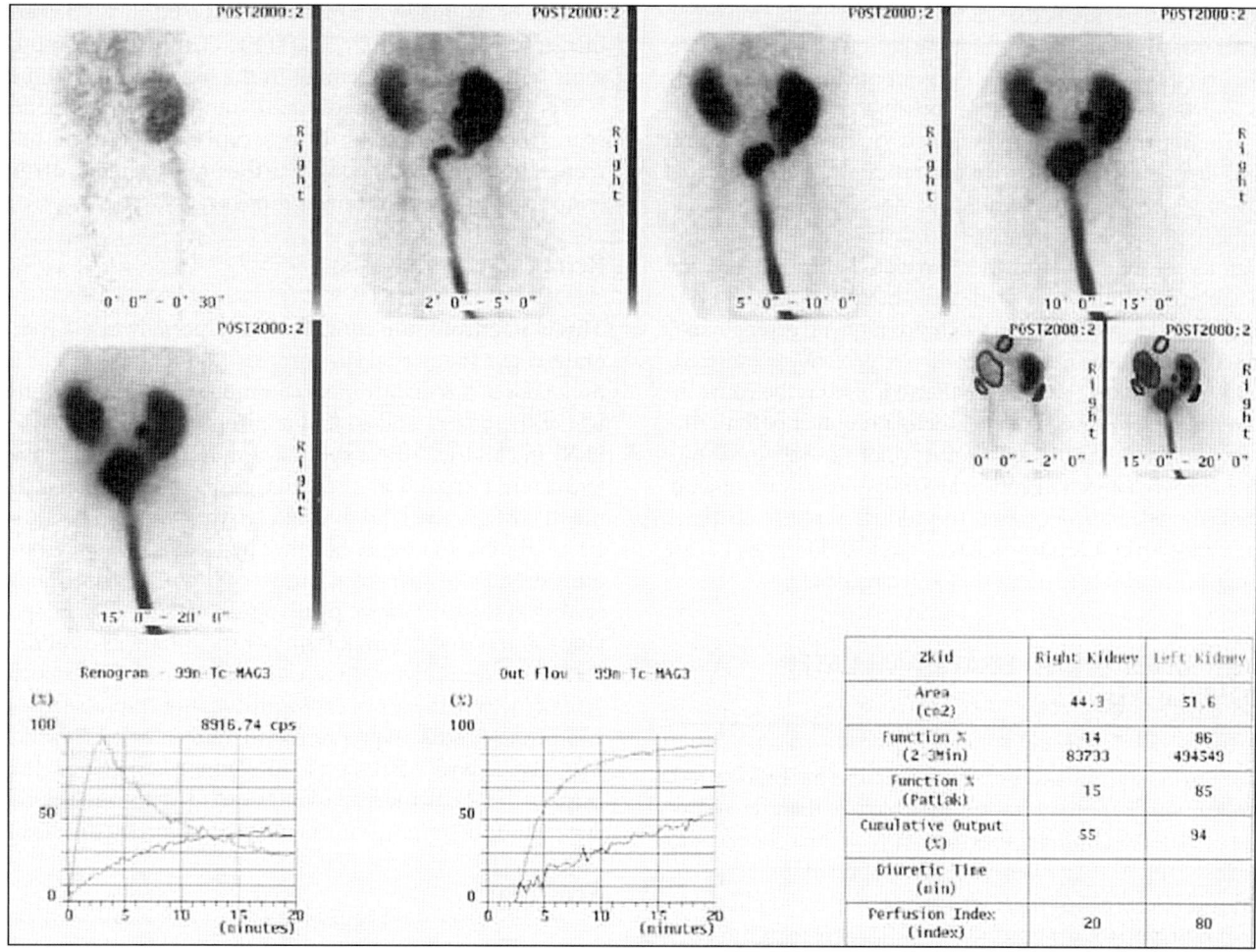

Figure 8F.1   *Results of a ^{99m}Tc-MAG$_3$ renogram performed in a 36-year-old male patient after a successful second kidney transplant.*

or catheter bag should always be obtained and recorded, even if it contains no activity.

THE LATER POSTOPERATIVE PERIOD

During the first 2 or 3 weeks following the operation, there is usually slow but definite resolution of the ATN. This is seen as a steady improvement in perfusion (shown as a fall in the perfusion index) accompanied by improving function as measured by a rising GFR, 2-min uptake or improved percentage of dose excreted during the study. However, it is not uncommon for an episode of rejection to develop, typically from about 5 or 7 days onwards. Since the introduction of cyclosporin A and other more advanced drugs as anti-rejection therapy this is less dramatic than it used to be in the earlier period when prednisolone and azathioprine were the only agents available (when a rejection episode could 'explode' in a matter of minutes). Now a typical timescale would be that a rejection will develop slowly over a day or so. This has taken much of the rush and drama out of management.

The features of a full-blown *rejection episode* are very characteristic, but it is also important to realize that it is relatively uncommon for all the features to be present. The most important feature is the impairment of perfusion, more easily detected when a measure of perfusion such as a perfusion index is used. Sometimes this may only be a failure of improvement of perfusion in a kidney with ATN.

The kidney may also swell, and in a functioning graft there may be deterioration of function. A feature that is often missed is the development of 'pseudo-obstruction'. This is a dilatation of the ureter, due to its rejection, with delay of entry of tracer into the bladder. One key feature is that in true obstruction there is dilatation of the renal calyces, whereas in rejection the calyces are compressed by edema of the renal pyramids and may not be visualized. With successful treatment of the rejection, the features should all reverse, but the perfusion may take up to 5 days to recover after treatment.

It is important to realize that renal blood flow falls following hemodialysis, so that in the oliguric patient on hemodialysis, the study must be performed at least 6 h after a dialysis session; in practice, this usually means carrying out the nuclear medicine study first thing in the morning before starting dialysis. During the period of postoperative oliguria it is helpful to study the graft once or twice a week to follow recovery and monitor possible complications.

The third major complication is *cyclosporin A toxicity*. This drug is used in lower concentrations than initially, and toxicity is less of a problem. At the dose levels now used, it initially produces a parenchymal impairment . If sustained high levels occur, then further vascular changes may occur. Therefore, as might be predicted, the initial feature on a nuclear medicine study is a deterioration in parenchymal function, as measured by uptake or percentage excreted, while perfusion is relatively unaffected.[6] This is the converse of rejection. However, if there is deterioration of both perfusion and parenchymal function it is not possible to distinguish between rejection and cyclosporin A toxicity on nuclear medicine grounds. However, to produce vascular changes, the cyclosporin A levels will have been high for several days, while for rejection to occur they will have been low.

THE FUNCTIONING GRAFT AND LATER COMPLICATIONS

Once urine output and excretory function have recovered, nuclear medicine studies are indicated if there is subsequent deterioration in function (which may be due to cyclosporin A toxicity or the development of acute or chronic rejection), or there is a suspicion of a complication.

It is helpful to carry out serial studies at regular intervals after transplantation: it is almost impossible to make helpful comments on a graft that has not been studied for several years, but where the function has suddenly deteriorated.

Ureteric complications

As mentioned above, ureteric obstruction is uncommon (indeed many surgeons deliberately do not implant the ureter with an anti-reflux incision because they are more worried about obstruction). Where it is suspected, an F-15 postfrusemide study may be carried out, but anecdotal experience is that this is unreliable, perhaps because the system is rigid, or because the diuresis is inadequate, and it may be necessary to arrange a formal radiological antegrade pyelogram. However, it is important to recognize the pseudo-obstruction of rejection (see above).

Lymphoceles

A lymphocele is the commonest fluid collection around a transplanted kidney. It may result from damage to the lymphatics in the hilum of the kidney or of the iliac vessels during the operation. It is seen as a photon-deficient area in relation to the kidney.[7] Rarely, it may cause obstruction of the ureter.

Very occasionally, a lymphocele may 'fill in' on delayed images, especially with ^{99m}Tc-DTPA.[8] This probably represents lymphatic fluid forming in the legs (and containing ^{99m}Tc-DTPA which has diffused into the extra-vascular space) taking some time to pass up into the groin and thence into the lymphocele. Further management of the lymphocele is by aspiration and/or surgery.

Renal artery stenosis

This is an uncommon complication, especially in cadaveric grafts where the arterial anastomosis is done using a patch of donor aorta. It is slightly more common in live-related grafts, where there is an end-to-end anastomosis. It is also more likely in children, where the anastomosis becomes fibrotic, and cannot expand as the child grows, and the required blood flow increases, producing a relative renal artery stenosis. Typically, it presents as either hypertension or a failing graft months to years after surgery. The nuclear medicine study will show deteriorating perfusion, but there are no specific features, and it is important to realize that this condition cannot be separated from rejection or chronic cyclosporin A toxicity. Even the use of captopril does not help, as all these conditions produce a pre-glomerular vascular lesion which may give a positive response to captopril challenge. It is important to remember the condition, and to be prepared to suggest arteriography, which will give the correct diagnosis.

Scarring

There is accumulating evidence that scarring of the renal transplant is commoner than was first thought, especially in patients with abnormal lower urinary tracts. SPECT studies using DMSA may show this clearly.[9]

INFECTION

In the later phases, apparent chronic infection may be a problem, presenting either as a pyrexia of unknown origin (PUO), or as recurrent urinary tract infections. In this setting, ^{67}Ga scintigraphy is often of value. Particular regions to be studied are the native kidneys and the peritoneum in patients who had been treated with chronic ambulatory peritoneal dialysis (CAPD) prior to transplantation.

Chronic infection in the native kidneys is a particular problem, especially in patients with polycystic kidneys. Typically, these patients present with infections every 2 or 3 months. In this setting, it is helpful to perform the gallium study some 4–6 weeks after an acute episode, rather than on admission, when the patient is usually on treatment.[10]

Patients on CAPD often develop a chronic low-grade chemical peritonitis, which may be seen on the gallium study, but which does not cause a pyrexia. On the other hand a focal accumulation may represent a localized collection. It is also important to look at bowel activity carefully, as small bowel and/or peritoneal uptake may be the only feature of tuberculosis in these patients.

TECHNICAL METHODOLOGY

The study is performed with the patient supine under the gamma camera, and is positioned so that the upper edge of the field of view is at the level of the aortic bifurcation (a marker on the umbilicus gives this level), and the lower edge is below the base of the bladder.

The computer is set for a frame rate of 1 per second for 30 or 40 s, followed by 1 per 20 s for 20 min. A minimum resolution of 64×64 is used, but 128×128 is preferred. In small patients or with large cameras, the camera should be zoomed so that the field of view is filled. An alternative approach, which is easily implemented on modern systems, is to acquire the study using a 256×256 matrix over the full field of the camera, then use software zooming on processing to select a 128×128 section of this dataset for processing.

A bolus of 300 MBq of ^{99m}Tc-DTPA or MAG$_3$ is injected, and the system started. For analysis, ROIs are defined over the graft, the iliac artery distal to the graft, and a background area. Activity–time curves are generated, and analyzed. It is essential to examine images as well as the curves. For further details, the reader is referred elsewhere.[4,11]

Case history

A 36-year-old patient had a failing renal transplant. A suitable donor became available before he needed to return to dialysis, and he was successfully transplanted. Because it was not clear how much of his renal function was coming from each kidney, a ^{99m}Tc-MAG$_3$ renogram was performed (Fig. 8F.1). This clearly shows the smaller right kidney with slow transit (due to chronic rejection) which contributes 15% of the total function, and the better-perfused, better-functioning (new) left kidney. Note that the bladder is on continuous drainage via the unclamped catheter.

REFERENCES

1 Gupta R, Birnbaum Y, Uretsky BF. The renal patient with coronary artery disease: current concepts and dilemmas. *J Am Coll Cardiol* 2004; **44**: 1343–53.

2 Patel AD, Abo-Auda WS, Davis JM, *et al.* Prognostic value of myocardial perfusion imaging in predicting outcome after renal transplantation. *Am J Cardiol* 2003; **92**: 146–51.

3 Fernando DCJ, Young KC. Scintigraphic patterns of acute vascular occlusion following renal transplantation. *Nucl Med Commun* 1985; **7**: 223–31.

4 Hilson AJW, Maisey MN, Brown CB, *et al.* Dynamic renal transplant imaging with Tc-99m DTPA (Sn) supplemented by a transplant perfusion index in the management of renal transplants. *J Nucl Med* 1978; **19**: 994–1000.

5 Dubovsky EV, Russell CD, Erbas B. Radionuclide evaluation of renal transplants. [Review]. *Semin Nucl Med* 1995; **25**: 49–59.

6 Kim EE, Pjura G, Lowry PA, *et al.* Cyclosporin-A nephrotoxicity and acute cellular rejection in renal transplant recipients: correlation between radionuclide and histologic findings. *Radiology* 1986; **159**: 443–6.

7 Bingham JB, Hilson AJ, Maisey MN. The appearances of renal transplant lymphocoeles during dynamic renal scintigraphy. *Br J Radiol* 1978; **51**: 342–6.

8 Fortenbery EJ, Blue PW, Van Nostrand D, Anderson JH. Lymphocele: the spectrum of scintigraphic findings in lymphoceles associated with renal transplant. *J Nucl Med* 1990; **31**: 1627–31.

9 Cairns HS, Spencer S, Hilson AJW, *et al.* ^{99m}Tc-DMSA imaging with tomography in renal transplant recipients with abnormal lower urinary tracts. *Nephrol Dial Transplant* 1994; **9**: 1157–61.

10 Tsang V, Lui S, Hilson AJW, *et al.* Gallium-67 scintigraphy in the detection of infected polycystic kidneys in renal transplant recipients. *Nucl Med Commun* 1989; **10**: 167–70.

11 Burke JR, Counahan R, Hilson AJW, *et al.* Serial quantitative imaging with ^{99m}Tc-DTPA in pediatric renal transplantation. *Clin Nephrol* 1979; **12**: 174–7.

Renal tumors

P. SHREVE

SCINTIGRAPHIC EVALUATION OF RENAL TUMORS USING SINGLE PHOTON TRACERS

Applications of nuclear medicine imaging techniques to renal tumors historically have been limited due to the absence of tracers specific for tumors commonly encountered in the kidney. Through the 1980s, imaging of a renal mass was chiefly the depiction of the photopenia secondary to the absent tracer uptake in a cyst or solid mass.[1] Renal masses in excess of 3 cm can be resolved on routine spot and whole body acquisitions both with renal specific tracers such as ^{99m}Tc-diethylenetriaminepentaacetic acid (^{99m}Tc-DTPA) and ^{99m}Tc-mercaptoacetyltriglycine (^{99m}Tc-MAG$_3$), and non-renal specific tracers such ^{99m}Tc-methylene diphosphonate (^{99m}Tc-MDP) (Fig. 8G.1). Using renal cortical specific tracers such as ^{99m}Tc-dimercaptosuccinimide (^{99m}Tc-DMSA), renal masses as small as 2 cm can be resolved using ^{99m}Tc-DMSA and single photon emission computed tomography (SPECT).[1] For many years ^{99m}Tc-DMSA with or without SPECT was used as a problem-solving technique to differentiate a space-occupying solid mass from a column of Bertin in response to a finding of calyceal displacement on intravenous pyelography or a sonographically demonstrated hypoechoic mass.

Gallium-67 citrate, the most widely used single photon tracer specific for neoplasm, can depict renal gallium-avid lymphomatous masses, generally when greater than 2 cm in diameter.[2] The hypervascularity of renal cell carcinoma has been reported as an incidental finding on a ^{99m}Tc-labeled red blood cell scan performed for evaluation of gastrointestinal bleeding.[3] Both antibody and peptide single photon radiopharmaceuticals have been of very limited value for the detection of primary renal neoplasms or metastases

to the kidney, in part due to the high nonspecific renal accumulation observed with these tracers.[4]

Perhaps the current most common current application of nuclear medicine imaging to renal tumors is the use of conventional renal scintigraphy with ^{99m}Tc-MAG$_3$ to quantify renal function and evaluate relative renal function prior to nephrectomy,[5,6] in order to predict postoperative renal insufficiency.

CLINICAL MANAGEMENT OF RENAL TUMORS

Radionuclide imaging had been used successfully to distinguish a space-occupying mass from normal variants in response to findings on excretory urography.[7] With the continued evolution of cross-sectional anatomic imaging modalities from the 1980s to present, however, the detection and characterization of a renal mass remains almost exclusively within the realm of anatomic imaging. A space-occupying renal mass includes simple cysts, complex cysts and solid masses. Cystic renal masses are commonly classified based on their contrast computed tomography (CT) and sonographic features according to the categories first described by Bosniak.[8] Simple renal cysts (Bosniak category I) are readily diagnosed on contrast CT or ultrasound,[9] are common, and unequivocally benign. Category II renal cysts can be managed by directed anatomic imaging follow-up, while category III and IV complex cysts, for which there is a possibility of malignancy, typically require surgical exploration, as no anatomic imaging method can reliably exclude malignancy.[10] Solid renal masses are nearly always malignant. Malignant solid renal masses include renal cell carcinoma, by far the most common, transitional cell carcinoma, lymphoma, squamous cell carcinoma and metastases (typically lung cancer or melanoma). Benign solid renal masses include angiomyolipomas, which can be reliably diagnosed on CT or ultrasound by demonstration of fat components within the mass,[11] and oncocytomas, which cannot be reliably differentiated from renal cell carcinomas on anatomic imaging.[12] Hence, solid renal masses and complex cystic masses which are not unequivocally benign on anatomic imaging are either removed or undergo biopsy. Percutaneous biopsy of a renal mass is limited by potential sampling errors and possibility of tracking of neoplastic cells along the needle tract,[13] but this is of less concern. Large renal masses, occupying more than one half of the kidney, are generally managed with nephrectomy. Small renal masses (generally those less than 3 cm in diameter) are increasingly common incidental findings on CT and ultrasound examinations of the abdomen.[14,15] Incidental small renal masses, especially in elderly or high surgical risk patients may be managed conservatively,[16] or in the setting of patients with compromised renal function nephron-sparing surgery may be considered.[17,18]

SCINTIGRAPHIC EVALUATION OF RENAL TUMORS USING POSITRON TRACERS

The development of positron emission tomography and its emergence as a clinical tool in the 1990s greatly expanded the capability of nuclear medicine imaging applications in oncology. The advantages of much higher counting statistics, the potential for quantitative tracer kinetics, and especially the versatility of positron radionuclide-based tracers apply to applications in nephrology and urinary tract oncology as well.[19] The alterations in glucose metabolism found in a wide range of malignant neoplasms was also noted in primary renal cell carcinoma and can be depicted with positron emission tomography (PET) imaging using the tracer 2-deoxy-2-[^{18}F]fluoro-D-glucose (^{18}F-FDG).[20] The loss of oxidative dominant metabolism and the availability of anabolic pathways on malignant transformation of renal parenchyma could also be depicted on PET imaging using the metabolic tracer ^{11}C-acetate.[21] Amino acid tracers and amino acid analogs have undergone limited investigation.[22]

In initial limited clinical studies, renal masses surgically proven as renal cell carcinoma were identified on FDG PET, although to a large extent due to the bulk of the masses.[23,24] Small renal masses proved difficult to identify both due to the well known confounding effect of urinary FDG tracer in the intrarenal collecting system[25,26] and the, on average, modest level of FDG tracer uptake in renal cell carcinoma. Among 68 renal cell carcinomas, the average standardized uptake value (SUV) at 60 min post-injection on filtered

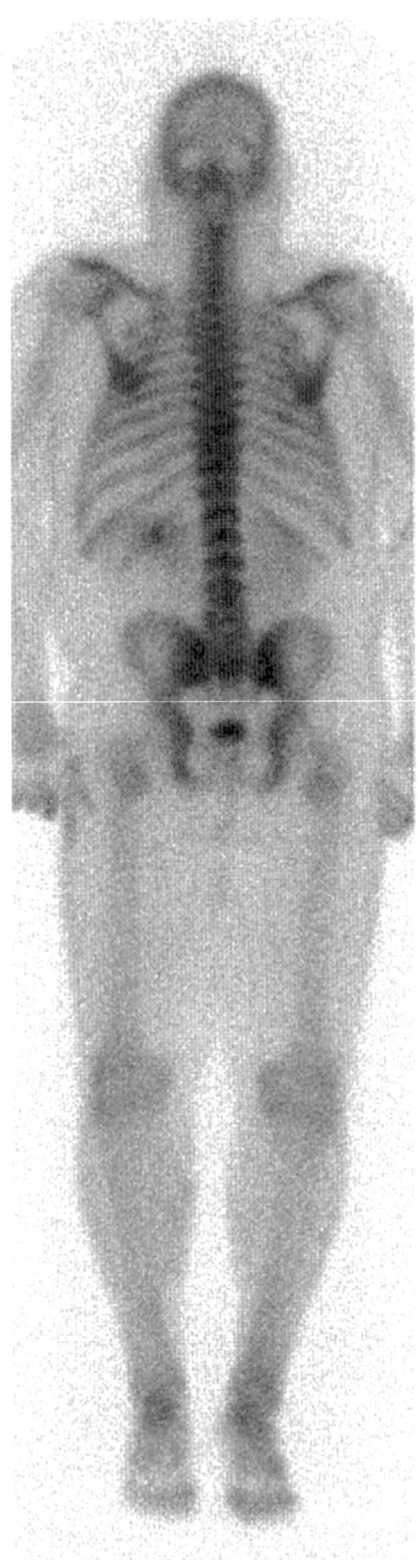

Figure 8G.1 *Bone scan of renal cell carcinoma. Posterior whole-body bone scan performed for 4 h following intravenous administration of 900 MBq ^{99m}Tc-MDP, depicts the primary renal mass as a photopenic area at the mid and inferior aspect of the right kidney.*

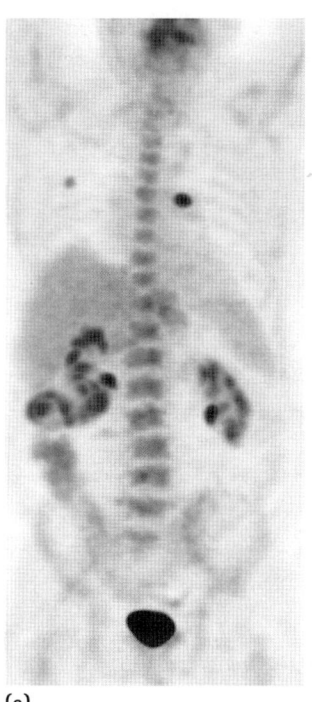

(a)

Figure 8G.2 *Primary renal cell carcinoma with pulmonary metastases on FDG PET. PET-CT performed for evaluation of pulmonary nodules. Whole torso attenuation corrected maximum intensity projection PET image (a) reveals two FDG-avid pulmonary nodules and an FDG-avid right retroperitoneal mass. Transaxial contrast enhanced CT (b) and attenuation corrected PET (c) images depict a large FDG avid heterogenously enhancing right renal mass reflecting the primary renal cell carcinoma.*

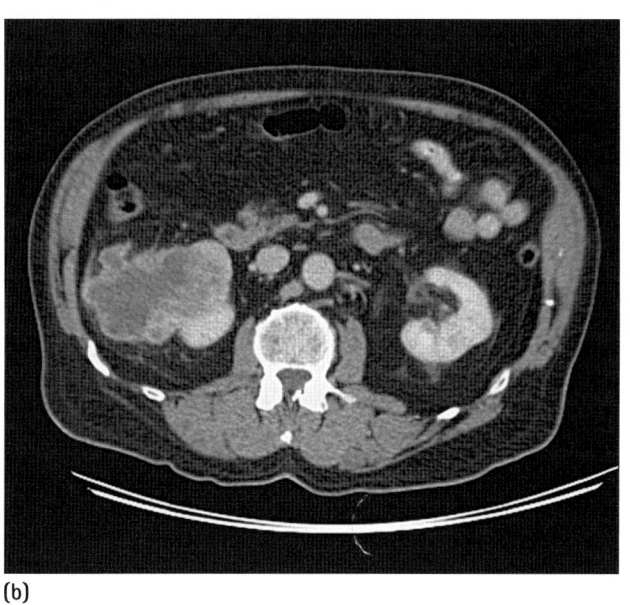

(b)

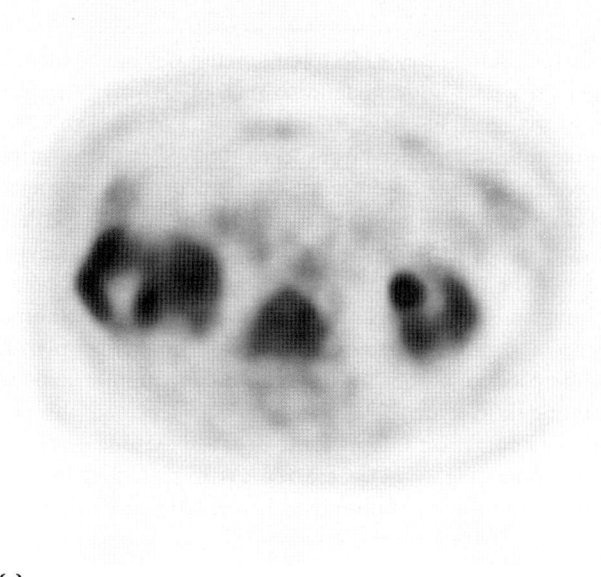

(c)

back-projection image reconstruction was 4.6, or slightly greater than adjacent renal parenchyma, although an SUV as high as 10 was observed in a few cases.[27] FDG uptake in oncocytomas fell within the range of renal cell carcinomas, and there was no correlation between histological grade or Fuhrman nuclear grade and measured SUVs.[28] In a prospective series of 35 patients FDG PET characterization of renal masses was 47% sensitive and 80% specific for malignancy.[29] A retrospective study of 66 patients with known or suspected renal cell carcinoma found FDG PET sensitivity for malignancy of the primary renal tumor of 60% compared to 92% for contrast CT.[30] Regarding evaluation of complex renal cysts, in a limited series of 11 Bosniak category III cysts, in which one contained renal cell carcinoma, all were negative on FDG PET.[23]

When renal cell carcinoma is FDG-avid, both primary renal tumor and metastatic deposits are well visualized on FDG PET (Fig. 8G.2). As with other neoplasms, when a

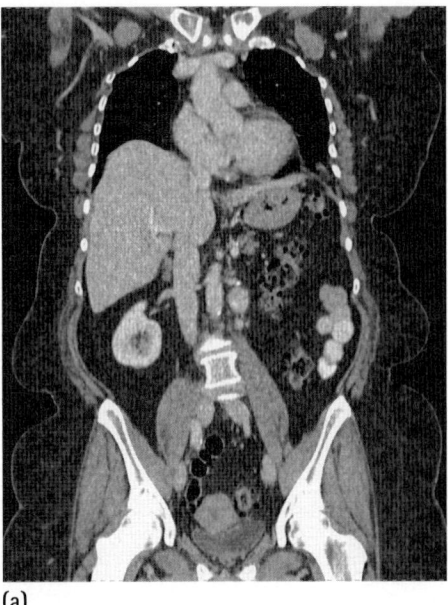
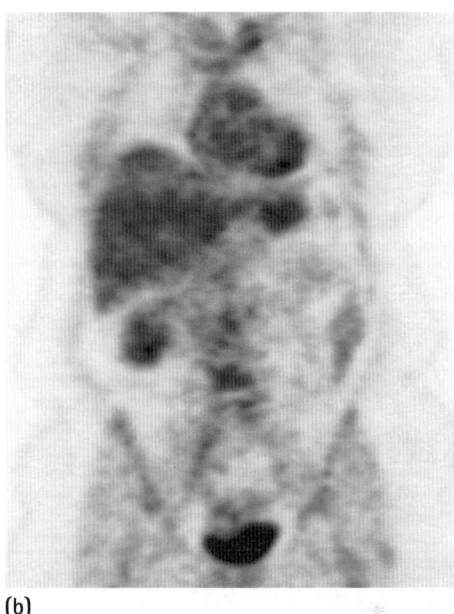

(a)   (b)

Figure 8G.3 *Recurrent renal cell carcinoma on FDG PET. PET-CT performed for assessment of recurrent renal cell carcinoma post nephrectomy. Coronal contrast enhanced CT (a) and PET (b) images demonstrate an enlarged enhancing left para-aortic lymph node metastasis of renal cell carcinoma which is not FDG-avid.*

renal cell carcinoma is FDG-avid, metastases can be identified on whole-body imaging, although sensitivity in the reported series has been limited, ranging from 63 to 77%, while specificity ranged from 75 to 100%.[28–31] The positive predictive value for detecting local recurrence or metastases on re-staging renal cell carcinoma with FDG PET was greater than 90% in one series.[32] The lack of sensitivity of FDG PET for both diagnosis of primary renal cell carcinoma and recurrent or metastatic renal cell carcinoma reflects the wide range of FDG uptake by this neoplasm, with up to roughly one third of renal cell carcinomas demonstrating little, if any, FDG tracer uptake. Hence the absence of FDG uptake on PET imaging does not exclude renal cell carcinoma (Fig. 8G.3). Case reports suggest that Wilms' tumor, the most common renal neoplasm in children, is FDG-avid,[33] but a series assessing diagnostic performance of FDG PET is not yet reported. While a series assessing the performance of FDG in the detection of metastatic neoplasm to the kidneys has not been reported, both lymphomatous involvement and metastases of lung cancer or melanoma have been reported (Fig. 8G.4).

Given the limitations of FDG as a tracer for renal malignancies, primarily the modest and variable FDG uptake and urinary excretory route, other tracers have been investigated, including amino acids and amino acid analogs.[22] Acetate is also retained by renal cell carcinoma but rapidly cleared from the renal parenchyma as CO_2, and no urinary excretion (Plate 8G.1). Higher average SUVs and tumor-to-renal-cortex values are obtained within 10 min of tracer injection than FDG at 1 h post-injection, and highest acetate

tracer accumulation was found in granulocytic tumors.[34,35] While such tracers of amino acid transport or lipid related metabolism may have a role in characterizing small renal mass or response to therapy, detecting RCC in complex renal masses and metastatic disease requires high consistent tracer uptake in the renal neoplasm, and such has not yet been demonstrated with this tracer.

RADIONUCLIDE TREATMENT OF RENAL TUMORS

Building on experience with radioimmunotherapy of lymphoma, radiolabeled monoclonal antibodies have been developed targeting renal tumors (cf. renal cell carcinoma). Monoclonal antibody G250 was found to have very high targeting (in terms of percent injected dose per gram) in primary and metastatic renal cell carcinoma in phase I clinical trials.[36] Similar high tumor targeting of renal cell carcinoma, but without evidence of anti-murine antibody immunogenicity, was demonstrated in clinical studies using a chimeric G250 (murine Fv-grafted human IgG1K), cG250.[37]

An advantage of chimeric monoclonal antibodies is the much reduced host immune response, allowing for dose fractionation, which can allow for proliferative recovery of bone marrow, ultimately enabling delivery of higher absorbed dose to the targeted tumor.

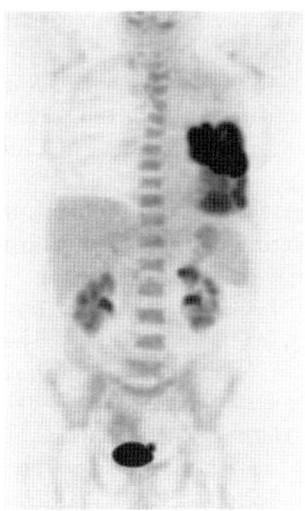

(a)

Figure 8G.4 *Renal mass secondary to metastatic non-small cell lung cancer on FDG PET. PET-CT performed for staging of large left lung non-small cell lung cancer. Whole torso attenuation corrected maximum intensity projection PET image demonstrates large FDG-avid mass in left hemithorax (a). Focus of abnormal FDG tracer uptake in upper pole of left kidney is partly obscured by normal urinary FDG tracer activity in renal calyces. Transaxial contrast enhanced CT (b) and PET images (c) reveal 1 cm FDG-avid renal mass reflecting the solitary metastasis.*

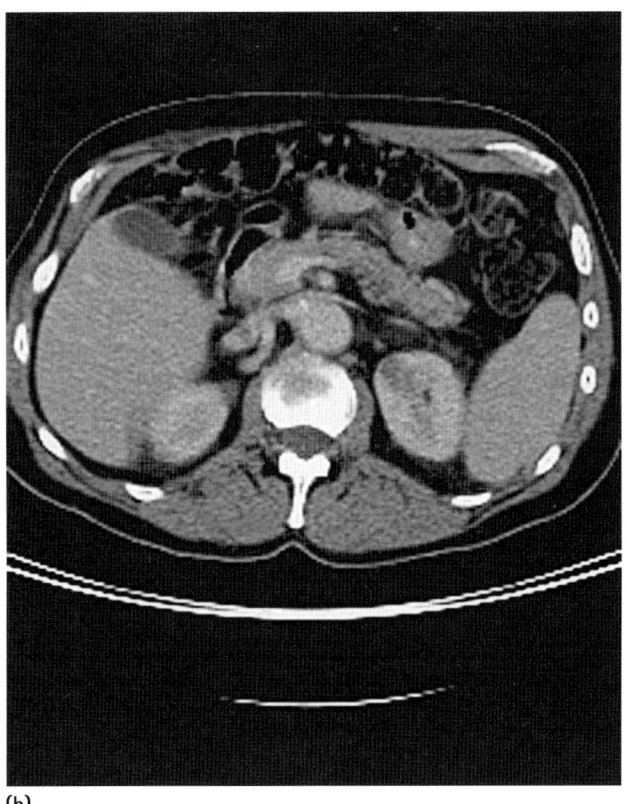

(b)

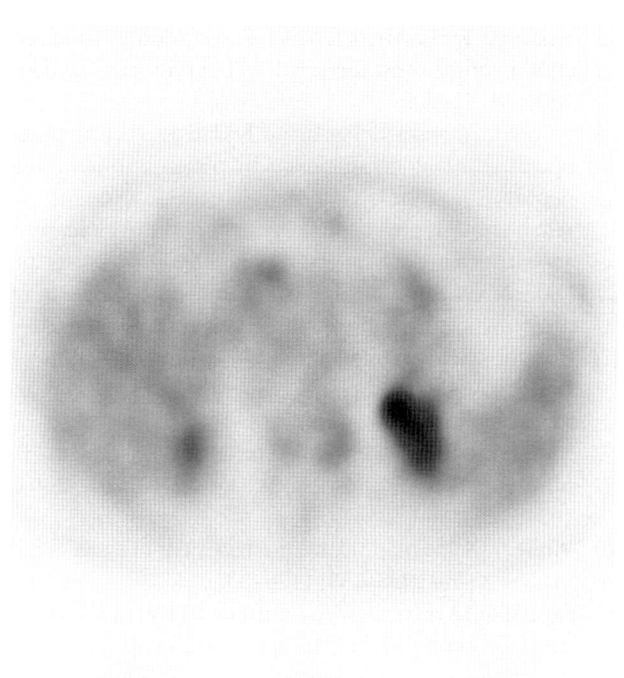

(c)

Initial results with a phase I fractionated dose clinical trial with ^{131}I labeled cG250, however, demonstrated no evidence for fractionation-induced sparing of the hematopoietic system; dose limiting toxicity was hematopoietic and the maximum tolerated dose per cycle was 0.75 Gy.[38] In a dose escalation clinical study using [131]I cG250 of 29 patients, disease in five patients stabilized while disease progressed in 14 of the 29 subjects.[39] Dose escalation was limited by hematopoietic toxicity and formation of anti-chimeric antibodies. Immunoscintigraphic images did depict good uptake of the labeled cG250, with tumor to background level of >1.5 in at least one lesion. To improve the delivered dose of radiation to tumors with a given targeting antibody, alternative radiolabeling methods, including the use of chelated radionuclides, have been investigated. Immunoscintigraphy of human subjects with metastatic renal cell carcinoma 4 days after administration of cG250 revealed more metastatic lesions with cG250 labeled with ^{111}In than ^{131}I, presumably due to internalization and retention of the chelated indium tracer.[40] Similarly, in a animal study the therapeutic efficiency of cG250 was higher with ^{177}Lu and ^{90}Y conjugates than ^{131}I, presumably due to improved residualizing of the chelate metallic radionuclides in the tumors.[41] Continued improvements in the targeting and residualization of radionuclide labeled antibodies likely will be required for effective radio-immunotherapy of renal tumors.

REFERENCES

1 Pjura GA, Lowry PA, Kim EE. Radionuclide imaging of the upper urinary tract. In: Gottschalk A, Hoffer PB, Potchen EJ. (eds.) *Diagnostic nuclear medicine.* Baltimore: Williams & Wilkins, 1979.

2 Taniguchi M, Higashi K, Ohguchi M, *et al.* Gallium-67-citrate scintigraphy of primary renal lymphoma. *Ann Nucl Med* 1998; **12**: 51–3.

3 Cortes J, Alonso JI, Ruis-Olivia F, *et al.* Renal cell carcinoma detected on Tc-99m-labeled red blood cell imaging. *Clin Nucl Med* 2003; **28**: 920–2.

4 Sharkey RM, Goldenberg DM. Perspective on cancer therapy with radiolabled monoclonal antibodies. *J Nucl Med* 2005; **46**: 115S–27S.

5 Shirasaki Y, Tsushima T, Saika T, *et al.* Kidney function after nephrectomy for renal cell carcinoma. *Urology* 2004; **54**: 43–7.

6 Shirasaki Y, Saika T, Tsushima T, *et al.* Predicting post-operative renal insufficiency in patients undergoing nephrectomy for renal malignancy: assessment by renal scintigraphy using 99m-technetium-mercapto-acetyltriglycine. *J Urol* 2005; **173**: 388–90.

7 Older RA, Korobkin M, Workman J, *et al.* Accuracy of radionuclide imaging in distinguishing renal masses from normal variants. *Radiology* 1980; **136**: 443–8.

8 Bosniak MA. The current radiographic approaches to renal cysts. *Radiology* 1986; **158**: 1–10.

9 Middleton WD, Kurtz AB, Hertzberg BS. *Kidney in ultrasound: the requisites.* St. Louis: Mosby, 2004: 103–51.

10 Wolfe Jr JS. Evaluation and management of cystic renal masses. *J Urol* 1998; **159**: 1120–33.

11 Bosniak MA, Megibow AJ, Hulnick DH, *et al.* CT diagnosis of renal angiomyolipoma: the importance of detecting small amounts of fat. *Am J Roentgenol* 1988; **151**: 497–501.

12 Licht MR. Renal adenoma and oncocytoma. *Semin Urol Oncol* 1995; **13**: 262–6.

13 Wehle MJ, Grebstald H. Contraindications of needle aspiration of a solid renal mass: tumor dissemination by renal needle aspiration. *J Urol* 1986; **136**: 446–8.

14 Smith SJ, Bosniak MA, Megibow AJ, *et al.* Renal cell carcinoma: earlier discovery and increased detection. *Radiology* 1989; **170**: 699–703.

15 Lightfoot N, Conlon M, Kreiger N, *et al.* Impact of non-invasive imaging on increased incidental detection of renal cell carcinoma. *Eur Urol* 2000; **37**: 6521–7.

16 Wehle MJ, Thiel DD, Petrou SP, *et al.* Conservative management of incidental contrast-enhancing renal masses as safe alternative to invasive therapy. *Urology* 2004; **64**: 49–52.

17 Butler BP, Novick AC, Miller DP, *et al.* Management of small unilateral renal cell carcinomas: radical versus nephron-sparing sugery. *Urology* 1995; **45**: 34–41.

18 Bosniak MA, Rofsky NM. Problems in the detection and characterization of small renal masses. *Radiology* 1996; **198**: 638–41.

19 Shreve PD. Renal imaging with positron emission tomography. In: Taylor A, Nally JV, Thomsen H. (eds.) *Radionuclides in nephrology*, third edition. Reston: Society of Nuclear Medicine, 1997: 200–205.

20 Wahl RL, Harney J, Hutchins G, Grossman HB. Imaging of renal cancer using positron emission tomography with 2-deoxy-2-(18F)-fluoro-D-glucose: pilot animal and human studies. *J Urol* 1991; **146**: 1470.

21 Shreve P, Chiao P-C, Humes HD, *et al.* Carbon-11 acetate PET imaging of renal disease. *J Nucl Med* 1995; **36**: 1595–601.

22 Langen K-J, Borner AR, Muller-Mattheis V, *et al.* Uptake of *cis*-4-[^{18}F]fluoro-L-proline in urologic tumors. *J Nucl Med* 2001; **42**: 752–4.

23 Goldenberg MA, Mayo-Smith WW, Papanicolaou N, *et al.* FDG PET characterization of renal masses: Preliminary experience. *Clin Radiol* 1997; **52**: 510–5.

24 Ramdave S, Thomas GW, Berlangieri SU, *et al.* Clinical role of F-18 fluorodeoxyglucose positron emission tomography for detection and management of renal cell carcinoma. *J Urol* 2001; **166**: 825–30.

25 Shreve PD, Anzai Y, Wahl RL. Pitfalls in oncologic diagnosis with FDG PET imaging: physiologic and benign variants. *Radiographics* 1999; **19**: 61–77.

26 Zhuang H, Duarte PS, Pourdehnad M, *et al.* Standardized uptake value as a unreliable index of renal disease on fluorodeoxyglucose PET imaging. *Clin Nuc Med* 2000; **25**: 358–60.

27 Shreve PD, Miyauchi T, Wahl RL. Characterization of primary renal cell carcinoma by FDG PET. *Radiology* 1998; **209**: P94.

28 Aide N, Cappele O, Bottet P, *et al.* Efficiency of [(18)F]FDG PET in characterizing renal cancer and detecting distant metastases: a comparison with CT. *Eur J Nucl Med Mol Imaging* 2003; **30**: 1236–45.

29 Safaei A, Figlin R, Hoh CK, *et al.* The usefulness of F-18 deoxyglucose whole-body positron emission tomography (PET) for re-staging of renal cell cancer. *Clin Nephrol* 2022; **57**: 56–62.

30 Kang DE, White RL Jr., Zuger JH, *et al.* Clinical use of fluorodeoxyglucose F-18 positron emission tomography for detection of renal cell carcinoma. *J Urol* 2004; **17**: 1806–9.

31 Majhail NS, Urbain JL, Albani JM, *et al.* F-18 fluorodeoxyglucose positron emission tomography in the evaluation of distant metastases from renal cell carcinoma. *J Clin Oncol* 2003; **21**: 3995–4000.

32 Jadvar H, Kherbache HM, Pinski JK, Conti PS. Diagnostic role of [F-18]-FDG positron emission tomography in restaging renal cell carcinoma. *Clin Nephrol* 2003; **60**: 395–400.

33 Shulkin BL, Chang E, Strouse PJ, *et al.* PET FDG studies of Wilms tumors. *Radiology* 1997; **19**: 334–8.

34 Shreve P, Chiao P-C, Humes HD, *et al.* Carbon-11 acetate PET imaging of renal disease. *J Nucl Med* 1995; **36**: 1595–1601.

35 Shreve PD, Wahl RL. Carbon-11 acetate PET imaging of renal cell carcinoma. *J Nucl Med* 1999; **40**: 257P.

36 Oosterwijk E, Bander NH, Divgi CR, *et al.* Antibody localization in human renal cell carcinoma: a phase I study of monoclonal antibody G250. *J Clin Oncol* 1993; **11**: 738–50.

37 Steffens MG, Boerman OC, Osterwijk-Wakka JC, *et al.* Targeting of renal cell carcinoma with iodine-131-labeled chimeric monoclonal antibody G250. *J Clin Oncol* 1997; **15**: 1529–37.

38 Divgi CR, O'Donoghue JA, Welt S, *et al.* Phase I clinical trial with fractionated radioimmunotherapy using ^{131}I-labeled chimeric G250 in metastatic renal cancer. *J Nucl Med* 2004; **45**: 1412–21.

39 Brouwers AH, Mulders PF, de Mulder PH, *et al.* Lack of efficacy of two consecutive treatments of radioimmunotherapy with ^{131}I-cG250 in patients with metastasized clear cell renal cell carcinoma. *J Clin Oncol* 2005; **20**: 6540–8.

40 Brouwers AH, Buijs WC, Oosterwijk E, *et al.* Targeting of metastatic renal cell carcinoma with chimeric monoclonal antibody G250 labled with ^{131}I or [111]In: an intra-patient comparison. *Clin Cancer Res* 2003; **9**: 3953S–60S.

41 Brouwers AH, van Eerd JE, Frielink C, *et al.* Optimization of radioimmunotherapy of renal cell carcimoma: labeling of monoclonal antibody cG250 with ^{131}I, ^{90}Y, ^{177}Lu or [186]Re. *J Nucl Med* 2004; **45**: 327–37.

9

Musculoskeletal radionuclide imaging

9A Skeletal physiology and anatomy applied to nuclear medicine

Introduction	331	Radionuclides and the skeleton	332
Skeletal structure and physiology	331	References	334

9B Skeletal malignancy

Introduction	337	Specific cancers	343
Skeletal metastases	337	PET and PET/CT in skeletal metastases	344
Radiopharmaceuticals for imaging skeletal metastases	338	Primary bone tumors	346
Scintigraphic patterns in imaging skeletal metastases		Specific primary bone tumors	347
and the role of correlative imaging	338	References	350

9C Metabolic bone disease

Introduction	355	Osteomalacia	358
Paget's disease	355	Renal osteodystrophy	359
Osteoporosis	357	References	360
Hyperparathyroidism	358		

9D Trauma and sports injuries

Background	363	Injuries in children	365
Pathophysiology	363	Non-sporting trauma	366
Biomechanics	363	Sports-related injuries	368
Clinical presentation	364	Complications in fracture healing	375
Prevalence of injuries by age and site	364	Conclusion	376
Principles of scintigraphy in trauma	365	References	376

9E Radionuclide evaluation of the failed joint replacement

Introduction	381	Summary	389
Radionuclide imaging	382	References	390

9F Rheumatology and avascular necrosis

Inflammatory arthropathies	393	Reflex sympathetic dystrophy syndrome	397
Osteoarthritis	394	Bone mass measurement	398
Ankylosing spondylitis	395	References	401
Avascular necrosis	396		

9G Pediatric indications

General and technical considerations   403   Reflex sympathetic dystrophy   408
Pediatric bone scintigraphy indications   405   Tumor imaging and response assessment   408
Trauma   406   References   411

Skeletal physiology and anatomy applied to nuclear medicine

GARY J.R. COOK

INTRODUCTION

The major functions of the skeleton are as a supporting and protective framework for the body and as a store of minerals, particularly calcium and phosphate. The skeleton is not a static organ but is in a dynamic state, constantly being broken down and rebuilt in a process known as remodeling. The adult skeleton consists of two major types of bone, cortical (compact) and trabecular (cancellous) bone, the proportions of which vary at different skeletal sites. The way that the skeleton behaves in health and disease is fundamental to the methods used in nuclear medicine approaches to investigating skeletal disease.

SKELETAL STRUCTURE AND PHYSIOLOGY

The basic constituents of the skeleton are an extracellular matrix, mineral, and cells. The extracellular matrix consists of collagen fibers and noncollagenous proteins and accounts for approximately 35% of bone. Type 1 collagen fibers make up more than 90% of the total protein and are usually laid down in an organized, lamellar pattern. Lamellae can be in parallel on flat surfaces, e.g. trabecular and periosteal bone, or concentrically surrounding a central blood vessel or Haversian system, in cortical bone.

Hydroxyapatite crystals, $Ca_{10}(PO_4)_6(OH)_2$, form the mineral phase of bone on and within the collagen fibers providing mechanical strength and rigidity, accounting for approximately 65% of bone. Alternatively, woven bone, which lacks this organized pattern, occurs in the embryo, fracture healing and in situations where there is highly accelerated bone remodeling.

Cortical bone forms the compact outer wall of bones and accounts for approximately 80% of total skeletal mass. It is most abundant in the diaphysis of long bones where it encircles the medullary cavity consisting of hemopoeitic bone marrow. Eighty to 90% of cortical bone is calcified and its function is predominantly mechanical.

Trabecular bone accounts for approximately 20% of the skeleton and only 15–25% is calcified. Trabecular bone occurs predominantly in the metaphyseal regions of long bones and the inner portion of flat bones and is particularly abundant in vertebrae. It consists of a network of trabeculae which contribute mechanical strength but has a large surface area in contact with bone marrow and therefore has a significant metabolic function. Most of bone turnover occurs at bone surfaces, predominantly the endosteal surface which is in contact with bone marrow.[1–3]

The predominant cells in bone include osteoblasts and osteoclasts. Osteoblasts are derived from local mesenchymal stem cells and synthesize bone matrix. They are cuboidal in shape and always found in clusters lining the layer of matrix being produced on the bone surface. The matrix is termed osteoid tissue before mineralization has taken place, which takes about 10 days. The plasma membrane of osteoblasts is rich in alkaline phosphatase (ALP), which increases local phosphate concentration and removes inhibitors of mineralization, thereby increasing the rate and extent of mineralization. Serum levels of this enzyme are used as an index of bone formation rate. Osteoblasts have receptors for parathyroid hormone (PTH) on the plasma membrane and for estrogens, vitamin D_3, and various cytokines in the nucleus.

The osteoclast is the cell that is predominantly responsible for bone resorption. It derives from mononuclear/phagocytic cell lineage, is a multinucleated giant cell which undergoes apoptosis after a cycle of resorption and is found in contact with calcified bone surfaces in lacunae which result from resorptive activity. It has a large number of osteocalcin receptors. Osteoclasts attach to the matrix by cell membrane receptors known as integrins at a peripheral clear zone, sealing off a central resorbing compartment. The ruffled border (foldings of the plasma membrane in the area facing the matrix) secretes hydrogen ions which dissolve bone mineral and proteolytic enzymes which digest the matrix. Osteoclasts and precursors are under the control of cytokines secreted by cells of osteoblastic lineage as well as hormones.[1–3]

Abnormalities in bone remodeling are found in many focal and global skeletal disorders including osteoporosis, Paget's disease, fractures, metastases, and hyperparathyroidism. Normal remodeling gives rise to bone growth and turnover and occurs continuously in the adult skeleton either on trabecular surfaces or Haversian systems in discrete packets or bone remodeling units.[4] Each unit normally takes a period of at least 3–4 months for the remodeling cycle to complete. The factors governing remodeling differ in cortical and trabecular bone. Trabeculae are in intimate association with bone marrow cells which produce a variety of osteotopic cytokines which control osteoblastic and osteoclastic function. Cortical bone cells are further removed from bone marrow and are under a greater influence by systemic hormones including PTH and vitamin D_3. Although trabecular bone only forms 20% of the skeletal mass, 80% of turnover occurs here. A number of local hormones are also implicated in regulation of bone remodeling, mediating osteoclast and osteoblast replication, differentiation, recruitment and function.[1,5–7]

RADIONUCLIDES AND THE SKELETON

The first description of the use of radionuclides to study the skeleton was by Chiewitz and Hevesy in 1935[8] where ^{32}P activity was measured in rat organs with a Geiger–Muller counter and where uptake of ^{32}P from blood to bone was noted suggesting that skeletal metabolism is a dynamic process.

The abundance of calcium in the skeleton in the form of hydroxyapatite, $Ca_{10}(PO_4)_6(OH)_2$, logically led to the use of calcium isotopes, including ^{45}Ca, ^{47}Ca, and ^{49}Ca or analogs, including ^{85}Sr and ^{87m}Sr, to study skeletal metabolism. ^{47}Ca appears to have been the most extensively utilized calcium isotope for evaluation of global skeletal kinetics from the late 1950s through to the 1980s and beyond.[9–11] Although it is possible to produce images with this isotope,[12] its high energy gamma ray (1.3 MeV) is not suitable for standard gamma cameras. More suitable physical properties of some of the rare-earth elements with respect to gamma camera imaging, including ^{177}Lu and ^{153}Sm, led to their evaluation as possible bone scanning agents but these were not frequently used.[13] Gallium and barium isotopes were also evaluated for this role.[14]

In 1961 the first radionuclide skeletal images were produced by Fleming and colleagues[15] using ^{85}Sr and this radioisotope was the most commonly used for bone scanning and the study of skeletal kinetics. Although ^{87m}Sr was introduced as an alternative bone scanning agent with a more suitable gamma ray energy of 388 keV and half-life of 2.8 h, the introduction of [^{18}F]fluoride and then ^{99m}Tc-labeled compounds superseded this.

The positron emitting ion, [^{18}F]fluoride, was first described as a scanning agent in 1962 by Blau et al.[16] Its rapid blood clearance, high skeletal uptake and convenient half-life showed advantages over previous scanning agents. The 511 keV annihilation photons are not ideal for conventional gamma cameras which are optimized for ^{99m}Tc (140 keV) and although the use of ^{99m}Tc bone-seeking agents has taken over in the last two decades, [^{18}F]fluoride was an important bone scanning agent in the early days of clinical nuclear medicine (Fig. 9A.1). There has been some renewed interest in its use with PET cameras following the description of skeletal kinetic quantification by Hawkins et al. in 1992.[17]

The availability and optimal physical characteristics (i.e. generator production, gamma energy 140 keV and half-life of 6 h) of ^{99m}Tc, together with the good skeletal-to-background ratios of various labeled phosphate-containing complexes, has led to these radiopharmaceuticals being used almost exclusively in modern clinical nuclear medicine.

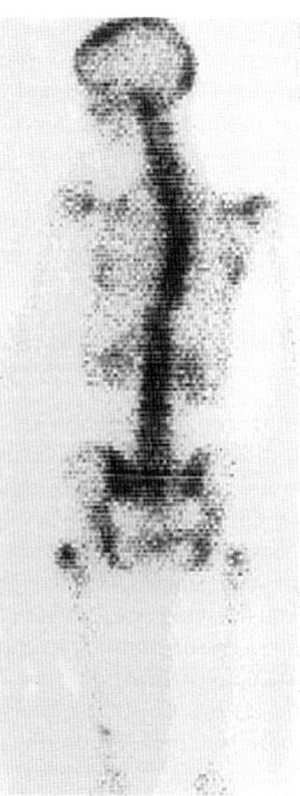

Figure 9A.1 [^{18}F]fluoride rectilinear bone scan performed at Guy's Hospital (1973) in a patient with breast cancer and bone metastases.

Initially ^{99m}Tc polyphosphates and pyrophosphates were employed[18,19] but subsequently diphosphonates such as hydroxyethylidene diphosphonate (HEDP) and methylene diphosphonate (MDP) were introduced[20,21] and ^{99m}Tc-MDP continues to be the most widely used bone radiopharmaceutical today (Fig. 9A.2).

The mechanism of accumulation of $[^{18}F]$fluoride in bone is thought to be by ion exchange with hydroxyl groups in hydroxyapatite to form fluoroapatite, although only partial substitution is thought to take place.[14,22]

$$2F^- + Ca_{10}(PO_4)_6(OH)_2 \rightarrow Ca_{10}(PO_4)_6F_2 + 2OH^- \quad (9A.1)$$

This reaction is thought to be limited to the surface of crystals. Fluoride ions therefore pass from plasma through bone ECF into a shell of bound water surrounding hydroxyapatite and then onto the crystal surface. The passage from plasma to bone ECF is rapid and once the ions have entered the water shell they are essentially part of bone mineral.[23] In animals and human pathological specimens fluoride has been shown to be preferentially deposited at bone surfaces where remodeling is greatest[24,25] and corresponds to tetracycline labeling.[26]

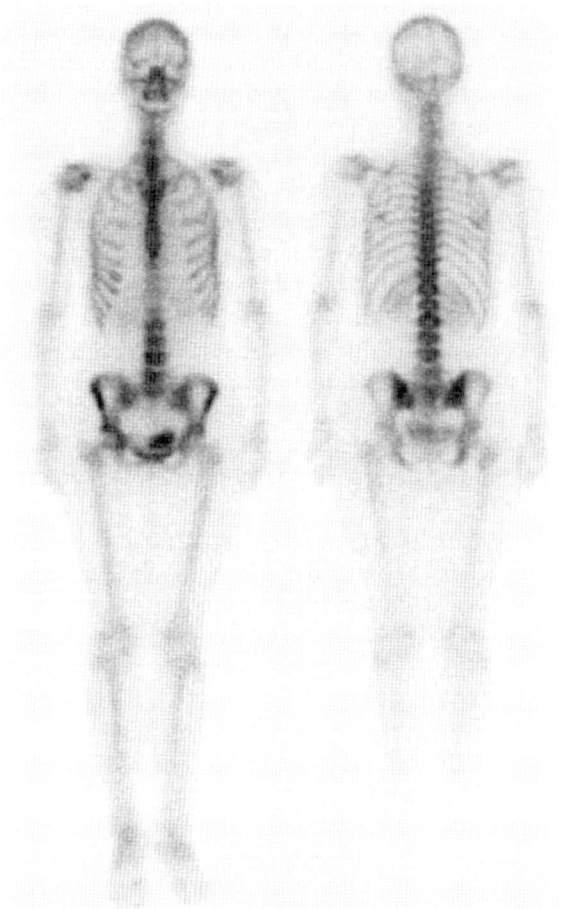

Figure 9A.2 *A normal ^{99m}Tc-methylene diphosphonate (^{99m}Tc-MDP) whole-body bone scan.*

The unidirectional extraction of $[^{18}F]$fluoride at low flow rates, e.g. as observed in cortical bone, approaches unity, explaining Wootton's observations in the rabbit hind limb.[27] In contrast, at higher flow rates, such as seen at trabecular sites, extraction falls and so first pass uptake underestimates true blood flow.[28] At very high flow rates it is predicted that tracer extraction becomes diffusion limited rather than perfusion limited across the continuous endothelium that is present in bone capillaries.[28]

Hawkins and colleagues, who first described the use of $[^{18}F]$fluoride and dynamic PET with nonlinear regression analysis, found that a three compartment model resulted in a significantly better fit of the data than a two compartment one.[17] This model includes a central extravascular compartment in addition to both plasma and bone mineral (or bound bone) compartments. Here it was possible to measure clearance of $[^{18}F]$fluoride to total bone tissue (K_1) within the ROI (extravascular and bound compartments) in ml min^{-1}ml^{-1}, rate constants describing the exchange of $[^{18}F]$fluoride both backwards and forwards from the central compartment (k_2, k_3 respectively) and release of $[^{18}F]$fluoride from the bound bone mineral compartment back to the central extravascular compartment (k_4). The clearance of $[^{18}F]$fluoride from plasma to the bone mineral compartment (K_i) is then calculated from

$$K_i = \frac{K_1 k_3}{k_2 + k_3}. \quad (9A.2)$$

Unlike the ionic exchange mechanism of $[^{18}F]$fluoride it is thought that the phosphate/phosphonate group of radiopharmaceuticals are chemi-adsorbed onto bone crystal surfaces.[14,29–31] It would seem that uptake of these tracers is primarily in areas of new bone formation where there is active mineralization rather than nonspecific uptake into mature bone.[14,32] It has also been postulated that uptake may be due to complexing with enzymes such as ALP but there seems little support for this and circumstances where ALP levels are either raised (e.g. Paget's disease) or diminished (e.g. hypophosphatasia) do not appear to alter diphosphonate kinetics.[30] It has also been suggested that much of the uptake of these compounds is associated with osteoid.[33–35] Initial studies[33] were criticized, however, as bone that was studied had undergone various chemical and physical traumas which may have accounted for these observations. Where ^{99m}Tc has been observed in osteoid it has been suggested that this may be in association with calcium phosphate present within the organic matrix.[32] The high uptake of ^{99m}Tc diphosphonate compounds in osteomalacia, where there is an excess of unmineralized osteoid, was also thought to support binding to osteoid but again this may be either due to calcium phosphate within osteoid or due to secondary hyperparathyroidism.

Although local blood flow has some effect on diphosphonate uptake, a series of studies has suggested that skeletal extraction related to local bone formation or osteoblastic activity is the predominant factor.[36,37] Following binding to bone surfaces and incorporation into hydroxyapatite, there is little subsequent release of tracer as these compounds are resistant to breakdown by tissue phosphatases. Uptake of these tracers is based on the fact that most focal skeletal lesions excite an osteoblastic reaction and an increase in vascularity although this response is not specific and does not necessarily allow the differentiation of benign from malignant lesions.

The observations regarding the relation of tracer uptake, to some extent on blood flow and to a larger extent on regional remodeling, as well as the description of kinetics, distribution and clearance of these tracers outside the skeleton, has obvious implications for the optimum use of these radiopharmaceuticals for bone imaging.[38] The clearance of background vascular and ECF activity by renal filtration has to be balanced with the skeletal activity and the physical decay of the ^{99m}Tc label to obtain optimal skeletal to background ratios for lesion detection. In practice bone scans with diphosphonates are obtained between 2 and 4 h after injection (and with [^{18}F]fluoride at 1–2 h) but if renal function is significantly impaired (without concomitant renal osteodystrophy and associated skeletal remodeling) then scans may be performed at a later time to allow further clearance of ECF and vascular activity.

A normal bone scan (Fig. 9A.2) will show higher activity concentration in the parts of the skeleton predominated by trabecular bone, e.g. spine, compared to the shafts of long bones that are predominantly cortical bone. To obtain optimum contrast in all areas of the skeleton, this variation in activity concentration may necessitate viewing images at different intensity settings to optimize contrast at different skeletal sites. Sites of muscle insertion may appear as focal areas of increased activity and are usually symmetrical. This is commonly seen at the deltoid insertion in the humerus and in the posterior ribs. Bladder and renal collecting system activity is usually appreciated even if patients void prior to scanning.

With the increase in availability of dual-headed gamma cameras it is now common to obtain both anterior and posterior whole-body skeletal acquisitions simultaneously with single or multiple spot views being reserved for further analysis of focal lesions or where only focal pathology is suspected. Localized dynamic acquisitions performed immediately after intravenous injection of bone-seeking radiopharmaceuticals can give further information on the blood flow and blood volume related to a skeletal lesion.

REFERENCES

- Seminal primary article
- Key review paper

1 Mundy GR. Factors regulating bone resorbing and bone forming cells. In: Mundy GR. (ed.) *Bone remodeling and its disorders*. London: Martin Dunitz, 1995: 39–65.

2 Fleisch, HA. Bone and mineral metabolism. In: Fleisch HA. (ed.) *Bisphosphonates in bone disease*. New York: Parthenon Publishing Group, 1997: 11–29.

3 Baron R. Anatomy and ultrastructure of bone. In: Favus MJ. (ed.) *Primer on the metabolic bone diseases and disorders of mineral metabolism*. 4th edition. Philadelphia: Lippincott Williams and Wilkins, 1999: 3–10.

● 4 Frost HM. Dynamics of bone remodeling. In: Frost HM. (ed.) *Bone biodynamics*. Boston: Little Brown, 1964: 315.

5 Canalis E. Insulin-like growth factors and osteoporosis. *Bone* 1997; **21**: 215–16.

6 Jilka RL. Cytokines, bone remodeling, and estrogen deficiency: a 1998 update. *Bone* 1998; **23**: 75–81.

7 Mundy GR. Bone remodeling. In: Favus MJ. (ed.) *Primer on the metabolic bone diseases and disorders of mineral metabolism*. 4th edition. Philadelphia: Lippincott Williams and Wilkins, 1999: 30–8.

● 8 Chiewitz P, Hevesy G. Radioactive indicators in the study of phosphorus metabolism in rats. *Nature* 1935; **136**: 754–5.

9 Charles P, Eriksen EF, Mosekilde L, *et al*. Bone turnover and balance evaluated by a combined calcium balance and ^{47}calcium kinetic study and dynamic histomorphometry. *Metab Clin Exp* 1987; **36**: 1118–24.

10 Reeve J, Arlot M, Bernat M, *et al*. Calcium-47 kinetic measurements of bone turnover compared to bone histomorphometry in osteoporosis: the influence of human parathyroid fragment (hPTH 1-34) therapy. *Met Bone Dis Rel Res* 1981; **3**: 23–30.

11 Bauer GCH, Carlsson A, Lindquist B. Bone salt metabolism in humans studied by means of radiocalcium. *Acta Med Scand* 1957; **158**: 143–50.

12 Weber DA, Greenberg EJ, Dimich A, *et al*. Kinetics of radionuclides used for bone studies. *J Nucl Med* 1969; **10**: 8–17.

13 O'Mara RE, McAfee JG, Subramanian G. Rare earth nuclides as potential agents for skeletal imaging. *J Nucl Med* 1969; **10**: 49–51.

◆ 14 Jones AG, Francis MD, Davis MA. Bone scanning: radionuclidic reaction mechanisms. *Semin Nucl Med* 1976; **6**: 3–18.

● 15 Fleming WH, McIraith JD, King ER. Photoscanning of bone lesions utilising strontium-85. *Radiology* 1961; **77**: 635–6.

● 16 Blau M, Nagler W, Bender MA. Fluorine-18: a new isotope for bone scanning. *J Nucl Med* 1962; **3**: 332–4.

● 17 Hawkins RA, Choi Y, Huang SC, *et al*. Evaluation of the skeletal kinetics of fluorine-18-fluoride ion with PET. *J Nucl Med* 1992; **33**: 633–42.

● 18 Subramanian G, McAfee JG. A new complex of ^{99m}Tc for skeletal imaging. *Radiology* 1971; **99**: 192–6.

19 Subramanian G, McAfee JG, Bell EG, *et al.* ^{99m}Tc-labeled polyphosphate as a skeletal imaging agent. *Radiology* 1972; **102**: 701–4.

20 Subramanian G, McAfee JG, Blair RJ, *et al.* ^{99m}Tc-EHDP: a potential radiopharmaceutical for skeletal imaging. *J Nucl Med* 1972; **13**: 947–50.

● 21 Subramanian G, McAfee JG, Blair RJ, *et al.* Technetium-99m-methylene diphosphonate – a superior agent for skeletal imaging: comparison with other technetium complexes. *J Nucl Med* 1975; **16**: 744–55.

22 Grynpas MD. Fluoride effects on bone crystals. *J Bone Miner Res* 1999; **5**: S169–75.

23 Blau M, Ganatra R, Bender, MA. ^{18}F-fluoride for bone imaging. *Semin Nucl Med* 1972; **2**: 31–7.

24 Ishiguro K, Nakagaki H, Tsuboi S, *et al.* Distribution of fluoride in cortical bone of human rib. *Calc Tissue Int* 1993; **52**: 278–82.

25 Narita N, Kato K, Nakagaki H, *et al.* Distribution of fluoride concentration in the rat's bone. *Calc Tissue Int* 1990; **46**: 200–4.

26 Bang S, Baud CA. Topographical distribution of fluoride in iliac bone of a fluoride-treated osteoporotic patient. *J Bone Miner Res* 1990; **5**: S87–9.

● 27 Wootton R, Dore C. The single-passage extraction of ^{18}F in rabbit bone. *Clin Physiol Phys Meas* 1986; **7**: 333–43.

28 Peters AM, Myers MJ. Body fluids, electrolytes and bone. In: Peters AM, Myers MJ. (eds.) *Physiological measurements with radionuclides in clinical practice.* New York: Oxford University Press, 1998: 270–7.

29 Francis MD. The inhibition of calcium hydroxyapatite crystal growth by polyphosphonates and polyphosphates. *Calc Tissue Res* 1969; **3**: 151–62.

◆ 30 Fogelman I. Skeletal uptake of diphosphonate: a review. *Eur J Nucl Med* 1980; **5**: 473–6.

31 Blake GM, Park-Holohan SJ, Cook GJ, Fogelman I. Quantitative studies of bone with the use of ^{18}F-fluoride and ^{99m}Tc-methylene diphosphonate. *Semin Nucl Med* 2001; **31**: 28–49.

32 Tilden RL, Jackson J, Enneking WF, DeLand FH, McVey JT. ^{99m}Tc-polyphosphate: histological localization in human femurs by autoradiography. *J Nucl Med* 1973; **14**: 576–8.

33 Kaye M, Silverton S, Rosenthall L. Technetium-99m-pyrophosphate: studies in vivo and in vitro. *J Nucl Med* 1975; **16**: 40–5.

34 Rosenthall L, Kaye M. Technetium-99m-pyrophosphate kinetics and imaging in metabolic bone disease. *J Nucl Med* 1975; **16**: 33–9.

35 Rosenthall L, Kaye, M. Observations on the mechanism of ^{99m}Tc-labeled phosphate complex uptake in metabolic bone disease. *Semin Nucl Med* 1976; **6**: 59–67.

36 Lavender JP, Khan RA, Hughes SP. Blood flow and tracer uptake in normal and abnormal canine bone: comparisons with Sr-85 microspheres, Kr-81m, and Tc-99m MDP. *J Nucl Med* 1979; **20**: 413–18.

37 Sagar VV, Piccone JM, Charkes ND. Studies of skeletal tracer kinetics. III. Tc-99m(Sn)methylenediphosphonate uptake in the canine tibia as a function of blood flow. *J Nucl Med* 1979; **20**: 1257–61.

38 Makler PT, Charkes ND. Studies of skeletal tracer kinetics. IV. Optimum time delay for Tc-99m(Sn) methylene disphosphonate bone imaging. *J Nucl Med* 1980; **21**: 641–5.

Skeletal malignancy

GARY J.R. COOK AND IGNAC FOGELMAN

INTRODUCTION

A variety of nuclear medicine techniques have been utilized in the diagnosis and management of musculo-skeletal tumors, including primary bone and soft tissue tumors as well as bone metastases from many cancers. In recent years there have been advances in anatomical imaging techniques, such as computed tomography (CT) and magnetic resonance imaging (MRI), as well as technological advances in nuclear medicine, including the use of single photon emission computed tomography (SPECT), the introduction of new radiopharmaceuticals and an increase in the availability of clinical positron emission tomography (PET). With a large choice of imaging modalities and with continually emerging new data there is inevitably a variation in imaging protocols in musculo-skeletal tumors between institutions and countries.

The role of nuclear medicine in the diagnosis and monitoring of bone metastases is accepted and is the most important contribution in musculo-skeletal oncology but the use of radiopharmaceuticals for primary bone and soft tissue tumors is less well established. This may be changing with the development of new single photon radiopharmaceuticals for gamma camera imaging and the wider availability and clinical experience with PET.

SKELETAL METASTASES

Skeletal metastases are far more commonly encountered than primary malignant bone tumors and between one third and two thirds of patients with some of the commoner malignancies, such as breast, lung, and prostate cancer, will have metastatic involvement of the skeleton at the time of death.[1] Metastatic deposits in bone are one of the most important factors for the morbidity and disability caused by cancer and are the commonest cause of pain in cancer patients. In addition to pain, complications include pathological fracture, hypercalcemia, myelosuppression, spinal cord compression, and nerve root lesions. These complications are more common in patients with osteolytic metastases compared to those with predominantly osteosclerotic disease, and indeed, the prognosis in the former group is worse.[2] In some cancers with skeletal metastases the clinical course may be relatively short (e.g. median survival of 3 months for lung cancer) but in others it may be prolonged (e.g. median survival of 24 months for those with breast cancer or 20 months with prostate cancer).[3]

Paralleling developments in imaging there have been enormous changes in the treatment options available for cancers that have metastasized to bone with the ability to reduce the frequency of skeletal related events. Bone-specific treatments, including therapeutic radionuclides, bisphosphonates, as well as high dose chemotherapy, provide potential improvement in disease control. There is also evidence that earlier treatment of bone metastases may prolong survival. The availability of effective treatments increases the need for efficient methods for detecting and monitoring of disease. The costs of treating bone metastases and associated complications make a major demand on health care resources[4] and it is therefore important that accurate methods are available to monitor therapy which can give an indication of success or failure early in the course of treatment. At present the most standardized way of assessing response is by comparing serial radiographs. The Union Internationale Contre le Cancer (UICC) defined a number of criteria that indicate response to treatment, including resolution of lesions and sclerosis of formerly lytic lesions.[5] Although standardization is improved by using these criteria, the method is otherwise relatively insensitive as it may take more than 6 months for radiographic evidence of response to be seen and the evaluation of metastases that are sclerotic at baseline may be especially problematic with this method. Interestingly, it has been noted that the response of skeletal metastases to systemic therapy may be less than that seen in soft tissue disease within the same individual.[6] Rather than there being a different biological response between skeletal and soft tissue metastases, it is likely that this phenomenon may simply reflect the relative insensitivity of the UICC radiographic skeletal assessment method.

RADIOPHARMACEUTICALS FOR IMAGING SKELETAL METASTASES

The mechanisms for the uptake and localization of bone-specific radiopharmaceuticals is discussed in more detail in Chapter 9A. Bone agents are preferentially localized at sites of new or reactive bone formation. Therefore, active osteoblastic metastases, causing a sclerotic radiographic appearance, in which newly formed bone is laid down without prior resorption, are associated with markedly increased uptake of bone tracers. This pattern is most commonly encountered in prostate cancer. Although osteolytic metastases, caused by osteoclastic bone resorption stimulated by tumor-derived cytokines, are more commonly seen in most cancers, this type of metastasis is nearly always accompanied by reactive bone formation leading to uptake of bone radiopharmaceuticals. In tumors where osteolysis predominates, such as myeloma, there may be little in the way of an osteoblastic response and hence there may be little or no abnormality visible on bone scintigraphy. It is rare for a bone scan to be completely normal in myeloma patients but a radiographic skeletal survey may be a better method to assess the extent of skeletal disease[7] and remains the method of choice in many institutions.

Other single photon radiopharmaceuticals have been used in the assessment of both primary and metastatic bone tumors and are most commonly nonspecific tumor agents rather than acting as bone tracers. Thallium-201, an analog of potassium, enters tumor cells via the Na^+/K^+ ATPase pump but as well as reflecting the metabolic status of the cell, uptake also depends on blood flow. Sestamibi labeled with ^{99m}Tc shows a similar distribution to ^{201}Tl but has a different mechanism of accumulation. It is thought to reflect cell viability and is mainly associated with mitochondria intracellularly. Uptake of ^{99m}Tc(V)-dimercaptosuccinic acid has also been described in bone metastases; the exact mechanism of uptake is uncertain.[8]

The majority of bone metastases initially seed in bone marrow and there is therefore the potential to use bone marrow scintigraphy as a method to detect bone metastases at an early stage by demonstrating focal areas of marrow replacement.[9] There are a number of limitations of this technique including difficulty in visualizing the spine because of overlying hepatic and splenic activity and the inability to assess areas of the skeleton where red marrow is scarce. Because of this the technique is unlikely to be used to routinely detect and determine the extent of skeletal metastases but may nevertheless be useful in certain cases in conjunction with ^{99m}Tc-methylene diphosphonate (^{99m}Tc-MDP) scintigraphy where the specificity for individual lesions may be improved.

A number of nuclear medicine tracers exist which are specific to a type or group of tumors. These localize in both skeletal and soft tissue metastases and are often valuable in assessing the total extent of disease. Examples include ^{131}I for differentiated thyroid cancers, ^{131}I- and ^{123}I-labeled meta-iodobenzylguanidine (MIBG), which behaves as a noradrenaline analog, localizing in a number of neuroendocrine tumors, and ^{111}In-labeled octreotide, which localizes in tumors bearing somatostatin receptors, also including a number of neuroendocrine tumors.

Positron emission tomography (PET) tracers that are currently available and have potential roles for assessing skeletal metastases include the [^{18}F]fluoride ion and 2-[^{18}F]fluoro-2-deoxy-D-glucose (^{18}F-FDG). Whilst [^{18}F]fluoride behaves as a bone-specific tracer, similar to ^{99m}Tc-labeled diphosphonates, tumor uptake of ^{18}F-FDG depends on tumor glycolysis and membrane glucose transporters. The uptake of ^{18}F-FDG is not restricted to tumor involving the skeleton and has the advantage of demonstrating all metastatic sites in a cancer patient, whether they are in soft tissue or bone.

SCINTIGRAPHIC PATTERNS IN IMAGING SKELETAL METASTASES AND THE ROLE OF CORRELATIVE IMAGING

Although uptake of labeled diphosphonate on a bone scan is not specific for metastases, by studying the pattern and distribution of lesions it is often possible to infer the etiology of abnormalities without requiring further correlative imaging. However, as uptake of bone tracers is not specific to malignant disease a number of cases will remain problematic and there remains a substantial role for correlative imaging.

The majority of bone metastases are distributed irregularly in the axial skeleton and ribs (Fig. 9B.1) and there is usually little doubt as to the cause of multiple scattered lesions in this distribution. A small proportion (<10%) affect the appendicular skeleton and this is most commonly seen in clinical practice in carcinoma of the lung, prostate, kidney and breast.[10,11] It is arguable whether scans should routinely include the peripheries in asymptomatic patients, but certainly if a patient being assessed for skeletal metastases has peripheral symptoms, then the distal limbs

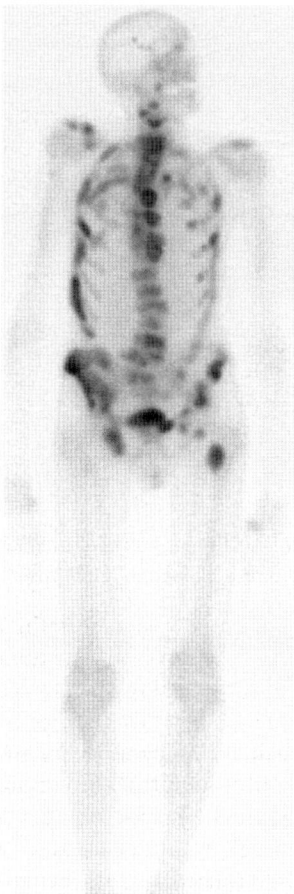

Figure 9B.1 *^{99m}Tc-methylene diphosphonate (^{99m}Tc-MDP) whole-body bone scan demonstrating the irregular distribution of skeletal metastases predominantly in the axial skeleton in a patient with prostate cancer.*

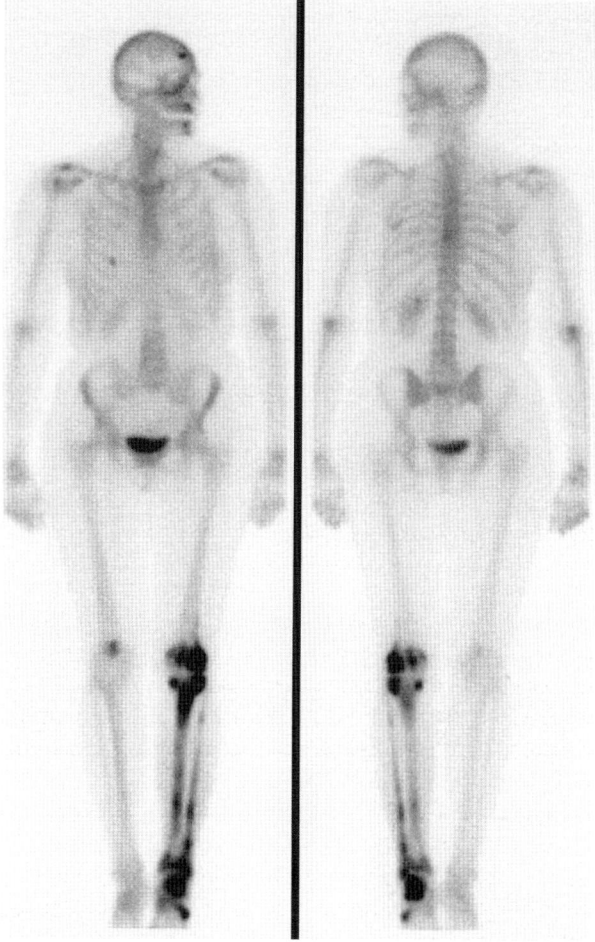

Figure 9B.2 *^{99m}Tc-MDP bone scan of a woman with metastatic breast cancer demonstrating an unusual pattern of peripheral skeletal metastatic disease in the left leg. A further metastasis is seen in the skull and an old healing anterior right rib fracture is also demonstrated.*

should be included. This is much easier with modern gamma cameras where a whole-body scan can be performed in less time than a scan comprising multiple spot views of the skeleton (Fig. 9B.2).

When bone metastases are very extensive, on first inspection a bone scan may appear normal due to the confluent nature of the lesions. However, the 'superscan', so called because of the apparent good quality of the scan because of diffusely increased skeletal uptake, has a number of distinguishing features. In addition to the apparent high quality of the scan, the soft tissues, including the kidneys, may be inconspicuous or invisible due to the increased ratio between skeletal and soft tissue accumulation. Metabolic bone diseases may also cause a superscan but that caused by malignancy may be differentiated on close inspection where some irregularity of uptake is usually visible. This is more apparent in the ribs or the ends of the long bones (Fig. 9B.3).

To increase the specificity of bone scan interpretation it is necessary to have a knowledge of normal variants that can mimic metastases and of other skeletal disorders that might cause confusion. One example is of increased tracer accumulation at the manubriosternal junction. This is a relatively common normal variant but may cause difficulty in patients with carcinoma of the breast as the sternum is a common site for early metastatic disease (Fig. 9B.4). Clues that a lesion at this site is not benign are asymmetry and/or lack of linearity. If doubt persists, or if there are local symptoms or signs, then further imaging may be required. The sternum is often difficult to adequately visualize with radiography and so localized CT or MRI are often more helpful in this circumstance. Other variants that should be recognized include activity at the confluence of sutures at the pterion in the skull, the deltoid muscle insertion on the humerus and symmetrical muscle insertion in the posterior ribs of paraspinal muscles causing a stippled appearance. On occasion, the tip of the scapula overlying a rib may mimic a focal abnormality. This can be easily distinguished by taking a further scan with the arms raised, thereby moving the tip of the scapula outside the line of the ribs.

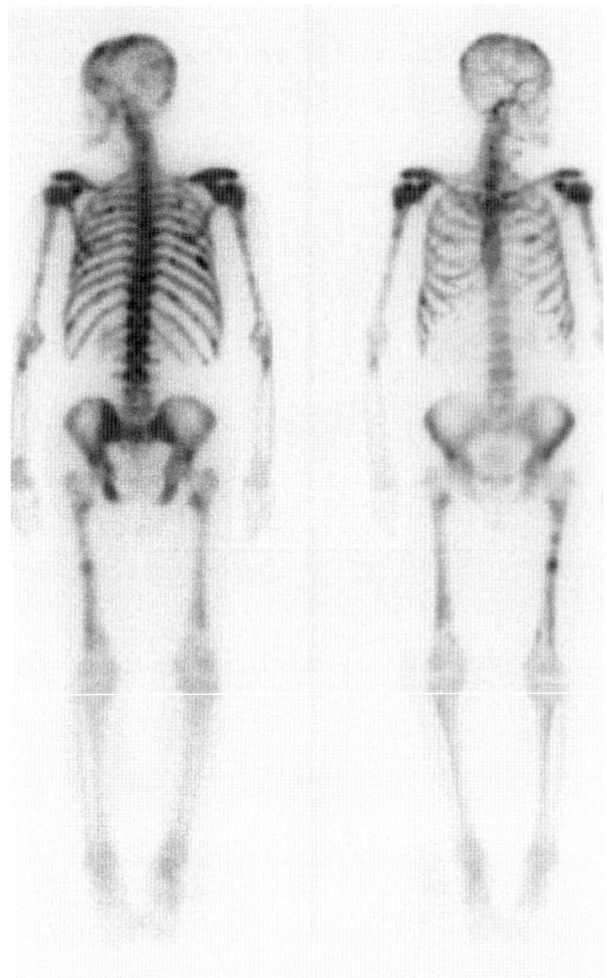

Figure 9B.3   *⁹⁹ᵐTc-MDP bone scan of a man with prostate cancer demonstrating widespread heterogeneously increased uptake throughout most of the skeleton in keeping with a malignant superscan.*

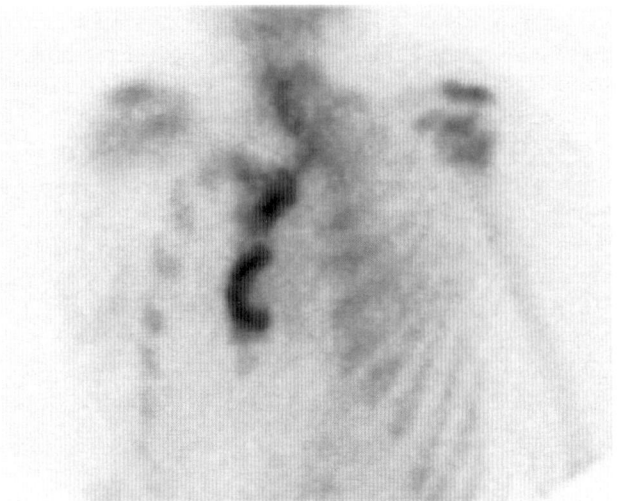

Figure 9B.4   *⁹⁹ᵐTc-MDP bone scan of a patient with breast cancer demonstrating sternal and manubrial infiltration. The appearance of the lower sternal lesion suggests an aggressive metastasis causing bone destruction (photopenic center with a rim of increased osteoblastic activity).*

The appearance of a single lesion may aid interpretation. A focal rib lesion is often the result of trauma that may not even be recalled by the patient but a lesion extending along the length of a rib is usually malignant in nature. However, Baxter and colleagues[12] have suggested that a single rib hot spot in a patient with a known malignancy may turn out to have a malignant etiology in a surprisingly large number of patients (41%). Even focal abnormalities at the anterior ends of ribs, a position where abnormalities are often considered to be benign in the majority of cases, showed a large number of confirmed metastases (36%). These findings differ from those previously reported by Tumeh *et al.*[13] in a similar retrospective study where only 10% of solitary rib lesions proved to be malignant. A linear array of rib lesions in adjacent ribs remains a situation where one can usually be confident of a traumatic etiology.

The interpretation of abnormal areas of increased activity, whether solitary or multiple, may be especially problematic in the spine as there is a high prevalence of benign abnormalities, such as degenerative disease, which may be indistinguishable without further investigation. In the situation of a single spinal hot spot in patients with a known primary tumor, Coakley and colleagues[14] found that just over one half (57%) turned out to be benign on subsequent clinical and imaging follow-up. These authors went on to classify distinguishing features and found that only complex areas of uptake were a useful feature with 11 out of 15 of such abnormalities being due to malignant disease. Conversely, all paravertebral abnormalities had a benign etiology. It is clear, however, that in many instances further imaging will be required to increase specificity.

When further evaluating a vertebral scintigraphic abnormality, plain X-rays are often the recommended next step. If a radiographically benign abnormality is evident in the position of a bone scan abnormality a metastasis is unlikely; less than 1% of such abnormalities subsequently developing malignant changes.[15] Unfortunately, the converse is not true, and if a radiograph of a solitary bone scan lesion is negative, further imaging is required. Computed tomography may be of some help and is certainly more sensitive than plain X-rays[16] but MRI is regarded as being more sensitive, as imaging of the bone marrow is possible, thereby often detecting metastases before there has been bone destruction.[17]

Vertebral body fractures have a characteristic appearance on bone scintigraphy showing a linear area of increased activity. However, it is not possible to differentiate fractures due to benign diseases such as osteoporosis from malignant collapse. A follow-up scan after a few months which shows reducing activity at a vertebral fracture site suggests a benign cause. Correlative imaging may be required prior to this, however. In this situation radiographs do not commonly add further information but merely confirm that the pattern seen on bone scan is due to collapse of a vertebra. MRI, where altered signal in the bone marrow or evidence of a soft tissue mass[18] confirms malignancy, is probably the most accurate, non-invasive next investigation.

The addition of SPECT to a bone scanning protocol may improve sensitivity and specificity but evidence is relatively limited at present. There is potential for increased accuracy with SPECT with an increased sensitivity for lesion detection because of the resultant improvement in contrast compared to planar imaging and a better three-dimensional localization of abnormalities which may aid specificity. Early reports have suggested that the use of SPECT may not only improve sensitivity in the spine but may also improve specificity as it may be possible to examine the pattern and position of abnormalities within the vertebra (Fig. 9B.5). For example, lesions involving the vertebral body and seen extending into the posterior elements or with pedicular involvement alone, are more likely to represent metastases than those in the facet joints, anterior vertebral body, and intervertebral disk space.[19–21]

Abnormalities seen at joints outside the spine on bone scanning are generally benign. An area of increased uptake that occurs either side of a joint is reassuring. This pattern is commonly seen in joints that are affected by degenerative disease, including the knee, hip, and shoulder. Another benign condition that may cause difficulty in interpretation is Paget's disease. This may be present in up to 5% of the population over 40 years of age in some areas and is asymptomatic in the majority and often an incidental finding in endemic regions.[22] Usually, the diffuse nature of increased diphosphonate accumulation due to osteoblastic activity and increased vascularity in pagetoid bone, together with the appearance of expansion of the affected bone, diffuse uptake throughout the bone or abnormality extending from a joint into the diaphysis of a long bone, will aid correct interpretation. Radiographic correlation is helpful for confirmation where typical radiologic features are usually apparent.

When using bone-specific tracers to assess response to treatment it must be noted that an increase in activity of lesions or even an apparent increase in the number of lesions does not always correspond to disease progression. The well recognized flare response on the bone scan, whereby an increase in uptake in responding metastases due to a local bone osteoblastic reaction in the early months following instigation of systemic therapy, has been described as a result of chemotherapy and hormone therapy in both breast and prostate cancer.[23,24] This may be indistinguishable from truly progressive disease. The appearance of new uptake in hitherto undetected lesions has also been described as part of this phenomenon.[25] The increased uptake as a result of the flare response may last for as long as 6 months after therapy before a subsequent decrease in uptake in individual lesions is noted but has been reported

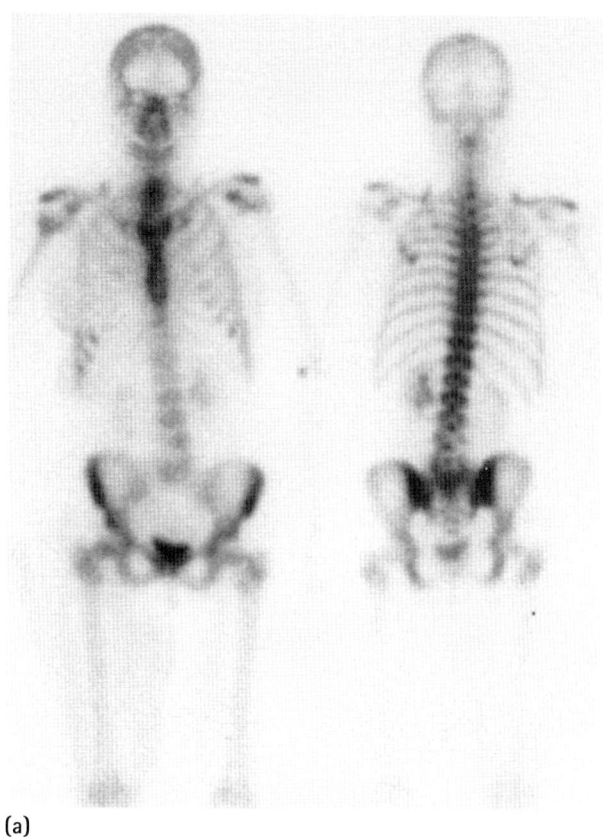

(a)

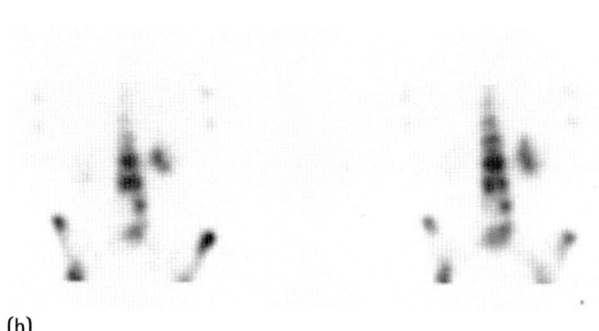

(b)

Figure 9B.5   *^{99m}Tc-MDP planar (a) and coronal single photon emission computed tomography (SPECT) (b) images of a patient with breast cancer and back pain. On the planar images there is subtle reduction in uptake in the lower lumbar spine of the right. SPECT images improve image contrast and show a clear area of reduced uptake corresponding to an aggressive bone metastasis that did not cause an osteoblastic reaction.*

to be associated with a more favorable prognosis.[26] An early reduction in uptake after treatment virtually always indicates a response (Fig. 9B.6) except in the instances where very aggressive osteolytic disease may continue to progress without an osteoblastic response, an observation that is rare, however.

If a bone scan is performed at a time beyond which the flare response can occur, then an increase in the number of

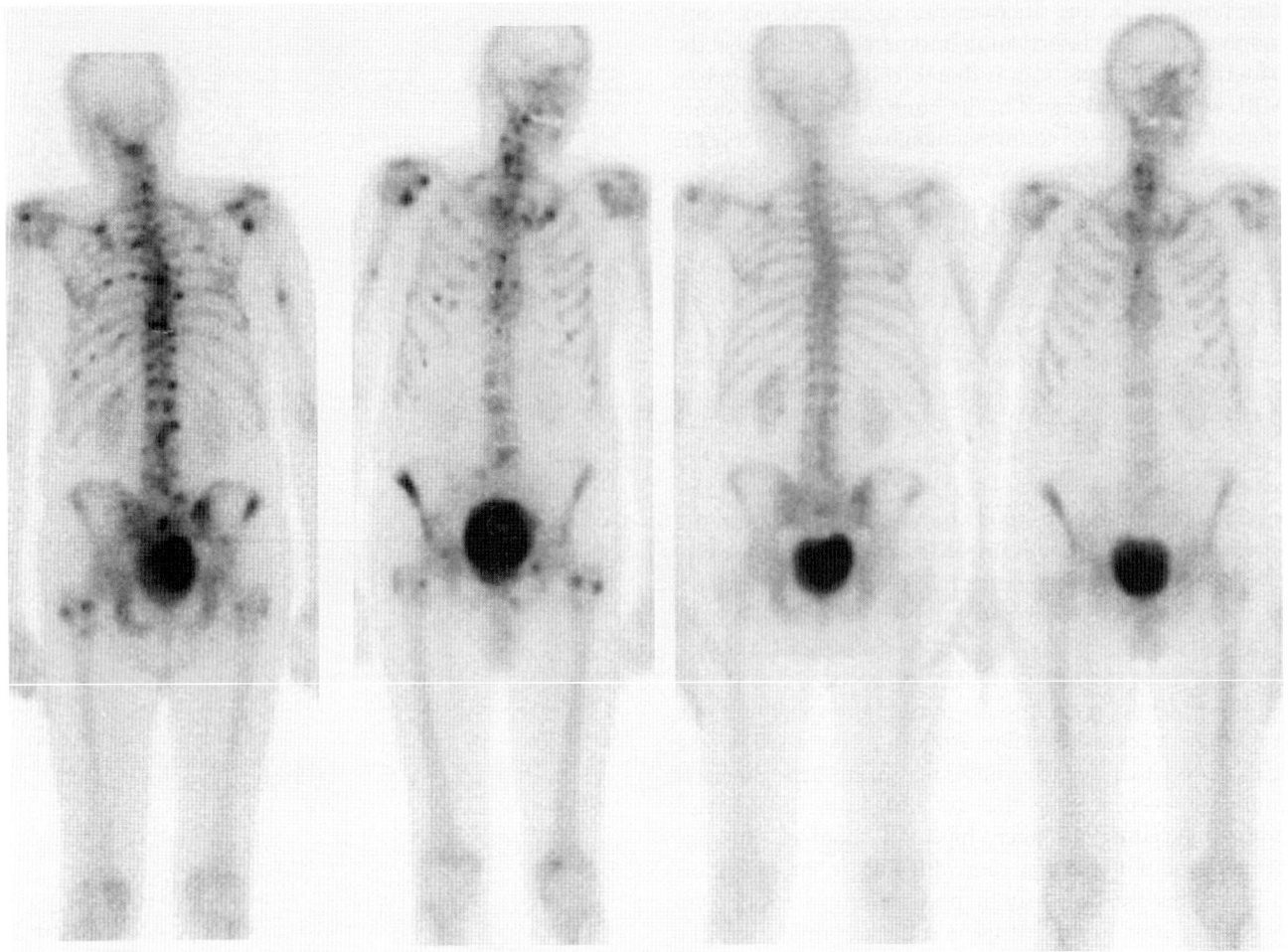

Figure 9B.6 *The pair of images on the left are ^{99m}Tc-MDP bone scans of a man with metastatic prostate cancer before treatment. The pair of images on the right, obtained after the patient had received chemotherapy, show near complete resolution of the skeletal metastases.*

skeletal lesions is usually taken as incontrovertible evidence of disease progression. Similarly, allowing for technical acquisition and display factors, an increase in intensity in known skeletal metastases is also generally regarded as evidence of disease progression,[27] although is not as reliable a sign[28] (Fig. 9B.7).

It is the functional nature of bone scintigraphy and the fact that most skeletal metastases are accompanied by an osteoblastic response, whether they are predominantly sclerotic or lytic in nature, that makes it such a sensitive technique. It has been estimated that at least 50% of bone must be destroyed before a lesion is evident radiographically.[29] Galasko reported a lead-time of between 12 and 18 months for bone scintigraphy over radiography,[30] and in a serial study of 6 monthly bone scans a median lead time of 4 months (range, 0–18 months) was found.[31] There is no doubt that some modern imaging techniques may be more sensitive for detecting skeletal metastases. MRI is especially sensitive for detecting altered bone marrow signal and

may detect metastases before they have caused a sufficient osteoblastic response required for detection with bone scintigraphy.[17] Previously, it has not been possible to easily evaluate the whole skeleton with MRI but with faster MRI scanning sequences now becoming available it is possible that this modality will play an increasing role in assessing the skeleton of patients with cancer in the future.

At the present time bone scintigraphy remains the most commonly used method for assessing the skeleton for metastatic spread. Radiographs are frequently employed to evaluate indeterminate lesions and when these reveal no abnormality to explain the scintigraphic findings then focused CT or MRI can be used. CT can detect deposits within the bone marrow and can also display bone destruction or sclerotic foci when present. MRI is probably more sensitive for assessing marrow involvement whilst visualizing cortical bone less well and is particularly helpful in the spine to evaluate cord compression or any soft tissue extent of a metastatic deposit.[32]

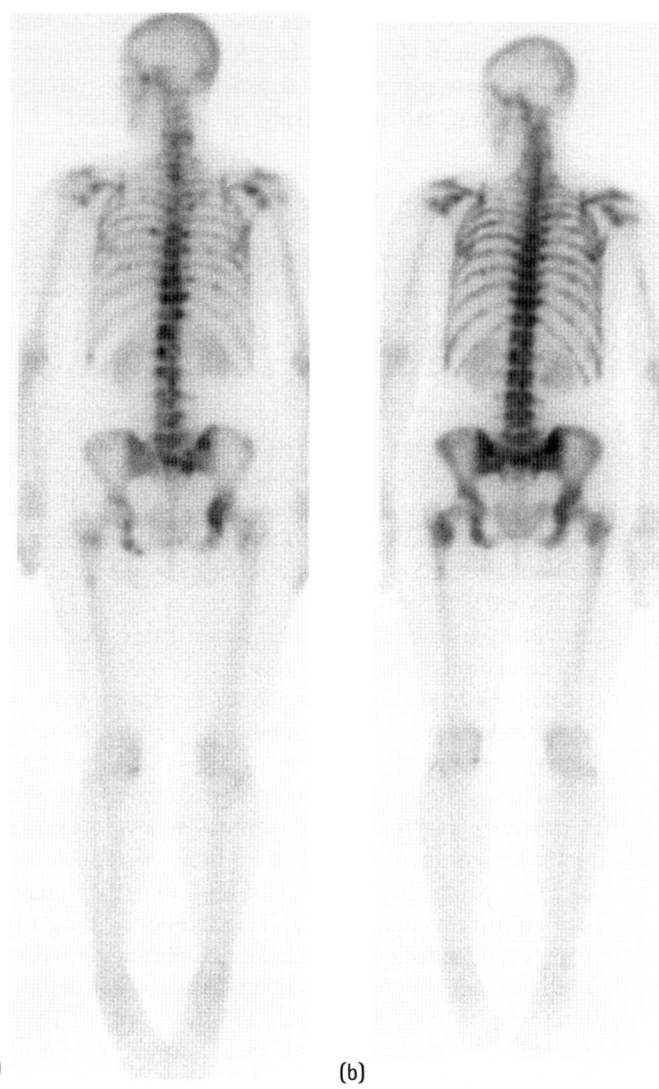

(a)   (b)

Figure 9B.7 *⁹⁹ᵐTc-MDP bone scans of a woman with metastatic breast cancer with an interval of 1 year between the scans. Whilst the initial scan (a) shows evidence of widespread metastatic disease, the follow-up scan (b) shows more confluent abnormal heterogeneous uptake more extensively in the skeleton confirming progression of skeletal involvement.*

SPECIFIC CANCERS

Whilst bone scintigraphy may play a role in the detection of skeletal metastases from virtually any primary tumor, it is most commonly used in those cancers that have a predilection for skeletal spread. Breast and prostate cancer are most frequently investigated with this technique but it may play a role in a number of miscellaneous tumors where bone involvement is common including lung cancer, other genitourinary cancers and neuroblastoma.

Breast cancer

Some controversy has existed as to the precise role of bone scanning in patients at different stages of breast cancer management and its use still varies between institutions. In one of the largest studies,[33] with clinical staging, imaging technique, and interpretation well standardized, and with

at least 1 year of follow-up in all patients ($n = 1267$) the scan positive rates for stages I to IV were 0, 3, 7, and 47%, respectively. When staging by tumor size alone it was found that T2 tumors were very unlikely to be associated with a positive scan (0.3%) but T3 and T4 tumors had scan detection rates of 8 and 13%, respectively. The authors concluded that routine scans are not required in those with tumors of less than 2 cm but were recommended for all those with stage II, III or IV disease.

Although the pick-up rate of new metastases in those being screened serially varies between reported studies, most authors conclude that follow-up scans in asymptomatic patients are unnecessary and not cost-effective. Rather than serially scanning all asymptomatic patients Coleman and colleagues tried to identify those with adverse prognostic factors that may make serial scanning worthwhile.[31] Using 6 monthly follow-up scans for 2 years in 560 patients they identified patients with T4 tumors, more than four axillary lymph nodes and inoperable tumors as having a high enough scan conversion (>6%) to justify serial scanning. Few would argue that a bone scan is justified in patients with new symptoms or in whom there are other worrying clinical, laboratory or radiological features and it may help in decisions on subsequent local or systemic palliative treatment and provide prognostic information.

As discussed above, the flare phenomenon limits the usefulness of bone scintigraphy in assessing treatment response in the skeleton but by only interpreting scans with a detailed knowledge of previous therapy the bone scan may provide a valuable objective measure of response not routinely available by other means and may also give prognostic information.[34]

Prostate cancer

Historically, at presentation, the proportion of patients with carcinoma of the prostate with skeletal metastases has been high, in the region of 30–50%.[35] More recently, with more frequent early detection of prostate cancer following screening prostate specific antigen (PSA) measurement, the proportion of patients presenting with bone metastases is now probably much less. Not surprisingly, the rate of positive bone scans at presentation has been found to vary with the stage of disease as measured by clinical stage,[36] T classification,[37] Gleason staging[38] or biochemical parameters such as PSA.[39] The most useful single parameter in deciding the need for a staging bone scan in asymptomatic patients appears to be PSA. Although there is some uncertainty whether a level of 10 or 20 ng mL^{-1} should be used as an upper threshold for performing scintigraphy, certainly a level of less than 10 ng mL^{-1} is very rarely associated with bone metastases. By combining the various parameters mentioned above we found that bone scans could be avoided if the PSA level is less than 20 ng mL^{-1}, clinical stage is less than T4 and Gleason score <8, and scans can be omitted unless the major Gleason pattern is 4.[40]

PSA measurement may also be helpful in deciding which asymptomatic patients to follow-up with bone scans. Although a relatively high conversion from bone scan negative at presentation to bone scan positive by the second year (20%) has been described,[41] patients with skeletal metastases soon developed clinical or biochemical evidence of metastases and so routine scanning was not endorsed. However, if the PSA level begins to rise then bone scintigraphy is justified[42] and if a patient has symptoms suggesting bone involvement then scintigraphy is valuable in confirmation and in assessing the extent of disease and prognosis.

Following treatment, bone scintigraphy is helpful to assess the effectiveness of therapy and infer prognosis. For those patients in whom bone scan appearances deteriorate despite therapy, prognosis is much worse. It has been shown that the 1-year survival for those with progression was only 7% compared to 60% in those without.[43]

The flare phenomenon may also occur with metastatic prostate cancer. Care must be taken to avoid interpreting this as disease progression as patients demonstrating this phenomenon are more likely to have a good clinical response.[44]

PET AND PET/CT IN SKELETAL METASTASES

[^{18}F]fluoride imaging

With modern PET scanners it is possible to acquire high-resolution, functional, tomographic images and with the high contrast that is achievable between normal and diseased bone as early as 1 h following injection of [^{18}F]fluoride, this method has been evaluated in the investigation of bone metastases.[45,46] More recently, with the advent of combined PET/CT scanners, [^{18}F]fluoride PET/CT has also been described with an improvement in specificity of interpretation of skeletal lesions.[47]

Both sclerotic and lytic bone metastases have been reported to show increased uptake of [^{18}F]fluoride in breast cancer patients[47,48] as is seen with ^{99m}Tc-labeled diphosphonates. Although PET shows superior quantitative accuracy over planar or SPECT gamma camera imaging it is unlikely that quantification of [^{18}F]fluoride uptake alone, as a nonspecific bone agent, would be able to differentiate benign from malignant focal skeletal lesions. Using a relatively crude index of uptake (lesion to normal ratios) it has not been possible to differentiate benign from malignant lesions.[49] By making dynamic measurements of regional skeletal [^{18}F]fluoride activity, including plasma clearance of [^{18}F]fluoride to bone mineral, metastases have been shown to have between three times[45] and five to ten times[48] higher values compared to normal bone but have not been directly compared to benign lesions. By obtaining dynamic acquisitions it is also possible to generate parametric images of regional indices, a process which may facilitate measurement of regional kinetic indices.[45] From the practical point of view it is much more likely that PET/CT [^{18}F]fluoride imaging will provide extra specificity rather than a quantitative approach.[47]

As [^{18}F]fluoride PET images are of better spatial resolution than conventional bone scintigraphy and the fact that tomographic images are required routinely, rather than as an additional acquisition of a localized area, it has potential advantages with regard to sensitivity and specificity in detecting bone metastases, even when not combined with CT. Schirrmeister and colleagues have compared [^{18}F]fluoride PET with ^{99m}Tc-MDP in 44 patients with varied primary cancers (prostate, lung, and thyroid), using CT, MRI, and ^{131}I scintigraphy as reference methods.[50] It was found that all known metastases were detected by [^{18}F]fluoride PET and overall, nearly twice as many benign and malignant

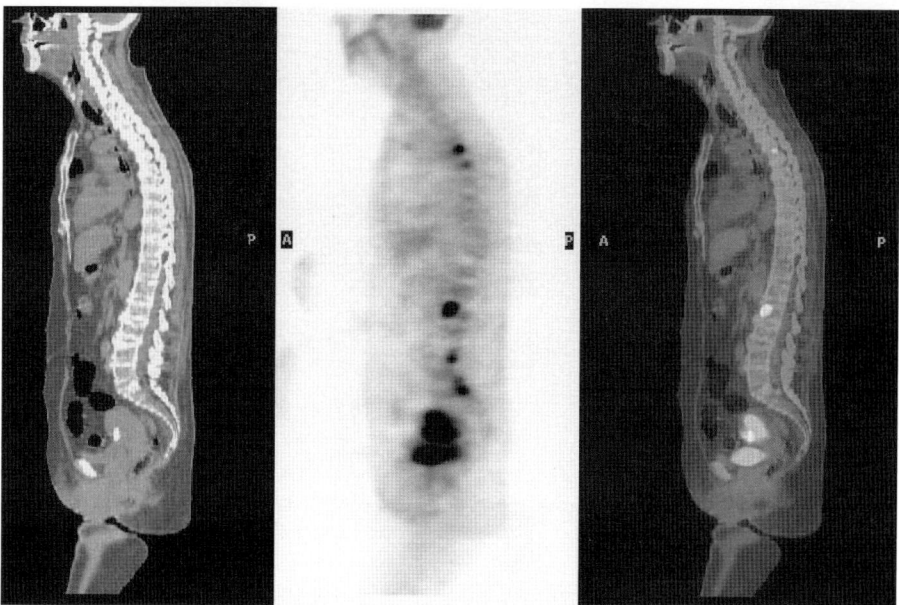

Figure 9B.8 *Sagittal positron emission tomography/computed tomography (PET/CT) images (left to right CT, PET, fused PET/CT) of a patient with uterine carcinoma (visible above the bladder) with skeletal metastases in the spine.*

lesions were identified compared to [99mTc]-MDP bone scans. It was also possible to correctly classify a larger number of benign and malignant lesions with [[18F]fluoride (97%) compared to [99mTc]-MDP (80.5%) because of the superior spatial localization of the former, particularly in the spine. However, it is possible that the observed differences would not have been as great if [99mTc]-MDP SPECT images had also been routinely available. In a subsequent study, [[18F]fluoride PET proved superior to planar bone scintigraphy but was not statistically significantly better with regards to accuracy when compared to bone scintigraphy supplemented by SPECT.[51] In a further study of patients with breast cancer, the greater accuracy of [[18F]fluoride PET led to a change of management in four out of 34 patients compared to conventional [99mTc]-MDP bone scans.[49]

[18F]-fluorodeoxyglucose imaging

With respect to skeletal metastases, uptake of [18F]-FDG is assumed to be within tumor cells rather than as a result of bone reaction, and there is therefore potential for [18F]-FDG PET imaging of the skeleton to be more sensitive and specific in the evaluation of the skeleton in metastatic disease (Fig. 9B.8). The possible role of [18F]-FDG in the evaluation of skeletal metastases has been explored in a number of studies. On a patient-by-patient basis, the sensitivity for detecting metastases was found to be the same as [99mTc]-MDP in subjects with non-small cell lung cancer but [18F]-FDG PET correctly confirmed the absence of bone metastases in a larger number of cases (87 out of 89 compared to 54 out of

89).[52] The most likely explanation for these observations is that uptake of [18F]-FDG is more specific for tumor and does not accumulate into coincidental benign skeletal disease such as osteoarthritis. In a similar study of 145 patients with a variety of cancers, [18F]-FDG PET demonstrated a higher sensitivity and specificity on a lesion-by-lesion basis.[53] The improved sensitivity may be due to direct imaging of tumor metabolism, leading to the detection of metastases at an earlier stage when only bone marrow is involved and before a significant bone reaction has taken place, this being necessary for bone tracers to localize. This probably accounts for the superiority of [18F]-FDG PET over conventional scintigraphy in malignancy that is primarily marrow-based, including lymphoma and myeloma.[54,55]

Greater accuracy of [18F]-FDG PET is not a universal finding for bone metastases. In breast cancer a higher false negative rate has been described in the skeleton compared to other metastases.[56] One possible explanation is that different types of bone metastasis behave differently with regard to uptake of [18F]-FDG. Although a significantly higher number of metastases has been reported with [18F]-FDG compared to planar [99mTc]-MDP in a group of patients with progressive advanced breast cancer, a subgroup with predominantly sclerotic disease had fewer lesions identified with [18F]-FDG PET but as a group had a more favorable prognosis than those with predominantly lytic disease.[2] In addition, sclerotic metastases showed lower uptake of [18F]-FDG in terms of standardized uptake values (SUVs). Similarly, there are reports that [18F]-FDG is less accurate in assessing skeletal disease in prostate cancer, a tumor which results in predominantly sclerotic bone metastases.[57,58] As

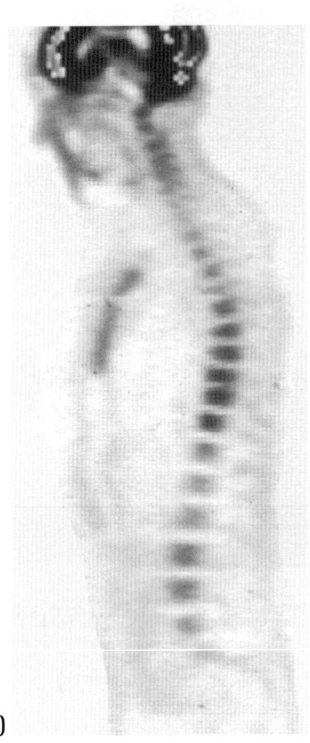

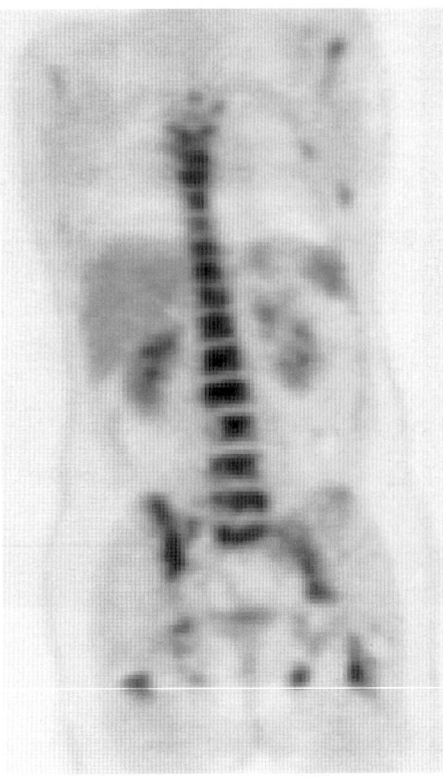

(a)   (b)

Figure 9B.9 *(a) Sagittal ¹⁸F-fluorodeoxy-glucose (¹⁸F-FDG) PET image of a patient with lymphoma. The image was obtained 3 weeks after the patient had received chemotherapy and demonstrates a diffuse benign reactive increase in bone marrow activity. (b) Coronal ¹⁸F-FDG PET image of a patient with non-Hodgkin's lymphoma. The image was obtained at presentation and demonstrates heterogeneous increased uptake in the bone marrow (see lower lumbar spine and pelvis in particular) indicating widespread marrow infiltration subsequently confirmed on bone marrow biopsy.*

an explanation for these findings, it is possible that sclerotic metastases have different biology and are less metabolically active. Alternatively, sclerotic metastases are relatively acellular and lower volumes of viable tumor within lesions may also account for the relative insensitivity of ¹⁸F-FDG in contrast to the florid osteoblastic activity resulting in uptake of nonspecific bone tracers.[59] In addition, more aggressive lytic disease might be expected to outstrip its blood supply, rendering the metastasis relatively hypoxic, a property which is associated with increased ¹⁸F-FDG uptake in some cell lines.[60]

In lymphoma, where skeletal metastases are predominantly marrow-based rather than purely osseous, ¹⁸F-FDG PET has shown greater sensitivity than conventional bone scintigraphy.[54] As bone marrow staging of lymphoma is limited to biopsy of the iliac crest only and therefore has potential sampling errors, it has also been suggested that ¹⁸F-FDG PET might be complementary to bone marrow biopsy as a staging procedure, with the advantage that nonskeletal tissues will also be assessed.[61,62] For assessing bone marrow response to treatment the situation may be more difficult with ¹⁸F-FDG as it is known that chemotherapy and granulocyte colony stimulating factors cause a benign, diffuse increase in marrow activity (Fig. 9B.9).[63,64] Similarly, in the staging of myeloma, ¹⁸F-FDG PET is more sensitive than conventional staging procedures and in one series revealed a greater extent of skeletal involvement than radiographs in 14 out of 23 patients.[55]

Overall, it would appear that ¹⁸F-FDG PET is more specific and at least as sensitive as bone scintigraphy for detection of skeletal metastases in most malignancies. In predominantly sclerotic disease the sensitivity may be less.

PRIMARY BONE TUMORS

With the advent of MRI and CT, nuclear medicine techniques have been used less widely in the investigation and management of primary bone tumors but a role exists, usually in conjunction with anatomic imaging, in some circumstances. With the development of clinical PET and new single photon radiopharmaceuticals clinical applications are likely to increase.

Bone scintigraphy is the initial investigation of choice when a bone lesion which cannot be characterized is seen incidentally on a radiograph. A bone scan may contribute to the characterization of a lesion and also determine whether it is solitary or multiple, the latter being likely to indicate metastatic disease. A negative bone scan greatly increases the chances that the lesion is benign and of no clinical consequence. Unfortunately, the converse is not true and an area of metabolic activity which corresponds to the radiographic abnormality does not confidently differentiate benign from malignant lesions. Dynamic scintigraphy with the three-phase bone scan may not be of sufficient help. Although malignant tumors are characteristically very vascular there are a number of benign bone tumors with similar appearances that may cause confusion e.g. osteoid osteoma or aneurysmal bone cyst.

Characteristic patterns of uptake have been described in some primary bone tumors[65,66] but in practice there is enough overlap of features for the radioisotope bone scan to be insufficiently reliable to differentiate types of tumor. Differential diagnosis will usually depend on anatomical imaging techniques such as radiography, CT or MRI, which may be very specific, and ultimately, histological examination. Improving the specificity in differentiating benign from malignant lesions may be possible with other tracers such as gallium, thallium, sestamibi, and ^{99m}Tc(V)-DMSA. For example, differential uptake of gallium between the majority of benign and malignant bone tumors except chondrosarcoma has been described.[67] Similar results were found with the use of thallium by Van der Wall *et al.*[68] The more optimal imaging characteristics of ^{99m}Tc have been successfully employed by using the radiopharmaceutical ^{99m}Tc-sestamibi in differentiating benign from malignant bone lesions but a number of malignant lesions (6/42) were negative.[69] Early work with the radiopharmaceutical ^{99m}Tc(V)-DMSA suggests that this may be able to differentiate benign from malignant chondrogenic tumors.[70] These results suggest that there may be a limited role for nuclear medicine techniques in this clinical situation particularly if anatomic imaging techniques are unhelpful, equivocal or unavailable but they are not routinely employed in most institutions.

Once a diagnosis of a primary bone lesion has been made, the use of bone scintigraphy in the initial evaluation of primary bone tumors prior to surgical resection is controversial. Although some authors have described a good correlation between activity and tumor extent this has not been supported by other studies.[71,72] Poor correlation between scintigraphic activity and actual tumor extent may be due to peritumoral reactive bone changes or to bone marrow and soft tissue extension. For this reason anatomical imaging with MRI is probably the most accurate method of delineating the extent of tumor tissue at present and is particulary effective at determining marrow involvement. The use of bone scintigraphy in the detection of skeletal metastases from primary bone tumors is accepted but the frequency of use will depend on the frequency of skeletal metastases at presentation in each individual tumor.

Nuclear medicine imaging has a potentially important role in the post-therapy evaluation of primary bone tumors. Although the bone scan is helpful in detecting skeletal metastases, it is less useful for assessing response of the primary tumor to chemotherapy. Thallium-201 has been found to be a better measure of tumor response than either gallium or ^{99m}Tc-MDP scintigraphy.[73] Thallium accumulation depends on ATPase activity and may therefore more accurately reflect tumor viability than ^{99m}Tc-MDP and gallium, both of which show some nonspecific bone localization.[74,75] ^{99m}Tc-MIBI has also been assessed post-therapy in a series where bone sarcomas predominated and was found to accurately differentiate active sarcoma from post-treatment changes.[76] In this same study ^{18}F-FDG PET was assessed and found to be superior to ^{99m}Tc-MIBI. Most work using PET has investigated soft tissue sarcomas rather than bone tumors but in another small series of mixed tumors Jones *et al.* describe reduction in FDG uptake in tumors responding to neoadjuvant therapy but also noted prominent accumulation

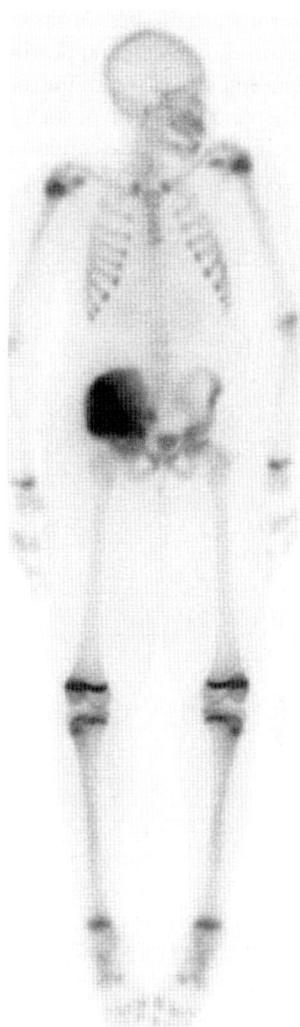

Figure 9B.10 *^{99m}Tc-MDP bone scan of an adolescent with osteosarcoma of the right iliac bone.*

corresponding to benign reactive tissues within and adjacent to tumor.[77] The timing of FDG PET scanning may therefore be of importance in treatment assessment.

SPECIFIC PRIMARY BONE TUMORS

Osteosarcoma

Osteosarcomas occur in two different age groups, in adolescents and in the elderly, the latter being frequently related to tumors complicating Paget's disease. Tumors are usually metaphyseal, most commonly around the knee. Treatment is primarily surgical but pre- and postoperative chemotherapy improve survival. Accurate preoperative staging and evaluation of response to chemotherapy are therefore important factors in the evaluation of osteosarcoma. Bone scintigraphy (Fig. 9B.10) may be limited in the ability to assess local tumor extent but is a sensitive method for assessing the rest of the skeleton for metastatic sites. At presentation skeletal metastases are relatively rare, only appearing in between 2 and 6% of patients and so this technique may be more useful in the post-treatment follow-up of such patients because at this stage skeletal metastases are common.[71,78] The lungs are a common site of metastatic spread and although uptake of bone radiopharmaceuticals such as ^{99m}Tc-MDP has been recorded in the chest, this is not a sufficiently reliable technique for staging, CT being the currently preferred technique both at presentation and as a follow-up investigation. The developing role of nuclear medicine tracers to examine tumor viability is discussed above and is relevant to osteosarcoma management.

Ewing's sarcoma

These tumors most frequently occur in children and adolescents arising in the diaphysis of long bones. The primary lesion shows avid uptake of ^{99m}Tc-MDP which is more uniform and shows less irregularity of contours than with osteosarcoma[65,71] but may not accurately demonstrate the true extent of tumor due to marrow involvement. Gallium also avidly accumulates into primary lesions[79] but surprisingly Caner *et al.* noted absent uptake in a number of Ewing's tumors using ^{99m}Tc-MIBI.[69] Skeletal metastases are commoner (>10%) than in osteosarcoma and so routine bone scintigraphy has a role in the initial staging of these patients[80,81] (Fig. 9B.11). Bone scintigraphy also has a role in routine surveillance of patients as more than one third subsequently develop skeletal metastases.

Osteoid osteoma

This benign bone tumor is most common in adolescents who may present with a classical history of night pain relieved by nonsteroidal anti-inflammatory drugs. The tumors are often small and may not be detected with conventional radiography,[82] the commonest sites of occurrence being the meta-diaphysis of long bones and the posterior elements of vertebral bodies in the spine. Bone scintigraphy has historically played an important role in localizing osteoid osteomas. They are characteristically very vascular and metabolically active and bone scintigraphy is extremely sensitive being helpful in radiographically occult lesions (Fig. 9B.12). Once located, further imaging, e.g. with CT, may lead to a specific diagnosis as an appearance of sclerotic cortical thickening and a radiolucent area within the sclerosis is a typical appearance. The high avidity for ^{99m}Tc-MDP in osteoid osteomas can also be used to accurately locate the tumor during surgery by the use of a probe and ensuring complete excision.[83]

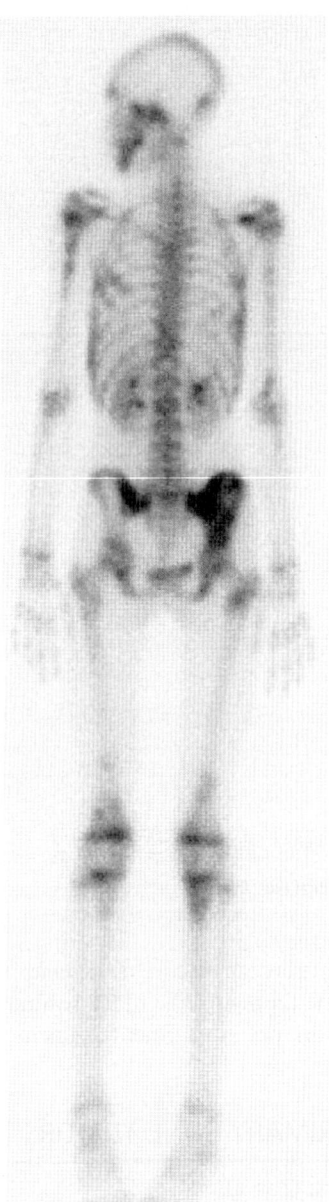

Figure 9B.11   *[99m]Tc-MDP bone scan of an adolescent with metastatic Ewing's sarcoma.*

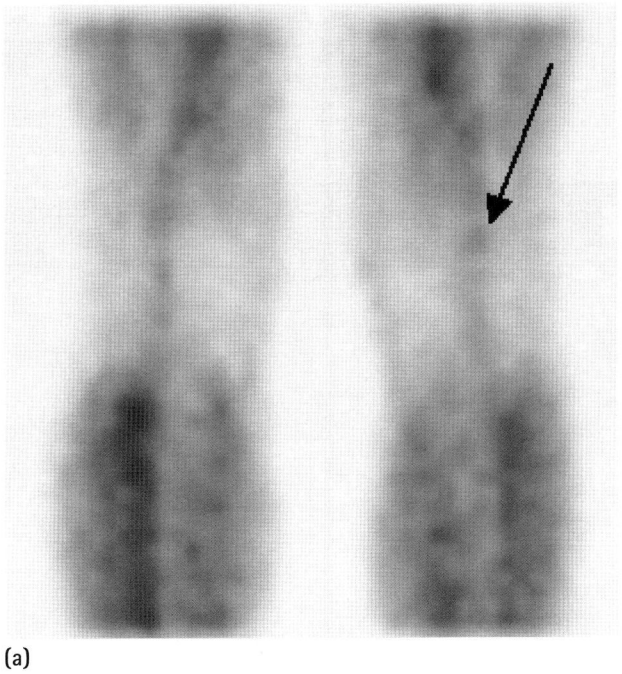

(a)

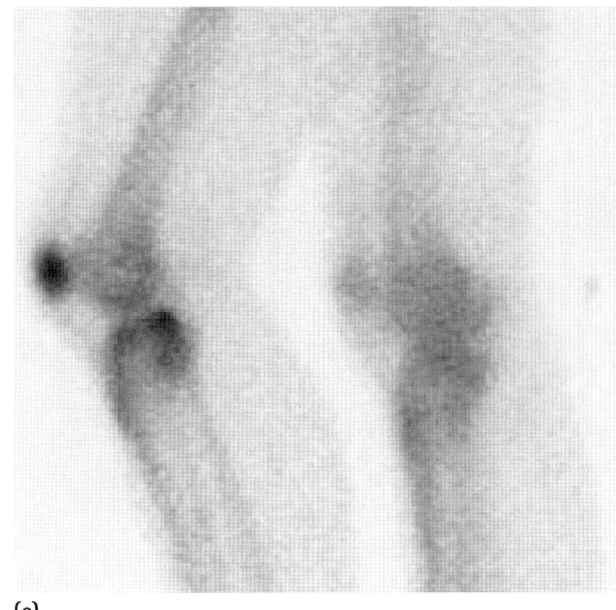

(c)

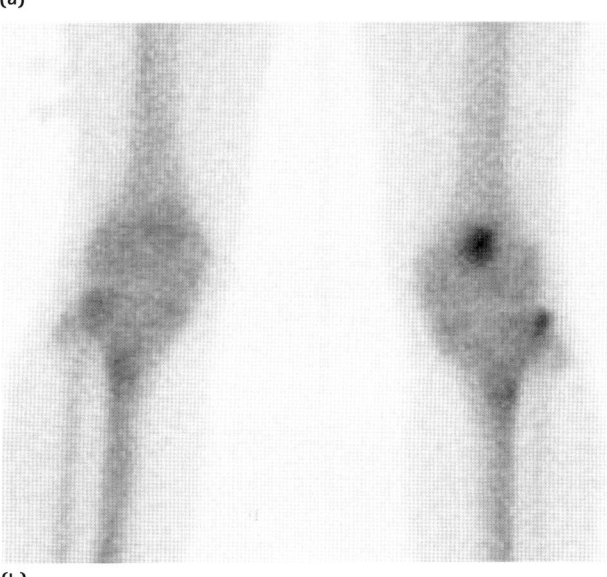

(b)

Figure 9B.12 *Dynamic ^{99m}Tc-MDP scan of the knees of a young woman who complained of nocturnal left knee pain. A vascular (a) metabolically active lesion (indicated by the arrow) is demonstrated in the left knee (b and c). The lesion proved to be an osteoid osteoma.*

Case history

An elderly man with newly diagnosed prostate cancer had a prostate specific antigen (PSA) level of 148 ng mL^{-1}. A staging bone scan (Fig. 9B.13(a)) revealed skeletal metastases affecting both sides of the pelvis but predominantly on the right. Due to pain in the right side of the pelvis the patient received radiotherapy with good symptomatic relief. Two years later the PSA level began to rise and on restaging (Fig. 9B.13(b)) the good response to radiotherapy is revealed in the right side of the pelvis but with local progression of disease in the left side of the pelvis.

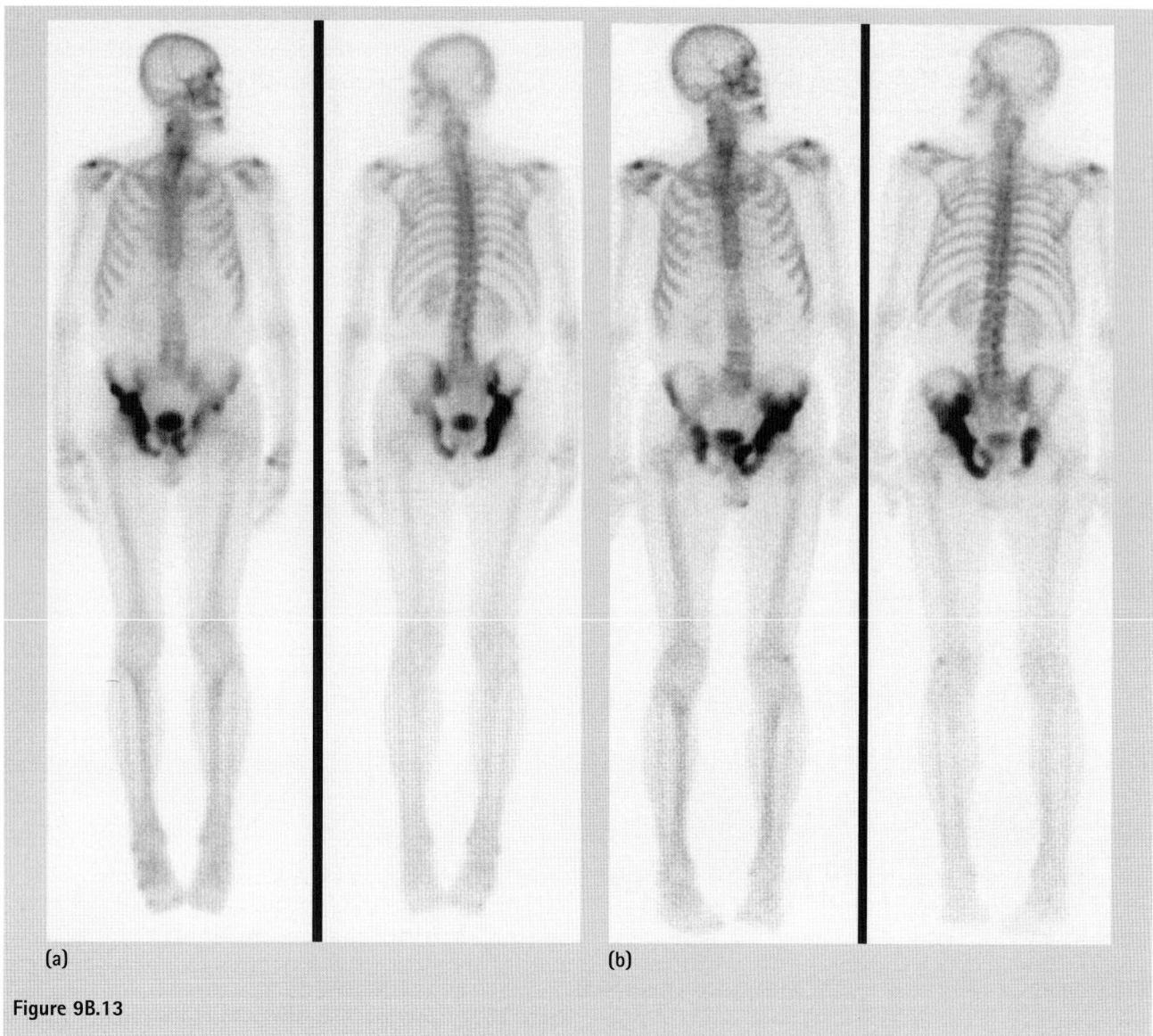

(a)

(b)

Figure 9B.13

REFERENCES

- Seminal primary article
- Key review paper

1 Galasko CSB. The anatomy and pathways of skeletal metastases. In: Weiss L, Gilbert AH. (eds.) *Bone metastases*. Boston: GK Hall, 1981: 49–63.

2 Cook GJ, Houston S, Rubens R, *et al*. Detection of bone metastases in breast cancer by ¹⁸FDG PET: differing metabolic activity in osteoblastic and osteolytic lesions. *J Clin Oncol* 1998; **16**: 3375–9.

3 Rubens RD. Bone metastases: incidence and complications. In: Rubens RD, Munday GR (eds.) *Cancer and the skeleton*. London: Martin Dunitz, 2000: 33–42.

4 Richards MA, Braysher S, Gregory WM, Rubens RD. Advanced breast cancer: use of resources and cost implications. *Br J Cancer* 1993; **67**: 856–60.

5 Hayward JL, Rubens RD, Carbone PP, *et al*. Assessment of response to therapy in advanced breast cancer. *Eur J Cancer* 1977; **13**: 89–94.

- 6 Coleman RE, Rubens RD. The clinical course of bone metastases from breast cancer. *Br J Cancer* 1987; **55**: 61–6.

7 Wolfenden JM, Pitt MJ, Durie BGW, Moon TE. Comparison of bone scintigraphy and radiology in myeloma. *Radiology* 1980; **134**: 723–8.

8 Lam AS, Kettle AG, O'Doherty MJ, *et al*. Pentavalent ⁹⁹Tcᵐ-DMSA imaging in patients with bone metastases. *Nucl Med Commun* 1997; **18**: 907–14.

9 Dunker CM, Carrio I, Bernal L, *et al*. Radioimmune imaging of bone marrow in patients with suspected bone metastases from primary breast cancer. *J Nucl Med* 1990; **31**: 1450–5.

- 10 Tofe AJ, Francis MD, Harvey WJ. Correlation of neoplasms with incidence and localisation of skeletal metastases. An analysis of 1355 diphosphonate bone scans. *J Nucl Med* 1975; **16**: 986–9.

11 Miric A, Banks M, Allen D, *et al.* Cortical metastatic lesions of the appendicular skeleton from tumors of known primary origin. *J Surg Oncol* 1998; **67**: 255–60.

12 Baxter AD, Coakley FV, Finlay DB, *et al.* The aetiology of solitary hot spots in the ribs on planar bone scans. *Nucl Med Commun* 1995; **16**: 834–7.

13 Tumeh SS, Beadle G, Kaplan WD. Clinical significance of solitary rib lesions in patients with extraskeletal malignancy. *J Nucl Med* 1985; **26**: 1140–3.

14 Coakley FV, Jones AR, Finlay DB, Belton IP. The aetiology and distinguishing features of solitary spinal hot spots on planar bone scans. *Clin Radiol* 1995; **50**: 327–30.

15 Jacobson AF, Stomper MD, Cronin EB, Kaplan WD. Bone scans with one or two new abnormalities in cancer patients with no known metastases: the reliability of interpretation of initial correlative radiographs. *Radiology* 1990; **174**: 503–7.

16 Muinidi J, Coombes RC, Golding S. The role of CT in the detection of bone metastases in breast carcinoma patients. *Br J Radiol* 1983; **56**: 233–6.

17 Daffner RH, Lupetin AR, Dash N, Deeb ZL, Sefczek RJ, Schapiro RL. MRI in the detection of malignant infiltration of bone marrow. *AJR* 1986; **146**: 353–358.

18 Yuh WT, Zachar CK, Barloon TJ, *et al.* Vertebral compression fractures: distinction between benign and malignant causes with MR imaging. *Radiology* 1989; **172**: 215–18.

19 Delpassand ES, Garcia JR, Bhadkamkar V, *et al.* Value of SPECT imaging of the thoracolumbar spine in cancer patients. *Clin Nucl Med* 1995; **20**: 1047–51.

20 Bushnell DL, Kahn D, Huston B, *et al.* Utility of SPECT imaging for determination of vertebral metastases in patients with known primary tumors. *Skeletal Radiol* 1995; **124**: 13–16.

21 Han LJ, Au-Yong TK, Tong WCM. Comparison of bone SPET and planar imaging in the detection of vertebral metastases in patients with back pain. *Eur J Nucl Med* 1998; **25**: 635–8.

22 Barker DJP, Clough PWL, Guyer PB, Gardner MJ. Paget's disease of bone in 14 British towns. *BMJ* 1977; **1**: 1181–3.

23 Schneider JA, Divgi CR, Scott AM, *et al.* Flare on bone scintigraphy following Taxol chemotherapy for metastatic breast cancer. *J Nucl Med* 1994; **35**: 1748–52.

24 Johns WD, Garrick MB, Kaplan WD. Leuprolide therapy for prostate cancer. An association with scintigraphic flare on bone scan. *Clin Nuc Med* 1990; **15**: 485–7.

25 Rossleigh MA, Lovegrove FT, Reynolds PM, *et al.* The assessment of response to therapy in bone metastases from breast cancer. *Aust NZ J Med* 1984; **14**: 19–22.

● 26 Coleman RE, Mashiter G, Whitaker KB, *et al.* Bone scan flare predicts successful systemic therapy for bone metastases. *J Nucl Med* 1988; **29**: 1354–9.

27 Jacobson AF, Cronin EB, Stomper EC, Kaplan WD. Bone scans with one or two new abnormalities in cancer patients with no known metastases: frequency and serial scintigraphic behaviour of benign and malignant lesions. *Radiology* 1990; **175**: 229–32.

28 Condon BR, Buchanan R, Garvie NW, *et al.* Assessment of progression of secondary bone lesions following cancer of the breast or prostate using serial radionuclide imaging. *Br J Radiol* 1981; **54**: 18–23.

29 Edelstyn GA, Gillespie PJ, Grebbel FS. The radiological demonstration of osseous metastases. Experimental observations. *Clin Radiol* 1967; **18**: 159–62.

30 Galasko CSB. The significance of occult skeletal metastases detected by scintigraphy in patients with otherwise early breast cancer. *Br J Surg* 1975; **56**: 757–64.

31 Coleman RE, Fogelman I, Habibollahi F, *et al.* Selection of patients with breast cancer for routine follow up bone scans. *Clin Oncol* 1990; **2**: 328–32.

◆ 32 Hamaoka T, Madewell JE, Podoloff DA, *et al.* Bone imaging in metastatic breast cancer. *J Clin Oncol* 2004; **22**: 2942–53.

● 33 Coleman RE, Rubens RD, Fogelman I. Reappraisal of the baseline bone scan in breast cancer. *J Nucl Med* 1998; **29**: 1045–9.

34 Bitran JD, Beckerman C, Desser RK. The predictive value of serial bone scans in assessing response to chemotherapy in advanced breast cancer. *Cancer* 1980; **45**: 1562–8.

35 McKillop JH. Bone scanning in metastatic disease. In: Fogelman I. (ed.) *Bone scanning in clinical practice.* Berlin: Springer-Verlag, 1987: 41–60.

36 Paulson DF, and the Uro-oncology Research Group. The impact of current staging procedures in assessing disease extent in prostatic adenocarcinoma. *J Urol* 1979; **121**: 300–2.

37 Biersack HJ, Wegner G, Distelmaier W, Krause U. Bone metastases of prostate cancer in relation to tumour size and grade of malignancy. *Nuklearmedizin* 1980; **19**: 29–32.

38 Shih WJ, Mitchell B, Wierzbinski B, *et al.* Prediction of radionuclide bone imaging findings by Gleason histologic grading of prostate carcinoma. *Clin Nucl Med* 1991; **16**: 763–6.

39 Chybowski FM, Keller JJL, Bergstralh EJ, Oesterling JE. Predicting radionuclide bone scan findings in patients with newly diagnosed, untreated prostate cancer: prostate specific antigen is superior to all other clinical parameters. *J Urol* 1991; **145**: 313–18.

40 O'Sullivan JM, Norman AR, Cook GJ, *et al.* Broadening the criteria for avoiding staging bone scans in prostate cancer: a retrospective study of patients at the Royal Marsden Hospital. *Br J Urol Intern* 2003; **92**: 685–9.

41 Huben RP, Schellhammer PF. The role of routine follow up bone scan after definitive therapy of localised prostatic cancer. *J Urol* 1982; **128**: 510–12.

42 Terris MK, Klonecke AS, McDougall IR, Stamey TA. Utilisation of bone scans in conjunction with prostate-specific antigen levels in the surveillance for recurrence of adenocarcinoma after radical prostatectomy. *J Nucl Med* 1991; **32**: 1713–17.

43 Pollen JJ, Gerber K, Ashburn WL, Schmidt JD. Nuclear bone imaging in metastatic cancer of the prostate. *Cancer* 1981; **47**: 2585–94.

44 Sundqvist CMG, Ahlgren L, Lilja B, Mattson S, Abrahamson PA, Wadstrom LB. Repeated quantitative bone scintigraphy in patients with prostatic carcinoma treated with orchidectomy. *Eur J Nucl Med* 1988; **14**: 203–6.

45 Hawkins RA, Choi Y, Huang SC, *et al.* Evaluation of the skeletal kinetics of fluorine-18-fluoride ion with PET. *J Nucl Med* 1992; **33**: 633–42.

46 Schirrmeister H, Guhlmann A, Kotzerke J, *et al.* Early detection and accurate description of extent of metastatic bone disease in breast cancer with fluoride ion and positron emission tomography. *J Clin Oncol* 1999; **17**: 2381–9.

47 Even-Sapir E, Metser U, Flusser G, *et al.* Assessment of malignant skeletal disease: initial experience with ^{18}F-fluoride PET/CT and comparison between ^{18}F-fluoride PET and ^{18}F-fluoride PET/CT. *J Nucl Med* 2004; **45**: 272–8.

48 Hoh CK, Hawkins RA, Dahlbom M, *et al.* Whole body skeletal imaging with [^{18}F]fluoride ion and PET. *J Comp Assist Tomog* 1993; **17**: 34–41.

49 Petren-Mallmin M, Andreasson I, Ljunggren O, *et al.* Skeletal metastases from breast cancer: uptake of ^{18}F-fluoride measured with positron emission tomography in correlation with CT. *Skeletal Radiol* 1998; **27**: 72–6.

50 Schirrmeister H, Guhlmann A, Elsner K, *et al.* Sensitivity in detecting osseous lesions depends on anatomic localization: planar bone scintigraphy versus ^{18}F PET. *J Nucl Med* 1999; **40**: 1623–9.

51 Schirrmeister H, Glatting G, Hetzel J, *et al.* Prospective evaluation of the clinical value of planar bone scans, SPECT, and (18)F-labeled NaF PET in newly diagnosed lung cancer. *J Nucl Med* 2001; **42**: 1800–4.

52 Bury T, Barreto A, Daenen F, Barthelemy N, Ghaye B, Rigo P. Fluorine-18 deoxyglucose positron emission tomography for the detection of bone metastases in patients with non-small cell lung cancer. *Eur J Nucl Med* 1998; **25**: 1244–7.

53 Chung JK, Kim YK, Yoon JK. Diagnostic usefulness of F-18 FDG whole body PET in detection of bony metastases compared to Tc-99m MDP bone scan. *J Nucl Med* 1999; **40**: 96P.

54 Moog F, Kotzerke J, Reske SN. FDG PET can replace bone scintigraphy in primary staging of malignant lymphoma. *J Nucl Med* 1999; **40**: 1407–13.

55 Schirrmeister H, Bommer M, Buck AK, *et al.* Initial results in the assessment of multiple myeloma using ^{18}F-FDG PET. *Eur J Nucl Med Mol Imaging* 2002; **29**: 361–6.

56 Moon DH, Maddahi J, Silverman DH, *et al.* Accuracy of whole body fluorine-18-FDG PET for the detection of recurrent or metastatic breast carcinoma, *J Nucl Med* 1998; **39**: 431–5.

57 Shreve PD, Grossman HB, Gross MD, *et al.* Metastatic prostate cancer: initial findings of PET with 2-deoxy-2-[F-18]fluoro-D-glucose. *Radiology* 1996; **199**: 751–6.

58 Yeh SD, Imbriaco M, Larson SM, *et al.* Detection of bony metastases of androgen-independent prostate cancer by PET-FDG. *Nucl Med Biol* 1996; **23**: 693–7.

59 Hiraga T, Mundy GR, Yoneda T. Bone metastases – morphology. In: Rubens RD, Mundy GR. (eds.) *Cancer and the skeleton.* London: Martin Dunitz, 2000: 65–74.

60 Clavo AC, Brown RS, Wahl RL. Fluorodeoxyglucose uptake in human cancer cell lines is increased by hypoxia. *J Nucl Med* 1995; **36**: 1625–32.

61 Moog F, Bangerter M, Kotzerke J, *et al.* 18-F-fluorodeoxyglucose-positron emission tomography as a new approach to detect lymphomatous bone marrow. *J Clin Oncol* 1998; **16**: 603–9.

62 Carr R, Barrington SF, Madan B, *et al.* Detection of lymphoma in bone marrow by whole-body positron emission tomography. *Blood* 1998; **91**: 3340–6.

63 Cook GJ, Fogelman I, Maisey MN. Normal physiological and benign pathological variants of 18-fluoro-2-deoxyglucose positron-emission tomography scanning: potential for error in interpretation. *Semin Nucl Med* 1996; **26**: 308–14.

64 Hollinger EF, Alibazoglu H, Ali A, *et al.* Hematopoietic cytokine-mediated FDG uptake simulates the appearance of diffuse metastatic disease on whole-body PET imaging. *Clin Nucl Med* 1998; **23**: 93–8.

65 McLean RG, Murray IP. Scintigraphic patterns in certain primary bone tumours. *Clin Radiol* 1984; **35**: 379–83.

66 Goodgold HM, Chen DC, Majd M, Nolan NG. Scintigraphy of primary bone neoplasia. *J Nucl Med* 1983; **24**: 57.

67 Simon MA, Kirchner PT. Scintigraphic evaluation of primary bone tumours. Comparison of technetium 99m phosphate and gallium citrate imaging. *J Bone Joint Surg Am* 1980; **62**: 758–64.

68 Van der Wall H, Murray IPC, Huckstep RL, Philips RL. The role of thallium scintigraphy in excluding malignancy in bone. *Clin Nucl Med* 1993; **18**: 551–7.

69 Caner B, Kitapel M, Unlu M, *et al.* Technetium-99m-MIBI uptake in benign and malignant bone lesions: a comparative study with technetium-99m-MDP. *J Nucl Med* 1992; **33**: 319–24.

70 Kobayashi H, Kotoura Y, Hosono M, *et al.* Diagnostic value of Tc-99m (V) DMSA for chondrogenic tumours with positive Tc-99m HMDP uptake on bone scintigraphy. *Clin Nucl Med* 1995; **20**: 361–4.

71 McKillop JH, Etcubanas E, Goris ML. The indications for and the limitations of bone scintigraphy in osteogenic sarcoma. *Cancer* 1981; **48**: 1133–8.

72 Chew FS, Hudson TM. Radionuclide bone scanning of osteosarcoma: falsely extended uptake patterns. *Am J Roentgenol* 1982; **139**: 49–54.

73 Ramanna L, Waxman A, Binney G, *et al.* Thallium-201 scintigraphy in bone sarcoma: comparison with gallium-67 and technetium-MDP in the evaluation of the chemotherapeutic response. *J Nucl Med* 1990; **31**: 567–72.

74 Kostakoglu L, Panicek DM, Divgi CR, *et al.* Correlation of the findings of thallium-201 chloride scans with those of other imaging modalities and histology following therapy in patients with bone and soft tissue sarcomas. *Eur J Nucl Med* 1995; **22**: 1232–7.

75 Ohtomo K, Terui S, Yokoyama R, *et al.* Thallium-201 scintigraphy to assess effect of chemotherapy in osteosarcoma. *J Nucl Med* 1996; **37**: 1444–8.

76 Garcia JR, Kim EE, Wong FCL. Comparison of fluoride-18-FDG PET and technetium-99m-MIBI SPECT in evaluation of musculoskeletal sarcomas. *J Nucl Med* 1996; **37**: 1476–9.

77 Jones DN, McCowage GB, Sostman HD, *et al.* Monitoring of neoadjuvant therapy response of soft tissue and musculoskeletal sarcoma using fluorine-18-FDG PET. *J Nucl Med* 1996; **37**: 1438–44.

78 Murray IPC, Elison BS. Radionuclide bone imaging for primary bone malignancy. *Clin Oncol* 1986; **5**: 141–58.

79 Frankel RS, Jones AE, Cohen JA, *et al.* Clinical correlations of 67-gallium and skeletal whole body radionuclide studies with radiography in Ewing's sarcoma. *Radiology* 1974; **110**: 597–603.

80 Goldstein H, McNeil BJ, Zufall E, Treves S. Is there a place for bone scanning in Ewing's sarcoma? *J Nucl Med* 1980; **21**: 10–12.

81 Nair N. Bone scanning in Ewing's sarcoma. *J Nucl Med* 1985; **26**: 349–52.

82 Smith FW, Gilday DL. Scintigraphic appearance of osteoid osteoma. *Radiology* 1980; **137**: 191–5.

83 Ghelman B, Thompson FM, Arnold WD. Intraoperative localisation of an osteoid osteoma. *J Bone Joint Surg* 1981; **63**: 826–7.

Metabolic bone disease

GARY J.R. COOK AND IGNAC FOGELMAN

INTRODUCTION

Since bone scintigraphy started to become a routine clinical imaging technique in the 1960s and 1970s both gamma cameras and radiopharmaceuticals have undergone substantial development. Gamma cameras are now able to perform high-resolution imaging in short scan times either as whole-body acquisitions or as a number of localized views of the skeleton. More recently, tomographic scintigraphic imaging has become more widely available, and its use has become routine in nuclear medicine, leading to improved sensitivity and specificity for lesion detection.

The most commonly used radiopharmaceuticals for bone imaging are labelled with ^{99m}Tc, therefore being easily available to all nuclear medicine departments and with physical properties that make them ideal for acquiring high-resolution image data. Diphosphonate compounds such as methylene diphosphonate (MDP), labelled with ^{99m}Tc, are the most commonly used radiopharmaceuticals for bone scintigraphy currently. These compounds are closely related to the group of antiresorptive drugs used in a number of metabolic bone diseases that are known as bisphosphonates.

The exact mechanism of localization of these compounds in bone is not fully understood. The degree of accumulation in bone is dependent on local blood flow but is influenced more strongly by the degree of osteoblastic activity, and hence bone formation. Most metabolic bone diseases result in altered bone turnover with both osteoblast and osteoclast activity being increased. A bone scan is therefore a functional map of bone turnover, which may affect the skeleton globally or focally in the metabolic bone diseases.

The use of bone scintigraphy may aid clinical management of a number of metabolic bone diseases including Paget's disease, osteoporosis, hyperparathyroidism, osteomalacia, and renal bone disease or renal osteodystrophy.[1,2]

PAGET'S DISEASE

The isotope bone scan has proven invaluable in the assessment of patients with Paget's disease, for diagnosis, to define the extent of skeletal involvement and to assess response to treatment. Paget's disease is most commonly a polyostotic disease in 80–90% of cases and is characterized by increased osteoblastic and osteoclastic activity as well as increased blood flow in affected bones. This may lead to bone that appears radiographically expanded with disorganized architecture including sclerosis and lysis and coarsened trabeculae. Many patients with Paget's disease are asymptomatic but the clinical features that may result include pain, deformity, pathological fracture, neural impingement and, very rarely, sarcomatous change.

Bone scintigraphy is a convenient way to evaluate the whole skeleton and has been shown to have a greater sensitivity for detecting affected sites in symptomatic patients than have radiographic skeletal surveys[3] (Fig. 9C.1). Characteristically, affected bones show intensely increased activity, which starts at the end of a bone and spreads either proximally or distally, often showing a 'V' or 'flame-shaped' leading edge. Another sign that a scintigraphic abnormality is due to Paget's disease rather than other focal skeletal pathology is that a whole bone is often involved, and this is most often seen in the pelvis, scapula, and vertebrae. In vertebrae, the characteristic finding is of abnormal tracer

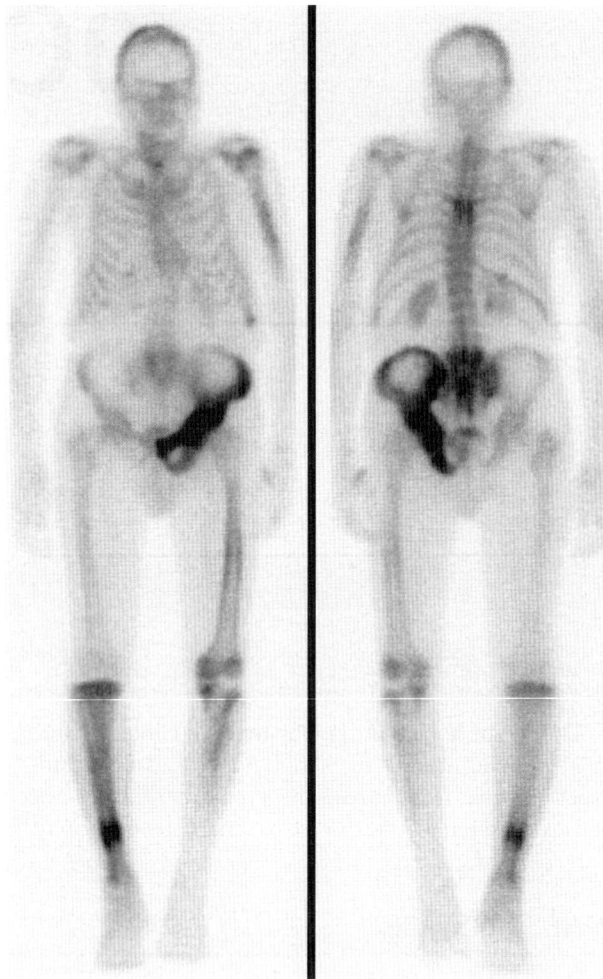

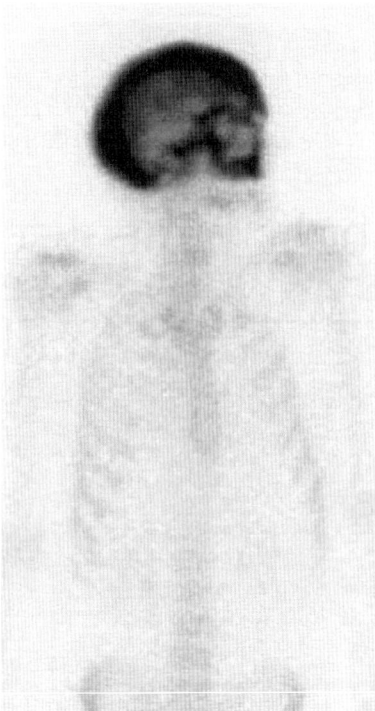

Figure 9C.2 *⁹⁹ᵐTc-MDP bone scan demonstrating Paget's disease of the skull.*

Figure 9C.1 *⁹⁹ᵐTc-methylene diphosphonate (⁹⁹ᵐTc-MDP) bone scan of a patient with polyostotic Paget's disease. There is a typical pattern of diffusely increased uptake in a number of bones including the left hemi-pelvis, T7, L5, sacrum, right 11th rib, left femur, left upper tibia and right tibia. A more intense linear focus of activity is seen in the right tibia representing a pathological stress fracture at this site.*

accumulation throughout the vertebral body and posterior elements, including the spinous and transverse processes. The skull may show a different pattern with a ring of increased activity only in the margins of the lesion, representing what is recognized radiologically as osteoporosis circumscripta (Fig. 9C.2).

As powerful treatments for Paget's disease in the form of bisphosphonates have become available in recent years, it is being recognized that preventive treatment with regard to possible complications is desirable, rather than simply treating symptomatic cases. It is therefore increasingly important to be able to accurately evaluate the extent of disease and response to treatment. Monitoring of pagetic activity is usually performed with serum bone markers, the most common being bone specific alkaline phosphatase, a marker of increased osteoblastic activity within the skeleton. Although

a relatively inexpensive and valuable measure of activity, the use of bone markers is limited when they lie within the normal range, e.g. monostotic or limited disease, or when the location of skeletal involvement needs to be assessed, particularly in multifocal disorders such as Paget's disease.[4,5] In these circumstances, bone scintigraphy can act as a valuable adjunctive measure of disease location and activity. Changes in activity can be sensitively measured qualitatively or quantitatively in these circumstances with bone scintigraphy. It has been recognized from the early days of bone scintigraphy that it has the potential to be a sensitive and reproducible quantitative measure of treatment response.[6-8] A number of groups have used a variety of quantitative indices to successfully monitor changes in metabolic activity in Paget's disease,[9-13] with some evidence to show that quantification is superior to qualitative assessment.[9]

A scan can be obtained approximately 3–6 months after therapy for comparison with a baseline study. It is recognized that pagetic lesions may often respond in a heterogeneous manner, even in individual patients.[14] After intravenous bisphosphonate therapy, some bones may completely normalize, whereas the majority show some improvement, and a small proportion remain unchanged. It is important to be aware that the bone scan appearances can be unusual after successful bisphosphonate treatment, resultant heterogeneous uptake sometimes mimicking metastatic disease and hence a complete clinical history is essential for correct interpretation. Persistent active disease evident on bone scan after initial treatment may be an indication for more aggressive therapy in selected cases to achieve optimal therapeutic and prognostic benefit. Subsequently, the bone scan may also act as a sensitive measure of reactivation of disease, influencing decisions on further treatment. Vallenga and colleagues reported that in some cases recurrent disease was evident on bone scintigraphy up to 6 months prior to biochemical relapse.[10]

The radionuclide bone scan may occasionally identify complications of Paget's disease. An incremental fracture on the convex surface of a bowed long bone may be shown as a linear area of increased activity running perpendicular to the cortex (Fig. 9C.1). Although osteosarcoma complicating Paget's disease is very rare, clues that sarcomatous change may have occurred include a change to heterogeneous and irregular uptake within an area of bone, perhaps with some photon-deficient areas corresponding to bone destruction. However, the bone scan may be misleading in the event of fracture or sarcomatous change or both, as it may prove difficult to identify focally increased tracer uptake against a high background of activity. It is therefore also important to perform radiographs of any symptomatic site when there is clinical suspicion of focal complications. Colarinha and colleagues reported a case of polyostotic Paget's disease that showed abnormal uptake of thallium in sarcomatous change of the iliac bone but no uptake in the remaining sites of benign active Paget's disease suggesting that this radiopharmaceutical may be helpful when sarcomatous degeneration is suspected.[15]

There have been early reports of the use of positron emission tomography (PET) radiopharmaceuticals including [18F]fluoride and 2-[18F]fluoro-2-deoxy-D-glucose (18F-FDG) in the study of Paget's disease. [18F]fluoride acts as a bone-specific tracer and by acquiring dynamic scans it is possible to quantify regional skeletal kinetic indices with the potential that this method could be used to more sensitively quantify regional treatment response in the future.[16,17] Unsurprisingly, parameters relating to regional blood flow and mineralization are increased in pagetic bones when compared to non-pagetic bones in the same individual.

It has also been noted that active benign Paget's disease may show significant uptake of 18F-FDG that would appear to correlate with disease activity as measured by biochemical markers such as alkaline phosphatase. The utility of this tracer to detect sarcomatous change in pagetic bone is likely to be limited.[18] Nevertheless, it is important that interpreters of 18F-FDG PET scans are aware of possible false positive uptake of this radiopharmaceutical into pagetic bone in patients being scanned to evaluate metastatic disease from other malignant tumors. A history of Paget's disease may be available from the patient but as many cases are asymptomatic there is the potential for misinterpretation.

Uptake of other radiopharmaceuticals, including labeled octreotide,[19] [67]Ga,[20] and [99m]Tc(V)-dimercaptosuccinic acid ([99m]Tc(V)-DMSA)[21] have also been reported in benign Paget's disease with dynamic pentavalent DMSA imaging having been assessed as a method to monitor the therapeutic effects of bisphosphonate therapy.[21]

OSTEOPOROSIS

In clinical management of the metabolic bone diseases, the isotope bone scan can be of utility in osteoporotic patients, in whom it has a valuable role in evaluation of complications and their treatment.[22] The bone scan has no role in the diagnosis of osteoporosis *per se* but is most often used in established osteoporosis to diagnose vertebral fracture.

Although not used in routine diagnosis, there is evidence that quantitative bone scintigraphic techniques may provide information on altered skeletal metabolism in osteoporotic patients. With whole-body retention measurements at 24 h after administration of a bone-seeking radiopharmaceutical, Fogelman and colleagues were not able to differentiate osteoporotic patients from normals, although a number of other metabolic bone diseases including renal osteodystrophy, osteomalacia and hyperparathyroidism showed higher values than normals, indicative of increased skeletal turnover.[23] However, using a similar technique it was possible to differentiate the low skeletal turnover of post-menopausal women on hormone replacement therapy from those with accelerated turnover without treatment.[24] In contrast, using quantitative single photon emission computed tomography (SPECT), Israel and colleagues reported a significant increase in cortical bone turnover and a nonsignificant increase in trabecular bone turnover compared to controls.[25]

When used in the evaluation of vertebral fractures, the characteristic appearance of this type of fracture on bone scintigraphy is of intense, linearly increased tracer uptake at the affected level (Fig. 9C.3). Although the bone scan may become positive immediately after a fracture, it can take up to 2 weeks for the scan to become abnormal, especially in the elderly. Subsequently, there is a gradual reduction in tracer uptake, with the scan normalizing between 3 and 18 months after the incident, the average being between 9 and 12 months.[26] Because of this, the bone scan also is extremely useful in assessing the age of fractures. If a patient complains of back pain with multiple vertebral fractures on radiographs, and the bone scan is normal, then this essentially excludes recent fracture as a cause of symptoms. Other causes of pain should then be considered. Currently a vertebral fracture is defined on the basis of morphometry,[27] but morphometric abnormalities are not specific to fracture and, for example, may be due to congenital vertebral anomalies or progressive degenerative changes. The bone scan may therefore have a role in the decision of whether a morphometric abnormality is related to a fracture, provided that it is acquired within several months of the start of symptoms. It is interesting to note that by comparing vertebral fractures identified with scinitigraphy with morphometric radiographic changes, that only in vertebrae with morphometric deformities greater than three standard deviations below the normal mean, can fractures be confidently diagnosed.[28] To date this approach has not been used in clinical practice, however.

Because of its sensitivity, the bone scan also is helpful in identifying unsuspected fragility fractures at other sites including the ribs, pelvis, and hip. It also has an important role in assessing suspected fractures where radiography is unhelpful, either because of poor sensitivity related to the anatomic site of the fracture (e.g. sacrum; Fig. 9C.3) or because adequate views are difficult to acquire due to the patient's discomfort.[22]

An isotope bone scan also may be valuable in patients in whom back pain persists for longer than one would expect after vertebral fracture. It is common to find that there has been additional unsuspected vertebral fracture. In addition, it is becoming increasingly apparent that osteoporotic patients with chronic back pain may have unsuspected abnormalities affecting the facet joints.[22,29] It is not known whether this is related to physical disruption of the joint at the time of vertebral collapse or is caused by subsequent

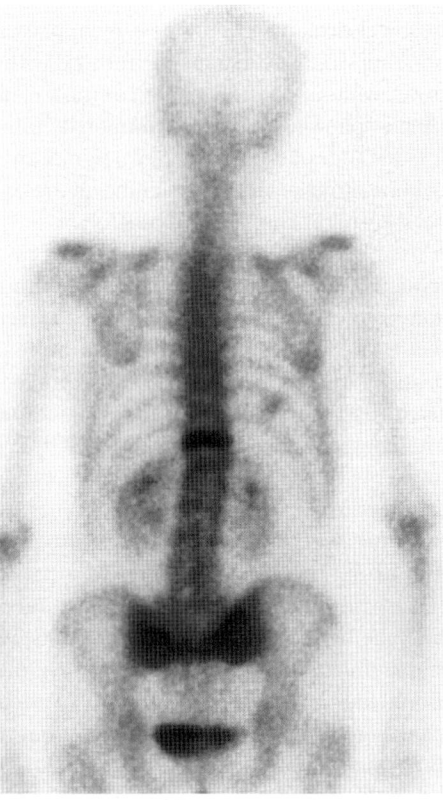

Figure 9C.3 *An elderly woman with back pain demonstrates abnormal linear uptake at T11 caused by osteoporotic vertebral collapse together with increased uptake within the sacrum as a result of a sacral insufficiency fracture.*

secondary degenerative or inflammatory changes. To identify abnormalities in the facet joints, SPECT imaging is essential. On planar imaging alone, it is not possible to separate activity in the facet joints from associated activity in the vertebral body caused by fracture, and the three-dimensional properties of this technique allow more confident anatomic placement of abnormal foci of increased activity. In the osteoporotic patient, it also is important to exclude secondary causes for pain, such as metastatic disease, infection, Paget's disease, and others.

HYPERPARATHYROIDISM

Most cases of primary hyperparathyroidism are asymptomatic and are unlikely to be associated with changes on bone scintigraphy unless the disease is advanced. The diagnosis is made biochemically and the bone scan therefore has no routine role in diagnosis. However, bone scans are often used to help differentiate the causes of hypercalcemia, in particular, hyperparathyroidism versus malignancy, and so typical features of metabolic bone disorders should be recognized to aid interpretation. In hyperparathyroidism there is increased turnover throughout the skeleton and in the more severe cases, commonly seen as part of renal osteodystrophy, this will be evident scintigraphically. A bone scan may show a number of features in hyperparathyroidism, but the most important is the generalized increased uptake throughout the skeleton which may be identified because of increased contrast between bone and soft tissues. Indeed, renal activity clearly seen on a normal bone scan may not be evident. The resultant appearance is of a metabolic superscan demonstrating apparent high-quality images due to the high bone uptake. Other typical features that have been described in bone scans in hyperparathyroidism and other metabolic bone diseases include a prominent calvarium and mandible, beading of the costochondral junctions, and a 'tie' sternum.[30]

Severe forms of hyperparathyroidism may be associated with ectopic calcification that may lead to uptake of bone radiopharmaceuticals into soft tissue, the most dramatic example being that of microcalcification in the lungs where a diffuse increase in parenchymal uptake of bone tracer may be demonstrated. Focal skeletal abnormalities may represent brown tumors that may be associated with hyperparathyroidism. Nuclear medicine is the most frequently used modality for imaging abnormal parathyroid glands before surgery but is covered in detail in Chapter 12B.

OSTEOMALACIA

Patients with osteomalacia usually demonstrate similar features of a bone scan as described in hyperparathyroidism, although in the early stages of the disease, it may appear normal.[31] The reason that osteomalacia shows these features remains uncertain. Tracer accumulation may reflect diffuse uptake in osteoid, although more likely it is due to the degree of secondary hyperparathyroidism that is present. In addition, the presence of focal lesions may represent pseudofractures or true fractures. Pseudofractures are characteristically found in the ribs, the lateral border of the scapula, the pubic rami, and the medial femoral cortices (Fig. 9C.4). Although osteomalacia is usually a biochemical and/or histologic diagnosis, the typical bone scan features can be helpful in suggesting the diagnosis. The detection of pseudofracutures with this technique is more sensitive than that with radiography.[32]

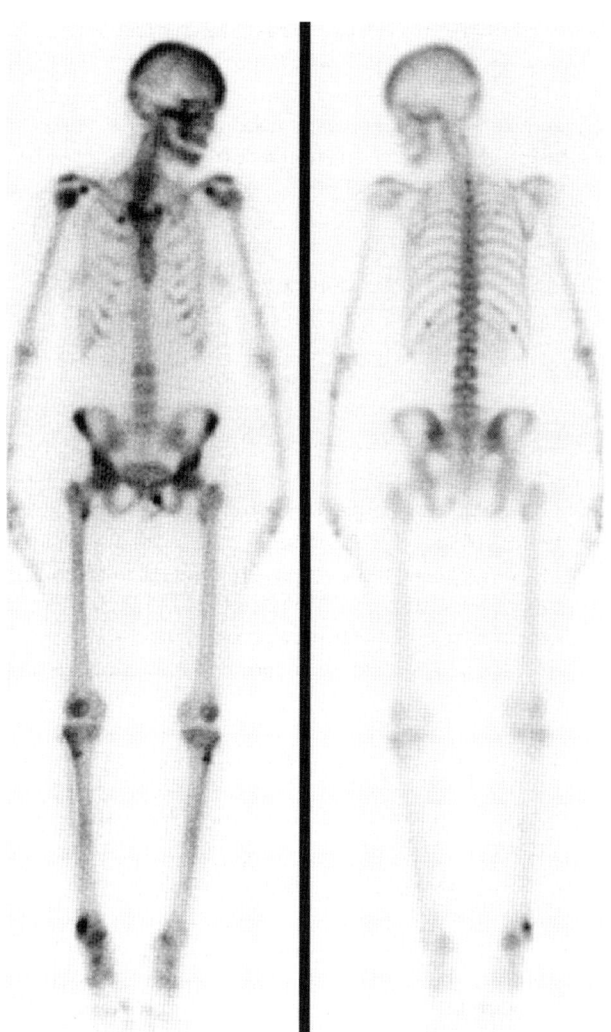

Figure 9C.4 *99mTc-MDP bone scan demonstrating a diffuse increase in skeletal activity (increased bone to soft tissue/renal ratio) together with some focal lesions in the ribs, pelvis and upper right femur representing pseudo fractures in a patient with osteomalacia. Further fractures were present in the right lower tibia and right humeral head following trauma.*

RENAL OSTEODYSTROPHY

Renal osteodystrophy is due to a combination of bone disorders as a consequence of chronic renal dysfunction and often demonstrates the most severe cases of metabolic bone disease. It may comprise osteoporosis, osteomalacia, secondary hyperparathyroidism, and adynamic bone in varying degrees. The commonest bone scan appearance is similar to a superscan from other metabolic bone disorders (Fig. 9C.5). Uptake of diphosphonate in areas of ectopic calcification also may be seen. A differentiating sign to distinguish this metabolic bone disease from others is that there may be a lack of bladder activity in view of renal failure. Although rarely seen now, aluminum toxicity from hemodialysis causes a poor-quality bone scan with reduced skeletal uptake and increased soft tissue activity, as aluminium blocks mineralization, and hence uptake of tracer. This pattern is applicable to other forms of adynamic bone disease and is clearly differentiated from renal osteodystrophy with a predominance of hyperparathyroidism and high turnover.[33]

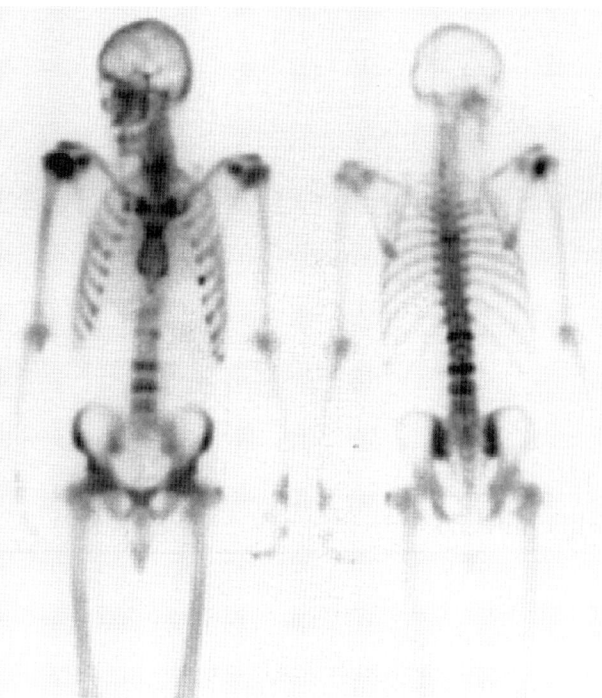

Figure 9C.5 *99mTc-MDP bone scan demonstrating diffusely increased uptake within the skeleton (increased bone to soft tissue/renal ratio) but with focal linear uptake at a number of levels in the spine and in the left anterior 5th rib. Focal uptake is also demonstrated in the right upper humerus with soft tissue activity over the left greater trochanter. This patient had chronic renal failure and renal osteodystrophy demonstrating a metabolic superscan, fragility fractures in the spine and rib, avascular necrosis of the right humeral head and soft tissue calcification over the hip.*

Case history

A 67-year-old Asian man presented with early prostate cancer and severe bone pain. A bone scan demonstrated widespread focal abnormalities, particularly in the ribs and an increased skeletal to soft tissue/renal activity. Although he was initially considered to have bone metastases his prostate specific antigen level was only 7.1 ng mL^{-1}. Blood biochemistry revealed almost unrecordable vitamin D levels, a low serum calcium, and raised alkaline phosphatase. A diagnosis of osteomalcia was made and the symptoms responded dramatically to vitamin D medication.

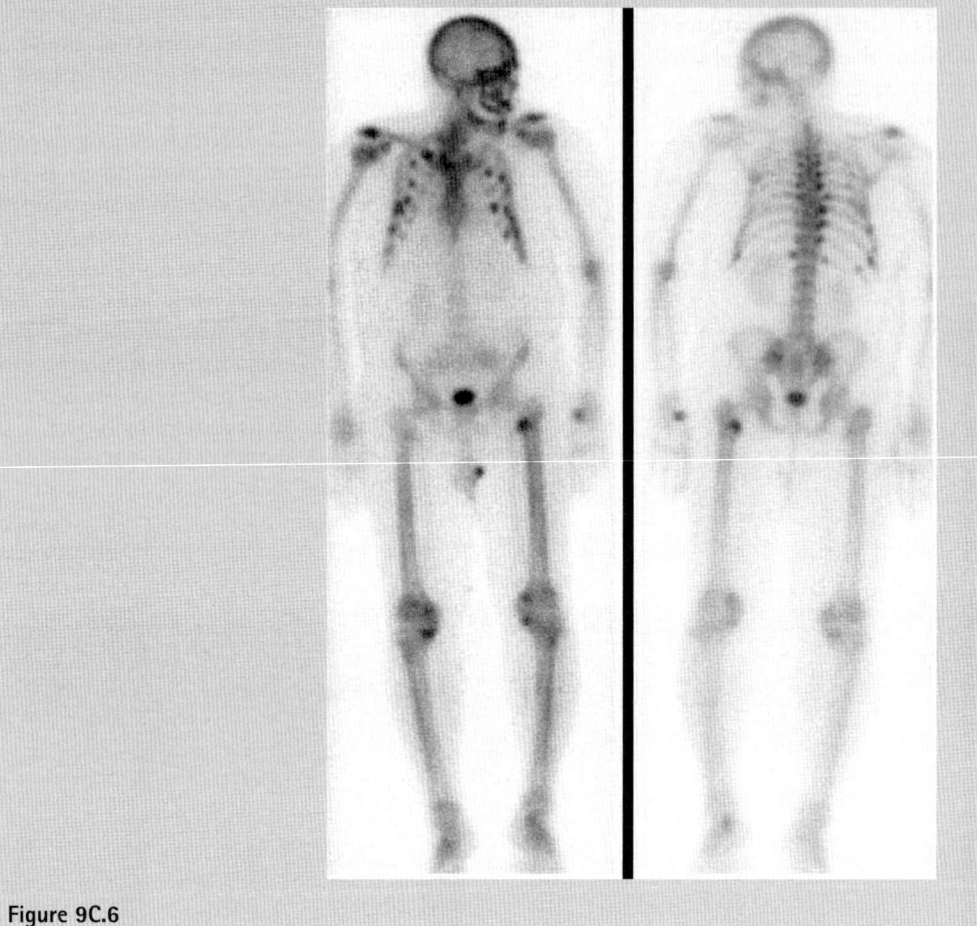

Figure 9C.6

REFERENCES

- ● Seminal primary article
- ◆ Key review paper
- ★ First formal publication of a management guideline

1 Mari C, Catafau A, Carrio I. Bone scintigraphy and metabolic disorders. *Q J Nucl Med* 1999; **43**: 259–67.
◆ 2 Ryan PJ, Fogelman I. Bone scintigraphy in metabolic bone disease. *Semin Nucl Med* 1971; **27**: 291–305.
3 Fogelman I, Carr D. A comparison of bone scanning and radiology in the assessment of patients with symptomatic Paget's disease. *Eur J Nucl Med* 1980; **5**: 417–21.
4 Patel S, Pearson D, Hosking DJ. Quantitative bone scintigraphy in the management of monostotic Paget's disease of bone. *Arthritis Rheum* 1995; **38**: 1506–12.

5 Ang G, Feiglin D, Moses AM. Symptomatic and scintigraphic improvement after intravenous pamidronate treatment of Paget's disease of bone in patients with normal serum alkaline phosphatase levels. *Endocr Pract* 2003; **9**: 280–3.
6 Goldman AB, Braunstein P, Wilkinson D, Kammerman S. Radionuclide uptake studies of bone: a quantitative method of evaluating the response of patients with Paget's disease to diphosphonate therapy. *Radiology* 1975; **117**: 365–9.
● 7 Lentle BC, Russell AS, Heslip PG, Percy JS. The scintigraphic findings in Paget's disease of bone. *Clin Radiol* 1976; **27**: 129–35.
● 8 Lavender JP, Evans IM, Arnot R, *et al.* A comparison of radiography and radioisotope scanning in the detection of Paget's disease and in the assessment of

response to human calcitonin. *Br J Radiol* 1977; **50**: 243–50.

9   Vellenga CJ, Pauwels EK, Bijvoet OL. Comparison between visual assessment and quantitative measurement of radioactivity on the bone scintigram in Paget's disease of bone. *Eur J Nucl Med* 1984; **9**: 533–7.

10 Vellenga CJ, Pauwels EK, Bijvoet OL, *et al*. Bone scintigraphy in Paget's disease treated with combined calcitonin and diphosphonate (EHDP). *Metab Bone Dis Relat Res* 1982; **4**: 103–11.

11 Vellenga CJ, Pauwels EK, Bijvoet OL, *et al*. Quantitative bone scintigraphy in Paget's disease treated with APD. *Br J Radiol* 1985; **58**: 1165–72.

12 Pons F, Alvarez L, Peris P, *et al*. Quantitative evaluation of bone scintigraphy in the assessment of Paget's disease activity. *Nucl Med Commun* 1999; **20**: 525–8.

13 Griffith K, Pearson D, Parker C, *et al*. The use of a whole body index with bone scintigraphy to monitor the response to therapy in Paget's disease. *Nucl Med Commun* 2001; **22**: 1069–75.

14 Ryan PJ, Gibson T, Fogelman I. Bone scintigraphy following pamidronate therapy for Paget's disease of bone. *J Nucl Med* 1992; **33**: 1589–93.

15 Colarinha P, Fonseca AT, Salgado L, Vieira MR. Diagnosis of malignant change in Paget's disease by Tl-201. *Clin Nucl Med* 1996; **21**: 299–301.

16 Cook GJR, Blake GM, Marsden PM, *et al*. Quantification of skeletal kinetic indices in Paget's disease using dynamic ^{18}F-fluoride positron emission tomography. *J Bone Min Res* 2002; **17**: 854–9.

17 Schiepers C, Nuyts J, Bormans G, *et al*. Fluoride kinetics of the axial skeleton measured in vivo with fluorine-18-fluoride PET. *J Nucl Med* 1997; **38**: 1970–6.

18 Cook GJR, Maisey MN, Fogelman I. Paget's disease of bone: appearances with 18-FDG PET. *J Nucl Med* 1997; **38**: 1495–7.

19 Kang S, Mishkin FS. Visualization of Paget's disease during somatostatin receptor scintigraphy. *Clin Nucl Med* 1999; **24**: 900–2.

20 Mills BG, Masuoka LS, Graham Jr CC, *et al*. Gallium-67 citrate localization in osteoclast nuclei of Paget's disease of bone. *J Nucl Med* 1988; **29**: 1083–7.

21 Kobayashi H, Shigeno C, Sakahara H, *et al*. Three phase ^{99}Tc^{m} (V)DMSA scintigraphy in Paget's disease: an indicator of pamidronate effect. *Br J Radiol* 1997; **70**: 1056–9.

22 Cook GJR, Hannaford E, Lee M, *et al*. The value of bone scintigraphy in the evaluation of osteoporotic patients with back pain. *Scand J Rheumatol* 2002; **31**: 245–8.

● 23 Fogelman I, Bessent RG, Turner JG, *et al*. The use of whole-body retention of Tc-99m diphosphonate in the diagnosis of metabolic bone disease. *J Nucl Med* 1978; **19**: 270–5.

24 Fogelman I, Bessent RG, Cohen HN, *et al*. Skeletal uptake of diphosphonate. Method for prediction of post-menopausal osteoporosis. *Lancet* 1980; **2**: 667–70.

25 Israel O, Lubushitzky R, Frenkel A, *et al*. Bone turnover in cortical and trabecular bone in normal women and in women with osteoporosis. *J Nucl Med* 1994; **35**: 1155–8.

● 26 Spitz J, Lauer I, Tittel K, Wiegand H. Scintimetric evaluation of remodeling after bone fractures in man. *J Nucl Med* 1993; **34**: 1403–9.

★ 27 Eastell R, Cedel SL, Wahner HW, *et al*. Classification of vertebral fractures. *J Bone Miner Res* 1991; **6**: 207–15.

28 Ryan PJ, Fogelman I. Osteoporotic vertebral fractures: diagnosis with radiography and bone scintigraphy. *Radiology* 1994; **190**: 669–72.

29 Ryan PJ, Evans PA, Gibson T, *et al*. Osteoporosis and chronic back pain: a study with single photon emission computed bone scintigraphy. *J Bone Min Res* 1992; **7**: 1455–9.

30 Fogelman I, Carr D. A comparison of bone scanning and radiology in the evaluation of patients with metabolic bone disease. *Clin Radiol* 1980; **31**: 321–6.

31 Fogelman I, McKillop JH, Bessent RG, *et al*. The role of bone scanning in osteomalacia. *J Nucl Med* 1978; **19**: 245–8.

32 Fogelman I, McKillop JH, Greig WR, *et al*. Pseudofractures of the ribs detected by bone scanning. *J Nucl Med* 1977; **18**: 1236–7.

33 Karsenty G, Vigneron N, Jorgetti V, *et al*. Value of the ^{99m}Tc-methylene diphosphonate bone scan in renal osteodystrophy. *Kidney Int* 1986; **29**: 1058–65.

Trauma and sports injuries

HANS VAN DER WALL AND SIRI KANNANGARA

BACKGROUND

The pathophysiology of trauma to bone or its attached soft-tissue structures such as the periosteum, ligaments, and tendons is highly conducive to the localization of the bone-seeking radiopharmaceuticals. The inherently high contrast resolution of bone scintigraphy leads to rapid detection of the changes following trauma at a nascent stage. Such changes precede structural abnormalities and therefore can be detected earlier than plain radiography and computed tomography (CT) and in a similar time course to magnetic resonance imaging (MRI). Scintigraphy allows the healing process to be assessed sequentially and is an ideal method for detecting complications such as the chronic regional pain syndrome (reflex sympathetic dystrophy) and non-union. The additional advantage of scintigraphy is the potential to image the entire skeleton, allowing the detection of unsuspected sites of trauma, particularly in the setting of polytrauma.

Bone scintigraphy is ideally suited to the detection of sporting injuries as the pathophysiology of such injuries is either acute, acute on chronic or chronic trauma.

PATHOPHYSIOLOGY

Three-phase bone scintigraphy detects soft-tissue and bony pathology. Damage to tissue leads to hemorrhage, necrosis, and calcification, which binds the phosphate complexes utilized in scintigraphy. Scintigraphy can detect bone bruising, an acute injury that results from direct trauma at a level of force that leads to trabecular microfractures without frank cortical disruption.[1] Histological evidence of fragments of hyaline cartilage impacted into the trabecular bone with hemorrhage and fat necrosis supports this concept.[2] It is usually detected by bone scintigraphy and MRI, but not by plain radiography or CT scanning. The greater force transmission involved in cortical fracture ensures early detection by three-phase scintigraphy.

Osteochondral fractures are an acute injury to the articular cartilage that usually occurs in the knee or talar dome in association with impaction, rotational or shearing forces. Stress fracture occurs as the result of repetitive or prolonged muscular action on bone that has not accommodated to the applied stress.[3,4] Repetitive stress causes periosteal resorption that outstrips the rate of remodeling, weakening the cortex and resulting in fracture.[5] The response to the fracture with hyperemia, formation of callus and remodeling leads to uptake of the scintigraphic agents.

BIOMECHANICS

Bone responds to stress according to Wolff's law.[6] As the stress applied increases, there is progressive deformity throughout an elastic range with return to its original state if stress ceases. If the elastic range is exceeded, a plastic deformity occurs due to microfractures. Progressive microfractures lead to cortical cracks and persistence of the stress will lead to propagation of the cracks and frank cortical fracture.[7]

Acute fracture repairs by formation of callus which reflects the normal growth of bone by apposition with formation of new bone in layers. The process of remodeling is coordinated with osteoclasts removing dying osteons and osteoblasts producing new osteoid. Osteoid is rapidly mineralized by calcium phosphate complexes with the development of hydroxyapatite. Osteoblasts eventually migrate into lacunae, becoming quiescent osteocytes as the process matures. The normal remodeling process accelerates following fracture. A periosteal response is evident within 48 h of injury, creating a partial callus of trabecular and cartilaginous tissue and leading to a soft-tissue response with angiogenesis and intense cellular activity. Calcification of the formed cartilage commences within days. Endochondral ossification follows, but at a slower rate. Trabecular bone gains a mature laminar structure that with appropriate remodeling possesses the mechanical strength of the original tissue.

Repetitive or minor trauma to osteoporotic or pathologically abnormal bone can lead to fracture at low levels of stress. Commonly, minor trauma can lead to compression fracture of the vertebrae. The subsequent response is, however, stereotypic of any acute fracture. Associated abnormalities of mineralization will be reflected by abnormally prolonged uptake of the scintigraphic agents.

CLINICAL PRESENTATION

The clinical presentation of fractures is almost always with localized pain that worsens with the intensity of activity. Eventually, the pain becomes so severe that the activity will be completely curtailed. Initially, pain diminishes with rest but recurs with activity at a progressively decreasing threshold. Limping or failure to move a limb may be the only manifestation of injury in childhood and infancy. Awareness of the child at risk is important, and suspicion should be aroused by unusual sites of injury or multiple injuries of various ages.

Physical examination may identify point tenderness or diffuse tenderness, depending on the site and co-existent conditions such as shin splints. It is also important to identify anatomical variants that may predispose to stress injuries such as pes planus or spastic flat foot. Other possibilities such as tumors or infection should also be considered, especially in young patients. Predisposing factors for reduced bone mineral content should be reviewed, particularly in female athletes with secondary amenorrhea or in adolescents with anorexia nervosa.

Regardless of the care with which the history and examination is conducted, the average time for a firm diagnosis after sporting injury remains at approximately 16 weeks.[8] There is some suggestion that this may be due to a normal plain radiograph which is found in 50% of patients with a stress fracture.

PREVALENCE OF INJURIES BY AGE AND SITE

The pattern and prevalence of injury in childhood has a loose dependence on progressive skeletal maturity, particularly affected by the growth plate and the physiological changes that occur. Thus, the occurrence of Perthe's disease, slipped capital femoral epiphysis (Fig. 9D.1) and apophyseal avulsions (Fig. 9D.2) will occur in distinct age groups. Distinct patterns of fracture also heighten suspicion in the child at risk.

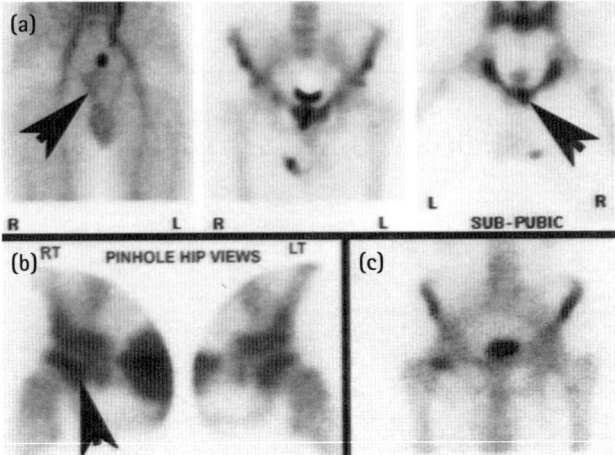

Figure 9D.1 *Hip and pelvis. (a) Osteitis pubis. Hyperemia in the right side of the pubic symphysis (arrowhead) and increased uptake in a soccer player complaining of severe anterior pelvic pain. Activity in the bladder and bladder neck can lead to false positive findings, unless the sub-pubic view is used, which clearly shows the activity to be in bone (arrow). (b) Slipped capital femoral epiphysis. The early change of a slip is usually increased uptake in the capital growth plate (arrow), leading to asymmetry between the hips. Collecting the images for a preset time is crucial to appreciating the asymmetry. (c) Sub-capital fracture of the right hip. Increased uptake is evident in the right sub-capital region of the hip in a patient who tripped on a carpet and felt pain in the right inguinal region. Plain films were reported as normal.*

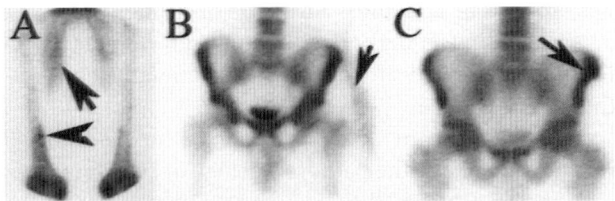

Figure 9D.2 *Pelvic injuries. (a) Rhabdomyolysis of the adductor muscles (arrow) and thigh splints (arrowhead) in a young man who accelerated an exercise program in order to reach peak fitness for a soccer game. (b) Uptake around a large hematoma (arrow) in a football player kicked quite hard in the left hip during a tackle. A fracture was suspected due to the degree of swelling around the hip. The large photopenic area medial to the uptake is the hematoma. (c) Apophyseal avulsion. Forced rotation of the trunk while playing football led to sudden onset of pain in the left upper pelvis. Intense uptake in the left anterior superior iliac crest due to avulsion of an apophysis by the oblique abdominal musculature.*

In the past, stress-related injuries were rarely reported in childhood, but have been reported with increasing prevalence. The relative incidence of stress fractures increases with age, with approximately 75% occurring before the age of 40 years.[8] Approximately 9% of fractures occur in children less than 15 years of age, 32% in the age range 16–19 years and 59% in patients older than 20 years.[9] The distribution of stress fractures in the pediatric population, based on 23 published reports is 51% in the tibia, 20% in the fibula, 15% in the pars interarticularis, 3% in the femur, and 2% in the metatarsals.[10] In adults, 50% occur in the tibia and 14% in the metatarsals with less than 1% in the pars interarticularis. Up to 17% of fractures will be bilateral.[8]

PRINCIPLES OF SCINTIGRAPHY IN TRAUMA

Planning of scintigraphic studies is essential for optimal imaging. A dynamic and blood pool study is almost invariably required as pain is the presenting symptom in most patients. An additional benefit of a three-phase study is the increased diagnostic yield with the chronic regional pain syndrome (reflex sympathetic dystrophy) (Fig. 9D.3). Positioning of the joint or limb is crucial and can only be determined by a good history and physical examination. In children, acquisition of blood pool images of the joint above and below the site of symptoms is important as pain can be referred from distant sites. It is also important to have the face of the camera perpendicular to the growth plates in order to examine the metaphyseal regions carefully and look for asymmetry in the growth plates, especially in the hips. The blood pool is important in the decision regarding a diagnosis of fracture versus soft-tissue injury. In the wrists, shoulders, hips, ankles, and feet, it can provide invaluable additional information on soft-tissue pathology involving the tendons, bursae, fasciae and synovial structures.

Creative positioning can aid substantially in the accurate localization of the sites of bony injuries. This can be performed relative to anatomical models,[11] plain radiographs[12] or CT.

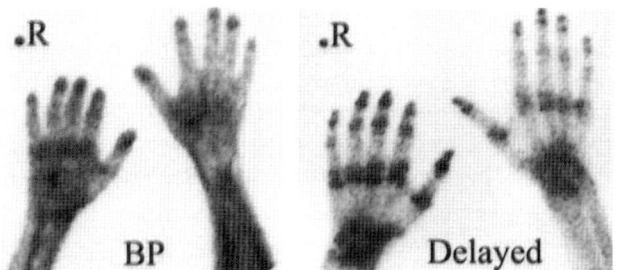

Figure 9D.3 *Chronic regional pain syndrome. Diffuse hyperemia in the right hand and diffuse peri-articular increase in uptake characterize the syndrome.*

INJURIES IN CHILDREN

Growth plate injury may attend acute trauma or chronic stress, as the physis is the weakest portion of the immature skeleton. These injuries usually occur through the zone of provisional calcification and although this zone heals well, extension into the germinal zones has the potential for growth arrest.[13] Included in this group of injuries is trauma to the apophysis, a growth plate that does not contribute to longitudinal growth. Important sites of growth plate injury are the distal radial (Fig. 9D.4) and proximal humeral physis in the upper limb and the distal femoral and distal tibial physis in the lower limb. Thus, although injuries to the distal femoral physis account for 2% of all physeal injuries, it accounts for nearly 40% of the causes of bony bridging.[14] Commonly affected apophyses are located in the medial epicondyle (Little leaguer's elbow), olecranon, coracoid, acromion, vertebrae, and around the pelvis (Fig. 9D.2). Radiographic evidence of damage includes widening of the growth plate and evidence of apophyseal separation. The scintigraphic equivalent is asymmetric increase in uptake in the affected growth plate (Fig. 9D.1).[13] These regions are

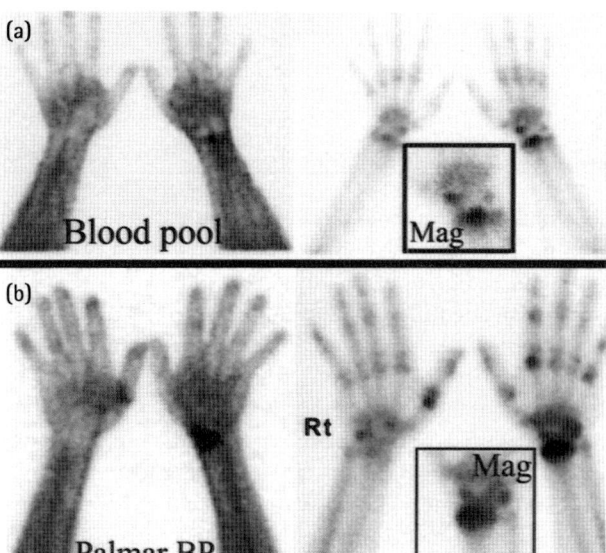

Figure 9D.4 *(a) Fracture of scaphoid and radial growth plate injury. Intense hyperemia is evident in the scaphoid with milder hyperemia in the adjacent distal radius. The delayed study confirms intense uptake in the scaphoid, as clinically suspected, but unexpected increase in uptake in the distal radial growth plate, suggesting significant injury. There were however no sequelae from either injury. (b) Occult fracture of radius. As plain radiography was normal, this patient was referred for bone scinitgraphy with a suspected scaphoid fracture, following a high-impact fall on to the hand. The flow study shows intense hyperemia in the distal radius and surrounding soft tissues. Delayed images show intense uptake in the distal radius and only mild increase in uptake in the other carpal bones, more readily apparent in the magnified view.*

affected by the osteochondroses, a disparate group of disorders characterized by a number of eponyms such as Kohler's disease (navicular), Freiberg's infraction (second metatarsal head), and Sever's disease (calcaneal apophysitis). Others include Osgood–Schlatter disease (tibial tubercle), Sinding–Larsen–Johansson disease (inferior pole of patella) and Panner's disease (capitellum).

NON-SPORTING TRAUMA

Traumatic fractures

In general, a high-impact injury will produce a fracture that is apparent on plain X-ray at most sites of trauma. Bone scintigraphy clearly has no role in such cases unless other occult fractures are suspected. This is illustrated by a study of 119 patients with forearm fractures where scintigraphy detected an unsuspected second injury in nine patients.[15] Scintigraphy has a greater utility in the polytraumatized patient, particularly where the patient is unconscious or unable to give a history. In a screening study of 162 patients, Spitz et al.[16] identified 50% more unexpected fractures in a group where plain radiography had identified 1536 fractures. An unexpected yield of 40% was also shown in 48 children with polytrauma.[17] This may relate to the differences in temporal and contrast resolution between plain radiography and scintigraphy.

FRACTURE OF THE SCAPHOID

Fractures of the scaphoid are usually apparent at 48–72 h after trauma in scintigraphic studies, compared to 2–3 weeks for the plain radiographic changes (Fig. 9D.4).[18] The injury can also be identified at a nascent stage with MRI which is not superior to scintigraphy.[19] The great advantage of MRI, however, is in the detection of associated carpal instability.[20] If untreated, the fracture may be complicated by pseudoarthrosis or avascular necrosis of the proximal fragment. Scintigraphy carries important prognostic information, in that focal decrease in uptake in the proximal fragment may suggest early avascular necrosis (Fig. 9D.5) and a poor outcome, as was shown in 3/50 patients by Bellmore et al.[21]

FRACTURE OF OTHER CARPAL BONES

In 50 patients studied by scintigraphy for suspected scaphoid injury, fracture was confirmed in 52%, with the rest showing injuries of other carpal bones or the distal radius (Figs 9D.5 and 9D.6).[22] A range of soft-tissue injuries such as tenosynovitis may also be detected by scintigraphy (Fig. 9D.6).[23]

FRACTURES OF THE HIP

The early detection and treatment of hip fractures is medically, socially, and legally important. Scintigraphic detection

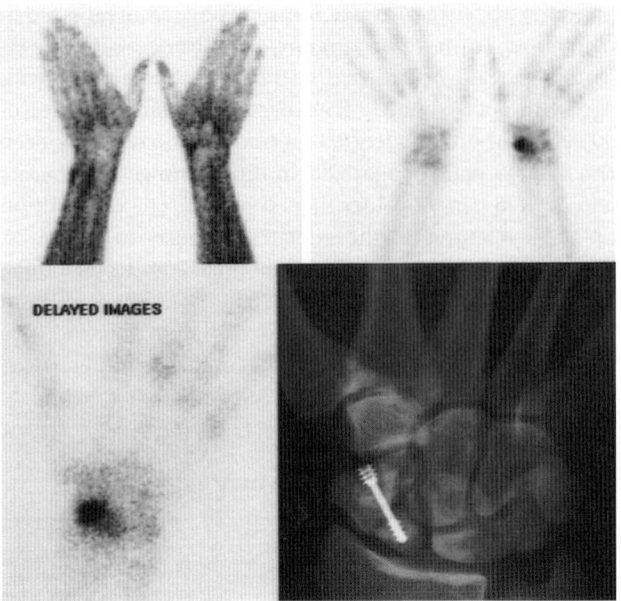

Figure 9D.5 *Post-operative scan after internal fixation of fractured scaphoid. The radiograph shows fracture reduction by a screw with some cortication of the edges of the fracture line suggestive of non-union. The bone scans shows hyperemia in the distal fragment, but relatively reduced flow to the proximal fragment. Delayed images confirm the finding of markedly decreased uptake in the proximal fragment, with increased uptake in the distal fragment. It confirms avascular necrosis of the proximal fragment as well as non-union which was apparent on the plain film.*

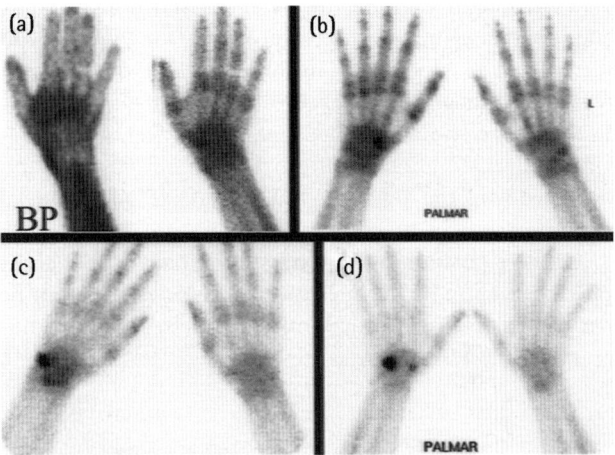

Figure 9D.6 *Hand injuries. (a) Tenosynovitis of the abductor and extensor pollicis tendons. Hyperemia is seen in the tendons with secondary increase in uptake in the adjacent radius. (b) Fracture of the trapezium. Intense uptake in the right trapezium. (c) Fracture of the right pisiform bone with intense uptake in the bone. (d) Fracture of the right hamate.*

of such fractures has been reported with some variability, largely due to a number of pitfalls that can be avoided if due care is taken with the timing and interpretation of images. Two false positive and two false negative studies were reported in 213 patients with equivocal radiographs (Fig. 9D.1), mainly in elderly patients.[24] However, Holder et al.[25] found a sensitivity of 93% with a specificity of 95% for fracture detection in 160 patients. In the false positive group, 3/7 had trochanteric fractures, which were correctly identified in another 33 patients. False negative studies occurred in four patients over 70 years of age, where studies were obtained within 72 h. As the delivery of tracer to the fracture site is dependent on blood flow, the reduction of blood supply in displaced femoral neck fractures coupled with age-related reduction in flow may warrant 3–4 h and 24 h imaging for optimization. Alternatively, a repeat study after several days may be indicated, particularly to distinguish a trochanteric fracture from an intertrochanteric fracture.[26] SPECT has the potential to improve the performance of scintigraphy, provided back-projection reconstruction artifacts from the bladder are overcome by techniques such as statistical reconstruction.

FRACTURES IN CHILDHOOD

Very young children may present with failure to move a limb or joint and a history may not be available, especially in pre-school children. Englaro et al.[27] identified focal abnormalities in 30 of 56 children under 5 years of age with leg pain or gait disturbances. Alternative imaging studies were abnormal in 9/56. The major scintigraphic abnormalities were located in the cuboid (9/56) and the calcaneum (4/56) in contrast to previous findings of the calcaneum as the most common site of trauma. The toddler's fracture involving a spiral fracture of the mid-shaft of the tibia has also been described[28] but carries the caution that this scan appearance is similar to the result of corner fractures with periosteal elevation, infection, and vascular occlusion.[29]

Child at risk (non–accidental trauma)

Unexpected polytrauma out of proportion to the forces of the injury, injuries of varying age or in specific locations should raise suspicion of the abused child (Fig. 9D.7), especially in children too young to give a history. Careful whole-body evaluation with pinhole or magnified views of the common sites of corner fractures in the femoral and tibial metaphyses is essential.[30] This study often accompanies a whole-body skeletal survey with plain radiographs and correlation is important. In a landmark paper, Sty and Starshak[31] demonstrated scintigraphic lesions in 120/261 children while radiography identified 95 with 32 false negatives in comparison to two false negatives for scintigraphy. In 15 patients, one or more of the fractures were demonstrated by scintigraphy alone, while in another 17 it identified additional sites of injury.

The most common injuries in over 50% of cases[32–34] are in the diaphysis, where twisting of the limb induces periosteal reaction and posterior rib fractures as the consequence of shaking an infant (Fig. 9D.7). Fractures of the first rib may be the only manifestation of abuse as shown

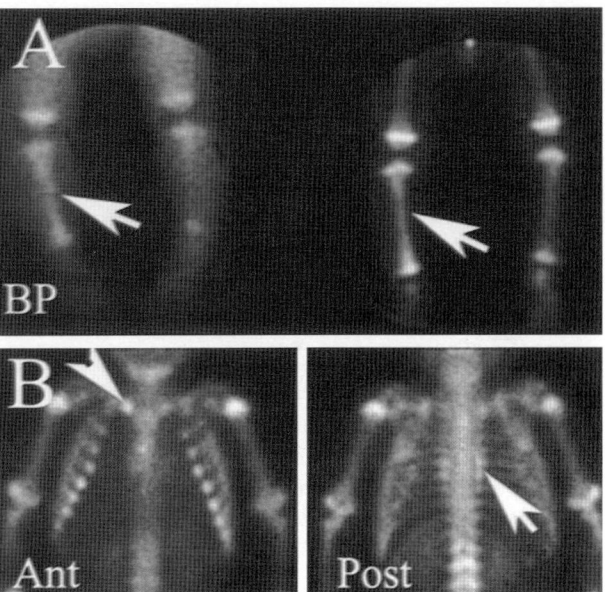

Figure 9D.7 *Child at risk. (a) There is diffuse hyperemia and uptake (arrows) in the right tibia in the characteristic pattern of a spiral fracture of the bone as a result of a shearing injury to the tibia during physical assault. This is also the appearance of the toddler's fracture at this site. (b) Anterior and posterior images of the thorax in a child with a fractured clavicle (arrowhead) due to direct trauma and posterior rib fractures (arrowheads) due to pressure from fingers against the posterior thorax while being shaken. Posterior rib fractures are highly specific for this type of injury. (Courtesy of Professor Monica Rossleigh, Prince of Wales Hospital, Sydney, Australia.)*

by Strouse and Owings.[35] Metaphyseal corner fractures and epiphyseal injury are easily visualized by scintigraphy but may be difficult to detect when bilateral.[36] Scintigraphy is less reliable than radiography in detecting skull fractures because of the poor contrast resolution in the skull, as Sty and Starshak[31] showed in 4/11 children. It is an area where radiography is essential. Scintigraphy has also been reported to show soft-tissue contusions and necrosis.

Insufficiency injuries

Insufficiency fractures are those that occur with minimal trauma in osteopenic or osteoporotic bone. Scintigraphic appearances are similar to fatigue fractures, but there may be reduced contrast resolution due to metabolic disturbances in uptake of the tracer. Weight-bearing structures such as the hip, spine, and pelvis are the major sites of these fractures. Any factor that alters normal bone structure will predispose to insufficiency fractures, as was shown by Abe et al.[37] in 27 of 80 women irradiated for uterine cancer.

PELVIC FRACTURES

Insufficiency fractures of the sacrum characteristically present as an H-shaped abnormality (Fig. 9D.8),[38] although a

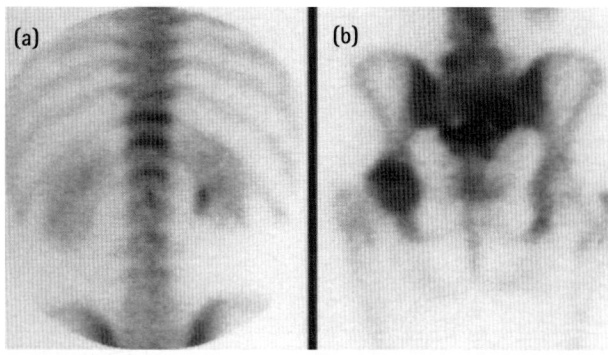

Figure 9D.8   *Insufficiency fractures. (a) Transverse linear increase in uptake is evident in the bodies of T11, T12 and mildly in L1 compatible with compression fractures. The milder uptake in L1 is suggestive of an older fracture. (b) Intense transverse increase in uptake from the left sacroiliac joint across the sacrum, characteristic of an insufficiency fracture of the sacrum.*

variety of alterations such as focal unilateral lesions in children have been documented.[39,40] Multiple insufficiency fractures of the pelvis may also occur, as was shown in 20 of 25 patients by Davies *et al.*[41]

VERTEBRAL FRACTURES

Osteoporosis is the most common cause of compression fractures of a vertebra.[42] The scintigraphic appearance is of loss of vertebral height and contour with intense linear uptake (Fig. 9D.8). The bone scan can confirm vertebral fracture as the cause of pain, as well as alternative diagnoses such as degenerative disease.[42] An additional advantage is in the dating of such fractures for both management and medicolegal reasons.[43]

SPORTS-RELATED INJURIES

Ankle and foot

The key to detection of soft-tissue injuries is the blood pool phase of the study which shows hyperemia in the affected structure with delayed uptake apparent only if there is close apposition of adjacent bony structures, as with the medial malleolus in tibialis posterior tendonitis.

SOFT-TISSUE INJURY

Injuries to the soft-tissues include the tendons, ligaments, joint capsule, and bursae. Bone scintigraphy is capable of showing either enthesitis or traction injury of the Achilles tendon (Fig. 9D.9), the most commonly injured tendon. The second most frequently injured tendon is tibialis posterior, usually in ballet dancers and gymnasts. Tibialis posterior tendonitis may also be seen in association with increased uptake in the accessory navicular bone, constituting the

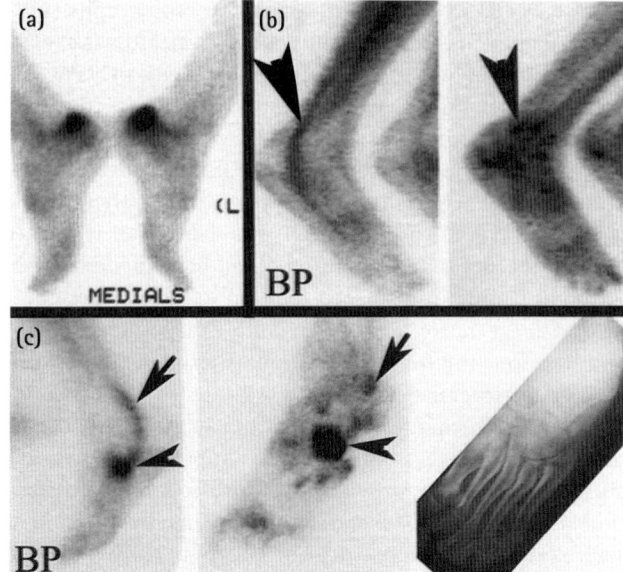

Figure 9D.9   *(a) Achilles' tendonitis. Intense uptake at the site of attachment of the distal Achilles tendons into the posterior calcanei. (b) Peroneal tenosynovitis. Intense hyperemia in the distribution of the peroneal tendons (arrowhead) with secondary increase in uptake in the adjacent posterior fibula. Extensive degenerative changes are present elsewhere in the foot. (c) Peroneal tenosynovitis and fracture of the left cuboid. Hyperemia is seen in the distribution of the peroneal tendons (arrow) and the cuboid (arrowhead). The delayed study shows secondary uptake in the fibula (arrow) and intense uptake in the cuboid (arrowhead).*

accessory navicular syndrome.[44] A similar pattern of blood pool activity in the distribution of the tendon has also been described with the peroneal tendons (Fig. 9D.9).[45]

Posterolateral pain is usually due to posterior impingement syndrome, impingement of the os trigonum or peroneal tendonitis (Fig. 9D.10). An os trigonum is present in approximately 3–13% of the population. Posterior impingement may occur with forced plantar flexion of the ankle, as happens in ballet dancers. Posterior impingement can also be caused by an enlarged posterior talar process, prominent posterior calcaneal process, loose bodies or avulsion of the posterior tibiotalar ligament.[46] The scintigraphic appearance[47] is characterized by intense uptake in the posterior talus (Fig. 9D.10).

The anterior impingement syndrome is caused by repeated traction of the anterior ankle joint capsule and impingement of the talus against the tibia. The chronic process leads to calcific deposits along the lines of the capsular fibers and spur formation on the dorsum of the anterior talus and tibia.[46] A pattern of intense increase in uptake of tracer is seen in the anterior aspect of the ankle (Fig. 9D.10).

PLANTAR FASCIITIS

Heel pain is one of the most common presentations in sports medicine, plantar fasciitis being the most common

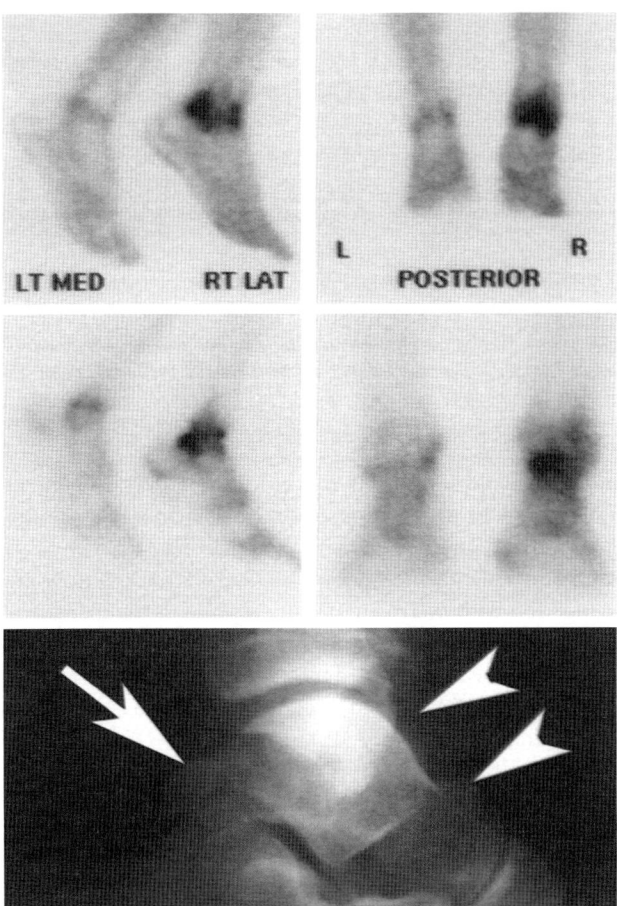

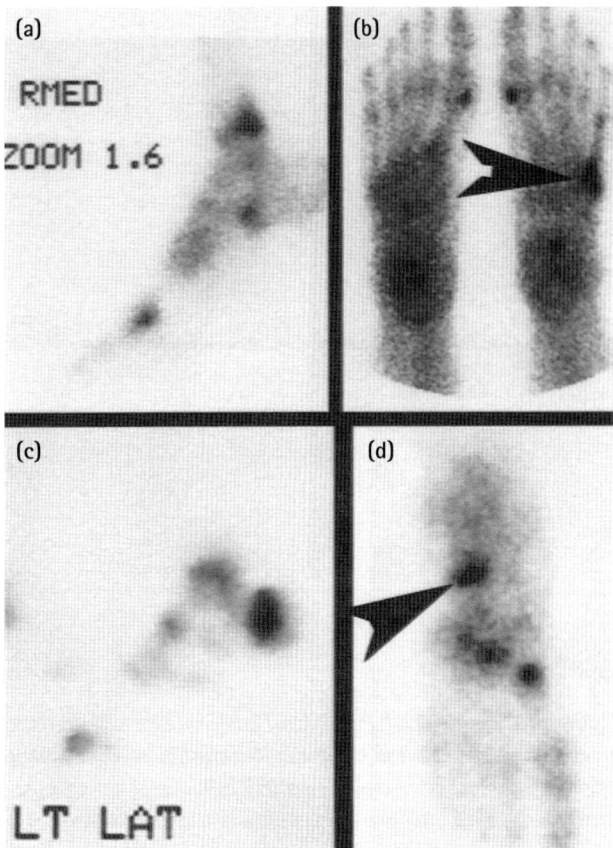

Figure 9D.10 *Impingement syndrome. Hyperemia is evident in the anterior and posterior aspects of the ankle. The delayed study shows intense increase in uptake at the anterior and posterior aspects of the right ankle corresponding to a spur on the anterior aspect of the talus and the edge of the plafond (arrowheads) and a large os trigonum (arrow) in the corresponding X-ray.*

Figure 9D.11 *Trauma to the foot. (a) Fracture of the tibial plafond. Increased accumulation in the posteromedial aspect of the plafond, distinct from talar dome accumulation. (b) Jones' fracture. Intense uptake of the base of the left 5th metatarsal bone (arrowhead) at a site of fracture. (c) Calcaneal fracture. Vertical increase in uptake through the posterior aspect of the calcaneum at a site of fracture. (d) Calcaneal fracture. Increased uptake in the anterior aspect of the calcaneum (arrowhead) at a site of fracture.*

cause.[48] Other causes of heel pain that may be elucidated by scintigraphy include Achilles tendonitis and bursitis, retrocalcaneal bursitis, apophysitis of the calcaneum and calcaneal stress fracture (Fig. 9D.11).

Bony and ligamentous injury

The ankle is the site of acute injury in up to 75% of participants in sport,[49] 15% having serious sequelae.[50] About 70% of acute injuries are inversion 'sprains' with injury to the lateral ligamentous complex of the ankle and less often to the medial ligamentous complex. In a small proportion, serious injuries will occur to the talus, tibio-fibular syndesmosis (Fig. 9D.12), cuboid (Fig. 9D.9), calcaneus (Fig. 9D.11) or navicular bones.

TALAR DOME FRACTURES

Osteochondral fractures occur in up to 6% of acute ankle sprains, most commonly in the posteromedial talar dome

followed by the anterolateral talar dome.[51] Plain X-ray may miss up to 33% of fractures.[52] Plain radiography has an accuracy of 25% when correlated with arthroscopy.[52] Scintigraphy is a good screening test in the presence of a normal radiograph (Fig. 9D.13), as was shown in a small series of 24 patients.[53] In a larger series of 122 patients, bone scintigraphy was shown to have a sensitivity of 94% and specificity of 76% for detecting talar dome fractures. Blood pool abnormalities were associated with higher grade fractures.

ACUTE FRACTURES OF THE PLAFOND AND INTEROSSEOUS MEMBRANE

In a review of 639 cases of ankle sprain, 15% had either avulsion or compression fractures and 5% had significant injuries to the interosseous membrane.[50] Scintigraphically, this is evident as hyperemia in the posterior aspect of the ankle, extending superiorly into the interosseous membrane.

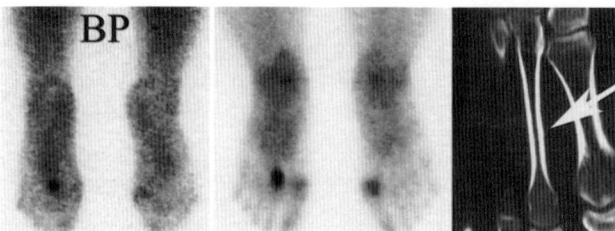

Figure 9D.14   *Stress fracture of 2nd metatarsal. Intense hyperemia and uptake in the left second metatarsal bone. The computed tomography scan was initially reported as normal but on review was shown to have a small area of periosteal reaction at the site of fracture (arrow).*

Figure 9D.12   *Injury to the tibio-fibular syndesmosis. Intense uptake is evident between the distal tibia and fibula, mainly along the lateral tibial cortex and the posterior tibial plafond. It represents injury to the inferior aspect of the posterior tibio-fibular ligament with an avulsion chip fracture at its attachment to the posterior tibial plafond.*

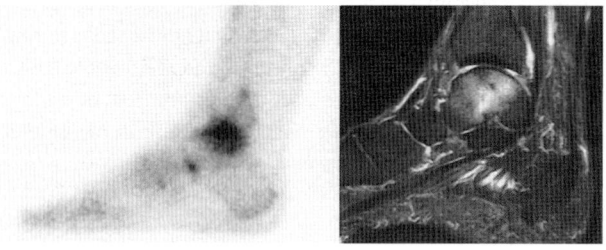

Figure 9D.13   *Talar dome fracture. Intense uptake in the postero-medial aspect of the talar dome. The magnetic resonance imaging study shows intense signal from the same site in the T2 study. Initial X-rays were reported as normal.*

Delayed images demonstrate increased uptake in the posterior plafond (avulsion or chip fracture), medial edge of the posterior fibula (avulsion fracture) and extension into the distal syndesmosis (Fig. 9D.12).[54] This injury is often associated with a fracture of the proximal fibula (Maisonneuve fracture).

FRACTURES OF THE TARSAL BONES

Stress fracture of the talus is rare (Fig. 9D.13). Although rare in overall terms, acute navicular fractures are the most common mid-foot fracture and require careful treatment in order to avoid long-term morbidity. The dorsal ligament avulsion fracture is the most common navicular fracture and presents with pinpoint tenderness after eversion or inversion injury on a plantar-flexed foot. Navicular stress fractures are being seen with increasing frequency due to the increasing participation of women and adolescents in various sports. Fractures are easily detected by scintigraphy, CT and MRI in nearly all cases.[55,56] Cuboid fractures are unusual and account for approximately 5% of all tarsal fractures (Fig. 9D.11).[57] Cuneiform fractures comprise approximately 4% of all mid-foot fractures.[57] Acute fractures of the anterior process of the calcaneus have been reported to account for up to 15% of all calcaneal fractures (Fig. 9D.11).[58]

Stress fractures of the calcaneus have been reported in approximately 20% of male and 40% of female military recruits undergoing basic military training.[59,60] The most common site of fracture is the posterior calcaneal tubercle (Fig. 9D.11).

METATARSAL STRESS FRACTURE

These are perhaps the most common form of stress injury in the foot and ankle. In a large series of 295 subjects with 339 stress fractures, 28% were in the metatarsals.[61] These injuries occur in athletes who participate in high-impact sports involving mainly running and jumping. Stress fractures predominantly (90%) occur in the second and third metatarsal bones (Fig. 9D.14). There is also a high level of stress through the fifth metatarsal, although less than in the second.[62] Fractures of the fifth metatarsal are usually through the shaft and more rarely, proximally located (Jones fracture) (Fig. 9D.11).[63]

SESAMOID INJURIES

The sesamoid bones beneath the first metatarsal head are within the capsule of the first metatarsophalangeal (MTP) joint and may be multipartite in 5–30% of people. Stress fractures may therefore be difficult to diagnose radiologically. Scintigraphy has been found to be useful in the diagnosis of injury to the sesamoids in case studies.[64]

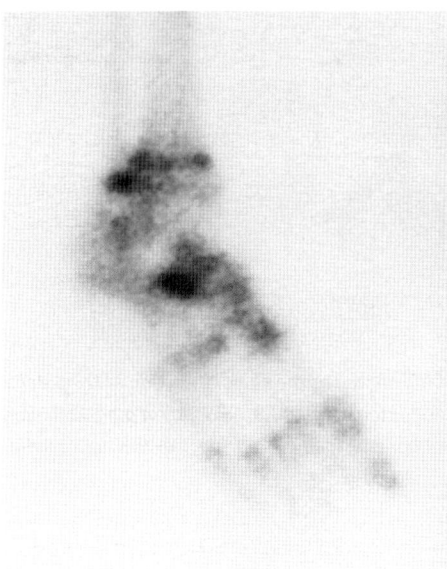
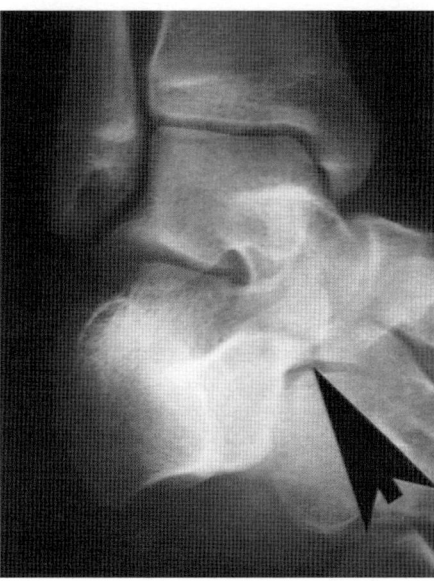

Figure 9D.15 *Calcaneonavicular coalition. Intense uptake is present extending from the anterior aspect of the calcaneus to the navicular. The radiograph shows beaking of the anterior calcaneus and an irregular bridging region with the navicular (arrow).*

TARSAL COALITION

A failure of segmentation of the mesenchymal anlage of the hindfoot bones in the embryo is thought to be the cause of tarsal coalition. An autosomal dominant inheritance pattern has been established and tarsal coalitions occur in approximately 1% of the population. Fifty percent will be bilateral and a significant proportion have multiple coalitions.[65] Coalitions of the talocalcaneal and calcaneonavicular bones (Fig. 9D.15) are the most common, followed by the talonavicular and calcaneocuboid bones. These coalitions may be fibrous, cartilaginous or bony. Symptoms usually occur when the coalitions ossify and present with pain in the early to middle teens with ankle pain in the lateral and anterolateral aspects of the ankle. Physical examination shows a valgus hindfoot and patients may have a flat foot. The flat foot is usually associated with peroneal muscle spasm due to hindfoot rigidity. Mandell *et al.*[66] reported the successful localization of 7/9 fibrous talocalcaneal coalitions using pinhole scintigraphy.

Tibial region

Stress fractures of the tibia are the single most common fracture in sports medicine.[4,67,68] The diagnosis must be distinguished from shin splints and compartment syndrome. Stress fractures of the fibula are less common, but may occur in association with other injuries.

SOFT-TISSUE INJURIES

The two major chronic soft-tissue injuries are shin splints and the chronic compartment syndromes. Other causes of pain include entrapment of arteries and nerves, deep venous thrombosis, rupture of the gastrocnemius muscle, fascial herniations, and muscle strains. Muscle strains are probably the single most common cause of acute pain in the lower limbs.[69]

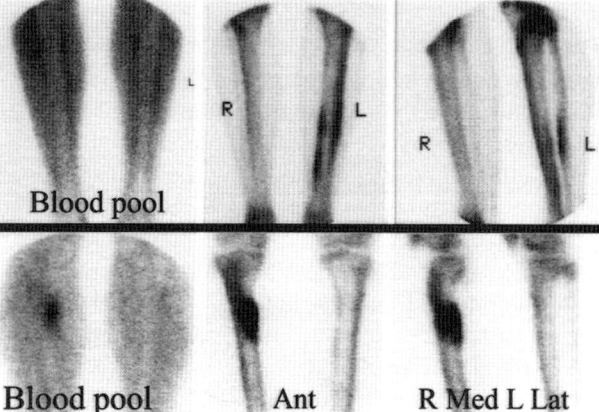

Figure 9D.16 *Shin splints versus stress fracture. The upper panel shows diffuse cortical increase in uptake along the posteromedial aspect of the left tibia and fibula without alteration in blood pool appearance at the sites. This is the well-described appearance of shin splints compared to the intense hyperemia and uptake in the proximal tibia, characteristic of a high-grade fracture (lower panel).*

SHIN SPLINTS

Shin splints have been called the medial tibial stress syndrome due to the localization of exercise-induced pain to the posteromedial aspect of the distal two thirds of the tibia.[69] Considerable controversy surrounds the etiology of so-called shin splints. Biopsy evidence shows inflammation of the crural fascia and increased bony metabolism with vascular ingrowth in the majority.[69] The triple-phase bone scan appearance was well described by Holder and Michael[70] as showing low-grade uptake in the distal posteromedial tibia on the delayed phase only, with no alterations in blood flow (Fig. 9D.16). Scintigraphic studies currently define the diagnosis.

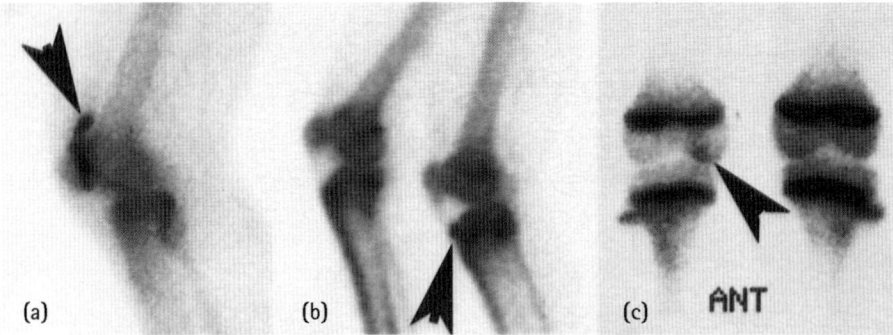

Figure 9D.17 *Knee injuries. (a) Reverse, jumper's knee. Intense uptake at the superior pole of the patella at the site of insertion of the patella tendon (arrowhead). (b) Enthesitis/avulsion injury at the insertion of the inferior patellar tendon into the tibia (arrowhead) in a basketballer. (c) Osteochondritis dissecans. Moderate increase in uptake of tracer is seen in the subchondral bone of the lateral aspect of the right medial femoral condyle (arrowhead).*

BONY INJURIES

TIBIAL STRESS FRACTURES

The incidence of tibial stress fractures has been reported from 4 to 31%, but accounts for over 50% of all stress fractures, particularly in military recruits.[4,68] Predisposing factors include altered biomechanics in the lower limb, changes in footwear or rapid acceleration in the level of activity.

The utility of bone scintigraphy in the early diagnosis of tibial stress fractures has been well established since the description of early detection compared to plain radiology in the mid-1970s.[71] The usual scan appearance is of hyperemia with intense transverse uptake at the site of fracture (Fig. 9D.16). More recent literature has shown an equivalence with MRI for early diagnosis,[72,73] with scan findings of periosteal and bone-marrow edema. The posterior aspect of the upper third of the shaft is the most common site of fracture in children and the elderly. The distal third is the most common site in long-distance runners.

In a large series,[74] 164 of 280 fractures occurred in the mid-shaft. This group described a classification of tibial stress fractures into four grades, extending from poorly defined cortical uptake (Grade I) to well-defined intra-medullary trans-cortical uptake (Grade IV). The scintigraphic grade of uptake gave valuable prognostic information regarding the period of rest required for healing, being more prolonged in the higher grades.

FIBULAR STRESS FRACTURES

Stress fractures of the fibula account for 20% of pediatric[10] and up to 30% of adult stress fractures.[75] The vast majority develop in the distal third, with the proximal and middle third being rare. Scintigraphy has been established as a reference standard since the earliest experiences with athletics injuries.[71]

Knee injuries

The knee is a joint capable of complex motion and prone to injury in any activity involving rapid changes in direction.

The menisci separate the femoral condyles from the tibial plateau. The cruciate ligaments, medial and lateral collateral ligaments, joint capsule, and muscles afford joint stability. Planar imaging can yield a number of diagnoses such as bursitis, enthesopathy, osteochondritis dissecans (Fig. 9D.17), bone bruises or fractures of the tibial plateau. Internal derangements of the knee may be detected by SPECT images.

ACUTE AND CHRONIC INJURY

Knee SPECT has a defined role in the assessment of both acute and chronic knee pain.[76–80] Good to excellent performance has been shown[78] in a variety of knee disorders in 158 patients in which knee SPECT made the correct diagnosis in 89%. Even if SPECT does not provide a specific diagnosis, it may be helpful in directing arthroscopy and shortening the examination.[77,78]

MENISCAL INJURY

Knee SPECT has been evaluated in the setting of chronic and acute meniscal tears.[76–79,81,82] Meniscal tears are characterized by peripherally increased uptake in a crescent in the tibial plateau as well as focal posterior femoral condylar uptake (Fig. 9D.18).[77,79,82] Ryan *et al.*[79] in a study of 100 patients with undiagnosed knee pain showed a sensitivity of 84%, specificity of 80%, positive predictive value of 88%, and negative predictive value of 76% for SPECT, with similar values for MRI.

CRUCIATE LIGAMENT INJURY

Knee SPECT can detect cruciate ligament injuries. The characteristic feature providing primary evidence of anterior cruciate ligament (ACL) injury is focal uptake at the insertion sites, more commonly at the femoral than the tibial attachment.[80,82] Corollary evidence is provided by uptake in the lateral femoral condyle or posterolateral tibial plateau due to bone bruising at these sites, which often occurs during

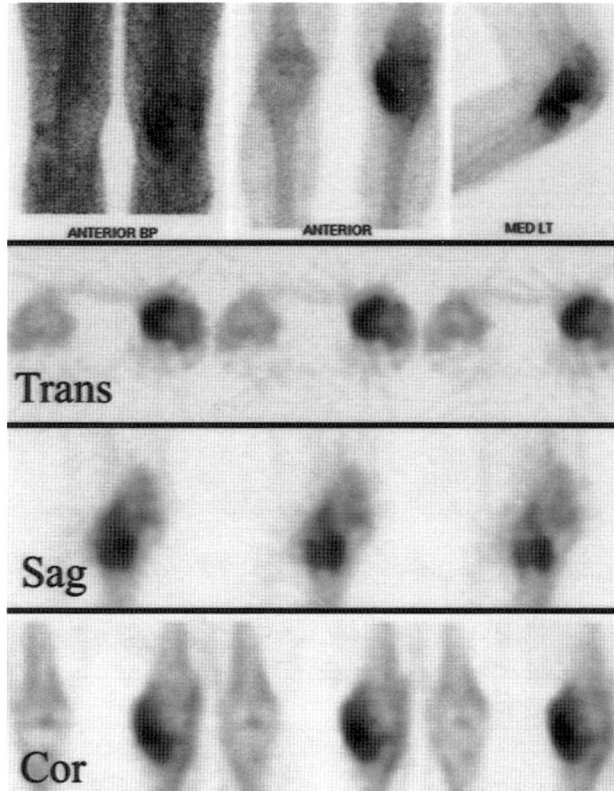

Figure 9D.18 *Knee single photon emission computed tomography (SPECT) in meniscal injury/bone bruising. Intense hyperemia and uptake are present in the medial aspect of the knee in the planar study (upper panel). The SPECT study shows crescentic increase in uptake in the medial tibial plateau in the distribution of the medial meniscus. There is less intense uptake in the medial femoral condyle and subcondral bone of the medial tibial plateau, consistent with bone bruising. A torn medial meniscus was found at arthroscopy with friability of the cartilage of the medial femoral condyle.*

the process which produces ACL injury.[80,82,83] So *et al.*[80] showed relatively poor results in ACL injury using primary or corollary evidence alone, but a sensitivity of 84% and positive predictive value of 81% when combined.

MISCELLANEOUS INJURIES

Collateral ligament injuries are characterized by focal uptake at both attachments of the ligament, often accompanied by an arc of blood pool activity around the centre of the knee.[77,82,84] Avulsion may lead to focal uptake in the proximal attachment, and is called Pellegrini–Stieda disease. Osteochondritis and focal condylar erosions are easily visualized with knee SPECT, perhaps better than by MRI.[82] Osteochondritis dissecans occurs at different sites, most frequently at the lateral aspect of the medial femoral condyle, to subchondral infractions which occur in weight-bearing regions, usually in the lateral compartment.[85]

Thigh, hip, and pelvis

SOFT-TISSUE INJURIES OF THE THIGH, HIP, AND PELVIS

A variety of soft-tissue injuries have been reported in the thigh. Adductor splints are an over-use injury of the adductor muscles, manifested by a periosteal reaction at the insertion into the cortex of the femur as with shin splints (Fig. 9D.2, page 364).[86] Direct muscular trauma with or without hematoma formation may also be detected due to muscular uptake at the sites of damage (Fig. 9D.2). In patients with symptomatic muscle pain after ultra-marathon competition, up to 90% will have evidence of rhabdomyolysis.[87]

Other causes of scintigraphic alterations in the region include bursitis of the iliopsoas bursa, greater trochanteric bursa, and ischial bursa. Numerous tendon insertion enthesopathies have also been described.[48]

BONY INJURIES OF THE HIP AND PELVIS

STRESS FRACTURES OF THE HIP

Stress fractures of the hip account for approximately 4.5% of all stress fractures.[88] There are two patterns that have been described: transverse and compression. Transverse fractures are in the superior or tension side of the femoral neck and occur in older individuals. The rate of complications is much higher with these fractures.[89] Compression fractures occur on the medial side of the femoral neck in younger patients. The fracture heals well with rest if undisplaced, but requires more aggressive therapy if displaced.[89]

AVULSION FRACTURES OF THE PELVIS

Avulsion fractures are a common injury in adolescent athletes. These injuries occur through the apophysis and are equivalent to physeal fractures (Fig. 9D.2, page 364). The usual mechanism involved is a sudden violent contraction of a large muscle attached to bone, resulting in tearing of the attached tendon and bone through its weakest point, the provisional zone of calcification.[89] Presentation is with sudden onset of localized pain. The degree of displacement of the fragment is important for prognosis.

PELVIC STRESS FRACTURE

Pelvic stress fracture is rare but positive when tested with bone scintigraphy.[90] Fracture of the inferior pubic ramus has been reported in female military recruits[91] and is thought to be due to repetitive strain of the large muscles on the pubic bones.[89]

OSTEITIS PUBIS

This is mainly reported in runners, soccer and football players and presents with groin, pubic, perineal or scrotal pain. The mechanism is thought to be due to the action of the large adductor muscles on the pubic bones as weight is

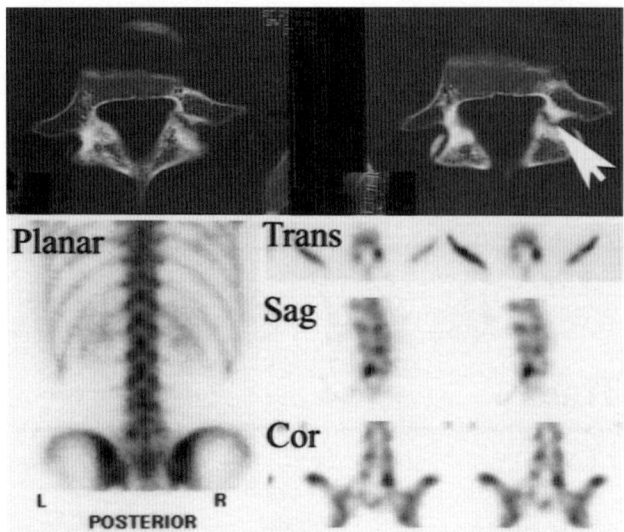

Figure 9D.19 *Injuries of the thorax and spine. (a) Rib fractures. Intense uptake in the right 5th and 6th ribs in a rower. (b) Fracture of the transverse process. Intense uptake in the left transverse processes of L2 and L3 in a footballer who fell hard onto the left loin during a tackle.*

transferred from one leg to the other during running. The diagnosis is easily made by scintigraphy (Fig. 9D.1),[92] and may often be diagnosed in the asymptomatic elite athlete.[93] A sup-pubic view is important in order to overcome confounding activity in the urinary bladder.[93]

Injuries of the chest

Rib stress fractures occur in 5.3% of all injuries in female and male rowers and account for 39.5% of chronic chest injuries in female rowers.[94] These injuries are readily apparent on bone scintigraphy (Fig. 9D.19).

Injuries of the vertebral column

CERVICAL AND THORACIC SPINE

The availability of multi-headed gamma cameras has led to major improvements in imaging of the cervical spine. The normal anatomy has been well defined,[95,96] and the utility assessed in the setting of acute neck trauma in a small series.[96] In 16 patients with abnormal results, SPECT detected occult fractures in seven of 35 patients (27%), including three with normal radiographs and four with equivocal radiographs. Recent fractures were excluded in 6/9(67%). None of the patients with normal SPECT studies had CT or MRI evidence of recent fractures.

Little work has been published about the utility of scintigraphy in the thoracic spine. Several case reports document detection of fractures of the vertebral bodies and posterolateral elements.

LUMBAR SPINE

Low back pain is common among athletes. The causes vary and must be distinguished from stress fracture of the pars

Figure 9D.20 *Spondylolysis. Intense uptake is present in the left posterolateral elements of L5 in the planar study, which is well localized to the pars interarticularis in the SPECT study. These findings are confirmed by the computed tomography scan, showing a fracture through the left pars interarticularis of L5.*

interarticularis which has an incidence of 6% in the general population and accounts for about 15% of pediatric stress fractures. Most pars fractures occur at the L5 and to a lesser degree, L4 levels of the spine. Young athletes are at most risk, particularly those involved in tennis, gymnastics, cricket (fast bowling), and throwing. Careful scintigraphic imaging is important as 15% of evolving fractures may not be evident on CT scanning.[97] Pars lesions must also be distinguished from facet joint pathology. The two entities may be distinguished by localizing the site of increased tracer uptake relative to the vertebral body and relative to the spinal canal which appears as a linear cold area running through the posterolateral elements (Fig. 9D.20).[11] The facet joint lies in the plane of the intervertebral disc while the pars is located further inferiorly, posterior to the vertebral body. Oblique reconstruction using 45° azimuth rotation may be useful to demonstrate the lesion's relationship to the vertebral body and intervertebral disc.[98] SPECT reveals 20–50% greater lesion detection than planar imaging.[99]

One of the major utilities of bone scintigraphy is in deciding if a pars fracture is of long standing and has no potential for healing, or is metabolically active and has capability for healing.[100] One study that examined surgical outcomes for spondylolysis based on pre-operative SPECT, clearly showed that those with positive studies had a better outcome than those with negative SPECT.[101] Rarely, rotational movements may lead to avulsion/traction injuries of the multifidus muscles of the lumbar spine, presenting as increased uptake in the spinous processes and posterolateral vertebral bodies.[102]

Shoulder and upper limb

THE SHOULDER

The shoulder is a difficult joint to study with scintigraphy due to its size and the dominance of soft-tissue injuries. One of the first attempts at systematic study was by Clunie et al.[103] Using a number of positioning techniques, they were able to identify a cause of the painful shoulder in 79% of patients.

ARM AND FOREARM

Injuries other than acute fractures are infrequently reported in the humerus, with occasional reports of muscle insertion splints at the proximal insertion of the brachioradialis.[104] Injuries around the elbow are more common, with scintigraphic reports of a number of soft-tissue manifestations such as triceps avulsion from the olecranon process, olecranon bursitis, medial and lateral epicondylitis, and distal biceps avulsion injury.[105] The majority of forearm injuries are due to acute or chronic fractures. Distal radial fractures are reported to account for one sixth of all acute fractures presenting to the emergency room,[106] with 50% involving dislocation and over 60% involving the radiocarpal or radioulnar joint.

Wrist and hand

SOFT-TISSUE INJURY

Scintigraphy can demonstrate evidence of soft-tissue and bony injury in the wrist. It can demonstrate tenosynovitis of the tendons of the wrist. De Quervain's tenosynovitis has been described as showing elongated hyperemia in the distribution of the tendons in the radial compartment of the wrist with delayed uptake in the radial styloid (Fig. 9D.6, page 366).[23] Post-traumatic pain due to the complex regional pain syndrome I (reflex sympathetic dystrophy) may be diagnosed accurately (Fig. 9D.3, page 365).

BONY INJURY

Reports of the scintigraphic detection of fractures of every bone in the carpus and hand have been made since the inception of the technique.[107,108] Scaphoid fractures are the most common, accounting for 60–70% of all carpal injuries (Figs 9D.4, page 365 and 9D.5, page 366).[109] Fractures of the lunate are rare but prone to avascular necrosis if not treated, as 20% of the population have only a single blood supply to the bone.[109] Injuries to the hamate usually affect the hook, although any portion of the bone may be involved (Fig. 9D.6).[109] Fractures of the hook are usually seen in sports that involve bats, clubs or racquets. Fractures of the triquetrum, pisiform, capitate, trapezium (Fig. 9D.6), and trapezoid may occur due to direct blows or compression of the wrist in falls. These are easily diagnosed by scintigraphy, with significant improvement in accuracy if the study is co-registered with the plain radiographs.[110]

COMPLICATIONS IN FRACTURE HEALING

The scintigraphic changes reflecting the remodeling of skeletal fractures persist for a considerable period. While diminution or even disappearance of the accumulation is to be expected by 6 months, the rate of change in the alterations is so variable that it is difficult to assess whether there is any significant delay in union. The site of fracture and the age of the patient will influence the rate of return to normality but many other factors will also be relevant, both systemic and local. Many of these, such as loss of blood supply, failure of immobilization with consequent poor contact of the fracture ends and infection, may be responsible for non-union. Subsequently, a pseudoarthrosis may form at the fracture site.

Fracture non-union

A number of attempts have been made to achieve a method to predict whether or not normal healing would proceed and thus permit early intervention. Auchinloss and Watt[111] suggested that a study at 6 weeks was justified in those who might have a healing problem (Fig. 9D.5). It may be difficult to separate delayed union from frank non-union, in particular from reactive non-union in which the scan will show persistent intense accumulation at the fragment ends despite the cessation of healing. These appearances differ from those in atrophic non-union in which there may be reduction of accumulation in one or both aspects of the fracture. In particular, visualization of a distinct photopenic gap between the fragment ends indicates a very low probability of union being achieved. Desai et al.[112] found that 59 of 62 fractures which showed intense uptake healed successfully with electrical stimulation whereas no healing could be identified in any of those in which an area of decreased activity was demonstrated.

Pseudoarthrosis

Pseudoarthrosis may also be identified by the demonstration of absent accumulation at the site of the false joint. Atrophic pseudoarthrosis, for which bone graft is essential, is characterized by the absence of peripheral accumulation in contrast with the intense uptake surrounding a hypertrophic pseudoarthrosis (Fig. 9D.21). The complication is a major clinical problem in patients who have undergone lumbar fusion but with continued post-operative low back pain. Slizofski et al.[113] studied 26 patients who had undergone a lumbar spinal fusion more than 6 months previously.

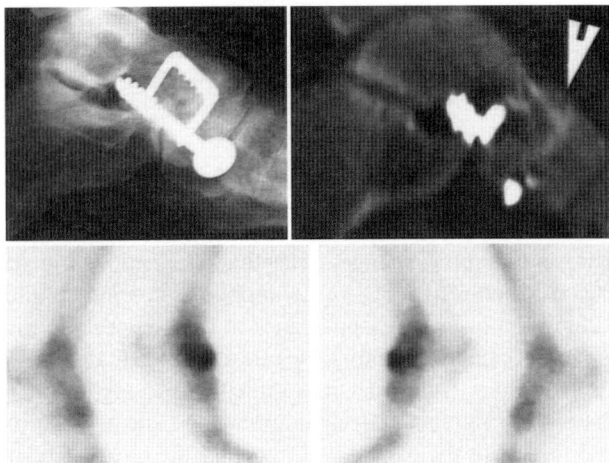

Figure 9D.21 *Pseodoarthrosis following fusion of talus and navicular. Persistent pain led to this study 2 years after fusion of the talus and navicular bone for arthritis. The bone scan showed intense uptake at the site of fusion. The plain film was unhelpful, but tomography showed a clear linear area of pseudoarthrosis (arrowhead).*

In 15 who were symptomatic, focal accumulation compatible with pseudoarthrosis was visualized, SPECT identifying a more focal area of intense activity within the area of increased accumulation at the fusion site. Six of 11 asymptomatic patients had focal areas of increased uptake. It was suggested that this might reflect painless pseudoarthrosis, reputed to occur in 50% of patients. Failed fusion was correctly identified by Even-Sapir *et al.*[114] in all six patients studied within 4 years of surgery but in only four of five who were investigated later than this.

Infection

Difficulties exist in identifying the presence of complicating infection, mainly because of the vascularity and intense metabolic activity at a fracture site and the consequent uptake, on occasion, of alternative imaging agents. Most attempts to use scintigraphy comparing the congruence of ^{99m}Tc and ^{67}Ga uptake have not been successful.[115] The experience with ^{111}In leukocytes has varied considerably. Kim *et al.*[116] reported a sensitivity of only 50% if marked uptake was the diagnostic criterion. Because of the incidence of false positives, the technique does appear most useful in excluding infection by observing a normal study.

CONCLUSION

Bone scintigraphy has extensive applications in the diagnosis and monitoring of bony and soft-tissue trauma. However, it requires a good history of the activity, possible mechanism of the injury, and a good working knowledge of anatomy in order to reach an accurate diagnosis. Correlative images should be used whenever available and these should be supplemented with anatomical models or a good anatomical atlas. The gamut of diagnostic possibilities encompasses soft-tissue and bony injuries, making the acquisition of high-quality blood pool phase images essential. When imaging children, special consideration needs to be given to positioning and anatomical variations.

REFERENCES

● Seminal primary article
◆ Key review paper

● 1 Mink JH, Deutsch AL. Occult cartilage and bone injuries of the knee: detection, classification and assessment with MR imaging. *Radiology* 1989; **170**: 823–9.
● 2 Rangger C, Kathrein A, Freund MC, *et al.* Bone bruise of the knee. Histology and cryosections in 5 cases. *Acta Orthop Scand* 1998; **69**: 291–4.
◆ 3 Daffner RH, Pavlov H. Stress fractures: current concepts. *Am J Roentgenol* 1992; **159**: 245–52.
  4 Devas MB. *Stress fractures.* London: Churchill Livingstone, 1975.
◆ 5 Knapp TP, Garrett Jr WE. Stress fractures: general concepts. *Clin Sports Med* 1997; **16**: 339–56.
● 6 Chamay A, Tschants P. Mechanical influence in bone remodelling: experimental research in Wolff's law. *J Biomech* 1972; **5**: 173–80.
● 7 Carter DR, Caler WE. Cycle-dependent and time-dependent bone fracture with repeated loading. *J Biomech Eng* 1983; **105**: 166–70.
◆ 8 Courtenay BG, Bowers DM. Stress fractures: clinical features and investigation. *Med J Aust* 1990; **153**: 155–6.
◆ 9 Orava S, Jormakka E, Hulkko A. Stress fractures in young athletes. *Arch Orthop Trauma Surg* 1981; **98**: 271–4.
  10 Yngve DA. Stress fractures in the pediatric athlete. In: Sullivan JA, Grana WA. (eds.) *The pediatric athlete.* Park Ridge, Illinois: American Academy of Orthopedic Surgeons, 1988: 235.
● 11 Van der Wall H, Storey G, Frater C, Murray P. Importance of positioning and technical factors in anatomic localization of sporting injuries in scintigraphic imaging. *Semin Nucl Med* 2001; **31**: 17–27.
  12 Hawkes DJ, Robinson L, Crossman JE, *et al.* Registration and display of the combined bone scan and radiograph in the diagnosis and management of wrist injuries. *Eur J Nucl Med* 1991; **18**: 752–6.
  13 Connolly SA, Connolly LP, Jaramillo D. Imaging of sports injuries in children and adolescents. *Radiol Clin North Am* 2001; **39**: 773–90.
◆ 14 Peterson HA. Physeal and apophyseal injuries. In: Rockwood CAJ, Wilkins KE, Beaty JH. (eds.)

Fractures in children. Philadelphia: JB Lippincott, 1996: 103–66.

15 Goldberg HD, Young JW, Reiner BI, *et al*. Double injuries of the forearm: a common occurrence. *Radiology* 1992; **185**: 223–7.

● 16 Spitz J, Becker C, Tittel K, Weigand H. Clinical relevance of whole body skeletal scintigraphy in multiple injury and polytrauma patients. *Unfallchirurgie* 1992; **18**: 133–47.

17 Heinrich SD, Gallagher D, Harris M, Nadell JM. Undiagnosed fractures in severely injured children and young adults. Identification with technetium imaging. *J Bone Joint Surg Am* 1994; **76**: 561–72.

18 Dias JJ, Thompson J, Barton NJ, Gregg PJ. Suspected scaphoid fractures. The value of radiographs. *J Bone Joint Surg Br* 1990; **72**: 98–101.

● 19 Tiel-van Buul MM, Roolker W, Verbeeten BW, Broekhuizen AH. Magnetic resonance imaging versus bone scintigraphy in suspected scaphoid fracture. *Eur J Nucl Med* 1996; **23**: 971–5.

20 Thorpe AP, Murray AD, Smith FW, Ferguson J. Clinically suspected scaphoid fracture: a comparison of magnetic resonance imaging and bone scintigraphy. *Br J Radiol* 1996; **69**: 109–13.

21 Bellmore MC, Cummine JL, Crocker EF, Carseldine DB. The role of bone scans in the assessment of prognosis of scaphoid fractures. *Aust NZ J Surg* 1983; **53**: 133–7.

22 Rolfe EB, Garvie NW, Khan MA, Ackery DM. Isotope bone imaging in suspected scaphoid trauma. *Br J Radiol* 1981; **54**: 762–7.

23 Sopov W, Rozenbaum M, Rosner I, Groshar D. Scintigraphy of de Quervain's tenosynovitis. *Nucl Med Commun* 1999; **20**: 175–7.

● 24 Lewis SL, Rees JI, Thomas GV, Williams LA. Pitfalls of bone scintigraphy in suspected hip fractures. *Br J Radiol* 1991; **64**: 403–8.

● 25 Holder LH, Schwartz L, Wernicke PG, *et al*. Radionuclide bone imaging in the early detection of fractures of the proximal femur (hip). *Radiology* 1990; **174**: 509–15.

26 Slavin Jr JD, Mathews J, Spencer RP. Bone imaging in the diagnosis of fractures of the femur and pelvis in the sixth to tenth decades. *Clin Nucl Med* 1986; **11**: 328–30.

27 Englaro EE, Gelfand MJ, Paltiel HJ. Bone scintigraphy in preschool children with lower extremity pain of unknown origin. *J Nucl Med* 1992; **33**: 351–4.

● 28 Miller JH, Sanderson RA. Scintigraphy of toddler's fracture. *J Nucl Med* 1988; **29**: 2001–3.

29 Park HM, Kernek CB, Robb JA. Early scintigraphic findings of occult femoral and tibial fractures in infants. *Clin Nucl Med* 1988; **13**: 271–5.

● 30 Kleinman PK, Marks Jr SC. A regional approach to the classic metaphyseal lesion in abused infants: the proximal humerus. *Am J Roentgenol* 1996; **167**: 1399–403.

● 31 Sty JR, Starshak RJ. The role of bone scintigraphy in the evaluation of the suspected abused child. *Radiology* 1983; **146**: 369–75.

* 32 Kleinman PK. Shaken babies. *Lancet* 1998; **352**: 815–16.

33 Kleinman PK, Marks Jr SC, Nimkin K, *et al*. Rib fractures in 31 abused infants: postmortem radiologic-histopathologic study. *Radiology* 1996; **200**: 807–10.

34 Kleinman PK, Nimkin K, Spevak MR, *et al*. Follow-up skeletal surveys in suspected child abuse. *Am J Roentgenol* 1996; **167**: 893–6.

35 Strouse PJ, Owings CL. Fractures of the first rib in child abuse. *Radiology* 1995; **197**: 763–5.

◆ 36 Nimkin K, Kleinman PK. Imaging of child abuse. *Radiol Clin North Am* 2001; **39**: 843–64.

37 Abe H, Nakamura M, Takahashi S, *et al*. Radiation-induced insufficiency fractures of the pelvis: evaluation with ^{99m}Tc-methylene diphosphonate scintigraphy. *Am J Roentgenol* 1992; **158**: 599–602.

38 Cooper KL, Beabout JW, Swee RG. Insufficiency fractures of the sacrum. *Radiology* 1985; **156**: 15–20.

39 Grier D, Wardell S, Sarwark J, Poznanski AK. Fatigue fractures of the sacrum in children: two case reports and a review of the literature. *Skeletal Radiol* 1993; **22**: 515–18.

◆ 40 Peh WC, Khong PL, Yin Y, *et al*. Imaging of pelvic insufficiency fractures. *Radiographics* 1996; **16**: 335–48.

41 Davies AM, Evans NS, Struthers GR. Parasymphyseal and associated insufficiency fractures of the pelvis and sacrum. *Br J Radiol* 1988; **61**: 103–8.

42 Cook GJ, Hannaford E, See M, *et al*. The value of bone scintigraphy in the evaluation of osteoporotic patients with back pain. *Scand J Rheumatol* 2002; **31**: 245–8.

43 Versijpt J, Dierckx RA, De Bondt P, *et al*. The contribution of bone scintigraphy in occupational health or medical insurance claims: a retrospective study. *Eur J Nucl Med* 1999; **26**: 804–11.

44 Crisp TA. Tibialis posterior tendonitis associated with os naviculare. *Med Sci Sports Exerc* 1998; **30**: 1183–90.

45 Sinha P, Kim A, Umans H, Freeman LM. Scintigraphic findings in peroneal tendonitis: a case report. *Clin Nucl Med* 2000; **25**: 17–19.

◆ 46 Umans H. Ankle impingement syndromes. *Semin Musculoskelet Radiol* 2002; **6**: 133–40.

47 Johnson RP, Collier BD, Carrera GF. The os trigonum syndrome: use of bone scan in the diagnosis. *J Trauma* 1984; **24**: 761–4.

48 Huang H, Qureshi A, Biundo J. Sports and other soft tissue injuries, tendinitis, bursitis, and occupation-related syndromes. *Curr Opin Rheumatol* 2000; **12**: 150–4.

49 Yeung MS, Chan KM, So CH, Yuan WY. An epidemiological survey on ankle sprain. *Br J Sports Med* 1994; **28**: 112–16.

- 50   Fallat L, Grimm DJ, Saracco JA. Sprained ankle syndrome: prevalence and analysis of 639 acute injuries. *J Foot Ankle Surg* 1998; **37**: 280–5.

51   Shea MP, Manoli A. Osteochondral lesions of the talar dome. *Foot Ankle* 1993; **14**: 48–55.

52   Stroud CC, Marks RM. Imaging of osteochondral lesions of the talus. *Foot Ankle Clin* 2000; **5**: 119–33.

53   Anderson IF, Crichton KJ, Grattan-Smith T, *et al.* Osteochondral fractures of the dome of the talus. *J Bone Joint Surg* 1989; **71A**: 1143–52.

- 54   Frater C, Van Gaal W, Kannangara S, Van Der Wall H. Scintigraphy of Injuries to the distal tibiofibular syndesmosis. *Clin Nucl Med* 2002; **27**: 625–7.

55   Boden BP, Osbahr DC. High-risk stress fractures: evaluation and treatment. *J Am Acad Orthop Surg* 2000; **8**: 344–53.

56   Orava S, Karpakka J, Hulkko A, Takala T. Stress avulsion fracture of the tarsal navicular. An uncommon sports-related overuse injury. *Am J Sports Med* 1991; **19**: 392–5.

57   Lee EW, Donatto KC. Fractures of the midfoot and forefoot. *Curr Opin Orthop* 1999; **10**: 224–30.

58   Hodge JC. Anterior process fracture or calcaneus secundarius: a case report. *J Emerg Med* 1999; **17**: 305–9.

59   Greaney RB, Gerber FH, Laughlin RL, *et al.* Distribution and natural history of stress fractures in US Marine recruits. *Radiology* 1983; **146**: 339–46.

60   Pester S, Smith PC. Stress fractures in the lower extremities of soldiers in basic training. *Orthop Rev* 1992; **21**: 297–303.

61   Brudvig TJ, Gudger TD, Obermeyer L. Stress fractures in 295 trainees: a one-year study of incidence as related to age, sex and race. *Milit Med* 1983; **148**: 666–7.

- 62   Donahue SW, Sharkey NA. Strains in the metatarsals during the stance phase of gait: implications for stress fractures. *J Bone Joint Surg* 1999; **81A**: 1236–44.

63   Hulkko A, Orava S, Nikula P. Stress fracture of the fifth metatarsal in athletes. *Ann Chir Gynaecol* 1985; **74**: 233–8.

64   Georgoulias P, Georgiadis I, Dimakopoulos N, Mortzos G. Scintigraphy of stress fractures of the sesamoid bones. *Clin Nucl Med* 2001; **26**: 944–5.

- ◆ 65   Bohne WH. Tarsal coalition. *Curr Opin Pediatr* 2001; **13**: 29–35.

- 66   Mandell GA, Harcke HT, Hugh J, *et al.* Detection of talocalcaneal coalitions by magnification bone scintigraphy. *J Nucl Med* 1990; **31**: 1797–801.

67   McBryde Jr AM. Stress fractures in athletes. *J Sports Med* 1975; **3**: 212–17.

68   McBryde AM. Stress fractures in runners. *Clin Sports Med* 1985; **4**: 737–52.

69   Kortebein PM, Kaufman KR, Basford JR, Stuart MJ. Medial tibial stress syndrome. *Med Sci Sports Exerc* 2000; **32**: S27–33.

- 70   Holder LE, Michael RH. The specific scintigraphic pattern of 'shin splints' in the lower leg: Concise communication. *J Nucl Med* 1984; **25**: 865–9.

71   Geslien GE, Thrall JH, Espinosa JL, Older RA. Early detection of stress fractures using ^{99m}Tc-polyphosphate. *Radiology* 1976; **121**: 683–7.

72   Brukner P, Bennell K. Stress fractures in female athletes. Diagnosis, management and rehabilitation. *Sports Med* 1997; **24**: 419–29.

73   Ishibashi Y, Okamura Y, Otsuka H, *et al.* Comparison of scintigraphy and magnetic resonance imaging for stress injuries of bone. *Clin J Sport Med* 2002; **12**: 79–84.

- 74   Zwas ST, Elkanovitch R, Frank G. Interpretation and classification of bone scintigraphic findings in stress fractures. *J Nucl Med* 1987; **28**: 452–7.

75   Bennell KL, Brukner PD. Epidemiology and site specificity of stress fractures. *Clin Sports Med* 1997; **16**: 179–96.

76   al-Janabi MA. The role of bone scintigraphy and other imaging modalities in knee pain. *Nucl Med Commun* 1994; **15**: 991–6.

- 77   Murray IPC, Dixon J, Kohan L. SPECT for acute knee pain. *Clin Nucl Med* 1990; **15**: 828–40.

78   Ryan PJ, Chauduri R, Bingham J, Fogelman I. A comparison of MRI and bone SPET in the diagnosis of knee pathology. *Nucl Med Commun* 1996; **17**: 125–31.

- 79   Ryan PJ, Reddy K, Fleetcroft J. A prospective comparison of clinical examination, MRI, bone SPECT, and arthroscopy to detect meniscal tears. *Clin Nucl Med* 1998; **23**: 803–6.

80   So Y, Chung JK, Seong SC, *et al.* Usefulness of ^{99}Tc^{m}-MDP knee SPET for pre-arthroscopic evaluation of patients with internal derangements of the knee. *Nucl Med Commun* 2000; **21**: 103–9.

- 81   Collier BD, Johnson RP, Carrera GF, *et al.* Chronic knee pain assessed by SPECT: comparison with other modalities. *Radiology* 1985; **157**: 795–802.

82   Ryan PJ. Bone SPECT of the knees. *Nucl Med Commun* 2000; **21**: 877–85.

83   Chung HW, Kim YH, Hong SH, *et al.* Indirect signs of anterior cruciate ligament injury on SPET: comparsion with MRI and arthroscopy. *Nucl Med Commun* 2000; **21**: 651–8.

84   Cook GJ, Fogelman I. Lateral collateral ligament tear of the knee: appearances on bone scintigraphy with single-photon emission tomography. *Eur J Nucl Med* 1996; **23**: 720–2.

85   Marks PH, Goldenberg JA, Vezina WC, *et al.* Subchondral bone infractions in acute ligamentous knee injuries demonstrated on bone scintigraphy and magnetic resonance imaging. *J Nucl Med* 1992; **33**: 516–20.

86   Charkes ND, Siddhivarn N, Schneck CD. Bone scanning in the adductor insertion avulsion syndrome ('thigh splints'). *J Nucl Med* 1987; **28**: 1835.

87 Matin P, Lang G, Carretta R, Simon G. Scintigraphic evaluation of muscle damage following extreme exercise: concise communication. *J Nucl Med* 1983; **24**: 308–11.

88 Volpin G, Hoerer D, Groisman G, *et al.* Stress fractures of the femoral neck following strenuous activity. *J Orthop Trauma* 1990; **4**: 394–8.

89 Amendola A, Wolcott M. Bony injuries around the hip. *Sports Med Arthroscopy Rev* 2002; **10**: 163–7.

90 Shah MK, Stewart GW. Sacral stress fractures: an unusual cause of low back pain in an athlete. *Spine* 2002; **27**: E104–8.

91 Hill PF, Chatterji S, Chambers D, Keeling JD. Stress fracture of the pubic ramus in female recruits. *J Bone Joint Surg Br* 1996; **78**: 383–6.

92 Le Jeune JJ, Rochcongar P, Vazelle F, *et al.* Pubic pain syndrome in sportsmen: comparison of radiographic and scintigraphic findings. *Eur J Nucl Med* 1984; **9**: 250–3.

93 Frater CJ. Importance of positioning and frequency of unexpected scintigraphic findings in a high impact sport. *Nucl Med Commun* 2001; **22**: 1231–5.

94 Hickey GJ, Fricker PA, McDonald WA. Injuries to elite rowers over a 10-yr period. *Med Sci Sports Exerc* 1997; **29**: 1567–72.

95 Murray IPC, Frater CJ. Prominence of the C2 vertebra on SPECT. A normal variant. *Clin Nucl Med* 1994; **19**: 855–9.

96 Seitz JP, Unguez CE, Corbus HF, Wooten WW. SPECT of the cervical spine in the evaluation of neck pain after trauma. *Clin Nucl Med* 1995; **20**: 667–73.

97 Congeni J, McCulloch J, Swanson K. Lumbar spondylolysis. A study of natural progression in athletes. *Am J Sports Med* 1997; **25**: 248–53.

98 Gates GF. Oblique angle bone SPECT imaging of the lumbar spine, pelvis and hips. *Clin Nucl Med* 1996; **21**: 359–62.

99 Gates GF. Bone SPECT imaging of the painful back. *Clin Nucl Med* 1996; **21**: 560–71.

100 Ryan PJ, Fogelman I. The role of nuclear medicine in orthopaedics. *Nucl Med Commun* 1994; **15**: 341–60.

101 Raby N, Matthews S. Symptomatic spondylolysis: correlation of CT and SPECT with clinical outcome. *Clin Radiol* 1993; **48**: 97–9.

102 Howarth D, Southee A, Cardew P, Front D. SPECT in avulsion injury of the multifidus and rotator muscles of the lumbar region. *Clin Nucl Med* 1994; **19**: 571–4.

103 Clunie G, Bomanji J, Ell PJ. Technetium-99m-MDP patterns in patients with painful shoulder lesions. *J Nucl Med* 1997; **38**: 1491–5.

104 Roach PJ, Cooper RA. Arm-splints seen on a bone scan in a volleyball player. *Clin Nucl Med* 1993; **18**: 900–1.

105 Van der Wall H, Frater CJ, Magee MA, *et al.* A novel view for the scintigraphic assessment of the elbow. *Nucl Med Commun* 1999; **20**: 1059–65.

106 Knirk JL, Jupiter JB. Intra-articular fractures of the distal end of the radius in young adults. *J Bone Joint Surg* 1986; **68A**: 647–59.

107 Maurer AH. Nuclear medicine in evaluation of the hand and wrist. *Hand Clin* 1991; **7**: 183–200.

108 Patel N, Collier BD, Carrera GF, *et al.* High-resolution bone scintigraphy of the adult wrist. *Clin Nucl Med* 1992; **17**: 449–53.

109 Sherman GM, Seitz WH. Fractures and dislocations of the wrist. *Curr Opin Orthop* 1999; **10**: 237–51.

110 Mohamed A, Ryan P, Lewis M, *et al.* Registration bone scan in the evaluation of wrist pain. *J Hand Surg (Br)* 1997; **22**: 161–6.

111 Auchincloss JM, Watt I. Scintigraphy in the evaluation of potential fracture healing: a clinical study of tibial fractures. *Br J Radiol* 1982; **55**: 707–13.

112 Desai A, Alavi A, Dalinka M, Brighton C, Esterhai J. Role of bone scintigraphy in the evaluation and treatment of nonunited fractures: concise communication. *J Nucl Med* 1980; **21**: 931–4.

113 Slizofski WJ, Collier BD, Flatley TJ, *et al.* Painful pseudarthrosis following lumbar spinal fusion: detection by combined SPECT and planar bone scintigraphy. *Skeletal Radiol* 1987; **16**: 136–41.

114 Even-Sapir E, Martin RH, Mitchell MJ, *et al.* Assessment of painful late effects of lumbar spinal fusion with SPECT. *J Nucl Med* 1994; **35**: 416–22.

115 Esterhai J, Alavi A, Mandell GA, Brown J. Sequential technetium-99m/gallium-67 scintigraphic evaluation of subclinical osteomyelitis complicating fracture nonunion. *J Orthop Res* 1985; **3**: 219–25.

116 Kim EE, Pjura GA, Lowry PA, *et al.* Osteomyelitis complicating fracture: pitfalls of ^{111}In leukocyte scintigraphy. *Am J Roentgenol* 1987; **148**: 927–30.

Radionuclide evaluation of the failed joint replacement

CHRISTOPHER J. PALESTRO

INTRODUCTION

The concept of reconstructing the failed human joint has existed for several thousand years, and sporadic attempts at joint arthroplasty were carried out in the nineteenth century. The era of modern joint replacement surgery, which revolutionized the treatment of advanced hip and knee disorders, did not begin in earnest until the second half of the twentieth century.[1]

Sir John Charnley, who has been called the father of the total hip replacement, developed the predecessors of today's hip replacements during the late 1950s and early 1960s. The hip prosthesis of today is a modular device, which allows the surgeon to modify the different components to suit an individual patient's needs. An arthroplasty that consists of both femoral and acetabular components is known as a 'total hip arthroplasty'; an arthroplasty in which the femoral component articulates with the native acetabulum is referred to as a 'hemiarthroplasty'. In addition to polymethylmethacrylate (PMMA), or surgical cement, there are several ways by which these devices, that are composed of metal (cobalt-chromium and titanium), and an ultrahigh molecular weight (UHMW) polyethylene plastic, can be secured to the native bone.[2,3] Fixation of the cementless, porous coated prosthesis is the result of bony ingrowth into a porous coating applied to the surface of the device. In some prostheses, the surface of the components is coated with a hydroxyapatite compound that stimulates new bone formation and serves as an attachment for newly formed osseous tissue around the hardware. Acetabular components can also be forced, or press-fit, into the acetabulum

and, if needed, can be further secured with orthopedic screws.[4]

If Sir John Charnley is the father of the hip replacement, then Dr John Insall is surely the father of the knee replacement. The prototype of the modern knee replacement, the total condylar knee replacement, was developed at the Hospital for Special Surgery in New York City, in the mid 1970s under Dr Insall's direction.[1] It was a fixed-bearing implant, consisting of a one-piece metallic femoral component, a polyethylene patellar component, and a polyethylene tibial tray with a central peg. The modern, mobile-bearing prosthesis offers greater joint mobility with less polyethylene breakdown than its fixed-bearing predecessor.[1,5]

Implant failure

Nearly 500 000 hip and knee arthroplasties are performed annually in the United States, and it is estimated that by the year 2030, this number may exceed 700 000.[4] Although the clinical results of joint replacement surgery are usually excellent, these implants do fail. Failures due to infection, fracture and dislocation are now relatively rare, while failure due to aseptic loosening has continued to increase in incidence. More than 25% of all prostheses will eventually demonstrate evidence of loosening, often necessitating revision arthroplasty.[4] While inappropriate mechanical load, fatigue failure at the bone prosthesis or cement prosthesis interface, implant motion, and hydrodynamic pressure are sometimes responsible, the most important cause of aseptic loosening is an inflammatory reaction to one or more of the prosthetic components.[6] Particulate debris, produced by component fragmentation, presumably attracts and activates the tissue phagocytes normally present around the prosthesis. This debris, impervious to regular enzymatic destruction, frustrates the degradative function of the inflammatory cells and leads to repeated, but futile, attempts at phagocytosis. This process, in turn, stimulates the secretion of proinflammatory cytokines and proteolytic enzymes that damage bone and cartilage and activate immune cells. The heightened inflammatory response leads to osteolysis, which, if unchecked, results in loss of supporting osseous tissues and, eventually, loosening of the prosthesis. Histopathologically, a synovial-like pseudomembranous structure develops at the cement–bone interface. The cellular composition of this pseudomembrane is variable: histiocytes are the most commonly identified cell (95% of specimens) in the pseudomembrane, followed by giant cells (80%), and lymphocytes and plasma cells (25%). Neutrophils are present in less than 10% of the cases.[7–9]

Though uncommon, infection is perhaps the most serious complication of joint arthroplasty surgery, ranging in frequency from about 1% to 2% for primary implants, to about 3–5% for revision implants.[10] Risk factors for infection include the characteristics of the operating room, quality of the native bone, and complexity of the surgery. Immunocompromised patients and those with diabetes mellitus and rheumatoid arthritis are at increased risk for infection.[6] Bacteria readily bind to most of the materials used in joint arthroplasty surgery. In fact, once attached to the implant, *Staphylococcus epidermidis*, one of the most commonly identified causative organisms, produces a surface glycocalyx to protect itself from the host inflammatory response.[6] Other organisms identified in joint replacement infections include *Staphylococcus aureus*, and less commonly, *Streptococcus viridans*, *Escherichia coli*, *Enterococcus faecalis*, and group B *Streptococcus*.[11] About one third of prosthetic joint infections develop within 3 months, another third within 1 year, and the remainder more than 1 year after surgery.[12] Histopathologically, the inflammatory reaction accompanying the infected prosthesis is similar to that present in aseptic loosening, with one important difference: neutrophils, usually absent in aseptic loosening, are invariably present in large numbers in infection.[11,12]

The treatment of infected hardware often requires multiple admissions. An excisional arthroplasty, or removal of the prosthesis, is performed, followed by a protracted course of antimicrobial therapy. Eventually, a revision arthroplasty is carried out. Aseptic loosening, in contrast, usually is managed with a single stage exchange arthroplasty requiring only one hospital admission and one surgical intervention.[4]

Because their treatments are so radically different, the importance of distinguishing infection from aseptic loosening of a prosthesis cannot be overemphasized. This distinction, unfortunately, can be challenging. Clinical signs of infection such as joint pain, swelling and erythema are often absent. Elevated peripheral blood leukocytes, an elevated erythrocyte sedimentation rate, and the presence of

C-reactive protein level are suggestive of, but are neither sensitive nor specific for, infection. The results of joint aspiration have been disappointing with large numbers of false positive and false negative results having been reported.[4,13–16] Plain radiographs are neither sensitive nor specific and the hardware-induced artifacts limit the utility of cross-sectional imaging modalities, such as computed tomography and magnetic resonance imaging.[4]

Radionuclide studies, which reflect physiologic processes, are not limited by the presence of metallic hardware and are extremely useful in the evaluation of the painful joint replacement, especially when infection is suspected.

RADIONUCLIDE IMAGING

Bone scintigraphy

Bone scintigraphy, widely available and easily performed, is a sensitive technique for detecting complications of prosthetic surgery. Gelman *et al.*[17] reported that bone scintigraphy had an accuracy of 85% for diagnosing loosening of a hip prosthesis. Weiss *et al.*[18] found that bone scintigraphy was 100% sensitive and 77% specific for diagnosing infection or loosening of the total hip replacement, and concluded that bone scintigraphy was a useful technique for identifying prostheses requiring surgical treatment. McInerney and Hyde[19] came to similar conclusions: bone scintigraphy is useful for identifying the failed joint prosthesis, but cannot distinguish among the causes for failure. Unfortunately, merely confirming that a prosthesis has failed is usually not sufficient; the cause of the failure must be determined, if appropriate treatment is to be instituted. Williamson *et al.*[20] suggested that it was possible, by analyzing periprosthetic uptake patterns, to distinguish aseptic loosening from infection of hip prostheses. They found that focal periprosthetic uptake was associated with loosening, while diffuse uptake around both the femoral and acetabular components was associated with infection (Fig. 9E.1). Williams *et al.*[21] reviewed 38 total hip replacements, 14 of which were infected. While all 14 infected prostheses demonstrated the diffuse pattern of periprosthetic uptake, diffuse periprosthetic activity was also present around 13 uninfected prostheses. Mountford *et al.*[22] found that, although the diffuse pattern of periprosthetic uptake was reasonably specific for infection, it was present in only five out of 11 (45%) infected joint replacements, and thus was not sensitive. Aliabadi *et al.*[23] reported that bone scintigraphy was moderately sensitive and very specific for diagnosing loosening with or without infection, but could not distinguish the loosened uninfected from the loosened, infected prosthesis. Lieberman *et al.*[24] reported that bone scintigraphy was sensitive and specific for identifying loosening of both the femoral and acetabular components of hip replacements. They excluded infected devices from

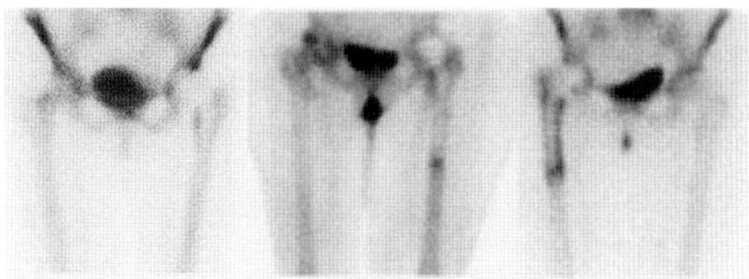

Figure 9E.1 *Left: Normal bone scan of a left total hip replacement. Periprosthetic activity is indistinguishable from activity in adjacent nonarticular bone. Middle: Focally increased uptake at the tip of the femoral component of a left hip replacement is often associated with aseptic loosening of cemented prostheses more than 1 year old. Unfortunately, during the first year after implantation this can be a normal finding. In the case of cementless devices, focal uptake at the distal tip of the femoral component, can persist for well beyond 1 year, even in asymptomatic patients. Right: Diffusely increased activity around the shaft of a right hip replacement has been ascribed to infection. This pattern is produced by periprosthetic osteolysis, which occurs not only in infection, but in aseptic loosening as well.*

their analysis, however. The interpretation of bone scintigraphy is further complicated by the numerous patterns of periprosthetic uptake associated with asymptomatic hip replacements. During the first year following implantation of a total hip replacement, periprosthetic uptake patterns are very variable; beyond 1 year, in the case of the cemented hip replacement, 10% of asymptomatic patients demonstrate persistent uptake, even in the absence of any complications.[25] In the case of the cementless or porous-coated hip replacement, persistent uptake beyond 1 year is even more frequent.[26–28] The use of hybrid, bipolar and hydroxyapatite coated devices further complicates matters, as few data are available about the evolution of normal periprosthetic uptake patterns around these devices.

Evaluation of knee replacements with bone scintigraphy is even more problematic than that of hip prostheses, as increased periprosthetic activity can persist for some time after implantation. Periprosthetic activity has been observed in more than 60% of the femoral components and nearly 90% of the tibial components of asymptomatic knee replacements more than 1 year after their implantation.[29] Palestro et al.[30] reviewed the role of bone scintigraphy for diagnosing infected total knee replacements and found that the study was neither sensitive nor specific. Hoffman et al.[31] studied asymptomatic cemented and cementless knee replacements with serial bone scans over a 2-year period. These investigators found that although, in general, periprosthetic activity decreased over time after implantation, there was considerable patient-to-patient variation. They concluded that a single study cannot reliably detect prosthetic failure, and that sequential scans are needed.

The majority of lower extremity joint replacement infections occur within 1 year after implantation, when, regardless of the type or location of the prosthesis, periprosthetic uptake is so variable that only a normal bone scan contributes useful information. The overall accuracy of radionuclide bone imaging in the evaluation of the painful prosthetic joint is about 50–70%.[32] Despite this, the study does have a high negative predictive value and can be used as an initial

screening test, or in conjunction with other diagnostic tests (see Case history 1 on page 389).

Bone–gallium imaging

Gallium-67 citrate has had an important role in the radionuclide diagnosis of infection ever since its propensity to accumulate in inflammation and infection was first recognized three decades ago. Several factors appear to be responsible for gallium uptake in infection. Following injection, approximately 99% of circulating gallium is in the plasma, bound primarily to transferrin. Inflammation is characterized by increased perfusion and increased vascular membrane permeability which result in increased delivery and increased accumulation of plasma proteins and hence, gallium, at inflammatory sites. At least some of this tracer is probably bound to circulating leukocytes that then migrate to foci of infection. Bacteria also affect gallium uptake in infection. Direct bacterial uptake of gallium has been demonstrated *in vitro*. Siderophores, low molecular weight chelating agents produced by bacteria, have a high affinity for gallium. Presumably, the siderophore–gallium complex is transported into the bacterium, from which it cannot be released without destruction of the entire molecule. The plasma protein lactoferrin is present in inflammatory exudates. It is thought that gallium, delivered to the site of infection primarily as a gallium–transferrin complex, dissociates from transferrin and complexes with lactoferrin.[33]

Although uptake of gallium in inflammatory conditions was first noted in the early 1970s, it was not until the latter half of that decade that extensive investigations of its role in musculoskeletal infection were conducted. In one series, 79 patients with painful lower extremity joint replacements underwent bone and gallium imaging. Bone scintigraphy was very sensitive (100%), but very nonspecific (15%). Gallium scintigraphy, in contrast, was both sensitive (95%) and specific (100%).[34] Rushton et al.[35] reported that all 13 patients with an infected hip prosthesis demonstrated

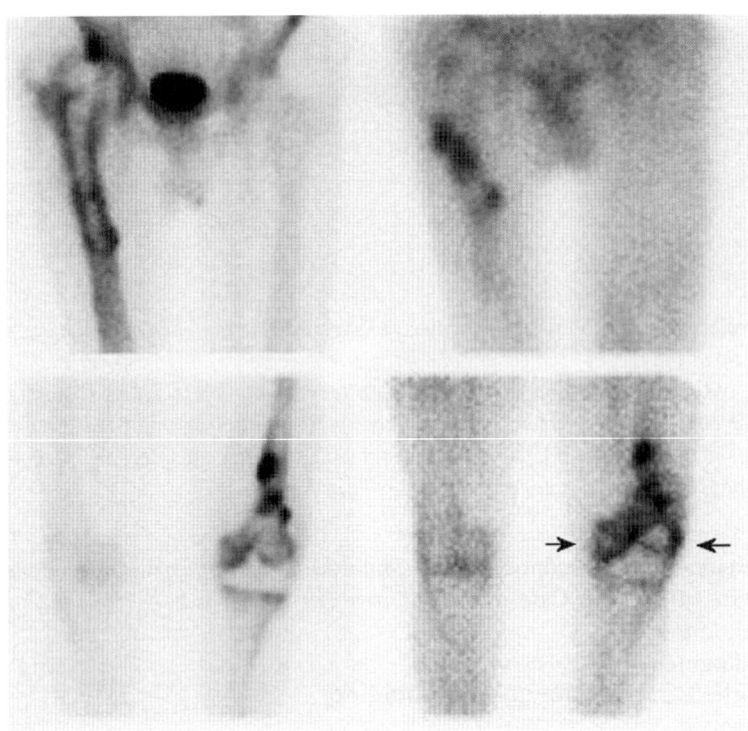

Figure 9E.2 *Top: The distribution of activity on the bone (left) and gallium (right) images is spatially incongruent, and the combined study is positive for infection. Bottom: The distribution of activity on the bone (left) and gallium (right) images is spatially congruent, but the intensity of periprosthetic uptake on the gallium image is greater than that on the bone image and the combined study is positive for infection.*

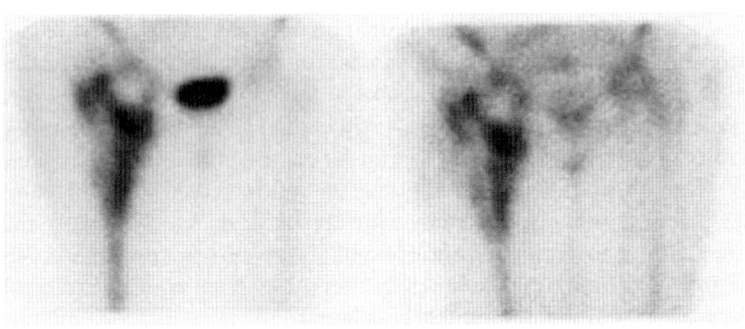

Figure 9E.3 *The distribution of activity on the bone (left) and gallium (right) images is congruent, both spatially and in intensity, and the combined study is equivocal for infection.*

abnormal periprosthetic accumulation of gallium, while none of 18 patients with aseptically loosened devices demonstrated abnormal periprosthetic activity (100% accuracy). McKillop *et al.*[36] reported that gallium images were abnormal in five of six infected joint replacements and normal in seven of nine uninfected prostheses (80% accuracy). Mountford *et al.*[22] also found that the accuracy of gallium scintigraphy for diagnosing prosthetic hip infection was about 80%. Aliabadi *et al.*[23] reported that gallium scintigraphy was only 37% sensitive, but 100% specific for prosthetic hip infection. Unfortunately, gallium accumulates in both septic and aseptic inflammation, as well as in the bone marrow, and in areas of increased bone mineral turnover in the absence of infection. In an effort to improve the accuracy of both bone and gallium imaging, the two studies are often interpreted together, according to standardized criteria.[37] Sequential bone–gallium imaging is:

- *Positive for infection* when the distribution of the two radiotracers is spatially incongruent or when their distribution is spatially congruent *and* the intensity of gallium uptake exceeds that of the bone agent (Fig. 9E.2)
- *Equivocal for infection* when the distribution of the two tracers is spatially congruent *and* the relative intensity of uptake of each tracer is similar (Fig. 9E.3)
- *Negative for infection* when gallium images are normal, regardless of the bone scan findings, or when the spatial distribution of the two tracers is congruent *and* the relative intensity of gallium uptake is less than that of the bone tracer (Fig. 9E.4)

Interestingly, interpreting bone and gallium images together has not resulted in a marked improvement in accuracy over either study alone. Although Tehranzadeh *et al.*[38] reported a 95% accuracy for the combined study, most other investigations have reported less satisfactory results. Williams *et al.*[21] investigated bone and gallium imaging in 30 patients with painful joint prostheses, 14 of which were infected. All 30 prostheses demonstrated increased periprosthetic activity on the bone images. While 13/14 infected joint replacements

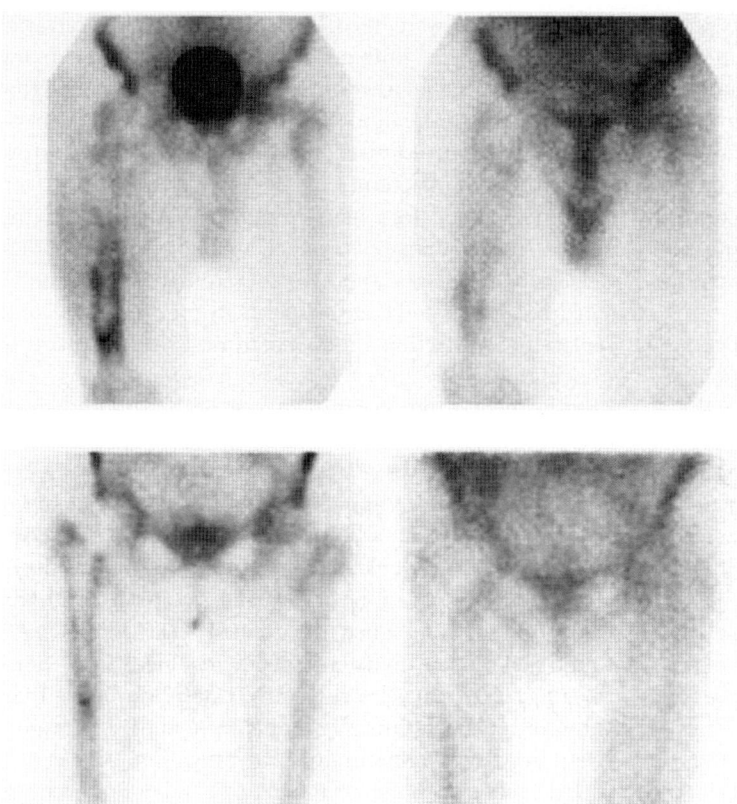

Figure 9E.4 *Top: The distribution of activity on the bone (left) and gallium (right) images is spatially congruent, but the intensity of periprosthetic uptake on the gallium image is less than that on the bone image and the combined study is negative for infection. Bottom: Focally increased activity is present at the tip of the femoral component on the bone image (left). The gallium image (right) is normal, and therefore the combined study is negative for infection.*

demonstrated abnormal gallium uptake, only 2/16 uninfected prostheses demonstrated abnormal gallium uptake. When these investigators interpreted bone and gallium images together, however, they found that only seven of the 14 infected joint replacements demonstrated spatially incongruent bone–gallium images; in the other seven infected joint replacements, the images were congruent. In a prospective investigation, Merkel *et al.*[39] evaluated bone–gallium imaging in a canine model, and found that the sensitivity, specificity and accuracy of the technique for diagnosing the infected joint replacement were 61%, 71% and 67%, respectively. These investigators, in a retrospective review of 130 patients with painful orthopedic prostheses, reported that sequential bone–gallium imaging was 66% sensitive, 81% specific, and 77% accurate for diagnosing the infected joint replacement.[40] Gomez-Luzuriaga *et al.*[41] evaluated 40 patients with painful total hip replacements, who subsequently underwent surgery, and reported a sensitivity, specificity and accuracy of 70%, 90% and 80%, respectively, for combined bone–gallium imaging. Kraemer *et al.*[42] reported 38% sensitivity, and 100% specificity for bone–gallium imaging for diagnosing prosthetic hip infection. With an accuracy that ranges from about 60% to about 80%, bone–gallium scintigraphy offers only a modest improvement over bone scintigraphy alone, and is of limited value for diagnosing prosthetic joint infection.

Scintigraphy using labeled leukocytes

The accumulation of labeled leukocytes at a focus of infection depends on intact chemotaxis, the number and types of cells labeled, and the principal cellular component of a given inflammatory response. Regardless of whether only granulocytes or a mixed population of leukocytes are labeled, the majority of cells labeled are neutrophils. Hence, imaging using labeled leukocytes is most sensitive for detecting neutrophil-mediated inflammatory processes.[32] Although neutrophils are almost always found in the infected joint prosthesis, the accuracy of labeled leukocyte imaging for diagnosing this entity has been the subject of controversy. Some investigators have found the study to be reasonably sensitive and specific. Merkel *et al.*[39] prospectively evaluated labeled leukocyte imaging in a canine model. Using periprosthetic uptake greater than surrounding bone activity, they reported a sensitivity of 94% and specificity of 86% for diagnosing infection. Pring *et al.*,[43] using labeled granulocytes, evaluated 50 prosthetic joints, and classified any periprosthetic activity as positive for infection. They reported that the test was 100% sensitive and 89.5% specific for diagnosing infection. They reported similar results in another investigation, observing that the intensity of periprosthetic uptake was always significant in the setting of infection; in 16/18 infected devices uptake was at least as intense as it was in normal marrow.[44] Rand and Brown[45] studied 38 painful knee replacements, and classified studies demonstrating moderately to markedly increased activity as positive for infection. They reported that labeled leukocyte imaging was 83% sensitive and 85% specific. Magnuson *et al.*[46] studied 98 patients with suspected orthopedic implant infection. When scans showing at least minimally increased activity were classified as positive for infection, the sensitivity and specificity of the technique were 88% and 73% respectively.

Some investigators have reported that labeled leukocyte scintigraphy is specific, but not sensitive. Mountford et al.[22] reported that using periprosthetic uptake more intense than the contralateral hip, labeled leukocyte imaging was only 78% sensitive, but 95% specific for prosthetic hip infection. McKillop et al.[36] reported 50% sensitivity and 100% specificity. The poor sensitivity of white cell imaging was attributed to the chronic nature of the process.

Still other investigators have reported that labeled leukocyte imaging is sensitive but not specific for diagnosing infected joint replacements. Wukich et al.[47] reported that the technique was 100% sensitive but only 45% specific for diagnosing prosthetic joint infection, and speculated that false positive studies may have resulted from nonspecific aseptic inflammation. Johnson et al.[48] reported that labeled leukocyte imaging was 100% sensitive, but only 50% specific for diagnosing the infected hip replacement.

What then is the explanation for these contradictory results? It must be recalled that the accuracy of labeled leukocyte imaging is directly related to the presence or absence of neutrophils in a given situation. The paucity of neutrophils in the aseptically loosened prosthesis, together with their invariable presence in infected hardware, rules against chronicity and nonspecific inflammation as explanations for the poor results that have been reported by some investigators. The explanation for the varying and often contradictory results that have been reported is related to the methods used for image interpretation. In these investigations, images were interpreted as positive for infection when the intensity of uptake in the region of interest exceeded that of some reference point or when activity outside the normal distribution of the tracer was observed. Unfortunately, the intensity of uptake in a focus of infection, as well as the normal distribution of labeled leukocytes, can be very variable. Palestro et al.[49] reported that the sensitivity and specificity of labeled leukocyte imaging for diagnosing infected hip replacements varied with the criteria used for interpretation of the images. When any periprosthetic activity was considered positive for infection, the test was 100% sensitive, but only 23% specific. When only activity more intense than the contralateral side was considered positive for infection, the specificity rose to 61%, but the sensitivity fell to 65%. These investigators observed similar changes in specificity when these same criteria were applied to knee replacements.[30]

The normal distribution of hematopoietically active marrow in an adult is limited to the axial skeleton and proximal humeri and femurs, with activity outside these regions interpreted as indicating osseous infection. There is, however, considerable individual-to-individual variation. Generalized marrow expansion, which may be either transient or permanent, is a response to a systemic process, such as tumor, various anemias, and myelophthisic states.[32] Localized marrow expansion, which is usually transient, is a response to a local stimulus, such as fracture, inflammation,

orthopedic hardware, the Charcot joint, and even calvarial hyperostosis.[32,50,51] Both generalized and localized marrow expansion can alter the 'normal' distribution of marrow making it very difficult to separate uptake of labeled leukocytes in atypically located, but otherwise normal, marrow from uptake in infection.

Some investigators have found that interpreting the labeled leukocyte images together with conventional radionuclide bone images improves the accuracy of the study. Wukich et al.[47] found that the specificity for diagnosing joint replacement infection improved from 45% for leukocyte imaging alone to 85% for leukocyte/bone imaging. The improvement came at the expense of sensitivity, which decreased from 100% to 85%. Johnson et al.[48] reported similar results in their study of total hip replacements. Combined leukocyte/bone imaging offered a higher specificity, 95% versus 50%, but a lower sensitivity, 88% versus 100%, than labeled leukocyte imaging alone. The results of subsequent investigations have been less satisfactory. In an evaluation of total knee replacements, Palestro et al.[30] found that the sensitivity and specificity of leukocyte–bone imaging, 67% and 78% respectively, were no better than those of leukocyte imaging alone, 89% and 75% respectively. Recently, in a preliminary investigation, Love et al.[52] found leukocyte–bone imaging to be no more accurate than leukocyte imaging alone for diagnosing the infected hip replacement. Work by Oswald et al.[26] also suggests that the leukocyte–bone technique has limitations. They found that in 15% of asymptomatic patients with porous-coated hip arthroplasties, leukocyte–bone images were incongruent and they concluded that, in patients with this type of hip replacement, incongruence of activity is of little clinical utility. A limitation of the leukocyte–bone technique is that, while diphosphonates accumulate in bone, labeled leukocytes accumulate in marrow. Conditions that affect marrow may or may not affect bone and vice versa. Even when a particular entity affects both bone and marrow, the effects may be dramatically different, such as in patients undergoing radiation therapy.[53]

While some investigators have combined labeled leukocyte imaging with bone scintigraphy in an effort to improve the accuracy of the technique for diagnosing the infected joint replacement, others have used labeled leukocyte imaging in conjunction with sulfur colloid marrow imaging for this same purpose. The principle of leukocyte–marrow imaging is very simple. Both labeled leukocytes and sulfur colloid accumulate in the reticuloendothelial cells, or fixed macrophages, of the bone marrow. The distribution of marrow activity on leukocyte and sulfur colloid images is similar in normal individuals as well as in those with underlying marrow abnormalities. The images are, in other words, spatially congruent. The exception to this is osteomyelitis, which exerts opposite effects on labeled leukocytes and sulfur colloid. While stimulating uptake of white cells, osteomyelitis suppresses uptake of sulfur colloid. In osteomyelitis, therefore, in contrast to other conditions that

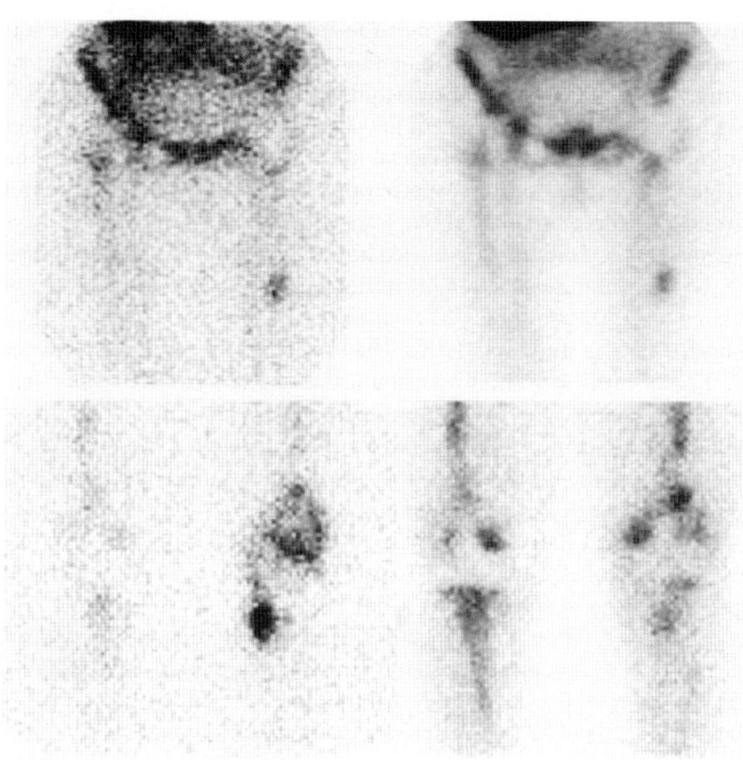

Figure 9E.5 *Top: Moderately intense labeled leukocyte activity (left) is present at the tip of the femoral component of a left hip prosthesis. Interpreted in isolation, this easily could be misconstrued as indicative of infection. Virtually the same distribution of activity is present on the marrow image (right), and the combined study is negative for infection. Bottom: The distribution of periprosthetic activity around a left knee replacement on the labeled leukocyte (left) and sulfur colloid marrow images (right) is spatially incongruent and the combined study is positive for infection. Notice, however, that the area of discordance is confined to the knee itself. The remainder of the activity in the distal femur and proximal tibia is due to marrow. It is important to be cognizant of the fact that the distribution of marrow is extremely variable, and that the presence of labeled leukocyte activity outside the expected 'normal' marrow distribution cannot automatically be equated with infection. Note the distribution of activity around the asymptomatic right knee replacement.*

affect the marrow, the leukocyte and marrow images are spatially incongruent (Fig. 9E.5).[32]

Mulamba *et al.*[54] reported a sensitivity of 92% and a specificity of 100% for diagnosing infected hip replacements with combined leukocyte marrow imaging. Palestro *et al.*[49] as part of a larger series, reviewed the results of labeled leukocyte–marrow imaging performed on 50 patients with painful total hip replacements, and found that the study was 100% sensitive and 97% specific for diagnosing infection. In a subsequent investigation of painful knee replacements, they obtained comparable results and found that leukocyte–marrow imaging was superior to bone scintigraphy, leukocyte imaging, and combined leukocyte–bone imaging.[30] In contrast to these uniformly excellent results, one recent investigation found that, though leukocyte–marrow imaging was 100% specific, it was only 46% sensitive for diagnosing prosthetic joint infection.[55] When a 'flow phase' was added to the marrow portion of the study, sensitivity improved to 66%, and specificity decreased to 98%. The reasons for the discordant results, according to the investigators, were related to lack of operative confirmation in all cases, and insufficient length of clinical follow-up in many patients in previous studies. There are, however, other equally important differences between this and previous investigations. First of all, these investigators used 370 kBq (10 μCi), rather than 370 MBq (10 mCi), of ^{99m}Tc sulfur colloid. Second, no information on the quality of the sulfur colloid preparation was given. Third, leukocytes were sent to an outside radiopharmacy for labeling. Fourth, and

perhaps most importantly, images were interpreted by a bone radiologist, with no indication of this individual's experience in interpreting radionuclide studies. Finally, no examples of false negative studies were provided. Love *et al.*[56] recently reviewed the results of leukocyte–marrow imaging performed on 59 patients with failed lower extremity joint replacements. In this series, experienced personnel labeled the leukocytes on-site, all patients received 370 MBq (10 mCi) of freshly prepared ^{99m}Tc sulfur colloid, and experienced nuclear physicians interpreted all images. Finally, all 59 patients had surgical and histopathogical/microbiological confirmation of the final diagnosis. In this investigation, the results of leukocyte–marrow imaging were comparable to what most previous studies have shown: 100% sensitivity, 91% specificity, and 95% accuracy for diagnosing joint replacement infection.

The importance of meticulous technique to the success of combined leukocyte–marrow scintigraphy cannot be overemphasized. When the combined study is performed with indium-111-labeled leukocytes and ^{99m}Tc sulfur colloid, the marrow part of the study can be performed either before (such as at the time of white cell labeling) or immediately after completion of the leukocyte study. Our preference is to perform marrow imaging immediately after completion of the leukocyte study. There are two reasons for this: first, if there is no labeled leukocyte activity around the prosthesis, marrow imaging need not be performed. The second reason is that, with state-of-the-art gamma cameras, it is possible to perform simultaneous dual isotope acquisition, allowing for more precise comparison of leukocyte and marrow images, as well as direct computer superimposition of one image on another, facilitating study interpretation. We recommend that the sulfur colloid be made just prior to use. We have observed that using sulfur colloid that is more than about 60 min old results in images of inferior quality, with persistently increased background and, often, considerable urinary bladder activity, which is especially troublesome when studying the hip.

The use of technetium-labeled leukocytes necessitates some modifications of the procedure. Obviously, since both parts of the study employ the same radionuclide, ^{99m}Tc, simultaneous acquisition is not possible. Although we have not rigorously evaluated the optimal interval between leukocyte and marrow imaging when using ^{99m}Tc-labeled leukocytes for both parts, we have observed persistent, and potentially confounding, activity on the leukocyte images up to 48 h after injection. On those occasions when we do use technetium-labeled leukocytes, therefore, we allow at least 72 h between the two phases.

Pelosi et al.[57] have recently suggested that, by acquiring labeled leukocyte images at multiple time points, it may be possible to avoid performing bone marrow scintigraphy. Early images are thought to reflect labeled leukocyte uptake in marrow while late images are thought to reflect labeled leukocyte uptake in infection. Incongruence between early and late images is indicative of infection. Using visual analysis, the accuracy of this 'dual time-point' imaging was only about 75%; using semiquantitative analysis, the accuracy improved to about 95%. Unfortunately, only about half the patients in this series had surgical confirmation of the final diagnosis, and therefore the true merits of this technique await further investigation.

Other agents

Its value notwithstanding, there are significant disadvantages to leukocyte–marrow scintigraphy. The *in vitro* labeling process is labor intensive, not always available, and requires direct contact with blood products. The need for marrow imaging adds to the complexity and cost of the study and is an additional inconvenience to patients, many of whom are elderly and debilitated. Thus, investigators continue to search for suitable alternatives. *In vivo* techniques for labeling leukocytes, including peptides and anti-granulocyte antibodies/antibody fragments, have been explored. One such agent that has been investigated in the United States is ^{99m}Tc-fanolesomab, a radiolabeled murine monoclonal M class immunoglobulin, which has a very high affinity for CD15 receptors present on the surface membrane of human polymorphonuclear leukocytes. Accumulation of this agent at sites of infection is thought to be due to binding of the antibody to circulating neutrophils which subsequently migrate to the nidus of infection, as

well as to diffusion of the antibody across capillary membranes with subsequent binding to neutrophils and neutrophil debris already sequestered in a focus of infection.[58] Although this agent has shown promising results for diagnosing musculoskeletal infection in general, its role in the evaluation of suspected prosthetic joint infection has not been established.[59]

Indium-111-labeled immunoglobulin has also been used in the evaluation of painful joint replacements. In a series of 102 prostheses, 85 total hip and 17 total knee, sensitivity of the study was 100%. The specificity, however, was 80% for hip and 50% for knee prostheses. False positive results were noted up to 14 months after implantation of cementless prostheses and in the presence of aseptic inflammation.[60] When it is considered that inflammation frequently accompanies aseptic loosening and nearly 70% of prosthetic joint infections occur within the first year after implantation, the role of this agent in the evaluation of the painful joint replacement, if any, is limited.

Several investigators have studied the role of fluorodeoxyglucose positron emission tomography (FDG PET) in the evaluation of painful lower extremity joint prostheses. The high-resolution tomographic images, availability of the agent, and rapid completion of the procedure are all very desirable traits. Although initial reports suggested that FDG PET could accurately identify the infected joint prosthesis, more recent studies are less encouraging.[56,61–64] FDG PET does not appear to be capable of distinguishing the inflamed aseptically loosened, from the infected, prosthesis.[56] This is not surprising when it is considered that FDG uptake is dependent on tissue metabolism. Inflammation and infection are both hypermetabolic states and will, therefore, both be manifest as areas of increased activity (Fig. 9E.6). Unfortunately for FDG PET, nuclear medicine is often called upon to distinguish infection from inflammation.

A novel approach to infection imaging is the use of radiolabeled antibiotics. The most extensively investigated tracer in this group is the radiolabeled fluoroquinolone, ^{99m}Tc-ciprofloxacin. Although it has been a source of controversy, the postulated uptake mechanism of this agent is the same as that for the unlabeled antibiotic: accumulation and binding by live bacteria with DNA-gyrase inactivation. Initial investigations indicated that ^{99m}Tc-ciprofloxacin is moderately sensitive but highly specific for infection. Recent data indicate that, at least in orthopedic infections, this agent may be more sensitive than specific.[65–67] Sarda et al.[67] reported that although the agent showed good sensitivity and had a high negative predictive value for detection of bone and joint infection, it could not discriminate between infected and aseptic osteoarticular disease. Although this study did not specifically address the prosthetic joint, the findings raise concerns about the role of this agent in the evaluation of the failed joint replacement and point to the need for focused investigations for this indication.

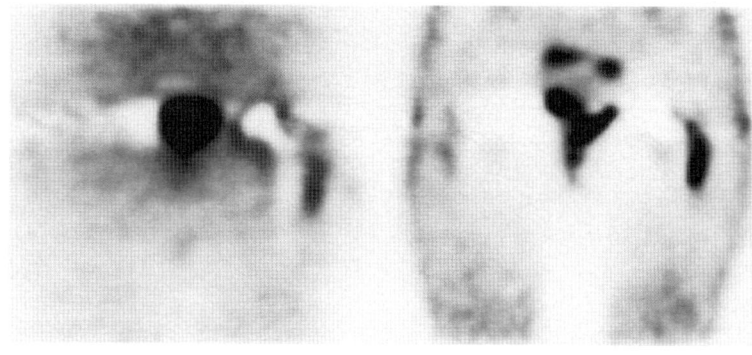

Figure 9E.6 *Fluorodeoxyglucose images of infected (left) and aseptically loosened (right) hip prostheses. Bone–prosthesis interface activity is present along the femoral component of both prostheses. Originally thought to be specific for infection, it is likely that this uptake is secondary to osteolysis, which may be present in both infection and aseptic loosening.*

SUMMARY

The primary role of nuclear medicine, differentiating aseptic loosening from infection of a prosthetic joint, remains a daunting task. The relationship between aseptic loosening and inflammation renders nonspecific indicators of inflammation nearly worthless. While bone scintigraphy may be used as a screening procedure, combined leukocyte–marrow scintigraphy, despite its disadvantages, remains the procedure of choice for diagnosing the infected joint replacement (see Case history 2, below). To replace leukocyte–marrow imaging, agents capable of differentiating infection from aseptic inflammation must be developed.

Case history 1

An 83-year-old woman with bilateral hip prostheses was referred to nuclear medicine for evaluation of persistent left lower quadrant/left hip pain. The orthopedic surgeon, who felt that infection was unlikely and that the patient's complaints might not be related to the prosthesis, requested a bone scan, as a screening test. The bone scan was completely normal, and no further evaluation of the prosthesis was performed. Subsequent work-up found that the patient's pain was due to diverticulitis.

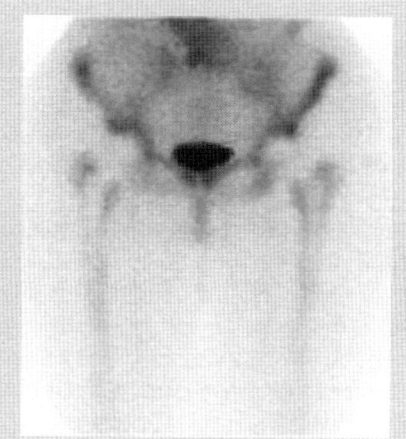

Figure 9E.7

Case history 2

A 64-year-old woman was referred to nuclear medicine because of suspected infection involving a painful 4-year-old cemented right total hip replacement. Although both the bone image alone and the combined bone–gallium images are consistent with infection, the leukocyte–marrow study is negative for infection. At surgery an aseptically loosened prosthesis was revised. Bone and gallium studies cannot reliably distinguish infection from aseptic loosening, and when infection is suspected leukocyte–marrow imaging should be performed.

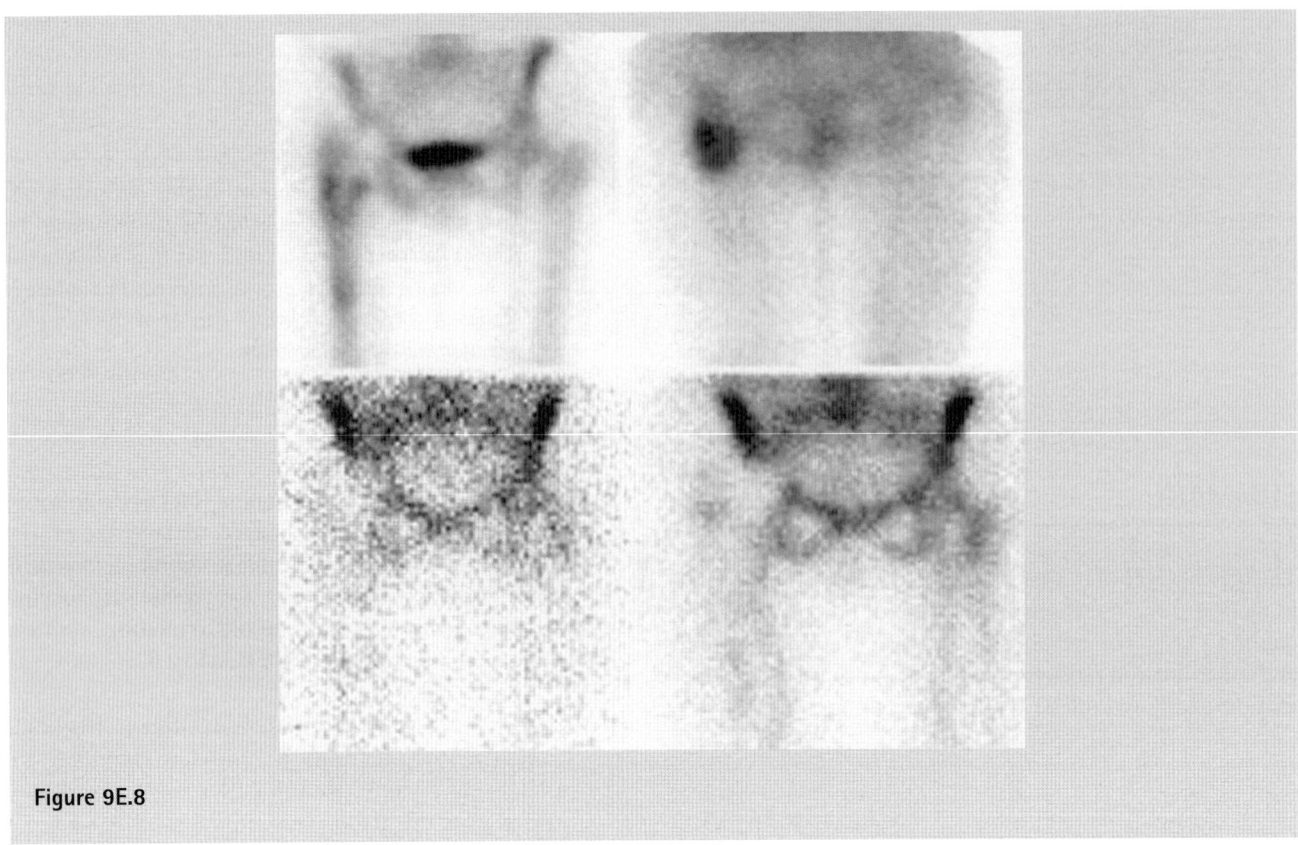

Figure 9E.8

REFERENCES

1   Steinberg DR, Steinberg ME. The early history of arthroplasty in the United States. *Clin Orthop* 2000; **374**: 55–89.

2   Daniels AU, Tooms RE, Harkess J. Arthroplasty. Introduction and overview. In: Canale ST. (ed.) *Campbell's operative orthopaedics*, 9th edition. St Louis: Mosby, 1998: 211–27.

3   Harkess JW. Arthroplasty of hip. In: Canale ST. (ed.) *Campbell's operative orthopaedics*, 9th edition. St Louis: Mosby, 1998: 296–456.

4   Love C, Tomas MB, Marwin SE, *et al.* Role of nuclear medicine in diagnosis of the infected joint replacement. *RadioGraphics* 2001; **21**: 1229–38.

5   Guyton JL. Arthroplasty of ankle and knee. In: Canale ST. (ed.) *Campbell's operative orthopaedics*, 9th edition. St Louis: Mosby, 1998: 232–85.

6   Bauer TW, Schils J. The pathology of total joint arthroplasty. II. Mechanisms of implant failure. *Skeletal Radiol* 1999; **28**: 483–97.

7   Maloney WJ, Smith RL. Periprosthetic osteolysis in total hip arthroplasty: the role of particulate wear debris. *J Bone Joint Surg* 1995; **77A**: 1448–61.

8   Wooley PH, Nasser S, Fitzgerald Jr RH. The immune response to implant materials in humans. *Clin Orthop* 1996; **326**: 63–70.

9   Toumbis CA, Kronick JL, Wooley PH, Nasser S. Total joint arthroplasty and the immune response. *Semin Arth Rheum* 1997; **27**: 44–7.

10 Hanssen AD, Rand JA. Evaluation and treatment of infection at the site of a total hip or knee arthroplasty. *J Bone Joint Surg* 1998; **80A**: 910–22.

11 Della Valle CJ, Bogner E, Desai P, *et al.* Analysis of frozen sections of intraoperative specimens obtained at the time of reoperation after hip or knee resection arthroplasty for the treatment of infection. *J Bone Joint Surg* 1999; **81A**: 684–9.

12 Tsukayama DT, Estrada R, Gustilo RB. Infection after total hip arthroplasty. *J Bone Joint Surg* 1996; **78A**: 512–23.

13 Feldman DS, Lonner JH, Desai P, Zuckerman JD. The role of intraoperative frozen sections in revision total joint arthroplasty. *J Bone Joint Surg* 1995; **77A**: 1807–13.

14 Spangehl MJ, Masri BA, O'Connell JX, Duncan CP. Prospective analysis of preoperative and intraoperative investigations for the diagnosis of infection at the sites of two hundred and two revision total hip arthroplasties. *J Bone Joint Surg* 1999; **81A**: 672–83.

15 Tobin EH. Prosthetic joint infections: controversies and clues. *Lancet* 1999; **353**: 770–1.

16 Spanghel MJ, Younger AS, Masri BA, Duncan CP. Diagnosis of infection following total hip arthroplasty. *J Bone Joint Surg* 1997; **79A**: 1578–88.

17 Gelman MI, Coleman RE, Stevens PM, Davey BW. Radiography, radionuclide imaging, and arthrography in the evaluation of total hip and knee replacement. *Radiology* 1978; **128**: 677–82.

18 Weiss PE, Mall JC, Hoffer PB, *et al.* ^{99m}Tc-methylenediphosphonate bone imaging in the evaluation of total hip prostheses. *Radiology* 1979; **133**: 727–9.

19 McInerney DP, Hyde ID. Technetium ^{99}Tc^m pyrophosphate scanning in the assessment of the painful hip prosthesis. *Clin Radiol* 1978; **29**: 513–17.

20 Williamson BRJ, McLaughlin RE, Wang GJ, *et al.* Radionuclide bone imaging as a means of differentiating loosening and infection in patients with a painful total hip prosthesis. *Radiology* 1979; **133**: 723–6.

21 Williams F, McCall IW, Park WM, *et al.* Gallium-67 scanning in the painful total hip replacement. *Clin Radiol* 1981; **32**: 431–9.

22 Mountford PJ, Hall FM, Wells CP, Coakley AJ. ^{99}Tc^m-MDP, ^{67}Ga-citrate and ^{111}In-leucocytes for detecting prosthetic hip infection. *Nucl Med Commun* 1986; **7**: 113–20.

23 Aliabadi P, Tumeh SS, Weissman BN, McNeil BJ. Cemented total hip prosthesis: radiographic and scintigraphic evaluation. *Radiology* 1989; **173**: 203–6.

24 Lieberman JR, Huo MH, Schneider R, *et al.* Evaluation of painful hip arthroplasties. *J Bone Joint Surg* 1993; **75B**: 475–8.

25 Utz JA, Lull R J, Galvin EG. Asymptomatic total hip prosthesis: natural history determined using Tc-99m MDP bone scans. *Radiology* 1986; **161**: 509–12.

26 Oswald SG, Van Nostrand D, Savory CG, Callaghan JJ. Three-phase bone scan and indium white blood cell scintigraphy following porous coated hip arthroplasty: a prospective study of the prosthetic tip. *J Nucl Med* 1989; **30**: 1321–31.

27 Oswald SG, Van Nostrand D, Savory CG, *et al.* The acetabulum: a prospective study of three-phase bone and indium white blood cell scintigraphy following porous-coated hip arthroplasty. *J Nucl Med* 1990; **31**: 274–80.

28 Ashbrooke AB, Calvert PT. Bone scan appearances after uncemented hip replacement. *J Roy Soc Med* 1990; **83**: 768–9.

29 Rosenthall L, Lepanto L, Raymond F. Radiophosphate uptake in asymptomatic knee arthroplasty. *J Nucl Med* 1987; **28**: 1546–9.

30 Palestro CJ, Swyer AJ, Kim CK, Goldsmith SJ. Infected knee prostheses: diagnosis with In-111 leukocyte, Tc-99m sulfur colloid, and Tc-99m MDP imaging. *Radiology* 1991; **179**: 645–8.

31 Hofmann AA, Wyatt RWB, Daniels AU, *et al.* Bone scans after total knee arthroplasty in asymptomatic patients. *Clin Orthop* 1990; **251**: 183–8.

32 Palestro CJ, Torres MA. Radionuclide imaging in orthopedic infections. *Semin Nucl Med* 1997; **27**: 334–45.

33 Palestro C. The current role of gallium imaging in infection. *Semin Nucl Med* 1994; **24**: 128–41.

34 Reing CM, Richin PF, Kenmore PI. Differential bone-scanning in the evaluation of a painful total joint replacement. *J Bone Joint Surg* 1979; **61A**: 933–6.

35 Rushton N, Coakley AJ, Tudor J, Wraight EP. The value of technetium and gallium scanning in assessing pain after total hip replacement. *J Bone Joint Surg* 1982; **64B**: 313–18.

36 McKillop JH, McKay I, Cuthbert GF, *et al.* Scintigraphic evaluation of the painful prosthetic joint: a comparison of gallium-67 citrate and indium-111 labelled leukocyte imaging. *Clin Radiol* 1984; **35**: 239–41.

37 Seabold JE, Palestro CJ, Brown ML, *et al. Society of Nuclear Medicine procedure guideline for gallium scintigraphy in inflammation.* Reston, Virginia: Society of Nuclear Medicine, 1997: 75–8.

38 Tehranzadeh J, Gubernick I, Blaha D. Prospective study of sequential technetium-99m phosphate and gallium imaging in painful hip prostheses (comparison of diagnostic modalities). *Clin Nucl Med* 1988; **13**: 229–36.

39 Merkel KD, Fitzgerald Jr RH, Brown ML. Scintigraphic examination of total hip arthroplasty: comparison of indium with technetium–gallium in the loose and infected canine arthroplasty. In: Welch RB. (ed.) *The hip. Proceedings of the Twelfth Open Scientific Meeting of the Hip Society*, Atlanta, Georgia, 1984: 163–92.

40 Merkel KD, Brown ML, Fitzgerald Jr RH. Sequential technetium-99m HMDP–gallium-67 citrate imaging for the evaluation of infection in the painful prosthesis. *J Nucl Med* 1986; **27**: 1413–17.

41 Gomez-Luzuriaga MA, Galan V, Villar JM. Scintigraphy with Tc, Ga and In in painful total hip prostheses. *Intern Orthop* 1988; **12**: 163–7.

42 Kraemer WJ, Saplys R, Waddell JP, Morton J. Bone scan, gallium scan, and hip aspiration in the diagnosis of infected total hip arthroplasty. *J Arthroplasty* 1993; **8**: 611–15.

43 Pring DJ, Henderson RG, Keshavarzian A, *et al.* Indium-granulocyte scanning in the painful prosthetic joint. *Am J Roentgenol* 1986; **146**: 167–72.

44 Pring DJ, Henderson RG, Rivett AG, *et al.* Autologous granulocytes scanning of painful prosthetic joints. *J Bone Joint Surg* 1986; **68B**: 647–52.

45 Rand JA, Brown ML. The value of indium-111 leukocyte scanning in the evaluation of painful or infected total knee arthroplasties. *Clin Orthop* 1990; **259**: 179–82.

46 Magnuson JE, Brown ML, Hauser MF, *et al.* In-111 labeled leukocyte scintigraphy in suspected orthopedic prosthesis infection: comparison with other imaging modalities. *Radiology* 1988; **168**: 235–9.

47 Wukich DK, Abreu SH, Callaghan JJ, *et al.* Diagnosis of infection by preoperative scintigraphy with indium-labeled white blood cells. *J Bone Joint Surg* 1987; **69A**: 1353–60.

48 Johnson JA, Christie MJ, Sandler MP, *et al.* Detection of occult infection following total joint arthroplasty using sequential technetium-99m HDP bone scintigraphy and indium-111 WBC imaging. *J Nucl Med* 1988; **29**: 1347–53.

49 Palestro CJ, Kim CK, Swyer AJ, *et al.* Total hip arthroplasty: periprosthetic indium-111-labeled leukocyte activity and complementary technetium-99m-sulfur colloid imaging in suspected infection. *J Nucl Med* 1990; **31**: 1950–5.

50 Torres MA, Palestro CJ. Leukocyte-marrow scintigraphy in hyperostosis frontalis interna. *J Nucl Med* 1997; **38**: 1283–5.

51 Palestro CJ, Mehta HH, Patel M, *et al.* Marrow versus infection in the Charcot joint: indium-111 leukocyte and technetium-99m sulfur colloid scintigraphy. *J Nucl Med* 1998; **39**: 346–50.

52 Love C, Tomas MB, Marwin SE, Palestro CJ. Diagnosing prosthetic hip infection: an intraindividual comparison of leukocyte, leukocyte/bone, and leukocyte/marrow imaging [Abstract]. *Eur J Nucl Med* 2002; **29**: P104.

53 Palestro CJ, Kim CK, Vega A, Goldsmith SJ. Acute effects of radiation therapy on indium-111-labeled leukocyte uptake in bone marrow. *J Nucl Med* 1989; **30**: 1989–91.

54 Mulamba L'AH, Ferrant A, Leners N, *et al.* Indium-111 leucocyte scanning in the evaluation of painful hip arthroplasty. *Acta Orthop Scand* 1983; **54**: 695–7.

55 Joseph TN, Mujitaba M, Chen AL, *et al.* Efficacy of combined technetium-99m sulfur colloid/indium-111 leukocyte scans to detect infected total hip and knee arthroplasties. *J Arthroplasty* 2001; **16**: 753–8.

56 Love C, Marwin SE, Tomas MB, *et al.* Diagnosing infection in the failed joint replacement: a comparison of coincidence detection fluorine-18 FDG and indium-111-labeled leukocyte/technetium-99m-sulfur colloid marrow imaging. *J Nucl Med* 2004; **45**: 1864–71.

57 Pelosi E, Baiocco C, Pennone M, *et al.* 99mTc-HMPAO-leukocyte scintigraphy in patients with symptomatic total hip or knee arthroplasty: improved diagnostic accuracy by means of semiquantitative evaluation. *J Nucl Med* 2004; **45**: 438–44.

58 Love C, Palestro CJ. 99mTc-fanolesomab. *Invest Drugs* 2003; **6**: 1079–85.

59 Palestro CJ, Kipper SL, Weiland FL, *et al.* Osteomyelitis: Diagnosis with 99mTc-labeled antigranulocyte antibodies compared with diagnosis with indium-111-labeled leukocytes – initial experience. *Radiology* 2002; **223**: 758–64.

60 Nijhof MW, Oyen WJ, van Kampen A, *et al.* Hip and knee arthroplasty infection. In-111-IgG scintigraphy in 102 cases. *Acta Orthop Scand* 1997; **68**: 332–6.

61 Zhuang H, Duarte PS, Pourdehnad M, *et al.* The promising role of 18F-FDG PET in detecting infected lower limb prosthesis implants. *J Nucl Med* 2001; **42**: 44–8.

62 Chacko TK, Zhuang H, Stevenson K, *et al.* The importance of the location of fluorodeoxyglucose uptake in periprosthetic infection in painful hip prostheses. *Nucl Med Commun* 2002; **23**: 851–5.

63 Manthey N, Reinhard P, Moog F, *et al.* The use of [18F]fluorodeoxyglucose positron emission tomography to differentiate between synovitis, loosening and infection of hip and knee prostheses. *Nucl Med Commun* 2002; **23**: 645–53.

64 Stumpe KD, Notzli HP, Zanetti M, *et al.* FDG PET for differentiation of infection and aseptic loosening in total hip replacements: comparison with conventional radiography and three-phase bone scintigraphy. *Radiology* 2004; **231**: 333–41.

65 Sonmezoglu K, Sonmezoglu M, Halac M, *et al.* Usefulness of 99mTc-ciprofloxacin (infecton) scan in diagnosis of chronic orthopedic infections: comparison with 99mTc-HMPAO leukocyte scintigraphy. *J Nucl Med* 2001; **42**: 567–74.

66 Yapar Z, Kibar M, Yapar YF, *et al.* The efficacy of technetium-99m ciprofloxacin (Infecton) imaging in orthopaedic infections: a comparison with sequential bone/gallium imaging. *Eur J Nucl Med* 2001; **28**: 822–30.

67 Sarda L, Cremieux AC, Lebellec Y, *et al.* Inability of 99mTc-ciprofloxacin scintigraphy to discriminate between septic and sterile osteo-articular diseases. *J Nucl Med* 2003; **44**: 920–6.

Rheumatology and avascular necrosis

P. RYAN

INFLAMMATORY ARTHROPATHIES

The role of nuclear medicine in the routine evaluation of the major arthropathies has been limited, but it is a field that is still under-explored and could play a more significant role in clinical practice.

In rheumatoid arthritis bone scanning will demonstrate increased activity in the active, affected joints on both the static and dynamic phases of imaging. Uptake will parallel other markers of disease activity. The bone scan is, of course, nonspecific and, in individual joints, cannot separate active rheumatoid arthritis from other forms of arthritis, including osteoarthritis when the latter has a significant inflammatory component. The pattern of uptake in different joints, however, may allow the distinction of different forms of arthritis; for example, rheumatoid arthritis typically affects the proximal interphalangeal, metacarpophalangeal and wrist joints in the hand and proximal interphalangeal, metatarsophalangeal and tarsal joints in the feet, with a symmetrical pattern between left and right limbs. On occasions in rheumatoid arthritis, and indeed in other arthropathies, the bone scan can be helpful in distinguishing arthralgia, where there is pain without inflammation, from an arthritis, where inflammation is present.[1] The bone scan may be helpful in selecting joints for further therapy, such as radioactive synovectomy, particularly if initial treatment has not been successful. It is also of note that joints with absent or minimal activity in newly diagnosed rheumatoid arthritis do not appear to erode.[2] Erosions are more likely to appear in joints with persistent and high scintigraphic activity.

Labeled white-cell imaging is a more specific test for joint inflammation, with the reduction in activity following intra-articular steroids paralleling the pain response.

At present in clinical practice joint inflammation is assessed by symptoms and signs and crude indices such as the erythrocyte sedimentation rate and C-reactive protein. Both the isotope bone scan and labeled white-cell imaging could be used as an adjunct to other measurements to assess the level of disease activity and the requirements for second line drugs, particularly with respect to individual joints that may be difficult to assess such as the hip. However, further research is needed to clearly demonstrate such a role.

More recent studies using ^{99m}Tc-labeled human immunoglobulin have shown it to be of value in imaging the active joints of rheumatoid arthritis (Fig. 9F.1). It is more sensitive and specific than the bone scan and has been demonstrated to reflect individual variation in disease activity in rheumatoid arthritis.[3,4] Human immunoglobulin imaging has also been shown to be more sensitive than physical examination in the detection of histologically determined synovitis.[5] Human immunoglobulin appears to reflect only local inflammation and not aspects of destructive arthritis. It probably binds to intra-articular protein in inflamed joints and may be more sensitive for active joints than labeled white cells.[6]

Other studies have examined the role of gallium-67 citrate, ^{99m}Tc-nanocoll, indium-111 chloride and labeled liposomes. All these techniques do have value but have not found a role in routine practice. More recently, labeled CD3 and CD4 lymphocyte antibodies and E selectin endothelial antibodies have shown promise as more selective agents to image inflammatory disorders[7] but, again, these approaches have not yet been taken further to become clinical tools.[7] Ciprofloxacin (Infecton) labeled with ^{99m}Tc is also taken up into inflamed joints and could represent another useful approach and an alternative to human immunoglobulin.[8]

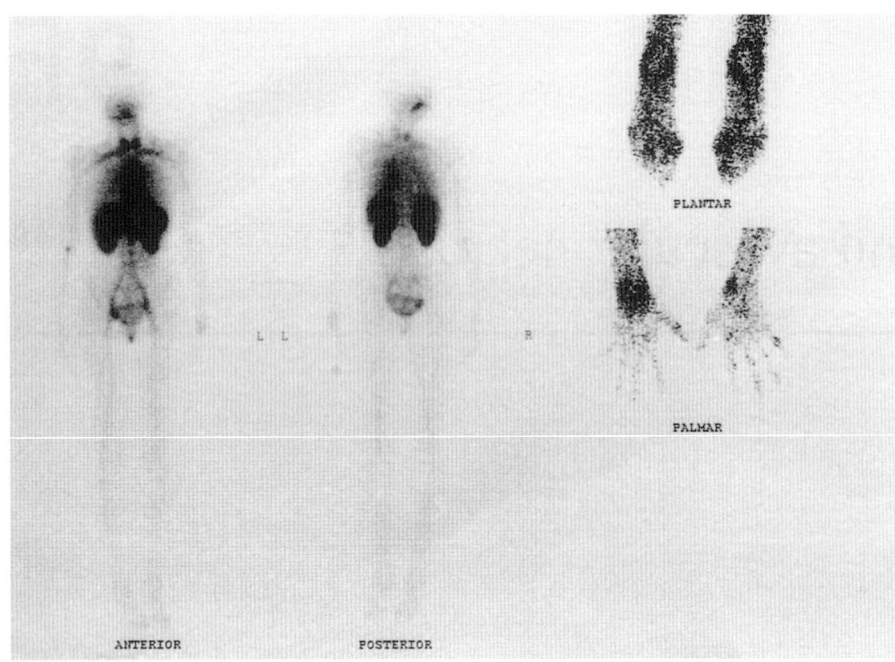

ANTERIOR   POSTERIOR

PLANTAR

PALMAR

Figure 9F.1 *Human immunoglobulin scan in rheumatoid arthritis. Whole-body and spot views of distal limbs. Abnormal uptake in the right carpus.*

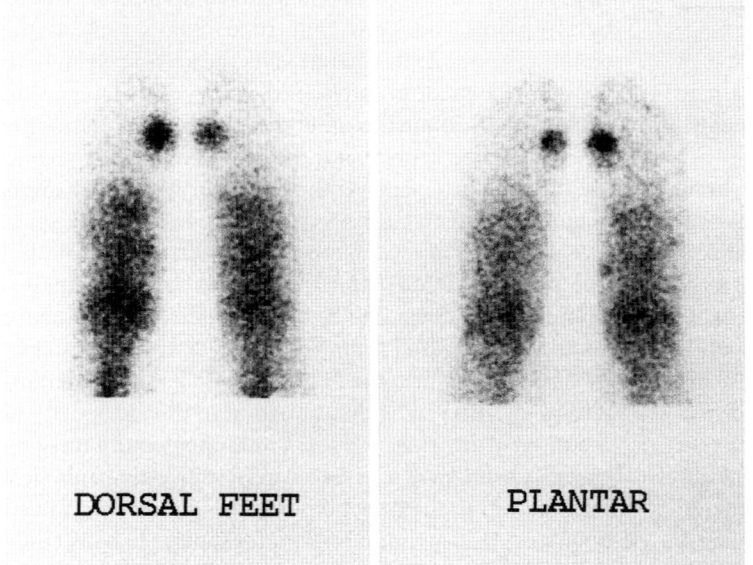

DORSAL FEET   **PLANTAR**

Figure 9F.2 *Bone scan delayed images of the feet showing uptake in osteoarthritis of the first metatarsophalangeal joints.*

OSTEOARTHRITIS

Bone scintigraphy in osteoarthritis is also of value (Figs 9F.2 and 9F.3). It is not routinely used for primary diagnosis but can be helpful in some difficult sites such as the ankles, mid tarsal joints, lumbar spine, and the hips. This is because scan activity may precede radiological change and also may be more dramatic than radiological change, enabling a confident diagnosis rather than a suspicion of the diagnosis. Scan activity can also predict radiological change with joints that are inactive on scan showing little or no radiological progression.[9] In the knees, the bone scan can be helpful in determining whether there is disease in one or both weight-bearing compartments. This is important as it can guide appropriate operative intervention (osteotomy, uni- or bicompartmental joint replacement). Bone scan changes may also resolve with an osteotomy presumably due to removal of stresses on the subchondral bone.[10] Planar scintigraphy has better resolution for patellofemoral osteoarthritis but sensitivity is enhanced by single photon emission computed tomography (SPECT), which is also useful in assessing the medial and lateral compartments and helping distinguish simple meniscal lesions from osteoarthritis. In the spine, planar and SPECT imaging can be useful to make a positive diagnosis of spondylolysis and facet joint disease, the latter usually being degenerative in origin.

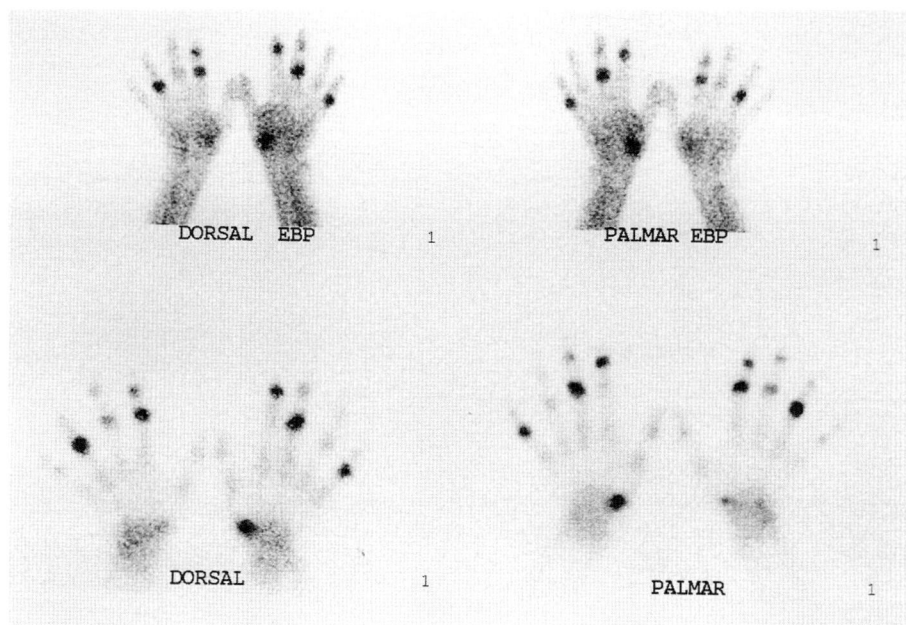

Figure 9F.3 *Two-phase bone scan of the hands and wrists with uptake in osteoarthritic joints.*

ANKYLOSING SPONDYLITIS

The bone scan has been used for many years in the investigation of ankylosing spondylitis (Fig. 9F.4). There are two main diagnostic issues where scintigraphy may be helpful in this condition. The first is at presentation where diagnosis may be uncertain; the second is later in the disease process, when the cause of non-inflammatory back pain may be unclear. For diagnosis, quantitative sacroiliac joint uptake (SIJ) has been used for almost three decades. The rationale for this is that in early disease there will be increased SIJ activity due to inflammation, which precedes radiological changes. The most common technique is to derive a profile of tracer uptake over the SIJs and sacrum, and to establish an SIJ to sacral ratio from the peaks. Initial studies were promising and the results enabled good separation of ankylosing spondylitis from other causes of back pain, although later studies were less conclusive and it is now apparent that other conditions such as rheumatoid arthritis, lumbosacral spondylitis, trauma or excessive activity can produce elevated SIJ to sacral ratios. It is also recognized that the sacrum may be involved in ankylosing spondylitis and improvements can be achieved by comparing SIJ activity to other bony areas or a trough of activity between the sacrum and the SIJ. Provided that other causes of elevated SIJ to sacral ratios are excluded, the test remains a valuable tool to identify patients who require further investigation or follow-up.[11] SPECT now appears more useful than planar or quantitiative techniques in initial diagnosis with high uptake in the inferior aspect of the joints, giving high sensitivity and specificity for the diagnosis of sacroiliitis. Hanley *et al.*[12] showed a sensitivity of 85% and specificity of 90% in 20 patients with clinical sacroiliitis and 20 controls. Respective

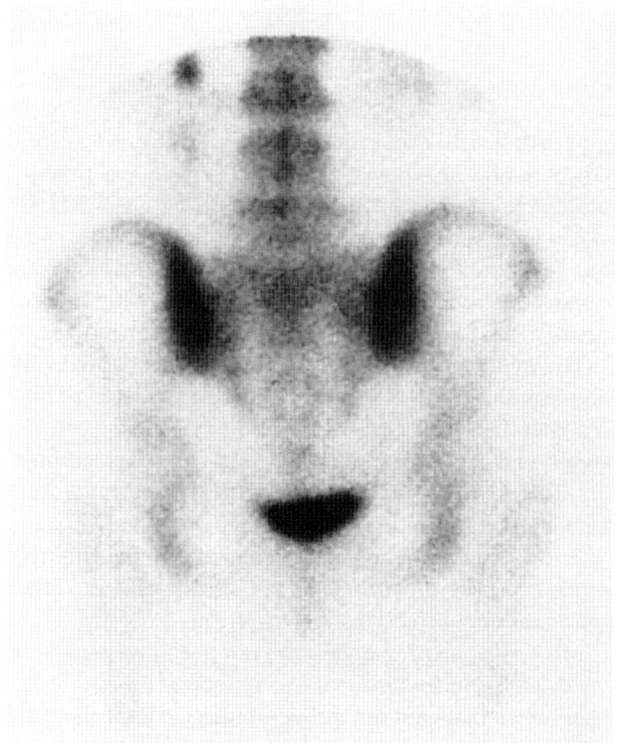

Figure 9F.4 *Ankylosing spondylitis. High uptake in the sacroiliac joints.*

findings for quantitative planar imaging were 25% and 95%. The view that SPECT is useful for diagnosis is supported by a study of Yildez *et al.*[13] who compared nanocolloid, quantitative bone scintigraphy, planar imaging and SPECT in 32 patients clinically with sacroiliac disease. The

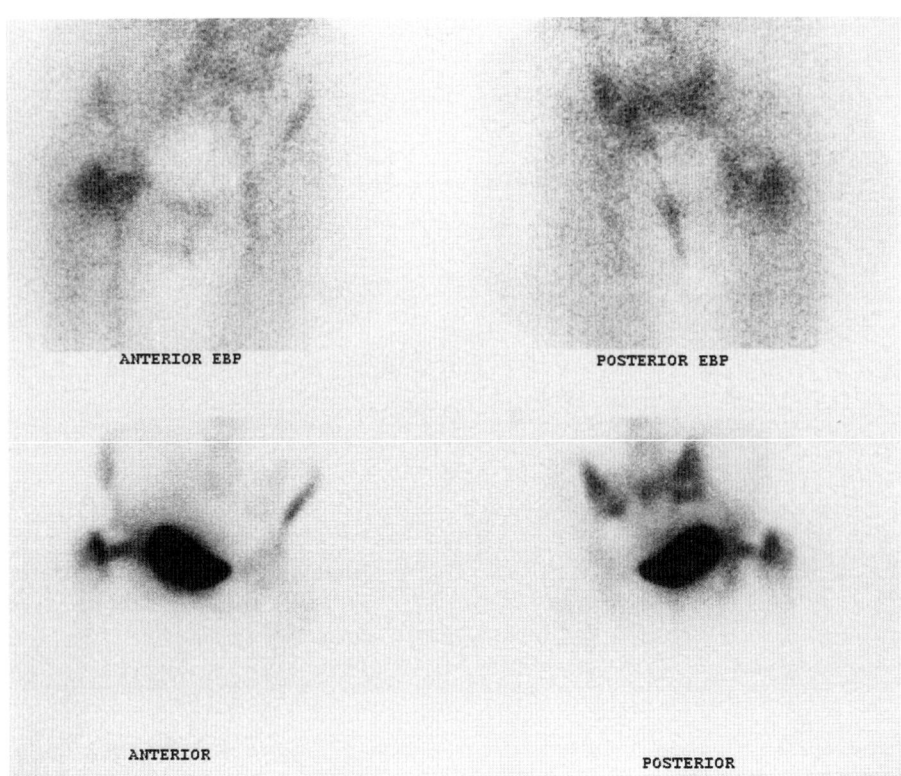

ANTERIOR EBP   POSTERIOR EBP

ANTERIOR   POSTERIOR

Figure 9F.5 *Two-phase bone scan of the hips showing a femoral neck fracture and avascular necrosis of the femoral head.*

respective sensitivities and specificities were 47%, 25%, 69%, 97% and 90%, 80%, 95% and 90%. In clinical practice radiography and magnetic resonance imaging (MRI) are widely used as imaging techniques and some studies show that MRI can be highly accurate[14] although not all papers support this conclusion.[15] However, the high clinical accuracy of SPECT suggests bone scanning is under-utilized.

The value of the bone scan in back pain associated with long-standing ankylosing spondylitis has only received limited attention. However, one study in 1984, using SPECT, suggested that sites of abnormal uptake could be identified. Other work has shown that many patients with ankylosing spondylitis have uptake in the facet joints and in some cases the uptake may be spectacular, involving multiple joints.[16] The use of bone imaging in sacroiliitis due to other causes has not been extensively investigated.

Most other arthropathies have not been investigated in any detail by nuclear medicine techniques. However, it has been shown that gout can mimic an infected joint clinically and may show increased activity on a three-phase bone scan as well as on gallium and white-cell scans.

Seronegative arthropathies are associated with enthesopathies where there is inflammation at the musculotendinous junction. These may be diagnosed clinically but sometimes a bone scan can be helpful. Typically, there is focal uptake at the relevant site on all three phases of the scan. An example is plantar fasciitis where bone scan imaging is useful particularly if the patient does not respond to initial therapy.

AVASCULAR NECROSIS

Bony infarction is a recognized complication of fracture although it may occur in other conditions, such as sickle cell disease and in patients on long-term oral corticosteroids. Early diagnosis is necessary to prevent long-term complications. The bone scan appearances are initially those of reduced uptake due to a diminished blood supply but when reparative processes begin increased uptake occurs and at this stage diagnosis is more difficult. Investigation should begin as soon as possible after suspicion of the diagnosis.

Imaging of the hip following fracture can be very helpful to detect avascular necrosis secondary to the fracture (Fig. 9F.5). Sensitivity is enhanced by SPECT of the hip which can sometimes allow identification of a photon-deficient center in an area of increased activity which is not apparent on planar imaging.[17] In practice, however, there is commonly an artifactual photopenic area in the femoral head on SPECT due to the distortional effects of bladder activity. Delayed imaging of the hip can be useful to assess whether patients will require a hip replacement with normal activity in the femoral head excluding persistant avascular necrosis.[18] MRI is sensitive and specific for avascular necrosis and sensitivity is better than planar bone imaging. However, when compared to bone SPECT, MRI does not appear to be better and bone SPECT is more sensitive.[19]

Other sites of avascular necrosis include the lunate (Keinbock's disease), talus (Kohler's disease), and the second metatarsal (Freiberg's disease). At all these sites, particularly

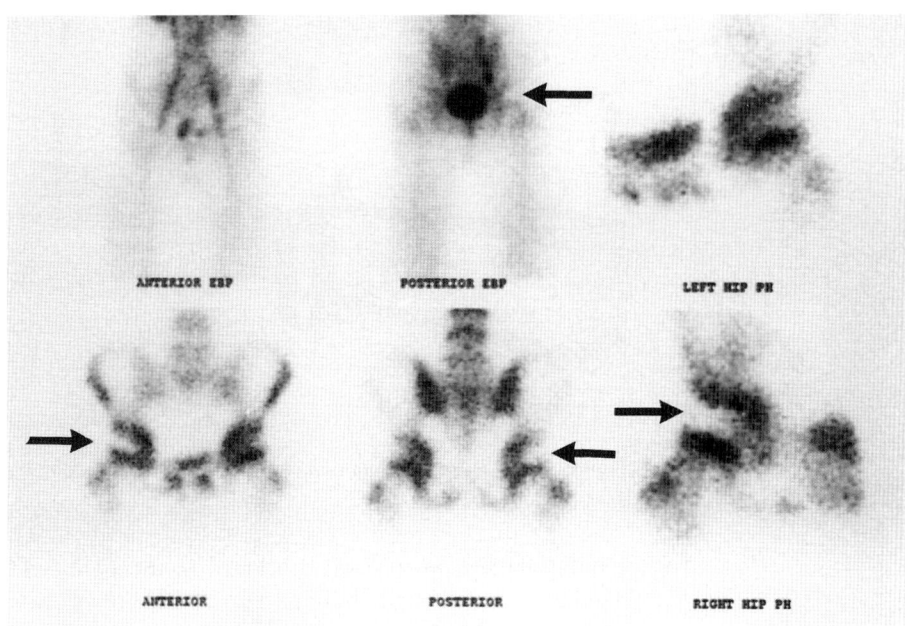

ANTERIOR EBP   POSTERIOR EBP   LEFT HIP PH

ANTERIOR   POSTERIOR   RIGHT HIP PH

Figure 9F.6 *Two-phase bone scan of the hips in a patient with Perthes' disease of the right hip.*

the second metatarsal head, the bone scan can be very useful as they can be difficult to assess radiologically. There is usually increased uptake on all three phases of the bone scan due to reparative process surrounding the avascular area. The typical site of uptake in the context of a relevant history usually secures the diagnosis. The scaphoid is another important site where avascular necrosis following fracture can occur. Blood supply to the scaphoid enters distally and then runs proximally leading to avascular necrosis of the proximal fragment following fracture in some cases. There may be a proximal scaphoid photon deficient area but commonly as at other sites of avascular necrosis there is increased uptake on all phases of the scan due to reparative processes around the avascular area. This may be difficult to distinguish from uptake related to the fracture itself but careful localization and greater uptake than expected given the age of fracture may be clues. The knees are also another important skeletal site of avascular necrosis usually involving the femoral condyles. Typically there is increased uptake on all three phases of the bone scan with the delayed images showing a well delineated abnormality. Smaller focal areas of osteochondritis may also be apparent on a bone scan usually related to the anterior femoral condyles and these are sometimes better defined on SPECT.[20]

In children, the bone scan is useful to detect Perthes' disease where the study has excellent sensitivity and specificity (Fig. 9F.6). The typical finding is absent uptake in the femoral head on blood pool and delayed images. In most cases the scan appearances are clear, though in mild cases the changes on bone scan can be subtle. Pinhole images should be acquired as they enhance diagnostic accuracy. Occasionally a 'cold' femoral head can be seen in transient synovitis, trauma, and septic arthritis but from experience

these causes are rare. MRI is also very sensitive for Perthes' disease and the choice of imaging test may well depend on availability and patient preference.

REFLEX SYMPATHETIC DYSTROPHY SYNDROME

Bone scintigraphy has an important role in the diagnosis of reflex sympathetic dystrophy syndrome, now usually called chronic regional pain syndrome. It is a condition which is relatively uncommon but seen not infrequently following fracture particularly those of the hand, wrist, foot, and ankle. It can be associated with a range of other conditions such as stroke, myocardial infarction or malignancy. The typical clinical features are those of pain, swelling, and vasomotor disturbance. High sensitivity and specificity for the bone scan has been found in several studies compared with relatively poor sensitivity for X-ray. Sensitivity is greater on the static images although there is usually increased blood flow and blood pool. McKinnon and Holder reported a 96% sensitivity and 98% specificity for the delayed images compared to 45% sensitivity for the blood flow and 52% for the blood pool images.[21] The characteristic feature on bone scan is increased activity throughout the extremity with particular periarticular uptake (Fig. 9F.7).[22] In chronic reflex sympathetic dystrophy syndrome the early phases normalize and in some patients there may be a reduced pattern of uptake. The late phase of the bone scan will also normalize and again there may be reduced uptake in chronic disease. Abnormal studies have shown a strong predictability of response to systemic corticosteroid therapy.[23]

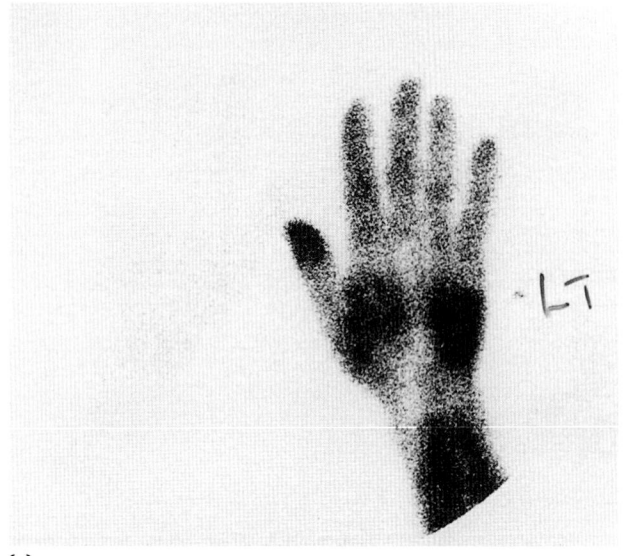

(a)

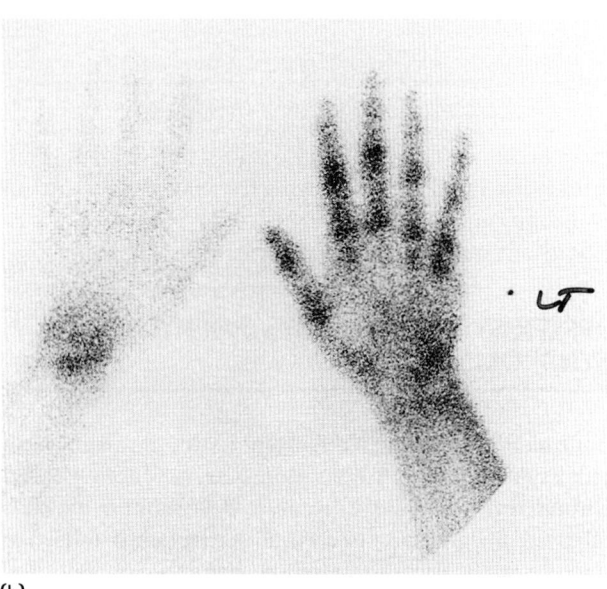

(b)

Figure 9F.7   *(a) and (b) Two-phase bone scan images showing reflex sympathetic dystrophy syndrome, left hand.*

BONE MASS MEASUREMENT

Introduction

There is a wide variety of non-invasive techniques available for the measurement of bone mass. In the past the most widely used approaches were single photon absorptiometry[24] and dual photon absorptiometry.[25] Single photon absorptiometry measured forearm bone mass using the transmission of a ^{125}I source through bone and soft tissue. The attenuation of the beam limited its use to appendicular sites and the need for constant soft tissue thickness required the use of a water bath to provide soft tissue equivalence. Dual

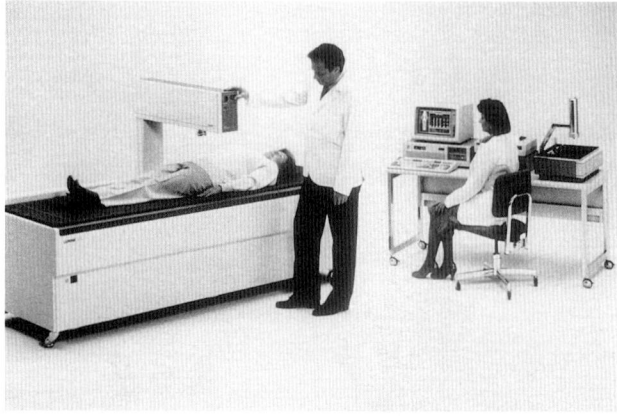

Figure 9F.8   *Patient having a dual-energy X-ray absorptiometry scan of the hips.*

photon absorptiometry was developed in the 1970s and allowed measurement at the important clinical sites of spine and hip. Gadolinium-153 was used as the transmission source which had the advantage of two energies, 44 keV and 100 keV, enabling the separate computation of soft tissue and bone mass. The use of [153]Gd allowed measurement at the axial sites where variable soft tissue thickness meant a single energy source could not be used.

However, these techniques are now obsolete and bone densitometry is most widely performed using dual energy X-ray absorptiometry (DXA) (Fig. 9F. 8). An X-ray rather than a radionuclide source is used to produce the photon beam. X-rays of two photon energies are generated either by rapid switching of a generator voltage between a high and low keV in synchrony with the mains supply or by using a constant potential generator with a rare earth filter with a K absorption edge of around 45 keV. The latter splits the polyenergetic X-ray spectrum into high and low energy components. The X-ray tube produces a much higher photon flux than [153]Gd, enabling the radiation beam to be highly collimated and resulting in high-resolution images, improved precision, shorter scanning times and reduced radiation dose. DXA is usually performed at the spine and hip but can be used to measure forearm, lateral spine, and total body (Fig. 9F.9). Some units will measure forearm bone mineral density (BMD), particularly in the elderly, where the spine is less reliable due to degenerative disease or where patients cannot be accommodated on the BMD couch. Software is also available to measure hand bone density and bone mass around prostheses. More recent DXA scanners use a fan beam X-ray source generated with a slit collimator combined with multiple solid state detectors which enable a scan to be acquired in a few seconds.[26] There is now increasing interest in instant vertebral assessment where a DXA scanner can be used to obtain a lateral spine X-ray at the same time as a BMD measurement for rapid assessment of vertebral fracture.[27]

DXA provision is still variable but increasingly most hospitals in the UK either have a scanner or access to a scanner

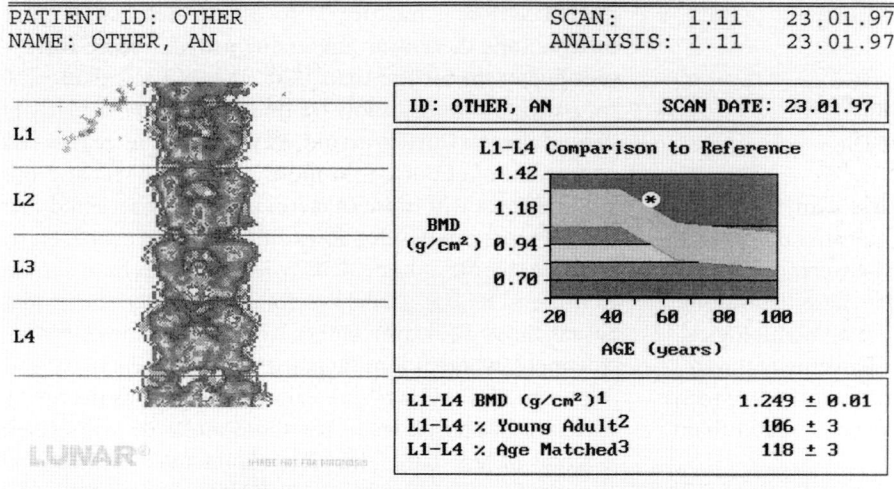

AP SPINE RESULTS
Medway Hospital
Medway N.H.S. Trust, Rochester

PATIENT ID: OTHER   SCAN: 1.11   23.01.97
NAME: OTHER, AN   ANALYSIS: 1.11   23.01.97

ID: OTHER, AN   SCAN DATE: 23.01.97

L1–L4 Comparison to Reference

BMD (g/cm^2)

L1–L4 BMD (g/cm^2)[1]	1.249 ± 0.01
L1–L4 % Young Adult[2]	106 ± 3
L1–L4 % Age Matched[3]	118 ± 3

Age (years)........	56	Large Standard......	280.40
Sex...............	Female	Medium Standard.....	209.75
Weight (Kg)........	80.0	Small Standard......	149.43
Height (cm)........	176	Low keV Air (cps)...	780084
Ethnic.............	White	High keV Air (cps)..	449145
System.............	8040	Rvalue (%Fat).......	1.353(19.5)

Scan Mode.......	Medium
Scan Type...........	DPX-Alpha
Collimation (mm).....	1.68
Sample Size (mm).....	1.2x 1.2
Current (uA)........	750

REGION	BMD[1] g/cm^2	Young Adult[2] %	Young Adult[2] Z	Age Matched[3] %	Age Matched[3] Z
L1	1.117	99	-0.11	111	0.90
L2	1.264	105	0.54	117	1.55
L3	1.271	106	0.59	118	1.60
L4	1.322	110	1.01	122	2.02
L1-L2	1.192	104	0.35	116	1.36
L1-L3	1.218	104	0.40	116	1.41
L1-L4	1.249	106	0.58	118	1.58
L2-L3	1.268	106	0.56	117	1.57
L2-L4	1.288	107	0.74	119	1.75
L3-L4	1.299	108	0.82	120	1.83

1 - See appendix E on precision and accuracy. Statistically 68% of repeat scans will fall within 1 SD.
2 - USA AP Spine Reference Population. Ages 20-45. See Appendices.
3 - Matched for Age. Ethnic.

Figure 9F.9 *Dual-energy X-ray absorptiometry result using a Lunar device in a normal patient.*

in a neighboring hospital trust. This has had an enormous impact on the development of osteoporosis services and hospitals with scanners are increasingly the pivot around which the management of osteoporosis occurs in the locality. An average DXA scanner should be performing around 4000–5000 scans per annum. There are also now a large variety of cheaper machines measuring bone mass at peripheral sites using DXA, ultrasound, digital radiogrammetry or computed tomography (CT). These techniques do have a predictive capacity for fracture but all have poor and individually varying relationships to axial BMD. In general their fracture prediction is less strong, particularly at the clinically important site of the hip. Furthermore, the therapeutic trials of drugs widely used in osteoporosis have been demonstrated to work on the basis of cohorts selected on axial BMD thresholds and the use of similar thresholds on

peripheral scanners for patient selection remains contentious. There is an attractive role, however, for peripheral scanners in the pre-selection of patients for full DXA. Quantitative CT can also be used to measure bone mass at axial sites and has the advantage of being able to isolate trabecular bone in the vertebral body for analysis. This is beneficial because of the high responsiveness of trabecular bone to aging and disease. However, existing CT scanners are usually in heavy demand for other medical usages and given that the capital costs of DXA scanners are vastly less and the technique has a lower radiation dose, it is unlikely CT will be used as a mainstay of providing a bone density measurement service.

The use of T scores is now the established method of reporting bone densitometry results with use of the WHO recommendations of spine and hip measurements in standard deviation units related to young normals. The T score is calculated by taking the difference between a patient's measured BMD and the mean of healthy young adults matched for gender and ethnic group and expressing the difference relative to young adult population SD:

$$\text{T score} = \frac{\text{BMD} - \text{young adult BMD}}{\text{young adult SD}}.$$

Osteoporosis is defined as a T score of less than -2.5 with an intermediate category between osteoporosis and normal defined as osteopenia with a T score between -1.0 and -2.5. It is important to remember that these definitions were developed for Caucasian women for epidemiological purposes and were not intended to establish treatment thresholds. Indeed the majority of 'osteoporotic fractures' are recognized to occur in people who are osteopenic rather than osteoporotic.[28,29]

Increasingly, it is realized that BMD is a measure of risk of fracture and being used to provide an assessment of relative and absolute fracture risk. The relative risk of fracture increases by 1.5- to 2-fold for every SD reduction in BMD, except for the hip where the relative risk is 2.5–3 for hip BMD. Because of the exponential relationship between fracture risk and BMD the risk of fracture multiplies for each SD reduction, i.e. a 2 SD reduction at the femoral neck gives up to a 9-fold increase in risk for hip fracture. It has been more recently recognized that for the same T score the risk of fracture is much greater for older patients than younger patients. Age therefore needs to be considered when identifying fracture risk for any T score. For example, a Caucasian woman age 50 with a T score of -2.5 has a 10-year fracture risk of about 3% but an 80-year-old with the same T score has a 10-year fracture risk of 20%. There is therefore now a trend to identify fracture risk in absolute rather then relative terms and data are emerging from large population cohorts to enable this to occur.[30]

The use of BMD to determine fracture risk in other ethnic groups has to be undertaken with caution unless there are good reference ranges. Even so it is not really possible to go beyond reporting in terms other than relative risk. Reporting of male patients also requires caution as although the relative risk of fracture changes with BMD in the same way as females the absolute fracture risk is less as men have a higher BMD. Data suggest that absolute fracture risk is the same for females as males for the same BMD. In men it is important therefore to consider T and Z scores for relative risk but BMD for absolute risk. The Z score has become less popular but is still helpful in the young and elderly. In premenopausal women, low Z scores without osteoporosis may alert the clinician to consider secondary causes of osteoporosis and institute measures to preserve BMD. Among the elderly over 75 years most patients will be osteoporotic and Z scores can help identify those who would most benefit from treatment.

In addition to age, other risk factors need to be considered when reporting scans. Prior low trauma fracture increases risk of future fracture approximately twofold independent of BMD. Prior vertebral fracture increases risk of further vertebral fracture 4- to 5-fold. Because of these observations there is an increasing use of T score thresholds higher than T less than -2.5 such as T less than -2.0 for patients with prior low trauma fracture, particularly in older patients. Corticosteroid users have an increased risk of fracture of about 2-fold independent of BMD and this risk increases with dose of steroid. It is now accepted that steroid users can develop low trauma fracture, particularly of the vertebrae at bone density levels greater than seen in non-users. Recent guidelines for steroid users have suggested those aged over 65 years who are commenced on treatment, where it is anticipated treatment will be at least 3 months, should be co-prescribed osteoporosis treatment, usually a bisphosphonate. For those under 65 years BMD T scores of less than -1.5 are recommended as treatment thresholds.

Follow-up scans

A common question is which patients should be offered follow-up studies? These can easily swamp any service provision but in some patients are critical to their management. For example, a young patient aged 35 on steroids may have a normal bone mass but is at risk of unusual accelerated bone loss and may require treatment if this occurs. Patients on aromatase inhibitors are recognized to be at some increased risk of fracture and accelerated bone loss and it would be good practice to monitor such patients. Similar comments apply to those who may be just above a treatment threshold but would cross it if greater bone loss than average occurred.

Monitoring patients on treatment can also be valuable to demonstrate an improvement to the patients and help guide the length of therapy. It is clearly not possible to keep monitoring everyone and selection of those most deserving is inevitably required. It has to be remembered that most patients on bisphosphonates do develop a significant rise in BMD and respond to therapy. The International Society of Clinical Densitometry has helpfully recently suggested that the main object of serial BMD measurements on treatment is to identify those who are losing bone mass who should be re-evaluated and assessed for compliance and previously undiagnosed secondary osteoporosis. When monitoring treatment with BMD, 18 months to 2 years is generally recommended as an appropriate time interval, in order to be able to demonstrate a significant change. This is about 4–5% at the spine which is the most responsive site to monitor on antiresorptive therapy.

There is now also increasing interest in using sensitive biochemical markers of bone turnover to monitor response to treatment and there are advantages of this approach as within 3 months of commencing a bisphosphonate a significant response can be identified.[31] Bone markers are not without their pitfalls, however, as other factors can of course affect them such as the presence of other skeletal disorders such as Paget's disease and the development of skeletal conditions such as a fracture occurring in the time interval between marker measurements. Although their use at present is still somewhat experimental, their value has been enhanced by the recognition that the benefit of treatment for antiresorptives appears now to be mainly through an improvement in bone quality rather than an increase in the physical amount of bone present. Indeed, antiresorptives do not appear histologically and on micro-quantitative CT (QCT) to produce new bone but rather to stabilize the trabecular network and produce more mineralized bone due to the reduction in activation frequency.[32] Bone quality cannot be measured in clinical practice in a meaningful way but bone markers are the best available approach.

Scans not required

Some patients do not necessarily require a BMD scan and these include the elderly with spinal or hip fractures where other conditions that could produce these have been excluded. Patients who are over 65 years of age and on steroids should be offered treatment without recourse to scanning. Patients with height loss or kyphosis should have an X-ray or perhaps instant vertebral assessment, with a DXA scan if fractures are present. Those with back pain should also be X-rayed first if there is suspicion of fracture and DXA performed if there is a vertebral fracture, where it would be helpful to confirm such a fracture is osteoporotic.

REFERENCES

1   Shearman J, Esdaile J, Hawkins D, Rosenthall L. Predictive value of radionuclide joint scintigrams. *Arthritis Rheum* 1982; **25**: 83–6.

2   Mottonen TT, Hannonen P, Toivanen J, *et al.* Value of joint scintigraphy in the prediction of erosiveness in early rheumatoid arthritis. *Ann Rheum Dis* 1988; **47**: 183–9.

3   De Bois MHW, Arndt JW, Van Der Velde EA, *et al.* Tc human immunoglobulin scintigraphy – a reliable method to detect joint activity in rheumatoid arthritis. *J Rheumatol* 1992; **19**: 1371–6.

4   De Bois MHW, Wesedt ML, Arndt JW, *et al.* Technetium 99m labelled polyclonal human immunoglobulin G scintigraphy before and 26 weeks after initiation of parenteral gold treatment in rheumatoid arthritis. *J Rheumatol* 1995; **22**: 1461–5.

5   Be Bois MHW, Tak PP, Arnddt JW. Joint scintigraphy for quantification of synovitis with ^{99m}Tc labelled human immunoglobulin G compared to histologic examination. *Clin Exp Rheumatol* 1995; **13**: 155–9.

6   De Bois MHW, Welling ML, Vewey CL. ^{99}Tc^{m} HIG accumulates in the synovial tissues of rats with adjuvant arthritis by binding to extra cellular matrix proteins. *Nucl Med Commun* 1996; **17**: 54–9.

7   Jamar F, Houssiau FA, Devogelar J-P, *et al.* Scintigraphy using a technetium 99m labelled anti-E-selectin Fab fragment in rheumatoid arthritis. *Rheumatology* 2002; **41**: 53–61.

8   Appelboom T, Emery P, Tant L, *et al.* Evaluation of technetium-99m-ciprofloxacin (Infecton) for detecting sites of inflammation in arthritis. *Rheumatology* 2003; **42**: 3211–20.

9   Dieppe P, Cushnaghan J, Young P, Kirwan J. Prediction of the progression of joint space narrowing in osteoarthritis of the knee by bone scintigraphy. *Ann Rheum Dis* 1993; **52**: 567–73.

10 Bruce W, Macdessi S, Van Der Wall H. Reversal of medial compartment osteoarthritis pattern after high tibial osteotomy. *Clin Nucl Med* 2001; **26**: 916–18.

11 Ryan P, Fogelman I. Sacroiliac quantitative bone scintigraphy. *Nucl Med Commun* 1993; **14**: 719–20.

12 Hanley JG, Barnes DC, Mitchell MJ, *et al.* Single photon emission computed tomography in the diagnosis of inflammatory spondyloarthropathies. *J Rheumatol* 1993; **20**: 2062–8.

13 Yildez A, Gungor F, Tuncer T, Karayalcin B. The evaluation of sacroiliitis using ^{99m}Tc-nanocolloid and ^{99m}Tc-MDP scintigraphy. *Nucl Med Commun* 2001; **22**: 785–94.

14 Puhakka KB, Jurik AG, Schiottz-Christiensen, *et al.* Magnetic resonance imaging of sacroiliitis in early seronegative spondyloarthropathy. Abnormalities correlated to clinical and laboratory findings. *Rheumatology* 2004; **42**: 234–7.

15 Marc V, Dromer C, Le Guennec P, *et al.* Magnetic resonance imaging and axial involvement in spondylarthropathies. *Rev Rheum (English Edition)* 1997; **64**: 465–73.

16 Ryan P, Chicanza I, Gibson T. Single photon emission computed tomography and the source of lumbar back pain in advanced ankylosing spondylitis. *J Clin Rheumatol* 1995; **1**: 323–7.

17 Collier BD, Carrera GF, Johnston RP, *et al.* Detection of femoral head avascular necrosis in adults by SPECT. *J Nucl Med* 1985; **26**: 979–87.

18 Lucie RS, Fuller S, Burdick DC, Johnston RM. Early prediction of avascular necrosis of the femoral head following femoral neck fractures. *Clin Orthop Rel Res* 1981; **161**: 207–14.

19 Ryu J-S, Kim JS, Moon DH, *et al.* Bone SPECT is more sensitive than MRI in the detection of early osteonecrosis of the femoral head after renal transplantation. *J Nucl Med* 2002; **43**: 1006–11.

20 Ryan P. Bone SPECT of the knees. *Nucl Med Commun* 2000; **21**: 877–85.

21 McKinnon SE, Holder SE. The use of three-phase radionuclide bone scanning in the diagnosis of reflex sympathetic dystrophy. *J Hand Surg* 1984; **9A**: 556–63.

22 Genant HK, Kozin F, Bekerman C, *et al.* The reflex sympathetic dystreophy syndrome. *Radiology* 1975; **117**; 21–32.

23 Kosin F, Soin JS, Ryan LM, *et al.* Bone scintigraphy in the reflex sympathetic syndrome. *Radiology* 1981; **138**: 437–43.

24 Cameron JR, Sorenson J. Measurement of bone mineral in vivo: an improved method. *Science* 1963; **142**: 230–2.

25 Wahner HW, Dunn WL, Riggs BL. Non-invasive bone mineral measurements. *Semin Nucl Med* 1983; **13**: 282–9.

26 Genant HK, Engelke K, Fuerst T, *et al.* Non invasive assessment of bone mineral and structure: state of the art. *J Bone Min Res* 1996; **6**: 707–30.

27 Greenspan SL, Von Stetten E, Emond SK, *et al.* Instant vertebral assessment. *J Clin Densitom* 2001; **4**: 373–80.

28 Guidelines for the provision of a clinical bone density service. National Osteoporosis Society, May 2002.

29 Position statement on the reporting of dual energy x-ray absorptiometry (DXA) bone mineral scans. National Osteoporosis Society, August 2002.

30 Kanis J. Diagnosis of osteoporosis and assessment of fracture risk. *Lancet* 2002; **359**: 1929–36.

31 Eastell R, Barton I, Hannon RA, *et al.* Relationship of early changes in bone resorption to the reduction in fracture risk with risedronate. *J Bone Min Res* 2003; **18**: 1051–6.

32 Borah B, Dufresne TE, Chmielewski PA, *et al.* Risedronate preserves trabecular architecture and increases bone strength in vertebra of ovariectomised minipigs as measured by three dimensional microcomputed tomography. *J Bone Min Res* 2002; **17**: 1139–47.

Pediatric indications

H.R. NADEL

GENERAL AND TECHNICAL CONSIDERATIONS

Bone scintigraphy is an extremely sensitive technique to assess musculoskeletal complaints in children. Whole-body scintigraphy and the liberal use of single photon emission computed tomography (SPECT) can provide a relatively simple screening for potential system disease even when the initial symptom complex may suggest focal disease. Tumor, trauma and infectious etiologies can be the cause of the abnormality seen on scintigraphy and therefore correlation with anatomic imaging as well as knowledge of the clinical presentation and other laboratory investigations is essential for improving diagnostic accuracy. The many advances in instrumentation, computer hardware and software and the introduction of new radiopharmaceuticals have contributed to an improvement in detection and diagnosis of musculoskeletal disease in children.

Techniques that allow a child to feel comfortable and unafraid while having their scintigraphic procedures are often employed in departments that perform pediatric nuclear medicine procedures. Parents and/or siblings can remain in the imaging room with the child and the child may be allowed to hold a favorite toy or a prized possession that parents have been instructed to bring with them for the test. The use of topical anesthetic creams as premedication to eliminate painful injections is routine. Immobilization techniques can include sleep deprivation, pre-examination feed, and bundling infants and young children. Distraction techniques that include videos and music can aid immensely in achieving cooperation of a young child. It is not our routine to sedate children, although occasionally this may be necessary. Children between the ages of 2 and 5 years, or who

are mentally handicapped or have severe attention deficit problems are more likely to require sedation. Usually, conscious sedation under the appropriate direction of a qualified physician will suffice. Many children's hospitals employ the services of the anesthesiology department to provide sedation services, using either conscious sedation or general anesthesia at their discretion. As a minimum, conscious sedation in children requires continuous monitoring of the patient and their oxygenation with pulse oximeter display by a nurse or physician during the time of the examination. The child then needs to be recovered sufficiently after the procedure to the point of discharge when fully awake. The cooperation of an older child can often be obtained if the procedure is carefully explained to them and their parents.[1–5]

The correct dosing for administration of radiopharmaceuticals to children can be based on either body surface area or the weight of the child relative to adult dosage. It is important to have some knowledge of what the absorbed dose would be for standard musculoskeletal scintigraphic examinations in children to enable the physician to give appropriate risk assessment when explaining the procedures.[6] The Pediatric Committee of the European Association of Nuclear Medicine has published guidelines for radiopharmaceutical dosing and for bone scintigraphy technique that are referenced below.[7]

Scanning is usually performed as a three-phase bone scan with immediate blood flow and blood pool imaging of the site of symptoms obtained after injection, followed by delayed imaging 1.5–3 h later. It is important that the children are well hydrated in order to have optimum visualization. In children who are suspected of a more systemic illness or who are under 2 years of age, whole-body blood pool imaging

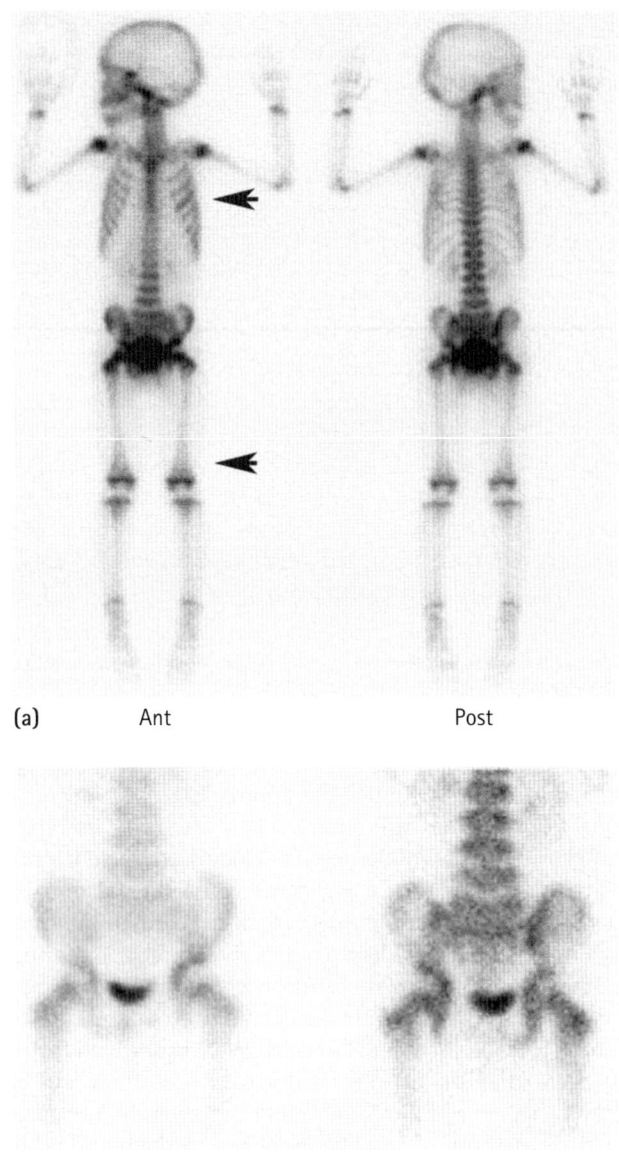

(a)   Ant   Post

(b)   Ant   Post

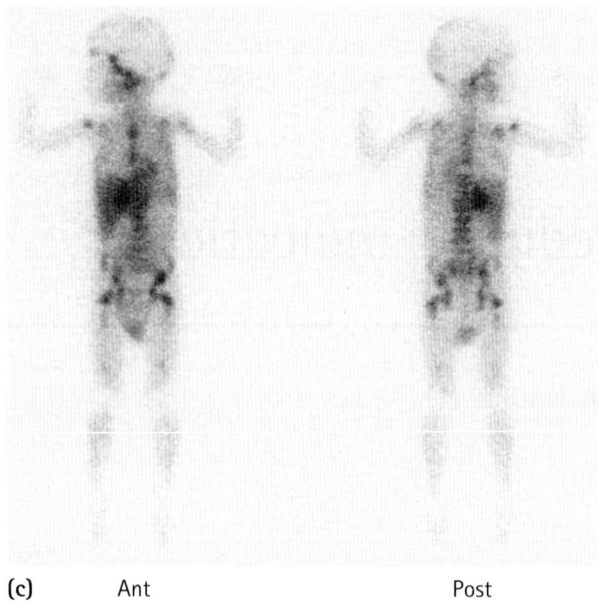

(c)   Ant   Post

Figure 9G.1 *Three-year-old boy referred from a pediatric orthopedic surgeon for suspected hip abnormality. There is no associated fever, but he has had general malaise according to the mother. (a) Methylene diphosphonate (MDP) bone scan of the whole body shows multiple abnormalities including areas of increased activity in the pelvis to include the right ilium, a rib (arrow), skull base and orbit, and patchy increased and decreased abnormality in the spine. There is also symmetrical metaphyseal increased activity in the long bones (arrow at knee). (b) The spot pelvic images with an empty bladder better delineate the diffuse abnormality in the pelvis and adjacent spine. The differential diagnosis includes leukemia, neuroblastoma and lymphoma. Ultrasound of the abdomen identified a right adrenal mass that was not easily palpated and bone marrow aspirate confirmed the diagnosis of metastatic neuroblastoma. (c) ^{123}I-MIBG scan confirmed widespread disease in keeping with stage 4 neuroblastoma with right adrenal primary that was not identified on the bone scan.*

can identify sites of hyperemia or hypoemia. Under 2 years of age, osteomyelitis with hematogenous spread can have a multifocal presentation. It is routine to perform whole-body delayed imaging in all children who present for bone scintigraphy, even if they have focal and localized symptoms. Systemic illnesses in children can present with focal symptoms such as refusal to weight-bear or unexplained bone pain. The diagnoses that might cause such multifocal abnormalities on bone scan would include tumor or tumor-like conditions such as neuroblastoma, lymphoma, leukemia, Langerhans' cell histocytosis, hematogenous osteomyeltis in child under 2 years of age, chronic recurrent multifocal osteomyelitis and fibrous dysplasia (Fig. 9G.1).

Proper positioning is important in pediatrics particularly in young infants. Although children are smaller it does not imply that more of a child can be imaged on a single scintigraphic view. In fact, examinations take longer in children and infants due to the requirement of 'joint-to-joint' images for detailed assessment. The examination may need additional delayed spot views and should be tailored as required to each individual patient's clinical presentation in order to confirm or exclude suspected diagnosis. Magnified spot views or even pinhole imaging may be required. Twenty-four hour delayed imaging to distinguish between suspected osteomyelitis and cellulitis can often be helpful. SPECT allows for improved image contrast and hence improved diagnostic accuracy. It is helpful in localizing and further defining most musculoskeletal abnormalities to include the extremities and is essential when assessing a child with the clinical problem of back pain. Correlative imaging with conventional radiographs and other cross-sectional imaging is essential when evaluating a child with musculoskeletal symptoms. Combined gamma camera/computed tomography (CT) devices allowing direct anatomic and physiologic correlation offer a further level of sophistication to the specificity of each modality and although still awaiting validation in the pediatric age group in a large series will surely further impact the care of the pediatric patient.[8]

The recognition of normal variations in the pediatric skeleton at various ages is important. Growth plates will be visualized as areas of increased activity when open. As the child grows, asymmetric closure of growth plates can sometimes be confounding but can be resolved when correlated with appropriate radiographs. It is important to be able to recognize subtle developmental variants that may mimic disease. Bone scintigraphy does not diagnosis syndromes in children, but certain syndromes may have characteristic appearances that should be able to be recognized on the scan images.[9,10]

PEDIATRIC BONE SCINTIGRAPHY INDICATIONS

In order to correctly diagnose an inflammatory process as being due to either osteomyelitis, septic arthritis, or cellulitis, a three-phase methylene diphosphonate (MDP) bone scan with blood flow, blood pool and delayed imaging is recommended. Occasionally, the flow phase may not be necessary but at least two phases are essential to show the distribution of soft tissue hyperemia. The above mentioned three inflammatory processes all demonstrate hyperemia and all three can co-exist. Hyperemia due to septic arthritis characteristically presents with involvement of both sides of the infected joint. In both cellulitis and septic arthritis, delayed bone images may be normal or show only a mild increase in bone uptake, or some persistence of soft tissue activity in a diffuse pattern without focal localization of the radiopharmaceutical on the delayed phase. Twenty-four hour delayed images in the presence of cellulitis without osteomyelitis will show clearing of mainly the soft tissue activity without focal abnormal bony localization that would be seen with osteomyelitis. Occasionally, the three-phase bone scan can help to identify subtle soft tissue abnormalities without bony involvement with careful attention to all three phases of the scan and correlation with appropriate clinical findings and other imaging studies.

Classically, osteomyelitis shows focal hyperemia on the blood flow and blood pool images with focal delayed increased uptake in bone on the delayed images. Some children presenting with acute virulent onset of disease, including high fever, rapid onset of symptoms and severe bone pain, may have 'cold' bone lesions with decreased uptake in bone on the initial imaging study delayed views.[11–13] Delayed 'cold' bone scans usually show evidence of increased hyperemia in the blood flow and blood pool phase of the study at the margins of the inflammatory process, however.

Regardless, all bone scans are positive by the end of the first week considerably earlier than radiographic change would be seen.

Whenever possible, it is ideal to obtain the bone scan prior to a joint aspiration, since the aspiration procedure itself may cause some bone reaction and increased activity on the scan images. There may be less reactive change on the scintigraphic examination if the scan is performed within a few hours of aspiration. A transient photopenic joint on the scan due to the inability of the radiopharmaceutical to reach the site of infection can be seen if there is increased joint pressure such as in the presence of a joint effusion.[14]

Because the bone scan may not become positive until 48–72 h after the onset of infection an early scan may be equivocal. The addition of specific inflammatory radiopharmaceutical imaging will increase the sensitivity in those patients in whom there is a convincing clinical suspicion of osteomyelitis. Sometimes a repeat bone scan in 48–72 h after the first scan may confirm the diagnosis and provide less of a radiation burden to the child. Imaging with white blood cells labeled with ^{111}In-oxine is not recommended in children because of the high radiation burden.[15]

Neonatal osteomyelitis was once thought to be poorly assessed with bone scintigraphy.[16] Age or size of the patient is no longer a deterrent to performing skeletal scintigraphy. Careful attention to technique with appropriate magnification spot views can result in extremely accurate images. In one study of 20 neonates scintigraphy had a 90% sensitivity for detection of focal skeletal involvement.[17]

Back pain is an uncommon symptom in childhood and vertebral scintigraphy with SPECT is an essential and sensitive means of assessing this area. After localizing the area of abnormality on scintigraphy, cross-sectional imaging with CT as either hybrid or stand-alone studies and magnetic resonance imaging (MRI) can define the abnormality. Diskitis, infection of the intervertebral disk space, is a specific inflammatory process that occurs in children. The usual pattern is delayed bone scan uptake in the vertebrae on either side of the affected disk space, but in adolescents the increase in uptake may affect only a single end plate. The differential diagnosis of acute back pain may be spondylolysis, with focal involvement of the pars interarticularis area best seen on the tomographic images.

Chronic recurrent multifocal osteomyelitis (CRMO) or chronic nonbacterial osteomyelitis is a distinct variant of osteomyelitis that occurs in children and adolescents. Its peak incidence is at age 14 years and it is more common in girls. Although an infectious agent is suspected no specific pathogen has been found and its etiology remains unknown. The clinical features include recurrent attacks of infection at multiple sites in the skeleton which are self-limited and eventually resolve after a few years of an unpredictable clinical course. Symptoms may be present from weeks to months. The child commonly presents with pain with or without swelling and fever and constitutional symptoms may or may not occur. The white blood cell count is

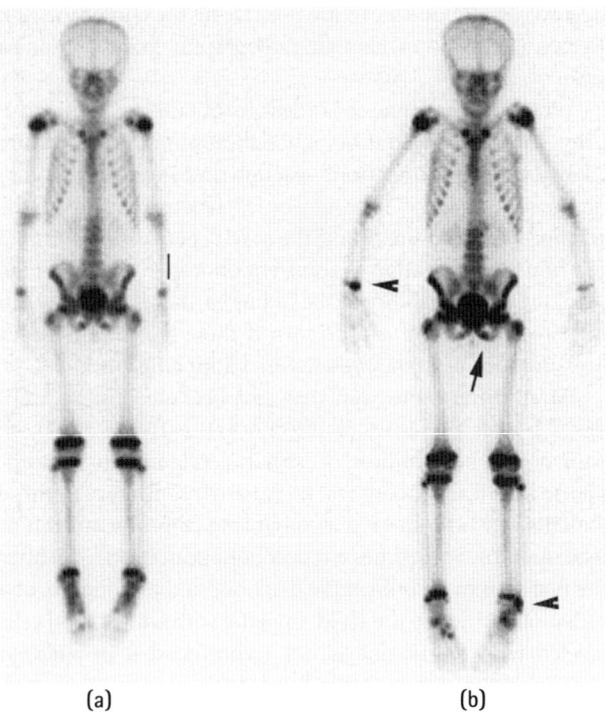

(a)   **(b)**

Figure 9G.2 *(a) Eight-year-old girl presents with recurrent episodes of pain in her left ankle. Initial bone scan is negative. (b) Repeat scan at time of recurrent symptoms in her left ankle identifies multifocal lesions including the left ankle and right wrist. No radiographic abnormality has been found. No organism has been cultured on biopsy. The diagnosis is chronic recurrent multifocal osteomyelitis.*

usually normal. The diagnosis is based on clinical, imaging and pathologic findings.[18,19] Variable radiographic appearances of mixed lytic and sclerotic lesions that involve any part of the skeleton can occur. Common sites of involvement are the metaphyseal portions of the long bones, medial ends of the clavicles, face, spine pelvis and upper extremities. Sequestra and sinus formation are uncommon. Antibiotics have no impact on the clinical course of this disease. Although CRMO and conventional osteomyelitis share a common histopathologic feature of chronic inflammation, they are different in that typically a predisposing cause is not found for CRMO in contrast to conventional osteomyelitis (Fig. 9G.2).

Bone scintigraphy can demonstrate the multifocal nature of this disease with identification of both symptomatic and asymptomatic foci. The findings on scintigraphy at typical sites are similar to that for conventional osteomyelitis. A three-phase abnormality is the hallmark at active sites, but non-active sites may not show abnormal activity. The differential diagnosis is however non-specific based on the scintigraphic findings alone and can include primary musculoskeletal neoplasm and Langerhan's cell histiocytosis.[20]

TRAUMA

In young children who are beginning to weight-bear, repetitive stress on normal bone may lead to a stress type injury complex that can involve the lower extremity. The classic toddler's fracture most commonly affects the tibia and is usually diagnosed by radiographs. Occasionally, the radiographs are equivocal, or they may involve less commonly affected bony structures such as the fibula or small bones of the feet. When a young child presents with limb pain without symptoms of infection and the radiographs are negative, bone scintigraphy may correctly and quickly localize the cause of the pain (Fig. 9G.3).

In a young child presenting with acute hip pain, bone scintigraphy may be helpful to detect avascularity of the femoral head due to Legg–Calvé–Perthes disease long before radiographic change occurs. In the healing phase various scintigraphic patterns have been described depending on whether healing occurs with a more rapid process and recanalization of existing vessels or by neovascularization with a more prolonged course. Scintigraphically, recanalization appears with visualization of a lateral column of activity after the whole head cold phase and has a better prognosis. The development of new vessels appears on bone scan as base filling and mushrooming and with the prolonged healing time may put the femoral head at greater risk for further complications and growth disturbances.[21,22]

In older children presenting with acute hip pain, the bone scan may show subtle findings that suggest the diagnosis of slipped capital femoral epiphysis. The bone scan may show characteristic increased activity involving the proximal femoral epiphyseal plate that is best seen from a posterior position and on a frog lateral positioned view. The bone scan will also identify patterns that may suggest avascular necrosis of the femoral head or chondrolysis.

Bone scintigraphy in the suspected case of child abuse can provide a quick assessment for defining and characterizing the extent and severity of trauma that is complementary to other radiologic investigations.[23] The major advantages of bone scintigraphy are its increased sensitivity (25–50%) in detecting evidence of soft tissue as well as bone trauma, and in the documentation of specific and characteristic sites of abuse such as in the ribs or the diaphyses of the extremities[24,25] (Fig. 9G.4). Scintigraphy may be particularly helpful in young infants when subtle areas of bony injury may be too early to detect on radiographs or completely healed areas may be radiographically normal. In both of these instances the bone scan may show areas of increased activity. The study is performed as a three-phase study to include whole-body blood pool imaging, and can include a 5 min renogram to assess unsuspected renal injury. SPECT of the thorax is particularly helpful in detecting the position of acute and healing rib fractures. Careful attention to technique and visualization of all bony structures with maximum zoom and in multiple projections is important. Scintigraphy is not

Blood pool   Delayed

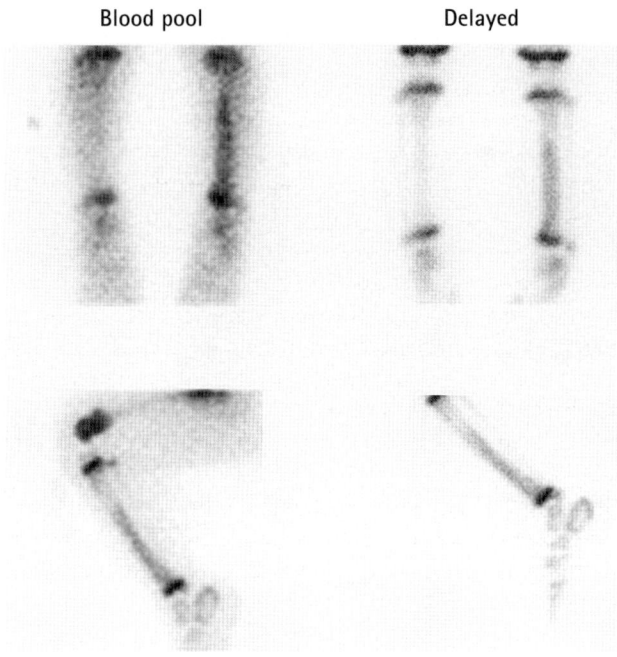

(a)

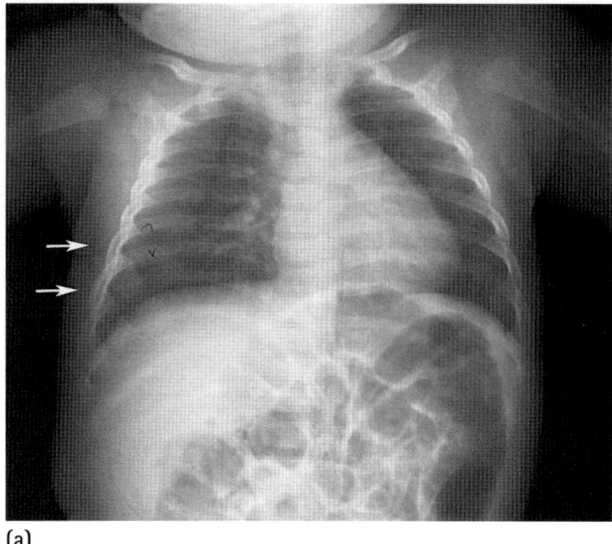

(a)

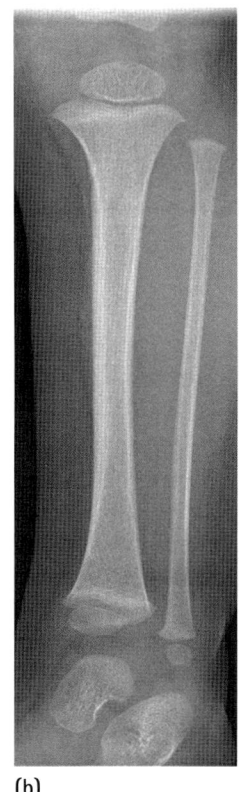

(b)

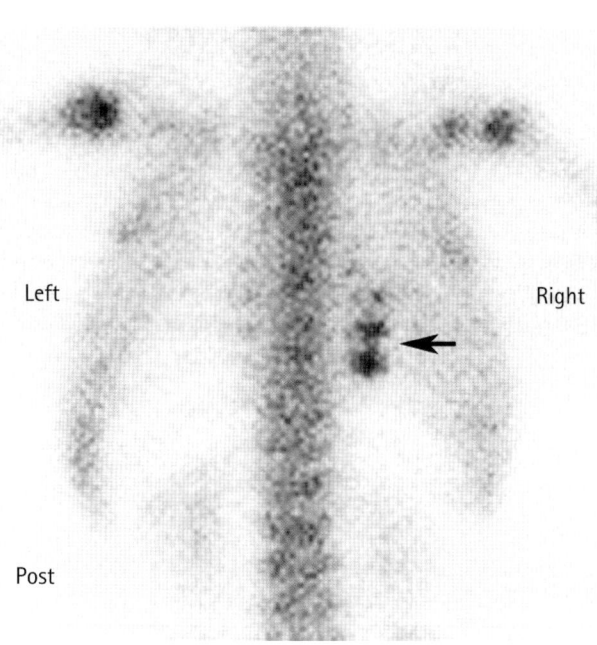

Left   Right

Post

(b)

Figure 9G.3 *(a) This 15-month-old boy presented with decreased weight-bearing on his left leg without fever. Blood pool and delayed methylene diphosphonate bone imaging shows hyperemia and corresponding obliquely oriented focal activity in the left tibia. (b) Corresponding radiograph of the left tibia was negative. The bone scan confirmed the clinical findings of a radiographically occult toddler's fracture in the left tibia.*

Figure 9G.4 *(a) Chest radiograph in a 6-month infant with suspected non-accidental injury. There were healing anterior right rib fractures identified in 7th and 8th rib (arrow). No posterior rib fractures were identified radiographically. (b) Methylene diphosphonate delayed bone scan image obtained 2 weeks after the initial radiograph shown in (a) shows increased activity in contiguous posterior right ribs in the costovertebral region which is a characteristic site for fractures of possible non-accidental injury. These fractures subsequently showed healing only on follow-up radiographs, thus confirming fractures of varying ages consistent with non-accidental injury. SPECT images (not shown) also revealed increased activity in right anterior contiguous ribs which did show radiographic appearance consistent with healing rib fractures.*

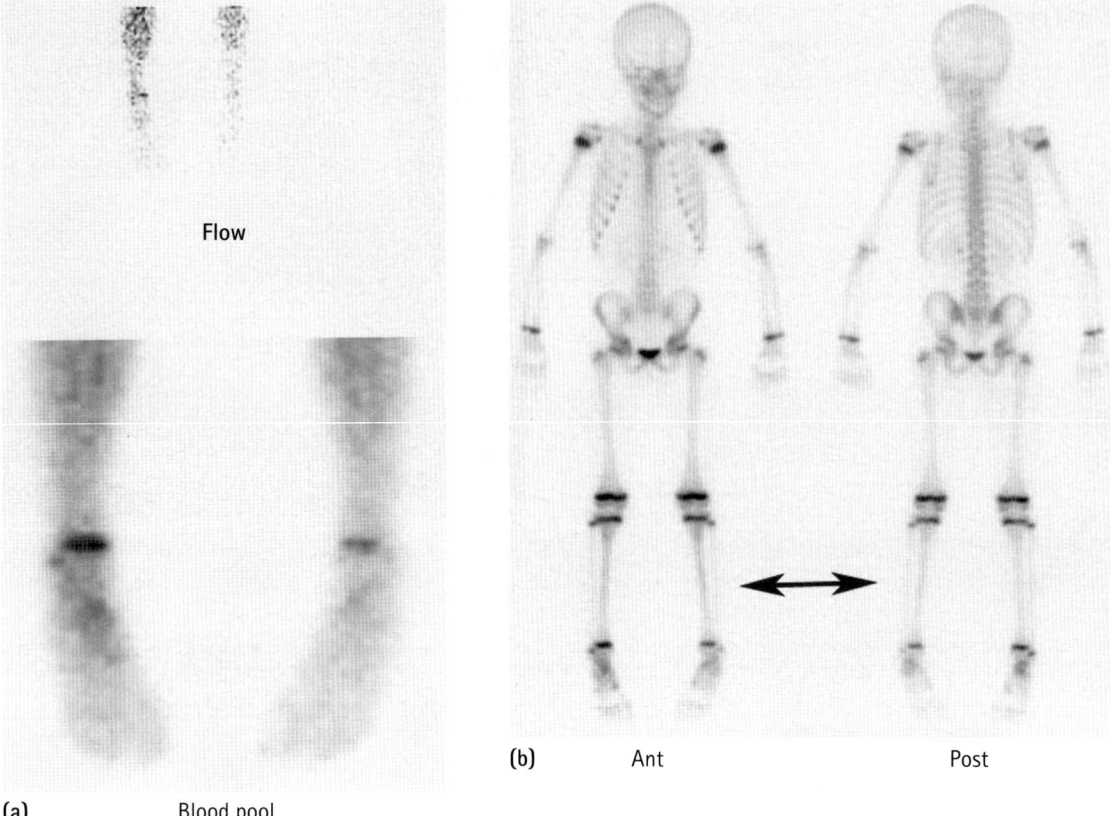

Flow

(a) Blood pool

(b) Ant   Post

Figure 9G.5 *(a) Anterior blood flow and blood pool images and (b) delayed whole body images in 14-year-old athlete with pain in the left leg. No known previous trauma. There is a three-phase cold abnormality involving the left leg and foot. Radiographs were normal. The findings are consistent with the cold form of reflex sympathetic dystrophy. The adolescent was treated supportively and with physiotherapy with relief of her symptoms.*

reliable for detection of skull fractures so conventional radiographs and or CT would be necessary for this evaluation.

REFLEX SYMPATHETIC DYSTROPHY

Reflex sympathetic dystrophy is the pain syndrome that has various clinical forms, precipitating factors, localizations, physiological, physiopathological hypotheses and diagnostic criteria and is now used to encompass all variants of the syndrome which include pain, hyperesthesia, vasomotor disturbances and dystrophic changes that usually improve with sympathetic denervation. Trauma that is acute or may also be remote by months or longer is the most common precipitating factor in the pain syndrome. Children may not have a defined antecedent event and the pain can be misdiagnosed as having a psychiatric cause and the diagnosis delayed.

The three-phase bone scan can play an important role in diagnosis of this syndrome as there are often few if any other radiologic modalities which will show an abnormality. The classic scintigraphic appearance includes intense periarticular

activity in an involved extremity on the delayed phase of the scan preceded by hyperemia in a similar distribution on the immediate post-injection blood flow and blood pool phases of the scan.[26] A cold scintigraphic form of the disease has been called *les formes froides*.[27] This cold variant is the more common form seen in children.[28] Bone scan findings in the cold variant of RSD include photopenic abnormalities on the delayed scan and hypoemia on the immediate blood flow and blood pool phase. The abnormality can be recognized in children who have open epiphyses by the incongruence of the involved epiphyseal activity compared to remote ipsilateral and contralateral epiphyseal plate activity[29] (Fig. 9G.5)

TUMOR IMAGING AND RESPONSE ASSESSMENT

Scintigraphic examinations can be used in the evaluation of musculoskeletal tumors in children to include osteogenic sarcoma, Ewing's sarcoma, rhabdomyosarcoma, neuroblastoma, lymphoma and occasionally leukemia. These tumors can be evaluated with conventional MDP bone scan or other tumor-specific radiopharmaceuticals that include ^{201}Tl, ^{99m}Tc-sestamibi, *meta*-iodobenzylguanidine (MIBG) and fluorodeoxyglucose (FDG) positron emission tomography (PET).

Primary malignant bone tumors such as osteogenic sarcoma, Ewing's sarcoma and rhadomyosarcoma involving bone will all show intense increased activity on MDP bone scans. In osteogenic sarcoma there may be soft tissue extension of the tumor detected as well. Rarely, bone lymphoma and leukemic lesions will appear photopenic. MDP scintigraphy is still the appropriate way to survey the skeleton for extent of disease including metastatic or multifocal disease including skip lesions. An 'extended pattern' of diffuse increased uptake can occur in other bones in the same extremity as the lesion, particularly in the adjacent joints. In osteogenic sarcoma pulmonary metastases can show uptake of ^{99m}Tc-MDP but the sensitivity for uptake is much less than the sensitivity for metastatic disease detected with CT scan. Bone marrow disease may show a diffuse marrow type pattern typically showing metaphyseal activity that is more diffuse and can be symmetrical usually around the hips and knees; but the bone scan is not specific for marrow disease. MDP bone scintigraphy is not useful for tumor response assessment, as the bone scan remains abnormal in bone tumors in the presence of healing bone lesions. Surveillance bone scans are used to re-screen for progressive metastatic disease or local recurrence after tumor resection. Whole-body scintigraphy and the liberal use of SPECT are routine for MDP bone scintigraphy.

Increased ^{99m}Tc-MDP activity not due to metastatic disease may be found after amputation of a lower limb and fitting of a prosthesis at various sites to include: the stump tip, in the ipsilateral hip joint and sacroiliac joint, in the soft tissues surrounding the prosthesis, and diffusely in the entire limb due to altered biomechanical stress. Allograft limb reconstruction following limb-sparing surgery for osteogenic sarcoma will show persistent increased ^{99m}Tc activity at the junction of the allograft and normal bone. Persistently decreased ^{99m}Tc-MDP activity is seen in the graft cortical bone and variable uptake is noted at the periphery of the graft. Similar to adults use of colony stimulating factors (CSFs) to reduce myelotoxicity in patients on chemotherapy can cause a pattern of nonspecific increased activity in the axial skeleton and/or juxta-articular areas on bone scintigraphy.

Between 10 and 25% of pediatric lymphoma patients may have bone involvement. The conventional bone scan, therefore, has been an important tool in the work-up of these patients. FDG PET is also very sensitive for detecting lymphomatous bone involvement. Between 35 and 100% of neuroblastoma patients show bone scan uptake into their soft tissue neuroblastoma primary tumors. Sixty-six percent of patients with stage 4 neuroblastoma have bone metastases at the time of presentation and 47% have bone metastases at first recurrence.[30] Therefore the nuclear

bone scan has been an important part of the diagnostic work-up of patients with neuroblastoma. The abnormal bony uptake on the bone scan can, however, be difficult to interpret due to the high frequency of symmetrical metaphyseal uptake. Particularly in those cases, the ^{123}I-MIBG scan may be more revealing about bone metastases.

The characteristic appearance of symmetrical metaphyseal activity on conventional bone scan can be subtle and difficult to interpret for those not used to viewing such scintigraphic images in children and if the abnormality is widespread in all or many long bones. Normal appearances of the growing metabolically active epiphysis on bone scan should appear as a linear area of increased activity with no surrounding 'blooming' into the metaphysis. The differential diagnosis of symmetrical metaphyseal abnormal appearance on bone scan can be due to marrow expansion from anemia or replacement with either tumor or fibrosis. Poor positioning can mimic this finding as well. Seeing the joint areas in two projections can often be helpful and the addition of SPECT may further clarify planar findings. This abnormal pattern can be seen in tumors to include neuroblastoma, lymphoma, leukemia and rhabdomyosarcoma or any other tumor that can have marrow involvement. The search for this pattern once ^{99m}Tc-MDP has been injected into a child to confirm systemic disease is another reason to perform whole-body scintigraphy and to avoid only regional bone scans in the pediatric age group. Also, pediatric tumors that affect bone as either primary or metastatic disease can have lesions that occur distal to the elbows and knees (Fig. 9G.6).

Histologic response assessment to presurgical adjuvant chemotherapy is one of the best predictors of overall survival in tumors such as osteosarcoma and Ewing's sarcoma.[31,32] Thallium and sestamibi scintigraphy have been used at diagnosis to determine tumor avidity for the radiopharmaceuticals in the hopes of using these radiopharmaceuticals as surrogate tumor markers of response. A decrease in tumor uptake by these radiopharmaceuticals indicates a good response, while persistence of radiopharmaceutical activity in the primary site signifies a poor response[33–38] (Fig. 9G.7).

FDG PET and FDG PET/CT imaging in primary malignant bone tumors is being evaluated and is showing good sensitivity in staging, prognosis evaluation and response assessment. Primary malignant bone tumors have increased FDG uptake in primary and metastatic bone and soft tissue disease. Pulmonary metastatic disease visualization is variable but may in part be due to small size of lesions. Response assessment and prognosis can be tied to a decrease in the maximum standardized uptake value (SUV$_{max}$) when evaluation at diagnosis is compared to early post treatment evaluation. Large studies in pediatric age groups have not as yet been validated in these tumor types. FDG PET and PET/CT studies often identify more lesions than conventional bone scan in primary malignant bone tumors as both bone and soft tissue lesions can be detected. Because of the significance

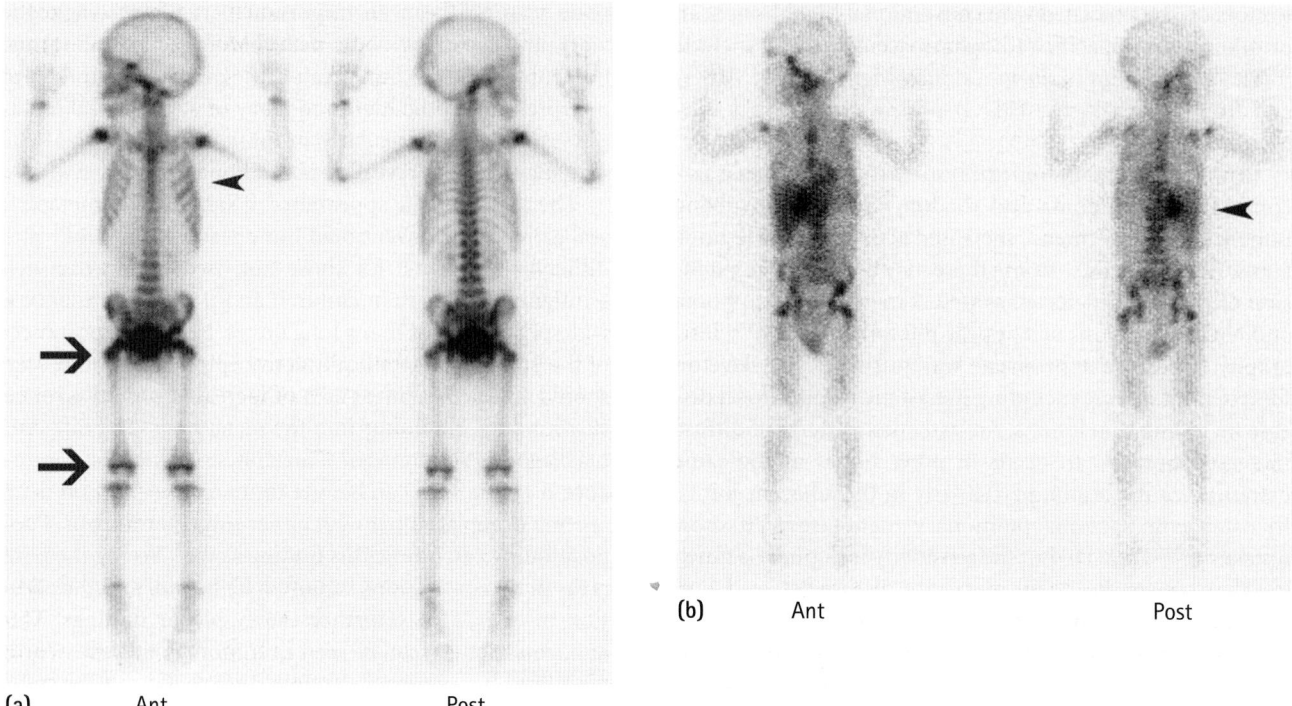

(a)   Ant   Post

(b)   Ant   Post

Figure 9G.6   *(a) Three-year-old boy presents with vague hip pain and inability to weight-bear. Whole-body methylene diphosphonate (MDP) bone scan identifies diffuse symmetrical metaphyseal abnormal activity (arrows showing representative metaphyseal abnormality at hips and knees on anterior view). Spot views of the pelvis with the bladder empty confirm abnormality diffusely in pelvis and patchy abnormal activity in the spine. More diffuse abnormality is also present on the whole-body bone images involving skull base and a left rib (arrowhead). SPECT imaging helped to further delineate the widespread abnormality. On further clinical evaluation blood and bone marrow aspirate confirmed the diagnosis of neuroblastoma. (b) ¹²³I-MIBG whole-body image shows diffuse involvement with stage 4 disease. The MIBG scan also identifies a right upper quadrant adrenal mass (arrowhead) that did not show soft tissue uptake on the MDP bone scan. If only regional bone scan of the hips had been performed, the widespread nature of the disease might have been more difficult to appreciate and there might have been a delay in obtaining the correct diagnosis in this patient.*

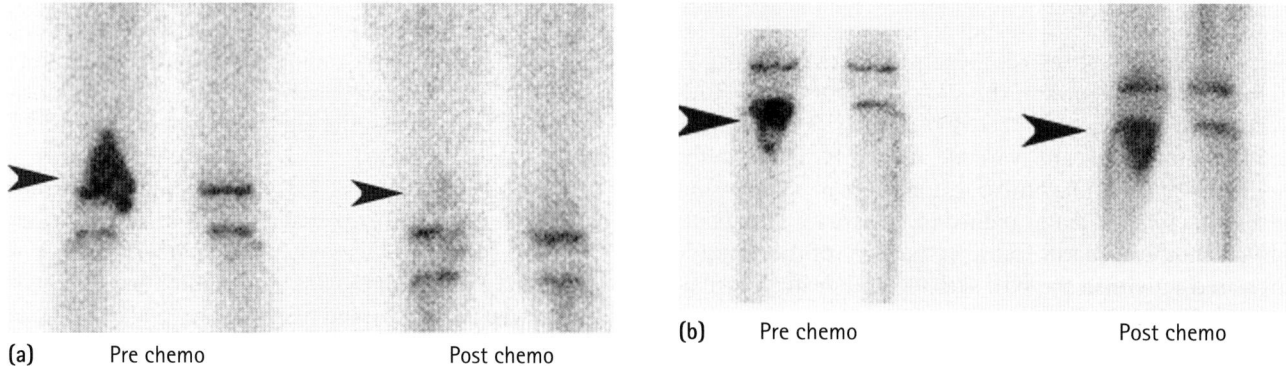

(a)   Pre chemo   Post chemo

(b)   Pre chemo   Post chemo

Figure 9G.7   *(a) Thallium-201 scan in a boy with osteogenic sarcoma of the right distal femur. Pre-chemotherapy there is intense thallium uptake in the primary lesion; post-adjuvant chemotherapy these is almost complete resolution of the previously noted thallium activity. This good response was confirmed at the time of definitive surgery with greater than 95% tumor histologic necrosis. This suggests that this patient will have a good prognosis for an event-free survival. (b) Patient who shows persistent thallium avidity in primary osteogenic sarcoma in the right proximal tibia both pre- and post-chemotherapy. This patient had persistent mitotic malignant cells in pathologic specimen confirmed after definitive surgery and would not be expected to have as good a prognosis for event-free survival.*

of a poor prognosis in the presence of microscopic bone marrow disease, FDG PET/CT studies can be helpful in directing sites of biopsy[39–43] (Plate 9G.1).

Future considerations for musculoskeletal scintigraphic imaging in children could potentially include the use of ^{18}F to replace conventional MDP bone scintigraphy. Fusion imaging with SPECT/CT will also better localize disease sites. The issues around hybrid imaging have not yet fully been worked out in children. Controversies include whether to perform diagnostic contrast-enhanced CT scans routinely with either PET/CT or SPECT/CT and the complete interpretation of both these studies routinely.

REFERENCES

1 American Academy of Pediatrics Committee on Drugs. Guidelines for monitoring and management of pediatric patients during and after sedation for diagnostic and therapeutic procedures. *Pediatrics* 1992; **89**: 1110–5.

2 Frush DP, Bisset 3rd GS, Hall SC. Pediatric sedation in radiology: the practice of safe sleep. *Am J Roentgenol* 1996; **167**: 1381–7.

3 Hopkins KL, Davis PC, Sanders CL, Churchill LH. Sedation for pediatric imaging studies. *Neuroimaging Clin N Am* 1999; **9**: 1–10.

4 Krauss B, Green SM. Sedation and analgesia for procedures in children. *N Engl J Med* 2000; **342**: 938–45.

5 Weiss S. Sedation of pediatric patients for nuclear medicine procedures. *Semin Nucl Med* 1993; **23**: 190–8.

6 Stabin MG, Gelfand MJ. Dosimetry of pediatric nuclear medicine procedures. *Q J Nucl Med* 1998; **42**: 95–112.

7 Hahn K, Fischer S, Colarinha P, *et al.* Guidelines for bone scintigraphy in children. *Eur J Nucl Med* 2001; **28**: BP42–7.

8 Horger M, Eschmann SM, Pfannenberg C, *et al.* The value of SPET/CT in chronic osteomyelitis. *Eur J Nucl Med Mol Imaging* 2003; **30**: 1665–73.

9 Gordon I, Hahn K, Fischer S. *Atlas of bone scintigraphy in the pathological paediatric skeleton.* Berlin: Springer Verlag, 1996.

10 Hahn K, Fischer S, Gordon I. *Atlas of bone scintigraphy in the developing paediatric skeleton.* Berlin: Springer Verlag, 1993.

11 Pennington WT, Mott MP, Thometz JG, *et al.* Photopenic bone scan osteomyelitis: a clinical perspective. *J Pediatr Orthop* 1999; **19**: 695–8.

12 Rosovsky M, FitzPatrick M, Goldfarb CR, Finestone H. Bilateral osteomyelitis due to intraosseous infusion: case report and review of the English-language literature. *Pediatr Radiol* 1994; **24**: 72–3.

13 Rosovsky M, Goldfarb CR, Finestone H, Ongseng F. 'Cold spots' in pediatric bone imaging. *Semin Nucl Med* 1994; **24**: 184–6.

14 Mandell GA. Nuclear medicine in pediatric orthopedics [Review]. *Semin Nucl Med* 1998; **28**: 95–115.

15 Gainey MA, Siegel JA, Smergel EM, Jara BJ. Indium-111 labeled white blood cells: Dosimetry in children. *J Nucl Med* 1988; **29**: 689–94.

16 Ash J, Gilday DL. The futility of bone scanning in neonatal osteomyelitis: concise communication. *J Nucl Med* 1980; **21**: 417–20.

17 Aigner RM, Fueger GF, Ritter G. Results of three-phase bone scintigraphy and radiography in 20 cases of neonatal osteomyelitis. *Nucl Med Commun* 1996; **17**: 20–8.

18 Chow LT, Griffith JF, Kumta SM, Leung PC. Chronic recurrent multifocal osteomyelitis: a great clinical and radiologic mimic in need of recognition by the pathologist. *APMIS* 1999; **107**: 369–79.

19 Trobs R, Moritz R, Buhligen U, *et al.* Changing pattern of osteomyelitis in infants and children. *Pediatr Surg Int* 1999; **15**: 363–72.

20 Mandell GA, Contreras SJ, Conard K, *et al.* Bone scintigraphy in the detection of chronic recurrent multifocal osteomyelitis. *J Nucl Med* 1998; **39**: 1778–83.

21 Conway JJ. A scintigraphic classification of Legg–Calve–Perthes disease. *Semin Nucl Med* 1993; **23**: 274–95.

22 Tsao AK, Dias LS, Conway JJ, Straka P. The prognostic value and significance of serial bone scintigraphy in Legg–Calve–Perthes disease. *J Pediatr Orthop* 1997; **17**: 230–9.

23 Kleinman PK. *Diagnostic imaging of child abuse.* St. Louis: Mosby Inc., 1998.

24 Conway JJ, Collins M, Tanz RR, *et al.* The role of bone scintigraphy in detecting child abuse. *Semin Nucl Med* 1993; **23**: 321–33.

25 Sty JR, Wells RG. Child abuse. Extraosseous abdominal bone imaging uptake. *Clin Nucl Med* 1994; **19**: 1011.

26 Kozin F, Soin JS, Ryan LM, *et al.* Bone scintigraphy in the reflex sympathetic dystrophy syndrome. *Radiology* 1981; **138**: 437–43.

27 Driessens M, Dijs H, Verheyen G, Blockx P. What is reflex sympathetic dystrophy? *Acta Orthop Belg* 1999; **65**: 202–17.

28 Oud CF, Legein J, Everaert H, *et al.* Bone scintigraphy in children with persistent pain in an extremity, suggesting algoneurodystrophy. *Acta Orthop Belg* 1999; **65**: 364–6.

29 McEachern AM, Nadel HR. Reflex sympathetic dystrophy: characteristic findings in children [Abstract]. *Pediatr Radiol* 1999; **29**: 941.

30 Cheung NK, Cohn SL. (eds.) *Neuroblastoma.* Berlin: Springer, 2005.

31 Picci P, Rougraff BT, Bacci G, *et al.* Prognostic significance of histopathologic response to chemotherapy in nonmetastatic Ewing's sarcoma of the extremities. *J Clin Oncol* 1993; **11**: 1763–9.

32 Provisor AJ, Ettinger LJ, Nachman JB, *et al.* Treatment of nonmetastatic osteosarcoma of the extremity with

preoperative and postoperative chemotherapy: a report from the Children's Cancer Group. *J Clin Oncol* 1997; **15**: 76–84.

33 Howman-Giles R, Uren RF, Shaw PJ. Thallium-201 scintigraphy in pediatric soft-tissue tumors. *J Nucl Med* 1995; **36**: 1372–6.

34 Imbriaco M, Yeh SD, Yeung H, *et al.* Thallium-201 scintigraphy for the evaluation of tumor response to preoperative chemotherapy in patients with osteosarcoma. *Cancer* 1997; **80**: 1507–12.

35 Nadel HR. Thallium-201 for oncological imaging in children. *Semin Nucl Med* 1993; **23**: 243–54.

36 Ohtomo K, Terui S, Yokoyama R, *et al.* Thallium-201 scintigraphy to assess effect of chemotherapy in osteosarcoma. *J Nucl Med* 1996; **37**: 1444–8.

37 Sumiya H, Taki J, Tsuchiya H, *et al.* Midcourse thallium-201 scintigraphy to predict tumor response in bone and soft-tissue tumors. *J Nucl Med* 1998; **39**: 1600–4.

38 Taki J, Sumiya H, Tsuchiya H, *et al.* Evaluating benign and malignant bone and soft-tissue lesions with technetium-99m-MIBI scintigraphy. *J Nucl Med* 1997; **38**: 501–6.

39 Brisse H, Ollivier L, Edeline V, *et al.* Imaging of malignant tumours of the long bones in children: monitoring response to neoadjuvant chemotherapy and preoperative assessment. *Pediatr Radiol* 2004; **34**: 595–605.

40 Franzius C, Daldrup-Link HE, Wagner-Bohn A, *et al.* FDG-PET for detection of recurrences from malignant primary bone tumors: comparison with conventional imaging. *Ann Oncol* 2002; **13**: 157–60.

41 Franzius C, Schober O. Assessment of therapy response by FDG PET in pediatric patients. *Q J Nucl Med* 2003; **47**: 41–5.

42 Hawkins DS, Rajendran JG, Conrad 3rd EU, *et al.* Evaluation of chemotherapy response in pediatric bone sarcomas by [F-18]-fluorodeoxy-D-glucose positron emission tomography. *Cancer* 2002; **94**: 3277–84.

43 Hawkins DS, Schuetze SM, Butrynski JE, *et al.* [^{18}F]Fluorodeoxyglucose positron emission tomography predicts outcome for Ewing sarcoma family of tumors. *J Clin Oncol* 2005; **23**: 8828–34.

10

Neuroimaging

10A Dementia

Introduction	415	Dementia of the Lewy body type	419
Alzheimer's disease	416	Future developments	420
Vascular dementia	418	Conclusion	421
Fronto-temporal dementia	418	References	421

10B Functional imaging in cerebrovascular disease and neuropsychiatry

Introduction	425	SPECT imaging in mood disorders	429
Clinical role of brain perfusion SPECT in cerebrovascular	426	Schizophrenia	429
disease		Anxiety disorders	430
Functional imaging in psychiatry	428	References	430

10C Epilepsy

Introduction	435	Pediatric epilepsies	439
SPECT imaging	436	Conclusion	440
Positron emission tomography	436	References	442

10D Neuro-oncology

Epidemiology	445	Other radiotracers for positron emission tomography	450
Histopathologic classification	446	Imaging protocol for brain FDG PET	452
Imaging of brain tumors	446	Image registration	452
SPECT imaging of brain tumors	447	Conclusion	453
FDG PET imaging of brain tumors	447	References	453

10E PET and SPECT imaging in movement disorders

Introduction	457	Dystonia	460
PET and SPECT studies		Choreatic disorders	460
in parkinsonism	458	References	461
Essential tremor	460		

Dementia

PAUL M. KEMP

INTRODUCTION

This chapter discusses the role of neuro-imaging in cognitive failure. In particular, the complementary modalities of functional and structural imaging are discussed in relation to the four most common types of dementia, namely Alzheimer's disease (AD), vascular, Lewy body and fronto-temporal dementia. With the potential development of therapies in Alzheimer's disease, which may halt the progress of this disease in a significant minority for up to 18 months, it is becoming increasingly important to be able to establish an accurate diagnosis in the earliest stages of the disease process.[1] Histopathological studies have shown that the clinical diagnosis can be incorrect in a substantial proportion of patients in the early stages[2] and therefore one needs to be aware of the contribution, and limitations, of imaging modalities to augment the clinical findings.

It is estimated that approximately 2–5% of people over the age of 65 years are demented, which increases exponentially with age. Indeed, over 40% of people older than 85 years of age are thought to be sufficiently cognitively impaired to warrant a diagnosis of dementia. Obviously, many more subjects may have minor cognitive problems which, as yet, do not fulfil the criteria for an established dementia. Clearly, with the aging population, the prevalence of disease is going to increase. Direct costs to the health and welfare systems in the UK for the estimated prevalence of 800 000 cases of dementia are estimated at approximately $10 billion (approximately equivalent to £6 billion/8 billion euros);[3] indirect costs may be at least three-fold these values. These vast sums reflect that demented patients require considerable nursing and social support over many years.

Types of dementia

It is clearly important to exclude potentially reversible causes, biochemical, inflammatory or structural, in any patient presenting with cognitive impairment. The primary neuro-degenerative dementias have four major etiologies. It is estimated that approximately 60% of all patients with dementia have Alzheimer's disease, a further 15–20% will have vascular and Lewy body dementia each and approximately 1% will have fronto-temporal dementia. Sporadic (i.e. nonfamilial) dementias can occur from the age of 40 onwards. Current terminology recommends the term early-onset disease if the dementia commences before retirement age (i.e. 65 years) and late-onset disease after this. Although this may appear an arbitrary cut-off it does have clinical relevance. The relative prevalence of the different types of dementias differs with age of presentation. The major difference is that in early-onset dementia the proportion of fronto-temporal cases increases to 25% (compared to 1% in the late-onset cases); of the remainder Alzheimer's disease and vascular dementia account for approximately 50% and 25% respectively.[4]

Clinical criteria have been developed for all these disease processes and there is a considerable range of values in the literature for the diagnostic accuracies. Obviously, patients with moderately severe disease are more easily categorized than those with mild impairment. Histopathological material is crucial for verifying the accuracy of the clinical diagnosis and investigations. This reflects that, as yet, there is no reliable 'gold standard' investigation whilst the patient is alive. Given the limitations of the clinical assessment, it is therefore important to establish whether neuro-imaging can contribute to formulating a more accurate diagnosis.

Imaging modalities

Neuro-imaging can be subdivided into functional (single photon emission computed tomography (SPECT) and positron emission tomography (PET)) and structural (computed tomography/magnetic resonance (CT/MR)) imaging. Given the expense of brain imaging and the limited facilities, it is important that these resources are used appropriately. It is also important to consider whether the patient can tolerate the techniques. Obviously CT is a relatively quick procedure and less prone to movement artifacts. MRI, SPECT and PET are relatively long acquisition procedures and it is important that the patient is able to remain motionless for the 15–30 min acquisitions. A substantial proportion of cognitively impaired patients find MRI too claustrophobic; unfortunately radiographic staff cannot be sufficiently close to reassure the patient. Functional and structural imaging should be regarded as complementary in the investigation of patients with suspected cognitive impairment. Structural imaging is essential in appropriate patients for the detection of infarcts, cerebral neoplasm, subdural hematoma and normal pressure hydrocephalus.

Since the late 1980s, there has been a deluge of studies assessing the relative merits of neuro-imaging in dementia. Unfortunately, very few of these studies have autopsy data. Given that demented patients can live for up to 15 years following diagnosis, there can be a considerable delay in establishing 'truth'. Consequently, accurate data can only be obtained up to a decade after the initial presentation and by this stage there have usually been significant developments in imaging hardware and software. Despite these limitations, it is still possible to derive trends from the plethora of studies in the literature.

ALZHEIMER'S DISEASE

This is the commonest dementia in the Western world and can be subclassified according to age of onset. Presentation before the age of 65 years is described as early onset, whereas those presenting after this age are termed late onset.

Late-onset (senile) Alzheimer's disease

HISTOPATHOLOGY

In the United Kingdom, it is believed that there are approximately 500 000 people fulfilling the criteria for late onset AD. Histopathological studies have demonstrated that the basic pathology appears to be related to the deposition of amyloid tangles and plaques in neural tissue and the vasculature (amyloid angiopathy). This amyloid protein is initially deposited in the region of the medial temporal lobe structures, namely the entorhinal cortex, the hippocampal, parahippocampal, and fusiform gyri.[5] These medial temporal structures are crucial links in short-term memory circuits and therefore destruction of this tissue leads to the clinical manifestation of forgetfulness. As there are numerous projections from this region to the posterior association cortices, namely the parieto-temporal association areas, then as these projections become disrupted this leads to synaptic loss in the target areas.[6] Consequently, after the initial presentation of amnesia, the patient usually develops cognitive problems related to these parieto-temporal association areas. It is important to emphasize that *initially* the parieto-temporal symptoms and signs are due to this disconnection phenomenon (diaschisis) and not due to direct amyloid infiltration *at this stage*.[7,8] As the disease progresses there is direct amyloid infiltration into these posterior association areas. Left-sided parieto-temporal symptoms in right-handed individuals (i.e. the dominant side of the brain) will present as language dysfunction. Right-sided parieto-temporal involvement will be heralded clinically by visuo-spatial impairment, i.e. patients will find themselves getting lost in familiar places and have difficulties with dressing, tying shoe laces etc. Finally, as the amyloid deposition progresses to the frontal lobes, patients will have behavioral and personality problems. Average life expectancy after presentation is approximately 7–8 years.

The clinical criteria for diagnosing Alzheimer's disease are generally based upon the findings of short-term memory impairment, due to medial temporal involvement, plus impairment in another cognitive domain, usually parietal. Clinical diagnosis using the NINCDS-ADRDA criteria[9] can be subdivided into 'possible' or 'probable' AD. The sensitivity of a *probable* diagnosis is approximately 50% against a specificity of 95%. However, for a *possible or probable* diagnosis, the sensitivity increases to 85%, but the specificity falls to around 60%.[2] This scenario typifies the trade-off between sensitivity and specificity observed in all areas of diagnostic medicine. Clearly, there would appear to be considerable scope for ancillary investigations to augment the clinical findings.

IMAGING STUDIES

There is a multitude of studies published in the literature assessing the accuracy of functional and structural imaging in Alzheimer's disease. One of the major factors for the variation in accuracies is the dementia severity of the population studied. Patients with advanced disease are more likely to have abnormalities on imaging, i.e. increased sensitivity. However, it is clearly important nowadays to be able to diagnose the disease at its earliest stages. The age of the population studied also needs to be taken into account when interpreting functional and structural imaging studies, as the physiological effects of healthy aging may overlap early pathological appearances.[10] In addition, group separation of demented cases from healthy controls gives more favorable results as opposed to differentiating the different types of dementia. Very few studies have histopathological follow-up; the vast majority rely on the clinical diagnosis as the gold standard. This is somewhat ironic, because it is the lack of accuracy of clinical criteria that necessitated the evaluation of imaging techniques. An important population-based prospective study with histopathological follow-up is the OPTIMA (Oxford Project to Investigate Memory and Ageing) trial.[8] This study commenced in the mid-1980s with patients undergoing serial clinical assessments, CT and hexamethylpropylene amine oxime (HMPAO) SPECT imaging annually. CT assessed for medial temporal atrophy and HMPAO SPECT assessed for parieto-temporal hypoperfusion (Plates 10A.1 and 10A.2). At death, post-mortem material was obtained in a highly creditable 95% of cases. A substantial publication by this group in 1998,[8] gave results for sensitivities and specificities of HMPAO SPECT and CT of the order of 75–90% which would appear to be more accurate than the clinical criteria.

These initial results clearly demonstrated that neural imaging may have a useful role in the diagnosis of Alzheimer's disease. However, it is important to address some of the shortcomings of the study. In particular, the results were based on the final imaging obtained and therefore the majority of the patients would have had a moderate severity of disease at that stage. Furthermore, the HMPAO SPECT scans were obtained on a single-headed gamma camera, which has now been superseded by multi-detector systems.

Most centers investigating patients with suspected AD will assess for bilateral deficits in perfusion to the parieto-temporal association areas. However, by definition, these patients will have progressed to a moderate disease severity. Unilaterally parietal temporal abnormalities need to be interpreted cautiously, as a substantial minority of these deficits could represent ischemia.[11] Bilateral parietal temporal deficits are not pathognomonic for AD and are also noted in dementia with Lewy bodies and vascular disease. In the latter case the presence of defects elsewhere is helpful.

THE ROLE OF THE MEDIAL TEMPORAL LOBE, PRECUNEUS, AND POSTERIOR CINGULATE GYRUS

Given that the disease commences in the medial temporal lobe structures, then some functioning imaging studies have focussed on the detection of hypoperfusion/hypometabolism to these regions (Plates 10A.3 and 10A.4). There have been conflicting reports in the literature as to the usefulness of identifying medial temporal abnormalities on functional imaging, but the consensus appears to favor the reliability of imaging these structures, although not agreed by all.[12–16] It is important to note that the finding of medial temporal lobe (MTL) hypoperfusion/hypometabolism on functional imaging may not be specific for AD as structural imaging studies have clearly implicated this region in vascular and Lewy body dementia.[8,17] In addition to the MTL structures, group comparative studies have shown that

hypoperfusion/metabolism of the precuneus (medial parietal lobe) and posterior cingulate gyrus may also be very useful markers of very early AD;[18,19] the usefulness of these findings when extrapolated to the individual case needs to be clarified.

The detection of atrophy on structural imaging of the medial temporal structures appears to have a similar accuracy to functional imaging, being of the order of 85%. Simple visual ratings or linear measures generally perform similar to undertaking more complex volumetric analysis.[20]

The advent of memory clinics means that more patients are presenting with minimal cognitive impairment. It is clearly essential to address whether imaging can predict which patients will progress to ultimately fulfil AD criteria as opposed to those who do not progress with their cognitive problems – the so called 'worried well'. Functional imaging studies with both SPECT and PET appear to have an accuracy of approximately 80%.[21,22] Similar results have been claimed for structural imaging based on hippocampal width.[23]

Sophisticated software programs have been developed to assist with the visual interpretation of functional and structural images. These have the obvious advantage of reducing observer bias. Programs to assess functional images include statistical parametric mapping (SPM),[24] surface projection mapping[25] and BRASS (brain registration and analysis of SPECT studies).[26] There are not many studies in the literature assessing the merits of these programs, but there is some evidence to suggest that they may play a useful role. In particular, the use of such programs to identify hypoperfusion to small areas of the brain, especially the hippocampi and posterior cingulate gyri/precuneus, may be extremely helpful to augment the confidence in the visual interpretation. More large-scale studies of these, and other, software programs are clearly required.

Early-onset (presenile) Alzheimer's disease

It is estimated in the UK that approximately 20 000 patients are diagnosed as suffering from dementia before the age of 65 years; appropriately half of these cases will have Alzheimer's disease. In contrast to the senile presentation of AD, it appears that younger AD patients have a tendency for presenting with symptoms referrable to the parieto-temporal association areas, as opposed to the characteristic amnesia reflecting medial temporal involvement. Consequently, younger patients are more likely to present with visuo-spatial and language problems.[27] On functional imaging younger patients tend to have parieto-temporal association area hypoperfusion/metabolism in the early stages of the disease process (Plate 10A.4) whereas in the older patient these areas may not be involved until the moderate stages of disease severity.[28–31] As the relatively larger parieto-temporal association areas are much more readily visualized on functional imaging than the medial temporal structures, functional imaging appears at its most sensitive in the diagnosis of the mildest stages of early-onset AD as opposed to late-onset AD. This is a fortunate situation as the younger patients may still be in employment, hence it is critically important to establish an accurate early diagnosis given the implications on occupational and subsequent financial and domestic matters.

VASCULAR DEMENTIA

It is convenient to sub-classify this disease as either large-vessel or small-vessel disease. Large-vessel infarction affects both gray and white matter, whereas small-vessel disease predominantly affects white matter. However, many patients may have a combination of small-vessel and large-vessel disease. Clinically, stepwise deterioration is highly suggestive of large-vessel disease, i.e. a multi-infarct dementia whereas co-existent small-vessel disease will produce a progressive decline (akin to Alzheimer's disease) and may complicate the clinical picture. Large-vessel infarcts are readily demonstrated on CT, MRI, and functional imaging. Previous transient ischemic attacks, which may have apparently resolved clinically, may leave evidence of permanent damage on neuro-imaging (Plate 10A.5). In contrast the detection of small-vessel vascular disease is more difficult.

Small-vessel vascular disease is associated with ischemia to the myelin sheaths of the nerve fibers constituting the cerebral white matter. This results in slowing of the neural transmission and patients present with psychomotor retardation, depression, and apathy.[32] CT attempts to depict low attenuation in the white matter, but interpretation is compounded by the fact that many apparently healthy cognitive people will have this finding also. However, the finding of extensive white matter low attenuation appears clinically helpful. MRI, with its greater resolution and sensitivity, attempts to demonstrate T_2 hyperintensities as a surrogate marker of ischemia to the white matter. Once again, this finding also appears to be found in many healthy individuals. Although there is considerable controversy as to the relationship of these CT and MRI findings with cognitive impairment, there does appear to be a significant, albeit weak, relationship.[32,33]

Functional imaging can readily detect large-vessel infarcts, although the ability to demonstrate the 'characteristic' patchy perfusion pattern associated with small-vessel vascular disease appears questionable. Given that the subfrontal circuits appear to be predominantly affected, some authors have demonstrated frontal hypoperfusion as an indicator of small-vessel vascular disease.[34] PET imaging appears slightly more reliable. In particular, the greater resolution of PET imaging allows the easier detection of multi-focal deficits which would be suggestive of widespread vascular disease. This most probably explains why PET is superior to SPECT in being able to differentiate the patterns of Alzheimer's and vascular disease.[35]

FRONTO–TEMPORAL DEMENTIA

Fortunately, fronto-temporal dementia (FTD) is a relatively rare dementia and accounts for less than 1% of all demented patients. However, it is more common in younger patients, accounting for approximately 25% of early-onset dementias. There is considerable heterogeneity on histopathology, including Pick's inclusion bodies, gliosis, and neuronal loss. Although it is convenient to subclassify fronto-temporal dementia, it must be realized that there is considerable overlap in clinical features. Moreover, although there may be differing initial presentations, all the features will eventually merge. FTD can be conveniently subclassified as follows:

- The frontal variant of FTD
- Semantic dementia
- Primary progressive aphasia

Frontal variant of fronto–temporal dementia (fvFTD)

Depending on the initial location of the underlying pathological process, patients can present in different ways. The dorso-lateral aspect of the frontal lobes control executive functions and damage in this area leads to the dysexecutive syndrome (associated with planning and organizational impairment). Damage to the medial frontal lobes/anterior cingulate gyrus is associated with apathy, whereas impairment of the orbital basal regions of the frontal lobes appears to be associated with behavior and personality disorders (Plate 10A.6).

Despite no large-scale prospective imaging studies with histopathological confirmation available in the literature, it is still possible to derive trends albeit based on the clinical diagnoses. HMPAO SPECT appears to be more sensitive than MRI, which in turn is more sensitive than CT, in a heterogeneous group of patients presenting with the frontal variants of FTD.[36] This is supported by the findings of a smaller study.[37]

A small, but poignant, study based on only two patients who presented with behavioral/apathy features and had longitudinal HMPAO SPECT and MRI investigations throughout the course of their illness, with subsequently autopsy confirmation of FTD, did not demonstrate abnormalities on imaging during the early stages of their illness. It appears that these patients presented with behavioral/apathetic features and, consequently, the orbito-basal and medial frontal regions of the frontal lobes may be difficult areas to identify abnormalities in the early stages of disease. This is in contrast to detecting abnormalities in the relatively larger dorsal–lateral aspects of the frontal lobes in those presenting clinically with dysexecutive features.[38]

In some patients presenting with the frontal variant of FTD it may be possible to identify bi-temporal hypoperfusion/atrophy even though the patient may not have overt clinical features to suggest antero-temporal involvement (viz. semantic memory impairment) at that stage. This can be extremely helpful in those patients presenting with behavioral problems or apathy in which the hypoperfusion to the orbital basal and medial frontal regions may be difficult to identify. Fluorodeoxyglucose (FDG) PET imaging appears to be sensitive in detecting frontal abnormalities in all types of frontal variant presentations.[39,40]

Semantic dementia

The lateral aspects of the temporal lobes are involved in semantic (naming) memory. Structural and functional imaging demonstrate abnormalities in the anterior and lateral aspects of the temporal lobe. Given that this is a relatively large area of the brain, functional imaging appears sensitive at detecting abnormalities. It appears that functional imaging is marginally more sensitive than structural imaging.[41,42] As the disease progresses, the frontal lobes will become involved. Parietal abnormalities on functional imaging have been noted, however these deficits are less than those seen elsewhere in the cortex.

Primary progressive aphasia

Histopathological processes involve the peri-Sylvian fissure region, in particular the inferior frontal lobe and anterior temporal lobe of the brain, with features of neuronal loss, gliosis, and mild spongiform changes. Patients come to medical attention with word finding difficulties, prominent spelling errors, and abnormal speech patterns.[43] The subsequent involvement of the frontal and temporal lobes produces the clinical picture of FTD. The peri-Sylvian fissure abnormalities are readily detected on PET and SPECT which are more sensitive than structural imaging.[41,44]

DEMENTIA OF THE LEWY BODY TYPE

Clinical aspects

It is thought that dementia of the Lewy body type (DLB) accounts for 10–20% of dementia cases. Histopathological diagnosis relies on the detection of cortical Lewy bodies. This dementia has many similarities to Alzheimer's disease and the differential diagnosis can be difficult clinically. In comparison to patients with Alzheimer's disease, DLB patients tend to have more detailed visual hallucinations, features of parkinsonism, a more fluctuant time course, and a history of falls. Obviously, if the patient volunteers the appropriate history, then the clinical diagnosis can be made with a high degree of confidence. Unfortunately, at presentation, approximately 65% of DLB patients will not have experienced visual hallucinations, 55% will not have features

of parkinsonism, 40% do not give a history of a fluctuant course, and 90% do not provide a history of falls.[45] It has also being noted at post-mortem that many patients who fulfil the histopathological criteria for DLB also have neurofibrillary tangles and plaques.[46] Consequently, the clinical distinction between DLB and AD may be blurred.[47]

Imaging studies

Given the similarities in the clinical presentations of DLB and AD, it is not surprising that the initial abnormalities on HMPAO SPECT and FDG PET are in the posterior association cortices of the brain, namely the parieto-tempero-occipital regions. Indeed, it can be difficult on HMPAO SPECT and FDG PET to differentiate DLB from AD. However, DLB patients appear to have a tendency for greater occipital involvement although this is not agreed by all.[48–51] Another feature to favor a diagnosis of DLB over late-onset AD is a greater degree of frontal hypoperfusion.[52,53] An FDG PET study comparing DLB and AD patients noted a lesser degree of hypometabolism to the medial temporal structures in the former although this did not attain significance.[50] Interestingly, an MRI study noted significantly less atrophy of the medial temporal lobe in DLB as compared to AD.[54] Note that the pattern of posterior cortical hypoperfusion/metabolism with relative preservation of medial temporal lobe function appears analogous to the appearances in early-onset AD – hopefully the age of the patient may assist with the differentiation (Plate 10A.7). Unfortunately, the preservation of medial temporal lobe structures may only be present in up to 40% of patients at presentation.[55]

It may be of considerable importance to accurately differentiate DLB from the other dementias. In particular, the administration of neuroleptics (possibly to treat the hallucinations) in DLB patients may exacerbate the parkinsonian features in approximately 80% of cases, of which 40% may be life threatening.[56] Interestingly, cholinergic therapy may be more beneficial in DLB patients, as compared to AD patients, most probably as a partial consequence of the greater cholinergic deficit in DLB.[57]

Although several studies have noted significant differences on FDG PET and HMPAO SPECT imaging between *groups* of patients with DLB and AD, extrapolation of these findings to the *individual* case needs to be interpreted with extreme caution given the potential for DLB patients to experience a life threatening parkinsonian crisis with neuroleptic treatment.

The relationship to Parkinson's disease

DLB and Parkinson's disease (PD) may be differing presentations of the same underlying disease process. Both entities are based on the histopathological evidence of Lewy bodies, with DLB patients having predominant cortical

Lewy bodies whereas PD patients have predominant brain stem Lewy bodies leading to striatal neuronal loss. Indeed, 40% of patients who initially present with PD will subsequently fulfil the clinical criteria for dementia and many of the remainder will have cognitive impairment.[58] Conversely, 75% of DLB patients will develop features of parkinsonism during the course of their illness.[44] In recent years, there has been considerable interest in imaging the presynaptic dopaminergic system for the diagnosis of Parkinson's disease. Consequently, given the shared histopathology of Parkinson's disease and DLB, the same imaging techniques maybe of relevance in the early diagnosis of DLB.

Imaging the dopaminergic system

Iodine-123-labeled tropanes (^{123}I-FP-CIT or ^{123}I-β-CIT) and ^{18}F-DOPA have been used in functional imaging to image the presynaptic dopaminergic system. The PET ligand ^{18}F-DOPA enters the pre-synaptic terminal and is metabolized in parallel with dopamine. The SPECT ligands, ^{123}I-FP-CIT and ^{123}I-β-CIT, are taken up by the dopamine active transporter mechanism into the presynaptic terminal; the compounds are very similar and the former is imaged at 3–6 h post-injection whereas the latter is imaged at 24 h. DaTSCAN is the trade name for ^{123}I-FP-CIT. In healthy individuals the images following the injection of either agent will be of the pre-synaptic dopaminergic terminals in the corpus striata (caudate and lentiform nuclei); these appear as 'commas' (Plate 10A.8). In patients with early PD there is loss of pre-synaptic dopaminergic terminals in the putamen and globus pallidus (lentiform nuclei) leaving visualization of the caudate nuclei only; these appear as 'full-stops' (Plate 10A.9).

In vitro histopathological studies have demonstrated significant depletion of dopamine and the active transporter mechanism both in PD and DLB patients.[59] Consequently ^{18}F-DOPA and ^{123}I-FP-CIT may assist with the diagnosis in both these disease states. Phase III trials have suggested that the accuracy of ^{123}I-FP-CIT in PD is of the order of 95–100%.[60] Unfortunately, there are no studies with histopathological follow-up yet and the clinical diagnosis has to be relied upon as the gold standard. The major reason that imaging the pre-synaptic terminal appears extremely sensitive in the detection of early PD is that there has to be a considerable loss of dopamine from the striata before the patient presents clinically with parkinsonism. Although the depletion of the active transporter mechanism from the striata in DLB is not as great as in PD, there is still a considerable loss from these nuclei and therefore the ^{123}I-FP-CIT should be abnormal in DLB patients, even in those who do not have any clinical features of parkinsonism (as yet). Most importantly, patients with AD do not have depletion of dopamine or the active transporter mechanism and therefore should have normal studies on imaging. A recent publication using ^{123}I-FP-CIT in the first 10 cases

of suspected DLB to come to post-mortem has demonstrated the considerable potential of this agent.[61] The results showed a sensitivity of 100% and a specificity of 85%; the one false positive study was due to infarction throughout the striatum which, arguably, should have been noted on MRI. These early results suggest a very useful role for ^{123}I-FP-CIT imaging in patients with suspected DLB.

Parkinson's dementia complex

It is worth mentioning that there appears to be some confusion about the relationship between Parkinson's dementia complex and Lewy body dementia. It would appear that in patients who present initially with features of Parkinson's disease there may be subsequent disconnection of the fibers from the striata to the frontal cortex, thereby giving rise to frontal symptomatology, namely apathy and dysexecutive features – the so-called Parkinson's dementia complex.[62] Convention dictates that this cognitive impairment commences at least 1 year after the initial presentation with Parkinson's disease. This most probably explains the reduced frontal metabolism and perfusion on FDG PET and HMPAO SPECT imaging noted in such patients.[52,53] This contrasts to the predominantly reduced perfusion/metabolism to the posterior association cortices associated with LBD. The distinction between the frontal involvement of Parkinson's dementia complex and the predominant posterior involvement of DLB may be somewhat academic as neuroleptic treatment must be used with caution in either case and, ultimately, the clinical features will merge into a final common pathway.

FUTURE DEVELOPMENTS

This is an extremely exciting era in dementia imaging. Many countries are realizing the enormous expense of this disease to the health and welfare system and are keen to fund research in this field.

Although MRI studies have a role in detecting appropriate atrophy, sequential imaging to assess for the rate of atrophy of critical areas may be more powerful. Indeed, one study noted good results from undertaking MRI scans at a time interval of less than 6 months.[63] This area clearly needs further exploration.

Future areas of research in functional imaging should include further evaluation of the diagnostic accuracy of voxel-by-voxel software programs in the very early diagnosis of dementia[24–26] and imaging with specific ligands.

The ^{123}I-FP-CIT SPECT ligand for imaging the dopaminergic system in suspected DLB appears highly promising, although it remains to be seen whether specific ligands can be developed to provide more useful diagnostic information in the other dementias than current perfusion and metabolic imaging. Neuroreceptor imaging certainly plays a major role in enhancing our understanding of the patho-physiological processes of dementia and the effects of treatment, in particular in the future of neuroprotective therapies. Given the predominant involvement of the cholinergic nervous system in AD, attempts have been made to image the pre- and post-synaptic muscarinic and nicotinic acetylcholinergic neural system. Pre-synaptic muscarinic imaging has been successfully undertaken using [^{123}I]iodo-benzovesamicol (^{123}I-IVBM).[64] Post-synaptic muscarinic imaging has also been carried out using ^{123}I-quinuclidinyl benzilate (^{123}I-QNB).[65,66] The PET ligand ^{11}C-nicotine has been successfully used to image the nicotinic system.[67]

Targeting the amyloid directly remains the 'holy grail' of AD imaging and there is recent excitement in using the fluorinated PET ligand fluoroethyl-methyl-ethylidene-malonitrile (^{18}F-DDNP).[68] The ligand PK11195 labeled with either ^{123}I for SPECT, or ^{11}C for PET, targets the benzo-diazepine receptor on activated microglia and thereby demonstrates cerebral inflammation. This may have a useful role in detecting abnormal patterns in early disease states[69] and, ultimately, may provide a useful tool for monitoring therapy.

CONCLUSION

It would appear that structural and functional imaging can play a useful role in the early and accurate diagnosis of cognitive impairment. However, it is crucially important to be aware of the capabilities, and limitations, of these imaging modalities in the various dementias.

REFERENCES

1   O'Brien JT. Drugs for Alzheimer's disease. Cholinesterase inhibitors have passed NICE's hurdle. [Editorial] *BMJ* 2000; **323**: 123–4.

2   Hogervost E, Barnetson L, Yobst KA, *et al.* Diagnosing dementia: interrater reliability assessment and accuracy of the NINCDS/ADRDA criteria versus CERAD histo-pathological criteria for Alzheimer's disease. *J Dementia Geriat Cognit Disorders* 2000; **11**: 107–13.

3   Bosenquet N, May J, Johnson N. *Alhzeimer's disease in the United Kingdom: burden of disease and future care.* Health Policy Review Paper No. 12. London: Imperial College of Science, Technology and Medicine, 1998.

4   Harvey RJ, Rosser MN, Skeleton-Robinson M, *et al. Young onset dementia: epidemiology, clinical symptoms, family burden, support and outcome.* Research on behalf of the NHS Executive, RFG045. London: The Dementia Research Group, Imperial College School of Medicine, 1998.

5   Braak H, Braak E. Neuropathological staging of Alzheimer related changes. *Acta Neuropath* 1991; **82**: 239–59.

6   Terry RD, Masliah E, Salmon DP, *et al.* Physical basis of cognitive alterations in Alzheimer's disease: synapse loss is the major correlate of cognitive impairment. *Ann Neurol* 1991; **30**: 572–80.

7   Mielke R, Schroder R, Fink GR, *et al.* Regional cerebral glucose metabolism and post-mortem pathology in Alzheimer's disease. *Acta Neuropath* 1996; **91**: 174–9.

8   Jobst KA, Barnetson LBD, Shepstone BJ. Accurate prediction of histologically confirmed Alzheimer's disease and the differential diagnosis of dementia; the use of NINCDS-ADRDA and DSM-III-R criteria, SPECT, x-ray CT, and Apo E4 in medial temporal lobe dementias. *Intern Psychogeriat* 1998; **10**: 271–302.

9   McKhann G, Drachman D, Folstein M, *et al.* Clinical diagnosis of Alzheimer's disease. *Neurology* 1984; **34**: 939–44.

10 Jobst KA, Sniff AD, Szatmari M, *et al.* Rapidly progressing atrophy of medial temporal lobe in Alzheimer's disease. *Lancet* 1994; **343**: 829–30.

11 Holman BL, Johnson KA, Geradaq B, *et al.* The scinti-graphic appearances of Alzheimer's disease: a prospective study using technetium 99-m-HMPAO SPECT. *J Nucl Med* 1992; **33**: 181–5.

12 Villa G, Cappa A, Tavolozza M, *et al.* Neuropsychological tests and Tc-99m HMPAO SPECT in the diagnosis of Alzheimer's dementia. *J Neurol* 1995; **242**: 349–66.

13 Ohnishi T, Hoshi H, Nagamochi S, *et al.* High-resolution SPECT to assess hippocampal perfusion in neuro-psychiatric diseases. *J Nucl Med* 1995; **36**: 1163–9.

14 Rodriguez G, Vitali P, Calvini P, *et al.* Hippocampal perfusion in mild Alzheimer's disease. *Psychiat Res* 2000; **100**: 65–74.

15 Nebu A, Ikeda M, Fukuhara R, *et al.* Utility of Tc99m HMPAO SPECT hippocampal image to diagnose early stages of Alzheimer's disease using semiquantitative analysis. *J Dementia Geriat Cognit Disorders* 2001; **12**: 153–7.

16 Kitayama N, Matsuda H, Ohnishi T, *et al.* Measurements of both hippocampal blood flow and hippocampal grey matter volumes in the same individuals with Alzheimer's disease. *Nucl Med Commun* 2001; **22**: 473–7.

17 O'Brien JT, Metcalfe S, Swann A, *et al.* Medial temporal lobe width on CT scanning in Alzheimer's disease: comparison with vascular dementia, depression, and dementia with Lewy bodies. *J Dementia Geriatr Cognit Disorders* 2000; **11**: 114–18.

18 Bradley KM, O'Sullivan VT, Soper NDW, *et al.* Cerebral perfusion SPECT correlated with Braak pathological stage in Alzheimer's disease. *Brain* 2002; **125**: 1772–81.

19 Sakamoto S, Matsuda H, Asada T, *et al.* Apolipoprotein E genotype and early Alzheimer's disease: a longitudinal SPECT study. *J Neuroimage* 2003; **13**: 113–23.

20 Frisoni GB. Structural imaging in the clinical diagnosis of Alzheimer's disease: problems and tools. [Editorial] *J Neurol Neurosurg Psychiat* 2001; **70**: 711–18.

(Erratum appears in *J Neurol Neurosurg Psychiat* 2001; **71**: 418.)

21 Johnson KA, Jones K, Holman BL, *et al*. Preclinical prediction of Alzheimer's disease using SPECT. *Neurology* 1998; **50**: 1563–71.

22 Silverman DH, Small GW, Chang CY, *et al*. Positron emission tomography in the evaluation of dementia. Regional brain metabolism and long-term outcome. *JAMA* 2001; **286**: 2120–7.

23 El Fakhri G, Fijewski MF, Johnson KA, *et al*. MRI-guided SPECT perfusion measures and volumetric MRI in prodromal alzheimer disease. *Arch Neurol* 2003; **60**:1066–72.

24 Soonawala D, Amin T, Ebmeirer KP, *et al*. Statistical parametric mapping of Tc-99m HMPAO SPECT images for the diagnosis of Alzheimer's disease: normalisation to cerebellar tracer uptake. *Neuroimage* 2002; **17**: 1193–202.

25 Minoshima S, Frey KA, Koeppe RA, *et al*. A diagnostic approach in Alzheimer's disease using three-dimensional stereotactic surface projection mapping of fluorine-18-FDG PET. *J Nucl Med* 1995; **36**: 1238–48.

26 Van Laere KJ, Warwick J, Versijpt J. Analysis of clinical brain SPECT data based on anatomic standardisation and references to normal data in ROC-based comparison of visual, semiquantitative, and voxel-based methods. *J Nucl Med* 2002; **43**: 458–69.

27 Roth M. Evidence on the possible heterogeneity of Alzheimer's disease and its bearing on future enquiries into aetiology and treatment. In: Butler RN, Bearne AG (eds). *The ageing process: therapeutic implications*. New York: Raven Press, 1984.

28 Salmon E, Collette F, Degueldre C, *et al*. Voxel-based analysis of confounding effects of age and severity on cerebral metabolism in Alzheimer's disease. *Human Brain Mapping* 2000; **10**: 39–48.

29 Sakamoto J, Ishii K, Sasaki M, *et al*. Differences in cerebral metabolic impairment between early and late onset types of Alzheimer's disease. *J Neurol Sci* 2002; **200**: 27–32.

30 Kemp PM, Holmes C, Hoffman SA, *et al*. Alzheimer's disease: differences in technetium 99m HMPAO SPECT scan findings between early onset and late onset dementia. *JNNP* 2003; **74**: 715–19.

31 Frisoni GB, Testa C, Sabattoli F, Beltramello A, Soininen H, Laakso MP. Structural correlates of early and late onset Alzheimer's disease: voxel based morphological study. *J Neurol Neurosurg Psychiatry* 2005; **76**: 112–114.

32 O'Brien JT, Erkinjuntti T, Reisberg B, *et al*. Vascular cognition impairment. [Review] *Lancet Neurology* 2003; **2**: 89–98.

33 Barber R, Ghokar A, Ballard C, *et al*. White matter lesions on MRI in dementia with Lewy bodies, Alzheimer's disease, vascular dementia and normal ageing. *JNNP* 1999; **67**: 66–72.

34 Toghi H, Chiba A, Hiroi S, *et al*. Cerebral perfusion patterns in vascular dementia of Biswanger's type

compared with senile dementia of the Alzheimer type: a SPECT study. *J Neurol* 1991; **238**: 365–70.

35 Mielke R, Piertrzyk U, Jacobs A, *et al*. HMPAO SPECT and FDG PET in Alzheimer's disease and vascular dementia: comparison of perfusion and metabolic pattern. *Eur J Nucl Med* 1994; **21**: 1052–60.

36 Varma AR, Adams W, Lloyd JJ. Diagnostic patterns of regional atrophy on MRI and regional cerebral blood flow change on SPECT in young onset patients with Alzheimer's disease, fronto-temporal dementia and vascular dementia. *Acta Neurol Scand* 2002; **105**: 261–9.

37 Miller BL, Ikonte BS, Ponton M. A study of the Lund–Manchester research criteria for fronto-temporal dementia: clinical and single photon emission CT correlations. *Neurology* 1997; **48**: 937–42.

38 Gregory CA, Serra-Mestres J, Hodges JR. The early diagnosis of the frontal variant of fronto-temporal dementia: how sensitive are standard neuro-imaging and neuro-psychological tests. *Neuropsychiat Neuropsychol Behav Neurol* 1999; **12**: 128–35.

39 Ischii K, Sakamoto S, Sasaki M, *et al*. Cerebral glucose metabolism in patients with fronto-temporal dementia. *J Nucl Med* 1998; **39**: 1875–8.

40 Jauss M, Herholz K, Kracht, *et al*. Fronto-temporal dementia: clinical, neuroimaging and molecular biological findings in 6 patients. *Eur Arch Psychiat Clin Neurosci* 2001; **251**: 225–31.

41 Sinnatamby R, Autoun NA, Miles KA, *et al*. Neuroradiological findings in primary progressive aphasia: CT, MRI and cerebral perfusion SPECT. *Neuroradiology* 1996; **38**: 232–8.

42 Garrard P, Hodges JR. Semantic dementia: clinical, radiological and pathological perspectives. *J Neurol* 2000; **247**: 409–22.

43 Mesulam MM. Primary progressive aphasia – a language based dementia. [Review] *N Engl J Med* 2003; **349**: 1535–42.

44 Nestor PJ, Graham NL, Fryer TD, *et al*. Progressive non-fluent aphasia associated with hypometabolism centred on the left anterior insula. *Brain* 2003; **126**: 2406–18.

45 McKeith IG, O'Brien JT. Dementia with Lewy bodies. *Aust NZ J Psychiat* 1999; **33**: 800–8.

46 Lansen L, Salmon D, Galasko D, *et al*. The Lewy body variant of Alzheimer's disease: a clinical and pathological entity. *Neurology* 1990; **40**: 1–8.

47 Merdes AR, Hansen LA, Jeste DV, *et al*. Influence of Alzheimer's pathology on clinical diagnostic accuracy in dementia with Lewy bodies. *Neurology* 2003; **60**: 1586–90.

48 Ishii K, Imamwa T, Sasaki M, *et al*. Regional cerebral glucose metabolism in dementia with Lewy bodies and Alzheimer's disease. *Neurology* 1998; **51**: 125–30.

49 Colloby SJ, Fenwick JD, Williams ED, *et al*. A comparison of Tc-99m HMPAO SPET changes in dementia with Lewy bodies and Alzheimer's disease using

statistical parametric mapping. *Eur J Nucl Med* 2002; **29**: 615–22.

50 Lobotesis K, Fenwick JD, Phipps A, *et al.* Occipital hypoperfusion on SPECT in dementia with Lewy bodies but not AD. *Neurology* 2001; **56**: 643–9.

51 Minoshima S, Foster NZ, Sima AA. Alzheimer's disease versus dementia with Lewy bodies: cerebral metabolic distinction with autopsy confirmation. *Ann Neurol* 2001; **50**: 358–65.

52 Defebvre LJ, Leduc V, Duhomel A, *et al.* Technetium HMPAO SPECT study in dementia with Lewy bodies, Alzheimer's disease and idiopathic Parkinson's disease. *J Nucl Med* 1999; **40**: 956–62.

53 Steinling M, De Febvre L, Duhamel A, *et al.* Is there a typical pattern of brain SPECT imaging in Alzheimer's disease? *J Dementia Geriat Cognit Disorders* 2001; **12**: 371–8.

54 Barber R, Gholkar A, Sheltens P, *et al.* Medial temporal lobe atrophy on MRI in dementia with Lewy bodies. *Neurology* 1999; **52**: 1153–8.

55 Pasquier F, Hamon M, Lebert F, *et al.* Medial temporal lobe atrophy in memory disorders. *J Neurol* 1997; **244**: 175–81.

56 McKeith IG, Fairbairn AF, Perry RH, *et al.* Neuroleptic sensitivity of patients with senile dementia of the Lewy body type. *BMJ* 1992; **305**: 673–8.

57 McKeith IG, Mintzer J, Aarsland D, *et al.* Dementia with Lewy bodies. *Lancet Neurology* 2004; **3**: 19–28.

58 Cummings JL. Intellectual impairment in Parkinson's disease: clinical, pathological and biochemical correlates. *J Geriatr Psychiat Neurol* 1988; **1**: 24–36.

59 Piggott MA, Marshall EF, Thomas N, *et al.* Striatal dopimenergic markers in dementia with Lewy bodies, Alzheimer's and Parkinson's disease; rostro-caudal distribution. *Brain* 1999; **122**: 1449–68.

60 Benamer HT, Patterson J, Grosset DG, *et al.* Accurate differentiation of Parkinsonism and essential tremor using visual assessment of I-123-FP-CIT SPECT imaging: the I-123-FP-CIT Study Group. *Movement Disord* 2000; **15**: 503–10.

61 Walker Z, Costa DC, Walker RWH, *et al.* Differentiation of dementia with Lewy bodies from Alzheimer's disease using a dopaminergic presynaptic ligand. *JNNP* 2002; **73**: 134–40.

62 Emre M. Dementia associated with Parkinson's disease. [Review] *Lancet Neurology* 2003; **2**: 229–37.

63 Bradley KM, Bydder GM, Budge MM, *et al.* Serial brain MRI at 3–6 months as a surrogate marker for Alzheimer's disease. *Br J Radiol* 2002; **75**: 506–13.

64 Kuhl DE, Minoshima P, Fessler JA, *et al.* In-vivo mapping of cholinergic terminals in normal ageing, Alzheimer's disease and Parkinson's disease. *Ann Neurol* 1996; **40**: 399–410.

65 Brown D, Chisholm JA, Owens J, *et al.* Acetylcholine muscarinic receptors and response to anti-cholinesterase therapy in patients with Alzheimer's disease. *Eur J Nucl Med* 2003; **30**: 296–300.

66 Kemp PM, Holmes C, Hoffmann SA, *et al.* A randomised placebo-controlled study to assess the effects of cholinergic therapy in Alzheimer's disease. *JNNP* 2003; **74**: 1567–70.

67 Nordberg A. Nicotinic receptor abnormalities of Alzheimer's disease; therapeutic implications. [Review] *Biol Psychiat* 2001; **49**: 200–10.

68 Shoghi-Jadid K, Small GW, Agdeppa ED, *et al.* Localisation of neurofibrillary tangles and beta-amyloid plaques in the brains of living patients with Alzheimer's disease. *Am J Geriatr Psychiat* 2002; **10**: 24–35.

69 Cagnin A, Brooks DJ, Kennedy AM, *et al.* In-vivo measurement of activated microglia in dementia. *Lancet* 2001; **358**: 461–7.

Functional imaging in cerebrovascular disease and neuropsychiatry

R. JAYAN AND S. VINJAMURI

INTRODUCTION

After heart disease and cancer, stroke is the third leading cause of mortality in developed countries. Brain perfusion single photon emission computed tomography (SPECT) is a functional imaging tool for the study of physiological and pathological events in the brain. This information is complementary to other neuro-imaging techniques such as computed tomography (CT) and magnetic resonance imaging (MRI). However, brain perfusion SPECT has clinical value by itself because functional impairment in cerebral diseases often precedes structural changes.[1] With the advent of newer therapies for stroke such as thrombolysis, there has been much interest in regional cerebral blood flow (rCBF) imaging in cerebrovascular disease.

Physiology of cerebral perfusion

The cerebral circulation is unique and has major differences to other circulatory systems in the body. The blood–brain barrier consists of special endothelial cells with tight junctions within brain capillaries which prevents the entrance of high-molecular-weight and hydrophilic substances to the central nervous system (CNS). Another difference is that the brain vascular system has an auto-regulatory mechanism to maintain cerebral blood flow (CBF).[1]

Regional cerebral blood flow is normally maintained at a constant level within given limits by the ability of the cerebral vasculature to autoregulate the blood flow in response to the metabolic needs of the cells through various stimuli. This mechanism of maintaining blood flow is called cerebro-vascular reserve (CVR).

Radiopharmaceuticals

The oldest agent used for estimating rCBF is ^{133}Xe, a lipophilic radioactive tracer that easily diffuses through the blood–brain barrier (BBB). ^{133}Xe was the radiopharmaceutical of choice to quantify CBF (mL min^{-1} 100 g^{-1} tissue) by means of brain perfusion SPECT.

The ^{99m}Tc-labeled compounds hexamethylenepropyl amine oxime (HMPAO) and L,L-ethyl cysteinate dimer (ECD) have been the most widely used for brain perfusion imaging, although neither fulfils all the characteristics of an ideal radiopharmaceutical for this purpose.[2]

The retention of HMPAO intracellularly is due to conversion from a lipophilic to a hydrophilic form that cannot diffuse freely across the cell membranes. The conversion probably occurs mainly inside mitochondria and is catalyzed by glutathione. As infarcted tissue lack mitochondria there is failure of HMPAO retention (hypo-fixation). This phenomenon lasts for up to 10 days after stroke onset. After 10 days the opposite phenomenon is observed with increased HMPAO retention (hyper-fixation). The exact mechanism for this is unclear. This affects infarct areas with reperfusion and hence a hot spot on the HMPAO image corresponding to a CT or MRI infarct is evidence of thrombolysis although the degree of 'luxury perfusion' is exaggerated by HMPAO. Following reperfusion the hyperemia gradually decreases and becomes less compared to the opposite hemisphere. This means that at one stage around day 14–20 there may not be any asymmetry and even a large infarct can potentially not be evident on SPECT images.[3]

The tracer ^{99m}Tc-labeled ECD has a retention mechanism slightly different from HMPAO. It is de-esterified enzymatically to become hydrophilic and is thereby retained intracellularly. This process is much reduced in infarct which hence shows low uptake regardless of the level of flow.[4] Hence, ECD may be considered as a marker of viability of brain tissue although there may be some uptake in massive infarcts with reperfusion even in the absence of viable tissue.

Hence both HMPAO and ECD have their advantages. HMPAO is more useful for determining blood flow to infarct tissue than assessing the infarct itself. If the aim is to outline the infarct, then ECD is better.

Positron emission tomography (PET) can also be utilized to estimate cerebral blood flow using a number of positron emitters but its role has been largely as a research tool. rCBF can be assessed by SPECT using a semiquantitative method comparing the counts in a given region of interest (ROI) with those in a comparable ROI in the opposite presumably normal hemisphere or the cerebellum.

CLINICAL ROLE OF BRAIN PERFUSION SPECT IN CEREBROVASCULAR DISEASE

The potential role of brain perfusion SPECT in cerebrovascular disease is illustrated in Table 10B.1.

Evaluation and management of acute ischemic stroke

Therapy for acute stroke depends on ensuring the diagnosis and excluding diseases that mimic cerebral ischemia, such as hypoglycemia, hyponatremia, seizure, or a mass lesion such as a tumor or subdural hematoma. The exclusion of a hemorrhagic rather than ischemic stroke can be determined rapidly and accurately with CT or MR imaging.[5] CT

Table 10B.1 *Role of perfusion brain SPECT in cerebrovascular disease*

- *Acute ischemic stroke*
- *Stroke rehabilitation and prediction of functional recovery*
- *Chronic cerebrovascular disease*
- *Transient ischemic attack*
- *Subarachnoid hemorrhage*
- *Head injury*
- *Determination of brain death*

is still the most widely used modality for imaging acute stroke. MRI for evaluating acute stroke is being studied and there is likely to be an increasing role in the future.

Perfusion patterns with HMPAO correlate with the extent, severity and short-term outcome of hemispheric stroke. Early severe hypo-perfusion within 6 h after onset was highly predictive of poor neurological outcome.[6] Spontaneous reperfusion after stroke was shown to be associated with improved clinical outcome.[7] Brain tissue metabolic recovery assessed with ^{99m}Tc-ECD SPECT after ischemic stroke was also shown to have a beneficial effect on clinical outcome[8] (Plate 10B.1).

The normal cerebral blood flow is 50–60 mL 100 g^{-1} brain tissue min^{-1}. The threshold of ischemia lies at about 25 mL 100 g^{-1} min^{-1}. CBF of less than 10 mL 100 g^{-1} min^{-1} cannot be tolerated beyond a few minutes before infarction occurs, but between 10 and 25 mL 100 g^{-1} min^{-1}, cell death requires many minutes to hours.[5] This region of milder ischemia is called the ischemic penumbra and consists of salvageable brain tissue if the infarct-related vessels are reperfused with thrombolysis. This period when thrombolysis can be useful in preventing irreversible damage is called the therapeutic window.

The evidence for the benefits of treating patients with acute stroke with thrombolytic therapy is increasing. The major problem with this therapy is intracerebral hemorrhage. Perfusion SPECT scanning may be useful in this setting to select patients who benefit most and screen out patients who are at higher risk of bleeding.

Assessing cerebral blood flow by perfusion SPECT can help determine the extent of the ischemic penumbral region. Fibrinolytic therapy must be implemented within the therapeutic window of 2–3 h, when no structural technique can reveal the extent and severity of ischemia. In this situation, brain perfusion SPECT patterns seem to forecast the outcomes of stroke patients[9] and thus could help in the selection of candidates for fibrinolytic therapy. The patients with the larger ischemic regions are likely to get maximum benefit from thrombolytic therapy.

The best candidates would be those patients presenting with an area of reduced tracer uptake (hypo-perfusion) on the SPECT image which is likely to point to significant salvageable tissue in the ischemic penumbra. A normal brain SPECT image implies a favorable prognosis as a result of effective collateral circulation and in this subset of patients the benefits of thrombolysis are likely to be limited. An area with no tracer uptake (cold area) seems to be associated with hemorrhagic complications if fibrinolysis is used as recanalization of arteries serving tissues that are severely ischemic or infarcted may increase the risk of edema and hemorrhage.[6] Ischemic tissue with CBF less than 35% of cerebellar flow has been shown to be at a higher risk for hemorrhage.[10]

Hence, the potential benefits of recanalization of arteries supplying injured but viable tissue must be weighed against the potentially increased morbidity and mortality.

Pre-treatment SPECT has been shown to provide useful parameters to increase the efficacy of thrombolysis by reducing hemorrhagic complications and improving neurologic outcome. Other imaging modalities such as CT or MRI are not yet able to give such prognostic information regarding the success of thrombolytic therapy.

Unfortunately, a precise relationship of rCBF level to the time available for tissue salvage has not been determined, and so the benefit of quantification of rCBF in acute stroke has not been proven.[11] Another limitation of this approach is that the therapeutic decision must be made in the emergency room, and brain SPECT should be performed and reported between the first 3–6 h after stroke onset.

SPECT has been used to assess the effect of therapeutic and nursing maneuvers during treatment of stroke. Ouchi et al. reported that cerebral blood flow is better for patients with stroke in the horizontal rather than upright position.[12] In our series of eight patients we found that cerebral perfusion was better in a semi-recumbent position rather than a supine position[13] (Plate 10B.2).

Evaluation of chronic cerebrovascular disease

A reduced CVR can indicate patients with occlusive cerebrovascular disease and compromised hemodynamics who may be at increased risk of cerebral ischemia. Such arteries are unable to increase their capacity in response to a stress such as hypotension or decreased cardiac output, and acute stroke may occur.[5]

Carotid artery endarterectomy reduces the risk of stroke in patients with severe stenosis of the internal carotid artery. Doppler ultrasound is the most widely used investigation for the diagnosis of carotid artery stenosis. However the hemodynamic significance of carotid artery stenosis cannot be assessed from the severity of the stenosis alone. A resting SPECT study by itself is of limited value in assessing this.[14] SPECT with vasodilator challenge using acetazolamide is useful in helping clinicians select patients with carotid artery stenosis who are the best candidates for surgery.[15,16] This also helps to identify the subset of patients who may require carotid shunting during carotid endarterectomy to prevent cerebral ischemia due to carotid clamping.[17] Other agents such as adenosine, dipyridamole or CO_2 have also been used to assess CVR.[18,19]

These challenge tests include the intravenous injection of 1 g of the vasodilating agent acetazolamide (Diamox). This produces an increase in CBF of 50–100% within 20–30 min. This is compared to a baseline scan which is performed on a separate day. A 1-day protocol with a double injection of ^{99m}Tc-ECD has also been tried.[20] The lack of flow augmentation indicates a loss of autoregulation and inadequate vascular reserves.[21] Such patients are at a higher risk of stroke and are most likely to benefit from an endarterectomy.[1] CVR has been shown to improve after successful endarterectomy.[22] Dynamic imaging of the inflow of HMPAO to the brain has been used to estimate the hemispherical CBF

using the Patlak plot.[23] These findings have also been replicated using positron emission tomography (PET) perfusion tracers.[24]

Impaired CVR has also been demonstrated in asymptomatic patients with high grade carotid artery stenosis[25] and in asymptomatic diabetic patients with no history of neurological disease.[26] Validation of this qualitative methodology for assessment of carotid stenosis has not been fully established. The precise ratios of rCBF that suggest an increased risk for future stroke and the potential need for surgical flow augmentation are yet to be determined.[5]

Transient ischemic attacks

Transient ischemic attacks (TIAs), by definition, produce transient neurological dysfunction which is resolved spontaneously by 24 h. Conventional imaging for TIA includes CT scanning to exclude cerebral infarction and exclude other causes that mimic stroke such as cerebral tumors. MRI has been less used due to limited availability but has the advantage of being able to detect smaller infarcts.

Several SPECT studies have demonstrated regional hypoperfusion in some TIA patients.[27] Focal hypo-perfusion on SPECT probably reflects previous or ongoing clinical and/or subclinical episodes of cerebral ischemia.[28] Perfusion SPECT may influence patient management by helping to define the vascular topography and by suggesting the probable mechanism (embolic or hemodynamic). Some studies report a link between persisting focal hypo-perfusion and recurrent stroke[29] but the evidence is limited. Further studies are needed to establish the potential role of SPECT in patients with TIA.

Subarachnoid hemorrhage

The standard algorithm for management of subarachnoid hemorrhage includes CT scan for initial diagnosis and magnetic resonance angiography for localization of the site of the aneurysm.

Subarachnoid hemorrhage (SAH) leads to vasospasm in up to 75% of cases[30] and is a major cause of morbidity and mortality in those patients who survive the initial event. Vasospasm produces ischemia and infarction in the territory distal to the involved vessels because of low flow. Perfusion imaging may aid in this early diagnosis by differentiating this from other causes of clinical worsening such as recurrent hemorrhage or metabolic disorders and helps to initiate rapid therapeutic intervention.[31]

Regional hypo-perfusion on SPECT due to vasospasm after SAH correlates with the presence and severity of delayed neurological deficits.[32] Seventeen percent of patients in a series of 162 were found to have basilar artery vasospasm with brain stem hypo-perfusion when imaged with ^{99m}Tc-ECD SPECT.[33]

Role in stroke rehabilitation and prediction of functional recovery

The mechanisms that are responsible for the remarkable potential for functional recovery from stroke in humans remain unclear, and functional neuro-imaging techniques increasingly are being used to investigate this issue. Such studies confirm that recovery of function is related to the volume of penumbra tissue that escapes infarction.[34] This was demonstrated by imaging with hypoxic imaging agent ^{99m}Tc-metronidazole and ^{99m}Tc-ECD SPECT.[35] Another hypothesis to explain functional recovery is the model of recovery of tissue not directly affected by stroke but affected by temporary cessation of function by deafferentation or diaschisis.[36]

Management following head injury

Hyperventilation is used therapeutically after head injury to reduce cerebral blood flow and hence intracranial volume to provide space for the swelling brain. However, if autoregulation is lost, the hyperventilation can result in vasoconstriction of the normal vessels and potential ischemia of normal brain, with a paradoxical increased flow in those arteries feeding the injured tissues, followed by increased swelling.[37] In this setting, perfusion imaging may provide information on appropriate ventilation management.[38]

Perfusion SPECT scanning is also useful in patients with persistent behavioral abnormalities after mild degrees of trauma when the CT and MR studies are normal. Sixty-eight percent of patients with mild head injury and normal CT had perfusion abnormalities on SPECT scan.[39]

A negative initial SPECT scan after trauma is a good predictor for a favorable clinical outcome[40] although a negative scan does not completely exclude hypoxic brain injury.[41] Conversely, patients with the greatest disability were found to have the greatest number of lesions and the lowest cerebral blood flow as determined by SPECT.[42] Perfusion abnormalities in the frontal and temporal lobes were associated with a poor outcome after rehabilitation.[43]

Areas of hypo-perfusion may be seen in patients who have abnormal neuropsychological tests.[44] Decreased blood flow to the frontal lobes was significantly correlated with disinhibitive behavior. There was also a significant correlation between decreased blood flow in the left cerebral hemisphere and increased social isolation.[45] In conclusion, SPECT plays a complementary role to CT and MRI. SPECT can reveal areas of hypo-perfusion that are not associated with anatomical abnormalities and is helpful in managing patients with head injury.[46]

Determination of brain death

When clinical determination of brain death is difficult due to concomitant hypnotic or sedative use, perfusion imaging may be useful to determine brain death by demonstrating absence of cerebral perfusion. Diagnosing brain death is important in managing the comatose patient for whom the continuation of life support is being questioned and when organ harvesting is being considered.[47] Perfusion SPECT with HMPAO appears to be highly sensitive and in addition 100% specific as a confirmatory test for brain death.[48]

Conclusion

Perfusion imaging with SPECT can play an important role in the assessment of stroke risk, selection of patients for newer therapies such as thrombolysis and also in predicting the success of rehabilitation by giving prognostic information about functional recovery. The role of brain perfusion SPECT in assessing rCBF is likely to increase with increasing use of thrombolytic therapy for ischemic stroke. It also yields additional information useful in the management of patients with subaracnoid hemorrhage and head injury.

FUNCTIONAL IMAGING IN PSYCHIATRY

With approximately 450 million people worldwide suffering from psychiatric diseases, there is a great need to understand and diagnose these disorders. Functional imaging of the brain yields complementary information to the data obtained from conventional brain imaging modalities such as CT and MRI. This information is potentially useful in the management of many psychiatric conditions.

Blood flow to different parts of the brain is closely coupled to the functional activity of these brain structures. SPECT using cerebral perfusion imaging agents such as ^{99m}Tc-HMPAO allows determination of rCBF. The parallelism between CBF, metabolism and neuronal activity (or cerebral function) is the basis for the use of brain perfusion SPECT in assessing cerebral function and, consequently, in detecting cerebral dysfunction. In the absence of cerebrovascular disease, hypo-perfusion detected in SPECT images can thus be related to impaired cerebral function, and a hyper-perfused area can be related to increased neuronal activity.[1] Changes in neuronal activity can hence be inferred from the changes in regional cerebral blood flow. Newer discoveries have led to a vast array of new radiolabeled ligands for investigation of neuroreceptor systems.

Interpretation of perfusion SPECT images

The normal adult brain shows bilaterally symmetrical tracer distribution, with higher activity in temporal, parietal, and occipital (primary visual) cortices, basal ganglia, thalami, and cingulate gyrus. Activity in the white matter and interhemispheric fissures is less.[2]

SPECT IMAGING IN MOOD DISORDERS

Unipolar depression

Depression is a common psychiatric illness and some reports have found reduction in global cerebral blood flow in patients free of medications.[49] This was found to be especially prominent in the frontal and parietal regions. This has also been demonstrated quantitatively using region of interest analysis and pixel-by-pixel comparison techniques.[50] The reduction was found to be more pronounced in the left hemisphere in some studies.[51] Other studies have also found reduced perfusion in the temporal cortex,[52,53] prefrontal cortex, limbic systems and paralimbic areas.[50] Galynker et al. reported that the finding of hypofrontality in major depressive disorder (MDD) is associated specifically with negative symptom severity[54] (Plate 10B.3).

Bipolar disorder

There are only a few studies with small numbers of patients which try to assess cerebral blood flow in bipolar disorder. Some studies found no difference in cerebral perfusion between bipolar depressives and normal controls.[55] Delvenne et al. reported an asymmetry of rCBF with reduced perfusion to the left cerebral hemisphere.[56]

In manic patients, a higher blood flow has been demonstrated globally.[57] Other studies have demonstrated hypofrontality, increased blood flow to the temporal regions and altered blood flow to the basal ganglia in manics and these are difficult to differentiate from patterns seen in schizophrenia.[55]

Effects of treatment

Although some studies have shown a variable response with medications, most studies demonstrate an increase in cerebral blood flow either globally or regionally after psychotropic antidepressant treatment.[56] Patients with severe depression on antidepressant medication and not responding to medications were found to have reduced blood flow to the frontal cortices bilaterally, anterior temporal cingulate gyrus and caudate nucleus.[58] Technetium-99m-HMPAO uptake was also shown to increase in patients who responded to electroconvulsive therapy and remain unchanged in patients who did not respond to the treatment.[59]

Serotonin transporter binding imaging

The serotonergic system is postulated to play an important role in the pathophysiology of major depressive disorder. Preliminary studies using ^{123}I-labeled 2-((2-((dimethylamino)methyl)phenyl)thio)-5-iodophenylamine (ADAM) and SPECT brain imaging suggest the possibility of decreased SERT binding in the midbrain region of patients with MDD, with the degree of decrease correlating with the severity of depressive symptoms.[60]

SCHIZOPHRENIA

Schizophrenia is a mental illness that is among the world's top ten causes of long-term disability. About 1% of the population is affected by schizophrenia with similar rates in different countries, cultural groups and sexes.[61]

Schizophrenia is characterized by disordered affect, behavior and thinking. Positive symptoms include auditory, tactile, visual or olfactory hallucinations, delusions, and aggressiveness and negative symptoms include poor eye contact, speech, apathy and inattentiveness.

Structural and functional neuro-imaging techniques have consistently demonstrated that abnormal lateralization of temporal lobes may be important in identifying the pathophysiologic processes in schizophrenia.[62] Brain SPECT most frequently shows hypofrontality, and temporal lobe hypoperfusion, usually on the left side which is frequently associated with ipsilateral frontal lobe hypo-perfusion. These findings are mostly seen in treated patients.[63] Hyperfrontality and hypertemporality have also been reported in untreated schizophrenics in the acute disease. These patients also did not show the increase in blood flow to the frontal lobes seen in normal controls during the Wisconsin card test activation test.[64]

Perfusional changes in the basal ganglia may be seen and are possibly related to the use of neuroleptic drugs. In patients who are not receiving medication, different positive symptoms may be associated with different rCBF values, some of which are related to hyper-perfusion, and some related to hypo-perfusion.[65] Injection of perfusion agents at the time of visual or auditory hallucinations have been reported to show hyper-perfusion of the primary visual or auditory cortex, respectively.[66]

Iodine-123-iodobenzamide (^{123}I-IBZM) SPECT has been used for assessment of dopamine D_2 receptor occupancy in schizophrenic patients treated with neuroleptics.[67] The concentration of striatal dopamine D_2 receptors has been shown to be significantly reduced on the left side in male schizophrenics compared with male controls.[68] Decreased D_2 striatal binding availability with certain medications also indicates higher D_2 receptor affinity and correlates with a higher risk of developing extrapyramidal symptoms. Semiquantitative analysis of IBZM SPECT images may help predict treatment outcome: the ratio of the basal ganglia to the frontal cortex decreased with therapy in good responders and increased in poor responders.[69]

Other receptors implicated include the glutamatergic N-methyl-D-aspartate (NMDA) receptor, gamma-aminobutyric acid (GABA) receptor and the serotoninergic receptors.

There is a large amount of research being carried out in developing and imaging using radiolabeled ligands to these receptors.

ANXIETY DISORDERS

Anxiety is a normal reaction to stress. However, when this is excessive and irrational it can be a disability. There are five major types of anxiety disorders:

- Generalized anxiety disorder
- Obsessive–compulsive disorder
- Panic disorder
- Post-traumatic stress disorder
- Social anxiety disorder (social phobia)

Obsessive–compulsive disorder

The essential feature of this disorder is recurrent obsessional thoughts or compulsive acts. Obsessional thoughts are ideas, images or impulses that enter the individual's mind again and again in a stereotyped form. Compulsive acts or rituals are stereotyped behaviors that are repeated again and again.

Recent neurobiological models of obsessive–compulsive disorder (OCD) suggest a dysfunction in orbitofrontal–subcortical circuitry. Results of a recent meta-analysis summarizing the results of SPECT and PET studies suggest that differences in radiotracer uptake between patients with OCD and healthy controls have been found consistently in the orbital gyrus and the head of the caudate nucleus. Most studies show hypermetabolism compared to controls but some show hypometabolism.[70] Studies investigating serotonin transporter availability in midbrain and brain stem have shown mixed results.[71,72] Low levels of dopaminergic D_2 receptor binding have also been reported.[73]

In patients responding to fluvoxamine treatment, reduced rCBF was demonstrated in the right thalamus[74] and frontal regions[75] compared to pre-therapy imaging.

Panic disorders

Brain perfusion studies have reported right left asymmetry in the inferior frontal region, occipital regions and abnormality in the perfusion to the caudate nuclei and hippocampus.[76,77] Hypo-perfusion in the frontal lobes of patients with panic disorder with yohimbine challenge was not seen in healthy volunteers.[78] Reduced benzodiazepine receptor binding was also demonstrated by iomazenil SPECT.[79] Serotonin receptors have also been implicated.

Post-traumatic stress disorder

This arises as a delayed and/or protracted response to a stressful event or situation (either short- or long-lasting) of an exceptionally threatening or catastrophic nature.[80] A previous SPECT study showed decreased central type benzodiazepine receptors in the prefrontal cortex in Vietnam War veterans with post-traumatic stress disorder. However this was not replicated in a study on 19 Gulf War veterans with post-traumatic stress disorder. Less severe symptoms and shorter duration of the illness in the latter group was given as the possible explanantion.[81]

Dysfunction of the medial prefrontal cortex, hippocampus and amygdala have been hypothesized to underlie symptoms of this disorder. Decreased medial prefrontal cortical function has been the most consistent finding on SPECT studies.[82,83] Other replicated findings include decreased inferior frontal gyrus and hippocampal function. Greater activation of the amygdala and anterior paralimbic structures (which are known to be involved in processing negative emotions such as fear) has also been reported.[84,85]

Social anxiety disorder (social phobia)

Social phobias often start in adolescence and are centered around a fear of scrutiny by other people in comparatively small groups (as opposed to crowds), leading to avoidance of social situations. Unlike most other phobias, social phobias are equally common in men and women.[80] Social phobia may be associated with low binding of ^{123}I-IBZM to D_2 receptors in the striatum.[86]

Although each of the anxiety disorders may be mediated by different neurocircuits, there is evidence of some overlap in the functional neuro-anatomy of their response to treatment with selective serotonin re-uptake inhibitors. The current data are consistent with previous work demonstrating the importance of limbic circuits in this spectrum of disorders.[87]

Conclusion

SPECT with perfusion tracers and other ligands has proved extremely useful in understanding the pathophysiology of various psychiatric disorders. Despite the sometimes overlapping and non-specific nature of the SPECT findings, perfusion and receptor imaging findings may be used as an additional diagnostic tool keeping in context the clinical possibilities to guide clinicians searching for a definite diagnosis.

REFERENCES

- ● Seminal primary article
- ◆ Key review paper
- ✱ First formal publication of a management guideline

◆ 1 Catafau AM. Brain SPECT in clinical practice: Perfusion. *J Nucl Med* 2001; **42**: 259–71.

◆ 2 Camargo EE. Brain SPECT in neurology and psychiatry. *J Nucl Med* 2001; **42**: 611–23.

◆ 3 Sperling B, Lassen NA. Cerebral blood flow by SPECT in ischaemic stroke. In: De Deyn PP, Dierckx RA, Alavi A, Pickut BA. (eds.) *SPECT in neurology and psychiatry.* London: John Libbey, 1997: 299–305.

● 4 Lassen NA, Sperling BK. Tc-99m bicisate reliably images CBF in chronic brain diseases but fails to show reflow hyperemia in subacute stroke: report of a multicenter trial of 105 cases. *J Cereb Blood Flow Metab* 1994; **14**: S44.

✳ 5 Latchaw RE, Yonas H, Hunter GJ, *et al.* AHA scientific statement – guidelines and recommendations for perfusion imaging in cerebral ischemia. *Stroke* 2003; **34**: 1084.

● 6 Alexandrov AV, Black SE, Ehrlich IE, *et al.* Simple visual analysis of brain perfusion on HMPAO SPECT predicts early outcome in acute stroke. *Stroke* 1996; **27**: 1537–42.

● 7 Barber PA, Davis SM, Infeld B, *et al.* Spontaneous reperfusion after ischemic stroke is associated with improved outcome. *Stroke* 1998; **29**: 2522–8.

● 8 Berrouschot J, Barthel H, Hesse S, *et al.* Reperfusion and metabolic recovery of brain tissue and clinical outcome after ischemic stroke and thrombolytic therapy. *Stroke* 2000; **31**: 1545–51.

● 9 Ueda T, Sakaki S, Kumon Y. Ohta S. Multivariable analysis of predictive factors related to outcome at 6 months after intra-arterial thrombolysis for acute ischemic stroke. *Stroke* 1999; **30**: 2360–5.

● 10 Ueda T, Sakaki S, Yuh WT, *et al.* Outcome in acute stroke with successful intra-arterial thrombolysis and predictive value of initial SPECT. *J Cereb Blood Flow Metab* 1999; **19**: 99–108.

11 Jezzard P. Advances in perfusion MR imaging. *Radiology* 1998; **208**: 296–9.

● 12 Ouchi Y, Nobezawa S, Yoshikawa E, *et al.* Postural effects on brain hemodynamics in unilateral cerebral artery occlusive disease: a positron emission tomography study. *J Cereb Blood Flow Metab* 2001; **21**: 1058–66.

● 13 Mayes C, Bhansali I, Prosser J, *et al.* Influence of body posture on cerebral blood flow in acute stroke. *Nucl Med Commun* 2002; **23**: 386.

● 14 Nakagawara J, Nakamura J, Takeda R, *et al.* Assessment of postischemic reperfusion and diamox activation test in stroke using ^{99m}Tc-ECD SPECT. *J Cereb Blood Flow Metab* 1994; **14(suppl)**: S49–S57.

● 15 Cikrit DF, Dalsing MC, Lalka SG, *et al.* The value of acetazolamide SPECT scans before and after carotid endarterectomy. *J Vasc Surg* 1999; **30**: 599–605.

● 16 Kuroda S, Houkin K, Kamiyama H, *et al.* Long term prognosis of medically treated patients with internal carotid or middle cerebral artery occlusion. Can acetazolamide test predict it? *Stroke* 2001; **32**: 2110–6.

● 17 Kim JS, Moon DH, Kim GE, *et al.* Acetazolamide stress brain perfusion SPECT predicts the need for carotid shunting during carotid endarterectomy. *J Nucl Med* 2000; **41**: 1836–41.

● 18 Hwang TL, Saenz A, Farrell JJ, Brannon WL. Brain SPECT with dipyridamole stress to evaluate cerebral blood flow reserve in carotid artery disease. *J Nucl Med* 1996; **37**: 1595–9.

● 19 Soricelli A, Postiglione A, Cuocolo A, *et al.* Effect of adenosine on cerebral blood flow as evaluated by single-photon emission computed tomography in normal subjects and in patients with occlusive carotid disease. A comparison with acetazolamide. *Stroke* 1995; **26**: 1572–6.

20 Hattori N, Yonekura Y, Tanaka F, *et al.* One-day protocol for cerebral perfusion reserve with acetazolamide. *J Nucl Med* 1996; **37**: 2057–61.

● 21 Yonas H, Pindzola RR, Meltzer CC, Sasser H. Qualitative versus quantitative assessment of cerebrovascular reserves. *Neurosurgery* 1998; **42**: 1005–12.

● 22 Russell D, Dybevold S, Kjartansson O, *et al.* Cerebral vasoreactivity and blood flow before and 3 months after carotid endarterectomy. *Stroke* 1990; **21**: 1029–32.

● 23 Garai I, Varga J, Szomjak E, *et al.* Quantitative assessment of blood flow reserve using ^{99m}Tc-HMPAO in carotid stenosis. *Eur J Nucl Med Mol Imaging* 2002; **29**: 216–20.

● 24 Firlik AD, Kaufmann AM, Jungreis CA, Yonas H. Effect of transluminal angioplasty on cerebral blood flow in the management of symptomatic vasospasm following aneurysmal subarachnoid hemorrhage. *J Neurosurg* 1997; **86**: 830.

● 25 Engelhardt M, Pfadenhauer K, Zentner J, *et al.* Impaired cerebral autoregulation in asymptomatic patients with carotid artery stenosis: comparison of acetazolamide-SPECT and transcranial CO(2)-dopplersonography. *Zentralbl Chir* 2004; **129**: 178–82.

● 26 Jimenez-Bonilla JF, Quirce R, Hernandez A, *et al.* Assessment of cerebral perfusion and cerebrovascular reserve in insulin-dependent diabetic patients without central neurological symptoms by means of ^{99m}Tc-HMPAO SPET with acetazolamide. *Eur J Nucl Med* 2001; **28**: 1647–55.

27 Laloux P. SPECT imaging in transient ischemic attacks and subarachnoid haemorrhage. In: De Deyn PP, Dierckx RA, Alavi A, Pickut BA. (eds.) *SPECT in neurology and psychiatry.* London: John Libbey, 1997: 323–34.

● 28 Marti-Fabregas JA, Catafau AM, Mari C, *et al.* Cerebral perfusion and haemodynamics measured by SPET in symptom-free patients with transient ischaemic attack: clinical implications. *Eur J Nucl Med* 2001; **28**: 1828–35.

● 29 Bogousslavsky J, Delaloye-Bischof A, Regli F, Delaloye B. Prolonged disturbances of regional cerebral blood flow in transient ischemic attacks. *Stroke* 1985; **16**: 932.

● 30 Davis S, Andrews J, Lichtenstein M, *et al.* A single photon emission computed tomography study of hypoperfusion after subarcahnoid haemorrhage. *Stroke* 1990; **21**: 252.

● 31 Davis SM, Andrews JT, Lichtenstein M, *et al.* Correlations between cerebral arterial velocities, blood flow, and delayed ischemia after subarachnoid haemorrhage. *Stroke* 1992; **23**: 492–497.

● 32 Imaizumi M, Kitagawa K, Oku N, *et al.* Clinical significance of cerebrovascular reserve in acetazolamide challenge – comparison with acetazolamide challenge H_2O-PET and gas-PET. *Ann Nucl Med* 2004; **18**: 369–74.

● 33 Sviri GE, Lewis DH, Correa R, *et al.* Basilar artery vasospasm and delayed posterior circulation ischemia after aneurysmal subarachnoid hemorrhage. *Stroke* 2004; **35**: 1867–72.

● 34 Herholz K, Heiss WD. Functional imaging correlates of recovery after stroke in humans. *J Cereb Blood Flow Metab* 2000; **20**: 1619–31.

● 35 Song HC, Bom HS, Cho KH, *et al.* Prognostication of recovery in patients with acute ischemic stroke through the use of brain SPECT with technetium-99m-labeled metronidazole. *Stroke* 2003; **34**: 982–6.

36 Mountz JM, Deutsch G, Hetherington HP, *et al.* Applications of rCBF brain SPECT and NMR imaging in the evaluation of stroke: implications in rehabilitation prognosis. In: De Deyn PP, Dierckx RA, Alavi A, Pickut BA. (eds.) *SPECT in neurology and psychiatry*. London: John Libbey, 1997: 335–46.

● 37 Darby JM, Yonas H, Marion DW, Latchaw RE. Local 'inverse steal' induced by hyperventilation in head injury. *Neurosurgery* 1988; **23**: 84–8.

● 38 Adelson PD, Clyde B, Kochanek PM, *et al.* Cerebrovascular response in infants and young children following severe traumatic brain injury: a preliminary report. *Pediatr Neurosurg* 1997; **26**: 200–7.

● 39 Abdel-Dayem HM, Abu-Judeh H, Kumar M, *et al.* SPECT brain perfusion abnormalities in mild or moderate traumatic brain injury. *Clin Nucl Med* 1998; **23**: 309–17.

● 40 Jacobs A, Put E, Ingels M, *et al.* Prospective evaluation of technetium-99m-HMPAO SPECT in mild and moderate traumatic brain injury. *J Nucl Med* 1994; **35**: 942–7.

● 41 Vinjamuri S, O'Driscoll K, Maltby P, *et al.* Identification of hypoxic regions in traumatic brain injury. *Clin Nucl Med* 1999; **24**: 891.

● 42 Newton MR, Greenwood RJ, Britton KE, *et al.* A study comparing SPECT with CT and MRI after closed head injury. *J Neurol Neurosurg Psych* 1992; **55**: 92–4.

● 43 Vinjamuri S, O'Driscoll K. Significance of white matter abnormalities in patients with closed head injury. *Nucl Med Commun* 2000; **21**: 645–9.

● 44 Ichise M, Chung DG, Wang P, *et al.* Technetium-99m-HMPAO SPECT, CT, and MRI in the evaluation of the patients with chronic traumatic brain injury: a correlation with neuropsychological performance. *J Nucl Med* 1994; **35**: 217–26.

● 45 Oder W, Goldenberg G, Spatt J, *et al.* Behavioral and psychosocial sequelae of severe closed head injury and regional cerebral blood flow. A SPECT study. *J Neurol Neurosurg Psych* 1992; **55**: 475–80.

◆ 46 Newberg AB, Alavi A. Neuroimaging in patients with head injury. *Semin Nucl Med* 2003; **33**: 136–47.

● 47 Richard K, Lai K, Kay-Yin BS. Tc-99m hexamethylpropylene amine oxime scintigraphy in the diagnosis of brain death and its implications for the harvesting of organs used for transplantation. *Clin Nucl Med* 2000; **25**: 7.

● 48 Conrad GR, Sinha P. Scintigraphy as a confirmatory test of brain death. *Semin Nucl Med* 2003; **33**: 312–23.

● 49 Lesser IM, Mena I, Boone KB, *et al.* Reduction of cerebral blood flow in older depressed patients. *Arch General Psychiatr* 1994; **51**: 677.

● 50 Ito H, Kawashima R, Awata S, *et al.* Hypoperfusion in the limbic system and prefrontal cortex in depression: SPECT with anatomic standardization technique. *J Nucl Med* 1996; **37**: 410–14.

● 51 Kawakatsu S, Komatani A. Xe-133 inhalation SPECT in manic depressive illness. *Nippon Rinsho* 1994; **52**: 1180.

● 52 Austin MP, Dougall N, Ross M, *et al.* Single photon emission tomography with Tc-99m exametazime in major depression and the pattern of brain activity underlying the psychotic/neurotic continuum. *J Affect Disord* 1992; **26**: 31.

● 53 Yazici KM, Kapucu O, Erbas B, *et al.* Assessment of changes in regional blood flow in patients with major depression using the Tc-99m HMPAO SPECT method. *Eur J Nucl Med* 1992; **19**: 1038.

● 54 Galynker II, Cai J, Ongseng F, *et al.* Hypofrontality and negative symptoms in major depressive disorder. *J Nucl Med* 1998; **39**: 608–12.

◆ 55 D'haenen HAH. SPECT imaging in primary mood disorders. In: De Deyn PP, Dierckx RA, Alavi A, Pickut BA. (eds.) *SPECT in neurology and psychiatry*. London: John Libbey, 1997: 107–15.

● 56 Delvenne V, Delecluse F, Hubain P, *et al.* Regional cerebral blood flow in patients with affective disorders. *Br J Psychiatr* 1990; **157**: 359.

- 57 Rush AJ, Schesler MA, Stokely E, *et al*. Cerebral blood flow in depression and mania. *Psychopharmacol Bull* 1982; **18**: 6.

- 58 Mayberg HS, Lewis PJ, Regenold W, Wagner HN. Paralimbic hypoperfusion in unipolar depression. *J Nucl Med* 1994; **35**: 929–34.

- 59 Bonne O, Krausz Y, Shapira B, *et al*. Increased cerebral blood flow in depressed patients responding to electroconvulsive therapy. *J Nucl Med* 1996; **37**: 1075–80.

- 60 Newberg AB, Amsterdam JD, Wintering N, Alavi A. ^{123}I-ADAM binding to serotonin transporters in patients with major depression and healthy controls: a preliminary study. *J Nucl Med* 2000; **46**: 973–7.

- 61 Mueser K, McGurk S, Schizophrenia. *Lancet* 2004; **363**: 2063–72.

- 62 Russell JM, Early TS, Patterson JC, *et al*. Temporal lobe perfusion asymmetries in schizophrenia. *J Nucl Med* 1997; **38**: 607–12.

- 63 Woods SW. Regional cerebral blood flow imaging with SPECT in psychiatric disease: focus on schizophrenia, anxiety disorders and substance abuse. *J Clin Psychiatry* 1992; **53(suppl)**: 20–5.

- 64 Catafau AM, Parellada E, Lomena FJ, *et al*. Prefrontal and temporal blood flow in schizophrenia: resting and activation technetium-99m-HMPAO SPECT patterns in young neuroleptic-naive patients with acute disease. *J Nucl Med* 1994; **35**: 935–41.

- 65 Sabri O, Erkwoh R, Schreckenberger M, *et al*. Correlation of positive symptoms exclusively to hyperperfusion or hypoperfusion of cerebral cortex in never-treated schizophrenics. *Lancet* 1997; **349**: 1735–9.

- 66 Musalek M, Podreka I, Walter H, *et al*. Regional brain function in hallucinations: a study of regional cerebral blood flow with ^{99m}Tc-HMPAO-SPECT in patients with auditory hallucinations, tactile hallucinations, and normal controls. *Compr Psychiatry* 1989; **30**: 99–108.

- 67 Dresel S, Tatsch K, Dahne I, *et al*. Iodine-123-iodobenzamide SPECT assessment of dopamine D2 receptor occupancy in risperidone-treated schizophrenic patients. *J Nucl Med* 1998; **39**: 1138–42.

- 68 Acton PD, Pilowsky LS, Costa DC, Ell PJ. Multivariate cluster analysis of dynamic iodine-123 iodobenzamide SPET dopamine D2 receptor images in schizophrenia. *Eur J Nucl Med* 1997; **24**: 111–8.

- 69 Schroöder J, Silvestri S, Bubeck B, *et al*. D2 dopamine receptor up-regulation, treatment response, neurological soft signs, and extrapyramidal side effects in schizophrenia: a follow-up study with ^{123}I-iodobenzamide single photon emission computed tomography in the drug-naive state and after neuroleptic treatment. *Biol Psychiatry* 1998; **43**: 660–5.

- 70 Whiteside SP, Port JD, Abramowitz JS. A meta-analysis of functional neuroimaging in obsessive-compulsive disorder. *Psychiatry Res* 2004; **132**: 69–79.

- 71 Stengler-Wenzke K, Muller U, Angermeyer MC, *et al*. Reduced serotonin transporter-availability in obsessive–compulsive disorder (OCD). *Eur Arch Psychiatry Clin Neurosci* 2004; **254**: 252–5.

- 72 Pogarell O, Hamann C, Popperl G, *et al*. Elevated brain serotonin transporter availability in patients with obsessive–compulsive disorder. *Biol Psychiatry* 2003; **54**: 1406–13.

- 73 Denys D, van der Wee N, Janssen J, *et al*. Low level of dopaminergic D-2 receptor binding in obsessive–compulsive disorder. *Biol Psychiatry* 2004; **55**: 1041–5.

- 74 Ho Pian KL, van Megen HJ, Ramsey NF, *et al*. Decreased thalamic blood flow in obsessive–compulsive disorder patients responding to fluvoxamine. *Psychiatry Res* 2005; **138**: 89–97.

- 75 Hoehn-Saric R, Pearlson G, Harris G, *et al*. Effects of fluoxetine on regional cerebral blood flow in obsessive–compulsive patients. *Am J Psychiatry* 1991; **148**: 1243–5.

- 76 De Cristofaro MT, Sessarego A, Pupi A, *et al*. Brain perfusion abnormalities in drug-naive, lactate-sensitive panic patients: a SPECT study. *Biol Psychiatry* 1993; **33**: 505–12.

- 77 Lucey JV, Costa DC, Adshead G, *et al*. Brain blood flow in anxiety disorders. OCD, panic disorder with agoraphobia, and post-traumatic stress disorder on ^{99m}Tc-HMPAO single photon emission tomography (SPET). *Br J Psychiatry* 1997; **171**: 346–50.

- 78 Devous Sr MD. Comparison of SPECT applications in neurology and psychiatry. *J Clin Psychiatry* 1992; **53(suppl)**: 13–19.

- 79 Bremner JD, Innis RB, White T, *et al*. SPECT [I-123]iomazenil measurement of the benzodiazepine receptor in panic disorder. *Biol Psychiatry* 2000; **47**: 96–106.

- 80 World Health Organization. *The ICD-10 classification of mental and behavioural disorders*. Geneva: WHO, 1992.

- 81 Fujita M, Southwick SM, Denucci CC, *et al*. Central type benzodiazepine receptors in Gulf War veterans with posttraumatic stress disorder. *Biol Psychiatry* 2004; **56**: 95–100.

- 82 Bremner JD. Neuroimaging studies in post-traumatic stress disorder. *Curr Psychiatry Rep* 2002; **4**: 254–63.

- 83 Zubieta JK, Chinitz JA, Lombardi U, *et al*. Medial frontal cortex involvement in PTSD symptoms: a SPECT study. *J Psychiatr Res* 1999; **33**: 259–64.

- 84 Pitman RK, Shin LM, Rauch SL. Investigating the pathogenesis of posttraumatic stress disorder with neuroimaging. *J Clin Psychiatry* 2001; **62(suppl 17)**: 47–54.

● 85 Sachinvala N, Kling A, Suffin S, *et al.* Increased regional cerebral perfusion by ^{99m}Tc hexamethyl propylene amine oxime single photon emission computed tomography in post-traumatic stress disorder. *Mil Med* 2000; **165**: 473–9.

● 86 Schneier FR, Liebowitz MR, Abi-Dargham A, *et al.* Low dopamine D(2) receptor binding potential in social phobia. *Am J Psychiatry* 2000; **157**: 457–9.

● 87 Carey PD, Warwick J, Niehaus DJ, *et al.* Single photon emission computed tomography (SPECT) of anxiety disorders before and after treatment with citalopram. *BMC Psychiatry* 2004; **4**: 30.

Epilepsy

S.F. BARRINGTON

INTRODUCTION

Epilepsy is characterized by recurrent seizures that are caused by spontaneous electrical discharges, which are propagated through brain tissue. Epilepsy may be 'partial' or 'generalized' depending on whether a single region of the brain can be identified as the source of the electrical discharges. It may be 'simple' or 'complex', depending on whether the patient retains or loses consciousness. The classification of epilepsy adopted by the International League against Epilepsy is shown in Table 10C.1.

Neuroimaging has an important role in the detection of focal abnormalities, responsible for complex partial seizures (CPS) if medical treatment is ineffective. It has been estimated that 'intractable' complex partial seizures occur in 1:1000 of the general population,[1] and if the focus can be identified then it may be amenable to resection. A recent randomized trial of surgical versus medical treatment for mesial temporal lobe epilepsy (TLE), which is the most common site of origin, reported that 58% of patients had significant improvement in seizures compared to 8% in the medical group at 1 year.[2] It has been estimated that a successful outcome with surgery occurs in 90% for patients with mesial TLE where there is hippocampal atrophy on magnetic resonance imaging (MRI) with concordant findings on electroencephalography (EEG).[3] The outcome for patients with extra-temporal epilepsy is less good, with approximately 50% rendered seizure-free provided a focus is defined.[4]

Initial investigation of patients with CPS considered for surgery would include scalp EEG with video telemetry and MRI, enabling the focus to be defined in the majority of

Table 10C.1 *Classification of epilepsy, as adopted by the International League against Epilepsy*

I. Partial (focal) seizures
- A. *Simple partial seizures*
- B. *Complex partial seizures*
- C. *Partial seizures evolving to secondarily generalized seizures*

II. Generalized seizures (convulsive or non-convulsive)
- A. *Absence seizures*
- B. *Myoclonic seizures*
- C. *Clonic seizures*
- D. *Tonic seizures*
- E. *Tonic-clonic seizures*
- F. *Atonic seizures*

III. Unclassified seizures

patients. MRI is used to detect structural abnormalities associated with epilepsy such as tumor, congenital developmental abnormalities, vascular malformations, acquired cortical damage and hippocampal atrophy (frequently with volumetric analysis).[5] The MRI and EEG findings are concordant and establish the focus in approximately 60% of patients with TLE[6] but if the MRI is normal or conflicts with the EEG findings then a functional imaging test such as single photon emission computed tomography (SPECT) or positron emission tomography (PET) may assist in localization.[7] The imaging findings should always be interpreted in the knowledge of the EEG findings as incidental structural or functional abnormalities can occur, which are not responsible for the generation of epileptiform activity. However, the use of neuroimaging over the last 10–15 years has reduced the need for invasive EEG in many patients[3,8] thereby reducing cost and associated morbidity such as infection and hemorrhage.[9]

The basis underlying the use of functional imaging techniques such as SPECT and PET is that perfusion and glucose metabolism may be increased during seizures and reduced immediately after and between seizures. The period during a seizure is referred to as 'ictal', the period immediately afterwards is referred to as 'post-ictal' and the period between seizures is referred to as 'inter-ictal'. There is high first pass extraction of perfusion tracers used for brain SPECT imaging such as ^{99m}Tc-hexamethylpropylene amine oxime (^{99m}Tc-HMPAO) and ^{99m}Tc-ethyl cysteinate dimer (^{99m}Tc-ECD). SPECT imaging is therefore suited to both 'ictal' and 'inter-ictal' imaging. As the tracers also have high retention in the brain the patient may be imaged several hours after a seizure, once in a stable condition. Most clinical PET studies use the tracer ^{18}F-fluorodeoxyglucose (^{18}F-FDG) which is taken up at a much slower rate and reaches steady state within brain tissue between 30 and 60 min. As most seizures last for less than 90 s, any increase in glucose metabolism during the seizure is likely to be masked by the reduced glucose metabolism that occurs around the epileptic focus in the inter-ictal state when the 'signal' is effectively averaged over 30–60 min. PET studies are therefore undertaken in the 'inter-ictal' state. 'Ictal' studies do arise fortuitously but are rare, especially in adult patients who are scanned on treatment.[10]

The area of hypoperfusion or hypometabolism usually includes the epileptic focus but is frequently more diffuse, reflecting distant effects, maybe due to diaschisis where there is a structural lesion or to reduced synaptic inhibition in areas of epileptic propagation. The latter is suggested by the association of inter-ictal spiking and slow wave activity on EEG thorough areas of hypometabolism demonstrated on PET, using FDG.[11] There is no relationship between neuronal loss and hippocampal gliosis at surgery with FDG hypometabolism.[12] SPECT and PET cannot therefore localize a focus precisely but may be useful aids to lateralize a focus.[13]

SPECT IMAGING

Inter-ictal SPECT imaging is less reliable than inter-ictal PET imaging as the measurement of metabolism is superior to blood flow in inter-ictal studies.[7,14] PET also has better resolution. Correct lateralization with SPECT occurs in approximately 45% of patients with TLE.[15,16] However, reliable results may be obtained with 'ictal' SPECT imaging. Typically, there is hyperperfusion in the region of the focus with surrounding hypoperfusion followed by a 'switch' to more profound hypoperfusion post-ictally before returning to the inter-ictal state when perfusion may be normal or reduced (Plate 10C.1). The drawbacks to ictal imaging are

that the patient requires admission to hospital, often needs withdrawal of antiepileptic medication and needs continuous EEG monitoring and video telemetry. The correct timing of the onset of the seizure is vital to interpretation of the SPECT data.[7] A relative usually stays with the patient to alert the staff to the onset of a seizure and a member of staff trained to inject radiopharmaceuticals is present on the ward 24 hourly. The best results are obtained when the tracer is injected during the seizure or within 30 s of its completion. Under these conditions, correct lateralization occurs in unilateral TLE in approximately 80–90% of cases and incorrect lateralization in only 2%.[6,17–19] When tracer injection is delayed the accuracy of the technique falls[20] and has been reported as 70% with a mean injection time of 4 min after seizure onset.[19] Subtraction maps of the ictal and inter-ictal SPECT images registered to the patient's MRI (SISCOM) have been reported to aid analysis.[21]

The accuracy of ictal SPECT imaging in extratemporal lobe epilepsy has also been reported in the region of 62–92%.[6,22–24] As the wide variation in the reported accuracy indicates, the localization of extratemporal foci is more difficult than for TLE and this also applies to other imaging modalities including MRI and PET. Nonetheless the site of an abnormality on SPECT may help to guide placement of intracranial subdural electrodes.[7,25]

POSITRON EMISSION TOMOGRAPHY

Fluorodeoxyglucose imaging

The typical pattern of unilateral hypometabolism with FDG PET in TLE correctly lateralizes the focus in 75–90%[6,26,27] (Plate 10C.2). One series comparing PET with ictal SPECT suggests PET was more sensitive than SPECT but that both techniques had high accuracy and either could be used.[6] Hypometabolism may extend beyond the region of the focus, from the medial temporal lobe into the anterior and lateral temporal lobes and diffuse changes do not preclude a good surgical outcome.[28] Hypometabolism may also extend beyond the temporal lobe into frontal and parietal cortex and into deep structures such as the thalamus. The implications of extratemporal hypometabolism in TLE is not certain with conflicting reports in the literature.[29–31] Bilateral hypometabolism may be associated with a worse prognosis in terms of medical treatment and surgical outcome.[32] It should prompt further investigation with intracranial EEG to rule out bitemporal epileptiform activity, which would preclude surgical resection.[33] Reports regarding the utility of FDG PET in extratemporal epilepsy are variable, with correct lateralization in the region of 30–78% in adults[6,23,26,34] (Fig. 10C.1). The sensitivity of the technique may depend on the underlying aetiology. FDG PET is more sensitive than MRI in the detection of extratemporal foci in association with neuronal migration disorders rather than tumors.[23]

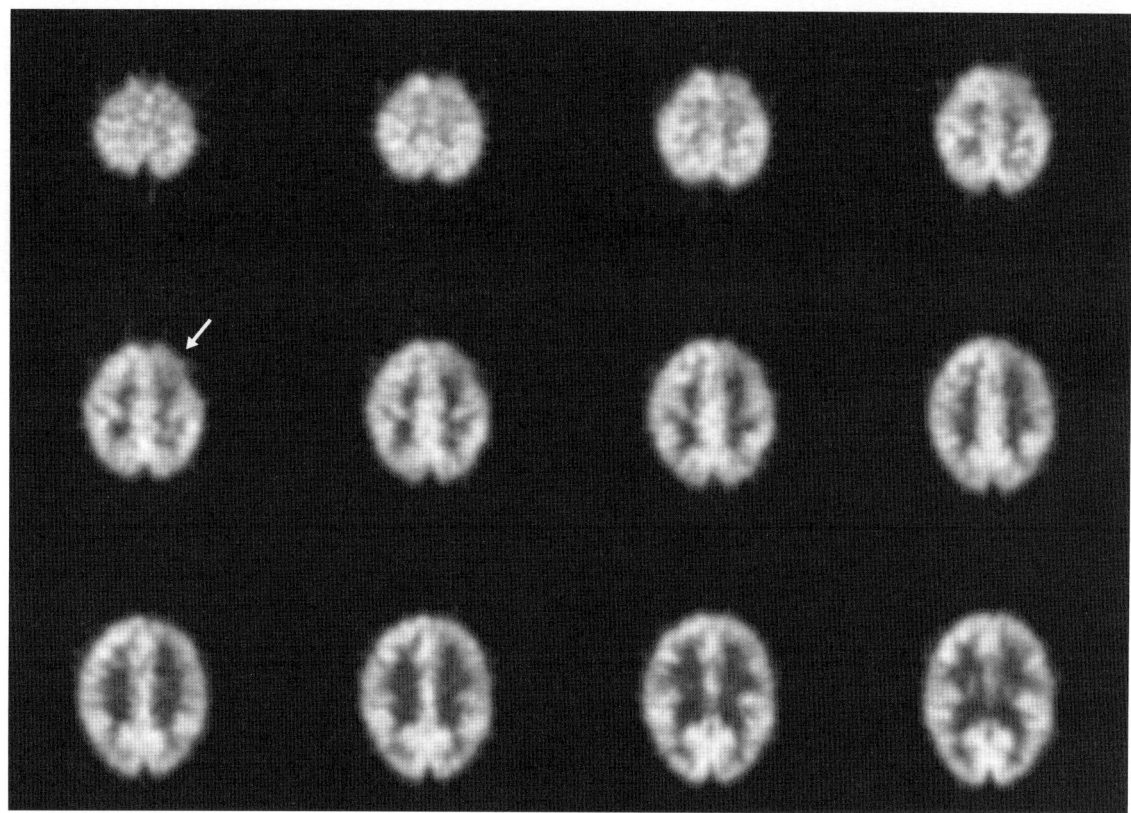

Figure 10C.1   *An example of left frontal hypometabolism is shown using fluorodeoxyglucose positron emission tomography in this series of transaxial slices.*

Quantification in positron emission tomography

There is considerable overlap between the rate of FDG uptake in normal brain and sites of epileptic foci.[35] Therefore absolute quantification is not applied clinically. Typically, asymmetry of greater than 10% is taken as representing significant hypometabolism and can be easily detected visually. An asymmetry index (AI), in percent, may be quoted as follows:

$$AI = \left(\frac{left - right}{(left + right)/2} \right) \times 100.$$

Use of asymmetry indices of 10–15% or more has been shown to be statistically significantly associated with a successful outcome to surgery.[28,30] Regions of interest can be placed over matching areas within the brain to calculate AIs (Fig. 10C.2) or a line profile may be drawn through a temporal lobe slice and the height of the two peaks in a histogram compared. The use of a color scale can be just as useful in the clinical situation (Plate 10C.2).

These sampling methods are relatively inefficient, however, as they sample only a part of the data and can be highly operator dependent. Voxel-based approaches may

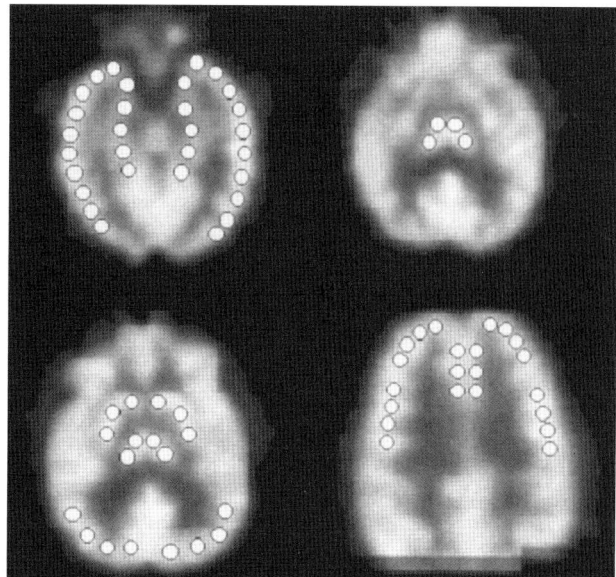

Figure 10C.2   *This shows regions of interest placed over corresponding areas in the cerebral hemispheres for calculation of asymmetry indices.*

be applied, in which the data are transformed to comply with an anatomical 'blueprint', the most commonly used of which is the Talairach space. An automatic pixel by pixel comparison is then made with reference to a 'control'

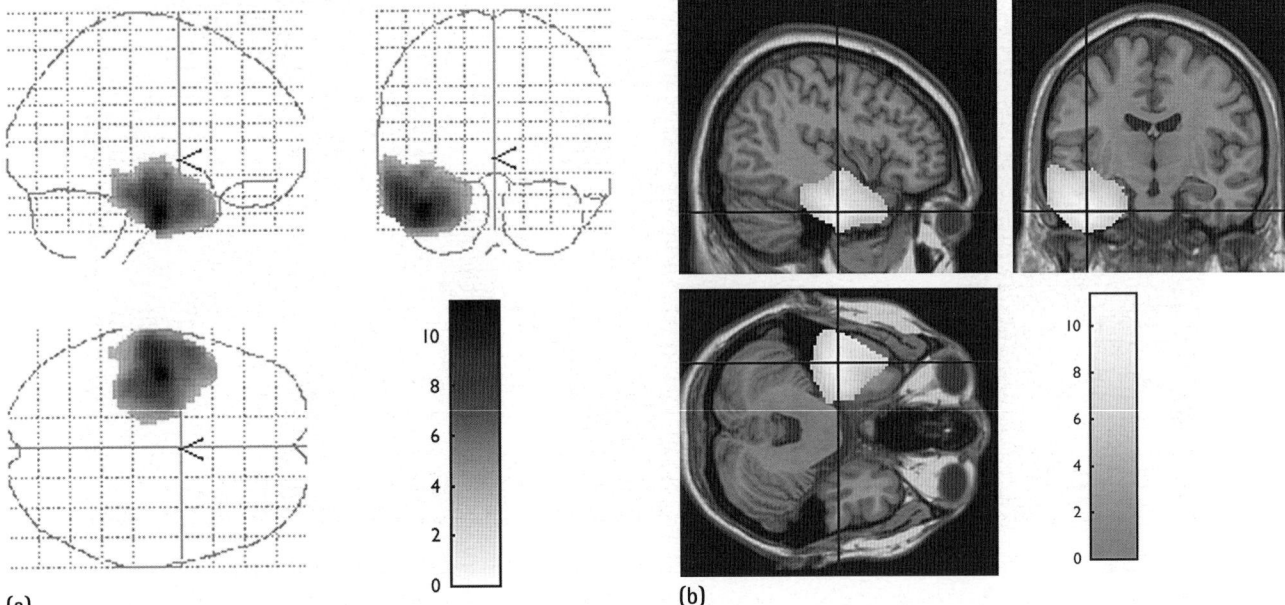

(a)   (b)

Figure 10C.3   *This figure shows a statistical parametric map of T values from a comparison between 20 healthy controls and a patient with left temporal lobe epilepsy. These maps are commonly displayed on the three orthogonal 'glass brain' image (a) and T1-weighted magnetic resonance imaging (b) using neurological convention according to which the left side of the brain is shown on the left side of the figures. Here, the hypothesis that the uptake in a given voxel is lower in this patient than in the control population was tested and the map was thresholded at a level of P = 0.001. Areas which are above this threshold indicate significant reduction of glucose uptake and are observed in the left temporal lobe as shown with a gray scale of T values. Image by courtesy of Dr Nozomi Akanuma, Department of Clinical Neurophysiology and Epilepsies, Guy's and St Thomas' Hospital, London.*

database to generate statistical images, usually superimposed on MRI images for anatomical definition. Statistical inference may be drawn from these statistical parametric maps (SPMs) with the generation of Z scores (Fig. 10C.3). In one study using this approach, statistical parametric analysis was no better than 'experienced' visual analysis at detecting the seizure onset zone in patients with temporal lobe epilepsy. However, it improved the sensitivity in extratemporal epilepsy but detected multiple abnormalities more often[36] so the cruder semi-quantitative methods described above are often sufficient for initial clinical interpretation.

Benzodiazepine receptor imaging

There is a reduction in the levels of the inhibitory neurotransmitter gamma aminobutyric acid (GABA) in epilepsy. Reduction in tracer uptake with ^{11}C-flumazenil which binds to benzodiazepine receptors within the benzodiazepine–GABA$_A$ complex has been reported in both temporal and extra-temporal epilepsy.[36–38] This is probably due to reduction in the density of GABA receptors at the site of the epileptic focus[39] which has been demonstrated in autoradiographic sections of brain excised for the treatment of frontal lobe epilepsy.[40] Reduced tracer uptake

maybe also be partly due to reduced binding affinity of the receptors.[41]

Initial reports suggested that the reduction in benzodiazepine binding imaged using ^{11}C-flumazenil appeared to be better circumscribed than change in flow or metabolism. The area of reduced flumazenil uptake also seemed to be closely correlated with the ictal onset zone[37,42,43] and perhaps with the outcome of temporal lobe surgery.[43] The largest series to date exploring the use of flumazenil reported on imaging findings in 100 patients undergoing evaluation for surgery. All patients had video telemetry and EEG, MRI, FDG and ^{11}C-flumazenil PET. Forty patients also had intracranial EEG with surgery performed in forty-four.[27] Carbon-11-flumazenil did not provide superior data to FDG PET overall, although flumazenil was slightly more sensitive than FDG in TLE. Carbon-11-flumazenil was falsely lateralizing, however, in some patients with TLE in whom the FDG scan was normal. Others have also found increases in binding outside the affected hippocampus in temporal lobe white matter and in frontal and parietal cortex.[44] In patients with cryptogenic frontal lobe epilepsy, flumazenil was more sensitive than FDG in the study by Ryvlin *et al.* but neither tracer was able to localize the lesion accurately enough to obviate the requirement for invasive EEG. However, the PET studies could be used to direct placement of intracranial electrodes.[27] In a small group of

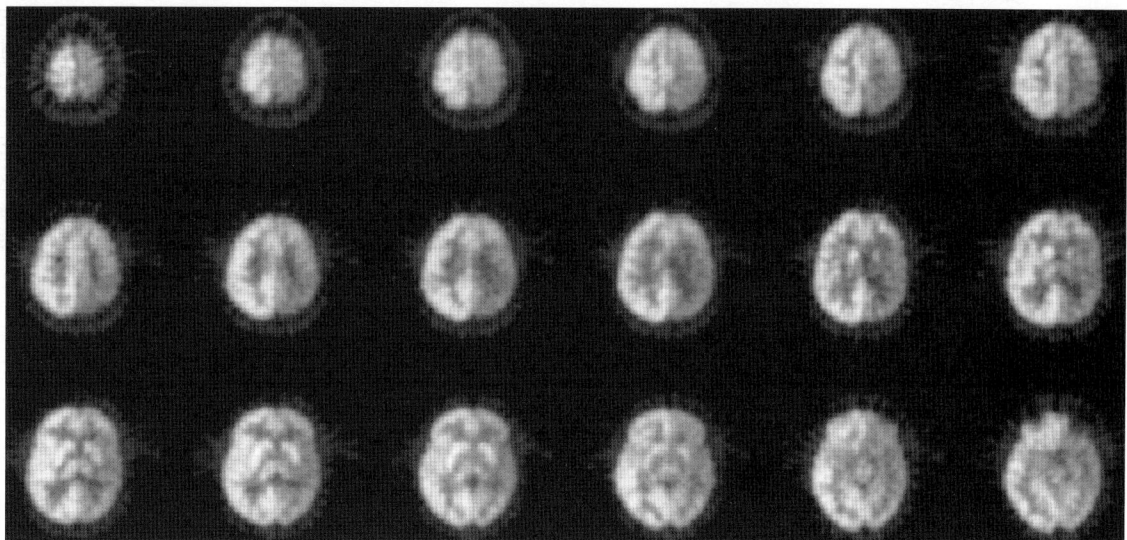

Figure 10C.4   *This shows diffuse hypometabolism in the left cerebral hemisphere in a previously healthy child presenting with seizures and a progressive right hemiparesis. The diagnosis of Rasmussen's encephalitis was confirmed at hemispherectomy. Reproduced with permission from Maisey MN, Wahl RW, Barrington SF. Atlas of clinical positron emission tomography. London: Arnold, 1999; p. 293.*

patients with bitemporal abnormalities ^{11}C-flumazenil helped to confirm bilateral involvement.

The data for benzodiazepine receptor imaging with PET are promising particularly for the evaluation of extra-temporal epilepsy and maybe for the detection of bitemporal epilepsy. These data are based, however, on small numbers and further prospective evaluation is needed before ^{11}C-flumazenil imaging can be considered to be part of the routine surgical work-up.[24]

PEDIATRIC EPILEPSIES

Partial epilepsies

Partial epilepsies account for up to half of childhood epilepsies. The management of children with intractable TLE is similar to adults, except that there may be greater pressure to suppress seizures earlier to avoid developmental consequences if seizures are truly 'intractable'.[45,46] The commonest surgical procedure, as in adults, is anterior temporal lobectomy. Extra-temporal focal resection is considered in the presence of a structural lesion, which is concordant with unifocal EEG findings. Hemispherectomy may be considered in the management of Rasmussen's syndrome or 'smouldering encephalitis' which occurs in a healthy child who develops partial seizures, progressive hemiplegia, and dementia.[47] Rasmussen's syndrome may have a viral etiology and diagnosis is difficult, often established only by brain biopsy. FDG PET and SPECT may show abnormal metabolism in the early stages unilaterally in the frontal and temporal lobes then diffuse hemispheric changes[48,49] and hence may be useful in facilitating diagnosis and guiding biopsy in

early stages when MRI can be normal (Fig. 10C.4). Early surgery may prevent progressive neurological deterioration.

Generalized epilepsies

Infantile spasms occur usually in the first 2 years of life and are associated with developmental delay or regression and the presence of hypsarrythmia on inter-ictal EEG. This triad makes up the syndrome referred to as 'West syndrome'.[47] The prognosis with medical treatment is poor. However, focal abnormalities may be present in up to 20% of patients on FDG PET. When focal PET abnormalities are concordant with EEG findings, surgery can result in a marked reduction in seizure frequency or abolition of seizures and improvements in development in approximately 75% of children.[50] The areas of focal abnormality on PET correlate with the presence of microscopic cortical dysplasia at surgery.[50] In very young children incomplete myelination may be a reason why it may be difficult to detect such lesions on MRI.[51]

Lennox–Gastaut syndrome is characterized by mixed seizure types including tonic, myoclonic, absence, and partial seizures that are associated with mental retardation and slow spike and wave pattern on the EEG. Seizure frequency is high and associated neurological abnormalities occur in many of these children.[47] A variety of patterns have been described in this condition on PET scanning[52,53] and focal abnormalities or diffuse unilateral abnormalities on PET may be a basis for further evaluation of children for focal resection or hemispherectomy if hemiparesis is present.[8]

In patients with Sturge–Weber syndrome, the presence of bilateral changes on PET indicate a worse prognosis[54] and a worse outcome following hemispherectomy.[55]

Wada test

The Wada test involves injection of sodium amytal into the internal carotid artery, which produces anesthesia of one cerebral hemisphere for several minutes. Language and memory testing are performed during the state of hemianesthesia, first in one cerebral hemisphere then the other. Impairment of memory function in the unaffected hemisphere may be considered a contraindication to surgery whilst memory impairment on the side considered for resection may indicate temporal lobe dysfunction on that side producing corroborative evidence for resection.[56]

CONCLUSION

Nuclear imaging is useful in the group of patients undergoing presurgical evaluation for TLE with normal MRI or where the MRI conflicts with EEG findings. SPECT imaging and PET imaging may then assist in lateralization. There is sufficient confidence in the accuracy of inter-ictal PET that if there is clear evidence of unilateral temporal hypometabolism which is concordant with scalp EEG findings and video telemetry, the patient may proceed for anterior temporal lobectomy without the need for presurgical intracranial EEG.[7] If the imaging findings are not in agreement with the EEG, however, or in most cases of extra-temporal epilepsy, invasive studies should be considered and the nuclear imaging may help to direct placement of intracranial electrodes[7] (Figs 10C.5 and 10C.6). In some children with malignant epilepsies, FDG PET may help to localize focal abnormalities with a potential for surgical resection, where structural lesions are not evident. Carbon-11-flumazenil shows promise for lateralization in extra-temporal epilepsy and in the detection of bitemporal epilepsies but its role requires further evaluation in larger series of patients.

Case history: Clinical case 1

This patient presented with complex partial seizures. Magnetic resonance imaging showed right occipital microgyria although scalp EEG and foramen ovale telemetry indicated bilateral seizure activity. Representative transaxial slices are shown of the FDG PET scan which show right occipital hypometabolism concordant with the MR abnormality. Subsequent subdural EEG confirmed the site of the epileptic focus as the right occipital lobe. The patient underwent resection with significant improvement in seizure frequency.

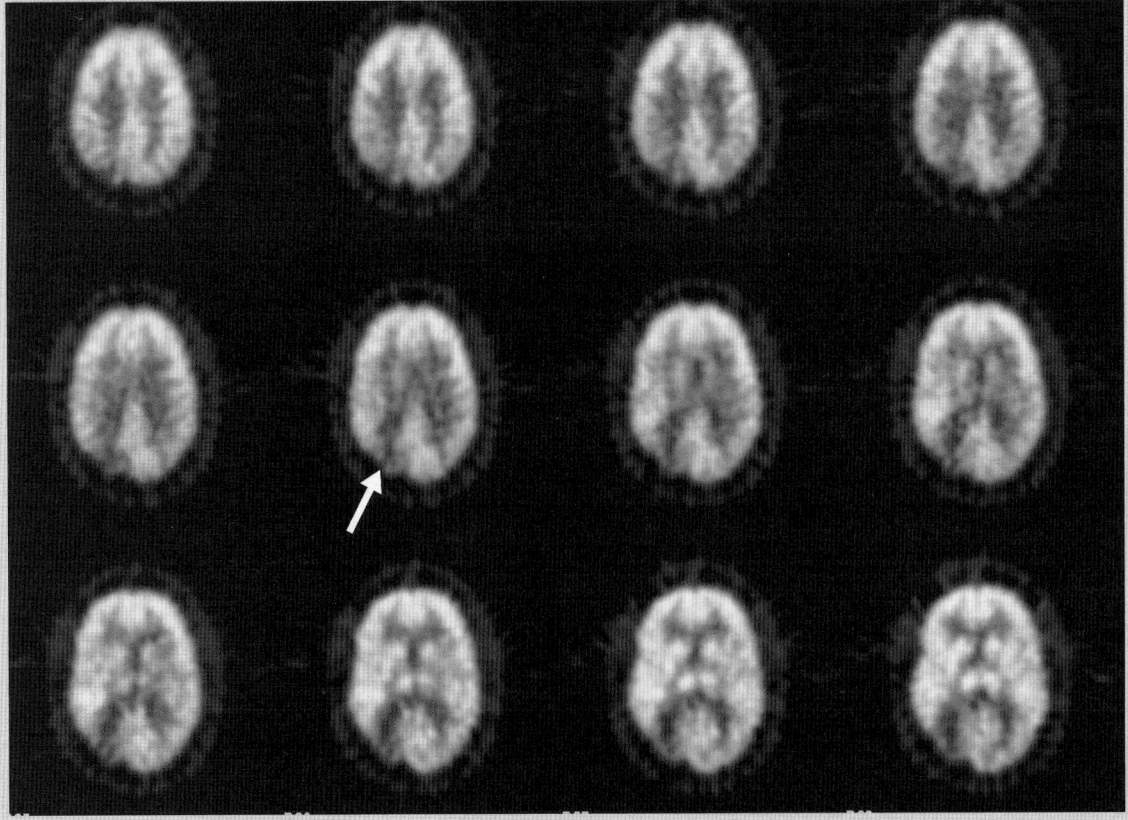

Figure 10C.5

Case history: Clinical case 2

This 7-year-old girl presented with occipital seizures and left lower quadrantinopia. Inter-ictal and ictal EEG (a) show clear localized abnormality over the occipital electrodes (O1, O2 with O2 (right) prominence). MR imaging had been reported as normal. Ictal ^{99m}Tc-HMPAO SPECT (b) was performed and showed hyperperfusion over the right occipital cortex. Repeat review of FLAIR and T2 coronal MR (c) showed a right medial occipital abnormality, suggestive of a localized malformation of cortical development. Case by courtesy of Dr Helen Cross, Epilepsy Unit, Department of Paediatric Neurology, Great Ormond Street Hospital for Children, London. See also Plate 10C.3 for color version of Fig. 10C.6(b).

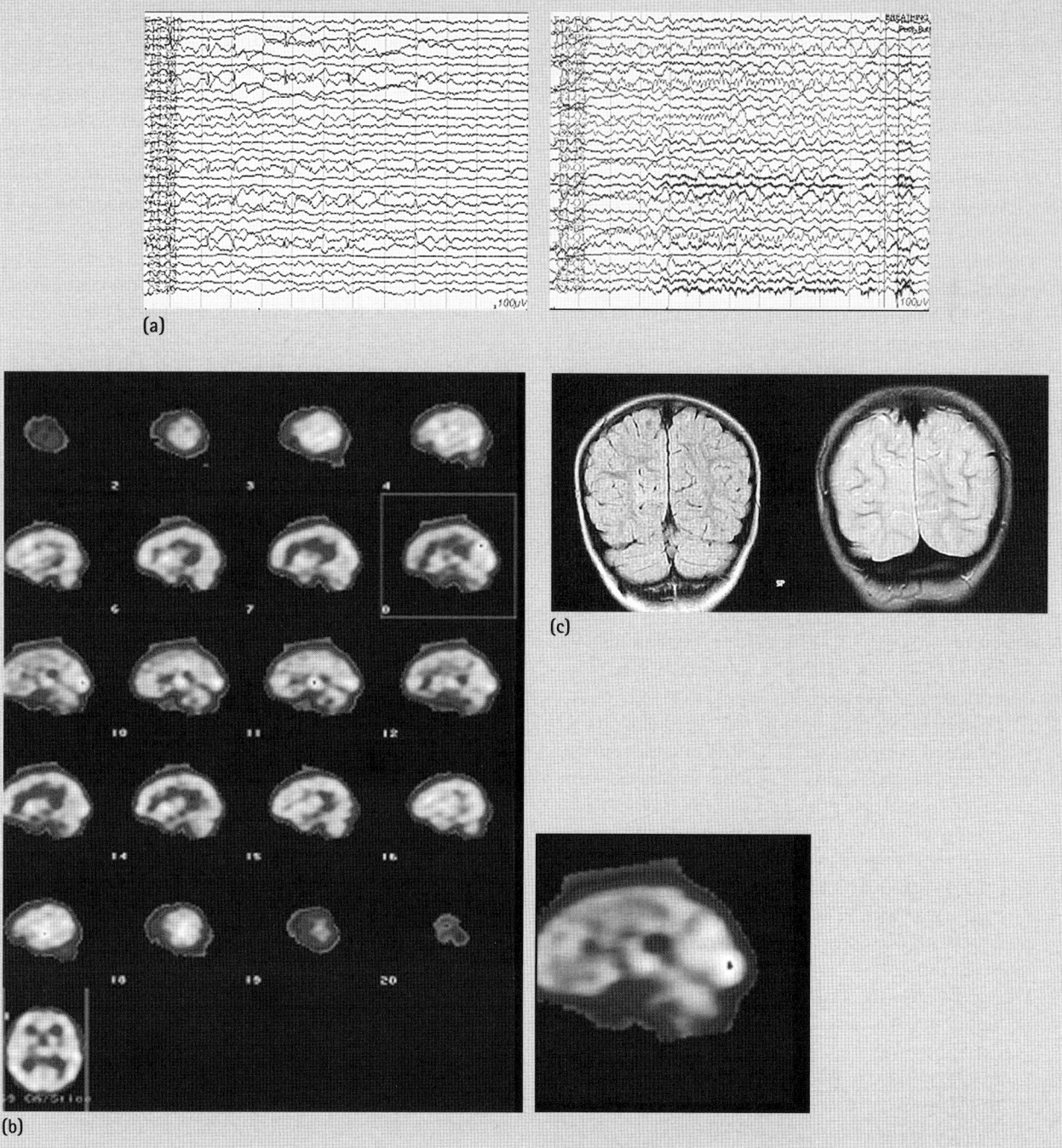

Figure 10C.6

REFERENCES

● Seminal primary article
◆ Key review paper
★ First formal publication of a management guideline

1　Shorvon S. Medical services for epilepsy. In: Richens A, Laidlaw J, Oxley J. (eds.) *A textbook of epilepsy*. 3rd edition. London: Churchill Livingstone, 1988: 611–30.

● 2　Wiebe S, Blume WT, Girvin JP, Eliasziw M. Effectiveness and Efficiency of Surgery for Temporal Lobe Epilepsy Study Group. A randomized, controlled trial of surgery for temporal-lobe epilepsy. *N Engl J Med* 2001; **345**: 311–18.

3　Spencer SS. When should temporal-lobe surgery be treated surgically? *Lancet Neurol* 2002; **1**: 375–82.

4　Crandall P, Rausch R, Engel J. Preoperative indicators for optimal surgical outcome for temporal lobe epilepsy. In: Wieser H, Elgar CE. (eds.) *Presurgical evaluation of epilepsies*. 9th edition. Berlin: Springer, 1987: 325–34.

◆ 5　Duncan JS. Positron emission tomography receptor studies. *Adv Neurol* 1999; **79**: 893–9.

6　Won HJ, Chang KH, Cheon JE, *et al.* Comparison of MR imaging with PET and ictal SPECT in 118 patients with intractable epilepsy. *Am J Neuroradiol* 1999; **20**: 593–9.

★ 7　Neuroimaging Subcommision of the International League Against Epilepsy. Commission on Diagnostic Strategies: recommendations for functional neuroimaging of persons with epilepsy. *Epilepsia* 2000; **41**: 1350–6.

8　Cummings TJ, Chugani DC, Chugani HT. Positron emission tomography in pediatric epilepsy. *Neurosurg Clin N Am* 1995; **6**: 465–72.

9　Engel Jr J, Henry T, Risinger M, Sutherling W, Chugani HT. PET in relation to intracranial electrode evaluations. *Epilepsy Res* 1992; **Suppl 5**: 111–20.

10　Barrington S, Koutroumanidis M, Agathonikou A, *et al.* Clinical value of 'ictal' FDG-PET and the routine use of simultaneous scalp EEG studies in patients with intractable partial epilepsies. *Epilepsia* 1998; **39**: 753–66.

11　Koutroumanidis M, Barrington S, Agathonikou A, *et al.* Interictal regional slow activity in temporal lobe epilepsy correlates with lateral temporal hypometabolism as imaged with FDG-PET. Neurophysiologic and metabolic implications. *J Neurol Neurosurg Psychiat* 1998; **65**: 170–6.

12　Foldvary N, Lee N, Hanson MW, *et al.* Correlation of hippocampal neuronal density and FDG-PET in mesial temporal lobe epilepsy. *Epilepsia* 1999; **40**: 26–9.

13　Koutroumanidis M, Binnie C, Panayiotopoulos C. Positron emission tomography in partial epilepsies: the clinical point of view. *Nucl Med Commun* 1998; **19**: 1123–6.

14　Gaillard WD, Fazilat S, White S, *et al.* Interictal metabolism and blood flow are uncoupled in temporal lobe cortex of patients with complex partial epilepsy. *Neurology* 1995; **45**: 1841–7.

15　Jack CRJ, Mullan BP, Sharbrough FW, *et al.* Intractable nonlesional epilepsy of temporal lobe origin: lateralization by interictal SPECT versus MRI. *Neurology* 1994; **44**: 829–36.

16　Devous MDS, Thisted RA, Morgan GF, *et al.* SPECT brain imaging in epilepsy: a meta-analysis. *J Nucl Med* 1998; **39**: 285–93.

17　Newton MR, Berkovic SF, Austin MC, *et al.* Ictal, postictal and interictal single-photon emission tomography in the lateralization of temporal lobe epilepsy. *Eur J Nucl Med* 1994; **21**: 1067–71.

18　Shen W, Lee BI, Park HM, *et al.* HIPDM-SPECT brain imaging in the presurgical evaluation of patients with intractable seizures. *J Nucl Med* 1990; **31**: 1280–4.

19　Rowe C, Berkovic S, Austin M. Patterns of postictal cerebral blood flow in temporal lobe epilepsy: qualitative and quantitative analysis. *Neurology* 1991; **41**: 1096–103.

20　Avery RA, Spencer SS, Spanaki MV, *et al.* Effect of injection time on postictal SPET perfusion changes in medically refractory epilepsy. *Eur J Nucl Med* 1999; **26**: 830–6.

21　Zubal IG, Spencer SS, Imam K, *et al.* Difference images calculated from ictal and interictal technetium-99m-HMPAO SPECT scans of epilepsy. *J Nucl Med* 1995; **36**: 684–9.

22　Newton MR, Berkovic SF, Austin MC, *et al.* SPECT in the localisation of extratemporal and temporal seizure foci. *J Neurol Neurosurg Psychiat* 1995; **59**: 26–30.

23　Hwang SI, Kim JH, Park SW, *et al.* Comparative analysis of MR imaging, positron emission tomography, and ictal single-photon emission CT in patients with neocortical epilepsy. *Am J Neuroradiol* 2001; **22**: 937–46.

24　Theodore WH. When is positron emission tomography really necessary in epilepsy diagnosis? *Curr Opin Neurol* 2002; **15**: 191–5.

25　Henry TR, Van Heertum R. Positron emission tomography and single photon emission computed tomography in epilepsy care. *Semin Nucl Med* 2003; **33**: 88–104.

26　Spencer S. The relative contributions of MRI, SPECT and PET imaging in epilepsy. *Epilepsia* 1994; **35**(**Suppl 6**): S72–89.

27　Ryvlin P, Bouvard S, Le Bars D, *et al.* Clinical utility of flumazenil-PET versus [^{18}F]fluorodeoxyglucose-PET and MRI in refractory partial epilepsy. A prospective study in 100 patients. *Brain* 1998; **121**(**Part 11**): 2067–81.

28　Manno EM, Sperling MR, Ding X, *et al.* Predictors of outcome after anterior temporal lobectomy: positron emission tomography. *Neurology* 1994; **44**: 2331–6.

29　Swartz BE, Tomiyasu U, Delgado-Escueta A, *et al.* Neuroimaging in temporal lobe epilepsy: test sensitivity and relationships to pathological and postoperative outcome. *Epilepsia* 1992; **33**: 624–34.

30 Theodore WH, Sato S, Kufta C, *et al.* Temporal lobectomy for uncontrolled seizures: the role of positron emission tomography. *Ann Neurol* 1992; **32**: 789–94.

31 Newberg AB, Alavi A, Berlin J, *et al.* Ipsilateral and contralateral thalamic hypometabolism as a predictor of outcome after temporal lobectomy for seizures. *J Nucl Med* 2000; **41**: 1964–8.

32 Blum DE, Ehsan T, Dungan D, *et al.* Bilateral temporal hypometabolism in epilepsy. *Epilepsia* 1998; **39**: 651–9.

33 Koutroumanidis M, Hennessy MJ, Seed PT, *et al.* Significance of interictal bilateral temporal hypometabolism in temporal lobe epilepsy. *Neurology* 2000; **54**: 1811–21.

34 Swartz BW, Khonsari A, Vrown C, *et al.* Improved sensitivity of 18FDG-positron emission tomography scans in frontal and 'frontal plus' epilepsy. *Epilepsia* 1995; **36**: 388–95.

35 Henry TR, Mazziotta JC, Engel JJ, *et al.* Quantifying interictal metabolic activity in human temporal lobe epilepsy. *J Cereb Blood Flow Metab* 1990; **10**: 748–57.

36 Drzezga A, Arnold S, Minoshima S, *et al.* ^{18}F-FDG PET studies in patients with extratemporal and temporal epilepsy: evaluation of an observer-independent analysis. *J Nucl Med* 1999; **40**: 737–46.

37 Savic I, Persson A, Roland P, *et al.* In-vivo demonstration of reduced benzodiazepine receptor binding in human epileptic foci. *Lancet* 1988; **2**: 863–66.

38 Savic I, Thorell JO, Roland P. [11]C]flumazenil positron emission tomography visualizes frontal epileptogenic regions. *Epilepsia* 1995; **36**: 1225–32.

39 Henry TR, Frey KA, Sackellares JC, *et al.* In vivo cerebral metabolism and central benzodiazepine-receptor binding in temporal lobe epilepsy. *Neurology* 1993; **43**: 1998–2006.

40 Arnold S, Berthele A, Drzezga A, *et al.* Reduction of benzodiazepine receptor binding is related to the seizure onset zone in extratemporal focal cortical dysplasia. *Epilepsia* 2000; **41**: 818–24.

41 Nagy F, Chugani DC, Juhasz C, *et al.* Altered in vitro and in vivo flumazenil binding in human epileptogenic neocortex. *J Cereb Blood Flow Metab* 1999; **19**: 939–47.

42 Juhasz C, Chugani DC, Muzik O, *et al.* Relationship of flumazenil and glucose PET abnormalities to neocortical epilepsy surgery outcome. *Neurology* 2001; **56**: 1650–8.

43 Lamusuo S, Pitkanen A, Jutila L, *et al.* [11]C]Flumazenil binding in the medial temporal lobe in patients with temporal lobe epilepsy: correlation with hippocampal MR volumetry, T2 relaxometry, and neuropathology. *Neurology* 2000; **54**: 2252–60.

44 Hammers A, Koepp MJ, Hurlemann R, *et al.* Abnormalities of grey and white matter ^{11}C]flumazenil binding in temporal lobe epilepsy with normal MRI. *Brain* 2002; **125**(**Part 10**): 2257–2271.

45 Cross J. Update on surgery for epilepsy. *Arch Dis Child* 1999; **81**: 356–9.

46 European Federation of Neurological Societies Task Force. Pre-surgical evaluation for epilepsy surgery – European standards. *Eur J Neurol* 2000; **7**: 119–22.

47 Pellock J. Treatment of seizures and epilepsy in children and adolescents. *Neurology* 1998; **51**(**5, Suppl 4**): S8–14.

48 Lee JS, Juhasz C, Kaddurah AK, Chugani HT. Patterns of cerebral glucose metabolism in early and late stages of Rasmussen's syndrome. *J Child Neurol* 2001; **16**: 798–805.

49 English R, Soper N, Shepstone B, *et al.* Five patients with Rasmussen's syndrome investigated by single-photon-emission computed tomography. *Nucl Med Commun* 1989; **10**: 105–14.

50 Chugani HT, Shields WD, Shewmon DA, *et al.* Infantile spasms: I. PET identifies focal cortical dysgenesis in cryptogenic cases for surgical treatment. *Ann Neurol* 1990; **27**: 406–13.

51 Chugani HT, Conti JR. Etiologic classification of infantile spasms in 140 cases: role of positron emission tomography. *J Child Neurol* 1996; **11**: 44–8.

52 Theodore WH, Rose D, Patronas N, *et al.* Cerebral glucose metabolism in the Lennox–Gastaut syndrome. *Ann Neurol* 1987; **21**: 14–21.

53 Ferrie CD, Marsden PK, Maisey MN, Robinson RO. Cortical and subcortical glucose metabolism in childhood epileptic encephalopathies. *J Neurol Neurosurg Psychiat* 1997; **63**: 181–7.

54 Lee JS, Asano E, Muzik O, *et al.* Sturge–Weber syndrome: correlation between clinical course and FDG PET findings. *Neurology* 2001; **57**: 189–95.

55 Rintahaka PJ, Chugani HT, Messa C, Phelps ME. Hemimegalencephaly: evaluation with positron emission tomography. *Ped Neurol* 1993; **9**: 21–8.

56 Akanuma N, Koutroumanidis M, Adachi N, *et al.* Presurgical assessment of memory-related brain structures: the Wada test and functional neuroimaging. *Seizure* 2003; **12**: 346–58.

Neuro-oncology

RONALD B. WORKMAN, TERENCE Z. WONG, WEN YOUNG, AND R. EDWARD COLEMAN

EPIDEMIOLOGY

Advances in medicine have resulted in improved prevention, detection, and treatment for cancer. The number of individuals living with cancer in the United States is expected to double from approximately 1.3 million presently to roughly 2.6 million over the next 50 years.[1] Not all malignancies, however, have benefited equally from these advances. In 2004, approximately 18 400 new cases of central nervous system (CNS) malignancy were diagnosed in the United States, with an estimated 12 690 deaths attributable to these neoplasms.[2] Although the incidence of CNS malignancies is low relative to other cancers, the mortality remains high with 2% of the overall cancer mortality due to primary brain tumors. Furthermore, the overall 5-year survival has only improved from 22% in the mid 1970s to 32% in the mid 1990s.[3] In the EUROCARE-3 project, which pooled cancer data from 20 European nations, 27 587 brain tumor cases were included from 1990 to 1994, with an average 5-year relative survival rate of less than 20%.[4]

Brain tumors can occur in the young and old, but the average age at diagnosis for all primary brain tumors is approximately 54 years. In adults, the most common primary brain tumors are gliomas and meningiomas, with gliomas constituting about half of all brain tumors and having a slight male predisposition. Lower-grade gliomas, such as oligodendrogliomas, tend to occur in younger patients, and higher grade gliomas, such as glioblastoma multiforme (GBM), tend to occur in older individuals. Prognosis is highly correlated with patient age and tumor grade, and the 2-year survival rates for those with GBM range from 30% for younger patients (i.e. those less than 20 years) to only 2% for those older than 65 years. Meningiomas

represent about 20% of all brain tumors; these extra-axial tumors occur more frequently in females and the elderly. Prognosis is generally good for these tumors, with an 81% overall 5-year survival, although this decreases to 55% overall 5-year survival if the tumors have undergone malignant degeneration.[3] Primary CNS lymphomas constitute about 4% of primary brain tumors and tend to occur in immunocompromised patients.

In pediatric patients, CNS tumors comprise approximately 16% of all malignancies, and are the most frequently occurring solid tumors. Roughly half of these tumors are astrocytomas, with medulloblastoma, primitive neuroectodermal tumors (PNET), other gliomas, and ependymomas following in frequency. Younger patients typically have a better prognosis than older patients, and the overall 5-year survival for children with brain tumors is 67%. Pediatric brain tumors are notoriously challenging to treat, with local recurrence being a long-term problem. Pediatric patients with brain tumors typically have a high morbidity, and the significant relapse rate confers a high late mortality.[5]

The etiology of brain tumors has both genetic and environmental components. Research has shown that overexpression of the gene coding for platelet-derived growth factor (PDGF), which results in increased proliferation and migration of glioma cells, coupled with a defect in the tumor suppressing *p53* gene may constitute a cooperative tumorigenic effect.[6] There are also hereditary syndromes such as tuberous sclerosis and neurofibromatosis that carry a high incidence of brain tumors. Despite these observations, only about 2–10% of patients with brain tumors have an identified genetic predisposition, and only approximately 5% of gliomas may be familial.[3] Previous exposure to radiation therapy has been shown to be a strong risk factor in the subsequent development of primary brain tumors. Some studies have also pointed to other environmental factors such as heavy metal and petrochemical exposure as presenting a possible increased risk.[7] Immune suppression, either due to HIV or immunosuppressive medication, has also been shown to confer an increased risk in the development of primary CNS lymphoma.[3] Recent years have seen a dramatic increase in the number of individuals using cellular phones but no clear link has been made between exposure to the electromagnetic radiation from cellular phone use and the development of primary brain tumors. With the exception of primary CNS lymphoma, the incidence of brain tumors has remained relatively stable over the time that cellular phones have been in use.[8]

HISTOPATHOLOGIC CLASSIFICATION

There is a wide variety of CNS tumors, and their classification is complex. The World Health Organization (WHO) organizes primary brain tumors according to their cell of origin. The most common class of brain tumors are those of neuroepithelial lineage, and these include the astrocytomas, oligodendrogliomas, ependymomas, and mixed gliomas. Less common are tumors of the choroid plexus, pineal parenchymal tumors, embryonal tumors, and primitive neuroectodermal tumors. Other CNS tumors include pituitary adenomas, craniopharyngiomas, primary CNS lymphomas, and extra-axial tumors such as meningiomas.[9] Tumor grade is typically assigned based on an assessment of conventional histological features such as the degree of cellular atypia, mitotic activity, necrosis, endothelial proliferation, and invasion. Grading of these tumors is also being based on an analysis of gene expression profiles which has been shown to parallel morphology-based assessments. This molecular-based classification using gene expression profiling has also been correlated with survival.[10]

The WHO has developed a tumor grading scheme ranging from I to IV, with grades I and II representing low-grade neoplasms, and grades III and IV assigned to high-grade lesions. Low-grade tumors include pilocytic astrocytomas (I) and well-differentiated astrocytomas and oligodendrogliomas (II). High-grade tumors include anaplastic astrocytomas and anaplastic oligodendrogliomas (III). The most common primary brain cancer of adults, GBM, is also the most aggressive, has the highest grade (IV), and has the worst prognosis. The high-grade gliomas (III and IV) can be further described as either primary or secondary malignant astrocytomas.[11] Primary malignant astrocytomas occur in older patients with no history of prior low-grade tumor. Secondary malignant astrocytomas arise from further malignant degeneration of pre-existing low-grade gliomas and tend to occur in younger patients. The occurrence of secondary malignant astrocytomas in younger patients is the main reason behind the previously mentioned prolonged morbidity and high late mortality often seen in children.

Brain tumors are microscopically heterogeneous, and the more dedifferentiated cell populations within a tumor tend to grow more aggressively than other, more well-differentiated cells. This heterogeneity results in a tumor which has varying grades within it, and ultimately accounts for the disease progression seen when low-grade tumors become high grade after a period of time. Primary and secondary malignant astrocytomas are considered distinct entities, and the mechanisms behind their malignant degeneration are being actively investigated. These mechanisms are known, in part, to be related to over-expression of growth regulating oncogenes, such as *EGFR* and *PDGFR* (typically seen in primary glioblastomas), coupled with eventual loss of tumor suppression by inactivation of tumor suppressor genes such as *p53* and *INK4a-ARF* (typically seen in secondary glioblastomas).[6,12,13]

IMAGING OF BRAIN TUMORS

Contrast-enhanced computed tomography (CT) and especially magnetic resonance imaging (MRI) are the mainstays of brain tumor imaging. MRI provides superb anatomic detail by allowing exceptional spatial resolution and delineation of gray and white matter structures. The most sensitive imaging modality for the detection of brain tumors can be found with standard T1- and T2-weighted magnetic resonance images. The administration of intravenous contrast assesses the integrity of the blood–brain barrier and further raises the sensitivity of MRI because many tumors, particularly those which are higher grade, show a corresponding increase in contrast enhancement. Lower-grade tumors may have low or minimal contrast enhancement, but typically do show increased signal on T2-weighted images. MRI frequently provides additional clinically important information such as the presence and/or degree of mass effect, hemorrhage, edema, and necrosis which often accompany brain tumors.[14]

MRI and CT provide primarily anatomic information. The tumor margins of high-grade gliomas are often not well defined due to their infiltrative nature. The degree of contrast enhancement can also provide information about the grade of tumor but this is limited. Advanced MRI techniques such as spectroscopy and rapid dynamic contrast-enhanced imaging show promise in providing additional functional information about tumor grade and vascularity, and these techniques will likely become more widely available in the future. Because brain tumors are heterogeneous and often grow in an infiltrative manner, accurate information regarding tumor grade is essential. Limitations in MRI may arise in the post-therapeutic setting in which patients treated with resection followed by radiotherapy show enhancement that may be due to post-therapy changes (i.e. radionecrosis) or residual tumor.[15] To address these limitations, much work has been done with single photon emission computed tomography (SPECT) and positron emission tomography (PET) as a way to gain important information regarding tumor grade.

SPECT IMAGING OF BRAIN TUMORS

While PET is considered the state-of-the-art for brain tumor imaging, SPECT has a few advantages. It is more widely available, is less expensive than PET, and a wider range of radiopharmaceuticals is available. Image resolution is lower, however, and accurate quantification is more difficult. In selected cases, SPECT imaging can provide similar or equivalent information as PET at lower cost.

Nuclear medicine efforts to address the limitations of anatomic imaging of brain tumors include the use of ^{201}Tl SPECT. Most brain imaging protocols recommend doses in the 75–150 MBq (2–4 mCi) range with early imaging possible at 10–15 min post-injection. Increased uptake of ^{201}Tl in brain tumors was demonstrated in the mid 1980s by Kaplan et al., and was felt to be related to a combination of perturbation of the blood–brain barrier, increased blood flow, and likely increased expression of the sodium/potassium ATPase pump.[16] In 1989, Black et al. described a quantitative technique to predict whether gliomas were high or low grade. Regions of interest were drawn over tumor and over normal, homologous contralateral tissue and an index was calculated based on the ratio of tumor uptake to normal (i.e. non-tumor) uptake. These values were then compared to histology following biopsy. Using an index threshold of 1.5, the investigators were able to predict high- or low-grade tumor with 89% accuracy.[17] In addition to confirming a strong positive correlation with histopathologic grade, more recent research by Higa et al. has actually shown ^{201}Tl uptake in tumors to be a stronger predictor of outcome than grade alone.[18]

In patients who have had prior radiation therapy, differentiation between radionecrosis and residual tumor is often very difficult. Studies have demonstrated the efficacy of differentiating high-grade gliomas from radionecrosis with ^{201}Tl; a shortcoming of ^{201}Tl imaging is that it may not be reliable in differentiating lower-grade gliomas from benign post-radiation change.[19–21] However, there is evidence that a dual-tracer approach combining ^{201}Tl imaging with a brain perfusion agent, such as ^{99m}Tc-hexamethylpropylene amine oxime (^{99m}Tc-HMPAO) can potentially improve this discrimination.[22,23]

SPECT imaging of brain tumors has also been performed using ^{99m}Tc-sestamibi (^{99m}Tc-MIBI). Like ^{201}Tl, ^{99m}Tc-MIBI has been utilized primarily as a myocardial perfusion agent. Technetium-99m has better imaging properties than ^{201}Tl, and anywhere from 370 to 1110 MBq (10–30 mCi) of ^{99m}Tc-MIBI can be injected intravenously. Its mechanism of uptake in brain tumors relies on increased flow, loss of integrity of the blood–brain barrier, and is also influenced by mitochondrial density. In 1993, O'Tuama

et al. compared ^{201}Tl and ^{99m}Tc-MIBI in 19 children with brain tumors and found a similar range of tumor avidity. This study reported similar sensitivity and specificity for ^{201}Tl and ^{99m}Tc-MIBI (67% sensitivity for both, and 91% specificity for ^{201}Tl and 100% specificity for ^{99m}Tc-MIBI). While lesion boundaries were more sharply defined with ^{99m}Tc-MIBI, problematic physiologic uptake was present in the choroid plexus which complicated evaluation of paraventricular tumors.[24]

Somatostatin-receptor imaging (SRI) has also been used to evaluate intracranial tumors.[25–28] Meningiomas express somatostatin receptors and can be imaged with radiolabeled somatostatin analogs such as ^{111}In-pentetreotide.[25] SRI can be especially helpful when MRI is inconclusive (e.g. differentiating postoperative scar versus recurrent meningioma) or when attempting to narrow the differential diagnosis of brain tumors, particularly at the skull base.[26,27] Astrocytomas can also been seen with SRI. Specifically, grade I and II astrocytomas frequently express somatostatin receptors, whereas high-grade astrocytomas do not. However, radiolabeled somatostatin analogs do not reach these tumors if the blood–brain barrier is intact; therefore, the many low-grade astrocytomas which do not disturb the blood–brain barrier yet express somatostatin receptors will not be seen with ^{111}In-pentetreotide imaging.[28] These significant limitations prevent SRI from being employed routinely in the evaluation of brain tumors.

FDG PET IMAGING OF BRAIN TUMORS

Some of the first research using positron emitting isotopes to visualize brain tumors began as early as the 1950s with Wrenn et al.[29] and Brownell and Sweet.[30] Currently, the most widely available PET radiotracer for brain and body imaging is 2-[^{18}F]fluoro-2-deoxy-D-glucose (^{18}F-FDG). Significant support for the clinical application of PET in brain tumor evaluation gained momentum in the 1980s, after the American College of Nuclear Physicians and the Society of Nuclear Medicine convened the Task Force on Clinical PET in 1987. This support was based primarily on the pioneering work of Di Chiro on the value of FDG PET for evaluation of brain tumors, at the National Institutes of Health.[31] Shortly thereafter, additional recommendations regarding the clinical application of PET in evaluating brain tumors came from the National Cancer Institute in 1988, and from the American Academy of Neurology later in 1991.[32,33] Clinical applications for FDG PET of the brain include work-up of dementia, surgical treatment planning for intractable seizure disorders, and evaluation of primary brain tumors.

FDG is a glucose analog and, like glucose, is actively transported into metabolically active cells. Once phosphorylated by hexokinase in the intracellular space, however, FDG-6-phosphate is essentially trapped within cells because it is not metabolized further in the glycolytic pathway. The disproportionately higher metabolic rate of glucose in high-grade malignant cells combined with FDG's resemblance to glucose is the basis behind tumor imaging with FDG PET. However, normal gray matter structures in the brain also have high glucose metabolism, and the major challenge for evaluating brain tumors by FDG PET is distinguishing this high background activity from high-grade tumor. Our institution (Duke University Medical Center in Durham, North Carolina) has a multidisciplinary Brain Tumor Center which attracts many brain tumor patients from all over the world. As a referral center, most of the patients come to DUMC already with a diagnosis to explore various therapeutic options. In 2003, the Duke PET Facility conducted 431 FDG PET studies for brain tumor evaluation. The majority of these studies were performed to follow the effectiveness of surgical resection, radiotherapy, and/or chemotherapy.

The main value of FDG PET in evaluating brain tumors is the correlation between FDG uptake and tumor grade. The degree of FDG accumulation in brain tumors also has prognostic significance. In 1983, work by Patronas *et al.* showed that FDG uptake is a more accurate representation of tumor grade than the degree of contrast enhancement by CT.[34] As previously mentioned, physiologic background FDG activity is high in gray matter and low in white matter. When evaluating the metabolic activity of a brain tumor, comparison of the FDG uptake within the tumor to contralateral homologous (and presumably more normal) brain allows a relatively simple and rapid qualitative assessment of grade. By this method, low-grade tumors have FDG accumulation similar to or less than normal white matter, and high-grade tumors have activity which is similar to or greater than normal gray matter.[14] Tumors may be difficult to locate on brain PET studies alone, particularly if they are small or adjacent to cortical structures. Low-grade tumors can be indistinguishable from adjacent white matter, and high-grade tumors can similarly blend in with adjacent normal cortex. Therefore, accurate localization of

the tumor is essential to make an accurate assessment of tumor grade. Our approach is to co-register the FDG PET images with anatomic imaging, usually MRI, for anatomic localization of the brain tumor. This image registration is performed routinely for all of our brain tumor patients, using software developed at our institution. This is discussed in more detail at the end of this chapter.

The FDG uptake in low- and high-grade tumors relative to normal white and gray matter has also been studied quantitatively. In 1995, Delbeke *et al.* studied 58 patients with brain tumors; 32 had biopsy proven high-grade disease (WHO III and IV), and 26 had biopsy proven low-grade tumor (WHO I and II). Regions of interest were used to assign tumor-to-white matter (T/WM) and tumor-to-gray matter (T/GM) ratios in an effort to determine an appropriate threshold value to distinguish high from low grade. They found that T/WM ratios greater than 1.5 and T/GM ratios greater than 0.6 were indicative of high-grade disease with a sensitivity of 94% and a specificity of 77%.[35] These findings support the qualitative approach described above in which FDG uptake in low-grade tumors resembles white matter and uptake in high-grade tumors resembles gray matter. An example of a low-grade tumor is shown in Fig. 10D.1. Note that the poorly enhancing abnormality in the left parietal lobe has low FDG activity, similar to that of normal white matter. Biopsy confirmed that this was a well-differentiated glioma.

Grading brain tumors by FDG PET can be especially important, because glial tumors have notoriously heterogeneous pathology. This was strikingly evident when Paulus and Peiffer studied the histologic features of 1000 samples from 50 brain tumors (20 samples per tumor to simulate multiple biopsies). They observed that different grades were detected in 82% of tumors, and a majority (62%) of the gliomas contained both low and high grade features (WHO grades II, III, and IV).[36] This heterogeneity helps to explain the problem of sampling error and under-staging often encountered in managing brain tumors. The emergence of high-grade disease within a previously low-grade lesion

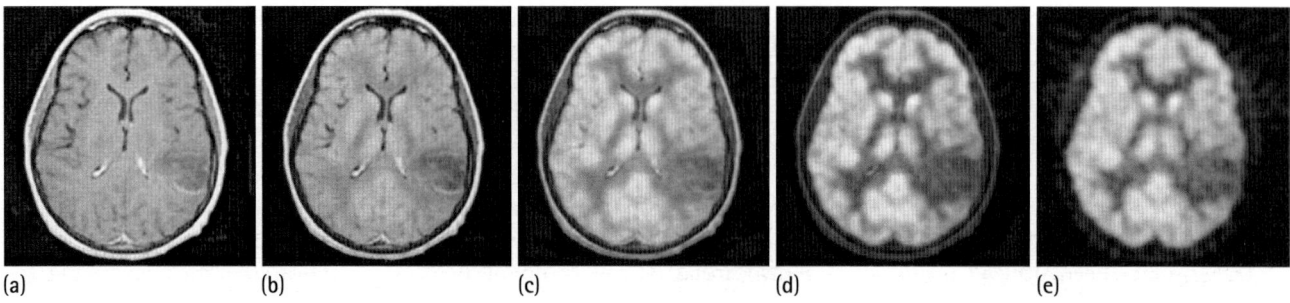

(a)   (b)   (c)   (d)   (e)

Figure 10D.1 *Low-grade tumor. Co-registered axial magnetic resonance (MR) and fluorodeoxyglucose (FDG) positron emission tomography (PET) images from a 35-year-old female patient who initially presented with a seizure. (a) 100% MRI, (b) 75% MRI, 25% PET, (c) 50% MRI, 50% PET, (d) 25% MRI, 25% PET, and (e) 100% PET. Tumor in the left parietal lobe demonstrates minimal contrast enhancement on T1W MRI (a). On FDG PET (e), the activity within the MRI-defined mass is similar to white matter, compatible with low-grade tumor. Biopsy revealed a well-differentiated glioma (WHO grade II).*

cannot be detected by MRI, but with FDG PET more hypermetabolic areas are more likely to have the highest grade and can be specifically targeted for stereotactic biopsy thereby improving the chances of accurately grading the tumor.[37–40]

The degree of FDG uptake in brain tumors also carries prognostic significance. One study of 29 patients with treated and untreated primary brain tumors found that patients with hypermetabolic tumors had a substantially worse prognosis than those with hypometabolic tumors.[41] Another study of 45 patients with high-grade tumors, showed that those with high metabolic activity had a mean survival of 5 months compared to a mean survival of 19 months for those with less metabolically active tumors.[42] Patients with low-grade tumors who subsequently develop hypermetabolic foci also have a poorer prognosis.[43,44] Figure 10D.2 shows FDG PET and MRI scans from the same patient as in Fig. 10D.1. These were taken 3 years later and demonstrate new contrast enhancement in the tumor region. There is corresponding hypermetabolic FDG activity, similar to gray matter, compatible with high-grade tumor (biopsy confirmed anaplastic astrocytoma). This is an example of high-grade transformation of an initially low-grade tumor. Note the heterogeneous nature of the contrast enhancement and FDG accumulation, which reflects the heterogeneous tumor grades within the mass.

For accurate interpretation of findings in FDG PET and MRI scans, the PET images must be correlated with areas of enhancement on MRI to differentiate post-therapy changes from residual tumor which may be indistinguishable by MRI alone. Post-surgical changes do not result in hypermetabolism, although, typically, there is a rim of enhancement on the MRI along the surgical resection cavity.[45] Hypermetabolic activity within the resection bed following surgery almost always represents residual tumor.

In patients who receive high-dose radiotherapy, the resulting radionecrosis is usually hypometabolic; however, hypermetabolism can occasionally be observed which can be difficult to distinguish from recurrent tumor. This post-therapy hypermetabolism is thought to be due to inflammatory changes brought on by accumulation of metabolically active macrophages at therapy sites. Similar post-therapy uptake is often also seen in other areas such as the thorax which can be subject to radiation-induced changes following treatment for pulmonary malignancies. While the typical post-radiotherapy hypermetabolism is uniform and intermediate (between white and gray matter) in activity, there can occasionally be nodular characteristics and/or hypermetabolism which approaches, or even exceeds, gray matter activity. In this event, radionecrosis cannot be differentiated from high-grade tumor recurrence. In 1997, Barker et al. looked at 55 patients with high-grade tumors who underwent surgery and radiation therapy and in whom recurrence was suspected because of enlarging areas of enhancement on MRI. Those who had FDG uptake equal to or exceeding gray matter had a significantly poorer prognosis than those without corresponding hypermetabolism.[46] In 2001, Chao et al. looked at 47 patients with primary and metastatic brain tumors who underwent stereotactic biopsy. The results revealed a 75% sensitivity and 81% specificity for detecting recurrent tumor as opposed to radionecrosis.[47] Seizures, either clinical or subclinical, during the uptake phase can result in a false positive FDG PET brain study.[48] Patients with documented or suspected seizure disorders can be scanned with EEG monitoring to minimize the impact on specificity. An example of a patient with seizure activity is illustrated in Fig. 10D.3. Focal, intense hypermetabolic activity is noted adjacent to low-grade tumor in the medial right temporal lobe, but note that there is no corresponding contrast enhancement on the co-registered MR image. Non-enhancing high-grade tumor could have a similar appearance.

At our institution, we are investigating high-dose brachytherapy with ^{131}I-labeled monoclonal antibodies directed against the glycoprotein tenascin expressed by gliomas. Patients receiving this treatment have undergone resection and placement of an indwelling reservoir which allows controlled access to the resection cavity.[49] The beta emission from the ^{131}I results in a very high local radiation dose delivered to the tumor cavity. The FDG PET images from patients who have had brachytherapy reveal a uniform

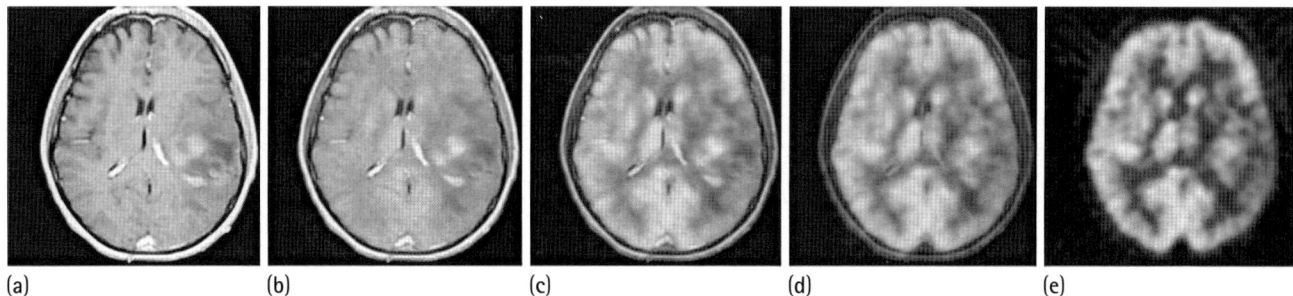

(a) (b) (c) (d) (e)

Figure 10D.2 *High-grade tumor. Same patient as in Fig. 10D.1 3 years later. New contrast enhancement has developed on MRI. (a) 100% MRI, (b) 75% MRI, 25% PET, (c) 50% MRI, 50% PET, (d) 25% MRI, 25% PET, and (e) 100% PET. FDG PET images demonstrate new corresponding hypermetabolic activity similar to that of gray matter, consistent with high-grade tumor. Biopsy was positive for anaplastic astrocytoma (WHO grade III). This progression typifies malignant degeneration of an initially low-grade tumor. (Abbreviations as in the legend to Fig. 10D.1.)*

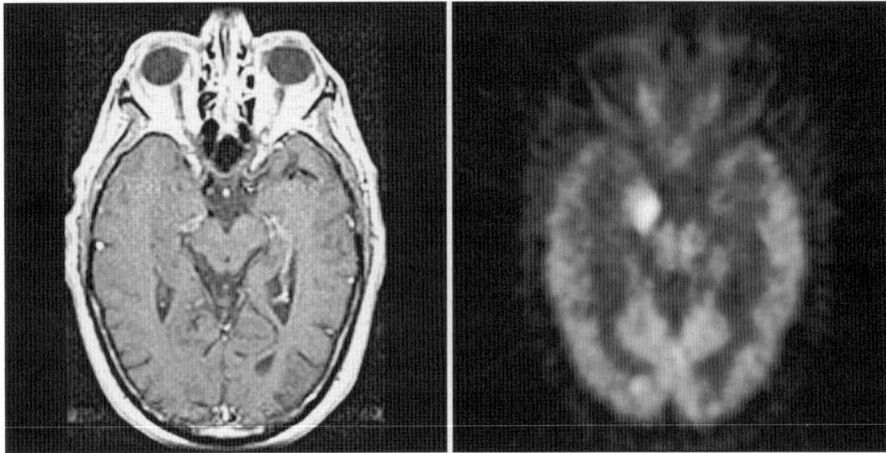

Figure 10D.3 *Seizure focus in a patient with low-grade tumor. Intense hypermetabolic focus (greater than normal gray matter in intensity) in the medial right temporal lobe without corresponding contrast enhancement on co-registered MRI. Non-enhancing high-grade tumor could have a similar appearance.*

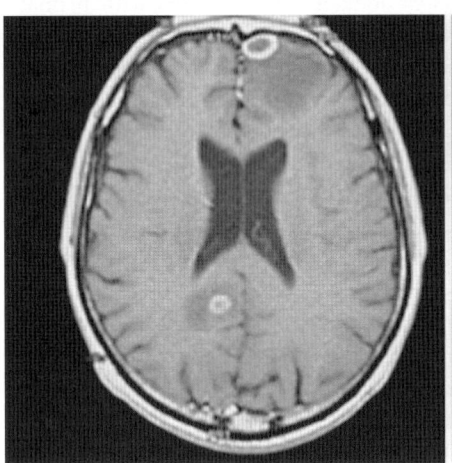
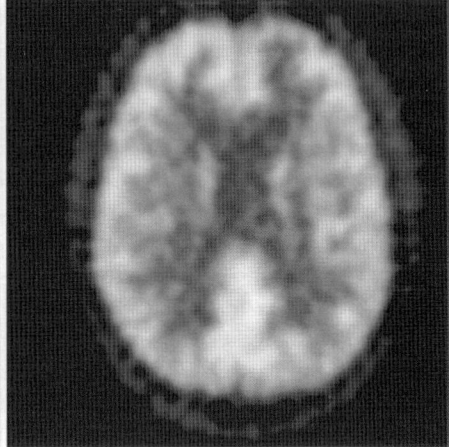

Figure 10D.4 *Metastases in a patient with lung cancer. Multiple ring enhancing lesions on MRI are obscured by adjacent gray matter on the co-registered FDG PET study. (Reprinted from Wong and Coleman[69] with permission from Springer-Verlag.)*

rim of intermediate level hypermetabolism along the resection margin. The development of hypermetabolic nodularity along this rim suggests recurrence.[50] Similar interpretive considerations can be made in patients following other forms of high-dose radiation therapy, such as stereotactic radiosurgery or brachytherapy.

The majority of the data with FDG PET and brain tumors involves the astrocytic tumors, but the correlation between FDG uptake and malignancy generally applies to other CNS tumors as well. Although usually benign, meningiomas can become aggressive and recur, and a positive correlation has been shown between glucose metabolism and aggressive behavior in these tumors.[51] CNS lymphomas are typically highly FDG avid, and FDG PET can accurately differentiate patients with CNS lymphoma from infectious etiologies like toxoplasmosis, which do not have avid FDG uptake.[52] Juvenile pilocytic astrocytomas are low-grade tumors which may have nodular enhancing components on MRI. However, because of their metabolically active fenestrated epithelial cells, they may demonstrate hypermetabolism which simulates high-grade tumor. Nonetheless, these tumors have low-grade behavior with a favorable prognosis.[53]

FDG PET is not as sensitive as MRI or contrast-enhanced CT imaging for detecting intracranial metastases. This is due to a number of factors, including the high normal gray matter activity, the propensity for metastases to occur at the gray–white junction, and the variable degree of FDG metabolism within the metastatic lesions. Brain metastases with hypermetabolic activity exceeding that of normal gray matter may be detected on FDG, but frequently the activity is iso-metabolic to gray matter. A lung cancer patient with intracranial metastases clearly evident on MRI is shown in Fig. 10D.4. These lesions are not apparent on the corresponding co-registered FDG PET image.

OTHER RADIOTRACERS FOR POSITRON EMISSION TOMOGRAPHY

FDG is currently the most commonly used radiopharmaceutical for brain PET imaging. A major reason is that FDG is generally used for PET body imaging and is widely available. The 2-h half-life of ^{18}F-based tracers makes same-day

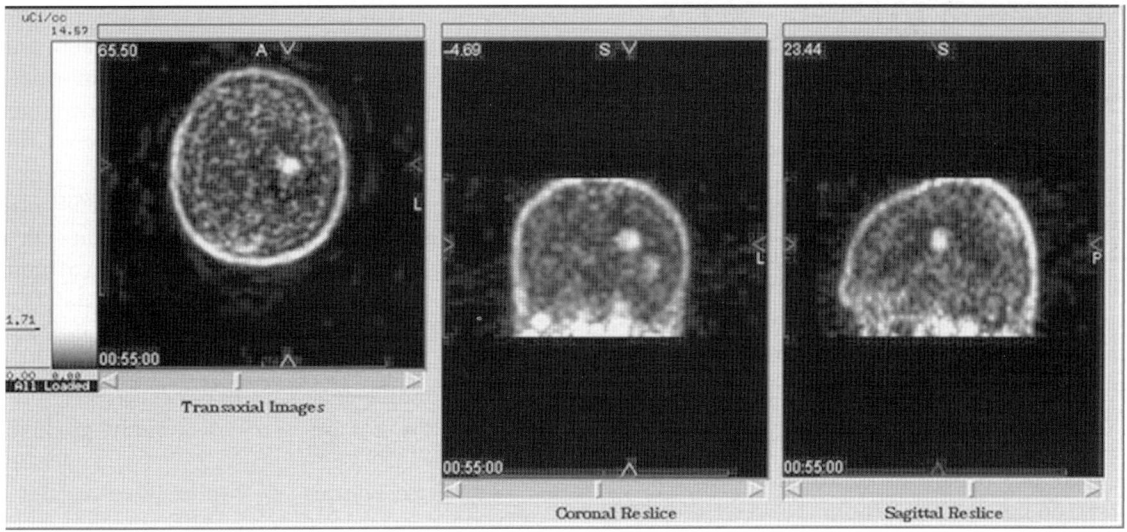

Figure 10D.5 *[^{18}F]fluorothymidine (FLT) PET images in a patient with glioblastoma multiforme. Unlike FDG, thymidine-, methionine-, and choline-based radiotracers do not have high background cortical activity, resulting in a high target-to-background ratio for brain tumors.*

shipping possible and facilitates commercial availability. As mentioned above, FDG PET is useful for indicating tumor grade. One disadvantage is that low-grade tumor (i.e. associated with little or no FDG accumulation) cannot be distinguished from other etiologies having low glucose metabolism, such as infection, infarction or radionecrosis.

Radiolabeled amino acid PET imaging using ^{11}C has been used clinically primarily with ^{11}C-methionine (MET) and ^{11}C-tyrosine.[54] A major advantage over FDG PET imaging is the low background amino acid uptake in the cerebral cortex; MET in particular has 1.2 to 3.5 times greater uptake in tumor than in normal brain. MET PET is better than FDG PET in delineating tumor margins, and in differentiating between tumor and radionecrosis because amino acid uptake is less influenced by inflammation.[54,55] In 1998, Sasaki *et al.* showed that MET PET is more sensitive than ^{201}Tl SPECT or FDG PET in detecting low-grade astrocytomas, and is able to reliably distinguish between low- and high-grade tumors.[56] Chung *et al.* recently looked at MET PET in the evaluation of brain lesions with low-level FDG uptake and found 89% sensitivity in detecting low-grade tumors, with 100% specificity in identifying benign processes.[57] MET PET may have a role in distinguishing low-grade tumors from entities in which FDG PET is inconclusive such as inflammation from radionecrosis, infection or benign tumors. However, one of the major limitations to the use of ^{11}C in clinical practice is its very short half-life (20 min) which makes it necessary for a cyclotron to be on site.

PET imaging using the positron emitter [15]O has been used to study cerebral blood volume (inhaled C[15]O), blood flow (H$_2$[15]O), and oxygen utilization (O[15]O).[58,59] Animal studies conducted by Raichle *et al.*, in 1983, found excellent correlation between cerebral blood flow measured by PET and true cerebral blood flow.[60] In 1994, Mineura *et al.* showed that patients with a higher value of regional cerebral blood flow, blood volume or metabolic rates of oxygen consumption had significantly longer survival times than those with lower values.[61] Furthermore, because cerebral perfusion to a particular area is related to cortical activation, PET studies using H$_2$[15]O can be obtained while the patient is performing various purposeful tasks thereby helping to localize eloquent cortical regions to be avoided during surgery.

[18]F-fluorocholine (^{18}F-FCH) and ^{11}C-choline are markers of membrane metabolism, and have also been used to image brain tumors, and the initial results are promising. Like MET, the low accumulation of these tracers in normal brain provides better tumor-to-normal brain ratios than available with FDG. A major advantage that ^{18}F-labeled compounds have over ^{11}C radiotracers is the longer half-life, which allows practical distribution to PET facilities which do not have on-site cyclotron facilities. Recently, ^{18}F-fluorothymidine (^{18}F-FLT) has been developed, which is a similar marker of cell proliferation.[62] An FLT PET scan in a patient with glioblastoma is shown in Fig. 10D.5. Radiolabeled thymidine, choline, and methionine compounds have relatively high radiotracer accumulation within tumor, and relatively low background activity in the surrounding normal brain. Co-registering these images with anatomic imaging can be challenging, and combined PET/CT imaging will likely play an important role for anatomic correlation; either the PET scans can be obtained in conjunction with contrast-enhanced CT, or the CT images can be used as a template for accurate co-registration with MR images.

IMAGING PROTOCOL FOR BRAIN FDG PET

Patients scheduled to undergo an FDG PET brain study are asked to avoid any caloric intake for at least 4 h prior to scanning, and we routinely measure blood glucose just prior to FDG injection. Frequently, patients with brain tumors are on corticosteroids, which can result in insulin resistance and hyperglycemia. Hyperglycemia leads to competitive inhibition of FDG uptake and can result in decreased differentiation between gray and white matter on the PET images. However, it has been shown that steroids do not significantly affect metabolism within brain tumors.[63] For adults, we inject 370 MBq (10 mCi) of FDG intravenously and instruct the patient to rest quietly for 30 to 40 min during the uptake phase. Patients are told to keep their eyes open, and we do not use ear occlusion. However, the uptake phase takes place in an environment where auditory and visual stimuli are minimized to avoid extraneous cortical activation. At our institution, brain imaging is performed on an Advance PET scanner (GE Medical Systems, Milwaukee, Wisconsin). An 8-min emission acquisition is obtained with three-dimensional mode with one table position, and the data are reconstructed using filtered back-projection. Attenuation correction is calculated rather than measured which eliminates the need for a separate transmission scan. By using three-dimensional acquisition and calculated attenuation correction, the scan time is minimized. Not only does this improve throughput, but it also reduces motion-induced artifacts. Often, pediatric patients or patients with altered mental status who may have difficulty obeying commands may require even shorter scan times, which can be accomplished with dynamic imaging. Once obtained, the resulting PET images have an axial slice thickness of 4.25 mm with a 25.6-cm field-of-view depicted in a 128×128 pixel matrix.

IMAGE REGISTRATION

In 1993, while investigating visceral tumors, Wahl et al. described the fusion of FDG PET images with CT or MRI and coined the resulting image an 'anatometabolic' fusion image.[64] This technique allows increased confidence in the interpretation of whole-body PET/CT images because the two contemporaneously acquired images from different modalities complement one another and can be fused. This technique is fast becoming the standard for whole-body PET imaging. Combining anatomic with functional imaging is even more crucial, if not essential, for evaluating brain tumors with FDG PET. The general paradigm for interpretation is (1) co-register the FDG PET images with MRI, (2) utilize MRI to accurately define the abnormality, and (3) interrogate the abnormal region on the co-registered PET image to determine whether low- or high-grade FDG activity is present. There are scenarios where formal image registration may not be necessary, such as when the tumors have high-grade activity which exceeds that of gray matter, or when the tumors are located well within white matter.[14] Both of these scenarios may avoid confusing tumor activity with physiologic gray matter activity. However, the absence of hypermetabolic abnormalities on PET alone does not exclude high-grade tumor, which is frequently obscured by adjacent gray matter. Therefore, correlation with anatomic imaging is essential for FDG PET evaluation of brain tumors. Side-by-side comparison of axial MRI and PET images can be done, but small lesions identified on MRI are difficult to localize on PET because the two scans are usually obtained at different angles. In our experience, formal image co-registration is necessary for accurate grading of brain tumors by FDG PET.

For these reasons, we routinely co-register all brain FDG PET images with recent MRI studies.[65] T1-weighted, gadolinium-enhanced images are used to localize enhancing brain lesions, while T2-weighted images can be used to localize non-enhancing abnormalities. Image registration is performed using a semi-automated surface fit technique that has been described by Turkington et al.[66,67] and Pelizzari et al.[68] and implemented by software developed at the Duke PET facility. In this process, digital images are gathered either by direct transfer in the case of in-house imaging, from recordings on digital media, or, in the case of hard copies, following digitization by a high resolution film digitizer (Vidar Systems Corporation, Herndon, Virginia). An example of an electronically co-registered data set is shown in Figure 10D.6. The volumetric FDG PET data is represented as dots, while the stacked circular contours represent the axial MR images. The PET volume is rotated and translated to minimize the error in the surface registration.

In-house software is also utilized to display the co-registered PET and magnetic resonance images. The software permits the reader to scroll through the axial MRI slices, and display the corresponding FDG PET images. The software offers the option of displaying the co-registered images by toggling between the corresponding PET and magnetic resonance images, or by observing a composite image displayed along an interactively controlled continuum ranging from 100% MRI to 100% PET, as illustrated in Figs 10D.1 and 10D.2. As an aid in interpretation, a mouse arrow, or any other pointing device, can be placed near an area of interest on MRI and physicians can toggle between 100% MRI and 100% PET or move along the continuum between the two modalities to evaluate the metabolic activity of the area in question.

For reasons mentioned above, a reliable method for anatomic/metabolic image registration is essential for evaluating brain tumors by FDG PET. Other radiotracers used to image the brain do not have high cortical activity, which can make image registration more difficult. In the future, PET/CT scanners will likely be used to provide intrinsically co-registered CT images which can be used for attenuation correction for the PET images as well as anatomic localization.

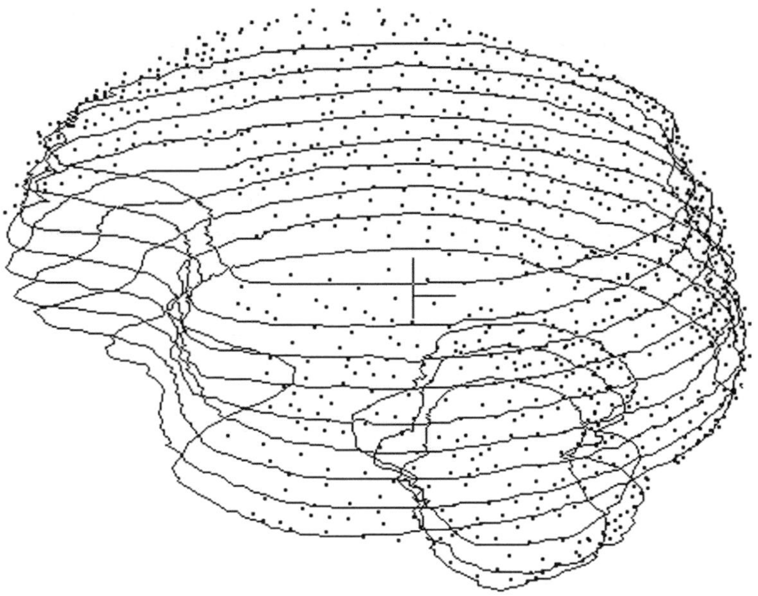

Figure 10D.6 *Semi-automated image registration. The three-dimensional FDG PET volume is depicted by the dots, while the axial MRI images are represented by the continuous circles. The PET image is rotated and translated so that the corresponding PET information correlates with each MRI slice.*

The CT can, in turn, be co-registered with MRI if necessary for additional tumor localization and characterization. The combined functional, anatomic, and attenuation data then can be incorporated into neuronavigation systems for surgical or radiation therapy treatment planning.

CONCLUSION

Primary brain tumors are relatively rare, but are frequently aggressive and associated with high morbidity and mortality. Local recurrence remains the primary problem when treating these tumors. Brain tumors are challenging to evaluate, because of their heterogeneous pathology and widely varying grade. FDG PET is useful for assessing tumor grade and can provide prognostic information. FDG PET is also useful for determining response to therapy. While FDG is currently the most widely available PET tracer, other radiopharmaceuticals, such as ^{11}C-MET can be useful for evaluating low-grade tumors. ^{11}C- and ^{15}O-based radiotracers have been utilized in brain PET imaging, but these studies can only be performed at centers with on-site cyclotrons. Newer ^{18}F-labeled compounds such as ^{18}F-choline and ^{18}F-thymidine have the potential to be commercially available due to their favorable half-lives.

Treating high-grade brain tumors also remains a challenge, due to the infiltrative nature of the tumor margins and the frequent proximity of tumors to important functional areas of the brain. In the future, functional imaging techniques such as PET may be useful for specifically directing therapy, such as radiation, to the most metabolically active portions of the tumor. Stereotactic and other navigation techniques are presently more advanced for the brain than for other areas of the body, and functional imaging such as PET may provide a metabolic map to improve local control of these devastating tumors, while preserving function and quality of life.

REFERENCES

1 Simmonds MA. Cancer statistics, 2003: further decrease in mortality rate, increase in persons living with cancer. *CA Cancer J Clin* 2003; **53**: 4.
2 Jemal A, Murray T, Samuels A, *et al.* Cancer statistics, 2003. *CA Cancer J Clin* 2003; **53**: 5–26.
3 Wrensch M, Minn Y, Chew T, *et al.* Epidemiology of primary brain tumors: current concepts and review of the literature. *Neuro-oncology* 2002; **4**: 278–99.
4 Coleman MP, Gatta G, Verdecchia A, *et al.* EUROCARE-3 summary: cancer survival in Europe at the end of the 20th century. *Ann Oncol* 2003; **14(suppl. 5)**: v128–49.
5 Sklar CA. Childhood brain tumors. *J Pediatr Endocrinol Metab* 2002; **15(suppl. 2)**: 669–73.
6 Hesselager G, Uhrbom L, Westermark B, Nister M. Complementary effects of platelet-derived growth factor autocrine stimulation and p53 or Ink4a-Arf deletion in a mouse glioma model. *Cancer Res* 2003; **63**: 4305–9.
7 Navas-Acien A, Pollan M, Gustavsson P, *et al.* Interactive effect of chemical substances and occupational electromagnetic field exposure on the risk of gliomas and meningiomas in Swedish men. *Cancer Epidemiol Biomarkers Prev* 2002; **11**: 1678–83.
8 Lonn S, Klaeboe L, Hall P, *et al.* Incidence trends of adult primary intracerebral tumors in four Nordic countries. *Int J Cancer* 2004; **108**: 450–5.
9 Kleihues P, Louis DN, Scheithauer BW, *et al.* The WHO classification of tumors of the nervous system.

J Neuropathol Exp Neurol 2002; **61**: 215–25; discussion 226–9.

10 Fuller GN, Hess KR, Rhee CH, *et al.* Molecular classification of human diffuse gliomas by multidimensional scaling analysis of gene expression profiles parallels morphology-based classification, correlates with survival, and reveals clinically-relevant novel glioma subsets. *Brain Pathol* 2002; **12**: 108–16.

11 Behin A, Hoang-Xuan K, Carpentier AF, Delattre JY. Primary brain tumours in adults. *Lancet* 2003; **361**: 323–31.

12 Kleihues P, Ohgaki H. Primary and secondary glioblastomas: from concept to clinical diagnosis. *Neuro-oncology* 1999; **1**: 44–51.

13 Mischel PS, Cloughesy TF. Targeted molecular therapy of GBM. *Brain Pathol* 2003; **13**: 52–61.

14 Wong T, van der Westhuizen GJ, Coleman RE. Brain tumors. In: Oehr P, Biersack HJ, Coleman RE. (eds) *PET and PET – CT in oncology.* Heidelberg: Springer, 2004: 113–25.

15 Nelson SJ. Imaging of brain tumors after therapy. *Neuroimaging Clin N Am* 1999; **9**: 801–19.

16 Kaplan WD, Takvorian T, Morris JH, *et al.* Thallium-201 brain tumor imaging: a comparative study with pathologic correlation. *J Nucl Med* 1987; **28**: 47–52.

17 Black KL, Hawkins RA, Kim KT, *et al.* Use of thallium-201 SPECT to quantitate malignancy grade of gliomas. *J Neurosurg* 1989; **71**: 342–6.

18 Higa T, Maetani S, Yoichiro K, Nabeshima S. Tl-201 SPECT compared with histopathologic grade in the prognostic assessment of cerebral gliomas. *Clin Nucl Med* 2001; **26**: 119–24.

19 Staffen W, Hondl N, Trinka E, *et al.* Clinical relevance of ^{201}Tl chloride SPET in the differential diagnosis of brain tumours. *Nucl Med Commun* 1998; **19**: 335–40.

20 de Vries B, Taphoorn MJ, van Isselt JW, *et al.* Bilateral temporal lobe necrosis after radiotherapy: confounding SPECT results. *Neurology* 1998; **51**: 1183–4.

21 Yoshii Y, Moritake T, Suzuki K, *et al.* Cerebral radiation necrosis with accumulation of thallium 201 on single-photon emission CT. *Am J Neuroradiol* 1996; **17**: 1773–6.

22 Schwartz RB, Carvalho PA, Alexander 3rd E, *et al.* Radiation necrosis vs high-grade recurrent glioma: differentiation by using dual-isotope SPECT with ^{201}Tl and ^{99m}Tc-HMPAO. *Am J Neuroradiol* 1991; **12**: 1187–92.

23 Carvalho PA, Schwartz RB, Alexander 3rd E, *et al.* Detection of recurrent gliomas with quantitative thallium-201/technetium-99m HMPAO single-photon emission computerized tomography. *J Neurosurg* 1992; **77**: 565–70.

24 O'Tuama LA, Treves ST, Larar JN, *et al.* Thallium-201 versus technetium-99m-MIBI SPECT in evaluation of childhood brain tumors: a within-subject comparison. *J Nucl Med* 1993; **34**: 1045–51.

25 Scheidhauer K, Hildebrandt G, Luyken C, *et al.* Somatostatin receptor scintigraphy in brain tumors

and pituitary tumors: first experiences. *Horm Metab Res (Suppl)* 1993; **27**: 59–62.

26 Bohuslavizki KH, Brenner W, Braunsdorf WE, *et al.* Somatostatin receptor scintigraphy in the differential diagnosis of meningioma. *Nucl Med Commun* 1996; **17**: 302–10.

27 Luyken C, Hildebrandt G, Krisch B, *et al.* Clinical relevance of somatostatin receptor scintigraphy in patients with skull base tumours. *Acta Neurochir Suppl (Wien)* 1996; **65**: 102–4.

28 Schmidt M, Scheidhauer K, Luyken C, *et al.* Somatostatin receptor imaging in intracranial tumours. *Eur J Nucl Med* 1998; **25**: 675–86.

29 Wrenn Jr F, Good M, Handler P. The use of positron emitting radioisotopes for localization of brain tumors. *Science* 1951; **113**: 525–7.

30 Brownell G, Sweet W. Localization of brain tumors with positron emitters. *Nucleonics* 1953; **11**: 40–5.

31 Di Chiro G. Positron emission tomography using [^{18}F]fluorodeoxyglucose in brain tumors. A powerful diagnostic and prognostic tool. *Invest Radiol* 1987; **22**: 360–71.

32 Al-Aish M, Coleman RE, Larson SM. Advances in clinical imaging using positron emission tomography. National Cancer Institute Workshop Statement. *Arch Intern Med* 1990; **150**: 735–9.

33 Mazziotta JC, Coleman RE, Di Chiro G, *et al.* Report of the Therapeutics and Technology Assessment Subcommittee of the American Academy of Neurology Assessment: positron emission tomography. *Neurology* 1991; **41**: 163–7.

34 Patronas NJ, Brooks RA, De La Paz RL, *et al.* Glycolytic rate (PET) and contrast enhancement (CT) in human cerebral gliomas. *Am J Neuroradiol* 1983; **4**: 533–5.

35 Delbeke D, Meyerowitz C, Lapidus RL, *et al.* Optimal cutoff levels of F-18 fluorodeoxyglucose uptake in the differentiation of low-grade from high-grade brain tumors with PET. *Radiology* 1995; **195**: 47–52.

36 Paulus W, Peiffer J. Intratumoral histologic heterogeneity of gliomas. A quantitative study. *Cancer* 1989; **64**: 442–7.

37 Hanson MW, Glantz MJ, Hoffman JM, *et al.* FDG–PET in the selection of brain lesions for biopsy. *J Comput Assist Tomogr* 1991; **15**: 796–801.

38 Pirotte B, Goldman S, Brucher JM, *et al.* PET in stereotactic conditions increases the diagnostic yield of brain biopsy. *Stereotact Funct Neurosurg* 1994; **63**: 144–9.

39 Pirotte B, Goldman S, Bidaut LM, *et al.* Use of positron emission tomography (PET) in stereotactic conditions for brain biopsy. *Acta Neurochir (Wien)* 1995; **134**: 79–82.

40 Pirotte B, Goldman S, David P, *et al.* Stereotactic brain biopsy guided by positron emission tomography (PET) with [F-18]fluorodeoxyglucose and [C-11]methionine. *Acta Neurochir Suppl (Wien)* 1997; **68**: 133–8.

41 Alavi JB, Alavi A, Chawluk J, *et al.* Positron emission tomography in patients with glioma. A predictor of prognosis. *Cancer* 1988; **62**: 1074–8.

42 Patronas NJ, Di Chiro G, Kufta C, *et al.* Prediction of survival in glioma patients by means of positron emission tomography. *J Neurosurg* 1985; **62**: 816–22.

43 Francavilla TL, Miletich RS, Di Chiro G, *et al.* Positron emission tomography in the detection of malignant degeneration of low-grade gliomas. *Neurosurgery* 1989; **24**: 1–5.

44 De Witte O, Levivier M, Violon P, *et al.* Prognostic value positron emission tomography with [¹⁸F]fluoro-2-deoxy-D-glucose in the low-grade glioma. *Neurosurgery* 1996; **39**: 470–6; discussion 476–7.

45 Hanson MW, Hoffman JM, Glantz MJ. FDG PET in the early postoperative evaluation of patients with brain tumor. [Abstract] *J Nucl Med* 1990; **31**: 799.

46 Barker 2nd FG, Chang SM, Valk PE, *et al.* 18-Fluorodeoxyglucose uptake and survival of patients with suspected recurrent malignant glioma. *Cancer* 1997; **79**: 115–26.

47 Chao ST, Suh JH, Raja S, *et al.* The sensitivity and specificity of FDG PET in distinguishing recurrent brain tumor from radionecrosis in patients treated with stereotactic radiosurgery. *Int J Cancer* 2001; **96**: 191–7.

48 Coleman RE, Hoffman JM, Hanson MW, *et al.* Clinical application of PET for the evaluation of brain tumors. *J Nucl Med* 1991; **32**: 616–22.

49 Reardon DA, Akabani G, Coleman RE, *et al.* Phase II trial of murine (131)I-labeled antitenascin monoclonal antibody 81C6 administered into surgically created resection cavities of patients with newly diagnosed malignant gliomas. *J Clin Oncol* 2002; **20**: 1389–97.

50 Marriott CJ, Thorstad W, Akabani G, *et al.* Locally increased uptake of fluorine-18-fluorodeoxyglucose after intracavitary administration of iodine-131-labeled antibody for primary brain tumors. *J Nucl Med* 1998; **39**: 1376–80.

51 Di Chiro G, Hatazawa J, Katz DA, *et al.* Glucose utilization by intracranial meningiomas as an index of tumor aggressivity and probability of recurrence: a PET study. *Radiology* 1987; **164**: 521–6.

52 Hoffman JM, Waskin HA, Schifter T, *et al.* FDG–PET in differentiating lymphoma from nonmalignant central nervous system lesions in patients with AIDS. *J Nucl Med* 1993; **34**: 567–75.

53 Roelcke U, Radu EW, Hausmann O, *et al.* Tracer transport and metabolism in a patient with juvenile pilocytic astrocytoma. A PET study. *J Neuro-oncol* 1998; **36**: 279–83.

54 Jager PL, Vaalburg W, Pruim J, *et al.* Radiolabeled amino acids: basic aspects and clinical applications in oncology. *J Nucl Med* 2001; **42**: 432–45.

55 Weber WA, Avril N, Schwaiger M. Relevance of positron emission tomography (PET) in oncology. *Strahlenther Onkol* 1999; **175**: 356–73.

56 Sasaki M, Kuwabara Y, Yoshida T, *et al.* A comparative study of thallium-201 SPET, carbon-11 methionine PET and fluorine-18 fluorodeoxyglucose PET for the differentiation of astrocytic tumours. *Eur J Nucl Med* 1998; **25**: 1261–9.

57 Chung JK, Kim YK, Kim SK, *et al.* Usefulness of ¹¹C-methionine PET in the evaluation of brain lesions that are hypo- or isometabolic on ¹⁸F-FDG PET. *Eur J Nucl Med Mol Imaging* 2002; **29**: 176–82.

58 Sadato N, Yonekura Y, Senda M, *et al.* PET and the autoradiographic method with continuous inhalation of oxygen-15-gas: theoretical analysis and comparison with conventional steady-state methods. *J Nucl Med* 1993; **34**: 1672–80.

59 Okazawa H, Yamauchi H, Sugimoto K, *et al.* Quantitative comparison of the bolus and steady-state methods for measurement of cerebral perfusion and oxygen metabolism: positron emission tomography study using ¹⁵O-gas and water. *J Cereb Blood Flow Metab* 2001; **21**: 793–803.

60 Raichle ME, Martin WR, Herscovitch P, *et al.* Brain blood flow measured with intravenous H₂(15)O. II. Implementation and validation. *J Nucl Med* 1983; **24**: 790–8.

61 Mineura K, Sasajima T, Kowada M, *et al.* Perfusion and metabolism in predicting the survival of patients with cerebral gliomas. *Cancer* 1994; **73**: 2386–94.

62 DeGrado TR, Baldwin SW, Wang S, *et al.* Synthesis and evaluation of (18)F-labeled choline analogs as oncologic PET traces. *J Nucl Med* 2001; **42**: 1805–14.

63 Roelcke U, Blasberg RG, von Ammon K, *et al.* Dexamethasone treatment and plasma glucose levels: relevance for fluorine-18-fluorodeoxyglucose uptake measurements in gliomas. *J Nucl Med* 1998; **39**: 879–84.

64 Wahl RL, Quint LE, Cieslak RD, *et al.* 'Anatometabolic' tumor imaging: fusion of FDG PET with CT or MRI to localize foci of increased activity. *J Nucl Med* 1993; **34**: 1190–7.

65 Wong TZ, Turkington TG, Hawk TC, Coleman RE. PET and brain tumor image fusion. *Cancer J* 2004; **10**: 234–42.

66 Turkington TG, Jaszczak RJ, Pelizzari CA, *et al.* Accuracy of registration of PET, SPECT and MR images of a brain phantom. *J Nucl Med* 1993; **34**: 1587–94.

67 Turkington TG, Hoffman JM, Jaszczak RJ, *et al.* Accuracy of surface fit registration for PET and MR brain images using full and incomplete brain surfaces. *J Comput Assist Tomogr* 1995; **19**: 117–24.

68 Pelizzari CA, Chen GT, Spelbring DR, *et al.* Accurate three-dimensional registration of CT, PET, and/or MR images of the brain. *J Comput Assist Tomogr* 1989; **13**: 20–6.

69 Wong TZ, Coleman RE. Brain tumors. In: Bender H, Palmedo H, Biersack H-J, Valk PE. (eds) *Atlas of clinical PET in oncology.* Berlin: Springer-Verlag, 2000: 153–70.

PET and SPECT imaging in movement disorders

JAN BOOIJ, JAN ZIJLMANS, AND HENK W. BERENDSE

INTRODUCTION

In recent decades, much progress has been made in the development of radiotracers as markers for various neurotransmitter systems or metabolic activity. Moreover, the accuracy of positron emission tomography (PET) and single photon emission computed tomography (SPECT) cameras has improved dramatically. This has stimulated the use of scintigraphic techniques to examine neurotransmitter systems as well as brain metabolic activity in health and disease. In particular, such studies have increased our understanding of the pathophysiology of movement disorders and contributed to the monitoring of treatment effects in these disorders. For example, a recent PET study using ^{11}C-PK11195 showed increased microglial activation in patients with corticobasal degeneration involving both cortical regions and the basal ganglia,[1] which may help to characterize in vivo the underlying disease activity. In a recent longitudinal study in Parkinson's disease (PD) patients, SPECT scans were used to monitor degeneration of the nigrostriatal projection with the aim of studying differential effects of treatment with a dopamine agonist or levodopa on the neurodegenerative process.[2]

The clinical diagnosis of movement disorders is often straightforward, obviating the need for scintigraphic tests, but when incomplete syndromes are present, a proper diagnosis of individual patients can be difficult at times.[3] In such cases scintigraphic imaging techniques may aid the diagnostic process. In this chapter, we will describe the scintigraphic techniques that are frequently used in routine clinical practice in patients with movement disorders: imaging of nigrostriatal dopaminergic terminals, dopamine D_2 receptors, and glucose metabolism.

In several movement disorders, including PD, there is a massive loss of dopaminergic nigrostriatal neurons. Since dopamine transporters (DATs) are positioned exclusively on the membrane of presynaptic dopaminergic neurons (Fig. 10E.1), imaging of these transporters can be used as an in vivo marker of the density of dopaminergic nerve terminals and, consequently, of the number of dopaminergic neurons. The DAT is presumably a unique constituent of dopaminergic nerve terminals.[4] Another possibility for measuring in vivo the integrity of dopaminergic neurons, is the use of ^{18}F-DOPA PET. This technique provides a measure of the structural as well as biochemical integrity of dopaminergic neurons; the uptake rate constant of DOPA is determined by the transfer of DOPA across the blood–brain barrier, its decarboxylation to fluoro-dopamine, and its retention in nerve terminals. In some movement disorders, such as multiple system atrophy (MSA), there is a loss of striatal neurons bearing dopamine D_2 receptors. PET as well as SPECT tracers have been developed successfully for these receptors. The vast majority of these D_2 receptors are located post-synaptically in the striatum (Fig. 10E.1). Therefore, imaging of these receptors is frequently referred to as imaging of post-synaptic striatal D_2 receptors. Finally, several centers routinely use ^{18}F-fluorodeoxyglucose (^{18}F-FDG) PET to measure regional glucose metabolism in patients suffering from movement disorders.

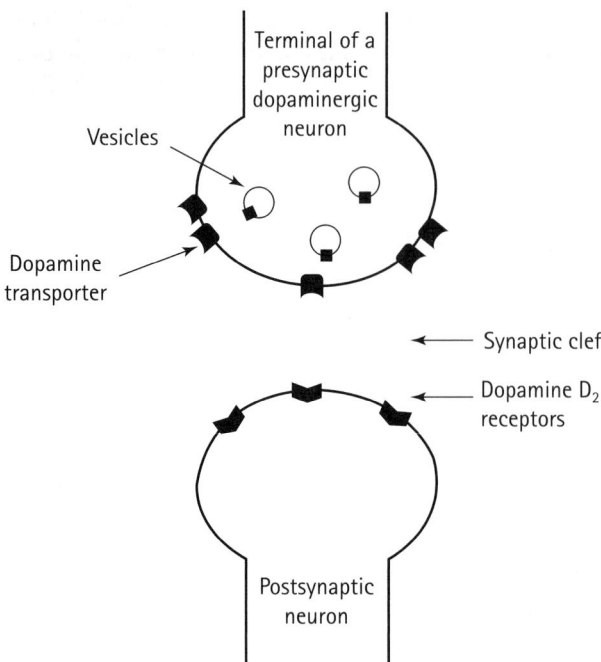

Figure 10E.1 *Schematic diagram of a dopaminergic nerve terminal, showing dopamine transporters in the cell membrane. These transporters are expressed exclusively in dopaminergic neurons, and are presumably confined to perisynaptic areas.[4] Among others, radioligands derived from cocaine (such as ^{123}I-FP-CIT or ^{123}I-β-CIT) bind in vivo to these transporters. The vast majority of dopamine D_2 receptors are located on postsynaptic neurons. Radioligands such as ^{123}I-IBZM and ^{11}C-raclopride bind in vivo to these receptors.*

PET AND SPECT STUDIES IN PARKINSONISM

Parkinson's disease

The major cause of parkinsonism is PD.[5] Dopaminergic projections from the substantia nigra to the striatum degenerate in PD, especially those to the putamen, while those to the caudate nucleus are relatively spared.[6] Degeneration of the nigrostriatal dopaminergic projection leads to loss of striatal DATs.[7] This degeneration is believed to be responsible, at least in part, for the motor deficits in PD such as rigidity and bradykinesia.[6]

Until recently, much research on the dopaminergic deficit in PD has been performed with ^{18}F-DOPA PET or radiotracers for the DAT.[8–11] A series of cocaine analogues has been developed successfully for imaging of DATs, e.g. ^{123}I-β-CIT, ^{123}I-FP-CIT, ^{123}I-IPT, ^{99m}Tc-TRODAT or ^{18}F-CFT.[12] Most of these radiotracers not only label dopamine but also serotonin transporters. However, since the vast majority of transporters within the striatum are dopaminergic, DAT ligands are very useful for clinical studies to detect a loss of striatal DATs. Of these radiotracers, ^{123}I-FP-CIT is registered in Europe as DaTSCAN.

In agreement with results from necropsy studies, ^{18}F-DOPA PET and DAT scintigraphy studies typically show a more pronounced reduction of striatal binding in the putamen than in the caudate nucleus in PD (Plates 10E.1 and 10E.2). Moreover, striatal binding of the radiotracer is asymmetric (in most PD patients, symptomatology starts unilaterally) and correlates with disease severity.[13–18] For clinical practice, results obtained in early PD patients are of special interest. SPECT imaging with ^{123}I-labeled or ^{99m}Tc-labeled cocaine analogs have shown a severe loss of striatal DATs in PD patients.[15,18] In addition, DAT scintigraphy techniques were able to discriminate completely between groups of PD patients and groups of controls.[14,16,19–21] The results of a recent study suggest that ^{123}I-FP-CIT may be more accurate than ^{99m}Tc-TRODAT in detecting loss of striatal DATs in early parkinsonism.[22] Using both DAT scintigraphy and ^{18}F-DOPA PET a bilateral loss of striatal DATs and DOPA uptake, respectively, has been demonstrated in hemiparkinsonian PD patients.[10,19,21,23] Interestingly, data from a recent longitudinal study have provided direct evidence that DAT is able to detect dopaminergic degeneration scintigraphically even before clinical motor signs of PD appear.[24,25] DAT scintigraphy thus appears to be very sensitive in detecting dopaminergic degeneration.

Recent reports describing the feasibility of detecting loss of extrastriatal DATs in PD,[26] and the development of several new and highly selective radiotracers for the DAT, e.g. PE2I,[27] are of little value in clinical practice at this point.

In agreement with necropsy studies, scintigraphic studies do not show a loss of dopamine D_2 receptors in PD.[28,29] In an early phase of PD, the binding of tracers for D_2 receptors may even be slightly increased.[12] Lastly, ^{18}F-FDG PET studies have shown a normal or slightly increased (on the contralateral side) striatal FDG uptake in PD.[30,31]

Multiple system atrophy

MSA may account for up to 10% of patients with parkinsonism.[32] It may present with any combination of extrapyramidal, pyramidal, autonomic, and cerebellar signs. The response to dopaminomimetics in MSA patients is often poor.[32] Neuropathologically, MSA is characterized by neuronal degeneration and gliosis in the basal ganglia, brain stem, cerebellum, and spinal cord.[33] As in PD, degeneration of the nigrostriatal dopaminergic pathway has been reported.[34] On the basis of the clinical presentation, MSA can be subdivided into those with prominent parkinsonism (MSA-p) and those with prominent cerebellar ataxia (MSA-c).

Initial ^{18}F-DOPA PET studies showed that MSA may present with a relatively stronger degeneration of the nigrostriatal projections to the caudate nucleus than PD[9] (Plate 10E.1). Consequently, it has been suggested that putamen-to-caudate nucleus ratios could be used in the differential diagnosis among different forms of parkinsonism. However, the results from more recent studies[30,35,36] showed that the pattern of presynaptic dopaminergic degeneration may be comparable in MSA and PD patients. Therefore, it is unlikely that it is possible to distinguish between MSA and PD in individual cases on the basis of the results of imaging studies of the nigrostriatal pathway alone. Although in a recent study the reduction of putamen DATs in a group of MSA-p patients was higher than in a group of MSA-c patients,[37] there was a clear overlap of uptake values between both groups.

Due to the loss of post-synaptic striatal neurons, MSA is characterized neuropathologically by an additional loss of dopamine D_2 receptors.[38] In agreement with this, PET and SPECT studies (Plates 10E.1 and 10E.2) have shown a loss of these receptors in MSA.[9,30,39,40] In several studies, a certain degree of overlap was found between the individual data of MSA and PD patients[39] or healthy controls.[28,40] Therefore, D_2 receptor densities in the 'low normal range' may not exclude MSA scintigraphically. There may be no difference between MSA-p and MSA-c patients in the extent of D_2 receptor loss.[39]

Recently, radiotracers with very high affinity for D_2 receptors have been developed, which offer the advantage to also assess extrastriatal D_2 receptors. Such radiotracers have recently been evaluated in parkinsonian syndromes.[41] For example, ^{123}I-epipride SPECT showed a markedly higher specific-to-nonspecific binding ratio in comparison to IBZM or other D_2 ligands. However, so far, this advantage has not resulted in a better discrimination between different basal ganglia disorders.[42]

FDG PET studies revealed a reduced FDG uptake in the striatum of MSA-p patients, but not in PD patients[30,31,43] (Plate 10E.1). In MSA, reduced FDG uptake is not restricted to the striatum, but also includes the frontal lobe.[43]

Progressive supranuclear palsy

Another akinetic–rigid syndrome is progressive supranuclear palsy (PSP) or Steele–Richardson–Olszewski syndrome. PSP is characterized clinically by increased axial tone, bulbar palsy, rigidity of the extensors of the neck, early postural instability, and supranuclear vertical gaze palsy. Necropsy studies showed neuronal loss in the basal ganglia, including the nigrostriatal pathway, and the brain stem nuclei associated with deposition of neurofibrillary tangles. In contrast to findings in PD, a similar degree of depletion of dopamine was found in both caudate nucleus and putamen.[44] In agreement with this post-mortem finding, striatal loss of ^{18}F-DOPA uptake in PSP involves the putamen and the caudate nucleus to the same extent.[45,46] This finding stands in contrast with the relative sparing of the caudate nucleus in PD.[9] More recent studies on the pattern of striatal DAT loss in PSP have produced conflicting results. Two studies[35,36] showed that the pattern of loss of striatal DATs in PSP is comparable to the pattern in PD. In contrast to this observation, other studies[47–49] showed a relatively uniform degree of DAT loss in the caudate nucleus and putamen in PSP. Although the pattern of striatal DAT loss may be different

from that in PD in a sample of patients with PSP, it does not seem possible to make a distinction in all individual cases on the basis of the results of imaging studies of the striatal DAT density alone.[35]

PSP is characterized scintigraphically by a loss of striatal D_2 receptors.[40,50] Moreover, FDG PET studies showed reduced FDG uptake in the striatum, the thalamus, parts of the frontal cortex, and the midbrain.[51]

Corticobasal degeneration

Corticobasal degeneration (CBD) is a rare movement disorder. Patients may present with motor signs (especially rigidity and hypokinesia), but also with signs of cortical dysfunction, which in typical cases are strongly asymmetrical. In CBD patients, an asymmetric degeneration of the cortex and basal ganglia can be visualized using MRI: DAT scintigraphy may show a slight loss of DAT binding on the side that corresponds to the side with the most pronounced cortical atrophy, the caudate and putamen being equally involved (Plate 10E.3).[52] FDG PET studies showed an asymmetrical reduction in glucose utilization, which may be characteristic for CBD.[53] Striatal D_2 receptor binding may be reduced in cases of CBD, although intact D_2 receptor binding has also been reported.[28,54]

Vascular parkinsonism

Vascular parkinsonism (VP) is characterized clinicopathologically in two ways: one by an insidious onset of parkinsonism with extensive subcortical white matter lesions affecting the thalamocortical loops, bilateral symptoms at onset, and the presence of early shuffling gait or early cognitive dysfunction; and another less common type of (sub)acute onset with strategic infarcts affecting putaminopallido-thalamic loops, i.e. in the globus pallidus, the ventrolateral nucleus of the thalamus and the substantia nigra area, and the parkinsonism at onset consisting of a contralateral bradykinetic rigid syndrome or shuffling gait.[55] DAT SPECT[56,57] tested normal in patients with VP associated with subcortical white matter lesions and has been used to differentiate this form of VP from PD at a group level. In contrast, DAT imaging and ^{18}F-DOPA PET in VP of (sub)acute onset due to basal ganglia infarction may show abnormalities comparable to PD,[58,59] or may reveal a 'punched-out' deficit in the striatum closely following the limits of the vascular lesion.[60] One unique ^{123}I-FP-CIT SPECT study reported diminished striatal binding in VP patients who had no basal ganglia infarcts.[61] A recent report on four different cases of VP showed loss of D_2 receptors.[62]

Drug–induced parkinsonism

Drug-induced parkinsonism occurs frequently, in particular as a result of treatment with dopamine antagonists (antipsychotics) or antiemetics. The clinical features may be quite indistinguishable from PD.[3] Recovery after drug withdrawal may take up to 15–18 months, or even longer.[63] DAT density is not altered by antipsychotics or antiemetics, because the D_2 receptors are the site of action of these drugs. DAT imaging may therefore help to confirm or refute an underlying dopaminergic deficit in uncertain cases.[63]

Psychogenic parkinsonism

Psychogenic movement disorders can mimic the entire spectrum of true movement disorders.[63] The diagnosis of psychogenic or pseudo-parkinsonism tends to be one of exclusion and is a protracted process, particularly when supporting features are not present.[3] DAT scans are presumably within the normal range, and may be of value to differentiate psychogenic movement disorder from its main differential of PD.[3,63]

ESSENTIAL TREMOR

Classically, patients with essential tremor (ET) suffer from a postural tremor of approximately 7 Hz, involving hands or forearms. A postural tremor similar to that seen in patients with ET may also occur in patients with PD, in addition to a resting tremor.[64] The reverse is true as well; the elderly patient with ET may also have slight resting tremor and mild parkinsonian features. Consequently, this may occasionally lead to difficulties in distinguishing ET from tremor-dominant PD.

SPECT and PET studies have shown that there is no loss of nigrostriatal dopaminergic neurons in patients with classical ET.[36,65,66] However, using ^{123}I-IPT SPECT in patients in whom a resting tremor developed after the onset of postural tremor, one study found a mild loss of striatal DATs.[65] Nevertheless, SPECT or PET is at least of value in discriminating classical ET from PD.

Orthostatic tremor may be considered as a special variant of ET,[67] although associations between orthostatic tremor, parkinsonism, and dopaminergic treatment effects have been reported. A recent ^{123}I-FP-CIT SPECT study showed a marked reduction in striatal tracer binding in patients suffering from orthostatic tremor.[68] Caudate and putamen were equally affected, yet tracer uptake was significantly higher and more symmetrical than in PD.

DYSTONIA

DOPA-responsive dystonia (DRD) is a rare genetic disorder involving the synthesis of dopamine. Both DRD and juvenile PD are young-onset disorders characterized clinically by parkinsonism and dystonia. Clinical distinction is quite important as prognosis and treatment benefit differ substantially. Juvenile PD is characterized by a loss of DATs, whereas DAT density is normal in DRD. In both disorders, D_2 receptor density is normal on slightly increased.[12]

Few PET and SPECT studies have been performed in other forms of dystonia. In one study a loss of DATs was found in idiopathic cervical dystonia.[69] Loss of D_2 receptors has been described in focal as well as in generalized dystonia.[70,71]

CHOREATIC DISORDERS

Huntington's disease (HD) is characterized by a severe loss of striatal neurons. Not surprisingly, PET and SPECT studies in HD showed a loss of striatal dopamine D_2 receptors, but normal ^{18}F-DOPA uptake.[72–74] Moreover, striatal FDG uptake is reduced in HD.[74] As genetic confirmation of a clinical diagnosis of HD is possible, scintigraphic studies are rarely performed in clinical practice.

In dentato-rubro-pallido-luysian atrophy and neuroacanthocytosis, loss of striatal FDG uptake has been described.[75,76] Reduced striatal D_2 receptors and striatal ^{18}F-DOPA uptake have been reported in neuroacanthocytosis.[77] In Wilson's disease, scintigraphic studies have revealed losses of both striatal D_2 receptors and striatal DATs.[78] In clinical practice, scintigraphy does not play a major role in the diagnostic process of these rare diseases.

Case history

A 62-year-old left-handed woman was referred to our neurology outpatient clinic with an 8-year history of slowly increasing motor dysfunction of the left hand which gradually involved the entire left arm. Over the years she had also experienced sensory loss in the left hand and a burning, sharp pain in the entire left half of the body. She had a history of repeated electroconvulsive therapy for severe depression and was using alprazolam and amitriptyline.

Neurological examination revealed left-sided hemiparkinsonism without tremor, increased tendon reflexes in the left arm, a slight sensory loss over the left side of the body and a slight sensory ataxia of the left arm and leg. Previous CT and MRI scans of the brain had not revealed abnormalities. In spite of the presence of atypical clinical features a tentative diagnosis of Parkinson's disease was made and treatment with a dopamine agonist was initiated. Over the next few months, treatment remained without effect and she developed a slight mixed-type aphasia and a focal myoclonus of the left hand muscles. A repeated MRI scan of the brain now revealed asymmetric atrophy of the right hemisphere (Plate 10E.3(c)). A ^{123}I-β-CIT SPECT scan showed a striking asymmetry of striatal DAT binding, with lower values for the right striatum, although both left and right striatal binding values were within the normal range (Plate 10E.3(b)). Based on the clinical features and the imaging data diagnosis was changed to corticobasal degeneration, a rare, progressive neurodegenerative disorder characterized by an asymmetrical degeneration of both cortical and subcortical structures. There is no causal treatment for this disorder and the effect of symptomatic treatment is usually disappointing. Cognitive and motor dysfunction rapidly increased in our patient, she was admitted to a nursing home and died within 3 years from diagnosis at the age of 65 years.

REFERENCES

♦ Key review paper

1 Gerhard A, Watts J, Trender-Gerhard I, *et al.* In vivo imaging of microglial activation with [^{11}C](*R*)-PK11195 PET in corticobasal degeneration. *Mov Disord* 2004; **19**: 1221–6.

2 Parkinson Study Group. Dopamine transporter brain imaging to assess the effects of pramipexole vs levodopa on Parkinson disease progression. *JAMA* 2002; **287**: 1651–61.

♦ 3 Marshall V, Grosset D. Role of dopamine transporter imaging in routine clinical practice [Review]. *Mov Disord* 2003; **18**: 1415–23.

4 Hoffman BJ, Hansson SR, Mezey E, Palkovits M. Localization and dynamic regulation of biogenic amine transporters in the mammalian central nervous system [Review]. *Frontiers Neuroendocrinol* 1998; **19**: 187–231.

5 Hughes AJ, Ben-Shlomo Y, Daniel SE, Lees AJ. What features improve the accuracy of clinical diagnosis in Parkinson's disease: a clinicopathologic study. *Neurology* 1992; **42**: 1142–6.

6 Kish SJ, Shannak K, Hornykiewicz O. Uneven pattern of dopamine loss in the striatum of patients with idiopathic Parkinson's disease. *N Engl J Med* 1988; **876**: 876–80.

7 Kaufman MJ, Madras BK. Severe depletion of cocaine recognition sites associated with the dopamine transporter in Parkinson's-diseased striatum. *Synapse* 1991; **9**: 43–9.

8 Leenders KL, Palmer AJ, Quinn N, *et al.* Brain dopamine metabolism in patients with Parkinson's disease measured with positron emission tomography. *J Neurol Neurosurg Psychiatry* 1986; **49**: 853–60.

9 Brooks DJ, Salmon EP, Mathias CJ, *et al.* The relationship between locomotor disability, autonomic dysfunction, and the integrity of the striatal dopaminergic system in patients with multiple system atrophy, pure autonomic failure, and Parkinson's disease, studied with PET. *Brain* 1990; **113**: 1539–52.

10 Ito K, Morrish PK, Rakshi JS, *et al.* Statistical parametric mapping with ^{18}F-dopa PET shows bilaterally reduced striatal and nigral dopaminergic function in early Parkinson's disease. *J Neurol Neurosurg Psychiatry* 1999; **66**: 754–8.

11 Lee CS, Samii A, Sossi V, *et al.* In vivo positron emission tomographic evidence for compensatory changes in presynaptic dopaminergic nerve terminals in Parkinson's disease. *Ann Neurol* 2000; **47**: 493–503.

♦ 12 Booij J, Tissingh G, Winogrodzka A, van Royen EA. Imaging of the dopaminergic neurotransmission system using single-photon emission tomography and positron emission tomography in patients with parkinsonism [Review]. *Eur J Nucl Med* 1999; **26**: 171–82.

13 Brücke T, Kornhuber J, Angelberger P, *et al.* SPECT imaging of dopamine and serotonin transporters with [^{123}I]β-CIT. Binding kinetics in the human brain. *J Neural Transm (General Section)* 1993; **94**: 137–46.

14 Frost JJ, Rosier AJ, Reich SG, *et al.* Positron emission tomographic imaging of dopamine transporter with ^{11}C-WIN 35,428 reveals marked declines in mild Parkinson's disease. *Ann Neurol* 1993; **34**: 423–31.

15 Tatsch K, Schwarz J, Mozley PD, *et al.* Relationship between clinical features of Parkinson's disease and presynaptic dopamine transporter binding assessed with [^{123}I]IPT and single-photon emission tomography. *Eur J Nucl Med* 1997; **24**: 415–21.

16 Seibyl JP, Marek KL, Quinlan D, *et al.* Decreased single-photon emission computed tomographic {^{123}I}β-CIT striatal uptake correlates with symptom severity in Parkinson's disease. *Ann Neurol* 1995; **38**: 589–98.

17 Booij J, Tissingh G, Boer GJ, *et al.* [^{123}I]FP-CIT SPECT shows a pronounced decline of striatal dopamine transporter labelling in early and advanced Parkinson's disease. *J Neurol Neurosurg Psychiatry* 1997; **62**: 133–40.

18 Huang WS, Lee MS, Lin JC, *et al.* Usefulness of brain ^{99m}Tc-TRODAT-1 SPET for the evaluation of Parkinson's disease. *Eur J Nucl Med Mol Imaging* 2004; **31**: 155–61.

19 Tissingh G, Booij J, Bergmans P, *et al.* Iodine-123-*N*-ω-fluoropropyl-2-β-carbomethoxy-3β-(4-iodophenyl)tropane SPECT in healthy controls and

early stage, drug-naive Parkinson's disease. *J Nucl Med* 1998; **39**: 1143–8.

20 Rinne JO, Bergman J, Ruottinen, *et al.* Striatal uptake of a novel PET ligand, [^{18}F]β-CFT, is reduced in early Parkinson's disease. *Synapse* 1999; **31**: 119–24.

21 Weng YH, Yen TC, Chen MC, *et al.* Sensitivity and specificity of ^{99m}Tc-TRODAT-1 SPECT imaging in differentiating patients with idiopathic Parkinson's disease from healthy subjects. *J Nucl Med* 2004; **45**: 393–401.

22 Van Laere K, De Ceuninck L, Dom R, *et al.* Dopamine transporter SPECT using fast kinetic ligands: ^{123}I-FP-β-CIT versus ^{99m}Tc-TRODAT-1. *Eur J Nucl Med Mol Imaging* 2004; **31**: 1119–27.

23 Marek KL, Seibyl JP, Zoghbi SS, *et al.* [^{123}I]β-CIT/SPECT imaging demonstrates bilateral loss of dopamine transporters in hemi-Parkinson's disease. *Neurology* 1996; **46**: 231–7.

24 Berendse HW, Booij J, Francot CMJE, *et al.* Subclinical dopaminergic dysfunction in asymptomatic Parkinson's disease patients' relatives with a decreased sense of smell. *Ann Neurol* 2001; **50**: 34–41.

25 Ponsen MM, Stoffers D, Booij J, *et al.* Idiopathic hyposmia as a preclinical sign of Parkinson's disease. *Ann Neurol* 2004; **56**: 173–81.

26 Ouchi Y, Yoshikawa E, Okada H, *et al.* Alterations in binding site density of dopamine transporter in the striatum, orbitofrontal cortex, and amygdala in early Parkinson's disease: compartment analysis for β-CFT binding with positron emission tomography. *Ann Neurol* 1999; **45**: 601–10.

27 Prunier C, Payoux P, Guilloteau D, *et al.* Quantification of dopamine transporter by ^{123}I-PE2I SPECT and the noninvasive Logan graphical method in Parkinson's disease. *J Nucl Med* 2003; **44**: 663–70.

28 Schwarz J, Tatsch K, Gasser T, *et al.* ^{123}I-IBZM binding compared with long-term clinical follow up in patients with de novo parkinsonism. *Mov Disord* 1998; **13**: 16–19.

29 Antonini A, Schwarz J, Oertel WH, *et al.* [^{11}C]raclopride and positron emission tomography in previously untreated patients with Parkinson's disease: influence of L-dopa and lisuride therapy on striatal dopamine D2-receptors. *Neurology* 1994; **44**: 1325–9.

30 Antonini A, Leenders KL, Vontobel P, *et al.* Complementary PET studies of striatal neuronal function in the differential diagnosis between multiple system atrophy and Parkinson's disease. *Brain* 1997; **120**: 2187–95.

31 Ghaemi M, Hilker R, Rudolf J, *et al.* Differentiating multiple system atrophy from Parkinson's disease: contribution of striatal and midbrain MRI volumetry and multi-tracer PET imaging. *J Neurol Neurosurg Psychiatry* 2002; **73**: 517–23.

32 Quinn N. Multiple system atrophy – the nature of the beast [Review]. *J Neurol Neurosurg Psychiatry* 1989; **52(Suppl)**: 78–89.

33 Fearnley J, Lees AJ. Striatonigral-degeneration: a clinico-pathological study. *Brain* 1990; **113**: 1823–42.

34 Spokes EGS, Bannister R, Oppenheimer DR. Multiple system atrophy with autonomic failure. Clinical, histological and neurochemical observations on four cases. *J Neurol Sci* 1979; **43**: 59–62.

35 Brücke T, Asenbaum S, Pirker W, *et al.* Measurement of dopaminergic degeneration in Parkinson's disease with [^{123}I]β-CIT and SPECT. Correlation with clinical findings and comparison with multiple system atrophy and progressive supranuclear palsy. *J Neural Transm* 1997; **50(Suppl)**: 9–24.

36 Benamer HTS, Patterson J, Grosset DG, *et al.* Accurate differentiation of parkinsonism and essential tremor using visual assessment of [^{123}I]-FP-CIT SPECT imaging: the [^{123}I]-FP-CIT study group. *Mov Disord* 2000; **15**: 503–10.

37 Lu CS, Weng YH, Chen MC, *et al.* ^{99m}Tc-TRODAT-1 imaging of multiple system atrophy. *J Nucl Med* 2004; **45**: 49–55.

38 Churchyard A, Donnan GA, Hughes A, *et al.* Dopa resistance in multiple-system atrophy: loss of postsynaptic dopamine D2 receptors. *Ann Neurol* 1993; **34**: 219–26.

39 Schulz JB, Klockgether T, Petersen D, *et al.* Multiple system atrophy: natural history, MRI morphology, and dopamine receptor imaging with ^{123}IBZM-SPECT. *J Neurol Neurosurg Psychiatry* 1994; **57**: 1047–1056.

40 van Royen E, Verhoeff NF, Speelman JD, *et al.* Multiple system atrophy and progressive supranuclear palsy. Diminished striatal D$_2$ dopamine receptor activity demonstrated by ^{123}I-IBZM single photon emission computed tomography. *Arch Neurol* 1993; **50**: 513–16.

41 Schreckenberger M, Hagele S, Siessmeier T, *et al.* The dopamine D$_2$ receptor ligand ^{18}F-desmethoxyfallypride: an appropriate fluorinated PET tracer for the differential diagnosis of parkinsonism. *Eur J Nucl Med Mol Imaging* 2004; **31**: 1128–35.

42 Pirker W, Asenbaum S, Wenger S, *et al.* Iodine-123-epidepride-SPECT: studies in Parkinson's disease, multiple system atrophy and Huntington's disease. *J Nucl Med* 1997; **38**: 1711–17.

43 De Volder AG, Francart J, Laterre C, *et al.* Decreased glucose utilization in the striatum and frontal lobe in probable striatonigral degeneration. *Ann Neurol* 1989; **26**: 239–47.

44 Kish SJ, Chang LJ, Mirchandani L, *et al.* Progressive supranuclear palsy: relationship between extrapyramidal disturbances, dementia, and brain neurotransmitter markers. *Ann Neurol* 1985; **18**: 530–6.

45 Brooks DJ, Ibanez V, Sawle GV, *et al.* Differing patterns of striatal ^{18}F-dopa uptake in Parkinson's disease, multiple system atrophy, and progressive supranuclear palsy. *Ann Neurol* 1990; **28**: 547–55.

46 Leenders KL, Frackowiak RS, Lees AJ. Steele–Richardson–Olszewski syndrome. Brain energy

metabolism, blood flow and fluorodopa uptake measured by positron emission tomography. *Brain* 1988; **111**: 615–30.

47 Messa C, Volonté MA, Fazio F, *et al.* Differential distribution of striatal [^{123}I]β-CIT in Parkinson's disease and progressive supranuclear palsy, evaluated with single-photon emission tomography. *Eur J Nucl Med* 1998; **25**: 1270–6.

48 Ilgin N, Zubieta J, Reich SG, *et al.* PET imaging of the dopamine transporter in progressive supranuclear palsy and Parkinson's disease. *Neurology* 1999; **52**: 1221–6.

49 Antonini A, Benti R, De Notaris R, *et al.* ^{123}I-Ioflupane/SPECT binding to striatal dopamine transporter (DAT) uptake in patients with Parkinson's disease, multiple system atrophy, and progressive supranuclear palsy. *Neurol Sci* 2003; **24**: 149–50.

50 Arnold G, Tatsch K, Kraft E, *et al.* Steele–Richardson–Olszewski syndrome: reduction of dopamine D$_2$ receptor binding relates to the severity of midbrain atrophy in vivo: ^{123}IBZM SPECT and MRI study. *Mov Disord* 2002; **17**: 557–62.

51 Garraux G, Salmon E, Degueldre C, *et al.* Comparison of impaired subcortico-frontal metabolic networks in normal aging, subcortico-frontal dementia, and cortical frontal dementia. *Neuroimage* 1999; **10**: 149–62.

52 Pirker W, Asenbaum S, Bencsits G, *et al.* [^{123}I]β-CIT SPECT in multiple system atrophy, progressive supranuclear palsy, and corticobasal degeneration. *Mov Disord* 2000; **15**: 1158–67.

53 Coulier IM, de Vries JJ, Leenders KL. Is FDG-PET a useful tool in clinical practice for diagnosing corticobasal ganglionic degeneration? *Mov Disord* 2003; **18**: 1175–8.

54 Plotkin M, Amthauer H, Klaffke S, *et al.* Combined ^{123}I-FP-CIT and ^{123}I-IBZM SPECT for the diagnosis of parkinsonian syndromes: study on 72 patients. *J Neural Transm* Published online: 14 September 2004.

55 Zijlmans J, Daniel S, Hughes A, *et al.* Lees A. A clinicopathological investigation of vascular parkinsonism (VP). Including clinical criteria for the diagnosis of VP. *Mov Disord* 2004; **19**: 630–40.

56 Tzen KY, Lu CS, Yen TC, *et al.* Differential diagnosis of Parkinson's disease and vascular parkinsonism by ^{99m}Tc-TRODAT-1. *J Nucl Med* 2001; **42**: 408–13.

57 Gerschlager W, Bencsits G, Pirker W, *et al.* [^{123}I]β-CIT SPECT distinguishes vascular parkinsonism from Parkinson's disease. *Mov Disord* 2002; **17**: 518–23.

58 Sibon I, Guyot M, Allard M, Tison F. Parkinsonism following anterior choroidal artery stroke. *Eur J Neurol* 2004; **11**: 283–4.

59 Boecker H., Weindl A, Leenders K, *et al.* Secondary parkinsonism due to focal substantia nigra lesions: a PET study with [^{18}F]FDG and [^{18}F]fluorodopa. *Acta Neurol Scand* 1996; **93**: 387–92.

60 Peralta C, Werner P, Holl B, *et al.* Parkinsonism following striatal infarcts: incidence in a prospective stroke unit cohort. *J Neural Transm* 2004; **111**: 1473–83.

61 Lorberboym M, Djaldetti R, Melamed E, *et al.* ^{123}I-FP-CIT SPECT imaging of dopamine transporters in patients with cerebrovascular disease and clinical diagnosis of vascular parkinsonism. *J Nucl Med* 2004; **45**: 1688–93.

62 Plotkin M, Amthauer H, Quill S, *et al.* Imaging of dopamine transporters and D2 receptors in vascular parkinsonism: a report of four cases. *J Neural Transm* 2005; **112**: 1355–61.

◆ 63 Tolosa E, Coelho M, Gallardo M. DAT imaging in drug-induced and psychogenic parkinsonism [Review]. *Mov Disord* 2003; **18**: S28–33.

64 Koller WC, Vetere-Overfield B, Barter R. Tremors in early Parkinson's disease. *Clin Neuropharmacol* 1989; **12**: 293–7.

65 Lee MS, Lim YD, Im JH, *et al.* ^{123}I-IPT brain SPECT study in essential tremor and Parkinson's disease. *Neurology* 1999; **52**: 1422–6.

66 Antonini A, Moresco RM, Gobbo C, *et al.* The status of dopamine nerve terminals in Parkinson's disease and essential tremor: a PET study with the tracer [^{11}C]FE-CIT. *Neurol Sci* 2001; **22**: 47–8.

67 Deuschl G, Bain P, Brin M. Consensus statement of the Movement Disorder Society on Tremor. Ad Hoc Scientific Committee. *Mov Disord* 1998; **13**(**Suppl 3**): 2–23.

68 Katzenschlager R, Costa D, Gerschlager W, *et al.* [^{123}I]-FP-CIT-SPECT demonstrates dopaminergic deficit in orthostatic tremor. *Ann Neurol* 2003; **53**: 489–96.

69 Naumann M, Pirker W, Reiners K, *et al.* Imaging the pre- and postsynaptic side of striatal dopaminergic synapses in idiopathic cervical dystonia: a SPECT study using [^{123}I]epidepride and [^{123}I]β-CIT. *Mov Disord* 1998; **13**: 319–23.

70 Horstink CA, Praamstra P, Horstink MW, *et al.* Low striatal dopamine D$_2$ recepotr binding as assessed by [^{123}I]IBZM SPECT in patients with writer's cramp. *J Neurol Neurosurg Psychiatry* 1997; **62**: 672–3.

71 Oertel WH, Tatsch K, Schwarz J, *et al.* Decrease of dopamine D$_2$ receptors indicated by ^{123}I-iodobenzamide single-photon emission computed tomography relates to neurological deficit in treated Wilson's disease. *Ann Neurol* 1992; **32**: 743–748.

72 Brücke T, Podreka I, Angelberger P, *et al.* Dopamine D$_2$ receptor imaging with SPECT: studies in different neuropsychiatric disorders. *J Cereb Blood Flow Metab* 1991; **11**: 220–8.

73 Turjanski N, Weeks R, Dolan R, *et al.* Striatal D1 and D2 receptor binding in patients with Huntington's disease and other choreas. A PET study. *Brain* 1995; **118**: 689–96.

74 Leenders KL, Frackowiak RS, Quinn N, Marsden CD. Brain energy metabolism and dopaminergic function in Huntington's disease measured in vivo using positron emission tomography. *Mov Disord* 1986; **1**: 69–77.

75 Dubinsky RM, Hallett M, Levey R, Di Chiro G. Regional brain glucose metabolism in neuroacanthocytosis. *Neurology* 1989; **39**: 1253–5.

76 Hosokawa S, Ichiya Y, Kuwabara Y, *et al.* Positron emission tomography in cases of chorea with different underlying diseases. *J Neurol Neurosurg Psychiatry* 1987; **50**: 1284–7.

77 Brooks DJ, Ibanez V, Playford ED, *et al.* Presynaptic and postsynaptic striatal dopaminergic function in neuroacanthocytosis: a positron emission tomographic study. *Ann Neurol* 1991; **30**: 166–71.

78 Barthel H, Hermann W, Kluge R, *et al.* Concordant pre- and postsynaptic deficits of dopaminergic neurotransmission in neurologic Wilson disease. *Am J Neuroradiol* 2003; **24**: 234–8.

Head and neck disease

11A Head and neck cancer

Clinical background   467
Diagnosis and morphologic imaging   467
Imaging with thallium-201 chloride and gallium-67 citrate   468
Imaging with ^{99m}Tc-labeled radiotracers   469
Radiopharmaceutical binding to receptors   469
Imaging with positron emission tomography   471

Positron emission tomography and lymph node metastases
    from an unknown primary   473
Sentinel node scintigraphy in head and neck squamous cell
    carcinoma   475
References   477

11B Salivary pathology

Introduction   483
Imaging of salivary gland function   483

Imaging of salivary gland tumors   484
References   484

11C Lachrymal studies

Dacryoscintigraphy   485
Other radiopharmaceuticals and the lachrymal gland   485

References   487

11

Head and neck cancer

GERHARD W. GOERRES

CLINICAL BACKGROUND

Head and neck cancers are most often squamous cell carcinomas (HNSCCs) originating from the mucosal membrane of the superior alimentary and respiratory tracts. HNSCCs are the eighth most common malignancies worldwide. The incidence depends on genetic factors, viruses, tobacco, alcohol use, immunologic, and occupational risk factors.[1] Other malignant lesions in the head and neck can originate from the lymphoid tissue, skin, salivary glands, bones, and soft tissues, causing lymphomas, melanomas, adenocarcinomas, primary bone tumors, and soft tissue sarcomas. The HNSCCs range from poorly differentiated to well differentiated histologies and also non-keratinizing and undifferentiated carcinomas (lymphoepithelioma) with infiltrating lymphocytes are possible.[2] Because the development of cancer on mucosal membranes is related to the exposure of carcinogens multiple anatomical sites may be at risk. Therefore, simultaneous or sequential malignant/premalignant lesions are a common finding. Premalignant lesions include leukoplakia and erythroplakia with histologic features of hyperplasia and dysplasia.

Symptoms depend on the location of the carcinoma and can be either functional or morphological. Common symptoms of patients with HNSCC are a sore throat, difficulties in swallowing, a painless lump in the neck, or an ulcer in the mouth which does not heal within a few weeks. Because the symptoms are often considered to be minor in the beginning, many patients will not take medical advice until the disease is in an advanced stage.

A wide spectrum of treatments is used for HNSCC depending on the initial stage and localization. Based on a recent analysis of US databases the use of combined chemotherapy and radiation treatment has increased thus improving functional outcome. Radical surgery has increasingly been abandoned.[3] Furthermore, the combination of radiation therapy with chemotherapy can significantly improve patient outcome.[4]

DIAGNOSIS AND MORPHOLOGIC IMAGING

Physical examination includes visual inspection of the mucosal membranes with pharyngoscopy and indirect laryngoscopy and palpation of the floor of the mouth and neck lymph node stations. Transnasal fiberendoscopy of the nasal cavity, the nasopharynx, oropharynx, hypopharynx, and larynx are usually performed and in many centers panendoscopy under anesthesia will be done early in the work-up. The primary will be histologically proven and often ultrasound guided fine-needle aspiration cytology (FNA) of suspicious lymph nodes is performed.[5,6] However, imaging with contrast-enhanced (high resolution helical) computed tomography (CT) or magnetic resonance imaging (MRI) from the skull base to the clavicles is usually acquired for staging and to plan surgical interventions or radiation therapy.

Imaging work-up is done to stage the patients according to the TNM classification system as described by the American Joint Committee of Cancer (or by a slightly adapted version).[7] The stage of cancer is defined by the primary tumor, the involvement of lymph nodes and the presence of distant metastases. At the level of the primary tumor in most regions of the head and neck, the size of the carcinoma decides whether the patient has a T1, T2 or T3 stage. In all areas T4 stage describes a tumor invading adjacent structures such as bones, cartilage, muscles or vessels and nerve sheaths. The risk of nodal metastasis is related to the primary site and stage of the tumor. It has been described to be low in patients presenting with glottic cancer and high in patients with SCC of the nasopharynx.[2] The identification of lymph node involvement is crucial for optimal therapy and has an important prognostic value. Structural imaging methods such as CT and MRI mainly rely on morphologic criteria to decide if a lymph node is probably involved by tumor spread or not.[6] For example, any lymph node larger than 10 mm in largest diameter, or any node having lost its normal oval-shaped appearance or with signs of central necrosis is usually considered to be malignant. When changing the critical size from 10 mm to 8 mm the sensitivity of lymph node assessment will increase but the specificity will be lowered at the same time. However, the size criterion is not good when compared with histology. Ultrasound has a reported accuracy for the identification of lymph node metastases of up to 89%.[6] Staging of distant disease is important in patients with HNSCC, because in approximately 12% distant metastases or secondary tumors will be found.[8–10] However, to date, no guidelines are available governing the use of imaging tests for M-staging. The morphological imaging techniques are limited in identifying unknown primary tumors, occult cervical metastases and in differentiating recurrent tumor from therapy-induced tissue changes. Because of these limitations there was always great interest in the use of functional imaging methods.

IMAGING WITH THALLIUM-201 CHLORIDE AND GALLIUM-67 CITRATE

The mechanism of uptake of thallium-201 chloride into the tumor cell is thought to be regulated by the Na^+/K^+ ATPase pump activity. Its uptake into tissues is nonspecific and in proportion to the regional perfusion. An examination with thallium-201 chloride is usually performed with a standard activity of approximately 150 MBq causing an effective dose equivalent of 37 mSv and a dose to the uterus of 6 mGy.[11] Uptake of thallium-201 chloride was first described as an incidental finding in a lung tumor of a patient undergoing myocardial scintigraphy.[12] In 1988 El-Gazzar et al. reported on the use of ^{201}Tl scintigraphy in five patients with advanced stage HNSCC.[13] A large primary, tumor persistence after chemotherapy, and lymph node and bone metastases were visualized. Other groups confirmed the value of ^{201}Tl single photon emission computed tomography (SPECT) imaging for assessing response after radiation treatment and to detect occult lesions.[14] However, ^{201}Tl SPECT is not better than CT or MRI for identification of lymph node involvement.[15] Valdes-Olmos

et al. reported on 79 patients undergoing staging for a histologically proven HNSCC. Thallium-201 SPECT had higher accuracy than CT/MRI for the depiction of involved neck sides, because of false positive findings with CT/MRI.[16] Mukherji et al. confirmed the high accuracy of thallium-201 chloride imaging for the detection of recurrent disease and the better discriminative ability between recurrence and postoperative changes.[17] However, the background activity within normal tissues is rather high because the salivary and thyroid glands take up thallium-201 chloride thus disguising pathologies.[18] The limited value of ^{201}Tl SPECT for the staging of a primary tumor was also described by Güney et al.[19] However, these authors showed that ^{201}Tl has the ability to differentiate malignant from benign neck masses (without malignant salivary gland tumors).[20]

Gallium-67 citrate has been used by several groups to examine patients with HNSCC at staging and for follow-up.[21–25] Gallium-67 citrate accumulates in areas with high lactoferrin content and therefore lachrymal and salivary glands and also the nasopharynx are regularly visualized. Gallium-67 citrate is a classical method for whole-body staging of patients with lymphoma but has not been widely used for imaging of patients with HNSCC. Scintigraphy for oncologic imaging is usually performed 48–72 h after injection of a standard activity of 150 MBq, which causes an effective dose equivalent of 17 mSv and a dose to the uterus of 12 mGy.[11] As with thallium-201 chloride the ability of gallium-67 citrate to visualize the primary is related to the size of the tumor. In a study by Onizawa and Yoshida it was shown that only large advanced carcinomas were seen and only 25% of lymph node metastases.[24] These authors concluded that ^{67}Ga scintigraphy is not helpful for initial staging of patients with oral cavity SCC. In contrast, in a smaller series of patients Murata et al. found that gallium-67 citrate is useful for restaging of patients and that the sensitivity and specificity for detection of a recurrence was better compared to CT (sensitivity 87% vs. 80%, specificity 91% vs. 62%).[23] However, these authors confirmed the observation of others that the sensitivity for the detection of lymph node metastases is rather low. In a prospective comparison Kitagawa et al. compared ^{67}Ga scintigraphy with morphological imaging (MRI and CT) and fluorodeoxyglucose (FDG) PET in HNSCC patients undergoing treatment with combined intra-arterial chemotherapy and radiotherapy.[25] They found it more difficult to identify a lesion with gallium-67 citrate than with CT, MRI, and PET. In this study the sensitivity of gallium-67 citrate for identification of the primary before treatment was 40% but 100% for FDG PET.[25]

However, using gallium-67 citrate and also thallium-201 chloride small primaries are often missed and also lymph node metastases and local recurrences are only identified when they are large. Both tracers have a rather long half-life and the physical properties for imaging are not excellent. Therefore, ^{99m}Tc-labeled radiotracers became more popular for routine clinical use.

IMAGING WITH ^{99m}TC–LABELED RADIOTRACERS

Technetium-99m-sestamibi and ^{99m}Tc-tetrofosmin have lipophilic and cationic properties and are bound in cells with a high number of mitochondria. For oncologic imaging a standard activity of 900 MBq sestamibi is given leading to an equivalent dose of 11 mSv and a uterus dose of 11 mGy.[11] Both radiopharmaceuticals were primarily designed to replace thallium-201 chloride as flow tracer for myocardial studies. They are rapidly taken up by the tumor cell and images are acquired early (5–10 min) after the injection. *In vitro* studies have shown that sestamibi reaches a steady state within the cell which is inversely proportional to the MDR1 P-glycoprotein, a membrane efflux transporter.[26] Therefore, sestamibi can be used for functional imaging of the P-glycoprotein-mediated multi-drug resistance.[27] In contrast, the efflux of thallium-201 chloride out of the cell is not influenced by P-glycoprotein.[28]

Sestamibi and tetrofosmin can be used to detect HNSCC of the nasopharynx and lymph node metastases.[29,30] In patients with nasopharyngeal HNSCC and equivocal MRI findings 4 months after the end of radiation treatment tetrofosmin SPECT has a high sensitivity and specificity for the identification of local recurrence.[31] SPECT imaging is also helpful in identifying lymph node metastases.[32] Wang *et al.* compared ^{201}Tl with sestamibi SPECT and found a higher sensitivity for the detection of nasopharyngeal carcinomas with sestamibi.[33] Both tracers show comparable performance for the detection of primary nasopharyngeal carcinomas and recurrences, but in a recent study sestamibi showed a higher sensitivity for the detection of lymph node metastases.[34] A comparison of tetrofosmin with CT and FDG PET revealed a worse sensitivity for tetrofosmin: sensitivity/specificity 64%/86% for tetrofosmin, 73%/83% for CT and 100%/97% for PET.[35] In patients with suspected local recurrence/residual cancer it is difficult to differentiate the malignancy from radiation-induced changes with CT and in this situation it has been shown that sestamibi imaging has a higher specificity than CT although the sensitivity is lower.[36] However, Kao *et al.* compared sestamibi with FDG PET and found that PET had a higher sensitivity in patients with suspected recurrent or persistent nasopharyngeal cancer.[37]

Another ^{99m}Tc-labeled radiotracer is ^{99m}Tc(V)-dimercaptosuccinic acid (^{99m}Tc(V)-DMSA), which has been used by several authors in HNSCC patients.[38] In contrast to sestamibi and tetrofosmin scintigraphy, a high uptake of ^{99m}Tc(V)-DMSA is found later after injection and the best image quality will be obtained when scanning after 4 h.[39] Imaging with a standard activity of 400 MBq ^{99m}Tc(V)-DMSA causes an equivalent dose of 3 mSv and a uterus dose of 2 mGy.[11] As with sestamibi and tetrofosmin the uptake in the tumor cells is nonspecific. However, most of the tracer is located in the cytosol of the cell.[39]

Technetium(V)-99m-DMSA imaging is not specific for HNSCC and uptake can be observed in inflammatory lesions and benign tumors. Furthermore, ^{99m}Tc(V)-DMSA SPECT is worse than clinical examination and CT imaging in patients with lymph node metastases and even the combination of CT with ^{99m}Tc(V)-DMSA SPECT does not offer an advantage to CT alone.[40] An example of planar imaging with bone scintigraphy and ^{99m}Tc(V)-DMSA in a patient with HNSCC is shown in Figure 11A.1.

RADIOPHARMACEUTICAL BINDING TO RECEPTORS

The use of radiopharmaceutical binding to receptors allows for selective imaging of tumor cells. Such radiopharmaceuticals not only increase specificity of imaging for diagnosis and follow-up, but also could be used for therapy when labeled with a beta- or alpha-emitting radionuclide since HNSCCs are radiosensitive cancers. Several groups have tested antibodies and antibody fragments against antigens present on HNSCC tumor cells. A range of different antibodies and fragments have been evaluated during the last few years, such as ^{111}In-labeled antibodies against carcinoembryonic antigen (CEA), ^{99m}Tc-labeled antibody U36 IgG, (E48 F(ab′)2), and Mab 174H.64 binding to a cytokeratin-associated antigen expressed by more than 90% of SCC.[41–45] Using radioimmunoscintigraphy, small lymph node metastases can be missed and also false positive findings are possible.[44,45] Adamietz *et al.* scanned 40 HNSCC patients with a murine ^{99m}Tc-labeled antibody before they underwent radiation therapy.[46] Radioimmunoscintigraphy detected metastases not identified by morphological imaging and thus had a relevant impact on further treatment.[46] To date, several animal and patient studies are available reporting on first results of treatment based on the use of antibodies labeled with beta-emitting radionuclides.[47,48]

m-[$^{123/131}$I]iodobenzylguanidine ($^{123/131}$I-MIBG) is specifically taken up by pheochromocytoma, neuroblastoma, carcinoid tumors, and nonfunctioning paraganglioma, also referred to as carotid body tumors, tympanic paragangliomas, glomus vagale tumors or chemodectomas.[49,50] In patients with disseminated metastases ^{131}I-MIBG is an effective systemic treatment. Since paragangliomas are neuroendocrine tumors with a high expression of somatostatin receptors they can be imaged with ^{111}In-DTPA-D-Phe-1-octreotide and analogs. In Figure 11A.2, a patient with small-cell carcinoma of the maxillary sinus scanned with ^{111}In-DOTATOC is shown. Many different derivatives have been evaluated for diagnostic use and, recently, agents suitable for therapy have also been introduced.[51–53] However, treatment of HNSCC patients with radiopharmaceutical binding to receptors is still in an experimental stage. Based on the results of available studies this treatment option cannot replace the standard therapy using surgery or (combined) radiation and chemotherapy. However, it has

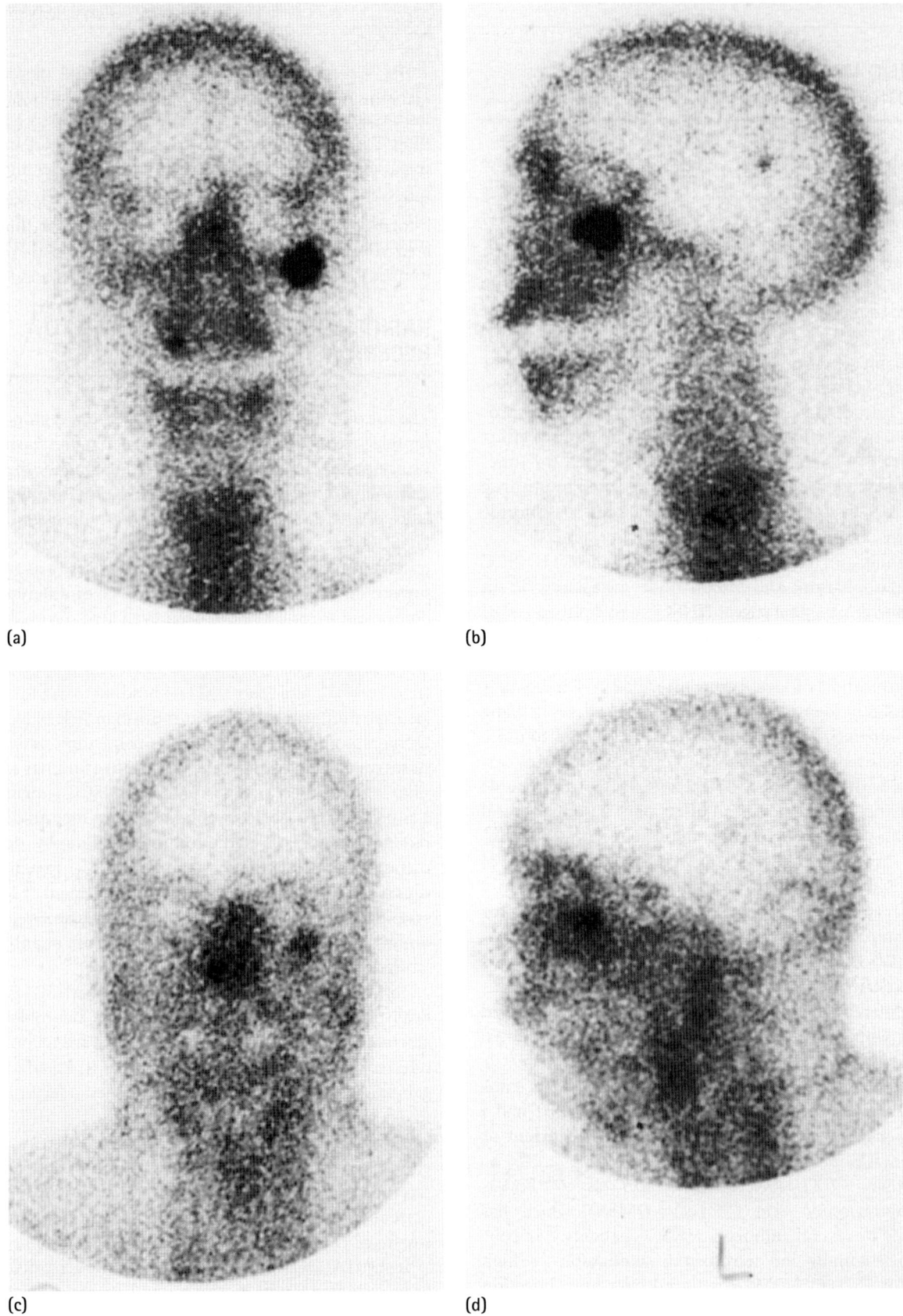

(a)

(b)

(c)

(d)

Figure 11A.1 *Skeletal scintigraphy and $^{99m}Tc(V)$-dimercaptosuccinic acid ($^{99m}Tc(V)$-DMSA) scintigraphy of a 64-year-old male patient who underwent surgery and radiation therapy for a squamous cell carcinoma of the epiglottis 2 years ago. He developed a secondary cancer in the left maxillary sinus. Planar scintigraphy in AP and left lateral projections (a and b) reveal intense uptake at the zygomatic bone with both tracers. Image quality is limited and lymph node metastases are not detected with $^{99m}Tc(V)$-DMSA (c and d). There is relatively high nonspecific tracer uptake in the soft tissues mainly in the nasal and nasopharyngeal region. This examination was done 15 years ago without the adjunct of SPECT.*

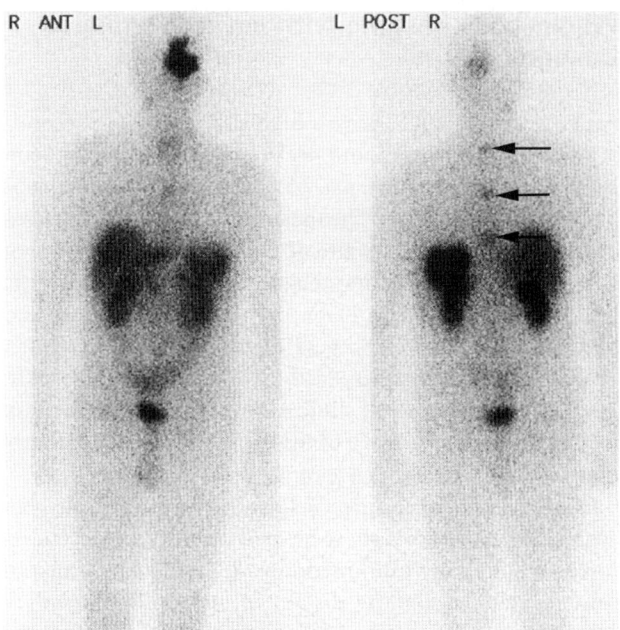

R ANT L   L POST R

Figure 11A.2 *Whole-body DOTATOC scintigraphy of a patient with a small-cell cancer of the nasal cavity and paranasal maxillary and ethmoidal sinuses. Image acquisition was done 6 h after the injection of 111 MBq ^{111}In-labeled DOTATOC. There is high uptake in the primary and in bone metastases in the thoracic vertebral spine (arrows). (Images courtesy of Prof. Jan Mueller-Brand, Nuclear Medicine, University Hospital Basel, Switzerland.)*

been suggested that such a treatment modality could be an interesting adjuvant systemic therapy in patients with locally advanced stage HNSCC.[47]

IMAGING WITH POSITRON EMISSION TOMOGRAPHY

Many different PET tracers have been tested for imaging such as ^{11}C-methionine, ^{11}C-tyrosine, ^{11}C-thymidine and [^{18}F]fluorodeoxyglucose (^{18}F-FDG). With these tracers different aspects of tumor metabolism can be evaluated. Methionine is a marker of amino acid transport.[54] Tyrosine can be used to determine protein synthesis activity and is suitable to assess protein synthesis rate and treatment effects in patients with HNSCC.[55–58] Thymidine is incorporated into nucleic acids; thus it is possible to measure proliferative activity of cancer cells. However, the metabolism of thymidine is rather complicated and the short half-life of ^{11}C makes it difficult to use this tracer in clinical routine.[59] Tumor hypoxia can be visualized with ^{18}F-misonidazole and [62]Cu(II)-diacetyl-bis[N(4)-methylthiosemicarbazone] ([62]Cu-ATSM) thus enabling improved planning of radiation therapy by delineating hypoxic regions in HNSCC.[60,61] FDG is the most important tracer used for PET imaging.

A first report of Minn *et al.* in 1988 showed that FDG is taken up by HNSCC tumor cells.[62] It has been shown that uptake of glucose is increased due to an upregulation mainly of GLUT-1 facilitated diffusion transport and that this transport is inversely proportional to the differentiation of the tumor.[63] Therefore, PET provides prognostic information: patients with moderately or poorly differentiated HNSCC have higher FDG uptake than patients with well-differentiated cancers and patients with high FDG uptake at staging have a worse prognosis.[64,65] For imaging HNSCC patients FDG PET is usually not acquired dynamically but after an uptake time between injection and the start of imaging of approximately 60 min. Because FDG is a glucose analog it is important that the patient fasts before scanning. The blood sugar level should be controlled because hyperglycemia can decrease tumor uptake. This can impair visualization and delineation of the primary or metastatic lymph nodes since neck muscles may show increased FDG uptake.[66] The injection of a standard activity of 400 MBq causes an effective equivalent dose of 10 mSv and an uterine dose of 7 mGy.[11] To better describe a lesion it is a common practice to measure FDG uptake by means of the standardized uptake value (SUV). The SUV measurement is easily done, but needs transmission scanning for attenuation correction. SUV values are not excellent discriminators between malignant lesions and benign tissues with high metabolic activity, such as active inflammation. Additionally, it has to be considered that SUV measurements can be corrupted by metal induced artifacts in patients with dental metalwork.[67,68]

Positron emission tomography imaging of the primary tumor

Because of the high FDG uptake in HNSCC it is possible to identify even small lesions which may be missed using structural imaging, such as MRI or CT.[69] PET can be used for the identification of a primary tumor, but is not able to correctly classify the T-stage of a lesion. T-staging needs anatomic information and the possibility to exactly measure tumor size. Wong *et al.* reported a sensitivity of up to 100% for the identification of the primary with visual assessment of PET images.[70] However, it is possible to miss small primary tumors (<1 cm), tumors with a superficial spreading growth pattern and lesions in the supraglottic area.[71,72] Furthermore, detection of a primary lesion is more difficult in the tonsils and at the base of the tongue, because of physiologic low to moderate FDG uptake of lymphatic tissue in Waldeyer's ring.[73] Furthermore, laryngeal cancers can be missed in patients who speak during the study.[74,75]

The most important prognostic information for a patient with HNSCC is the exact localization of lymph node involvement and the identification of distant metastases or a secondary tumor. Because T-staging is not possible without morphological imaging, PET focuses on N- and M-staging of the patient.

Positron emission tomography imaging of lymph node involvement

Correct lymph node staging is the key to an optimal treatment strategy since HNSCC mainly spread regionally. In patients with pathologically N0 neck treated for oral cancer the 5-year survival will be 73%, in patients with pathologically positive lymph nodes 50%, and in patients with extracapsular spread of lymph node involvement 30%.[76] FDG PET is better than clinical examination and CT for the detection of lymph node metastases.[77,78] The reported sensitivity for lymph node detection ranges from 50 to 94% and the specificity from 82 to 100% being regularly better than CT or MRI.[69,70,73,77,79-85]

An advantage of PET is the high negative predictive value, i.e. FDG PET is able to exclude the presence of disease with a high probability. Lymph nodes may reactively be enlarged on morphologic images but should not show relevant FDG uptake. In contrast, high FDG uptake can be seen in normal sized lymph nodes when they are involved with metastatic spread. Note that up to 40% of lymph node metastases are localized in normal-sized lymph nodes.[5] Therefore, sensitivity and specificity of PET is regularly better than with morphologic imaging.[69,77,79-81]

False negative findings are possible for example in (large) necrotic lymph nodes, where the active tumor tissue is located in a thin rim around an FDG negative necrosis. This can avoid visualization of the metastasis, because the number of FDG-avid tumor cells is too low to produce enough signal for detection by the PET camera. Furthermore, some tumors do not show high FDG uptake. This has been reported for adenoid cystic carcinomas and adenocarcinomas.[86] Inflammation is the main reason for false positive findings and is due to activated white blood cells taking up FDG. False positive and false negative PET findings are possible early after the end of radiation treatment.[87] Therefore, it is important to choose the best time point for scanning after the end of treatment.[88,89] Another potential source of false positive findings is dental problems, which are common in patients with HNSCC. If infectious disease of dental roots and/or periodontal space is present, normally the teeth will be surgically removed before radiation treatment is scheduled. This will cause an inflammation reaction which can be visible for several weeks.[90]

It has been suggested that PET can be successfully used in patients with clinical N0 neck. The sensitivity of FDG PET appears to be much higher than that of morphologic imaging, but it should be remembered that PET, like other imaging methods, cannot detect microscopic metastases.[91] In a recent study it has been shown that FDG PET has limited value in these patients compared to sentinel lymph node scintigraphy.[92]

Whole-body imaging with positron emission tomography

Patients with HNSCC have a high risk to develop secondary cancers in the head and neck, esophagus or lung. Léon et al. reported an incidence of developing a second neoplasm of 4% per year.[93] The incidence of distant metastases depends on the primary site of the lesion and the stage of disease at the time of first diagnosis. For example, glottic cancers spread rarely and later in the course of disease and patients with nasopharyngeal carcinoma relatively often show distant metastases at the time of first diagnosis. Furthermore, the overall clinical status of a patient and risk factors influence the stage of disease at the time of primary diagnosis and the incidence of secondary cancers.

Many secondary cancers such as bronchogenic and esophageal carcinoma show increased FDG uptake. Therefore, a whole-body examination is routinely performed in some centers to identify distant metastases or secondary tumors in the same examination. Stokkel et al. performed dual-head positron emission tomography in 68 patients with a primary tumor in the oral cavity or oropharynx and found a simultaneous malignancy in 12 of 68 patients (18%).[94] In contrast, Keyes et al. examined 56 patients, including the head, neck, and chest, and found secondary malignancies in only 5%.[95] Two of the three cases where increased FDG uptake corresponded to tumors were obvious from other routine examinations. Therefore, these authors concluded that there is no indication for including the chest in PET studies of HNSCC patients.[95] In contrast, other authors found PET for screening of distant metastases most useful in patients with advanced stage disease.[10,96] Findings of whole-body PET outside the head and neck area can impact on treatment decisions in between 10 and 20% of all patients.[10,97,98] Because secondary carcinomas are not only a problem at initial staging but may arise during the later disease course, whole-body imaging can be recommended also for follow-up examinations.

Fluorodeoxyglucose positron emission tomography for follow-up examinations

A local recurrence is most often found within the first 2 years after treatment. After surgical and/or radiation treatment the soft tissues of the neck are altered and interpretation of CT and MRI findings is difficult. Several authors recommend to wait 4 months after the end of treatment before scanning patients to identify residual cancer/early recurrence.[87] In contrast, in a recent study it has been shown that at 6 weeks after the end of a combined chemotherapy and radiation treatment a reliable assessment of residual vital cancer tissue is possible with >90% sensitivity and specificity.[89] However, the best time point for follow-up PET depends on both the therapy performed and the clinical situation of the patient.

Many authors have shown that FDG PET has a high sensitivity and a high negative predictive value for the evaluation of suspected recurrence or residual tumor.[99,100] The reported sensitivity for the detection of a local recurrence using FDG PET ranges from 80 to 100% with a specificity ranging from 57 to 100% being regularly better than CT or MRI.[69,83,99–106] However, it is possible that after radiation therapy a small number of carcinoma cells remain viable, but will be invisible on a PET scan due to the low number of FDG-avid cells. In case of postoperative inflammation or infection FDG uptake will be increased. Early after therapy an increased FDG uptake can be found in patients with radiation induced mucositis of the pharynx and esophagus.[90] Another possible treatment-induced pitfall is FDG uptake in the bone marrow as a sign of rebound in patients who underwent previous chemotherapy. Figure 11A.3 shows a patient with HNSCC undergoing PET imaging for staging and restaging. Color versions of the figure are shown in Plate 11A.1.

Combined positron emission tomography/computed tomography imaging

It has been questioned whether PET alone is suitable for routine evaluation of head and neck cancer patients, because of the lack of anatomic information.[74] For staging and planning of surgery or radiotherapy morphological information is essential. Early publications have shown that with image co-registration of PET with CT or MRI, HNSCC can be evaluated better.[107,108] However, the co-registration of data sets obtained on different devices at different time points has major drawbacks, such as patient repositioning and intercurrent anatomic changes. With the recent introduction of combined PET/CT scanners both imaging modalities can be obtained in the same imaging session. The combined information facilitates interpretation of equivocal findings, reduces erroneous interpretation and improves the confidence of image reading.[109] The discrimination of benign from malignant lesions and thus the specificity of PET findings is improved by the structural information of CT. However, to date, no studies are available evaluating the impact of PET/CT imaging on the management of HNSCC patients.

The CT data of a PET/CT scan can be used for attenuation correction.[110] This shortens imaging time, because no additional conventional transmission scan is needed. However, the potential problems with attenuation correction based on CT transmission data are somewhat different from conventional transmission scanning. Artifacts due to dental metalwork such as nonremovable metal dentures, bridgework, and fillings can look different from the artifacts generated with conventional transmission scanning and can appear more evident.[67,68] Furthermore, artifacts on the CT image can reduce the quality of the co-registered PET/CT images. Although artifacts mimic FDG uptake, it has been shown that artifacts do not prevent identification of the primary tumor.[71]

The CT data of a PET/CT scan can also be used for radiation treatment planning and the PET data help to better define the target volume. To date, few studies report on the use of FDG PET and PET/CT to improve radiation therapy.[111,112] If the CT scan is used for planning, the patient has to be positioned in exactly the same way as for the radiation treatment and the CT scan has to be acquired with a sufficiently high value for the product of tube current × exposure time (in milliamp seconds, mAs) to reliably calculate the attenuation values. To date, more studies are needed to evaluate the effects PET/CT-based radiation therapy planning on local cancer control and patient outcome. In Plate 11A.2 a case of whole-body PET/CT for staging and planning of the radiation field is shown.

POSITRON EMISSION TOMOGRAPHY AND LYMPH NODE METASTASES FROM AN UNKNOWN PRIMARY

The cervical lymph nodes are a common site for the manifestation of a carcinoma of an unknown primary.[113,114] Histologic analysis of such metastases predominantly reveals squamous cell carcinoma (SCC) followed by adenocarcinoma.[115]

A metastasis of an unknown primary was defined by Abbruzzese et al. in 1995 as a biopsy-confirmed malignancy for which the site of origin was not identified by routine clinical work-up.[116] However, to date no consensus has been established on how a routine clinical work-up should be done in patients with a neck metastasis from an unknown primary tumor. This is one reason for the reported differences in detection rate of an unknown primary with true positive findings in between 8 and 45% of patients.[117–121] In most publications patients with various histologies, such as squamous cell carcinoma, adenocarcinoma, large-cell carcinoma, melanoma, plasmocytoma, and other nondefined or undifferentiated cancers were included. In a patient with a metastasis from an SCC the primary is located more likely in the head and neck itself, while patients with a metastasis from an adenocarcinoma more often have a primary in the thorax or abdomen. Furthermore, if the upper jugular lymph nodes are involved it is more likely that the primary is located in the head neck region and tumors from the abdomen spread more often to lymph nodes in the lower neck such as Virchow's lymph node. The work-up of the patient should thus be adapted to the histology and the localization of the lymph node metastasis.[122]

In the case of SCC, the primary tumor has to be thoroughly searched for in the entire upper aerodigestive tract, since the detection of the primary site has great impact on the treatment and the prognosis of the patient. This allows identification of the primary in up to 50% of cases.[123]

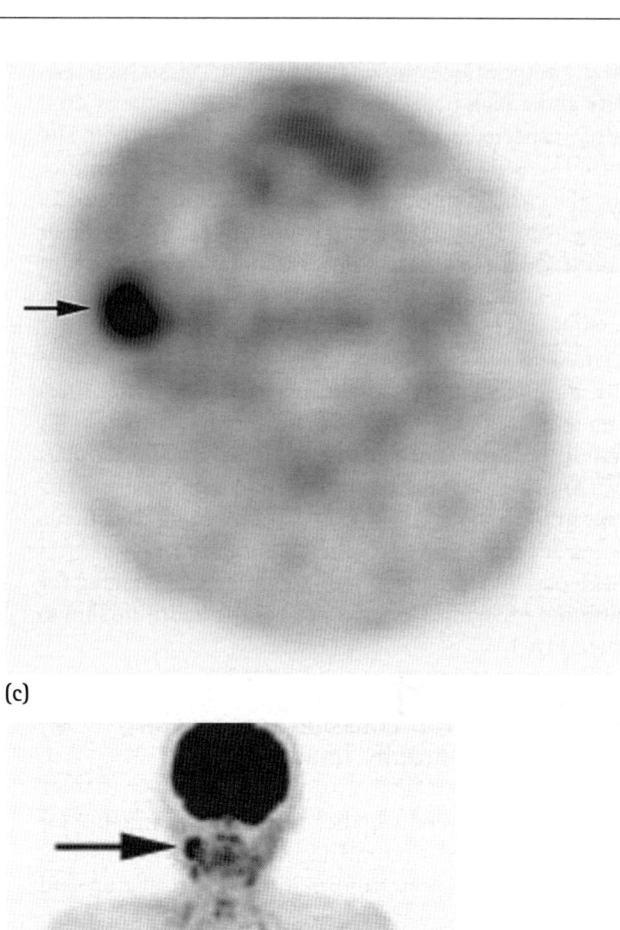

(a)

(c)

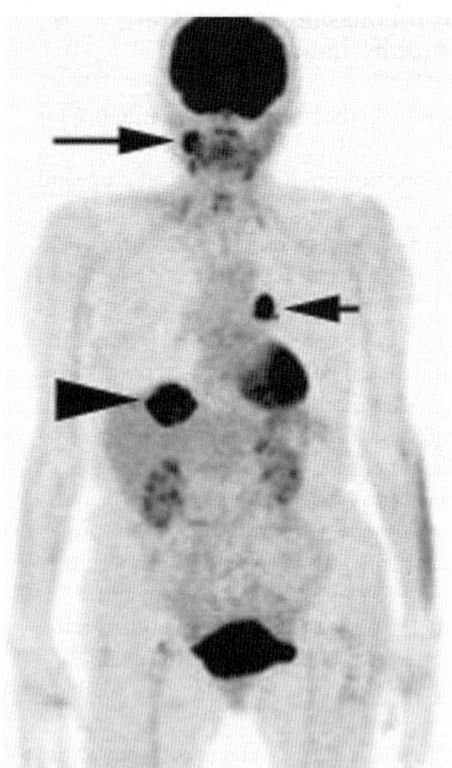

(b)

(d)

Figure 11A.3 *The clinical case history. PET coronal maximum intensity projection image (MIP) and two transverse images at the level of the primary tumor and a lymph node metastasis (arrows) in a 67-year-old female patient (staging PET) (a, b, and c). This woman had a clinical T4 head and neck squamous cell carcinoma with high uptake of fluorodeoxyglucose (FDG) at the cheek with extension to the mandibular angle and invasion of the bone and adjacent pterygoid muscle. The ipsilateral solitary lymph node (arrows) corresponds to an N1 situation. No distant metastases were found. The patient underwent radiation treatment with concomitant chemotherapy (62 Gy with cisplatin) and then a resection of the tumor with neck dissection of the ipsilateral side was performed.*

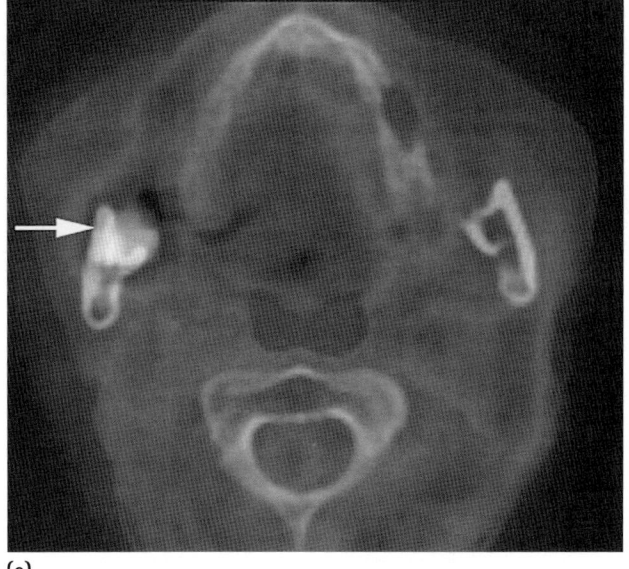

(e)

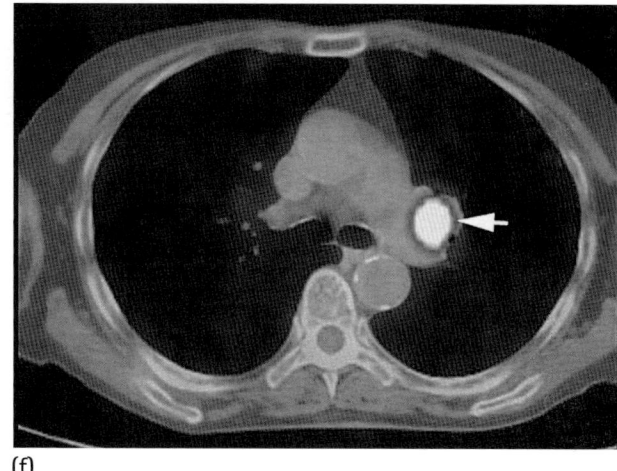

(f)

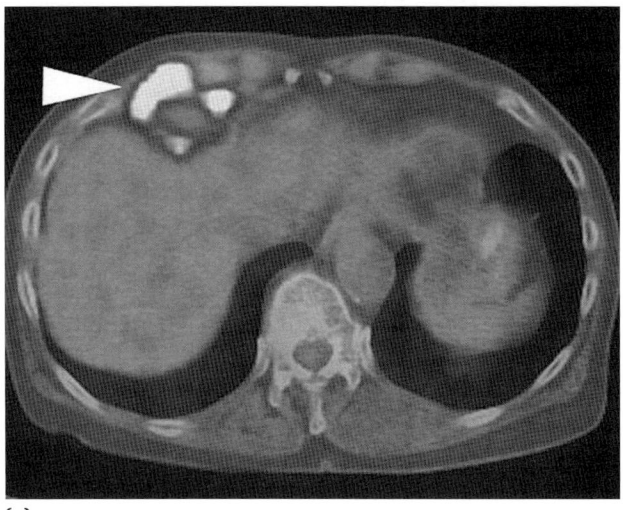

(g)

Figure 11A.3 *(Continued)   A partial resection of the lower jaw with reconstruction using a combined technique with radial flap and osteosynthesis and pectoral flap to cover the defect was performed. After 18 months a local recurrence was suggested and the patient underwent PET/CT scanning for restaging (d to g). On the MIP image (d), the local recurrence (long arrow), a hilar lesion (short arrow), and a lung metastasis in projection on the liver are visible (arrowhead). The transverse co-registered PET/CT images make it easy to delineate the metastases and to identify bone invasion of the local recurrence (e to g). See also Plate 11A.1 for color versions of parts (e) to (g).*

During endoscopic procedures clinically and radiologically inapparent primary SCC are most often found hidden in the tonsilar fossa, in the nasopharynx or the pyriform sinus.[118,124] In a patient who has already undergone a work-up with clinical evaluation, morphological imaging or panendoscopy the performance of FDG PET will likely be worse than in a patient where PET is done at the beginning of the work-up.[122] It has therefore been suggested that PET could be a good first line imaging tool before more invasive procedures such as panendoscopy under anesthesia are performed.[122] However, an important advantage of PET is the ability to provide whole-body imaging in patients where a primary in the thorax or abdomen is more likely.

SENTINEL NODE SCINTIGRAPHY IN HEAD AND NECK SQUAMOUS CELL CARCINOMA

In patients with evident lymph node metastases it will be easier to decide on further surgical or radiation therapy than in patients with equivocal findings. Many studies have described the distribution of metastatic spread depending on the primary site and stage of disease.[125–128] Because imaging methods cannot identify micrometastases, one can never be sure that a clinical N0 neck would remain negative if the patient underwent neck dissection and the pathological specimen was carefully analyzed. It has been shown that neck dissection performed in patients with clinical N0 neck reveals lymph node metastases in more than 30%.[124]

In this situation sentinel lymph node (SLN) scintigraphy can identify nodes draining a particular site in an individual patient in order to guide a surgical procedure and to describe patterns of unusual lymphatic flow. SLN scintigraphy is a relatively cheap and available method and has also been used for cutaneous melanomas of the head and neck and thyroid tumors.[129,130] The radiotracer is injected superficially around the tumor and uptake in the SLN is visible within minutes (Fig. 11A.4).[131] The SLN can be visualized by immediate gamma camera images to document the first visualized node. A delay between the injection and

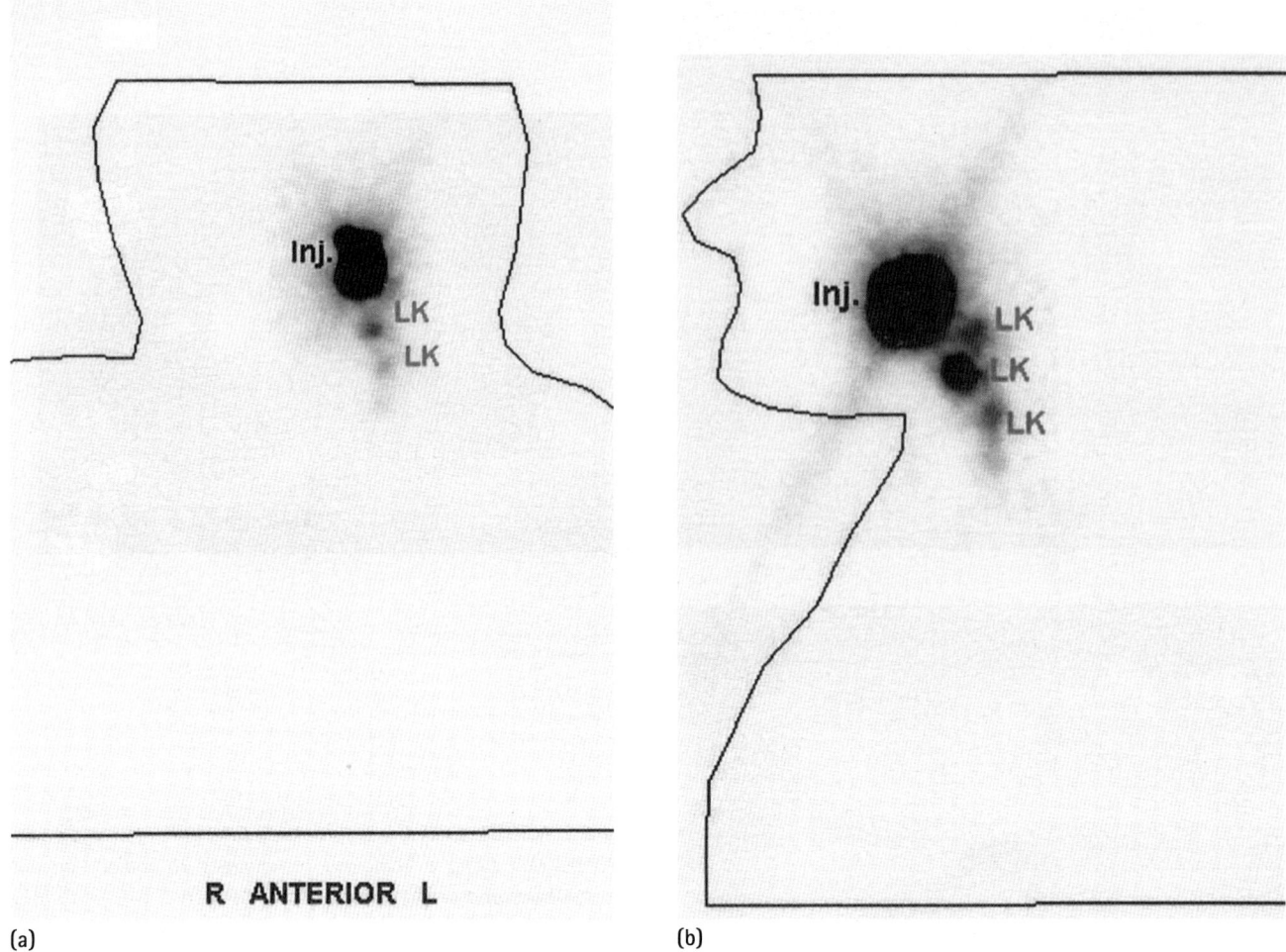

(a)   R ANTERIOR L

(b)

Figure 11A.4 *Sentinel node scintigraphy in AP and left lateral projection of a 57-year-old female patient with a clinical T1N0 oropharyngeal carcinoma. On the planar images several ipsilateral lymph nodes are visualized, but an angular lymph node (level II) was the first visible on sequential images. Four lymph nodes were resected and histological work-up did not reveal cancer. A neck dissection was not performed. LK = lymph node.*

scintigraphy (or the beginning of surgery) will influence the number of identified lymph nodes. Therefore, some authors perform intra-operative injection and in some centers a combination of blue dye and radioactive colloid will be injected. The combination of both markers increases sensitivity and specificity, because some nodes will become blue but not radioactive and vice versa.[132–134]

A limitation of the SLN concept is the possibility of soft tissue metastases in the neck without evident relationship to a lymph node. Soft tissue deposits can be found in neck dissection specimens of patients with a clinical N0 neck.[135,136] Furthermore, metastases may spread to another lymph node than the one identified as SLN. Such skip metastases have previously been described in HNSCC.[137]

However, this technique is promising in patients with a unilateral primary and N0 neck, in patients with a primary in the midline and bilateral N0 or only unilateral N-positive neck. The labeling of the SLN allows for an intra-operative search, guided by a gamma probe, thus limiting the surgical procedure to the relevant site of disease. When performing

a fast histological work-up the decision to continue with neck dissection can be done intra-operatively. If no metastatic involvement is found, the surgeon could stop. This decreases the morbidity as a consequence of a more extensive surgical procedure which will only be done when the SLN is affected by tumor. Another possibility would be to first perform a minimally invasive procedure to excise the SLN, then histologically evaluate the specimen using serial sectioning and immunohistochemistry and in a second intervention perform the neck dissection, if necessary. In a recent study SLN evaluation in patients with clinically N0 neck was compared with the ability of PET to identify lymph node metastases.[92] The SLN concept was superior to FDG PET because micrometastases can be detected using this approach as shown also by others.[138] The overall sensitivity of the SLN procedure is 90% as reported at the Second International Conference on Sentinel Node Biopsy in Mucosal Head and Neck Cancer (Zurich, Switzerland, 12–13 September 2003). The SLN technique is still under investigation and studies to validate the impact on clinical outcome of patients with HNSCC are under way.[139] Further studies are needed to determine whether the concept of SLN biopsy is as accurate as neck dissection in patients with N0 neck and if this technique is cost-effective in clinical routine.[140] Because this method is relatively new, it has been recommended that SLN biopsy is performed within the context of clinical trials.[92,133]

REFERENCES

● Seminal primary article
◆ Key review paper

1 Decker J, Goldstein JC. Risk factors in head and neck cancer. *N Engl J Med* 1982; **306**: 1151–5.

2 Vokes EE, Weichselbaum RR, Lippman SM, Hong WK. Head and neck cancer. *N Engl J Med* 1993; **328**: 184–94.

3 Hoffman HT, Karnell LH, Funk GF, *et al.* The National Cancer Data Base report on cancer of the head and neck. *Arch Otolaryngol Head Neck Surg* 1998; **124**: 951–62.

● 4 Forastiere AA, Goepfert H, Maor M, *et al.* Concurrent chemotherapy and radiotherapy for organ preservation in advanced laryngeal cancer. *N Engl J Med* 2003; **349**: 2091–8.

5 van den Brekel MW, Castelijns JA, Stel HV, *et al.* Occult metastatic neck disease: detection with US and US-guided fine-needle aspiration cytology. *Radiology* 1991; **180**: 457–61.

◆ 6 van den Brekel MW, Castelijns JA, Snow GB. Imaging of cervical lymphadenopathy. *Neuroimaging Clin N Am* 1996; **6**: 417–34.

7 AJCC. American Joint Committee on Cancer. *Cancer staging handbook.* New York: Springer, 2002.

8 Calhoun KH, Fulmer P, Weiss R, Hokanson JA. Distant metastases from head and neck squamous cell carcinomas. *Laryngoscope* 1994; **104**: 1199–205.

9 Troell RJ, Terris DJ. Detection of metastases from head and neck cancers. *Laryngoscope* 1995; **105**(3 Pt 1): 247–50.

10 Goerres GW, Schmid DT, Gratz KW, *et al.* Impact of whole body positron emission tomography on initial staging and therapy in patients with squamous cell carcinoma of the oral cavity. *Oral Oncol* 2003; **39**: 547–51.

11 ARSAC. Administration of Radioactive Substances Advisory Committee. Notes for guidance on the clinical administration of radiopharmaceuticals and use of unsealed radioactive sources. *Nucl Med Commun* 2000: Supplement.

● 12 Cox PH, Belfer AJ, van der Pompe WB. Thallium 201 chloride uptake in tumours, a possible complication in heart scintigraphy. *Br J Radiol* 1976; **49**: 767–8.

● 13 el-Gazzar AH, Sahweil A, Abdel-Dayem HM, *et al.* Experience with thallium-201 imaging in head and neck cancer. *Clin Nucl Med* 1988; **13**: 286–90.

14 Togawa T, Yui N, Kinoshita F, *et al.* Visualization of nasopharyngeal carcinoma with Tl-201 chloride and a three-head rotating gamma camera SPECT system. *Ann Nucl Med* 1993; **7**: 105–13.

15 Gregor RT, Valdes-Olmos R, Koops W, *et al.* Preliminary experience with thallous chloride T1 201-labeled single-photon emission computed tomography scanning in head and neck cancer. *Arch Otolaryngol Head Neck Surg* 1996; **122**: 509–14.

16 Valdes Olmos RA, Balm AJ, Hilgers FJ, *et al.* Thallium-201 SPECT in the diagnosis of head and neck cancer. *J Nucl Med* 1997; **38**: 873–9.

17 Mukherji SK, Gapany M, Phillips D, *et al.* Thallium-201 single-photon emission CT versus CT for the detection of recurrent squamous cell carcinoma of the head and neck. *Am J Neuroradiol* 1999; **20**: 1215–20.

18 Mukherji SK, Drane WE, Tart RP, *et al.* Comparison of thallium-201 and F-18 FDG SPECT uptake in squamous cell carcinoma of the head and neck. *Am J Neuroradiol* 1994; **15**: 1837–42.

19 Guney E, Yigitbasi OG, Tutus A, *et al.* Value of thallium-201 scintigraphy for primary tumour detection in patients with malignant neck masses. *Eur J Nucl Med* 1998; **25**: 431–4.

20 Yigitbasi OG, Tutus A, Bozdemir K, *et al.* 201Tl imaging for differentiating between malignant and benign neck masses. *Nucl Med Commun* 1998; **19**: 555–60.

21 Edeling CJ. Observations on the sequential use of Tc-99m phosphonate and Ga-67 imaging in untreated primary and secondary malignant tumors of the head and neck. *Clin Nucl Med* 1983; **8**: 107–111.

● 22 Poublon RM. Evaluation of head and neck tumours before and after radiotherapy of 40 Gy using gallium-67-citrate. A pilot study. *Clin Otolaryngol* 1982; **7**: 181–4.

23 Murata Y, Ishida R, Umehara I, *et al.* 67Ga whole-body scintigraphy in the evaluation of head and neck squamous cell carcinoma. *Nucl Med Commun* 1999; **20**: 599–607.

24 Onizawa K, Yoshida H. Evaluation of 67Ga citrate and 99mTc bone scintigraphy at initial examination for primary oral squamous cell carcinoma. *J Oral Maxillofac Surg* 2003; **61**: 913–7.

25 Kitagawa Y, Nishizawa S, Sano K, *et al.* Prospective comparison of 18F-FDG PET with conventional imaging modalities (MRI, CT, and 67Ga scintigraphy) in assessment of combined intraarterial chemotherapy and radiotherapy for head and neck carcinoma. *J Nucl Med* 2003; **44**: 198–206.

26 Piwnica-Worms D, Rao VV, Kronauge JF, Croop JM. Characterization of multidrug resistance P-glycoprotein transport function with an

organotechnetium cation. *Biochemistry* 1995; **34**: 12210–20.

27 Piwnica-Worms D, Chiu ML, Budding M, *et al.* Functional imaging of multidrug-resistant P-glycoprotein with an organotechnetium complex. *Cancer Res* 1993; **53**: 977–84.

♦ 28 Ballinger JR, Sheldon KM, Boxen I, *et al.* Differences between accumulation of ^{99m}Tc-MIBI and ^{201}Tl-thallous chloride in tumour cells: role of P-glycoprotein. *Q J Nucl Med* 1995; **39**: 122–8.

29 Shen YY, Kao CH, Changlai SP, *et al.* Detection of nasopharyngeal carcinoma with head and neck Tc-99m tetrofosmin SPECT imaging. *Clin Nucl Med* 1998; **23**: 305–8.

30 Kao CH, Wang SJ, Lin WY, *et al.* Detection of nasopharyngeal carcinoma using ^{99m}Tc-methoxy-isobutylisonitrile SPECT. *Nucl Med Commun* 1993; **14**: 41–6.

31 Weng YC, Yen RF, Tsai MH, *et al.* Detection of recurrent nasopharyngeal carcinomas after radiotherapy with technetium-99m tetrofosmin single photon emission computed tomography in patients with indeterminate magnetic resonance imaging findings. *Cancer Invest* 2003; **21**: 695–700.

32 Tai CJ, Liu FY, Liang JA, *et al.* Detection of cervical lymph node metastases in nasopharyngeal carcinomas: comparison with technetium-99m tetrofosmin single photon emission computed tomography and with magnetic resonance imaging. *Anticancer Res* 2003; **23(1B)**: 719–22.

33 Wang SJ, Hsu CY, Lin WY, *et al.* Comparison of Tl-201 and Tc-99m MIBI SPECT imaging in nasopharyngeal carcinoma. *Clin Nucl Med* 1995; **20**: 800–2.

● 34 Kostakoglu L, Uysal U, Ozyar E, *et al.* A comparative study of technetium-99m sestamibi and technetium-99m tetrofosmin single-photon tomography in the detection of nasopharyngeal carcinoma. *Eur J Nucl Med* 1997; **24**: 621–8.

● 35 Kao CH, Tsai SC, Wang JJ, *et al.* Comparing 18-fluoro-2-deoxyglucose positron emission tomography with a combination of technetium-99m tetrofosmin single photon emission computed tomography and computed tomography to detect recurrent or persistent nasopharyngeal carcinomas after radiotherapy. *Cancer* 2001; **92**: 434–9.

36 Shiau YC, Tsai SC, Ho YJ, Kao CH. Comparison of technetium-99m methoxyisobutylisonitrile single photon emission computed tomography and computed tomography to detect recurrent or residual nasopharyngeal carcinomas after radiotherapy. *Anticancer Res* 2001; **21(3C)**: 2213–7.

● 37 Kao CH, Shiau YC, Shen YY, Yen RF. Detection of recurrent or persistent nasopharyngeal carcinomas after radiotherapy with technetium-99m methoxy-isobutylisonitrile single photon emission computed tomography and computed tomography: comparison

with 18-fluoro-2-deoxyglucose positron emission tomography. *Cancer* 2002; **94**: 1981–6.

38 Ohta H, Endo K, Fujita T, *et al.* Imaging of head and neck tumors with technetium(V)-99m DMSA. A new tumor-seeking agent. *Clin Nucl Med* 1985; **10**: 855–60.

● 39 Watkinson JC, Allen S, Higgins M, *et al.* Subcellular biodistribution of [99m]Tc[m](V) DMSA in squamous carcinoma: a comparative study in humans and in an animal tumour model. *Nucl Med Commun* 1990; **11**: 547–55.

40 Watkinson JC, Lazarus CR, Todd C, *et al.* Metastatic squamous carcinoma in the neck: an anatomical and physiological study using CT and SPECT [99m]Tc[m] (V) DMSA. *Br J Radiol* 1991; **64**: 909–14.

41 Timon CI, McShane D, Hamilton D, Walsh MA. Head and neck cancer localization with indium labelled carcinoembryonic antigen: a pilot project. *J Otolaryngol* 1991; **20**: 283–7.

● 42 de Bree R, Roos JC, Quak JJ, *et al.* Radioimmunoscintigraphy and biodistribution of technetium-99m-labeled monoclonal antibody U36 in patients with head and neck cancer. *Clin Cancer Res* 1995; **1**: 591–8.

43 de Bree R, Roos JC, Verel I, *et al.* Radioimmunodiagnosis of lymph node metastases in head and neck cancer. *Oral Dis* 2003; **9**: 241–8.

● 44 Baum RP, Adams S, Kiefer J, *et al.* A novel technetium-99m labeled monoclonal antibody (174H.64) for staging head and neck cancer by immuno-SPECT. *Acta Oncol* 1993; **32**: 747–51.

● 45 van Dongen GA, Leverstein H, Roos JC, *et al.* Radioimmunoscintigraphy of head and neck cancer using ^{99m}Tc-labeled monoclonal antibody E48 F(ab′)2. *Cancer Res* 1992; **52**: 2569–74.

46 Adamietz IA, Baum RP, Schemman F, *et al.* Improvement of radiation treatment planning in squamous-cell head and neck cancer by immuno-SPECT. *J Nucl Med* 1996; **37**: 1942–6.

47 Colnot DR, Quak JJ, Roos JC, *et al.* Radioimmunotherapy in patients with head and neck squamous cell carcinoma: initial experience. *Head Neck* 2001; **23**: 559–65.

● 48 Postema EJ, Borjesson PK, Buijs WC, *et al.* Dosimetric analysis of radioimmunotherapy with [186]Re-labeled bivatuzumab in patients with head and neck cancer. *J Nucl Med* 2003; **44**: 1690–9.

● 49 Macfarlane DJ, Shulkin BL, Murphy K, Wolf GT. FDG PET imaging of paragangliomas of the neck: comparison with MIBG SPET. *Eur J Nucl Med* 1995; **22**: 1347–50.

50 Mandigers CM, van Gils AP, Derksen J, *et al.* Carcinoid tumor of the jugulo-tympanic region. *J Nucl Med* 1996; **37**: 270–2.

51 Muros MA, Llamas-Elvira JM, Rodriguez A, *et al.* ^{111}In-pentetreotide scintigraphy is superior to ^{123}I-MIBG scintigraphy in the diagnosis and location of chemodectoma. *Nucl Med Commun* 1998; **19**: 735–42.

52 Duet M, Sauvaget E, Petelle B, *et al*. Clinical impact of somatostatin receptor scintigraphy in the management of paragangliomas of the head and neck. *J Nucl Med* 2003; **44**: 1767–74.

53 Waldherr C, Pless M, Maecke HR, *et al*. The clinical value of [^{90}Y-DOTA]-D-Phe^1-Tyr^3-octreotide (^{90}Y-DOTATOC) in the treatment of neuroendocrine tumours: a clinical phase II study. *Ann Oncol* 2001; **12**: 941–5.

54 Ishiwata K, Kubota K, Murakami M, *et al*. Re-evaluation of amino acid PET studies: can the protein synthesis rates in brain and tumor tissues be measured in vivo? *J Nucl Med* 1993; **34**: 1936–43.

55 Kole AC, Pruim J, Nieweg OE, *et al*. PET with L-[1-carbon-11]-tyrosine to visualize tumors and measure protein synthesis rates. *J Nucl Med* 1997; **38**: 191–5.

56 de Boer JR, van der Laan BF, Pruim J, *et al*. Carbon-11 tyrosine PET for visualization and protein synthesis rate assessment of laryngeal and hypopharyngeal carcinomas. *Eur J Nucl Med* 2002; **29**: 1182–7.

57 De Boer JR, Pruim J, Burlage F, *et al*. Therapy evaluation of laryngeal carcinomas by tyrosine-PET. *Head Neck* 2003; **25**: 634–44.

58 Braams JW, Pruim J, Nikkels PG, *et al*. Nodal spread of squamous cell carcinoma of the oral cavity detected with PET-tyrosine, MRI and CT. *J Nucl Med* 1996; **37**: 897–901.

59 Shields AF, Coonrod DV, Quackenbush RC, Crowley JJ. Cellular sources of thymidine nucleotides: studies for PET. *J Nucl Med* 1987; **28**: 1435–40.

60 Koh WJ, Rasey JS, Evans ML, *et al*. Imaging of hypoxia in human tumors with [F-18]fluoromisonidazole. *Int J Radiat Oncol Biol Phys* 1992; **22**: 199–212.

61 Chao KS, Bosch WR, Mutic S, *et al*. A novel approach to overcome hypoxic tumor resistance: Cu-ATSM-guided intensity-modulated radiation therapy. *Int J Radiat Oncol Biol Phys* 2001; **49**: 1171–82.

62 Minn H, Joensuu H, Ahonen A, Klemi P. Fluorodeoxyglucose imaging: a method to assess the proliferative activity of human cancer *in vivo*. Comparison with DNA flow cytometry in head and neck tumors. *Cancer* 1988; **61**: 1776–81.

63 Reisser C, Eichhorn K, Herold-Mende C, *et al*. Expression of facilitative glucose transport proteins during development of squamous cell carcinomas of the head and neck. *Int J Cancer* 1999; **80**: 194–8.

64 Reisser C, Haberkorn U, Strauss LG. [Diagnosis of energy metabolism in ENT tumors – a PET study]. *HNO* 1992; **40**: 225–31.

65 Minn H, Lapela M, Klemi PJ, *et al*. Prediction of survival with fluorine-18-fluoro-deoxyglucose and PET in head and neck cancer. *J Nucl Med* 1997; **38**: 1907–11.

66 Lindholm P, Minn H, Leskinen-Kallio S, *et al*. Influence of the blood glucose concentration on FDG uptake in cancer – a PET study. *J Nucl Med* 1993; **34**: 1–6.

67 Goerres GW, Hany TF, Kamel E, *et al*. Head and neck imaging with PET and PET/CT: artefacts from dental metallic implants. *Eur J Nucl Med* 2002; **29**: 367–70.

68 Kamel EM, Burger C, Buck A, *et al*. Impact of metallic dental implants on CT-based attenuation correction in a combined PET/CT scanner. *Eur Radiol* 2003; **13**: 724–8.

69 Bailet JW, Abemayor E, Jabour BA, *et al*. Positron emission tomography: a new, precise imaging modality for detection of primary head and neck tumors and assessment of cervical adenopathy. *Laryngoscope* 1992; **102**: 281–8.

70 Wong WL, Chevretton EB, McGurk M, *et al*. A prospective study of PET-FDG imaging for the assessment of head and neck squamous cell carcinoma. *Clin Otolaryngol* 1997; **22**: 209–14.

71 Goerres GW, Eyrich GK. Do hardware artefacts influence the performance of head and neck PET scans in patients with oral cavity squamous cell cancer? *Dentomaxillofac Radiol* 2003; **32**: 365–71.

72 McGuirt WF, Greven KM, Keyes Jr JW, *et al*. Positron emission tomography in the evaluation of laryngeal carcinoma. *Ann Otol Rhinol Laryngol* 1995; **104(4 Pt 1)**: 274–8.

73 Kau RJ, Alexiou C, Laubenbacher C, *et al*. Lymph node detection of head and neck squamous cell carcinomas by positron emission tomography with fluorodeoxyglucose F 18 in a routine clinical setting. *Arch Otolaryngol Head Neck Surg* 1999; **125**: 1322–8.

74 Keyes Jr JW, Watson Jr NE, Williams 3rd DW, *et al*. FDG PET in head and neck cancer. *Am J Roentgenol* 1997; **169**: 1663–9.

75 Kostakoglu L, Wong JC, Barrington SF, *et al*. Speech-related visualization of laryngeal muscles with fluorine-18-FDG. *J Nucl Med* 1996; **37**: 1771–3.

76 Myers JN, Greenberg JS, Mo V, Roberts D. Extracapsular spread. A significant predictor of treatment failure in patients with squamous cell carcinoma of the tongue. *Cancer* 2001; **92**: 3030–6.

77 Laubenbacher C, Saumweber D, Wagner-Manslau C, *et al*. Comparison of fluorine-18-fluorodeoxyglucose PET, MRI and endoscopy for staging head and neck squamous-cell carcinomas. *J Nucl Med* 1995; **36**: 1747–57.

78 McGuirt WF, Williams 3rd DW, Keyes Jr JW, *et al*. A comparative diagnostic study of head and neck nodal metastases using positron emission tomography. *Laryngoscope* 1995; **105(4 Pt 1)**: 373–5.

79 Jabour BA, Choi Y, Hoh CK, *et al*. Extracranial head and neck: PET imaging with 2-[F-18]fluoro-2-deoxy-D-glucose and MR imaging correlation. *Radiology* 1993; **186**: 27–35.

80 Braams JW, Pruim J, Freling NJ, *et al*. Detection of lymph node metastases of squamous-cell cancer of the head and neck with FDG-PET and MRI. *J Nucl Med* 1995; **36**: 211–6.

81　Benchaou M, Lehmann W, Slosman DO, *et al.* The role of FDG-PET in the preoperative assessment of N-staging in head and neck cancer. *Acta Otolaryngol* 1996; **116**: 332–5.

82　Adams S, Baum RP, Stuckensen T, *et al.* Prospective comparison of ^{18}F-FDG PET with conventional imaging modalities (CT, MRI, US) in lymph node staging of head and neck cancer. *Eur J Nucl Med* 1998; **25**: 1255–60.

83　Nowak B, Di Martinbo E, Janicke S, *et al.* Diagnostic evaluation of malignant head and neck cancer by F-18-FDG PET compared to CT/MRI. *Nuklearmedizin* 1999; **38**: 312–8.

84　Di Martino E, Nowak B, Hassan HA, *et al.* Diagnosis and staging of head and neck cancer: a comparison of modern imaging modalities (positron emission tomography, computed tomography, color-coded duplex sonography) with panendoscopic and histopathologic findings. *Arch Otolaryngol Head Neck Surg* 2000; **126**: 1457–61.

85　Stuckensen T, Kovacs AF, Adams S, Baum RP. Staging of the neck in patients with oral cavity squamous cell carcinomas: a prospective comparison of PET, ultrasound, CT and MRI. *J Craniomaxillofac Surg* 2000; **28**: 319–24.

86　Bui CD, Ching AS, Carlos RC, *et al.* Diagnostic accuracy of 2-[fluorine-18]fluoro-2-deoxy-D-glucose positron emission tomography imaging in nonsquamous tumors of the head and neck. *Invest Radiol* 2003; **38**: 593–601.

87　Greven KM, Williams 3rd DW, Keyes Jr JW, *et al.* Positron emission tomography of patients with head and neck carcinoma before and after high dose irradiation. *Cancer* 1994; **74**: 1355–9.

88　Conessa C, Clement P, Foehrenbach H, *et al.* [Value of positron-emission tomography in the post-treatment follow-up of epidermoid carcinoma of the head and neck]. *Rev Laryngol Otol Rhinol (Bord)* 2001; **122**: 253–8.

♦ 89　Goerres GW, Schmid DT, Bandhauer F, *et al.* Positron emission tomography in the early follow-up of advanced head and neck cancer. *Arch Otolaryngol Head Neck Surg* 2004; **130**: 105–9; discussion 120–1.

90　Goerres GW, Von Schulthess GK, Hany TF. Positron emission tomography and PET CT of the head and neck: FDG uptake in normal anatomy, in benign lesions, and in changes resulting from treatment. *Am J Roentgenol* 2002; **179**: 1337–43.

● 91　Myers LL, Wax MK. Positron emission tomography in the evaluation of the negative neck in patients with oral cavity cancer. *J Otolaryngol* 1998; **27**: 342–7.

92　Stoeckli SJ, Steinert H, Pfaltz M, Schmid S. Is there a role for positron emission tomography with ^{18}F-fluorodeoxyglucose in the initial staging of nodal negative oral and oropharyngeal squamous cell carcinoma. *Head Neck* 2002; **24**: 345–9.

● 93　Leon X, Quer M, Diez S, *et al.* Second neoplasm in patients with head and neck cancer. *Head Neck* 1999; **21**: 204–10.

94　Stokkel MP, Moons KG, ten Broek FW, *et al.* ^{18}F-fluorodeoxyglucose dual-head positron emission tomography as a procedure for detecting simultaneous primary tumors in cases of head and neck cancer. *Cancer* 1999; **86**: 2370–7.

95　Keyes Jr JW, Chen MY, Watson Jr NE, *et al.* FDG PET evaluation of head and neck cancer: value of imaging the thorax. *Head Neck* 2000; **22**: 105–10.

96　de Bree R, Deurloo EE, Snow GB, Leemans CR. Screening for distant metastases in patients with head and neck cancer. *Laryngoscope* 2000; **110(3 Pt 1)**: 397–401.

97　Kitagawa Y, Nishizawa S, Sano K, *et al.* Whole-body (18)F-fluorodeoxyglucose positron emission tomography in patients with head and neck cancer. *Oral Surg Oral Med Oral Pathol Oral Radiol Endod* 2002; **93**: 202–7.

● 98　Schwartz DL, Rajendran J, Yueh B, *et al.* Staging of head and neck squamous cell cancer with extended-field FDG-PET. *Arch Otolaryngol Head Neck Surg* 2003; **129**: 1173–8.

99　Lapela M, Grenman R, Kurki T, *et al.* Head and neck cancer: detection of recurrence with PET and 2-[F-18]fluoro-2-deoxy-D-glucose. *Radiology* 1995; **197**: 205–11.

● 100　Fischbein NJ, Assar OS, Caputo GR, *et al.* Clinical utility of positron emission tomography with ^{18}F-fluorodeoxyglucose in detecting residual/recurrent squamous cell carcinoma of the head and neck. *Am J Neuroradiol* 1998; **19**: 1189–96.

101　Greven KM, Williams 3rd DW, Keyes Jr JW, *et al.* Can positron emission tomography distinguish tumor recurrence from irradiation sequelae in patients treated for larynx cancer? *Cancer J Sci Am* 1997; **3**: 353–7.

102　Kao CH, ChangLai SP, Chieng PU, *et al.* Detection of recurrent or persistent nasopharyngeal carcinomas after radiotherapy with 18-fluoro-2-deoxyglucose positron emission tomography and comparison with computed tomography. *J Clin Oncol* 1998; **16**: 3550–5.

103　Mitsuhashi N, Hayakawa K, Hasegawa M, *et al.* Clinical FDG-PET in diagnosis and evaluation of radiation response of patients with nasopharyngeal tumor. *Anticancer Res* 1998; **18(4B)**: 2827–32.

104　Farber LA, Benard F, Machtay M, *et al.* Detection of recurrent head and neck squamous cell carcinomas after radiation therapy with 2-^{18}F-fluoro-2-deoxy-D-glucose positron emission tomography. *Laryngoscope* 1999; **109**: 970–5.

105 Haenggeli CA, Dulguerov P, Slosman D, *et al.* [Value of positron emission tomography with 18-fluorodeoxyglucose (FDG-PET) in early detection of residual tumor in oro-pharyngeal-laryngeal carcinoma]. *Schweiz Med Wochenschr Suppl* 2000; **116**: 8S–11S.

106 Lonneux M, Lawson G, Ide C, *et al.* Positron emission tomography with fluorodeoxyglucose for suspected head and neck tumor recurrence in the symptomatic patient. *Laryngoscope* 2000; **110**: 1493–7.

107 Chisin R, Pietrzyk U, Sichel JY, *et al.* Registration and display of multimodal images: applications in the extracranial head and neck region. *J Otolaryngol* 1993; **22**: 214–9.

● 108 Wong WL, Hussain K, Chevretton E, *et al.* Validation and clinical application of computer-combined computed tomography and positron emission tomography with 2-[^{18}F]fluoro-2-deoxy-D-glucose head and neck images. *Am J Surg* 1996; **172**: 628–32.

● 109 Hany TF, Steinert HC, Goerres GW, *et al.* PET diagnostic accuracy: improvement with in-line PET-CT system: initial results. *Radiology* 2002; **225**: 575–81.

● 110 Burger C, Goerres G, Schoenes S, *et al.* PET attenuation coefficients from CT images: experimental evaluation of the transformation of CT into PET 511-keV attenuation coefficients. *Eur J Nucl Med* 2002; **29**: 922–7.

● 111 Dizendorf EV, Baumert BG, von Schulthess GK, *et al.* Impact of whole-body ^{18}F-FDG PET on staging and managing patients for radiation therapy. *J Nucl Med* 2003; **44**: 24–9.

112 Rahn AN, Baum RP, Adamietz IA, *et al.* [Value of ^{18}F fluorodeoxyglucose positron emission tomography in radiotherapy planning of head – neck tumors]. *Strahlenther Onkol* 1998; **174**: 358–64.

113 Wang RC, Goepfert H, Barber AE, Wolf P. Unknown primary squamous cell carcinoma metastatic to the neck. *Arch Otolaryngol Head Neck Surg* 1990; **116**: 1388–93.

114 Leipzig B, Winter ML, Hokanson JA. Cervical nodal metastases of unknown origin. *Laryngoscope* 1981; **91**: 593–8.

● 115 Nordstrom DG, Tewfik HH, Latourette HB. Cervical lymph node metastases from an unknown primary. *Int J Radiat Oncol Biol Phys* 1979; **5**: 73–6.

116 Abbruzzese JL, Abbruzzese MC, Lenzi R, *et al.* Analysis of a diagnostic strategy for patients with suspected tumors of unknown origin. *J Clin Oncol* 1995; **13**: 2094–103.

117 Bohuslavizki KH, Klutmann S, Kroger S, *et al.* FDG PET detection of unknown primary tumors. *J Nucl Med* 2000; **41**: 816–22.

118 Mendenhall WM, Mancuso AA, Parsons JT, *et al.* Diagnostic evaluation of squamous cell carcinoma metastatic to cervical lymph nodes from an unknown head and neck primary site. *Head Neck* 1998; **20**: 739–44.

119 Kole AC, Nieweg OE, Pruim J, *et al.* Detection of unknown occult primary tumors using positron emission tomography. *Cancer* 1998; **82**: 1160–6.

120 Jungehulsing M, Scheidhauer K, Damm M, *et al.* 2-[^{18}F]fluoro-2-deoxy-D-glucose positron emission tomography is a sensitive tool for the detection of occult primary cancer (carcinoma of unknown primary syndrome) with head and neck lymph node manifestation. *Otolaryngol Head Neck Surg* 2000; **123**: 294–301.

121 Mukherji SK, Drane WE, Mancuso AA, *et al.* Occult primary tumors of the head and neck: detection with 2-[F-18] fluoro-2-deoxy-D-glucose SPECT. *Radiology* 1996; **199**: 761–6.

122 Stoeckli SJ, Mosna-Firlejczyk K, Goerres GW. Lymph node metastasis of squamous cell carcinoma from an unknown primary: impact of positron emission tomography. *Eur J Nucl Med* 2003; **30**: 411–6.

123 de Braud F, al-Sarraf M. Diagnosis and management of squamous cell carcinoma of unknown primary tumor site of the neck. *Semin Oncol* 1993; **20**: 273–8.

124 Jones AS, Phillips DE, Helliwell TR, Roland NJ. Occult node metastases in head and neck squamous carcinoma. *Eur Arch Otorhinolaryngol* 1993; **250**: 446–9.

125 Buckley JG, MacLennan K. Cervical node metastases in laryngeal and hypopharyngeal cancer: a prospective analysis of prevalence and distribution. *Head Neck* 2000; **22**: 380–5.

126 Mukherji SK, Armao D, Joshi VM. Cervical nodal metastases in squamous cell carcinoma of the head and neck: what to expect. *Head Neck* 2001; **23**: 995–1005.

127 Tomik J, Skladzien J, Modrzejewski M. Evaluation of cervical lymph node metastasis of 1400 patients with cancer of the larynx. *Auris Nasus Larynx* 2001; **28**: 233–40.

128 Shah JP. Patterns of cervical lymph node metastasis from squamous carcinomas of the upper aerodigestive tract. *Am J Surg* 1990; **160**: 405–9.

129 Davison SP, Clifton MS, Kauffman L, Minasian L. Sentinel node biopsy for the detection of head and neck melanoma: a review. *Ann Plast Surg* 2001; **47**: 206–11.

130 Dixon E, McKinnon JG, Pasieka JL. Feasibility of sentinel lymph node biopsy and lymphatic mapping in nodular thyroid neoplasms. *World J Surg* 2000; **24**: 1396–401.

131 Pitman KT, Ferlito A, Devaney KO, *et al.* Sentinel lymph node biopsy in head and neck cancer. *Oral Oncol* 2003; **39**: 343–9.

132 Pitman KT, Johnson JT, Brown ML, Myers EN. Sentinel lymph node biopsy in head and neck squamous cell carcinoma. *Laryngoscope* 2002; **112**: 2101–13.

133 Shoaib T, Soutar DS, Prosser JE, *et al.* A suggested method for sentinel node biopsy in squamous cell carcinoma of the head and neck. *Head Neck* 1999; **21**: 728–33.

134 Werner JA, Dunne AA, Ramaswamy A, *et al.* Sentinel node detection in N0 cancer of the pharynx and larynx. *Br J Cancer* 2002; **87**: 711–5.

135 Coatesworth AP, MacLennan K. Squamous cell carcinoma of the upper aerodigestive tract: the prevalence of microscopic extracapsular spread and soft tissue deposits in the clinically N0 neck. *Head Neck* 2002; **24**: 258–61.

◆ 136 Violaris NS, O'Neil D, Helliwell TR, *et al.* Soft tissue cervical metastases of squamous carcinoma of the head and neck. *Clin Otolaryngol* 1994; **19**: 394–9.

137 Ferlito A, Shaha AR, Rinaldo A, *et al.* 'Skip metastases' from head and neck cancers. *Acta Otolaryngol* 2002; **122**: 788–91.

138 Hyde NC, Prvulovich E, Newman L, *et al.* A new approach to pre-treatment assessment of the N0 neck in oral squamous cell carcinoma: the role of sentinel node biopsy and positron emission tomography. *Oral Oncol* 2003; **39**: 350–60.

139 Ross GL, Soutar DS, MacDonald DG, *et al.* Improved staging of cervical metastases in clinically node-negative patients with head and neck squamous cell carcinoma. *Ann Surg Oncol* 2004; **11**: 213–8.

140 Kosuda S, Kusano S, Kohno N, *et al.* Feasibility and cost-effectiveness of sentinel lymph node radiolocalization in stage N0 head and neck cancer. *Arch Otolaryngol Head Neck Surg* 2003; **129**: 1105–9.

Salivary pathology

GERHARD W. GOERRES

INTRODUCTION

The major salivary glands include the parotid and submandibular glands. They produce saliva to clean and protect the mouth and upper digestive tract. They excrete digestive enzymes, antibodies, heavy metals (and other poisonous substances), and iodine. The salivary gland concentrates pertechnetate, as do other organs, i.e. gastric mucosa, thyroid gland, and choroid plexus. Pertechnetate is excreted in saliva and therefore the excretion of saliva can be measured with dynamic imaging. The intravenous application of 40 MBq [^{99m}Tc]pertechnetate causes an effective dose of approximately 0.5 mSv and a dose to the uterus of 0.3 mGy.[1] Salivary gland scintigraphy is easily performed and well tolerated yielding quantitative parameters for parenchymal and excretory function. Scintigraphy is done in patients with pathologies involving the gland and the duct, such as suspected calculi, strictures, and sialectasia. Furthermore, the accumulation of pertechnetate in the glands and excretion after the administration of a sialogogue (lemon juice) can be disturbed in patients after radiation treatment of head and neck tumors. Other pathologies involving the salivary glands are infections/inflammations, tumors and systemic diseases disturbing function, such as mumps, sarcoidosis, and Sjögren's syndrome, all potentially causing xerostomy.

For the assessment of salivary gland pathologies ultrasound is performed and conventional radiography with or without application of contrast medium by a canula inserted into the salivary gland duct. Magnetic resonance imaging and computed tomography will be used in patients with malignant disease for the assessment of size and invasion into adjacent structures and better delineation of the pathology for therapy planning. In malignant salivary gland pathology fluorodeoxyglucose (FDG) positron emission tomography (PET) imaging has been used, too.

IMAGING OF SALIVARY GLAND FUNCTION

After the intravenous injection of pertechnetate the accumulation within the salivary glands can be seen and measured using dynamic planar AP images with the region of interest (ROI) in the area of both parotid and submandibular glands. After stimulation with lemon juice the activity in the ROI decreases as saliva is excreted. The normal pattern of the salivary gland scintigraphy shows adequate accumulation in all four glands with rapid clearance after lemon juice stimulation and a subsequent rise again (Plate 11B.1).

The salivary glands are very sensitive to radiation. Radiation sialadenitis causes tenderness of the salivary gland and dry mouth. Xerostomy is a common side-effect of radiation therapy and scintigraphy can be used for monitoring and documentation. Salivary glands that have been irradiated show an inadequate uptake and a reduced clearance of pertechnetate. Dysfunction of the salivary glands has also been described in patients undergoing combined radiation and chemotherapy.[2]

An increased uptake of gallium-67 citrate as a sign of inflammation has been described after radiation therapy which may persist for several years.[3] Additionally, in patients undergoing treatment with ^{131}I for thyroid cancer, xerostomy has been described as a side-effect in up to 12% of patients.[4] In this situation radiation exposure of the glands can be reduced by using foods that increase the flow of saliva. A recent study[5] has described a reduction of salivary gland parenchymal damage and xerostomy by amifostine, an organic thiophosphate. However, it is not clear if this treatment could influence the uptake of ^{131}I in the thyroid cancer itself.

A bilateral enlargement of the salivary glands is sometimes found in patients with inflammation, granulomatous disease, and diffuse neoplastic involvement (lymphoma/leukemia) but is preferably evaluated with ultrasound. It has been reported that in patients with Warthin's tumor a focally increased uptake can be found probably due to retention of the pertechnetate. This has also been described in oxyphilic adenoma.[6]

IMAGING OF SALIVARY GLAND TUMORS

Salivary gland tumors are a heterogeneous group of neoplasms with a wide spectrum of biological behavior. Most occur in the parotids, with over two thirds representing mixed or pleomorphic adenomas. The major prognostic factor is the histopathological type of the tumor.[7] Warthin's tumor is a benign proliferation of lymphoid cells (papillary cystadenoma lymphomatosum) often found bilaterally in smokers. Therefore Warthin's tumor shows very avid uptake of FDG.[8] The more common malignant tumors include mucoepidermoid carcinoma, adenocarcinoma, and squamous cell carcinoma. The reported experience with FDG PET indicates that PET cannot reliably distinguish between benign and malignant salivary gland lesions.[9] Keyes et al. were able to correctly identify only 18 of 26 salivary gland tumors (69%) since false positive readings were obtained in eight patients.[10] Primary salivary gland tumors can be missed because of physiologic FDG uptake in the glands. However, the uptake of FDG is related to the histology of the primary: adenoid cystic carcinoma shows low uptake while squamous cell carcinomas have an intense FDG accumulation.[11] Although the identification within the salivary gland is difficult, FDG PET based lymph node staging could be useful in tumors with a histology known to show high FDG uptake.

REFERENCES

● Seminal primary article

1 Administration of Radioactive Substances Advisory Committee. Notes for guidance on the clinical administration of radiopharmaceuticals and use of unsealed radioactive sources. *Nucl Med Commun* 2000; **Suppl**: S1–S95.

● 2 Kosuda S, Satoh M, Yamamoto F, *et al.* Assessment of salivary gland dysfunction following chemoradiotherapy using quantitative salivary gland scintigraphy. *Int J Radiat Oncol Biol Phys* 1999; **45**: 379–84.

● 3 Bekerman C, Hoffer PB. Salivary gland uptake of ^{67}Ga-citrate following radiation therapy. *J Nucl Med* 1976; **17**: 685–7.

● 4 Allweiss P, Braunstein GD, Katz A, Waxman A. Sialadenitis following I-131 therapy for thyroid carcinoma: concise communication. *J Nucl Med* 1984; **25**: 755–8.

● 5 Bohuslavizki KH, Klutmann S, Brenner W, *et al.* Salivary gland protection by amifostine in high-dose radioiodine treatment: results of a double-blind placebo-controlled study. *J Clin Oncol* 1998; **16**: 3542–9.

● 6 Fiori-Ratti L, de Campora E, Senin U. Sequenced scintigraphy: a morphological and functional study of the salivary glands. *Laryngoscope* 1977; **87**: 1086–94.

7 Wahlberg P, Anderson H, Biorklund A, *et al.* Carcinoma of the parotid and submandibular glands – a study of survival in 2465 patients. *Oral Oncol* 2002; **38**: 706–13.

8 Goerres GW, Von Schulthess GK, Hany TF. Positron emission tomography and PET CT of the head and neck: FDG uptake in normal anatomy, in benign lesions, and in changes resulting from treatment. *Am J Roentgenol* 2002; **179**: 1337–43.

9 McGuirt WF, Keyes Jr JW, Greven KM, *et al.* Preoperative identification of benign versus malignant parotid masses: a comparative study including positron emission tomography. *Laryngoscope* 1995; **105**: 579–84.

10 Keyes Jr JW, Harkness BA, Greven KM, *et al.* Salivary gland tumors: pretherapy evaluation with PET. *Radiology* 1994; **192**: 99–102.

11 Bui CD, Ching AS, Carlos RC, *et al.* Diagnostic accuracy of 2-[fluorine-18]fluoro-2-deoxy-D-glucose positron emission tomography imaging in non-squamous tumors of the head and neck. *Invest Radiol* 2003; **38**: 593–601.

Lachrymal studies

GERHARD W. GOERRES

DACRYOSCINTIGRAPHY

Scintigraphy of lachrymal drainage (dacryoscintigraphy) can be used to evaluate the normal pathway of drainage of tears from the eye to the nasopharynx. Problems with this drainage, i.e. epiphora, or a dry eye are not uncommon ophthalmologic problems. For example, it has been shown that kerato-conjunctivitis sicca, which causes a dry eye, can be found in patients after therapy with ^{131}I for thyroid cancer.[1] With scintigraphy the function of the lachrymal drainage apparatus will usually be tested by the application of ^{99m}Tc-colloid or pertechnetate as eye drops. It is possible to image the flow of tears by placing a drop of radioactive fluid in the eye and taking a series of sequential images. The use of a high-resolution pinhole collimator is recommended for this study. In contrast to other radiological studies where the lachrymal ducts are filled with contrast medium (dacryo-cystography), the nuclear medicine study is simple, safe, and much more physiologic. The test is indicated in patients with epiphora and suspected obstruction of the nasolachrymal drainage system and most useful when radiological methods are not conclusive.[2,3] Furthermore, it is a good test in patients who have already undergone surgery to relieve obstruction without success. It has been shown that this study can be used to assess treatment-induced changes in patients after radiation therapy of tumors located adjacent to the eye.[4] Dacryoscintigraphy can assess the drainage of tears and the pump function of the drainage apparatus in patients with an open lachrymal duct system as shown with radiological techniques.[5]

For a diagnostic lachrymal drainage study the application of 4 MBq as eye drops will cause an effective dose of approximately 0.05 mSv and a dose to the uterus of 0.1 mGy.[6]

In a normal dacryoscintigraphy the lachrymal sac will be visualized after 5–10 s. During the next 40 s a good filling of the canaliculi, the nasolachrymal sac, and nasolachrymal duct can be documented. With regions of interests the time–activity curves of different parts of the lachrymal duct system can be documented. Abnormalities consist of obvious lack of filling and obstruction or when the clearance of the radiotracer is prolonged beyond 5 min.

OTHER RADIOPHARMACEUTICALS AND THE LACHRYMAL GLAND

Like the salivary glands the lachrymal glands take up pertechnetate and are usually seen in ^{67}Ga and ^{131}I whole-body scans. Intense accumulation was reported with [99m]Tc(V)-DMSA but only low uptake is seen in a normal lachrymal gland with FDG.[7] In patients with Graves' disease and thyroid dysfunction an increased uptake of ^{111}In-labeled somatostatin analog is found in retro-orbital inflammation. This can also involve the lachrymal gland.[8] Additionally, such uptake has been described in lymphoma.[9]

However, due to the small structure of the lachrymal gland and the low specificity of flow tracers, pathologies within the orbit are mainly examined by means of morphological imaging methods. To date no studies in large patient groups are available regarding the use of conventional nuclear medicine techniques and PET or PET/CT for the assessment of lachrymal gland or intraorbital pathologies. PET and PET/CT have been used to assess patients with carcinomas from paranasal sinuses infiltrating into the orbit. In such a case the combination of the structural imaging information obtained by CT or MRI

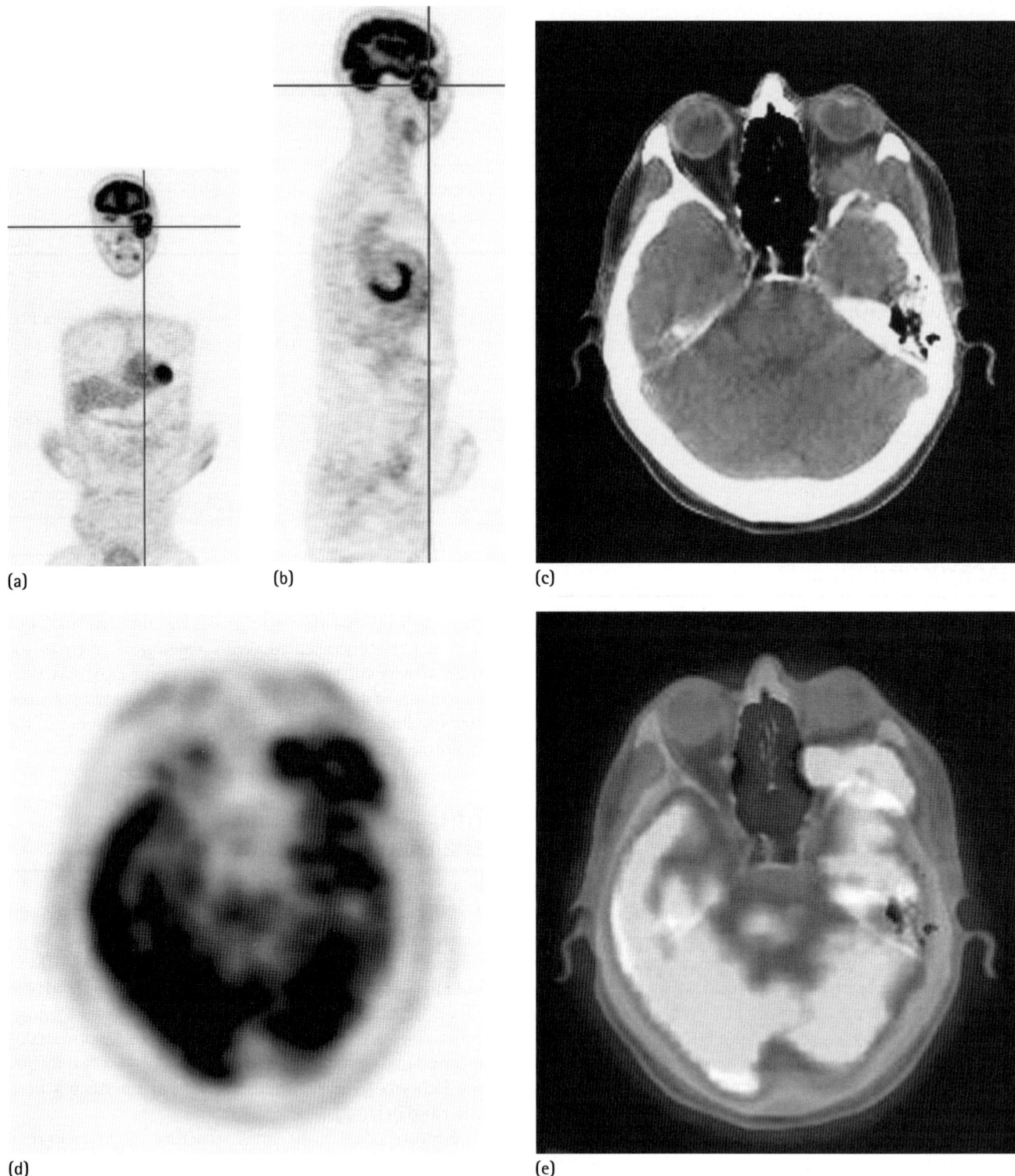

(a)

(b)

(c)

(d)

(e)

Figure 11C.1 *Coronal and sagittal positron emission tomography (PET) images (a and b) and transverse computed tomography (CT), PET and co-registered PET/CT images (c to e) of a 56-year-old male patient with a HNSCC of the maxillary sinus. The patient had had trigeminal pain for 2 years and recently had experienced difficulties in opening the mouth. In this staging examination a large tumor is identified infiltrating from the maxillary sinus into the orbital cavity and cranially extending through the skull base into the cavernosus sinus. Combined treatment with radiation and chemotherapy was planned.*

and the functional information of FDG uptake can help to better delineate the lesion allowing for a more precise planning of surgical or radiation therapy. However, this has to be confirmed in future studies. Figure 11C.1 shows a case of HNSCC with invasion into the orbit.

REFERENCES

◆ Key review paper

◆ 1 Solans R, Bosch JA, Galofre P, *et al.* Salivary and lacrimal gland dysfunction (sicca syndrome) after radioiodine therapy. *J Nucl Med* 2001; **42**: 738–43.

2 Weber AL, Rodriguez-DeVelasquez A, Lucarelli MJ, Cheng HM. Normal anatomy and lesions of the lacrimal sac and duct: evaluated by dacryocysto-graphy, computed tomography, and MR imaging. *Neuroimaging Clin N Am* 1996; **6**: 199–217.

3 Ziccardi VB, Charron M, Ochs MW, Braun TW. Nuclear dacryoscintigraphy: its role in oral and maxillofacial surgery. *Oral Surg Oral Med Oral Pathol Oral Radiol Endod* 1995; **80**: 645–9.

4 Brizel HE, Sheils WC, Brown M. The effects of radio-therapy on the nasolacrimal system as evaluated by dacryoscintigraphy. *Radiology* 1975; **116**: 373–81.

5 Hanna IT, MacEwen CJ, Kennedy N. Lacrimal scintigra-phy in the diagnosis of epiphora. *Nucl Med Commun* 1992; **13**: 416–20.

6 Administration of Radioactive Substances Advisory Committee. Notes for guidance on the clinical adminis-tration of radiopharmaceuticals and use of unsealed radioactive sources. *Nucl Med Commun* 2000; **Suppl**: S1–S95.

7 Sakurai H, Mitsuhashi N, Hayakawa K, *et al.* Ectopic lacrimal gland of the orbit. *J Nucl Med* 1997; **38**: 1498–1500.

8 Moncayo R, Baldissera I, Decristoforo C, *et al.* Evaluation of immunological mechanisms mediating thyroid-associated ophthalmopathy by radionuclide imaging using the somatostatin analog ^{111}In-octreotide. *Thyroid* 1997; **7**: 21–9.

9 Raderer M, Traub T, Formanek M, *et al.* Somatostatin-receptor scintigraphy for staging and follow-up of patients with extraintestinal marginal zone B-cell lym-phoma of the mucosa associated lymphoid tissue (MALT)-type. *Br J Cancer* 2001; **85**: 1462–6.

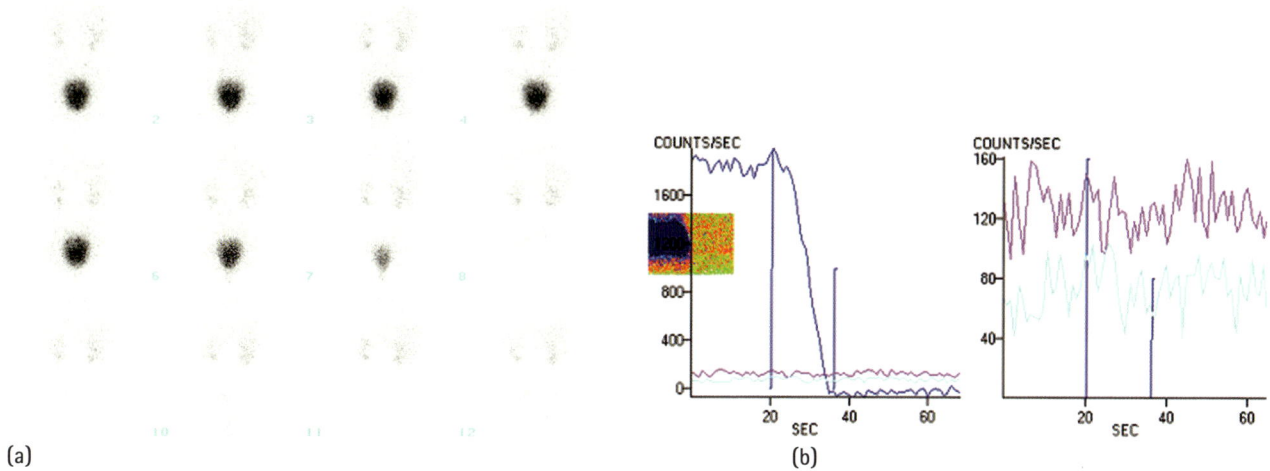

(a)

(b)

Plate 8C.1 *A normal indirect radionuclide cystography scan with complete and prompt bladder emptying (a) and no evidence of reflux. The time–activity curves (b) both on the bladder and the kidneys confirm the findings. See page 285.*

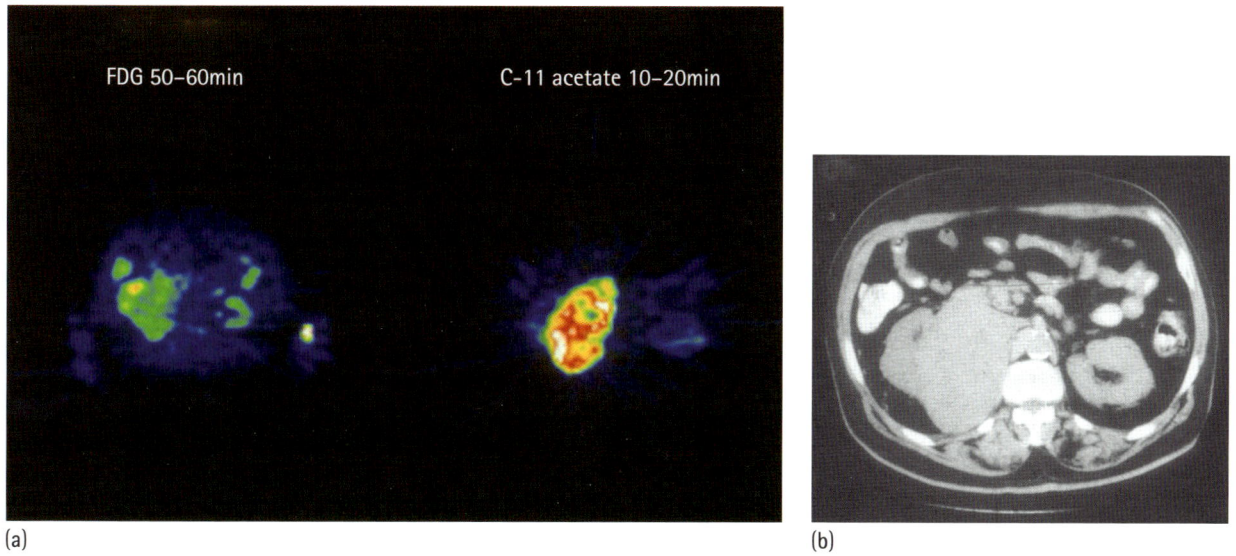

(a)

(b)

Plate 8G.1 *Carbon-11 acetate PET images at 10–20 minutes and FDG PET images at 50–60 minutes (a) of a large solid right renal mass (b), corresponding to a mixed granular-clear cell histology renal cell carcinoma. There is intense retention of the carbon-11 tracer in the renal carcinoma reflecting the anabolic dominent metabolism of the aceate, while the renal cortical tracer activity has cleared reflecting the oxidative dominent metabolism in the non-neoplastic renal cortical tissue. There is also no urinary tracer excretion of the carbon-11 acetate tracer. See page 324.*

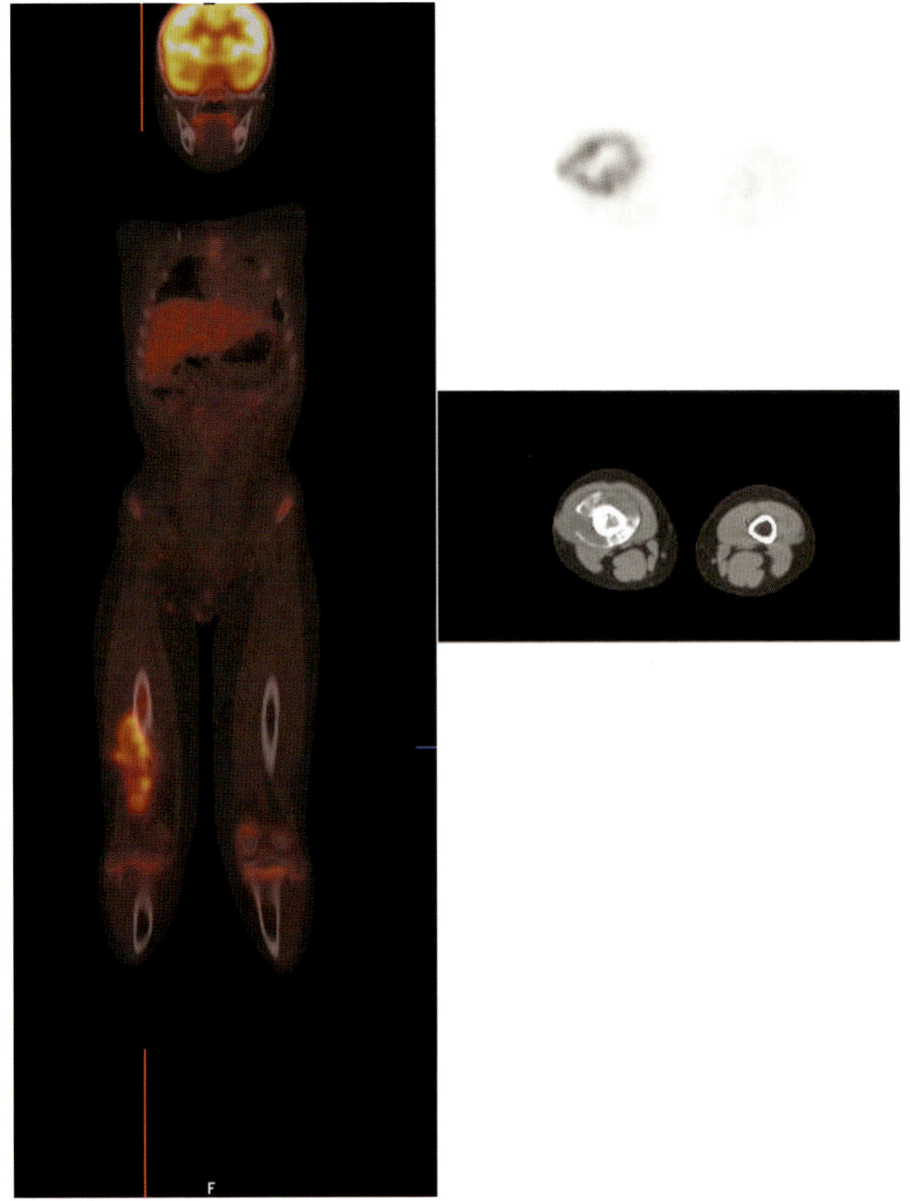

Plate 9G.1 *Nine-year-old boy with osteogenic sarcoma of the right distal femur. FDG PET/CT fused whole-body image shows the tumor FDG uptake overlayed on the large characteristic tumor appearance on the CT. The transaxial slices to the right are of the FDG PET uptake (upper) through the tumor mass on CT (lower). See page 411.*

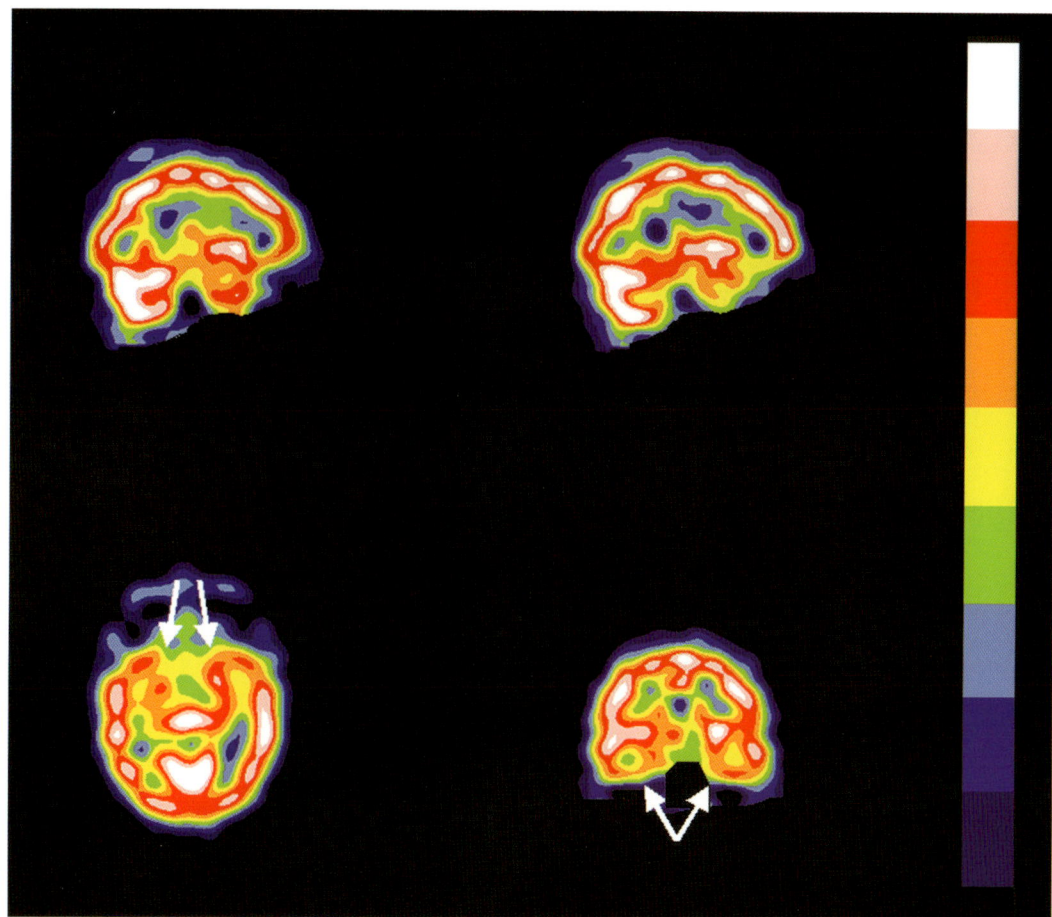

Plate 10A.1 *Typical example of a HMPAO SPECT scan in a healthy volunteer. Format of the images: first row left – a right parasagittal slice; first row right – a left parasagittal slice; second row left – the critical temporal lobe slice; second row right – a coronal slice cut through the anterior aspect of the temporal lobes. The arrows indicate the perfusion to the medial temporal lobes critical for short-term memory. A color bar is displayed; all images are normalized to cerebellum. White/red coloration indicates good perfusion; orange/yellow indicates moderate perfusion and green/blue indicates reduced perfusion. It may aid the reader to think of the hot colors (white/red) as demonstrating good perfusion, warm colors indicate moderate perfusion, and cold colors indicating diminished perfusion. See page 417.*

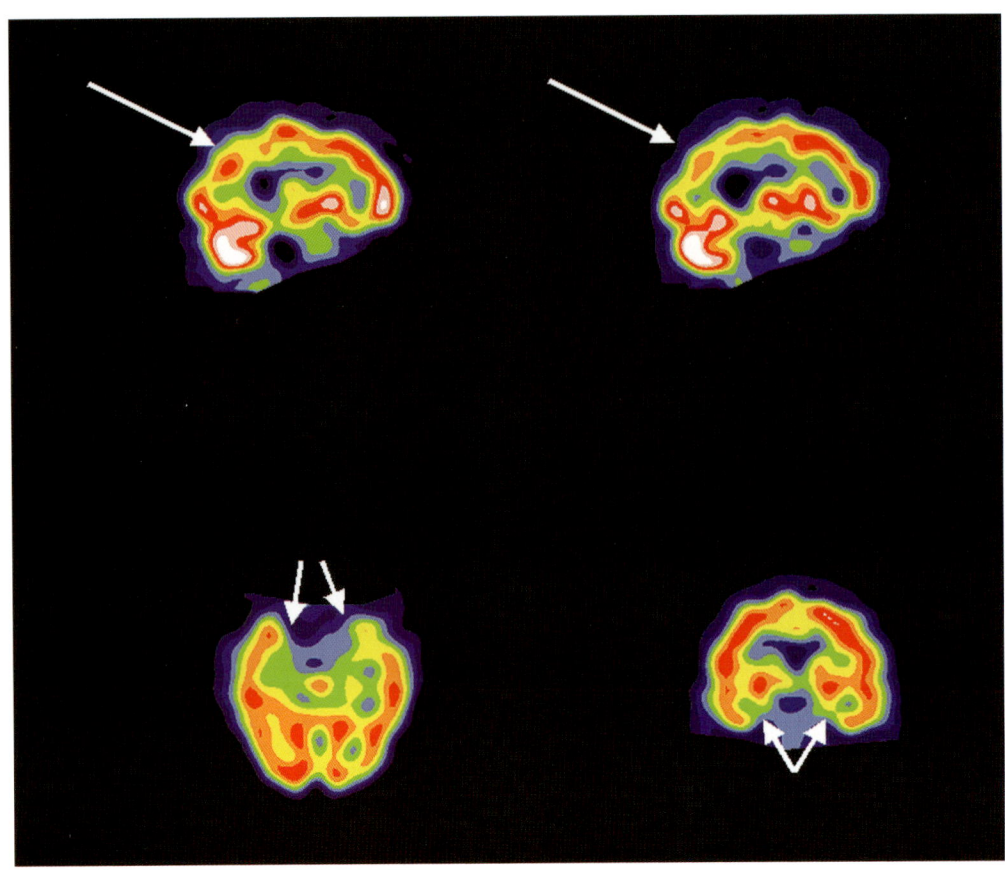

Plate 10A.2 *A typical HMPAO SPECT scan appearance of a 79-year-old patient (MMSE 20) with late-onset Alzheimer's disease of mild/ moderate severity demonstrating markedly reduced perfusion to the medial temporal lobe structures bilaterally and mildly reduced perfusion to the left anterolateral temporal lobe (short arrows), and a mild reduction to the parietal association areas (long arrows). See page 417.*

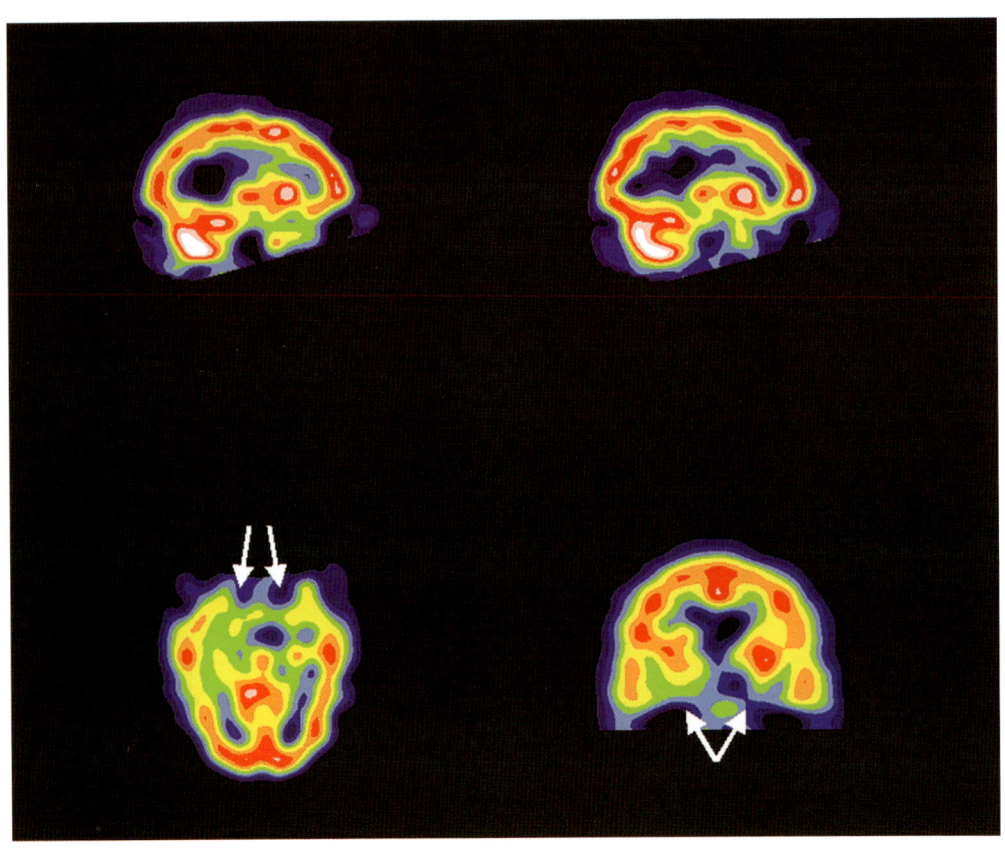

Plate 10A.3 *Example of a 78-year-old patient (MMSE 26) presenting with amnesia who subsequently progressed to fulfil the criteria for late-onset Alzheimer's disease. Perfusion to the medial temporal lobe structures is markedly reduced (arrows) and there is mildly reduced perfusion to the anterolateral temporal lobes; parietal perfusion is still intact at this stage. See page 417.*

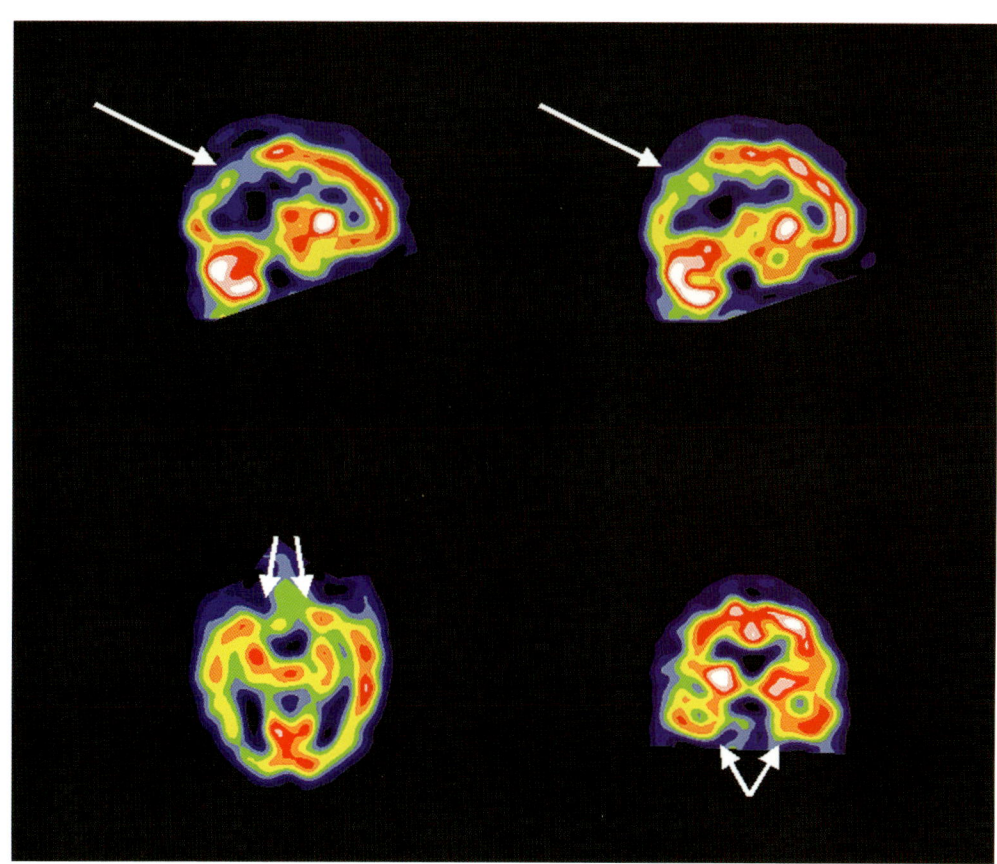

Plate 10A.4 *Example of a 57-year-old patient (MMSE 20) with early-onset Alzheimer's disease. Note the markedly reduced perfusion to the parietal association areas (long arrows) with relative preservation of perfusion to the medial temporal structures (short arrows). See page 417.*

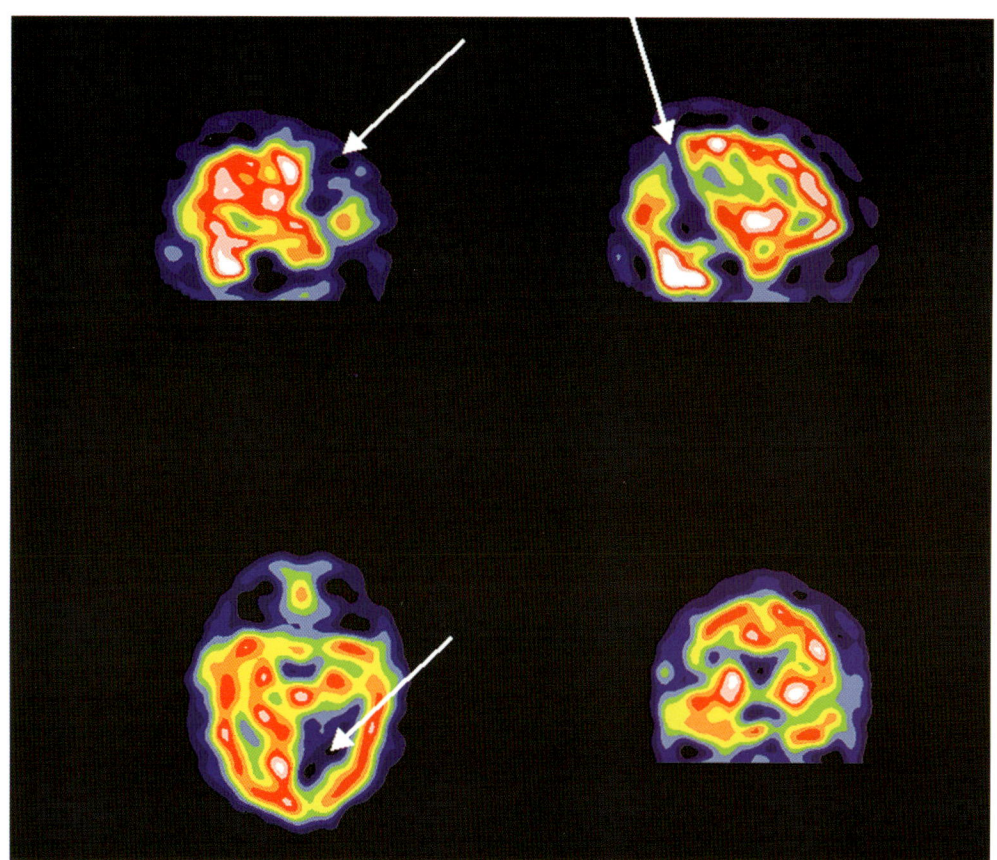

Plate 10A.5 *Example of a 70-year-old patient with multi-infarct dementia. Note the wedge-shaped infarcts (arrows). The patient gave a history of three previous transient ischemic attacks. Although these episodes may have been clinically transient the defects on imaging are permanent and cumulative, eventually giving rise to overt cognitive impairment. See page 418.*

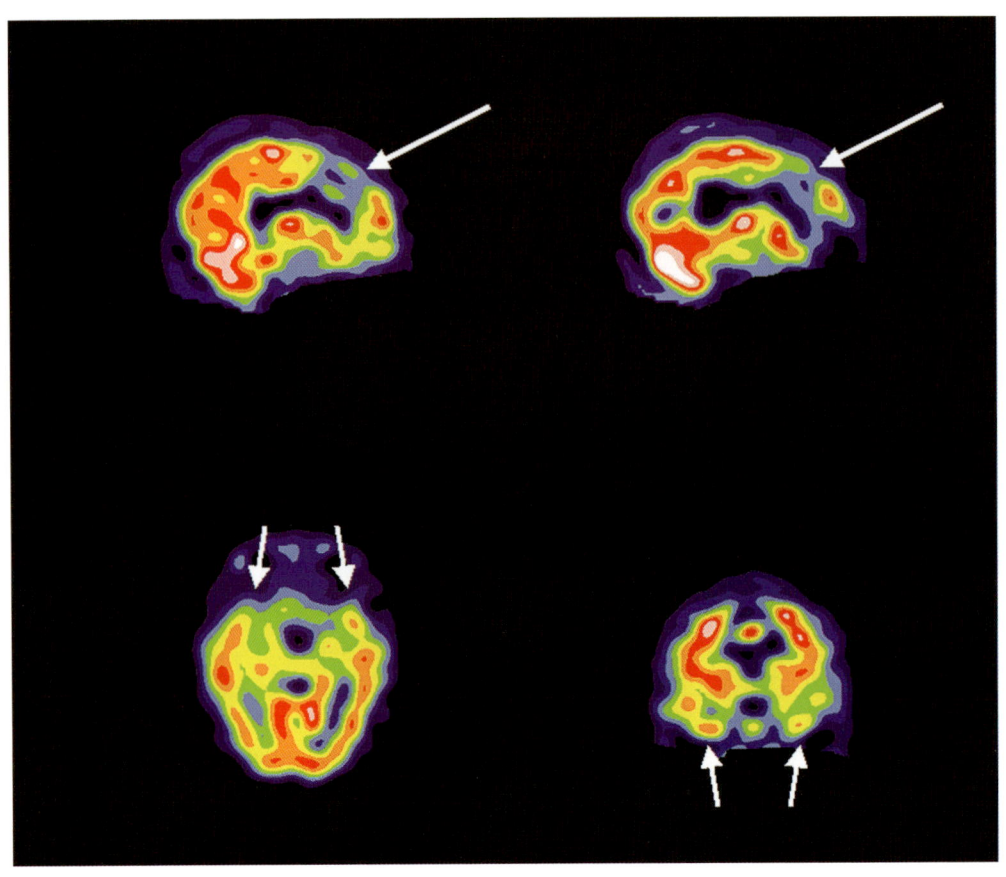

Plate 10A.6 *Example of a 73-year-old patient with fronto-temporal dementia. Note the markedly reduced perfusion bilaterally to the dorsal aspects of the frontal lobes (long arrows) and the orbito-basal region on the left, and the reduced perfusion to the anterior aspects of the temporal lobes (short arrows). See page 418.*

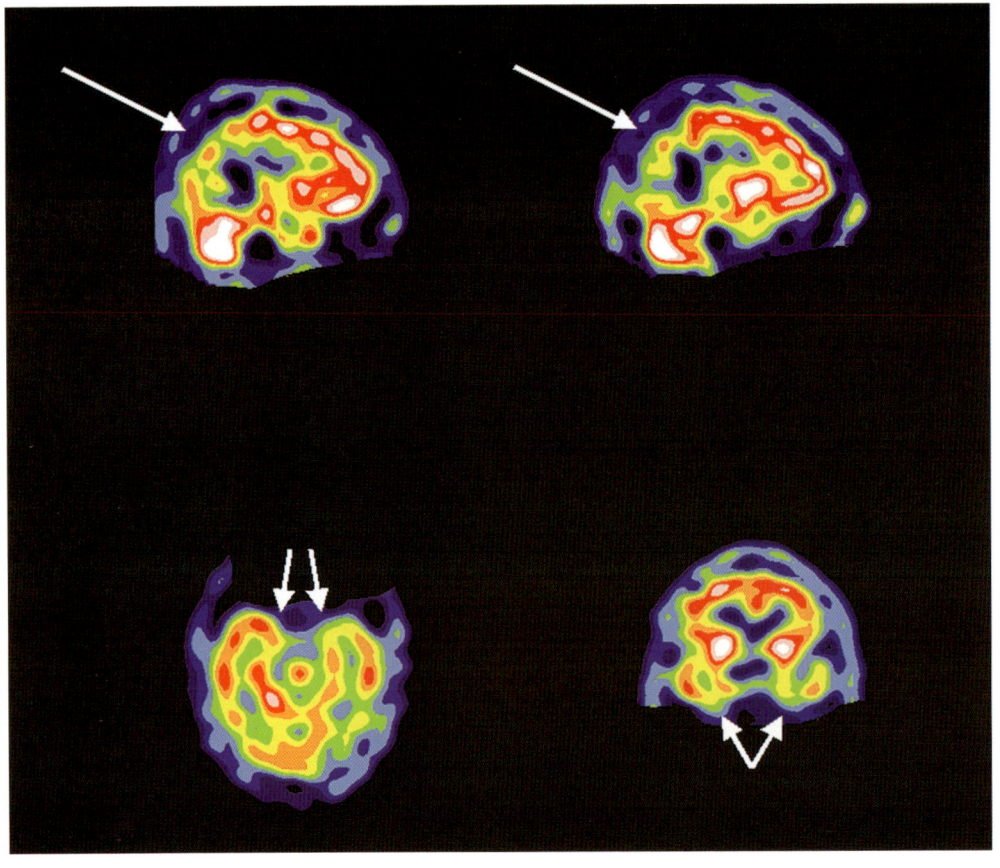

Plate 10A.7 *Example of a 79-year-old patient with Lewy body dementia. Note the reduced perfusion of the posterior association areas (long arrows) compared with the perfusion to the medial temporal lobe structures (short arrows). The preservation of perfusion to the medial temporal lobes may aid the differentiation from late-onset Alzheimer's disease. Unfortunately, only a minority of patients with dementia of the Lewy body type will have this appearance at presentation. See page 419.*

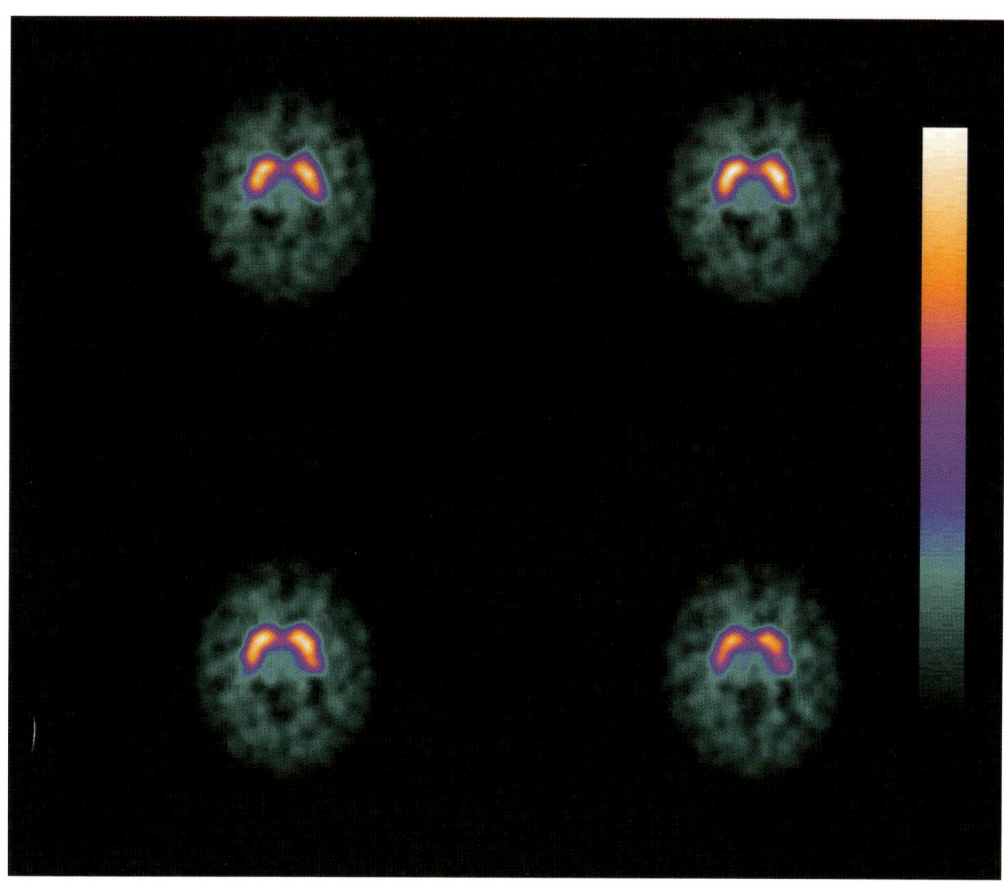

Plate 10A.8 *Example of a DaTSCAN demonstrating the normal appearances of uptake of ^{123}I-FP-CIT. The normal appearance is of two mirror imaged commas and represents uptake in the caudate and lentiform nuclei. Patients with Alzheimer's disease will have this normal appearance. See page 420.*

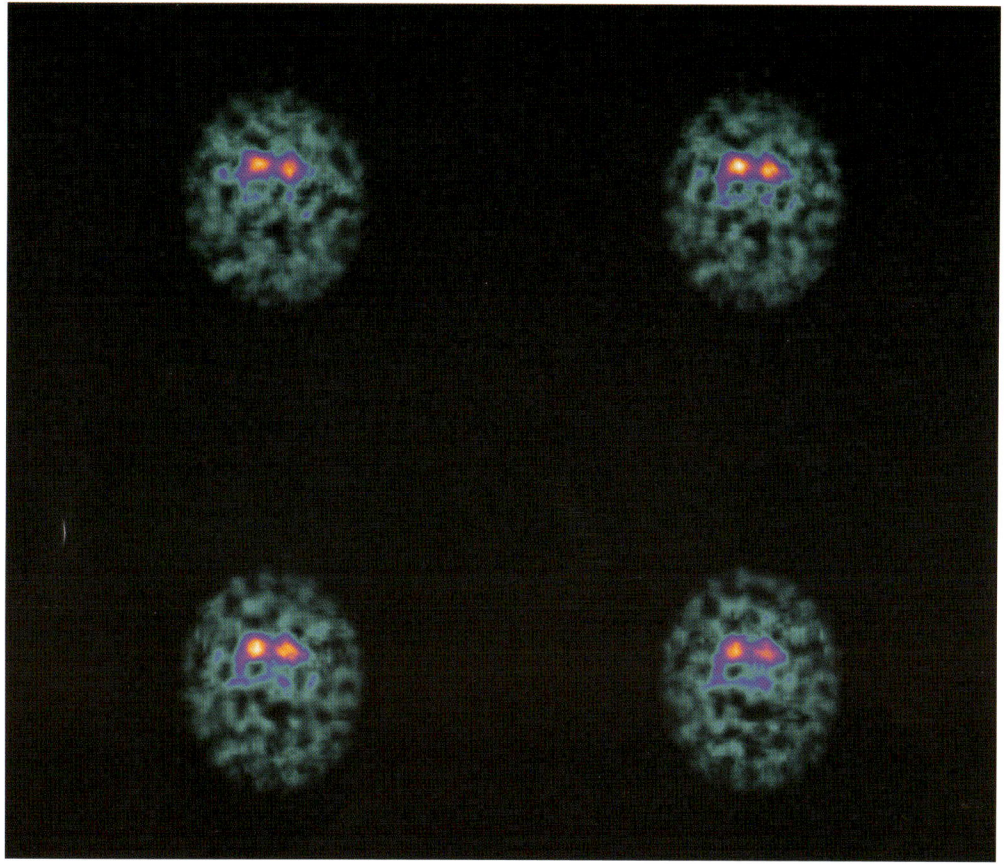

Plate 10A.9 *Example of an abnormal DaTSCAN of a patient with Lewy body dementia whose HMPAO scan is shown in Plate 10A.7. Note that there is reduced uptake in the lentiform nuclei (the tail of the 'comma') with uptake only in the caudate nuclei. This has the appearance of two 'full stops'. See page 420.*

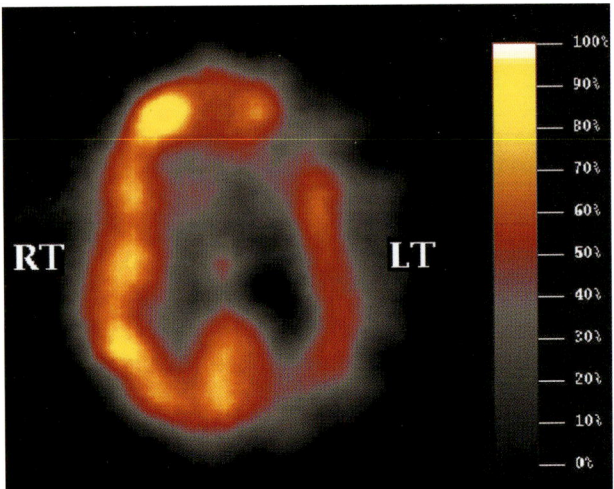

Plate 10B.1 *Technetium-99m-HMPAO brain perfusion SPECT shows reduced perfusion to the left temporo-parietal region of the brain. Patient presented with right sided weakness. The demonstration of reduced perfusion in the acute phase of stroke (less than 3 h) with normal CT scanning enables the administration of thrombolytic therapy within the therapeutic window. See page 426.*

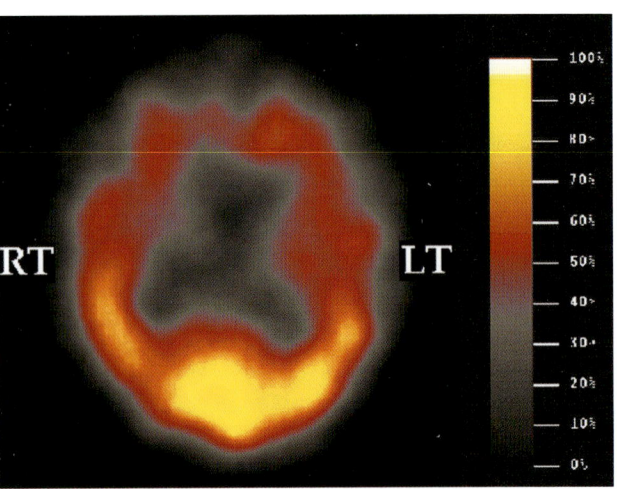

Plate 10B.3 *Technetium-99m-HMPAO brain perfusion SPECT shows reduced perfusion to the frontal and temporal lobes bilaterally. There is intact perfusion posteriorly. The findings are more likely to represent depression in an elderly patient with a possible diagnosis of pseudo-dementia. See page 429.*

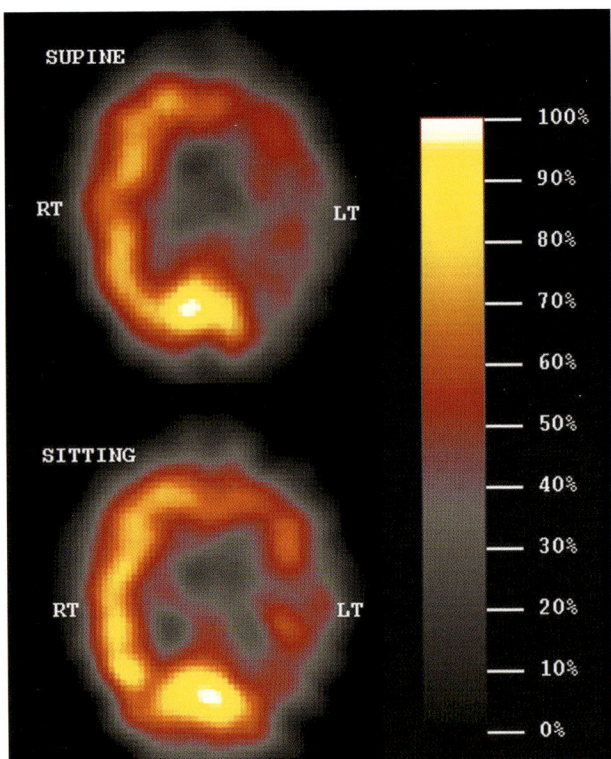

Plate 10B.2 *Two serial registered ^{99m}Tc-HMPAO brain perfusion SPECT performed in two postures (supine and semi-recumbent) 3–4 h apart show more than 30% improvement in perfusion to part of the left temporal lobe in the semi-recumbent posture in comparison to the supine posture. See page 427.*

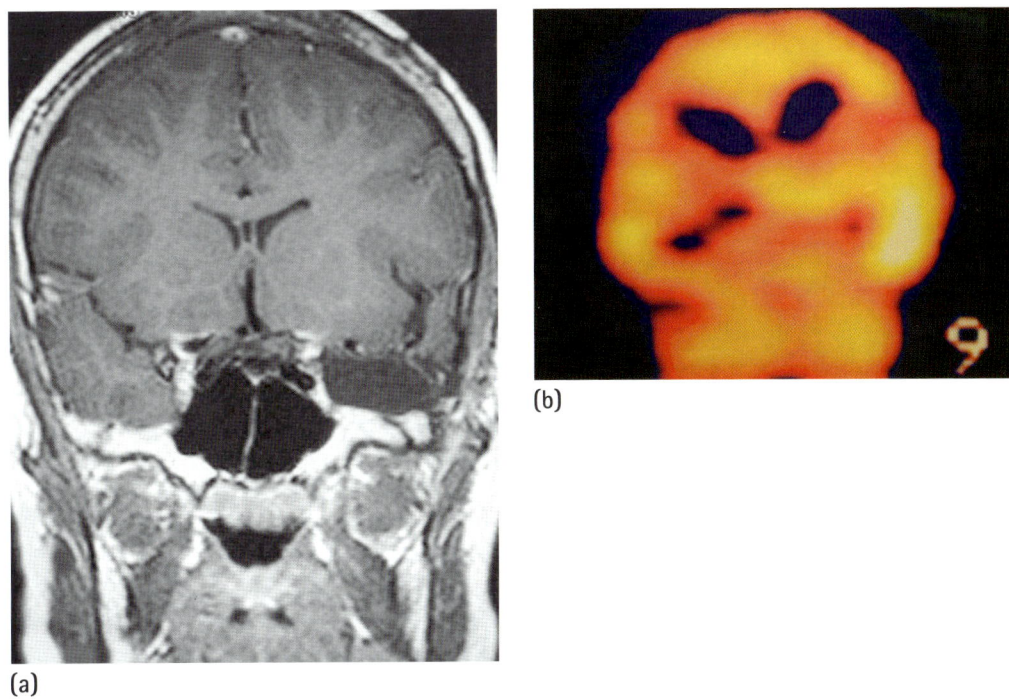
(a)

(b)

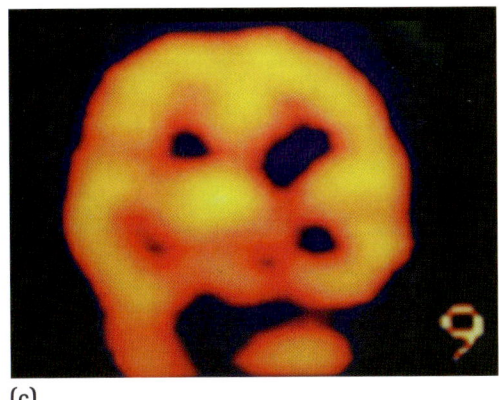
(c)

Plate 10C.1 *This shows coronal T1-weighted views of a magnetic resonance imaging scan performed on a child with seizures of left temporal origin (a). Changes seen in the left temporal lobe were highly suggestive of a dysembryoplastic epithelial tumour with cystic change. Ictal single photon emission computed tomography (SPECT) shows hyperperfusion of this area (b), when compared to interictal SPECT (c). Image by courtesy of Dr Helen Cross, Epilepsy Unit, Department of Paediatric Neurology, Great Ormond Street Hospital for Children, London. See page 436.*

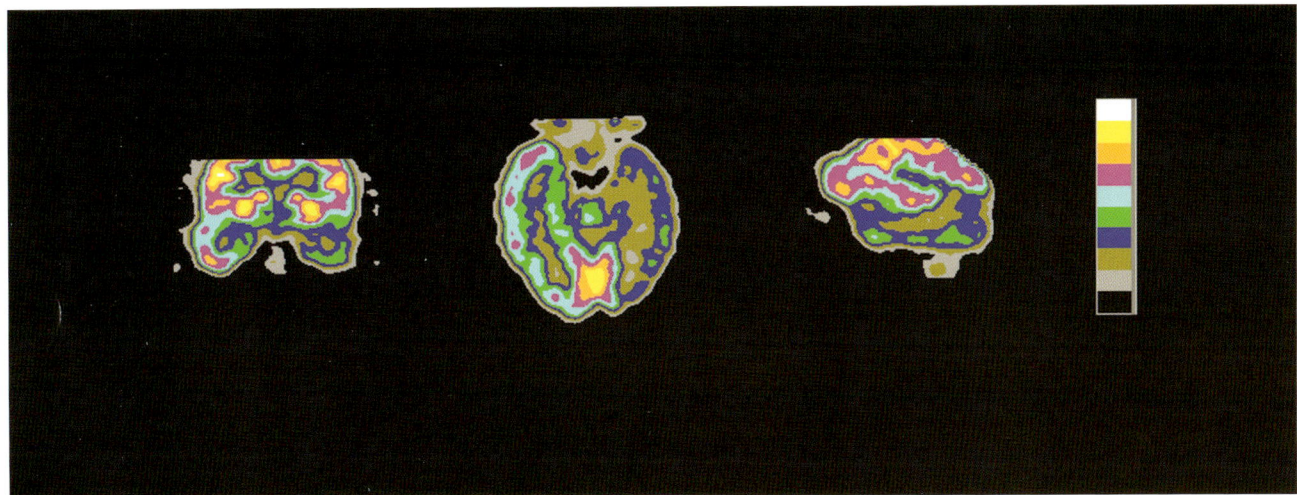

Plate 10C.2 *This is an example of left temporal hypometabolism using fluorodeoxyglucose (FDG) positron emission tomography. Orthogonal planes are shown of the temporal lobes: coronal (left) axial (middle) and sagittal (right). The color scale chosen is a discontinuous scale with ten color bars each representing a 10% change in counts relative to the maximum uptake in the brain. Uptake of FDG in the left temporal lobe is 20–30% lower than in the right temporal lobe. See page 436.*

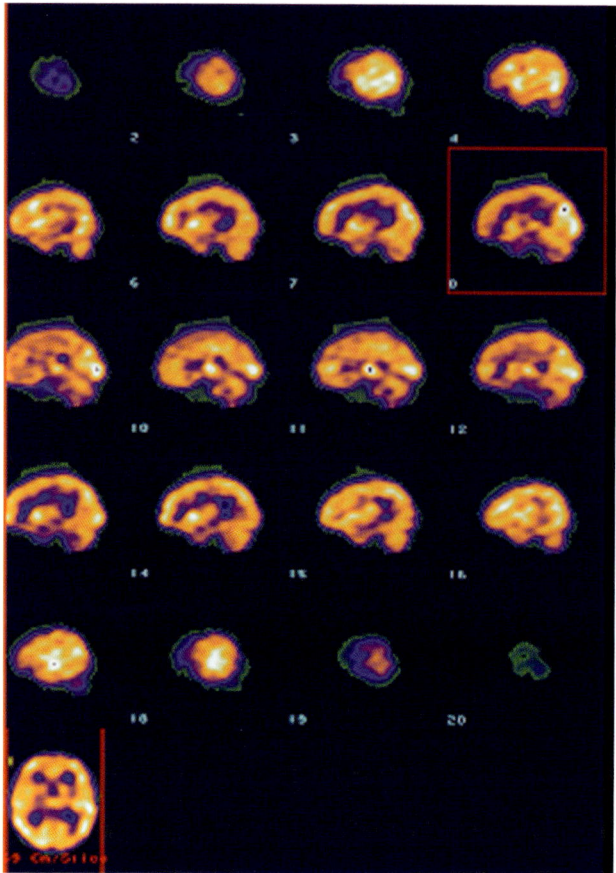

Plate 10C.3 *This 7-year-old girl presented with occipital seizures and left lower quadrantinopia. Ictal ^{99m}Tc-HMPAO SPECT was performed and showed hyperperfusion over the right occipital cortex. This is a color version of Fig. 10C.6(b): see complete figure on page 441.*

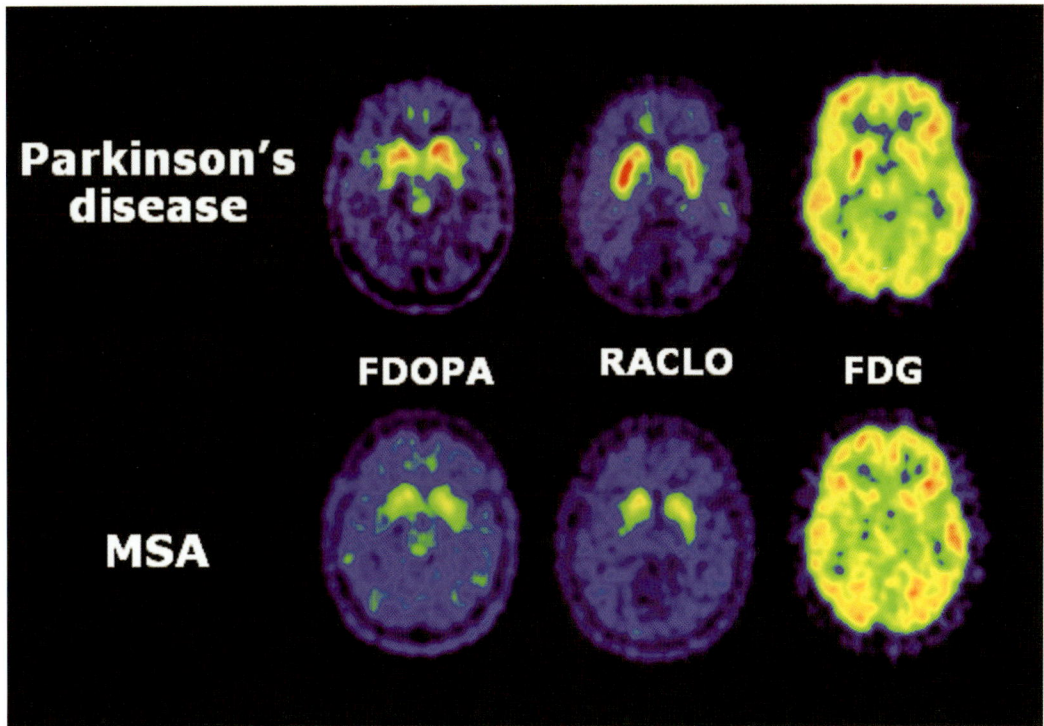

Plate 10E.1 *Representative positron emission tomography images of FDOPA (^{18}F-DOPA), RACLO (^{11}C-raclopride) and FDG (^{18}F-FDG) at the midstriatal level from a patient suffering from Parkinson's disease and a patient with multiple system atrophy (MSA). The FDOPA scan is abnormal in both patients, whereas the RACL and FDG scans are abnormal in the MSA patient only. (Reprinted from Antonini et al.,[30] with permission from Oxford University Press, UK.) See page 458.*

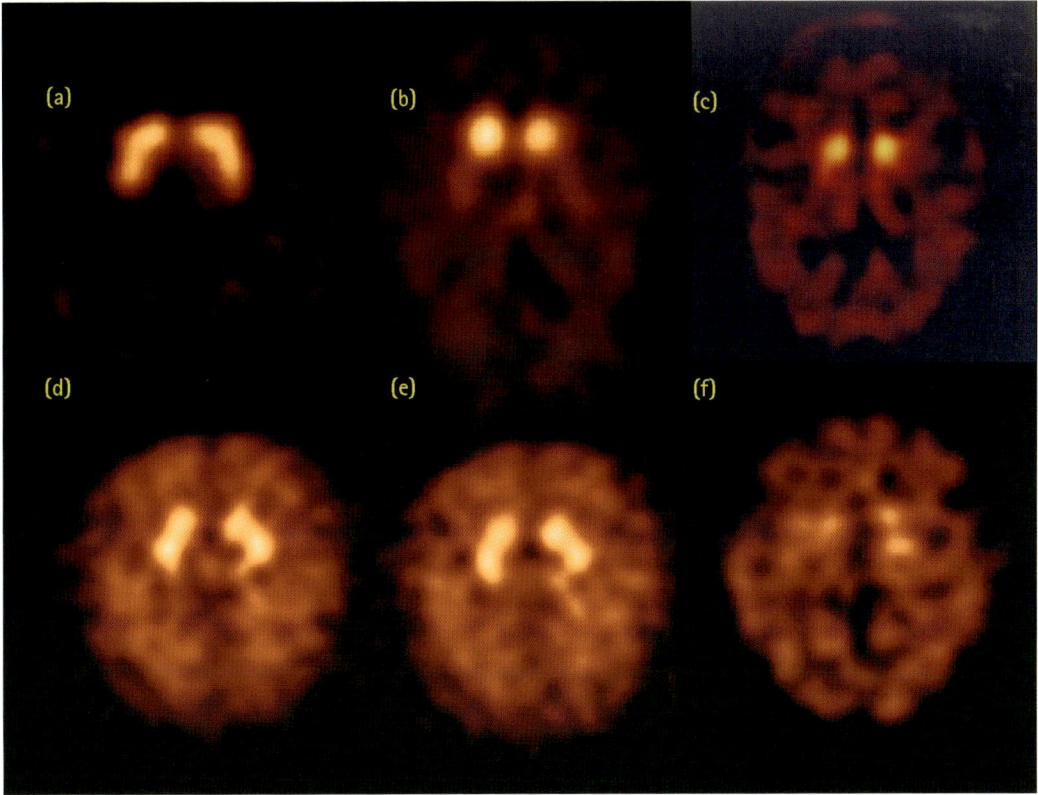

Plate 10E.2 *^{123}I-FP-CIT (a–c) and ^{123}I-IBZM (d–f) SPECT scans of a healthy control (a and d), a patient with Parkinson's disease (PD) (b and e) and a patient suffering from multiple system atrophy (MSA) (c and f). The ^{123}I-FP-CIT SPECT scan of the PD patient shows loss of striatal ^{123}I-FP-CIT binding due to degeneration of nigrostriatal dopaminergic neurons (b), while the D_2 receptor binding, which relates to the integrity of postsynaptic striatal neurons, is normal (e). The scans of the MSA patient show loss of presynaptic dopamine transporters (c) as well as loss of the postsynaptic element (f) of the nigrostriatal dopaminergic system. (Reprinted, with permission, from Bewegingsstoornissen. E.Ch. Wolters and T. van Laar (eds.) Amsterdam: VU uitgeverij, 2002.) See page 458.*

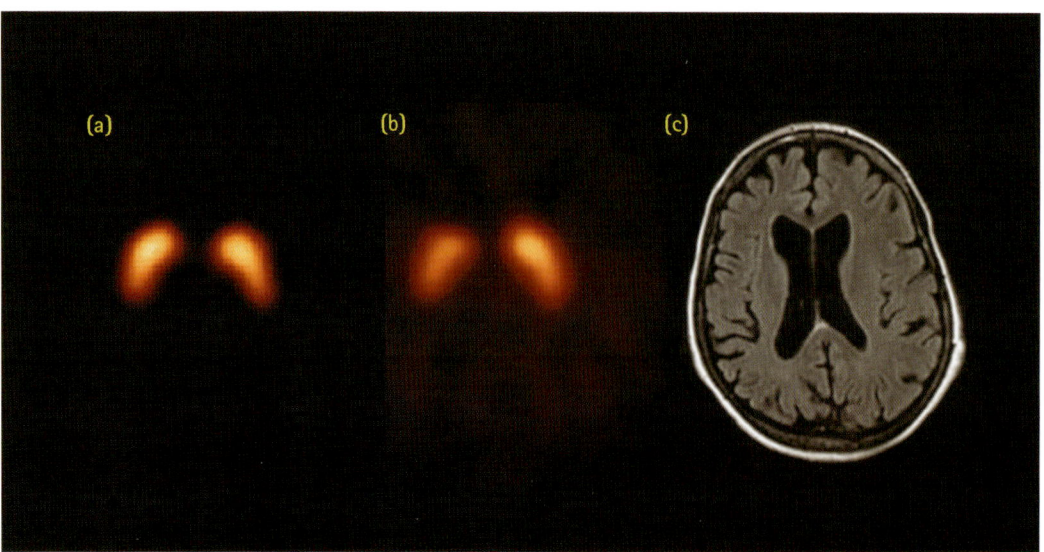

Plate 10E.3 ^{123}I-β-CIT $SPECT$ $scan$ of a $healthy$ $control$ (a) and a $patient$ $suffering$ $from$ $corticobasal$ $degeneration$ (b), as $well$ as a $magnetic$ *resonance image of the same patient (c). The corticobasal degeneration has led to an asymmetrical degeneration of the nigrostriatal pathway (b) and a unilateral atrophy of the brain (c), both contralateral to the body side that showed clinical motor signs. (Reprinted, with permission, from* Bewegingsstoornissen. *E.Ch. Wolters and T. van Laar (eds.) Amsterdam: VU uitgeverij, 2002.) See page 459.*

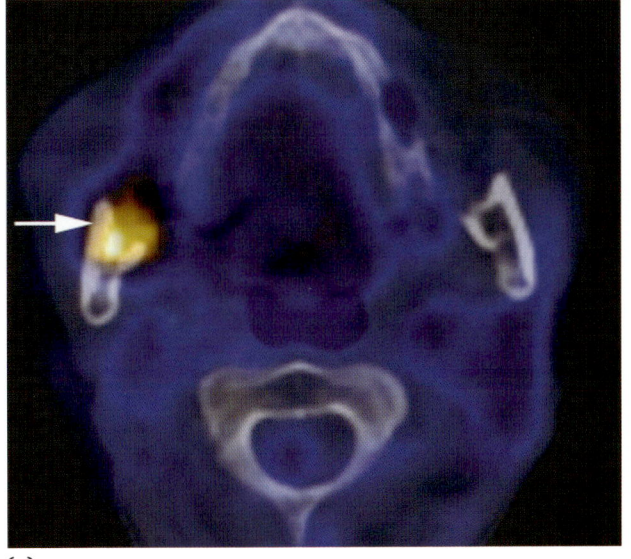

(a)

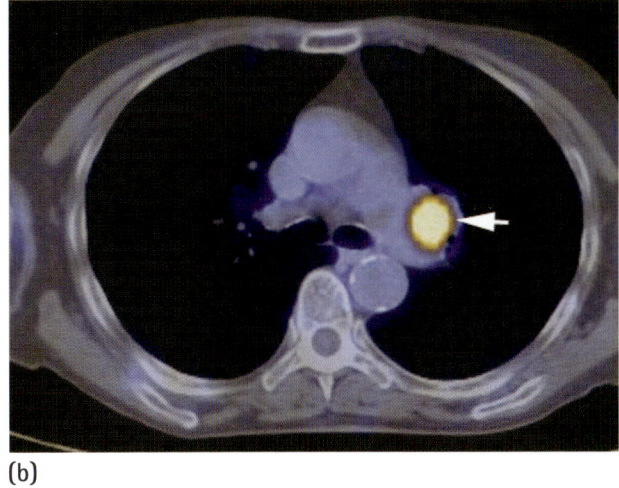

(b)

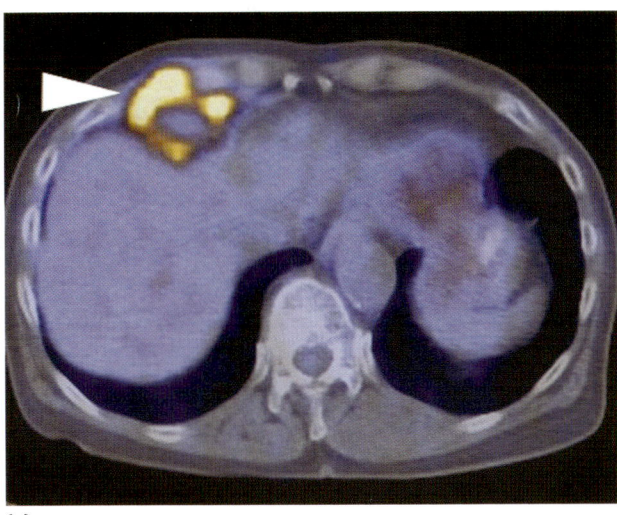

(c)

Plate 11A.1 *The transverse co-registered positron emission tomography/computed tomography (PET/CT) images (a to c) make it easy to delineate the metastases and to identify bone invasion of the local recurrence. These are color versions of Fig. 11A.3(e to g). See complete figure on page 473.*

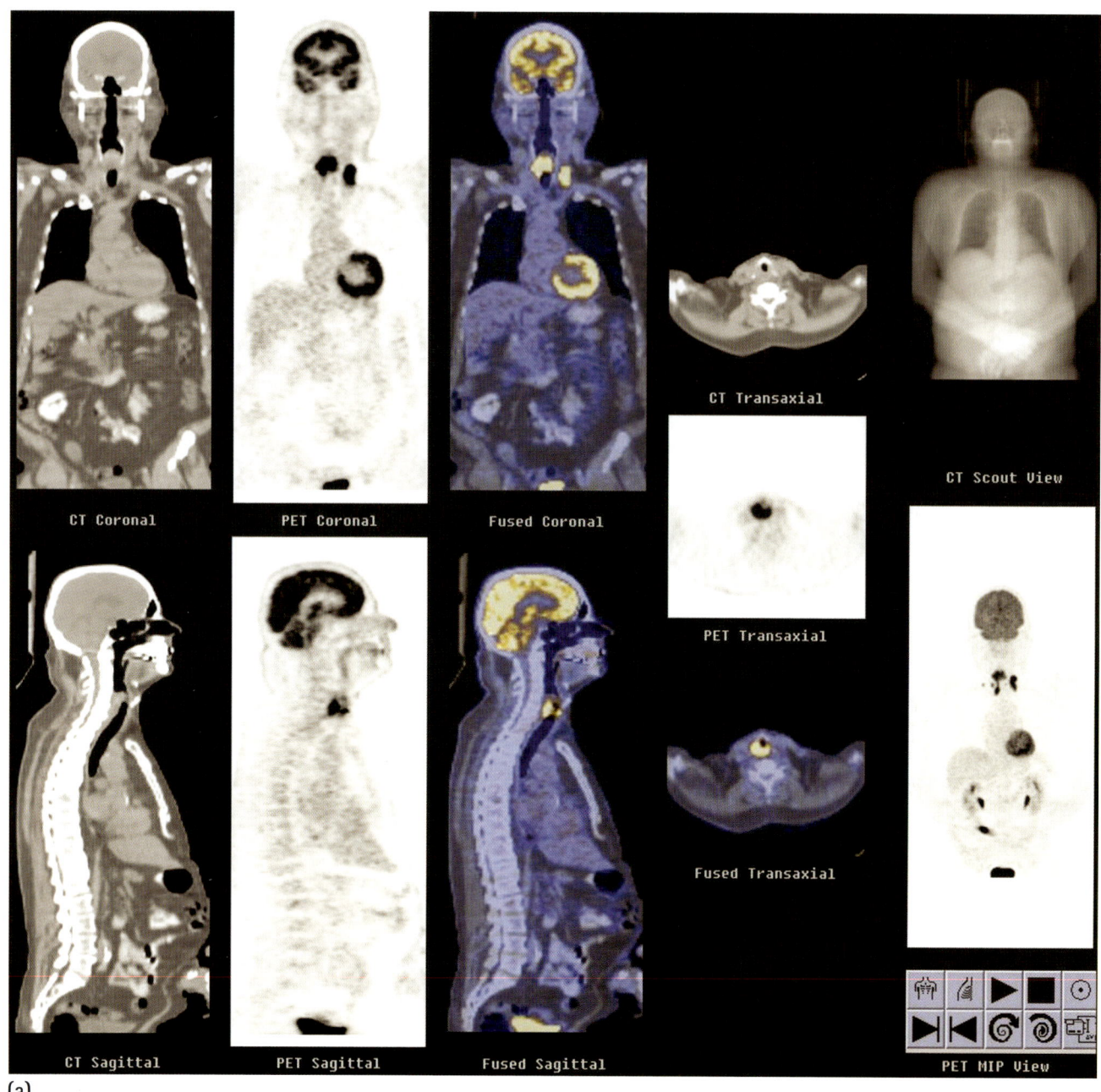

CT Coronal

PET Coronal

Fused Coronal

CT Transaxial

CT Scout View

PET Transaxial

Fused Transaxial

CT Sagittal

PET Sagittal

Fused Sagittal

PET MIP View

(a)

Plate 11A.2 *Overview of PET/CT images (a) and transverse PET, CT, and PET/CT images. See page 473.*

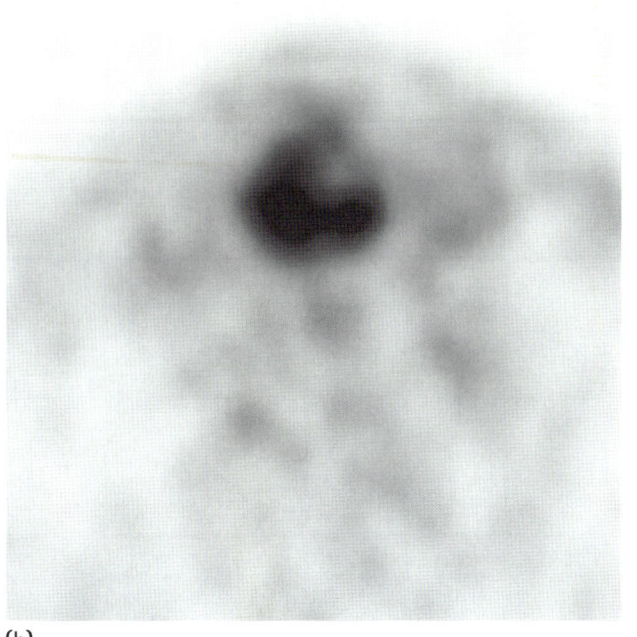

(b)

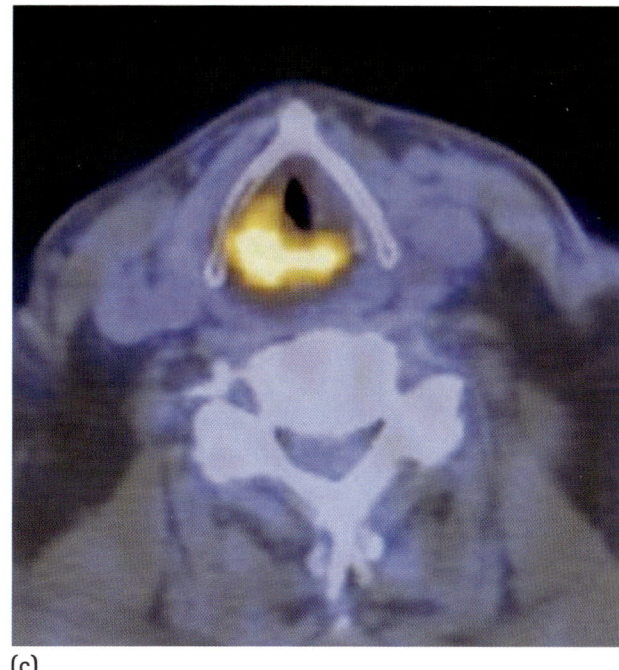

(c)

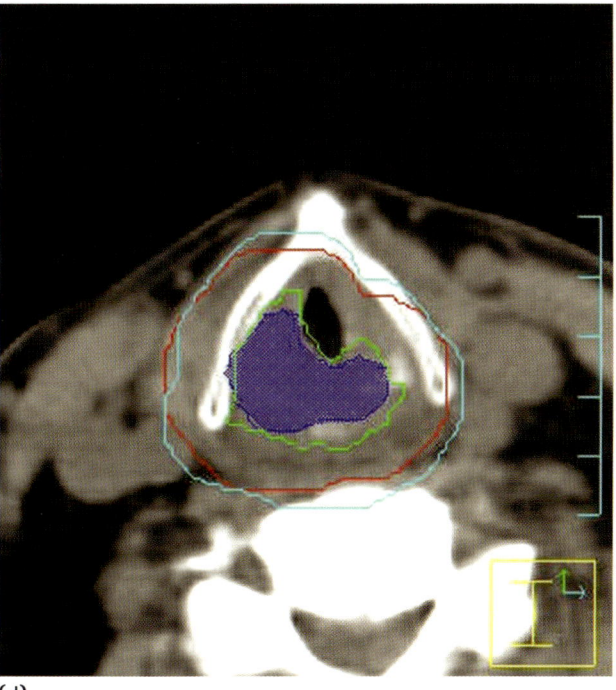

(d)

Plate 11A.2 *(Continued)* *(b to d) for radiation treatment planning of a 65-year-old male patient. This patient underwent laser therapy 1 year ago for a T2 N0 glottic cancer. He now presents with a large recurrent tumor with infiltration into adjacent structures such as the thyroid gland. The tumor reaches the esophagus with a cranio-caudal extension of 2.8 cm. Lymph node metastases were clinically evident ipsilaterally but on PET images bilateral lymph node involvement is found paratracheally. No distant metastases were found. The PET data were used for the planning of the radiation treatment. PET information is co-registered on CT information and used to better delineate the area which should receive maximum radiation dose. The fluorodeoxyglucose-avid area is blue on the planning CT (only one transversal slice is shown).* *See page 473.*

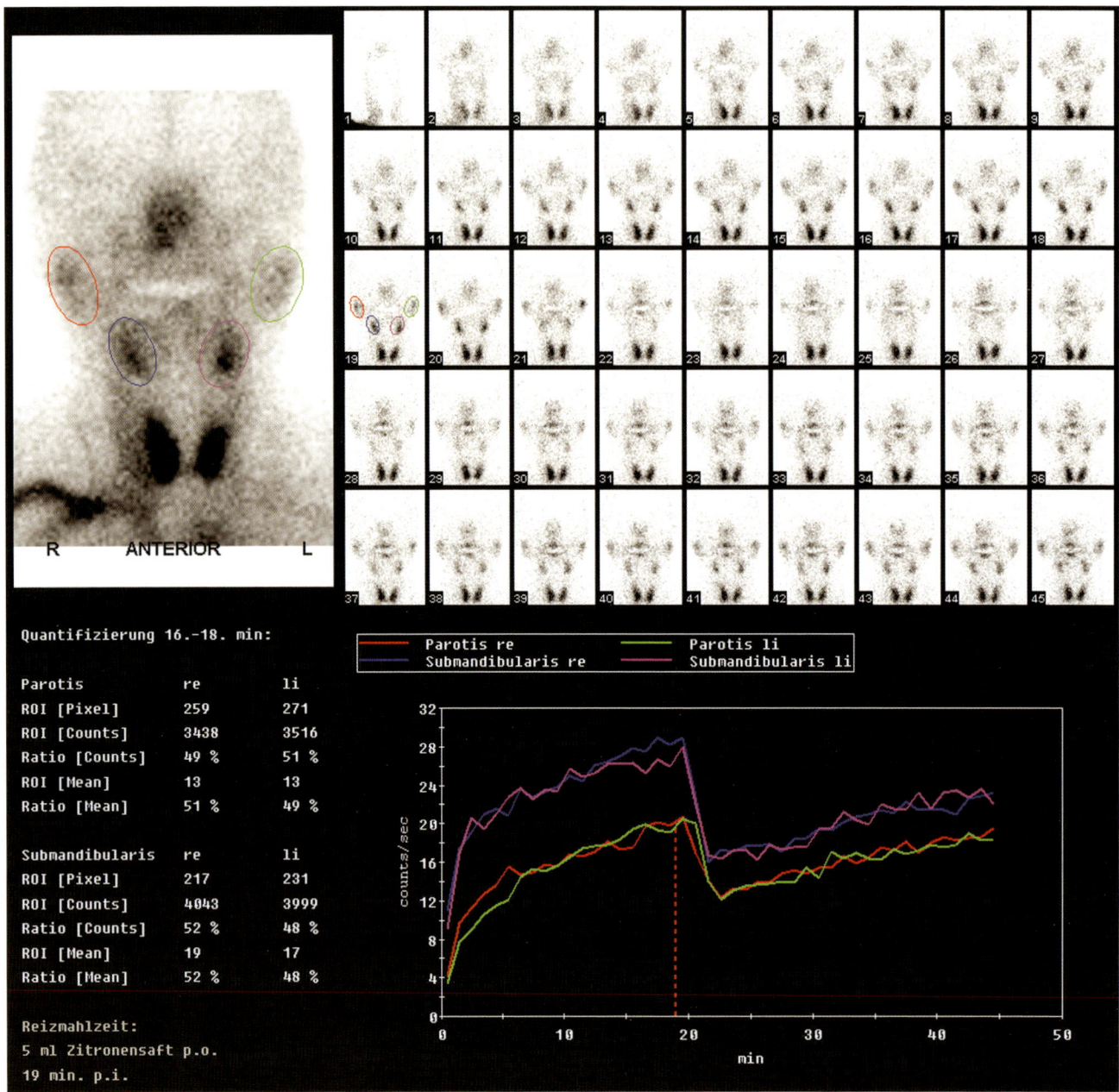

Quantifizierung 16.-18. min:

Parotis	re	li
ROI [Pixel]	259	271
ROI [Counts]	3438	3516
Ratio [Counts]	49 %	51 %
ROI [Mean]	13	13
Ratio [Mean]	51 %	49 %

Submandibularis	re	li
ROI [Pixel]	217	231
ROI [Counts]	4043	3999
Ratio [Counts]	52 %	48 %
ROI [Mean]	19	17
Ratio [Mean]	52 %	48 %

Reizmahlzeit:
5 ml Zitronensaft p.o.
19 min. p.i.

Plate 11B.1 *Salivary gland study of a 70-year-old female patient with tonsilar carcinoma before radiation therapy was started. There is a normal appearance of both parotid and submandibular glands with adequate ^{99m}Tc uptake and good excretion after stimulation with lemon juice. See page 483.*

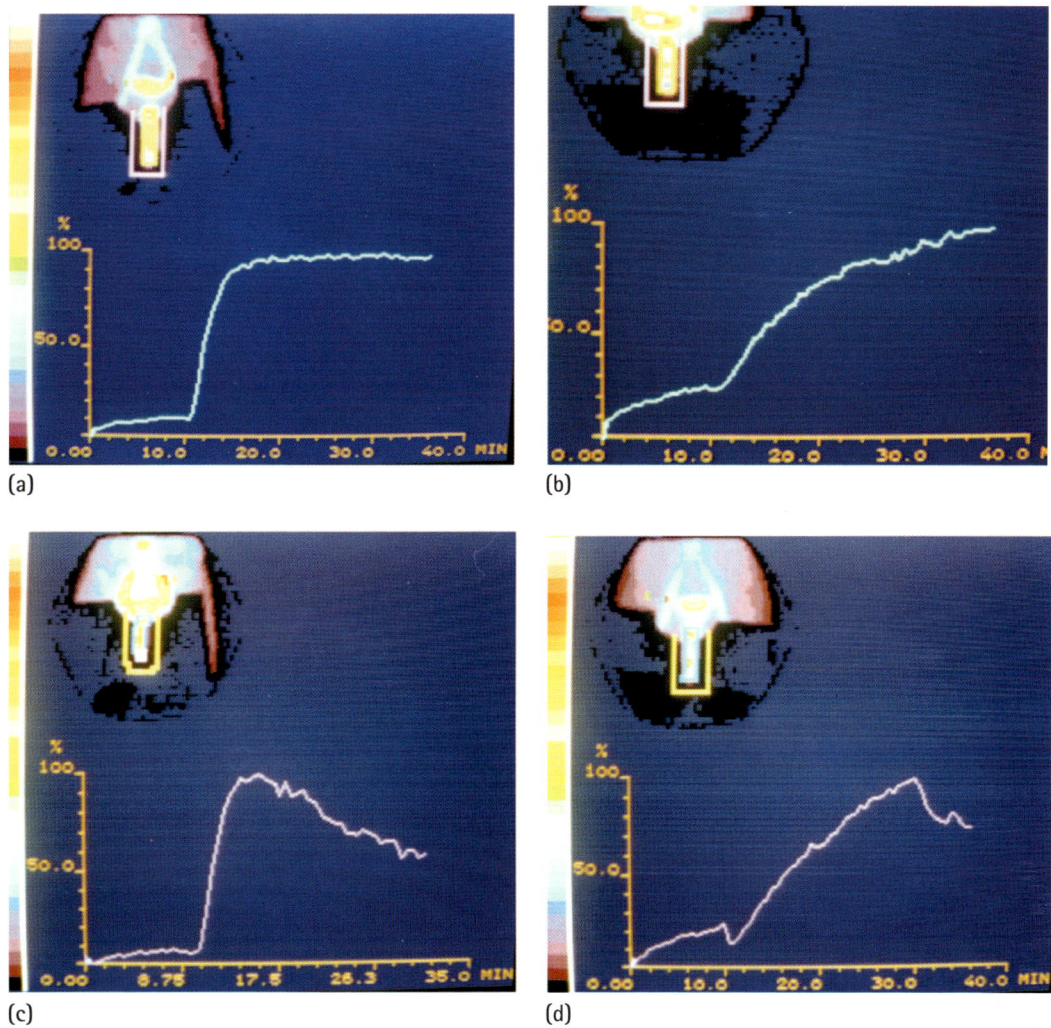

Plate 13D.1 *Erection phallogram curves of (a) a subject with normal erectile response, (b) an arteriogenic impotence patient, (c) a venous leakage patient, and (d) a patient with arteriotegenic impotence with secondary venous–occlusive dysfunction. See page 581.*

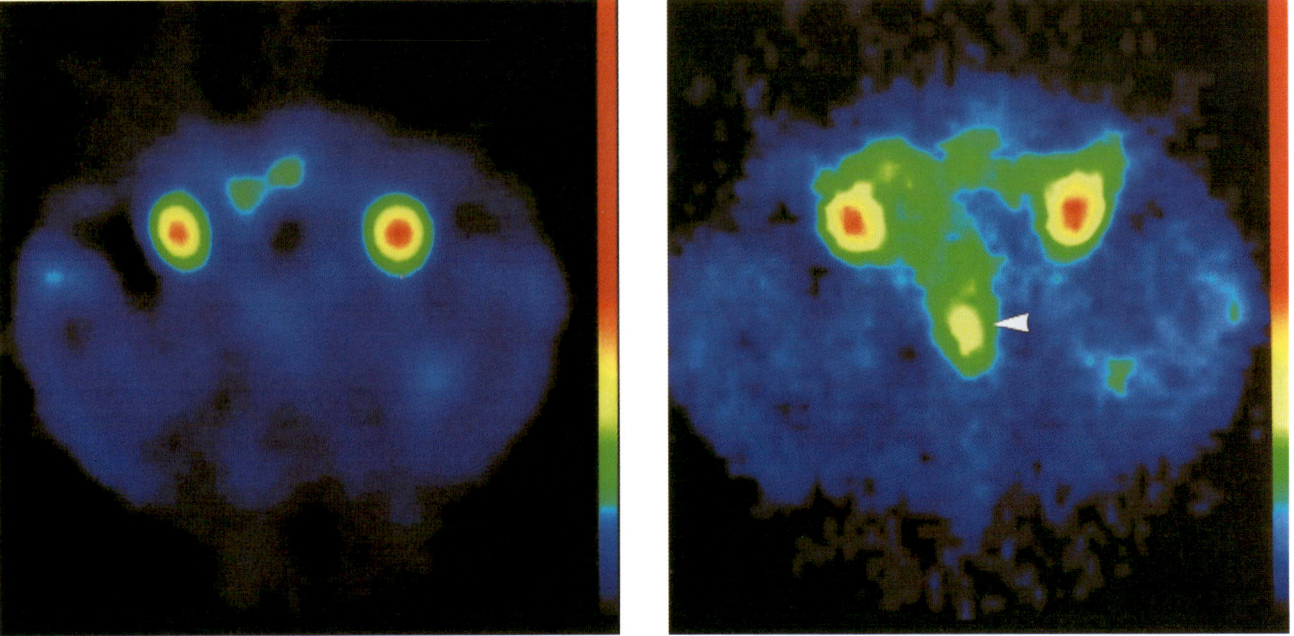

Plate 13H.1 *Prostate transverse SPECT radioimmunoscintigraphy with* ^{99}*mTc-CYT-351 in recurrent prostate cancer. Left: image at 1 hour, right: image at 26 hours showing the appearance of specific uptake in the pre-rectal recurrence (arrowhead pointing left). See page 611.*

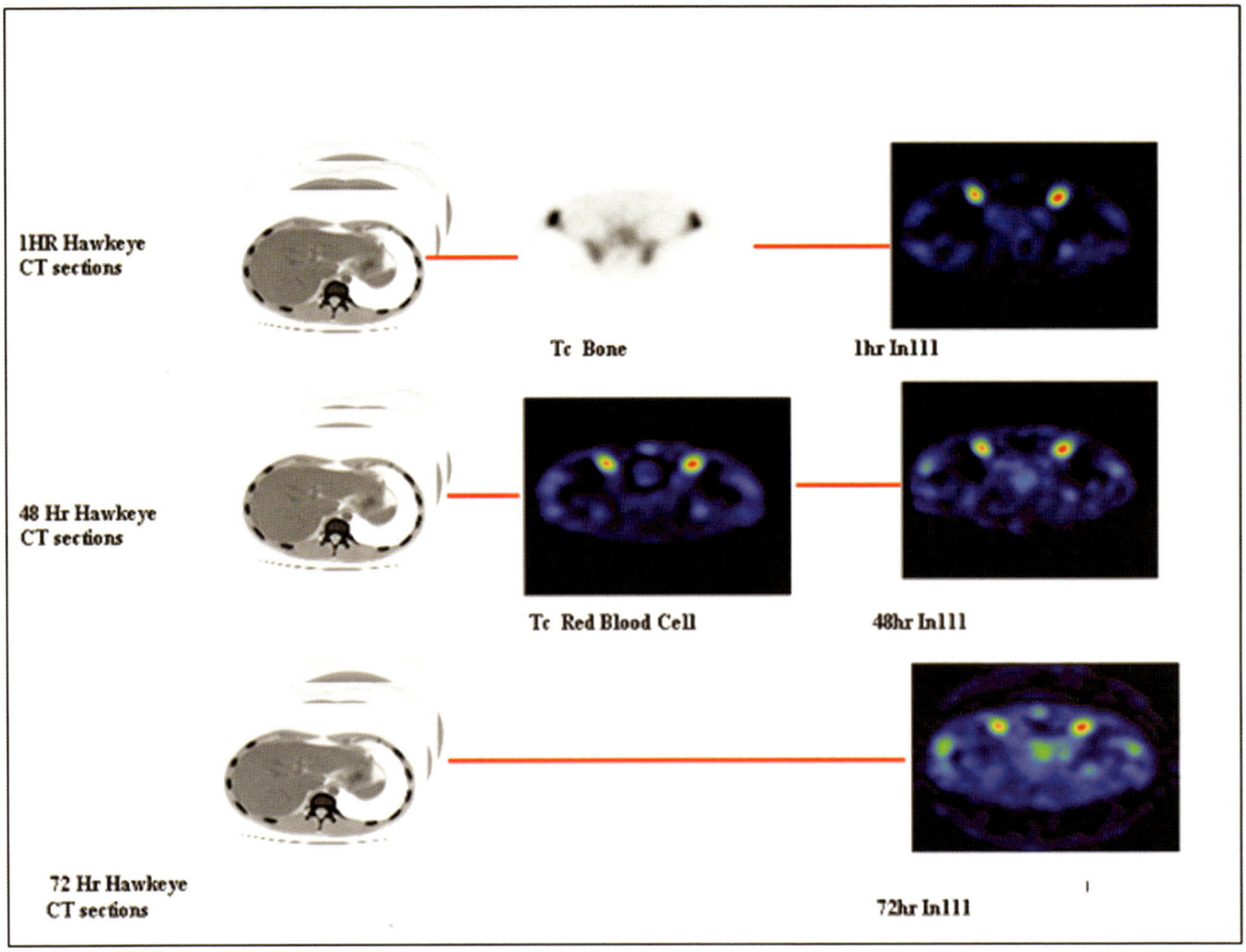

1HR Hawkeye
CT sections

Tc Bone

1hr In111

48 Hr Hawkeye
CT sections

Tc Red Blood Cell

48hr In111

72 Hr Hawkeye
CT sections

72hr In111

Plate 13H.2 *Prostascint-related data sets. Left: computed tomography scans at the three time points. Centre: bone scan at 1 h; red cell scan at 48 h. Right: Prostascint scans at the three time points. See page 612.*

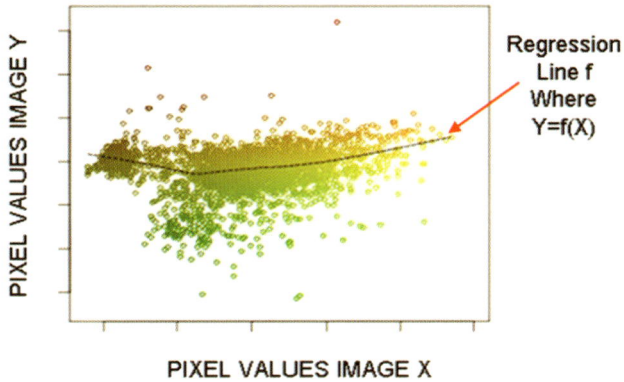

Plate 13H.3 *Example of an image based scattergram with associated nonparametric regression line. See page 613.*

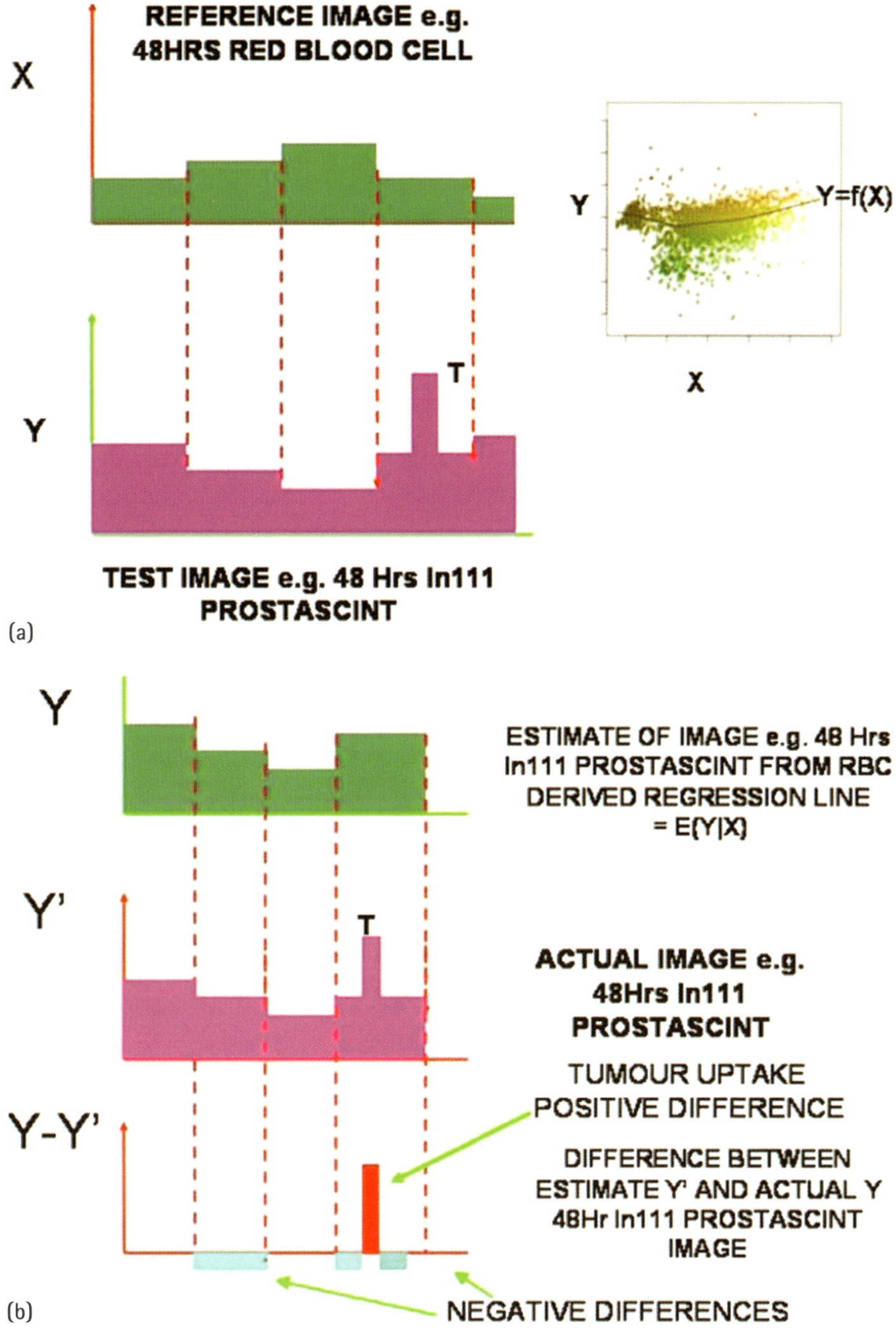

REFERENCE IMAGE e.g. 48HRS RED BLOOD CELL

X

Y=f(X)

Y

X

T

Y

TEST IMAGE e.g. 48 Hrs In111 PROSTASCINT

(a)

Y

ESTIMATE OF IMAGE e.g. 48 Hrs In111 PROSTASCINT FROM RBC DERIVED REGRESSION LINE = E{Y|X}

Y'

T

ACTUAL IMAGE e.g. 48Hrs In111 PROSTASCINT

TUMOUR UPTAKE POSITIVE DIFFERENCE

Y-Y'

DIFFERENCE BETWEEN ESTIMATE Y' AND ACTUAL Y 48Hr In111 PROSTASCINT IMAGE

(b)

NEGATIVE DIFFERENCES

Plate 13H.4 *(a) Dual energy ^{99m}Tc-RBC and ^{111}In-Prostascint acquisitions with associated scattergram and nonparametric regression curve. (b) Expected ^{111}In-Prostascint image Y derived from the nonparametric regression of ^{99m}Tc- RBC and ^{111}In-Prostascint image data is compared to actual Prostascint image Y'. The difference gives rise to areas of positive and negative charge, and hence detection of the tumor signal T. See page 614.*

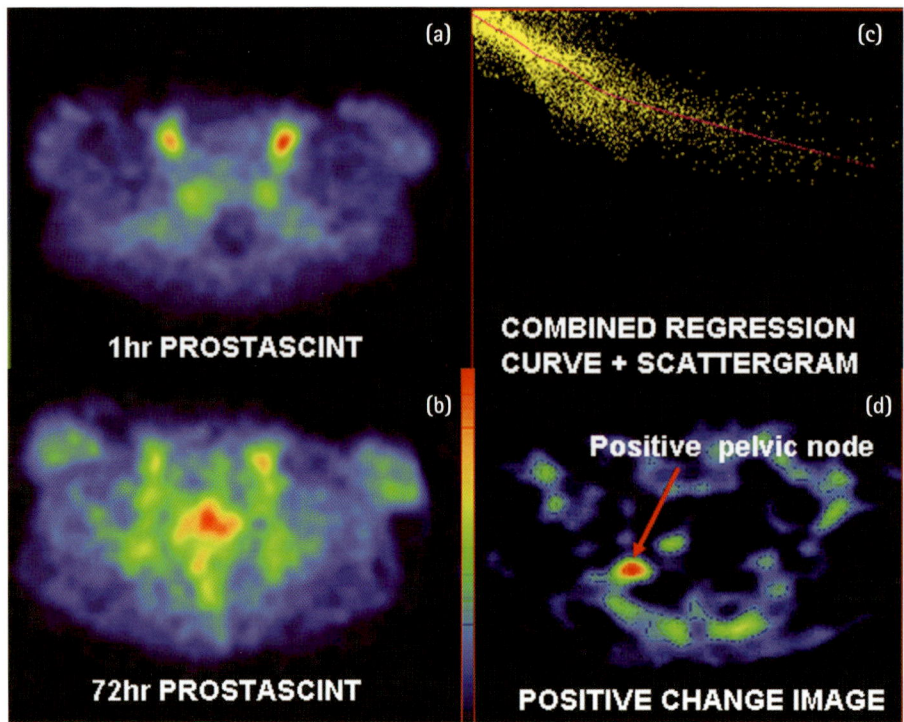

Plate 13H.5 *An example of statistical change detection showing homologous transverse sections at (a) 1 h and (b) 72 h. (c) The associated scattergram and nonlinear regression curve. (d) The detection of a Prostascint positive lymph node. See page 614.*

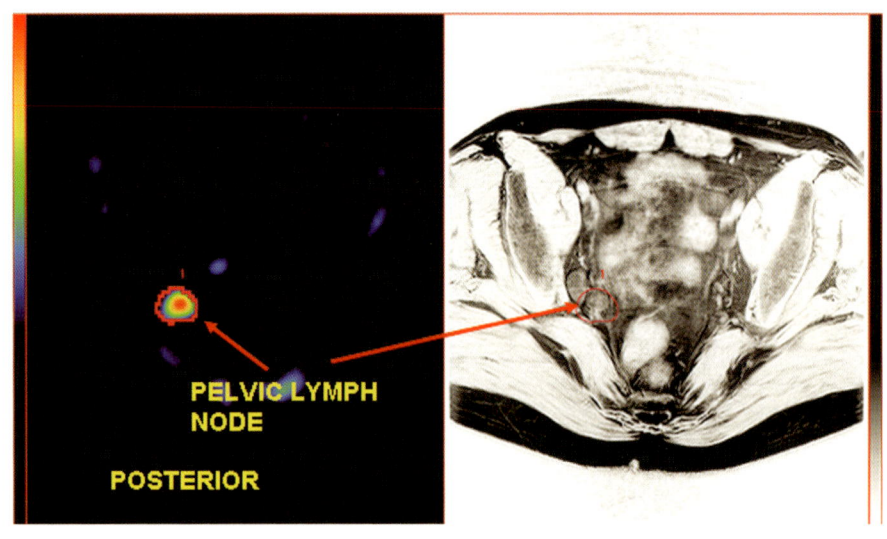

Plate 13H.6 *Example of image fusion demonstrating mapping of a Prostascint positive lymph node from the change detection image onto the corresponding T1 magnetic resonance imaging transverse section and identifying which of the two nodes shown on the magnetic resonance image is involved. See page 614.*

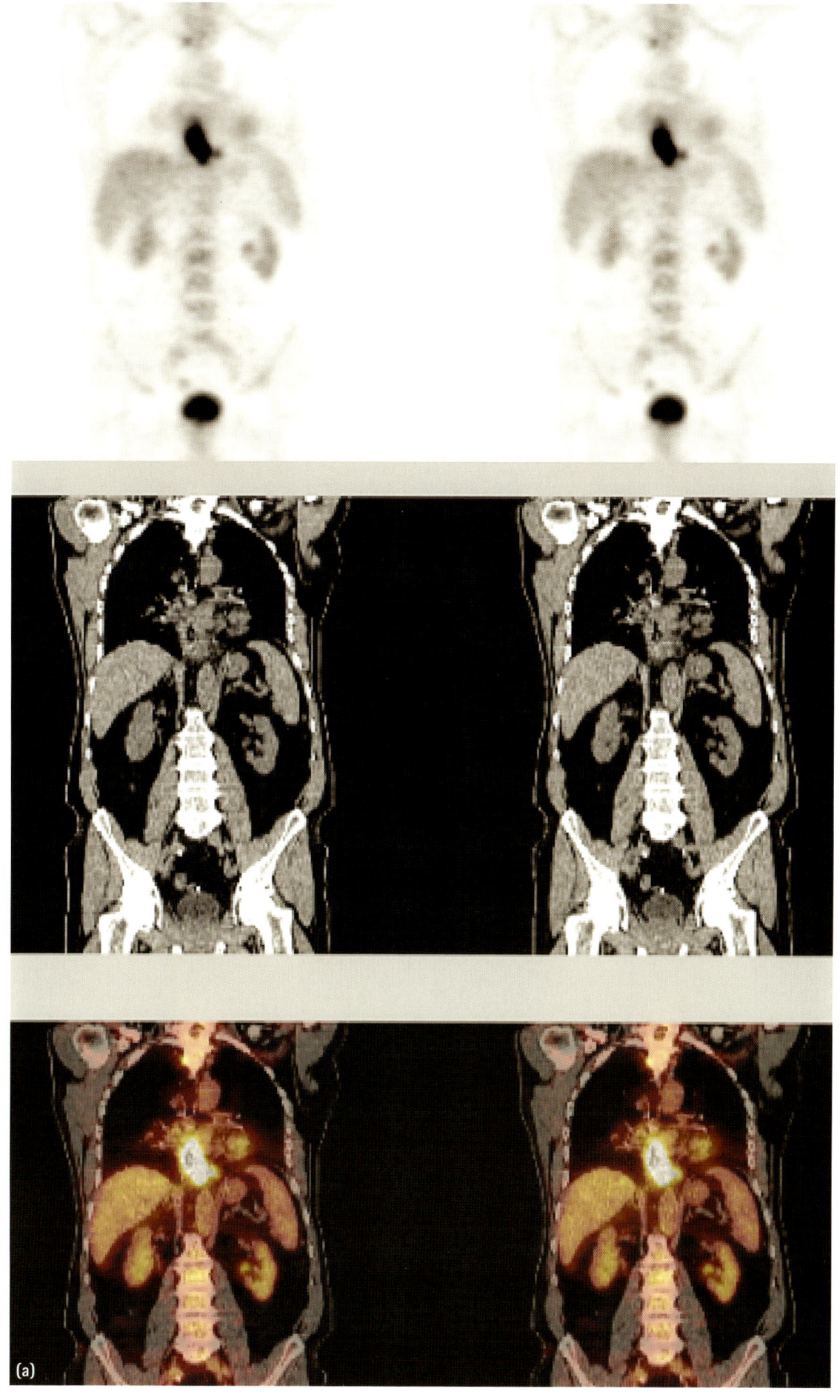

Plate 14D.1 *Coronal ¹⁸F–FDG PET/CT images demonstrating a primary esophageal carcinoma with peri-esophageal (a), See page 645*

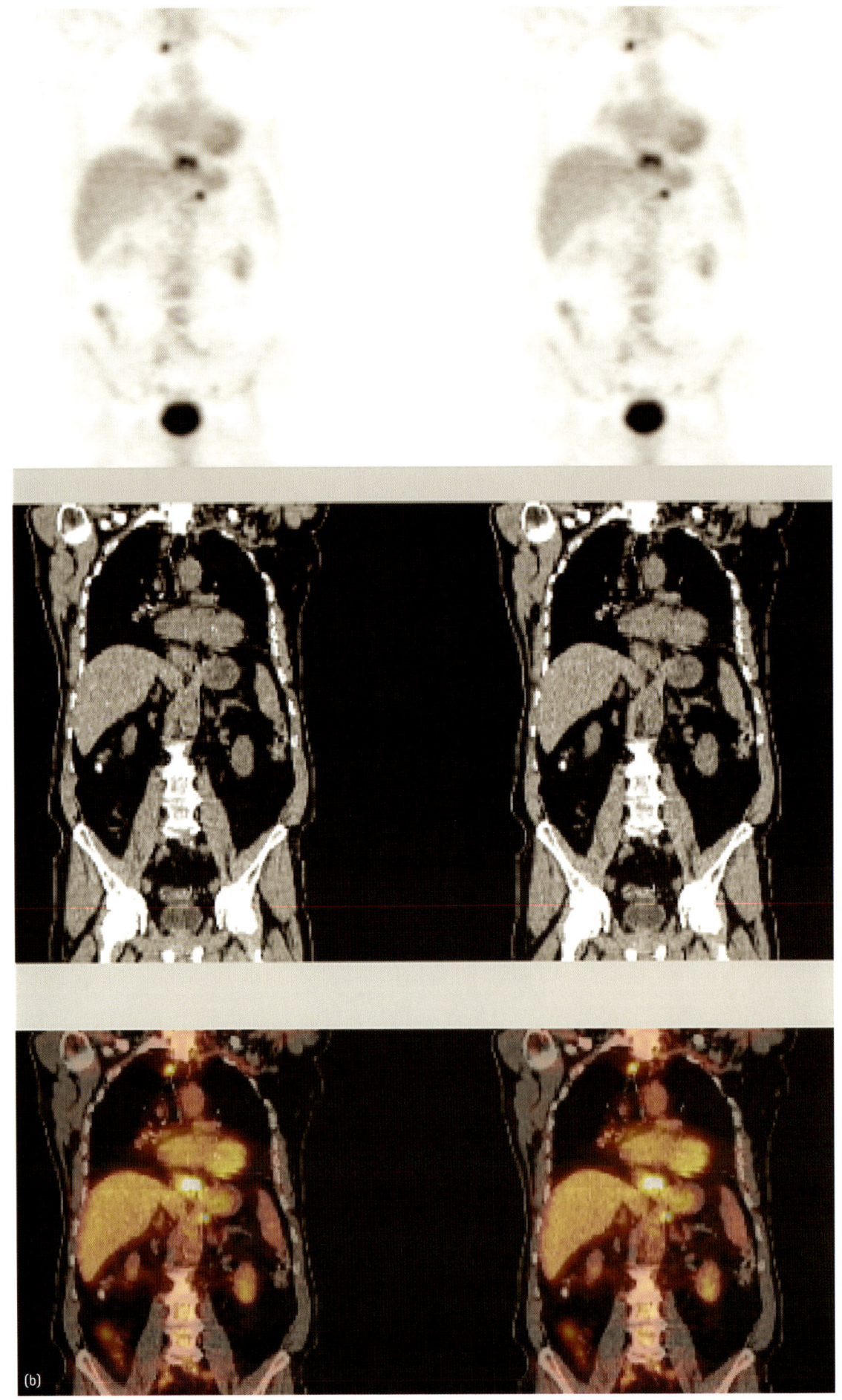

Plate 14D.1 *(Continued)*   *nodal and distant metastases (b). See page 645.*

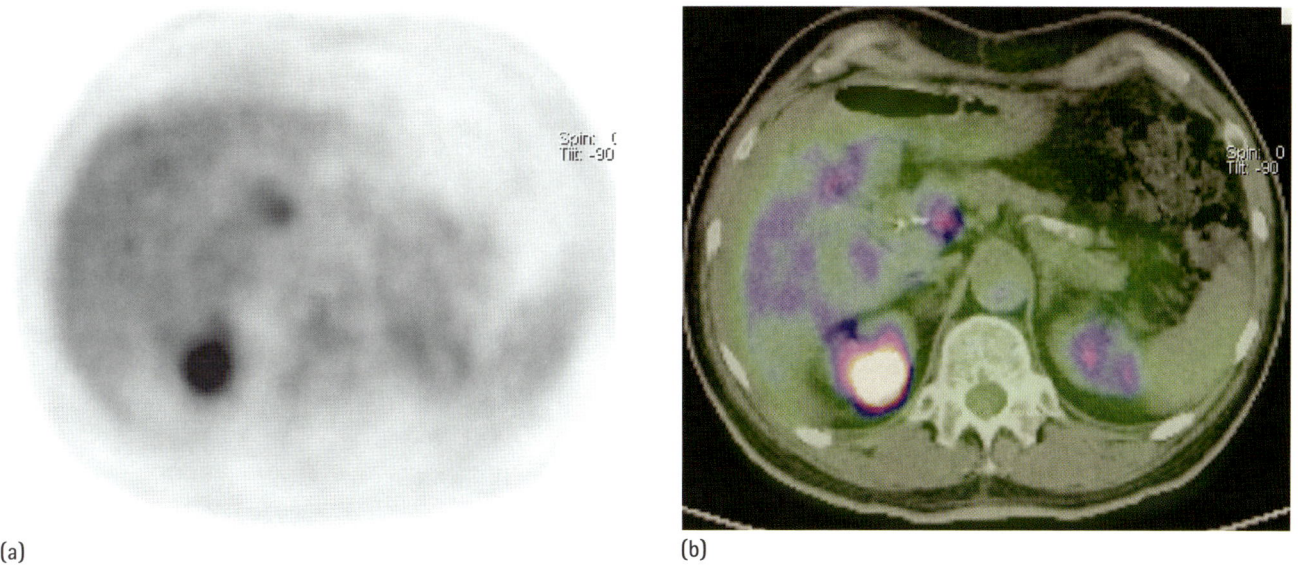

(a)   (b)

Plate 14D.2 *Transaxial* ^{18}*F-FDG PET/CT images of a patient who had undergone pancreatic resection for pancreatic carcinoma but on follow-up was found to have rising tumor markers (CA 19-9). Images show an area of focal uptake in the surgical resection bed indicating a small area of recurrent tumor. See page 646.*

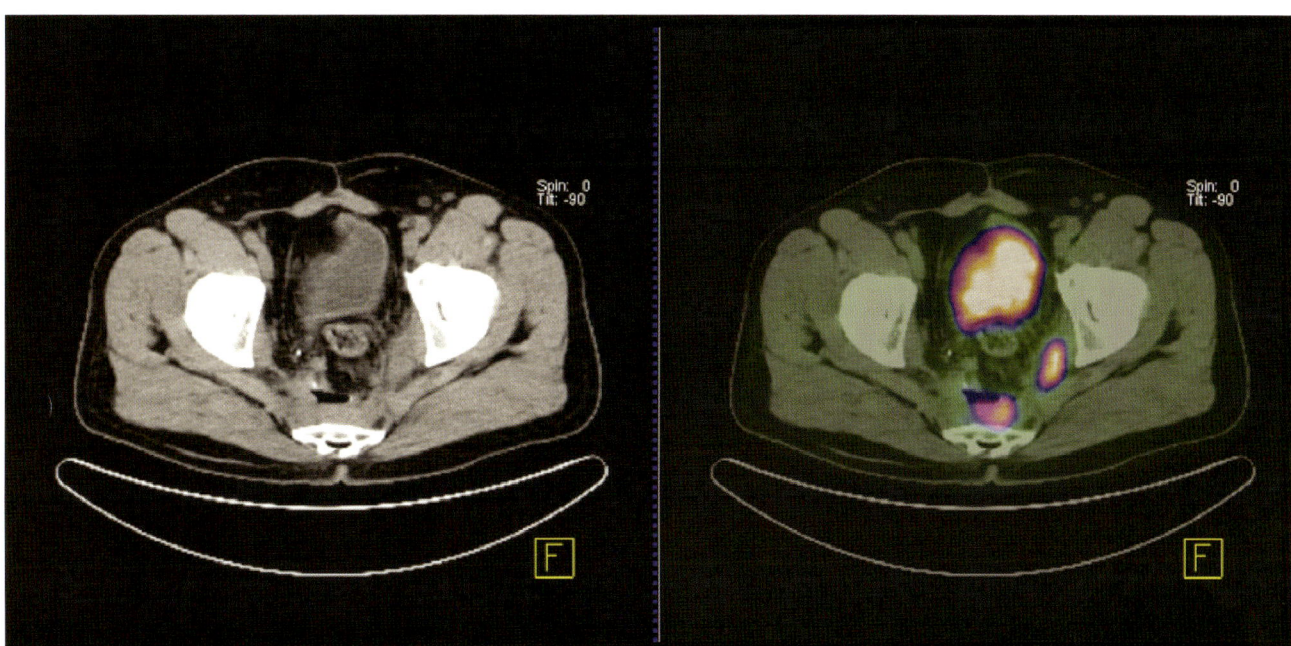

Plate 14D.3 *The transaxial images (left CT and right fused PET/CT) demonstrate abnormal uptake of* ^{18}*F-FDG not only in the presacral soft tissue thickening but also in abnormal soft tissue in the left pelvic sidewall. (See case study, page 648.)*

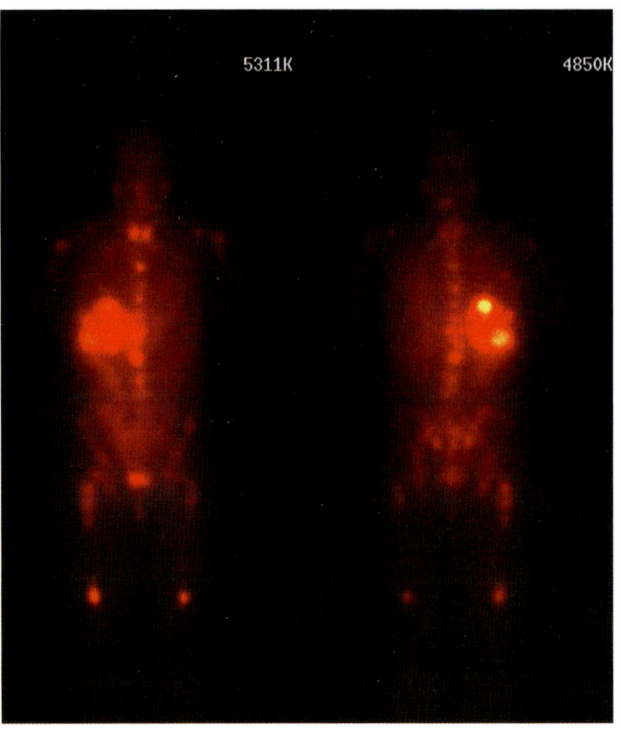

Plate 14E.1 *Anterior and posterior whole-body ^{111}In-octreotide images in a patient with a malignant insulinoma. There is extensive disease within the liver but also within the spine, humeral heads, femora, and both patellae. See page 656.*

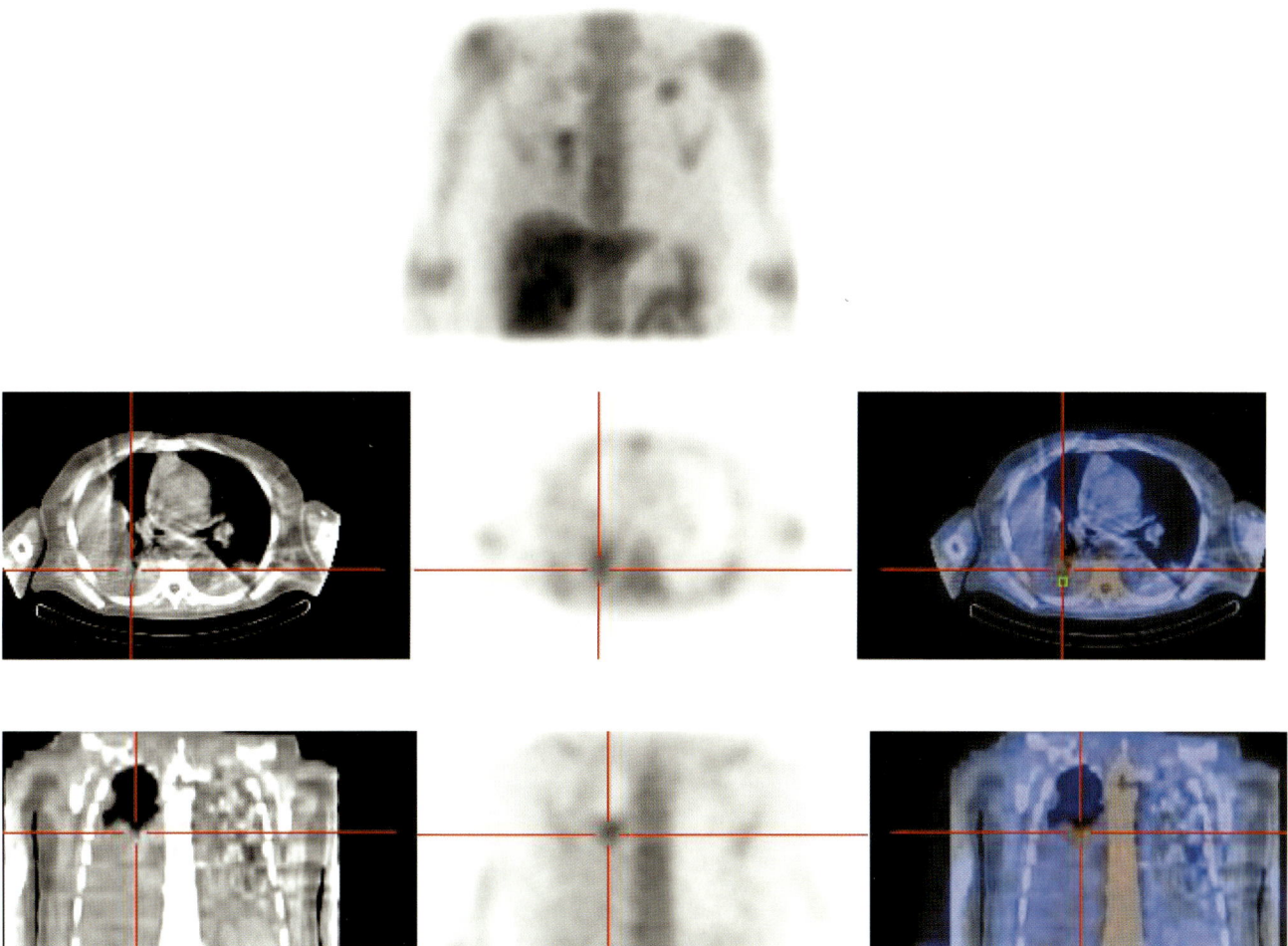

Plate 16C.1 *64-year-old male recently diagnosed with non-Hodgkin's lymphoma underwent a pre-therapy ^{67}Ga imaging study. Anterior planar image (top panel) reveals two foci of increased radiotracer uptake in the right middle chest and left upper chest. Further evaluation with SPECT imaging study simultaneously acquired with a CT scan demonstrates that on both axial (middle panel) and coronal (lower panel) sections, the focus on the right corresponds to the consolidated lung fields in the apical segment of the right lower lung, consistent with lymphoma of the lung. See page 699.*

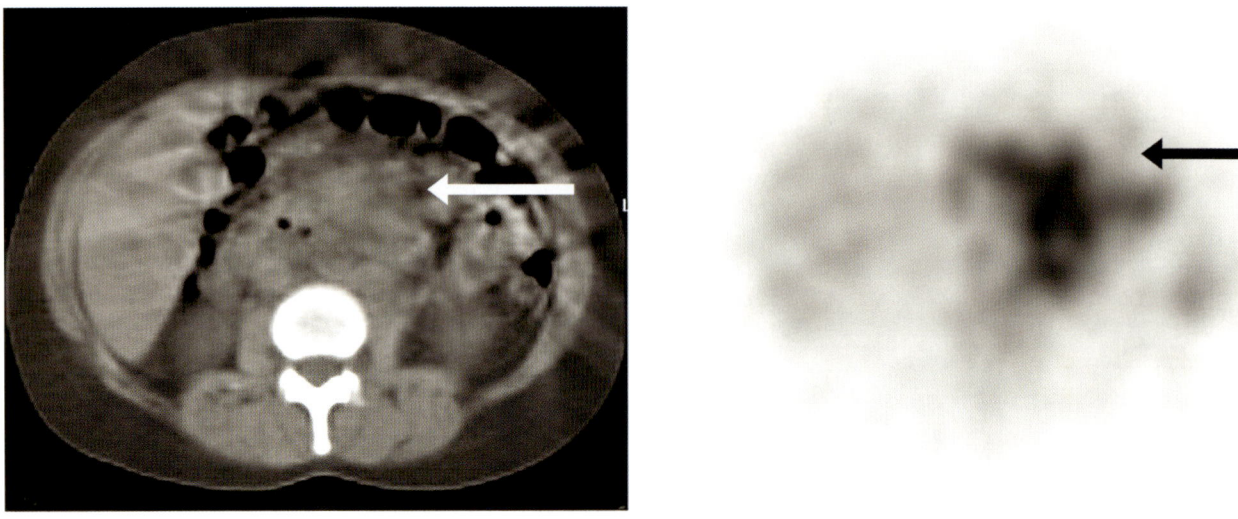

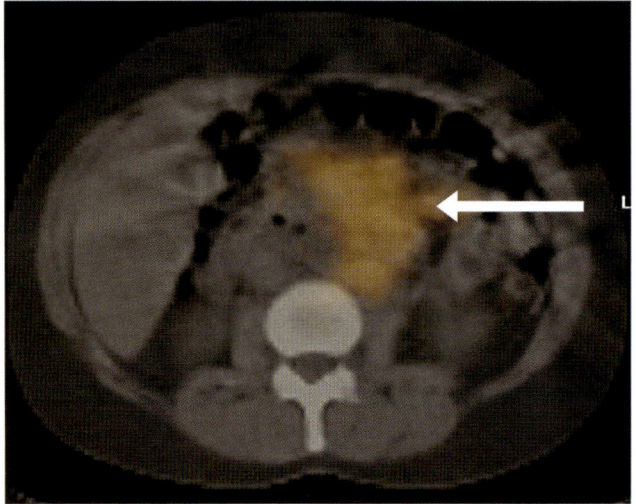

Plate 16C.2 *Patient with a diagnosis of diffuse large cell lymphoma underwent a pre-therapy* ^{67}*Ga SPECT/CT imaging, to evaluate for the extent of disease. Axial images of low dose CT (top left),* ^{67}*Ga (top right) and SPECT-CT fusion (lower panel) demonstrate intense increased* ^{67}*Ga uptake in a mass involving the retroperitoneal and mesenteric lymph nodes (arrows) , consistent with active lymphoma. See page 699.*

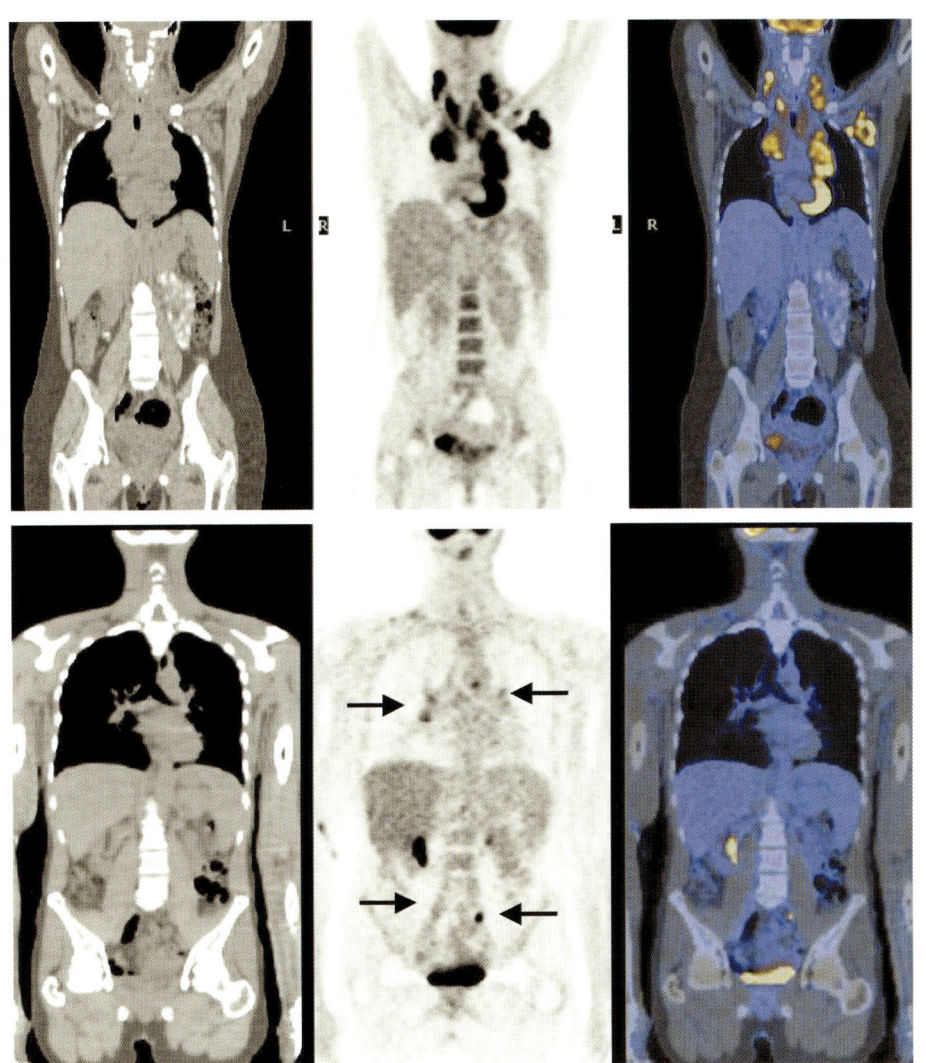

Plate 16C.3 *Patient diagnosed with Hodgkin's disease (upper panel) underwent a pre-therapy FDG-PET imaging study simultaneously acquired with a CT scan, to evaluate for the extent of disease. Coronal FDG-PET/CT images demonstrate multiple small foci of abnormal FDG uptake distributed in a contiguous fashion in the lower neck, anterior mediastinum and the left axilla, consistent with Hodgkin's disease (SUVmax 11). Patient diagnosed with follicular lymphoma (lower panel) underwent a pre-therapy FDG-PET imaging study simultaneously acquired with a CT scan. Coronal FDG-PET/CT images demonstrate multiple small foci of abnormal FDG uptake in the precarinal, bilateral hilar, paraaortic and bilateral iliac lymph nodes (arrows) (SUVmax 4.8). Note the difference in FDG avidity between these two cases due to differences in grades (high grade vs low grade). See page 702.*

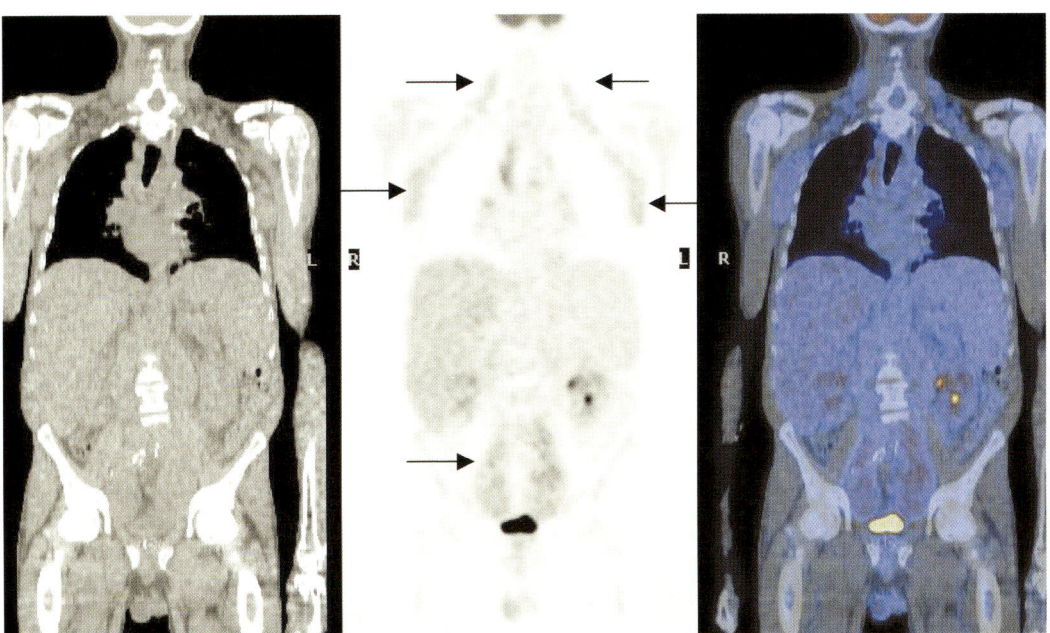

Plate 16C.4 *Patient diagnosed with small lymphocytic non-Hodgkin's lymphoma (CLL/SLL) underwent a pre-therapy FDG-PET imaging study simultaneously acquired with a CT scan, to evaluate for the extent of disease. Coronal FDG-PET/CT images demonstrate multiple small foci of abnormal FDG uptake in the bilateral lower cervical, axillary, paratracheal, hilar and iliac lymph nodes (arrows) (SUVmax: 3.5), consistent with CLL/SLL. Note the difference in metabolic activity between this case and those in Plate 16C.7. See page 702.*

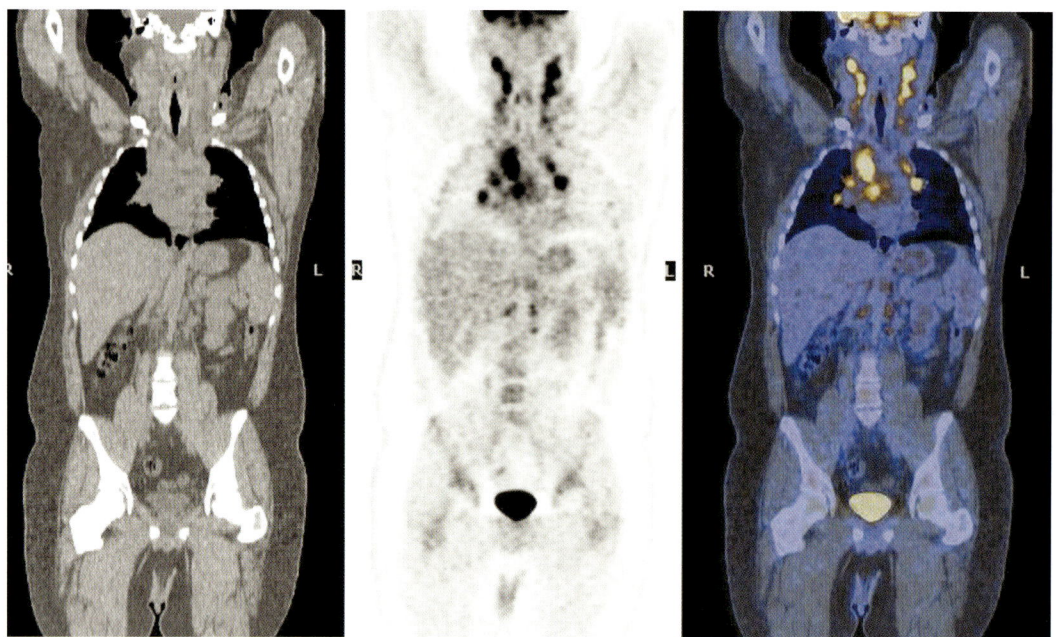

Plate 16C.5 *Patient with a diagnosis of non-Hodgkin's lymphoma underwent a pre-therapy FDG-PET imaging study simultaneously acquired with a CT scan, for staging. Coronal images of CT (left), PET (middle) and PET-CT fusion (right) demonstrate increased FDG uptake in multiple lymph nodes in the bilateral cervical stations, anterior mediastinum, and bilateral hila. Additionally, several unenlarged proximal paraaortic lymph nodes (arrow) demonstrate increased uptake, consistent with lymphoma and upgrading the stage from II to III. See page 702.*

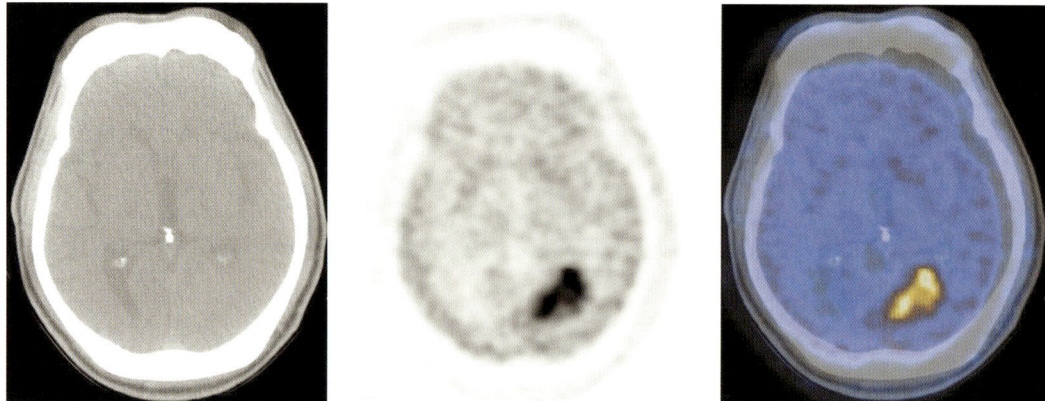

Plate 16C.6 *The patient with a history of AIDS recently found to have a brain lesion in the left parietooccipital lobe, referred for FDG-PET imaging to differentiate between toxoplasmosis from CNS lymphoma. There is intense FDG uptake in a lesion corresponding to the left posterior parietooccipital cortex consistent with CNS lymphoma (arrow). The patient was subsequently started on chemotherapy rather than continued on antibiotherapy. See page 703.*

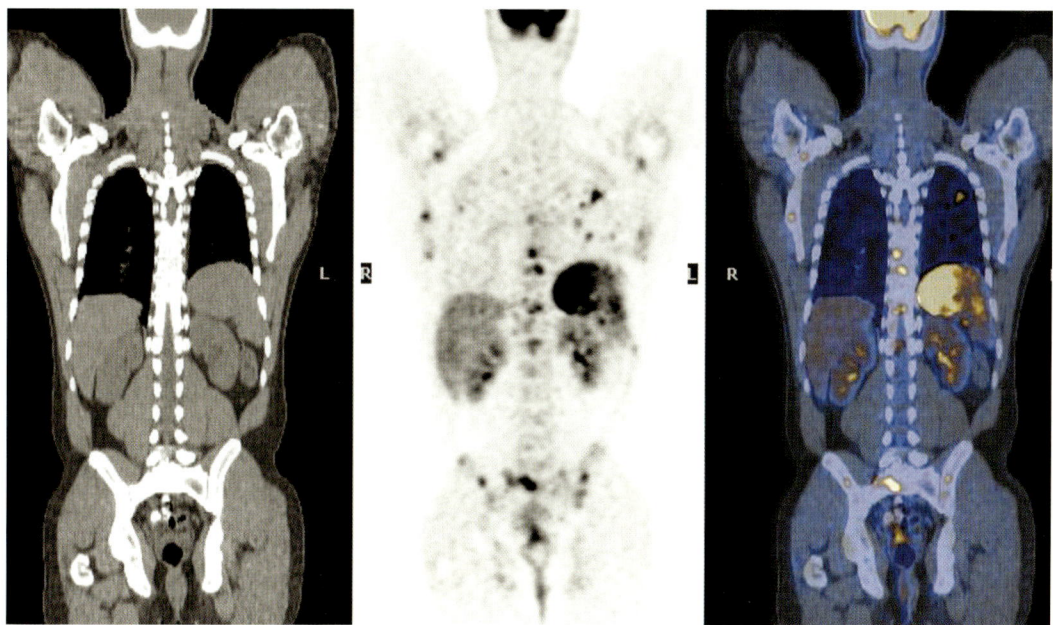

Plate 16C.7 *The patient with a recent diagnosis of aggressive non-Hodgkin's lymphoma referred for evaluation of extent of disease, staging prior to chemotherapy. Coronal images of CT (left), PET (middle), PET-CT fusion (right) demonstrate innumerable foci of increased FDG uptake in the axial and visualized appendicular skeleton, consistent with bone/bone marrow involvement. Note the heterogeneously increased uptake in the medial aspect of the spleen, consistent with splenic involvement. See page 703.*

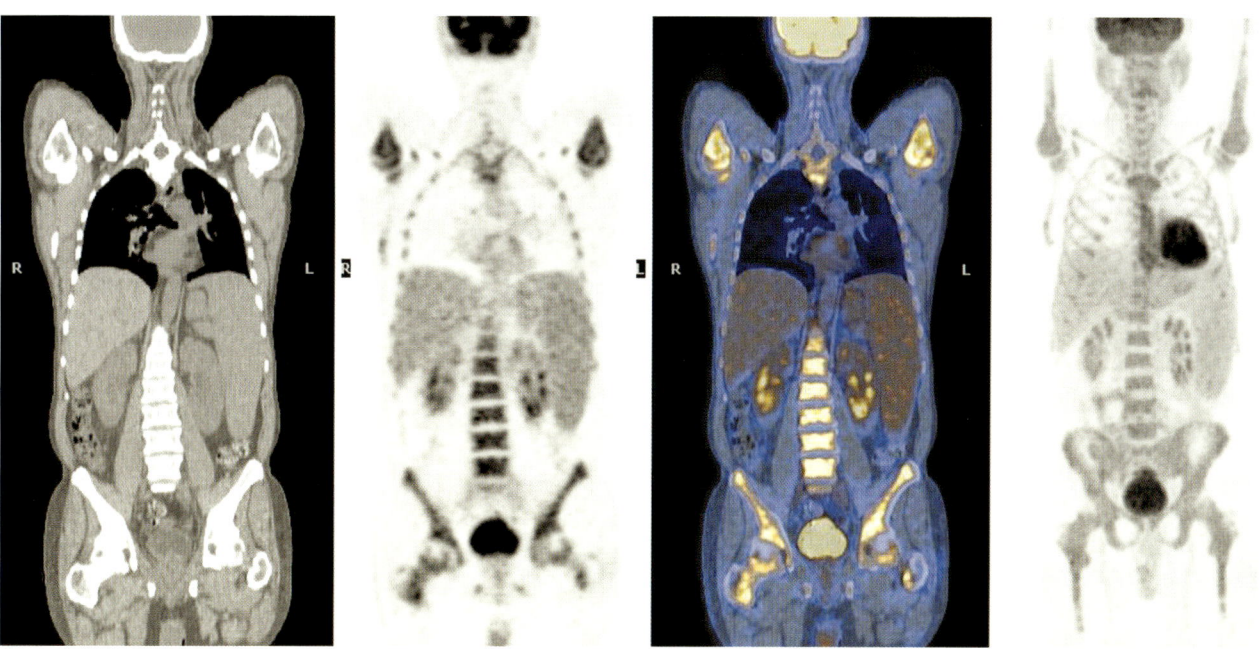

Plate 16C.8 *Coronal images of CT (left), PET (middle), PET-CT fusion (right) and the volume rendered image (right most) demonstrate diffusely increased FDG uptake in the entire vertebral column, ribs, pelvis and proximal femora, consistent with reactive bone marrow changes secondary to recent administration of colony stimulators (G-CSF). Due to the reactive changes in the bone marrow, possible involvement of the bone marrow cannot be evaluated with certainty. Note the increased FDG uptake in the spleen which may be due to extrameduallry hematopoiesis incited by the colony stimulators. However splenic lymphoma cannot be evaluated, if the initial presentation was with splenic involvement. See page 703.*

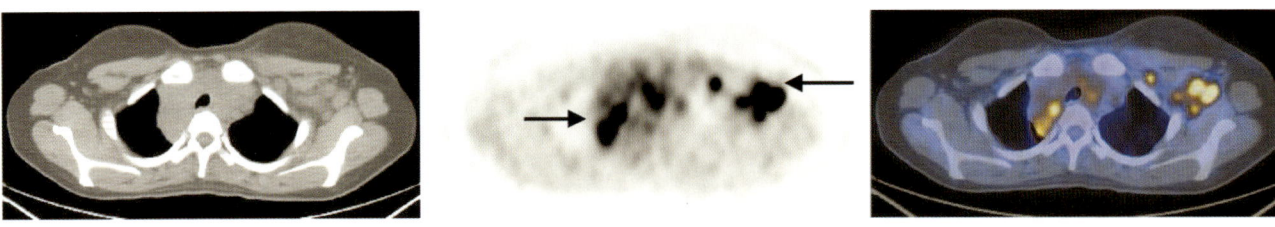

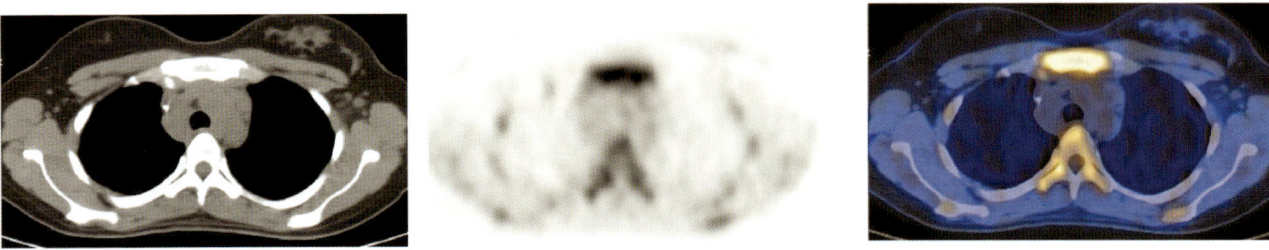

Plate 16C.9 *Patient with non-Hodgkin's lymphoma underwent a PET-CT study prior to and immediately following completion of therapy to evaluate response to therapy. Pre-therapy coronal images (upper panel) of CT (left), PET (right) demonstrate increased FDG uptake in multiple lymph nodes in the anterior mediastinum and the left axilla, consistent with active lymphoma (arrows). Post-therapy coronal images (lower panel) of CT (left), PET (right) demonstrate complete resolution of disease in the mediastinum and the left axilla with no evidence of residual uptake. These findings are consistent with favorable response to therapy. The PFS has not been reached for this patient after a follow up of 36 months. See page 704.*

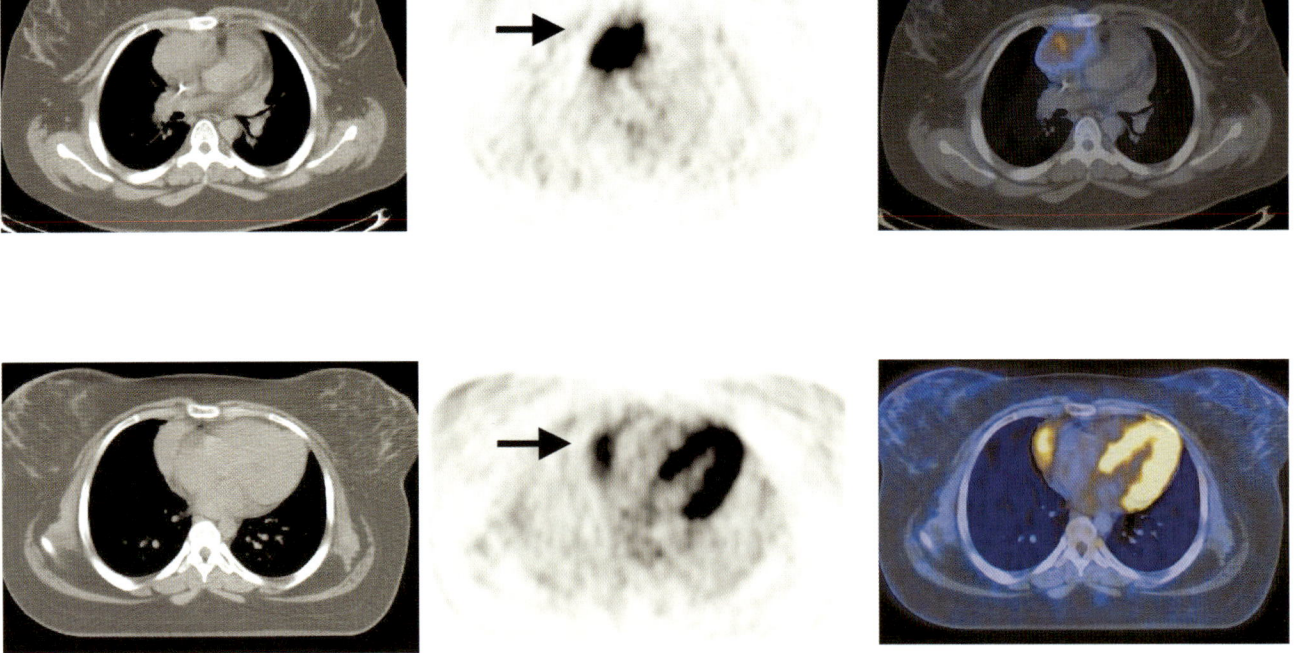

Plate 16C.10 *Patient with non-Hodgkin's lymphoma underwent a PET-CT study prior to and immediately following completion of therapy to evaluate response to therapy. Pre-therapy axial images (upper panel) of CT (left), PET (right) demonstrate increased FDG uptake in the anterior mediastinum, consistent with lymphoma (arrow). Post-therapy axial images (lower panel) of CT (left), PET (right) demonstrate persistent FDG uptake in the anterior mediastinum in the region of original disease (arrow). These findings are consistent with unfavorable response to therapy. The patient was subsequently placed on an alternative therapy. Note the physiologic uptake in the myocardium in the post-therapy image. See page 704.*

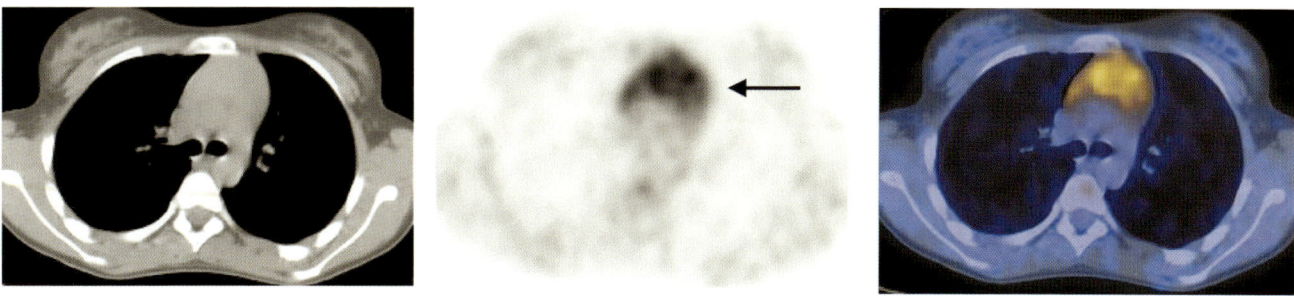

Plate 16C.11 *17-year-old female with a history of Hodgkin's disease underwent a PET-CT study 3 months following completion of therapy to evaluate disease status. Axial images of CT (left), PET (right) demonstrate increased FDG uptake in a crescent shaped soft tissue mass in the anterior superior mediastinum corresponding to the thymus (arrow), consistent with thymic rebound. Of note thymic rebound may persist for 18 months after therapy. See page 706.*

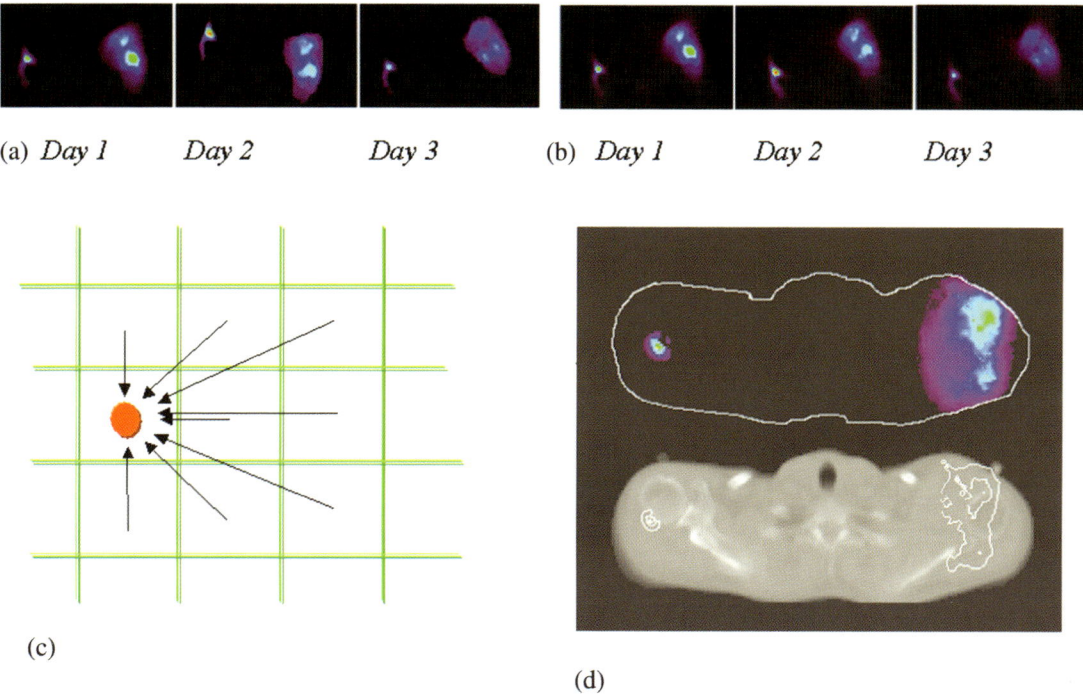

Plate 17F.1 *(a) Pre-registration SPECT. (b) Post-registration SPECT. (c) Dose to target voxel from source voxels. Process repeated for all voxels. (d) Absorbed dose map. See page 786.*

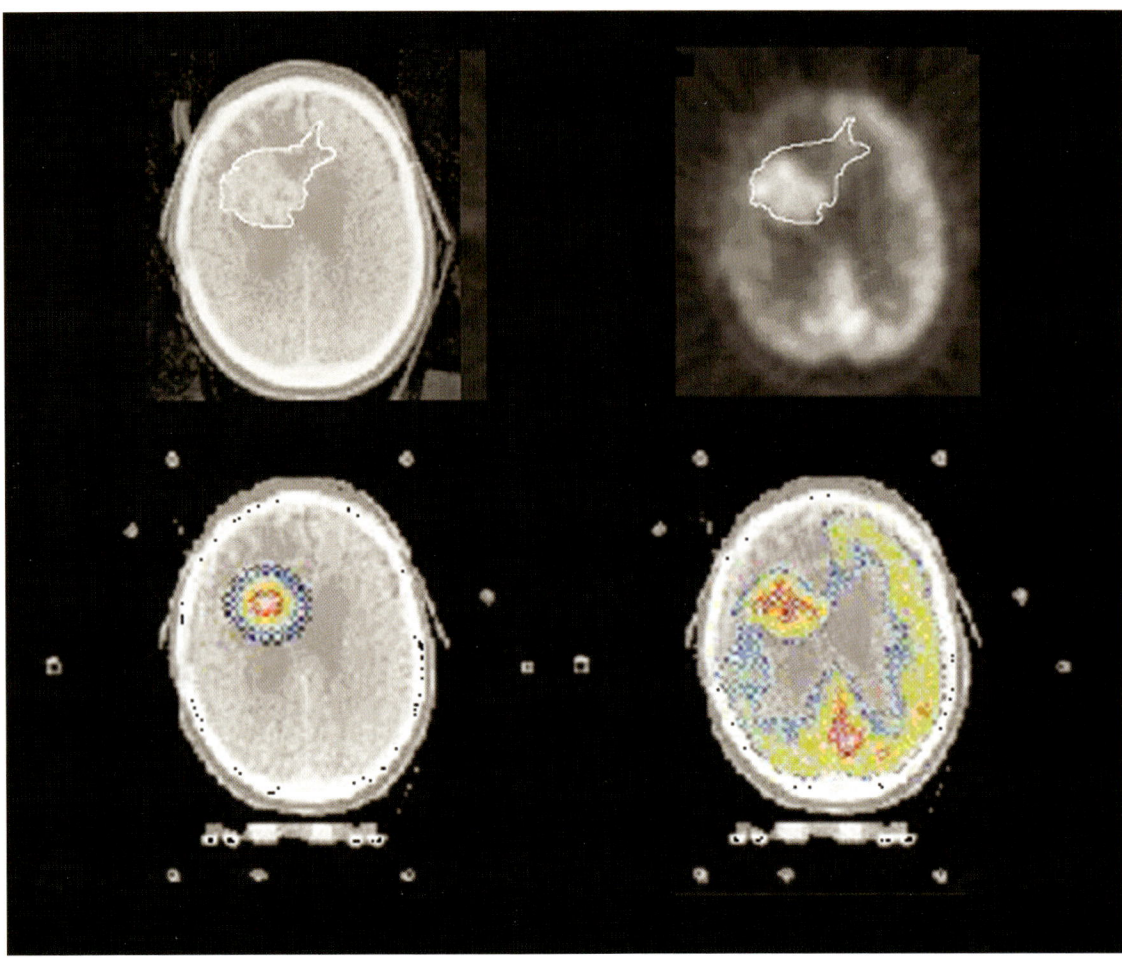

Plate 21B.1 *Top row: Malignant glioma outlined using registered computed tomography (CT) (left) and fluorodeoxyglucose (FDG) positron emission tomography (PET) (right). Bottom row: absorbed dose map following uptake of ^{131}I-anti-tenascin monoclonal antibody from direct infusion (left) and pseudocolor scale depiction of FDG PET overlaid onto CT using a 'chessboard' display to aid delineation. See page 864.*

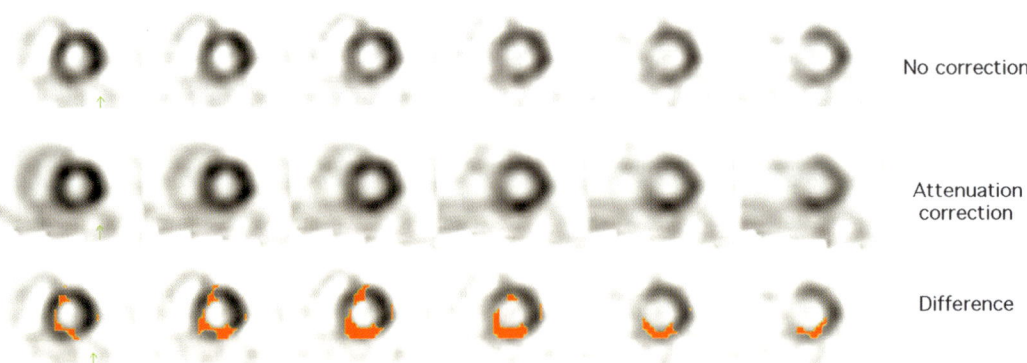

No correction

Attenuation correction

Difference

Plate 21C.1 *An example of the application of attenuation correction in myocardial perfusion SPECT shows (top row) the short-axis reconstruction with no attenuation correction, (middle) the same data after attenuation correction on a system which uses scanning line sources of [153]Gd, and (bottom) the differences between the two sets of data superimposed on the non-attenuation corrected images. See page 875.*

12

Endocrine disease

12A Thyroid

Introduction	491	Nontoxic goiters	506
Diagnosis of thyroid dysfunction	492	Ectopic thyroid	508
Hyperthyroidism	495	Neonatal hypothyroidism	509
Solitary thyroid nodules	503	References	510
Painful goiter	505		

12B Parathyroid localization

Introduction	511	Imaging methodology	513
Anatomy and physiology	511	Clinical role of parathyroid localization	517
Preoperative localizing techniques	512	References	518

12C The adrenal gland

Introduction	521	Adrenal medulla	530
Adrenal cortex	522	References	536

Thyroid

M.N. MAISEY

INTRODUCTION

The prevalence of diseases of the thyroid is high. In 1956, Perlmutter and Slater[1] estimated that 4–12% of the population of the USA had palpable thyroid nodules of which 2–5% were probably malignant. In a cohort of adolescents there was a 3.7% incidence of thyroid disorders rising to 10.5% when they were followed up after 20 years.[2,3] In a population study of north-east England, Tunbridge et al.[4] reported that in adult females, the prevalence of hyperthyroidism was 1.9–2.7%, of overt hypothyroidism 1.4–1.9%, of subclinical hypothyroidism 7.5%, and of nontoxic goiters 8.6% although the prevalence of these conditions was much lower in males and in a recent follow-up from the original survey the incidence of thyroid disease was well documented.[3] A classification of thyroid diseases is shown in Table 12A.1.

The correct management of thyroid diseases depends on accurate diagnosis, appropriate treatment and careful monitoring. Radionuclides have always played a leading part in all aspects of the management of thyroid diseases: radioimmunoassay techniques revolutionized the investigation of thyroid dysfunction while radionuclide scanning has long been the main method for investigating the thyroid gland *in vivo*. The role of thyroid scanning in clinical practice expanded with the introduction of new radiopharmaceuticals (Table 12A.2). The increasing use of other diagnostic imaging techniques, including ultrasound, computed tomography (CT), and magnetic resonance imaging (MRI), has had considerable impact on the way we use radionuclides for the investigation of thyroid disease, but radionuclide scanning remains key to the optimal management of many clinical situations. Radioactive iodine is well

Table 12A.1 *Classification of thyroid disease*

I. Diseases primarily characterized by euthyroidism

   A. Nontoxic diffuse goiter
      1. Sporadic
      2. Endemic
      3. Compensatory, following subtotal thyroidectomy

   B. Nontoxic uninodular goiter
      1. Functional nodule
      2. Nonfunctional

   C. Nontoxic multinodular goiter due to causes under IA
      1. Functional nodules
      2. Nonfunctional nodules
      3. Functional and nonfunctional nodules

   D. Tumors
      1. Adenoma and teratoma
      2. Carcinoma
      3. Lymphoma
      4. Sarcoma

   E. Acute thyroiditis
      1. Suppurative
      2. Subacute, nonsuppurative

   F. Chronic thyroiditis
      1. Lymphocytic (Hashimoto's)
      2. Invasive fibrous (Riedel's)
      3. Suppurative
      4. Nonsuppurative

   G. Degeneration or infiltration
      1. Hemorrhage or infarction
      2. Amyloid
      3. Hemochromatosis

   H. Congenital anomaly

(Continued)

Table 12A.1   *(Continued)*

II. Diseases primarily characterized by hyperthyroidism

    A.   *Toxic diffuse goiter (Graves', Basedow's disease)*

        1.   *With eye changes (ophthalmopathy)*

        2.   *With localized dermopathy or acropachy*

        3.   *Neonatal or congenital*

        4.   *With incidental nonfunctional nodule(s)*

        5.   *With euthyroidism and eye changes*

    B.   *Toxic uninodular goiter*

    C.   *Toxic multinodular goiter*

        1.   *Functional nodules, nonfunctional parenchyma*

        2.   *Functional nodules, functional parenchyma*

    D.   *Nodular goiter with hyperthyroidism due to exogenous iodine (Jod–Basedow)*

    E.   *Exogenous thyroid hormone excess*

        1.   *Thyrotoxicosis factitia*

        2.   *Thyrotoxicosis medicamentosa*

    F.   *Tumors*

        1.   *Adenoma of thyroid, follicular*

        2.   *Carcinoma of thyroid, follicular*

        3.   *Thyrotrophin-secreting tumors*

III. Diseases primarily characterized by hypothyroidism

    A.   *Idiopathic hypothyroidism*

        1.   *Myxedema*

        2.   *Cretinism*

    B.   *Iatrogenic destruction*

        1.   *Surgery*

        2.   *Radioiodine*

        3.   *X-ray*

    C.   *Thyrotrophin deficiency*

        1.   *Isolated*

        2.   *Panhypopituitarism*

    D.   *Thyrotrophin-releasing factor deficiency due to hypothalamic injury or disease*

established as a simple, cheap, and effective method of treating thyrotoxicosis, and in most cases will represent the treatment of choice.

In this chapter we discuss systematic and practical approaches to the management of the most important clinical problems in thyroid disease with emphasis on the role of nuclear medicine techniques.

DIAGNOSIS OF THYROID DYSFUNCTION

Pathophysiology

A knowledge of the changes that occur in hyperthyroidism and hypothyroidism is fundamental to an understanding of the laboratory investigations of these conditions. The basic abnormality in hyperthyroidism and hypothyroidism is an increased or decreased concentration of circulating free thyroid hormones with a corresponding change in the total serum concentration of these hormones.

In hyperthyroidism, both serum thyroxine (T4) and tri-iodothyrorine (T3) are usually raised, and therefore it is not usually necessary to measure both hormones routinely, but in about 10% of hyperthyroid patients, serum total T3 concentration may be abnormally raised at presentation when serum T4 lies within the normal range; elevated serum T4 with normal T3 has rarely been reported. These discrepancies occur less often with free T3 (fT3) and free T4 (fT4) measurements. Other factors beside hyperthyroidism such as a co-existing severe nonthyroidal illness, which impairs peripheral conversion of T4 to T3, may also account for some disparities in hormone concentrations. For most patients with hyperthyroidism, the rise in serum T3 is much greater than that of serum T4, therefore measurement of serum T3 is a more sensitive and reliable investigation for diagnosing hyperthyroidism than serum T4. Assays of thyroid-stimulating hormone (TSH) have increased in

Table 12A.2   *Radiopharmaceuticals used in the investigation of thyroid diseases*

Radiopharmaceutical	Application(s)
[^{99m}Tc]pertechnetate	*Routine thyroid scanning*
Sodium [^{123}I]iodide	*Thyroid scanning when a radioisotope of iodine is required*
Sodium [^{131}I]iodide	*The investigation of thyroid cancer*
[^{67}Ga]Gallium citrate	*Investigation of thyroid lymphoma, silent thyroiditis, thyroid infection and amyloid*
[^{201}Tl]Thallous chloride	*Investigation of thyroid cancer, thyroid nodules, demonstration of suppressed thyroid tissue*
^{99m}Tc(V)-DMSA	*Investigation of medullary thyroid carcinoma*
^{131}I/^{123}I-MIBG	*Investigation of medullary thyroid carcinoma*
^{18}F-FDG	*All forms of thyroid cancer*

DMSA, dimercaptosuccinic acid; MIBG, *meta*-iodobenzylguanidine; FDG, fluorodeoxyglucose.

sensitivity, and low suppressed levels of serum TSH that occur in hyperthyroidism can be distinguished from normal levels. A combination of a raised T3 with suppressed TSH levels is the best marker of hyperthroidism.

In hypothyroidism there is a greater and earlier fall in serum T4 compared with serum T3, which may often remain within the normal range. Thus, while serum T3 is the investigation of choice for hyperthyroidism, serum T4 is generally a better screening test for hypothyroidism. Thyroid failure may be a primary abnormality of the thyroid gland, or rarely may be secondary to impaired secretion of TSH by the pituitary gland. In primary hypothyroidism, the low serum T4 is accompanied by a raised serum TSH, whereas in secondary hypothyroidism the low serum T4 is associated with a low serum TSH. Measurement of serum TSH is therefore essential for distinguishing between primary and secondary hypothyroidism. A low serum TSH is not always sufficient to confirm hypothyroidism due to pituitary failure, and it may be necessary to show that serum TSH concentration is unresponsive to thyrotrophin-releasing hormone (TRH) stimulation. Lately, TSH assays have increased in sensitivity, and low suppressed levels of serum TSH that occur in hyperthyroidism can be distinguished from normal levels.

Changes in serum total T3 (tT3) and T4 (tT4) levels may be due not only to altered thyroid function but also to altered concentrations of carrier proteins, especially thyroxine-binding globulin (TBG) in the absence of any thyroid dysfunction. Since over 99% of the total circulating thyroid hormones are bound to serum proteins, an increase or decrease in serum TBG is accompanied by a corresponding increase or decrease in bound and total serum T3 and T4 in the presence of normal concentrations of free hormones. In such cases, serum total T3 and T4 levels may not reflect the patient's true thyroid status. The widespread adoption of free hormone measurements has now made these considerations of less importance.

Clinical situations

HYPERTHYROIDISM

The single most reliable test for hyperthyroidism is a serum TSH level which will be suppressed below the normal range $(0.3–3\,\mathrm{mU\,L^{-1}})$. A serum free T3 level will provide increased diagnostic certainty, and in the absence of an available sensitive TSH assay, the T3 measurement is the primary test for hyperthyroidism. Rarely, the serum T4 will be elevated when the serum T3 is normal, but when a normal T3 is found with a suppressed TSH this should not present a problem.

HYPERTHYROID PATIENTS RECEIVING TREATMENT

BETA BLOCKERS

Propranolol or other beta-blocking drugs that are used for symptomatic treatment of hyperthyroidism may slightly lower serum T3 concentrations, probably by interfering with peripheral conversion of T4 to T3. However, the fall is quantitatively minimal, and does not account for the main therapeutic effect of the drugs, and is unlikely to cause confusion in the laboratory assessment of thyroid function.

ANTITHYROID DRUGS

Patients receiving treatment with antithyroid drugs should have serum T3 and T4 levels measured regularly to assess whether they are being under- or overtreated, as it may be difficult to assess the clinical status. During treatment, there is a tendency for an earlier and greater fall in serum T4 compared with serum T3, and measurement of one hormone may be misleading. A persistently raised serum T3 with raised or normal serum T4 means that the patient is still hyperthyroid. A normal serum T3 and T4, or a borderline high serum T3 with normal or borderline low T4, usually indicates that the patient is euthyroid. A low serum T4 with normal or low serum T3 suggests that the patient is becoming hypothyroid. The dose of antithyroid drugs will be adjusted in the light of the thyroid function results and the patient's clinical state. The TSH level may be helpful in indicating excess treatment if it is elevated, but the reverse does not always apply – the patient may be euthyroid or hypothyroid with a persistently suppressed TSH level.

RADIOIODINE AND THYROIDECTOMY

Both serum T3 and TSH should be routinely measured during the first few months (usually at 6-weekly intervals) following radioiodine treatment or subtotal thyroidectomy, to determine whether the patient remains hyperthyroid, or is becoming euthyroid or hypothyroid. When the T3 has become normal, the TSH and T4 measurements are used to detect developing hypothyroidism. Hypothyroidism occurring within the first 6 months of radioiodine or surgical treatment may be transient and revert spontaneously, especially when the fall in T4 is not accompanied by a rise in TSH. On the other hand, late onset hypothyroidism is usually permanent. Early asymptomatic or mild hypothyroidism may be left untreated and followed-up with TSH measurements to allow recovery to occur. If the patient becomes symptomatic, thyroid replacement should not be withheld but it may be advisable to stop treatment for 4–6 weeks at the end of the first year to confirm that hypothyroidism is permanent. All patients who have been treated with ^{131}I or had surgery for hyperthyroidism due to Graves' disease must have long-term follow-up to detect late hypothyroidism. In the absence of any specific symptoms or signs, annual serum T4 estimation is the best and easiest routine follow-up investigation for screening. If T4 is below normal, hypothyroidism can be confirmed by measurement of serum TSH. If recurrent hyperthyroidism is suspected clinically, serum T3 should be estimated. The addition of a TSH measurement to the follow-up protocol improves the effectiveness of the assessment but will increase the cost.

BLOCK/REPLACEMENT REGIME

The best tests for assessing the effectiveness of a thyroid hormone replacement therapy regime where antithyroid drugs and thyroid hormones are given together will depend on which thyroid hormone (T3 or T4) is given in combination with the antithyroid drug. The TSH level should ideally be maintained in the normal range during treatment. If T4 is given, both the T3 and T4 should be measured and maintained in the normal range although a better regime is to give T3 as the replacement hormone, and keep the TSH and T3 in the normal range. Under these circumstances, the T4 level should be almost undetectable and will establish whether the antithyroid drug-blocking effect is complete.

HYPOTHYROIDISM – DIAGNOSIS

When hypothyroidism is suspected clinically, laboratory investigations should be performed not only to confirm the diagnosis but also to differentiate between primary and secondary thyroid failure. The distinction is important as in addition to thyroid replacement secondary hypothyroidism requires further investigation for the diagnosis and subsequent management of the underlying cause.

Serum T4 is usually the initial investigation of choice as it is a more sensitive and reliable test of hypothyroidism than serum T3; better results are obtained if this is combined with TSH, which should always be measured when T4 levels are found to be low.

NORMAL SERUM THYROXINE

If the serum T4 is within the normal range, the diagnosis of hypothyroidism is practically excluded and no further investigation is necessary unless the clinical suspicion of thyroid failure remains high, when further confirmatory investigations should be performed.

LOW OR BORDERLINE LOW SERUM THYROXINE

If the serum T4 is below or near the lower limit of the normal range, serum TSH concentration should be measured on serum stored from the same blood specimen. Raised serum TSH and low or borderline low serum T4 confirms mild primary hypothyroidism. It is useful to measure serum thyroid auto-antibodies in these patients, as their presence in significant titers indicates primary hypothyroidism due to autoimmune thyroiditis (Hashimoto's disease), which usually requires life-long thyroid replacement. This should be distinguished from the transient hypothyroidism, which may be associated with De Quervain's thyroiditis, radioiodine therapy or subtotal thyroidectomy.

If the TSH is not elevated in spite of a low T4, the patient may have secondary hypothyroidism. If total T4 is used a low TBG should be excluded by measuring serum TBG or free T4. A TRH stimulation test may be performed to confirm or exclude pituitary hypothyroidism. An absent TSH response to TRH with a low serum T4 will confirm pituitary hypothyroidism. Further investigations will include full pituitary function tests and radiographs and CT of the pituitary fossa should be carried out to establish the nature and extent of the pituitary abnormality.

HYPOTHYROIDISM – TREATMENT

Thyroid function tests should be used to monitor thyroid hormone replacement in hypothyroid patients. L-Thyroxine (T4) is the usual preparation used and the normal replacement dose is 0.1–0.2 mg daily (100–200 µg). A low dose is used initially (0.05 mg T4 daily), increasing gradually by small increments every 2–4 weeks until the full replacement dose is achieved. In elderly patients, and subjects with prolonged hypothyroidism or associated heart disease, the starting dose should be even lower – 0.025 mg (25 µg) daily, and increased very slowly every 4 weeks, to avoid the risk of precipitating tachycardia and/or myocardial ischemia.

The dose of thyroid hormone is adjusted until the elevated serum TSH has fallen to normal levels, but not suppressed below the normal range. It is important to remember that the TSH levels may continue to fall for several weeks after a change of dose; thyroid function tests should not be performed until the patient has been on the same dose of thyroxine for at least 4 weeks. When the serum TSH has returned to normal, serum T4 is usually found to be in the upper normal range or slightly elevated, whereas T3 is usually in the mid-normal range. In all patients receiving thyroid replacement, it is advisable to check the serum TSH concentration once a year, in order to ensure that their requirements have not changed.

With pituitary hypothyroidism, since serum TSH is not elevated, serum T4 estimations are used to monitor the dose of thyroid replacement, which is increased until the serum T4 concentration is within the upper normal range.

It may be necessary to assess whether thyroxine treatment need be continued in patients who were started on hormone replacement without a definitive diagnosis of hypothyroidism. Thyroid medication is withheld for 4–6 weeks and serum T4 and TSH measured. If the patient is unwilling to withhold the full treatment dose for the test, the dose is halved for 6 weeks and serum T4 and TSH are measured. If the patient is found biochemically to be hypothyroid on half doses, medication can then be withheld completely and the tests repeated.

NEONATAL HYPOTHYROIDISM

Congenital hypothyroidism is an important cause of severe mental retardation, with an estimated incidence of one in every 3000–6000 live births in non-endemic areas. Early diagnosis and treatment significantly affects the prognosis for mental development. Routine biochemical screening of all newborn babies for congenital hypothyroidism is now considered essential for the early diagnosis and treatment of this condition.

Measurement of serum T4 alone will miss many cases of neonatal hypothyroidism, including particularly those with 'compensated hypothyroidism', i.e. normal T4 and high TSH at or shortly after birth, which may occur with ectopic thyroids. If the condition is not diagnosed and remains untreated, frank hypothyroidism and associated mental retardation may develop subsequently. Measurement of serum TSH alone is a more sensitive screening test than serum T4 but will miss secondary hypothyroidism, which contributes only 3–5% of all cases of congenital hypothyroidism. Measurement of serum T4 and TSH both will detect all cases, but the increased workload and cost make it a less practical proposition, particularly since the detection rate is only improved by 3–5% over that of screening with serum T4 or TSH alone.

It is intended that the screening program will permit the diagnosis of congenital hypothyroidism to be made as quickly as possible after birth, preferably within 2 weeks so that patients can be recalled for assessment and further testing if necessary and treatment started with minimum delay. It has also been shown that hypothyroidism may be transient in about 10% of cases, so that the need to continue permanent thyroid replacement should be reviewed at a suitable time when treatment may be safely withheld for a few weeks for repeat thyroid function tests.

PREGNANCY AND ESTROGEN THERAPY

Due to high circulating estrogen concentrations, pregnant women and those on the contraceptive pill or other estrogen preparations have raised serum TBG concentrations, which may spuriously increase serum tT3 and tT4 levels, even when they are euthyroid. Therefore, free thyroid hormones should always be used to assess thyroid function in this group of patients; however, if total T3 and T4 are used, serum TBG needs to be measured, and the serum T3 and T4 results interpreted carefully in the light of the serum TBG value. Sensitive serum TSH measurements are the most useful measurements together with the free hormones.

ELDERLY SICK PATIENTS

Serum T3 falls slightly but significantly in old age, even in the absence of any thyroid dysfunction. On the other hand, serum T4 either remains unchanged or shows a comparatively lesser age-related decrease. The fall in serum T3 becomes more marked in elderly patients who are seriously ill for whatever reason, probably due to failure of peripheral conversion of T4 to T3. Consequently, the serum concentration of these hormones, particularly serum T3, may not reflect the true thyroid status. Serum TSH will always be necessary to confirm or exclude thyroid dysfunction in elderly sick patients, particularly since clinical diagnosis is often difficult in this age group.

HYPERTHYROIDISM

The diagnosis of hyperthyroidism is incomplete without establishing the cause, since the choice of management and prognosis will depend on the underlying cause. A brief discussion of the etiology and mechanism of hyperthyroidism is important for understanding the method(s) of investigation and diagnosis. Table 12A.3 lists the most important causes of hyperthyroidism.

Excess thyroid hormone secretion is usually associated with the presence of an abnormal 'thyroid-stimulating immunoglobulin' (TSI or TSab) directed against the TSH receptor. This thyroid stimulator is found in patients with a toxic diffuse goiter (Graves' disease), and results in diffuse hyperplasia of thyroid tissue. If the gland contains pre-existing nonfunctioning nodular areas, cysts or scars, only the paranodular tissue will be stimulated and the gland may be nodular. The cause of hyperthyroidism is then Graves' disease superimposed on a previous nodular goiter, i.e. Graves' disease with incidental nonfunctioning nodules.

Hyperthyroidism may also occur if a localized area of the thyroid has changed in such a way that the follicular cells secrete thyroid hormones independently of TSH control. This is an autonomous functioning nodule, and as the nodule grows in size, it may secrete sufficient hormones to exceed the physiological requirements and the patient becomes hyperthyroid. The rest of the gland may be normal but have function suppressed due to secondary suppression of TSH. The gland may also contain pre-existing nonfunctioning nodules if the autonomous change has occurred in a pre-existing nodular goiter. Hyperthyroidism caused by one or more such autonomous functioning

Table 12A.3   *Causes of hyperthyroidism*

1. *Graves' disease (diffuse or nodular variants)*

2. *Solitary or multiple toxic autonomous nodules (toxic adenoma, Plummer's disease)*

3. *Thyroid hormone 'leakage'*

    (a) Subacute (De Quervain's) thyroiditis

    (b) Painless (silent) thyroiditis

    (c) Hashimoto's thyroiditis

    (d) Post-partum thyroiditis

4. *Iodide-induced hyperthyroidism (Jod–Basedow's phenomenon)*

5. *Excess thyroid hormone ingestion*

6. *Rare causes including:*

    (a) Pituitary TSH-dependent hyperthyroidism

    (b) Ectopic TSH-secreting tumor

    (c) Extensive functioning differentiated thyroid cancer

    (d) Trophoblastic tumor

    (e) Struma ovarii

nodules is also referred to as single or multiple toxic adenomas (Plummer's disease), and sometimes, toxic nodular goiter. The last terminology is the least satisfactory and should be avoided, as it is a descriptive clinical term for a nodular goiter associated with hyperthyroidism, which may be due to either autonomous functioning nodules or nonfunctioning nodules in a diffuse toxic goiter as discussed above.

Hyperthyroidism may also occur if stored hormones leak out of the thyroid due to an inflammatory process which damages the follicles. This may be related to viral infection (subacute De Quervain's thyroiditis) or an autoimmune process (Hashimoto's disease) or post-partum thyroiditis. In each case, hyperthyroidism is usually mild and transient.

Hyperthyroidism may be precipitated by excess iodide or thyroid hormone ingestion or drugs such as amiodarone and very rarely may be due to extensive functioning papillary or follicular thyroid carcinoma or excess TSH production. In practice, Graves' disease and single or multiple autonomous toxic nodules (uninodular or multinodular Plummer's disease) account for the majority of cases of thyrotoxicosis. Nevertheless, the remaining causes are clinically important and should always be borne in mind because their management and clinical course are different.

Diagnosing the cause of hyperthyroidism

The history and physical examination will often suggest the cause of hyperthyroidism in patients with Graves' disease, but a clinical diagnosis can only be made with certainty in the presence of pathognomonic ocular or cutaneous signs, i.e. exophthalmos or other infiltrative eye signs, localized pretibial myxedema and acropachy. However, this classical presentation of Graves' disease is rare, and investigations are usually necessary to confirm or establish the etiology. A diffuse goiter although most commonly associated with Graves' disease is not by itself diagnostic of the condition as it may occur in patients with subacute or painless thyroiditis or in those who are ingesting excessive thyroid hormones for a nontoxic goiter.

The finding of a thyroid nodule or a multinodular goiter in a hyperthyroid patient does not establish the cause of hyperthyroidism since the diagnosis may be either Plummer's disease or variants of Graves' disease (as discussed above). In a proportion of hyperthyroid patients, the thyroid gland is not palpable, which may make the clinical diagnosis of the underlying cause even more difficult. The patient should be carefully questioned for the possibility of iodide or thyroid hormone-induced hyperthyroidism, but most commonly the cause of hyperthyroidism is found on investigation to be a small diffuse toxic goiter or a nonpalpable toxic nodule.

Hyperthyroidism associated with subacute thyroiditis typically presents with a short history of painful tender goiter often accompanied by fever, anorexia, and other constitutional symptoms. The clinical picture is often atypical, and in most cases investigations are necessary to confirm or establish the diagnosis. Painless thyroiditis as a cause of hyperthyroidism can only be diagnosed by appropriate investigations, although a proportion of these occurring in epidemics have been shown to be due to the incorporation of beef thyroid into hamburger meat. It is thus apparent that investigations are usually necessary to establish the cause of hyperthyroidism.

Management of thyrotoxicosis

The appropriate management of patients with hyperthyroidism depends in many instances on an accurate initial diagnosis, and the thyroid scan has an important role in thyrotoxicosis. The radionuclide scan has three main uses in managing hyperthyroidism: (1) establishing the cause of thyrotoxicosis; (2) the measurement of tracer uptake and gland size for the selection of an appropriate ^{131}I therapy regime; and (3) for the follow-up of patients after treatment.

ESTABLISHING THE CAUSE OF THYROTOXICOSIS

There are a large number of patients in whom the diagnosis cannot be made clinically, and without the thyroid scan an incorrect diagnosis may often be assumed. This can result in inappropriate treatment; in a review, we found that 22% of patients with toxic nodules (Plummer's disease) had received long-term antithyroid medication before the correct diagnosis was established and appropriate treatment instituted.[5]

THE SOLITARY THYROID NODULE AND THYROTOXICOSIS

When a patient with thyrotoxicosis is found to have a solitary thyroid nodule on clinical examination, this is usually due to an autonomous toxic nodule (Fig. 12A.1). However, clinical examination is unreliable, in up to one third of patients. Other causes may be identified by subsequent investigations; for example, a solitary nonfunctioning nodule in a patient with Graves' disease (Fig. 12A.2), an asymmetrically enlarged thyroid (Fig. 12A.3), or diffuse enlargement of a single lobe with agenesis of the other lobe, may all simulate a toxic nodule. It may not always be possible to differentiate between these on the initial scan: for example, differentiating a large toxic nodule with complete suppression of

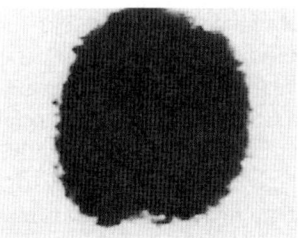

Figure 12A.1 *A typical left-sided thyroid toxic nodule with complete suppression of the right lobe.*

the other lobe from agenesis of a lobe in a patient with Graves' disease may require further investigations, and a repeat scanning with ^{201}Tl may often show uptake in tissue that is not accumulating ^{99m}TcO$_4$ or ^{123}I/^{131}I (Fig. 12A.4); ultrasound will demonstrate a lobe which is present but not taking up tracer, or a hypoplastic or aplastic lobe; the use of fluorescent X-ray establishes the presence of ^{127}I-containing tissue on the contralateral side but is not often used clinically. Even a simple method of shielding the active nodule with lead on routine thyroid scanning may be sufficient to show uptake in the other lobe. The importance of making the correct diagnosis lies in the choice of treatment and subsequent follow-up. Patients with toxic nodules respond well to radioiodine treatment, and the nodule usually decreases in size to 50–60% of the original volume, with complete cure being the normal outcome and hypothyroidism a rare sequel,[5–7] whereas a single lobe with Graves' disease will usually be treated in a conventional manner – initially with antithyroid drugs, and is followed by ablative radioiodine therapy only when a relapse occurs. However, some centers prefer to treat these nodules surgically, but this now represents a minority view. Children with toxic nodules will still usually be treated surgically. A patient with Graves' disease who has an incidental non-functioning nodule on the radionuclide scan is usually treated by subtotal thyroidectomy in order to identify possible malignancy, which has an incidence similar to a cold nodule in a normal gland. An alternative approach is fine needle aspiration cytology examination of the nodule followed by radioiodine treatment of the toxic diffuse goiter, after which some nonfunctioning nodules that are TSH dependent (Marine–Lenhart syndrome), will function following resolution of disease (Fig. 12A.5). These nodules probably do not require surgical treatment.

NODULAR GOITER ASSOCIATED WITH THYROTOXICOSIS

When thyrotoxic patients present with a multinodular goiter, they are often labelled as having a toxic nodular goiter. However, there are three possible causes for this: (1) multiple toxic nodules developing in a long-standing multinodular goiter (Plummer's disease); (2) Graves' disease occurring in a patient with a previous nontoxic multinodular goiter; and (3) a patient with Graves' disease in whom the enlarged gland has become nodular. The latter two can be differentiated by the presence or absence of a previous history of nodular goiter. The scan appearances of Plummer's disease may vary from a single toxic nodule to multiple clearly defined nodules throughout the gland. Occasionally, the nodules appear almost confluent when the scan may be difficult to differentiate from Graves' disease in a multinodular gland (Fig. 12A.6). Most often, the diagnosis can be made from the scan, although appearances do overlap and further investigations may be necessary. These include the measurement of serum thyroid-stimulating antibody, and repeating the scan after the serum TSH rises with antithyroid drugs.[8] Alternatively, a diagnosis may be established

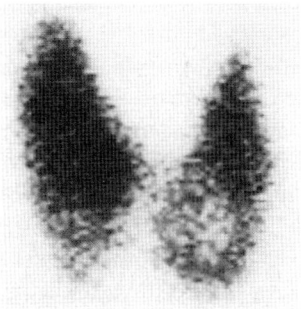

Figure 12A.2 *Scan of a patient with a diffuse toxic goiter (Graves' disease) and an incidental cold nodule in the left lower pole.*

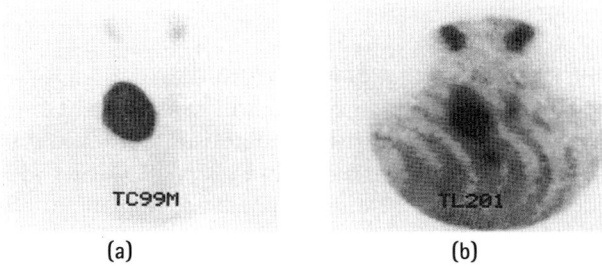

(a)   (b)

Figure 12A.4 *(a) [^{99m}Tc]pertechnetate scan with virtually no uptake on the left side. (b) ^{201}Tl scan shows the presence of metabolically active thyroid tissue on the left.*

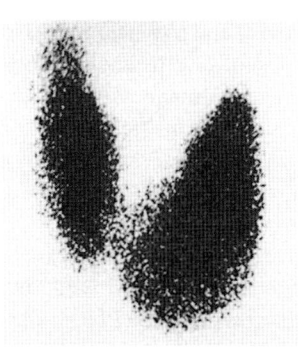

Figure 12A.3 *Graves' disease presenting with an asymmetrical goiter simulating a single nodule on clinical examination.*

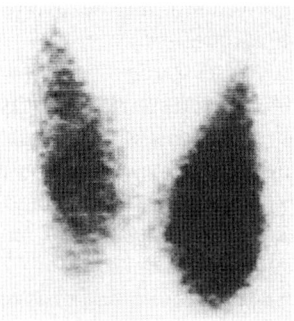

Figure 12A.5 *The non-functioning nodule in Fig. 12A.2 is now taking up the tracer: the Marine–Lenhart syndrome.*

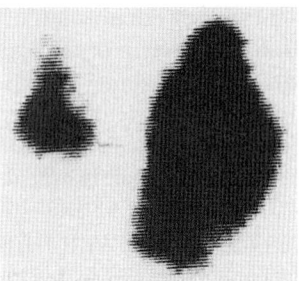

Figure 12A.6 *Confluent nodules in a patient with multiple autonomous toxic thyroid nodules.*

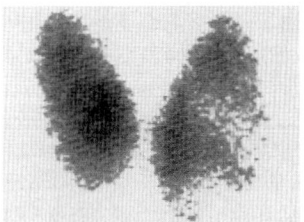

Figure 12A.7 *After treatment with* [131]*I of the patient, whose scan is shown in Fig. 12A.6, there is a quite different distribution of uptake, confirming the original diagnosis.*

retrospectively when patients are re-scanned after radio-iodine treatment (Fig. 12A.7). As mentioned previously for the single nodule, ^{201}Tl can be used to demonstrate tissue in which the uptake function but not the metabolic activity is suppressed and may demonstrate the suppressed perinodular thyroid tissue.

THE IMPALPABLE GLAND AND THYROTOXICOSIS

If the thyroid is small it may be difficult to palpate and when it is not obviously enlarged in thyrotoxicosis, a thyroid scan should always be performed. In a series of patients with toxic nodules, 10% were impalpable and some of these nodules could not be palpated even after identification on the scan.[5] The scan may demonstrate any of the recognized patterns associated with thyrotoxicosis such as diffuse uptake, low uptake or functioning nodules. This is particularly important in elderly patients with atrial fibrillation, who should have a scan to detect toxic nodules that may not be producing obvious clinical disease, as these can be easily treated with radioiodine.

LOW TRACER UPTAKE AND THYROTOXICOSIS

The thyroid scan in patients with thyrotoxicosis may have low uptake. This finding may indicate a cause for thyro-toxicosis, which could be self-limiting and avoid unnecessary and ineffective administration of radioiodine. These conditions are shown in Table 12A.4.

Amiodarone, an iodine-rich drug, has recently been recognized to be a frequent cause of thyrotoxicosis through a number of mechanisms, and is almost always associated with low uptake of tracer and non-visualization of the thyroid on

Table 12A.4   *Causes of low tracer uptake in hyperthyroidism*

- *Subacute thyroiditis*
- *Iodine-induced thyrotoxicosis (Jod–Basedow)*
- *Amiodarone-induced thyrotoxicosis*
- *Ectopic thyroid tissue*
- *Thyrotoxicosis factitia (excess thyroid hormone administration)*
- *Recent high iodine load (due to dilutional effects)*

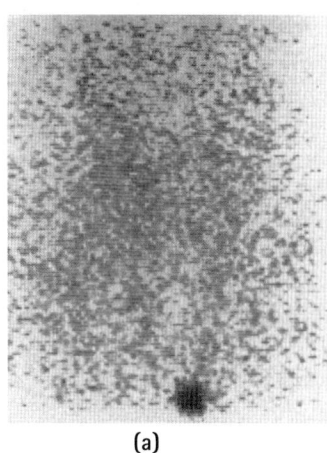
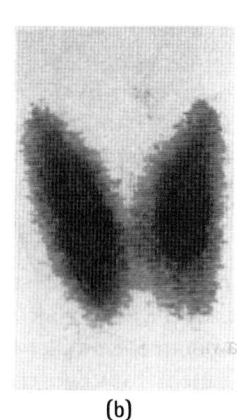

(a)   (b)

Figure 12A.8 *(a) Subacute thyroiditis causing thyrotoxicosis. (b) With resolution of the hyperthyroidism the scan returns to normal.*

the scan. In an early review of 35 patients with amiodarone-induced thyrotoxicosis,[8,9] 24-h ^{131}I uptake was less than 4% in 12 patients who had no palpable abnormality but was more than 8% in the 17 patients with goiters.

Ectopic tissue may occasionally cause hyperthyroidism with nonvisualization of the 'normal' thyroid on routine scanning. This may rarely be due to thyrotoxicosis caused by metastatic follicular cancer, or a retrosternal goiter with a toxic nodule, or an intrathoracic goiter causing Graves' thyrotoxicosis. In each case, the cervical thyroid uptake was low or absent, either due to suppression or absence of tissue. In females, a scan in such cases should include the pelvis to identify the rare struma ovarii. Post-partum thyroiditis is being increasingly recognized and may be associated with both hypo- and hyperthyroidism (or occasionally both), which is usually transient. In both situations, the scan reveals low tracer uptake.

Subacute thyroiditis continues to be a regular cause of transient hyperthyroidism. This is usually diagnosed clinically in a patient with a painful thyroid and a low technetium or iodine uptake on the scan (Fig. 12A.8). Occasionally, the diagnosis may be more difficult, and cases of subacute thyroiditis have been demonstrated while being investigated for pyrexia of unknown origin (PUO), and the cause of the PUO and hyperthyroidism was identified with intense ^{67}Ga scan uptake in the thyroid. While subacute thyroiditis is occasionally painless, what was initially thought to be a

Table 12A.5 *Treatment of Graves' disease: advantages and disadvantages of each type of treatment*

	Drugs	Surgery	Radioiodine
Relapse or recurrence	*High*	*Low*	*Low (dose-related)*
Hypothyroidism	*Low*	*Intermediate*	*High (dose-related)*
Complications	*Rare*	*Low but significant mortality and morbidity*	*Rare*
Ease of treatment and cost	*Intermediate*	*Least favorable*	*Simple and cheap*
Onset of therapeutic effect	*Moderate (1 or 2 weeks)*	*Rapid after pre-op. preparation*	*Slow (few weeks)*

mini-epidemic of such cases was shown to result from the addition of bovine thyroid tissue to hamburgers – the so-called 'hamburger thyrotoxicosis'.

Treatment of hyperthyroidism

The diagnosis of hyperthyroidism should be confirmed biochemically and its cause established (as discussed in preceding sections) before specific therapy is advised. While awaiting laboratory investigations, provided there are no contraindications such as asthma, a beta-adrenergic blocking drug such as propranolol may be prescribed to relieve sympathetic symptoms such as sweating, tremors, palpitations or irritability. Specific treatment can subsequently be instituted when the diagnosis is confirmed.

The importance of diagnosing the cause of hyperthyroidism is stressed as it determines the choice of therapy, the clinical course of the condition and the likelihood of hypothyroidism or recurrent hyperthyroidism. The tendency of some physicians to initiate therapy with antithyroid drugs routinely in every patient with hyperthyroidism is open to criticism as they may be ineffective in certain types of hyperthyroidism, such as that associated with thyroiditis, or may not represent the treatment of choice in other cases, such as elderly patients or those with Plummer's disease.

GRAVES' DISEASE (TOXIC DIFFUSE GOITER)

The conventional treatments for hyperthyroidism due to Graves' disease include antithyroid drugs, subtotal thyroidectomy and radioactive iodine. The advantages and disadvantages of each form of therapy are summarized in Table 12A.5, and should always be weighed against each other when selecting the most appropriate treatment for an individual patient. The treatment of choice for a particular patient depends on several factors: the patient's age; the presence of any associated cardiovascular problems such as atrial fibrillation, heart failure, ischemic heart disease or other major medical problems; a previous history of hyperthyroidism and the type of treatment received; local medical facilities such as the availability of an experienced thyroid surgeon or an adequately equipped nuclear medicine department; the physician's personal experience and preference, and the patient's willingness to undergo the particular form of therapy advised.

For a young patient with uncomplicated Graves' disease, the conventional treatment is a course of antithyroid drug therapy for 6 months to 2 years. Drugs such as propylthiouracil and carbimazole or methimazole are effective in reducing thyroid hormone production and release, but in at least 50% of patients there is an early relapse or later recurrence of hyperthyroidism when treatment is stopped even after a prolonged course. Side-effects of antithyroid drugs are uncommon and usually become manifest within a few weeks of starting treatment. Allergic skin reactions are the most common, but the most serious is agranulocytosis, which has been reported in 0.2–0.3% of patients.

Subtotal thyroidectomy offers a higher chance of cure in a much shorter time but requires admission, an experienced thyroid surgeon and the patient's fitness and willingness to undergo surgery. Complications of subtotal thyroidectomy depend on the surgeon's experience and the adequacy of the patient's pre-operative preparation. They include post-operative hemorrhage, recurrent laryngeal nerve palsy, and transient or permanent hypoparathyroidism; the morbidity ranges between 0.2 and 1%. It is now used only for patients with very large goiters where there is a suspicion of malignancy or when the patient is particularly keen to avoid radioiodine therapy.

Radioactive iodine provides the highest rate of cure, approaching 100%, although the effective dose is variable and more than one treatment dose may be necessary. Radioiodine has the advantage of being a very simple and cheap form of therapy. In the past, radioiodine treatment has been confined entirely to hyperthyroid patients over the reproductive age, owing to the fear of radiation-induced cancer or genetic complications. As experience with radioiodine treatment has increased, many thyroidologists now feel that the use of ^{131}I need no longer be restricted but may be extended to younger adults and children. The major disadvantage of radioiodine therapy for Graves' disease is the high incidence of post-treatment hypothyroidism. With moderate doses of ^{131}I the incidence of hypothyroidism is about 20% in the first year of treatment, with an additional annual increase of 3% over subsequent years, and by 10 years up to 50% of treated patients may be hypothyroid. The risk of hypothyroidism is less with smaller doses of radioiodine but the chance of successful therapy is also reduced. Large single doses of ^{131}I, e.g. 555 MBq (15 mCi), achieve a high cure rate in Graves' hyperthyroidism, with 70–90% requiring T4 replacement.

CHOICE OF THERAPY FOR HYPERTHYROIDISM

CHILDREN AND ADOLESCENTS

Antithyroid drugs are the treatment of choice in very young patients with Graves' disease, but the duration of therapy may be a problem. The aim of therapy is to continue with antithyroid drugs in yearly courses as necessary until the patient has reached the late teens or early twenties. Clinical and biochemical evidence of persistent or recurrent hyperthyroidism is sought at the end of each course of antithyroid drugs before resuming a new course of treatment.

ADULTS

In general, a course of antithyroid drugs for 6 months to 2 years is recommended for most adults with newly diagnosed Graves' disease. At the end of the course of treatment, if the disease is still active or if it recurs subsequently, they are referred for ^{131}I therapy. In a small proportion of patients, hyperthyroidism is not satisfactorily controlled with a regular maintenance dose of antithyroid drugs. The problem can usually be overcome by keeping these patients on a 'block-replace' regime, which consists of a full dose of antithyroid drugs to completely block endogenous thyroid hormone production, supplemented by a replacement dose of exogenous thyroid hormone, e.g. 20–40 µg of T3 or 0.1–0.2 mg of T4 daily. Replacement with exogenous T3 is preferred so that the block of endogenous hormone production can be assessed by measuring serum T4 which comes only from endogenous secretion and should be very low. Patients with associated disease such as cardiac disease or diabetes are best treated with ^{131}I.

PREGNANCY AND LACTATION

The whole issue of thyroid disease and pregnancy is complex and has been reviewed.[10] Radioiodine treatment or investigation is absolutely contraindicated during pregnancy and lactation owing to irradiation of the fetus or newborn, from radioiodine transferred across the placenta and in the milk as well as from indirect exposure from the radioiodine in the mother. The choice of treatment therefore lies between surgery and antithyroid drugs. Surgery should in any case be avoided during the first and third trimester of pregnancy owing to the risk of abortion or premature labor. The middle trimester is thus the safest period for thyroidectomy if considered necessary. Hypothyroidism after surgery should be detected and treated as soon as possible as it increases the risk of spontaneous abortion and fetal death. Many clinicians recommend that thyroxine therapy should routinely be given after surgery and the dose subsequently adjusted rather than wait until the patient is hypothyroid.

The preferred treatment during pregnancy is antithyroid drugs but it is essential to avoid over-treatment, which may increase fetal mortality from maternal hypothyroidism, and as antithyroid drugs cross the placenta they may induce fetal goiter and hypothyroidism particularly when used in larger doses. It is therefore safer to maintain the mother in a slightly hyperthyroid state using the smallest possible dose of antithyroid drugs. Thyroid function tests including serum T3, T4, and TSH should be carried out frequently.

Iodide treatment and propranolol should be avoided during pregnancy. The former crosses the placenta, blocks the fetal thyroid and may induce goiter or hypothyroidism; the latter increases uterine muscle tone, which may result in a small placenta and growth retardation of the fetus. Propranolol can also induce bradycardia in the newborn baby, hypoglycemia and impaired response to hypoxia.

As antithyroid drugs are secreted in breast milk, they should either be stopped whenever possible if the mother wishes to breast-feed, or if treatment needs to be continued artificial feeding should be advised. It is essential to check babies born of mothers with Graves' disease for neonatal hyperthyroidism or hypothyroidism, which is usually transient (due to placental transfer of maternal thyroid-stimulating immunoglobulins) and may be prolonged. When treatment of the baby is indicated, it usually involves antithyroid drugs and propranolol but great care should be taken to avoid hypothyroidism in the newborn child owing to the risk of subsequent mental and physical retardation.

THYROTOXICOSIS IN THE ELDERLY

Hyperthyroidism in the elderly constitutes a more serious problem, with an increased mortality and morbidity rate, particularly due to cardiovascular complications such as heart failure and atrial fibrillation, with the added risk of arterial embolism. The aim of treatment in these patients is to cure hyperthyroidism promptly and permanently, when they first present, in order to avoid or reverse any cardiovascular problems and prevent recurrence of the hyperthyroid state, and its associated complications. In view of the increased risk of surgery in this age group and the high relapse rate after antithyroid drugs, this is best achieved with radioiodine. Elderly patients and those with cardiac complications or other associated serious medical problems, irrespective of age, should be treated with a short course (usually 4–8 weeks) of antithyroid drugs in full dosage, until they are clinically and biochemically euthyroid. The drug is then stopped for 48–72 h, after which the patient is given a single large oral dose of ^{131}I (e.g. 550 MBq), which will result in a 70–90% cure rate of Graves' hyperthyroidism, albeit at the risk of permanent hypothyroidism. It is advisable to resume the antithyroid drug at a suitable dosage 2–3 days after the radioiodine drink for another 4–6 weeks to cover the period before the ^{131}I has its full therapeutic effect. Patients under the age of 65 years with atrial fibrillation may also be anticoagulated prophylactically against thromboembolism, but this remains controversial. Digoxin and/or beta blockers may be used to control the heart rate, and diuretics may be needed to control heart failure. Treated in this way, many patients with atrial fibrillation will revert to sinus rhythm spontaneously while being treated. Those who are still in atrial fibrillation after having become euthyroid or hypothyroid should be advised DC cardioversion, which will often restore sinus rhythm. Anticoagulants and digoxin may be stopped if sinus rhythm is maintained for a few weeks after the patient has become euthyroid or hypothyroid.

THE THYROID SCAN BEFORE ^{131}I TREATMENT

One of the major factors involved in calculating the radiation from a therapeutic dose of ^{131}I is the measurement of thyroid mass. There have been a number of formulae proposed for calculating the thyroid mass derived from the thyroid scan, which make assumptions about the geometry of the lobe. Thyroid volume is best calculated using a combined radionuclide and ultrasound method. However, with regard to calculating the dose for ^{131}I for therapy, the functional tissue volume as opposed to the total tissue volume is likely to be much more important.

The second important factor in dose calculation is the peak uptake of ^{131}I. However, it is not certain that in the absence of detailed measurements of ^{131}I turnover and possibly some measure of tissue sensitivity the results from these measurements can significantly improve upon the results achieved using the much more convenient approach of an arbitrary choice of dose.

It has been suggested that the thyroid scan, together with an uptake measurement, may be used to assess thyroid activity during antithyroid drug treatment to provide an indication as to the likelihood of a relapse when the patient discontinues treatment. However, the ^{99m}Tc uptake is a poor predictor of relapse in patients with Graves' disease.

TREATMENT OF TOXIC AUTONOMOUS NODULES (PLUMMER'S DISEASE)

Treatment of hyperthyroidism caused by single or multiple autonomous nodules is similar, but differs in several important aspects from that of Graves' disease. First, long-term antithyroid drugs should not be used to treat Plummer's disease, as functioning nodules rarely go into spontaneous remission. Second, hyperthyroidism due to Plummer's disease is more resistant to radioiodine and usually requires larger therapeutic doses, but despite this, post-radiation hypothyroidism is rarely observed. This is explained on the basis that in Graves' disease, the whole of the gland concentrates radioiodine and becomes irradiated, which subsequently leads to hypothyroidism. In contrast, in Plummer's disease, radioiodine concentrates only in the autonomous nodules, which are destroyed, while the suppressed extranodular tissue takes up little radioiodine and returns to normal function after the nodules have been destroyed. It is important to note that this is only true if at the time of radioiodine treatment, the extranodular tissue has not been stimulated by a rise in TSH as a result of preceding antithyroid drug therapy. Radioiodine has the added advantage that it also destroys functioning micronodules and thus prevents recurrence of hyperthyroidism. Patients who refuse ^{131}I may be treated with surgery.

It is important to obtain a thyroid scan before giving radioiodine for treating autonomous toxic nodules (Plummer's disease), particularly in those who have received antithyroid drug therapy, because in order to prevent subsequent hypothyroidism it is important to ensure that the normal thyroid tissue is fully suppressed at the time of ^{131}I administration. When patients with toxic nodules are treated in this way, the likelihood of hypothyroidism is very low. In a series of 48 patients treated with 500 MBq of ^{131}I, not a single patient developed hypothyroidism in the follow-up period (mean 37 months).[7] The only patients who are likely to become hypothyroid have received antithyroid drugs before treatment without first establishing that the normal tissue was suppressed and the TSH was not elevated. If the normal thyroid tissue is not fully suppressed because the TSH has risen during treatment, then a further period of time off antithyroid drugs is required or, alternatively, thyroid hormone replacement therapy may be instituted, if clinically acceptable, and the thyroid scan repeated before giving ^{131}I dose.

Radioiodine treatment usually consists of a single large dose of ^{131}I (standard adult dose, 400–500 MBq). Unless the patient is seriously ill with thyrocardiac complications such as heart failure or atrial fibrillation, pre-treatment with antithyroid drugs should be avoided, as it increases the risk of post-radioiodine hypothyroidism. A course of propranolol for 2–4 weeks may be helpful in providing symptomatic relief until the radioiodine starts to have a therapeutic effect. If the patient has received antithyroid drugs, these should be stopped and radioiodine treatment postponed for 4 weeks (Fig. 12A.9).

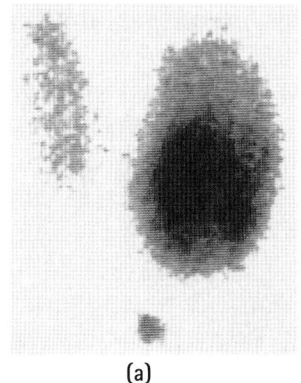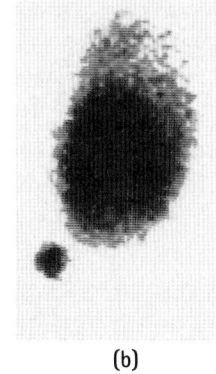

(a)   (b)

Figure 12A.9 *Patient with thyrotoxicosis who has received treatment with antithyroid drugs. (a) The use of these drugs has permitted some tracer uptake into the normally suppressed perinodular tissue. (b) After discontinuing the drugs for a few weeks, there is a return to the suppressed state.*

After radioiodine treatment, patients are usually reviewed at 1, 3, 6, 9, and 12 months. A repeat thyroid scan is carried out after 6 months, at which time most patients with Plummer's disease will be clinically and biochemically euthyroid and have a normal TSH. The thyroid scan can be used to establish that radioiodine therapy has been completely successful in destroying autonomous nodule(s) (Fig. 12A.10). Successfully treated nodules will be nonfunctional on the scan by 6 months after treatment, but those with a liability to relapse will retain some functional activity. The scan at 6 months can thus be valuable as an indicator of prognosis because residual activity in the nodule predisposes to a subsequent relapse of thyrotoxicosis and these patients should be followed-up. Those who are not cured at 6 months are given a second dose of ^{131}I and followed as before. Once the patient is cured an annual examination is sufficient since post-radiation hypothyroidism is quite rare.

TREATMENT OF OTHER TYPES OF HYPERTHYROIDISM

The management of hyperthyroidism due to causes other than Graves' disease and Plummer's disease depends on the underlying condition, but in general, treatment with antithyroid drugs, subtotal thyroidectomy or radioiodine, is not applicable to these conditions.

SUBACUTE THYROIDITIS AND HASHIMOTO'S THYROIDITIS

Hyperthyroidism is usually mild, transient, and requires no specific therapy, except possibly symptomatic treatment with a beta-sympathetic blocking drug such as propranolol. Since the raised serum hormones in these conditions are due to leakage of stored thyroid hormones accompanying the inflammatory process rather than excess production, the conventional treatment for Graves' disease is ineffective. In subacute thyroiditis and occasionally with Hashimoto's thyroiditis, pain and tenderness over the neck, with or without constitutional symptoms, may require symptomatic relief with an anti-inflammatory analgesic. In more severe cases, steroid treatment in moderate doses, for a few weeks, may be necessary. Subacute thyroiditis is a self-limiting condition and complete recovery after a few weeks or months is the rule. Mild hypothyroidism may occur in

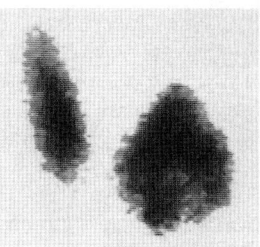

Figure 12A.10 *Complete destruction of the toxic nodule shown in Fig. 12A.1 has resulted in a return to normal function of the previously suppressed tissue.*

the recovery stage but this is usually transient. On the other hand, permanent hypothyroidism is common with Hashimoto's thyroiditis, and long-term thyroid replacement is usually necessary.

HYPERTHYROIDISM ASSOCIATED WITH EXCESS IODIDE

Hyperthyroidism precipitated by acute excess iodide such as administration of radiological contrast media is also usually mild and remits spontaneously without any specific treatment. Rarely, if the condition is severe, a course of antithyroid drugs may be necessary, but surgery and radioiodine treatment are not used. The low uptake of radioiodine in this condition, as in thyroiditis, precludes the use of radioiodine. In the case of chronic excess iodide ingestion, appropriate dietary advice should also be given to avoid persistence of the condition. One of the most common causes of iodine-induced hyperthyroidism is now the anti-arrhythmic cardiac drug, amiodarone. Initial treatment with antithyroid drugs together with withdrawal of amiodarone, and followed by ^{131}I when the uptake is high enough, is generally advised but it can be difficult to control and steroids or carbimazole with potassium perchlorate have been recommended.[11,12]

HYPERTHYROIDISM ASSOCIATED WITH EXCESS THYROID HORMONE

If the patient is on an excessive dose of thyroid hormone for documented hypothyroidism, the dose should be adjusted until the patient is clinically and biochemically euthyroid. The usual therapeutic dose of thyroxine is 100–200 µg daily. Occasionally, a patient may have been put on thyroid replacement for unrecognized transient hypothyroidism, and may subsequently produce adequate or even excess endogenous hormone; therefore, in such cases thyroid hormone medication should be stopped and the patient's thyroid status assessed to determine the need for continuation of thyroid hormone replacement. Patients taking excess thyroid hormones of their own accord should also be advised to discontinue the drug, and their thyroid status should be reassessed clinically and biochemically. Some of these patients may also need psychiatric assessment and advice.

HYPERTHYROIDISM ASSOCIATED WITH THYROID CANCER

This is a rare complication of extensive metastatic functioning papillary or follicular thyroid cancer, which may secrete excess endogenous thyroid hormones due to the large mass of functioning tumour. The management is essentially that of the underlying carcinoma, involving large ablation doses of radioiodine. If hyperthyroidism is severe, treatment with antithyroid drugs and beta blockers may be necessary. Exogenous thyroid hormone medication should not be given while hyperthyroidism from tumor secretion persists.

Hyperthyroidism may also occur if patients with thyroid cancer are put on excess suppressive doses of thyroid hormone. The optimal dose is that which suppresses the TSH below normal; in the average patient this is 150–300 µg of thyroxine daily. Patients with functioning metastases producing significant amounts of endogenous hormones will of course need smaller doses of thyroid hormone.

Hyperthyroidism associated with pituitary or ectopic TSH hypersecretion, trophoblastic tumors and ectopic thyroid tissue in ovarian tumors is exceedingly rare, and will be treated by removing the primary cause.

SOLITARY THYROID NODULES

This is a common clinical problem, and as many as 15.5% of the population may have palpable nodules,[4] with a 3.2% incidence of solitary nodules in women and 0.8% in men in England. In the USA, the incidence of thyroid nodules has been reported at 4–7%.[13] The various causes of solitary thyroid nodules are shown in Table 12A.6.

The likelihood of malignancy occurring in a single nodule is 2–10%, but varies considerably from series to series, depending on selection criteria. The problem is compounded by the frequency with which nodules are found in normal adults (up to 50% in those over 50 years of age). There is an increased risk of thyroid cancer associated with previous external radiation to the head or neck, although the clinical course of the cancer is the same as thyroid cancers found in other settings. Schneider *et al.*[14] identified 318 cases of thyroid cancer in 5379 patients given radiotherapy for benign conditions of head, neck and upper

Table 12A.6   *Causes of solitary thyroid nodules*

- *Thyroid cyst*
- *Local subacute thyroiditis*
- *Local Hashimoto's disease*
- *Functioning adenoma (hot nodule)*
- *Benign adenoma*
- *Colloid nodule*
- *Thyroid cancer*
- *Metastatic deposit*

thoracic area. Metastases frequently occur in the thyroid, but rarely present clinically as thyroid nodules.

The clinical problem is how to detect the small number of solitary thyroid nodules due to cancer, without the need to perform unnecessary operations on the other 90%, and it has been this goal, i.e. to identify benign disease with a high degree of accuracy without loss of sensitivity in detecting cancer, that has driven the diagnostic developments in this area. Certain clinical features increase the probability of malignancy in a solitary nodule:

- The presence of an invasive tumor may be suggested by hoarseness, fixation, and hardness of the nodule, rapid or painful enlargement, cervical lymphadenopathy or distant metastases. These clinical features are usually absent at the time of presentation of most differentiated thyroid carcinomas.
- A previous history of irradiation to the head or neck should be specifically asked for, as this will increase the likelihood of malignancy in a solitary nodule.
- Symptoms and signs that are characteristic of a medullary thyroid carcinoma, such as diarrhea, mucosal neuromas, a history or suspicion of associated pheochromocytoma or hyperparathyroidism, and a known family history of any of these conditions.
- Age and sex of the patient, e.g. a solitary nodule in a man over 40 years has a higher probability of being malignant than in a young woman.

Investigation and management of solitary nodules

The thyroid scan has been the most widely used method for investigating a thyroid nodule, on the basis that finding a solitary cold nodule increases the probability of malignancy, whereas finding a functioning nodule or a simple multinodular goiter without a single dominant nodule decreases the chance of malignancy to low levels.

Ultrasound provides a valuable tool for demonstrating thyroid abnormalities, and in particular for discriminating between solid and cystic lesions (Fig. 12A.11). It can be

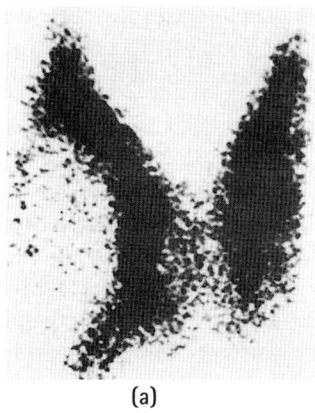
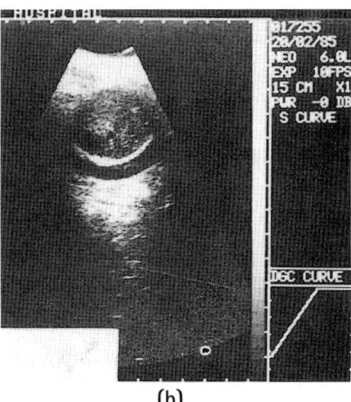
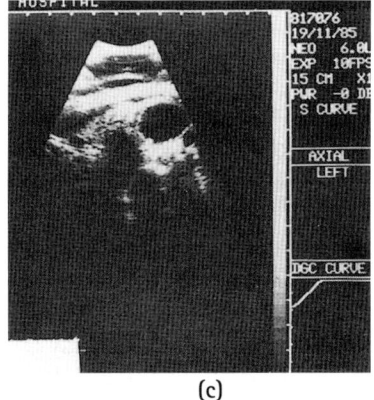

(a)   (b)   (c)

Figure 12A.11   *Non-functioning nodule in the right lobe (a) shown to be solid on ultrasound (b) compared with a cyst on ultrasound (c).*

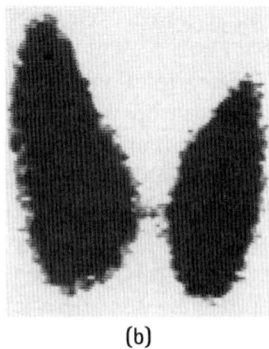

(a)   (b)

Figure 12A.12 *Patient who presented with a cold nodule in the right lobe (a) due to a cyst. A follow-up scan after aspiration (b) confirms complete aspiration with no recurrence.*

used to measure thyroid volumes, detect nodules, and direct needle biopsy. Most malignancies are solid and calcification increases the risk of malignancy in a nodule,[15] but ultrasound cannot differentiate between functioning and nonfunctioning nodules, and even cystic lesions seen on ultrasound may be functional on a radionuclide scan.

The most important adjunct to imaging is fine needle aspiration (FNA) of a nodule for cytological examination, and this is now widely available.[16,17] The thyroid scan can be regarded as a supplement to physical examination and serving as a guide to FNA in pre-operative selection of patients. The problem of nondiagnostic or suspicious lesions will probably always remain. In a review of the Mayo Clinic experience, it was found that 20% of the results were nondiagnostic, and on follow-up of these cases about one fifth of them were found malignant.[16] However, in a review and follow-up of 6226 cases a sensitivity of 93% and specificity of 96% was reported when the samples were considered adequate.[16,18–21]

It has been suggested that all patients with a solitary nodule should have FNA as their initial investigation and a thyroid scan is not required. However, clinical examination may fail to detect that the 'clinically solitary nodule' is the more easily palpable nodule of a multinodular goiter. The combination of FNA and thyroid scan is an efficient method for detecting cancer in patients who have a cold nodule on the thyroid scan (Fig. 12A.12). The thyroid scan is of value in the follow-up of patients who have had thyroid cysts aspirated.

Other methods are used to reduce the surgical rate for thyroid nodules. X-ray fluorescence, which measures [127]I, is accurate for the identification of benign disease but the technique is not widely available. More controversial is the use of ^{201}Tl or ^{99m}Tc-sestamibi (^{99m}Tc-MIBI)[22,23] or ^{18}F-fluorodeoxyglucose (^{18}F-FDG) for evaluating the thyroid nodule. Although ^{18}F-FDG is not currently recommended for diagnosis the high uptake in thyroid malignancies does mean that when it is noted incidentally on a PET scan further investigation is essential.[24] While these tracers are taken up into malignant nodules they may also accumulate in benign lesions, and do not separate these entities sufficiently.

It is generally agreed that the correct management of a nonfunctioning nodule is surgical resection and not suppressive therapy with thyroxine as has been used in the past.

FUNCTIONING 'HOT' NODULE

If the thyroid scan shows the solitary nodule to be functioning or 'hot', the probability of malignancy is reduced to less than 1%, since most hot nodules are benign autonomously functioning adenomas; however, there have been occasional reports of malignancy. Three problems can be identified from these reports. The first is that some malignancies, while they do not organify the isotopes, do trap ^{99m}Tc-pertechnetate and iodine, and appear as hot or warm nodules on ^{99m}Tc scans or early ^{123}I scans. If we only consider those nodules that suppress TSH or remain hot on a ^{123}I scan after a perchlorate discharge test or delayed imaging as 'functioning', then the likelihood of malignancy remains very low. The second consideration is that nodules often occur in multinodular glands and the 'hot nodule' may be close to an 'incidentally' found malignancy, which may behave differently from the cancers that present clinically. Third, many adenomas and carcinomas have a good blood supply and it is the blood volume which 'creates' a 'warm' nodule rather than the true uptake of tracer.

There is no consensus on the investigation of this common clinical problem. Routine removal of all clinically apparent thyroid nodules no longer seems justified, and results in a great deal of unnecessary surgery. A reasonable policy (Fig. 12A.13) remains that of a ^{99m}Tc or ^{123}I scan in the first instance, which is a cheap, accurate, and widely available test. Functioning nodules are identified and these patients should have a sensitive TSH to confirm true biological function with subsequent follow-up and treatment for thyrotoxicosis as necessary. The evidence for any significant likelihood of malignancy in this group is not convincing. If reliable cytology is available then all nonfunctioning solitary nodules should have FNA cytology because of the well-documented reduction in unnecessary surgery. Ultrasound is only necessary as an adjunct to the scan when FNA is not available; simple cysts can then be aspirated and recurrences may be considered for injection with sclerosants. [201]Tl, ^{99m}Tc-MIBI or ^{18}F-FDG can be used when there is a relative contraindication to surgery, and when a negative or positive scan will help in making a decision, but it is probably not justified otherwise.

MULTINODULAR GOITER

A proportion of patients who are thought to have a solitary nodule on palpation are shown to have a multinodular goiter on scanning. The frequency with which this is noted depends on the experience of the clinician in palpating the thyroid, the ease with which the patient's thyroid can be palpated and the technique of the scan. Approximately 30–40% of clinically diagnosed solitary nodules can be shown to be multiple on scan; an even higher percentage

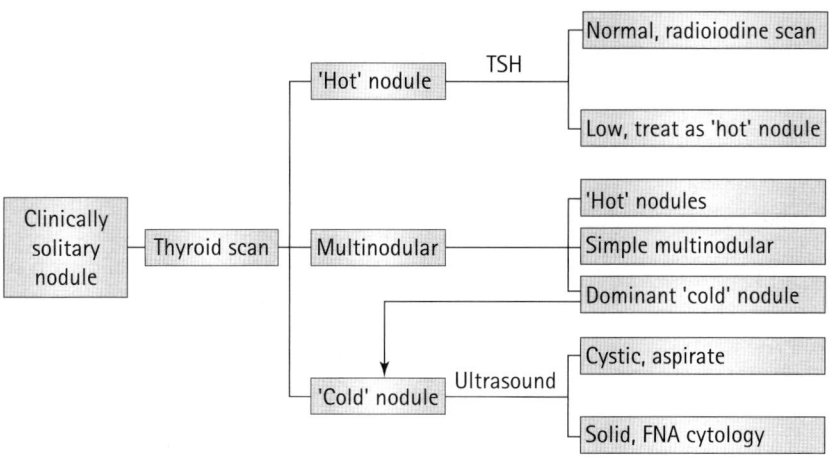

Figure 12A.13 *Scheme for the investigation of thyroid nodules.*

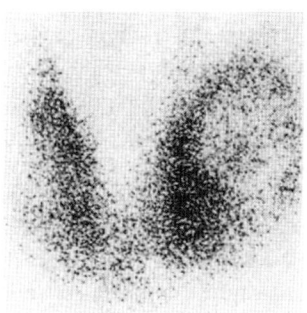

Figure 12A.14 *An example of a dominant nonfunctioning nodule in the left lobe of a multinodular gland.*

has been found at operation or autopsy.[25] It is often possible to palpate previously unsuspected nodules in the light of the scan findings.

The scintigraphic finding of a multinodular goiter, when a solitary nodule was suspected clinically, considerably decreases the probability of thyroid cancer in the absence of any clinical suspicion. Probably less than 1% of all multinodular goiters are malignant. Unless there is clinical suspicion of malignancy or local symptoms, a solitary nodule that is found to be part of a multinodular goiter on scanning does not need surgical excision.

The presence of a dominant cold nodule (Fig. 12A.14) in a gland with otherwise generally irregular uptake on scanning does not reduce the probability of malignancy to that of a typical multinodular goiter. Such dominant cold nodules should therefore be investigated with ultrasound and FNA cytology as for a solitary nodule, and excised if indicated.

PAINFUL GOITER

Pain originating from the thyroid associated with palpable enlargement may be due to one of the following conditions:

- Subacute (De Quervain's) thyroiditis
- Subacute or acute onset of Hashimoto's thyroiditis

- Hemorrhage into a thyroid nodule or cyst
- Thyroid cancer, particularly anaplastic carcinoma
- Acute suppurative thyroiditis (rare)

A careful history and clinical examination will often suggest the diagnosis, but should always be supplemented with appropriate investigations for confirmation. The most useful investigations include a full blood count and erythrocyte sedimentation rate, thyroid function tests, a radionuclide thyroid scan with ^{99m}Tc or ^{123}I, a perchlorate discharge test, and serum thyroid antibodies. Rarely, a biopsy may be necessary. Sudden onset of pain in the thyroid is most often caused by hemorrhage in a thyroid nodule or cyst, which may either be solitary or part of a multinodular goiter; thyroid function tests are normal and the thyroid scan shows a solitary cold nodule or a multinodular goiter with one or more cold nodules. Pain due to hemorrhage into a thyroid nodule usually lasts only a few days, and the nodule appears very rapidly, usually over a few hours. The nodule becomes smaller and may disappear completely after a few weeks. The patient should therefore be reviewed after 2 or 3 months and the thyroid scan repeated to confirm resolution or reduction of the nodule. If symptoms persist and the nodule enlarges, excision is advisable to exclude malignancy.

Subacute onset of pain over the neck, often described as a sore throat by the patient, associated with a recent upper respiratory infection, fever, malaise, anorexia, and a tender diffuse goiter, are characteristic of subacute thyroiditis. However, similar features may sometimes be caused by subacute onset of Hashimoto's thyroiditis. Investigations will establish the correct diagnosis. A mild leucocytosis and moderately elevated erythrocyte sedimentation rate may occur in both conditions, but subacute thyroiditis is characterized by mild biochemical hyperthyroidism in the early stages, a diffusely low uptake on ^{99m}Tc scan and absence of thyroid antibodies or only a transient rise. On the other hand, in Hashimoto's thyroiditis, thyroid function tests usually show frank or compensated hypothyroidism (high TSH with low or low-normal serum T4); thyroid scan characteristically, though not always, shows a high ^{99m}Tc uptake but a low radioiodine uptake, indicating trapping of iodine without organic binding. This can also be shown by a perchlorate discharge test, which will have an increased discharge of radioiodine. Hashimoto's thyroiditis may occasionally be associated with a normal or raised radioiodine uptake. Thyroid antibodies are present in high titers and persist in Hashimoto's thyroiditis. The differential diagnosis of Hashimoto's and subacute thyroiditis is important because their clinical course is quite different. In subacute thyroiditis, the thyroid usually recovers spontaneously after a few weeks or months without any sequelae, whereas Hashimoto's thyroiditis usually results in permanent hypothyroidism requiring long-term thyroid replacement.

It is important to distinguish atypical cases of thyroiditis with minimal or absent constitutional symptoms and a painful goiter, from a rapidly enlarging anaplastic thyroid carcinoma. The latter condition usually affects older patients and is often associated with evidence of local invasion such as hoarseness, Horner's syndrome, upper respiratory or esophageal obstruction, or distant metastases. The goiter is usually asymmetrical and hard, and the thyroid scan shows a focal area of low uptake with areas of normal uptake. Thyroid function tests are usually normal.

Acute suppurative thyroiditis due to bacterial or tuberculous infection is rare. The patient is very ill with marked constitutional symptoms, high fever, and a very tender goiter. Biopsy may be necessary to establish the diagnosis and provide culture material for antibiotic sensitivity. Confusion may be caused when subacute thyroiditis involves only one lobe with the characteristic low uptake in that lobe only on the scan. This may then resolve and the other lobe may be affected; this may occur in as many as 20% of the cases.

NONTOXIC GOITERS

Investigation and treatment of nontoxic goiters

The goiter may be diffuse or multinodular on examination, although occasionally it may be difficult to describe it clearly as one type or the other. Outside endemic areas of iodine deficiency, the main causes of a nontoxic goiter and the scan appearances are shown in Table 12A.7.

Certain points in the history and clinical examination of the patient are helpful in the diagnosis. They include the age of onset and duration of the goiter, a family history of goiter (suggesting Hashimoto's thyroiditis or familial dyshormonogenesis), the regular ingestion of goitrogens or a low iodine intake, the presence of nerve deafness in the patient (Pendred's syndrome), and the type of goiter on palpation (e.g. a soft diffuse simple colloid goiter, a simple multinodular goiter with several discrete nodules, or a bosselated firm goiter of Hashimoto's thyroiditis). Recent rapid enlargement of a long-standing goiter should raise a suspicion of malignancy, especially lymphoma or anaplastic carcinoma.

The basic investigations of a nontoxic goiter consist of thyroid function tests, particularly serum T4 and TSH, estimation of serum thyroid antibodies, and a thyroid scan with quantitative uptake. Further investigations that may be necessary include a perchlorate discharge test *in vivo*, studies of iodine kinetics and a thyroid biopsy.

SIMPLE COLLOID GOITER AND SIMPLE MULTINODULAR GOITER

These are the most common causes of a sporadic diffuse or nodular nontoxic goiter. The exact cause of these goiters is

Table 12A.7 *The thyroid scan in the assessment of goiter*

Scan findings	Cause	Comment
Diffuse, normal uptake of tracer	Diffuse nontoxic (simple) goiter	
Diffuse, with high uptake of tracer	Diffuse toxic goiter (Graves' disease)	May be first indication of hyperthyroidism
	Lymphocytic thyroiditis (Hashimoto's disease)	Occurs in early disease
	Iodine deficiency	
	Organification defects (inherited or goitrogens)	May be difficult to distinguish
Diffuse, low uptake of tracer	Subacute thyroiditis (De Quervain's)	
	Iodine-induced goiter	May be indistinguishable on the scan but
	Hashimoto's disease	presentation is entirely different
	Lymphoma	
Multifocal irregularity	Simple multinodular	Detection of autonomous nodule is important
Normal uptake of tracer	Hashimoto's disease	Diagnosis by antibodies
Irregular replacement of thyroid tissue	Diffuse cancer	Usually clinically apparent, but may be confused with multinodular goiter

uncertain, but they are thought to represent different stages of the same pathological process. Thyroid function tests including TSH are usually normal and thyroid antibodies are usually absent or in low titer. Uptake of ^{99m}Tc or radioiodine is normal. The distribution of uptake on the scan is diffuse in a simple colloid goiter, but markedly irregular often with discrete areas of diminished uptake in a multinodular goiter. Oblique views may be helpful. Occasionally, the goiter may contain one or more areas of increased uptake indicating developing autonomous functioning nodules. The TSH level will be suppressed. These autonomous nodules may give rise to frank hyperthyroidism (Plummer's disease) as the disease progresses.

No specific treatment is usually necessary for asymptomatic simple colloid or multinodular goiters. A large multinodular goiter causing tracheal or esophageal compression, as shown by radiography of the thoracic inlet or a barium swallow, should be resected although some of these patients may be treated with ^{131}I.[16,19–21] The average reduction in volume with ^{131}I is approximately 50%.[26] Thyroid hormone therapy in suppressive doses is rarely helpful in reducing goiter size, but may be tried in moderate-sized goiters if serum TSH is elevated. Multinodular goiters with autonomous nodules should be followed up regularly for signs of developing hyperthyroidism, which should then be treated with radioiodine or surgery. Recent rapid enlargement of a long-standing multinodular goiter should raise the possibility of malignancy and an aspiration biopsy or ^{201}Tl scan should be performed, followed by surgical excision if indicated.

The appearance of two symmetrical solitary nodules in a goiter should raise the suspicion of a medullary thyroid cancer (Fig. 12A.15) (although this is an uncommon tumor) and will further increase the likelihood of it being the familial type that has arisen from symmetrically distributed C-cell hyperplasia. Serum calcitonin measurement in addition to FNA cytology may be helpful in making a pre-operative diagnosis as may uptake of ^{99m}Tc(V)-dimercaptosuccinic acid (^{99m}Tc(V)-DMSA) or *meta*-[^{123}I/^{131}I]iodobenzylguanidine (^{123}I/^{131}I-MIBG).[25,27,28] This will be of particular value in cases of multiple endocrine neoplasias, and clearly pheochromocytoma must be identified prior to initial surgery. First-degree family screening is undertaken in all patients with diagnosed medullary thyroid cancers to establish whether or not it is the inherited type. When an elevated calcitonin is detected in a relative of the patient investigation of the thyroid is necessary. Because most surgeons prefer to know if there is a nodule present rather than simply perform a prophylactic total thyroidectomy, it will also be necessary to use the radionuclide thyroid scan and ultrasound or CT.

A thyroid lymphoma may develop spontaneously, with the patient usually presenting with a rapidly enlarging diffuse goiter, or may occur in a patient with Hashimoto's disease where there is recognized to be an increased risk of lymphoma. A radionuclide thyroid scan is not helpful because in the latter situation the patient will be hypothyroid and receiving thyroxine treatment, and in the former case the scan will usually show diffuse enlargement with an overall low uptake due to the diffuse infiltration. In these instances it is usual to proceed directly to surgical biopsy but there are clinical circumstances, e.g. if the patient is too anxious or has other pathology, when this is not advised and then a ^{67}Ga or ^{18}F-FDG PET scan, which shows avid accumulation in lymphoma, may provide valuable information (Fig. 12A.16). Finally, De Quervain's subacute thyroiditis if it is localized or initially involves only one lobe may simulate a malignant lesion.[29] Repeat thyroid scans show recovery of function in one area with appearance of the typical low uptake in the other lobe, confirming the diagnosis of thyroiditis and not malignancy.

HASHIMOTO'S THYROIDITIS

The diagnosis of this condition depends on three main features: (1) the presence of a goiter which is typically bosselated and firm on palpation; (2) subclinical or frank hypothyroidism, i.e. raised TSH with borderline low or low serum T4; and (3) serum thyroid antibodies which are usually strongly positive although they have been reported to be negative in a small proportion of biopsy-proven Hashimoto's thyroiditis. Other investigations are of limited diagnostic value, e.g. thyroid scan may show high, normal

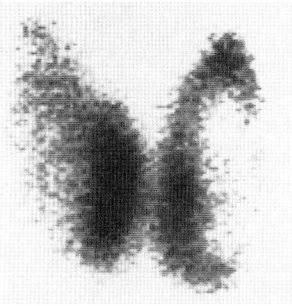

Figure 12A.15 *A patient discovered by family screening to have a medullary thyroid cancer, showing the symmetrical cold areas due to bilateral medullary cancers.*

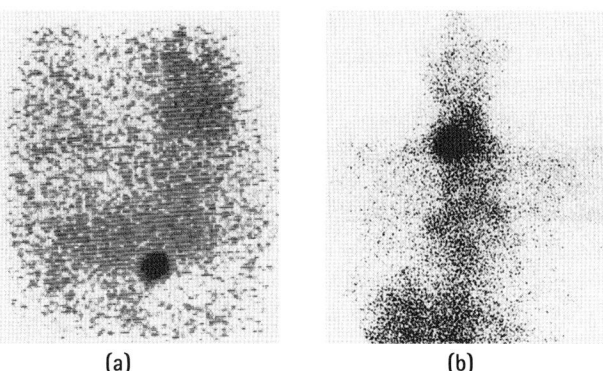

(a) (b)

Figure 12A.16 *Scans of a patient with lymphoma with markers; (a) shows a large gland with low uptake (^{99m}TcO$_4$), but the ^{67}Ga scan (b) shows avid accumulation.*

or low uptake of radionuclide with varying distribution (uniform, irregular or nodular) according to the degree of fibrosis. We have reviewed 32 cases, and a wide variety of scan patterns were obtained.[25,29] The most common scan appearances were either of an enlarged gland with diffusely increased tracer uptake similar to Graves' disease or those of a multinodular gland. However, other scans appeared normal, or showed a focal defect, or reduced tracer uptake throughout one lobe, or generally low uptake by the whole gland. Perchlorate discharge test shows excess discharge of radioiodine in most of the cases. Cytology or biopsy may be helpful in equivocal cases.

Hashimoto's thyroiditis is treated with long-term suppressive doses of thyroid hormones (e.g. thyroxine 100–200 mg daily). If treatment is started in the early stages of the condition considerable reduction in size of the goiter can be expected, whereas if diagnosis is made late, when considerable fibrosis is present in the gland, little or no improvement in goiter size may occur.

DYSHORMONOGENESIS

This refers to a group of genetic abnormalities, each involving a specific enzyme defect in the metabolic pathway of thyroid hormones. Most are transmitted by autosomal recessive inheritance and are rare. The best known and least rare is Pendred's syndrome, in which a familial goiter is associated with nerve deafness. Familial dyshormonogenesis should be considered in the differential diagnosis of goiter in the younger patient with a family history of goiter, absent thyroid antibodies and subclinical or frank hypothyroidism. From the point of view of clinical investigation, dyshormonogenesis may be divided into three groups.

ABNORMALITY OF IODIDE TRANSPORT INTO THE THYROID CELL

This condition is characterized by a very low iodine uptake in the thyroid as well as in the salivary glands, which share the same iodide trapping mechanism. The salivary glands should therefore be included in the field-of-view when the thyroid scan is performed.

ABNORMALITY OF ORGANIFICATION OF IODINE TO TYROSINE

This defect is characterized by a normal iodine uptake in the gland but the perchlorate discharge test reveals an excess discharge of unorganified iodide. The best-known and most common condition in this group is Pendred's syndrome. The organification defect is usually only partial, as indicated by normal or slightly low serum T4 with raised serum TSH and excess radioiodine discharge on perchlorate discharge test.

OTHER ENZYME DEFECTS

Familial goiters with a normal or high iodine uptake and normal perchlorate discharge may result from an abnormality in the metabolic pathway beyond the organification stage of iodine. Various types have been described, all of which are rare and depend on more detailed biochemical investigation for diagnosis.

ECTOPIC THYROID

Thyroid tissue may occur in other than the normal anatomical positions, when it may constitute a diagnostic or therapeutic problem. The most common places are at the back of the tongue (lingual thyroid), in the mid-line position of the upper neck (sublingual or subhyoid thyroid), inside the thoracic cavity (anterior or posterior mediastinal goiter) and in ovarian tumors (struma ovarii).

Lingual and sublingual thyroid

Failure or incomplete descent of the thyroid gland from its embryological mid-line position at the back of the tongue results in a lingual or sublingual thyroid. Either may contain the whole or only part of the patient's thyroid tissue. These ectopic thyroids usually present as a mid-line swelling at the back of the tongue or upper neck or as congenital hypothyroidism. Failure to recognize and diagnose a lingual or sublingual thyroid swelling may lead to inadvertent excision and permanent hypothyroidism requiring lifelong thyroid replacement.

A mid-line swelling at the back of the tongue or upper neck should therefore always be investigated for the possibility of an ectopic thyroid before excision. The presence or absence of a normally situated thyroid gland should also be confirmed. The sublingual or subhyoid ectopic thyroid is particularly likely to be mistaken clinically for a thyroglossal cyst or other nonthyroid swelling.

Thyroid function tests are performed to assess the patient's thyroid status and a radionuclide scan is carried out. Iodine-123 is better because of the higher uptake which avoids confusion with saliva and salivary glands on a ^{99m}Tc scan. The radiation dose with either radionuclide is small compared with ^{131}I, and the scan can therefore be used in infants, children or adolescents. The whole area from the mouth to the sternal notch should be imaged and reference markers placed on any palpable nodule and appropriate anatomical landmarks (e.g. the sternal notch). In the case of a lingual thyroid, a lateral view is important for accurate three-dimensional localization. Radionuclide uptake in the nodule confirms the presence of ectopic thyroid whereas other types of nodule (e.g. a thyroglossal cyst) appear cold. The presence or absence of a normal thyroid is also established at the same time. Rarely, if the normal thyroid is not visualized the scan should be repeated after TSH stimulation to exclude the possibility that its function may be suppressed.

A nodule that shows no uptake of ^{99m}Tc or ^{123}I can be excised. A functioning ectopic thyroid nodule can also be excised if the scan confirms the presence of a normal thyroid in addition in the normal site. However, a sublingual thyroid that contains the entire functioning thyroid tissue should be preserved. For cosmetic reasons the ectopic thyroid can be divided and relocated.

In patients who have undergone previous thyroid surgery, congenital remnants of thyroid tissue along the thyroglossal tract may hypertrophy to produce a mid-line swelling in the upper neck, particularly with recurrence of Graves' disease. This can be confirmed on a thyroid scan.

Intrathoracic (mediastinal) goiters

A normally situated thyroid gland may enlarge downward into the anterior mediastinum to produce a retrosternal goiter, or less commonly it may extend downwards behind the trachea and esophagus, as a posterior mediastinal goiter. These intrathoracic goiters are most commonly caused by nontoxic nodular goiters. Rarely, they are congenitally ectopic glands which have migrated with the primitive heart into the mediastinum. They may be asymptomatic and come to light incidentally in the differential diagnosis of an upper mediastinal opacity noted on routine chest radiography, or they may cause symptoms due to compression of the trachea, esophagus or superior vena cava. Occasionally, a large diffuse toxic goiter or toxic nodule may extend retrosternally or in the posterior mediastinum and cause similar symptoms in addition to those of hyperthyroidism.

Most retrosternal goiters are associated with palpable enlargement of the cervical thyroid and the diagnosis of retrosternal goiter can be inferred if the lower border of the goiter cannot be felt in the neck.

To confirm the intrathoracic goiter and assess its extent, a radiograph of the thoracic inlet and a thyroid scan with ^{123}I or ^{131}I should be performed. Although the presence of radioiodine uptake below the sternal notch confirms the diagnosis of intrathoracic goiter, its absence does not exclude a nonfunctioning intrathoracic goiter. In such cases, mediastinoscopy and tissue biopsy or a formal thoracotomy may be necessary to confirm the diagnosis. Mediastinal CT or MRI may be necessary to assess the extent and to evaluate tracheal compression.

Retrosternal or posterior intrathoracic goiters should be removed surgically if there is evidence of increasing tracheal or oesophageal compression as the goiter enlarges. If the patient is also thyrotoxic, initial treatment with antithyroid drugs until the patient is euthyroid, followed by surgery, is usually advised. However, if the patient is considered a poor surgical risk, antithyroid drugs followed by radioiodine therapy under close supervision in hospital may be preferable.

NEONATAL HYPOTHYROIDISM

If congenital hypothyroidism remains undiscovered, the neurological and skeletal sequelae can be irreversible and devastating. Over the past decade, the usefulness of the introduction of widespread screening programs for the detection of neonatal hypothyroidism has been confirmed. The incidence of disease in most countries is about 1 in 4000 with a female preponderance of around 4:1. The diagnosis of primary congenital hypothyroidism is based on the finding of a low thyroxine together with an elevated TSH level. This however, fails to distinguish between the presence of an ectopic or hypoplastic thyroid, athyreosis, dyshormonogenesis, and transient hypothyroidism. Neonatal hypothyroidism represents a spectrum of disease ranging from transient under-activity to complete absence of a thyroid gland. It is in this context that the question of the role of the thyroid scan in the investigation and management of these patients continues to be discussed.

The thyroid scan accurately delineates the anatomy in infants with congenital hypothyroidism, and in addition provides functional information. A scan should be obtained before commencing treatment with thyroxine. The anatomical findings may be broadly characterized into four groups based on scan findings:

- A normal gland
- Ectopic location
- No detectable thyroid activity
- Normal location with increased size of gland or increased tracer uptake.

An ectopic thyroid gland is found in approximately 45% of cases and athyreosis in 35%. Some 10% will have a normal gland and 10% other abnormalities. In the latter cases it is presumed that there is a disorder of thyroid hormonogenesis and a number will have defects of thyroid hormone synthesis. A perchlorate discharge test will identify those cases with an organification defect. There is some controversy as to the role of inhibitive immunoglobulins ('blocking' antibodies) as these may cause transient hypothyroidism. Further, the scan findings in isolation are misleading in terms of prognosis as there is no tracer uptake by the thyroid and will suggest athyreosis. The role of transplacental passage of maternal immunoglobulins may be important in the pathogenesis of sporadic congenital hypothyroidism.

The thyroid scan has prognostic significance as those with anatomical defects will have permanent hypothyroidism. Information obtained from a scan may also aid in genetic counselling as an ectopic thyroid or athyreosis occurs spontaneously while impaired biosynthesis of thyroid hormones implies an inherited defect. Thyroid scan data presented in a form that patients find easy to understand and accept is important with long-term therapy, as good patient compliance is required. Where an ectopic thyroid is present, a scan may avoid an unnecessary operation for a base of tongue swelling.

While in the great majority of cases of neonatal hypothyroidism the disease is permanent, some will have transient hypothyroidism, and clearly it is desirable to identify these cases. It has been found, however, that those with an anatomic defect or a secondary rise in TSH after the TSH has been initially suppressed by thyroxine therapy have permanent hypothyroidism. Thus, only approximately one third of cases will qualify for a trial off therapy. Thyroxine should be discontinued for a 3-week period after 3 years of age, and this is adequate and safe to confirm that hypothyroidism is permanent. Only 1–2% of newborn cases of hypothyroidism identified on screening will have transient disease.

REFERENCES

1 Perlmutter M, Slater SL. Which nodular goiters should be removed – physiologic plan for the diagnosis and treatment of nodular goiter. *N Engl J Med* 1956; **255**: 65–71.

2 Rallison ML, Dobyns BM, Meikle AW, *et al.* Natural history of thyroid abnormalities – prevalence, incidence, and regression of thyroid diseases in adolescents and young adults. *Am J Med* 1991; **91**: 363–70.

3 Vanderpump MPJ, Tunbridge WMG, French JM, *et al.* The incidence of thyroid disorders in the community – a 20-year follow-up of the Whickham survey. *Clin Endocrinol* 1995; **43**: 55–68.

4 Tunbridge WMG, Evered DC, Hall R, *et al.* Spectrum of thyroid disease in a community – Whickham survey. *Clin Endocrinol* 1977; **7**: 481–93.

5 Cooke SG, Ratcliffe GE, Fogelman I, Maisey MN. Prevalence of inappropriate drug treatment in patients with hyperthyroidism. *Br Med J* 1985; **291**: 1491–2.

6 Ratcliffe GE, Cooke S, Fogelman I, Maisey MN. Radioiodine treatment of solitary functioning thyroid nodules. *Br J Radiol* 1986; **59**: 385–7.

7 Ratcliffe GE, Fogelman I, Maisey MN. The evaluation of radioiodine therapy for thyroid patients using a fixed-dose regime. *Br J Radiol* 1986; **59**: 1105–7.

8 Reschini E, Peracchi M. Thyroid scintigraphy during antithyroid treatment for autonomous nodules as a means of imaging extranodular tissue. *Clin Nucl Med* 1993; **18**: 597–600.

9 Martino E, Aghinilombardi F, Lippi F, *et al.* 24 Hour radioactive iodine uptake in 35 patients with amiodarone associated thyrotoxicosis. *J Nucl Med* 1985; **26**: 1402–7.

10 Becks GP, Burrow GN. Thyroid disease and pregnancy. *Med Clin N Am* 1991; **75**: 121–50.

11 Bartalena L, Brogioni S, Grasso L, *et al.* Treatment of amiodarone-induced thyrotoxicosis, a difficult challenge: results of a prospective study. *J Clin Endocrinol Metabol* 1996; **81**: 2930–3.

12 Bogazzi F, Bartalena L, Gasperi M, *et al.* The various effects of amiodarone on thyroid function. *Thyroid* 2001; **11**: 511–19.

13 Rojeski MT, Gharib H. Nodular thyroid disease – evaluation and management. *N Engl J Med* 1985; **313**: 428–36.

14 Schneider AB, Bekerman C, Leland J, *et al.* Thyroid nodules in the follow-up of irradiated individuals: comparison of thyroid ultrasound with scanning and palpation. *J Clin Endocrinol Metabol* 1997; **82**: 4020–7.

15 Kakkos SK, Scopa CD, Chalmoukis AK, *et al.* Relative risk of cancer in sonographically detected thyroid nodules with calcifications. *J Clin Ultrasound* 2000; **28**: 347–52.

16 Gharib H. Subspecialty clinics – endocrinology/metabolism – fine-needle aspiration biopsy of thyroid nodules: advantages, limitations, and effect. *Mayo Clinic Proc* 1994; **69**: 44–9.

17 Woeber KA. Cost-effective evaluation of the patient with a thyroid nodule. *Surg Clin N Am* 1995; **75**: 357–63.

18 Amrikachi M, Ramzy I, Rubenfeld S, Wheeler TM. Accuracy of fine-needle aspiration of thyroid – a review of 6226 cases and correlation with surgical or clinical outcome. *Arch Pathol Lab Med* 2001; **125**: 484–8.

19 Huysmans D, Hermus A, Barentsz J, *et al.* Successful treatment of large, compressive multinodular goiters with radioiodine and L-thyroxine. *J Nucl Med* 1994; **35**: 165.

20 Huysmans D, Hermus A, Edelbroek M, *et al.* Radioiodine for non-toxic multinodular goiter. *Thyroid* 1997; **7**: 235–9.

21 Huysmans DA, Nieuwlaat WA, Hermus AR. Towards larger volume reduction of nodular goiters by radioiodine therapy: a role for pretreatment with recombinant human thyrotropin? *Clin Endocrinol* 2004; **60**: 297–9.

22 Sundram FX, Mack P. Evaluation of thyroid nodules for malignancy using $^{99}Tc^m$-sestamibi. *Nucl Med Commun* 1995; **16**: 687–93.

23 Wei JP, Burke GJ. Characterization of the neoplastic potential of solitary solid thyroid lesions with Tc-99m-pertechnetate and Tc-99m-sestamibi scanning. *Ann Surg Oncol* 1995; **2**: 233–7.

24 Cohen MS, Arslan N, Dehdashti F, *et al.* Risk of malignancy in thyroid incidentalomas identified by fluorodeoxyglucose positron emission tomography. *Surgery* 2001; **130**: 941–6.

25 Maisey MN, Moses DC, Hurley PJ, Wagner HN. Improved methods for thyroid scanning – correlation with surgical findings. *JAMA* 1973; **223**: 761–3.

26 Le Moli R, Wesche MFT, Tiel-van Buul MMC, Wiersinga WM. Determinants of longterm outcome of radioiodine therapy of sporadic non-toxic goiter. *Clin Endocrinol* 1999; **50**: 783–9.

27 Clarke SEM, Lazarus C, Fogelman I, Maisey MN. The role of Tc-99m(V) DMSA imaging in the management of patients with medullary carcinoma of the thyroid. *J Endocrinol* 1987; **112**: 91.

28 Clarke SEM, Lazarus CR, Wraight P, *et al.* Pentavalent [Tc-99m] DMSA, [I-131] MIBG, and [Tc-99m] MDP – an evaluation of 3 imaging techniques in patients with medullary carcinoma of the thyroid. *J Nucl Med* 1988; **29**: 33–8.

29 Ramtoola S, Maisey MN, Clarke SEM, Fogelman I. The thyroid scan in hashimotos thyroiditis – the great mimic. *Nucl Med Commun* 1988; **9**: 639–45.

Parathyroid localization

A.G. KETTLE, C.P. WELLS, AND M.J. O'DOHERTY

INTRODUCTION

The curative management of hyperparathyroidism is the surgical removal of abnormal parathyroid glands.[1] This surgical treatment may require bilateral neck exploration, unilateral neck exploration or minimally invasive parathyroidectomy.[2] This latter approach has been refined and improved over recent years by using probes, endoscopic directed methods or video assisted removal, such that selective removal of individual glands can be achieved in some cases using minimally invasive surgery.

The ability to perform surgical exploration or minimally invasive surgery is dependent on the presence of an experienced parathyroid surgeon and accurate preoperative localization of the parathyroid abnormality. The variable anatomical siting of the parathyroids means that their localization at operation can be difficult, and a strong case can be made for parathyroidectomy to be performed only by surgeons with specialized training and experience in the procedure.[1] A wide variety of preoperative localizing techniques have been described to assist the surgeon find the glands, particularly if these are at ectopic sites or when the patient has had previous neck surgery. This chapter gives an account of radionuclide and other techniques available for preoperative localization, and indicates the role of these in the management of hyperparathyroidism.

ANATOMY AND PHYSIOLOGY

There are normally four parathyroid glands (the range is from two to six), situated in close proximity to the thyroid, posterior to the upper and lower poles of the right and left lobe of the thyroid. Five percent of patients have more than four glands, and another 5% have only three glands.[2,3] The complicated embryological development of the parathyroids results in a number of variations in the normal anatomy, and glands may be sited in a number of ectopic sites in the neck or upper mediastinum. The upper glands may be found posterior to the esophagus or occasionally in the carotid sheath, the lower glands may be found in the thymus but are usually found within a centimeter or two below the lower pole if ectopic (Fig. 12B.1).

Parathormone (PTH) is the active peptide produced by the parathyroid. It causes a rise in ionized calcium in the blood by increasing calcium release from bone, promoting re-absorption from the renal tubules, and increasing synthesis of the active compound 1,25-dihydroxycholecalciferol. Both primary and secondary hyperparathyroidism are recognized. In primary hyperparathyroidism there is endogenous hypersecretion of PTH which may be due to:

- A parathyroid adenoma (80–85% of cases). Rarely there may be more than one adenoma.
- Hyperplasia involving more than one gland, usually with all four glands involved. This occurs in 10–15% of primary cases.
- Parathyroid carcinoma, which occurs in 3–4% of cases.

Secondary hyperparathyroidism occurs when there is a tendency to hypocalcemia resulting in increased stimulation of the parathyroid glands and increased PTH production. The most common clinical cause is renal failure but the condition can occasionally be seen with malabsorption or renal tubular disorder. In some cases of secondary hyperparathyroidism one or more of the glands can become autonomous, so that even when the primary disease causing hyperparathyroidism to develop is treated the glands continue to hypersecrete PTH; this is termed tertiary hyperparathyroidism.

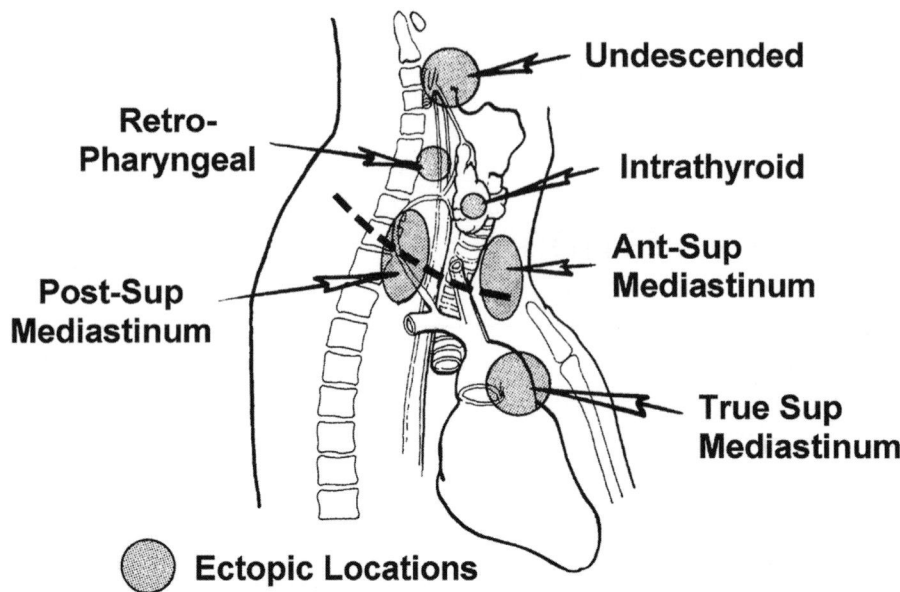

Figure 12B.1 *Distribution of the ectopic sites of parathyroid adenomas. (Adapted from Edis AJ, Sheedy PF, Beahrs OH, van Heerden JA. Results of re-operations for hyperparathyroidism, with evaluation of pre-operative localisation studies. Surgery 1978; 84: 384–393, with permission.)*

PREOPERATIVE LOCALIZING TECHNIQUES

A variety of anatomical and functional localizing techniques for parathyroid tissue have been used. The functional techniques have included [75Se]selenomethionine, 57Co-vitamin B_{12}, 131I-toluidine blue, and 123I-methylene blue with little success[4]. The breakthrough in functional imaging occurred with the use of [201Tl]thallous chloride and a subtraction technique in combination with pertechnetate.[5] This proved to have a major advantage over all the previous techniques with an improvement in sensitivity in the localization of primary parathyroid adenomas of between 42 and 96%, with a mean of 72%.[6] For secondary hyperparathyroidism there was a lower detection rate, varying from 32 to 81% with a mean of 43%. The next major change occurred with the recognition that 99mTc-sestamibi accumulated in parathyroid tissue and had a differential washout compared to underlying thyroid.[7,8] Following this observation a variety of scanning protocols were assessed and will be discussed below. Technetium-99m-tetrofosmin was the next compound to be considered for parathyroid imaging but the retention is similar in parathyroid tissue and thyroid tissue and therefore only subtraction techniques can be used.[9–11] Positron emission tomography has also been explored using both [18F]fluorodeoxyglucose and 11C-methionine with varying success.[12–15]

Anatomical imaging methods have included computerized tomography (CT), magnetic resonance imaging (MRI), arteriography, and high resolution ultrasound.[16–18] The use of CT in the localization of parathyroid tissue is primarily reserved for prior to the first operation with sensitivities for localization between 43 and 92%,[19–21] the lower sensitivities are found when re-exploration patients are scanned. Similar limitations are found with MRI with sensitivities found of 50–93%.[19,21–23] High resolution ultrasound is a technique which does need further exploration and the combination of this technique with sestamibi imaging may be the optimum combination prior to surgical exploration.[19]

Technetium-99m-sestamibi

Technetium-99m-sestamibi is a cationic complex developed as an alternative to thallium for studying myocardial blood flow. It has been shown to localize parathyroid tissue and is now the imaging agent of choice. The uptake and retention of sestamibi is different in parathyroid and thyroid tissue.[8] This allows the imaging at an early and late phase (dual-phase imaging) to localize parathyroid adenomas (Fig.12B.2(a) and (b)). The alternative to dual-phase imaging is the subtraction technique using either 123I or [99mTc]pertechnetate to localize the thyroid and sestamibi to localize the parathyroid tissue (Figs 12B.3 and 12B.4 (a) and (b)) (see (below). The uptake of sestamibi or tetrofosmin may be influenced by a number of biological factors. These include the size of the adenoma, the cell type, the P-glycoprotein expression, and the mitochondrial structure.[24] There are a variety of studies that have demonstrated that the identification of parathyroid adenomas is related to the increase in adenoma volume but not necessarily related to the weight of the tumor. The uptake tends to be concentrated in the mitochondria of the parathyroid cells and therefore those cells rich in mitochondria, the oxyphil cells, rather than

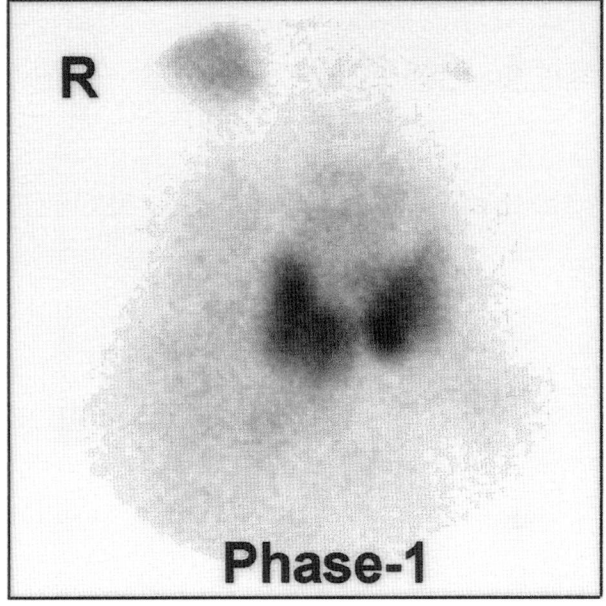
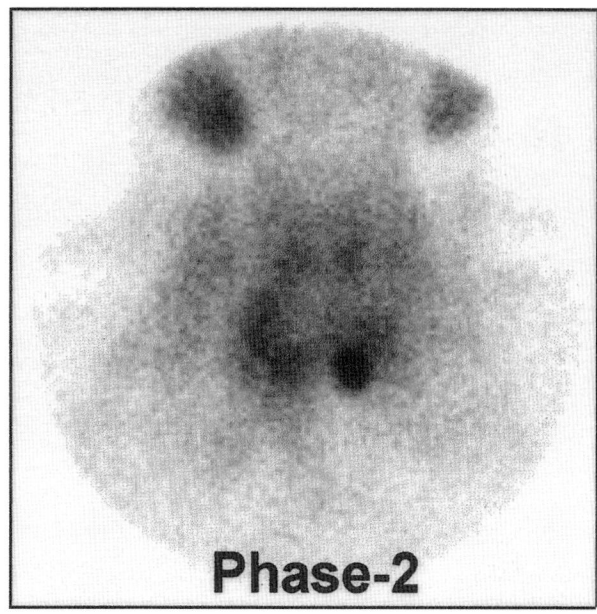

(a)

Figure 12B.2 *(a) Dual-phase technique. Technetium-99m-sestamibi images viewed at 20 min and 2 h post-injection of sestamibi. The early image on the left shows the distribution of sestamibi in the thyroid and parathyroid tissue, with a small area of slight increased uptake seen at the lower pole of the left lobe of the thyroid. This is seen more clearly at 2 h when the thyroid activity has 'washed out'.*

the chief cells tend to be more apparent in the tumors that are visualized. This expression of cell type has not been found by all observers, however.[24] In secondary hyperparathyroidism the accumulation of sestamibi has been found to be related to the cell cycle with the highest uptake found in the growth phase and not the resting phase.[25] The parathyroid tumors can also express multidrug resistance proteins or P-glycoprotein that result in efflux of sestamibi from the tumor and therefore hamper visualization of tumors and therefore result in false negative scans.

All of the functional techniques can result in false positive (Fig. 12B.4(a)) and false negative scans (Fig. 12B.5, page 516). The optimization of the techniques needs to be considered. Consideration has to be given to whether dual-phase or subtraction techniques are used, what collimation – parallel hole or pinhole, planar imaging or tomography (parallel hole or pinhole) or the combined use of gamma camera–CT imaging.

IMAGING METHODOLOGY

Planar subtraction method

The basis of this method is that the thyroid gland is visualized either by [^{99m}Tc]pertechnetate or ^{123}I and is subtracted from an image of the ^{99m}Tc-sestamibi (or ^{99m}Tc-tetrofosmin) uptake within the thyroid and parathyroid gland(s). It is more common to administer the thyroid imaging agent first

and image the thyroid before administration of sestamibi. If ^{123}I is used, correction for cross-talk between the ^{123}I and ^{99m}Tc windows is required. Rather than an image subtraction based on normalization of the images it is diagnostically helpful to create a subtraction loop where incremental amounts of the thyroid image are subtracted from the ^{99m}Tc-sestamibi distribution until the point of over subtraction.

Planar washout method

O'Doherty *et al.*[8] observed that ^{99m}Tc-sestamibi uptake in thyroid tissue cleared more quickly than that in parathyroid tissue and Taillefer *et al.*[26] proposed a washout method, dual-phase imaging, to exploit this finding. This technique is not applicable when ^{99m}Tc-tetrofosmin is used. An image of the distribution of ^{99m}Tc-sestamibi within the neck is obtained within a few minutes of its administration and then a delayed image obtained 1–2 h later. The method relies on clearance from the thyroid and not from the parathyroid(s) but there is increasing evidence that in some patients clearance from the parathyroid is similar to that of the thyroid and therefore the false negative rate is higher than with the subtraction method.

For both planar imaging methods pinhole views of the neck are preferred for optimum spatial resolution[27] and an additional full field of view image of the anterior neck/thorax to exclude an ectopic site in the chest. Pinhole imaging also can be acquired as an oblique image further improving sensitivity.[28]

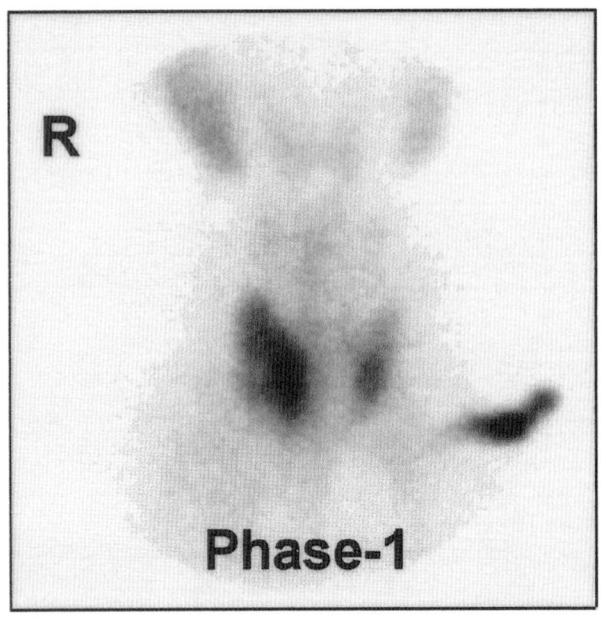
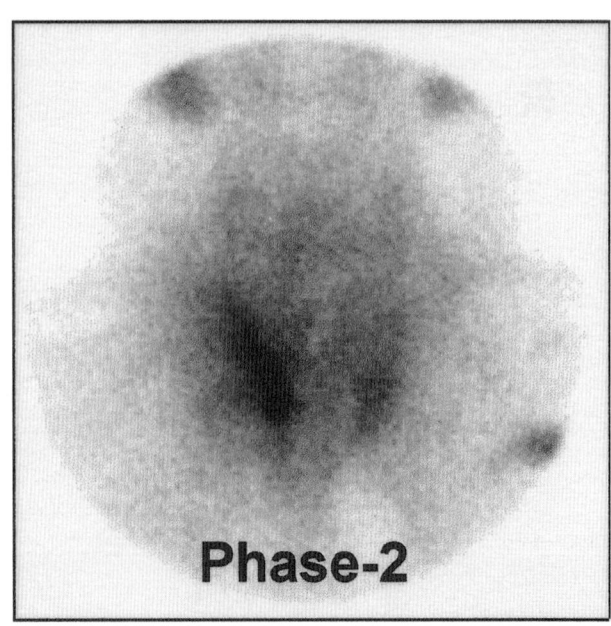

(bi)

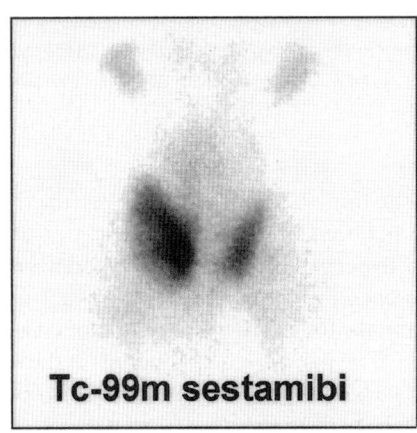
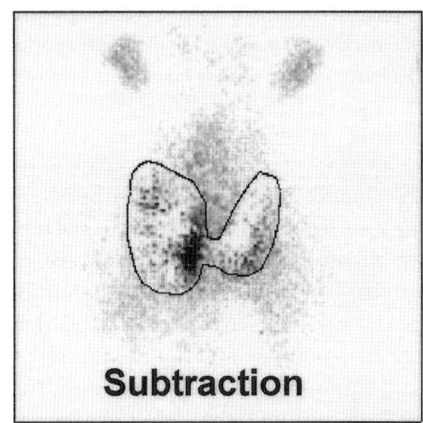

(bii)

Figure 12B.2 *(Continued)* *(b) A patient who had both a dual-phase and a subtraction image performed. The dual-phase images (bi) show a smaller left lobe of the thyroid than the right at 20 min (phase1) and then on the washout image performed at 2 h (phase2) there is an area of uptake seen in the lower pole of the right lobe of the thyroid. The subtraction scan (bii), on the same patient, shows a multinodular thyroid with a smaller left lobe than right on the ^{123}I image. The subtraction image clearly demonstrates an abnormal area of uptake at the level of the isthmus in the right lobe of the thyroid. This was the site of the parathyroid adenoma.*

Tomographic imaging

Dual isotope, ^{123}I/^{99m}Tc-sestamibi SPECT after the completion of planar imaging has been found beneficial in providing three-dimensional localization in patients who have suffered a failed parathyroidectomy. Some centers advocate single photon emission tomography (SPET) imaging for the two phases of the washout method. Increasingly, SPET imaging is being used for the initial localization procedure since this method gives better identification of the site of the adenoma such that minimally invasive surgery can be used to remove the adenoma.[29,30] The additional value of combined gamma camera–CT imaging has not yet been

explored in sufficient studies to identify a role for this methodology.

Other imaging techniques

Ultrasound evaluation of parathyroid glands varies with reported sensitivities of 38–92% and a specificity of 60–80% for adenomas in the neck. Ultrasound cannot detect mediastinal disease and has a lower sensitivity after neck exploration when the vascular anatomy and relationship to tissue planes have been altered. As with scintigraphy, ultrasound imaging cannot distinguish parathyroid from thyroid

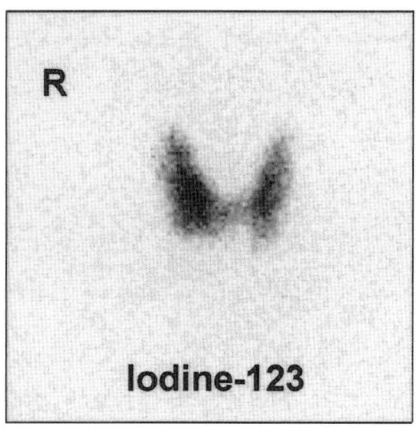
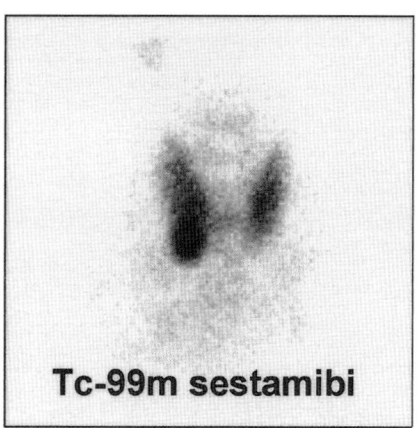
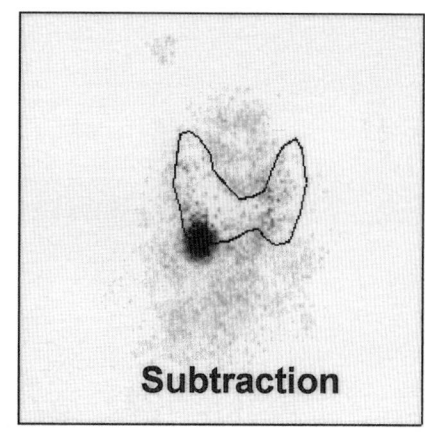

Figure 12B.3   *The patient had a subtraction scan performed. The iodine scan demonstrates normal distribution in the thyroid. The sestamibi scan demonstrates an abnormal area of accumulation at the lower pole of the right lobe of the thyroid, without the need for subtraction. The subtraction scan confirms this site of abnormality.*

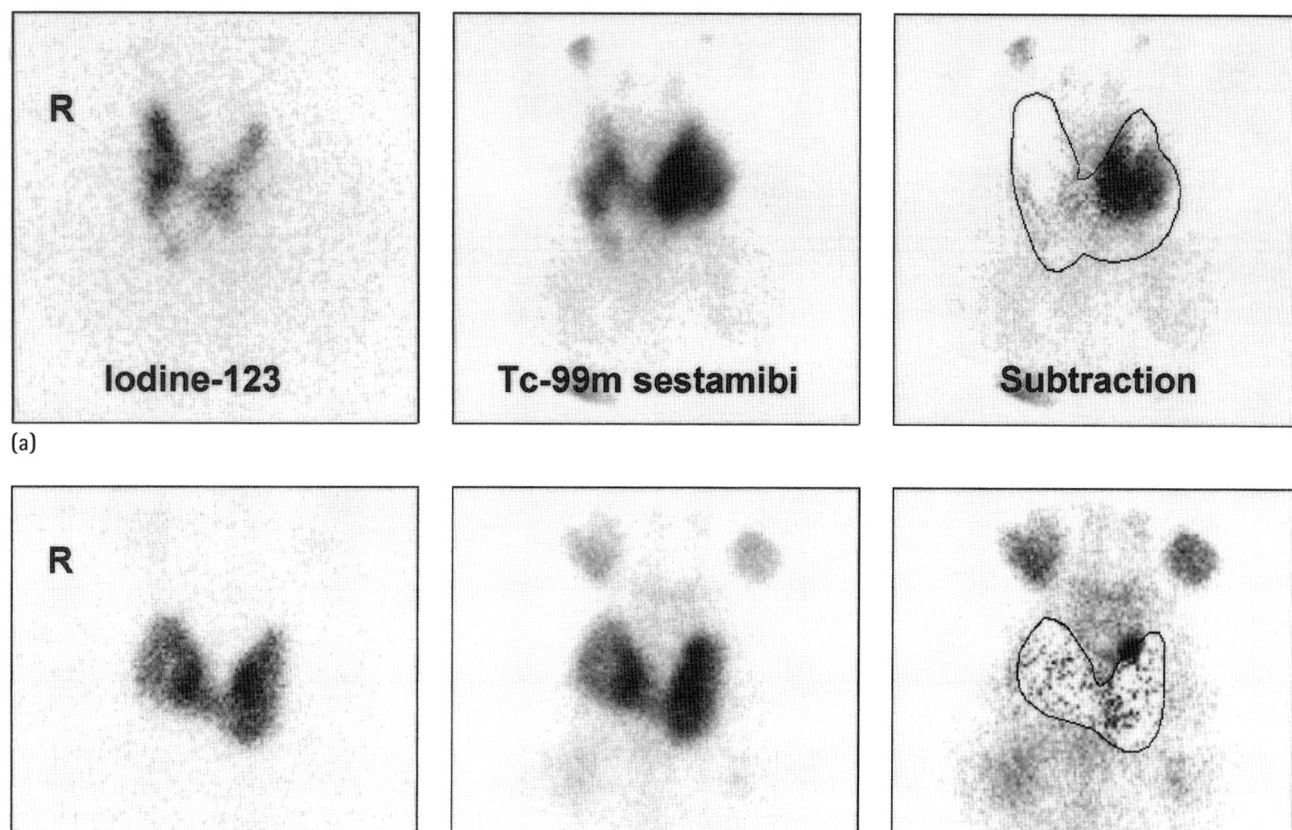

Figure 12B.4   *(a) The iodine scan demonstrates a multinodular thyroid, with cold nodules at the lower pole of the right lobe of the thyroid (cyst on ultrasound) and in the left lobe of the thyroid (solid nodule on ultrasound). The subtraction scan shows increased uptake of sestamibi in the left lobe of the thyroid. The medial uptake is within a parathyroid adenoma and the lateral uptake in a thyroid adenoma. (b) A multinodular thyroid shown on the iodine scan. The subtraction scan demonstrates the site of the parathyroid adenoma at the upper pole of the left lobe of the thyroid. This can also be seen on the sestamibi study.*

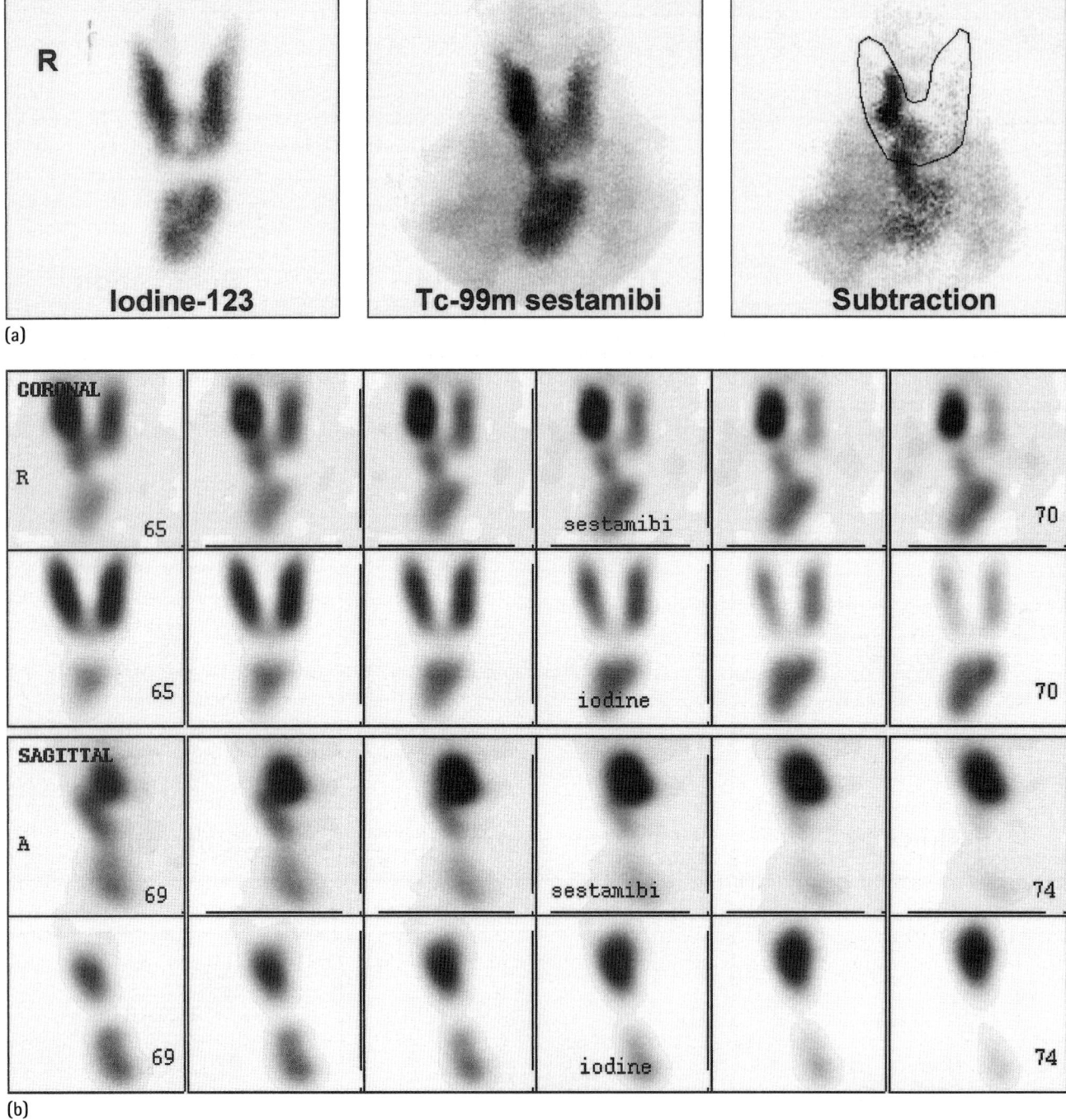

(a)

(b)

Figure 12B.5   *Planar and tomographic scan on a patient who had a retrosternal goiter and four-gland hyperplasia. (a) The iodine scan shows the nodular appearance of the thyroid and a retrosternal extension. The sestamibi study demonstrates abnormal uptake in the right lobe of the thyroid and uptake of a lower grade in the isthmus and between the thyroid and the retrosternal thyroid. (b) The tomographic scan shows marked increased uptake of sestamibi behind the right lobe of the thyroid on the coronal and sagittal images. The uptake between the 'normal' thyroid and the retrosternal thyroid was in a further hyperplastic gland smaller than the upper pole gland. The low grade uptake in the isthmus was in a benign thyroid nodule (false positive). The two glands on the left side measuring 200 mg were not visualized.*

nodules. If diffuse thyroid enlargement is present posteriorly placed parathyroid glands can be more difficult to identify when high resolution transducers are used. The technique is very operator dependent.

Despite the high resolution of CT, results for parathyroid localization have been generally disappointing. The sensitivity of detection appears higher for upper mediastinal glands than elsewhere in the neck, and again problems are encountered with co-existing thyroid disease. The sensitivity of the technique is 40–80%, specificity 85–98%, with the higher sensitivities in patients who have not had previous surgery and those with disease in the mediastinum.

Magnetic resonance imaging (MRI), while not having the intrinsic resolution of CT, has fewer streak artifacts and superior soft tissue contrast. The potential of MRI in parathyroid localization has not yet been fully explored, sensitivities between 64 and 88% and specificities of 88–95% have been found in small series of patients. The application of T1, T2, and short tau wave inversion recovery (STIR) images improve the recognition of adenomas and the separation of scar tissue and therefore potentially allow the improvement of identification of abnormalities for re-operation.[23]

Selective venous sampling, with or without prior arteriography, has the advantage of high specificity and can allow parathyroid glands to be distinguished from thyroid nodules.[19] This is an invasive technique available only in a few specialized centers. It has largely been replaced by the other techniques, although is still occasionally used for re-operative cases.

CLINICAL ROLE OF PARATHYROID LOCALIZATION

Surgical management of primary hyperparathyroidism is the most effective treatment although other techniques such as direct injection of the parathyroid adenoma with alcohol to destroy the gland have been tried. The approach to surgery has changed over the years but still the majority of surgeons use the bilateral neck exploration with a success rate of 95% and a complication rate of 1–2%.[2] This approach is under scrutiny because 85% of patients will have single gland disease and sestamibi scanning has a specificity of 90.7% and a sensitivity of 98.9%, suggesting that with correct pre-scanning selection the majority of patients should be suitable for limited surgical approach. These approaches fall under the umbrella of minimally invasive parathyroidectomy with or without the use of aids such as a radionuclide probe, an endoscope or a video assisted technique. The minimally invasive technique is performed through a small lateral incision in the neck, dependent on the preoperative localization of the adenoma, as a day case either using a general anesthetic or cervical block. The advantage over conventional surgery is the shortened operation time, shortened anesthetic, reduced complications, reduced inpatient stay and, if combined with intraoperative PTH assays, a 100% success rate, although this utility has been questioned.[31] The other techniques on the whole have longer operative times than this technique. The use of a probe to localize the parathyroid tissue requires the injection of the radiotracer approximately 2 h before the surgery. The value of the probe at surgery is to localize the parathyroid adenoma and confirm the removal of the correct gland by measuring the radioactivity within

the adenoma and over the remaining surgical bed after adenoma removal. Removal of a single adenoma can also be confirmed by intraoperative PTH levels, these should fall providing there is only a single adenoma present.

The value of preoperative localization is to be able to perform minimally invasive surgery in the majority of patients. Therefore there would appear to be little value in the assessment of patients with secondary hyperparathyroidism when preoperative tests have lower sensitivity and there is a requirement to explore all four glands. If primary hyperparathyroidism is the most likely diagnosis then the most accurate technique should be used to identify the site of the adenoma. The present evidence would suggest that a subtraction technique has a slight advantage over dual phase imaging.[30,32–34] If patients have no thyroid present either due to surgery or a known thyroiditis or administration of thyroxine then there is no added value of a subtraction technique and the dual phase technique should be used. The combination of planar imaging of the thyroid and mediastinum are the minimum assessments. The additional value of SPET to give more precise anatomical localization is a reasonable option and may be performed using dual energy SPET if ^{123}I and ^{99m}Tc-sestamibi are the agents used. The value of pinhole SPET or oblique views has been suggested and certainly may improve localization.[35] With minimally invasive surgery being offered the units performing such surgery should have access to intraoperative PTH measurements which should obviate the need for frozen section assessment of the removed gland. It is also reasonable to suggest that at least in equivocal radionuclide imaging studies a confirmatory test such as an ultrasound examination should be performed and if the two tests agree surgery should proceed. The additional value of radioguided and endoscopic surgery still remains to be proven.

In patients undergoing re-operation, whether because of a failed primary operation or because of recurrence of hyperparathyroidism, there is a strong case for preoperative localization. This is because second operations have a higher morbidity and a lower chance of establishing normocalcemia. Some surgeons would advise that the localization should definitely be confirmed by at least two techniques. The value of positron emission tomography (PET) would probably be reserved for these cases.

The recent summary statement by a consensus panel on asymptomatic primary hyperparathyroidism states 'preoperative localization testing is mandatory when the MIP procedure is used. Preoperative localization tests should not be used to make, confirm, or exclude the diagnosis of primary hyperparathyroidism.'[1] It also concludes that the key elements are an experienced parathyroid surgeon and an experienced imaging unit which result in the highest success in identifying and removing abnormal parathyroid tissue.[1] In today's health economic environment there can be no doubt that the value of preoperative localization is cost-effective by reducing inpatient stay and reducing the incidence of complications.[36]

REFERENCES

● Seminal primary article
◆ Key review paper

◆ 1 Bilezikian JP, Potts Jr JT, Fuleihan Gel-H, *et al.* Summary statement from a workshop on asymptomatic primary hyperparathyroidism: a perspective for the 21st century. *J Clin Endocrinol Metab* 2002; **87**: 5353–61.

◆ 2 Thomas SK, Wishart GC. Trends in surgical techniques. *Nucl Med Commun* 2003; **24**: 115–19.

3 Edis AJ, Sheedy PF, Beahrs OH, van Heerden JA. Results of re-operation for hyperparathyroidism, with evaluation of pre-operative localisation studies. *Surgery* 1978; **84**: 384–93.

◆ 4 O'Doherty MJ, Kettle AG. Parathyroid imaging: pre-operative localization. *Nucl Med Commun* 2003; **24**: 125–31.

5 Ferlin G, Borsato N, Camerani M, *et al.* New perspectives in localising enlarged parathyroids by technetium–thallium subtraction scan. *J Nucl Med* 1983; **24**: 438–41.

6 Sandrock D, Dunham RG, Neumann RD. Simultaneous dual energy acquisition for $^{201}Tl/^{99}Tc^m$ parathyroid subtraction scintigraphy: physical and physiological considerations. *Nucl Med Commun* 1990; **11**: 503–10.

● 7 Coakley AJ, Kettle AG, Wells CP, *et al.* ^{99m}Tc-sestamibi new agent for parathyroid imaging. *Nucl Med Commun* 1989; **10**: 791–4.

● 8 O'Doherty MJ, Kettle AG, Wells PC, *et al.* Parathyroid imaging with technetium-99m-sestamibi: preoperative localisation and tissue uptake studies. *J Nucl Med* 1992; **33**: 313–18.

9 Fjeld J G, Erichson K, Pfeffer P F, *et al.* Tc-99m-tetrofosmin for parathyroid imaging: comparison with sestamibi. *J Nucl Med* 1997; **38**: 831–4.

● 10 Giordano A, Meduri G, Marozzi P. Parathyroid imaging with $^{99}Tc^m$-tetrofosmin. *Nucl Med Commun* 1996; **17**: 706–10.

11 Froberg AC, Valkema R, Bonjer HJ, Krenning EP. ^{99m}Technetium-tetrofosmin or ^{99m}technetium-sestamibi for double-phase parathyroid scintigraphy. *Eur J Nucl Med Mol Imaging* 2003; **30**: 193–6.

12 Neumann DR, Esselstyn Jr CB, MacIntyre WJ, *et al.* Primary hyperparathyroidism: preoperative parathyroid imaging with regional body FDG PET. *Radiology* 1994; **192**: 509–12.

13 Melon P, Luxen A, Hamoir E, *et al.* Fluorine-18-fluorodeoxyglucose positron emission tomography for pre-operative parathyroid imaging in primary hyperparathyroidism. *Eur J Nucl Med* 1995; **22**: 556–8.

14 Cook GJ, Wong JC, Smellie WJ, *et al.* [^{11}C]Methionine positron emission tomography for patients with persistent or recurrent hyperparathyroidism after surgery. *Eur J Endocrinol* 1998; **139**: 195–7.

15 Sundin A, Johansson C, Hellman P, *et al.* PET and parathyroid l-[carbon-11] methionine accumulation in hyperparathyroidism. *J Nucl Med* 1996; **37**: 1766–70.

16 De Feo ML, Colagrande S, Biagini C, *et al.* Parathyroid glands: combination of ^{99m}Tc MIBI scintigraphy US for demonstration of parathyroid glands nodules. *Radiology* 2000; **214**: 393–402.

17 Casara D, Rubello D, Pelizzo MR, Shapiro B. Clinical role of ^{99m}TcO$_4$/MIBI scan, ultrasound and intra-operative gamma probe in the performance of unilateral and minimally invasive surgery in primary hyperparathyroidism. *Eur J Nucl Med* 2001; **28**: 1351–9.

18 Ammori BJ, Madan M, Gopichandran TD, *et al.* Ultrasound-guided unilateral neck exploration for sporadic primary hyperparathyroidism: is it worthwhile? *Ann R Coll Surg Engl* 1998; **80**: 433–7.

19 Lumachi F, Ermani M, Basso S, *et al.* Localization of parathyroid tumours in the minimally invasive era: which technique should be chosen? Population-based analysis of 253 patients undergoing parathyroidectomy and factors affecting parathyroid gland detection. *Endocrine-Related Cancer* 2001; **8**: 63–9.

20 Stark DD, Gooding GAW, Moss AA, *et al.* Parathyroid imaging: comparison of high-resolution CT and high-resolution sonography. *Am J Roentgenol* 1983; **141**: 633–8.

21 Dijkstra B, Healy C, Kelly LM, *et al.* Parathyroid localisation – current practice. *J R Coll Surg Edin* 2002; **47**: 599–607.

22 Miller DL, Doppman JL, Krudy AG, *et al.* Localisation of parathyroid adenomas in patients who have undergone surgery. Part 1. Non-invasive imaging methods. *Radiology* 1987; **162**: 133–7.

23 Delbridge LW, Dolan SJ, Hop TT, *et al.* Minimally invasive parathyroidectomy: 50 consecutive cases. *Med J Aust* 2000; **172**: 418–22.

◆ 24 Pons F, Torregrosa JV, Fuster D. Biological factors influencing parathyroid localization. *Nucl Med Commun* 2003; **24**: 121–4.

25 Torregrosa J-V, Fernandez-Cruz L, Canalejo A, *et al.* ^{99m}Tc-sestamibi scintigraphy and cell cycle in parathyroid glands of secondary hyperparathyroidism. *World J Surg* 2000; **24**: 1386–90.

● 26 Taillefer R, Boucher Y, Potviuc C, Lambert R. Detection and localisation of parathyroid adenomas in patients with hyperparathyroidism using a single radionuclide imaging procedure with ^{99m}Tc sestamibi (double phase study). *J Nucl Med* 1992; **33**: 1801–7.

27 Arveschoug AK, Bertelsen H, Vammen B. Presurgical localization of abnormal parathyroid glands using a single injection of Tc-99m sestamibi comparison of high resolution parallel hole and pinhole collimators, and interobserver and intraobserver variation. *Clin Nucl Med* 2002; **27**: 249–54.

28 Ho Shon IA, Bernard EJ, Roach PJ, Delbridge LW. The value of oblique pinhole images in pre-operative localisation with ^{99m}Tc-MIBI for primary hyperparathyroidism. *Eur J Nucl Med* 2001; **28**: 736–42.

29 Wanet PM, Sand A, Abramovici J. Physical and clinical evaluation of high-resolution thyroid pinhole tomography. *J Nucl Med* 1996; **37**: 2017–20.

30 Hindie E, Melliere D, Jeanguillame C, *et al*. Parathyroid imaging using simultaneous double window recording of technetium-99m-sestamibi and iodine-123. *J Nucl Med* 1998; **39**: 1100–5.

31 Palazzo FF, Sadler GP, Reene TS. Minimally invasive parathyroidectomy. *BMJ* 2004; **328**: 849–50.

32 Neumann DR, Esselstyn Jr CB, Go RT, *et al*. Comparison of double-phase ^{99m}Tc-sestamibi with ^{123}I–^{99m}Tc-sestamibi subtraction SPECT in hyperparathyroidism. *Am J Roentgenol* 1997; **169**: 1671–4.

33 Leslie WD, Dupont JO, Bybel B, Riese KT. Parathyroid ^{99m}Tc-sestamibi scintigraphy: dual-tracer subtraction is superior to double-phase washout. *Eur J Nucl Med Mol Imaging* 2002; **29**: 1566–70.

34 Chen CC, Holder LE, Scovill WA, *et al*. Comparison of parathyroid imaging with Tc-99m pertechnetate/sestamibi subtraction, double phase Tc-99m sestamibi and Tc-99m sestamibi SPECT. *J Nucl Med* 1997; **38**: 834–9.

35 Spanu A, Falchi A, Manca A, *et al*. The usefulness of neck pinhole SPECT as a complementary tool to planar scintigraphy in primary and secondary hyperparathyroidism. *J Nucl Med* 2004; **45**: 40–8.

36 Udelsman R. Six hundred fifty-six consecutive explorations for primary hyperparathyroidism. *Ann Surg* 2002; **235**: 665–70.

The adrenal gland

R.T. KLOOS, M.D. GROSS, AND B. SHAPIRO

INTRODUCTION

The adrenal glands are paired retroperitoneal organs which lie superomedial to each kidney with the right adrenal gland positioned more cephaloposterior as compared to the position the left adrenal. Each gland consists of an outer cortex and an embryologically, histologically, and functionally distinct inner medulla. The adrenal cortex can be considered as an amalgamation of two organs, a subcapsular zona glomerulosa, which synthesizes mineralocorticoids, principally aldosterone, under the control of the renin–angiotensin system, and a deeper zona fasciculata and reticularis that secrete glucocorticoids, principally cortisol and the weak androgens dehydroepiandrosterone (DHEA), its sulfate (DHEA-S), and androstenedione, and estrogens under the control of adrenocorticotrophic hormone (ACTH) (Fig. 12C.1). The adrenal medulla shares its neural crest origin with the sympathetic ganglia, paraganglia, and other adrenergic tissues. Like those organs, it synthesizes and stores noradrenaline (norepinephrine), but its ability to convert noradrenaline to adrenaline (epinephrine) is unique.

Abnormal secretion of adrenal hormones may give rise to well-known clinical syndromes (Table 12C.1). Collectively, these syndromes may result from benign or malignant adrenal tumors, adrenal hyperplasia or, less frequently, from extra-adrenal disease. Differentiating these possibilities is

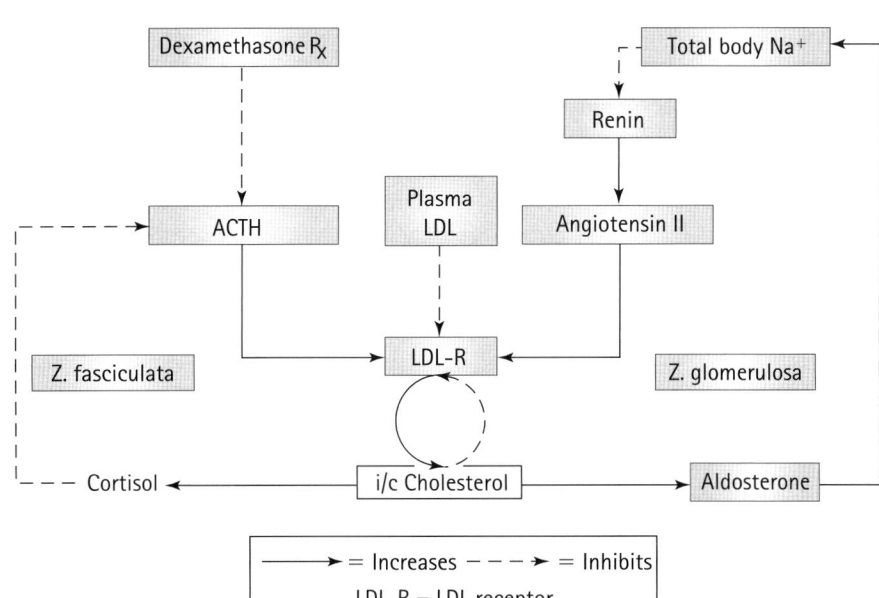

Figure 12C.1 *Regulation of the adrenocortical intracellular (i/c) cholesterol pool and hormone biosynthesis.*

Table 12C.1 *Syndromes of adrenal hormone excess*

Organ	Zone	Hormone	Syndrome
Cortex	Glomerulosa and outermost fasciculata	Aldosterone	Primary aldosteronism
	Fasciculata (and reticularis less importantly)	Cortisol	Cushing's syndrome
	Fasciculata and reticularis	Androgens	Masculinization
		Estrogens	Congenital adrenal hyperplasia
			Feminization
Medulla		Adrenaline and noradrenaline	Pheochromocytoma
Paraganglia		Noradrenaline	Extra-adrenal pheochromocytoma

Noradrenaline = norepinephrine.

often impossible on clinical or biochemical grounds alone. The noninvasive evaluation of adrenal anatomy is routinely made by either computed tomography (CT) or magnetic resonance imaging (MRI) and both can reliably resolve masses greater than 5 mm in diameter. Despite their high resolution, CT and MRI are relatively insensitive for smaller lesions, for recognizing subtle contour changes in bilateral hyperplasia and for identifying extra-adrenal disease. Both may be difficult to interpret postoperatively, particularly in the presence of surgical clips. The functional significance of anatomic abnormalities cannot be readily determined by CT or MRI and the widespread use of high-resolution anatomic imaging has led to the frequent finding of incidentally discovered adrenal masses (incidentalomas). The differential diagnosis of these lesions is extensive and includes hypersecreting and nonhypersecreting, as well as benign and malignant lesions. Incorporation of specific radiopharmaceuticals into normal or abnormal tissues, allows scintigraphic localization and functional characterization with a high degree of efficacy in each of the adrenal disorders outlined above and thus, adrenal scintigraphy can direct and complement anatomic imaging studies obviating the need for invasive diagnostic procedures in most cases.[1]

ADRENAL CORTEX

Physiology and radiopharmacology

Cholesterol is the precursor for steroid hormone biosynthesis. The major source of adrenal cholesterol is circulating cholesterol carried by low-density lipoproteins (LDLs). Adrenal cortical cells bear specific, high-affinity cell membrane receptors for LDLs. After the receptor–LDL complex is internalized, cholesterol is liberated, and that which is surplus to requirements for membrane maintenance is re-esterified by acyl-CoA:cholesterol acyltransferase (ACAT) and stored.

Cholesterol labeled with ^{131}I (19-[^{131}I]iodocholesterol) was the first clinically successful radiopharmaceutical for adrenocortical scintigraphy.[2] It has been superseded by the cholesterol analogs 6β-[^{131}I]iodomethyl-19-norcholesterol (NP-59)[3] and 6β-[^{75}Se]selenomethyl-19-norcholesterol (SMC),[4] both of which have greater affinity for the adrenal cortex and more favorable target-to-background activity ratios. Following uptake, the radiocholesterol analogs may be esterified by ACAT but are not significantly further metabolized. The major pathway of radiocholesterol excretion is hepatobiliary.

Both NP-59 and SMC appear to behave identically *in vivo*. Potential advantages and disadvantages of each radiopharmaceutical are listed in Table 12C.2. The adrenocortical uptake of the radiocholesterol analogs parallels that of cholesterol (Fig. 12C.1). Thus, ACTH stimulation enhances radiocholesterol accumulation while suppression of ACTH secretion (e.g. by dexamethasone) reduces adrenocortical radiocholesterol uptake by 50%.[5] Similarly, sodium loading with resultant extracellular volume expansion inhibits renin secretion and angiotensin II production and reduces adrenal radiocholesterol uptake by a further 10%. Thus, 40% of adrenocortical radiocholesterol uptake appears independent of either ACTH or angiotensin II stimulation. Hypercholesterolemia, by expansion of the extracellular cholesterol pool and down-regulating LDL receptors, reduces adrenal radiocholesterol uptake and enhances hepatobiliary excretion.[6]

It follows that several drugs may modify the uptake of adrenocortical scintigraphic agents (Table 12C.3). Clinically, these effects are only important in the setting of primary aldosteronism and syndromes of sex hormone excess when the timing of adrenocortical visualization under dexamethasone suppression (DS) is important to scan interpretation. Medications that increase adrenal radiocholesterol uptake may lead to bilateral early adrenal visualization and falsely suggest a bilateral process (e.g. hyperplasia). In most cases, the drug effect can be predicted from its known actions on the simplified schema in Figure 12C.1. Important exceptions are spironolactone and combination oral contraceptives (OCPs). Spironolactone, in addition to its well-known aldosterone antagonism in the kidney, inhibits aldosterone biosynthesis in aldosterone-producing adenomas (APAs), at least in the first month of therapy.[7,8] The combination OCPs also have dual effects: estrogen increases hepatic synthesis of the renin substrate, angiotensinogen, and increases plasma renin activity, while the progestagen induces a natriuresis, which further promotes renin secretion. The net result is an increase in angiotensin II levels.[9] It is not known whether the currently marketed low-dose OCPs cause a similar phenomenon. As a result, proper adrenocortical scintiscan interpretation is critically dependent not only on a confirmed biochemical diagnosis, but also on a careful drug history and exclusion of interfering medications when relevant.

Radiocholesterols are dissolved in an alcoholic vehicle containing Tween-80 and should be injected intravenously over 2–3 min to avoid extremity pain or discomfort. Repeated flushing of the syringe ensures complete delivery of the dose. Iodine-containing preparations are given to block thyroidal uptake of free [131]I (Table 12C.2). A laxative is used to decrease bowel background radioactivity (Table 12C.2). Images are obtained with a gamma camera interfaced to a dedicated, digital computer (>50 000 counts/image) after an appropriate delay after injection of the radiotracer (Tables 12C.2 and 12C.3, page 526). Additional images may be obtained daily or on alternate days for several weeks, but rarely are more than 1–2 days of imaging necessary. The posterior view affords the best adrenal gland visualization and is often the only image necessary for diagnostic interpretation. The normal posterior image demonstrates equal or slightly greater and cephalad radiotracer accumulation in the right adrenal gland compared with the left. A lateral view may assist in differentiating adrenal gland from liver, or the right adrenal from activity in the gallbladder. An anterior pelvic view should be obtained in cases of suspected ovarian or testicular hypersecretion. NP-59 and/or SMC are widely available worldwide as a routine, clinical imaging agent. In the United States, NP-59 is available as an investigational new drug (IND) and can be obtained from the University of Michigan Nuclear Pharmacy after filing an abbreviated Physician Sponsored IND Application with the US Food and Drug Administration.

Alternative adrenocortical imaging agents are low-density lipoproteins (LDLs) that have been labeled with a variety of radioisotopes (e.g. [111]In or ^{99m}Tc metal chelates) and demonstrate specific LDL–receptor mediated adrenocortical uptake.[10] Alternatively, inhibitors of adrenocortical hormone biosynthesis, ^{11}C-etomidate and ^{11}C-metomidate, have been used to image the adrenal cortex and some neoplasms of adrenocortical origin, and a metabolic intermediate of aerobic metabolism, ^{11}C-acetate, has been reported to image adrenal adenomas.[11,12]

Cushing's syndrome

Cushing's syndrome (CS) is due to excessive glucocorticoid secretion, usually associated to a greater or lesser extent with androgen excess. The syndrome may arise from several possible disorders: bilateral, generally symmetrical adrenocortical hyperplasia due to ACTH stimulation from the anterior pituitary (Cushing's disease) or from an extra-pituitary, benign or malignant neoplasm (ectopic ACTH and/or corticotrophin-releasing hormone); or as a result of a benign or malignant adrenocortical tumor autonomously secreting excess cortisol. Rarely, CS results from autonomous cortical nodular hyperplasia (CNH), which, although bilateral, is often anatomically asymmetric. ACTH-secreting pituitary tumors are responsible for two thirds of CS cases. Ectopic ACTH secretion accounts for about 15% of cases, half of which are due to small-cell lung carcinoma and the remainder are due to carcinoids, medullary thyroid carcinomas, pheochromocytomas, and other neuroendocrine tumors. Adrenal cortical adenomas account for 10% of CS cases and adrenal carcinomas and CNH each account for approximately 5%.

The scintigraphic patterns of radiocholesterol uptake in the various forms of CS reflect the underlying pathophysiology (Fig. 12C.2, page 527 and Table 12C.4, page 526). In ACTH-dependent adrenal hyperplasia, radiocholesterol uptake is bilaterally increased, and the degree of uptake correlates closely with the 24-h UFC excretion.[13] Thus, radiocholesterol uptake in the ectopic ACTH syndrome is generally higher than in Cushing's disease.

Autonomous adrenal cortical adenoma will demonstrate a pattern of unilateral uptake; the suppression of pituitary ACTH secretion inhibits tracer uptake by the contralateral adrenal cortex (and the ipsilateral normal cortical tissue). Similarly, inhibition of contralateral radiocholesterol uptake occurs with functioning adrenal carcinomas but because the uptake of radiocholesterol per gram of tissue in these tumors is usually very low,[14] the primary tumor is not visualized. Other causes of 'bilateral nonvisualization' such as severe hypercholesterolemia and subcutaneous extravasation of the radiotracer dose must be excluded. Radiocholesterol uptake by both primary and metastatic adrenocortical carcinoma has rarely been reported. Finally, ACTH-independent CNH produces bilaterally but usually asymmetrically increased radiocholesterol uptake.

In clinical practice, adrenal cortical scintigraphy for CS is indicated only in patients with the ACTH-independent form of the disease.[15] Once the biochemical diagnosis of the condition is made, abdominal CT is usually performed to locate the disease and define the surgical anatomy. In tumors without clear-cut CT signs of malignancy, scintigraphy will be helpful since bilateral nonvisualization will indicate the malignant nature of the tumor and allow appropriate surgical planning. More importantly, scintigraphy will reliably distinguish between adenoma and CNH. CNH should be suspected if CT has identified no tumor, only a small tumor, more than one tumor, any suggestion of a contralateral adrenal abnormality; in children and the young; when CS is associated with blue nevi, pigmented lentigines, myxomas, acromegaly or testicular or

Table 12C.2 Techniques of adrenal scintigraphy

	Radiopharmaceutical					
	NP-59	SMC	^{131}I–MIBG	^{123}I–MIBG[a]	^{111}In–pentetreotide	^{18}F–FDG
Thyroid blockade (SSKI 1 drop or Lugol's 2 drops in beverage t.i.d.)[b]	Start 2 days before injection and continue for 14 days	Not required	Start 2 days before injection and continue for 6 days	Start 2 days before injection and continue for 4 days	Not required	Not required[c]
Adult dose (i.v.)	37 MBq	9.25 MBq	18.5–37 MBq	370 MBq	222 MBq	555 MBq
Shelf-life	2 weeks; frozen	6–8 weeks; room temp	2 weeks; 4°C	24 h; 4°C	6 h; room temp	110 min; room temp
Percent uptake/adrenal	0.07–0.26%	0.07–0.30%	0.01–0.22%	0.01–0.22%	–	–
Dosimetry (cGy/dose)	–	–	From package insert	From package insert	–	–
Adrenal	28–88	6.1	0.38–0.75	8–28	1.51	0.12
Ovaries	8.0	1.9	0.14–0.27	0.35	0.98	0.11
Liver	2.4	3.5	1.45–2.90	0.32	2.43	0.24
Kidneys	2.2	–	0.16–0.32	–	10.83	0.21
Spleen	2.7	–	1.10–2.20	–	14.77	0.15
Urinary bladder	–	–	1.40–2.80	–	6.05	0.73
Thyroid	150	0.43	0.17–0.33	17.7	1.49	0.12
Whole body	1.2	1.4	–	0.29	–	0.12
Effective dose equivalent	–	–	0.35–0.70	–	2.61	0.19
Beta emission	Yes	No	Yes	No	No	No
Laxatives (e.g. bisacodyl 5–10 mg p.o. b.i.d.)	Begin 2 days before and continue during imaging	No	Begin post-injection	Begin post-injection	Begin post-injection	2 days pre-inj.

Imaging interval post-radiotracer administration	Non-DS; 1 or more days 5, 6 or 7 post-injection	7 (14) days post-injection	24, 48 (72) h post-injection	2–4, 24 (48) h post-injection	4–6, 24, (48) h post-injection	60 min post-inj
(optional additional imaging times)	DS: one or more early: (3), 4 and one or more late: 5, 6 or 7 days post-injection	(No published experience with DS scans)				None
Collimator	High-energy, parallel-hole	Medium-energy, parallel-hole	High energy, parallel-hole	Low-energy, parallel-hole	Medium-energy, parallel-hole	None
Principal photopeak (abundance)	364 keV (81%)	137 keV (61%), 265 keV (59%), 280 keV (25%)	364 keV	159 keV	172 keV (90%), 245 keV (94%)	511 keV positron tomography
Window	20% window	20% window	20% window	20% window	20% window	
Imaging time and counts (per view)	20 min/100 kcounts	20 min/200 kcounts (± SPECT)	20 min/100 kcounts	10 min (at 3 h); 20 min/1 million counts (± SPECT)	Head and neck: 10–15 min/300 kcounts (at 4–24 h) and 15 min/200 kcounts (at 48 h) Chest and abdomen: 10 min/500 kcounts (± SPECT)	5 min/bed position × 4 positions 3-D images

DS: dexamethasone suppression. NP59: 6β-$[^{131}I]$iodomethyl-19-norcholesterol; SMC: 6β-$[^{75}Se]$selenomethyl-19-norcholesterol; MIBG: m-iodobenzylguanidine; FDG: fluorodeoxyglucose.

[a] 0–1.4% ^{125}I contamination.

[b] Patients allergic to iodine may be given potassium perchlorate 200 mg every 8 h after meals or triiodothyronine 20 mg every 8 h.

[c] Maintain euglycemia; may require supplemental insulin/glucose.

Table 12C.3 *Clinically important modifiers of adrenocortical uptake of radiocholesterol analogs*

Drug	Effect on uptake	Mechanism	Drug withdrawal interval
Dexamethasone/glucocorticoids	Decrease (zona fasciculata/reticularis)	ACTH suppression	None[a]
Spironolactone	Increase (zona glomerulosa)	Naturesis, decreased aldosterone action (± secretion) cause PRA and AII increases	4–6 weeks
Diuretics	Increase (zona glomerulosa)	Naturesis causes PRA and AII increases	4–6 weeks
Oral contraceptives	Increase (zona glomerulosa)	Naturesis and increased angiotensinogen cause PRA and AII increases	4–6 weeks
Cholestyramine and other lipid-lowering drugs	Increase (all zones)	Decreased plasma cholesterol decreases radiotracer dilution and up-regulates LDL receptors	4–6 weeks
Minoxidil/hydralazine	Increase (zona glomerulosa)	Vasodilatation causes PRA and AII increases	1–2 weeks

[a] Studies may be intentionally performed with dexamethasone suppression.

PRA, plasma renin activity; AII, angiotensin II.

Table 12C.4 *Summary of scintigraphic findings in adrenocortical disorders*

Disorder	Pathology	Scintigraphy
Cushing's syndrome	Adenoma	Concordant, unilateral increased uptake, normal suppressed
	Hyperplasia	Bilateral increased uptake (may be asymmetrical)
	Carcinoma	Bilateral non-visualization, or very rarely concordant, unilateral increased uptake
Primary aldosteronism[a]	Adenoma	Concordant, unilateral adrenal imaging before day 5
	Hyperplasia	Bilateral adrenal imaging before day 5 (may be asymmetrical)
	Carcinoma (very rare)	Discordant image day 5 or later, or concordant, unilateral adrenal image before day 5
Masculinization[a]	Adrenal adenoma	Concordant, unilateral adrenal imaging before day 5
	Adrenal carcinoma	Discordant image day 5 or later, or concordant, unilateral adrenal image before day 5
	Adrenal hyperplasia	Bilateral adrenal imaging before day 5 (may be asymmetrical)
	Ovarian	Ovarian visualization
Incidental adrenal mass	Non-hypersecretory benign adenoma	Concordant, increased uptake
	Non-adenoma (e.g. metastasis or primary adrenal carcinoma)	Discordant, decreased uptake

[a] Dexamethasone suppression imaging with 1 mg orally four times per day starting 7 days before radiotracer administration and continuing though the 'early visualization' imaging period (see Table 12C.2).

other tumors; and in the very rare patient with intermittent or cyclical CS. In patients whose CS has relapsed after bilateral adrenalectomy for primary or secondary adrenocortical hyperplasia, scintigraphy is valuable for locating the functioning remnant(s).[16]

Primary aldosteronism (Conn's syndrome)

Excess aldosterone secretion by an adrenal cortical tumor (almost always benign and <2 cm) or by diffuse or nodular hyperplasia of the zona glomerulosa is characterized by hypertension and usually hypokalemia. Adenomas (aldosteronomas) account for little more than half of all cases. High circulating aldosterone levels result in kaliuresis, sodium retention and expansion of extracellular fluid volume with secondary inhibition of renin release. It is essential to exclude more common causes of hypokalemia among hypertensive patients, such as overt or covert use of diuretics and laxatives. The diagnosis of primary aldosteronism is confirmed by the demonstration of suppressed plasma renin activity (PRA) with an elevated plasma or urinary aldosterone

CUSHING' SYNDROME (CS)   SCAN PATTERN

A. ACTH – DEPENDENT – CS
   1. Bilateral hyperplasia
     (hypothalamic, pituitary,
     ectopic)

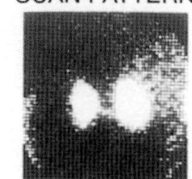

Bilateral symmetric
activity

B. ACTH – INDEPENDENT – CS
   1. Bilateral nodular
     hyperplasia

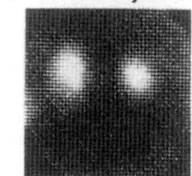

Bilateral asymmetric
activity

   2. Adrenocortical adenoma

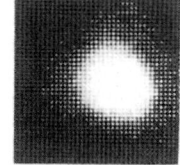

Unilateral activity

   3. Adrenocortical carcinoma

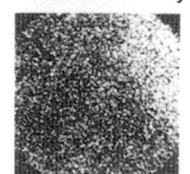

Bilateral
non-visualization

Figure 12C.2 *Patterns of adrenocortical scintigraphy in Cushing's syndrome (NP-59 posterior scintiscans, no dexamethasone suppression. (Reproduced, with permission, from* Urol Radiol *1981; 3: 241–4.)*

level, regardless of the presence of drugs, which may interfere with the renin–angiotensin system. However, because many drugs interfere with this system, it is critical to stop all potentially interfering medications for an appropriate interval before proceeding with diagnostic testing, or to be aware of how they may alter the results so that the biochemical tests may be interpreted appropriately.[17] If antihypertensive therapy cannot be interrupted, peripheral alpha- and beta-blocking agents or clonidine are generally acceptable.[17]

The vexing distinction between an aldosterone-producing adenoma (APA) and bilateral adrenal hyperplasia (BAH) as the cause of primary aldosteronism is important, since the treatment is primarily surgical in the former and medical in the latter.

As anticipated from the autonomous pathophysiology of primary aldosteronism, patients with APA have increased radiocholesterol uptake in the affected adrenal and nearly normal uptake on the unaffected side, since ACTH-dependent uptake by the zona fasciculata and reticularis is unaffected. In BAH, radiocholesterol uptake is increased bilaterally, and often asymmetrically. However, since ACTH-dependent tissue normally accounts for 50% of adrenal

radiocholesterol uptake (see above) and the normal range of radiocholesterol uptake is broad with a significant overlap between normal adrenals and primary aldosteronism due to BAH.[5] The dexamethasone suppression (DS) adrenal scan was introduced to suppress the ACTH-dependent component of radiocholesterol uptake. In normal individuals, dexamethasone (1 mg every 6 h) for 7 days before injection of NP-59 and throughout the imaging period delays visualization of the normal adrenal cortex for at least 5 days after injection.[18] Visualization at or beyond 5 days presumably reflects the 50% of normal radiocholesterol uptake that is ACTH-independent. Unilateral or bilateral visualization earlier than 5 days after injection under DS in biochemically proven primary aldosteronism suggests adenoma or hyperplasia, respectively (Fig. 12C.3; Table 12C.4). Drugs that increase adrenal radiocholesterol uptake must be discontinued for an appropriate time interval before scintigraphy (Table 12C.3). While quantification of NP-59 uptake on the DS adrenal scan has been shown to correlate with 24-h urinary aldosterone excretion,[19] the qualitative endpoint of early unilateral or bilateral visualization better separates APA from BAH, since hyperplasia can produce such marked asymmetry of quantitative uptake as to suggest unilateral disease.[20] In the rare, autosomal dominant variant, glucocorticoid-suppressible aldosteronism, early adrenal visualization will not occur and the biochemical (high PA and low PRA) and physiological (hypertension) manifestations resolve with DS.

If a convincing majority of noninvasive evidence suggests a unilateral adenoma, adrenalectomy can proceed without recourse to adrenal vein sampling. However, it has been stated that patients with APA do not benefit from adrenalectomy when their hypertension does not respond to a 3-week trial of high-dose spironolactone (400 mg day^{-1}).[21]

Hyperandrogenism

Apparent disorders caused by an excess of sex hormones (androgens and estrogens) are not uncommon clinical problems. Excessive androgens in women cause masculinization (e.g. hirsutism, menstrual disturbances) with frank virilization in more severe cases (e.g. clitoromegaly, male body habitus, voice deepening, fronto-temporal balding). The differential diagnosis of masculinization is extensive.[22,23] However, pathological conditions associated with morbidity and mortality makes up <10% of cases. The rapid onset of severe masculinization should suggest an androgen-secreting tumor. Anatomical and functional imaging is reserved for the very small minority of patients whose history, examination or biochemical testing suggests a tumor.

The ovaries accumulate cholesterol as a precursor for steroid hormone biosynthesis in a similar fashion to the adrenals. The ratio of ovarian to adrenal uptake is increased by glucocorticoid suppression of adrenal cortical radiocholesterol uptake. Thus, in women with hyperandrogenism,

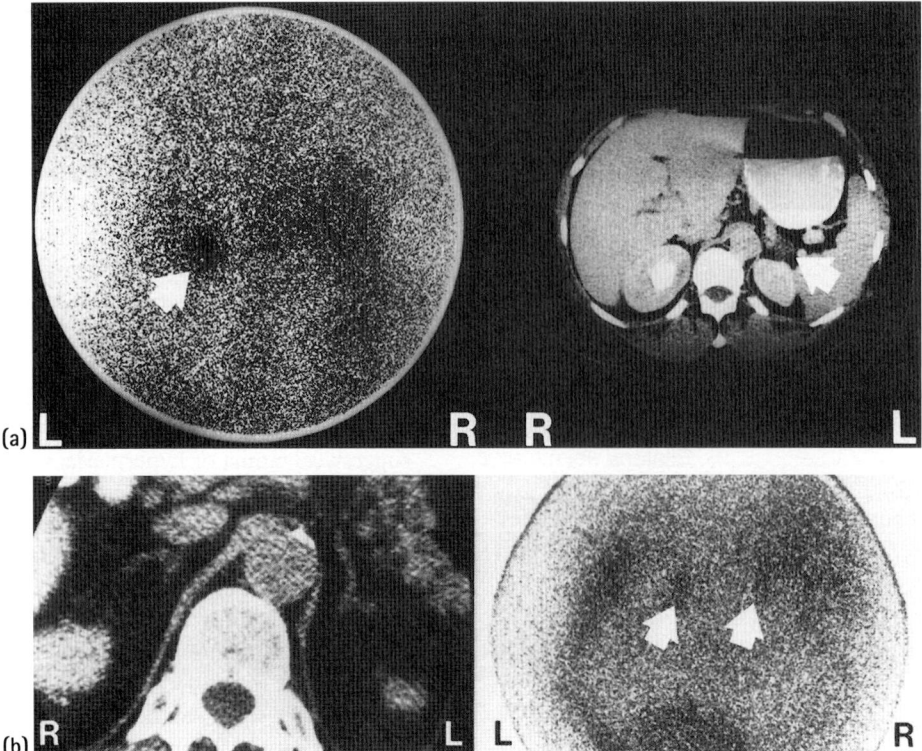

Figure 12C.3 *Dexamethasone suppression adrenocortical scans in primary aldosteronism (NP-59 posterior scintiscans 4 days after injection). (a) Two centimeter left aldosteronoma (arrows) on NP-59 (left panel) and CT images (right panel). Right adrenal NP-59 uptake is suppressed by dexamethasone. (b) Bilateral adrenal hyperplasia. The adrenals appeared morphologically normal on CT (left panel). Bilateral early uptake of NP-59 (right panel, arrows) despite dexamethasone.*

radiocholesterol scintigraphy may be performed using the same DS regimen with the exclusion of potential modifiers of radiocholesterol uptake as described for primary aldosteronism (Tables 12C.3 and 12C.4). Dexamethasone suppression scintigraphy has also been useful for defining the functional significance of ovarian enlargement discovered by ultrasonography or CT during the evaluation of hyperandrogenism. Indeed, the limited comparative data available indicated that DS scintigraphy may be more accurate than either CT or selective adrenal/ovarian vein sampling in the differential diagnosis of hyperandrogenism.[24]

The most common identifiable disorder in hyperandrogenic, oligomenorrheic or amenorrheic women is the polycystic ovary (Stein–Leventhal) syndrome (PCOS). The pathogenesis of PCOS is obscure, and abnormal adrenal androgen metabolism has frequently been demonstrated, although the majority of evidence favors the ovary as the primary source of excess androgen.[25,26] Adrenal radiocholesterol uptake (without DS) tends to be bilaterally increased in these patients, with the mean uptake being similar to that found in patients with Cushing's disease.[27]

The 'incidentally discovered' adrenal mass

The incidentally discovered adrenal mass (adrenal incidentaloma) is recognized as a common clinical problem due to

the widespread use of high-resolution abdominal imaging (MRI and CT) which identify an asymptomatic adrenal mass in approximately 0.35–5% of patients imaged for reasons other than suspected adrenal disease.[28] In the absence of a known extra-adrenal malignancy, 70–94% of these masses are nonhypersecretory benign adenomas.[23] Benign adenomas are more common with advancing age, hypertension, blacks compared with whites, diabetes mellitus (2- to 5-fold), obesity, heterozygote carriers of CAH, multiple endocrine neoplasia, and McCune–Albright syndrome.[17,23] In the setting of a known extra-adrenal malignancy the incidence of adrenal masses approximately doubles, with roughly 50% being adrenal metastases. Further, in this setting, malignancy rates in adrenal masses <3 cm are from 0 to 50%, while in adrenal masses >3 cm malignancy rates have ranged from 43 to 100%.[23] The adrenal is a frequent site of metastasis, particularly for carcinomas of the lung, breast, stomach, ovary, and kidney, as well as leukemias, lymphomas and melanomas. The distinction between a metastasis and other causes of adrenal masses may be critical in patients who may benefit from curative surgery if the primary malignancy is not disseminated.

It is suggested that hormonal hypersecretory states be initially excluded; the benign versus malignant nature of those deemed nonhypersecretory can then be investigated.[29] Hypersecretory masses usually require surgical excision, although adrenalectomy is not generally indicated for CAH, primary aldosteronism due to bilateral adrenal hyperplasia, or ACTH-dependent Cushing's syndrome with secondary macronodular adrenal hyperplasia. History and physical examinations must consider hypersecretion of cortisol, androgens, estrogen, mineralocorticoids, and catecholamines. However, the need for biochemical screening of all adrenal masses lacking an obvious radiological diagnosis – regardless of the history and physical examination – cannot be overemphasized, as clinically silent hypersecretory lesions are common.[17,23] Partially cystic lesions also warrant complete evaluations of their secretory status and malignant potential.

The prevalence of pheochromocytoma in patients with classic symptoms of episodic headache, palpitations, and diaphoresis is similar to the 0–11% incidence of pheochromocytomas among adrenal incidentalomas.[23] Some 65% of pheochromocytomas overlap with adrenal metastases in relative signal intensity on T2-weighted spin-echo MRI, and percutaneous adrenal biopsy of pheochromocytoma may precipitate hypertensive crisis, severe retroperitoneal bleeding, and death.[23] Plasma or urinary catecholamines and metanephrines, and urinary vanillylmandelic acid (VMA) are of approximately equal diagnostic utility, but the latter may be the least sensitive.[23,30]

The CT appearance of most adrenal incidentalomas is nonspecific (e.g. no clear evidence of spread beyond the adrenal to indicate malignancy, or the presence of a simple thin-walled cyst, hemorrhage or myelolipoma). Further, some CT morphological features are more common in malignancy and no single feature – or combination of features – can reliably distinguish a metastasis from an adenoma. Malignancies tend to be large, less well defined, have inhomogeneous attenuation, and a thick irregular enhancing rim. Adenomas tend to be smaller with a homogeneous density. However, even when >6 cm in maximal diameter, adenomas are more common than non-adenomatous lesions in the absence of a known extra-adrenal malignancy.[23] Because morphologic CT features alone do not usually allow an unequivocal differentiation of adrenal adenoma from malignancy, recent attention has centered on the value of CT densitometry. Using a threshold value of <10 Hounsfield units (H), there is a 73% sensitivity and 96% specificity for the diagnosis of adrenal adenoma by unenhanced CT. At <0 H, specificity is 100% but sensitivity is reduced to 33–47%.[23,31] Unlike unenhanced CT attenuation values, immediate post-injection contrast enhanced CT values cannot accurately differentiate adrenal adenomas from non-adenomas.[31] However, combining two independent CT properties of adrenal adenomas, rapid contrast enhancement washout and a propensity for intratumoral lipid, leads to a protocol that spares most adenomas from contrast enhancement. Korobkin et al. have reported the accuracy of combined unenhanced and delayed enhanced CT densitometry for characterization of adrenal masses.[32] One hundred and sixty-six adrenal masses were prospectively studied with unenhanced CT; those with attenuation values greater than 10 H underwent contrast-enhanced and 15 min delayed enhanced CT and correctly characterized 160 of the 166 (96%) masses. Excluding five non-adenomas that were not metastases, the sensitivity and specificity for characterizing a mass as adenoma versus metastasis using delayed CT densitometry were 98% (124/127) and 97% (33/34), respectively.[32]

There has been extensive investigation of MRI features of benign and malignant adrenal lesions, with initial studies demonstrating a diagnostic overlap in about 20–30% of cases. MRI chemical shift imaging takes advantage of the different hydrogen atom resonant frequency peaks in water and triglyceride (lipid) molecules, this technique demonstrates a decreased signal intensity (SI) of tissue containing both lipid and water compared with tissue without lipid. This technique was described by Mitchell et al. to detect the significant amount of lipid often present in adrenal adenomas and typically absent in most metastases and other non-adenomatous adrenal masses.[32,33] Korobkin et al. compared quantitive to qualitative assessment of opposed-phase images; only adenomas showed a visible decrease in relative signal intensity ratio (100% specificity), with a sensitivity of 81%; with a quantitative relative SI loss of 12% compared with liver, specificity was 100% and sensitivity was 84%.[34]

The incidental adrenal mass is one of the best clinical applications of adrenal scintigraphy as the currently available data suggest it has the highest accuracy and lowest cost in this setting.[35] Adrenal scintigraphy is comparable to thyroid scanning for characterizing lesions as nonfunctioning ('cold', and possibly malignant) versus functioning ('hot', and probably benign).[23] However, unlike thyroid scanning, the majority of adrenal images offer a diagnostic result without need for further investigation. Non-adenomas demonstrate decreased, distorted or absent radiocholesterol uptake in the affected adrenal gland (Fig. 12C.4(a)). Hormonally nonhypersecretory adrenal adenomas demonstrate increased NP-59 accumulation (concordant image; Fig. 12C.4(b)). With over 25 years of experience to date, in the setting of a normal biochemical screening evaluation and the absence of interfering medications, NP-59 avidity has been a highly accurate ($\approx$100%) predictor of benignity, while discordant imaging has been a 100% accurate predictor of a non-adenomatous lesion.[23,36–40] Similar accuracy has been reported with SMC.[41] Symmetrical, bilateral NP-59 uptake (normal, or nonlateralizing scan pattern) is seen in all peri-adrenal and pseudo-adrenal masses. Unfortunately, nonlateralizing scans also occur in some patients harboring either benign or malignant adrenal masses <2 cm. Nonhypersecretory masses <1 cm, and >1 to <2 cm have yielded diagnostic (e.g. lateralizing) images in 52% and 89% of patients, respectively. Non-adenomatous lesions, including malignancies, <1 cm, >1 to <2 cm and >2 to <3 cm were present in 0%, 9%, and 10% of patients, respectively.[42]

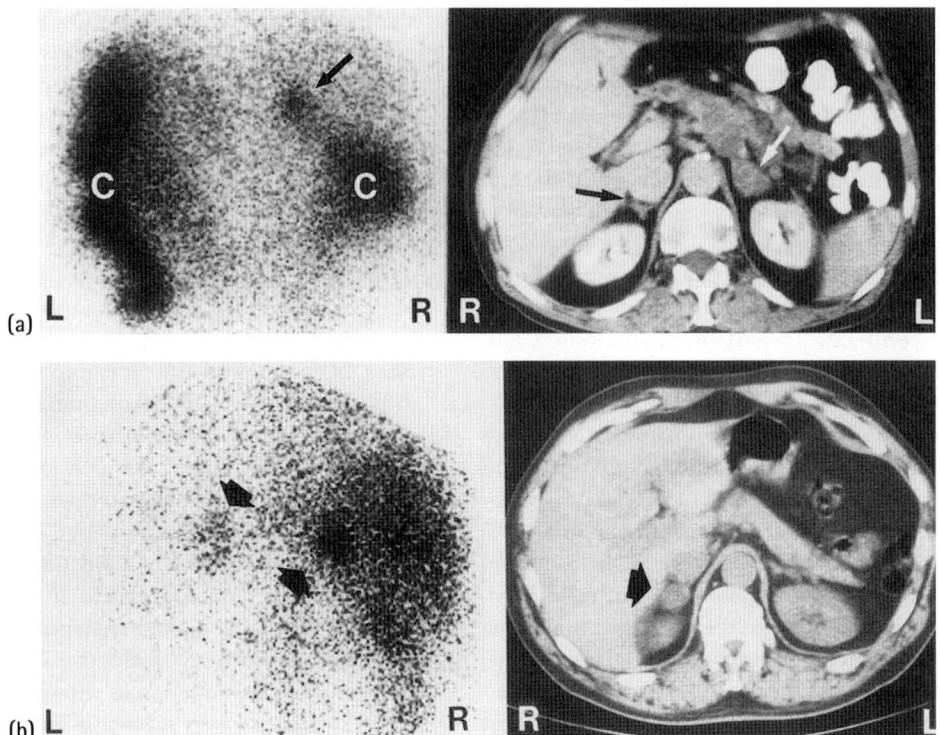

Figure 12C.4 *Incidental adrenal masses (NP-59 posterior scintiscans 5 days after injection, no dexamethasone suppression). (a) Discordant scintigraphy (left panel) with less NP-59 uptake on the side of the left adrenal mass seen on CT (right panel, white arrow) relative to the morphologically and scintigraphically normal right adrenal (black arrows). CT-guided biopsy diagnosed metastatic adenocarcinoma. (C, NP-59 in colon). (b) Concordant scintigraphy (left panel) with greater NP-59 uptake on the side of the 2 cm right adrenal mass seen on CT (right panel, arrow) than on the side of the morphologically normal left adrenal gland. No biochemical evidence of adrenocortical dysfunction (including adrenal vein sampling). (Reproduced, with permission, from* Ann Intern Med *1988; 109: 613–18.)*

Adrenal masses are bilateral in 11–16% of incidentaloma cases.[17] NP-59 uptake equal to or greater than the contralateral adrenal gland and/or liver (as a normal reference tissue) by visual inspection is compatible with a benign process, while NP-59 uptake markedly less than the contralateral adrenal gland and/or liver is compatible with a non-adenomatous lesion. In this setting, Gross *et al.* reported that NP-59 scintigraphy may identify bilateral benign adrenal masses, as well as the gland toward which further evaluation should be directed.[43] Clinical and biochemical evaluations in this setting are critical given the probable increased incidence of CAH, and the rare occurrence of primary adrenal insufficiency from bilateral adrenal destruction by metastases, hematological malignancy, hemorrhage, infection or granulomatous diseases.

Positron emission tomography (PET) with 2-[18F]fluoro-2-deoxy-D-glucose (18F-FDG) has also been used to characterize adrenal masses in patients with cancer.[44] PET tumor-to-background ratios (standardized uptake value, SUV) correctly differentiated benign (0.2–1.2 SUV) from all malignant lesions (2.9–16.6 SUV). However, adrenal masses <1.5 cm were excluded, and the estimated spatial resolution is 1 cm (possibly less for lesions with intense FDG uptake). More recent studies confirm that [18F]fluorodeoxyglucose can be used to successfully distinguish benign from malignant incidentally discovered adrenal masses.[45] In addition, the 11β-hydroxylase inhibitor etomidate and analogs have been used to image the adrenal cortex and to depict adrenocortical neoplasms.[11,46]

ADRENAL MEDULLA

Physiology

Catecholamines are derived from the amino acid L-tyrosine. The first committed (and rate determining) step in the catecholamine biosynthetic pathway is the hydroxylation of tyrosine to dihydroxyphenylalanine (DOPA), catalyzed by tyrosine hydroxylase. DOPA is decarboxylated in the cytosol to dopamine, which is taken up into the catecholamine storage vesicles, where it is hydroxylated to noradrenaline (norepinephrine). This pathway is common to both adrenergic neurons and the adrenal medulla. The major blood supply to the adrenal medulla is via an adrenal portal system, which is derived from the cortical sinusoidal plexus. The resulting high medullary level of cortisol induces and maintains the activity of phenylethanolamine-N-methyltransferase (PNMT), which catalyses the methylation of noradrenaline to adrenaline (epinephrine). Noradrenaline and adrenaline are stored in membrane-bound storage vesicles in association with soluble proteins (chromogranins) and nucleotides. Stimulation of the adrenal medulla by the preganglionic, cholinergic splanchnic nerves or by other secretagogues (angiotensin, serotonin, histamine, bradykinin) releases the vesicle contents by exocytosis. Some of the released catecholamines diffuse from the medullary interstitium (or, in the case of adrenergic neurons, from the synaptic cleft) into the general circulation. However, most of the catecholamines are inactivated locally by re-uptake via a stereospecific, sodium- and energy-dependent, saturable pathway (uptake-1), following which they are stored or, if unstored, are rapidly degraded by monoamine oxidase (MAO) to dihydroxymandelic acid. Circulating catecholamines are inactivated predominantly in extra-neuronal, extra-adrenal tissues by uptake via a nonspecific, sodium-independent mechanism (uptake-2), rapidly followed by metabolism by catechol-O-methyl-transferase (COMT) to metanephrines normetadrenaline (normetanephrine) and metadrenaline (metanephrine). Dihydroxymandelic acid and the metanephrines are both metabolized further (by COMT and MAO, respectively) to 3-methoxy-4-hydroxymandelic acid (vanillylmandelic acid, VMA). Dopamine undergoes a similar metabolic sequence to homovanillic acid (HVA).

Pheochromocytoma

Pheochromocytomas are neoplasms arising from mature adrenal medullary cells (pheochromocytes). They produce the well-described syndrome of hypertension associated with a classical triad of paroxysmal headache, palpitations (with relative bradycardia), and sweating attributable to episodic hypersecretion of catecholamines. The same syndrome can be produced by catecholamine-secreting tumors arising from the extra-adrenal paraganglia (functioning paragangliomas, 'extra-adrenal pheochromocytomas') that include the organ of Zuckerkandl (caudal to the origin of the inferior mesenteric artery) and the 'chemoreceptor' organs such as the carotid bodies.

While hypertension is a virtually constant feature of the pheochromocytoma syndrome, it is paroxysmal in fewer than half of the cases. Most patients have sustained hypertension with or without further paroxysmal increases. A high index of suspicion is essential, since these tumors have potentially life-threatening cardiovascular effects and their resection is curative. Important clinical clues include orthostatic hypotension in an untreated hypertensive, hypertension resistant to standard therapy (including exacerbation by beta blockers due to unopposed α-adrenergic peripheral vasoconstriction), and failure of the blood pressure to fall at night. The diagnosis can be established

biochemically in most cases of pheochromocytoma, as described above under incidental adrenal masses.

More recently, an increased number of pheochromocytomas have come to clinical attention as adrenal incidentalomas. This is consistent with the fact that the classic pheochromocytoma syndrome is present in an estimated 0.1% of hypertensive patients and yet an estimated 0.1% of the general population is found at autopsy to harbor a pheochromocytoma.[23] These tumors demonstrate biochemical profiles ranging from normal to only several-fold elevations as opposed to the typical >5- to 10-fold elevations seen with classically symptomatic pheochromocytomas.

Most pheochromocytomas arise in the adrenal medulla. However, this condition has been referred to as 'the 10% disease' since approximately 10% of adrenal tumors are bilateral, 10% are extra-adrenal, and 10% are malignant (defined by local invasion or distant metastases). Some 10% of cases are associated with one of the following autosomal dominant syndromes; multiple endocrine neoplasia (MEN) type 2a (Sipple's syndrome) or 2b (the mucosal neuroma syndrome); neurofibromatosis (von Recklinghausen's disease); von Hippel–Lindau disease (angioma of the retina, cerebellar hemangioblastoma, renal-cell carcinoma, pancreatic cysts, and epididymal cystadenoma); or the syndrome of familial pheochromocytomas with or without paragangliomas. Finally, 10% of pheochromocytomas occur in children, among whom bilaterality, multiplicity, and malignancy are more frequent than in adults. Bilateral pheochromocytomas should always raise the strong suspicion of a familial syndrome and prompt a search for medullary thyroid carcinoma (MTC), characteristic of MEN-2a and 2b, as well as screening of family members for MEN, pheochromocytoma, and MTC. The RET proto-oncogene mutations associated with MEN-2a, 2b, and familial medullary thyroid cancer have led to improved genetic counseling for these families.[47]

The first successful scintigraphic demonstration of pheochromocytomas in humans was reported in 1981 using m-[131I]iodobenzylguanidine (131I-MIBG).[48] Since that report, extensive worldwide experience with this agent in large series of patients has shown uniformly high sensitivity (87%) and specificity (97%) of 131I-MIBG for locating adrenal (Fig. 12C.5) and extra-adrenal (Fig. 12C.6) tumor sites and metastases of malignant pheochromocytoma.[49–51] Whereas the sensitivity of CT approached 100% for adrenal tumors >2 cm in diameter, 131I-MIBG has greater specificity and has clearly superior sensitivity for smaller tumors and extra-adrenal sites. It can also detect pre-neoplastic adrenal medullary hyperplasia in asymptomatic affected relatives of patients with MEN-2a or 2b.[52]

Radiopharmacology

MIBG is an aralkylguanidine, which structurally resembles noradrenaline sufficiently to be recognized by the uptake-1

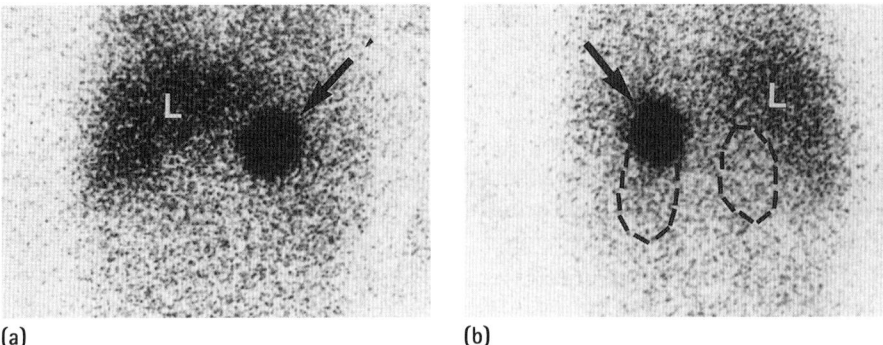

(a)   (b)

Figure 12C.5   *Left adrenal pheochromocytoma (arrows). (a) Anterior and (b) posterior* ^{131}*I-MIBG scintiscans 48 h after injection. The renal outlines are transferred from a* ^{99m}*Tc-DTPA renal scan. Note the displacement of the left kidney. L = liver.*

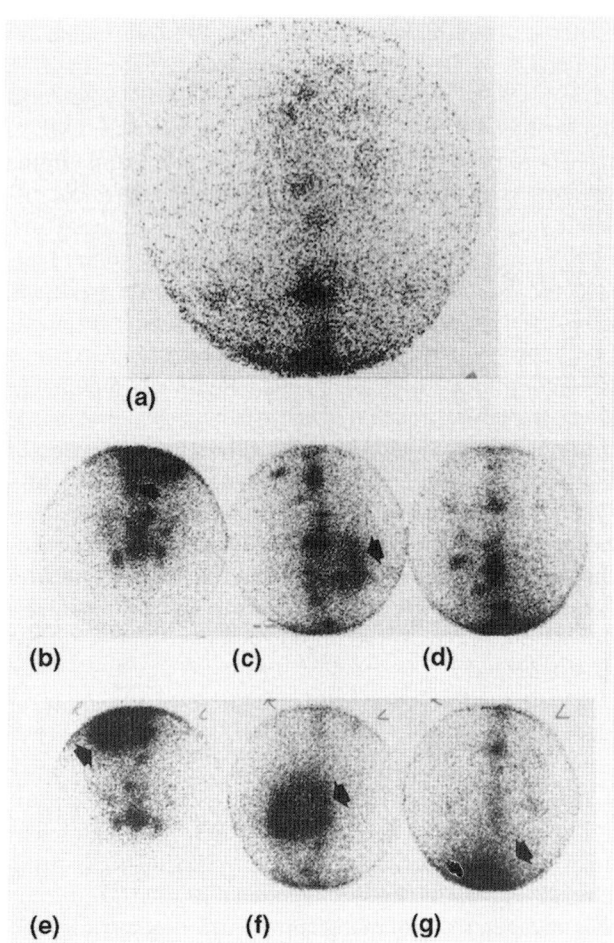

Figure 12C.6   *Malignant pheochromocytoma. Widespread skeletal metastases demonstrated with* ^{131}*I-MIBG. (a) Anterior head and neck; (b) posterior pelvis; (c) posterior abdomen; (d) posterior chest; (e) anterior pelvis; (f) anterior abdomen; (g) anterior chest. Arrows indicate right adrenal primary. Note photopenic, necrotic center. (Reproduced, with permission, from Shapiro et al.[50])*

mechanism and to be stored in the catecholamine storage vesicles.[53] Whereas unstored noradrenaline is rapidly degraded, the halogenated benzyl ring of MIBG confers resistance to COMT while its guanidine side-chain is resistant

to MAO. After intravenous injection of ^{131}I-MIBG, approximately 50% of the administered radioactivity appears in the urine by 24 h and 70–90% is recovered within 4 days; 75–90% of the urinary activity is in the form of unaltered MIBG, with *m*-iodohippuric acid and free iodide accounting for most of the remainder. There is thus little *in vivo* metabolism of MIBG.[54]

Uptake of MIBG is inhibited both *in vitro* and *in vivo* by uptake-1 inhibitors (Table 12C.5). Phenylpropanolamine and other sympathomimetics are frequent constituents of nonprescription 'decongestants', cough remedies, and anorectic 'diet aids', the use of which should be specifically ruled out before radiotracer administration.

MIBG should be slowly injected intravenously over 2–3 min. If tracer uptake is to be quantified, the activity in the syringe should be measured before and after injection for accurate calculation of the administered dose. ^{131}I-MIBG is normally taken up by liver, spleen, myocardium, salivary glands, colon, and occasionally by the lungs and brain.[38,55–57] Thyroid uptake of liberated radioiodide will occur unless blocked with stable iodide (Table 12C.2, page 524). The normal adrenal glands are usually not seen, but faint uptake may be visible 48–72 h after injection in up to 16% of cases. Laxative administration decreases intraluminal colonic radiotracer activity seen in 15–20% of cases, which may mimic or obscure tumor activity (Table 12C.2). Splenic, myocardial, and salivary gland uptake reflect the rich sympathetic innervation of these organs – thus, salivary gland uptake cannot be blocked by perchlorate or iodide, but is reduced on the affected side in patients with Horner's syndrome or stellate ganglion blockade. The degree of myocardial uptake (and, to a lesser extent, salivary gland uptake) is inversely related to circulating noradrenaline levels, so that cardiac uptake is frequently reduced or absent in patients with pheochromocytomas.[58]

Dosimetric considerations limit the dose of ^{131}I-MIBG for diagnostic studies (Table 12C.2). This, coupled with the low detection efficiency of gamma cameras for the 364 keV photon of ^{131}I, led to the introduction of ^{123}I-MIBG. The 159 keV photon of ^{123}I is efficiently detected, and the 20-fold larger dose yields sufficiently high counting statistics to

Table 12C.5 *Drug interactions with pheochromocytomas and their diagnosis*

Drug	Contraindicated with possible pheochromocytoma	Increase catecholamines and metabolites	Reduce MIBG uptake	Interval of drug withdrawal before MIBG imaging
Acute clonidine or alcohol withdrawal, beta blockers, minoxidil, hydralazine	Yes	Yes	No	None
Phenoxybenzamine, phentolamine, prazosin, doxazosin, diuretics, spironolactone, amiloride, levodopa, methyldopa	No	Yes	No	None
Cocaine, sympathomimetics	Yes	Yes	Yes	1 week
Dopamine, dopaminergic drugs	Yes	Yes	Possible	1 week
Clonidine, ACE inhibitors	No	No	No	None
Butyrophenones, amphetamines	No	Yes	Possible	1 week
Labetalol	No	Yes	Yes	4 weeks
Guanethidine, guanadrel	Yes	No	Possible	1 week
Phenothiazines	Possible	Variable	Possible	1 week
Tricyclic antidepressants	No	Variable	Yes	4 weeks
Calcium-channel blockers	No	No	Possible	1 week
Methylglucamine (component of iodinated contrast)	No	False normal up to 72 h	No	None
Reserpine	No	No	Yes	4 weeks

Table reproduced, with permission, from Kloos R, Korobkin M, Thompson NW, *et al.* Incidentally discovered adrenal masses. In: Arnold A. (ed.) *Endocrine neoplasms*. Kluwer Academic Publishers, 1997.

improve spatial resolution, permit single photon emission computed tomography (SPECT), and improve lesion detection.[58] The shorter imaging time is beneficial, especially in children. In spite of high circulating catecholamines, the normal adrenal medullary output of catecholamines is not suppressed.[57] The normal adrenal medulla, lacrimal glands and even the uterus are more frequently visualized with ^{123}I-MIBG compared with ^{131}I-MIBG images.[59–61] The disadvantages of ^{123}I-MIBG are its cost, limited availability, and limited shelf life.

In spite of these difficulties, ^{123}I-MIBG is the ideal imaging agent for pheochromocytoma. A sensitivity of 93% and specificity of 100% for ^{123}I-MIBG compared with 86% and 100%, respectively for X-ray CT was reported in a comparative study.[61] It is proposed that, after the initial biochemical investigation for a suspected pheochromocytoma, the first imaging screen should be with ^{123}I-MIBG. In those with equivocal clinical and biochemical findings, a negative ^{123}I-MIBG excludes the need for further investigation. If there is strong clinical or biochemical evidence and a negative ^{123}I-MIBG scan, then X-ray CT or MRI of the neck, chest, abdomen and pelvis should be performed. A positive ^{123}I-MIBG scan for a primary tumor showing no metastases may lead to a tailored X-ray CT of the site to accurately delineate the mass and help plan the appropriate surgical intervention. Where ^{123}I-MIBG shows metastatic disease, X-ray CT is mainly helpful when considering surgical debulking.

Because MIBG is excreted in the urine, normal bladder activity may obscure pelvic or bladder tumor foci. Thus, pelvic views are best obtained immediately after the patient has voided. Alternatively, simultaneous dual-window data acquisition following the injection of 74 MBq of ^{99m}Tc-diethylenetriaminepentaacetic acid (^{99m}Tc-DTPA) with subsequent computer-assisted subtraction of urinary tract activity may be used. The same principle, using the appropriate ^{99m}Tc-labeled radiopharmaceutical, has been used to clarify the relationship of abnormal MIBG uptake to bone, liver or cardiac blood pool.

Somatostatin is a naturally occurring neuropeptide with a wide range of physiological actions and a half-life of 2–3 min. A high concentration of somatostatin receptors (of which there are at least five subtypes) has been demonstrated on many neuroendocrine tumors and these may be exploited for imaging with the long-acting somatostatin peptide analog ^{111}In-pentetreotide (OctreoScan) (Fig. 12C.7).[38,62] Unlike MIBG, ^{111}In-pentetreotide does not have an extensive list of potentially interfering medications. It is recommended that concurrent octreotide therapy be discontinued 24–48 h before radiotracer administration, so as to not saturate the receptors. However, pre-treatment with octreotide in a small group of patients has been reported to

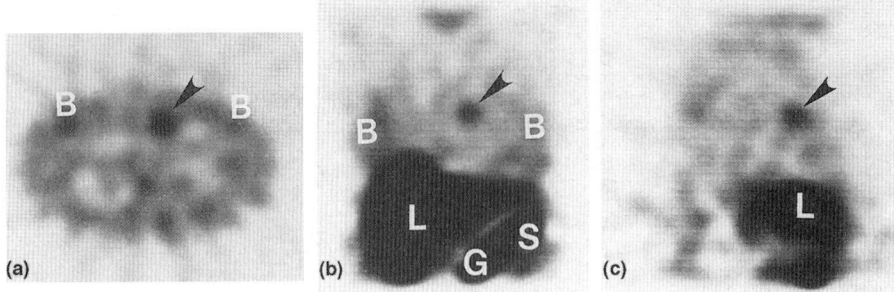

Figure 12C.7 *Indium-111-pentetreotide SPECT images 24h after injection of radiotracer into a patient with a retrosternal pulmonary pheochromocytoma metastasis (arrow), status post-left adrenalectomy and nephrectomy. (a) Transverse; (b) coronal; (c) sagittal sections. B = breast; L = liver; G = gut; S = spleen.*

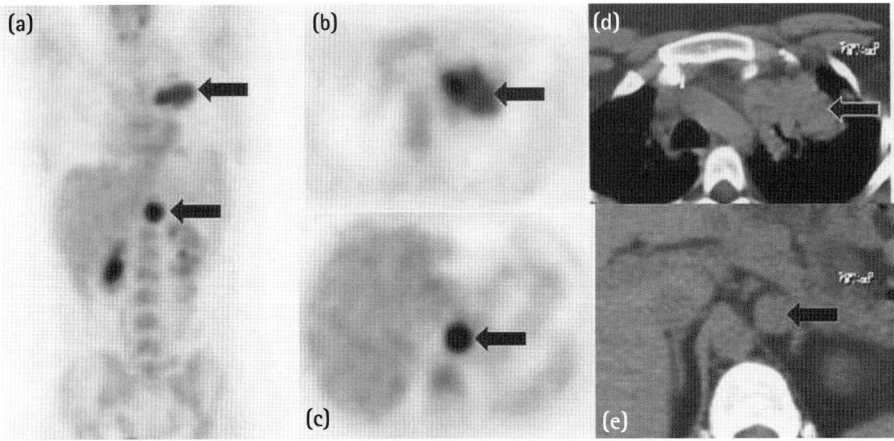

Figure 12C.8 *Unsuspected pheochromocytoma in a 24-year-old woman with Hodgkin's disease (HD) studied with fluorodeoxyglucose (FDG) for post-therapy evaluation. The FDG PET (a–c)/CT (d–e) depicts recurrent HD in a mediastinal mass (arrow) and intense uptake in the left adrenal (arrow), which was later demonstrated to be a pheochromocytoma.*

improve visualization of hepatic metastases.[63] After binding, the somatostatin–receptor complex may become internalized with subsequent somatostatin detachment and removal from the cell. While binding properties of ^{111}In-pentetreotide to somatostatin receptors are similar to those of somatostatin, they are not identical. ^{111}In-pentetreotide is cleared rapidly from the blood with 68–85% excreted unaltered in the urine by 24 h.[62] Normal tissue accumulation of ^{111}In-pentetreotide includes intense uptake in the spleen, liver, and kidneys, with more modest uptake in the pituitary, thyroid, urinary bladder, colon, breast (variable), and occasionally the gallbladder (Fig. 12C.7). ^{111}In-pentetreotide imaging lacks specificity for neuroendocrine tumors as a number of non-neuroendocrine tumors, granulomatous diseases, autoimmune diseases, and inflammatory conditions may also be imaged. [123]I- or ^{131}I-MIBG and ^{111}In-pentetreotide detect pheochromocytomas almost equally.[62] MIBG offers the advantages of absent or minimal confounding of normal renal and hepatic radiotracer accumulation, and the potential for therapy should the tumor be malignant.[55,61,62] Some data suggest that [123]I- or ^{111}In-pentetreotide may serve complementary roles.[23,62] More recently other analogs of octreotide labeled with various isotopes, e.g. [68]Ga, ^{90}Y, and ^{99m}Tc have been offered as diagnostic and potential therapeutic agents for somatostatin-expressing neoplasms.[64,65]

Positron emission tomography (PET) ^{18}F-FDG, ^{11}C-hydroxyephedrine (^{11}C-HED), ^{18}F-DOPA and ^{18}F-dopamine (^{18}F-DA) have been used to localize pheochromocytoma and neuroblastoma.[66–68] High quality PET images of these tumors can be obtained as early as 10 min following injection and are comparable to SPECT images obtained 24 h following ^{123}I-MIBG (Figs 12C.8 and 12C.9).[69,70] The fluorinated DOPA and dopamine analogs have identified metastases of pheochromocytomas not depicted by ^{131}I-MIBG.[71,72] As described earlier, adrenaline is an endogenous substrate for the uptake-1 mechanism. PET imaging with ^{11}C-adrenaline suggests that most pheochromocytomas accumulate the radiotracer. However, it appears that MIBG and ^{11}C-adrenaline are not handled identically, as one tracer may locate

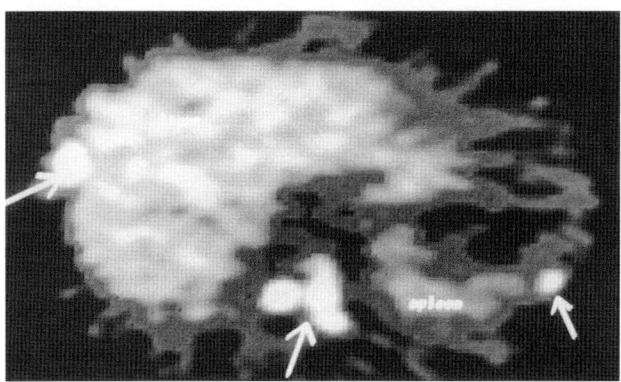

Figure 12C.9 *Carbon-11-hydroxyephedrine (¹¹C-HED) PET scan in a patient with malignant pheochromocytoma. Multiple areas of increased ¹¹C-HED uptake are seen in the liver, abdomen and spleen (arrows). (Reprinted, with permission, from Gross MD, Shapiro B. Adrenal scintigraphy. In: Khalkhali et al. (eds.) Nuclear oncology. Philadelphia: Lippincott, Williams & Wilkins, 2000: 473.)*

tumors when the other does not and rapid intravesicular metabolism of epinephrine by monoamine oxidase may decrease its imaging efficacy.[73]

Other 'neuroendocrine' tumors

Neuroblastomas and their metastases regularly show MIBG uptake with 92% sensitivity compared with 77% for ¹¹¹In-pentetreotide.[51,64,74,75] MIBG uptake in the extremities is a more sensitive index of skeletal involvement than conventional ⁹⁹ᵐTc-labeled MDP bone scans (Fig. 12C.10), bone marrow aspiration and biopsy, and plain radiographs.[76] PET imaging with ¹¹C-hydroxyephedrine has also been used to localize neuroblastoma.[77]

A number of tumors other than pheochromocytomas and neuroblastomas image with MIBG and ¹¹¹In-pentetreotide with varying frequency. MIBG appears to be more sensitive to detect ganglioneuroma (100%), schwannoma, and retinoblastoma.[51] Indium-111-pentetreotide appears more sensitive for carcinoid tumors (86% vs. 70%), medullary thyroid cancer (66% vs. 35%), endocrine pancreatic tumors (70% vs. 60%), paraganglioma (97% vs. 89%), small-cell lung cancer (95% vs. 15%), Merkel cell tumors (80% vs. 50%), and several pituitary tumor types (GH, TSH and non-secretory).[51] Although several of these tumors do not actively secrete catecholamines, they originate from the neural crest and retain the mechanisms for amine precursor uptake and decarboxylation (hence, 'APUDomas') and have typical dense core neurosecretory granules on electron microscopy. Uptake of MIBG by these tumors is likely to be via a mechanism similar or identical to uptake-1.

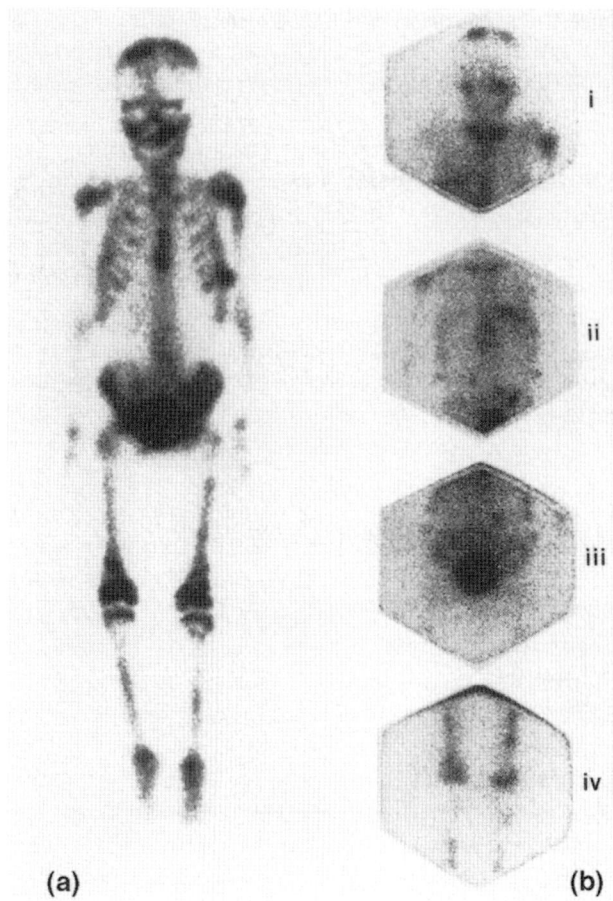

(a)   **(b)**

Figure 12C.10 *Metastatic neuroblastoma. (a) Technetium-99m-labeled MDP bone scan showing multiple skeletal metastases. (b) Iodine-131-MIBG scan showing more extensive skeletal and bone marrow involvement than suggested by the bone scan. i = anterior head and neck; ii = anterior chest and abdomen; iii = anterior pelvis and proximal femurs; iv = anterior lower limbs. (Reproduced, with permission, from J Nucl Med 1985; 26: 736–42.)*

Radiopharmaceutical therapy of neuroendocrine tumors

Following the demonstration of ¹³¹I-MIBG uptake by metastases of tumors derived from the neural crest, it was hypothesized that MIBG would be a useful therapeutic agent for these conditions. The cautious optimism raised by early reports[78,79] has been borne out for a minority of malignant pheochromocytomas and paragangliomas, which are relatively radioresistant tumors. Currently, therapy with high doses (e.g. 7.4 GBq per dose) of ¹³¹I-MIBG is indicated only in patients with progressive disease who have failed conventional therapy or with intractable bone pain from skeletal metastases, and only if a previous dosimetric study has predicted a delivered tumor dose of >0.5 cGy MBq⁻¹. A summary of ¹³¹I-MIBG therapy is given in Table 12C.6. The use of MIBG as a radiotherapeutic agent is discussed in Chapter 2.

Table 12C.6 *Summary of ^{131}I-MIBG therapy^a*

	Range	Number or %	Mean ± SD	Median
Number of doses administered	*1–11*	–	*3.3 ± 2.2*	^{b}
Age at MIBG therapy (years)	*12–76^d*	–	–	–
Site of primary (%)				
adrenal	–	77	–	–
extra-adrenal	–	21	–	–
both sites	–	2	–	–
Sites of metastases (%)				
soft tissue	–	39	–	–
bone	–	13	–	–
both sites	–	48	–	–
Specific activity of dose (mCi mmol^{-1})	*10–15*	–	–	–
Radiation dose to tumor (when calculated^e) (rads)	*100–19 790*	–	–	–
Individual dose activity (mCi)	–	–	*158*	–
Cumulative dose activity (mCi)	*98–2322*	–	*490 ± 350*	–
Initial response rate (%)	–			
symptomatic	–	78	–	–
hormonal	–	45^{b,c}	–	–
tumor volume	–	30^{b,c}	–	–
complete response	–	4.3	–	–
Adverse effects (no. of cases) total (radiation sickness)				
marrow	–	47	–	^{b}
liver	–	25	–	–
hypertensive	–	4	–	–
crisis	–	1	–	–
Duration of follow-up (months)	*13–108*	–	*30.9 ± 23.1*	^{b}
Fraction of responders relapsing or progressing (%) in study period	–	45	–	–
Interval from response to relapse or progression (months)	–	–	*29.3 ± 31.1*	*19*
Fraction of responders eventually dying (%) in study period	–	33	–	–
Interval from response to deaths (months)	–	–	*23.2 ± 8.1*	*22*
Fraction of nonresponders eventually dying (%) in study period	–	45	–	–
Interval from therapy to death in nonresponders (months)	–	*14.3 ± 8.3*	*13*	

^{a} Data (24 centers in 10 countries from 1983 to 1996) derived from Lohk L, *et al. Endocrinol Invest* 1997; **20**: 648–58, with permission.

^{b} There were five complete, durable hormonal and tumor responders (4.3%).

^{c} Soft tissue lesions were more responsive than those in bone.

^{d} Seventeen of 116 patients were ≤18 years of age.

^{e} Available in only 35 of 116 cases.

REFERENCES

● Seminal primary article

1 Gross MD, Rubello D, Shapiro B, *et al.* Is there a future for adrenal scintigraphy? *Nucl Med Commun* 2002; **23**: 197–202.

2 Beierwaltes WH, Lieberman LM, Ansari AN, *et al.* Visualization of human adrenal glands in vivo by scintillation scanning. *JAMA* 1971; **216**: 275–7.

3 Sarkar SD, Cohen EL, Beierwaltes WH, *et al.* A new and superior adrenal imaging agent, ^{131}I-6-beta-iodomethyl-19-nor-cholesterol (NP-59): evaluation in humans. *J Clin Endocrinol Metab* 1977; **45**: 353–62.

4 Hawkins LA, Britton KE, Shapiro B, *et al.* Selenium 75 selenomethyl cholesterol: a new agent for quantitative functional scintigraphy of the adrenals: physical aspects. *Br J Radiol* 1980; **53**: 883–9.

● 5 Gross MD, Valk TW, Swanson DP, *et al.* The role of pharmacologic manipulation in adrenal cortical scintigraphy. *Semin Nucl Med* 1981; **11**: 128–48.

6 Lynn MD, Gross MD, Shapiro B, *et al.* The influence of hyper-cholesterolaemia on the adrenal uptake and metabolic handling of ^{131}I-6-beta-iodomethyl-19-norcholesterol (NP-59). *Nucl Med Commun* 1986; **7**: 631–7.

7 Conn JW, Hinerman DL, *et al.* Spironolactone-induced inhibition of aldosterone biosynthesis in primary aldosteronism: morphological and functional studies. *Metabolism* 1977; **26**: 1293–307.

8 Kater CE, Biglieri EG, Schambelan M, *et al.* Studies of impaired aldosterone response to spironolactone-induced renin and potassium elevations in adenomatous but not hyperplastic primary aldosteronism. *Hypertension* 1983; **5**: V115–21.

9 Cain MD, Walters WA, Catt KJ, *et al.* Effects of oral contraceptive therapy on the reninangiotensin system. *J Clin Endocrinol Metab* 1971; **33**: 671–6.

10 Isaacsohn JL, Lees AM, Lees RS, *et al.* Adrenal imaging with technetium-99m-labeled low-density lipoproteins. *Metabolism* 1986; **35**: 364–6.

11 Bergstrom M, Bonasma TA, Bergstrom E, *et al.* In vitro and in vivo primate evaluation of carbon-11 etomidate and carbon-11 metomidate as potential tracers for PET imaging of the adrenal cortex and its tumors. *J Nucl Med* 1998; **39**: 982–7.

12 Shreve P, Kloos RT, Shapiro B, *et al.* Nonhypersecretory adrenal adenomas show marked uptake and retention of C-11 acetate. *J Nucl Med* 1996; **37**: 15.

13 Gross MD, Valk TW, Freitas JE, *et al.* The relationship of adrenal iodomethylnorcholesterol uptake to indices of adrenal cortical function in Cushing's syndrome. *J Clin Endocrinol Metab* 1981; **52**: 1062–6.

14 Seabold JE, Haynie TP, DeAsis DN, *et al.* Detection of metastatic adrenal carcinoma using ^{131}I-6-beta-iodomethyl-19-norcholesterol total body scans. *J Clin Endocrinol Metab* 1976; **45**: 788–97.

● 15 Fig LM, Gross MD, Shapiro B, *et al.* Adrenal localization in the adrenocorticotropic hormone-independent Cushing syndrome. *Ann Intern Med* 1988; **109**: 547–53.

16 Shapiro B, Britton KE, Hawkins LA, *et al.* Clinical experience with ^{75}Se-selenomethylcholesterol adrenal imaging. *Clin Endocrinol (Oxford)* 1981; **15**: 19–27.

17 Kloos RT, Korobkin M, Thompson NW, *et al.* Incidentally discovered adrenal masses. In: Arnold A. (ed.) *Endocrine neoplasms.* Boston: Kluwer Academic Publishers, 1996: 263–92.

18 Gross MD, Freitas JE, Swanson DP, *et al.* The normal dexamethasone-suppression adrenal scintiscan. *J Nucl Med* 1979; **20**: 1131–5.

● 19 Gross MD, Shapiro B, Grekin RJ, *et al.* The relationship of adrenal gland iodomethylnorcholesterol uptake to zona glomerulosa function in primary aldosteronism. *J Clin Endocrinol Metab* 1983; **57**: 477–81.

20 Gross MD, Shapiro B, Freitas JE, *et al.* Limited significance of asymmetric adrenal visualization on dexamethasone-suppression scintigraphy. *J Nucl Med* 1985; **26**: 43–8.

21 Melby JC, Azar ST, *et al.* Adrenal steroids and hypertension: new aspects. *The Endocrinologist* 1993; **3**: 344–51.

22 Kloos RT, Khafagi F, Shapiro B, *et al.* Four case histories of androgen excess: pitfalls of diagnosis. *The Endocrinologist* 1996; **6**: 1–13.

● 23 Kloos RT, Gross MD, Francis IR, *et al.* Incidentally discovered adrenal masses. *Endocrine Review* 1995; **16**: 460–84.

24 Taylor L, Ayers JW, Gross MD, *et al.* Diagnostic considerations in virilization: iodomethylnorcholesterol scanning in the localization of androgen secreting tumors. *Fertil Steril* 1986; **46**: 1005–10.

25 Soulez B, Dewailly D, Rosenfield RL, *et al.* Polycystic ovarian syndrome: a multidisciplinary challenge. *The Endocrinologist* 1996; **6**: 19–29.

● 26 Franks S, *et al.* (1995) Polycystic ovary syndrome. *N Engl J Med* 1995; **333**: 853–61. (Erratum appears in *N Engl J Med* 1995; **333**: 1435.)

27 Gross MD, Wortsman J, Shapiro B, *et al.* Scintigraphic evidence of adrenal cortical dysfunction in the polycystic ovary syndrome. *J Clin Endocrinol Metab* 1986; **62**: 197–201.

28 Kloos RT, Shapiro B, Gross MD, *et al.* The adrenal incidentaloma. *Curr Opin Endocrinol Diabetes* 1995; **2**: 222–30.

29 Grumbach MM, Biller BMK, Braunstein GD, *et al.* Management of the clinically inapparent adrenal mass ('incidentaloma'). *Ann Intern Med* 2003; **138**: 424–9.

30 Lenders JW, Keiser HR, Goldstein DS, *et al.* Plasma metanephrines in the diagnosis of pheochromocytoma. *Ann Intern Med* 1995; **123**: 101–9.

31 Korobkin M, Brodeur FJ, Yutzy GG, *et al.* Differentiation of adrenal adenomas from nonadenomas using CT attenuation values. *Am J Roentgenol* 1996; **166**: 531–6.

32 Caoili EM, Korobkin M, Francis IR, *et al.* Combined unenhanced and delayed enhanced CT for characterization of adrenal masses. *Radiology* 2002; **222**: 629–33.

33 Mayo-Smith WW, Boland GW, Noto RB, *et al.* State-of-the art adrenal imaging. *Radiographics* 2001; **21**: 995–1012.

34 Mitchell DG, Outwater EK, Matteucci T, *et al.* Adrenal gland enhancement at MR imaging with Mn-DPDP. *Radiology* 1995; **194**: 783–7.

35 Korobkin M, Lombardi TJ, Aisen AM, *et al.* Characterization of adrenal masses with chemical shift and gadolinium-enhanced MR imaging. *Radiology* 1995; **197**: 411–18.

● 36 Dwamena BA, Kloos RT, Fendrick AM, *et al.* The adrenal incidentaloma: decision and cost effectiveness analyses of diagnostic management strategies [Abstract]. *J Nucl Med* 1996; **37**: 158P.

● 37 Gross MD, Shapiro B, Bouffard JA, *et al.* Distinguishing benign from malignant euadrenal masses. *Ann Intern Med* 1988; **109**: 613–18.

38 Rubello D, Bui C, Casara D, *et al.* Functional scintigraphy of the adrenal gland. *Eur J Endocrinol* 2003; **147**: 13–28.

39 Kurtaran A, Traub T, Shapiro B, *et al.* Scintigraphic imaging of the adrenal glands. *Eur J Radiol* 2002; **41**: 123–30.

40 La Cava G, Imperiale A, Olianti C, *et al.* SPECT semiquantitative analysis of adrenocortical ^{131}I-6β-iodomethyl-norcholesterol uptake to discriminate subclinical and preclinical functioning adrenal incidentaloma. *J Nucl Med* 2003; **44**: 1057–64.

41 Dominguez-Gadea L, Diez L, Bas C, *et al.* Differential diagnosis of solid adrenal masses using adrenocortical scintigraphy. *Clin Radiol* 1994; **49**: 796–9.

42 Kloos RT, Gross MD, Shapiro B, *et al.* The diagnostic dilemma of small incidentally discovered adrenal masses: a role for ^{131}I-β-iodomethyl-norcholesterol (NP-59) scintigraphy. *World J Surg* 1997; **21**: 36–40.

43 Gross MD, Shapiro B, Francis IR, *et al.* Incidentally discovered bilateral adrenal masses. *Eur J Nucl Med* 1995; **22**: 315–21.

44 Boland GW, Goldberg MA, Lee MJ, *et al.* Indeterminate adrenal mass in patients with cancer: evaluation at PET with 2-[F-18]-fluoro-2-deoxy-D-glucose. *Radiology* 1995; **194**: 131–4.

45 Maurea S, Mainolfi C, Bazzicalupo L, *et al.* Imaging of adrenal tumors using FDG PET: comparison of benign and malignant lesions. *Am J Roentgenol* 1999; **173**: 25–9.

46 Bergstrom M, Juhlin C, Bonasera TA, *et al.* PET imaging of adrenal cortical tumors with the 11β-hydroxylase tracer ^{11}C-metomidate. *J Nucl Med* 2000; **41**: 275–82.

47 Hofstra RM, Landsvater RM, Ceccherini I, *et al.* A mutation in the RET proto-oncogene associated with multiple endocrine neoplasia type 2B and sporadic medullary thyroid carcinoma. *Nature* 1994; **367**: 375–6.

● 48 Sisson JC, Frager MS, Valk TW, *et al.* Scintigraphic localization of pheochromocytoma. *N Engl J Med* 1981; **305**: 12–17.

49 Shapiro B, Sisson J, Kalff V, *et al.* The location of middle mediastinal pheochromocytomas. *J Thorac Cardiovasc Surg* 1984; **87**: 814–20.

● 50 Shapiro B, Sisson JC, Lloyd R, *et al.* Malignant phaeochromocytoma: clinical, biochemical and scintigraphic characterization. *Clin Endocrinol (Oxford)* 1984; **20**: 189–203.

51 Hoefnagel CA, *et al.* Metaiodobenzylguanidine and somatostatin in oncology: role in the management of neural crest tumors. *Eur J Nucl Med* 1994; **21**: 561–81.

● 52 Valk TW, Frager MS, Gross MD, *et al.* Spectrum of pheochromocytoma in multiple endocrine neoplasia. A scintigraphic portrayal using ^{131}I-metaiodobenzylguanidine. *Ann Intern Med* 1986; **94**: 762–7.

53 Tobes MC, Jaques Jr S, Wieland DM, *et al.* Effect of uptake-one inhibitors on the uptake of norepinephrine and metaiodobenzylguanidine. *J Nucl Med* 1985; **26**: 897–907.

54 Mangner TJ, Tobes MC, Wieland DW, *et al.* Metabolism of iodine-131 metaiodobenzylguanidine in patients with metastatic pheochromocytoma. *J Nucl Med* 1986; **27**: 37–44.

55 Nakajo M, Shapiro B, Copp J, *et al.* The normal and abnormal distribution of the adrenomedullary imaging agent m-[I-131] iodobenzylguanidine (I-131 MIBG) in man: evaluation by scintigraphy. *J Nucl Med* 1983; **24**: 672–82.

56 Shapiro B, Copp JE, Sisson JC, *et al.* Iodine-131 metaiodobenzylguanidine for the locating of suspected pheochromocytoma: experience in 400 cases. *J Nucl Med* 1985; **26**: 576–85.

57 Nakajo M, Shapiro B, Glowniak J, *et al.* Inverse relationship between cardiac accumulation of meta-[^{131}I]iodobenzylguanidine (I-131 MIBG) and circulating catecholamines in suspected pheochromocytoma. *J Nucl Med* 1983; **24**: 1127–34.

58 Lynn MD, Shapiro B, Sisson JC, *et al.* Pheochromocytoma and the normal adrenal medulla: improved visualization with I-123 MIBG scintigraphy. *Radiology* 1985; **155**: 789–92.

59 Bomanji J, Bouloux PM, Levison DA, *et al.* Observations on the function of normal adrenomedullary tissue in patients with phaeochromocytomas and other paragangliomas. *Eur J Nucl Med* 1987; **13**: 86–9.

60 Bomanji J, Britton KE, *et al.* Uterine uptake of iodine-123 metaiodobenzylguanidine during the menstrual phase of uterine cycle. *Clin Nucl Med* 1987; **12**: 601–3.

61 Bomanji J, Conry BG, Britton KE, *et al.* Imaging neural crest tumors with ^{123}I-metaiodobenzylguanidine and X-ray computed tomography: a comparative study. *Clin Radiol* 1988; **39**: 502–6.

● 62 Van der Harst E, de Herder WW, Bruining HA, *et al.* 123(I)Metaiodobenzylguanidine and 111 (In)octreotide uptake in benign and malignant pheochromocytoma. *J Clin Endocrinol Metab* 2000; **86**: 685–93.

63 Dorr U, Rath U, Sautter-Bihl ML, *et al.* Improved visualization of carcinoid liver metastases by indium-111 pentetreotide scintigraphy following treatment with cold somatostatin analogue. *Eur J Nucl Med* 1993; **20**: 431–3.

● 64 DeJong M, *et al.* Therapy of neuroendocrine tumors with radiolabeled somatostatin analogues. *Q J Nucl Med* 1999; **43**: 356–66.

65 Tiensu JE, *et al.* Treatment with high dose [(111)In-DTPA-D-Phe-1]-octreotide in patients with neuro-endocrine tumors: evaluation of therapeutic and toxic effects. *Acta Oncol* 1999; **38**: 373–7.

66 Shulkin BL, Thompson NW, Shapiro B, *et al.* Pheochromocytomas imaging with 2-fluorine-18-fluoro-2-deoxy-D-glucose PET. *Radiology* 1999; **212**: 35–41.

67 Shulkin BL, Wieland DM, Baro ME, *et al.* PET studies of neuroblastoma with carbon 11-hydroxyephedrine. *J Nucl Med* 1993; **33**: 220.

68 Virgolini I, *et al.* New radiopharmaceuticals for receptor scintigraphy and radionuclide therapy. *Q J Nucl Med* 2000; **44**: 50–58.

● 69 Shulkin BL, Wieland DM, Schwaiger M, *et al.* PET scanning with hydroxyephedrine: an approach to the localization of pheochromocytoma. *J Nucl Med* 1992; **33**: 1125–31.

70 Shulkin BL, Koeppe RA, Francis IR, *et al.* Pheochromo-cytomas that do not accumulate metaiodoben-zylguanidine: localization with PET and administraton of FDG. *Radiology* 1993; **186**: 711–15.

● 71 Ilias L, Yu J, Carrasquillo JA, *et al.* Superiority of 6-[^{18}F]-Fluorodopamine positron emission tomo-graphy versus [^{131}I]-metaiodobenzylguanidine scintigraphy in the localization of metastatic pheochromocytoma. *J Clin Endocrinol Metab* 2003; **88**: 4083–7.

72 Pacak K, Eisenhofer G, Carrasquillo JA, *et al.* 6-[^{18}F]Fluorodopamine emission tomographic (PET) scanning for diagnostic localization of pheochromocytoma. *Hypertension* 2001; **38**: 6–8.

73 Shulkin BL, Wieland DM, Shapiro B, *et al.* PET epi-nephrine studies of pheochromocytoma [Abstract]. *J Nucl Med* 1995; **36**: 229P.

74 Matthay KK, *et al.* Neuroblastoma: a clinical chal-lenge and biologic puzzle. *CA: Cancer J Clin* 1995; **45**: 179–92.

75 Erikson B, Oberg K, *et al.* Summing up 15 years of somatostatin analog therapy in neuroendocrine tumors: future outlook. *Ann Oncol* 1999; **10(Suppl 2)**: S31–38.

76 Gelfand MJ, *et al.* Meta-iodobenzylguanidine in children. *Semin Nucl Med* 1993; **23**: 231–42.

77 Shulkin BL, Wieland DM, Baro ME, *et al.* PET hydroxyephedrine imaging of neuroblastoma. *J Nucl Med* 1996; **37**: 16–21.

78 Sisson JC, Shapiro B, Beierwaltes WH, *et al.* Radiopharmaceutical treatment of malignant pheochromocytoma. *J Nucl Med* 1984; **25**: 197–206.

79 Fischer M, Winterberg B, Zidek W, *et al.* [Nuclear medical therapy of pheochromocytoma.] *Schweiz Med Wochenschr* 1984; **114**: 1841–3.

13

The breast and genital disease

13A Breast cancer

Breast cancer	543	Scintimammography	545
Detection of primary breast tumors	544	Positron emission tomography imaging of breast cancer	549
Radionuclide imaging of the breast	545	References	554

13B Breast disease: Single photon and positron emission tomography

Introduction	559	Receptors	564
Scintimammography	559	Positron emission tomography	564
Sentinel nodes	562	Conclusion	565
Radionuclide occult lesion localization	564	References	565

13C Testicular tumors

Introduction	569	Tumor recurrence and follow-up	570
Diagnosis and staging	569	Conclusion	572
Imaging at diagnosis	570	References	573

13D Impotence

Introduction	575	Blood pool techniques	579
Penile anatomy and physiology of erection	575	Evaluation of vasculogenic impotence by flaccid and	
Etiology and pathogenesis of vasculogenic impotence	576	erection phallography	579
Investigation of vasculogenic impotence: Nonradionuclide		Erection phallography protocol	581
techniques	577	Clinical diagnostic role	582
Radionuclide investigation of vasculogenic impotence:		Conclusion	582
early studies	578	References	583
Radionuclide investigation of impotence: current methods	578		

13E Infertility

Introduction	585	Hysterosalpingoscintigraphy	588
Relevant anatomy and physiology	585	References	591
Investigations	587		

13F Testicular perfusion imaging

Introduction	593	Scintigraphic technique and interpretation	596
Acute scrotum: clinical presentation and pathogenesis	593	Other imaging modalities for evaluating testicular perfusion	598
Testicular torsion	593	References	599

13G Gynecological cancer

Introduction   601   Patients and radioimmunoscintigraphy methodology   602
Radioimmunoscintigraphy   602   References   605

13H Prostate cancer

Introduction   609   Conclusion   614
Prostate cancer imaging   609   References   615
[111]In-Prostascint antibody: New methods   612   Appendix: Prostate immune study with ^{111}In-prostascint   617

Breast cancer

NORBERT AVRIL, MAREN BIENERT, AND JOERG DOSE SCHWARZ

BREAST CANCER

Breast cancer is the most common female malignancy in most European countries, North America, and Australia, while it is less frequent in Asia and in Africa. In Europe, one out of every 10–15 women will develop breast cancer in her lifetime and the risk is even higher in the United States, where it is one out of every eight women. Approximately 95% of breast cancer cases occur sporadically without any known genetic mutation and the causal mechanisms underlying this disease have yet to be fully elucidated. Overall, 5-year survival rates are approximately 75% with ranges of 92% for stage I (pT1, pN0, M0) to 15% for stage IV (M1) disease.[1]

The main prognostic factors in patients with breast cancer are lymph node status, grading, and the presence of distant metastases. Most patients with locally advanced disease have axillary lymph nodes involved with their tumors, but a subset of patients has large primary tumors without lymph node involvement. For patients with lymph node metastases, more than four lymph nodes involved predict poorer survival.[2] The College of American Pathologists has recently considered prognostic and predictive factors in breast cancer and stratified them into categories reflecting the strength of published evidence.[3] Factors ranked in category I included TNM staging, histologic grade, histologic type, mitotic figure counts, and hormone receptor status. Category II factors included c-erbB-2 (Her2-neu), proliferation markers, lymphatic and vascular channel invasion, and p53. Factors in category III included DNA ploidy analysis, microvessel density, epidermal growth factor receptor, transforming growth factor-alpha, bcl-2, pS2, and cathepsin D.

Both mammary glands are composed of approximately 15 to 20 lobes, each of which includes a series of branching ducts and lobules. Most breast cancer arises in the terminal duct lobular unit. Invasive ductal carcinoma is the most common histological type (70–80%), followed by invasive lobular carcinoma (6–10%), and medullary carcinoma (≈3%). The remaining tumors comprise a variety of histological types that are generally less malignant. Invasive breast cancer may be present as a single tumor, or multifocal if tumors are growing in the same quadrant of the breast, and multicentric if they are detected in different quadrants. The disease can occur in any part of the breast but most frequently occurs in the upper outer quadrant. Locally advanced breast cancer remains a particular challenge as the majority of patients with this diagnosis develop distant metastases despite appropriate therapy. Patients with locally advanced disease include advanced primary tumors (stage T4), advanced nodal disease, such as fixed axillary nodes or involvement of ipsilateral supraclavicular, infraclavicular, or internal mammary nodes, and inflammatory carcinomas.

Noninvasive breast cancer consists of two histological and clinical subtypes, ductal (DCIS) and lobular (LCIS) *in situ* carcinomas. The carcinoma cells are confined within the terminal duct lobular unit and the adjacent ducts, but have not yet invaded through the basement membrane. Generally, lobular *in situ* carcinoma does not present as a palpable tumor and is usually found incidentally in breast biopsies, often multifocal and bilateral. Ductal *in situ* carcinoma is increasingly diagnosed due to microcalcifications seen on mammograms and is more likely to be confined to one breast or even to one quadrant of the breast.

If breast cancer is suspected, a biopsy is necessary to confirm the diagnosis. The National Comprehensive Cancer Network has published guidelines for the work-up of women with newly diagnosed breast cancer. The recommendations include history and physical examination, diagnostic bilateral mammogram and ultrasound, and optional breast magnetic resonance imaging (MRI), pathology review, determination of estrogen receptor, progesterone receptor, nuclear grade and HER-2/neu status. The latter can all be determined from either fine-needle aspiration or core biopsy. To evaluate distant metastases, chest X-ray, ultrasound of the abdomen, bone scintigraphy and computed tomography (CT) or magnetic resonance imaging (MRI) might be indicated.

DETECTION OF PRIMARY BREAST TUMORS

Improved methods to detect and diagnose breast cancer early are required to achieve a significant impact on morbidity and mortality. More than 80% of cancers are detected because of a suspicious mass, either by self-examination or routine breast examination. Clinical signs are asymmetry of the breast contour, a protrusion, or a subtle dimpling of the skin (*peau d'orange*). Depending on the size of the breast and the density of breast tissue, most tumors are not palpable smaller than 1 cm in diameter. Breast carcinomas are often present as irregularly shaped, firm or hard, yet painless nodules or masses. Physical examination typically does not allow an accurate differentiation between a malignant and nonmalignant mass. Therefore, imaging modalities are used to improve the diagnostic accuracy and various new and innovative technologies are being investigated for advancing the early detection and diagnosis of breast cancer.

Screening mammography allows the detection of breast cancer earlier than breast self-examination, and seems to reduce the risk of death from breast cancer by approximately 30% in women over 50 years of age. Mammography localizes and assesses the extent of a lesion as well as identifying other suspicious masses. Studies in large series have shown that mammography, using mediolateral oblique and craniocaudal projections, is a useful tool to improve early detection of breast cancer. Depending on the lesion size and the radiographic appearance and breast tissue density, sensitivity ranges from 54 to 58% in women under the age of 40 and from 81 to 94% in those over 50.[4,5] Malignant and benign breast lesions often display similar radiographic appearance, resulting in a major limitation of mammography.[6] In some studies approximately six to eight out of 10 patients with suspicious lesions in mammography, who undergo surgery, have benign histology.[6,7] In modern mammography centers the relation between benign and malignant tumors is 1:1 or 1:2.

About 10% of breast carcinomas are not identified in mammography even when they are palpable.[8] One reason is that mammography is limited because cancer can have similar photon absorption as normal breast tissue especially in younger women with radiographic dense breasts. Despite these limitations, mammography is viewed as the best tool currently available for screening and early diagnosis.

Ultrasound has become an important imaging modality in evaluating the breast. Ultrasound is often used in addition to mammography and provides differentiation between cystic lesions and solid tumors. In younger patients with dense breasts, ultrasound can be superior in the detection of breast cancer in comparison to mammography. Breast cancer typically shows irregular shaped hypoechoic masses, posterior acoustical shadowing, and ill-defined demarcation against the surrounding tissue. Doppler ultrasound may help distinguish benign from malignant breast disease. However, the diagnostic accuracy is often not sufficient enough to accurately characterize abnormal tissue and specifically to exclude malignancy. Another common application of ultrasound is to provide guidance for interventional procedures. Less common uses include assisting in staging of breast cancer and evaluating patients with implants. Recently, there has been an interest in using ultrasound to screen asymptomatic women for breast cancer, as is done with mammography. Further studies must be performed to assess if this reduces mortality from breast cancer. Although primarily used to image the female breast, ultrasound also can be used to evaluate breast-related concerns in men. Uses of contrast-enhanced ultrasound are still experimental and would add an invasive component to an otherwise noninvasive study.

Magnetic resonance imaging has become a valuable tool in breast disease, especially in cases that are difficult to diagnose. Recent progress in both spatial and temporal resolutions, the imaging sequences used, pharmacokinetic modeling of contrast uptake, the use of dedicated and, more recently, phased-array breast coils, and gadolinium-based contrast agents have contributed to the advancement of this imaging technique. MRI has several distinct advantages for breast imaging. These include three-dimensional visualization of breast tissue, information about tissue vascularity, and chest wall visualization. Moreover, MRI allows evaluation of dense breast parenchyma that often limits the detection of breast cancer in mammography. The use of paramagnetic contrast agents has been found to be essential in identifying breast masses. Signal enhancement following intravenous contrast is a highly sensitive criterion to detect breast cancer and sensitivity is in most studies more than 90%. However, specificity of MRI is reported to be even less in comparison to mammography. MRI of the breast offers higher sensitivity for the detection of multifocal or multicentric cancer, which is important in selecting patients appropriately for breast-conserving surgery. It is also a valuable tool for the screening of patients with a high risk of breast cancer or where there is axillary disease or nipple discharge and conventional imaging has not revealed the primary focus. Techniques are also now available to biopsy lesions only apparent on MRI of the breast. MRI can differentiate scar tissue from tumor and is specifically useful in patients suspected for local recurrent disease. Studies suggest that MRI can identify responders and nonresponders to (neoadjuvant) chemotherapy with more accuracy. It is the modality of choice for the assessment of breast implants for rupture with accuracy higher than X-ray mammography and ultrasound. The most important limitations of MRI beside the low specificity are patient compliance, scan time, and cost.

RADIONUCLIDE IMAGING OF THE BREAST

Numerous radionuclides and radiopharmaceuticals have been shown to accumulate in breast tissue and breast cancer. In 1946, Low-Beer and colleagues[9] reported increased uptake of ^{32}P in an ulcerating breast carcinoma. Later, potassium-42,[10] rubidium-86,[11] bismuth-206 citrate,[12] and mercury-197 chloromerdin[13] were found to accumulate in breast cancer. Other radiopharmaceuticals used for breast imaging include ^{99m}Tc-pertechnetate,[14] ^{99m}Tc-labeled bisphosphonates[15] and gallium-68 citrate.[16] Wendt and colleagues[17] studied 31 patients with suspicious findings on mammography with ^{99m}Tc-diethylenetriaminepentaacetic acid (^{99m}Tc-DTPA) and found increased tracer uptake in benign and malignant breast abnormalities. However, the low specificity was a pivotal limitation of the radiotracers described above. A more specific binding was found using radiolabeled monoclonal antibodies, but most tumors smaller than 2 cm were not visualized.[18,19] Frequently, breast cancer demonstrates increased somatostatin receptor expression and ^{111}In-labeled octreotide showed positive uptake in about 75% of the breast cancer cases.[20] The receptor binding was found to be higher in invasive ductal breast cancer compared to invasive lobular breast cancer. In the early 1970s, thallium-201 chloride was used as myocardial perfusion agent and was also found to accumulate in breast cancer. Lee and colleagues studied 30 patients suspected of having breast cancer with thallium-201 chloride and found a sensitivity of 80% and a specificity of 96%.

The first abstract on the application of ^{99m}Tc-sestamibi for tumor imaging is dated in 1987, describing a thyroid cancer patient with lung metastases.[21] ^{99m}Tc-sestamibi was initially developed as myocardial perfusion agent, and provided a better target-to-background ratio compared to thallium-201 chloride when used for tumor imaging. Maublant *et al.*[22] compared the *in vitro* uptake of thallium-201 chloride and ^{99m}Tc-sestamibi in carcinoma cell lines and found that the uptake of sestamibi was four times higher compared to cultured normal cells whereas the uptake of ^{201}Tl was about only twice. The *in vivo* distribution of ^{99m}Tc-sestamibi is similar to ^{201}Tl with accumulation in the thyroid and the salivary glands, in the myocardium, liver, gastrointestinal tract, and the kidneys. Sestamibi passes the cell membrane and mitochondrial membrane via passive diffusion. The electrical potential within cells and mitochondria plays an important role for subsequent accumulation. Data from rat myocardium suggest that approximately 90% of sestamibi is concentrated in the mitochondria in an energy-dependent manner as a free cationic complex.[23] Cellular clearance of

sestamibi is related to energy (ATP) dependent transmembrane transporter proteins, which include the P-glycoprotein pump system and the multidrug resistence protein.[24] Tumor cells with a higher concentration of these transmembrane proteins demonstrate a faster rate of sestamibi clearance and, hence, less tracer accumulation. Cutrone and colleagues[25] studied the relationship between the degree of sestamibi uptake in benign and malignant breast lesions and histopathologic features. Immunohistochemical staining was performed for neovascularity targeting the factor VIII antigen, the alpha-actin antigen for desmoplasia, the mitochondrial antigen for mitochondrial density, and the MIB-1 antigen for cellular proliferation. They found a poor correlation between MIBI uptake and the degrees of neovascularity and intracellular mitochondrial density and a moderate correlation with cellular proliferation and desmoplasia. These findings suggest that the degree of MIBI uptake in breast lesions is multifactorial, but appears to be related more to the degree of desmoplastic activity and cellular proliferation than neovascularity and mitochondrial density.

Technetium-99m-tetrofosmin was initially developed as myocardial perfusion agent and also found to accumulate in tumors. Tetrofosmin is a phosphine ligand containing an ether group, which forms a complex with [99m]Tc. As a lipophilic cationic molecule it accumulates intracellularly and has a faster clearance from lungs and liver. This radiotracer demonstrates positive uptake and retention in various tumors including lung cancer, thyroid cancer, and breast cancer.[26–28] The diagnostic accuracy for detecting breast cancer is reported to be similar to that of sestamibi.[29,30]

SCINTIMAMMOGRAPHY

Scintimammography is a relatively new, noninvasive diagnostic modality in the evaluation of breast cancer. Sestamibi is the only agent that has been approved by the US Food and Drug Administration (FDA) for breast cancer detection. To perform the imaging procedure, no specific patient preparation is necessary. An activity of approximately 700–800 MBq (20–22 mCi) ^{99m}Tc-sestamibi is injected into the patient's arm opposite of the breast being studied. Patients may experience a brief metallic taste after the tracer is injected. After 5–10 min uptake period, a gamma camera is used to image the breast. The procedure takes approximately 45 min to 1 h. Several techniques have been proposed for scintimammography. Simulating the mammography projections by compressing the breast in the craniocaudal position has not been successful. Also, imaging the breast in the supine position was less effective than in the prone position. Prone dependent-breast imaging has several advantages including reduced respiratory motion and optimal separation of breast tissue from organs with high tracer uptake such as the liver and the myocardium. This technique also allows for a more natural breast contour and evaluation of the deep breast tissue adjacent to the chest wall. Both breasts should be imaged and planar images of the lateral aspect of the breast with the suspected abnormality should be acquired first. The recommended acquisition time is 10 min for each view. For better evaluation of posterior lesions, images in the 30° posterior oblique position can be obtained which also helps to define lesions in the axilla. The axilla can be imaged in supine position or in upright position with the arms around the detector. The images are best interpreted on a computer monitor using a linear grayscale display. Khalkhali et al.[31] found a very high interobserver correlation (97%) for the analysis of scintimammography. It is important to note that scintimammography should be delayed 2–3 days following cyst aspiration or fine-needle aspiration, 2 weeks following core biopsy, and at least 4–6 weeks following excisional breast biopsy or major breast injury to avoid false positive results.[32] The sestamibi uptake in normal breast tissue varies with the menstrual cycle with lower uptake in the mid-menstrual cycle period. Initial reports showed that imaging beyond 60–90 min improved the target-to-background ratio. However, delayed imaging may result in a higher number of false negative results caused by increased sestamibi washout from breast cancers expressing the multidrug resistance gene (*MDR1*). Another technical consideration is the use of single photon emission computed tomography (SPECT) imaging. The use of routine SPECT imaging for the detection of breast cancer in addition to planar imaging is still under debate. In a study by Tiling et al.[33] the sensitivity of planar scintimammography was 80% and the specificity was 83%, compared to a sensitivity of 71% for iterative reconstructed SPECT and 69% for filtered back-projection SPECT. SPECT provided additional information to planar scintimammography with respect to the exact localization of sestamibi uptake, the tumor extent, and improved diagnostic accuracy and detection of axillary nodes. Generally, SPECT acquired in the prone position allows for direct comparison to the lateral planar gamma camera images, but high quality SPECT imaging can only be achieved with the arms raised, which is often not possible in the prone position.

Detection of primary breast cancer with scintimammography

The first reports on the use of ^{99m}Tc-sestamibi for imaging breast cancer are dated in 1992.[34,35] In the following years, the clinical application of scintimammography has been studied extensively and led to a rich body of literature including several multicenter trials. In 1994, the group from Khalkhali[36] reported that in patients with abnormal mammograms scintimammography was true positive in 23 patients and true negative in 33 patients. However, five patients with benign breast lesions had false positive scans. The resulting sensitivity of scintimammography was 95.8% with a corresponding specificity of 86.8%. The positive predictive value was 82.1% but, more importantly, the negative predictive value for the

detection of carcinoma of the breast was 97.1%. The authors concluded that scintimammography was a highly sensitive test that improved the specificity of conventional mammography. In 1998, Palmedo et al.[37] published the results from a prospective European multicenter trial, which included 246 patients with suspicious breast masses or abnormal mammograms. Patients had a total of 253 lesions, 195 palpable and 58 nonpalpable, and subsequent histology revealed 165 malignant and 88 benign lesions. The overall sensitivity in this study was 71% and the specificity was 69%. For palpable lesions, the sensitivity and specificity were 83% and 91%, respectively. Another important result of this multicenter trial was that sensitivity was not dependent on the radiographic density of the breast tissue, which is an important limitation for mammography. Invasive ductal and invasive lobular cancers were detected with similar sensitivity. Technetium-99m-sestamibi was true positive in 60% of the false negative mammograms. Numerous studies have been published so far and a recent meta-analysis revealed an overall sensitivity for scintimammography of 85.2%, a specificity of 86.6%, a positive predictive value of 88.2%, a negative predictive value of 81.8%, and an accuracy of 85.9%.[38] This analysis included 64 published studies until end of 1999, with 5340 patients and a total of 5354 breast lesions identified as malignant and 2330 lesions as benign. A higher sensitivity for scintimammography was found in a recent prospective multicenter clinical trial.[39] A total of 1734 women were enrolled of whom 1243 had complete data upon study completion. Scintimammography was positive for 322 (26%) of the patients and negative for 921 (76%). Histopathology showed malignancy for 201 (16%) of the patients. Sensitivity and specificity of scintimammography were 93% and 87%, respectively; the positive predictive value 58% and the negative predictive value 98%. These results are important since the study had a lower prevalence of patients with cancer compared to previous studies.

Some studies indicated that scintimammography might be specifically helpful as an adjunct to physical examination and mammography in the detection of breast cancer in women with dense and fatty breasts. To further evaluate the role of scintimammography in these patients, a total of 558 women from 42 centers in North America were enrolled prospectively.[40] The results were based on 580 breasts with an abnormality out of which 276 breasts were dense and 228 had a malignant lesion. Comparing scintimammography of fatty versus dense breasts, the sensitivity was 72% vs 70%, the specificity was 80% vs 78%, the positive predictive value was 72% vs 67%, the negative predictive value 81% vs 81%, and the accuracy 77% vs 75%. Scintimammography led to significant changes in the post-test likelihood of cancer and was similar for both dense and fatty breasts. This study also clearly showed that the diagnostic accuracy of scintimammography was not affected by breast density.

Due to the limited spatial resolution of conventional gamma camera systems, the detectability of breast carcinomas is significantly influenced by the tumor size. Hermans et al.[41] studied 240 consecutive women referred to surgery and all false negative sestamibi scans occurred in cancers less than 1 cm. Tolmos *et al.*[42] evaluated scintimammography in 70 women with nonpalpable breast abnormalities and found a sensitivity of 56% and a specificity of 87%. Four of nine breast cancers were not detected by scintimammography. This is an important limitation and the authors concluded that scinti-mammography is not currently recommended as a screening test in patients with nonpalpable positive mammographic findings. In a three-center study including 420 patients, sensitivity in palpable masses was 98% and specificity was 89%.[43] In contrast, nonpalpable masses were detected with a sensitivity of 62% and a comparable specificity of 91%. In an analysis based on tumor stage, the sensitivity was 26% for tumors smaller than 0.5 cm (T1a), 56% for tumors between 0.5 and 1 cm (T1b) and 95% for tumors between 1 and 2 cm (T1c). Stage T2 tumors, which include carcinomas more than 2 cm but not more than 5 cm, were detected with a sensitivity of 97%. Recently, Tiling *et al.*[44] found similar results in a group of 219 patients. Overall sensitivity was 82.1% and specificity was 87.5%. The sensitivity for palpable lesions was 91.7% compared to 64.9% for nonpalpable lesions. With respect to tumor size, sensitivity ranged between 65.2% for breast cancer with a diameter of less than 1 cm and 93.7% for carcinoma larger than 1 cm in diameter.

Since the tumor size is an important factor for visualization of increased tracer uptake, the use of dedicated high-resolution breast-specific gamma cameras has been evaluated. Fifty patients with a total of 58 breast lesions were studied both with a clinical general purpose gamma camera and a prototype of a high-resolution breast-specific gamma camera.[45] The study group included 28 malignant and 30 benign lesions and all lesions were confirmed by pathology. Using the conventional gamma camera, the sensitivity for detection of breast cancer was 64.3% compared to 78.6% using the high-resolution breast-specific gamma camera. The specificity with both systems was 93.3%. The dedicated high-resolution gamma camera was specifically superior in the detection of small lesions. Four lesions with a median size of 8.5 mm were only detected with the dedicated high-resolution gamma camera. Seven out of 15 lesions up to 1 cm in diameter were detected with the general purpose camera compared to 10 out of 15 with the high-resolution gamma camera. For 18 nonpalpable lesions, sensitivity was 55.5% with the general purpose camera and 72.2% with the high-resolution gamma camera.

There is only limited information available regarding the detection of multifocal and multicentric breast cancer with scintimammography. In a retrospective review of 353 women who underwent mastectomy, 40 women had multifocal disease (*n* = 34) or multicentric (*n* = 6) breast cancer.[46] Scintimammography correctly identified the presence of cancer in 39 patients and the multifocal or multi-centric character in 22 (52%) of these patients. In contrast, anatomical imaging identified cancer in 28 patients (70%) and the combination of mammography and ultrasound

identified correctly multifocal or multicentric breast cancer only in eight patients (22%). This study suggested that scintimammography might be able to identify more cases of multifocal and multicentric cancer than mammography and/or ultrasound. In another study, multicentric disease was present in eight out of 58 patients who were treated by mastectomy. Scintimammography revealed a sensitivity of 62.5% and a specificity of 96% in detecting multicentric disease.[47] Although the overall sensitivity of scinti-mammography was higher compared to conventional mammography, this study also indicated some limitations for identification of muticentric disease.

Although the specificity of scintimammography is relatively high, there are a considerable number of benign changes that demonstrate positive sestamibi uptake. False positive findings occur in benign lesions such as fibroadenomas, papillomas, epithelial hyperplasia, fibrocystic breast disease, and inflammation. The sestamibi uptake in nonmalignant tissue seems to correlate with histopathological features, specifically a higher cellularity and increased cell proliferation and patients with atypical hyperplasia also showed a higher incidence of false positive findings.[48] In 97 women, Marini *et al.*[49] explored the use of scintimammography in breast micro-calcifications seen on conventional mammography. Using the receiver operating characteristic (ROC) statistical technique, combined mammography–scintimammography was superior to mammography alone. The authors stated that scintimammography provides additional information to mammography in the characterization of an isolated cluster of microcalcifications, but invasive procedures cannot be replaced.

Detection of lymph node metastases with scintimammography

Increased ^{99m}Tc-sestamibi uptake is not only observed in primary breast cancer but also in axillary lymph node metastases. The major limitation however, is the inability to detect small tumor involved lymph nodes. Lam *et al.*[50] studied 36 patients with primary untreated breast carcinoma and found true positive results in seven of 11 cases (64%) of axillary lymph node metastases and true negative results in 18 of 20 cases (90%). In another study, including 100 breast cancer patients, 52 had no axillary lymph node involvement with a total of 611 negative nodes and 48 patients had at least one axillary lymph node metastasis in axillary dissection.[51] The sensitivity of scintimammography in detecting metastatic axillary lymph node involvement was 79.2% and the specificity was 84.6%. Although scintimammography has a good diagnostic accuracy for detecting axillary lymph node involvement, the accuracy seems not to be sufficient to replace axillary lymph node dissection. This limitation is also shown in a series of 239 women, where sensitivity and specificity of sestamibi scintigraphy were 82.3% and 94.1%, respectively.[52] Sensitivity was 69.7% in 33 patients with fewer than three axillary node metastases and only one out of six patients with a single axillary node metastasis had a positive scan.

Monitoring response to treatment

Primary (neoadjuvant) chemotherapy is increasingly the treatment for patients with locally advanced breast cancer. Due to the preoperative reduction of tumor volume, the rate of breast preserving surgery has increased. Additionally, patients with complete pathological response have significantly higher disease-free and overall survival rates than nonresponders.[53,54] Approximately 70% of the patients undergoing primary chemotherapy show clinical response, but only 20–30% have partial or complete regression in histopathological tissue analysis. Therefore, the therapeutic effect cannot be accurately determined until definitive breast surgery is performed.

There are only a few studies available addressing the role of scintimammography for assessment of response after chemotherapy as well as for prediction of response during treatment. For semi-quantitative evaluation of scintimammography, the sestamibi uptake in treated primary breast cancer is measured by the region-of-interest technique and compared to the pre-treatment scan. Changes in sestamibi uptake are used to determine response to treatment. In 1997, Maini et al.[55] evaluated serial scintimammography for the assessment of neoadjuvant chemotherapy in 29 patients with locally advanced breast cancer. Patients were studied at baseline and after three cycles of chemotherapy. Approximately 1 day after the third cycle of chemotherapy patients underwent surgery. The sensitivity for the prediction of tumor presence after chemotherapy was 65% for scintimammography, 35% for clinical evaluation, and 69% for mammography. The specificity, however, for the prediction of the absence of tumor was 100% for scintimammography, 67% for clinical evaluation, and 33% for mammography. Mankoff et al.[56] used scintimammography to predict therapeutic response during chemotherapy. A total of 32 patients, in whom the response of the primary tumor was assessable, were studied before therapy, after 2 months of therapy, and close to the completion of chemotherapy prior to surgery. The sestamibi uptake ratio for tumor-to-normal breast was used for tracer quantification. The uptake ratio decreased by 35% in clinical responders but increased on average by 17% in nonresponders. Patients achieving a macroscopic complete response in histopathology had a mean decrease of 58% compared to only 18% in patients with a partial response. Using a cut-off value of 40%, decrease in the uptake ratio allowed the identification of a complete response with 100% sensitivity and 89% specificity. In a small series of nine patients, Tiling et al.[57] performed scintimammography before, during, and after neoadjuvant chemotherapy. In three patients who had complete response, the sestamibi uptake decreased 8 days after initiation of chemotherapy and

reached background levels in the following course. The decrease in sestambi uptake in another three patients with partial response was less marked and three patients without response showed a persisting high tumor activity even after chemotherapy was completed. On the other hand, Wilczek et al.[58] recently found that although there was a strong reduction of the relative tumor activity after finishing chemotherapy, there was no correlation with therapy effect as assessed by histology. They also did not observe a significant reduction of the relative tumor uptake after one course of chemotherapy.

Current clinical status of scintimammography

Scintimammography has been shown to contribute to the work-up of patients suspected of having breast cancer. It has been proposed that it is helpful as a complementary technique in patients with equivocal mammography, dense breast tissue, breast implants, doubtful microcalcifications, and suspected recurrent breast cancer. The detection of multicentric disease was improved by scintimammography. A general limitation of many studies addressing the diagnostic role of scintimammography is the inclusion of pre-selected patients with a high incidence of breast cancer. Scintimammography has a higher specificity compared to conventional mammography, with a lower number of false positive findings. However, the sensitivity is in the range between 60 and 80%, which is not sufficient to exclude breast cancer. Therefore, scintimammography should not be used to determine whether or not patients with mammographic abnormalities should undergo invasive procedures. Scintimammography is also not indicated in the further evaluation of small or uncertain mammographic findings and should not be used whenever histopathological clarification of suspicious lesions is necessary. The diagnostic accuracy also depends on tumor size and the detection rate of breast cancer smaller than 1 cm is low. The use of dedicated breast gamma cameras might improve the sensitivity of scintimammography in the future. With the current technology, scintimammography should not be used for screening of asymptomatic women or for early diagnosis of breast cancer.

The use of scintimammography has to be carefully stratified specifically with respect to improvements in other breast imaging modalities such as digital mammography, ultrasound, and magnetic resonance imaging. Depending on the availability, the higher spatial resolution of these imaging modalities has to be taken into consideration. Scintimammography may be helpful in selected patients who have a high risk of developing breast cancer, where conventional breast imaging is difficult to interpret. Also, the uptake of sestamibi in breast tissue seems to be little influenced by previous treatments, specifically chemotherapy or radiation therapy. Initial results for using scintimammography to assess response to treatment are promising but confirmation from studies that include larger patient populations is still needed. There is currently no role for axillary lymph node staging with sestamibi scintigraphy. The sentinel lymph node biopsy has an accuracy of higher than 90% and the sentinel lymph node concept is becoming more and more the standard of care in breast surgery. It is of note that incidental findings of positive sestamibi uptake in the breast or axilla, e.g. in nuclear cardiology studies, warrant further evaluation.

POSITRON EMISSION TOMOGRAPHY IMAGING OF BREAST CANCER

Positron emission tomography (PET) is a noninvasive imaging technique that measures the concentration of positron emitting radiopharmaceuticals within the body. Depending upon the radiolabeled tracer used, PET can be used to determine various physiological and biochemical processes *in vivo*. PET is highly sensitive, with the capacity to detect subnanomolar concentrations of radiotracer and provides superior image resolution compared to conventional nuclear medicine imaging with gamma cameras. Currently, PET imaging can target several biological features of cancer including glucose metabolism, cell proliferation, perfusion, and hypoxia. Following malignant transformation, various tumors are characterized by elevated glucose consumption and subsequent increased uptake and accumulation of the radiolabeled glucose analog 2-[^{18}F]fluoro-2-deoxy-D-glucose (^{18}F-FDG). PET imaging using ^{18}F-FDG provides more sensitive and more specific information about the extent of disease than morphological/anatomical imaging alone. FDG PET has become a standard imaging procedure for staging and restaging of many types of cancer. In the United States, insurance coverage currently includes head and neck cancer, thyroid cancer, solitary pulmonary nodules, lung cancer, breast cancer, esophageal cancer, colorectal cancer, lymphoma, and melanoma. The metabolic activity of neoplastic tissue assessed by PET offers additional information about cancer biology and can be used for the differentiation between benign and malignant lesions, identification of early disease and staging of metastases, assessment of therapeutic effectiveness as well as to determine tumor aggressiveness. The uptake mechanism and biochemical pathway of FDG has been extensively studied both *in vitro* and *in vivo*. The transport of the radiotracer through the cell membrane via glucose transport proteins (GLUTs) and subsequent intracellular phosphorylation by hexokinase (HK) have been identified as key steps for subsequent tissue accumulation. As FDG-6-phosphate is not a suitable substrate for glucose-6-phosphate isomerase, and the enzyme level of glucose-6-phosphatase is generally low in tumors, FDG-6-phosphate accumulates in cells and is visualized by PET when the ^{18}F-FDG is used.

Positron emission tomography imaging procedure and image analysis in the breast

To ensure a standardized metabolic state including low plasma glucose levels, it is necessary that oncology patients have fasted for at least 4–6 h prior to administration of ^{18}F-FDG. The blood glucose level prior to tracer injection should not exceed 200 mg/100 mL. Intravenous administration of about 300–400 MBq ($\approx$10 mCi) ^{18}F-FDG is used in most studies, although Adler *et al.* reported a higher breast cancer detection rate using up to 750 MBq ($\approx$20 mCi) ^{18}F-FDG.[59,60] To avoid artificial tracer retention in the axilla region, the tracer should be injected into an arm vein contralateral to the suspected tumor. Most of the studies reported in literature are done in the two-dimensional mode data acquisition and the influence of the three-dimensional mode on the results of breast imaging still needs to be studied. Imaging in the prone position with both arms at the side and the breast hanging free is recommended to avoid compression and deformation of the breast. Data acquisition should be started approximately 60 min after tracer injection. Boerner *et al.*[61] showed increasing target-to-background ratios over time suggesting a benefit of longer waiting periods between tracer injection and data acquisition. However, a lower image quality, due to radionuclide decay, has to be taken into account. Attenuation correction is recommended for optimal tumor localization as well as subsequent quantification of regional tracer uptake. The use of iterative reconstruction algorithms results in better image quality: an increase in diagnostic accuracy has not yet been reported. Visual image interpretation should include analysis of transaxial, coronal, and sagittal views. Breast cancer is typically present with focally increased FDG uptake, whereas benign tumors are negative in PET imaging. Proliferative mammary dysplasia may result in moderate, but diffuse increased tracer uptake.

Attenuation corrected PET images provide quantitative information about the tracer concentration in tissue. Various approaches of different complexity can be applied for quantitative PET analysis. Standardized uptake values (SUVs) are frequently being calculated providing a semi-quantitative measure of FDG accumulation in tissue by normalizing the tissue radioactivity concentration measured with PET to injected dose and patient's body weight. Quantitative methods may be used to complement visual image analysis for differentiation between benign and malignant breast tumors, i.e. by using a SUV normalized scale for image display.[62] In particular, SUV correction for partial volume effects and normalization to blood glucose has been shown to yield the highest diagnostic accuracy for breast imaging. Corresponding threshold values for optimal tumor characterization have been published for various quantification methods.[62] Dynamic data acquisition allows calculation of the tracer influx constant, although this procedure is more complex and did not increase diagnostic accuracy.

Whole-body imaging can be improved by intravenous injection of furosemide (20–40 mg) to reduce tracer retention in the urinary system and by scopolamine (20–40 mg) to reduce FDG uptake in the bowel.[63] Image evaluation requires an appreciation of the normal physiologic FDG uptake distribution and variation between individuals as well as consideration of artifacts and benign conditions that can mimic malignancy. Increased FDG uptake is found within the brain cortex, the myocardium, and the urinary tract. Low to moderate uptake is seen in the base of the tongue, salivary glands, thyroid, liver, spleen, gastrointestinal tract, bone marrow, musculature, and reproductive organs. Of particular importance is the inconsistent amount of normal uptake in glandular breast tissue. The most common normal cause of misinterpretation is related to muscle activity. Muscle tension may lead to increased FDG uptake and physical activity immediately before or after tracer injection can lead to spurious muscle activity. In some patients, supraclavicular uptake has been shown to represent brown fat. Inflammatory and infectious processes also demonstrate increased FDG uptake as well as some benign diseases, such as Paget's disease, Graves' disease, granulomatous disorders, healing fractures, post-radiation changes, and a few benign tumors.

Positron emission tomography imaging of the breast

The first FDG imaging in breast cancer patients was reported in 1989 by Minn and Soini using a collimated gamma camera.[64] Shortly afterwards, Kubota et al.[65] reported on PET imaging with ^{18}F-FDG in one case with local recurrence. In a first series of 10 patients with locally advanced breast cancer, Wahl et al. successfully identified all breast carcinomas.[66] Subsequent studies including a limited number of patients predominantly with advanced stages of disease suggested a high accuracy of FDG PET for the detection of primary breast carcinomas.[59,64–66] The largest patient group reported to date includes 144 patients with 185 histologically confirmed breast tumors.[67] PET detected breast cancer with an overall sensitivity of 64.4% by conservative image reading (regarding only definite FDG uptake as positive) and 80.3% by sensitive image reading (regarding equivocal as well as definite FDG uptake as positive). However, when applying sensitive image reading specificity decreased from 94.3 to 75.5%.[67,68] Schirrmeister et al. found similar results, with a sensitivity of 93% and specificity of 75%, in 117 patients.[69] The use of non-attenuation corrected PET imaging combined with sensitive imaging reading may have contributed to the higher sensitivity and lower specificity in this study. A recent study compared MRI of the breast with FDG PET and found in 32 patients a comparable diagnostic accuracy (88% vs 84%) for both methods.[70] The sensitivity of FDG PET was 79% whereas MRI detected all primary breast carcinomas. However, the specificity of FDG PET was higher (94 vs 72%). Baslaim et al.[71] evaluated the usefulness of FDG PET for diagnosing and staging of inflammatory breast cancer. All seven patients studied presented with diffuse breast enlargement, redness, and *peau d'orange*. PET showed diffuse FDG uptake in the involved breast with intense uptake in the primary tumor as well as increased FDG uptake in the skin.

The ability of PET to detect breast cancer greatly depends on tumor size. Regarding small tumors, only 30 (68.2%) out of 44 breast carcinomas at stage pT1 (<2 cm) were correctly identified, compared to 57 (91.9%) out of 62 at stage pT2 (>2–5 cm).[67] Sensitivity for tumors less than 1 cm (pT1a and b) was only 25% compared to 84.4% for tumors between 1 and 2 cm in diameter (pT1c). Invasive lobular carcinomas were more often false negative (65.2%) than invasive ductal carcinomas (23.7%). These results are consistent with a previous report from Crippa et al.[72] who found higher glucose metabolism for invasive ductal carcinomas (median SUV of 5.6) versus invasive lobular carcinomas (median SUV of 3.8). This is of particular importance in the clinical application of PET since lobular carcinomas are more difficult to diagnose by imaging procedures such as mammography, sonography, and MRI.[73–75] The identification of multifocal or multicentric breast cancer plays an important role in the decision of therapy, as it limits breast conserving surgery. Only nine (50%) out of 18 patients with multifocal or multicentric breast cancer were identified by PET.[67] Nevertheless, Schirrmeister et al. found that PET was twice as sensitive in detecting multifocal lesions (sensitivity 63%, specificity 95%) than the combination of mammography and ultrasound (sensitivity 32%, specificity 93%).[69]

The diagnosis of *in situ* carcinomas has increased over the past decade, mainly due to increased use and technological improvements of mammography. There is little information available about the ability of PET imaging to detect noninvasive breast cancer. Tse et al.[76] studied 14 patients and found that one out of two false negative cases had predominantly intraductal cancer with microscopic invasive foci. In 12 patients, (10 DCIS and two LCIS) none out of six *in situ* carcinomas smaller than 2 cm could be identified.[67] For larger *in situ* carcinomas, three (50%) out of six displayed increased FDG uptake. Although the number of patients studied is small, this data suggests that PET imaging cannot contribute to an improved diagnosis of noninvasive breast cancer.

Vranjesevic et al.[77] evaluated the influence of the breast tissue density on FDG uptake of normal breast tissue and found significantly lower SUVs for primarily fatty breasts than for dense breasts. Benign conditions of the breast are more common and are often difficult to differentiate from breast cancer in conventional imaging modalities. In general, benign breast masses display low FDG uptake. Only three out of 53 benign breast masses presented with focally increased tracer uptake including: one rare case of a ductal adenoma, one case with dysplastic tissue, and one fibroadenoma.[67] Fibroadenomas are common benign tumors and only one out of nine displayed increased tracer uptake. Moreover, dysplastic tissue often accounts for false positive results in MRI predominantly showing a diffuse pattern of little or moderate FDG uptake.

Loco-regional staging

The axillary lymph node status is still considered the single most important prognostic indicator in patients with breast cancer. Clinical examination is generally unreliable for staging the axilla.[78] Lack of conventional imaging techniques to determine the axillary lymph node involvement with acceptable accuracy has been the main reason for axillary lymph node dissection. However, up to 70% of patients with stage T1 and T2 tumors have negative axillary lymph nodes.[79] The extent, morbidity, and cost of the staging procedure of axillary lymph node dissection are often greater than the surgical treatment of the primary tumor. In anatomical based imaging modalities, such as computed tomography, ultrasound, and MRI, the size of a particular lymph node is of crucial importance in determining tumor involvement. Generally, lymph node enlargement over 1 cm in diameter is the decisive criterion. In contrast, metabolic imaging with FDG PET is suggested to provide more specific information based on detecting increased glucose consumption of cancer tissue. In 1991, Wahl et al. studied 12 patients with locally advanced breast cancer and found increased FDG uptake in axillary metastases.[66] In 50 patients, Adler et al. reported a sensitivity of 95%, a negative predictive value of 95%, and an overall accuracy of 77% for axillary PET imaging.[60] Greco et al.[80] studied 167 consecutive breast cancer patients and axillary involvement was detected in 68 of 72 patients resulting in a sensitivity of 94.4% and specificity of 86.3%; overall accuracy of lymph node staging with PET was 89.8%. However, there is some controversy about the sensitivity of axillary PET imaging.[81] It is a well-known phenomenon that due to the limited spatial resolution of current PET devices, (approximately 6–8 mm), the true FDG uptake is underestimated in small cancer deposits. Therefore, it cannot be expected that PET provides visualization of micrometastases. Avril et al. studied 51 patients and found an overall sensitivity and specificity for detection of axillary lymph node metastases of 79% and 96%, respectively.[82] In patients with primary breast tumors larger than 2 cm (larger than stage pT1), the sensitivity increased to 94%, with a corresponding specificity of 100%. However, PET could not identify lymph node metastases in four out of six patients with small primary breast cancer (stage pT1), which led to a sensitivity of only 33% in this group. Although the number of patients studied is small, this study clearly points out that the current achievable spatial resolution of PET imaging limits the detection of micrometastases and small tumor-infiltrated lymph nodes. This conclusion is also supported by others, e.g. by Schirrmeister et al. who studied 117 breast cancer patients and found similar results (sensitivity 79%, specificity 92%).[69] In a prospective multicenter study representing the largest patient cohort so far, 360 women with newly diagnosed invasive breast cancer underwent PET imaging.[83] Three experienced readers blindly interpreted PET images and the results from 308 axillae were compared with histopathology. If at least one probably or definitely abnormal axillary focus was considered positive, the sensitivity for PET was 61% and the specificity

was 80%. Patients with false negative PET had significantly smaller and fewer tumor-positive lymph nodes than true positive cases. Semiquantitative analysis of axillary FDG uptake showed that a nodal standardized uptake value (lean body mass) more than 1.8 had a positive predictive value of 90% but a sensitivity of only 32%. Finding two or more intense foci of tracer uptake in the axilla was highly predictive of axillary metastasis but had a sensitivity of only 27%.

Sentinel node biopsy has become accepted as a reliable method of predicting the status of the axilla in early stages of breast cancer.[79] There are few studies available directly comparing the diagnostic accuracy of PET with sentinel node biopsy in breast cancer patients. In one study, five out of 15 patients had sentinel lymph node metastases, but PET identified only one of these patients.[84] The size of missed metastases ranged from a small micrometastasis identified only by immunohistochemistry to an 11 mm tumor involved lymph node. Another study included 24 clinically node-negative breast cancer patients with primary tumors smaller than 3 cm and axillary staging by PET was accurate in 15 of 24 patients (62.5%).[85] PET was false negative in eight of 10 node-positive patients and false positive in one patient. The sensitivity and specificity of FDG PET were 20% and 93%, respectively. The mean diameter of false negative axillary lymph node metastases was 7.5 mm and ranged from 1 to 15 mm. In 32 breast cancer patients with clinically negative axillary nodes, sentinel lymph node biopsy was false negative in one patient whereas PET missed lymph node metastases in 11 patients resulting in a sensitivity of 20%.[86] These studies clearly indicate the limitation of FDG PET for axillary staging of small primary tumors. FDG PET is not accurate enough in clinically node-negative breast cancer patients qualifying for sentinel lymph node dissection. On the other hand, in patients with larger tumors sentinel biopsy can be avoided in patients with positive FDG PET, in whom complete axillary lymph node dissection should be the primary procedure. FDG PET cannot replace the axillary dissection, not only because of the limited sensitivity but also because the number of involved lymph nodes and extranodal extension cannot be determined. However, in patients with locally advanced disease who are undergoing primary chemotherapy, FDG PET seems to be a reliable method to determine the extent of disease.

Recently, the intrathoracic lymph node status has been retrospectively analyzed comparing CT and PET.[87] In 73 consecutive patients with recurrent or metastatic disease, PET was able to correctly identify 40% of the patients with intrathoracic lymph node metastases, resulting in a sensitivity of 85% and specificity of 90%. Only 23% of the patients had suspiciously enlarged lymph nodes in CT, leading to a sensitivity of 54% and specificity of 85%. PET and CT were both positive in 22% of the cases. Therefore, overall diagnostic accuracy of PET was higher (88%) than that of CT (73%). Despite the limitation in detection of small tumor deposits, FDG PET is currently the most sensitive imaging modality to detect lymph node metastases including parasternal and mediastinal nodes.

Diagnosis of distant metastases and recurrent disease

Distant metastases of breast cancer are frequently found in lymph nodes, lungs, liver, and bones. Therefore, chest X-ray, abdominal ultrasound, and bone scintigraphy are routinely performed for staging. Additionally, CT and MRI are used to further evaluate suspicious findings. Comparing the diagnostic accuracy of PET with CT and/or MRI, Bender et al.[88] studied 75 patients with suspected recurrent or metastatic disease. PET imaging correctly identified 28 (97%) out of 29 patients with lymph node involvement, 15 (100%) out of 15 patients with bone metastases, five (83%) out of six with lung metastases, and two patients with liver metastases. In addition, PET detected eight lymph node and seven bone metastases that had not been diagnosed by conventional imaging techniques. Even though CT and MRI show superior spatial resolution, PET provides more accurate information in discriminating between viable tumor, fibrotic scar, or necrosis. Moon et al. also found a high diagnostic accuracy of whole-body PET imaging in patients with suspected recurrent or metastatic breast carcinoma.[89] Based on the number of lesions, the sensitivity to detect distant metastases was 85% and specificity 79%. On a per patient basis, sensitivity and specificity were 93% and 79%, respectively. Bone metastases were more often false negative than other malignant sites. FDG PET is often superior to conventional imaging modalities as more lesions are detected in different sites. Recently, Dose et al.[90] compared FDG PET in 50 breast cancer patients for detection of metastatic disease with chest X-ray, bone scintigraphy, and ultrasound of the abdomen. FDG PET identified metastatic disease with a sensitivity and specificity of 86% and 90% as compared to 36% and 95%, respectively, for conventional imaging procedures. With respect to the location of metastases, the sensitivity of FDG PET was superior in the detection of pulmonary metastases and especially of lymph node metastases of the mediastinum in comparison to chest X-ray, whereas the sensitivity of FDG PET in the detection of bone and liver metastases was of the same magnitude when compared with bone scintigraphy and ultrasound of the abdomen. In a retrospective analysis of 62 patients, sensitivity and specificity for detecting local recurrence or distant metastases were 97% and 82% for FDG PET versus 84% and 60% for conventional imaging.[91] On a lesion-based analysis, FDG PET detected significantly more lymph nodes, namely 84 vs 23 but fewer bone metastases (61 vs 97). FDG PET increased the extent of disease in six patients (9.7%) and decreased it in eight patients (12.9%), leading to a change in therapeutic regimen in 13 patients (21%). Siggelkow et al.[92] studied 57 patients and PET was true positive for metastatic or recurrent disease in 25 out 27 cases. PET correctly diagnosed the absence of disease in 35 out of 38 scans. The overall sensitivity and specificity for PET were 80.6% and 97.6%, respectively. The use of FDG PET in patients with locally advanced breast cancer frequently results in the detection of unexpected distant metastases and has shown to change the clinical management.[93]

Brachial plexopathy is difficult to assess on conventional anatomical imaging. To address this issue, FDG PET and MRI was performed in 10 patients with clinical findings suggestive of breast cancer metastases.[94] Out of nine patients who had loco-regional breast cancer metastases, MRI was positive in five and indeterminate in four, whereas PET was positive in all patients. Similar results were found from Ahmad et al. in 19 breast cancer patients with symptoms referable to the brachial plexus.[95] These studies suggest that MRI or CT imaging and FDG PET are complementary in detecting and characterizing brachial plexopathy, specifically if other imaging studies are normal. PET may be particularly useful in distinguishing between radiation-induced and metastatic plexopathy.

The skeleton is a common site for distant metastases in breast cancer. Bone scintigraphy is being used for screening bony metastases and allows the extent of disease to be determined. Tracer uptake in bone scintigraphy reflects osteoblastic activity and is therefore limited in the detection of osteolytic lesions. Cook et al.[96] studied 23 breast cancer patients with known skeletal metastases and FDG PET was able to detect more lesions than bone scintigraphy overall. Higher FDG uptake was observed for osteolytic than osteoblastic disease and PET detected fewer bone metastases than bone scintigraphy in patients with osteoblastic metastases. In a larger series including 48 breast cancer patients, a total of 127 bone lesions including 105 metastatic and 22 benign lesions were found by either FDG PET or bone scintigraphy.[97] The diagnostic sensitivity and accuracy of FDG PET were 95.2% and 94.5% versus 93.3% and 78.7% for bone scintigraphy. Another study with 51 breast cancer patients revealed a sensitivity, specificity, and accuracy for the detection of bone metastases of 77.7%, 80.9%, and 80.3% for bone scintigraphy and 77.7%, 97.6%, and 94.1%, respectively for FDG PET.[98] Although the overall sensitivity for bone scintigraphy and PET are reported to be comparable, bone scintigraphy seems to be superior in the detection of osteoblastic disease and FDG PET in osteolytic metastases, suggesting a complementary role for both imaging procedures. The advantage of whole-body PET imaging is its ability to detect metastases in different sites and organs, whereas various other methods need to be applied by using conventional imaging. Further data is needed to prove a PET based staging strategy in breast cancer patients.

Positron emission tomography/ computed tomography

There are exciting new developments in the field of PET instrumentation. PET/CT is a new imaging modality that allows the acquisition of spatially registered PET and CT data in one imaging procedure.[99] This hardware solution overcomes limitations of software fusion methods such as alignment problems due to internal organ movement, variations in scanner bed profile, and positioning of the patient for the scan, thus improving sensitivity and specificity of PET imaging. PET/CT is unique because it provides combined anatomical and functional imaging information, which allows tissue characterization as well as assessment of the exact localization and the extent of tumor tissue. The diagnostic accuracy of PET/CT is higher compared to the single imaging procedures because of the exact anatomical correlation of abnormal FDG uptake and the functional correlation of suspected morphological abnormalities. The accuracy of PET is specifically increased in the neck and abdomen by distinguishing physiological from pathological uptake. Several abstracts indicate a distinct advantage of PET/CT also in breast cancer.

Monitoring response to treatment

There are several studies addressing the role of FDG PET in predicting response early in the course of therapy. In 1993, Wahl et al.[100] studied 11 women with newly diagnosed locally advanced primary breast cancers undergoing chemohormonotherapy with sequential FDG PET imaging. Patients underwent a baseline and four follow-up PET scans during the first three cycles of treatment. Tumor response was determined histopathologically after nine cycles of treatment. The FDG uptake in eight patients with partial or complete pathologic responses decreased promptly with treatment while the tumor diameter did not significantly decrease. On day 8 of therapy, tumor FDG uptake was 78% of baseline and decreased further to 68% at day 21, 60% at day 42 and 52% at day 63. In contrast, three patients with nonresponding tumors did not show a significant decrease in FDG uptake. The authors concluded that FDG PET has substantial promise as an early noninvasive metabolic marker of the efficacy of cancer treatment. Similar findings were also observed by Jansson et al.[101] in 12 patients with locally advanced or metastatic breast cancer treated with chemotherapy. In 30 patients with noninflammatory, large (>3 cm), or locally advanced breast cancers who received eight doses of primary chemotherapy the mean reduction in FDG uptake after the first cycle of chemotherapy was significantly higher in lesions with partial, complete macroscopic or complete microscopic response assessed by histopathologic examination.[102] After a single cycle of chemotherapy, PET predicted complete pathologic response with a sensitivity of 90% and specificity of 74%. In another study, Schelling et al.[103] compared results from PET imaging with pathological response using distinct histopathological criteria, namely minimal residual disease and gross residual disease, previously identified to provide prognostic information.[53,54] FDG uptake in breast cancer after the first and second cycle of chemotherapy was compared to baseline PET. Patients classified as a responder by histopathology had a significantly more pronounced decrease of FDG

uptake than nonresponding patients. Therefore, as early as after the first course of therapy, responding and nonresponding tumors could be differentiated by PET. By a threshold defined as a SUV decrease below 55% compared to the baseline, all responders were correctly identified after the first course (sensitivity 100%, specificity 85%). Accuracy to predict histopathological response was 88% and 91% after the first and second course of therapy. In the clinical setting FDG PET may be helpful in improving patient management by avoiding ineffective chemotherapy and unnecessary side effects, as well as supporting the decision to continue dose intensive preoperative chemotherapy in responding patients. In contrast, in 35 patients with breast cancer Mankoff et al.[104] found a large overlap between changes in metabolic activity in histopathological responders and nonresponders. This discrepant finding may be explained by the different timing of the PET scans comparing baseline with PET 2 months after completion of chemotherapy. After that period of time, histopathological nonresponding tumors may demonstrate a relatively large decrease in tumor size and FDG PET may therefore be unable to differentiate between small absolute differences in the amount of viable tumor cells. Consistent with this explanation, Smith et al. also observed a higher accuracy of FDG PET for prediction of tumor response after the first cycle of chemotherapy than at later points in time.[102]

It is important to note that a transient increase in glucose utilization has been found in responding tumors treated with hormonotherapy. In a first series, Dehdashti et al.[105] performed FDG PET in 11 women before and 7–10 days after initiation of therapy with tamoxifen. In all patients, clinical and radiological follow-up was performed with a median interval of 12 months. Seven patients responded and all showed an increase of FDG uptake 1 week after therapy. This 'metabolic flare' effect is a recognized side-effect of anti-estrogen therapy, which is clinically characterized by pain and erythema in soft tissue lesions and increased pain in osseous metastases. An explanation for this metabolic flare effect is that anti-estrogen therapy first has an agonist effect before the antagonist effect overrules. This agonist effect occurs within 7–10 days after the beginning of a treatment and is usually followed by disease remission. Recently, the same group confirmed their findings in a larger series including 40 patients.[106] In the responders, the tumor FDG uptake increased after tamoxifen by 28.4% with only five of these patients having evidence of a clinical flare reaction. In nonresponders, there was no significant change in tumor FDG uptake from baseline. There are no reports so far about metabolic flare in more aggressive chemotherapeutic regimes. Serial PET imaging can also be used for treatment monitoring of bone metastases.[107] In 24 women with stage IV bone-dominant breast carcinoma whole-body FDG PET imaging was performed at serial time points during the course of therapy. The changes in SUV with therapy correlated well with the overall clinical assessment of response.

Current clinical status of FDG PET in breast cancer

Breast cancer often displays only moderately increased FDG uptake and considering the limited spatial resolution of FDG PET, metabolic imaging results in a low sensitivity to detect small breast carcinomas, micrometastases and small tumor infiltrated lymph nodes. The restricted sensitivity of FDG PET does not allow the screening of asymptomatic women for breast cancer. Moreover, negative PET results in patients with suspicious breast masses or abnormal mammography do not exclude breast cancer. Therefore, PET imaging may not be used as a routine application for evaluation of primary breast tumors and currently cannot significantly reduce unnecessary invasive procedures in patients suspected of having breast cancer. Advances in technology such as the development of dedicated breast imaging devices may improve the detection of primary tumors with PET in the future. In patients with locally advanced breast cancer, PET accurately determines the extent of disease, particularly the loco-regional lymph node status. In smaller tumors, the sentinel node biopsy has become standard of care in many institutions. Several studies indicate that PET has a comparable or higher diagnostic accuracy when compared to conventional imaging modalities used for staging and restaging of breast cancer patients. Recent advances in instrumentation, with the introduction of combined PET/CT imaging, might become the most important single imaging modality for staging of breast cancer patients. Initial data suggest a complementary role of PET to bone scintigraphy in that PET might detect additional osteolytic breast cancer metastases, whereas osteoblastic metastases are better identified by bone scintigraphy. PET imaging was found to be highly useful for monitoring the effects of preoperative chemotherapy. Assessment of therapy response is possible earlier than with any other method. Monitoring chemotherapy may improve patient management by early identification of nonresponding patients.

REFERENCES

1 Sant M, Allemani C, Berrino F, et al. Breast carcinoma survival in Europe and the United States. *Cancer* 2004; **100**: 715–22.

2 Banerjee M, George J, Song EY, et al. Tree-based model for breast cancer prognostication. *J Clin Oncol* 2004; **22**: 2567–75.

3 Fitzgibbons PL, Page DL, Weaver D, et al. Prognostic factors in breast cancer. College of American Pathologists Consensus Statement 1999. *Arch Pathol Lab Med* 2000; **124**: 966–78.

4 Sickles EA. Breast masses: mammographic evaluation. *Radiology* 1989; **173**: 297–303.

5 Kopans DB, Feig SA. False positive rate of screening mammography. *N Engl J Med* 1998; **339**: 562–4.

6 Kopans DB. The positive predictive value of mammography. *Am J Roentgenol* 1992; **158**: 521–6.

7 Meyer JE, Eberlein TJ, Stomper PC, et al. Biopsy of occult breast lesions. Analysis of 1261 abnormalities. *J Am Med Ass* 1990; **263**: 2341–3.

8 Bird RE, Wallace TW, Yankaskas BC. Analysis of cancer missed at screening mammography. *Radiology* 1992; **184**: 613–17.

9 Low-Beer BV, Bell HG, McCorkle HJ, et al. Measurement of radioactive phosphorus in breast tumors in situ: a possible diagnostic procedure; preliminary report. *Radiology* 1946; **47**: 492–3.

10 Baker WH, Nathanson IT, Selverstone B. Use of radioactive potassium (K-42) in the study of benign and malignant breast tumors. *N Engl J Med* 1955; **252**: 612–15.

11 Sklaroff DM. The uptake of radioactive rubidium (Rb-86) by breast tumors. *Am J Roentgenol Radium Ther Nucl Med* 1958; **79**: 994–8.

12 Jacobstein JG, Quinn JL. Uptake of Bi-206 citrate in carcinomas of the breast. *Radiology* 1973; **107**: 677–9.

13 Sodee BD, Renner RR, Di Stefano B. Photoscanning localization of tumor, utilizing chlormerodrin mercury-197. *Radiology* 1965; **84**: 873–5.

14 Richman SD, Brodey PA, Frankel RS, et al. Breast scintigraphy with Tc99m-pertechnetate and Ga-67 citrate. *J Nucl Med* 1974; **16**: 293–9.

15 McDougall R, Pistenma DA. Concentration of Tc-99m diphosphonate in breast tissue. *Radiology* 1974; **112**: 655–7.

16 Richman SD, Ingle JN, Levenson SM, et al. Usefulness of gallium scintigraphy in primary and metastatic breast carcinoma. *J Nucl Med* 1975; **16**: 996–1001.

17 Wendt T, Büll U, Kessler M, et al. Diagnostik benigner und maligner Tumoren der weiblichen Brust durch Single Photon Emissions-Computertomographie mit Tc-99m DTPA. *Nuklearmedizin* 1984; **6**: 283–6.

18 Lamki LM, Buzdar AU, Singletary SE, et al. Indium-111 labeled B72.3 monoclonal antibody in the detection and staging of breast cancer: a phase I study. *J Nucl Med* 1991; **32**: 1326–32.

19 Lind P, Smola MG, Lechner P, et al. The immunoscintigraphic use of Tc99m-labeled monoclonal antibodies (BW 431/26) in patients with suspected primary, recurrent and metastatic breast cancer. *Int J Cancer* 1991; **47**: 865–9.

20 van Eijck CH, Krenning EP, Bootsma A, et al. Somatostatin-receptor scintigraphy in primary breast cancer. *Lancet* 1994; **343**: 640–3.

21 Mueller ST, Guth-Tougelides B, Creutzig H. Imaging of malignant tumors with Tc99m MIBI [Abstract]. *J Nucl Med* 1987; **28**: 562P.

22 Maublant JC, Zhang Z, Rapp M, *et al.* In vitro uptake of technetium-99m-teboroxime in carcinoma cell lines and normal cells: comparison with technetium-99m-sestamibi and thallium-201. *J Nucl Med* 1993; **34**: 1949–52.

23 Carvalho PA, Chiu ML, Kronauge JF, *et al.* Subcellular distribution and analysis of technetium-99m-MIBI in isolated perfused rat hearts. *J Nucl Med* 1992; **33**: 1516–22.

24 Kostakoglu L, Elahi N, Kiratli P, *et al.* Clinical validation of the influence of P-glycoprotein on technetium-99m-sestamibi uptake in malignant tumors. *J Nucl Med* 1997; **38**: 1003–8.

25 Cutrone JA, Yospur LS, Khalkhali I, *et al.* Immunohistologic assessment of technetium-99m-MIBI uptake in benign and malignant breast lesions. *J Nucl Med* 1998; **39**: 449–53.

26 Matsunari I, Kinuya S, Nishikawa T, *et al.* Technetium-99m tetrofosmin uptake in lung cancer: comparison with thallium-201. *Ann Nucl Med* 1996; **10**: 143–5.

27 Basoglu T, Sahin M, Coskun C, *et al.* Technetium-99m-tetrofosmin uptake in malignant lung tumours. *Eur J Nucl Med* 1995; **22**: 687–9.

28 Rambaldi PF, Mansi L, Procaccini E, *et al.* Breast cancer detection with Tc-99m tetrofosmin. *Clin Nucl Med* 1995; **20**: 703–5.

29 Obwegeser R, Berghammer P, Rodrigues M, *et al.* A head-to-head comparison between technetium-99m-tetrofosmin and technetium-99m-MIBI scintigraphy to evaluate suspicious breast lesions. *Eur J Nucl Med* 1999; **26**: 1553–9.

30 Horne T, Pappo I, Cohen-Pour M, *et al.* [99]Tc[m]-tetrofosmin scintimammography for detecting breast cancer: a comparative study with [99]Tc[m]-MIBI. *Nucl Med Commun* 2001; **22**: 807–11.

31 Khalkhali I, Cutrone JA, Mena IG, *et al.* Scintimammography: the complementary role of Tc-99m sestamibi prone breast imaging for the diagnosis of breast carcinoma. *Radiology* 1995; **196**: 421–6.

32 Romero L, Khalkhali I, Vargas HI. The role of nuclear medicine in breast cancer detection: a focus on technetium-99 sestamibi scintimammography. *Curr Oncol Rep* 2003; **5**: 58–62.

33 Tiling R, Tatsch K, Sommer H, *et al.* Technetium-99m-sestamibi scintimammography for the detection of breast carcinoma: comparison between planar and SPECT imaging. *J Nucl Med* 1998; **39**: 849–56.

34 Campeau RJ, Kronemer KA, Sutherland CM. Concordant uptake of Tc-99m sestamibi and Tl-201 in unsuspected breast tumor. *Clin Nucl Med* 1992; **17**: 936–7.

35 Aktolun C, Bayhan H, Kir M. Clinical experience with Tc-99m MIBI imaging in patients with malignant tumors. Preliminary results and comparison with Tl-201. *Clin Nucl Med* 1992; **17**: 171–6.

36 Khalkhali I, Mena I, Jouanne E, *et al.* Prone scintimammography in patients with suspicion of carcinoma of the breast. *J Am Coll Surg* 1994; **178**: 491–7.

37 Palmedo H, Biersack HJ, Lastoria S, *et al.* Scintimammography with technetium-99m methoxyisobutylisonitrile: results of a prospective European multicentre trial. *Eur J Nucl Med* 1998; **25**: 375–85.

38 Liberman M, Sampalis F, Mulder DS, *et al.* Breast cancer diagnosis by scintimammography: a meta-analysis and review of the literature. *Breast Cancer Res Treat* 2003; **80**: 115–26.

39 Sampalis FS, Denis R, Picard D, *et al.* International prospective evaluation of scintimammography with (99m)technetium sestamibi. *Am J Surg* 2003; **185**: 544–9.

40 Khalkhali I, Baum JK, Villanueva-Meyer J, *et al.* (99m)Tc sestamibi breast imaging for the examination of patients with dense and fatty breasts: multicenter study. *Radiology* 2002; **222**: 149–55.

41 Hermans J, Bodart F, Francois D, *et al.* Scintimammography: a new imaging technique for diagnosis and follow-up of breast cancer. *Bull Cancer* 2000; **87**: 334–40.

42 Tolmos J, Cutrone JA, Wang B, *et al.* Scintimammographic analysis of nonpalpable breast lesions previously identified by conventional mammography. *J Natl Cancer Inst* 1998; **90**: 846–9.

43 Scopinaro F, Schillaci O, Ussof W, *et al.* A three center study on the diagnostic accuracy of ^{99m}Tc-MIBI scintimammography. *Anticancer Res* 1997; **17**: 1631–4.

44 Tiling R, Linke R, Kessler M, *et al.* Breast scintigraphy using ^{99m}Tc-sestamibi – use and limitations. *Nuklearmedizin* 2002; **41**: 148–56.

45 Brem RF, Schoonjans JM, Kieper DA, *et al.* High-resolution scintimammography: a pilot study. *J Nucl Med* 2002; **43**: 909–15.

46 Cwikla JB, Buscombe JR, Holloway B, *et al.* Can scintimammography with ^{99m}Tc-MIBI identify multifocal and multicentric primary breast cancer? *Nucl Med Commun* 2001; **22**: 1287–93.

47 Vargas HI, Agbunag RV, Kalinowski A, *et al.* The clinical utility of Tc-99m sestamibi scintimammography in detecting multicentric breast cancer. *Am Surg* 2001; **67**: 1204–8.

48 Waxman AD. The role of ^{99m}Tc methoxyisobutylisonitrile in imaging breast cancer. *Semin Nucl Med* 1997; **27**: 40–54.

49 Marini C, Cilotti A, Traino AC, *et al.* Tc-99m-sestamibi scintimammography in the differentiation of benign and malignant breast microcalcifications. *Breast* 2001; **10**: 306–12.

50 Lam WW, Yang WT, Chan YL, *et al.* Detection of axillary lymph node metastases in breast carcinoma by technetium-99m sestamibi breast scintigraphy, ultrasound and conventional mammography. *Eur J Nucl Med* 1996; **23**: 498–503.

51 Taillefer R, Robidoux A, Turpin S, *et al.* Metastatic axillary lymph node technetium-99m-MIBI imaging in primary breast cancer. *J Nucl Med* 1998; **39**: 459–64.

52 Lumachi F, Ferretti G, Povolato M, *et al.* Usefulness of 99m-Tc-sestamibi scintimammography in suspected breast cancer and in axillary lymph node metastases detection. *Eur J Surg Oncol* 2001; **27**: 256–9.

53 Machiavelli MR, Romero AO, Perez JE, *et al.* Prognostic significance of pathological response of primary tumor and metastatic axillary lymph nodes after neoadjuvant chemotherapy for locally advanced breast carcinoma. *Cancer J Sci Am* 1998; **4**: 125–31.

54 Honkoop AH, van Diest PJ, de Jong JS, *et al.* Prognostic role of clinical, pathological and biological characteristics in patients with locally advanced breast cancer. *Br J Cancer* 1998; **77**: 621–6.

55 Maini CL, Tofani A, Sciuto R, *et al.* Technetium-99m-MIBI scintigraphy in the assessment of neoadjuvant chemotherapy in breast carcinoma. *J Nucl Med* 1997; **38**: 1546–51.

56 Mankoff DA, Dunnwald LK, Gralow JR, *et al.* Monitoring the response of patients with locally advanced breast carcinoma to neoadjuvant chemotherapy using [technetium 99m]-sestamibi scintimammography. *Cancer* 1999; **85**: 2410–23.

57 Tiling R, Kessler M, Untch M, *et al.* Breast cancer: monitoring response to neoadjuvant chemotherapy using Tc-99m sestamibi scintimammography. *Onkologie* 2003; **26**: 27–31.

58 Wilczek B, von Schoultz E, Bergh J, *et al.* Early assessment of neoadjuvant chemotherapy by FEC-courses of locally advanced breast cancer using ^{99m}Tc-MIBI. *Acta Radiol* 2003; **44**: 284–7.

59 Adler LP, Crowe JP, al-Kaisi NK, *et al.* Evaluation of breast masses and axillary lymph nodes with [F-18] 2-deoxy-2-fluoro-D-glucose PET. *Radiology* 1993; **187**: 743–50.

60 Adler LP, Faulhaber PF, Schnur KC, *et al.* Axillary lymph node metastases: screening with [F-18]2-deoxy-2-fluoro-D-glucose (FDG) PET. *Radiology* 1997; **203**: 323–7.

61 Boerner AR, Weckesser M, Herzog H, *et al.* Optimal scan time for fluorine-18 fluorodeoxyglucose positron emission tomography in breast cancer. *Eur J Nucl Med* 1999; **26**: 226–30.

62 Avril N, Bense S, Ziegler SI, *et al.* Breast imaging with fluorine-18-FDG PET: quantitative image analysis. *J Nucl Med* 1997; **38**: 1186–91.

63 Stahl A, Weber WA, Avril N, *et al.* Effect of *N*-butylscopolamine on intestinal uptake of fluorine-18-fluorodeoxyglucose in PET imaging of the abdomen. *Nuklearmedizin* 2000; **39**: 241–5.

64 Minn H, Soini I. F-18 fluorodeoxyglucose scintigraphy in diagnosis and follow up of treatment in advanced breast cancer. *Am J Clin Pathol* 1989; **91**: 535–41.

65 Kubota K, Matsuzawa T, Amemiya A, *et al.* Imaging of breast cancer with F-18 fluorodeoxyglucose and positron emission tomography. *J Comput Assist Tomogr* 1989; **13**: 1097–8.

66 Wahl RL, Cody RL, Hutchins GD, *et al.* Primary and metastatic breast carcinoma: initial clinical evaluation with PET with the radiolabeled glucose analogue 2-[F-18]-fluoro-2-deoxy-D-glucose. *Radiology* 1991; **179**: 765–70.

67 Avril N, Rose CA, Schelling M, *et al.* Breast imaging with positron emission tomography and fluorine-18 fluorodeoxyglucose: use and limitations. *J Clin Oncol* 2000; **18**: 3495–502.

68 Avril N, Dose J, Jänicke F, *et al.* Metabolic characterization of breast tumors with positron emission tomography using F-18 fluorodeoxyglucose. *J Clin Oncol* 1996; **14**: 1848–57.

69 Schirrmeister H, Kuhn T, Guhlmann A, *et al.* Fluorine-18 2-deoxy-2-fluoro-D-glucose PET in the preoperative staging of breast cancer: comparison with the standard staging procedures. *Eur J Nucl Med* 2001; **28**: 351–8.

70 Goerres GW, Michel SC, Fehr MK, *et al.* Follow-up of women with breast cancer: comparison between MRI and FDG PET. *Eur Radiol* 2003; **13**: 1635–44.

71 Baslaim MM, Bakheet SM, Bakheet R, *et al.* 18-Fluorodeoxyglucose-positron emission tomography in inflammatory breast cancer. *World J Surg* 2003; **27**: 1099–104.

72 Crippa F, Seregni E, Agresti R, *et al.* Association between F-18 fluorodeoxyglucose uptake and post-operative histopathology, hormone receptor status, thymidine labelling index and p53 in primary breast cancer: a preliminary observation. *Eur J Nucl Med* 1998; **25**: 1429–34.

73 Krecke KN, Gisvold JJ. Invasive lobular carcinoma of the breast: mammographic findings and extent of disease at diagnosis in 184 patients. *Am J Roentgenol* 1993; **161**: 957–60.

74 Gilles R, Guinebretière J-M, Lucidarme O, *et al.* Nonpalpable breast tumors: diagnosis with contrast-enhanced subtraction dynamic MR imaging. *Radiology* 1994; **191**: 625–31.

75 Paramagul CP, Helvie MA, Adler DD. Invasive lobular carcinoma: sonographic appearance and role of sonography in improving diagnostic sensitivity. *Radiology* 1995; **195**: 231–4.

76 Tse NY, Hoh CK, Hawkins RA, *et al.* The application of positron emission tomographic imaging with fluorodeoxyglucose to the evaluation of breast disease. *Ann Surg* 1992; **216**: 27–34.

77 Vranjesevic D, Schiepers C, Silverman DH, *et al.* Relationship between ^{18}F-FDG uptake and breast density in women with normal breast tissue. *J Nucl Med* 2003; **44**: 1238–42.

78 Sacre RA. Clinical evaluation of axillar lymph nodes compared to surgical and pathological findings. *Eur J Surg Oncol* 1986; **12**: 169–73.

79 Veronesi U, Paganelli G, Galimberti V, *et al.* Sentinel-node biopsy to avoid axillary dissection in breast cancer with clinically negative lymph-nodes. *Lancet* 1997; **349**: 1864–7.

80 Greco M, Crippa F, Agresti R, *et al.* Axillary lymph node staging in breast cancer by 2-fluoro-2-deoxy-D-glucose-positron emission tomography: clinical evaluation and alternative management. *J Natl Cancer Inst* 2001; **93**: 630–5.

81 Torrenga H, Licht J, van der Hoeven JJ, *et al.* Axillary lymph node staging in breast cancer by 2-fluoro-2-deoxy-D-glucose-positron emission tomography: clinical evaluation and alternative management. *J Natl Cancer Inst* 2001; **93**: 1659–61.

82 Avril N, Dose J, Jänicke F, *et al.* Assessment of axillary lymph node involvement in breast cancer patients with positron emission tomography using radiolabeled 2-(fluorine-18)-fluoro-2-deoxy-D-glucose. *J Natl Cancer Inst* 1996; **88**: 1204–9.

83 Wahl RL, Siegel BA, Coleman RE, *et al.* Prospective multicenter study of axillary nodal staging by positron emission tomography in breast cancer: a report of the staging breast cancer with PET Study Group. *J Clin Oncol* 2004; **22**: 277–85.

84 Kelemen PR, Lowe V, Phillips N. Positron emission tomography and sentinel lymph node dissection in breast cancer. *Clin Breast Cancer* 2002; **3**: 73–7.

85 Fehr MK, Hornung R, Varga Z, *et al.* Axillary staging using positron emission tomography in breast cancer patients qualifying for sentinel lymph node biopsy. *Breast J* 2004; **10**: 89–93.

86 Barranger E, Grahek D, Antoine M, *et al.* Evaluation of fluorodeoxyglucose positron emission tomography in the detection of axillary lymph node metastases in patients with early-stage breast cancer. *Ann Surg Oncol* 2003; **10**: 622–7.

87 Eubank WB, Mankoff DA, Takasugi J, *et al.* [18]Fluorodeoxyglucose positron emission tomography to detect mediastinal or internal mammary metastases in breast cancer. *J Clin Oncol* 2001; **19**: 3516–23.

88 Bender H, Kirst J, Palmedo H, *et al.* Value of F-18 fluorodeoxyglucose positron emission tomography in the staging of recurrent breast carcinoma. *Anticancer Res* 1997; **17**: 1687–92.

89 Moon DH, Maddahi J, Silverman DH, *et al.* Accuracy of whole-body fluorine-18-FDG PET for the detection of recurrent or metastatic breast carcinoma. *J Nucl Med* 1998; **39**: 431–5.

90 Dose J, Bleckmann C, Bachmann S, *et al.* Comparison of fluorodeoxyglucose positron emission tomography and 'conventional diagnostic procedures' for the detection of distant metastases in breast cancer patients. *Nucl Med Commun* 2002; **23**: 857–64.

91 Gallowitsch HJ, Kresnik E, Gasser J, *et al.* F-18 fluoro-deoxyglucose positron-emission tomography in the diagnosis of tumor recurrence and metastases in the follow-up of patients with breast carcinoma: a comparison to conventional imaging. *Invest Radiol* 2003; **38**: 250–6.

92 Siggelkow W, Zimny M, Faridi A, *et al.* The value of positron emission tomography in the follow-up for breast cancer. *Anticancer Res* 2003; **23**: 1859–67.

93 van der Hoeven JJ, Krak NC, Hoekstra OS, *et al.* ^{18}F-2-fluoro-2-deoxy-D-glucose positron emission tomography in staging of locally advanced breast cancer. *J Clin Oncol* 2004; **22**: 1253–9.

94 Hathaway PB, Mankoff DA, Maravilla KR, *et al.* Value of combined FDG PET and MR imaging in the evaluation of suspected recurrent local-regional breast cancer: preliminary experience. *Radiology* 1999; **210**: 807–14.

95 Ahmad A, Barrington S, Maisey M, *et al.* Use of positron emission tomography in evaluation of brachial plexopathy in breast cancer patients. *Br J Cancer* 1999; **79**: 478–82.

96 Cook GJ, Houston S, Rubens R, *et al.* Detection of bone metastases in breast cancer by F-18 FDG PET: differing metabolic activity in osteoblastic and osteolytic lesions. *J Clin Oncol* 1998; **16**: 3375–9.

97 Yang SN, Liang JA, Lin FJ, *et al.* Comparing whole body (18)F-2-deoxyglucose positron emission tomography and technetium-99m methylene diphosphonate bone scan to detect bone metastases in patients with breast cancer. *J Cancer Res Clin Oncol* 2002; **128**: 325–8.

98 Ohta M, Tokuda Y, Suzuki Y, *et al.* Whole body PET for the evaluation of bony metastases in patients with breast cancer: comparison with ^{99}Tc^{m}-MDP bone scintigraphy. *Nucl Med Commun* 2001; **22**: 875–9.

99 Townsend DW, Carney JP, Yap JT, *et al.* PET/CT today and tomorrow. *J Nucl Med* 2004; **45**: 4–14S.

100 Wahl RL, Zasadny K, Helvie M, *et al.* Metabolic monitoring of breast cancer chemohormonotherapy using positron emission tomography: initial evaluation. *J Clin Oncol* 1993; **11**: 2101–11.

101 Jansson T, Westlin JE, Ahlstrom H, *et al.* Positron emission tomography studies in patients with locally advanced and/or metastatic breast cancer: a method for early therapy evaluation? *J Clin Oncol* 1995; **13**: 1470–7.

102 Smith IC, Welch AE, Hutcheon AW, *et al.* Positron emission tomography using [(18)F]-fluorodeoxy-D-glucose to predict the pathologic response of breast cancer to primary chemotherapy. *J Clin Oncol* 2000; **18**: 1676–88.

103 Schelling M, Avril N, Nährig J, *et al.* Positron emission tomography using [F-18]fluorodeoxyglucose for monitoring primary chemotherapy in breast cancer. *J Clin Oncol* 2000; **18**: 1689–95.

104 Mankoff DA, Dunnwald LK, Gralow JR, *et al*. Changes in blood flow and metabolism in locally advanced breast cancer treated with neoadjuvant chemotherapy. *J Nucl Med* 2003; **44**: 1806–14.

105 Dehdashti F, Flanagan FL, Mortimer JE, *et al*. Positron emission tomographic assessment of 'metabolic flare' to predict response of metastatic breast cancer to antiestrogen therapy. *Eur J Nucl Med* 1999; **26**: 51–6.

106 Mortimer JE, Dehdashti F, Siegel BA, *et al*. Metabolic flare: indicator of hormone responsiveness in advanced breast cancer. *J Clin Oncol* 2001; **19**: 2797–803.

107 Stafford SE, Gralow JR, Schubert EK, *et al*. Use of serial FDG PET to measure the response of bone-dominant breast cancer to therapy. *Acad Radiol* 2002; **9**: 913–21.

Breast disease: Single photon and positron emission tomography

JOHN BUSCOMBE

INTRODUCTION

Breast imaging has become an important part of the use of nuclear medicine in oncology. New techniques have evolved in both the diagnosis and staging of breast cancer. There have been advances in both single photon and positron emission tomography (PET) techniques. However, there has been concern that these methods have not become widely adopted, maybe with the exception of sentinel node studies which in many centers is considered routine. The reason for this remains unclear, possibly related to established practice and imaging pathways but also nuclear medicine has not developed in a vacuum and there have been advances in digital mammography, ultrasound with power Doppler and magnetic resonance imaging (MRI) over the past 10 years. All these have competed for the attention of the breast care physician/surgeon.

SCINTIMAMMOGRAPHY

Scintimammography was a term coined by Professor Iraj Khalkhali, a breast and nuclear medicine radiologist working in UCLA Torrance in California. It is a method by which the breast may be imaged using functional nuclear medicine techniques. Though previous groups had attempted to use cancer-localizing radiopharmaceuticals before[1,2] the results had been disappointing. The reason for this was all too clear and demonstrated a clear lack of understanding of anatomy. Nuclear medicine imaging is

traditionally performed with the patient supine. In women, especially those who are older, part of the breast tissue on the right will tend to overly the liver and on the left the heart. This is important as almost all the cancer localizing agents available rely on the increased metabolic turnover of the cancer to have higher uptake than surrounding normal tissues. As both the liver and heart are metabolically active tissues they will have uptake physiologically of the same agents. Also, excretion of these radiopharmaceuticals, at least in part, tends to be via the liver.[1,2] This means that it may not be possible to see a small tumor overlying the heart or liver.

Professor Khalkhali and his senior technologist, Linda Diggles, had the idea of prone imaging. Using a board with a cut-out the breast being imaged drops away from the chest wall by gravity and allows a clear lateral image of the breast tissue to be performed.[3] The opposite breast is compressed and out of the field of view. The board is then turned round and the contralateral breast imaged. Recently, more comfortable scintimammography mattresses have been developed. Therefore the imaging position is similar to that obtained in breast MRI and the 'Mammotest' system.

The radiopharmaceuticls used have included thallium-201 chloride, ^{99m}Tc-sestamibi and ^{99m}Tc-tetrofosmin. Most work has been done with the latter two agents and they appear to produce similar results.[4] As the image quality using the ^{99m}Tc agents is much better than thallium, as are the clinical results, it is recommended that these are the radiopharmaceuticals which should be used.

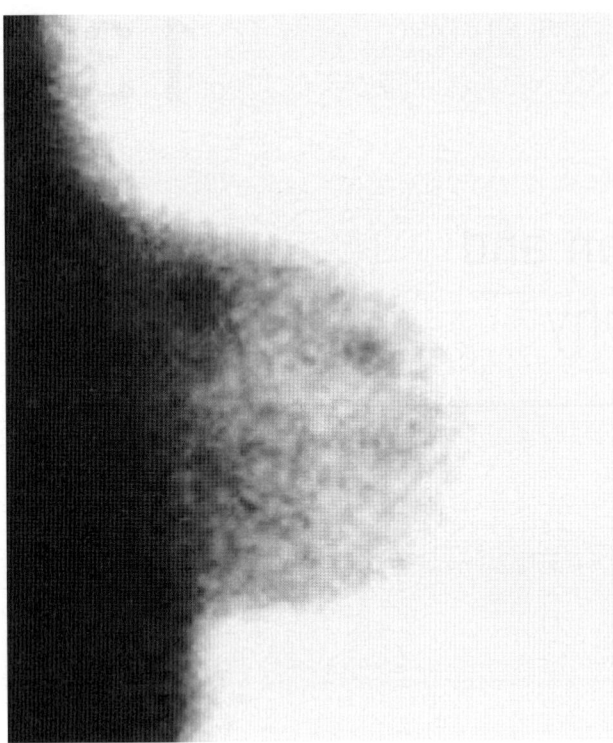

Figure 13B.1 *Prone lateral view of the right breast performed 25 min after injection of 740 MBq of* ^{99m}*Tc-MIBI showing two sites of breast cancer in the upper half of the breast, the larger being close to the chest wall: both were missed on X-ray mammography.*

Results

Scintimammography has proved to be a robust and consistent imaging system. Two multicenter trials have been performed and multiple single-center trials.[4–12] In single-center trials, where scans are normally read with some clinical knowledge of the patient, sensitivities of 90% can be obtained (Fig. 13B.1). In the multicenter trials the overall sensitivities tend to be less but all reading was performed using readers blinded to all clinical information. As both breasts are imaged in the protocol they were even unaware of which side was meant to contain the suspect lesion. From the North American study it was also noted that there was a high level of agreement between readers of the scintimammography scans.[12] There appears to be some limitations to the technique. It is better at finding small ductal carcinomas and less good at identifying lobular and papillary cancers.[13] Smaller cancers (less than 10 mm) may be missed by the technique,[11,12] although we have been able to find invasive ductal carcinomas of 5 mm and even less. It is also possible to identify carcinoma *in situ* and it appears to find over 90% of such tumors. This compares well with mammography where a carcinoma *in situ* may not calcify and be missed.[14]

How to perform scintimammography

The technique itself is fairly simple and involves the injection of a tumor-seeking radiopharmaceutical. The most commonly used agent is ^{99m}Tc-sestamibi[15–17] which is licensed for breast imaging in the USA and most EU countries. An alternative method has been to use a similar radiopharmaceutical, ^{99m}Tc-tetrofosmin. Early indications are that there is little difference between the two agents[17,18] but most experience has been gathered with ^{99m}Tc-sestamibi. Therefore, unless stated otherwise, the term scintimammography will refer to the use of ^{99m}Tc-sestamibi.

We recommend the use of a foot vein injection, the reason being that any extravasated activity in the arm can lodge in axillary lymph nodes giving a false positive result.

The patient is then taken to the special imaging mattress and lies prone, with the breast being imaged pendulent. A lateral image is performed with the contralateral breast either compressed against the mattress or shielded by a lead insert. Imaging is normally performed for 10 min, and this is followed by a 2–3 min view with a ^{99m}Tc or ^{57}Co marker placed on the nipple. The other breast is then imaged. Finally the mattress is removed and the patient has an image performed lying supine with arms elevated above the head so that the axillary tail and axilla can be seen.

When displaying the images, the influence of the counts in the chest and liver are reduced using a logarithmic scale or truncation. Finally, it may be possible, depending on the computer system available, to provide a zoomed image of the breasts. These can all be displayed on a single film.

When to use scintimammography?

Breast imaging is an emotive topic, clearly there are social and psychological implications to promoting a new technique and, as such, scintimammography should be seen not as a method which stands alone but one that complements the imaging arm of the standard triple assessment of the patient with a suspected breast cancer. In a retrospective review of over 350 patients, we have shown that adding scintimammography to mammography can improve the sensitivity of breast imaging from 69 to 93%.[19] Using receiver operator characteristic (ROC) curve analysis it was shown that this could be done whilst maintaining a specificity of just under 80%. However, whilst this study reflected the clinical use of scintimammography it must be noted that the patients studied were highly selected as they where those in whom the results of mammography (and ultrasound) had been inconclusive or the triple assessment had been discordant and further information was required. Would there be any advantage if used in a group of all patients in a prospective trial? The answer is clearly yes. In a study from Sweden it was shown that the sensitivity of both triple assessment and scintimammography were similar.[20] However, the greatest advantage was in those patients with mammographically dense breasts where using a combination of triple assessment and scintimammography found all cancers. Therefore clearly in any patient in whom there is doubt about the results of mammography or triple assessment scintimammography provides added value.

Other areas where scintimammography may be of use

As uptake of ^{99m}Tc-sestamibi is increased in both invasive cancer and carcinoma *in situ*, it may offer increased sensitivity in finding ductal and lobular carcinoma *in situ* (DCIS and LCIS). There is a single comparison published, in patients with pure DCIS or LCIS, which showed that mammography found 53% of DCIS and LCIS, the tumors missed being those without calcification.[14] ^{99m}Tc-sestamibi alone found 80% and, when combined, 93% of all DCIS and LCIS were found. This work must be confirmed in larger studies but clearly this may be an area in which scintimammography may have a significant role to play. It is not uncommon, especially in younger women, for there to be sites of DCIS around an invasive tumor. These areas may be easily seen on scintimammography. Therefore, clearly, it may be possible to identify multicentric or multifocal tumor. In a single-site study a retrospective survey was performed in 40 women who had undergone mastectomy, mammography, and scintimammography.[21] There were 40 patients with multiple tumor sites. Mammography identified cancer in 67% of these patients but only found the multiple sites of tumor in 25%. Scintimammography was positive in 92% of the cancers and identified the multifocal or multicentric nature of the cancer in 58%. Though this figure is not as high as would be wished it still offers a significant advantage over mammography alone and could result in significant changes in surgical management. It may also be of use in situations where use of mammography is problematical such as around a breast prosthesis (Fig. 13B.2).

Possible recurrence

This is another area of potential use of scintimammography in patients with smaller cancers who have been offered breast conservation surgery. Normally, it would be expected that there would be a recurrence rate of 1–5% per annum.[22–25] The latter figure would mean that by 5 years 25% of all women could have recurrence. There is a difficulty in diagnosis, however. Previous surgery and radiotherapy can distort mammography and ultrasound, and increased signal occurs on MRI from the post-surgical and post-radiotherapy breast. Therefore a method such as scintimammography which does not depend on breast anatomy would be ideal. There have been case reports of uptake of ^{99m}Tc-sestamibi in recurrence.[26] However, there is only one good comparative study. When looking at 63 women with suspected recurrence it was found that mammography and ultrasound were insensitive in finding recurrence; the sensitivity was 53%.[27] However, scintimammography was able to find 78%. The combination of both tests were able to find 90% of breast recurrences, a doubling of sensitivity over mammography and ultrasound. There has been some work showing that the cost

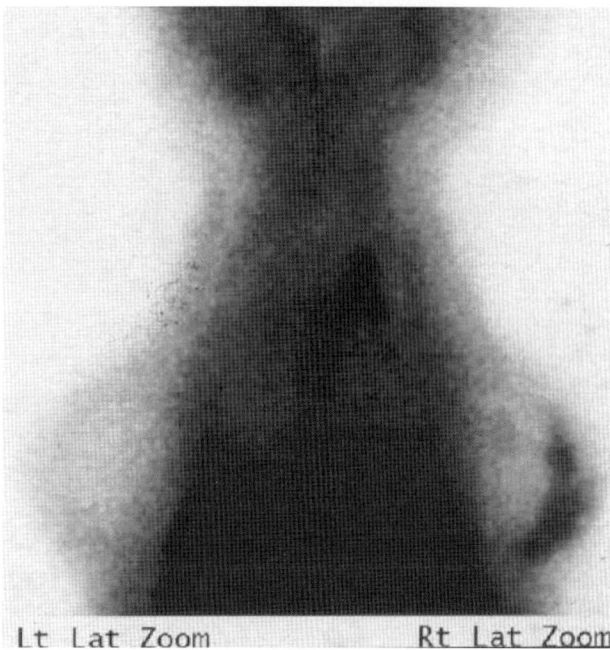

Figure 13B.2 *Both prone lateral views of a woman of 33 years with bilateral cosmetic breast implants showing intense uptake of ^{99m}Tc-MIBI in an extensive breast cancer in the right breast.*

per cancer found is cheaper by 33% if scintimammography is used as the first test.[28] In addition to recurrence within the breast, abnormal additional information is found in 60% of patients about axillary and loco-regional recurrence[27] (Fig. 13B.3).

Use of scintimammography in locally advanced breast cancer

Patients with locally advanced breast cancer (LABC) (normally T3 or T4) are often treated with neo-adjuvant chemotherapy. It may be difficult to assess the response to treatment as the tumor can be replaced by fibrous tissue, therefore affecting the results of palpation and mammography.[29] Scintigraphic techniques using a variety of tracers have been found to be of use in this scenario.[30,31] Therefore, it is logical to look at paired ^{99m}Tc-sestamibi scintimammography scans performed before and after the last cycle of chemotherapy. There was additional interest as it was known that ^{99m}Tc-sestamibi acted as a substrate for P-glycoptrotein (Pgp) which is encoded by the multi-drug resistance gene type 1 (*MDR1*).[32] Therefore it may be possible that the induction of *MDR1* would be seen, resulting in an efflux of the ^{99m}Tc-MIBI from the cells, rather than a response to therapy.

However, work on small numbers of patients has shown a good correlation between a reduction of uptake of ^{99m}Tc-sestamibi and the pathological response to chemotherapy.[33,34] Therefore it seems that ^{99m}Tc-sestamibi is able to monitor closely the effect of chemotherapy on LABC.

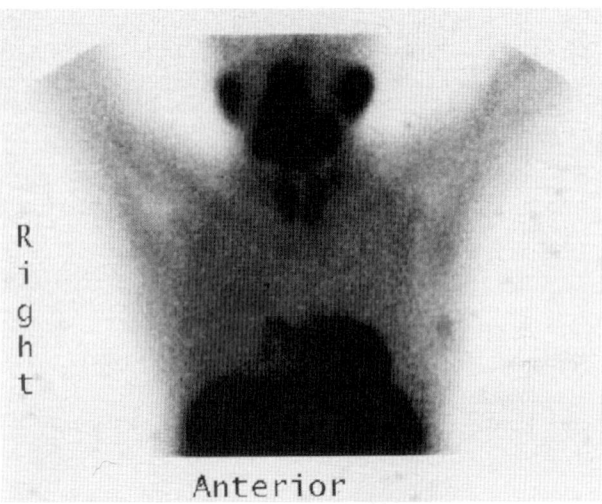

Figure 13B.3 *Anterior view of a ^{99m}Tc-MIBI scintimammography in a patient who had a wide local excision of a right breast cancer 3 years before. Focal uptake consistent with axillary nodal recurrence can be seen on the right side. However, unexpected and not seen on mammography was the new cancer in the outer part of the left breast.*

Could this method be used to predict response? A group from the USA has shown that ^{99m}Tc-sestamibi imaging before chemotherapy, and after the second cycle, was a good predictor of response. All patients where the uptake of ^{99m}Tc-sestamibi increased between the first and second scan had evidence for disease progression at 6 months. If uptake dropped by 40% between the two scans then 89% showed a good pathological response.[35] If the results of this study can be confirmed by a multicenter trial it may be possible to use sestamibi to predict response so that an increasing amount of ^{99m}Tc-sestamibi could result in changing the chemotherapy used or moving straight to surgery.

SENTINEL NODES

The sentinel node principle was first postulated by Morton in penile cancer and has since spread into melanoma and breast care. The reason why sentinel node studies are so important is that they provide information on staging the axilla without a high level of morbidity. It has been shown that in women with tumors of less than 2.5 cm only 10% of axillae contain lymph nodes which contain cancer. Therefore the vast majority of patients will undergo unnecessary axillary clearance which can result in lymphedema, arm pain, and stiffness. To try to reduce this possibility the Morton principle will state that the first draining lymph node (the sentinel) will collect cancer cells before any other lymph nodes; conversely, if there are no cancer cells in the sentinel lymph node there is little chance

that there is cancer elsewhere and no further treatment is needed.

Dye or radioactivity

Much of the original work on sentinel nodes was performed using methylene blue injected intratumorally or peritumorally about 30 min pre-operatively. During the operation the lymphatic channels to the axilla are identified and the first hopefully blue node seen is removed and assessed. This technique has been able to identify a sentinel node in around 90% of cases.[36–38] Using techniques developed in melanoma, radiocolloids were then used, initially injected intratumorally but more recently both peritumorally and subdermally. Imaging could be performed to identify any sentinel node which could take 1–4 h depending on a number of factors including the size of the colloid used and injection site. Then intraoperatively a probe is used to identify the node with the highest level of radioactivity. This is then removed and examined as the sentinel node. Using this technique it has been possible to achieve accuracies of 98% though there is a significant learning curve and this technique should only be performed in centers with sufficient training and throughput of patients to maintain competence.[39] Most observers now agree a combination of both techniques yields the fastest and most accurate method by which to find sentinel nodes within the axilla.

Technical points

There are many requirements for good practice in breast sentinel node localization but they are simple to follow and should allow singular success. The first and most important factor is that this is a team approach needing the participation of breast surgeon, breast radiologist (to help identify sites of nonpalpable tumor), physicists, technical staff, operating room staff, and pathologists. If all are trained and competent the technique becomes simple and reproducible. The type of probe used should be optimized to ^{99m}Tc with a collimator to prevent side-shine from activity at the injection site being picked up by the probe. Surgeons tend to favor a probe with an angled head and about 1–2 cm diameter. It should be light and well balanced to aid its use. There are electrical safety factors as these probes will be in contact with body fluids and it may be important to know who will deal with adjacent diathermy. The size of injection has been varied over time[40,41] but most users agree that a small volume (<0.5 mL) seems optimal. The site of injection may have a lesser bearing on the result, although intratumoral injections may result in slower clearance of tracer and a prolonged study. There is also some question of seeding along the track of the needle if an intratumoral injection is used. Other groups have reported an increased number of internal mammary nodes seen with intra- or peritumoral injections compared to subdermal injections

Controversies

Like many new techniques there remains some controversy as to the optimal method. However, when looking at published results it is clear that any method should be at least 95% accurate. It is important that each center, after training, sets up an audit system so that it is possible to determine if that particular center is obtaining and maintaining standards.

The main discussion has been over the type of colloid used. The problem being that there is no colloid that has been designed for the purpose of breast sentinel node localization.[42] The smaller the colloid, the faster it will run through the lymphatics and reach the sentinel node, but it may well have a short residency within that node, especially if less than 200 nm in diameter. This means that if operation is delayed for more than 6 h it may be possible that the sentinel node no longer contains the highest counts. This may mean that a number of nodes are identified and removed, one of which is the true sentinel node.[43] Imaging will assist in this process as it may be possible to track the colloid and warn the surgeon if it is likely the sentinel node is no longer the most active. Larger colloids (>500 nm) have been suggested as they tend to stick in the sentinel node and not pass through. This means that any operation can be delayed for up to 20 h with reasonable results. This would allow the operation to be performed the morning after injection and imaging. The choice of colloid, at present however, is actually made for the clinician as normally one or two types are available, and the availability changes country by country.

There have been discussions about when the operation should be performed, but once there is an understanding of how each type of colloid runs it is easier to work out when the operation should be performed. This may mean the way nuclear medicine works will have to change to accommodate the requirements of the surgical team.

The methods used to assess the histology of the removed sentinel nodes has also provide much debate.[44] Some centers will perform a 'frozen section' and the result, if positive, will result in a full axillary clearance. Other centers will look at the stained specimens, often with immunohistochemistry, and any further required operation will occur on a separate occasion.

Since its inception sentinel node scintigraphy has shown much more about the lymph drainage of the breast than was previously known. The drainage can be both variable and not logical. In small numbers of patients drainage to the contralateral axilla and to internal mammary nodes have been noted. Whilst these are clearly interesting there are few clinical protocols designed to deal with these anomalies. The anomalies seem more common in multicentric tumors and those with vascular invasion.[45]

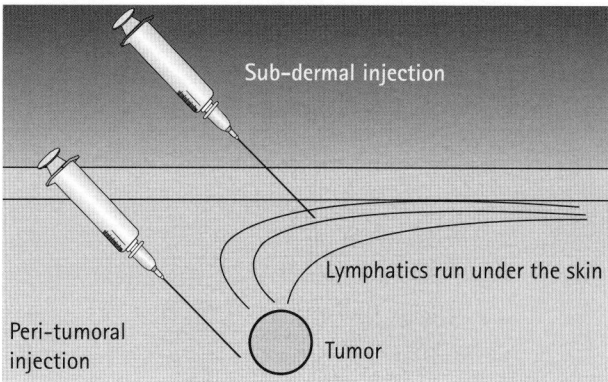

Figure 13B.4 *Cartoon showing the site for subdermal and peritumoral injection in sentinel node localization.*

There is some evidence that the classical subdermal or peritumoral approach may not work in patients who have had recent or significant breast surgery, chemotherapy or radiotherapy, or may have multifocal disease.[46] This multifocal disease can be identified by ^{99m}Tc-MIBI, PET or MRI. Some workers have suggested, however, that a peri-areolar technique may be useful in these circumstances and even advocate it for all sentinel nodes.[47]

Practical protocol

A typical protocol for a breast sentinel node scintigraphy includes the following. The patient should be prepared by receiving a full explanation of the test. With them sitting in a comfortable position about 0.4 mL containing 30–40 MBq of ^{99m}Tc-colloid is injected subdermally or peritumorally. For subdermal injection (Fig. 13B.4) we find an insulin syringe works best. If the lesion is nonpalpable the injection may need to be done under ultrasound control. After injection the area is gently massaged for 1–2 min. Imaging then commences, ensuring that the breast, ipsilateral axilla, and the sternum are all in the field of view. Imaging should continue until the sentinel node is seen. We image with the arm abducted by 90° as this is the position during the operation. It may be helpful to place a small lead shield over the injection site to aid imaging but remember the sentinel node may be no more than 1–2 cm from the primary cancer in lateral lesions. Anterior and lateral oblique images are best. The skin over any sentinel node found is then marked to aid the surgeon. Images are performed and a 'shadowgram' using a ^{60}Co source or very low activity ^{99m}Tc flood source is performed with the patient between the source and the gamma camera (Fig. 13B.5). The patient will attenuate the gamma rays from the flood source so an outline of the patient and, hopefully, the sentinel node appears.

Once in the operating room methylene blue dye is injected. A small insicion is made over the suspected lymphatic channel which is blue in color. This is then followed

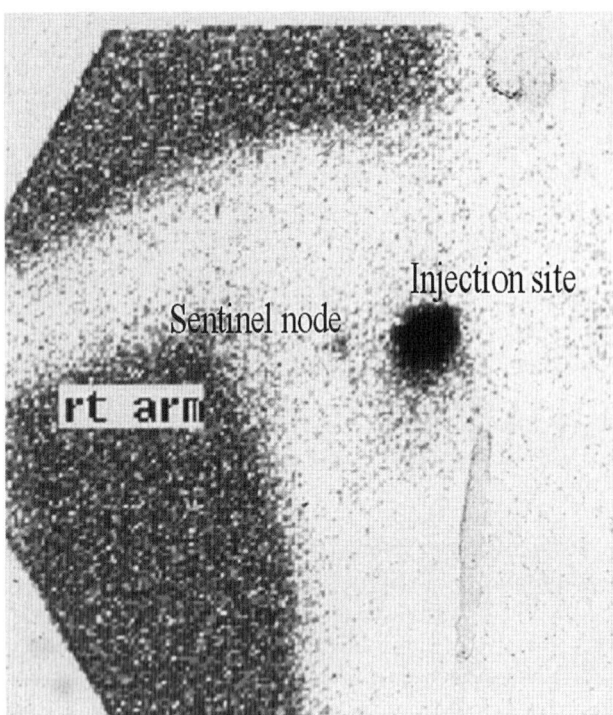

Figure 13B.5 *'Shadowgram' showing injection of colloid around a cancer near the axillary tail of the right breast and subsequent sentinel node adjacent to the tumor.*

by the probe until the radioactive lymph node is found and removed.

RADIONUCLIDE OCCULT LESION LOCALIZATION

Using the intraoperative probe it should be possible to identify any site of injection. Therefore it has been shown that to localize a nonpalpable lesion in the breast about 0.3 mL of 10 MBq of ^{99m}Tc-macro-aggregated albumin (^{99m}Tc-MAA) with a size >1000 nm will stay at the injection site. This can be identified by the probe intra-operatively and the suspicious area excised. This has been shown to compare favorably with the Kopan's wire.[48]

RECEPTORS

Over the past 20 years there have been various attempts to image both primary and metastatic breast cancer using receptor-based imaging methods. About 70% of breast cancers may express somatostatin subtype 2 receptors allowing identification with ^{111}In-pentetreotide.[49] Antibody imaging using the CEA and human milk fat globulin (HMFG) targets have also been reported on[50] but these techniques have not proved to be clinically useful.

POSITRON EMISSION TOMOGRAPHY

Whilst there is no doubt that positron emission tomography (PET) is able to identify both primary and metastatic breast cancer with a high level of accuracy[51] its role in clinical care is less clear. PET is clearly able to image the whole body easily (though the head is often not imaged in most clinical scenarios) which may not be appropriate in breast as isolated brain metastasis is not uncommon. This enables the load of both soft tissue and bone disease to be clearly elucidated and would therefore be ideal both for staging, restaging, and looking at response to specific treatments. Again, the reason that PET has not been widely adopted appears to be more related to inertia to new techniques by the breast cancer clinicians than to technical reasons or the availability of PET.

Staging

There has been much work looking at the accuracy of ^{18}F-fluorodeoxyglucose (^{18}F-FDG) in accurately identifying axillary disease and allowing precise noninvasive staging as an alternative to intra-operative probing and other surgical techniques. Accuracies of about 90% have been reported in locoregional nodal disease.[52–54] False negatives occur with microinvasion of the lymph nodes. The clinical significance of these micrometastases remains unclear and clearly will only be identified by histological investigation of samples. Therefore ^{18}F-FDG PET may not fully replace sentinel node localization and probe localization but may be able to offer an alternative in those patients for whom an operation is not ideal. Outside the loco-regional area the ability to see both bone and soft tissue disease makes ^{18}F-FDG PET the optimal single staging method and, probably, much more accurate than chest X-ray and liver ultrasound, which is chosen in many centers for staging, not because it is accurate but because it is cheap.

Restaging

The evidence for restaging is probably less clear but this is an area where functional imaging is likely to have a higher utility as most patients with breast cancer have been treated with surgery, and some with chemotherapy, radiotherapy, and endocrine therapy, all of which may result in changes to the structure of the breast and surrounding tissues. In this situation the use of ^{18}F-FDG PET may be invaluable. Examples include the use of brachial flexopathy where it is important to differentiate tumor from fibrosis.

PET techniques have been used to monitor the effect of therapy, with changes in uptake, as measured by the standardized uptake value (SUV), being able to predict outcome to chemotherapy.[55] There has also been work to show that uptake of ^{18}F-FDG correlated closely with the concentration of mutant p53, which is related to the mechanism of chemo-resistance.[56]

^{18}F-FDG can be a nonspecific marker in PET and will have uptake at sites of inflammation, therefore it has been suggested that in some breast cancers there could be an inflammatory response to endocrine or chemotherapy. These inflammatory changes would result in non-tumor specific uptake of ^{18}F-FDG. To provide better imaging of active cancer cells ^{18}F-labeled estrogens such as ^{18}F-FES have shown a much closer correlation to final tumor response than ^{18}F-FDG alone.[57]

General nuclear medicine

Though this section has concentrated on tests that are specific for breast cancer, nuclear medicine may have a significant contact with breast cancer patients without any of the tests described above being used. Many patients will have bone scintigraphy, isotopic glomerular filtration rate analysis, and gated ventriculography in assessing efficacy and side-effects of treatment. We have found that in patients on endocrine manipulation bone densitometry is of use and in patients with painful bone metastasis radionuclide pain palliation can be offered.

CONCLUSION

Scintimammography has an increasing role in nuclear medicine: it can aid diagnosis and localization of breast cancer. It can be used to find multifocal, multicentric disease. It has a new role in loco-regional recurrence and in monitoring chemotherapy. PET may yet have a role but more evaluation is needed. Before too long it may be possible to use nuclear medicine techniques to both diagnose and treat some cancers.

REFERENCES

1 Lee VW, Sax EJ, McAneny DB, *et al*. A complementary role for thallium-201 scintigraphy with mammography in the diagnosis of breast cancer. *J Nucl Med* 1993; **34**: 2095–100.

2 Waxman AD, Ramanna L, Memsic LD, *et al*. Thallium scintigraphy in the evaluation of mass abnormalities of the breast. *J Nucl Med* 1993; **34**: 18–23.

3 Khalkhali I, Mena I, Diggles L. Review of imaging techniques for the diagnosis of breast cancer: a new role of prone scintimammography using technetium-99m sestamibi. *Eur J Nucl Med* 1994; **21**: 357–62.

4 Obwegeser R, Berghammer P, Rodrigues M, *et al*. A head-to-head comparison between technetium-99m-tetrofosmin and technetium-99m-MIBI scintigraphy to evaluate suspicious breast lesions. *Eur J Nucl Med* 1999; **26**: 1553–9.

5 Khalkhali I, Cutrone J, Mena I, *et al*. Technetium-99m-sestamibi scintimammography of breast lesions: clinical and pathological follow-up. *J Nucl Med* 1995; **36**: 1784–9.

6 Taillefer R, Robidoux A, Lambert R, Turpin S, Laperriere J. Technetium-99m-sestamibi prone scintimammography to detect primary breast cancer and axillary lymph node involvement. *J Nucl Med* 1995; **36**: 1758–65.

7 Tiling R, Sommer H, Pechmann M, *et al*. Comparison of technetium-99m-sestamibi scintimammography with contrast-enhanced MRI for diagnosis of breast lesions. *J Nucl Med* 1997; **38**: 58–62.

8 Prats E, Carril J, Herranz R, *et al*. A Spanish multicenter scintigraphic study of the breast using Tc 99m MIBI. Report of results. *Rev Esp Med Nucl* 1998; **17**: 338–50.

9 Paz A, Melloul M, Cytron S, *et al*. The value of early and double phase [99]Tcm-sestamibi scintimammography in the diagnosis of breast cancer. *Nucl Med Commun* 2000; **21**: 341–8.

10 Prats E, Aisa F, Abos MD, *et al*. Mammography and ^{99m}Tc-MIBI scintimammography in suspected breast cancer. *J Nucl Med* 1999; **40**: 296–301.

11 Palmedo H, Biersack HJ, Lastoria S, *et al*. Scintimammography with technetium-99m methoxy-isobutylisonitrile: results of a prospective European multicentre trial. *Eur J Nucl Med* 1998; **25**: 375–85.

12 Khalkhali I, Villanueva-Meyer J, Edell SL, *et al*. Diagnostic accuracy of ^{99m}Tc-sestamibi breast imaging: multicenter trial results. *J Nucl Med* 2000; **41**: 1973–9.

13 Buscombe JR, Cwikla JB, Thakrar DS, Hilson AJ. Uptake of Tc-99m MIBI related to tumour size and type. *Anticancer Res* 1997; **17**: 1693–4.

14 Cwikla JB, Buscombe, JR, Hilson AJW. Detection of DCIS using Tc-99m MIBI scintimammography in patients with suspected primary breast cancer, compared with conventional mammography. *Nuc Med Review* 2000; **3**: 41–5.

15 Kabasakal L, Ozker K, Hayward M, *et al*. Technetium-99m sestamibi uptake in human breast carcinoma cell lines displaying glutathione-associated drug-resistance. *Eur J Nucl Med* 1996; **23**: 568–70.

16 Ballinger JR, Bannerman J, Boxen I, Firby P, Hartman NG, Moore MJ. Technetium-99m-tetrofosmin as a substrate for P-glycoprotein: in vitro studies in multidrug-resistant breast tumor cells. *J Nucl Med* 1996; **37**: 1578–82.

17 de Jong M, Bernard BF, Breeman WA, *et al*. Comparison of uptake of ^{99m}Tc-MIBI, ^{99m}Tc-tetrofosmin and ^{99m}Tc-Q12 into human breast cancer cell lines. *Eur J Nucl Med* 1996; **23**: 1361–6.

18 Rodrigues M, Chehne F, Kalinowska W, Berghammer P, Zielinski C, Sinzinger H. Uptake of ^{99m}Tc-MIBI and ^{99m}Tc-tetrofosmin into malignant versus nonmalignant breast cell lines. *J Nucl Med* 2000; **41**: 1495–9.

19 Buscombe JR, Cwikla JB, Holloway B, Hilson AJ. Prediction of the usefulness of combined mammography and scintimammography in suspected primary breast cancer using ROC curves. *J Nucl Med* 2001; **42**: 3–8.

20 Danielsson R, Reihner E, Grabowska A, Bone B. The role of scintimammography with ^{99m}Tc-sestamibi as a complementary diagnostic in the detection of breast cancer. *Acta Radiol* 2000; 41: 441–5.

21 Cwikla JB, Kolasinska AD, Buscombe JR, *et al.* Detecting multiple sites of primary breast cancer with Tc-99m MIBI. *Eur J Nucl Med* 2000; **27**: 928.

22 Clark RM, Whelan T, Levine M, *et al.* Randomized clinical trial of breast irradiation following lumpectomy and axillary dissection for node-negative breast cancer: an update. Ontario Clinical Oncology Group. *J Natl Cancer Inst* 1996; **88**: 1659–64.

23 Tartter PI, Kaplan J, Bleiweiss I, *et al.* Lumpectomy margins, reexcision, and local recurrence of breast cancer. *Am J Surg* 2000; **179**: 81–5.

24 Halyard MY, Grado GL, Schomberg PJ, *et al.* Conservative therapy of breast cancer. The Mayo Clinic experience. *Am J Clin Oncol* 1996; **19**: 445–50.

25 van Dongen JA, Voogd AC, Fentiman IS, *et al.* Long-term results of a randomized trial comparing breast-conserving therapy with mastectomy European Organization for Research and Treatment of Cancer 10801 trial. *J Natl Cancer Inst* 2000; **92**: 1143–50.

26 Buscombe JR, Cwikla JB, Thakrar DS, Parbhoo SP, Hilson AJ. Prone SPET scintimammography. *Nucl Med Commun* 1999; **20**: 237–45.

27 Cwikla JB, Kolasinska A, Buscombe JR, Hilson AJ. Tc-99m MIBI in suspected recurrent breast cancer. Cancer Biother Radiopharm 2000; **15**: 367–72.

28 Kolasinska AD, Cwikla JB, Buscombe JR, *et al.* Scintimammography: the most cost effective way to find breast cancer recurrence after mastectomy. *Eur J Nucl Med* 2000; **27**: 984.

29 Huber S, Wagner M, Zuna I, *et al.* Locally advanced breast carcinoma: evaluation of mammography in the prediction of residual disease after induction chemotherapy. *Anticancer Res* 2000; **20**: 553–8.

30 Sumiya H, Taki J, Tsuchiya H, *et al.* Midcourse thallium-201 scintigraphy to predict tumor response in bone and soft-tissue tumors. *J Nucl Med* 1998; **39**: 1600–4.

31 Romer W, Hanauske AR, Ziegler S, *et al.* Positron emission tomography in non-Hodgkin's lymphoma: assessment of chemotherapy with fluorodeoxyglucose. Blood 1998; **91**: 4464–71.

32 Holmes JA, West RR. The effect of MDR-1 gene expression on outcome in acute myeloblastic leukaemia. *Br J Cancer* 1994; **69**: 382–4.

33 Cwikla JB, Buscombe JR, Barlow RV, *et al.* The effect of chemotherapy on the uptake of technetium-99m sestamibi in breast cancer. *Eur J Nucl Med* 1997; **24**: 1175–8.

34 Reyes R, Parbhoo SP, Cwikla JB, *et al.* The role of scintimammography in prediction of response to primary chemotherapy. *Eur J Cancer* 2000; **36**: S136.

35 Mankoff DA, Dunnwald LK, Gralow JR, *et al.* Monitoring the response of patients with locally advanced breast carcinoma to neoadjuvant chemotherapy using [technetium 99m]-sestamibi scintimammography. *Cancer* 1999; **85**: 2410–23.

36 Giuliano AE, Kirgan DM, Guenther JM, Morton DL. Lymphatic mapping and sentinel lymphadenectomy for breast cancer. *Ann Surg* 1997; **225**: 126–7.

37 Veronesi U, Paganelli G, Galimberti V, *et al.* Sentinel-node biopsy to avoid axillary dissection in breast cancer with clinically negative lymph-nodes. *Lancet* 1997; **349**: 1864–7.

38 Tanis PJ, Nieweg OE, Valdes Olmos RA, Hoefnagel CA. An original approach in the diagnosis of early breast cancer: use of the same radiopharmaceutical for both non-palpable lesions and sentinel node localisation. *Eur J Nucl Med Mol Imaging* 2002; **29**: 436–7.

39 Krag D, Weaver D, Ashikaga T, *et al.* The sentinel node in breast cancer – a multicenter validation study. *N Engl J Med* 1998; **339**: 941–6.

40 Gulec SA, Moffat FL, Carroll RG, *et al.* Sentinel lymph node localization in early breast cancer. *J Nucl Med* 1998; **39**: 1388–93.

41 De Cicco C, Chinol M, Paganelli G. Intraoperative localization of the sentinel node in breast cancer: technical aspects of lymphoscintigraphic methods. *Semin Surg Oncol* 1998; **15**: 268–71.

42 Mariani G, Erba P, Villa G, *et al.* Lymphoscintigraphic and intraoperative detection of the sentinel lymph node in breast cancer patients: the nuclear medicine perspective. *J Surg Oncol* 2004; **85**: 112–22.

43 Paganelli G, De Cicco C, Cremonesi M, *et al.* Optimized sentinel node scintigraphy in breast cancer. *Q J Nucl Med* 1998; **42**: 49–53.

44 Veronesi U, Zurrida S, Mazzarol G, Viale G. Extensive frozen section examination of axillary sentinel nodes to determine selective axillary dissection. *World J Surg* 2001; **25**: 806–8.

45 De Cicco C, Cremonesi M, Luini A, *et al.* Lymphoscintigraphy and radioguided biopsy of the sentinel axillary node in breast cancer. *J Nucl Med* 1998; **39**: 2080–4.

46 Cohen LF, Breslin TM, Kuerer HM, *et al.* Identification and evaluation of axillary sentinel lymph nodes in patients with breast carcinoma treated with neoadjuvant chemotherapy. *Am J Surg Pathol* 2000; **24**: 1266–72.

47 Pelosi E, Bello M, Giors M, *et al.* Sentinel lymph node detection in patients with early-stage breast cancer: comparison of periareolar and subdermal/peritumoral injection techniques. *J Nucl Med* 2004; **45**: 220–5.

48 De Cicco C, Pizzamiglio M, Trifiro G, *et al.* Radioguided occult lesion localisation (ROLL) and surgical biopsy in

breast cancer. Technical aspects. *Q J Nucl Med* 2002; **46**: 145–51.

49 Alberini JL, Meunier B, Denzler B, *et al.* Somatostatin receptor in breast cancer and axillary nodes: study with scintigraphy, histopathology and receptor autoradiography. *Breast Cancer Res Treat* 2000; **61**: 21–32.

50 Britton KE, Jan H, al-Yasi AR, *et al.* Efficacy of immunoscintigraphy for detection of lymph node metastases. *Recent Results Cancer Res* 2000; **57**: 3–11.

51 Eubank WB, Mankoff DA. Current and future uses of positron emission tomography in breast cancer imaging. *Semin Nucl Med* 2004; **34**: 224–40.

52 Crippa F, Gerali A, Alessi A, *et al.* FDG-PET for axillary lymph node staging in primary breast cancer. *Eur J Nucl Med Mol Imaging* 2004; **31(Suppl 1)**: S97–102.

53 Greco M, Crippa F, Agresti R, *et al.* Axillary lymph node staging in breast cancer by 2-fluoro-2-deoxy-D-glucose-positron emission tomography: clinical evaluation and alternative management. *J Natl Cancer Inst* 2001; **93**: 630–5.

54 Wahl RL, Siegel BA, Coleman RE, Gatsonis CG. PET Study Group. Prospective multicenter study of axillary nodal staging by positron emission tomography in breast cancer: a report of the staging breast cancer with PET Study Group. *J Clin Oncol* 2004; **22**: 277–85.

55 Stafford SE, Gralow JR, Schubert EK, *et al.* Use of serial FDG PET to measure the response of bone-dominant breast cancer to therapy. *Acad Radiol* 2002; **9**: 913–21.

56 Crippa F, Seregni E, Agresti R, *et al.* Association between [^{18}F]fluorodeoxyglucose uptake and postoperative histopathology, hormone receptor status, thymidine labelling index and p53 in primary breast cancer: a preliminary observation. *Eur J Nucl Med* 1998; **25**: 1429–34.

57 Mortimer JE, Dehdashti F, Siegel BA, *et al.* Metabolic flare: indicator of hormone responsiveness in advanced breast cancer. *J Clin Oncol* 2001; **19**: 2797–803.

Testicular tumors

SHARON F. HAIN

INTRODUCTION

Testicular tumors are a relatively uncommon cancer, representing only 1% of all tumors but are important as they constitute the commonest malignancy in young men and the incidence is increasing.[1] Vast improvements in management have been made over the past 20 years so that now 95% of patients are cured. The morbidity of this is high, however, and more recent efforts have focused on decreasing the cost to morbidity of the treatments. Imaging has always played a part in the assessment and follow-up of patients but is primarily based on anatomical imaging. The advances of positron emission tomography with functional imaging have added a new dimension to prognosis and assessment of these tumors.

DIAGNOSIS AND STAGING

The commonest presentation of testicular cancer is a lump in the testis which should be urgently referred for assessment by specialists and orchidectomy. Although histology can be complex the basic pathology of testicular cancer is the distinction between seminomas and non-seminomatous germ cell tumors. The presence of other factors such as vascular invasion or involvement of the rete testes (in seminoma) is also important for prognosis and management decisions. All patients should have serum tumor markers (alpha-fetoprotein, human chorionic gonadotrophin, and lactate dehydrogenase) measured as these help to determine prognosis, help assess response to treatment and assess long-term follow-up.[2,3] Alpha-fetoprotein is raised in about 50% of nonseminomatous germ cell tumors (NSGCTs), and human chorionic gonadotrophin (HCG) in 30–35% of NSGCTs, and 10–15% of seminomas. Testicular cancer

spreads first to the para-aortic regions and hematogenous spread is more common in NSGCTs. Metastases commonly occur in the lung, brain, liver, and bone. Thus, anatomical imaging of the chest, abdomen, and pelvis must be performed for staging. One commonly used international staging system is the Royal Marsden staging system[4] (Table 13C.1) and patients should be classified on this basis.

Table 13C.1 *Staging of testicular cancer*

Stage	Description
I	No evidence of metastases
IM	*Rising concentrations of serum markers with no other evidence of metastases*
II	Abdominal node metastases
A	*<2 cm in diameter*
B	*2–5 cm in diameter*
C	*>5 cm in diameter*
III	Supradiaphragmatic nodal metastasis
M	*Mediastinal*
N	*Supraclavicular, cervical or axillary*
O	*No abdominal node metastasis*
ABC	*Node stage as defined in stage II*
IV	Extralymphatic metastasis
Lung	
L1	*<3 metastases*
L2	*>3 metastases, all <2 cm in diameter*
L3	*>3 metastases, one or more >2 cm in diameter*
H+, Br+, Bo+	*Liver, brain or bone*

Patients are also stratified by risk of metastases based on the factors including vascular invasion and raised markers in NSGCT. This classifies them as low risk or high risk and each has alternative treatments, strategies, and problems. Low-risk patients can be treated by either a surveillance protocol or immediate treatment with two courses of chemotherapy followed by surveillance. Both of these have good cure rates.[3,5] Undoubtedly, the risk strategy is not perfect, and some patients with metastases may miss out on treatment and some without metastases may undergo unnecessary treatment. There has been some concern recently over the toxicity of treatments including long-term effects, e.g. cardiovascular and second malignancies.[6] Seminomas are treated with para-aortic radiotherapy. Therefore, a tool which would assist in more accurate assessment of patients at diagnosis as truly stage I may limit toxicity to those who do not need treatment and improve treatment for those who do. Imaging techniques, especially functional imaging, have the potential to achieve this.

IMAGING AT DIAGNOSIS

Computed tomography (CT) scanning has been the mainstay of imaging at the initial staging of testicular tumors. This relies primarily on size criteria with a cut-off level of 1 cm being the differentiating factor between benign and malignant involvement of regional lymph nodes. This, however, has severe limitations as it is known that at least 25–30% of patients with normal-sized nodes on CT criteria will have tumor present and a similar number will have enlarged CT nodes but are in fact tumor free.[7–9] The key interest of a metabolic technique such as PET would be to discover if it improves the staging. There have been a few small studies in this area which have all shown sensitivities of 67–87% and specificities of 94–100% for fluorodeoxyglucose (FDG) positron emission tomography (PET).[10–12] All studies were limited somewhat by lack of complete histological follow-up and both PET and CT missed small retroperitoneal disease.

The issue of imaging and understaging is particularly important in NSGCT where true stage I disease could undergo surveillance and save the morbidity of chemotherapy. Lassen et al.[13] performed a prospective analysis in 40 patients with NSGCT clinical stage I and FDG PET. As they were clinically stage I all patients underwent surveillance and 10 relapsed, of which seven had positive PET scans. This implies a clear role for PET detection of occult disease in these patients. If this could be confirmed in larger studies PET could contribute significantly to the management of stage I NSGCT (Fig. 13C.1). In the UK, a multi-center trial has been started to evaluated this, supported by the Medical Research Council. This should establish the role of PET in this circumstance. Additional citations may be desirable indicating other trials as well.

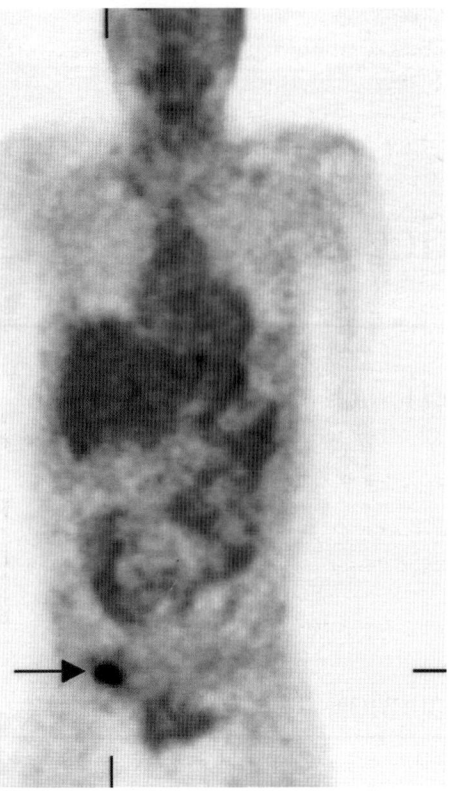

Figure 13C.1   *A coronal FDG PET in a patient with clinical stage I NSGCT. There is uptake in a right groin node (arrow) which was not detected on other imaging. Histology proved this to be metastatic disease.*

At staging, PET has also been found to define disease not found on other imaging including bone and viscera. While important this may make minor changes in initial management especially if patients are having adjuvant chemotherapy.[10]

TUMOR RECURRENCE AND FOLLOW-UP

Those patients with metastatic disease and NSGCT will be treated with chemotherapy. After this about 30% of these will have residual masses. These masses may contain fibrosis, active tumor or, in the case of NSGCT, mature teratoma differentiated (MTD). Those with fibrosis require no further treatment whilst those with residual disease do require it, and often surgical removal at the earliest opportunity is advisable. MTD is a benign tumor that is unstable and can lead to later relapse and therefore must be removed. However, the timing of surgery could be delayed to decrease the co-morbidity of recent chemotherapy and surgery if the histological of the mass is accurately known.

In patients with seminoma radiotherapy is performed as standard and if more widespread disease is apparent then chemotherapy can be added. These patients may also have residual masses following treatment that contain either fibrosis/necrosis or active tumor.

There are some patients who undergo multiple relapses, have persistent disease or become unresponsive to chemotherapy. Often combinations of chemotherapy, surgery, and radiotherapy are necessary to try to obtain a cure or to control the disease. Deciding which treatment is of most value at each time can be difficult as this depends on which sites contain active disease and which do not.

Imaging in residual/recurrent disease

RESIDUAL MASSES

Computed tomography and the change in the size of masses has been the mainstay for assessing residual masses following treatment. Functional imaging techniques using ^{67}Ga or ^{201}Tl, for example, have been applied to assess the presence of disease, with variable and inconsistent results.[14,15] There are now many studies evaluating the use of FDG PET in the post-treatment residual masses.[16–19] Clearly, PET can identify residual active disease with a higher sensitivity and specificity than CT and with positive predictive accuracies up to 96%. Standard FDG PET imaging in NSGCT clearly differentiates fibrosis/necrosis and MTD from active tumor but cannot differentiate between fibrosis/necrosis and MTD. As surgical removal of all MTDs is necessary, this suggests a limited role for PET in this circumstance. However, MTD can be left for a while and so the value of PET may be that it allows surgery to be delayed in a patient with morbidity from recent chemotherapy or radiotherapy. Sugwara et al.[20] have performed dynamic PET imaging and, by using analysis of rate constants, can successfully distinguish MTD from fibrosis/necrosis.

PET may be of more value in the assessment of residual masses in seminoma rather than NSGCT. Residual seminoma masses will contain either necrosis/fibrosis or active tumor. In these patients, radiotherpy following the chemotherapy has not been proven to be of value.[21] The major papers in the literature so far have all shown good results for seminoma,[17,18] although in smaller numbers than for NSGCT. De Santis et al.,[22] in a well conducted multi-center trial, reviewed the value in seminoma specifically and found high positive predictive values of 100% and negative predictive values of 97%, concluding that PET is a clinically useful predictor of viable tumor in post-chemotherapy residual masses of pure seminoma. This was particularly true for those greater than 3 cm.

Two problems with scanning emerged from these studies. Firstly, PET did miss very small volume active disease. Secondly, the timing of the PET scan in relation to the chemotherapy is important. Scans within 10–14 days of the last dose of chemotherapy showed false negative results.[17,18]

RAISED MARKERS

Throughout follow-up of patients, the concentrations of tumor markers should be measured and these remain an important indicator of relapse and response to treatment.[2,3] They do have some inherent problems including that recurrence can be marker negative even if the original disease was marker positive; some patients have persistently raised markers despite no evidence of disease as well as other factors leading to elevation.[23,24] Two scenarios are possible with raised markers. The first is the patient with raised markers suggesting recurrence and normal conventional imaging including CT. The second is a patient with multiple previous areas of disease and residual masses with raised markers and the question is which, if any, contain disease. This is important to establish in the latter case as management can be affected. If only one area is involved, then surgery may be the appropriate treatment whereas multiple areas would involve treatment with chemotherapy. Cremerius et al.[18] tried to address the issue of markers finding that in the cases where they had marker information PET improved the accuracy of the markers. Hain et al.[17] had information on markers in all 70 of their patients. In patients with raised markers PET was positive in all but one. More problematic were the patients with raised markers and negative PET scans. In three of the five, though, all other imaging was normal as well and follow-up PET studies were the first studies to identify the sites of the recurrence. This suggests a very clear role for PET in this circumstance.

EFFECT ON MANAGEMENT

In relapsed/residual disease, PET is useful in identifying the contents of post-treatment residual masses, identifying the site of recurrence in CT negative or CT stable disease and also where localized disease has been identified on other imaging and before starting local treatment to identify other sites of disease (Fig. 13C.2). Certainly, in staging, PET changes the stage in patients but especially where chemotherapy or radiotherapy was planned will change the management in fewer patients. In relapsed/residual disease PET also has the potential to change management. Hain et al.[17] found that PET resulted in a change of management in 57% of patients. These involved changes from local control to systemic therapy or surveillance and vice versa. Many of the patients in the study had multiple recurrence and some were chemo-resistant. This suggests PET is useful in this area but this needs further confirmation.

PREDICTION OF RESPONSE TO TREATMENT

PET has been found to be predictive of response to chemotherapy and immediate and long-term outcome during chemotherapy in other tumors including lymphoma and breast.[25–27] One study has evaluated PET compared to

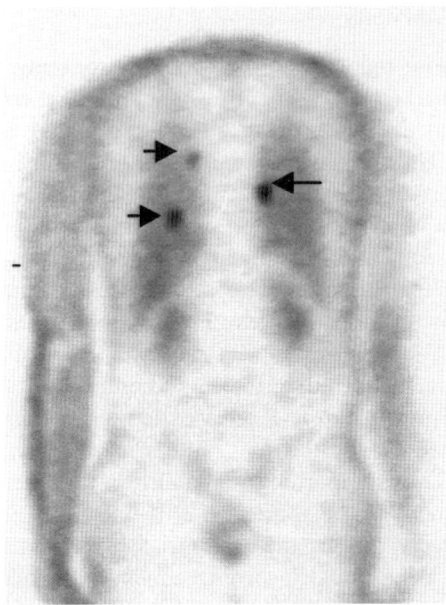

Figure 13C.2 *Coronal FDG PET studies. The patient had a known history of testicular cancer. Conventional imaging on follow-up showed a single small peripheral right lung lesion of questionable significance. The FDG PET study shows multiple areas of abnormal uptake in the lung fields (arrows) confirmed as metastatic disease.*

markers and CT/MR after two to three cycles of chemotherapy in patients with testicular cancer.[28] They found that in those patients who showed response to induction chemotherapy according to CT scans or serum tumor marker evaluation, PET added information to detect patients with an overall unfavorable outcome. It also identified patients most likely to achieve a favorable response to subsequent high-dose chemotherapy. They suggested it would be a valuable addition to the prognostic model of low-, intermediate- and high-risk patients; particularly in the low and intermediate groups for further selection of patients who would profit from high-dose chemotherapy.

CONCLUSION

FDG PET is a promising tool in testicular cancer. It has been shown to differentiate tumor from fibrosis and find active sites of disease with higher sensitivity and specificity than CT. It can appropriately alter management decisions in a number of patient-focused scenarios. More studies need to be performed particularly for stage I disease where PET could potentially have major management implications.

Case history

A young man had a history of testicular cancer and was being appropriately followed-up by markers and conventional imaging. The concentrations of his tumor markers began to rise and the imaging including CT showed a para-aortic mass that was stable over time and therefore reported as a residual fibrotic mass with evidence of disease. An FDG PET study (shown) was performed. This shows two areas of increased uptake in the para-aortic area (arrows), one corresponding to the mass and one lymph node <1 cm on CT. This illustrates that (1) PET can be used to locate disease where the markers are raised and the CT is normal or stable; (2) PET may overcome the size constraints of conventional imaging to define disease in a long-term stable residual mass as well as (3) in areas within normal limits on CT; and (4) PET may alter management by finding the site of disease and defining additional disease.

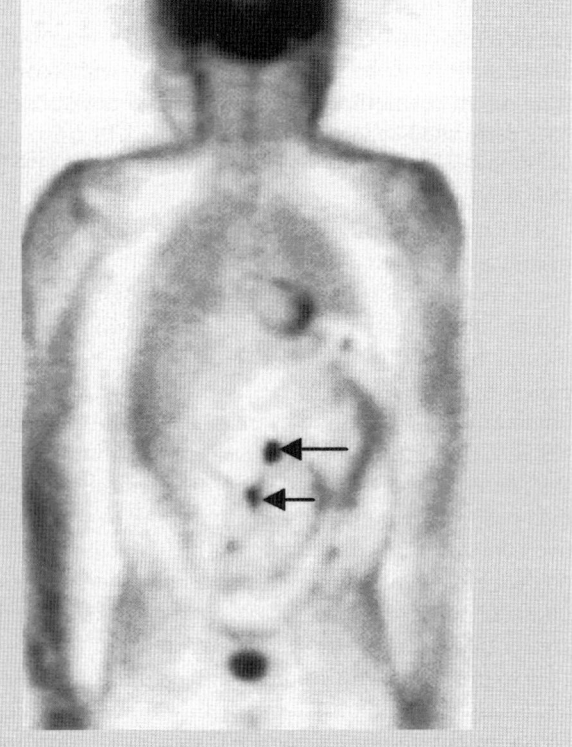

Figure 13C.3

REFERENCES

● Seminal primary article
✱ First formal publication of a management guideline

1 Cancer Research Campaign. *Testicular cancer – UK. Factsheet 16.* London: Cancer Research Campaign, 1998.

● 2 Wishnow KI, Johnson DE, Swanson DA, *et al.* Identifying patients at low risk clinical stage I testicular tumours who should be treated by surveillance. *Urology* 1989; **34**: 339–43.

✱ 3 Read G, Stenning SP, Cullen MH, *et al.* Medical Research Council prospective study of surveillance for stage I testicular teratoma. *J Clin Oncol* 1992; **10**: 1762–8.

4 Horwich A. Testicular cancer. In: Horwich A (ed.). *Oncology – a multidisciplinary textbook.* London: Chapman and Hall, 1995; pp. 485–98.

5 Cullen MH. Adjuvant chemotherapy in high risk stage I non-seminomatous germ cell tumours of the testis. In: Horwich A (ed.). *Testicular cancer – investigation and management.* London: Chapman and Hall, 1996; pp.181–91.

● 6 Huddart R, Norman A, Shahidi M, *et al.* Cardiovascular disease as a long-term complication of treatment for testicular cancer. *J Clin Oncol* 2003; **21**: 1513–23.

7 Nichols C. Testicular cancer. *Curr Probl Cancer* 1998; **22**: 187–274.

8 Aass N, fossa SD, Ous S, *et al.* Is routine retroperitoneal lymph node dissection still justified in patients with low stage non-seminomatous testicular cancer? *Br J Urol* 1990; **65**: 385–90.

9 Aass N, Hatun DE, Thoresen M, Fossa D. Prophylactic use of tropisetron or metoclopromide during adjuvant abdominal radiotherapy of seminoma stage I: a randomised, open trial in 23 patients. *Radiother Oncol* 1997; **45**: 125–8.

10 Hain SF, O'Doherty MJ, Timothy, *et al.* Fluorodeoxyglucose PET in the initial staging of germ cell tumours. *Eur J Nucl Med* 2000; **27**: 590–4.

11 Cremerius U, Wildberger JE, Borchers H, *et al.* Does positron emission tomography using 18-fluoro-2-deoxyglucose improve clinical staging of testicular cancer? Results in 50 patients. *Urology* 1999; **54**: 900–4.

12 Albers P, bender H, Yilmaz H, *et al.* Posiron emission tomography in the clinical staging of patients with stage I and II testicular germ cell tumours. *Urology* 1999; **53**: 808–11.

✱ 13 Lassen U, Daugaard G, Eigtved A, *et al.* Whole body FDG-PET in patients with stage I non-seminomatous germ cell tumours. *Eur J Nucl Med Mol Imaging* 2003; **30**: 396–402.

14 Warren GP. Gallium scans in the evaluation of residual masses after chemotherapy for seminoma. *J Clin Oncol* 1995; **13**: 2784–8.

15 Uchiyama M, Kantoff PW, Kaplan WD. Gallium-67 citrate imaging extragonadal and gonadal seminomas: relationship to radiologic findings. *J Nucl Med* 1994; **35**: 1624–30.

● 16 Stephens AW, Gonin R, Hutchins GD, Einhorn LH. Positron emission tomography of residual radiological abnormalities in postchemotherapy germ cell tumour patients. *J Clin Oncol* 1996; **14**: 1637–41.

✱ 17 Hain SF, O'Doherty MJ, Timothy AR, *et al.* Fluorodeoxyglucose positron emission tomography in the evaluation of germ cell tumours at relapse. *Br J Cancer* 2000; **83**: 863–9.

18 Cremerius U, Effert PJ, Adam G, *et al.* FDG PET for detection and therapy control of metastatic germ cell tumour. *J Nucl Med* 1998; **39**: 815–22.

19 Tsatalpas P, Beuthien-Baumann B, Kropp J, *et al.* Diagnostic value of ^{18}F-FDG positron emission tomography for detection and treatment control of malignant germ cell tumors. *Urol Int* 2002; **68**: 157–63.

● 20 Sugawara Y, Zasadny KR, Grossman HB, *et al.* Germ cell tumour: differentiation of viable tumor, mature teratoma and necrotic tissue with FDG PET and kinetic modelling. *Radiology* 1999; **211**: 249–56.

21 Duchesne GM, Stenning SP, Aass N, *et al.* Radiotherapy after chemotherapy for metastatic seminoma – a diminishing role. MRC Testicular Working Party. *Eur J Cancer* 1997; **33**: 829–35.

✱ 22 De Santis M, Bokemeyer C, Becherer A, *et al.* Predictive impact of 2-18fluoro-2-deoxy-D-glucose positron emission tomography for residual postchemotherapy masses in patients with bulky seminoma. *J Clin Oncol* 2001; **19**: 3740–4.

23 Rathmall AJ, Brand IR, Carey BM, Jones WG. Early detection of relapse after treatment for metastatic germ cell tumour of the testis: an exercise in medical audit. *Clin Oncol R Coll Radiol* 1993; **5**: 34–8.

24 Coogan CL, Foster RS, Rowland RG, *et al.* Postchemotherapy retroperitoneal lymph node dissection is effective therapy in selected patients with elevated tumor markers after primary chemotherapy alone. *Urology* 1997; **50**: 957–62.

25 Mikhaeel NG, Timothy AR, O'Doherty MJ, *et al.* 18-FDG-PET as a prognostic indicator in the treatment of aggressive non-Hodgkin's lymphoma – comparison with CT. *Leuk Lymphoma* 2000; **39**: 543–53.

● 26 Schelling M, Avril N, Nahrig J, *et al.* Positron emission tomography using [(18)F]fluorodeoxyglucose for monitoring primary chemotherapy in breast cancer. *J Clin Oncol* 2000; **18**: 1689–95.

● 27　Smith IC, Welch AE, Hutcheon AW, *et al.* Positron emission tomography using [(18)F]-fluorodeoxy-D-glucose to predict the pathologic response of breast cancer to primary chemotherapy. *J Clin Oncol* 2000; **18**: 1676–88.

● 28　Bokemeyer C, Kollmannsberger C, Oechsle K, *et al.* Early prediction of treatment response to high-dose salvage chemotherapy in patients with relapsed germ cell cancer using [(18)F]FDG PET. *Br J Cancer* 2002; **86**: 506–11.

Impotence

Q.H. SIRAJ

INTRODUCTION

Impotence, an inability to achieve or maintain an erection suitable for sexual intercourse, has a reported incidence of 25% at 65 years of age.[1] Erectile dysfunction may be caused by psychogenic, endocrine, neurologic, pharmacologic or vascular factors. It has now been established that only about one quarter of subjects have purely functional impotence and over 85% of patients with organic impotence have a vasculogenic etiology.[2]

Improvements in the understanding of erectile dysfunction have spurred the development of new radionuclide tests along with the fresh application of old procedures for evaluating vasculogenic impotence. This chapter reviews the various penile radionuclide studies in the light of the present concepts of the neuro-physiological, physio-pharmacological and hemodynamic processes that regulate penile function; highlighting the unique and specific contribution of radionuclide methods; defining the clinical role of the available scintigraphic techniques for evaluating erectile dysfunction; and outlining the basic methodology and the underlying theoretical principles of the current scintigraphic tests with emphasis on guidelines for interpretation.

PENILE ANATOMY AND PHYSIOLOGY OF ERECTION

Gross anatomy

The penis is composed of three fibroelastic cylinders: the paired corpora cavernosa lying dorsolaterally, and the corpus spongiosum positioned ventrally in the mid-line.

Corpora cavernosa comprise the main body of the penis and are fused with each other in the median plane, but their proximal ends separate to form the crura that attach to the sides of the pubic arch. A strong fibroelastic capsule, the tunica albuginea, surrounds the corpora cavernosa forming a lattice of cavernous spaces in the erectile tissue. The corpus spongiosum is traversed by the urethra and its distal end expands to form the glans penis. All three corpora are surrounded by a deep fascia (Buck's fascia) and a superficial fascial layer (Colle's fascia).

Arterial supply

Penile arterial supply arises from the internal iliac artery via the internal pudendal artery, which continues as the penile artery after giving off the superficial perineal branch. The penile artery terminates by dividing into the dorsal and the deep (cavernous) penile arteries. The cavernous arteries arborize into numerous tortuous helicine arteries that open directly into the cavernous spaces via short end-arterioles. They also provide nutrient vessels to the trabeculae and tunica, anastomotic branches that cross the septum, a few branches that end in capillaries within the corpora cavernosa, and small shunt arteries to veins in the corpus spongiosum, which are thought to be responsible for diverting blood away from the cavernosum in the flaccid state.

Each dorsal penile artery courses distally on the dorsum of the penis on either side of the mid-line superficial to the tunica albuginea. Its branches primarily supply the glans penis; the circumflex branches of the dorsal artery may provide blood to the cavernosal bodies through collaterals to the deep arteries on either side.

Venous drainage

The superficial, intermediate and deep penile venous drainage systems carry the venous efflux from the penis. The superficial system, comprising the single superficial dorsal vein mainly drains the superficial tissues and empties into the external iliac vein via the external pudendal vein. The intermediate system comprises the deep dorsal vein, the emissary and the circumflex veins. The emissary veins arise from the sub-tunical venous plexuses and pass through the tunica albuginea to emerge from the dorsolateral surface of the corpus cavernosum; compression of these venules during erection between the non-compliant tunica albuginea and the dilated sinusoids is thought to be responsible for venous outflow restriction. The distal portion of the corpus cavernosum empties predominantly through emissary or circumflex veins into the deep dorsal vein of the penis, which also drains the pendulous part of the corpus spongiosum, and empties via the peri-prostatic and peri-vesical plexuses into the internal iliac vein. The deep venous system (cavernous and crural veins) drains the proximal portions of the corpus spongiosum and the corpora cavernosa into the internal pudendal vein.

Nervous control

There are three sets of nerves subserving sexual function: somatic, sympathetic and parasympathetic. Somatic innervation of the penis is through the mixed motor-sensory pudendal nerve, which carries somatic afferent fibres from the penis and efferent nerves to the perineal striated musculature. The autonomic erection centre is located in the intermediolateral gray matter of the spinal cord at S2–4 and T11–L2 levels. The pelvic plexus, formed by the parasympathetic visceral efferent pre-ganglionic fibers from the sacral centre (S2–4) and sympathetic fibers from the thoracolumbar center (T11–L2), provides autonomic innervation to the pelvic organs and the external genitalia. Some sympathetic fibers coming from the sacral sympathetic chain are included in the pudendal nerve. Cavernous nerves (nervi erigentes) from the pelvic plexus represent the final common route for autonomic pathways: its terminal branches innervate the helicine arteries and the trabecular smooth muscles, and are responsible for the vascular events that result in penile erection. The thoracolumbar sympathetic nerves are responsible for ejaculation.

Erection can be psychogenic, elicited by supraspinal stimuli, or reflexogenic caused by local genital and/or visceral stimulation. The former is by sympathetic and parasympathetic pathways and the latter by sacral parasympathetic reflexes. Normally, the psychic and reflexogenic stimuli act synergistically to produce erection. However, psychogenic factors, endocrine disturbances that influence libido, or the supraspinal centers may interfere with the erectile reflex.

Mechanism of erection

Erection is a hemodynamic response to nervous stimuli: non-adrenergic non-cholinergic nerves in the penis are thought to elaborate a relaxant neurotransmitter (nitric oxide), which together with simultaneous withdrawal or counteraction of the smooth muscle contraction produced by noradrenaline, induces a chain of vascular events resulting in erection. During the flaccid state, cavernosal arterial flow bypasses the cavernosal sinusoids. Neurostimulation results in arterial dilatation, an increased penile arterial inflow exceeding the venous outflow, diversion of blood through the helicine arteries into the cavernosal spaces due to constriction of shunt arteries, relaxation of the cavernosal sinusoids, and cavernous venous outflow occlusion due to compression of the outflow venules between the expanding sinusoids and the rigid tunica albuginea.

ETIOLOGY AND PATHOGENESIS OF VASCULOGENIC IMPOTENCE

Either an inadequacy of the arterial inflow or an excess of venous outflow may result in erectile failure. Arteriogenic impotence is caused by small- or large-vessel occlusion and venogenic impotence results from venous-occlusive insufficiency. The majority of patients with organic impotence (about 50–70%) have combined arterial and venous dysfunction; arterial insufficiency alone accounts for about 30% of the cases; isolated venous leakage with normal arterial function is even rarer, occurring in approximately 15% of cases.[2]

Arteriogenic impotence

In 1923, Leriche first documented the relationship between impotence and the limitation of pelvic arterial inflow.[3] Numerous studies have subsequently confirmed the association between impotence and aortoiliac occlusive disease. A link between arterial risk factors (age, smoking, diabetes, hypertension and hyperlipidemia) and impotence has been well established.[4] Atheromatous disease of the penile arterial tree, post-traumatic alterations, sequelae of local infection and even congenital dysplasia, are etiologies of vascular alterations that may give rise to clinically isolated erectile impotence. Vascular damage caused by irradiation of the pelvis in malignancies may also result in impotence. Vascular surgical procedures that produce a reduction of blood flow in the internal pudendal artery can result in impotence; internal iliac ligation or transcatheter embolization for uncontrolled pelvic hemorrhage, and renal transplant surgery with end-to-end anastomosis of the internal iliac and the renal arteries, may compromise penile perfusion.

Venogenic impotence

Penile venous-occlusive insufficiency can prevent cavernous pressure from rising sufficiently for rigid erection. Venous leakage may cause primary erectile dysfunction in young men. Its incidence increases with age. Surgical procedures for treating priapism such as anastomosis of the saphenous vein to corpus cavernosum or the creation of cavernous–spongiosal shunts can result in venous–occlusive insufficiency. Significant post-traumatic venous leakage may occur due to rupture of tunica albuginea or by mechanical disruption of the delicate structures responsible for cavernosal venous-occlusion.

INVESTIGATION OF VASCULOGENIC IMPOTENCE: NONRADIONUCLIDE TECHNIQUES

Early studies

Among the early nonradionuclide screening techniques for the functional evaluation of penile circulatory status, penile pulse–volume recording using strain-gauge plethysmography, penile blood pressure measurement by various methods, and Doppler ultrasound estimation of flaccid penile blood flow are among the better known tests. Although useful, these techniques had an unacceptably low sensitivity and specificity. The most popular and widely employed tests are briefly discussed.

NOCTURNAL PENILE TUMESCENCE

Nocturnal penile tumescence (NPT) is a physiological phenomenon with normal healthy males experiencing sleep-related erections, accounting for about one third of the total sleep time. NPT testing has been a widely popular non-invasive screening technique. However, the accuracy of the NPT test is low: there is a high incidence of false positive test results in potent men; depression may cause a temporary reduction or inhibition of NPT; and false negative NPT responses may be seen in subjects with sensory neuropathies, pelvic steal syndrome and corporal leakage impotence.

PENILE BLOOD FLOW MEASUREMENTS

The average velocity of a column of red cells coursing through a vessel can be measured by a Doppler device. Malvar et al., first used the Doppler flowmeter to record the flow through the penile arteries in the flaccid penis.[5] In an attempt to quantify flow, a penile blood flow index was later derived, which showed a poor correlation with angiographic abnormalities, however. The technique is of limited value in the diagnosis of vasculogenic impotence.

Current studies

PHARMACOLOGICALLY INDUCED PENILE ERECTIONS

The achievement of a normal erection following intracavernosal injection of vasoactive drugs is useful in differentiating between vascular and functional impotence: rapid onset of an adequately rigid and durable erection obviates the need for further invasive investigations. Intracavernosal injections of papaverine (with or without an alpha-receptor blocker) or prostaglandin E_1 are commonly used for this purpose. A normal response is consistent with psychogenic or neurogenic etiology, whereas vasculogenic impotence patients show impaired penile tumescence. One limitation of this test is its inability to differentiate between arteriogenic and venogenic causes, but the main drawback of the technique is an anxiety-related poor erectile response in patients without organic erectile dysfunction due to psychological factors.

PELVIC AND INTERNAL PUDENDAL ANGIOGRAPHY

The current technique involves performing pelvic angiography with selective internal pudendal arteriography in conjunction with intracavernosal and/or intra-arterial vasoactive agents. Arteriography confirms the underlying pathology, provides anatomic localization of the site of occlusion, and may help direct any possible surgical intervention. However, the technique is invasive, has a potentially high risk of complications, requires special skills and equipment, is generally difficult to interpret, and provides no physiologic information. Further, the extent of the disease demonstrated arteriographically may bear little relation to the symptoms: aortic or bilateral internal iliac occlusion is not invariably accompanied by impotence, and short symptomatic lesions of the pudendal arteries are not demonstrable on arteriography. Therefore, this investigation is not used as a routine diagnostic test, but is indicated in selected cases of pelvic injury, in patients with a suspicion of isolated arterial disease, and in patients being considered for penile revascularization surgery.

CAVERNOSOMETRY AND CAVERNOSOGRAPHY

Dynamic pharmacocavernosometry and cavernosography are employed for the functional evaluation of the corporeal venous-occlusive mechanism. The technique involves intracavernosal injection of a vasoactive drug, followed by infusion of saline into the cavernosa at a controlled variable rate with concomitant recording of intracavernosal pressure. The flow rate required to obtain and sustain an erection adequate for intromission (cavernosal pressure $\geqslant 90\,mmHg$) is determined; this maintenance flow rate correlates with the degree of corporeal leakage. Dynamic cavernosography is next performed by infusion of diluted iodinated contrast and may allow visualization of the site(s) of venous leakage.

DOPPLER FLOW IMAGING OF PHARMACOLOGICAL ERECTION

Pulsed duplex sonography is performed for real-time imaging and measurement of flow through the cavernosal arteries during drug-induced erection. Arterial insufficiency is suggested by a failure of the arteries to dilate and the flow velocity to increase. An abnormally increased venous outflow can also be documented. Although the peak velocities show a wide variability and are strongly influenced by technical factors, despite these limitations it is currently widely used for vasculogenic screening.

RADIONUCLIDE INVESTIGATION OF VASCULOGENIC IMPOTENCE: EARLY STUDIES

Radionuclide penile vascular studies were pioneered by Shirai and Nakamura from Japan in the 1970s, who employed non-imaging probes for monitoring penile radioactivity changes following injection of blood pool radiopharmaceuticals.[6,7]

In 1982, Fanous and associates performed dynamic flaccid penile blood pool imaging using [99mTc]pertechnetate and quantified the change in the penile blood volume induced by an intravenous vasodilator, which parameter reportedly correlated well with the penile blood pressure index.[8] Although the data presented by the investigators did not substantiate their claim;[9] nonetheless, the technique offered an objective method for the assessment of penile vascular status.

Measurement of the rate of washout of a diffusible tracer such as ^{133}Xe is the standard radionuclide method for assessing organ perfusion. Clearance of ^{133}Xe following subcutaneous injection into the dorsal coronal sulcus of the flaccid penis was first reported by Nseyo et al.[10] and subsequently by other investigators. Lower flow rates were seen in patients with penile arterial insufficiency and in patients with mixed arteriogenic–venogenic impotence, with normal results in subjects with isolated venous leakage and nonvasculogenic impotence. The subcutaneous ^{133}Xe washout rate reflects superficial penile perfusion and can potentially identify major arterial disease. However, it is a crude and nonspecific technique, which does not provide any information about cavernosal flow.

Nevertheless, the major contribution of the original radionuclide investigations was the application and elaboration of innovative radionuclide methodologies, providing archetypes for later developments.

RADIONUCLIDE INVESTIGATION OF IMPOTENCE: CURRENT METHODS

The current radionuclide techniques used for the diagnosis and quantification of the arteriogenic and venous elements in vasculogenic erectile dysfunction commonly employ two main strategies:

- Estimation of penile arterial inflow using blood pool agents
- Assessment of the venous outflow by measuring the rate of clearance of an intracavernosally injected diffusible tracer (usually ^{133}Xe)

The studies can be performed both in the flaccid state and in conjunction with drug-induced erections.

Clearance studies

FLACCID [133]XE CLEARANCE STUDIES

The clearance rate of ^{133}Xe following an intracavernosal (IC) injection in the flaccid penis reflects basal cavernosal blood flow. Wagner and Uhrenholdt reported lower penile washout rates of IC ^{133}Xe in patients with arteriogenic impotence with no difference in the washout rates between normal subjects and patients with venous leakage.[11] Other investigators have reported slower flaccid penile washout rates of IC ^{133}Xe in venous leakage patients, compared with that in normal controls or nonvenous impotence, which factor was attributed to incompetent venous valves with backflow of blood into the penis.[12] However, this hypothesis is not supported by current medical opinion: venous restriction during erection is not dependent upon the presence or the absence of venous valves.

The discordant findings by different workers, together with the lack of a plausible explanation for the abnormal clearance results in venous impotence patients and an inability to differentiate between arteriogenic and venogenic forms of vasculogenic impotence, has caused an uncertainty about the relevance and clinical value of flaccid IC ^{133}Xe clearance test.

ERECTION [133]XE CLEARANCE STUDIES

Washout of IC ^{133}Xe from the erect penis reflects the egress of blood during tumescence. Erection IC ^{133}Xe clearance studies generally show decreased penile washout during erection in normal subjects, whereas an increased clearance rate is documented in patients with venous disease.

DIAGNOSTIC ROLE

Flaccid state cavernosal ^{133}Xe clearance rate is predominantly dependent on the arterial inflow. During the induction phase of erection, the arterial inflow and the venous outflow both influence the xenon clearance times; after achievement of full erection at steady-state or maintenance arterial flow rates, the measure mainly reflects venous outflow. Technical factors, such as a variable dilution of the cavernosal blood pool caused by the nonradioactive vasodilator injection together with the volume of the injected xenon with different energy may be a source of error.[13]

These confounding physiological variables and technical factors undermine the significance and reliability of xenon clearance studies for an objective evaluation of penile venous outflow or venous–occlusive mechanism.

BLOOD POOL TECHNIQUES

Flaccid studies

Siraj et al. developed the Fanous technique by performing dynamic penile scintigraphy (radionuclide phallography) using ^{99m}Tc-red blood cells (^{99m}Tc-RBCs).[14,15] Penile arterial inflow function was objectively evaluated by quantifying the hemodynamic response to intravenous vasodilator stress: the change in penile blood volume was quantified using a modification of the Fanous index, which improved the diagnostic accuracy; a quantitative parameter of blood flow was also derived. This non-invasive technique was effective in screening impotent patients for penile arterial insufficiency.[9,14,15]

Pilot radionuclide blood pool studies without pharmacological intervention were conduced by Siraj who recorded the flaccid penile blood flow patterns in normal individuals and patients with impotence. These studies provided new physiological insights into the normal penile hemodynamic changes during the flaccid state and the observations on patients with different etiologies of impotence helped further our understanding of the underlying basis of erectile dysfunction.[9,16,17]

Erection studies

The main limitation of penile vascular studies in the flaccid state was their inability to exclude venous leakage. To evaluate penile vascular function during the process of erection, Siraj et al. performed dynamic erection phallography, which allowed continuous monitoring of the penile circulatory changes during the various stages of drug-induced erections.[18] The technique provided an objective assessment of the normal erectile hemodynamic response and yielded specific data, which was helpful in the differential diagnosis of psychogenic, arteriogenic and venous leakage patients.

Penile blood volume can be estimated by measuring the activity of a venous blood sample taken from the patient.[14,19] This allowed absolute quantification of peak arterial flow rates (mL min^{-1}) following papaverine injection by calculating the maximal rate of change in penile activity from the slope of the penile time–activity curve,[20] which parameter showed a good correlation with the angiographic extent of penile arterial disease. Another estimate of arterial inflow during early erection, calculated from the ratio of penile blood volume 60 s before and 60 s after the peak flow, further improved the correlation with angiographic scoring.[21] This latter parameter, which measures the

relative difference between the flaccid and erection flow rates, is basically similar to the flow index described by Siraj et al.[18] In this context there appears no clear-cut benefit of venous sampling.

COMBINATION TESTS

Dual-isotope combination studies using a blood pool agent for estimating arterial inflow and the clearance of intracavernosally injected ^{133}Xe or ^{127}Xe for assessing venous outflow, have been employed for evaluating the penile hemodynamic status during pharmacologically induced erection. Schwartz and Graham performed a dual-isotope (^{127}Xe/^{99m}Tc-RBCs) study for calculating arterial and venous flow following papaverine-induced erection.[21] Their results, however, showed that measurement of xenon clearance alone was unreliable in predicting the competency of venous–occlusive mechanism. In a combination blood pool (^{99m}Tc-RBCs) and washout (^{133}Xe) study, Miraldi et al. estimated the peak arterial and venous flow rates after induction of pharmacological erection; the vascular flow parameters were reported to be helpful in differentiating normal, arteriogenic and venous leakage subjects.[22] However, the relevance of the venous outflow parameter for evaluating the erectile venous–occlusive integrity has been questioned on the basis that xenon was injected in the flaccid state before the papaverine injection.[23] Using a similar dual-isotope (^{133}Xe/^{99m}Tc-RBCs) technique, Kursh et al. computed arterial and venous flow rates in the flaccid and erect states and described specific patterns for distinguishing normal subjects from patients with arterial insufficiency and venous leakage.[24]

DIAGNOSTIC ROLE

In theory, the dual-isotope combination studies can potentially be used for simultaneous measurement of penile arterial inflow and venous outflow, and should ideally provide a continuous record of arterial and venous flow rates in the flaccid state and during various phases of erection. However, the full potential of the technique is yet to be realized. In view of the technical complexity of the test, it is unlikely to become a routine clinical nuclear medicine test for evaluating impotent patients.

EVALUATION OF VASCULOGENIC IMPOTENCE BY FLACCID AND ERECTION PHALLOGRAPHY

Most of the currently available penile vascular tests are still evolving, and their diagnostic efficiency and clinical role is yet to be fully established.[23] Radionuclide penile vascular tests, like their nonradionuclide counterparts, are also in the evolutionary stages. However, on the basis of the familiarity and long experience with the techniques used for studying a large number of patients with erectile dysfunction, and the practicality and ease of performance of the tests, an effective investigative approach is presented, which is based on contemporary physiological principles and provides maximum diagnostic information for minimum patient discomfort.

Flaccid phallography protocol

PROCEDURE AND DATA ANALYSIS

The study is performed using ^{99m}Tc-RBCs labeled *in vivo*; potassium perchlorate (400 mg) is administered orally to block the thyroid and improve labeling efficiency. Scintigraphy is performed using a standard field-of-view, computer-linked, gamma camera equipped with a low-energy, all-purpose collimator. The patient is positioned supine on the imaging couch and a lead mask is placed under the penis to shield background activity from the scrotum and thighs. The camera computer is programmed for a dynamic 64×64 matrix (word mode) acquisition with appropriate magnification set to cover the region extending from the umbilicus to the proximal one third of the thighs. Serial 30-s images are obtained for 55 min following a bolus injection of [^{99m}Tc]pertechnetate (dose 10 MBq kg^{-1}); an intravenous vasodilator such as isoxsuprine hydrochloride (dose 10 mg) is administered after 10 min.

Computer processing involves generating time–activity curves (TACs) from a background-subtracted penile region-of-interest and computation of quantitative indices of penile volume and flow. The methods of calculating the various numerical indices are detailed elsewhere: the maximum increase in the penile blood volume in response to the vasodilator stress is estimated through the penogram index,[8,14,15] and the magnitude of change in penile blood flow quantified through flow indices.[9,14,15]

FINDINGS AND INTERPRETATION

Early flow images may help in assessing the gross morphology of the internal iliac vasculature: there is generally better visualization of the internal iliac blood pool in the non-arteriogenic patients (Fig. 13D.1a) than in patients with advanced atherosclerotic disease of the internal iliac vessels (Fig. 13D.1b).

The penile TACs (phallogram curves) are assessed qualitatively and their general shape and pattern noted. Visual curve assessment reveals fairly characteristic patterns. Normal subjects and most patients with psychogenic impotence show rising curves with secondary pulsations, consistent with phasic increase in penile blood pool due to concomitant penile vascular and trabecular smooth muscle relaxation. There is also an appreciable increase in the steepness of the slope after the vasodilator injection reflecting increased arterial flow (Fig. 13D.2a). Patients with arteriogenic impotence typically show a convex-shaped curve with an insignificant change in the slope after the vasodilator

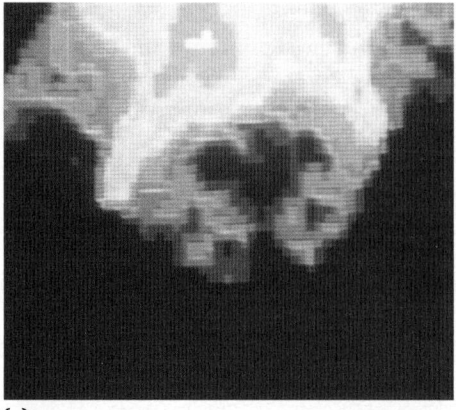

(a)

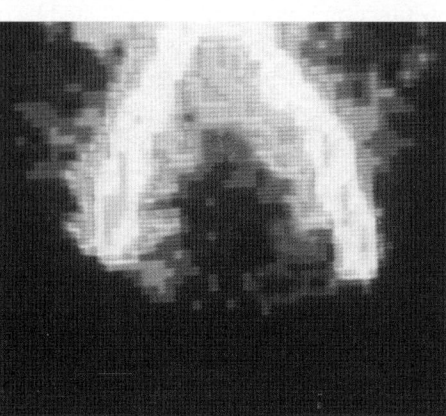

(b)

Figure 13D.1 *Early flow images showing: (a) clear visualization of the internal iliac vascular flow in a patient with psychogenic impotence; (b) poor internal iliac blood pool in a patient with advanced atherosclerotic disease of the internal iliac vessels.*

injection, suggesting a poor flow response; there is also an impairment of the normal rhythmic pulsations (Fig. 13D.2b), which may be attributed both to an inadequacy of resting penile arterial inflow and to sinusoidal dysfunction subsequent to penile ultrastructural damage brought about by an altered nutritive environment associated with chronic penile arterial insufficiency.[9,16,17] The phallogram curves of patients with cavernous–sinusoidal dysfunction show absence of pulsatile activity, whereas patients with isolated venous incompetence due to mechanical venous leakage display preserved pulsatile flow.[9,16,17] Hence, early subclinical sinusoidal dysfunction can be documented by the absence of normal cavernosal pulsatile flow, which also helps explain the delayed flaccid state cavernosal xenon clearance reported in patients with venogenic impotence.[12]

Quantitative hemodynamic parameters allow an objective evaluation of the penile vascular response to the systemic vasodilator injection; the penile volume and flow indices have a high accuracy (>90%) for the diagnosis of arteriogenic impotence.[9,15,17]

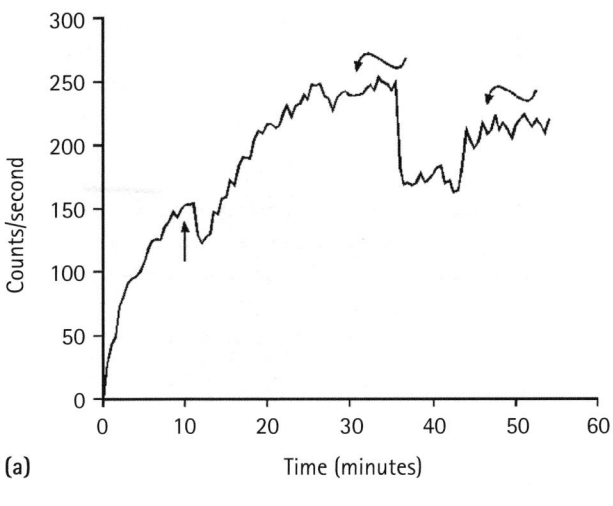

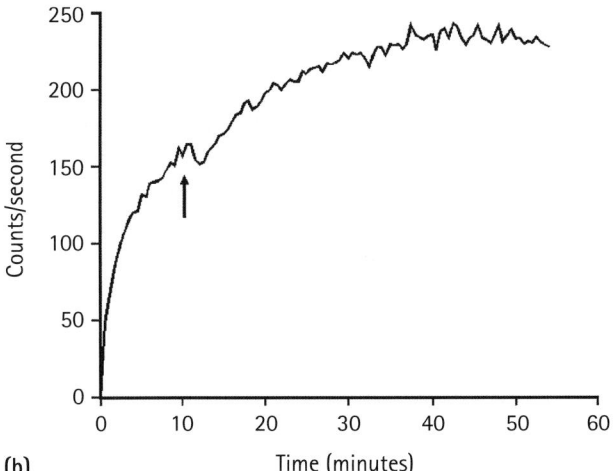

Figure 13D.2 *Representative flaccid phallogram curves: (a) of a psychogenic impotence patient showing normal pulsatile activity (curved arrows) as well as increased penile activity following vasodilator injection (straight arrow); (b) of an arteriogenic impotence patient showing impairment of secondary pulsations and no significant change in curve slope after intravenous vasodilator stress (arrow).*

ERECTION PHALLOGRAPHY PROTOCOL

Procedure and data analysis

The radiopharmaceutical, methodology and analysis of erection and flaccid phallography techniques are essentially similar; the erection test can be performed either following completion of the flaccid study or on a separate occasion. To minimize the affect of anxiety, the study is performed in a quiet and private atmosphere; diazepam (10 mg) may be injected intramuscularly to relax the patient. The penis is loosely but securely strapped by means of strips of adhesive tape to the lead mask covering the scrotum and upper thighs. A 21-gauge butterfly needle is inserted in the lateral aspect of the mid-shaft of the penis into either cavernosum and the patient positioned under the gamma camera. Following a bolus injection of [^{99m}Tc]pertechnetate, the computer is activated to acquire a dynamic study comprising of 60 frames, each of 30-s duration; 10 min later, 10 μg PGE$_1$ or 60 mg papaverine HCl is injected into the corpus cavernosum via the indwelling butterfly needle. The attending nuclear physician should note the time of onset of erection and periodically assess the erectile response during the acquisition period. After completion of the study, the erection is graded by: manual palpation, assessing penile tumescence by recording the penile circumference change, and penile rigidity by measuring the erectile angle.

The data may be analyzed in a variety of ways. A background-subtracted, decay-corrected, penile TAC is generated. The erectile hemodynamic function may be quantified through parameters of flow and volume: the penogram index calculated from the amplitude of the TAC provides a measure of the peak change in penile blood volume, and a flow index derived from the slope of the TAC estimates the relative change in penile flow following intracavernosal vasodilator injection compared with the resting flow rate.[18]

Findings and interpretation

The characteristics of the normal erectile hemodynamic response are evaluated qualitatively through the phallogram curves. In normal subjects and psychogenic impotence patients with good erectile response, the penile TACs characteristically show a sharp increase in the upslope immediately after the injection of the vasoactive drug followed by a plateau (Plate 13D.1a). The technique is helpful in differentiating between primarily arteriogenic and venous etiologies: in patients with mild-to-moderate arterial insufficiency the penile TAC shows a slowly rising curve with delayed time-to-plateau; when the arterial inflow is severely compromised, there is a gradually rising curve that fails to plateau (Plate 13D.1b). The penile TACs of patients with isolated venous leakage typically show an initial rapid rise succeeded by a fall (Plate 13D.1c), since the increase in cavernosal blood volume secondary to an increased arterial inflow cannot be maintained due to venous–occlusive insufficiency. In patients with co-existing arterial insufficiency and venous leakage, the penile TAC shows a poor upslope due to concomitantly reduced inflow and increased outflow, and a failure to plateau because of venous–occlusive dysfunction (Plate 13D.1d).

There is a good correlation between the flow index (FI) and the erectile angle, a physical measure of penile rigidity.[18] The FI provides an accurate and objective assessment of the rapid penile arterial flow during early tumescence. Erection is achieved by greater than five-fold increase in the penile blood flow over the resting state as judged by the FI values. Patients with arteriogenic impotence have low FI values indicative of poor arterial inflow, whereas venous leakage patients with short-lived erections have higher FI values indicating adequate arterial inflow.[18]

An anxiety-related, false positive response may be seen in some psychogenic impotence patients with poor drug-induced erections: the penile TAC patterns may be similar to that seen in arteriogenic impotence with low FI values.[18] However, a normal inflow rate and pattern documented on the flaccid phallogram helps differentiate these cases.[17]

CLINICAL DIAGNOSTIC ROLE

In current clinical practice, most patients seeking a cure for their erectile dysfunction are first treated at primary care level by the new cGMP inhibitor drugs such as sildenafil (type 5-cGMP inhibitor), which inhibits the breakdown of cGMP in erectile tissues and therefore aids the action of the nitric oxide/cGMP-induced erection. Patients who respond poorly to these drugs and those deemed clinically unsuitable for oral therapy are referred for specialist investigation into the cause of their impotence.

A pharmacological erection test is now routinely performed to test patients being investigated for erectile dysfunction. A normal response effectively excludes significant vasculogenic dysfunction, but a false positive response is seen in a large number of subjects without organic disease, due to anxiety-related increased sympathetic activity,[25] which reduces the arterial inflow and increases the venous outflow.[13,19] Further, the increase in penile blood flow after intracavernous vasodilator injection depends not only on the integrity of the penile arterial supply but also on the cavernosal smooth muscle function. Congenital fibrosis and atrophy of cavernosal smooth muscle,[26] and alteration of the fibroelastic properties of the corporal smooth muscle induced by hypercholesterolemia, ischemia or hypertension,[27] may result in a noncompliant sinusoidal compartment. Poor sinusoidal compliance may impair the erectile hemodynamic response by secondarily diminishing penile arterial inflow along with inadequate restriction of venous outflow.

Techniques that rely solely on evaluating penile hemodynamic parameters following intracavernosal injections, may not be able to differentiate poor responders due to anxiety, patients with primary venous–sinusoidal disease and subjects with cavernosal dysfunction secondary to penile arterial insufficiency. Therefore, functional evaluation of penile arterial inflow during the flaccid state appears a more rational approach since the measured response is not dependent on cavernosal compliance.[9,25] However, the current nonradionuclide penile vascular techniques are limited in their technical ability to provide a sensitive record of the flaccid penile vascular function.

Flaccid radionuclide phallography with intravenous vasodilator stress is a sensitive test for evaluating penile arterial insufficiency, which also provides supplementary information about cavernous sinusoidal function. In patients who show a poor erectile response to intracavernosal injection but with normal arterial function on flaccid radionuclide phallography, cavernous-venous incompetence can be assumed by default.[9,28] This can be further confirmed by erection phallography, which will show an inability to achieve a sustained increase in cavernous blood volume due to venous leakage. Patients showing evidence of cavernous–venous dysfunction on phallography are candidates for further evaluation by cavernosography and cavernosometry.

CONCLUSION

Arteriogenic impotence and/or cavernous–venous insufficiency are the major vasculogenic causes of impotence. The clinical management of patients in these categories differs significantly: isolated arteriogenic impotence patients with normal cavernosal smooth muscle function are suitable candidates for intracavernous pharmacotherapy or revascularization surgery, venous incompetence patients with cavernosographically documented leakage sites are likely candidates for venous ligation surgery, whereas in patients with venous–sinusoidal dysfunction or mixed vascular disease, implantation of a penile prosthesis is a more suitable option. Non-invasive vascular screening techniques must therefore be capable of reliably distinguishing between the various etiologies of vasculogenic impotence.

Currently, the Doppler ultrasound technique is the prime contender against radionuclide penile vascular studies as a front-line test for screening impotent patients for vasculogenic erectile dysfunction. Despite improvements in equipment design, the sonographic technique is limited by inherent technical factors. High ultrasound frequencies provide better spatial resolution at the cost of poor depth selectivity, with a proportional increase in the imprecision of the measurement at high blood flow velocities. Also, the physical measurement of flow is highly affected by variations in the transducer angle and inherent diffraction and side-lobe artifacts. Furthermore, Doppler devices measure velocities, not the actual blood flow rates, and the recording is not altogether dynamic, since measurements are made in a specific segment of a particular vessel at certain points during the development of erection. On the other hand, the radionuclide phallography technique can objectively measure whole-organ blood flow and continuously monitor penile blood volume changes from flaccidity through various phases of erection. Evidence of a sustained increase in the penile blood pool seen during erection helps in differentiating hemodynamically significant venous leakage from minor leaks, which when compensated by an increased arterial inflow following pharmacological vasodilation and aided by sexual stimulation, will still allow adequate performance.[28]

Radionuclide phallography of the flaccid penis with intravenous pharmacological stress in combination with erection phallography is helpful in differentiating between psychogenic, primary arteriogenic, venous, venous–sinusoidal, and mixed arteriogenic–venogenic etiologies. The two tests can be performed on a single outpatient visit, minimizing radiation exposure, time and expense.

REFERENCES

1 Kinsey AC, Pomeroy WB, Martin CE. Age and sexual outlet. In: Kinsey AC, Pomeroy WB, Martin CE (eds.) *Sexual Behaviour in the Human Male*. Philadelphia & London: WB Saunders Co., 1948: 218–62.

2 Krysiewicz S, Mellinger BC. The role of imaging in the diagnostic evaluation of impotence. *AJR Am J Roentgenol* 1989; **153**: 1133–9.

3 Leriche R. Des obliteration artérielles hautes obliteration de la termination de l'aorte comme cause d'une insuffisance circulatoire des membres inferiers. *Bull Soc Chir (Paris)* 1923; **49**: 1404.

4 Virag R, Bouilly P, Frydman D. Is impotence an arterial disorder? *Lancet* 1985; **I**: 181–4.

5 Malvar T, Baron T, Clark SS. Assessment of potency with the Doppler flowmeter. *Urology* 1973; **2**: 396–400.

6 Shirai M, Nakamura M. Differential diagnosis of organic and functional impotence by the use of ^{131}I-human serum albumin. *Tohoku J Exp Med* 1970; **101**: 317–24.

7 Shirai M, Nakamura M. Diagnostic discrimination between organic and functional impotence by radioisotope penogram with ^{99m}TcO$_4$. *Tohoku J Exp Med* 1975; **116**: 9–15.

8 Fanous HN, Jevtich MJ, Chen DCP, Edson M. Radioisotope penogram in the diagnosis of vasculogenic impotence. *Urology* 1982; **20**: 499–502.

9 Siraj QH, Hilson AJ. Diagnostic value of radionuclide phallography with intravenous vasodilator stress in the evaluation of arteriogenic impotence. *Eur J Nucl Med* 1994; **21**: 651–7.

10 Nseyo UO, Wilbur HJ, Kang SA, *et al.* Penile xenon (^{133}Xe) washout: a rapid method of screening for vasculogenic impotence. *Urology* 1984; **23**: 31–4.

11 Wagner G, Uhrenholdt A. Blood flow measurement by the clearance method in the human corpus cavernosum in the flaccid and erect states. In: Zorgniotti AW, Rossi G. (eds.) *Vasculogenic Impotence*. Springfield: Thomas, 1980: 41–6.

12 Yeh SH, Liu RS, Lin SN, *et al.* Radionuclide imaging clinical study. Corporeal ^{133}Xe washout for detecting venous leakage in impotence. *Nucl Med Commun* 1991; **12**: 203–9.

13 Siraj QH, Hilson AJW, Bomanji J, Ahmed M. Volume-dependent intracavernous hemodilution during pharmacologically induced penile erections. *J Urol* 1992; **148**: 1441–3.

14 Siraj QH. *Radioisotope Studies of Penile Blood Flow.* MSc thesis, University of London, 1984.

15 Siraj QH, Hilson AJ, Townell NH, *et al.* The role of the radioisotope phallogram in the investigation of vasculogenic impotence. *Nucl Med Commun* 1986; **7**: 173–82.

16 Siraj QH, Hilson AJW, Bomanji J, Ahmed M. A pilot study of flaccid penile blood flow patterns in normal subjects and patients with erectile dysfunction. *Nucl Med Commun* 1993; **14**: 976–82.

17 Siraj QH. *The Study of Penile Vascular Physiology and Pathology using Radiotracer Techniques.* PhD thesis, University of London, 1993.

18 Siraj QH, Bomanji J, Akhtar MA, *et al.* Quantitation of pharmacologically induced penile erections: the value of radionuclide phallography in the objective evaluation of erectile haemodynamics. *Nucl Med Commun* 1990; **11**: 445–58.

19 Shirai M, Nakamura M, Ishii N, *et al.* Determination of intrapenial blood volume using ^{99m}Tc-labeled autologous red blood cells. *Tohoku J Exp Med* 1976; **120**: 377–83.

20 Schwartz AN, Graham MM, Ferency GF, Miura RS. Radioisotope penile plethysmography: a technique for evaluating corpora cavernosal blood flow during early tumescence. *J Nucl Med* 1989; **30**: 466–73.

21 Schwartz AN, Graham MM. Combined technetium radioisotope penile plethysmography and xenon washout: a technique for evaluating corpora cavernosal inflow and outflow during early tumescence. *J Nuc Med* 1991; **32**: 404–10.

22 Miraldi F, Nelson AD, Jones WT, *et al.* A dual-radioisotope technique for the evaluation of penile blood flow during tumescence. *J Nucl Med* 1992; **33**: 41–6.

23 Seftel AD, Goldstein I. Vascular testing for impotence [Editorial]. *J Nucl Med* 1992; **33**: 46–8.

24 Kursh ED, Jones WT, Thompson S, *et al.* A dynamic dual isotope radionuclear method of quantifying penile blood flow. *J Urol* 1992; **147**: 1524–9.

25 Kim SC, Oh MM. Norepinephrine involvement in response to intracorporeal injection of papaverine in psychogenic impotence. *J Urol* 1992; **147**: 1530–2.

26 Aboseif SR, Baskin LS, Yen TSB, Lue TF. Congenital defect in sinusoidal smooth muscles: a cause of organic impotence. *J Urol* 1992; **148**: 58–60.

27 Azadzoi KM, Goldstein I. Erectile dysfunction due to atherosclerotic vascular disease – the development of an animal model. *J Urol* 1992; **147**: 1675–81.

28 Siraj QH, Hilson AJ. Penile radionuclide studies in impotence: an overview [Editorial]. *Nucl Med Commun* 1993; **14**: 517–9.

Infertility

M.P. ITURRALDE, QAISAR H. SIRAJ, AND FIDA HUSSAIN

INTRODUCTION

Infertility is commonly defined as a failure to conceive after 12 months of unprotected intercourse with an incidence of about 10–15% of all couples.[1] The European Society for Human Reproduction and Embryology considers infertility as the lack of pregnancy within 2 years despite regular coital exposure with an incidence of 5–6%.[2] For those who are affected it can become a major tragedy with significant psychological and physical disturbances. The number of infertile couples has increased in the past decade, due to both a larger population and an increase in sexually transmitted disease. This has caused a greater demand for specialized services in the diagnosis and management of male and female infertility.

Etiologies of infertility include problems of spermatozoa and oocyte availability and tubal occlusion.[2] A significant number of couples will have more than one cause, requiring that the diagnostic investigation be complete and thorough in each case. The single most common gynecological disorder relating to infertility is the high (30–50%) prevalence of tubal factors.[1–3] Congenital or acquired anatomical (various malformations, synechia, post-inflammatory occlusion, etc.) or functional (periodical spastic occlusion, decreased peristaltic activity, spasmus of the isthmus, etc.) tubal lesions are reported to be the cause. Male abnormalities are essentially those involving sperm production and transportation. Although the diagnostic evaluation of the male partner of the infertile couple is of extreme importance, imaging techniques are generally of only secondary importance as assessment of the semen is the most valuable diagnostic element in this evaluation.

The diagnosis of infertility is primarily made by serologic and radiologic means. However, about 15% of the infertile couples suffer from 'unexplained infertility' where the cause for infertility cannot be identified utilizing the currently available and acceptable diagnostic techniques. The possibility of a tubal factor in these patients has spurred an interest in functional studies of the tube as fundamental in the investigation of the infertile couple, primarily to assess patency, but also to determine the possibility of patent but 'nonfunctional' oviducts.[4]

RELEVANT ANATOMY AND PHYSIOLOGY

The fallopian tubes

Each fallopian tube is about 12 cm long and opens medially into the uterine cavity's superior angle and laterally into the peritoneal cavity near the corresponding ovary. The uterine ostium is small whilst the peritoneal opening or abdominal ostium, is deep within a trumpet-shaped expansion of the uterine tube. The infundibulum and its circumference is prolonged by a varying number of fimbriae. The fimbriae are lined by mucosa with longitudinal folds continuous with those in the infundibulum. The infundibulum opens into the ampulla, which is thin-walled, has a tortuous lumen and is more than half the tube's length. The ampulla leads into the isthmus, which is rounded and firm, and forms approximately the tube's medial third. The intramural uterine part is about 3 cm long.[5]

The fallopian tube has an external serosa, an intermediate muscular stratum and an internal mucosa. The serosa is

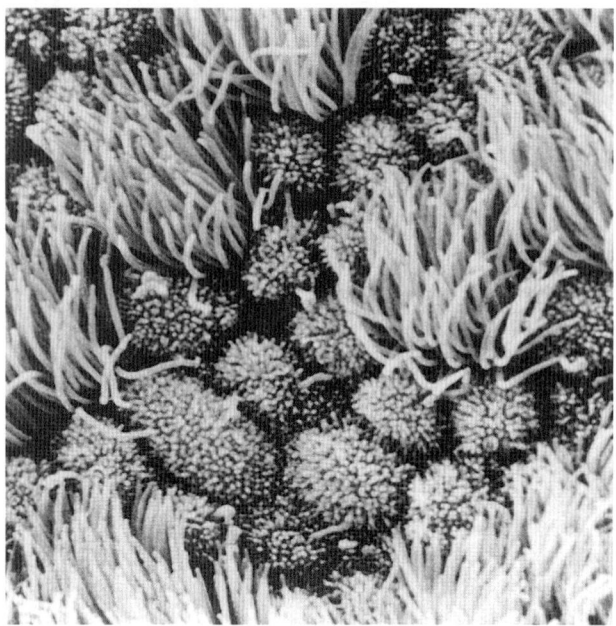

Figure 13E.1 *Electron microscopy of the ciliated epithelium of the fallopian tubes.*

a fold of the peritoneum with subjacent connective tissue. The muscular layer has external longitudinal and internal circular layers of non-striated muscle. A labyrinth of mucosal folds projects into the lumen with a smaller number of simpler longitudinal folds. The tubal mucosa has an epithelium and underlying connective tissue containing a rich substrate of blood, lymph vessels, and nerves. The simple columnar epithelial lining of the uterine tube is made up of ciliated cells interspersed with intercalated (indifferent) and nonciliated secretory cells that are believed to produce a nutritive secretion. The ciliated cells of the oviduct have a common structural and functional pattern of internal tubules, with propulsive action as that of most of the respiratory tract, some of the tympanic cavity and auditory tube, efferent ductules of the testis and spermatozoid flagellum (Fig. 13E.1).

Ciliated cells in the fallopian tubes are most prominent in the epithelial surface of the fimbriated infundibulum where they form dense arrays while large numbers of cilia may also be found in the ampulla. In general, ciliated cells are less frequent in the isthmus.

Growth of the ciliated epithelium appears to be under the influence of ovarian hormones, and data from humans and animals indicate that growth of these ciliated cells is promoted by estrogens. Ciliated and secretory cells begin to increase in height shortly after menstruation, and by the time of ovulation they are approximately 30 μm high.

The ciliary beat frequency changes at different stages of ovulation as the fallopian tubes prepare for ovum pick-up and transport under the influence of sex hormones. The normal ciliary beat frequency is about 5.6 Hz, which rises

to 6 Hz in the late follicular phase before ovulation and decreases to 4.9 Hz after ovulation.[6] There is a good correlation between the ciliary beat frequency and the percentage of ciliated cells in the fallopian tubes – the 'ciliary index'.

Fertilization

Upon ejaculation into the anterior vagina, the pool of highly concentrated semen bathes the external cervical os and spermatozoa gain access to the mucus-filled cervical canal largely under the influence of their own motility. Contractions of smooth muscle in the vagina and cervical walls as well as active directional beating of some ciliated cells in the cervical canal may assist this surprisingly rapid process. Migration of spermatozoa through the uterus to the fallopian tubes depends on myometrial contractions while sperm motility, which maintain the spermatozoa in suspension in the uterine fluids prevent their adhesion within the uterus (Fig. 13E.2). The existence of upward transportation processes at the time of conception implies that the motility of spermatozoa may not be the only relevant factor for their ascension. Indeed, the union of spermatozoon and oocyte depends not only on the active role of spermatozoa, but also on actions of the female reproductive tract. Muscular peristalsis and rate of beat of cilial activity in the fallopian tubes respond to the circulating concentrations of ovarian steroid hormones, although the autonomic nervous system directly regulates the myosalpinx. The rate of cilial beat and muscular contraction seems to be greatest just at or after the time of ovulation, thereby ensuring effective transport of eggs to the site of fertilization. However, progression of eggs to the ampullary–isthmic junction is not continuous, but rather consists of intermittent waves of contraction in the ampulla. Just after ovulation and around the time of fertilization when eggs are descending the ampulla while spermatozoa are ascending the isthmus the fallopian tube becomes birectional. Male and female gametes are transported in the tube and must meet at a specific site within well-defined time limits for fertilization to take place. Because of the key role of ovarian steroids in regulating these events, anomalous levels of estrogens and progesterone would certainly upset the normal mechanisms and timing of gamete transport. But most of all, healthy and patent oviducts facilitate conception.

Following fertilization the principal mechanisms regulating the passage of embryos into the uterus involve activity of myosalpinx and cilia, the reduction of edema in the mucosa, and the directional flow of fluid in the tubal lumen.

Seen in the context of their structure the fallopian tubes appear to be modest passive uterine appendages. Functionally, they are extremely sensitive organs responding to hormonal, biochemical, and neural stimulation that facilitates the process of fertilization. On the few special occasions

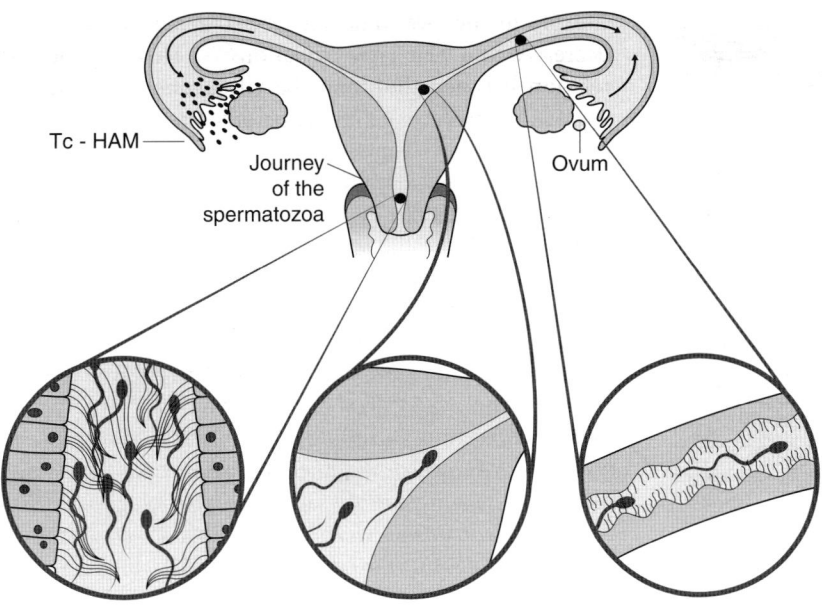

Figure 13E.2 *The journey of the spermatozoa through the female reproductive tract showing ciliated epithelium of the cervix and the tubes facilitating this migratory process. The same mechanism possibly occurs for the migration of radiolabeled microspheres during hysterosalpingoscintigraphy (HSS).*

that the oviducts are required to act, they constitute the most important element in the process of life creation. In simple terms, life begins in the fallopian tubes; they are the 'avenues of life'.

Physiopathology

In the adult female, the peritoneal cavity communicates with the outside via the fallopian tubes, the uterus, and the vagina and there is evidence for the migration of different substances in either direction. For example, malignant cells from ovarian carcinoma can be demonstrated in the posterior fornix of the vagina.[7] Retrograde menstruation is also a well-known phenomenon.[8] Peritonitis is said to occur more frequently in females because infection of the vagina, uterus or the uterine tube may spread directly to the peritoneum, via the abdominal ostium. Tubal inflammation (salpingitis), which is the most common cause of infertility, is usually secondary, having spread from the vagina or the uterus. For pregnancy to occur, spermatozoa have to move up the uterus as the ova moves down the tube. After insufflation, air and gases pass easily from the vagina into the peritoneal cavity up to the diaphragm. Radio-opaque contrast media are introduced through the uterus and tubes into the peritoneal cavity, and tubal patency is demonstrated during laparoscopy by injection of a dye through the cervix and into the fallopian tubes (chromopertubation).

If transit can take place so easily, it is probable that the same happens with chemical substances used for hygienic, cosmetic or medicinal purposes, many of which may have potential carcinogenic or irritating properties. Such migration could well explain the etiologic role of chemical substances in certain gynecologic diseases, and especially in carcinoma of the ovary and infertility.[9,10]

INVESTIGATIONS

Diagnostic procedures where gases, fluids, dyes, and contrast medium are introduced through manual interventions under positive pressure from the uterine cervix into the peritoneum are anatomically accurate and safe in the hands of those performing them regularly, but do not fully portray fallopian tube patency or function.

Laparoscopy under general anesthesia provides visual information about the gross anatomy of the pelvis. Pelvis adhesions, endometriosis, and post-surgical scarring limiting tubal motility, are the most common findings which are not necessarily diagnosed radiographically.[1]

Hysterosalpingography (HSG) is an important outpatient radiological procedure for evaluating uterine, tubal, and peritoneal causes of infertility. Its advantages include immediate information about proximal and distal occlusion and cornual lesions, and the assessment of intratubal architecture. A major limitation of HSG is its inability to demonstrate peritubal disease with consistency, and to evaluate the status of the tubal fimbria.[3,4] HSG is indicated early in the investigation of the infertile female particularly in those with a history of previous abdominal surgery, known episodes of pelvic inflammatory disease, post-partum infection, and/or palpable adnexal pathology compatible with hydrosalpinges or endometriosis. It is also indicated in women with previous sterilization who request tubal ligation reversal, or to confirm tubal occlusion after tubal sterilization.

Transcervical hysteroscopy has been utilized to visualize the tubal ostium and intramural portion of the fallopian tubes. Evidence of proximal tubal occlusion, polyps, adhesions and salpingitis isthmica nodosa may be found.

All the above are invasive procedures, uncomfortable for the patient, at times painful, and restricted under certain conditions. HSG is not free of risks of hypersensitivity reactions, uterine perforation and tubal rupture, hemorrhage, endometriosis, shock, granuloma formation, or pulmonary oil embolism.

Ultrasonography does not use radiation but the tubes are difficult to visualize during ultrasonographic examination of a normal pelvis. The difficulties are probably due to their small diameter, variable position within the pelvis and absence of fluid/tissue interfaces. Blockages at, or near, the junction of the uterus and oviduct may not give rise to any ultrasonographically detectable alteration.

HYSTEROSALPINGOSCINTIGRAPHY

Clinical studies

The inherent physiological nature of the nuclear medicine techniques potentially allows a study of the functional integrity of the female genital tract. This has been explored over the last 25 years by various investigators by introducing and developing hysterosalpingoscintigraphy (HSS), a new radionuclide technique for evaluating fallopian tube function.

In 1981, Iturralde and Venter first described spontaneous migration and imaging of particulate radioactive tracer from posterior vaginal fornix to the ovaries and peritoneal cavity.[11] The main aim of their study was to demonstrate the potential movement of suspected carcinogens like asbestos and talc from the vagina to the ovaries. ^{99m}Tc-labeled human albumin microspheres (HAM) were instilled in the posterior vaginal fornix pre-surgically in a group of patients undergoing gynecologic surgery and the retrograde migration of these 10–35 μm particles was demonstrated by *in vitro* counting of surgically removed uterine and adenexal specimens.

This encouraged the researchers to employ their technique in a group of patients referred from an infertility clinic. Anterior pelvic imaging was performed by using a large field-of-view gamma camera at 1, 2, 3, and 24 h post-deposition of 74–100 MBq of ^{99m}Tc-HAM at the posterior vaginal fornix. The study was interpreted as normal when activity was noted in one or both of the fallopian tubes or fimbria. The study was compared with contrast hystosalpingography (HSP) and peritoneoscopy. The researchers believed that their scintgraphic procedure provided a correct diagnosis since it depicted the functional state of the fallopian tubes in contrast to HSP.

Venter[12] later reported results obtained on a third group of patients with presumed normal fallopian tubes who were scheduled for tubal ligation for conservative reasons. Patients in this group showed evidence of a hormonal regulatory process of tubal ciliary function as migration of ^{99m}Tc-HAM was faster during the period of ovulation and slower in the luteal phase. During the time patients were using oral contraceptives migration was also slower. Later, Wildt *et al.*[13] performed HSS in a large group (580) of infertile women using ^{99m}Tc-labeled macroaggregates of human serum albumin (^{99m}Tc-MAA). They studied the rate and site of migration of activity applied to the posterior vaginal fornix, using sequential gamma-camera imaging. There was lateralization of MAA transport to the oviduct leading to the dominant follicle with a strong correlation to the follicular size. In 79% of patients studied during the follicular phase, radioactivity entered the fallopian tubes either unilaterally (64%) or bilaterally (15%) with the radioactivity staying in the uterine cavity in the remaining 21% of the patients.

In a prospective HSS study of 26 patients referred from an infertility clinic, McCalley *et al.*[14] introduced some procedural modifications including reduction of the administered dose to 37 MBq which was instilled directly onto the cervical mucosa thereby potentially sacrificing physiological fidelity. Anterior pelvic images were acquired after 15–30 min using pinhole collimation with caudal angulation to improve visualization of the region behind the uterus. Lateral oblique views were also obtained when needed. Imaging was terminated as soon as the study was interpreted as being normal or after 4 h in cases where obstruction was suspected. Patency of a fallopian tube was inferred if a relatively intense focus of activity was seen in the area of the adjacent adnexa. If no such activity was evident on images 1 h or more after radiotracer administration, then that tube was considered obstructed. Direct observations of surgical pathology, peritoneoscopy, and contrast HSG were used as comparison studies. Efficiency of HSS for evaluation of fallopian tube patency was over 94%. Two tubes that appeared obstructed on HSS but were judged patent by correlative examination, were found to be immotile at surgery with peritubal and periadnexal adhesions, which probably rendered them functionally incapable of transporting radiolabeled particles. These results lent further support to the contention that the radionuclide study is a more physiologic indicator of tubal function than the radiographic contrast study.

McQueen *et al.*,[15] following strict criteria for the classification of infertility, prospectively studied 96 infertile women with HSS and compared the findings of the radionuclide study with laparoscopy and contrast hysterosalpingography. The radionuclide test correlated with laparoscopy in the diagnosis of patency or blockage in 83 cases (86%). In nine patients, where 'blockage' was diagnosed on the radionuclide test but patency found at laparoscopy, a higher prevalence of pelvic abnormality was found, compared to the 78 patients where both tests demonstrated patency ($P < 0.02$). They concluded that HSS may facilitate detection of diseased but patent tubes and, as an adjunct to laparoscopy and chromopertubation, may provide useful information about tubal function.

A similar study conducted by Steck *et al.*[16] reported congruent findings between tubal patency on contrast HSG and tubal migration on HSS. For the detection of tubal obstruction, the sensitivity of radionuclide imaging was 86% and the specificity 66% when using the HSG as the standard, and the percentage of tubes correctly classified was 67%. For the detection of tubal occlusion, the figures for sensitivity and specificity of HSS were 91 and 60%, respectively, with an overall efficiency of 69%.

Uzler et al.,[17] studying a series of 46 infertile patients, reported that no patient whose tubes were nonfunctional on HSS became pregnant without in vitro fertilization (IVF), and five live, healthy births resulted in patients showing function of at least one tube. HSS is the only method that allows visual assessment of fallopian tube function and therefore plays a unique role in aiding infertility evaluation.

Recently, Schmiedehausen et al.[18] performed dynamic HSS to investigate the velocity and direction of sperm transport to the dominant follicle in patients with anatomically patent tubes. They demonstrated a rapid transit rate of transport of ^{99m}Tc-MAA to the dominant follicle with 67% in the first 30 s and nearly 80% with in the first minute with the transport directed to the fallopian tube leading to the dominant oocyte.

Brundin et al.[19] claimed to evaluate the active transportation capacity of the luminal epithelium lining the human uterus and fallopian tubes by HSS. The results were compared to the findings at normal hysterosalpingography. By using this method it was possible to verify active passage in cases of tubal spasm at HSG, lack of transport in cases of normal patent oviducts at HSG as well as presence or absence of active transport through sactosalpinges with or without fimbrial passages to the abdominal cavity as seen at normal HSG. Congruent findings between HSG and HSS were observed in 49%. The studied oviducts were found to be patent with normal HSG but lacked transportation capacity when studied by HSS in 41%. None of the patients with impaired oviductal transportation capacity but with a normal contrast HSG conceived, thereby implying that the capacity of transporting luminal content in those patients with damaged, but apparently patent tubes on HSG, on whom microsurgery is performed to restore luminal passage, could be seriously questioned.

Recent developments in physiological and surgical approaches to infertility could be aided by knowledge of fallopian tube function, and because of its functional nature, HSS could constitute an important tool for referring the infertile patient to an optimal choice of therapy for infertility due to a 'tubal factor'. If ciliary function is normal, the infertile patient should be directed to an in vitro fertilization programme. If a woman is found to have pelvic adhesions, but HSS shows normal ciliary function, she may require surgery. However, for women with abnormal tubal ciliary function HSS tells the gynecologist that gamete or zygote intra-fallopian transfer will not work and in vitro fertilization and embryo transfer will be needed instead.

Since the initial description of the procedure, extensive evaluation has taken place to determine the role of HSS in the investigation of tubal dysfunction compared to other diagnostic examinations. Technical refinements have been introduced to improve the imaging quality, reduce the radiation dose and increase the awareness of the radionuclide technique amongst the nuclear medicine professionals and the referring clinicians.

Hysterosalpingoscintigraphy protocol

SCINTIGRAPHIC TECHNIQUE

The study is undertaken during the pre-ovulatory phase of the cycle as close as possible to the ovulation. Scintigraphy is performed by using 10–15 MBq of ^{99m}Tc-labeled HAM or 10–25 MBq MAA in 0.5–1 mL normal saline. The radiotracer is instilled via a catheter into the posterior vaginal fornix or cervical canal. With the patient lying supine on the imaging table, dynamic study (30–60 s frames for 20 min) is performed in the anterior projection using a large-field-of-view gamma camera equipped with a low-energy all-purpose collimator. Serial static images of anterior pelvis are obtained at 1, 2, and 3 h with additional lateral or lateral–oblique views when required. Computer processing of the static images and dynamic studies allow for image enhancement and quantification.

FINDINGS AND INTERPRETATION

The normal and abnormal scintigraphic appearances and findings are described. Depending on the site of instillation, a central elongated area of high activity will be normally visualized over the vagina, with a narrow stretch of activity corresponding to the endocervix directly on top of this area. The uterus is seen as a smaller area of varying size, position, and shape appearing triangular in most of the cases. Visualization of large elongated uterine cavity signifies the follicular phase of the cycle, while broad area of radioactivity distribution signifies the luteal phase (Figs 13E.3 and 13E.4).

The fallopian tubes are seen extending laterally or upward in a diverging angle with a distal 'hot' spot of high intensity corresponding to the fimbriae and ovaries. Activity in the region of the tubal isthmus may not be visualized in some cases. Some investigators have used the term 'cornu cut-off sign' for a discontinuity of activity from the region of the cornu to the ipsilateral fallopian tube. Activity progression through one or both tubes within the 1–3 h should be taken as normal. Scans should be interpreted as abnormal if there is no activity in one or both tubes and especially if the distal focal area of high activity in the fimbriae or in the pelvic cavity up to 4 h after deposition (Fig. 13E.5).

RADIATION DOSIMETRY

The gonadal radiation doses received during the radionuclide procedure are comparable to those received during the radiographic contrast examination, not including the dose due to fluoroscopy. During radiographic fallopian tube recanalization, the average absorbed dose to the ovaries was calculated at 8.5 mGy.

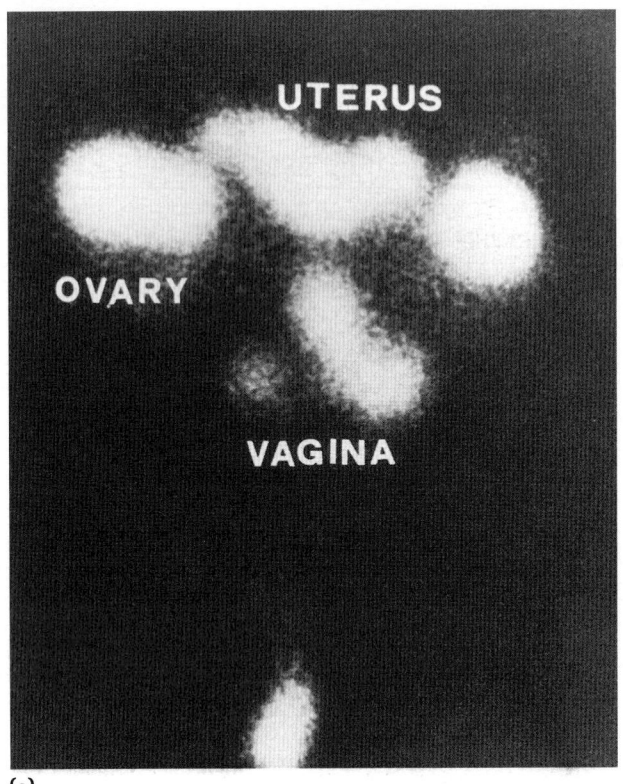

(a)

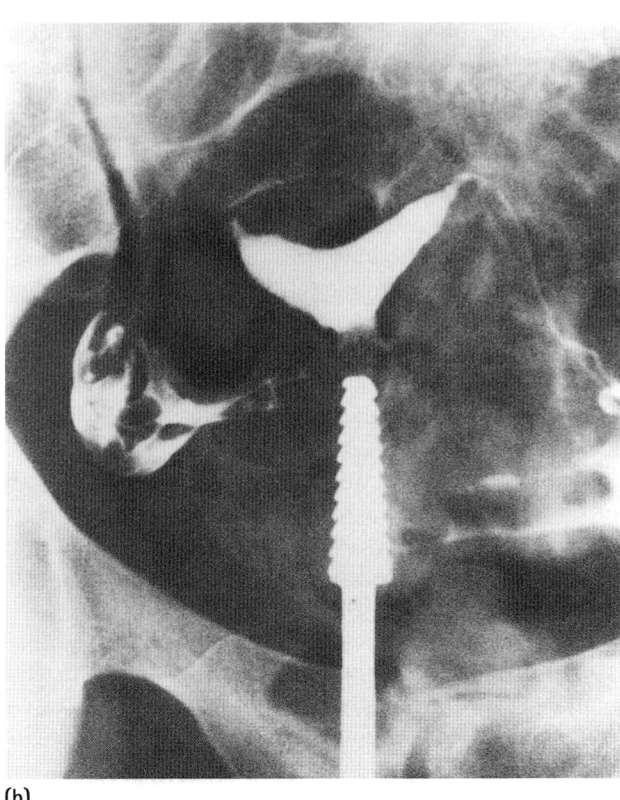

(b)

Figure 13E.3 *(a) Normal hysterosalpingoscintigraphy (HSS) showing the pattern of flow of radiolabeled microspheres from vagina, through the uterus to the fimbriated peritoneal opening of the patent fallopian tubes, and (b) contrast spillage into the peritoneal cavity during hysterosalpingography.*

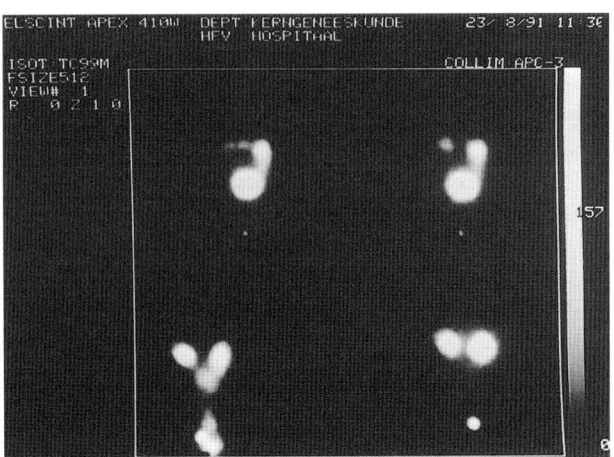

Figure 13E.4 *Normal hysterosalpingoscintigraphy at 30 min (top left), 60 min (top right), and 90 min (lower left), with asymmetric migration of radiolabeled microspheres appearing early in the left fimbriae, to bilateral tubal patency at 3 h (lower right).*

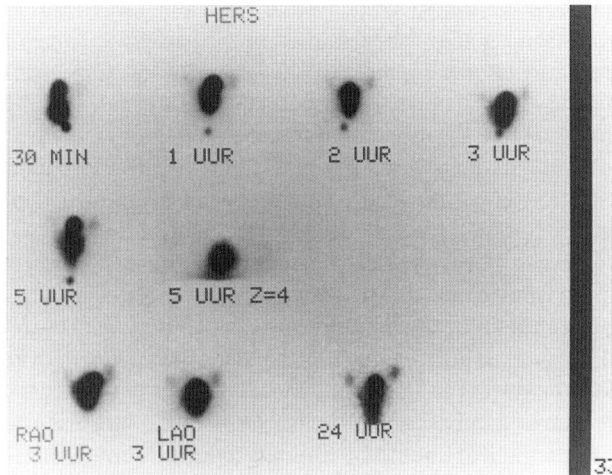

Figure 13E.5 *Abnormal HSS with images obtained for up to 24 h. Bilateral tubal obstruction (faint activity is portrayed bilaterally in ampulla of fallopian tubes).*

McCalley *et al.*[20] and van der Weiden and van Xil[21] have estimated an ovarian dose of 0.75 mGy MBq^{-1} (1.8 rad mCi^{-1}) for HSS, assuming that 5% of the administered dose resides on each ovary for the duration of the physical decay of ^{99m}Tc ($T_{1/2}$ 6 h). Stabin[22] (at the Oak Ridge

Radiopharmaceutical Internal Dose Information Center) corrected this dose estimate, suggesting that the actual dose to each ovary is 1.5 mGy MBq^{-1}. Kennedy *et al.*[23] estimated the dose to be much lower because the maximum uptake in the ovaries was found to be 4.6% of the administered activity, giving a maximum dose of 2.35 mGy per ovary. Using ^{99m}Tc-pertechnetate Yang *et al.*[24] reported a dose of 1.08 mGy (108 mrad) per study.

Clinical role

The mechanism by which the migration of spermatozoa or radiolabeled particles takes place is poorly understood, but it is assumed that it is a combination of muscular peristaltic movements, changes in peritoneal pressure, and ciliary motion. There also appears to be a cyclical hormonal component regulating this process, and it is suggested that migration is facilitated during the period of ovulation.[2,7]

Although ^{99m}Tc-MAA molecules are biochemically and immunologically different from human spermatozoa, their diameter roughly approximates the size of human spermatozoa. It has therefore been suggested that radiolabeled tracer molecules are transported by the same natural mechanisms supporting spermatozoal migration to the ovum during the period of fertilization and that tubal migration of the radionuclide reflects the ascending flow of spermatozoa. (Fig. 13E.5)

There are some clinical circumstances where HSS seems particularly attractive. The increasing number of sterilizations being performed on relatively young women of low parity, together with the availability of improved microsurgery techniques has led to an increased demand for reversal. Patients who have had surgical reanastomosis for previously ligated or fibrosed tubes are at an unacceptable risk (3.3%) of developing tubo-ovarian abscess or granuloma as a complication of contrast HSG performed during the first few weeks following surgery or being deceived by the diagnosis of tubal patency when in fact the tubes may be patent but nonfunctional due to deciliation in the blind loop resulting from ligation, while HSS is a simple method used to confirm the success of a tubal ligation for sterilization purposes.[25] This is a practical problem with potential legal implications for the surgeon (Fig. 13E.6).

When compared with the 'gold standard' of laparoscopy and direct observation of tubal motility at surgery, hysterosalpingoscintigraphy has a reported sensitivity of 93% and a specificity of 94% for the detection of tubal patency, with a sensitivity of 94% and the specificity of 93% for the detection of tubal obstruction. The overall predictive value of the test for tubal patency was 96% and 90% for tubal obstruction. The overall efficiency (percent of tubes correctly diagnosed for obstruction or patency) was 97%.[26]

Although it is encouraging to find a close correlation between HSS and HSG or LPC, this comparison between HSS and contrast HSG and LPC seems inappropriate since these procedures are fundamentally different in nature. Further, several studies have shown a marked discrepancy between HSG and LPC, with only about 50% correlation between these two techniques in the study of infertile women.[1,2,27,28] HSS functionally reflects the dynamic state

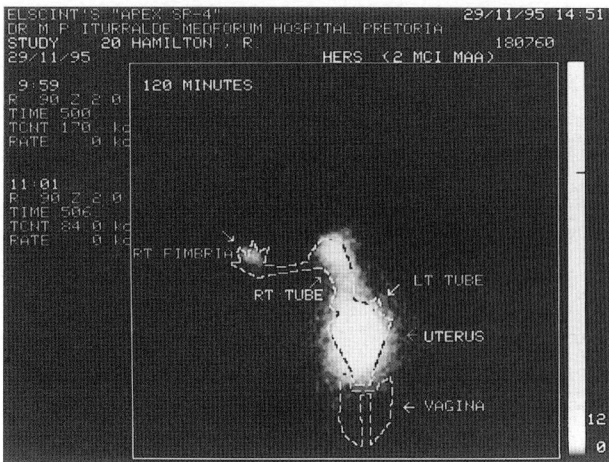

Figure 13E.6 *Hysterosalpingoscintigraphy of a patient who underwent tubal ligation, showing radiolabeled microsphere migration through the right tube to the fimbriae beyond the level of migration.*

Table 13E.1 *Indications for hysterosalpingoscintigraphy*

- *Normal fertility work-up including contrast hysterosalpingography*
- *To evaluate results of re-anastomosis/reconstructive surgery*
- *Assessment of sperm transport function*
- *Evaluation of tubal ligation to decide appropriate technique*
- *Choice of artificial insemination technique*
- *To determine the effect of fertility medicines*
- *In cases of repeated ectopic pregnancies*
- *To evaluate the cause of repeated unexplained peritoneal/pelvic infections*

of the female reproductive system by showing particulate migration, which is not the case of the other anatomically dependent diagnostic modalities used to evaluate tubal patency. The current indications for the HSS are listed in Table 13E.1.

HSS is the only currently available noninvasive technique that can reveal actual tubal function and if the functional nature of HSS could be shown to predict outcome better than contrast HSG, then gynecologists may be willing to exchange the superior spatial resolution of contrast HSG for the functional superiority of HSS.

REFERENCES

1 Winfield AC, Fleischer AC, Moore DE. Diagnostic imaging of fertility disorders. *Curr Probl Diagn Radiol* 1990; **19**: 1–38.

2 Jaffe R, Pierson RA, Abramowicz JS. *Imaging in infertility and reproduction endocrinology.* Philadelphia: JB Lippincott, 1994: 335.

3   Wiswede K, Allen DA. Infertility factors at the Groote Schuur Hospital fertility clinic. *S Afr Med J* 1989; **76**: 65–6.

4   Gurgan T, Kisnisci HA, Yarali H, *et al.* Evaluation of the functional status of the fallopian tubes in unexplained infertility with radionuclide hysterosalpingography. *Gynecol Obstet Invest* 1991; **32**: 224–6.

5   Hunter RHF. *The fallopian tubes.* Berlin: Springer-Verlag, 1988.

6   Paltieli Y. New laser technique can help pinpoint infertility due to fallopian tube pathology. *Med Chronicle* 1994; 7.

7   Greenfeld EF. Ovarian tumours. *Clin Obstet Gynecol* 1975; **18**: 61–86.

8   Schwarz RH. Acute pelvic inflammation disease. In: Monif GRG. (ed.) *Diseases in obstetrics and gynaecology.* London: Harper and Row, 1974: 381–95.

9   Howe JR. A method of recognising carcinogens in the laboratory. *Lab Prac* 1975; **24**: 457–6.

10 Lingeman CH. Etiology of cancer of the human ovary [Review]. *J Natl Cancer Inst* 1974; **53**: 1603–18.

11 Iturralde MP, Venter PF. Hysterosalpingo-radionuclide scintigraphy (HERS). *Semin Nuc Med* 1981; **11**: 301–14.

12 Venter PF. Epiteeltumore vand die Ovarium. Doctoral thesis, University of the Orange Free State, South Africa, 1979.

13 Wildt L, Kissler S, Licht P, Becker W. Sperm transport in the human female genital tract and its modulation by oxytocin as assessed by hysterosalpingoscintigraphy, hysterotonography, electrohysterography and Doppler sonography. *Human Reprod Update* 1998; **4**: 655–66.

14 McCalley MG, Braunstein P, Stone S, Henderson P, Egbert R. Radionuclide hysterosalpingography for evaluation of fallopian tube patency. *J Nucl Med* 1985; **26**: 868–74.

15 McQueen D, McKillop JH, Gray HW, Bessent RG, Black WP. Investigation of tubal infertility by radionuclide migration. *Human Reprod* 1991; **6**: 529–32.

16 Steck T, Wurfel W, Becker W, Albert PJ. Serial scintigraphic imaging for visual passive transport processes in the human fallopian tube. *Human Reprod* 1991; **6**: 1186–91.

17 Uzler M, Jacobson A, Warnich A, Nassor G. Radionuclide hysterosalpingography – appropriate for the new assisted reproduction techniques. *J Nucl Med* 1993; **164**: 797.

18 Schmiedehausen K, Kat S, Albert N, *et al.* Determination of velocity of tubar transport with dynamic hysterosalpingoscintigraphy. *Nucl Med Commun* 2003; **24**: 865–70.

19 Brundin J, Dahlborn M, Ahlber-Ahre E, Lundberg HJ. Radionuclide hysterosalpingography for measurement of human oviductal function. *Int J Gynecol Obstet* 1989; **28**: 53–9.

20 McCalley MG, Braunstein P, Stone S, *et al.* Radionuclide hysterosalpingography for evaluation of fallopian tube patency. *J Nucl Med* 1985; **26**: 868–74.

21 van der Weiden RMF, van Xil J. Radiation exposure of the ovaries during hysterosalpingography. Is radionuclide hysterosalpingography justified? *Br J Obstet Gynaecol* 1989; **96**: 471–2.

22 Stabin M. Radiation dosimetry in radionuclide hysterosalpingography [Letter]. *J Nucl Med* 1989; **30**: 415–16.

23 Kennedy SH, Mojiminiyi OA, Soper MDW, *et al.* Radiation exposure of the ovaries during hysterosalpingography. Is radionuclide hysterosalpingography justified? *Br J Obstet Gynaecol* 1989; **69**: 1359.

24 Yang KTA, Chiang J-H, Chen B-S, *et al.* Radionuclide hysterosalpingography with ^{99m}TcO; application and radiation dose to ovaries. *J Nucl Med* 1992; **33**: 282–6.

25 Strauss SA. Unsuccessful sterilisation of woman – doctor liable for child-raising cost. *S Afr Med J* 1990; **75**: 557.

26 Iturralde MP, Venter PF. Comparison of diagnostic accuracy of laparoscopy, hysterosalpingography and radionuclide hysterosalpingography in the evaluation of female infertility. Proceedings 4th Asia and Oceania Congress of Nuclear Medicine, Taipei, Taiwan, 1988.

27 Brosens IA, Gordon AG. *Tubal infertility.* Philadelphia: JB Lippincott, 1990.

28 Lindequest S, Justesen P, Larsen C, Rasmussen F. Diagnostic quality and complications of hysterosalpingography. *Radiology* 1991; **179**: 69–74.

Testicular perfusion imaging

Q.H. SIRAJ

INTRODUCTION

The use of perfusion scintigraphy in the evaluation of acute scrotal disease, particularly for reliable and accurate diagnosis of testicular torsion, has been the most widely employed clinical application of radionuclide testicular imaging. Scintigraphic evaluation of testicular perfusion in a patient presenting with an acute hemi-scrotum is one of the few emergency nuclear medicine procedures, and impacts significantly on clinical decision-making and patient management.

Nadel *et al.* pioneered perfusion scintigraphy with [^{99m}Tc]pertechnetate for investigating the acute scrotum.[1] The procedure primarily aims at differentiating inflammatory hypervascular conditions from the avascular scrotal lesion caused by compromised testicular perfusion due to spermatic cord torsion. A substantial number of studies with added refinements and modifications in the original methodology have been reported.[2–6] Testicular perfusion scintigraphy is now well established and is a widely validated noninvasive technique reputed for its high diagnostic efficiency. In acute or missed testicular torsion, testicular perfusion scintigraphy has a reported sensitivity of 96%, specificity of 89% and an overall accuracy of 96%.[7]

ACUTE SCROTUM: CLINICAL PRESENTATION AND PATHOGENESIS

The clinical evaluation of a young patient presenting with an acute onset of unilateral scrotal symptoms, poses a diagnostic dilemma. The nonspecificity of symptoms and inadequacy of clinical examination in a poorly compliant, distressed, pediatric patient suffering from extreme local discomfort, quite often contributes towards an indeterminate clinical conclusion; clinical diagnosis may be incorrect in up to 50% of the patients.[2]

The common causes of an acute scrotum include bacterial epididymitis and epididymo-orchitis, viral orchitis, testicular torsion, torsion of a testicular appendage, acute hydrocele and retention cysts (e.g. spermatocele and epididymal cysts). Uncommon differential diagnoses include testicular tumor, strangulated inguinal hernia, testicular trauma, scrotal deep vein thrombosis, idiopathic scrotal edema, inflammation of the scrotal sac, hemorrhage in a testicular tumor or associated with trauma, scrotal fat necrosis, and acute testicular inflammation associated with tuberculosis, Buerger's disease or Henoch–Schönlein purpura.

Epididymitis is the most frequent etiology of acute scrotum, which is easily treatable by drugs. In contrast, testicular torsion is a true medical emergency requiring immediate surgery to preserve testicular viability and prevent development of ischemic necrosis. Since clinical distinction between these two entities is usually unreliable, therefore prompt and accurate diagnosis through evaluation of testicular perfusion is pivotal in implementing appropriate therapy and avoiding unnecessary surgery.

TESTICULAR TORSION

Clinical features

EXTRAVAGINAL TESTICULAR TORSION

There are two distinct clinical types of testicular torsion, intravaginal and extravaginal. The extravaginal form is uncommon, found almost exclusively in neonates. The condition is caused by the rotation of the testis and its covering fascia, above the level of tunica vaginalis. Neonatal testicular torsion may occur during late intrauterine life or the early post-partum period. Clinical examination of the neonate reveals a firm, smooth and painless scrotal mass with a variable scrotal reaction. The presentation is fairly specific, which makes clinical diagnosis easy and straightforward. Unilateral orchiectomy is the current treatment for extravaginal testicular torsion, since at the time of surgical exploration the testis is invariably necrotic. In this clinical scenario, evaluation of testicular perfusion appears superfluous and the condition will not be discussed further.

INTRAVAGINAL TESTICULAR TORSION

Intravaginal testicular torsion is the most common acute scrotal ailment in the pediatric and young adult age group. Torsion of the spermatic cord, or that of a testicular appendage, develops in one out of 160 males before the age of 25 years, with a peak incidence at puberty between the ages of 12 and 20 years.[8] The patient with testicular torsion usually presents clinically with an acutely painful, swollen and tender scrotum, accompanied by nausea or vomiting. With time, the scrotal skin becomes increasingly congested and edematous. Frequently, there is co-existing inguinal or abdominal pain causing a delay in the diagnosis.

In suspected testicular torsion, timely surgical intervention is crucial in preserving testicular viability: the testicular salvage rates being inversely proportional to the degree and the duration of spermatic cord torsion. The majority of gonads are salvageable until 6 h, the critical gray zone is the 6- to 12-h period and a delay of more than 24 h produces only anecdotal salvage.[9]

It must be emphasized that testicular viability is not synonymous with preserved testicular function. Despite successful surgical restoration of testicular perfusion, a large proportion of the affected testes reportedly suffer histological injury with subsequent decrease in fertility.[10]

APPENDAGE TORSION

Torsion of testicular or gonadal appendages accounts for roughly 5% of acute scrotal pathology.[11] Unlike testicular torsion, the condition is relatively uncommon in young adults, with the result that a much higher percentage (around 20%) is encountered in the pediatric age population.[12] The majority (about 85%) of cases of appendage torsion have been reported in patients aged 7–14 years.[13] Clinically, the patient usually presents with an abrupt onset of moderate scrotal or groin pain. Usually, the pain is less intense than in testicular torsion and the tenderness more focal – at the upper pole of the testis. The clinical features of appendix testis and appendix epididymis torsions are similar as are the scan appearances.

Relevant anatomy and embryology

A basic knowledge of the testicular developmental anatomy and its blood supply is helpful in understanding the etiology of testicular torsion.

NORMAL DEVELOPMENTAL ANATOMY

During normal fetal development, the intra-abdominal testes, situated retroperitoneally near the kidneys, descend through the inguinal rings, into the scrotum. Relative shortening of a fibromuscular band, the gubernaculum testis, which attaches the caudal pole of the testis to the scrotal remnant, accomplishes this descent. The descending testis is preceded by the distal end of a tubular extension of the peritoneum, the processus vaginalis, which herniates into the scrotum approximately at birth (Fig. 13F.1a). The abdominal connection closes, leaving the testis enclosed by a serous sac, the tunica vaginalis testis (Fig. 13F.1b). On the posterolateral aspect of the testis, the visceral layer of tunica vaginalis encloses the epididymis between its two layers and helps anchor the testis by reflecting back to line the scrotum as the parietal layer. In addition, the testes are also anchored posterolaterally by the gubernaculum and the broad epididymal mesorchium.

BLOOD SUPPLY

The blood supply of the male genitalia stems from two distinct sources that follow separate routes. The cremasteric, testicular and deferential arteries running along the spermatic cord nourish the testis and are essential to its survival. Spermatic cord torsion may occlude these vessels causing testicular death. The spermatic cord and epididymis, the testis, and the tunica vaginalis are respectively supplied by the deferential, testicular and cremasteric arteries. The internal pudendal, the superficial and the deep external pudendal arteries supply the scrotum and penis. Testicular torsion does not affect scrotal or penile viability by virtue of their separate blood supply.

TESTICULAR APPENDAGES

After birth, vestigial remnants of various structures persist as five testicular appendages including the appendix testis, a müllerian or paramesonephric duct remnant at the superior pole of the testis; the appendix epididymis, a wolffian or mesonephric duct remnant at the head of the epididymis; the paradidymis and the superior and inferior vas aberrans, remnants of paragenital tubules. The pedunculated appendages, i.e. the appendix testis and the appendix epididymis are more prone to torsion, representing 98% of the reported cases.[14] Torsion of the appendix testis is about 10 times more frequent than that of the appendix epididymis, accounting for 92–95% of the total cases.[3,14]

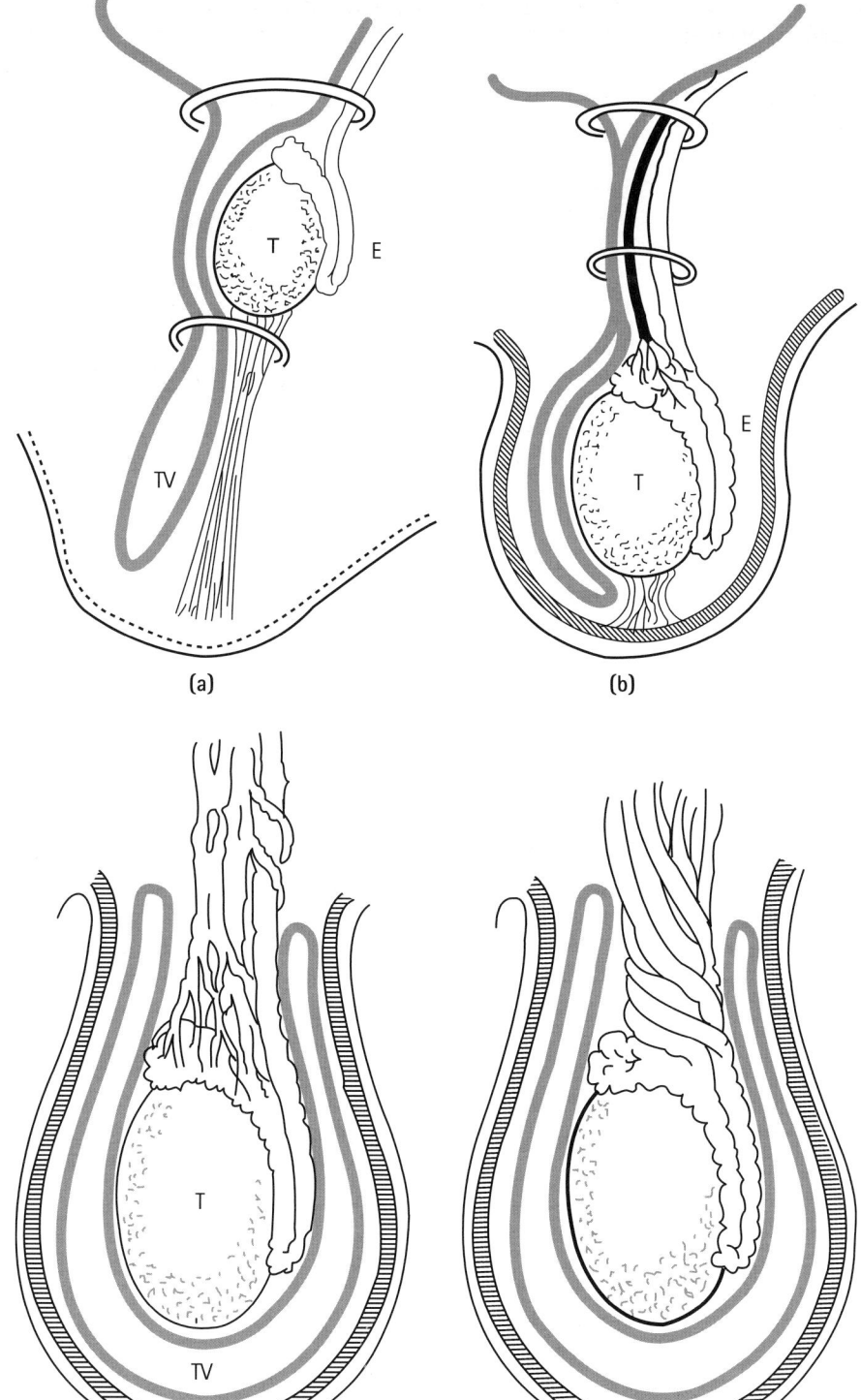

Figure 13F.1 *Diagram illustrating (a) descent of the testes from the abdomen through the inguinal rings into the scrotum, and (b) the formation of tunica vaginalis. (T, testis; TV, tunica vaginalis; E, epididymis).*

Figure 13F.2 *'Bell clapper' deformity with complete investation of the testis and epididymis by the tunica vaginalis leaving the testis anchored in the scrotum solely by the spermatic cord (a); the untethered testis is highly prone to torsion (b). (T, testis; TV, tunica vaginalis; E, epididymis).*

ABNORMAL DEVELOPMENTAL ANATOMY

Occasionally, the visceral layer of the tunica vaginalis encloses the entire testis and the epididymis so that the testis hangs within the scrotum like a bell – the so-called 'bell clapper' deformity (Fig. 13F.2a), which is the major cause of testicular torsion. Patients with this usually bilateral anatomic anomaly have a predisposition to torsion; such testes may rotate and the associated twisting of the spermatic cord (Fig. 13F.2b) compromises testicular and the epididymal perfusion with resultant infarction of the epididymis and loss of testicular viability and/or gonadal atrophy.

A less common developmental abnormality predisposing to torsion (accounting for about one third of testicular torsions) is an anomalous mesorchium, which is either elongated, incomplete or has a narrow area of attachment to the testis. Other uncommon anatomic abnormalities that may cause torsion include: partial or total separation of the epididymis and testis, an unusually bulky tunica vaginalis, an abnormally long spermatic cord, and atypical cremasteric muscle fibres that extend more distally than normal – contraction of the muscle, especially during sleep, may cause the cord to shorten and twist.

SCINTIGRAPHIC TECHNIQUE AND INTERPRETATION

The procedure is fairly simple and involves recording early (flow phase) and delayed (tissue phase) images of the scrotal region following an intravenous bolus injection of [^{99m}Tc]pertechnetate. The entire study is usually completed in 15–20 min.

Radiopharmaceuticals and equipment

Before the start of the study potassium perchlorate may be administered orally to block the thyroid. Scintigraphy is performed in adults using an intravenous injection activity of 555–740 MBq (15–20 mCi) of [^{99m}Tc]pertechnetate. The activity is reduced proportionately in young patients (7–10 MBq kg^{-1} or 200–250 μCi kg^{-1}) with a minimum activity of 55–74 MBq (1.5–2 mCi). The radiation dose to the patient is comparable to that of a chest X-ray.[15]

Imaging is performed using a standard or large field-of-view gamma camera with an on-line dedicated computer. For the adult and teenage patients, a general-purpose, low-energy collimator is used whereas a pinhole collimator is needed for pediatric patients.

Procedure

Immediately before the start of the study, the patient is instructed to empty his bladder to reduce the bladder activity. The patient is positioned supine on the imaging table, and the penis is turned upwards and taped to the pubic region to avoid overlapping of penile and scrotal activity. To obtain a technically satisfactory study, it is important to optimize scrotal visualization by minimizing the distance between the scrotum and the camera head, and reducing the background activity. Scrotal elevation is achieved either by means of a towel placed between the thighs, or through a tape sling under the scrotum stretching from thigh to thigh. In adults, the background radioactivity from the thighs is easily avoided by abducting the thighs. In children, a lead shield interposed between the sling and the scrotum

may be used to block background activity. To facilitate interpretation of flow images, the lead shield may be placed under the scrotum after completion of the dynamic phase of the study prior to the acquisition of the blood pool image, or alternatively a narrow lead shield that allows visualization of the femoral vessels may be used for both phases of the study.

The attending nuclear physician should conduct a brief physical examination of the scrotum and record relevant clinical findings. Examination may reveal testis redux, i.e. superior retraction of the testis induced by involuntary contraction of the cremasteric muscle associated with testicular torsion or inflammation. In the presence of testis redux, the testis should be gently retracted downwards and taped to the shield. Where the median raphe is displaced by a markedly asymmetric scrotal enlargement, it should be manually realigned and secured in the mid-line position by paper tapes attached to the shield and sideways to the ipsilateral thigh. For the static images, a lead-strip marker placed over the median raphe forms a useful demarcation line between the two halves of the scrotum.

Data acquisition

The gamma camera is programmed for dynamic 64 × 64 matrix word mode acquisition with appropriate computer magnification set to zoom in the field of view extending from below the umbilicus to the proximal one third of the thighs. Following a bolus injection of [^{99m}Tc]pertechnetate into a suitable ante-cubital vein, serial images are obtained for 1 min at a frame rate of 2–5 s. When a pinhole collimator is being used, the dynamic multi-frame study is substituted by a 60-s static blood-flow phase image. Immediately after the flow study, a static 500–1000 k count (word mode, 128 × 128 matrix or larger) tissue-phase image is obtained with a lead shield placed under the scrotum. Further static images may be obtained with appropriate markers.

Interpretation of scintigraphic findings

NORMAL SCAN

The early dynamic images show iliac and femoral vessels followed by occasional identification of activity in the regions corresponding to the scrotal and spermatic cord vascular trunks. The late dynamic frames show a very low-grade capillary and venous phase blush of scrotal activity. Tissue-phase images show homogeneous activity in the scrotum, with testicular activity either similar to or slightly less than activity in the adjacent thigh. The testicular, dartos and epididymal activities are indistinguishable.

TESTICULAR TORSION

Scrotal image patterns in testicular torsion vary according to the duration of the symptoms. The scan findings can be

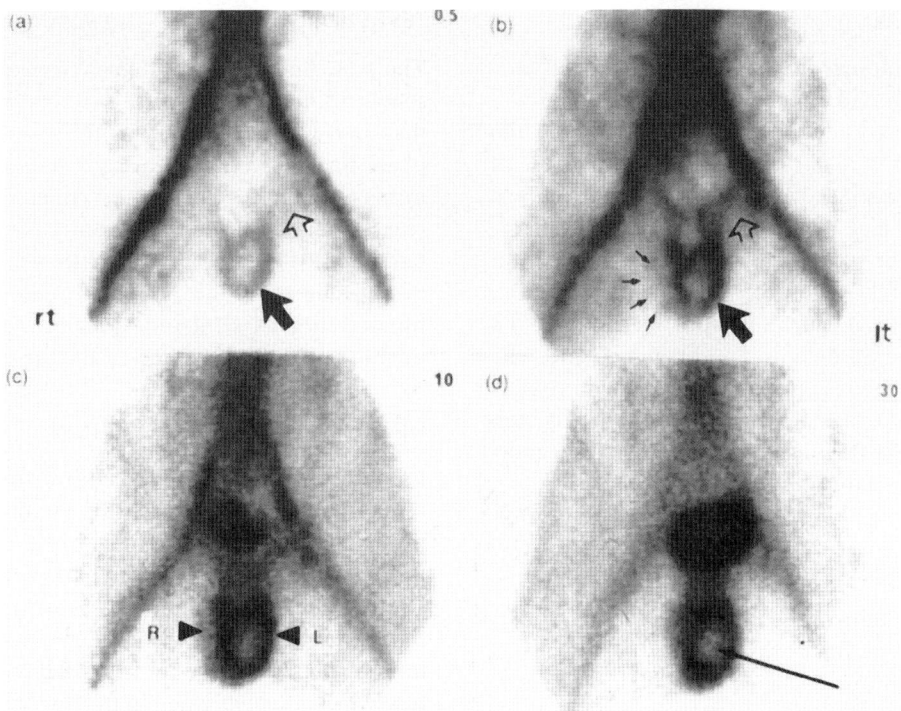

Figure 13F.3 *[^{99m}Tc]pertechnetate testicular perfusion scan of a 16-year-old boy with 3 days of left scrotal pain and swelling following trauma. The patient was afebrile with a normal urinalysis. Physical examination demonstrated an enlarged tender left testis. Blood flow phase image (a) and blood pool-tissue phase image at 2 min (b) show pudendal vascular hyperemia (open arrows) and rim of increased dartos activity (arrows) on the left; the right testis is outlined by small arrows (b). The late tissue-phase images at 10 min (c) and at 30 min (d) show markedly increased peri-testicular uptake (with a higher intensity compared to the activity in femoral vessels), a photopenic left testis (long arrow) and displacement of the right testis. The scan appearance is consistent with mid-phase 'missed torsion' and suggests testicular necrosis. Exploratory surgery revealed hemorrhagic infarction of the left testis due to spermatic cord torsion.*

graded into three stages: early-, mid- and late-phase torsion. Soon after the event, the twisting of the spermatic vascular pedicle occludes the venous return. Even when the degree of twisting is insufficient to occlude the lumen of the testicular artery, compression exerted by the congested veins within the rather rigid sheath of the spermatic cord secondarily blocks the arterial flow. On the flow images, this pooling of blood in the veins and the arterial occlusion may occasionally be seen as the 'nubbin sign', i.e. increased activity in the vascular pedicle of the cord up to the level of the twist; the pudendal vascular trunk is inconspicuous.[3] The late dynamic and the tissue-phase images show absence of activity in the affected testis.

In undiagnosed or untreated torsion, the ischemic injury progresses and scintigraphy performed in the mid-phase or early 'missed torsion' stage shows a hyperemic pudendal vascular trunk with increased activity in the dartos on the affected side (Fig. 13F.3a). This reactive hyperemic response in the scrotal tissues is induced by testicular necrosis and is seen as a loop of increased dartos activity surrounding a photopenic testis forming the scrotal bull's-eye or halo sign.[16] If spontaneous detorsion occurs prior to scintigraphy, the scan may be normal or may show increased activity in the blood-flow and tissue-phase images because of reactive hyperemia. A similar pattern may be seen in incomplete torsion.

The intensity of the peri-testicular rim of activity is inversely proportional to testicular salvage rates and forms a useful objective parameter for predicting surgical viability: where the scrotal activity equals or exceeds the activity in the femoral artery in blood pool-tissue phase images (Fig. 13F.3b–d), the chances of successful surgical salvage are poor.[5] Eventually, the testis undergoes atrophy with resolution of the surrounding hyperemia and a negative scan pattern ensues.

The predominant majority of missed torsions will typically demonstrate the rim sign. With time, the intensity of the peri-testicular rim of activity increases and in the late 'missed torsion' stage, a further increase in this activity is evident on the blood-flow and tissue-phase images. Emergency surgery may be deferred as testicular viability in late-phase missed torsion is low at ≤20%.[12,17] Since immune-mediated anti-spermatogenic effects of an infarcted testis left *in situ* pose a definite threat to the contralateral testis,[10] elective surgical exploration is still indicated.

APPENDAGE TORSION

The scintigraphic findings in appendage torsion are variable, with the affected side showing either normal, increased or decreased activity. In most of the cases, the scan shows normal activity. In a smaller proportion of patients, focally increased activity is seen near the upper pole of the testis, which may be misinterpreted for an inflammatory condition, in particular with focal inflammation involving only the head of the epididymis. However, the scan finding of focal hyperemia does not influence the clinical management, which is non-operative since the usual clinical outcome is appendage atrophy with resolution of symptoms. Occasionally, decreased uptake is seen on the scan, and it is these patients who are likely candidates for exploratory surgery.

INFLAMMATORY DISEASE

In acute bacterial epididymitis, the flow images show unilaterally augmented perfusion through the spermatic cord vessels and a crescentic or C-shaped area of increased activity located laterally in the scrotum, reflecting increased epididymal hyperemia. In the static images, there is increased uptake corresponding to the inflamed epididymis. The adjacent non-inflamed testis shows normal activity. On occasion, due to a medially displaced epididymis, the curvilinear activity is seen to be located in the medial scrotal region. Infective, traumatic and reactive forms of epididymitis have identical scintigraphic appearance. When there is associated orchitis, the involved testis also shows increased uptake. In viral epididymo-orchitis, there is comparatively a modest increase in activity seen on the flow and static images.

HYDROCELE, HEMATOCELE AND SPERMATOCELE

Collections of fluid or blood within the tunica vaginalis are the respective causes of hydroceles and hematoceles. These two conditions are scintigraphically indistinct, with a normal flow-phase and a curvilinear photopenic defect on the tissue-phase images. However, a hydrocele will transilluminate on physical examination. In spermatoceles, the vascular studies are normal and static images show a photopenic defect in the region corresponding to the location of the cyst, usually above the testis.

TESTICULAR ABSCESS

Classically, the flow study shows dramatically increased perfusion with enhanced visualisation of the spermatic trunk arterial vessels. On the static tissue-phase images, the scrotal abscess is visualized as photopenic or photo-deficient region(s) with surrounding hyperemia. The scan findings are similar to missed torsion, i.e. increased flow with a scrotal bull's-eye sign.

TESTICULAR TUMORS

The scan findings are variable. Generally, the flow study shows a diffuse mild increase in scrotal perfusion (less than that seen with epididymo-orchitis or abscess); the tissue-phase image reveals an enlarged testicle with moderately increased uptake, which may either be homogeneously (e.g. seminomas) or heterogeneously distributed (e.g. teratomas). The latter pattern reflects the relative avascular necrotic areas in the tumor. Certain vascular testicular tumors such as seminomas exhibit comparatively more intense activity in the perfusion and the tissue-phase images.

OTHER ACUTE SCROTAL CONDITIONS

In addition to those listed above, testicular perfusion scintigraphy can also identify inguinal hernia, scrotal trauma, varicoceles, scrotal involvement by Henoch–Schönlein purpura, etc. In inguinal hernia, the perfusion study is normal and the tissue-phase image shows a photopenic area extending from the involved hemi-scrotum to level of the inguinal ring. In scrotal trauma, there is diffusely increased perfusion in the flow study and the tissue-phase images show increased uptake with areas of diminished activity due to associated hematoma, hematocele or hydrocele formation.

OTHER IMAGING MODALITIES FOR EVALUATING TESTICULAR PERFUSION

Technological advancements in medical imaging have resulted in the application of nonradionuclide imaging modalities for the evaluation of scrotal pathology. It is therefore important to briefly comment on the current clinical role, the advantages and the inherent technical limitations of the individual techniques. The newer diagnostic methods include ultrasonography (US), color Doppler sonography (CDS) and magnetic resonance imaging (MRI).

Conventional gray-scale US provides high-resolution images of the scrotum and testis. US diagnosis of testicular torsion is based on the presence of equivocal, nonspecific and inconsistent morphological changes such as a reduction in testicular echogenicity with an increase in testicular size and the identification of small hydroceles. These US abnormalities are similar to those observed in epididymo-orchitis.[18] Further, the method provides no information on testicular perfusion and is therefore of limited value in this clinical context. The sensitivity of US for torsion is poor (47–50%) compared with scintigraphy (94–100%).[19] In the evaluation of scrotal disease, the US technique has different applications such as differentiating between intra- and extra-testicular conditions (e.g. epididymitis from a testicular abscess). For the evaluation of chronic or painless disorders of the scrotum, scintigraphic imaging is not the primary modality and by merits of its higher specificity, US is the preferred screening test. In selected cases, supplementing scintigraphy with sonography may reduce the incidence of false positive scans caused by spuriously decreased perfusion (e.g. hernia, hydrocele and hematocele), and when the perfusion scintigraphic findings are equivocal, US may help in identifying abnormality or substantiate normalcy.[20]

CDS potentially provides the facility to differentiate torsion of the testis from scrotal inflammatory diseases; several studies have reported the use of CDS as a useful imaging modality in children presenting with acute scrotal ailments, particularly for confirming the clinical diagnosis of epididymo-orchitis or testicular torsion.[21–23] However, the detection of testicular blood flow by CDS may be difficult in the pediatric age group due to the small size of the blood vessels.[22,23] The results of a recent CDS study report absence of testicular blood flow in one third of boys with normal testes.[24] Although CDS is a rapid non-invasive technique that may be helpful in diagnosing testicular torsion but has a limited clinical role due to its high false positive rate.

MRI and US are most useful in the evaluation of acute disorders that cause morphological alterations such as acute hydroceles, hematomas or testicular trauma.[25] Scrotal inflammatory diseases, such as epididymitis or orchitis, may be diagnosed by CDS,[26] US[27] or perfusion scintigraphy. The Doppler study is more specific and accurate than US with sensitivity comparable with that of scintigraphy.

In the assessment of testicular perfusion, these newer imaging modalities may in certain circumstances complement testicular perfusion scintigraphy with improvement in diagnostic specificity. However, in the context of spermatic cord torsion, the clinical effectiveness of these techniques remains to be established, and at present, none of these methods can be considered a reliable substitute for testicular perfusion scintigraphy. The scintigraphic patterns of various acute scrotal conditions are well documented and the technique remains the mainstay imaging modality of choice for the diagnosis of testicular torsion.

REFERENCES

1 Nadel NS, Gitter MH, Hahn LC, Vernon AR. Preoperative diagnosis of testicular torsion. *Urology* 1973; **1**: 478–9.

2 Riley TW, Mosbaugh PG, Coles JL, *et al.* Use of radioisotope scan in evaluation of intrascrotal lesions. *J Urol* 1976; **116**: 472–4.

3 Holder LE, Melloul M, Chen D. Current status of radionuclide scrotal imaging. *Semin Nucl Med* 1981; **11**: 232–49.

4 Chen DC, Holder LE, Melloul M. Radionuclide scrotal imaging: further experience with 210 patients. Part I: Anatomy, pathophysiology, and methods. *J Nucl Med* 1983; **24**: 735–42.

5 Chen DC, Holder LE, Melloul M. Radionuclide scrotal imaging: further experience with 210 new patients. Part 2: Results and discussion. *J Nucl Med* 1983; **24**: 841–53.

6 Mendel JB, Taylor GA, Treves S, *et al.* Testicular torsion in children: Scintigraphic assessment. *Paediatr Radiol* 1985; **15**: 110–5.

7 Tanaka T, Mishkin FS, Datta NS. Radionuclide imaging of scrotal contents. In: Freeman LM, Weissman HS. (eds.) *Nuclear Medicine Annual.* New York: Raven Press, 1981: 195–221.

8 Vogt LB, Miller MD, McLeod DG. To save a testis. *Emerg Med* 1988; **XX**: 69–76.

9 Sharer WC. Acute scrotal pathology. *Surg Clin North Am* 1982; **62**: 955–70.

10 Nagler HM, White R. The effect of testicular torsion on the contralateral testis. *J Urol* 1982; **128**: 1343–8.

11 Moharib NH, Krahn HP. Acute scrotum in children with emphasis on torsion of spermatic cord. *J Urol* 1970; **104**: 601.

12 Williamson RCN. Torsion of the testis and allied conditions. *Br J Surg* 1976; **63**: 465.

13 Fischman AJ, Palmer EL, Scott JA. Radionuclide imaging of sequential torsions of the appendix testis. *J Nucl Med* 1987; **28**: 119–21.

14 Skoglund RW, McRoberts JW, Radge H. Torsion of testicular appendages: Presentation of 43 new cases and a collective review. *J Urol* 1970; **104**: 598–600.

15 Blacklock ARE, Kwok HKY, Mason GR, *et al.* Radionuclide imaging in scrotal swellings. *Br J Urol* 1983; **55**: 749–53.

16 Dunn EK, Macchia RJ, Soloman NA. Scintigraphic pattern in missed testicular torsion. *Radiology* 1981; **139**: 175–80.

17 Skoglund RW, McRoberts JW, Radge H. Torsion of spermatic cord: A review of the literature and an analysis of 70 new cases. *J Urol* 1970; **104**: 604–7.

18 Arger PH, Mulhern CB, Coleman BG, *et al.* Prospective analysis of the value of scrotal ultrasound. *Radiology* 1981; **141**: 763–6.

19 Lutzker LG, Zuckier LS. Testicular scanning and other applications of radionuclide genital tract [Review]. *Semin Nucl Med* 1990; **20**: 159–88.

20 Mueller DL, Amundson GM, Rubin SZ, Wesenberg RL. Acute scrotal abnormalities in children: Diagnosis by combined sonography and scintigraphy. *AJR Am J Roentgenol* 1988; **150**: 643–6.

21 Middleton WD, Siegel BA, Melson GL, *et al.* Acute scrotal disorders: prospective comparison of color Doppler US and testicular scintigraphy. *Radiology* 1990; **177**: 177–81.

22 Burks DD, Markey BJ, Burkhard TK, *et al.* Suspected testicular torsion and ischaemia: evaluation with colour Doppler sonography. *Radiology* 1990; **175**: 815–21.

23 Atkinson GO, Partick LE, Ball TI, *et al.* Normal and abnormal scrotum in children: evaluation with color Doppler sonography. *Am J Radiol* 1992; **158**: 613–7.

24 Ingram S, Hollman AS. Colour Doppler sonography of the normal paediatric testis. *Clin Radiol* 1994; **49**: 266–7.

25 Thurnher S, Hricak H, Carroll PR, *et al.* Imaging the testis: comparison between MR imaging and US. *Radiology* 1988; **167**: 631–6.

26 Ralls PW, Jensen MC, Lee KP, *et al.* Color Doppler sonography in acute epididymitis. *J Clin Ultrasound* 1990; **18**: 383–6.

27 Fowler RC, Chennells PM, Ewing R. Scrotal ultrasonography: a clinical evaluation. *Br J Radiol* 1987; **60**: 649–54.

Gynecological cancer

K.E. BRITTON AND M. GRANOWSKA

INTRODUCTION

Cancers of the ovary, cervix, and uterus are becoming increasingly common. Ovarian cancer is one of the most malignant tumors and accounts for 6% of deaths from cancer in women in the Western world.[1] Ovarian malignancy accounts for almost 25% of all gynecological cancers of the female genital tract and has the highest case to mortality ratio. In spite of radical surgery coupled with the introduction of many new cytotoxic drugs, which may produce significant remissions, the overall 5-year survival rate remains at around 30%. Whereas screening for cervical cancer has benefits and uterine cancer demonstrates itself usually with post-menopausal bleeding, ovarian cancer typically remains concealed until late in its course.

Methods for screening women for ovarian cancer included abdominal or trans-vaginal ultrasound and serum markers such as CA125. Both have their limitations. In the original survey of 5000 women with trans-abdominal ultrasound, 234 abnormal masses were discovered in the pelvis. All these women were operated upon, and 225 of them did not have ovarian cancer.[2] The incidence of ovarian cancer is more than doubled if there is a family history in a close relative. Such patients at risk are being screened with trans-vaginal ultrasound with approximately 1 in 60 pick-up rate of ovarian cancer.[3] The CA125 marker by itself is insufficient to diagnose early ovarian cancer, since a certain tumor mass has to be present to release enough antigen to increase the blood level over its normal value and its biological variation.[4] For the same reason, it is a relatively insensitive marker of early recurrent ovarian cancer.

A pelvic 'adnexal' mass can represent a number of different benign and malignant conditions and the traditional strategy for establishing a final diagnosis has been to perform an exploratory laparotomy. Many women with advanced ovarian cancer undergo insufficient primary surgery at local hospitals. The amount of residual malignant tissue after primary surgery is an important prognostic factor in ovarian cancer.[5,6] This surgery demands specific skills and experience. Therefore, a method for better preoperative discrimination of patients with a pelvic mass is needed. The risk of malignancy index (RMI), based on the menopausal status, ultrasound findings, and the serum level of CA125, was introduced by Jacobs et al.[7,8] The RMI was derived from logistic regression analysis and was defined as follows:

$$\text{RMI} = U \times M \times c$$

where U is an ultrasound score of 0–3, increasing with the likelihood of malignancy; $M = 1$ if pre-menopausal and 3 if post-menopausal, and c is the value of the serum CA125 level. This combination has improved the preoperative diagnostic accuracy for ovarian cancer.[7,8]

Radiological techniques rely on detecting cancer as a physical entity. Features of ovarian cancer on magnetic resonance imaging, computed tomography (CT) or ultrasound include a thick irregular cyst wall, solid areas in a cyst, irregular septa, papillary-like projections from the cyst wall or evidence of metastases or ascites associated with malignancy. Color Doppler improves the specificity of transvaginal ultrasound by using the increased flow of an ovarian cancer as the basis of its detection. However, other ovarian masses such as a corpus luteum cyst, which is benign and usually self-limiting, and ovarian infection or abscess also increase flow to the mass. Trans-vaginal gray scale and color Doppler have difficulty in distinguishing primary from metastatic tumors to the ovary.[9] Color Doppler and power Doppler have been compared and have similar diagnostic accuracy.[10] Pattern recognition and logistic regression methods have not yet improved the discrimination bet-ween benign and malignant pelvic masses.[11] CT scanning is widely used, but is relatively insensitive and often inconclu-sive in the preoperative diagnosis of ovarian cancer.[12] It is also relatively insensitive for recurrent disease.[13] MRI is gaining ground as a means for assessing primary and recur-rent ovarian cancer.[13–15] Our recent MRI study showed an overall diagnostic accuracy for malignancy of 91%.[16] We also showed that radioimmunoscintigraphy (RIS) has par-ticular benefit in discriminating between benign and malig-nant adnexal masses of less than 10 cm diameter.[17]

RADIOIMMUNOSCINTIGRAPHY

The intention here is to use a property of the surface of the cancer cell, which differs qualitatively and quantitatively from that of the benign ovarian tumor and the normal ovary, so that malignancy can be distinguished. Because of the rela-tive vascularity of ovarian cancer ensuring good antibody delivery, RIS has generally been successful. There is a wide range of antibodies used to detect this cancer[18–40] (Table 13G.1).

Many monoclonal antibodies have been used for target-ing gynecological cancer. Anti-HCG has been used to detect the choriogonadotrophic hormone.[41] The polymor-phic epithelial mucin antigen has many different mono-clonal antibodies made against it. It is a normal constituent of the lining of the ducts of the breast or the follicles of the ovary. Such antigens are remote from the bloodstream, so a monoclonal antibody against them will not normally react *in vivo*. However, the architectural disruption caused by the cancerous process brings large quantities of such cell-bound antigens into contact with the blood where they are detectable using RIS. HMFG1 and HMFG2, both antibodies against the human milk fat globules, surface-lining protein of the milk duct and ovarian follicles, are in this class. SM3, a monoclonal antibody against the stripped mucin core pro-tein has a high specificity for breast and ovarian cancer and a low reactivity with normal tissues and benign tumors. SM3 (stripped mucin 3) is produced by Cancer Research UK[17,22–24] and has a high specificity for breast and ovarian cancers and a low reactivity with normal tissues and benign tumors. It is labeled with [99m]Tc. Whereas the malignant-to-benign uptake ratio for an HMFG antibody is about 8:1, that for SM3 is about 17:1 and this enables it to be used for distinguishing malignant from benign tumors in addition to detecting the tumor.[42] Some cancer cell proteins are pro-duced in larger amounts in the cancer cell than in normal cells. These include anti-placental alkaline phosphatase PLAP (H17-E2), which reacts with ovarian cancers and seminomas,[19,39,40] OVTL3,[35,36] OC-125, which is also used as a tumor marker,[37,38] and MoV-18.[25–27] The importance of the degree of antigen expression on the cancer cell is emphasized by Buist *et al.*[43] The intraperitoneal route has also been used.[44] Synthetic antigens have been created with

Table 13G.1   *Radioimmunoscintigraphy of ovarian cancer*

Cancer–associated antigen	Monoclonal antibody	References
Polymorphic epithelial	HMFG1 and HMFG2	18, 19, 20
Stripped mucin antigen	SM3	17, 22, 23, 24
Folate binding protein	MoV-18	25, 26, 27
TF antigen	170 H.82	28, 29, 30, 31
TAG72	B72.3, CC49, Oncoscint (satumab pendetide)	32, 33, 34
Released antigen	OVTL3	35, 36
Released antigen	OC125	37, 38
Placental alkaline phosphatase	PLAB, Hu2PLAB	39, 40

monoclonal antibodies such as 170-H82, which is called a panadenocarcinoma monoclonal antibody because of its wide range of reactivity.[28–31]

Radioimmunoscintigraphy is generally limited by a low tumor-to-background ratio, low percentage of the injected dose per gram taken up by the tumor and heterogeneity of the antigen. To overcome this problem change detection analysis algorithms have been used to detect small changes of uptake of antibody. Specific uptake increases with time, whereas nonspecific uptake decreases with time after an initial distribution.[45,46]

The success of imaging using radionuclide-labeled mono-clonal antibodies in the detection of recurrent ovarian can-cer has been demonstrated in a correlative imaging study by Peltier *et al.*[47] Intra-operative probe studies may be helpful.[48]

It may be concluded that RIS is a reasonable way of imaging primary and recurrent ovarian cancer and evalu-ating the effects of chemotherapy without 'second-look' laparotomy. It is also able to demonstrate that a mass seen on X-ray, CT or ultrasound contains or does not contain viable tumor. The combination of clinical examination, tumor markers, ultrasonogram, RMI, along with the aid of RIS and MRI is promising to help the surgical oncologist to take the appropriate steps regarding the diagnosis and management of a woman with a pelvic mass.

PATIENTS AND RADIOIMMUNOSCINTIGRAPHY METHODOLOGY

The patient protocol requires an explanation of the whole procedure to the patient before she enters the camera room. Such studies are usually carried out under ethics committee approval. No thyroid blockade is required and provided that 1 mg (or less) of whole monoclonal antibody is used, a patient reaction is no more common than for a bone scan or kidney agent. However, it is an absolute rule that patients with a known allergy to foreign protein or severe atopy should be excluded. Skin testing is useless and only sensitizes the patient to the monoclonal antibody. Human anti-mouse antibody (HAMA) responses may occur and may be detectable in the serum. Their presence is not directly related to clinical reactions. After about the third imaging injection, there may be an increased rate of clearance of the antibody, but in only a very small percentage of subjects does this interfere with tumor detectability.[49] An ^{111}In-labeled agent will show high uptake in the liver and usually quite marked bowel and marrow activity, whereas the ^{99m}Tc-labeled agent usually shows mainly renal excretion (the compound is usually a dicysteine complex of ^{99m}Tc) with low activity in the liver, marrow and bowel. Typically, 120 MBq (3 mCi) of ^{111}In or 600 MBq (15 mCi) of ^{99m}Tc-labeled monoclonal antibody (0.5 mg) is injected.

There are some important rules for imaging and image interpretation. First, specific uptake increases with time, so if a blood pool image is taken at 10 min, it will usually show no specific antibody (whole antibody) uptake in any tumor. Images taken at 6 and 24 h for ^{99m}Tc, or at 24 and 48 h for ^{111}In-labeled monoclonal antibodies, will show increasing tumor uptake with time. This should be contrasted with nonspecific uptake, e.g. in a uterine fibroid, which after the initial distribution decreases with time during the first 24 h. The initial blood pool image at 10 min acts as a template with which later images may be compared. This allows the detection of (visually and subsequently by image analysis) very small lesions that may not be detected without the blood pool image as a guide. Thus, a series of images, at least a pair or preferably a triplet, separated in time give the best visual interpretation for RIS.

The count content of the image is important and a minimum of 800 kcounts should be obtained per image, using a general-purpose or preferably a high-resolution, low-energy, parallel-hole collimator and the camera peaked at 140 keV with a ± 15% window for [99m]Tc. In order to provide comparable contrasts for the two images, a repositioning protocol for the patient is advised, whereby an image of markers on prominent body landmarks is taken before and for each set of images, so that on the second and third visits the patient can be repositioned in the same place. The markers are positioned on the costal margins, xiphisternum, iliac crests, and symphysis pubis. In this way the same amount of liver appears on an abdominal image giving the same image contrast, which allows comparisons to be made much more easily. SPET images are essential for the pelvis and often helpful for the liver and para-aortic regions in patients with ovarian cancer. Serial squat views may be of benefit in examining the pelvis. Accurate repositioning of the patient between images is a requirement for image analysis protocols using change detection algorithms, kinetic analysis, and probability mapping.[17,46] The challenge for RIS in patients with ovarian cancer is in distinguishing benign from malignant disease, for which SM3, OC-125 and MoV-18 appear the preferred antibodies. It is expected that 75% of women with lesions diagnosed by using ultrasound could be demonstrated not to have cancer using ^{99m}Tc-SM3,[24] if RIS were to be interposed between the ultrasound investigation and the laparotomy. Using an advanced change detection algorithm, the accuracy is increased to 92% for small tumors.[17]

Case history

A 19-year-old woman developed ascites and an ovarian mass due to poorly differentiated serous cystadenocarcinoma FIGO 3c. At operation, it was disseminated in the pelvis and related peritoneal lymph nodes.

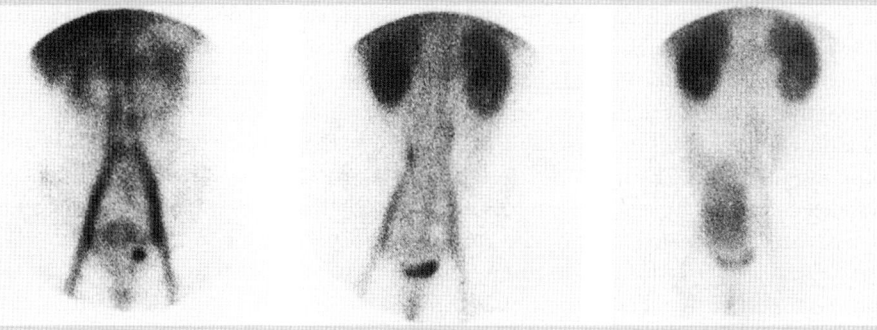

(a)

Figure 13G.1   *Radioimmunoscintigraphy with ^{99m}Tc-stripped mucin 3 (^{99m}Tc-SM3) before and after surgery. (a) Radioimmunoscintigraphy with ^{99m}Tc-SM3 before surgery. Anterior view at 10 min (left), 6 h (centre) and 24 h (right). The 10 min image shows initial vascular, uterine, renal and bladder activity. At 6 h, the non-specific vascular activity has faded. At 24 h, irregular increased uptake is seen in the center and right of the pelvis with some lateral extension of uptake on each side of the abdomen.*

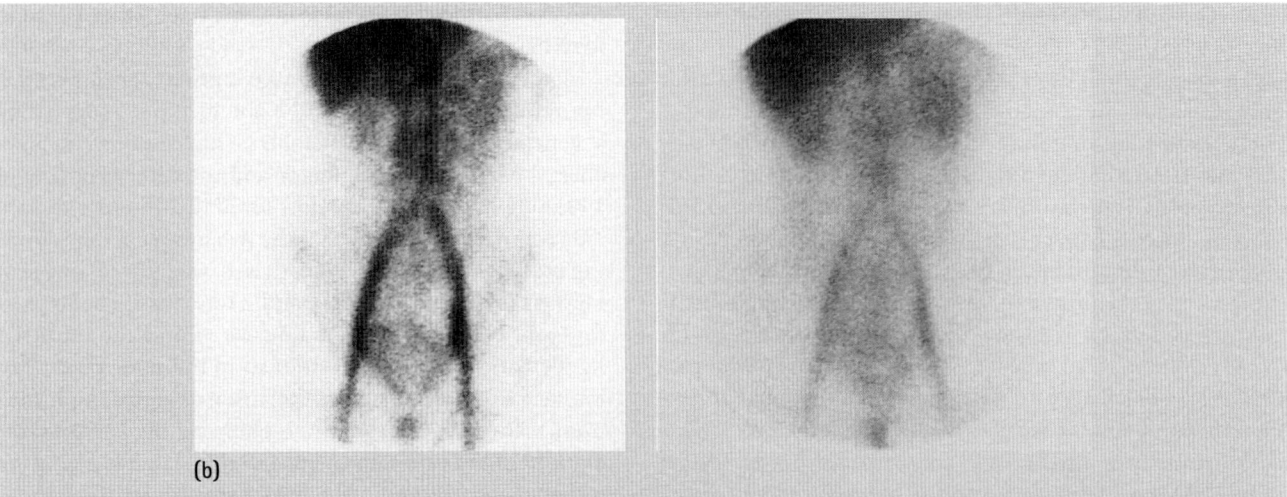

(b)

Figure 13G.1 *(Continued)* *(b) Radioimmunoscintigraphy was repeated after surgery and full chemotherapy with intravenous carboplatin and intraperitoneal cisplatin. Anterior views at 10 min (top) and 24 h (bottom) show no residual abnormal uptake. Second-look surgery showed no microscopic disease. (Reproduced courtesy of the* European Journal of Nuclear Medicine, 1993.)

Positron emission tomography

^{99m}Tc-sestamibi (^{99m}Tc-MIBI) is an all-purpose tumor imaging agent with increased mitochondrial uptake in malignancy. It may also be useful in the evaluation of pelvic masses.[50] It has been largely replaced by positron emission tomography (PET) which is showing its potential in the diagnosis of adnexal masses. A study by Fenchel *et al.*[51] where 85 asymptomatic women were evaluated by using ^{18}F-FDG PET revealed that the overall sensitivity and specificity of FDG PET were 50% and 78% respectively. They found that FDG PET was no better than transvaginal ultrasound in the evaluation of asymptomatic adnexal masses.[52] Grab *et al.*[53] showed that the specificity of FDG PET in detection of ovarian cancer in asymptomatic adnexal masses to be 80%. Rieber *et al.*[54] compared MRI, trans-vaginal sonography, PET, and a consensus diagnosis, and found sensitivities, respectively, of 83%, 92%, 58%, and 92%; specificities 84%, 59%, 78%, and 84%; and diagnostic accuracies of 83%, 63%, 76%, and 85%, respectively. The false negative findings were mainly with borderline tumors. PET/CT has been used to detect recurrent ovarian cancer with an accuracy of 82%.[55,56] In comparison with X-ray CT it is useful in the assessment of tumor response.[57–59] Chang *et al.*[60] found 93% accuracy in the detection of recurrent ovarian cancer suspected on the basis of an elevated serum CA-125. Choline labeled with ^{11}C has been used for PET in comparison with FDG[61] but was no better than FDG. Additionally, ^{11}C-labeled estrogens have been described.[62]

Ovarian cancer radionuclide therapy

The intraperitoneal (i.p.) route is the usual approach, traditionally with ^{198}Au,[63] ^{32}P,[64,65] or ^{125}I implants.[66] All suffer from the problem that many i.p. recurrences are subserosal rather than intraperitoneal and so are less accessible for therapy. Van Zanten-Przybysz *et al.*[67] showed that targeting ovarian cancer i.p. versus intravenously with chimeric cMov18 showed no targeting benefit. Nevertheless i.p. radioimmunotherapy (RIT) with ^{131}I-cMov18 achieved stable disease.[68] A range of radionuclide labels for RIT have and are being explored, previously ^{131}I, for example ^{131}I-B72.3 in pseudomyxoma[69] and recently combined with chemotherapy, ^{90}Y-CC49[70] or ^{177}Lu-CC49[71] with interferon alpha and Taxol. Experimental work has been undertaken in mice with ^{86}Y-trastuzumab, antiHer2/Neu, for ^{90}Y-trastuzumab dosimetry using microPET[72] and with alpha emitters ^{211}At-labeled to MoV-18[73] and ^{225}Ac-labeled to antiHer2/Neu.[74]

Nicholson *et al.*[75] have produced the best results for i.p. RIT in an adjuvant setting in patients after complete remission of ovarian cancer after receiving standard management. The patients received i.p. 25 mg ^{90}Y-HMFG1 in a single dose of 666 MBq m^{-2} (18 mCi m^{-2}). Their outcome was matched to a contemporaneous control group in complete remission, who had received only standard management. Survival of the adjuvant RIT group was 80% at 5 years versus 55% ($P = 0.0035$) and estimated at 80% at 10 years versus 32% for the control group ($P = 0.003$). It is likely that two- or three-step targeting will be more effective than i.p. therapy for recurrent disease in the future.

Residual ovarian teratoma containing malignant thyroid tissue has been successfully managed with repeated ^{131}I therapy.[76]

In conclusion, RIS has an important clinical role in the management of patients with suspected or known ovarian cancer, particularly in identifying whether surgery and chemotherapy have been successful (Table 13G.2). RIS is an important identifier of the suitability of a tumor for

Table 13G.2 *Management of ovarian cancer with radioimmunoscintigraphy*

Detection of primary	Clinical examination
	Ultrasound transabdominal
	Trans-vaginal
	Doppler color
Distinction of benign	Ultrasound, X-ray CT, MRI
from malignant	^{99m}Tc-SM3
	^{99m}Tc-MoV-18
Extent of surgery	Preoperative probe
Detection of recurrences	Serum markers
	Radioimmunoscintigraphy
Localization of recurrence	Radioimmunoscintigraphy
	MRI
Effect of chemotherapy	Radioimmunoscintigraphy
	Radiology: liver CT, ultrasound, pelvis MRI
	'Second-look' surgery, Laparoscopy
Confirmation of suitability for radioimmunotherapy	Radioimmunoscintigraphy

CT, computed tomography; MRI, magnetic resonance imaging; SM3, stripped mucin 3.

radioimmunotherapy and contributes to doismetry. Its wider application is limited by manmade problems, including over-regulation, which contributes over half the expense of commercializing these techniques and prevents them from becoming readily available.

REFERENCES

● Seminal primary article
◆ Key review paper

1 Williams C. Ovarian and cervical cancer. *Br Med J* 1992; **304**: 1501–4.
● 2 Campbell S, Bhan V, Royston P, *et al*. Transabdominal ultrasound screening for early ovarian cancer. *Br Med J* 1989; **299**: 1363–7.
3 Bourne TH, Whitehead MI, Campbell S, *et al*. Ultrasound screening for familial ovarian cancer. *Gynecol Oncol* 1991; **43**: 92–7.
● 4 Kenemans P, Yedema CA, Bon GG, von Mensdorff-Pouilly S. CA 125 in gynaecological pathology [Review]. *Eur J Obstet Gynecol Reprod Biol* 1993; **49**: 115–24.
5 Hacker NF, Van der Burg MEL. Debulking and intervention surgery. *Ann Oncol* 1993; **4(Suppl)**: 17–22.
6 Kehoe S, Powell J, Wilson S, *et al*. The influence of the operating surgeon's specialisation on patient survival in ovarian carcinoma. *Int J Cancer* 1994; **70**: 1014–17.

● 7 Jacobs I, Oram D, Fairbanks J, *et al*. A risk of malignancy index incorporating CA125, ultrasound and menopausal status after the accurate pre-operative diagnosis of ovarian cancer. *Br J Obstet Gynaecol* 1990; **97**: 922–9.
● 8 Davies AP, Jacobs I, Woolas R, *et al*. Adnexal mass: benign or malignant? Evaluation of a risk of malignant index. *Br J Obstet Gynaecol* 1993; **100**: 927–31.
9 Alcazar JL, Galan MJ, Ceamanos C, Garcia-Manero M. Transvaginal grey scale colour Doppler sonography in primary ovarian cancer and metastatic tumours to the ovary. *J Ultrasound Med* 2003; **22**: 243–7.
● 10 Guerriero S, Alcazar JL, Ajossa S, *et al*. Comparison of conventional colour Doppler imaging and power Doppler imaging for the diagnosis of ovarian cancer: results of a European Study. *Gynaecol Oncol* 2002; **84**: 352–3.
11 Valentin L, Hagen B, Tingulstad S, Eik-Nes S. Comparison of pattern recognition and logistic regression for discrimination between benign and malignant pelvic masses: a prospective cross validation. *Ultrasound Obstet Gynecol* 2001; **18**: 357–65.
12 Petru E, Schmidt F, Mikosch P, *et al*. Abdominopelvic computed tomography in the preoperative evaluation of suspected ovarian masses. *Int J Gynecol Cancer* 1992; **2**: 252–5.
13 Buist, MR, Golding RP, Burger CW, *et al*. Comparison and evaluation of diagnostic methods in ovarian carcinoma with emphasis on CT and MRI. *Gynecol Oncol* 1994; **52**: 191–8.
14 Stevens SK, Hricak H, Stern JL. Ovarian lesions – detection and characterization with gadolinium-enhanced MR imaging at 1.5 T. *Radiology* 1991; **181**: 481–8.
15 Semelka RC, Lawrence PH, Shoenut JP, *et al*. Primary ovarian cancer: prospective comparison of contrast-enhanced CT and pre- and post-contrast, fat-suppressed MR imaging, with histologic correlation. *J Magn Reson Imaging* 1993; **3**: 99–106.
● 16 Sohaib SA, Sahdev A, Van Trappen P, *et al*. Characterisation of adenexal mass lesions on MR imaging. *Am J Roentgenol* 2003; **180**: 1297–304.
● 17 Ali N, Jan H, Van Trappen P, *et al*. Radioimmunoscintigraphy with Tc-99m-labelled SM3 in differentiating malignant from benign adnexal masses. *Br J Obstet Gynaecol* 2003; **110**: 508–14.
● 18 Taylor-Papadimitrou J, Paterson JA, Arkie J, *et al*. Monoclonal antibodies to epithelium specific components of the human milk fat globule membrane, production and reaction with cells in culture. *Int J Cancer* 1981; **28**: 17–21.
● 19 Epenetos AA, Britton KE, Mather SJ, *et al*. Targeting of iodine-123 labelled tumour-associated monoclonal

antibodies to ovarian, breast and gastrointestinal tumours. *Lancet* 1982; **ii**: 999–1005.

20 Kalofonos HP, Karamouzis MV, Epenetos AA. Radioimmunoscintigraphy in patients with ovarian cancer. *Acta Oncol* 2001; **40**: 549–57.

21 Burchell J, Taylor-Papadimitrou J, Boshell M, *et al.* A short sequence, within the amino acid repeat of a cancer-associated mucin, contains immunodominant epitopes. *Int J Cancer* 1989; **44**: 691–6.

22 Girling A, Bartkora J, Burchell J, *et al.* A core protein epitope of the polymorphic epithelial mucin detected by monoclonal antibody SM3 is selectively exposed in a range of primary carcinomas. *Int J Cancer* 1989; **3**: 1072–6.

23 Burchell J, Gendler S, Taylor-Papadimitriou J, *et al.* Development and characterisation of breast cancer reactive monoclonal antibodies directed to the core protein of the human milk mucin. *Cancer Res* 1987; **47**: 5476–82.

24 Granowska M, Britton KE, Mather SJ, *et al.* Radioimmunoscintigraphy with technetium-99m monoclonal antibody, SM3, in gynaecological cancer. *Eur J Nucl Med* 1993; **20**: 483–9.

25 Crippa F, Buraggi GL, Di Re E, *et al.* Radioimmunoscintigraphy of ovarian cancer with the MoV-18 monoclonal antibody. *Eur J Cancer* 1991; **27**: 724–9.

26 Crippa F. Radioimmunotherapy of ovarian cancer. *Int J Biol Mark* 1991; **8**: 187–91.

27 Magnani P, Fazio F, Grana C, *et al.* Diagnosis of persistent ovarian carcinoma with three-step immunoscintigraphy. *Br J Cancer* 2000; **82**: 616–20.

28 McEwan AJB, Maclean GD, Hooper HR, *et al.* Mab 170 H.82: an evaluation of a novel panadenocarcinoma monoclonal antibody labeled with ^{99m}Tc and with ^{111}In. *Nucl Med Commun* 1992; **13**: 11–19.

29 Alexander C, Villena-Heinsen CE, Trampert K, *et al.* Radioimmunoscintigraphy of ovarian tumours with technetium-99m labelled monoclonal antibody-170: first clinical experience. *Eur J Nucl Med* 1995; **22**: 645–51.

30 Alexander C, Villena-Heinsen CE, Schaefer A, *et al.* Monoclonal antibody MAb-170 for immunoscintigraphic detection of ovarian tumors. *Am J Obstet Gynecol* 1999; **181**: 513–17.

31 Lieberman G, Buscombe JR, Hilson AJ, *et al.* Preoperative diagnosis of ovarian carcinoma with a novel monoclonal antibody. *Am J Obstet Gynecol* 2000; **183**: 534–40.

32 Jusko WJ, Kung LP, Schmelter RP. Immunopharmacokinetics of ^{111}In-CYT-103 in ovarian cancer patients. In: Maguire RT, Van Nostrand D. (eds.) *Diagnosis of colorectal and ovarian carcinoma.* New York: Marcel Dekker, 1992: 177–90.

33 McIntosh DG, Colcher D, Seemayer T, Smith ML. The intraoperative detection of ovarian adenocarcinoma using radiolabeled CC49 monoclonal anti-

body and a hand-held gamma-detecting probe. *Cancer Biother Radiopharm* 1997; **12**: 287–94.

34 Bohdiewicz PJ. Indium-111 satumomab pendetide: the first FDA-approved monoclonal antibody for tumor imaging. *J Nucl Med Technol* 1998; **26**: 155–63.

35 Tibben JB, Massuger LFAG, Claessens RAMJ, *et al.* Tumour detection and localization using 99Tcm-labelled OV-TL-3Fab′ in patients suspected of ovarian cancer. *Nucl Med Commun* 1992; **13**: 885–93.

36 Tibben JB, Massuger LFAG, Claessens RAMJ, *et al.* Clinical experience with radiolabelled monoclonal antibodies in the detection of colorectal and ovarian carcinoma recurrence. *Nucl Med Commun* 1999; **20**: 689–96.

37 Maughan TS, Haylock B, Hayward M, *et al.* OC 125 immunoscintigraphy in ovarian carcinoma: a comparison with alternative methods of assessment. *J Clin Oncol* 1990; **2**: 199–205.

38 Osmers RG, Rybicki T, Meden H, Kuhn W. Does an immunoscintigraphy with OC 125 affect the prognosis of ovarian cancer? *Eur J Gynaecol Oncol* 1997; **18**: 177–82.

39 Epenetos AA, Snook D, Hooker G, *et al.* Indium-111 labelled monoclonal antibody to placental alkaline phosphatase in the detection of neoplasms of testis, ovary and cervix. *Lancet* 1995; **ii**: 350–53.

40 Kosmas C, Kalofonos HP, Hird V, Epenetos AA. Monoclonal antibody targeting of ovarian carcinoma. *Oncology* 1998; **55**: 435–46.

41 Begent RHJ, Stanway G, Jones BE, *et al.* Radioimmunolocalisation of tumours by external scintigraphy after administration of ^{131}I antibody to human gonadotrophin. Preliminary communication. *J R Soc Med* 1980; **73**: 624–50.

42 Van Dam PA, Watson JV, Shepherd JH, Lowe DG. Flow cytometric quantification of tumour-associated antigens in solid tumors. *Am J Obstet Gynecol* 1990; **163**: 698–9.

43 Buist MR, Kenemans P, Molthoff CF, *et al.* Tumour uptake of intravenously administered radiolabelled antibodies in ovarian carcinoma patients in relation to antigen expression and other tumour characteristics. *Int J Cancer* 1995; **64**: 92–8.

44 Qian H, Feng J, Cui H. Clinical evaluation of radioimmunoimaging with 131-I-CE0C18 monoclonal antibody against ovarian carcinoma by intraperitoneal injection. *Gynaecol Oncol* 1992; **47**: 216–22.

45 Britton KE, Granowska M. Radioimmunoscintigraphy in tumour identification. *Cancer Surv* 1987; **6**: 247–67.

46 Granowska M, Nimmon CC, Britton KE, *et al.* Kinetic analysis and probability mapping applied to detection of ovarian cancer by immunoscintigraphy. *J Nucl Med* 1988; **29**: 599–607.

- 47 Peltier P, Wiharto K, Dutin J-P, *et al.* Correlative imaging study in the diagnosis of ovarian cancer recurrences. *Eur Nucl Med* 1992; **19**: 1006–1010.

- 48 Ind TEJ, Granowska M, Britton KE. Peroperative radioimmunodetection of ovarian carcinoma using a hand held gamma detection probe. *Br J Cancer* 1994; **70**: 1263–6.

49 Hertel A, Baum RP, Auerbach B, *et al.* Klinische Relevanz Humaner Anti-Maus-Antikorper (HAMA) in der Immunszintigraphie. *Nucl Med* 1990; **29**: 221–7.

50 Krolicki L, Cwikla J, Timorek A, *et al.* Technetium-99m MIBI imaging in the diagnosis of pelvic and abdominal masses in patients with suspected gynaecological malignancy. *Nucl Med Rev Cent East Eur* 2002; **5**: 131–7.

51 Fenchel S, Kotzerke J, Stohr I, *et al.* Preoperative assessment of asymptomatic adnexal tumors by positron emission tomography and F18 fluorodeoxyglucose. *Nuklearmedizin* 1999; **38**: 101–7.

- 52 Fenchel S, Grab D, Nuessle K, *et al.* Asymptomatic adnexal masses: correlation of FDG PET and histopathologic findings. *Radiology* 2002; **223**: 780–8.

53 Grab D, Flock F, Stohr I, *et al.* Classification of asymptomatic adnexal masses by ultrasound, magnetic resonance imaging, and positron emission tomography. *Gynecol Oncol* 2000; **77**: 454–9.

54 Rieber A, Nussle K, Stohr I, *et al.* Preoperative diagnosis of ovarian tumors with MR imaging: comparison with transvaginal sonography, positron emission tomography, and histologic findings. *Am J Roentgenol* 2001; **177**: 123–9.

- 55 Bristow RE, Simpkins F, Pannu HK, *et al.* Positron emission tomography for detecting clinically occult surgically resectable metastatic ovarian cancer. *Gynecol Oncol* 2002; **85**: 196–200.

56 Bristow RE, del Carmen MG, Pannu HK, *et al.* Clinically occult recurrent ovarian cancer: patient selection for secondary cytoreductive surgery using combined PET/CT. *Gynecol Oncol* 2003; **90**: 519–28.

- 57 Picchio M, Sironi S, Messa C, *et al.* Advanced ovarian carcinoma: usefulness of [(18)F]FDG-PET in combination with CT for lesion detection after primary treatment. *Q J Nucl Med* 2000; **47**: 77–84.

- 58 Baum RP, Przetak C. Evaluation of therapy response in breast and ovarian cancer patients by positron emission tomography (PET). *Q J Nucl Med* 2001; **45**: 257–68.

- 59 Rose PG, Faulhaber P, Miraldi F, Abdul-Karim FW. Positive emission tomography for evaluating a complete clinical response in patients with ovarian or peritoneal carcinoma: correlation with second-look laparotomy. *Gynecol Oncol* 2001; **82**: 17–21.

60 Chang WC, Hung YC, Kao CH, *et al.* Usefulness of whole body positron emission tomography (PET) with ^{18}F-fluoro-2-deoxyglucose (FDG) to detect recurrent ovarian cancer based on asymptomatically elevated serum levels of tumor marker. *Neoplasma* 2002; **49**: 329–33.

61 Torizuka T, Kanno T, Futatsubashi M, *et al.* Imaging of gynecologic tumors: comparison of (11)C-choline PET with (18)F-FDG PET. *J Nucl Med* 2003; **44**: 1051–6.

62 Dence CS, Napolitano E, Katzenellenbogen JA, Welch MJ. Carbon-11-labeled estrogens as potential imaging agents for breast tumors. *Nucl Med Biol* 1996; **23**: 491–6.

- 63 Patyanik M, Mayer A, Polgar I. Results of ovary tumor treatment with abdominally administered ^{198}Au evaluated on the basis of long term follow up. *Pathol Oncol Res* 2002; **8**: 54–7.

64 Condra KS, Mendenhall WM, Morgan LS, Marcus Jr RB. Consolidative ^{32}P after second-look laparotomy for ovarian carcinoma. *Radiat Oncol Investig* 1998; **6**: 97–102.

- 65 Varia MA, Stehman FB, Bundy BN, *et al.* Intraperitoneal radioactive phosphorus (^{32}P) versus observation after negative second-look laparotomy for stage III ovarian carcinoma: a randomized trial of the Gynecologic Oncology Group. *J Clin Oncol* 2003; **21**: 2849–55.

- 66 Monk BJ, Tewari KS, Puthawala AA, *et al.* Treatment of recurrent gynecologic malignancies with iodine-125 permanent interstitial irradiation. *Int J Radiat Oncol Biol Phys* 2002; **52**: 806–15.

- 67 van Zanten-Przybysz I, Molthoff CF, Roos JC, *et al.* Influence of the route of administration on targeting of ovarian cancer with the chimeric monoclonal antibody MOv18: i.v. vs. i.p. *Int J Cancer* 2001; **92**: 106–14.

- 68 van Zanten-Przybysz I, Molthoff CF, Roos JC, *et al.* Radioimmunotherapy with intravenously administered ^{131}I-labeled chimeric monoclonal antibody MOv18 in patients with ovarian cancer. *J Nucl Med* 2000; **41**: 1168–76.

69 Laitinen JO, Tenhunen M, Kairemo KJ. Absorbed dose estimates for ^{131}I-labelled monoclonal antibody therapy in patients with intraperitoneal pseudomyxoma. *Nucl Med Commun* 2000; **21**: 355–60.

- 70 Alvarez RD, Huh WK, Khazaeli MB, *et al.* A Phase I study of combined modality ^{90}yttrium-CC49 intraperitoneal radioimmunotherapy for ovarian cancer. *Clin Cancer Res* 2002; **8**: 2806–11.

- 71 Meredith RF, Alvarez RD, Partridge EE, *et al.* Intraperitoneal radioimmunochemotherapy of ovarian cancer: a phase I study. *Cancer Biother Radiopharm* 2001; **16**: 305–15.

- 72 Palm S, Enmon Jr RM, Matei C, *et al.* Pharmacokinetics and biodistribution of ^{86}Y-trastuzumab for ^{90}Y dosimetry in an ovarian carcinoma model: correlative MicroPET and MRI. *J Nucl Med* 2003; **44**: 1148–55.

● 73 Andersson H, Lindegren S, Back T, *et al.* The curative and palliative potential of the monoclonal antibody MOv18 labelled with [211]At in nude mice with intraperitoneally growing ovarian cancer xenografts – a long-term study. *Acta Oncol* 2000; **39**: 741–5.

● 74 Borchardt PE, Yuan RR, Miederer M, *et al.* Targeted actinium-225 in vivo generators for therapy of ovarian cancer. *Cancer Res* 2003; **63**: 5084–90.

● 75 Nicholson S, Gooden CS, Hird V, *et al.* Radioimmunotherapy after chemotherapy compared to chemotherapy alone in the treatment of advanced ovarian cancer: a matched analysis. *Oncol Rep* 1998; **5**: 223–6.

76 Suga K, Hirabayashi A, Motoyama K, *et al.* Repeated ^{131}I treatment of a residual ovarian teratoma containing malignant thyroid tissue. *Br J Radiol* 1999; **72**: 1110–13.

Prostate cancer

K.E. BRITTON, M.J. CARROLL, AND V.U. CHENGAZI

INTRODUCTION

Cancer of the prostate is the most common cancer in men and second after lung carcinoma in order of cancer-related deaths. Prostate cancer has a multiplicity of genetic changes associated with it.[1] Having a relative with prostate cancer doubles the likelihood of prostate cancer. Benign prostate hypertrophy appears not to be a risk factor. High vitamin A and vitamin C intake and cadmium are thought to be predisposing dietary factors. Protective effects of vitamin D, selenium, and lycopene, for example in tomato sauce, have been demonstrated. Prostate cancer may be discovered incidentally during digital rectal examination or following symptoms of bladder dysfunction. Its frequency and incidence are both increasing, as they are age-related. About 50% of patients present with cancer localized to the prostate. The cancer is in the peripheral zones in about 70% and central or anteriorly placed in 30%. In up to 20% of cases transurethral prostatectomy may reveal malignancy within the excised tissue. About 50% present with or have disease outside the prostate. The primary cancer may be undetected with the patient presenting as a consequence of bone metastases.

Prostate cancer spreads by the lymphatic route to the periprostatic and obturator lymph nodes, followed by internal and external iliac nodes. Iliac, hypogastric, para-aortic, and even Virchow nodes may be involved as the disease progresses. The prognosis falls from an 80% 5-year survival to a 35% 5-year survival, if a single related node is found to show microscopic involvement. Radioimmunoscintigraphy (RIS) has shown that nodal extension to the para-aortic glands and into the mediastinum is more frequent than previously expected. The blood-borne spread of prostate cancer particularly to the bone is well recognized. The bone scan is widely used, either actively for symptoms or passively to monitor therapy at regular intervals. The recognition of the fact that it is the soft tissue metastases rather than the bone metastases that usually kill the patient and that this may be shown by a rising prostate-specific antigen (PSA) in the patient with a negative bone scan, has increased the need for identification of such soft tissue metastases. Bone metastases are described in Chapter 9B. Palliation of pain due to bone metastases using ^{89}Sr and, more recently, ^{153}Sm and ^{186}Re phosphonate derivatives is discussed in Chapter 17D.

PROSTATE CANCER IMAGING

Primary prostate cancer may be staged using transrectal ultrasound, pelvic X-ray, transmission computed tomography (CT) and/or magnetic resonance imaging (MRI). All these techniques identify an abnormal node by its size rather than by its cancerous involvement. Thus enlarged nodes >1 cm diameter due to nonspecific inflammatory causes may be called malignant and normal-sized nodes with small metastases may be called benign. Resultant sensitivities of the order of 50% for accurate staging of prostate cancer when compared with the findings at radical prostatectomy are current.[2,3] Transrectal ultrasound and needle biopsy are the mainstay of the diagnosis of the primary tumor, but detecting the degree of local spread remains an important clinical problem. Treatment of primary prostate cancer by brachytherapy with ^{125}I seeds or by cryotherapy requires the knowledge that the cancer is confined to the prostate.

There have been several approaches to imaging of prostate cancer: the use of a metal, such as ^{65}Zn, which appears in higher concentration in the prostate than in the tissues; the use of substrates for prostate uptake such as [^{75}Se]seleno-methionine or positron emitters such as [^{18}F]fluorodeoxyglucose[4] or ^{11}C-choline;[5] the use of tumor-associated enzymes and antigens such as prostatic acid phosphatase (PAP),[6] PSA, and prostate specific membrane antigen (PSMA); and the use of hormone-receptor-related agents such as fluorinated androgens and androgen analog. An alternative approach is to use pelvic lymphoscintigraphy with a transrectal injection of ^{99m}Tc-antimony sulfide colloid or phytate. These can delineate the sites of nodes in the pelvis and the 'sentinel' node,[7] but not directly whether they are involved.

PSA is widely used as the most important serum marker of prostate cancer. It needs a sufficient size of tumor (or tumor metastases) to release sufficient antigen so that the rate of production of PSA exceeds its rate of metabolism. Then an elevated PSA is detected in the blood. The use of serum PSA as a screening test for prostate cancer is being advocated but remains controversial. Refinements include the measurement of free PSA and the ratio of bound to free PSA. Its use is established as a marker once prostate cancer has been diagnosed to indicate recurrence or assess the effects of therapy.[8–13] In particular, a PSA of less than 10 ng mL^{-1} makes it unlikely that a bone scan will be positive and a value over 20 ng mL^{-1} may be used as an indication for bone imaging. Imaging with anti-PSA monoclonal antibody has been tried, but found unsatisfactory because circulating PSA mops up the injected antibody.

PSMA is found in membranes of benign and malignant prostate cancer with much greater expression in the malignant cell.[14] The degree of expression of PSMA in the primary cancer correlates with the likelihood of subsequent recurrence.[15] It is not generally found in other human organs but may be expressed in the neovascular tissue of some tumors.[16] The antigen is a 100 kDa transmembrane glycoprotein with an internal and external domain.[17] It is thought to have neuropeptidase[18] and folate reductase functions.[19] The internal domain is recognized by an antibody, 7E11C5. This antibody is an IgG$_1$ of murine origin, produced by a hybridoma immunized against an LNCaP cell line. It has been labeled with ^{111}In and presented by the Cytogen Corporation as ^{111}In-CYT-356, Prostascint, now named capromab pendetide. It has received FDA approval so it is commercially available in the USA but not in Europe. The indium conjugate consists of a DTPA–GYK linker (the GYK standing for glycine, tyrosine and lysine) which takes the diethylenetriaminepentaacetic acid (DTPA) group a little away from the antibody so that the addition of indium does not affect its immunoreactivity. This antibody has the potential disadvantage of requiring internalization, which does occur[20] or else exposure of the internal domain of PSMA externally with damaged, leaky, apoptotic or necrosing cells. As a result a new antibody MUJ 591was developed against the external domain of PSMA by

Professor Bander,[16,20] which would overcome this potential problem by giving easier and more rapid access to the antigen. MUJ 591 has been labeled with ^{131}I and ^{90}Y with a view to prostate cancer diagnosis and therapy.[21,22] We received the supply of MUJ591, which we labeled with ^{99m}Tc for clinical assessment of prostate cancer by serial imaging over 24 h. In comparison, ^{111}In-Prostascint imaging is undertaken over 1–5 days after injection. ^{99m}Tc-MUJ 591 imaging proved no better than ^{111}In-Prostascint imaging.[23]

Growing experience with RIS using radiolabeled antibody to PSMA has been shown to help in the staging, monitoring, and response to the treatment of prostate cancer.[24] Neil and Meis[3] showed that ^{111}In-CYT-356 correctly identified negative nodes in 42 out of 44 patients and correctly identified positively involved nodes in 11 of 21 patients, as compared with CT images, which were positive in only 4/21. Babaian et al.[25] showed similar success in involved pelvic nodes. A particular feature of these studies has been the identification of unsuspected para-aortic, mediastinal and even left neck nodes involved by prostate cancer in patients with normal bone scans, revealing an extent of disease previously unexpected. Over 80 000 patients have been studied using this monoclonal antibody labeled with ^{111}In for imaging prostate cancer in the USA. Minor side-effects have been reported in 4% of patients, which may be reduced by excluding patients with allergy to foreign protein. The absorbed radiation dose is at the high end of the diagnostic range – 25–40 mSv per dose injected.[26]

Difficulties in the interpretation of these scans were reduced by undertaking early single photon emission computed tomography (SPECT) during the first hour to provide the blood pool image, since in the age group of these patients tortuous arteries and veins are more frequent. This aids interpretation of subsequent SPECT images at 3 and 4 days. A revision of pelvic anatomy may be required by the nuclear medicine physician to distinguish obturator and other nodes from the normal internal and external iliac vessels and to distinguish the bulb of the penis below the prostate from the prostate and the base of the bladder above. A definite learning curve is required to undertake reliable reporting of these images. The Cytogen Corporation has recognized this and have implemented a 'Partners in excellence' program, whereby physicians starting to interpret these examinations have their images and reports re-read initially by others with experience until such time that the physicians become confident in their reporting.

Disadvantages of ^{111}In include a considerable bone marrow uptake, occasional activity in the rectum because of bowel excretion, expense, and the need to order the indium. For these reasons, ^{99m}Tc has been evaluated as an alternative label, either using the direct reduction method of Mather and Ellison[27] called CYT-351, 'Prostatec' or using a Cytogen linker[28] called CYT-422. With ^{99m}Tc there is no bowel activity, much less marrow uptake, a higher count-rate suitable for SPET and a low absorbed radiation dose. The study can be arranged and completed within 24 h. The main disadvantage is increased urinary excretion of ^{99m}Tc-labeled peptides as a result of metabolism of the antibody. Feneley et al.[29] found about 13% of the injected dose excreted in the urine within 24 h with a mean blood clearance half-life of 33 h. The success of this approach to imaging primary and recurrent prostate cancer was confirmed by Chengazi et al.[30] in 39 patients, with 92% accuracy. An example of recurrent prostate cancer is shown in Plate 13H.1. The problem of rising PSA with a normal bone scan in a patient with known prostate cancer is usually solved by anti-PSMA RIS.

FDG with positron emission tomography (PET) detection has been considered. However, for prostate cancer the rate of glucose utilization is generally low, particularly in the early stages. Primary prostate cancer and its metastases tend to have weak uptake of FDG so FDG PET is not a good method for detecting early prostate cancer.[4,31,32] Aggressive metastatic prostate cancer shows good FDG uptake and the presence of FDG uptake may be correlated with a poor prognosis and indicate the need for combination chemotherapy.[33] ^{11}C-acetate[34,35] and ^{11}C-choline[5,36] give much better results but require a cyclotron on site for the study.

Primary prostate cancer

Prostate cancer is diagnosed by digital rectal examination and/or a rising PSA. Then a transrectal ultrasound is used to guide prostate biopsy and six to eight specimens are obtained. The number and histological grading of the positive biopsies is used to make a Gleason score. The higher the score the more likely is the spread to local lymph nodes and the worse the prognosis. Patients with localized disease thought to be confined to the prostate have a choice of treatment: radical prostate surgery, cryosurgery, implantation of ^{125}I seeds[37,38] or external-beam radiotherapy. Current tests make the diagnosis of suitability for these treatments by exclusion. A bone scan is performed to exclude bone metastases. CT and MRI may be performed to try to identify whether local lymph nodes are enlarged or whether there is involvement of seminal vesicles, as well as information about the prostate itself. However, a normal-sized node does not exclude the presence of cancer. Nodal involvement adversely alters prognosis. Patients may also undergo a pelvic lymph node dissection as a sampling procedure by laparoscopy, particularly in the USA, before proceeding to radical surgery, but in about a quarter of cases the sampling procedure fails to identify an involved node subsequently found at radical surgery.

Prostate RIS is, in principle, able to show that the cancer is confined to the prostate. RIS is able to show that there is evidence of extension through the capsule either posteriorly or towards the seminal vesicles or that the obturator node is involved on one or both sides. It is able to show that there is evidence of lymph node involvement in the iliac chain, or related to the aorta, or in the presacral region.[39–51] In practice, it can only detect macroscopic rather than microscopic histology so that clear capsular invasion with

extension posteriorly of the uptake in the prostate may be demonstrated, but histopathological evidence of micropathological invasion cannot. Obturator node involvement down to 2 mm disease can be demonstrated but micrometastases cannot. The technique needs very careful attention to detail and a top quality, well-maintained, double-headed, gamma camera system, preferably with a thick crystal. Slow rotation speed, accurate repositioning of the patient at each study time and the same count content on the late images as on the early ones are required. Interpretation may be difficult and requires a careful comparison of the early image, which often shows tortuous vascular structures, and a late image where the activity in the vessels is reduced. Nodes that occur in relation to blood vessels may be then demonstrated.

An alternative approach is to combine the imaging with ^{99m}Tc-labeled red cells.[52] We used a double radionuclide setting of the gamma camera for ^{99m}Tc-methylene diphosphonate (^{99m}Tc-MDP) bone scan on the first day and with ^{99m}Tc-labeled blood cells on the third day of the ^{111}In-Prostascint imaging. Comparison of the two images with co-location protocols allows the demonstration from the bone scan of the anatomical relationships and the bladder position and from the blood pool scan that a site of uptake is in a lymph node and not a tortuous blood vessel. Co-location of Prostascint imaging with a separate X-ray CT is helpful. The requirements for interpreting prostate RIS have been reviewed.[49] A technique is outlined in the Appendix on page 617.

Local recurrence

After primary surgery or radiotherapy, the serum PSA is monitored regularly. A common problem after radical surgery to the prostate or radical radiotherapy to the prostate for cancer is a rise in the PSA from zero, where it should be (probably with a precision of ± 0.03 unit). The normal range is up to 4 units. Patients and their surgical or radiotherapy clinicians become worried if, for example, there is a change from 0.4 to 0.8 of the PSA. Although this remains well within the normal range, it appears as 100% increase. We have even been asked to image patients where there is a change from 0.1 to 0.3 unit. Even in such patients, we and Raj et al.[48] have successfully demonstrated recurrence in the prostate bed or not, as the case may be, and/or node involvement. Unfortunately, the validation of this finding is difficult since most patients have radiotherapy without a prior nodal biopsy.

Metastastic prostate cancer

Demonstration of bone metastases using the bone scan and/or MRI is relatively straightforward. Many recurrences occur in soft tissue either in the prostate bed, pre-sacral or along the lymph node chain. Serial prostatic RIS is being investigated in this situation.[39,40,47] The response to salvage radiotherapy after failed radical prostatectomy could be predicted using ^{111}In-Prostascint.[41,43,47]

A negative prostate immunoscintigraphy would be a reason to delay radiotherapy which is sometimes given just in case. A patient with a rising PSA and a negative bone scan and radiology should therefore undergo RIS to determine the presence of lymph node involvement.[45,53] Liver, spleen,[54] and even brain metastases may be demonstrated. While there may still be no change in management, the identification of the source of a rising PSA level helps the surgeon and the patient to explain the phenomenon, which may be a major source of anxiety. Demonstration that a single lymph node was involved lead to direct surgery in one of our cases, which was followed by a fall in PSA. Radioimmunotherapy with these antibodies labeled with a beta-emitting radionuclide is under evaluation.[21,22,55]

Bone metastases are generally only positive on RIS during the active invasion stage when the PSA level is rising. Local radiotherapy or hormone ablation treatment impairs antibody uptake. Bone scan changes in patients who receive a variety of therapies and whose PSA is typically falling, may be positive due to changes related to healing and scarring, but negative on RIS. Local lymph node involvement has been shown by RIS in relation to a bone scan positive site for bone metastasis. This would suggest direct spread from node to bone may occur as well as the blood-borne route to bone metastasis.

^{111}In-PROSTASCINT ANTIBODY: NEW METHODS

[111]In-Prostascint SPET imaging may be combined with double radionuclide, dual energy ^{99m}Tc/^{111}In discrimination studies. A ^{99m}Tc-MDP bone scan may be done first (if not recently performed) followed by injection of ^{111}In-Prostascint with SPET of the pelvis. The bone scan provides the anatomical landmarks for co-registration of the prostate SPET images with a separate CT of the pelvis. On the third day a ^{99m}Tc blood pool study with dual energy SPET is performed. The combination of ^{99m}Tc-labeled red blood cell (RBC) imaging at 3 days with the ^{111}In imaging using the different energies of the two radionuclides to separate the images allows an accurate comparison of the lymph node uptake with blood vessel uptake. It also enables prostatitis or post-surgery inflammation blood pool uptake to be compared with the prostate antibody uptake to avoid misinterpreting an increased nonspecific antibody uptake.

The combined SPET/CT attachment to the Varicam two-headed camera (Elgems Ltd, Haifa, Israel) enables a direct physical co-location with a low resolution CT scan at the same attendance. This enables robust attenuation correction and defines the anatomical landmarks and some CT

detail to which the radionuclide images are fused (Plate 13H.2). The fusion Prostascint/low resolution CT image in turn allows the direct co-location of the image to either high resolution CT or MRI in a straightforward way, as the anatomical landmarks are in place. In this way the combination of biological and physical imaging can be incorporated into the external beam radiotherapy plan. All these advances have helped to put RIS of prostate cancer back in the staging and post-operative management of these patients. The techniques are set out in the Appendix on page 617.

In primary prostate cancer the applications are, firstly, to confirm operability and, secondly, to assess possible recurrence when the serum PSA, after radical prostatectomy or radical radiotherapy, rises above zero but within the normal range.[49] In the first case operative findings and histology provide the data with which the imaging can be compared. In the second case as operation or biopsy is rare, only the effect of therapy on reducing the PSA level could be used as a surrogate marker of the existence of recurrent cancer on imaging when radiotherapy is directed to the image-positive site. The benefit of image-directed radiotherapy was an up to 10-fold fall in PSA in CT and MRI (without contrast) negative recurrences of prostate cancer.[56] MRI with the new nanoparticle contrast agents performs well in this situation.[57] A further approach is to use three-dimensional (3-D) change detection analysis.[58]

Jani et al.[59] have demonstrated the influence of radioimmunoscintigraphy on post-prostatectomy radiotherapy treatment decision making.

The application of three-dimensional change detection to prostate cancer imaging

The automatic detection of subtle changes between ^{111}In-labeled Prostascint tomographic data sets acquired at 1 h, 48 h, and 72 h post-injection by means of 3-D statistical change detection is an important tool in staging both primary and recurrent prostate cancer. The 1 h post-injection data set may be taken to represent a tumor-free normal template against which to compare later image data sets. The real strength of statistical change detection lies in the objective detection of small areas of significant positive change representing antibody uptake within tumor sites over time and associating with each site of uptake a probability or significance value.

This detection process is further enhanced by the availability of a combined SPET/CT system (GE Systems, Hawkeye), a low-resolution CT system integral to the nuclear medicine gamma camera permitting the acquisition and subsequent fusion of CT data. These fused CT data sets contribute vital additional information including anatomical context and attenuation correction to the tumor detection process. Attenuation correction may be made in other ways by using moving linear or flood radiation sources.

The combined SPET/CT system provides the potential for multi-modal 3-D change detection. The term 'multi-modal change detection' in this case refers to the ability to detect change simultaneously both between nuclear medicine data sets and between associated homologous CT data sets.

Conventional ^{111}In-Prostascint imaging has relatively poor overall accuracy, 68% and 63% for primary and recurrent prostate disease, respectively. This poor accuracy is a consequence of confounding uptake of ^{111}In within gut, vascular structures, and marrow. It is in this arena that the power of statistical change detection applied to serial RIS image data combined with SPET/CT anatomical localization is able to improve the accuracy and detectability of both primary and recurrent prostate disease. Tomographic data are acquired in dual isotope serially as set out in the Appendix and the image data in Plate 13H.2.

Data analysis by the change detection process may be divided into three main steps: (1) body outline extraction, (2) iterative affine registration, and (3) single or multimodal statistical change detection tests.

Body outline extraction. Accurate image registration is critical to the change detection process and, in fact, may be the limiting factor with respect to detectability. The objective of accurately registering inter-patient nuclear medicine SPET tomographic data sets is vastly facilitated by the presence of CT data. These fused CT sections may be taken as being accurately registered to their homologous nuclear medicine data sets. Hence by determining the 3-D geometric transformation that maps respective SPET/CT data sets onto each other, then the selfsame transformation applies to the associated nuclear medicine data. Within these sections the patient's arms are visible as is the scanning couch. Prior to image registration potential sources of noise that will degrade the image matching process are removed including the patient's arms and the couch by using the Hawkeye data to form a binary mask. This mask further aids the efficiency of the matching process by acting as a look-up table and delineating only those image voxels that are required to participate in the matching process. This is important as a 3-D scan of the body contains a significant number of voxels containing useless information in that they contain only air, the scanning couch etc.

Iterative affine registration. Analysis of multi-temporal images requires accurate geometric alignment of the image data in order to compare corresponding regions in each image volume. Currently only rigid affine geometric transformations consisting of three dimensional rotations, translations and scale are considered. In the current analysis a voxel based approach is combined with the concept of maximization of mutual information. Mutual information is a basic concept from information theory that is applied to image registration to measure the amount of information that one image contains about the other. The maximization of mutual information registration concept states that the mutual information is maximal when images are correctly aligned and can be applied automatically and very reliably in routine clinical practice.

Single or multi-modal statistical change detection tests. Once the homologous image sets are registered then they must be compared to detect changes. These changes arise as a result of the pharmacokinetics of the radiolabeled antibody. Between early, e.g. 1 h post-injection, and later, e.g. 72 h, image data sets there will be a complex pattern of both positive and negative uptake of the antibody. Sites of positive uptake may include sites of both primary and secondary prostate cancer but will also include other sites of confounding uptake primarily in the gut and bone marrow.

The early (1 h) image set is taken to represent a normal tumor-free template against which later changes may be detected, although this assumption may not hold if a gross tumor burden is present. A further tumor-free template data set is available in this work in the form of the 48 h ^{99m}Tc-labeled RBCs.

The approach to statistical change detection implemented in this work is based upon the concept of nonparametric regression. Regression is one of the most widely used of all statistical tools, particularly in the form of linear regression. But in many real-world data sets such parametric models cannot be applied because of intrinsic nonlinearity in the data. In these cases nonparametric regression provides a means for modeling such data by letting the data speak for itself. Such a nonlinear data set arises when attempts are made to compare multi-temporal image data sets, as in Prostascint imaging.

A scattergram is calculated where the respective images' pixel intensity values are used to index into a two-dimensional or potentially higher order array. A suitable model for these data is given by

$$y = f(x) + \varepsilon,$$

where y denotes the response variable, e.g. a 72 h Prostascint data set; x is the covariate variable, e.g. a 1 h Prostascint data set; f is a function; and ε denotes an independent error term with a mean of zero and a variance σ^2. In the case of parametric regression analysis a linear relationship may be assumed to describe the relationship between the images Y and X, i.e.

$$y = a + bx.$$

In reality a linear relationship does not describe the relationship between the image X and image Y, as shown in Plate 13H.3.

In the case of nonparametric regression the regression expression is usually expressed as

$$y_i = m(x_i) + \varepsilon$$

within the statistical literature, where the designation m for the function f emphasizes that the regression curve $m(x)$ is the conditional expectation $m(x) = E(Y|X = x)$, i.e. the expected value of the dependent variable Y given that X takes the value x. The expected value, E, of the noise term ε, $E(\varepsilon|X = x) = 0$, i.e. zero mean with a variance $V(\varepsilon|X = x) = \sigma^2(x)$, which is not necessarily constant. Plate 13H.3 shows an example scattergram with a nonparametric regression line for images $Y = m(X)$ where the regression line is seen to adapt to the local structure within the data.

Initially, only nonparametric simple regression is considered where there is a response variable, e.g. a later image data set Y in this application and a single predictor variable X, i.e. a single earlier or tumor-free reference image data set. Subsequently, generalized nonparametric regression models are considered, where several predictor variables in the form of multiple reference image data sets are applied to the task of tumor detection.

The smooth curve in Plate 13H.3, which estimates the underlying regression curve $m(x)$, can be derived using several different approaches including nonparametric regression-based change detection.

Consider an image data set, e.g. a 48 h Prostascint tomographic data set, $Y(i,j,k)$ where i, j, and k represent the voxel coordinates, which contains potential sites of tumor uptake and background and a second co-registered tumor-free data set, e.g. 1 h Prostascint tomographic data containing only background data. Then the goal is to estimate the background component of the new image data as a function of the reference image, i.e. $\hat{y}(i,j,k) = m(x(i,j,k)) + \varepsilon$, using the principles of nonparametric regression.

Plate 13H.4(a) and (b) illustrates the nonparametric-based approach to change detection in a one-dimensional case. In this case the image sets are acquired simultaneously using different radionuclide energies rather than the same radionuclide at different times but the approach based on nonparametric regression is equally applicable. The dual-energy approach has the added advantage that both images are geometrically registered by virtue of their simultaneous acquisition. Plate 13H.4 shows a tumor-free reference image in the form of a 48 h RBC image along with a potential tumor-bearing 48 h ^{111}In image. Both images are seen to be spatially correlated but differ in intensity in a potentially complex manner which would be difficult to model explicitly, hence the role of nonparametric regression in letting the data speak for itself. Plate 13H.5 illustrates the change detection process in practice. Here the expected or predicted image $E(Y|X)$ is the 72 h Prostascint image predicted from the nonparametric regression curve derived from the 1 h to 72 h scattergram. When this expected 72 h image is compared with that of the actual observed 72 h Prostascint image then those areas that manifest positive errors represent areas of positive change including the tumor signal, T. Areas of negative error represent areas of negative change for example clearance of the pharmaceutical from the vascular system.

A probability measure is then calculated to give the significance of the difference between the predicted image and the observed image producing three dimensional parametric images or significance probability maps representing positive and negative changes.

Plate 13H.6 illustrates an example of fusing external high resolution imaging modalities, in this case MRI, onto the positive change detection map using the SPET/CT as a vehicle for multi-modality image registration.

Case history

A 55-year-old man with a T3bN1M0 carcinoma of the prostate, Gleeson grade 7, had a recent MRI scan suggesting pelvic lymph node involvement. These nodes measured 14–15 mm in diameter in the right internal iliac, left internal iliac, and presacral regions. He was therefore inappropriate for a radical prostatectomy. A Prostascint scan, Plate 13H.5, shows a single Prostascint positive lymph node. This was then co-located to the MRI scan, Plate 13H.6. This fusion image shows that only one of two nodes in the right iliac chain on the MRI was in fact involved and none of the other pelvic nodes showed any uptake. The patient is being reconsidered for surgery.

^{99m}Tc–bombesin

Bombesin receptors, which are gastrin-releasing peptide (GPR) receptors, have been demonstrated on prostate cancer cells.[60] Bombesin binds with high affinity to prostate cancer and to several other tumors, such as breast, lung, and neuroendocrine tumors. Bombesin has been radiolabeled with ^{99m}Tc via mercaptoacetyltriglycine (MAG$_3$) coupling[61] or by direct linkage via leucine[62] and with ^{111}In through DOTA linkage.[63] Scopinaro et al.[64] have shown that ^{99m}Tc-bombesin has clinical utility in planar and SPET imaging of prostate cancer. It has the advantage that imaging is limited to 1 and 3 h after injection. The technique looks promising.

CONCLUSION

Radioimmunoscintigraphy provides cancer-specific imaging of the prostate, with information about local involvement of nodes required for an assessment of radical prostatectomy, its spread to soft tissues and in untreated cases to bone. Once there is wide availability of the ^{111}In capromab pendetide kit and/or the efficacy of the ^{99m}Tc-bombesin is established, it will take its place in the regular clinical evaluation of prostate cancer. Advanced SPET/CT/MRI co-location systems will make it suitable for direct radiotherapy planning.

REFERENCES

● Seminal primary article
◆ Key review paper

◆ 1 Britton KE. The kidney and genital system. In: Feinendegen LE, Shreeve WW, Eckelman WC, *et al.* (eds.) *Molecular nuclear medicine.* Berlin: Springer, 2003: 583–5.

2 Gulfo JV. Clinical utility of monoclonal antibodies in prostate cancer. In: *Prostate cancer.* New York: Wiley Liss, 1994: 77–94.

◆ 3 Neil CE, Meis LC. Correlated imaging and monoclonal antibodies in colorectal, ovarian and prostate cancer. *Semin Nucl Med* 1994; **24**: 272–85.

● 4 Effert PJ, Bares R, Handt S, *et al.* Metabolic imaging of untreated prostate cancer by positron emission tomography with ^{18}fluorine labelled deoxyglucose. *J Urol* 1996; **155**: 994–8.

● 5 Hara T, Kosaka N, Kishi H. Development of F-18 fluoro ethyl choline for cancer imaging with PET: Synthesis, biochemistry and prostate cancer imaging. *J Nucl Med* 2002; **43**: 186–99.

● 6 Vihko P, Heikkila J, Konturri M, *et al.* Radioimaging of the prostate and metastases of prostate carcinoma with Tc-99m labelled prostate acid phosphatase specific antibodies and their Fab fragments. *Ann Clin Res* 1984; **16**: 51–2.

● 7 Wawroschek F, Vogt H, Wengenmair H, *et al.* Prostate lymphoscintigraphy and radio-guided surgery for sentinel lymph node identification in prostate cancer. Technique and results of the first 350 cases. *Urol Int* 2003; **70**: 303–10.

8 Lightner DJ, Lange PH, Reddy PK, *et al.* Prostate specific antigen and local recurrence after radical prostatectomy. *J Urol* 1990; **144**: 921–5.

● 9 Crook J, Robertson S, Collin G, *et al.* Clinical relevance of transrectal ultrasound, biopsy, and serum prostate-specific antigen following external beam radiotherapy for carcinoma of the prostate. *Int J Radiat Oncol Biol Phys* 1993; **27**: 31–7.

10 Foster LJ, Jagodi P, Fornier G, *et al.* The value of prostate specific antigen and transrectal ultrasound guided biopsy in detecting prostatic fossa recurrences following radical prostatectomy. *J Urol* 1993; **149**: 1024–8.

11 Partin AW, Kattan MW, Subong EN, *et al.* Combination of prostate-specific antigen, clinical stage, and Gleason score to predict pathological stage of localised prostate cancer. A multi institutional update. *J Am Med Assoc* 1997; **277**: 1445–8.

12 Crook JM, Cohan E, Perry GA, *et al.* Serum prostate specific antigen profile following radiotherapy for prostate cancer: implications for patterns of failure and definition of cure. *Urology* 1998; **51**: 556–70.

13 Gregorakis AK, Homes EH, Murphy GP. Prostate-specific membrane antigen: current and future utility. *Semin Urol Oncol* 1998; **16**: 2–12.

● 14 Wright GL, Haley C, Beckett ML, *et al.* Expression of prostate specific membrane antigen in normal benign and malignant prostate tissues. *Urol Oncol* 1995; **1**: 18–29.

15 Ross JS, Sheehan CE, Fisher HA, *et al.* Correlation of primary tumor prostate-specific membrane antigen expression with disease recurrence in prostate cancer. *Clin Cancer Res* 2003; **9**: 6357–62.

● 16 Liu H, Moy P, Kim A, *et al.* Monoclonal antibodies to the extracellular domain of prostate-specific membrane antigen also react with tumour vascular epithelium. *Cancer Res* 1997; **57**: 3629–34.

● 17 Troyer JK, Feng Q, Beckett ML, *et al.* Biochemical characterisation and mapping of the 7E11C5 epitope of the prostate specific membrane antigen. *Urol Oncol* 1995; **1**: 29–37.

18 Carter RE, Feldman AR, Coyle JT. Prostate-specific membrane antigen is a hydrolase with substrate and pharmacological characteristics of a neuropeptidase. *Proc Natl Acad Sci USA* 1996; **93**: 749–53.

19 Pinto JT, Suffoletto BP, Berzin TM, *et al.* Prostate-specific membrane antigen: a novel folate hydrolase in human prostatic carcinoma cells. *Clin Cancer Res* 1996; **2**: 1445–51.

● 20 Liu H, Rajasekaran AK, Moy P, *et al.* Constitutive and antibody induced internalisation of prostate-specific membrane antigen. *Cancer Res* 1998; **58**: 4055–60.

◆ 21 Bander NH, Nanus DM, Milowsky MI, *et al.* Targeted systemic therapy of prostate cancer with a monoclonal antibody to prostate-specific membrane antigen. *Semin Oncol* 2003; **30**: 667–76.

● 22 Bander NH, Trabulsi EJ, Kostakoglu L, *et al.* Targeting metastatic prostate cancer with radiolabeled monoclonal antibody J591 to the extracellular domain of prostate specific membrane antigen. *J Urol* 2003; **170**: 1717–21.

23 Britton KE, Gordon SJ, Mather SJ, *et al.* Tc-99m MUJ591 monoclonal antibody, MoAb, against the external domain of the prostate specific membrane antigen, PSMA: a pilot imaging study in prostate cancer [Abstract]. *J Nucl Med* 2001; **42**: 294P.

24 Horoszcewicz JS, Kawinski E, Murphy GP. Monoclonal antibodies to a new antigenic marker in epithelial prostate cells and serum of prostatic cancer patients. *Anticancer Res* 1987; **7**: 927–36.

● 25 Babaian RJ, Sayer J, Podoloff DA, *et al.* Radioimmunoscintigraphy of pelvic lymph nodes with ^{111}indium labelled monoclonal antibody CYT-356. *J Urol* 1994; **152**: 1952–55.

● 26 Mardirossian G, Brill AB, Dwyer KM, *et al.* Radiation absorbed dose from indium-111-CYT 356. *J Nucl Med* 1996; **37**: 1583–8.

● 27 Mather SJ, Ellison D. Reduction-mediated technetium-99m labelling of monoclonal antibodies. *J Nucl Med* 1990; **31**: 692–7.

28 Stalteri MA., Mather SJ, Chengazi VU, *et al.* Site specific conjugation and labelling of prostate antibody 7E11C5 with Tc-99m [Abstract]. *Nucl Med Commun* 1995; **15**: 241.

29 Feneley MR, Chengazi VU, Kirby RS, *et al.* Prostatic radioimmunoscintigraphy: preliminary results using technetium-labelled monoclonal antibody CYT-351. B*r J Urol* 1996; **77**: 373–81.

● 30 Chengazi VU, Feneley M, Nimmon CC, *et al.* Prostate cancer imaging with the monoclonal antibody Tc-99m-CYT-351. *J Nucl Med* 1997; **38**: 675–81.

● 31 Shreve PD, Grossman HB, Gross MD, Wahl RL. Metastatic prostate cancer; initial findings of PET with 2-deoxy-2 (F-18) fluoro-D-glucose. *Radiology* 1996; **199**: 751–6.

32 Hoh CK, Seltzer MA, Franklin J, *et al.* Positron emission tomography in urological oncology. *J Urol* 1998; **159**: 347–56.

33 Morris MJ, Akhurst T, Osman I, *et al.* Fluorinated deoxyglucose positron emission tomography imaging in progressive metastatic prostate cancer. *Urology* 2002; **59**: 913–18.

● 34 Oyama N, Miller TR, Dehdashti F, *et al.* C-11-acetate PET imaging of prostate cancer: detection of recurrent disease at PSA relapse. *J Nucl Med* 2003; **44**: 549–55.

35 Fricke E, Machtens S, Hofmann M. Positron emission tomography with C-11-acetate and F-18-FDG in prostate cancer patients. *Eur J Nucl Med* 2003; **30**: 607–11.

● 36 DeJong IJ, Pruim J, Elsinga PH, *et al.* Pre operative staging of pelvic lymph nodes in prostate cancer by C-11-choline PET. *J Nucl Med* 2003; **44**: 331–5.

● 37 Ragde H, Elgamal A-AA, Snow PB, *et al.* Ten year disease free survival after transperineal sonography-guided I-125 brachytherapy with or without 45-gray external beam irradiation in the treatment of patients with clinically localised, low to high Gleason grade prostate carcinoma. *Cancer* 1998; **83**: 989–1001.

38 Ellis RJ, Vertocnik A, Kim E, *et al.* Four-year biochemical outcome after radioimmunoguided transperineal brachytherapy for patients with prostate adenocarcinoma. *Int J Radiat Oncol Biol Phys* 2003; **57**: 362–70.

● 39 Kahn D, Haseman MK, Libertino J, *et al.* Indium-111 capromab pendetide (Prostascint) imaging of patients with rising PSA post-prostatectomy. *J Urol* 1997; **158**: 157–204.

40 Murphy GP, Maguire RT, Rogers B, *et al.* Comparison of serum PSMA, PSA levels with results of Cytogen-356 Prostascint scanning in prostatic cancer patients. *Prostate* 1997; **33**: 281–5.

41 Kahn D, Williams RD, Haseman MK, *et al.* Radioimmunoscintigraphy with In-111 labelled capromab pendetide predicts prostate cancer response to salvage radiotherapy after failed radical prostatectomy. *J Clin Oncol* 1998; **16**: 284–9.

● 42 Hinkle GH, Burgers JK, Neal CE, *et al.* Multicentre radioimmunoscintigraphic evaluation of patients with prostate carcinoma using indium-111 capromab pendetide. *Cancer* 1998; **83**: 739–47.

● 43 Levesque PE, Nieh PT, Zinman LN, *et al.* Radiolabelled monoclonal antibody indium-111-labelled CYT-356 localises extraprostatic recurrent carcinoma after prostatectomy. *Urology* 1998; **51**: 978–84.

44 Manyak MJ, Hinkle GH, Olsen JO, *et al.* Immunoscintigraphy with indium-111-capromab pendetide: evaluation before definitive therapy in patients with prostate cancer. *Urology* 1999; **54**: 1058–63.

● 45 Polascik TJ, Manyak MJ, Haseman MK, *et al.* Comparison of clinical staging algorithms and 111-indium-capromab pendetide immunoscintigraphy in the prediction of lymph node involvement in high risk prostate carcinoma patients. *Cancer* 1999; **85**: 1586–92.

● 46 Feneley MR, Jan H, Granowska M, *et al.* Imaging with prostate specific membrane (PSMA) in prostate cancer. *Prostate Cancer and Prostatic Diseases* 2000; **2**: 47–52.

● 47 Sodee DB, Malguria N, Faulhaber P, *et al.* Multicenter ProstaScint imaging findings in 2154 patients with prostate cancer. The ProstaScint Imaging Centers. *Urology* 2000; **56**: 988–93.

● 48 Raj GV, Partin AW, Polascik DJ. Clinical utility of indium-111 capromab pendetide. Immunoscintigraphy in the detection of early, recurrent prostate carcinoma after radical prostatectomy. *Cancer* 2002; **94**: 987–96.

◆ 49 Britton KE, Feneley MR, Jan H, Chengazi VU, Granowska M. Prostate cancer: the contribution of nuclear medicine. *Br J Urol Intern* 2000; **86(Suppl 1)**: 135–42.

● 50 Thomas CT, Bradshaw PT, Pollock BH, *et al.* Indium-111-capromab pendetide radioimmunoscintigraphy and prognosis for durable biochemical response to salvage radiation therapy in men after failed prostatectomy. *J Clin Oncol* 2003; **21**: 1715–21.

51 Ellis RJ, Kim EY, Conant R, *et al.* Radioimmunoguided imaging of prostate cancer foci with histopathological correlation. *Int J Rad Oncol Biol Phys* 2001; **49**: 1281–6.

● 52 Quintana JC, Blend MJ. The dual-isotope ProstaScint imaging procedure: clinical experience and staging results in 145 patients. *Clin Nucl Med* 2000; **25**: 33–40.

53 Berry MG, Feneley MR, Domizio P, *et al.* Evaluating the return of prostate adenocarcinoma. *J R Soc Med* 1998; **91**: 641–3.

54 Naseem MS, Jan HA, Britton KE, Nargund VH. Splenic metastases from adenocarcinoma of the prostate. *Br J Urol* 1998; **82**: 597–8.

● 55 Kahn D, Austin JC, Maguire RT, *et al.* A phase II study of [^{90}Y]yttrium-capromab pendetide in the treatment of men with prostate cancer recurrence following radical prostatectomy. *Cancer Biother Radiopharm* 1999; **14**: 99–111.

56 Hashimi D, Carroll MJ, Elnaas ST, *et al.* Multimodality imaging of prostate cancer, PC, with In-111 Prostascint [Abstract]. *Eur J Nucl Med Mol Imaging* 2003; **30**: S158.

● 57 Harisinghani MG, Barentsz J, Hahn PF, *et al.* Noninvasive detection of clinically occult lymph-node metastases in prostate cancer. *N Engl J Med* 2003; **348**: 2491–9.

58 Carroll MJ, Britton KE. Fusing anatomical data to SPECT – application to 3D statistical change detection [Abstract]. *Eur J Nucl Med Mol Imaging* 2003; **30**: S330.

● 59 Jani AB, Blend MJ, Hamilton R, *et al.* Influence of radioimmunoscintigraphy on post-prostatectomy radiotherapy treatment decision making. *J Nucl Med* 2004; **45**: 571–8.

● 60 Reubi JC, Wenger S, Schmuckli-Maurer J, Schaer JC, Gugger M. Bombesin receptor subtypes in human cancers: detection with the universal radioligand (125)I-[D-TYR(6), beta-ALA(11), PHE(13), NLE(14)] bombesin(6-14). *Clin Cancer Res* 2002; **8**: 1139–46.

● 61 Okarvi SM, al-Jammaz I. Synthesis, radiolabelling and biological characteristics of a bombesin peptide analog as a tumor imaging agent. *Anticancer Res* 2003; **23**: 2745–50.

62 Varvarigou AD, Scopinaro F, Leondiadis L, *et al.* Synthesis, chemical, radiochemical and radio-biological evaluation of a new ^{99m}Tc-labelled bombesin-like peptide. *Cancer Biother Radiopharm* 2002; **17**: 317–26.

● 63 Hoffman TJ, Gali H, Smith CJ, *et al.* Novel series of ^{111}In-labeled bombesin analogs as potential radio-pharmaceuticals for specific targeting of gastrin-releasing peptide receptors expressed on human prostate cancer cells. *J Nucl Med* 2003; **44**: 823–31.

● 64 Scopinaro F, De Vincentis G, Varvarigou AD, *et al.* ^{99m}Tc-bombesin detects prostate cancer and invasion of pelvic lymph nodes. *Eur J Nucl Med Mol Imaging* 2003; **30**: 1378–82.

APPENDIX: PROSTATE IMMUNE STUDY WITH ^{111}In-PROSTASCINT

Patients should be given a full explanation and should sign a consent form. Patients who are allergic to foreign protein, i.e. reaction to innoculation, are excluded. Vital signs may be monitored before and after injection. The requirements are as follows:

Radiopharmaceutical: ^{111}In-CYT-356 (capromab pende-tide monoclonal antibody, also known as Prostascint)
Energy: 171 and 245 keV
Activity: 200–400 MBq
Collimator: Medium energy
Post-injection time: 1–2, 24, 48 or 72 h. The 24 h image may be omitted.

The planar and SPET images are best done with a double-head 'thick' crystal camera system and the squat view with a single-head camera.

Procedure

1. Inject 185–300 MBq ^{111}In-Prostascint into an ante-cubital vein.
2. The patient empties his bladder, then at 60 min post-injection, the following planar views are taken in order anterior and posterior pelvis, anterior and posterior upper abdomen (128 × 128 matrix, 800 kcounts).
3. The patient again empties his bladder. Position the patient for squat views, having the single-head camera as low as possible, tilted backwards at an angle of 45°. The patient sits on a stool and leans forward, resting on a pillow on a lower stool. Check the position so that the kidneys and liver are not in the field of view. Take the squat view, 128 × 128 matrix, without markers, for 400 kcounts.
4. The patient again empties his bladder. Then SPET of the pelvis, 360°, 20 s per slice is undertaken.
5. Repeat steps 2 to 4 at 48 h and 72 h; SPET, 60 s per slice.

Improved procedure using a SPET/CT system

1a. Prior to the injection of ^{111}In-Prostascint, undertake a ^{99m}Tc-MDP bone scan. Immediately after completion of the 3 h bone scan, inject the 185–300 MBq ^{111}In-Prostascint and set up SPET for dual radionuclide capture of ^{99m}Tc and ^{111}In followed by the low-resolution CT for attenuation correction and fusion imaging.
5a. Prior to the 48 h SPET, perform the ^{99m}Tc blood pool scan. Inject a pyrophosphate/stannous kit intravenously, then 20 min later draw blood back into a large syringe containing 370 MBq (10 mCi) [^{99m}Tc]pertechnetate. Allow the solution to mix and re-inject for blood pool imaging. Set up SPET for ^{99m}Tc and ^{111}In dual radio-nuclide capture followed by CT.
5b. Undertake the 72 h SPET/CT imaging.
6. Compare the bone scan SPET with early ^{111}In-Prostascint for anatomical registration.

Compare early ^{111}In-Prostascint SPET/CT with late ^{111}In-Prostascint SPET/CT.

Compare early ^{111}In-Prostascint SPET/CT with ^{99m}Tc blood pool SPET/CT.

Compare late ^{111}In-Prostascint SPET/CT with ^{99m}Tc blood pool SPET/CT.

Compare 72 h ^{111}In-Prostascint SPET/CT with the 48 h ^{111}In-Prostascint SPET/CT.

The comparison is best made by co-registration of the images with transfer of a region of interest around an abnormality or suspected abnormality on the late ^{111}In-Prostascint SPET to the ^{99m}Tc blood pool SPET, to the bone scan and to the early ^{111}In-Prostascint SPET and the low resolution CT.

7. Apply attenuation correction to the RIS SPET images. Fuse these with the CT images. Co-locate the Hawkeye CT images with high-quality CT or MRI images transferred on-line or by disk from the radiology department.

Co-report with a radiological specialist.

Anatomical co-registration of these images, which combine the physical and biological extent of the cancer, should aid radiotherapy planning.

14

The gastrointestinal tract

14A Gastrointestinal bleeding

Introduction	621	Meckel's diverticulum	624
The role of scintigraphy	621	References	627
Techniques and interpretation	621		

14B Inflammatory bowel disease

Introduction	629	Applications and results	630
Techniques	629	References	634
Interpretation	629		

14C Functional studies of the gastrointestinal tract

Introduction	637	Protein loss	643
Gastrointestinal transit	637	Gastrointestinal blood loss	643
Malabsorption tests	641	Biliary scintigraphy	643
Breath tests	642	References	644

14D Positron emission tomography in gastrointestinal cancers

Introduction	645	Hepatobiliary tumors	648
Esophageal cancer	645	Gastrointestinal stromal tumors	648
Pancreatic cancer	646	Miscellaneous	648
Colorectal cancer	646	References	649

14E Gastrointestinal neuroendocrine tumors

Introduction	653	Staging	654
Sites of disease	653	Restaging	654
Functionality	653	Radionuclides used for imaging	655
Secretory syndromes	654	Therapy	657
Diagnosis	654	Conclusion	659
Localization	654	References	659

Gastrointestinal bleeding

PHILIP J.A. ROBINSON

INTRODUCTION

The clinical spectrum of gastrointestinal bleeding has evolved considerably since the introduction, three decades ago, of scintigraphic methods for localizing bleeding sites. In patients with acute bleeding, the choice of medical, surgical or radiological interventions and the role of nuclear imaging procedures largely depends on the rate of blood loss and the presence of co-morbidities in the patient, and some aspects remain controversial. In about 80% of patients, the source of acute bleeding is in the esophagus, stomach or duodenum and early endoscopy allows both diagnosis and an opportunity for therapeutic intervention, such as injection or banding of bleeding varices.[1,2] Most of the remaining 20% of acute bleeds originate in the colon, with small bowel hemorrhage accounting for a minority of cases.[3] Colonoscopy may be successful in identifying large bowel pathology, but the confirmation of active bleeding at the site of a colonic abnormality is often difficult since stigmata of recent bleeding are seen much less often than in the upper gastrointestinal (GI) tract. Adequate bowel preparation is often difficult, and blood in the lumen may obscure the colonoscopist's view. Diverticular disease and angiodysplasias may be found at colonoscopy for rectal bleeding, but are also common incidental findings in patients who have never bled. When rigorous diagnostic criteria are applied, the site of colonic bleeding remains uncertain in a substantial proportion of patients.[4]

THE ROLE OF SCINTIGRAPHY

Patients with bleeding sites in the upper GI tract will usually be diagnosed by endoscopy. Colonoscopy, or at least flexible sigmoidoscopy, will usually be used after a negative upper GI endoscopy and only if the cause still remains unclear will scintigraphic methods be appropriate. In patients with continuing rapid bleeding which is life-threatening, urgent angiography or surgery is required. The majority of patients with GI bleeding stop spontaneously with supportive therapy alone, and some of these never bleed again.[5] The morbidity of surgical procedures for GI bleeding is reduced if the site of bleeding is established preoperatively.[6] In an increasing proportion of patients, GI bleeding is a secondary presentation in patients already under treatment for other conditions,[7] so many of the patients who present in this way have co-morbidities that increase the risks of surgery.

Scintigraphic studies are fairly sensitive in detecting acute hemorrhage in the GI tract. The amount of bleeding required to produce a positive scintigraphic result equates approximately to the volume of blood which will result in a melena stool. Patients whose only evidence of GI bleeding is a positive chemical test for occult blood in the stools will produce negative results on scintigraphy. The patients in whom nuclear imaging is most likely to be helpful are those with the following characteristics:

- Upper GI endoscopy negative or inconclusive
- Colonoscopy inconclusive or inappropriate
- Prolonged or recurrent bleeding in spite of initial conservative therapy
- Bleeding sufficient to produce melena, but not torrential hemorrhage

TECHNIQUES AND INTERPRETATION[8]

Two different approaches have been described, each with particular advantages and drawbacks.

Radiolabeled red cells technique[9]

Autologous red cells can be labeled *in vivo* with ^{99m}Tc by injection of sodium [^{99m}Tc]pertechnetate after previous injection of a reducing agent, usually stannous chloride. However, this method is unsuitable for bleeding studies because the labeling efficiency is limited and free pertechnetate may be excreted not only in the urinary tract but also secreted by the gastric and colonic mucosa. More efficient labeling of autologous red cells is carried out *in vitro* where the residual free pertechnetate can be removed from the cell preparation before re-injecting into the patient. Following injection of about 400 MBq of labeled red cells, a first pass dynamic series may be obtained, to highlight vascular abnormalities in the abdomen and pelvis. Subsequent images are then obtained, preferably in dynamic mode to allow subsequent cine-replay, up to 1–2 h. If no bleeding site is found, further imaging is undertaken at intervals up to 24 h.

INTERPRETATION

After the first pass vascular phase, blood pool activity outlines the heart, liver, spleen, kidneys and major vessels (Fig. 14A.1). Small bowel and uterus often show a vascular blush and the portal vein is usually visible. This activity within the vascular compartment remains stable over the next 24 h although even with *in vitro* labeling, some free pertechnetate is released from the cells and excreted via the urinary tract, so it is important to empty the bladder to improve visualization of the pelvis. Bleeding sites are recognized as areas of locally increased activity, which are distinct from the main anatomic landmarks and vascular structures (Fig. 14A.2). Clues to the localization of the bleeding site are given by the position within the abdomen at which the extravasation is first seen, and the rate and direction of its

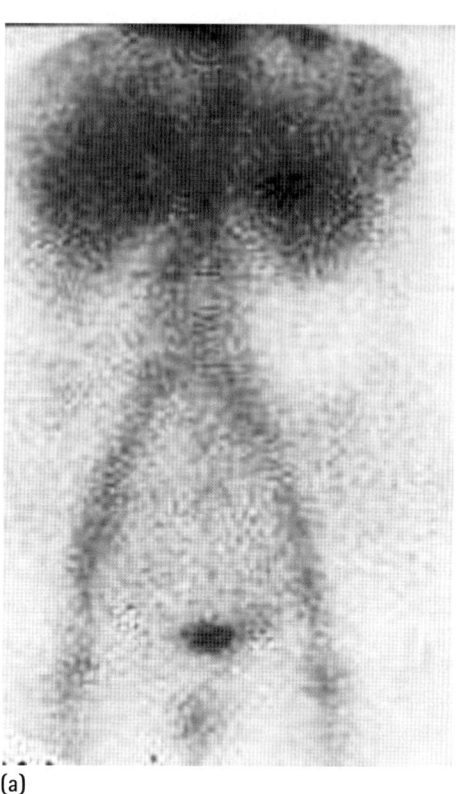

(a)

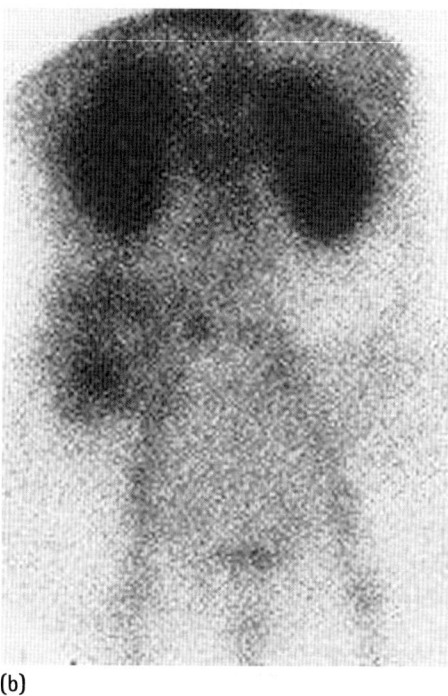

(b)

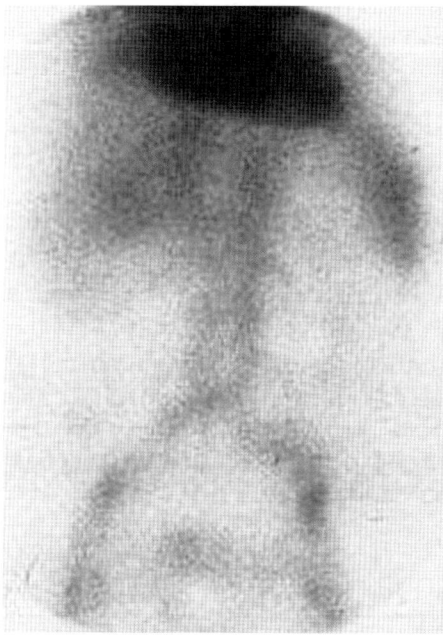

Figure 14A.1 *Normal distribution of ^{99m}Tc-labeled autologous red blood cells 2 h after re-injection.*

Figure 14A.2 *Bleeding into the cecum shown at 60 min (b), but only faintly visible at 15 min (a).*

subsequent movement on later images. It is often helpful to display the dynamic acquisition in a cine-loop to visualize the direction and speed of movement of extravasated activity in the bowel lumen.[10,11] Further assistance may be obtained by correlation with an abdominal radiograph or previous barium enema, which will help to confirm the disposition of the various sections of the colon. Colonic bleeding is often first seen near the periphery of the abdomen, and tends to move quite slowly along the lumen (Fig. 14A.3). Small bowel bleeding moves more briskly and is often first identified in a more central position in the abdomen or pelvis. When bleeding is visualized within 1–2 h after injection of labeled cells, localization of the site is usually accurate. However, when extravasation is only identified on later images, it is possible that the extravasated blood may have originated at a more proximal site. This is particularly likely if bleeding is very slow, or intermittent. In such cases the confidence of localization is reduced although it is usually still possible to give an indication of either small bowel or large bowel origin.

Radiolabeled colloid technique[12]

An alternative technique which is less widely used involves the injection of colloidal tin, sulfur or albumin labeled with [^{99m}Tc]pertechnetate. With a particle size of 30–1000 nm, the tracer is rapidly cleared into the reticulo-endothelial cells of the liver, spleen, and bone marrow. With a blood half-life of only a few minutes, background activity is rapidly cleared and sites of extravasation become readily visible within the abdomen or pelvis. About 400 MBq of labeled colloid is injected, and a rapid first pass dynamic sequence of images is obtained. This is followed by images at 1 min

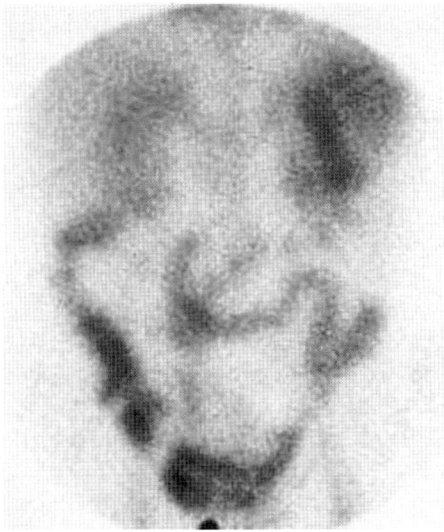

Figure 14A.3 *Extensive bleeding in large bowel shown at 6 h after re-injection of ^{99m}Tc-labeled red blood cells.*

intervals up to 5 min, then at 5 min intervals up to 60 min. The examination may be terminated sooner if a positive identification is made.

INTERPRETATION

As with red cells studies, localization of the bleeding site depends on the demonstration of extravasated activity in the bowel lumen. The rapid disappearance of the tracer from the circulation allows visualization of a relatively small volume of extravasated blood (<1 mL in animal studies), but the patient must be bleeding at the time of injection for a positive result to be obtained. Bleeding in the lower abdomen is usually visualized within the first few minutes after injection (Fig. 14A.4), but since uptake of the tracer by the liver and spleen may obscure bleeding sites in the stomach, proximal duodenum, splenic flexure, and transverse colon, it is important to continue up to 60 min in order to allow time for blood extravasated into these sections of bowel to move along the lumen far enough to become visible. As with red cells studies, identification of the bleeding site depends not only on the point at which the extravasation is first seen, but on the direction, speed, and pattern of its subsequent movement along the bowel lumen. A small amount of activity will normally escape into the urinary tract, so the bladder should be emptied from time to time to improve visualization of the pelvis.

Choice of technique

When positive, the colloid technique gives a quick and reliable localization of bleeding points. Its major disadvantage is the requirement for the patient to be actively bleeding at the time of injection. Since much GI bleeding is intermittent and episodic, negative colloid results may be obtained in patients who bleed again subsequently. Using labeled red cells allows observation of the patient over a longer period, with the possibility of detecting intermittent or slow bleeding. However, the accuracy of localization is reduced when bleeding is only detected on delayed images. With colloid, the appearance of extravasation depends on the rate of bleeding in the first few minutes after injection, whilst with labeled red cells detection depends on the volume of blood accumulating in the bowel lumen at the bleeding site. Studies with volunteers have shown that as little as 5 mL of labeled blood could be visualized in the stomach,[13] but under the less favorable conditions of clinical practice the volume required is likely to be considerably more than this.

Accuracy of the techniques

Many correlative studies have assessed the accuracy of scintigraphic localization of bleeding sites with subsequent

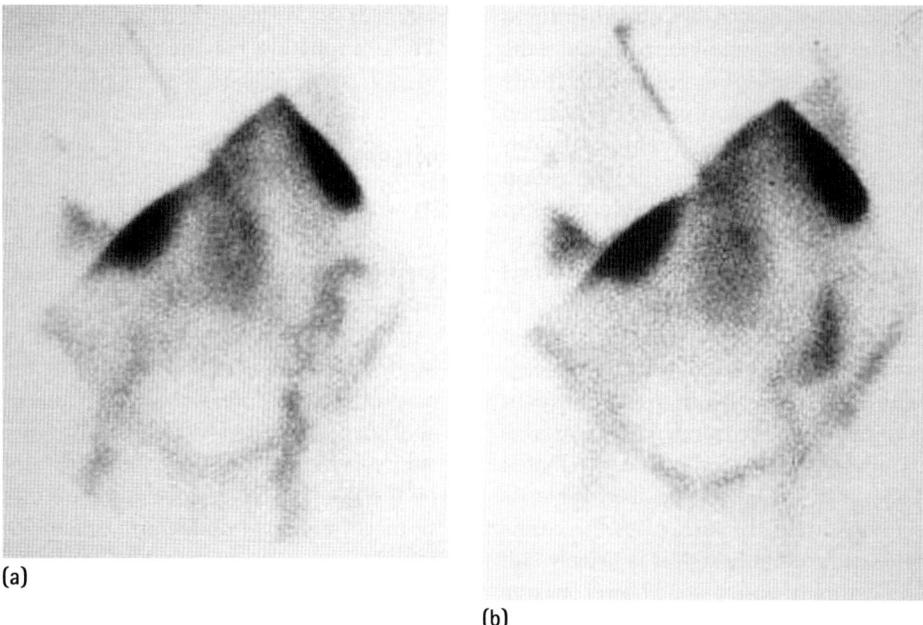

(a)

(b)

Figure 14A.4   *Bleeding site in sigmoid colon identified on images obtained (a) 3 min and (b) 10 min after injection of ^{99m}Tc-labeled colloid.*

arteriography and surgery.[14–23] Published results must be treated with caution for two main reasons. Firstly, the selection of patients for inclusion varies between different studies, and the population of patients presenting with acute GI bleeding is heterogeneous. Secondly, the problem of assigning the cause of bleeding to any colonic pathology which may be present has already been referred to above, and unless the patient was still actively bleeding at the time of surgery or arteriography, such attributions may be unreliable. Even with these reservations, it appears that the sensitivity of nuclear imaging techniques for localizing GI bleeding sites is in the region of 80–90%, but it must be emphasized that the indiscriminate use of these techniques in inappropriate patients will produce much less effective results. Direct comparisons of colloid and red cell techniques have usually favored the latter.[24,25] Patients whose labeled red cell studies are negative are less likely to rebleed, require less transfusion, and less often undergo surgery than those with positive studies.[26–28]

MECKEL'S DIVERTICULUM

Persistence of the enteric end of the omphalomesenteric duct – which is normally obliterated by the time of birth – results in Meckel's diverticulum in 1–3% of otherwise normal individuals. The condition is usually silent, only a small proportion of patients presenting with symptoms, most often in childhood or adolescence, less commonly in later life. About 60% of patients with Meckel's diverticulum contain areas of gastric mucosa which may undergo

ulceration and scarring. The most common mode of presentation in children is abdominal pain and bleeding, whilst obstruction, inflammation, and intussusception are more frequent presentations in adults. Scintigraphic detection relies upon the specific uptake of [^{99m}Tc]pertechnetate in the ectopic gastric mucosa, probably in the mucus-secreting cells.[29,30]

Technique and interpretation[8]

Adults and older children should starve overnight, but with infants and small children it is sufficient to withhold one feed. Pertechnetate is not only taken up by the gastric mucosa (Fig. 14A.5) but also secreted into the lumen of the stomach. To avoid difficulty in interpretating the images which may result if pertechnetate moves along the lumen of the small bowel (Fig. 14A.6), patients should be pretreated with an H2 blocker overnight. This does not inhibit the uptake of pertechnetate into the mucosa, but blocks its subsequent secretion into the lumen.[31]

After injection of 200–400 MBq of [^{99m}Tc]pertechnetate (scaled down appropriately for children), images of the abdomen and pelvis are obtained at intervals up to 1 h. Because of renal excretion of the tracer, it is important to empty the bladder towards the end of the procedure. Although other intra-abdominal sites have been described, the majority of Meckel's diverticula lie in the right iliac fossa or in the right side of the pelvis (Fig. 14A.7). Oblique or even lateral views may be helpful to distinguish possible abnormalities from pertechnetate in the ureters. Intra-abdominal structures with a large blood pool and extracellular space

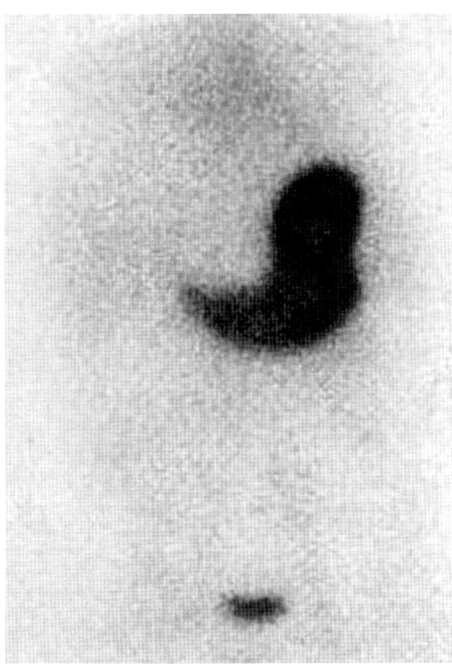

Figure 14A.5 *Normal gastric mucosa and a little urinary excretion in bladder outlined 30 min after injection of [⁹⁹ᵐTc]pertechnetate.*

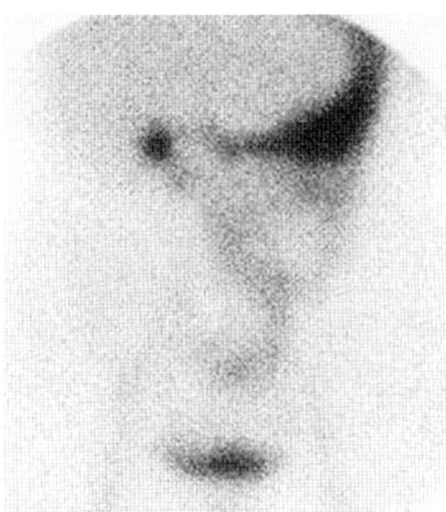

Figure 14A.6 *Normal study showing secretion of [⁹⁹ᵐTc]pertechnetate into small bowel loops which is usually prevented by premedication with H2 blockade.*

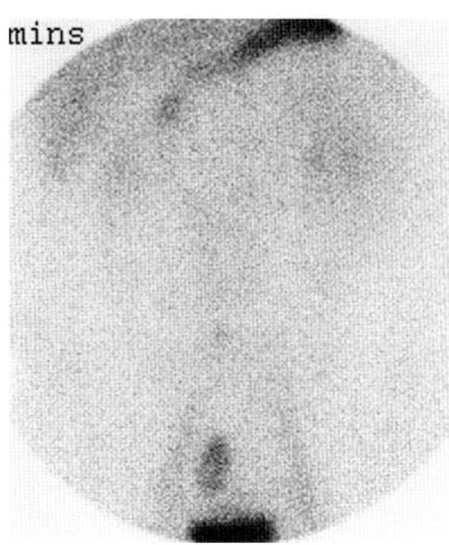

Figure 14A.7 *Meckel's diverticulum identified in the pelvis at 20 min after injection of [⁹⁹ᵐTc]pertechnetate.*

(e.g. small bowel, uterus, tumors, inflammatory masses) may show an early accumulation of the tracer, but gastric mucosa shows a gradually increasing concentration over the period of the study. Foci of activity outside the stomach which show a similar gradual increase in uptake should be regarded as probable sites of ectopic gastric mucosa, which may also be found in neurenteric or duplication cysts. Hormonal enhancements using glucagon, which paralyses the bowel, or pentagastrin, which increases the uptake of pertechnetate by the gastric mucosa, have been proposed, but the benefits of these additional agents have not been sufficiently established to recommend their general use.

Results

Multicentre series report the sensitivity for detecting clinically significant Meckel's diverticula in children with confirmed surgical findings to be about 90%.[32,33] In adults, positive results are less specific since the range of presentations is greater than in children and false positive results may be obtained with vascular tumors and malformations, areas of intussusception, focal inflammatory disease or abscesses. However, in a very large series of surgically confirmed adult cases, the sensitivity of scintigraphy in preoperative recognition of Meckel's diverticula was considerably better than barium studies and angiography.[34]

Case history: Case 1

A 76-year-old man presented acutely with large volume melena. No bleeding was visible at upper GI endoscopy. Scintigraphy using ^{99m}Tc-labeled colloid showed a small bowel bleeding site in the left mid abdomen (Fig. 14A.8(a) and (b)). Angiography with selective injection of jejunal branches identified a bleeding point which was successfully embolized (Fig. 14A.8(c) and (d)).

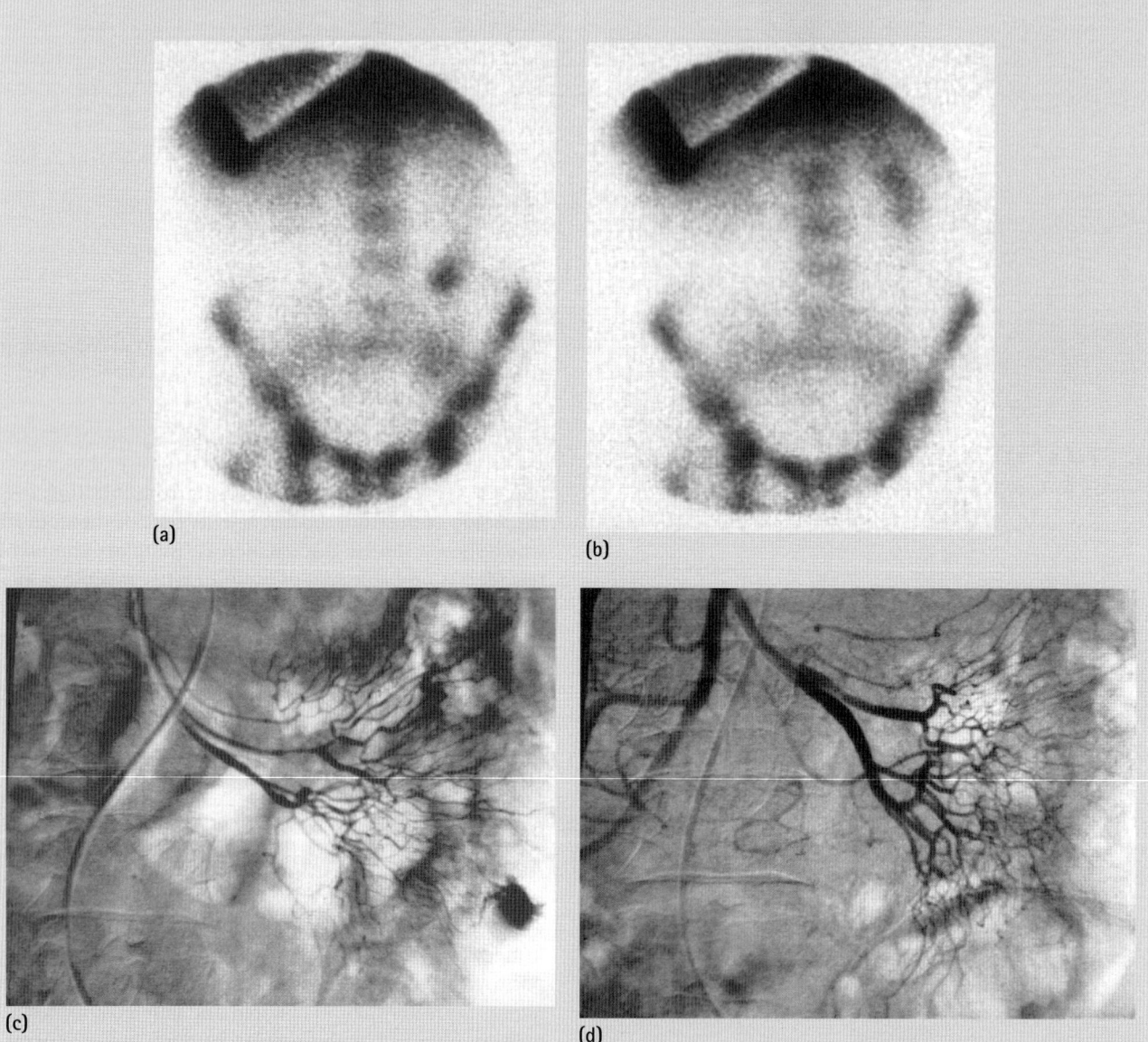

(a)

(b)

(c)

(d)

Figure 14A.8   *Small bowel hemorrhage identified in the left mid abdomen at 5 min (a) and 10 min (b) after injection of ^{99m}Tc-labeled colloid. Subsequent angiography identified a small bowel bleeding site (c) which was successfully embolized (d).*

Case history: Case 2

A 26-year-old man with a history of recurrent abdominal pain presented with a single, but severe episode of dark red rectal bleeding. Upper GI endoscopy and colonoscopy after stabilization showed no abnormality. [^{99m}Tc]pertechnetate scintigraphy identified ectopic gastric mucosa in the pelvis (Fig. 14A.9(a)). Angiography confirmed the persistent terminal branch of the superior mesenteric artery associated with a Meckel's diverticulum (Fig. 14A.9(b)) which was surgically removed.

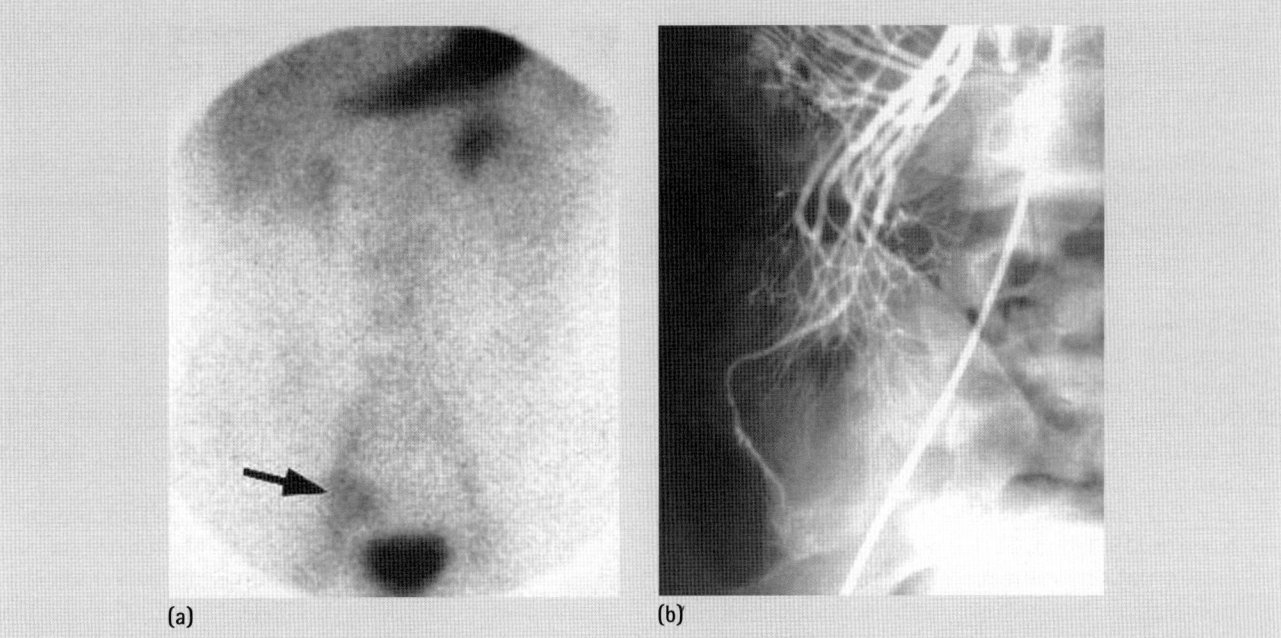

(a)   (b)

Figure 14A.9   *Ectopic gastric mucosa identified in the pelvis (arrow) (a) 30 min after [⁹⁹ᵐTc]pertechnetate injection; subsequent angiography (b) identified the abnormal termination of the superior mesenteric artery associated with a Meckel's diverticulum.*

REFERENCES

- Seminal primary article
- Key review paper

1 Kohler B, Riemann JF. Upper GI bleeding – value and consequences of emergency endoscopy and endoscopic treatment. *Hepatogastroenterol* 1991; **38**: 198–200.

2 Sacks HS, Chalmers TC, Blum AL. Endoscopic haemostasis: an effective therapy for bleeding peptic ulcers. *JAMA* 1990; **264**: 494–9.

3 Lau WY, Yuen WK, Chu KW, *et al.* Obscure bleeding in the gastrointestinal tract originating in the small intestine. *Surg Gyn Obst* 1992; **174**: 119–24.

4 Jaramillo E, Slezak P. Comparison between double contrast barium enema and colonoscopy to investigate lower gastrointestinal bleeding. *Gastrointest Radiol* 1992; **17**: 81–3.

5 Fleisher D. Aetiology and prevalence of severe persistent upper gastrointestinal bleeding. *Gastroenterology* 1983; **84**: 538–43.

6 Hunt PS, Hansky J, Korman MG. Mortality in patients with haematemesis and melaena: a prospective study. *Br Med J* 1979; **1**: 1238–40.

7 Gostout CJ, Wang KK, Ahlquist DA, *et al.* Acute gastrointestinal bleeding – experience of a specialised management team. *J Clin Gastroenterol* 1992; **14**: 260–7.

★ 8 Ford PV, Bartold SP, *et al.* Procedure guideline for gastrointestinal bleeding and Meckel's diverticulum scintigraphy. 1.0: *Society of Nuclear Medicine Procedure Guidelines Manual 2001–2002*. Reston, Viriginia: Society of Nuclear Medicine, 2001: 41–8.

9 McKusick KA, Froelich J, Callaghan RJ, *et al.* Tc99m red cells for detection of gastrointestinal bleeding. *AJR* 1981; **137**: 1013–18.

10 Maurer AH, Rodman MS, Vitti RA, *et al.* Gastrointestinal bleeding: improved localization with cine scintigraphy. *Radiology* 1992; **185**: 187–92.

11 O'Neill BB, Gosnell JE, Lull RJ, *et al.* Cinematic nuclear scintigraphy reliably directs surgical intervention for patients with gastrointestinal bleeding. *Arch Surg* 2000; **135**: 1076–82.

● 12 Alavi A, Dann RW, Baum S, Biery DN. Scintigraphic detection of acute gastrointestinal bleeding. *Radiology* 1977; **124**: 753–6.

13 Smith RK, Arteburn JG. Detection and localisation of gastrointestinal bleeding using Tc99m-pyrophosphate in vivo labelled red blood cells. *Clin Nucl Med* 1980; **5**: 55–60.

◆ 14 Winzelburg GG, Froelich J, McKusick KA, Strauss HW. Scintigraphic detection of gastrointestinal bleeding: review of current methods. *Am J Gastroenterol* 1983; **78**: 324–7.

15 Kester RR, Welch JP, Sziklas JP. The ⁹⁹ᵐTc labelled red cell scan: a diagnostic method for lower gastrointestinal bleeding. *Dis Colon Rectum* 1984; **27**: 47–52.

16 Gupta S, Luna E, Kingsley S, *et al.* Detection of gastro-intestinal bleeding by radionuclide scintigraphy. *Am J Gastroenterol* 1984; **9**: 26–31.

17 Szasz IJ, Morrison RT, Lystr DN. Technetium 99m-labelled red blood cell scintigraphy to diagnose occult gastrointestinal bleeding. *Can J Surg* 1985; **28**: 512–14.

18 Dusold R, Burke K, Carpentier W, Dyck WP. The accuracy of technetium-99m-labeled red cell scintigraphy in localizing gastrointestinal bleeding. *Am J Gastroenterol* 1995; **89**: 345–8.

19 Kouraklis G, Misiakos E, Karatzas G, *et al.* Diagnostic approach and management of active lower gastrointestinal hemorrhage. *Int Surg* 1995; **80**: 138–40.

20 Nicholson ML, Neoptolemos JP, Sharp JF, *et al.* Localization of lower gastrointestinal bleeding using in vivo technetium-99m-labelled red blood cell scintigraphy. *Br J Surg* 1989; **76**: 358–61.

21 Suzman MS, Talmor M, Jennis R, *et al.* Accurate localization and surgical management of active lower gastrointestinal hemorrhage with technetium-labeled erythrocyte scintigraphy. *Ann Surg* 1996; **224**: 29–36.

22 Rantis Jr PC, Harford FJ, Wagner RH, Henkin RE. Technetium-labelled red blood cell scintigraphy: is it useful in acute lower gastrointestinal bleeding? *Int J Colorectal Dis* 1995; **10**: 210–15.

23 Sommer A, Wetzel E, Loose R, *et al.* The role of colloid and labelled red blood cell scintigraphy in the investigation of acute or intermittent gastrointestinal bleeding. *Rofo Fortschr Geb Rontgenstr Neuen Blidgebenden Verfahren* 1996; **16**: 64–9.

24 Bunker SR, Lull RJ, Tenasescu DE, *et al.* Scintigraphy of gastrointestinal haemorrhage: superiority of ^{99m}Tc red blood cells over ^{99m}Tc sulfur colloid. *Am J Radiol* 1984; **143**: 543–8.

25 Siddiqui AR, Schauwecker DS, Wellman HN, Mock BH. Comparison of technetium 99m sulfur colloid and in vitro labelled technetium 99m RBCs in the detection of gastrointestinal bleeding. *Clin Nucl Med* 1985; **8**: 546–9.

26 Orechia PM, Hensley EK, Macdonald PT, Lull RJ. Localisation of lower gastrointestinal haemorrhage. *Arch Surg* 1985; **120**: 621–4.

27 Markisz JA, Front D, Royal HD, *et al.* An evaluation of ^{99m}Tc-labeled red blood cell scintigraphy for the detection and localization of gastrointestinal bleeding sites. *Gastroenterology* 1982; **83**: 394–8.

28 Winzelburg GG, McKusick KA, Froelich JW, *et al.* Detection of gastrointestinal bleeding with ^{99m}Tc labelled red blood cells. *Semin Nucl Med* 1982; **12**: 139–46.

29 Harden R, Mack G, Alexander WD, Kennedy I. Isotope uptake and scanning of stomach in man with ^{99m}Tc pertechnetate. *Lancet* 1967; **i**: 1305–7.

30 Jewett Jr TC, Duszynski DO, Allen JE. The visualisation of Meckel's diverticulum with ^{99m}Tc pertechnetate. *Surgery* 1970; **68**: 567–70.

31 Petrokubi RJ, Baum S, Rohrer GV. Cimetidine administration resulting in improved imaging of Meckel's diverticulum. *Clin Nucl Med* 1978; **3**: 385–8.

32 Conway JJ. Radionuclide diagnosis of Meckel's diverticulum. *Gastrointest Radiol* 1980; **5**: 209–13.

● 33 Sfakianakis GN, Conway JJ. Detection of ectopic gastric mucosa in Meckel's diverticulum and in other aberrations by scintigraphy. II: Indications and methods – a 10 year experience. *J Nucl Med* 1981; **22**: 732–8.

34 Kusumoto H, Yoshida M, Takahashi I, *et al.* Complications and diagnosis of Meckel's diverticulum in 776 patients. *Am J Surg* 1992; **164**: 382–3.

Inflammatory bowel disease

PHILIP J.A. ROBINSON

INTRODUCTION

The range of radiopharmaceuticals and techniques which have been used for scintigraphic investigation of inflammatory bowel disease is similar to that used in seeking evidence of infection or inflammation elsewhere in the body, which is discussed in Chapter 3. Initially promising results with labeled colloids, human immunoglobulin, dextran, porphyrins and polyethylene glycol-liposomes remain unconfirmed. The use of gallium-67 citrate has been overtaken by the development of labeled autologous leukocyte techniques. Technetium-labeled anti-granulocyte antibodies such as sulesomab have been tried, but so far results have been inferior to those obtainable with labeled leukocytes.[1,2] A novel approach involves the use of ^{99m}Tc-labeled interleukin-2, which is a cytokine that binds to receptors mainly expressed on activated T lymphocytes and monocytes. Initial studies suggest this agent may have a role in detecting areas of chronic inflammatory disease as well as areas of active inflammation.[3] Promising results have also been obtained in early studies using pentavalent (V) ^{99m}Tc-labeled DMSA,[4] and finally the possibility of identifying segments of inflamed bowel using ^{18}F-fluorodeoxyglucose and positron emission tomography has had some initial success.[5] Currently, however, clinical techniques center around the use of autologous leukocytes labeled with either ^{111}In or ^{99m}Tc using nonpolar lipophilic chelating agents which penetrate the cell membranes.

TECHNIQUES[6,7]

The chelating agents enter all blood cells, so the labeling procedure must be carried out *in vitro* using the leukocytes separated from 40–60 mL of whole blood. Difficulty will be encountered if the circulating granulocyte count is less than 2×10^9 cells per liter. The currently used chelating agents are tropolone for ^{111}In labeling and exametazime (hexamethylpropylene amine oxime, HMPAO) for ^{99m}Tc. After *in vitro* labeling, the cells are suspended in plasma and re-injected into the patient. Careful attention to technique and a quality assurance program are required to ensure a high labeling efficiency is achieved without damage to the leukocytes. Both ^{111}In and ^{99m}Tc chelates enter the cells readily, but once inside the cell their structure changes to become hydrophilic (^{99m}Tc) or bound to intracellular proteins (^{111}In) so the tracers remain trapped within the cells.

With ^{111}In (half-life 67.4 h, photopeaks at 171 and 247 keV, usual activity for adults 10–20 MBq) images are obtained at 1–3 h and 18–24 h after injection. With ^{99m}Tc (half-life 6 h, photopeak at 140 keV, usual activity 200 MBq) images are obtained at 30–60 min and at 2–4 h after injection. For most purposes, ^{99m}Tc-exametazime-labeled leukocytes are preferred because of their superior counting statistics, the lower radiation dose to the patient, more rapid results, and readier availability of the agent. There may still be a case for the use of ^{111}In chelates in patients with more chronic disease, and for those in whom ^{99m}Tc studies are inconclusive.

INTERPRETATION

The blood clearance of labeled white cells is fairly slow and early images show blood pool activity as well as uptake into the liver, bone marrow and particularly into the spleen. Abnormal bowel activity may become visible 30–60 min after injection and usually becomes more conspicuous on delayed images. With ^{99m}Tc-exametazime, hydrophilic secondary complexes may be excreted via the kidney or via the liver into the biliary tract and bowel lumen. Physiologic activity is often faintly visible in the bowel at 4 h after

[99m]Tc-exametazime injection, and occasionally the gall-bladder will be visualized. Normal bowel activity in children appears sooner. Early migration of tracer into the bowel is less marked with ^{111}In-labeled cells, but is often visible on 24-h images, probably due to the normal shedding of epithelial cells and leukocytes into the bowel lumen. Transient retention of labeled cells in the lung is seen on early images, but this normally clears within 3–4 h; persistent lung retention indicates diffuse pulmonary disease or possibly damage to the leukocytes during the labeling procedure.

Bowel uptake is seen not only in Crohn's disease and ulcerative colitis, but also in other inflammatory colitides, ischemia, and infection. The distribution and intensity of abnormal activity indicates the extent and severity of inflammation. The localization of diseased bowel segments is easier if correlation can be made with previous barium studies, plain abdominal radiographs or computed tomography, particularly in patients who have undergone previous bowel resection. Positive results are more likely in patients with an elevated circulating leukocyte count, and false negatives may occur in patients who are immunosuppressed, or undergoing steroid therapy. Focal activity which appears to be outside the lumen of the bowel may indicate abscess formation, but could also be the result of infections outside the gastrointestinal tract, or inflammation associated with tumors or hematomas.

APPLICATIONS AND RESULTS

Diagnosis of inflammatory bowel disease

In detecting the presence and extent of inflammatory changes in the large bowel, the 'gold standard' method is colonoscopy with biopsy and histology. Early studies with ^{111}In-labeled leukocytes showed very good correlation with colonoscopy and histology, and equivalent results have been obtained using ^{99m}Tc-exametazime-labeled cells.[8–11] In the detection of early disease, ^{99m}Tc-leukocyte scintigraphy has been shown to be at least as sensitive as colonoscopy and barium studies in both Crohn's colitis[12] and ulcerative colitis (UC)[13] (Figs 14B.1 and 14B.2). Because the technique is noninvasive and relatively simple for the patients, it may be preferable as the initial imaging procedure, particularly in children.[14,15] However, in the chronic stages of disease the scintigraphic methods are less helpful and may be negative during periods of quiescence. Whilst both ^{111}In and ^{99m}Tc techniques provide equivalent results in large bowel disease,

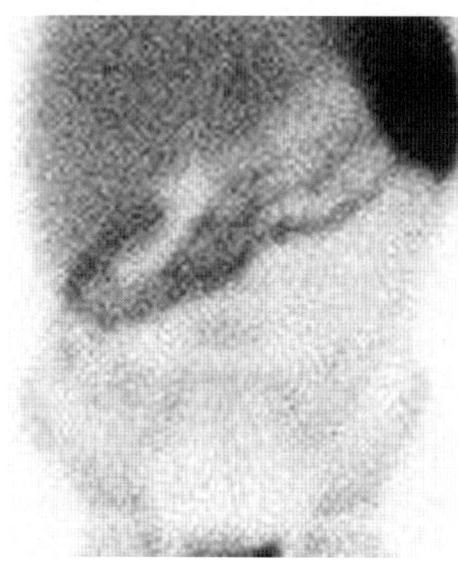

Figure 14B.1   *Diffuse involvement of the transverse and descending colon shown on ^{99m}Tc-leukocyte scintigraphy.*

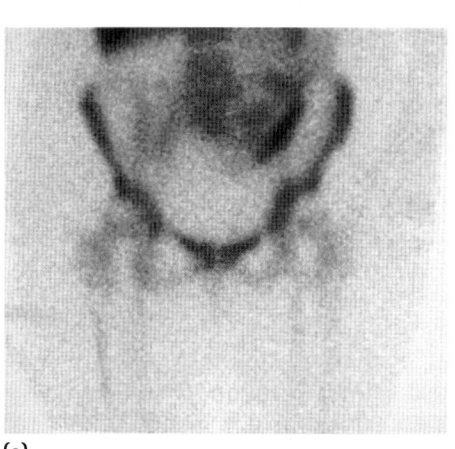

(a)

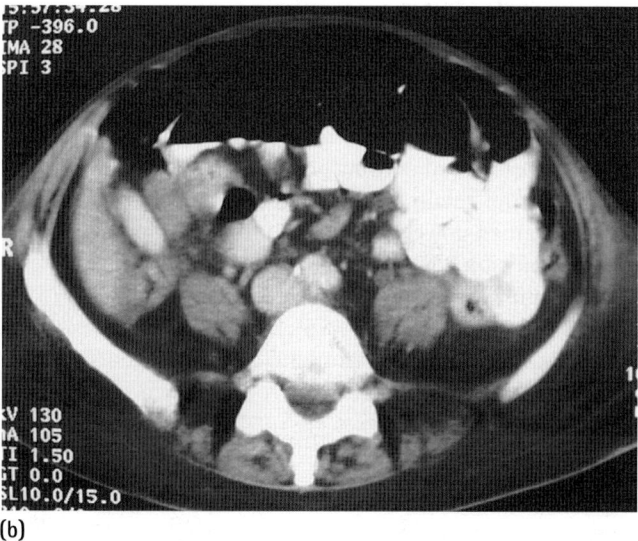

(b)

Figure 14B.2   *Abnormality localized to the descending colon shown on ^{99m}Tc-leukocyte scintigraphy in a 53-year-old female patient (a); subsequent computed tomography scan (b) showed thickening of the descending colon.*

small bowel involvement in Crohn's disease is best shown by ^{99m}Tc imaging, whereas ^{111}In studies have been disappointing.[16–18]

Severity of disease

Quantitative assessment of the uptake of labeled leukocytes in affected areas of the bowel has been shown to correlate well with clinical and histological indicators of disease severity in ulcerative colitis in adults,[19] but not in children.[20] In Crohn's disease, ^{99m}Tc-leukocyte scintigraphy correlates fairly well with clinical activity of disease and with biological markers in both children[20] and adults.[21] Quantitative analysis with SPECT may further improve the correlation of scintigraphy with other indices of disease activity.[22] During active episodes of inflammatory bowel disease, leukocytes are shed into the bowel lumen, and good correlation with disease severity has been achieved by measuring the activity of ^{111}In in a 4-day stool collection.[23]

Differential diagnosis

The distribution of abnormality on the labeled leukocyte image may make a valuable contribution to the differentiation of ulcerative colitis and Crohn's disease.[24–26] Although there is overlap in some cases, the distal colon and rectum are almost invariably involved in UC. In Crohn's disease the rectum is often spared, skip lesions may be seen, the disease is often predominantly right-sided, peri-anal sepsis may be a feature and the small bowel is often involved (Figs 14B.3 and 14B.4).

Follow-up and complications

Once the diagnosis has been made, leukocyte scintigraphy offers a fairly simple and noninvasive approach for monitoring the progress of disease and in particular for assessing the effects of therapy in both Crohn's disease and UC, although long term UC patients will still need colonoscopy to screen for malignant change. Patients with the surgical complications of

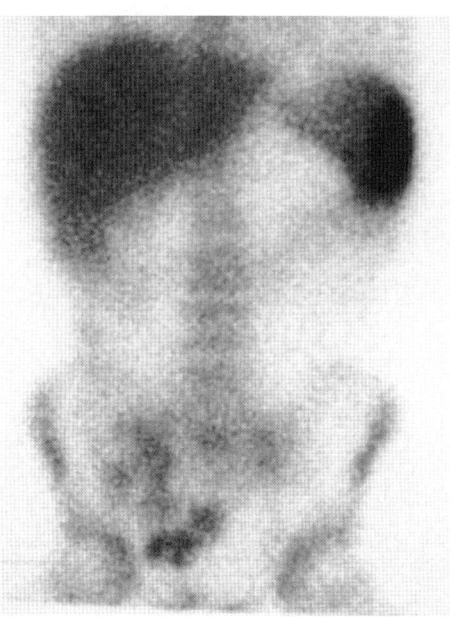

(a)

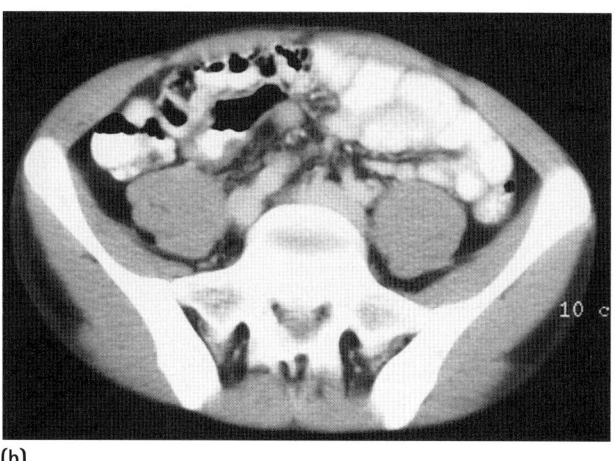

(b)

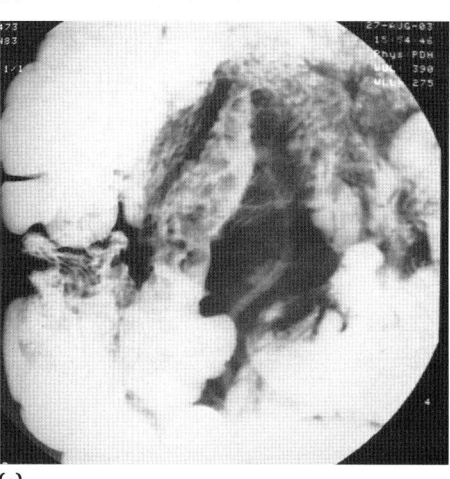

(c)

Figure 14B.3 *Distal ileal abnormality shown on ^{99m}Tc-leukocyte scintigraphy (a) in a 16-year-old boy with abdominal pain and anemia; subsequent computed tomography (b) and small bowel barium study (c) showed typical changes of Crohn's disease.*

inflammatory bowel disease (strictures, abscesses, and fistulae) will usually require anatomic imaging with contrast studies or computed tomography, but scintigraphy can often make an important contribution in these cases. With small-bowel strictures, evidence of active disease on ^{99m}Tc-leukocyte studies suggests the acute problem may be reversible with medical treatment. If there is no increased activity on scintigraphy, strictures are probably fibrotic and more likely to need surgical intervention. Scintigraphy may also be helpful in differentiating between infected collections or abscesses, and pockets of sterile fluid or isolated dilated bowel loops which may be confusing on sonography or computed tomography.

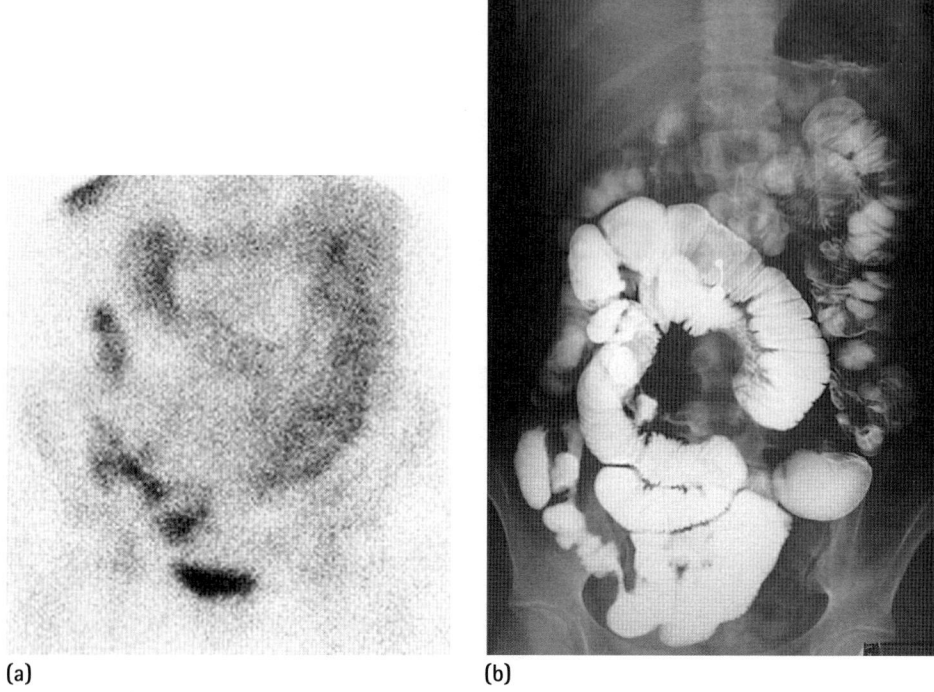

(a)   (b)

Figure 14B.4   *Multiple small bowel lesions shown on ^{99m}Tc-leukocyte scintigraphy (a) in a 16-year-old girl; subsequent small bowel barium study showed Crohn's disease with skip lesions (b).*

Case report 1

A 52-year-old patient had symptoms suggestive of inflammatory bowel disease, but normal clinical and biochemical findings. Colonoscopy was normal, but white cell scintigraphy (Fig. 14B.5) showed distal ileal abnormality. In spite of medical therapy, more severe symptoms ensued and subsequent CT and small bowel barium studies showed chronic changes of Crohn's disease.

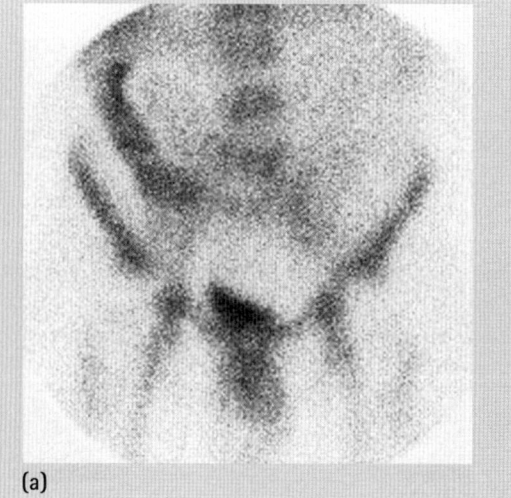

Figure 14B.5   *^{99m}Tc-leukocyte scintigraphy in a 52-year-old man showing localized disease in the right iliac fossa (a);*

(a)

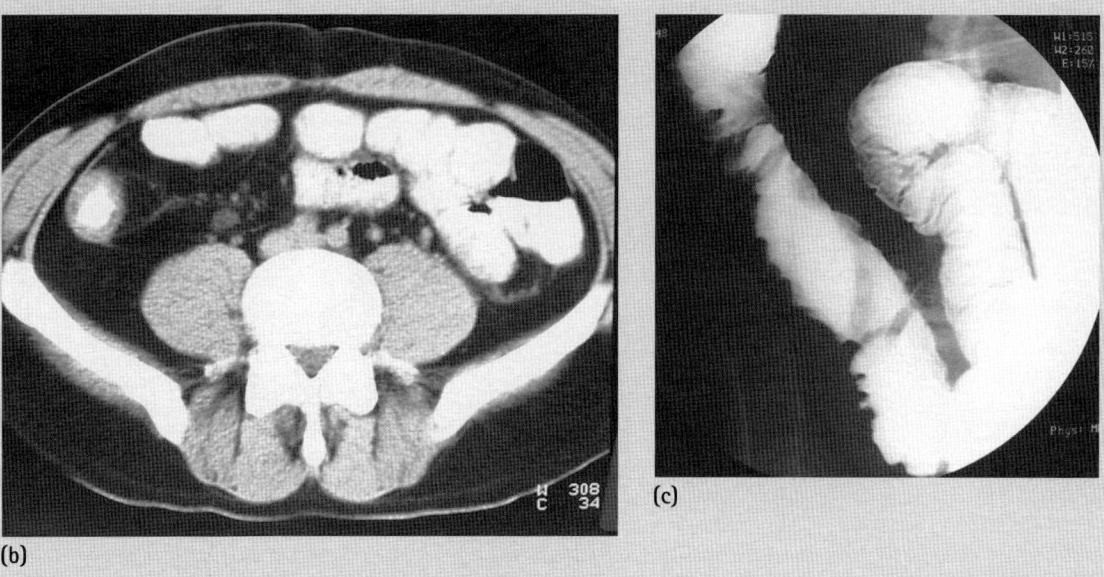

(b)

(c)

Figure 14B.5 *(Continued)*   *a computed tomography scan carried out 3 years after initial presentation showed localized thickening of the bowel wall in the affected area (b) and subsequent small bowel barium study showed typical Crohn's changes affecting the mesenteric border of the terminal ileum (c).*

Case report 2

A 19-year-old girl presented with abdominal pain, weight loss and low grade pyrexia. Leukocyte scintigraphy showed extensive abnormality suggesting widespread Crohn's disease of the small bowel and ascending colon (Fig. 14B.6). The patient responded well to medical therapy but re-presented 4 years later with a severe exacerbation of symptoms and an ill-defined pelvic mass on clinical examination. Computed tomography revealed a small pelvic abscess involving several loops of small and large bowel.

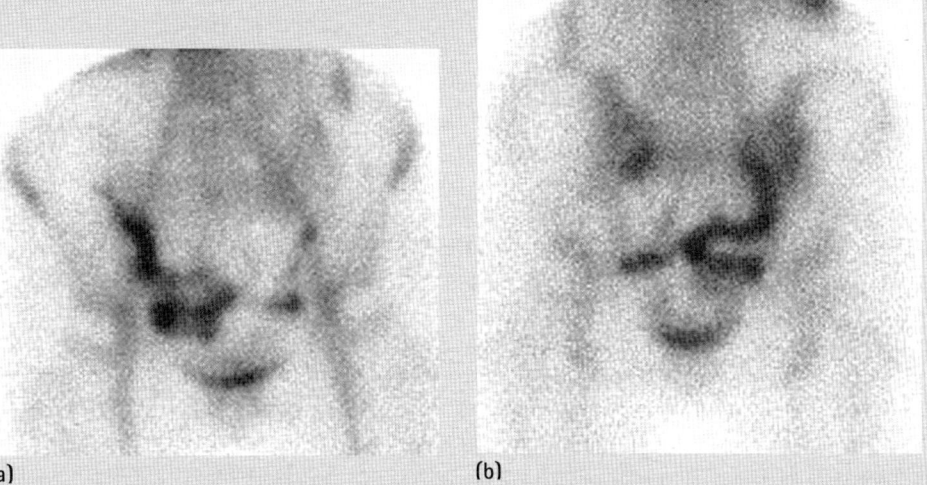

(a)

(b)

Figure 14B.6   *Anterior (a) and postenior (b) images from ^{99m}Tc–leukocyte scintigraphy showed disease in small bowel and ascending colon (a, b). Subsequent small bowel barium study showed typical changes of Crohn's disease in distal ileum and cecum*

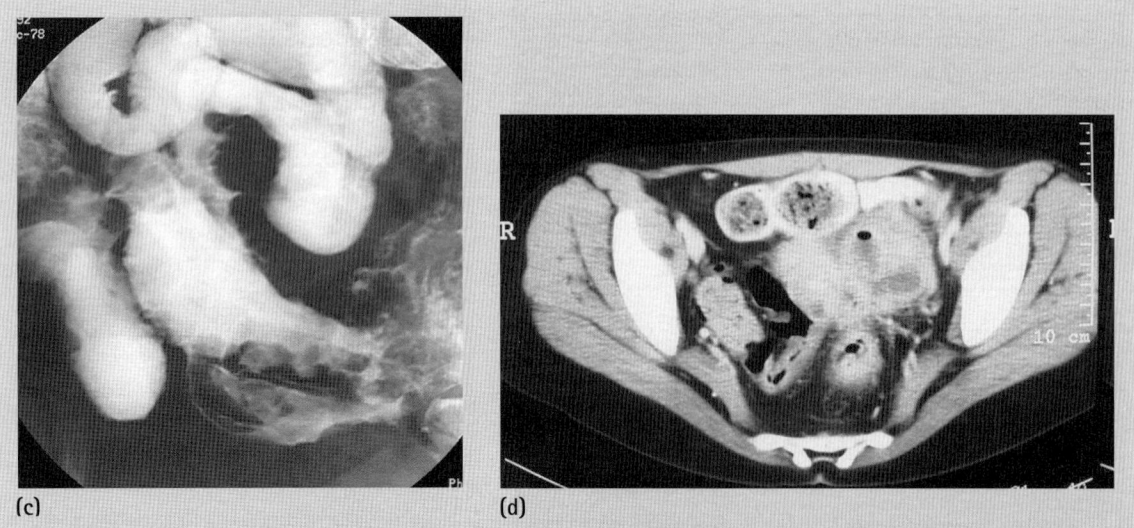

(c) (d)

Figure 14B.6 *(Continued)* *(c); later computed tomography showed a small pelvic abscess associated with thickened loops of both small and large bowel (d).*

REFERENCES

● Seminal primary article
◆ Key review paper
★ First formal publication of a management guideline

1 Stokkel MPM, Reigman HIE, Pauwels EKJ. Scintigraphic head-to-head comparison between ^{99m}Tc-WBCs and ^{99m}Tc-Leukoscan in the evaluation of inflammatory bowel disease: a pilot study. *Eur J Nucl Med* 2002; **29**: 251–4.

2 Charron M, Di Lorenzo C, Kocoshis SA, *et al.* (99m)Tc antigranulocyte monoclonal antibody imaging for the detection and assessment of inflammatory bowel disease newly diagnosed by colonoscopy in children. *Pediatr Radiol* 2001; **31**: 796–800.

3 Annovazzi A, Biancone L, Caviglia R, *et al.* ^{99m}Tc-interleukin-2 and ^{99m}Tc-HMPAO granulocyte scintigraphy in patients with inactive Crohn's disease. *Eur J Nucl Med* 2003; **30**: 374–382.

4 Koutroubakis IE, Koukouraki SI, Dimoulios PD, *et al.* Active inflammatory bowel disease: evaluation with ^{99m}Tc(V) DMSA scintigraphy. *Radiology* 2003; **229**: 70–4.

5 Mernagh JR, Thompson M, Jacobson, *et al.* Assessment of inflammation in inflammatory bowel disease with PET. 1998 Scientific Assembly and Annual Meeting of the Radiological Society of North America. *Radiology* 1998; **209(suppl)**: 172.

★ 6 Palestro CJ, Brown ML, Forstrom LA, *et al. Procedure guideline for 111 In-leukocyte scintigraphy for suspected infection/inflammation.* Society of Nuclear Medicine, Reston, Virginia. Published online, 2004.

★ 7 Palestro CJ, Brown ML, Forstrom LA, *et al. Procedure guideline for ^{99m}Tc-exametazime (HMPAO) – labelled leukocyte scintigraphy for suspected infection/inflammation.* Society of Nuclear Medicine, Reston, Virginia. Published online, 2004.

● 8 Saverymuttu S, Camilleri M, Rees H, *et al.* Indium-111 granulocyte scanning in the assessment of disease extent and disease activity in inflammatory bowel disease. A comparison with colonoscopy, histology, and faecal indium-111 granulocyte excretion. *Gastroenterology* 1986; **90**: 1121–8.

● 9 Becker W, Schomann E, Fischbach W, *et al.* Comparison of ^{99m}Tc-HMPAO and ^{111}In-oxine labelled granulocytes in man: first clinical results. *Nucl Med Commun* 1988; **9**: 435–47.

10 Middleton SJ, Li D, Wharton S, *et al.* Validation of ^{99m}Tc-HMPAO leucocyte scintigraphy in ulcerative colitis by comparison with histology. *Br J Radiol* 1995; **68**: 1061–6.

11 Lantto EH, Lantto TJ, Vorne M. Fast diagnosis of abdominal infections and inflammations with technetium-99m-HMPAO labelled leukocytes. *J Nucl Med* 1991; **32**: 2029–34.

12 Molnar T, Papos M, Gyulai C, *et al.* Clinical value of technetium-99m-HMPAO-labelled leukocyte scintigraphy and spiral computed tomography in active Crohn's disease. *Am J Gastroenterol* 2001; **96**: 1517–21.

13 Bennink R, Peeters M, D'Haens, *et al.* Tc-99m HMPAO white blood cell scintigraphy in the assessment of the extent and severity of an acute exacerbation of ulcerative colitis. *Clin Nucl Med* 2001; **26**: 99–104.

14 Jewell FM, Davies A, Sandhu B, *et al.* Technetium-99m-HMPAO labelled leucocytes in the detection

and monitoring of inflammatory bowel disease in children. *Br J Radiol* 1996; **69**: 508–14.

◆ 15 Charron M, del Rosario FJ, Kocoshis S. Pediatric inflammatory bowel disease: assessment with scintigraphy with ^{99m}Tc white blood cells. *Radiology* 1999; **212**: 507–13.

16 Park RH, McKillop JH, Duncan A, *et al.* Can 111-indium autologous mixed leucocyte scanning accurately assess disease extent and activity in Crohn's disease? *Gut* 1998; **29**: 821–5.

● 17 Saverymuttu SH, Peters M, Hodgson JH, *et al.* 111-Indium leukocyte scanning in small bowel Crohn's disease. *Gastrointest Radiol* 1983; **8**: 157–61.

18 Crama-Bohbouth GI, Arndt JW, Pena AS, *et al.* Value of indium-111 granulocyte scintigraphy in the assessment of Crohn's disease of the small intestine: prospective investigation. *Digestion* 1988; **40**: 227–36.

19 Lantto E, Jarvi K, Krekela I, *et al.* Technetium-99m hexamethylpropylene amine oxine leucocytes in the assessment of disease activity in inflammatory bowel disease. *Eur J Nucl Med* 1992; **19**: 14–18.

● 20 Charron M. Inflammatory bowel disease activity assessment with biological markers and ^{99m}Tc-WBC scintigraphy: are there different trends in ileitis versus colitis? *J Nucl Med* 2003; **44**: 1586–91.

21 Spinelli F, Milella M, Sara R, *et al.* The Tc-99m HMPAO leukocyte scan: an alternative to radiology and endoscopy in evaluating the extent and the activity of inflammatory bowel disease. *J Nucl Biol Med* 1991; **35**: 82–7.

22 Weldon MJ, Masoomi AM, Britten AJ, *et al.* Quantification of inflammatory bowel disease activity using technetium-99m HMPAO labelled leukocyte single photon emission computerised tomography (SPECT). *Gut* 1995; **36**: 243–50.

23 Saverymuttu SH, Peters AM, Crofton ME, *et al.* 111-Indium autologous granulocytes in the detection of inflammatory bowel disease. *Gut* 1985; **26**: 955–960.

24 Saverymuttu SH, Chadwick VS, Joseph AE, *et al.* Distinction between Crohn's colitis and ulcerative colitis by 111-indium granulocyte scanning. *Gut* 1988; **29**: A707.

25 Weldon M, Joseph A, Maxwell J. Technetium (Tc^{99m}) HMPAO white cell scanning can distinguish between Crohn's and ulcerative colitis. *Gut* 1992; **33**: S67.

26 Charron M, del Rosario JF, Kocoshis S. Use of technetium-tagged white blood cells in patients with Crohn's disease and ulcerative colitis: is differential diagnosis possible? *Pediatr Radiol* 1998; **28**: 871–7.

Functional studies of the gastrointestinal tract

ALP NOTGHI

INTRODUCTION

The gastrointestinal (GI) tract is a complex organ which stretches from mouth to anus and is primarily involved in the breakdown of food and absorption of nutrients. Food is broken down initially into small particles during its transit and then by different enzymes and chemicals into absorbable particles, and finally the waste material is excreted. The proper function of the GI tract depends on synchronized action of not only the GI tract but also other organs such as the salivary glands, liver, and pancreas. Nuclear medicine is well suited to the investigation of the GI tract as it allows quantitative and semiquantitative measurement of various functions. In the first part of this chapter imaging investigations that give a semiquantitative measure of transit of the contents through the GI tract are described. In the second part, the nonimaging nuclear investigations that look at different aspects of GI function such as bile reabsorption, terminal ileum malabsorption, bacterial overgrowth, and GI blood loss are explored.

GASTROINTESTINAL TRANSIT

The GI tract comprises several functional segments. Transit through each of these segments is regulated to allow for digestion and absorption of food. Hormones, the nervous system, and luminal content regulate coordinated movements of smooth muscle and sphincters. Disease processes may disturb this function. Endoscopy and radiographic examinations give detailed anatomical information and are crucial for detecting anatomical lesions. Nuclear medicine on the other hand gives functional information that can elicit physiological

or functional abnormalities of the GI tract. In this section the more common nuclear medicine tests for measuring transit through the GI tract are described.

Esophageal transit

The esophagus is approximately 25 cm long, connecting pharynx to stomach. Its function, primarily, is the transit of food. In some animals transit depends entirely on gravity, but in most animals, including human beings, peristaltic movement of the esophageal smooth muscle propels food into the stomach. There is some gravity dependence, however. Thus it is crucial to perform the test consistently in either supine, sitting or semirecumbent positions. Different meals have been used. Semisolid meals are more likely to show transit abnormalities than liquid meals. For liquid esophageal transit 40 MBq of ^{99m}Tc-colloid is mixed with 30 mL of water. The patient is asked to hold 10 mL of the prepared liquid and swallow after start of the data acquisition (100 frames, each of 1 s). For semisolid transit measurements 40 MBq of ^{99m}Tc-colloid cooked in scrambled egg (an egg and a spoonful of milk) can be used to produce three dessert spoonfuls of radiolabeled egg. The patient is then asked to swallow one spoonful at a time and a dynamic acquisition is performed. Three consecutive studies are performed for consistency. Markers either side of the sternum are used (outside the esophageal region of interest) for movement correction if required. The field of view must include the region from the mouth to stomach. Traditionally, three regions of interest are drawn around the esophagus (upper, middle, and lower third of the esophagus). Three dynamic curves are generated, representing the transit of activity through each region (Fig. 14C.1). Normal transit

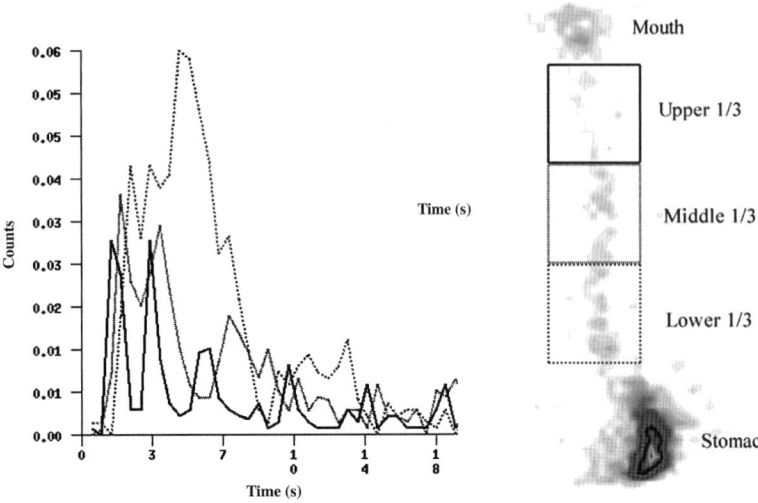

Figure 14C.1 *Time–activity curves for three regions of the esophagus. Transit through the oesophagus is normally less than 12 s.*

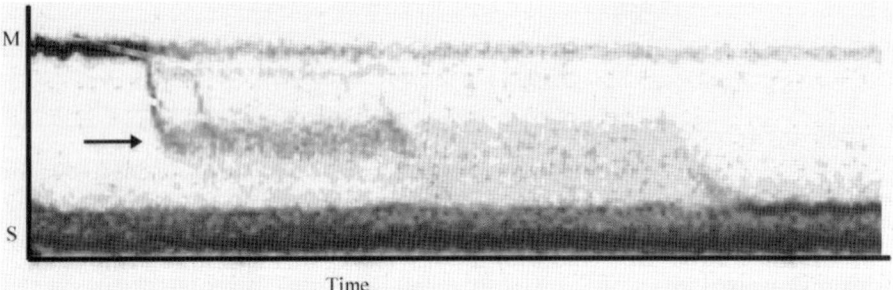

Figure 14C.2 *Condensed images of esophageal transit in a patient with hold-up in the mid esophagus. M = mouth, S = stomach and the arrow shows the area of hold-up.*

for the esophagus is less than 12 s (2, 4, and 6 s for upper, middle, and lower thirds, respectively, for a semisolid meal). An alternative approach is to create a condensed image from the dynamic sequence. For each frame the esophageal counts for each row of pixels between the mouth and stomach are summed to form a single column of pixels. These columns are then placed in time sequence order to create a condensed image. On this image the *y* axis represents the esophagus from mouth to stomach and the *x* axis represents time (Fig. 14C.2). Condensed images are easier to interpret and different patterns of transit can be recognized for different conditions. Hold-up in the esophagus, achalasia, reflux, and esophageal spasm can be readily recognized using this technique. Condensed images are also used to assess progression of disease or response to treatment.

Gastric emptying studies

The stomach is composed of two main parts, antrum and pylorus. However, in practice transit is measured through both parts simultaneously. Food is mixed in the stomach and broken down by acid and enzymes. Delayed gastric emptying may lead to a feeling of indigestion and fullness. Gastric emptying is influenced by the consistency of the food (liquid, solid), content of the food (caloric content, fat content, presence of spices) and gravity (whether the patient is supine or standing). The causes of delayed gastric emptying include diabetic neuropathy, surgery, and drugs.

The first recorded study of gastric emptying dates back to Roman times. An emperor measured the effect of exercise on gastric emptying by feeding two slaves. One slave was forced to exercise while the other rested. The slaves were then beheaded and the stomach contents examined. The emperor concluded that rest after a meal facilitates gastric emptying.[1] Nuclear medicine provides a noninvasive method of measuring gastric emptying; both liquid and solid meals can be used. Liquid meals have a very fast emptying time and have limited use, mainly for assessment of post-surgical dumping syndrome. A variety of solid meals are used. The most commonly used meals are egg-based recipes, including pancakes. The meal should be simple to prepare and have a good labeling efficiency so that the activity is not released into the gastric juices causing bi-phasic (liquid and solid) emptying curves. It is important to have a consistent meal and determine a normal range for the meal used, as the caloric, fat and protein content, volume and physical properties of the meal affect gastric emptying. For solid meal gastric emptying, a meal labeled with up to 12 MBq ^{99m}Tc-diethylenetriaminepentaacetic acid (^{99m}Tc-DTPA) is prepared, usually weighing approximately 300 g. The patient is asked to consume the food within 5 min and is imaged standing or sitting. Consecutive 120-s anterior and posterior images are acquired for the first 40 min so that a geometric mean of gastric activity can be obtained. If required, additional 120-s images are acquired every 10 min at least until the time to half emptying ($t_{1/2}$) is

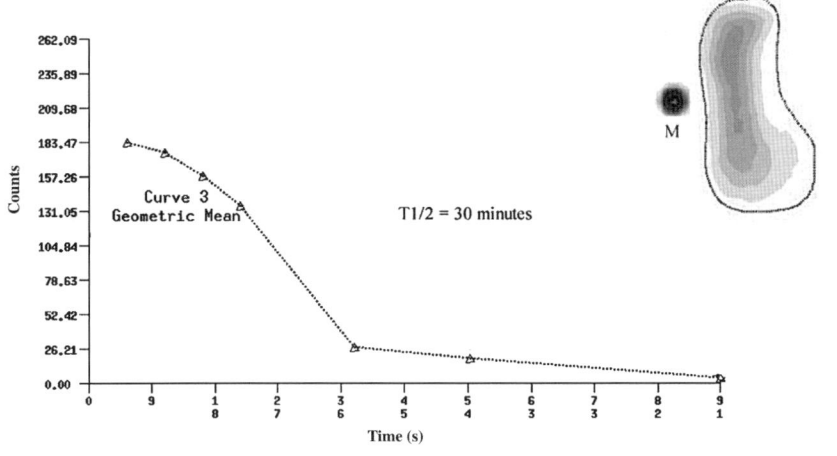

Figure 14C.3 *Normal gastric emptying. Markers (M) are used to align the images. The half-life (T½) is calculated from the geometric mean time–activity curve.*

reached. Two radioactive skin markers should be used for positioning of the patient and movement correction of the data. Solid gastric emptying is usually expressed in $t_½$ (Fig. 14C.3). Normal $t_½$ varies according to the meal used (30 min for pancake, up to 80 min for a meal of mince and potato). In children where milk is used, the milk curdles and the result is a combination of liquid and solid phase emptying. Therefore the result is expressed as a percentage of retained activity at 60 min (normal 65% at the age of 3 months to 50% at the age of 5 years).[2]

Small-bowel transit

The small bowel is a complex organ. Food, which is predominantly in liquid form in the small bowel, is further broken down by bile and pancreatic juices during its slow passage through the small bowel. Products are then transferred or absorbed through the lumen into the lymphatic system and blood and enter the portal circulation. The small bowel is a long organ (over 3.5 m in adults) and together with the surface folding and intestinal villi, provides a large surface for the absorption of digested materials. The passage of food through the small bowel usually takes about 4 h. It is then temporarily stored in the terminal ileum before release into the cecum and large bowel. Absorption occurs throughout the small bowel but certain chemicals are absorbed at different sites. Iron, minerals, vitamins, and fat are predominantly absorbed in the proximal small bowel, amino acids in the jejunum, and B_{12} and bile acids are absorbed exclusively at the terminal ileum (last 100 cm of the small bowel). Motility of the intestine and the individual movement of the intestinal villi regulate transit of food. Accelerated transit of a meal may lead to malabsorption, which in turn may result in bacterial overgrowth or delivery of irritant material to the large bowel. There is growing evidence that movement disorders of the gut affect the gut in its entirety (stomach, small, and large bowel). Small-bowel

transit can conveniently be measured together with a standard gastric emptying study. Following solid meal gastric emptying, hourly 120-s anterior and posterior images are obtained until the activity is clearly visible in the cecum, identifiable by its distinct shape and position. Small-bowel transit time is defined as the time it takes from 10% gastric emptying to 10% cecal filling or the time when the cecum is first visualized. The median for normal small-bowel transit is 190 min ranging from 45 to 350 min in adults. More than 6 h is clearly abnormal. It is also possible to detect specific sites of hold-up in the small bowel, that may be useful in conditions such as Crohn's disease. However, due to lack of anatomical markers it is often difficult to pinpoint the exact location within the bowel.

Large-bowel transit

The large bowel acts both as a reservoir for waste products as well as a major site of absorption of water and electrolytes. One to two liters of semiliquid material is delivered to the colon from the small bowel every day. The colon is capable of absorbing up to 8 L of fluid a day and absorbs over 90% of the delivered semiliquid material in the ascending and transverse colon. Large-bowel disorders account for one of the most common ailments, often presenting with constipation and bloating. These disorders can be so severe that surgical resection of part of the colon may be contemplated. It is imperative that constipation and lack of normal bowel movement is verified before such surgery. There are several methods for estimating colonic transit, radiographic techniques being the most popular. However, nuclear medicine techniques are the most physiological and quantifiable. Due to slow colonic transit, a radionuclide with a long (in radiopharmaceutical terms) half-life is used. Indium-111 is well suited for this test as it has a half-life of 2.7 days and its higher energy gamma rays are less affected by the depth of the activity in the abdomen. A dose of 7–10 MBq is

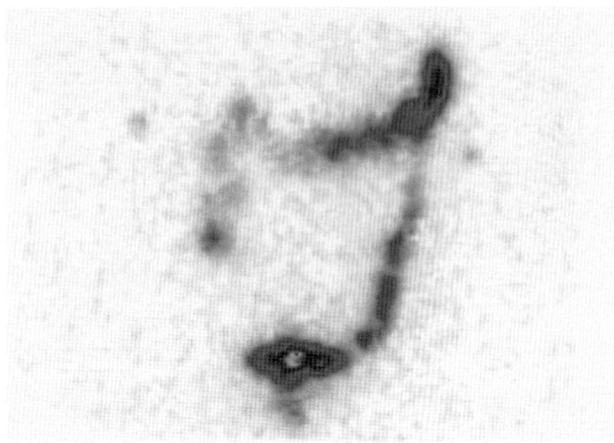

Figure 14C.4   *Raw image of colonic transit at 25 h after ingestion of the activity.*

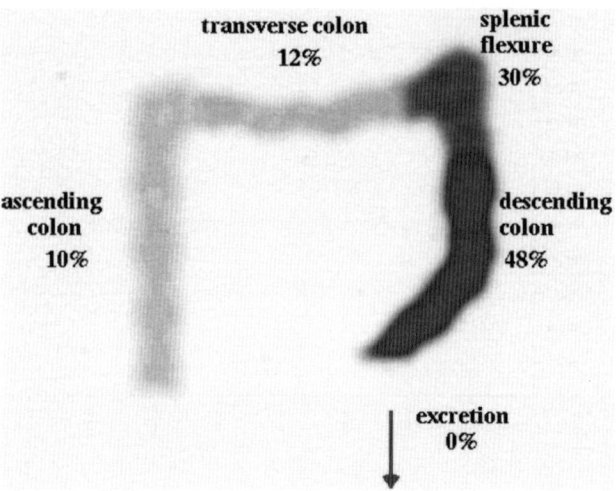

Figure 14C.5   *Percentage of baseline administered activity is calculated for each region of the colon in a patient 25 h after the ingestion of capsule. The lost activity compared to baseline would represent fecal excretion. This patient had no activity excreted by this time.*

sufficient for a study lasting up to a week. The activity can be given in liquid form. Gastric emptying is rapid and the activity is more or less delivered as a bolus into the small bowel. The activity can also be given in the form of labeled resin in an enteric-coated capsule. This ensures bolus delivery of the activity in the small bowel. If this is followed through, the activity normally accumulates in the terminal ileum and then empties into the cecum as a bolus. The activity is by then well mixed with the meal in the small bowel. At later stages it may spread throughout the colon and is eventually emptied. For practical purposes there is no need to acquire more than one image a day for up to 6 days. It is crucial to use radiolabeled markers (positioned lateral to the anterior iliac crests) so that the images can be positioned relative to each other for analysis. A set of anterior and posterior supine abdominal images are acquired at the end of day 1 ($\approx$8 h) and for the following 3 days (Fig. 14C.4). If the activity persists then further images may be acquired. The total decay-corrected geometric mean count for each image is calculated and the percentage excretion calculated by comparing it to the first set of images (100% activity). In the normal subject most of the activity is excreted by the third day. By drawing regions of interest in the colon (ascending colon and hepatic flexure, transverse colon, splenic flexure, descending colon, and rectum) and calculating the decay-corrected geometric mean counts for each time point, it is possible to calculate the transit through segments of the colon (Fig. 14C.5).[3] Colonic delay could be generalized, right sided or left sided. In a left-sided delay the transit through the colon is normal, but the patient cannot excrete activity for several days. This may denote a pelvic floor problem.

Defecography

Radionuclide defecography is a complementary test to X-ray proctography, providing quantitative information

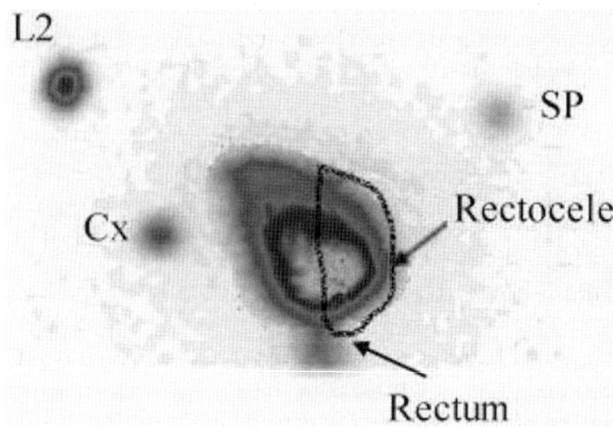

Figure 14C.6   *Radionuclide defecography shows a large rectocele. A region of interest around the rectocele is drawn to calculate the time–activity curve for the rectocele. Size and emptying of the rectocele can be assessed. Three markers on L2, coccyx (Cx) and symphysis pubis (SP) are used for movement correction.*

about rectal function. It is often requested in patients with difficulty in rectal evacuation and in patients with rectoceles before surgery is contemplated. The camera room has to be set up to provide patient privacy. A commode is positioned in front of the gamma camera, preferably with the patient's left side against the camera. A dose of 100 MBq of ^{99m}Tc-DTPA is mixed in 150 mL of porridge and made to the consistency of soft stool. Three radiolabeled markers are positioned at L2, the tip of the sacrum and the pubic bone. The 'meal' is introduced into the rectum via a rectal catheter. The patient is then positioned in front of the camera. A dynamic acquisition of 5 s per frame is commenced. After 30 s the patient is asked to evacuate the rectum. The acquisition is continued until the patient has either evacuated

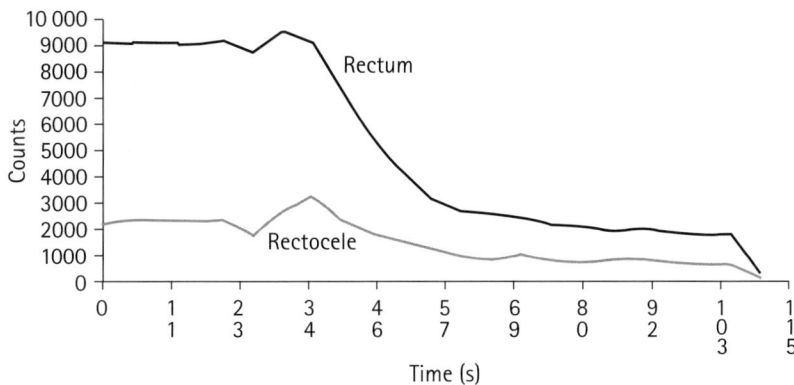

Figure 14C.7 *Time–activity curve shows normal rectal emptying with minimal retention in the rectocele.*

or is unable to evacuate any further. The anal canal is identified in the summed view. Any activity anterior to the canal is due to a rectocele (Fig. 14C.6). A region of interest is drawn around the rectum and one around the rectocele, if present. The percentage of rectal evacuation and rectocele emptying can be measured (Fig. 14C.7).[4] Normal rectal evacuation is more than 70%. Retention in the rectocele (poor rectocele evacuation) is abnormal. Various other parameters such as recto-anal angle and pelvic floor descent can be calculated.

MALABSORPTION TESTS

Bile acid malabsorption

Bile acids are excreted by the liver and released into the gut to assist in digestion of food. Most of the conjugated bile acids entering the small bowel are reabsorbed at the terminal ileum. Ninety-five percent of the bile acid secreted by the liver comes from the reabsorbed bile acids (enterohepatic circulation). Bile acid malabsorption may occur secondary to terminal ileal disease. 23-[^{75}Se]Seleno-25-homotaurocholic acid (SeHCAT) is a conjugated bile acid which is given orally. This is then absorbed in the terminal ileum and enters the enterohepatic circulation. Bile acids circulate through the enterohepatic circulation about five times a day. Normally, approximately 5% is lost per circulation. After 1 week (35 circulations) around 15–20% of the administered 23-seleno-25-homotaurocholic acid should still be in the circulation. This is the basis for the terminal ileal malabsorption test using SeHCAT. A whole-body count is obtained (either using an uncollimated gamma camera or whole-body counter) 5–10 min following administration of the capsule containing SeHCAT. The patient is then sent home and returns a week later and another whole-body count obtained under identical conditions. If the remaining activity is below 10% of the original count, severe terminal ileal malabsorption is indicated. More than 15% retention is normal. A value in between is indeterminate and may signify mild terminal ileal malabsorption.

Vitamin B$_{12}$ malabsorption

Vitamin B$_{12}$ cannot be synthesized in the human body. The main dietary source of this vitamin is animal products (meat and dairy food). In the stomach during digestion, B$_{12}$ is released and immediately bound to gastric R binder (a glycoprotein). This complex is then digested in the duodenum. The released B$_{12}$ is then bound to intrinsic factor (IF). Intrinsic factor is produced by parietal cells in the stomach together with hydrochloric acid. The B$_{12}$-IF complex is resistant to proteolytic digestion and thus travels to the distal ileum. There are specific IF receptors in the terminal ileum which bind B$_{12}$-IF complex and then B$_{12}$ is transported into the blood to be carried in the blood stream by binding to transport protein (transcobalamine II). B$_{12}$ malabsorption can occur as a result of IF deficiency or terminal ileal malabsorption. The Schilling test is used to diagnose B$_{12}$ malabsorption or IF deficiency. The most common cause of B$_{12}$ deficiency in temperate climates is pernicious anemia which is due to IF deficiency secondary to gastric atrophy. Clinical manifestations are those of megaloblastic anemia, GI problems (sore tongue, diarrhea) and in severe cases neurological manifestations (secondary to demyelination and axonal degeneration).

For a Schilling test, the patient is prepared by an intramuscular injection of 1000 μg of nonradiolabeled B$_{12}$. This saturates B$_{12}$ storage sites in the body so that any subsequently absorbed B$_{12}$ is excreted in the urine. Within 2 h of the nonradiolabeled B$_{12}$ injection the patient is administered a capsule containing 18.5 kBq ^{57}Co-B$_{12}$. This would normally be absorbed and mostly excreted in the urine. A 24-h urine collection is then commenced. Normally 14% or more of the administered activity should be excreted in the 24-h urine collection. In the presence of intrinsic factor deficiency or terminal ileal malabsorption, less than 14% of the radiolabeled B$_{12}$ will be excreted. Then a week later, part two of the Schilling test is performed. The patient returns and following 1000 μg i.m. B$_{12}$ injection, the test is repeated using a capsule containing 18.5 kBq ^{57}Co-B$_{12}$+IF. The recovered B$_{12}$ in 24-h urine collection should be 14% or more if the malabsorption in the first part was due to IF deficiency (pernicious anemia). However, the recovered radiolabeled B_{12} will be below 14% if it is due to terminal ileal malabsorption.

BREATH TESTS

Helicobacter pylori infection

Helicobacter pylori is a bacterium which infects the stomach and it has been associated with active chronic gastritis, gastric ulcers, and increased risk of gastric carcinoma. In Western countries 30% of the adult population is infected (50% in the over-60 age group) and this is more common in Third World countries. Infection is thought to be transmitted via the oro-fecal route. The individual can carry the infection indefinitely unless treated so it is important to diagnose and treat this infection. When a patient first presents with upper GI symptoms, endoscopy is usually the first investigation to be performed. It can be used to diagnose gastritis, active ulcers, and malignant growth. During endoscopy multiple biopsy samples are obtained. There are several methods of identifying the organism in the biopsy sample. Histological examination, cytological analysis, and culture may confirm *H. pylori* infection. Rapid urease testing (CLO test) on a sample would indicate bacterial presence. As sampling may miss the infected areas the biopsy may be negative even in the presence of *H. pylori* infection. Serological assay (anti-*H. pylori* IgG) would be positive if a patient had an infection, but may remain positive after treatment. Antigens in the feces have also been measured. A urea breath test using labeled urea is often the preferred test as the ingested urea is spread over the entire stomach and is not prone to sampling errors. The *H. pylori* bacterium breaks down urea into bicarbonate and ammonium ion. The ammonium ion neutralizes stomach acid forming a neutralized zone around the bacterium. The urea breath test (as well as the CLO test) relies on the ability of *H. pylori* to cause rapid breakdown of urea, which can be labeled with either ^{13}C (a nonradioactive nuclide) or ^{14}C (a beta-emitting radionuclide). Ingested urea is broken down by *H. pylori* in the stomach into ammonia and carbonic acid. The body excretes the carbonic acid in the form of carbon dioxide, which is released in the lungs. Up to 200 kBq of ^{14}C-urea in capsule or liquid form is given to the patient orally. In the presence of *H. pylori* infection this is broken down and absorbed. Breath samples are collected 10–30 min after administration of the activity. One millimole of total bicarbonate is trapped in hyamine solution and the percentage of $^{14}CO_2$ in the total collected sample is calculated. Nonradioactive CO_2 is produced as a result of body metabolism, the heavier the patient the higher the nonradioactive CO_2 production. Thus $^{14}CO_2$ is expressed as percent $^{14}CO_2$ multiplied by body weight (in kg) to correct for this. Normally a negligible amount (less the 0.2%) of $^{14}CO_2$ corrected for body weight is recovered.

In *H. pylori* infection the recovered $^{14}CO_2$ is usually more than 1%. The test is noninvasive with a low radiation dose to the patient (effective dose less than 0.02 mSv). It is a suitable test for follow-up of patients after treatment to assess the effectiveness of treatment or recurrence of infection.

Small-bowel bacterial overgrowth

Normally there is little bacterial growth in the small bowel (less than 10^4 colony forming units/mL) as compared to the colon (10^{10} to 10^{12} colony forming units/mL). This low count can be maintained because of acid in the stomach, rapid transit, and the ileocecal valve. Small-bowel bacterial overgrowth can occur in those with intestinal dysmotility syndromes associated with systemic disease (e.g. diabetes, scleroderma, intestinal pseudo-obstruction) and those with anatomical disorders following surgery (e.g. terminal ileal resection) or strictures of the small bowel. Gastric surgery and, in particular, that involving a blind loop is associated with a high prevalence of small-bowel bacterial overgrowth. Overgrowth can occur as the acidity of stomach falls (old age or antacids) or as the result of slow small-bowel transit or hold-ups (e.g. surgery, diabetes, Crohn's disease) leading to various symptoms such as bloating, pain, diarrhea, and various malabsorption syndromes. Small-bowel bacterial overgrowth may not be associated with any clinical symptoms. Its diagnosis can be difficult and several methods are available. Direct sampling and culture of the small bowel content is the 'gold standard'. It is relatively invasive and not readily available. There are several noninvasive tests available based on the breakdown of carbohydrates or bile acids. The most commonly used test is the hydrogen and methane breath test following a glucose or lactulose meal. The ^{14}C-glycocholate breath test and ^{14}C-xylose test are also used. In nuclear medicine the most commonly performed test is the ^{14}C-glycocholate breath test.

One of the first tests to be developed was the bile acid breath test. Following ingestion, ^{14}C-glycocholate is broken down to glycine by anaerobic bacteria and then metabolized to $^{14}CO_2$ which is then measured in the expired breath. However, it has a low sensitivity with a false negative rate of up to 30%, partly because it will not detect aerobic micobacterial overgrowth.

A dose of 185 kBq of ^{14}C-glycocholic acid in 200 mL liquid (orange juice) is administered orally. Breath samples are collected and 2 mmol of CO_2 from the sample is trapped in hyamine solution. An immediate sample (baseline) followed by hourly samples for up to 8 h are collected. The percent of $^{14}CO_2$ is calculated in each sample. In normal subjects the expired $^{14}CO_2$ percent of total CO_2 should not exceed 0.15% in each sample. In total, no more than 4% of the administered dose is exhaled in 6 h period. Different patterns of $^{14}CO_2$ exhaled may indicate different disease entities.

PROTEIN LOSS

Protein-losing enteropathy is secondary to lymphatic obstruction or mucosal disease of the gastrointestinal tract usually presenting with peripheral edema or GI symptoms such as diarrhea and malabsorption. Blood tests show reduced plasma albumin and globulins. There are several radionuclide tests used for diagnosing this condition. The commonly performed test is ^{51}Cr-labeled albumin or ^{51}CrCl$_3$ (chromium chloride) test. Alternatively indium-111 chloride can be used, which has the advantage that imaging can also be performed. Both ^{51}CrCl$_3$ and indium-111 chloride immediately bind irreversibly to transferrin in the blood. The fraction of recovered ^{51}Cr in a 4-day stool collection is normally less than 0.7% of the administered activity (3–4 MBq). In protein-losing enteropathy 2–40% of the administered activity may be recovered in the stool. The main problem with this test is urine contamination of the feces which may give false positive results. If indium-111 chloride is used (up to 10 MBq) then whole-body counts can be used for estimation of protein loss. Uncollimated whole-body images are acquired at 4 h (baseline) and 7 days. Loss of more than 10% of activity signifies protein loss. In addition, images obtained at 24 and 48 h using a medium energy collimator may show activity in the small intestine and colon which confirms excessive loss of protein into the gut.

GASTROINTESTINAL BLOOD LOSS

Gastrointestinal blood loss can be imaged using colloid or technetium-labeled red cells. In chronic blood loss and anemia GI loss can be quantified using chromium-labeled red cells. This topic is covered in detail in Chapter 14A.

In the assessment of anemia, *in vitro* ^{51}Cr-labeled red cells are used. Following injection of up to 4 MBq of ^{51}Cr-red blood cells, stool samples are collected for 5 consecutive days and the recovered activity compared to the counts from blood samples to calculate the blood loss in mLs. Normal fecal blood loss is usually less than 1.5 mL per day, more than 3 mL a day is abnormal.

BILIARY SCINTIGRAPHY

Biliary scintigraphy is a well established investigation for assessing biliary tract and gallbladder function. One can also assess the presence of entero-gastric reflux (bile reflux). Several iminodiacetic acid (IDA) compounds are used for biliary imaging, collectively known as HIDA compounds. ^{99m}Tc-labeled mebrofenin is a preferred agent that has rapid liver clearance even in the presence of jaundice. Following intravenous administration of HIDA compounds, there is rapid uptake by hepatocytes and subsequent excretion into the biliary tract and duodenum. Patients must fast overnight as gallbladder uptake may be diminished for several hours after a meal resulting in a false positive test.

For gallbladder function assessment, images are acquired 30 min after injection to allow gallbladder concentration of the agent. After baseline images, the gallbladder is stimulated either directly by intravenous infusion of synthetic cholecystokinin (CCK or Sincalide) or by oral administration of a fatty meal. Gallbladder ejection fraction is measured from the dynamic curves created from a gallbladder region of interest (Fig. 14C.8). The response to a fatty meal is delayed but stronger (normal ejection fraction >55%). With CCK there is a less intense but immediate gallbladder response (normal EF >40%). If CCK is used, it is possible to assess enterogastric reflux of bile. Image acquisition is ususally continued for 45 min.

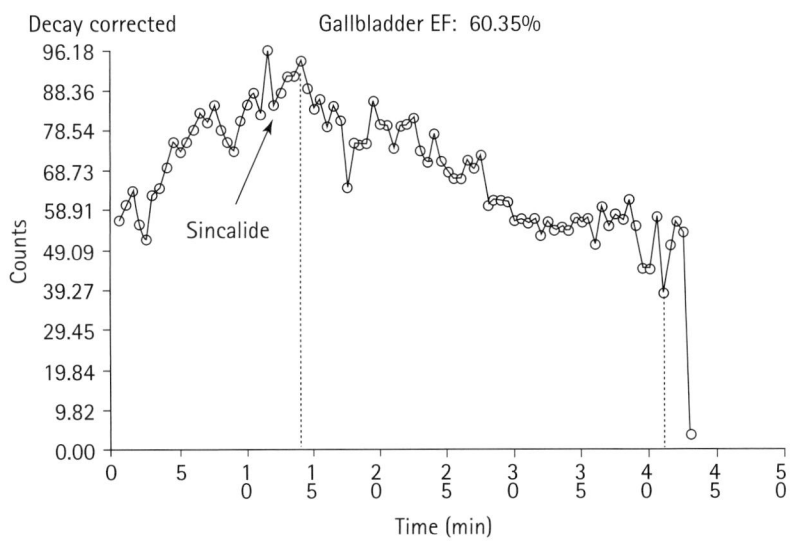

Figure 14C.8 *HIDA study showing a normal gallbladder response following sincalide infusion.*

For the investigation of suspected acute cholecystitis, a lack of gallbladder visualization by 1 h is consistent with this diagnosis. In chronic cholecystitis there can be delayed uptake but a poor response to CCK or a fatty meal.

If assessing neonatal jaundice when extrahepatic biliary atresia is suspected, either mebrofenin or the di-isopropyl derivative (DISIDA) are preferred agents as both have good hepatic clearance in patients with jaundice. Premedication with phenobarbitone is usually employed for 5 days prior to imaging in neonates to enhance liver enzyme induction, thereby maximizing uptake and excretion. Excretion of the radiopharmaceutical into the bowel by 24 h excludes extrahepatic biliary atresia.

Other indications for HIDA scintigraphy includes the demonstration of biliary leaks following surgical intervention or trauma or in the demonstration of other congenital biliary disorders including choledocal cysts.

REFERENCES

● Seminal primary article

1 McDowall TJS. *Handbook of physiology*, 43rd edition. London: John Murray, 1960.

● 2 Di Lorenzo C, Piepsz A, Ham H, Cardanel S. Gastric emptying with gastro-oesophageal reflux. *Arch Dis Child* 1987; **62**: 449–53.

● 3 Notghi A, Hutchinson R, Kumar D, Smith NB, Harding LK. A simplified method for the measurement of segmental colonic transit time. *Gut* 1994; **35**: 976–81.

● 4 Hutchinson R, Mostafa AB, Grant EA, *et al*. Scintigraphic defaecography: quantitative and dynamic assessment of anorectal function. *Dis Colon Rectum* 1993; **36**: 1132–8.

Positron emission tomography in gastrointestinal cancers

GARY J.R. COOK

INTRODUCTION

There are a number of areas in the clinical management of gastrointestinal malignancy where 2-[^{18}F]fluoro-2-deoxy-D-glucose (^{18}F-FDG) positron emission tomography (PET) has been shown to have complementary or incremental value compared to conventional noninvasive imaging methods. There is evidence to support the use of PET in esophageal, pancreatic, colorectal, and primary and secondary hepatic cancers. There has also been interest in the use of ^{18}F-FDG PET to monitor therapy in gastrointestinal stromal tumors (GISTs) and early interest in the use of alternative tracers such as ^{18}F-fluorothymidine and ^{18}F-fluorodopa as well as PET radionuclide labeled octreotide analogs in colorectal and neuroendocrine tumors, respectively.

ESOPHAGEAL CANCER

Esophageal cancer is related to smoking and alcohol consumption and is the third most common gastrointestinal cancer. Cancers in the upper two thirds of the esophagus are usually squamous cell carcinomas whilst those in the lower third and the gastro-esophageal junction are most often adenocarcinomas. Early stage esophageal cancers are potentially curable by surgery, or radical radiotherapy in the case of squamous cell carcinomas. More advanced stages may be amenable to chemotherapy downstaging before radical attempts at cure, whilst metastatic disease is usually only suitable for palliative treatments. Conventionally, staging of esophageal cancer has relied on computed tomography (CT) and endoscopic ultrasound but a high recurrence rate after

radical treatment infers suboptimal sensitivity for these modalities alone.

The vast majority of malignant esophageal tumors are ^{18}F-FDG avid and it is therefore rare to not see uptake at the primary site.[1–9] Small T1 tumors may not be resolved. However, diagnosis of the primary tumor is largely the task of endoscopy and as it is relatively common to see moderate uptake of ^{18}F-FDG in the lower esophagus, or stomach, as a result of inflammation, it is unlikely that there will be a role for ^{18}F-FDG PET in diagnosis or screening.

At present the most important role for PET is the staging of esophageal cancers prior to radical curative treatment, including surgery and radiotherapy. Most studies have shown that the sensitivity for detecting periesophageal malignant lymph nodes is relatively poor and both the T and local nodal staging are best performed by a combination of CT and endoscopic ultrasound.[1–9] However, the sensitivity for detecting distant nodes and metastases is very good and in most published series approximately 10–20% of patients deemed operable by conventional techniques will have metastatic disease identified by ^{18}F-FDG PET requiring a change from operative management as first line (Plate 14D.1).

Another area in which ^{18}F-FDG PET has a promising role is in the evaluation of neoadjuvant chemotherapy. Weber and colleagues performed ^{18}F-FDG PET scans at baseline and at 14 days after commencing chemotherapy for tumors at the gastro-esophageal junction and used clinical response at 3 months (reduction of tumor length and wall thickness by >50% by conventional imaging and endoscopy) as the standard for reference.[10] Responding tumors showed significantly greater reduction in standardized uptake value (SUV) compared to nonresponding tumors ($-54\% \pm 17\%$

compared to −15% ± 21%). An optimal cut-off of −35% predicted a clinical response with a sensitivity of 93% and specificity of 95%. A metabolic ^{18}F-FDG PET response also demonstrated prognostic value in that these patients showed a significantly longer time to progression and improved survival.[10–12] Similar results have been recorded by using ^{18}F-FDG PET at baseline and 3 weeks in squamous cell tumors following neoadjuvant chemoradiotherapy.[11]

In patients with clinical or radiological suspicion of recurrence conventional techniques including CT and endoscopic ultrasound were more accurate in diagnosing perianastomotic tumor recurrence.[13] Although ^{18}F-FDG PET detected all tumor recurrences there were a number of false positives (specificity 57%) in patients with progressive anastomotic restenoses. ^{18}F-FDG PET was more accurate than conventional techniques in detecting regional and distant metastases although this did not reach statistical significance. Twenty-seven percent of patients had additional information provided by PET imaging.

PANCREATIC CANCER

After colorectal and esophageal cancer, carcinoma of the pancreas is associated with the highest mortality rate from gastrointestinal cancers. Unfortunately, 5-year survival is appallingly low, at less than 5%. Surgical resection may be attempted but seldom results in cure or long-term survival. The biggest issues related to imaging are in the differential diagnosis of pancreatic masses and in accurate presurgical staging.

It is known that pancreatic carcinomas over-express membrane glucose transporters (GLUT-1) compared to mass forming pancreatitis and that uptake as measured by SUV is significantly greater (2.98 ± 1.23 vs 1.25 ± 0.51).[14] In a number of studies ^{18}F-FDG PET has resulted in reasonable sensitivity and specificity in the diagnosis of primary pancreatic carcinomas (85–94% and 84–97%, respectively)[15–19] but occasional false negatives and false positives have been described. The majority of false negatives appear to be associated with raised blood glucose levels,[19,20] one group noting a reduction in sensitivity from 86 to 42% in normoglycemic compared to hyperglycemic individuals.[19] In spite of greater GLUT-1 expression in pancreatic cancers compared to mass forming pancreatitis, false positives occur in inflammatory pancreatic lesions, particularly when there is serological evidence of inflammation such as a raised C-reactive protein level.[20] By scanning at a delayed time point at 2 h it may be possible to reduce the number of false positives by including both the SUV and a retention index between 1 and 2 h scans.[21] The majority of cancers show an increase in SUV between 1 and 2 h whilst the opposite occurs in benign masses.

The results for staging pancreatic cancer by conventional imaging are relatively poor and similarly the detection of regional lymph nodes by ^{18}F-FDG PET has been reported with a sensitivity of 49% and specificity of 63%.[20] In the detection of liver metastases ^{18}F-FDG PET has been reported to have an overall diagnostic accuracy of 90%, similar to CT and ultrasound.[22] The sensitivity becomes lower (≈70%) in liver metastases of less than 1 cm.

There are few published data on the use of ^{18}F-FDG PET in recurrent pancreatic cancer but it would appear to give additional information in a number of patients, particularly when conventional imaging is negative and there is evidence of rising tumor markers such as CA 19-9 (Plate 14D.2).[23] As a measure of treatment response to chemotherapy it has been shown that absence of ^{18}F-FDG uptake after 1 month from starting treatment is associated with an improved survival and that PET is a better predictor of response than CT.[24]

COLORECTAL CANCER

Colon cancer is the third commonest cancer and the second commonest cause of cancer death in men and women, having a 5-year survival rate of approximately 50%. Many patients are cured by primary surgery but approximately 30% will demonstrate recurrence within the first 2 years, of whom approximately 25% will have an isolated focus of recurrence that may be amenable to curative surgery. The liver is a common site for recurrence and may be resected with curative intent, often in combination with neoadjuvant and/or adjuvant chemotherapy, although the presence of extrahepatic disease is usually regarded as a contraindication.

There is unlikely ever to be a role for the use of ^{18}F-FDG PET for the screening of colorectal cancer as it is a relatively expensive technique and the presence of variable physiological uptake of tracer, particularly in the colon, is likely to reduce both sensitivity and specificity. There is some evidence to suggest that the use of ^{18}F-FDG PET may have incremental value over CT when used in the primary staging of colorectal cancer.[25,26] Although the local T and N staging for rectal cancers is best performed by magnetic resonance imaging (MRI) and by CT for colon cancers, PET is probably more accurate in detecting distant metastases, upstaging four out of 37 patients in one study.[25] Despite some evidence of its complementary nature in staging colorectal cancers at diagnosis, it is not widely used in this regard, perhaps because PET still has limited availability in many countries and the evidence is less strong than on the use of PET in recurrent colorectal cancer.

It is in the evaluation of recurrent colorectal cancer that ^{18}F-FDG PET has its most established role.[27–30] Diagnosis of local recurrence of rectal carcinoma may be problematic with anatomic imaging following surgery and radiotherapy where post-treatment changes may be indistinguishable from recurrent tumor. A number of studies have shown the

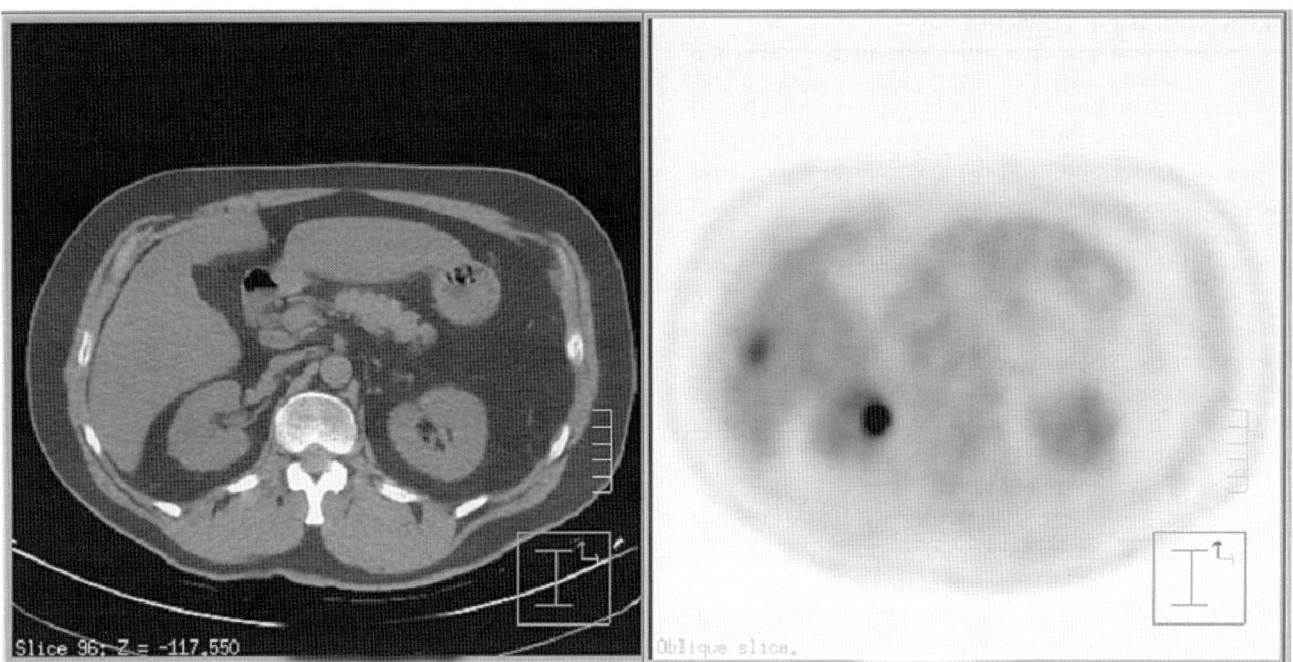

Figure 14D.1 *Transaxial ^{18}F-FDG PET and corresponding CT images from a combined PET/CT acquisition in a patient with a rising CEA level 6 months after primary surgery for colorectal cancer. A small ^{18}F-FDG-avid lesion is clearly seen on the PET component but is invisible on the unenhanced CT. A contrast-enhanced CT also failed to demonstrate the lesion but it was subsequently confirmed with MRI before the patient went forward for hepatic resection.*

superiority of PET over CT in detecting local recurrence.[28–30] Potential weaknesses of PET include false positive uptake for up to 6 months following radiotherapy, related to a inflammatory reaction[31,32] and a lower sensitivity for detecting mucinous carcinoma recurrence (58%) compared to nonmucinous recurrence (92%).[29]

Most studies have shown a small advantage in accuracy of ^{18}F-FDG PET compared to CT in the detection of hepatic metastases (Fig. 14D.1).[28–30,33,34] In more recent studies where ^{18}F-FDG PET has been compared to spiral CT differences are relatively small and at the present time there are no large studies comparing PET with new MRI techniques using novel hepatic contrast agents. Results with conventional MRI are similar to PET.[35,36] Compared to CT portography, PET has been reported to be slightly less sensitive but more specific and accurate (92% vs 80%).[33] PET is limited in sensitivity[37] in lesions of less than 1 cm and it is possible that the incremental value over conventional imaging with CT and MRI is not so much in the detection of hepatic metastases but in the detection of occult extrahepatic that can radically affect management. Most studies have shown superiority in this regard where on average, more than 25% of patients have occult disease detected.[27,28,30]

It is not uncommon for the first suspicion for colorectal cancer recurrence to be due to an increase in tumor markers such as carcinoembryonic antigen (CEA). When the volume of disease recurrence is small it may not be detected by conventional cross-sectional anatomical imaging but it would appear that ^{18}F-FDG PET may detect the recurrent site in approximately two thirds of cases.[28,38] When assessing the cost-effectiveness of PET and CT combined to CT alone in patients with raised CEA using a decision-tree analysis it has been found that the inclusion of PET is cost-effective, particularly in patients with liver metastases who are potentially curable with hepatic resection.[39]

Overall, a meta-analysis of 11 studies investigating the use of ^{18}F-FDG PET in recurrent colorectal cancer found a PET-directed change in patient management in 29%. Throughout the whole body the sensitivity for detecting recurrence was 97% with a specificity of 76%.[40]

Early data suggest that ^{18}F-FDG PET may be a good tool in the evaluation of treatment response in patients with colorectal cancers and liver metastases. Findlay *et al.* were able to predict response to 5-fluorouracil infusion at 4–5 weeks with a sensitivity of 100% and specificity of 90%.[41] Responding lesions had a greater reduction in uptake (67% of baseline level) compared to nonresponding metastases (99% of baseline level). In a further small study response was predicted as early as 72 h after starting 5-fluorouracil although reductions in ^{18}F-FDG uptake were smaller.[42]

When assessing the effects of radiofrequency ablation of colorectal liver metastases, continued activity in the periphery of a metastasis at one week and at 1 month with ^{18}F-FDG PET indicates incomplete tumor ablation that may not be detectable using CT criteria.[43]

HEPATOBILIARY TUMORS

Cholangiocarcinomas can either be intra- or extrahepatic in location and the intrahepatic types can occur peripherally or as central tumors at the liver hilum. In one study peripheral cholangiocarcinomas showed higher avidity for ^{18}F-FDG than hilar tumors although uptake in the latter was slightly higher than background liver activity.[44] Unexpected distant metastases were detected in four of 21 patients. In another study it was noted that the sensitivity for nodular cholangiocarcinomas was greater than that for infiltrating tumors (85% vs 18%).[45] False positive uptake was noted in cholangitis and surrounding biliary stents and surgical management was changed in 30% due to detection of unsuspected metastases. It was also noted that ^{18}F-FDG PET is useful in detecting residual gallbladder carcinoma following cholecystectomy.

In primary hepatocellular carcinomas the sensitivity of ^{18}F-FDG is only about 50%. It is thought that this is due to high levels of glucose-6-phosphatase in these tumors allowing dephosphorylation of ^{18}F-FDG-6-phosphate and hence release from the intracellular compartment.[46] The less well differentiated tumors are more likely to be detected than those that are well differentiated.[47] The role in the evaluation and differentiation of benign from malignant lesions in the liver is supported by a number of studies where apart from false negatives in hepatocellular carcinoma and a few false positives due to liver abscesses PET remains an accurate noninvasive technique.[33,48]

GASTROINTESTINAL STROMAL TUMORS

Gastrointestinal stromal tumors are rare soft tissue sarcomas that can occur anywhere in the gastrointestinal tract but most commonly in the stomach. Although rare, they are worthy of separate mention as they are particularly ^{18}F-FDG avid and commonly respond extremely well to the tyrosine kinase inhibitor, imatinib mesylate. This response can be sensitively detected by reduction in ^{18}F-FDG activity long before tumor shrinkage occurs and has been reported as early as 1 week after commencing treatment.[49–51] It would appear that ^{18}F-FDG PET and CT are of similar accuracy in the initial staging of GISTs but that early prediction of disease response to this drug is best measured by PET. It has also been noted that combined PET/CT imaging may provide additional information when measuring response in some cases.[52]

MISCELLANEOUS

Although ^{18}F-FDG remains the most commonly used clinical tracer in oncological imaging of the gastrointestinal tract, some tumors, e.g. of neuroendocrine origin, are not best imaged with this radiopharmaceutical due to low glycolytic activity.[53] It is also argued that changes in ^{18}F-FDG activity do not predict tumor response as well as the measurement of change in other biological parameters such as proliferation imaged with ^{18}F-fluorothymidine (FLT).[54] Another potential weakness of ^{18}F-FDG is its nonspecific accumulation in inflammatory processes and in animal models it would appear that FLT is more specific for tumor activity.[55] It is possible that radiopharmaceuticals such as ^{18}F-fluorodopa are more sensitive in staging neuroendocrine tumors than somatostatin receptor scintigraphy[56] although the latter remains a valuable method to confirm receptor status before radiolabeled somatostatin analog radionuclide therapy. It is also possible to use PET radionuclides to label somatostatin analogs with the possibility of improved image quality and resolution of small lesions.[57]

It is likely that as PET becomes more established as a clinical tool further radiopharmaceuticals will be developed and will become more routinely available for the evaluation of different tumors and different aspects of tumor biology with respect to baseline status and in response to modern anticancer agents.

Case history

A 54-year-old patient with rectal cancer was treated with neoadjuvant chemo-radiotherapy and then surgically with an anterior resection. In the year following surgery the CEA levels slowly rose from within the normal range ($<5\,\mathrm{ng\,ml^{-1}}$) to $6\,\mathrm{ng\,ml^{-1}}$. Diagnostic CT scans had shown stable appearances in the pelvis with some unchanging presacral soft tissue thickening interpreted as representing post-radiotherapy and post-surgical effects. A ^{18}F-FDG PET/CT scan was requested to determine possible sites of recurrent tumor to explain the rise in CEA. See Plate 14D.3.

The transaxial images (left CT and right fused PET/CT) demonstrate abnormal uptake of ^{18}F-FDG not only in the presacral soft tissue thickening but also in abnormal soft tissue in the left pelvic sidewall. No abnormalities were noted in the liver or elsewhere.

These results confirmed active tumor in two sites in the pelvis allowing appropriate further therapy to be planned.

REFERENCES

● Seminal primary article

● 1 Lerut T, Flamen P, Ectors N, *et al.* Histopathologic validation of lymph node staging with FDG-PET scan in cancer of the esophagus and gastro-esophageal junction: a prospective study based on primary surgery with extensive lymphadenectomy. *Ann Surg* 2000; **232**: 743–52.

● 2 Flamen P, Lerut A, Van Cutsem E, *et al.* Utility of positron emission tomography for the staging of patients with potentially operable esophageal carcinoma. *J Clin Oncol* 2000; **18**: 3202–10.

3 Yeung HW, Macapinlac HA, Mazumdar M, *et al.* FDG-PET in esophageal cancer. Incremental value over computed tomography. *Clin Positron Imaging* 1999; **2**: 255–60.

4 Rankin SC, Taylor H, Cook GJ, Mason R. Computed tomography and positron emission tomography in the pre-operative staging of oesophageal carcinoma. *Clin Radiol* 1998; **53**: 659–65.

5 Choi JY, Lee KH, Shim YM, *et al.* Improved detection of individual nodal involvement in squamous cell carcinoma of the esophagus by FDG PET. *J Nucl Med* 2000; **41**: 808–15.

6 Kole AC, Plukker JT, Nieweg OE, Vaalburg W. Positron emission tomography for staging of oesophageal and gastroesophageal malignancy. *Br J Cancer* 1998; **78**: 521–7.

7 Flanagan FL, Dehdashti F, Siegel BA, *et al.* Staging of esophageal cancer with ^{18}F-fluorodeoxyglucose positron emission tomography. *Am J Roentgenol* 1997; **168**: 417–24.

8 Ott K, Weber WA, Fink U, *et al.* Fluorodeoxyglucose-positron emission tomography in adenocarcinomas of the distal esophagus and cardia. *World J Surg* 2003; **27**: 1035–9.

9 Yoon YC, Lee KS, Shim YM, *et al.* Metastasis to regional lymph nodes in patients with esophageal squamous cell carcinoma: CT versus FDG PET for presurgical detection prospective study. *Radiology* 2003; **227**: 764–70.

● 10 Weber WA, Ott K, Becker K, *et al.* Prediction of response to preoperative chemotherapy in adenocarcinomas of the esophagogastric junction by metabolic imaging. *J Clin Oncol* 2001; **19**: 3058–65.

● 11 Brucher BL, Weber W, Bauer M, *et al.* Neoadjuvant therapy of esophageal squamous cell carcinoma: response evaluation by positron emission tomography. *Ann Surg* 2001; **233**: 300–9.

12 Flamen P, Van Cutsem E, Lerut A, *et al.* Positron emission tomography for assessment of the response to induction radiochemotherapy in locally advanced oesophageal cancer. *Ann Oncol* 2002; **13**: 361–8.

13 Flamen P, Lerut A, Van Cutsem E, *et al.* The utility of positron emission tomography for the diagnosis and staging of recurrent esophageal cancer. *J Thorac Cardiovasc Surg* 2000; **120**: 1085–92.

14 Reske SN, Grillenberger KG, Glatting G, *et al.* Over-expression of glucose transporter 1 and increased FDG uptake in pancreatic carcinoma. *J Nucl Med* 1997; **38**: 1344–8.

15 Sperti C, Pasquali C, Chierichetti F, *et al.* Value of 18-fluorodeoxyglucose positron emission tomography in the management of patients with cystic tumors of the pancreas. *Ann Surg* 2001; **234**: 675–80.

16 Keogan MT, Tyler D, Clark L, *et al.* Diagnosis of pancreatic carcinoma: role of FDG PET. *Am J Roentgenol* 1998; **171**: 1565–70.

17 Zimny M, Bares R, Fass J, *et al.* Fluorine-18 fluorodeoxyglucose positron emission tomography in the differential diagnosis of pancreatic carcinoma: a report of 106 cases. *Eur J Nucl Med* 1997; **24**: 678–82.

18 Bares R, Klever P, Hauptmann S, *et al.* F-18 fluorodeoxyglucose PET in vivo evaluation of pancreatic glucose metabolism for detection of pancreatic cancer. *Radiology* 1994; **192**: 79–86.

19 Diederichs CG, Staib L, Glatting G, *et al.* FDG PET: elevated plasma glucose reduces both uptake and detection rate of pancreatic malignancies. *J Nucl Med* 1998; **39**: 1030–3.

● 20 Diederichs CG, Staib L, Vogel J, *et al.* Values and limitations of ^{18}F-fluorodeoxyglucose-positron-emission tomography with preoperative evaluation of patients with pancreatic masses. *Pancreas* 2000; **20**: 109–16.

21 Nakamoto Y, Higashi T, Sakahara H, *et al.* Delayed (18)F-fluoro-2-deoxy-D-glucose positron emission tomography scan for differentiation between malignant and benign lesions in the pancreas. *Cancer* 2000; **89**: 2547–54.

22 Nakamoto Y, Higashi T, Sakahara H, *et al.* Contribution of PET in the detection of liver metastases from pancreatic tumours. *Clin Radiol* 1999; **54**: 248–52.

23 Franke C, Klapdor R, Meyerhoff K, Schauman M. 18-FDG positron emission tomography of the pancreas: diagnostic benefit in the follow-up of pancreatic carcinoma. *Anticancer Res* 1999; **19**: 2437–42.

24 Maisey NR, Webb A, Flux GD, *et al.* FDG-PET in the prediction of survival of patients with cancer of the pancreas: a pilot study. *Br J Cancer* 2000; **83**: 287–93.

25 Abdel-Nabi H, Doerr RJ, Lamonica DM, *et al.* Staging of primary colorectal carcinomas with fluorine-18 fluorodeoxyglucose whole-body PET: correlation with histopathologic and CT findings. *Radiology* 1998; **206**: 755–60.

26 Gupta NC, Falk PM, Frank AL, *et al.* Pre-operative staging of colorectal carcinoma using positron emission tomography. *Nebr Med J* 1993; **78**: 30–5.

27 Delbeke D, Vitola JV, Sandler MP, *et al*. Staging recurrent metastatic colorectal carcinoma with PET. *J Nucl Med* 1997; **38**: 1196–201.

28 Valk PE, Abella-Columna E, Haseman MK, *et al*. Whole-body PET imaging with [18F]fluorodeoxyglucose in management of recurrent colorectal cancer. *Arch Surg* 1999; **134**: 503–11.

29 Whiteford MH, Whiteford HM, Yee LF, *et al*. Usefulness of FDG-PET scan in the assessment of suspected metastatic or recurrent adenocarcinoma of the colon and rectum. *Dis Colon Rectum* 2000; **43**: 759–67.

30 Schiepers C, Penninckx F, De Vadder N, *et al*. Contribution of PET in the diagnosis of recurrent colorectal cancer: comparison with conventional imaging. *Eur J Surg Oncol* 1995; **21**: 517–22.

31 Moore HG, Akhurst T, Larson SM, *et al*. A case-controlled study of 18-fluorodeoxyglucose positron emission tomography in the detection of pelvic recurrence in previously irradiated rectal cancer patients. *J Am Coll Surg* 2003; **197**: 22–8.

32 Haberkorn U, Strauss LG, Dimitrakopoulou A, *et al*. PET studies of fluorodeoxyglucose metabolism in patients with recurrent colorectal tumors receiving radiotherapy. *J Nucl Med* 1991; **32**: 1485–90.

33 Delbeke D, Martin WH, Sandler MP, *et al*. Evaluation of benign vs malignant hepatic lesions with positron emission tomography. *Arch Surg* 1998; **133**: 510–15.

34 Vitola JV, Delbeke D, Sandler MP, *et al*. Positron emission tomography to stage suspected metastatic colorectal carcinoma to the liver. *Am J Surg* 1996; **171**: 21–6.

35 Yang M, Martin DR, Karabulut N, Frick MP. Comparison of MR and PET imaging for the evaluation of liver metastases. *J Magn Reson Imaging* 2003; **17**: 343–9.

36 Kinkel K, Lu Y, Both M, *et al*. Detection of hepatic metastases from cancers of the gastrointestinal tract by using noninvasive imaging methods (US, CT, MR imaging, PET): a meta-analysis. *Radiology* 2002; **224**: 748–56.

37 Fong Y, Saldinger PF, Akhurst T, *et al*. Utility of ^{18}F-FDG positron emission tomography scanning on selection of patients for resection of hepatic colorectal metastases. *Am J Surg* 1999; **178**: 282–7.

38 Flanagan FL, Dehdashti F, Ogunbiyi OA, *et al*. Utility of FDG-PET for investigating unexplained plasma CEA elevation in patients with colorectal cancer. *Ann Surg* 1998; **227**: 319–23.

39 Park KC, Schwimmer J, Shepherd JE, *et al*. Decision analysis for the cost-effective management of recurrent colorectal cancer. *Ann Surg* 2001; **233**: 310–19.

40 Huebner RH, Park KC, Shepherd JE, *et al*. A meta-analysis of the literature for whole-body FDG PET detection of recurrent colorectal cancer. *J Nucl Med* 2000; **41**: 1177–89.

41 Findlay M, Young H, Cunningham D, *et al*. Noninvasive monitoring of tumor metabolism using fluorodeoxyglucose and positron emission tomography in colorectal cancer liver metastases: correlation with tumor response to fluorouracil. *J Clin Oncol* 1996; **14**: 700–8.

42 Bender H, Bangard N, Metten N, *et al*. Possible role of FDG-PET in the early prediction of therapy outcome in liver metastases of colorectal cancer. *Hybridoma* 1999; **18**: 87–91.

43 Donckier V, Van Laethem JL, Goldman S, *et al*. [F-18] fluorodeoxyglucose positron emission tomography as a tool for early recognition of incomplete tumor destruction after radiofrequency ablation for liver metastases. *J Surg Oncol* 2003; **84**: 215–23.

44 Kim YJ, Yun M, Lee WJ, *et al*. Usefulness of ^{18}F-FDG PET in intrahepatic cholangiocarcinoma. *Eur J Nucl Med Mol Imaging* 2003; **30**: 1467–72.

45 Anderson CD, Rice MH, Pinson CW, *et al*. Fluorodeoxyglucose PET imaging in the evaluation of gallbladder carcinoma and cholangiocarcinoma. *J Gastrointest Surg* 2004; **8**: 90–7.

46 Torizuka T, Tamaki N, Inokuma T, *et al*. In vivo assessment of glucose metabolism in hepatocellular carcinoma with FDG-PET. *J Nucl Med* 1995; **36**: 1811–17.

47 Trojan J, Schroeder O, Raedle J, *et al*. Fluorine-18 FDG positron emission tomography for imaging of hepatocellular carcinoma. *Am J Gastroenterol* 1999; **94**: 3314–19.

48 Hustinx R, Paulus P, Jacquet N, *et al*. Clinical evaluation of whole-body ^{18}F-fluorodeoxyglucose positron emission tomography in the detection of liver metastases. *Ann Oncol* 1998; **9**: 397–401.

49 Jager PL, Gietema JA, van der Graaf WT. Imatinib mesylate for the treatment of gastrointestinal stromal tumours: best monitored with FDG PET. *Nucl Med Commun* 2004; **25**: 433–8.

50 Gayed I, Vu T, Iyer R, *et al*. The role of ^{18}F-FDG PET in staging and early prediction of response to therapy of recurrent gastrointestinal stromal tumors. *J Nucl Med* 2004; **45**: 17–21.

51 Stroobants S, Goeminne J, Seegers M, *et al*. [18]FDG-Positron emission tomography for the early prediction of response in advanced soft tissue sarcoma treated with imatinib mesylate (Glivec). *Eur J Cancer* 2003; **39**: 2012–20.

52 Antoch G, Kanja J, Bauer S, *et al*. Comparison of PET, CT, and dual-modality PET/CT imaging for monitoring of imatinib (STI571) therapy in patients with gastrointestinal stromal tumors. *J Nucl Med* 2004; **45**: 357–65.

53 Adams S, Baum R, Rink T, *et al*. Limited value of fluorine-18 fluorodeoxyglucose positron emission tomography for the imaging of neuroendocrine tumours. *Eur J Nucl Med* 1998; **25**: 79–83.

54 Francis DL, Freeman A, Visvikis D, *et al.* In vivo imaging of cellular proliferation in colorectal cancer using positron emission tomography. *Gut* 2003; **52**: 1602–6.

55 van Waarde A, Cobben DC, Suurmeijer AJ, *et al.* Selectivity of ^{18}F-FLT and ^{18}F-FDG for differentiating tumor from inflammation in a rodent model. *J Nucl Med* 2004; **45**: 695–700.

56 Becherer A, Szabo M, Karanikas G, *et al.* Imaging of advanced neuroendocrine tumors with (18)F-FDOPA PET. *J Nucl Med* 2004; **45**: 1161–7.

57 Kowalski J, Henze M, Schuhmacher J, *et al.* Evaluation of positron emission tomography imaging using [^{68}Ga]-DOTA-D-Phe(1)-Tyr(3)-octreotide in comparison to [^{111}In]-DTPAOC SPECT. First results in patients with neuroendocrine tumors. *Mol Imaging Biol* 2003; **5**: 42–8.

Gastrointestinal neuroendocrine tumors

JOHN BUSCOMBE AND GOPINATH GNANASEGARAN

INTRODUCTION

Neuroendocrine tumors are a wide range of neoplasms that have certain characteristics in common. They are defined not by site but by molecular characteristics. They can exist in any tissue of embryonic gut origin and therefore whilst most appear in the gastrointestinal (GI) system it is possible to find neuroendocrine tumors in other tissues such as the lung, kidneys, and genitalia. The most common forms arise in the mid and hind gut. In most subjects these can be benign and asymptomatic with some reports suggesting that at post-mortem 5% of the population may have such a tumor.[1] In a smaller number these tumors may grow and produce a mass effect or secrete hormones that produce a characteristic group of symptoms. Over the past 100 years since their discovery different forms of nomenclature have been used and even now the terms commonly used can be confusing. Most of the cell types making up neuroendocrine tumors contain granules of secretory material. The earliest characteristic noted was the ability to take up amine dyes with subsequent decarboxylation and so for many years they were known as APUDOMAs (amine precursor uptake and decarboxylation). Recognition that these cells are of neural crest origin but often secrete hormones has resulted in the term neuroendocrine tumors (NETs). Different secretory syndromes have also resulted in certain subtypes receiving names such as carcinoid if they produce serotonin, insulinoma if they produce insulin etc. In our practice 50% are described as non-secretors. This probably means that the products they produce are not pharmacologically active or not recognized. However, all of these cell types excrete chromogranins to some degree and these can be used as a tumor marker.[2] The tumors that present clinically are rare, with the incidence of clinically apparent carcinoid being 4 per million per year.[1]

SITES OF DISEASE

Although there are neuroendocrine tumors which are not directly gut-related, such as medullary cell carcinoma of the thyroid or small-cell lung cancer, the scope of this chapter is to discuss those which arise in the gastrointestinal tract. Here again we come across problems of definition. Carcinoid tumors occurring in the pancreas and cecum may both produce serotonin but the cellular characteristics and prognosis of the two tumors can be very different. Except for some gastric carcinoids, most fore-gut neuroendocrine tumors are found in the pancreas. About 50% seem to be secretory, of which carcinoids are the most common, then gastrinomas and then other types of secretory tumors such as insulinomas and VIPomas. The latter two may produce significant symptoms despite being small and solitary. In contrast, as serotonin is broken down in the liver, the carcinoid syndrome only occurs when the tumor has metastasized to the liver, so the endocrine products can be released directly into the systemic circulation.

In the mid and hind-gut, neuroendocrine tumors are normally carcinoid tumors, some of which may be non-secretory. These tend to present in an advanced state either with a mass causing bowel obstruction or other mass effects, including pain, or with liver metastases causing the carcinoid syndrome.

FUNCTIONALITY

These tumors share some common tumor genetics in that over 85% of carcinoids express the gene for the somatostatin type 2 receptor. A similar percentage of most pancreatic neuroendocrine tumors express this receptor except for insulinomas where only 50% may be positive. A significant number of carcinoids and gastrinomas also express *VMAT1* (vesicular monoamine transporter gene) and *VMAT2*, allowing uptake of *meta*-iodobenzyl guanidine (MIBG).[3] The secretory status of a tumor does not appear to correlate with expression of these receptors.

SECRETORY SYNDROMES

The carcinoid syndrome is caused by episodic release of serotonin into the systemic circulation and is characterized by flushing of the face and neck that may last up to 30 min. Triggers include alcohol, spicy foods, anxiety or the symptoms may arise spontaneously. In untreated patients this may occur many times a day. The attacks may be accompanied by palpitations and wheezing. If severe and continuous it is described as a carcinoid crisis which is a medical emergency. In the long term the patient may develop a characteristic facial rash and right-sided heart valve disease. They may have signs of liver failure and vitamin B group deficiency syndromes. It is a slow growing tumor but once there are liver and bone metastases most patients die within 5 years, although some remain well for much longer despite massive tumor loads.

Gastrinomas produce the Zollinger–Ellison syndrome, which is characterized by persistent gastric and duodenal ulceration and is diagnosed by a high fasting gastrin level. The disease is nearly always of pancreatic origin, and the tumor can grow rapidly and involve the liver. Treatment is directed towards reducing the effect of gastrin on the gut with proton pump inhibitors and attempting to treat the tumor mass.

Insulinomas are very rare and present with episodes of spontaneous hypoglycemia. Diagnosis depends on finding a high insulin and low glucose level, normally needing at least a 2-h fast and high C-peptide levels. Most of the tumors are small (<1 cm) and solitary. Occasionally, they are malignant and associated with liver and bone metastases. These patients may need to eat at 30-min intervals day and night to avoid death.

VIPomas (vasoactive intestinal peptide) are also rare tumors and characterized by continuous watery diarrhea which may require the patient to be placed on intravenous fluids as they can lose 5–6 L of fluid per day.

Multiple neuroendocrine neoplasia type 1 can be familial or sporadic with half of the patients occurring in each group. The pattern of disease includes a pancreatic neuroendocrine tumor, a parathyroid adenoma and a pituitary adenoma. These may appear concurrently or sequentially and must be sought in any patient with a proven pancreatic neuroendocrine tumor.

DIAGNOSIS

Diagnosis is normally established by clinical suspicion or after an acute medical or surgical emergency resulting in operation or imaging of the liver and upper abdomen, the common sites for metastases. In secreting tumors the identification of endocrine products in the blood from a fasting sample is normally diagnostic, although at present the serum serotonin assays are not so reliable. Therefore the breakdown product of serotonin, 5-hydroxy-indolacetic acid (5-HIAA), is measured over 24 h in the urine. For non-secretors, a raised chromogranin A can be a suspicious sign but normally a mass lesion must be identified.

LOCALIZATION

Unless the patient presents with a mass lesion it may be possible to identify that a patient has a tumor but not its site. The tumors can be small and isodense with surrounding tissue. The mainstay of localization is the computed tomography (CT) scan and for the pancreas a 3–5 m slice triple phase CT should be considered. If liver lesions are suspected then magnetic resonance imaging (MRI) may have a role in isodense tumors. In the pancreas, endoscopic ultrasound has a high sensitivity[4] and also allows for biopsy. If these investigations are unhelpful then somatostatin scintigraphy should be used but in insulinomas only 50% may be positive. In mid and hind-gut tumors often only the metastatic tumors are found with the primaries having involuted or remaining occult.

STAGING

In most neuroendocrine tumors the presence or absence of liver disease is important, therefore triple phase spiral CT of the upper abdomen should be performed. We would recommend the next test should be a whole-body ^{111}In-octreotide scan with tomography of the upper abdomen to help delineate tumors around the liver and spleen (Fig. 14E.1). If any unexpected sites of tumor are found these should be further investigated with CT or other imaging as appropriate. Bone scintigraphy may help stage bone disease but may be less sensitive than ^{111}In-octreotide imaging as it will not identify bone marrow infiltration. In foregut tumors there is evidence that 2-[^{18}F]fluoro-2-deoxy-D-glucose (^{18}F-FDG) positron emission tomography (PET) may be of use[5] especially if the tumors are ^{111}In-octreotide negative. PET using ^{18}F-DOPA and ^{68}Ga-DOTA octreotate has also shown promise.[6,7]

RESTAGING

Many neuroendocrine tumors show intense desmoplastic response to injury, therefore the use of radiologically based imaging to measure response is limited. If the patient has a complete response to treatment, a rare occurrence, then

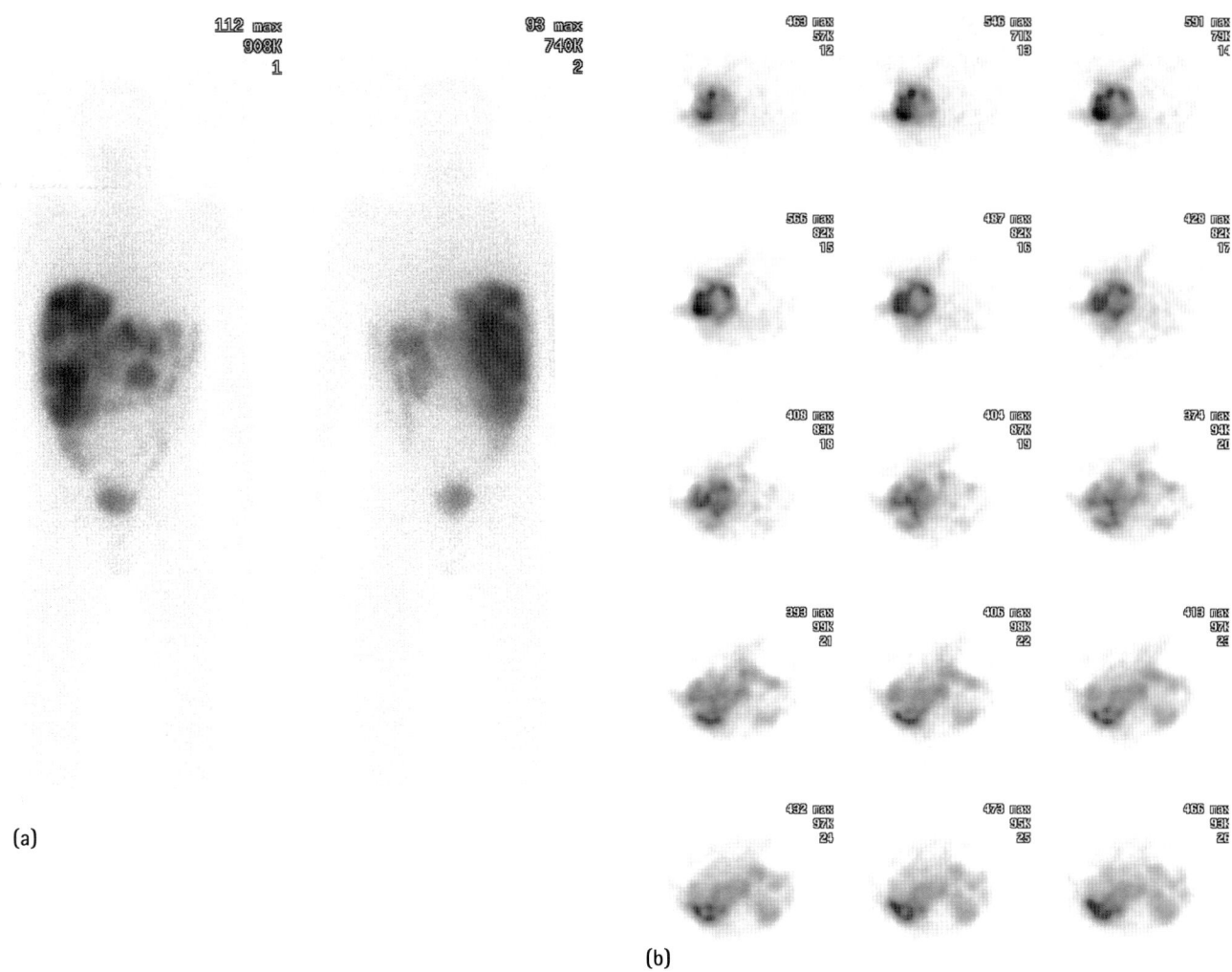

(a)

(b)

Figure 14E.1 *(a) Whole-body images of a patient with a malignant gastrinoma showing activity primarily in the tumor within the liver. (b) Transaxial tomographic slices through the liver allowing the site and extent of the liver tumor to be more clearly seen.*

anatomical imaging is more valuable. However, the complex nature of the tumor, containing both the cancer cells and fibrosis, normally means that radiological imaging may be of limited use. Normally in nuclear medicine we would look at PET techniques. The problem with neuroendocrine tumors is that the majority have little or no uptake of ^{18}F-FDG, the most commonly available PET pharmaceutical. This means that semiquantitative methods using single photon emission computed tomography (SPECT) have proven to be the most useful method in monitoring tumor response.[8]

RADIONUCLIDES USED FOR IMAGING

meta-Iodobenzylguanidine

Radioiodinated MIBG has been used for imaging neuroendocrine tumors for over 20 years.[9] Uptake is dependent on the expression of the *VMAT1* and *VMAT2* genes. These are expressed in most cells of neural crest origin. The technique used in imaging neuroendocrine tumors differs little from that used for other types of tumor imaging. Up to 300 MBq of ^{123}I-MIBG or 70 MBq of ^{131}I-MIBG can be administered. The patient's thyroid should be blocked with potassium iodide for 1 day before and 4 days after the procedure. With ^{123}I-MIBG, imaging can be performed up to 48 h and with ^{131}I-MIBG, up to 7 days. The normal distribution of the agent includes liver, heart, some lung and gut uptake as well as free iodine in the salivary glands. Image quality may appear poor (Fig. 14E.2), but this is due to high levels of background activity and may be assisted by the use of SPECT. The rates of positivity for MIBG imaging in most neuroendocrine tumors appears to be about 60%. Whilst this means it is not sufficient to use for staging, it will determine whether the patient's tumor will be likely to respond to high activities of therapeutic ^{131}I-MIBG. There are some drugs that interfere with the uptake of MIBG and these should be stopped if possible prior to imaging or therapy.[10]

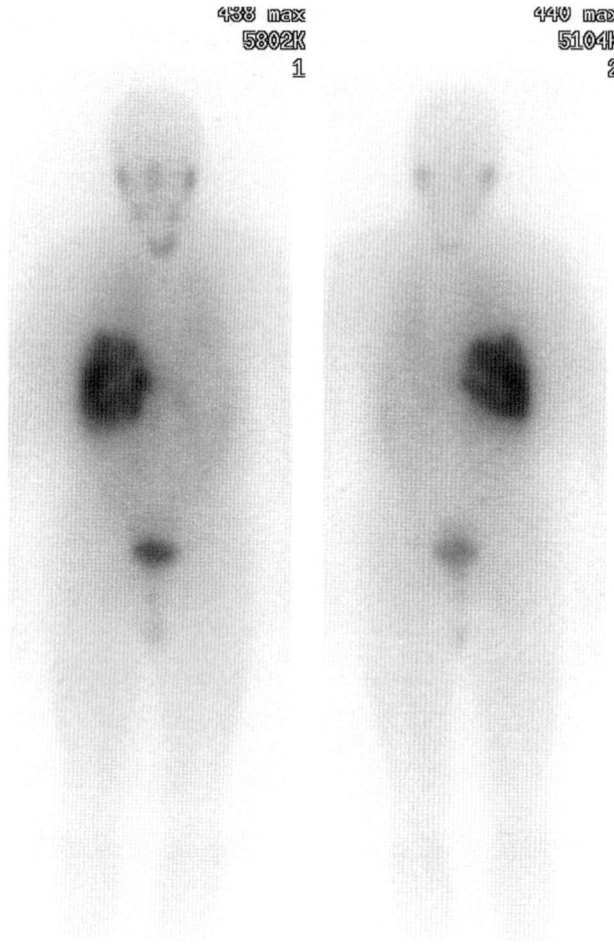

Figure 14E.2 *Whole-body* meta-[¹²³I]iodobenzylguanidine (¹²³I-MIBG) image showing a patient with carcinoid metastases in the right lobe of the liver, note the background activity is greater than with the* ¹¹¹*In-octreotide image (Fig. 14E.1).*

¹¹¹In–octreotide

¹¹¹In-octreotide has high affinity for the type-2 somatostatin receptor, which is over-expressed in most neuroendocrine tumors. Patient preparation is important as patients receiving somatostatin analogs as a treatment for their neuroendocrine tumor may find that uptake of the radiolabeled version is blocked by the administration of the cold therapeutic peptide. If the patient is taking subcutaneous octreotide then this should be stopped, if possible, for 24 h before the injection of ¹¹¹In-octreotide and for 6 h afterwards. It may not be possible to stop the treatment in very symptomatic patients. Imaging whilst still receiving cold octreotide can then occur. Those patients on long-acting analogs such Sandostatin LAR® and lanreotide should be imaged once they have been stabilized on at least 3 months of treatment. However, it may be noted that if all the receptors are saturated then the tumor may not be seen on scintigraphy.

Table 14E.1 *Reported positivities of* ¹¹¹*In-octreotide imaging in different neuroendocrine tumors*

Tumor type	Positivity (%)
Pancreatic neuroendocrine	75–100 (except for insulinomas 50–60)
Carcinoid	86–95
Small-cell lung cancer	80–100
Medullary cell thyroid cancer	65–70
Pheochromocytoma, paraganglioma, and neuroblastomas	85

Patients should be imaged with up to 300 MBq of ¹¹¹In-octreotide up to 48 h post-injection. In the earlier images performed up to 12 h, renal and urinary activity may be present and later there may be colonic and gallbladder activity. Thyroid, and to a lesser extent thymic, and pituitary activity are variable and should not be confused with pathology. We would recommend whole-body imaging at each time point. As all neuroendocrine tumors can metastasize to the skeleton this should be performed from head to feet (Plate 14E.1). SPECT should always be performed in the upper abdomen as other sites of physiological uptake include the liver, spleen, and kidneys. Therefore, smaller lesions in the pancreas or para-aortic lymph nodes may be more clearly appreciated with the inclusion of SPECT. In our experience SPECT is also very useful in the head and may help to localize lesions for correlation of images with CT and MRI in the chest and pelvis. Some camera systems now combine SPECT with CT enabling both sets of images to be performed simultaneously.

Up to 90% of patients with neuroendocrine tumors will be positive for ¹¹¹In-octreotide[11] (Table 14E.1), the caveat being in insulinoma where the low uptake of ¹¹¹In-octreotide may be related to little or no expression of somatostatin-2 receptors as well as the small size of the tumors, which may be less than 10 mm.

The role of these agents is primarily for staging. However, it is also possible to use these agents to help determine treatment either with somatostatin analogs but also with radio-labeled versions. Over the past 5 years therapeutic options using either high activity ¹¹¹In , ⁹⁰Y or ¹⁷⁷Lu have been developed and positivity on the ¹¹¹In-octreotide scan is essential before treatment can be given.

Other peptide systems

Although not used regularly clinically, other peptides have been shown to be valuable in neuroendocrine tumors. These have been based on the wish to produce a ⁹⁹ᵐTc-labeled octreotide such as ⁹⁹ᵐTc-HYNICTATE, which has been shown to have a high affinity for neuroendocrine

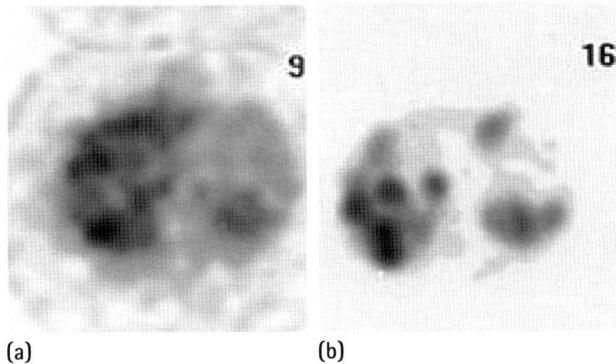

(a)   (b)

Figure 14E.3 *(a) Transverse tomographic meta-[^{123}I]iodobenzyl-guanidine (^{123}I-MIBG) slice through the liver showing multiple metastases in both right and left lobes. (b) Transverse tomographic ^{111}In-octreotide slice at the same level as Fig. 14E.4(a), again showing uptake in liver metastases but with a different distribution than that seen in Fig. 14E.4(a), showing some tumors have uptake of both tracers and some, one or other of the tracers used, suggesting three subpopulations of cells are present in the same patient.*

tumors. Alternatively, other peptides such as ^{99m}Tc-depreotide, normally used for non-small cell lung cancer, can also be used to image somatostatin recepetor positive tumors. This may have more action against subtypes 3 and 5 than ^{111}In-octreotide.[12] Radiolabeled gastrins have been shown to localize in some pancreatic and gut neuroendocrine tumors, although the relationship between gastrin and somatostatin receptors is less clearly understood. None of these agents are likely to be in routine clinical use in neuroendocrine tumors for the next few years.

meta-Iodobenzylguanidine or somatostatin imaging

It would appear from the published literature that there is no competition; ^{111}In-octreotide images are of higher quality than that seen on MIBG imaging and the sensitivity for tumor detection is higher.[13] However, within these broad statements lies a different truth. It would appear that not all patients imaged with these agents present receptors for one of both of these agents on all their cells. There appears to be a nonhomogeneous phenotypic expression of these receptors and this can be seen in some patients where there are some lesions which localize only ^{111}In-octreotide or only ^{123}I-MIBG and some which localize both (Fig. 14E.3).[14] It seems that ^{111}In-octreotide will usually be superior to ^{123}I-MIBG but in our experience a significant minority of patients have tumors that only localize ^{123}I-MIBG. This may have a crucial bearing on treatment as ^{131}I-MIBG can only be expected to treat the tumors which are positive for that agent and if the patients have multiple lesions, some of which are positive for MIBG and some for ^{111}In-octreotide, combinations of treatments may be needed.

Dimercaptosuccinic acid

Although ^{99m}Tc(V)-labeled dimercaptosuccinic acid (DMSA) has a high sensitivity for medullary cell carcinoma of the thyroid[15] its role in other forms of neuroendocrine tumors remains unproven.

Radionuclides for bone scanning

As with any tumor that metastasizes to the skeleton it may be possible to identify bone metastases in neuroendocrine tumors with ^{99m}Tc-diphosphonate bone scans, although in early disease the ^{111}In- octreotide scan may detect metastases in the bone earlier than the bone scan alone.

THERAPY

Non-nuclear methods

There is only one proven treatment in the cure of neuroendocrine tumor and that is surgery, with a high success rate in small, non-metastatic panreatic lesions and in appendicular carcinoids. All other forms or treatment are palliative. Therefore, before any treatment is initiated, it is essential that the medical team and the patient understand that the treatment is palliative only and that its aim is directed towards the alleviation of symptoms such as pain or flushing.

Chemotherapy and radiotherapy

Generally, these techniques have little place in the treatment of the disseminated neuroendocrine tumor. Small-field radiotherapy may help in the treatment of a single painful bone metastasis. Chemotherapy has a poor response rate except in fore-gut carcinoids (including those of pancreatic origin) where streptozocin-based regimes have proved to have a response rate of close to 50%.[16]

Biotherapy

The main treatment method in neuroendocrine tumors has been the use of biotherapy, normally based on somatostatin analogs. These may be given either as a short-term subcutaneous injection, maybe three to four times a day, or in one of the two long-acting preparations Sandostatin LAR and lanreotide autogel.[17] Both of the latter allow injections every 3–4 weeks. The addition of interferon may help reduce tumor size but many patients cannot tolerate the side effects.

Embolization

As most metastases are within the liver and the liver has a joint blood supply, it may be possible to treat liver metastases

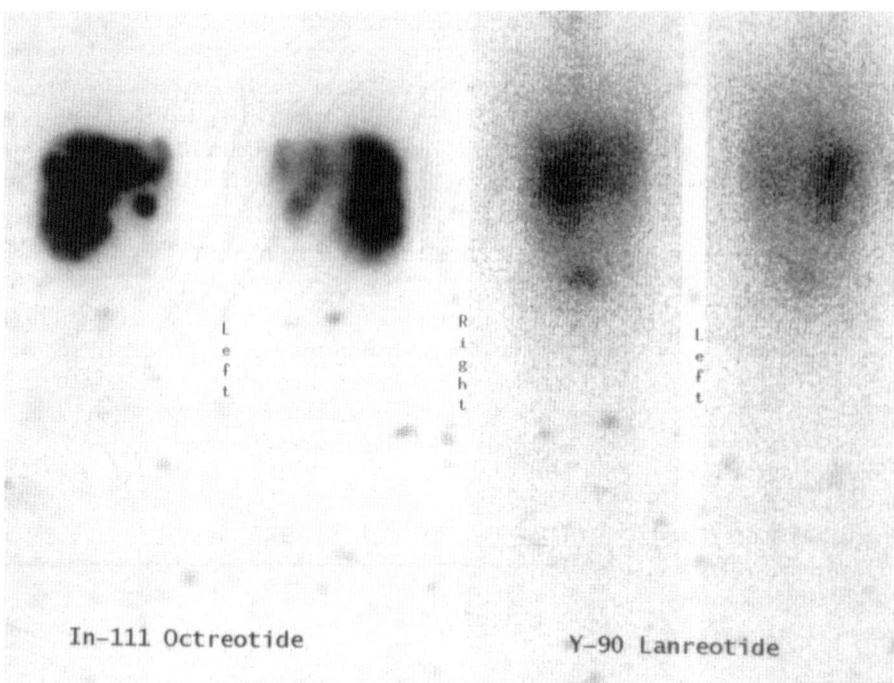

In-111 Octreotide   Y-90 Lanreotide

Figure 14E.4 *Whole-body imaging of a patient with disseminated carcinoid in the liver and left adrenal gland. The post-therapy Bremsstrahlung image shows similar uptake in the liver. (a) ^{111}In-octreotide; (b) ^{90}Y-lanreotide.*

with trans-arterial embolization techniques. The tumors are fed by the hepatic artery and the normal liver by the portal vein. Particle or gel-foam embolization can result in a significant reduction in liver disease load and may be combined with chemotherapy in fore-gut tumors.

Radionuclide therapy

Because of the failure of other treatment forms and the uptake of functional agents such as MIBG and somatostatin agents there have been attempts to treat neuroendocrine tumors with radionuclide therapy either on its own or in combination with other techniques.

meta-IODOBENZYLGUANIDINE

Although only 60% of neuroendocrine tumors show uptake of MIBG, where there is specific uptake it should be considered for treatment. There are a few reported trials[18–20] but most suggest that about 50% of patients either have some reduction in tumor bulk or at least reduction in symptoms such as flushing and diarrhea. The normal activities given include single high activities of 11 GBq of ^{131}I-MIBG or more, to three or more doses of 2.7 GBq over a 6-month period. As with imaging it is important that all drugs interfering with MIBG uptake are stopped. The patient should be well hydrated and started on iodide or perchlorate to protect their thyroid. Administration normally occurs in a specially prepared room and the patient will need to stay there until activity drops to the safe maximum for discharge home. When the retained activity is calculated at about 1 GBq the patient is imaged to demonstrate tumor localization. Side effects are normally trivial with some nausea in the first 2–3 days. This may be treated as required or by giving a prophylactic anti-emetic such as domperidone. There has been less reported bone marrow toxicity than seen with children and there is no maximum tolerated dose. However, both temporary and persistent bone marrow and renal toxicity have been noted.

RADIOPEPTIDE THERAPY

The ability of these tumors to concentrate radiopeptides directed towards the somatostatin type 2 receptor have resulted in attempts to treat tumors with therapeutic radiopeptides. The first such treatment depended on the Auger electron emitted from ^{111}In and therefore high activities (e.g. 7 GBq) were given on a frequent basis with some reasonable therapeutic response and minimal toxicity.[21,22] The use of DOTA linking meant that it was possible to chelate ^{90}Y to octreotide and later octreotate. Early studies with up to 4.4 GBq of ^{90}Y-octreotide showed about 50% of patients had a significant therapeutic response but renal toxicity was observed.[23] The renal damage was due to binding of the ^{90}Y-octreotide to the renal tubules. This binding can be reduced significantly by co-administration of lysine-containing amino acid solutions.[24] Various phase II trials have been performed and reported but as yet no phase III trial. Although a pure beta emitter, it is possible to use Bremsstrahlung imaging to identify localization (Fig. 14E. 4). Once the kidney is protected, bone marrow toxicity remains dose limiting and occurs mainly in those patients pre-treated with chemotherapy.

Table 14E.2 *Physical characteristics of the main isotopes used or proposed in treatment of neuroendocrine tumors*

Parameter	^{111}In	^{90}Y	^{177}Lu
Type of radiation	Auger electrons, gamma	Beta radiation	Beta, gamma
Therapeutic range	10 mm	12 mm	0.2 mm
Half-life (h)	64	67	106
Chelator	DTPA	DOTA	DOTA
Renal protection needed	No	Yes	Yes
Typical activity (GBq/cycle)	5	4.4	5.5

Recently, there have been attempts to vary the radiopharmaceutical, with ^{177}Lu being a viable alternative as the beta range is less than that with ^{90}Y (Table 14E.2).[25] Alternatively, variations on the peptide chain such as substituting lanreotide for octreotide have also been suggested with similar results but without the renal toxicity problems.[26] Future directions will result in specially designed radiopeptides for therapy of specific tumor types.

DOUBLE TARGETING

As most patients with metastatic neuroendocrine have disease within the liver and commonly only the liver, it may be more logical to direct treatment into the liver to treat the tumor at this site only, producing effectively a radionuclide version of chemoembolization. Although this approach is new it has been tried with ^{131}I-Lipiodol, ^{90}Y-impregnated resin beads and ^{90}Y-lanreotide. Early results are encouraging although much further work will be needed to verify this approach.

CONCLUSION

Nuclear medicine has developed a key role in the management of patients with neuroendocrine tumors and may be involved in the process from diagnosis, staging, therapeutics to re-staging. This role will expand as new agents become available and provide a model for the use of nuclear medicine in other tumor groups.

REFERENCES

1 Caplin ME, Buscombe JR, Hilson AJ, *et al.* Carcinoid tumour. *Lancet* 1998; **352**: 799–805.

2 O'Connor DT, Deftos LJ. Secretion of chromogranin A by peptide-producing endocrine neoplasms. *N Engl J Med* 1986; **314**: 1145–51.

3 Kolby L, Bernhardt P, Levin-Jakobsen AM, *et al.* Uptake of meta-iodobenzylguanidine in neuroendocrine tumours is mediated by vesicular monoamine transporters. *Br J Cancer* 2003; **89**: 1383–8.

4 Fidler JL, Johnson CD. Imaging of neuroendocrine tumors of the pancreas. *Int J Gastrointest Cancer* 2001; **30**: 73–85.

5 Adams S, Baum R, Rink T, *et al.* Limited value of fluorine-18 fluorodeoxyglucose positron emission tomography for the imaging of neuroendocrine tumours. *Eur J Nucl Med* 1998; **25**: 79–83.

6 Hoegerle S, Schneider B, Kraft A, *et al.* Imaging of a metastatic gastrointestinal carcinoid by F-18-DOPA positron emission tomography. *Nuklearmedizin* 1999; **38**: 127–30.

7 Hofmann M, Maecke H, Borner R, *et al.* Biokinetics and imaging with the somatostatin receptor PET radioligand (68)Ga-DOTATOC: preliminary data. *Eur J Nucl Med* 2001; **28**: 1751–7.

8 Gopinath G, Ahmed A, Buscombe JR, *et al.* Prediction of clinical outcome in treated neuroendocrine tumours of carcinoid type using functional volumes on ^{111}In-pentetreotide SPECT imaging. *Nucl Med Commun* 2004; **25**: 253–7.

9 Fischer M, Kamanabroo D, Sonderkamp H, Proske T. Scintigraphic imaging of carcinoid tumours with ^{131}I-metaiodobenzylguanidine. *Lancet* 1984; **2**: 165.

10 Hoefnagel CA, Schornagel J, Valdes Olmos RA. ^{131}I metaiodobenzylguanidine therapy of malignant pheochromocytoma: interference of medication. *J Nucl Biol Med* 1991; **35**: 308–12.

11 Krenning EP, Kwekkeboom DJ, Bakker WH, *et al.* Somatostatin receptor scintigraphy with [^{111}In-DTPA-D-Phe1]- and [^{123}I-Tyr3]-octreotide: the Rotterdam experience with more than 1000 patients. *Eur J Nucl Med* 1993; **20**: 716–31.

12 Menda Y, Kahn D. Somatostatin receptor imaging of non-small cell lung cancer with ^{99m}Tc depreotide. *Semin Nucl Med* 2002; **32**: 92–6.

13 Ramage JK, Williams R, Buxton-Thomas M. Imaging secondary neuroendocrine tumours of the liver: comparison of I123 metaiodobenzylguanidine (MIBG) and In111-labelled octreotide (Octreoscan). *QJM* 1996; **89**: 539–42.

14 Buscombe JR, Gopinath G. Neuroendocrine tumours part 1: the role of nuclear medicine in imaging neuroendocrine tumours. *World J Nucl Med* 2003; **2**: 232–40.

15 Clarke S, Lazarus C, Maisey M. Experience in imaging medullary thyroid carcinoma using ^{99m}Tc(V) dimercaptosuccinic acid (DMSA). *Henry Ford Hosp Med J* 1989; **37**: 167–8.

16 Oberg K. Chemotherapy and biotherapy in the treatment of neuroendocrine tumours. *Ann Oncol* 2001; **12(Suppl 2)**: S111–14.

17 Garland J, Buscombe JR, Bouvier C, *et al.* Sandostatin LAR (long-acting octreotide acetate) for malignant

carinoid syndrome: a 3-year experience. *Aliment Pharmacol Ther* 2003; **17**: 437–44.

18   Taal BG, Hoefnagel CA, Valdes Olmos RA, *et al.* Palliative effect of metaiodobenzylguanidine in metastatic carcinoid tumors. *J Clin Oncol* 1996; **14**: 1829–38.

19   Mukherjee JJ, Kaltsas GA, Islam N, *et al.* Treatment of metastatic carcinoid tumours, pheochromocytoma, paraganglioma, and medullary carcinoma of the thyroid with ^{131}I-meta-iodobenzylguanidine (^{131}I-mIBG). *Clin Endocrinol* 2001; **55**: 47–60.

20   Bomanji JB, Wong W, Gaze MN, *et al.* Treatment of neuroendocrine tumours in adults with ^{131}I-MIBG therapy. *Clin Oncol* 2003; **15**: 193–8.

21   Capello A, Krenning EP, Breeman WA, *et al.* Peptide receptor radionuclide therapy in vitro using [^{111}In-DTPA[0]]octreotide. *J Nucl Med* 2003; **44**: 98–104.

22   Buscombe JR, Caplin ME, Hilson AJW. Long-term efficacy of high-activity ^{111}In-pentetreotide therapy in patients with disseminated neuroendocrine tumours. *J Nucl Med* 2003; **44**: 1–6.

23   Otte A, Herrmann R, Heppeler A, *et al.* Yttrium-90 DOTATOC: first clinical results. *Eur J Nucl Med* 1999; **26**: 1439–47.

24   Bushnell D, Menda Y, O'Dorisio T, *et al.* Effects of intravenous amino acid administration with Y-90 DOTA-Phe1-Tyr3-octreotide (SMT487OctreoTher) treatment. *Cancer Biother Radiopharm* 2004; **19**: 35–41.

25   Kwekkeboom DJ, Bakker WH, Kam BL, *et al.* Treatment of patients with gastro-entero-pancreatic (GEP) tumours with the novel radiolabelled somatostatin analogue [^{177}Lu-DOTA(0),Tyr3]octreotate. *Eur J Nucl Med Mol Imaging* 2003; **30**: 417–22.

26   Virgolini I, Britton K, Buscombe J, *et al.* In- and Y-DOTA-lanreotide: results and implications of the MAURITIUS trial. *Semin Nucl Med* 2002; **32**: 148–55.

15

Hepatobiliary disease: Primary and metastatic liver tumors

ROLAND HUSTINX AND OLIVIER DETRY

Introduction	661	Liver metastases	666
Hepatocellular carcinoma	661	References	670
Cholangiocarcinoma	665		

INTRODUCTION

Malignant tumors are often found in the liver, which is the solid organ most frequently invaded by metastases from solid tumors, especially those arising in the gastrointestinal tract. Moreover, the incidence of primary hepatic malignancies has been increasing along with the progressing incidence of cirrhosis, both in the western and eastern worlds. Hepatocellular carcinoma (HCC) is now the fifth most common cancer worldwide,[1] and intra- or extrahepatic cholangiocarcinomas (CCs) are also more often diagnosed with the improvement of the means of detection.

The time is long gone since liver scintigraphy using radiolabeled albumin derivatives was the most popular noninvasive method for imaging liver tumors. The advent of ultrasonography (US), computed tomography (CT) and magnetic resonance imaging (MRI) has dramatically improved the oncological evaluation of the liver. These advances have further accelerated in recent years, with the development of fast, high-resolution helical multislice CTs or tissue-specific contrast agents for MRI. Nevertheless, we shall see in this chapter that there is still an important role for nuclear medicine techniques in the assessment of liver tumor involvement. Most if not all of the recent progress relates to positron emission tomography (PET), even though SPECT agents such as ^{111}In-pentetreotide are very useful in selected clinical indications.

HEPATOCELLULAR CARCINOMA

HCC ranks third among the cancer-related deaths worldwide.[1] Its incidence has increased in the United States over the past two decades, from 1.4/100 000 between 1986 and 1990 to 3/100 000 between 1996 and 1998.[2] Risk factors are well known and vary according to the geographical distribution of the disease. The majority of HCC occurs in cirrhotic liver. In Europe and the United States, hepatitis C virus (HCV) infection and alcohol abuse are the primary predisposing factors for cirrhosis and HCC. In Asia, hepatitis B virus (HBV) infection is a more frequent cause of cirrhosis. The incidence of HCC is expected to continue to increase, as a consequence of further exposure to hepatitis C virus.[2]

Various HCC staging systems co-exist, none of them being unanimously accepted. These systems were recently thoroughly reviewed and discussed by Befeler and Di Disceglie.[3] Diverse parameters are considered, such as the number of lesions and their size, the underlying hepatic function and the plasma level of α-fetoprotein (AFP). Prognosis of HCC patients depends on both the stage of the cancerous disease and the degree of cirrhotic liver failure at diagnosis. Long-term survival may reach 93% in the best situation, that is in patients with unique and centimetric HCC, preserved liver function and who are treated by surgery.[4] On the other hand, patients diagnosed with inoperable, advanced HCC and severe liver failure (Child B or C) have a 3-year survival rate of only 8%.[5] Curative HCC treatment options include liver transplantation, surgical resection, radio-frequency ablation, and percutaneous ethanol injection.[3] Palliation may be obtained in advanced HCC with preserved liver function by transarterial embolization or chemoembolization.

Cross-sectional imaging procedures play a key role in the diagnosis and staging of HCC. Liver US remains extensively used for screening, but developments in CT and MRI techniques have considerably modified the work-up of the disease. Triple phase CT (non-enhanced, arterial phase, portal phase) performed with helical, multislice devices is effective at detecting large lesions but its sensitivity remains limited for diagnosing small lesions (<2 cm)[6]. MRI is increasingly used, with a relatively high accuracy but there is a high variability in the appearance of HCC on both the T1- and the T2-weighted images.[7] Newer contrast agents such as the superparamagnetic iron oxide may be useful for grading HCC but they are not superior to gadolinium-based agents for diagnosis.[8] It is generally considered that 20–30% of the lesions are missed by all imaging techniques, and this figure increases as the size of the lesions diminishes.[1,7]

Fluorodeoxyglucose positron emission tomography imaging

Initial fluorodeoxyglucose positron emission tomography (FDG PET) studies were conducted using dynamic imaging and calculation of dynamic rate constants. Determination of microparameters was felt important because of the particularities of liver and HCC metabolism. In contrast with other organs, the liver is characterized by relatively high concentrations of glucose-6-phosphatase, an enzyme that dephosphorylates intracellular FDG-6-phosphate and thus allows leakage of the tracer from the cells. In HCC, the glyconeogenesis decreases and the glycolysis increases following malignant transformation.[9,10] Glycolytic rate, and hexokinase activity, may thus vary according to tumor grade. On the other hand, histopathological studies have shown low expression of the glucose transporter GLUT-1 in the majority of HCC.[11,12] Using a three-compartment model and dynamic imaging, Torizuka et al. showed high k_3 values, reflecting high hexokinase activity, in high grade lesions. k_4 values, corresponding to tracer efflux, were variable, with lower k_4/k_3 ratios in high-grade lesions.[13] Okazumi et al. also showed a high variability in k_4 values, with approximately 45% of HCC displaying similar values to the normal liver, whereas in metastases from other cancers it was virtually zero.[14] These preliminary results suggested that PET could distinguish HCC from other liver tumors but also characterize the degree of differentiation of the lesions. Recent investigations further support these results. Lee et al. correlated tumor uptake, as measured using the standardized uptake value (SUV) with the gene expression profiles of 10 HCCs.[15] They found that lesions with high FDG uptake also expressed molecular markers associated with tumor spread and aggressiveness.

Dynamic studies, however, are cumbersome and difficult to implement in a routine clinical fashion. Using visual analysis and SUV measurements, Trojan et al. found a 50% sensitivity (7/14) for detecting HCC, with increased FDG uptake associated with large tumor burden, moderate or poor differentiation and high serum levels of AFP.[16] Khan et al. similarly obtained 55% sensitivity (11/20). PET studies were evaluated using a visual analysis and 8/11 moderately or poorly differentiated lesions showed increased uptake as

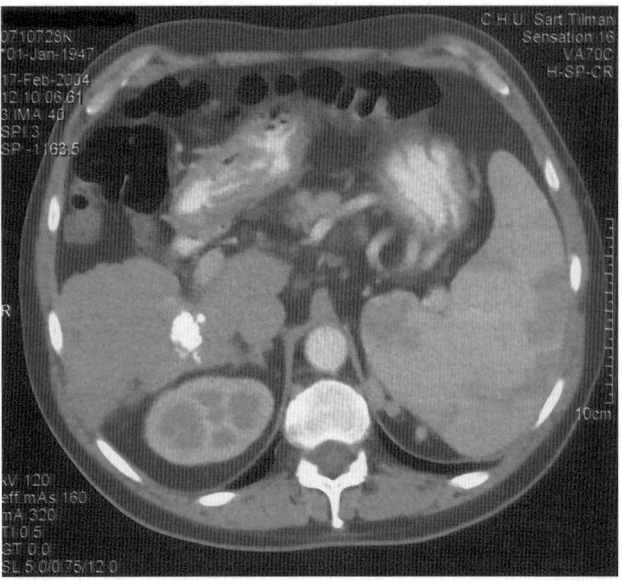

(a)

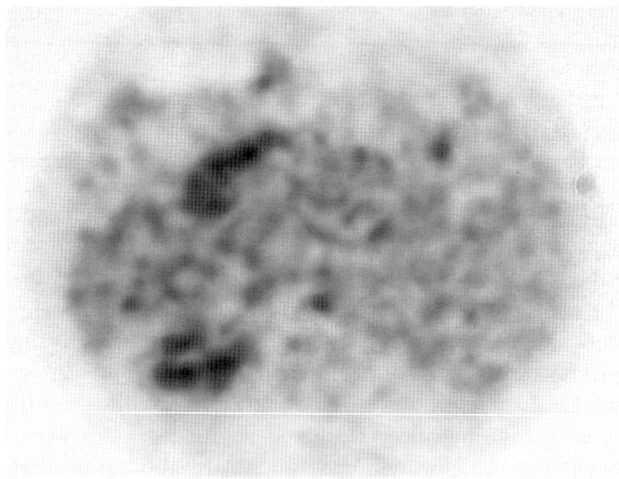

(b)

Figure 15.1 *Recurrent hepatocarcinoma, previously treated with lipiodol, visualized on computed tomography (CT) (a). There is no abnormal uptake in the liver on the fluorodeoxyglucose (FDG) positron emission tomography images (PET) (b). This was a false negative result, as surgery confirmed recurrent disease. Additionally, several centimetric lesions were discovered, which were missed by both techniques.*

compared to the surrounding liver[17] (Figs 15.1 and 15.2). The largest series to date was published in 2003 by Wudel et al.[18] The authors reported a 64% sensitivity (43/67 lesions evaluated prior to any treatment), but unfortunately the interpretation criteria of the PET studies were not detailed in the article. In 6/24 patients evaluated during follow-up, PET identified recurrent or metastatic disease. As for most cancer types, a major advantage of PET is its ability to survey the whole body and detect additional, unsuspected metastases (Fig. 15.3). Again, there was a correlation between tumor grade and FDG uptake. Overall, PET results had a

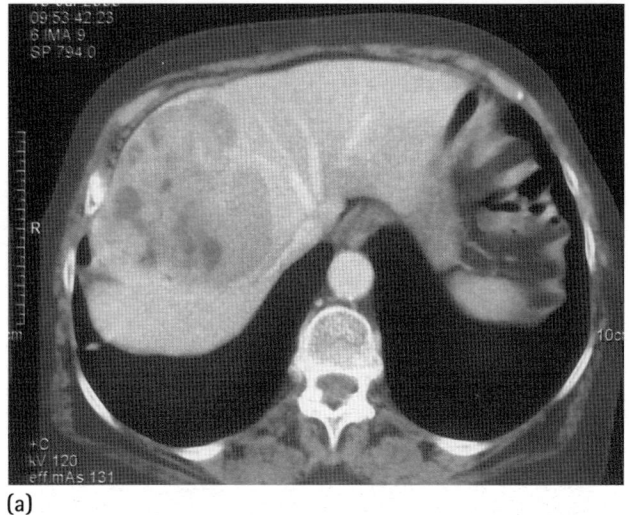

(a)

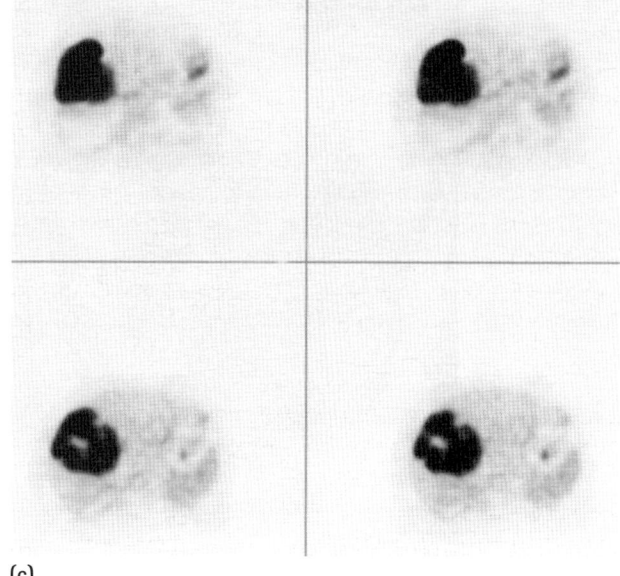

(c)

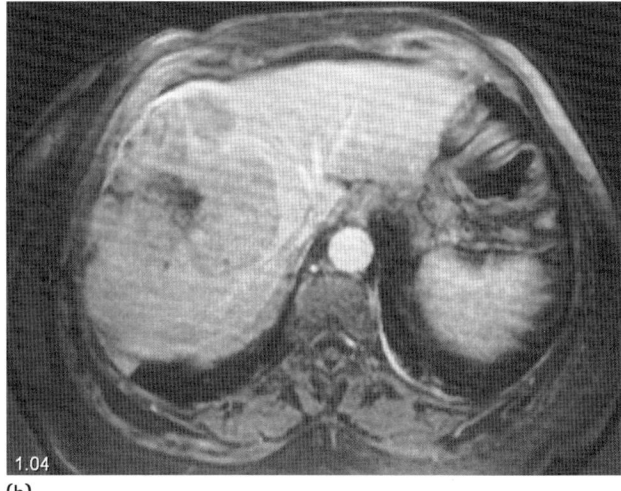

(b)

Figure 15.2   *Poorly differentiated hepatocarcinoma, in a patient without any history of cirrhosis or hepatitis. Both CT (a) and magnetic resonance imaging (b) show a large lesion in the right lobe of the liver. This lesion is highly hypermetabolic on the FDG PET study (c). (Abbreviations as in the legend to Fig. 15.1.)*

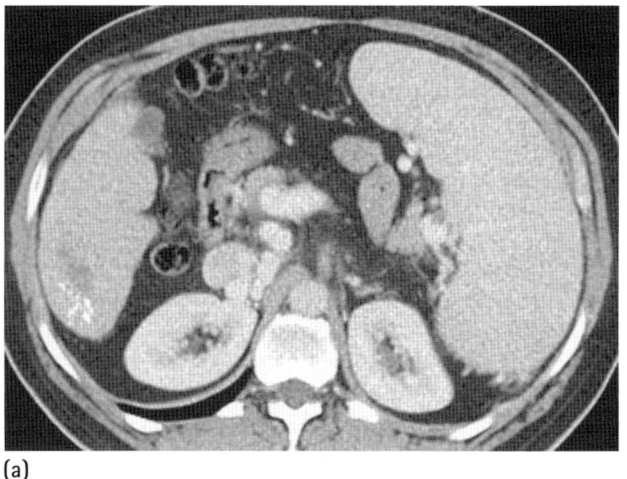

(a)

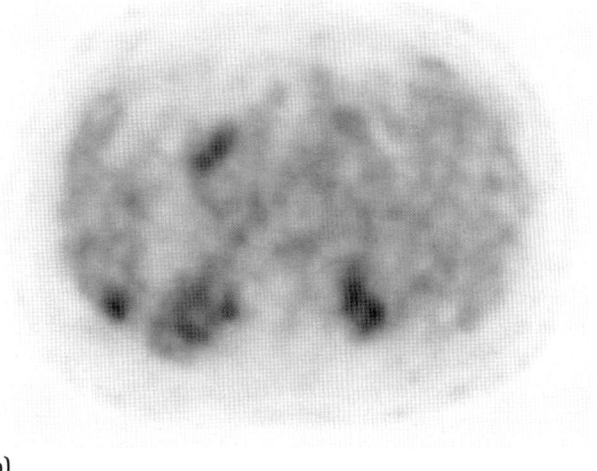

(b)

Figure 15.3   *Recurrent hepatocarcinoma, treated by surgery and intra-arterial infusion of lipiodol. The liver recurrence is clearly seen on both the CT (a) and the FDG PET images (b).*

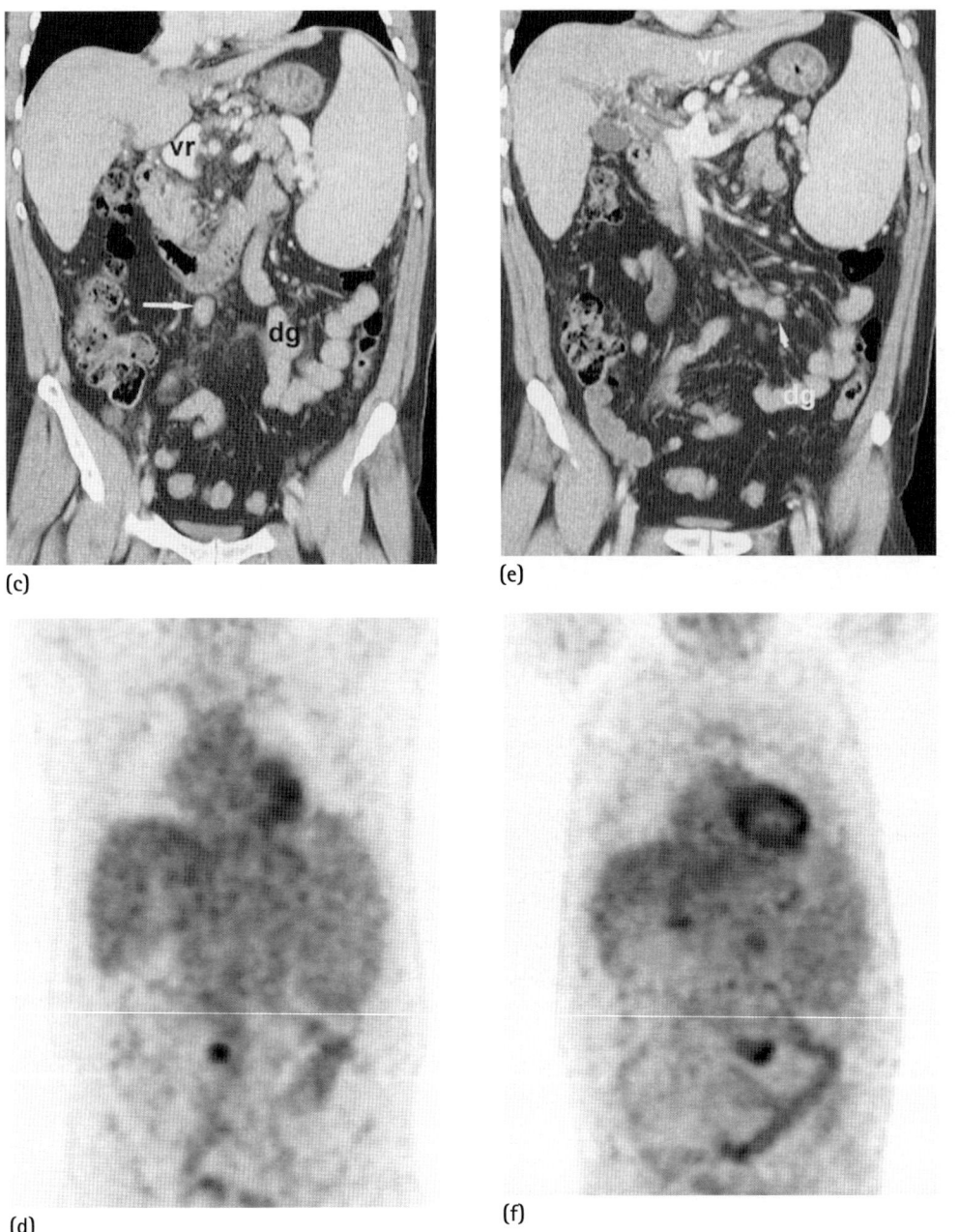

Figure 15.3 *(Continued)* *Nodal spread to the aorticocaval and mesenteric areas (white arrows on the CT images, c and e) is also identified with both PET (d and f) and CT, although the CT was initially read as negative for extrahepatic disease. The nodes are not easily distinguished from the digestive tract (dg on the CT images), whereas they clearly appear as foci of increased activity on the PET images. (Abbreviations as in the legend to Fig. 15.1.)*

clinical impact in 28% of the patients (26/91). Similar results were obtained for characterizing focal liver lesions in hepatitis B carriers with elevated AFP serum levels. PET was positive in 20/36 HCCs and negative in all 12 benign lesions.[19] The specificity of FDG PET is usually very high in the liver as very few benign lesions, apart from infectious ones, accumulate FDG. For instance, Kurtaran *et al.* reported no increased uptake in eight cases of focal nodular hyperplasia.[20] The prognostic value of FDG PET was evaluated in a series of 48 patients, most with multiple liver lesions.[21]

Interestingly, the SUV ratio (tumor to nontumor) was found to be predictive for both the cumulative survival rate and the tumor-volume doubling time, whereas the SUV was not, in either case. Iwata *et al.* also reported a correlation between the SUV ratio and the number of lesions: the median value was higher in multiple HCC than in patients with a single lesion, but the SUVs were comparable in both groups.[22]

Results were disappointing when PET was performed as a screening tool for occult HCC in patients with end-stage liver disease. In two series of eight and 25 patients, respectively,

Table 15.1 *Fluorodeoxyglucose positron emission tomography for diagnosing cholangiocarcinoma*

Reference	Date	Patients	Sensitivity	Specificity	Method of analysis
34	1998	21	100% (6/6)	100% (15/15)	Patlak
37	2001	15	77% (10/13)	0% (0/2)	Visual and activity ratios
74	2001	54	92% (24/26)	93% (26/28)	Visual > activity ratios > SUV
35	2003	21	57% (12/21)	NA	SUV_{max} (cut-off value of 4)
36	2004	36	61% (19/31)	80% (4/5)	Visual
Pooled data		147	73% (71/97)	90% (45/50)	

SUV, standardized uptake value.

PET failed to identify any of the HCCs diagnosed with other techniques (two and nine, respectively).[23,24]

PET imaging with other tracers

Few data are available and the use of these tracers remains limited to a small number of research centers. For instance, pharmacokinetic studies were performed using PET with ^{11}C-ethanol in patients with HCC and who were considered for treatment with percutaneous ethanol injection.[25] Such studies provided useful information as regard to the drug distribution, and may help treatment planning. Similarly, dynamic PET with ^{13}N-ammonia can assess the arterial blood flow of primary and metastatic liver tumors, which may in turn help to characterize the lesions and possibly contribute to assess the effects of treatment.[26]

SPECT imaging

The advent of US, CT and MR has rendered obsolete the use of colloid liver scintigraphy in oncology. Several attempts were made using alternative single photon emission computed tomography (SPECT) tracers to characterize focal liver lesions that remained questionable following CT or MRI. Two studies reported encouraging results with ^{201}Tl and ^{99m}Tc-colloid SPECT. The latter was used to identify the lesions, which appeared as photophenic areas. HCCs showed increased ^{201}Tl uptake in these areas, as compared to the surrounding liver.[27,28] Only 20 patients were studied however, and these initial results were not further confirmed. SPECT with ^{99m}Tc-methoxyisobutylisonitrile (MIBI) or ^{99m}Tc-tetrofosmin showed a sensitivity ranging from 9 to 44%.[29–32] A total of 87 patients were studied, and the highest sensitivity was found in the smallest series (eight subjects).[29] Like in other tumors, MIBI uptake was associated with the expression of the P-glycoprotein encoded by the multidrug-resistance genes (*MDR1*). In a series of 35 patients, 30 HCCs did not accumulate MIBI and showed variable expression levels of P-glycoprotein, whereas the five lesions that were seen on the SPECT studies did not express P-glycoprotein.[30] Again, these findings have yet to be confirmed in larger series.

In summary, because of its low sensitivity (about 50%), PET is not a useful screening or even diagnostic tool for HCC. However, as for other cancers, PET may survey the whole body and detect metastases not demonstrated by MRI or CT (Fig. 15.3). Moreover, as the presence and intensity of FDG uptake may be related to the HCC differentiation and grading, PET might be used in the future for HCC prognosis determination, but this hypothesis has to be further investigated.

CHOLANGIOCARCINOMA

The term 'cholangiocarcinoma' (CC) initially referred to tumors of the intrahepatic bile ducts. However, the term now includes tumors of the perihilar and distal extrahepatic bile duct as well.[33] These cancers are infrequent, slightly more in men than in women, and the majority arise in the perihilar area of the bile duct. The tumors are mostly adenocarcinomas, with a wide range of differentiation and pathological subtypes such as papillary carcinomas and mucinous carcinomas. Primary sclerosing cholangitis is an important risk factor for the development of cholangiocarcinoma. The staging system follows the TNM classification. Surgery is the only potentially curative treatment, but except for stage I disease, the prognosis is very poor. As most patients are diagnosed at an advanced stage, the overall 5-year survival does not exceed 10%.[33]

FDG PET imaging

Data regarding FDG PET imaging and cholangiocarcinoma are recent and remain relatively scarce. The available results are very encouraging, however, following the initial report from Keiding *et al.* who showed high FDG uptake in six CC lesions.[34] These data are summarized in Table 15.1. The pooled sensitivity is 73% but it greatly varies with the tumor type: hilar CCs, infiltrating lesions and mucinous tumors were poorly detected in comparison with peripheral [Ccs,35] nodular lesions,[36] and tumors of the tubular pathological type, with high cell density and limited mucin production,[37]

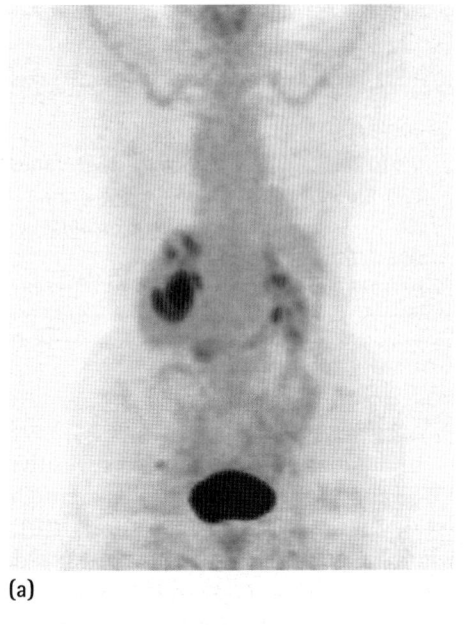

(a)

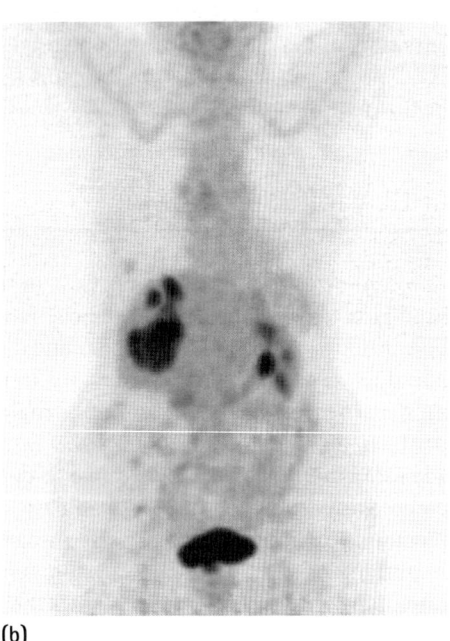

(b)

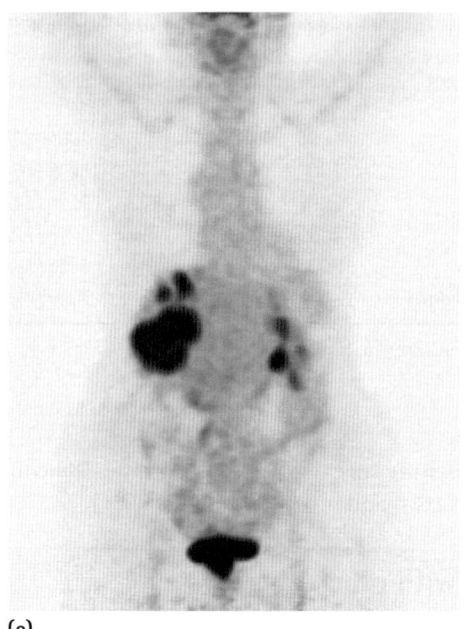

(c)

Figure 15.4 *Multifocal intrahepatic cholangiocarcinoma. Repeated FDG PET studies show slowly progressing disease, despite systemic treatment.*

respectively. In addition, PET may detect distant lesions, either nodal or organ metastases. Anderson *et al.* reported a sensitivity of 65% for metastatic disease.[36] This figure may seem low but is nonetheless clinically valuable, as these lesions were undetected according to the initial conventional staging. In this series, PET accordingly changed management in 30% of the patients. An example of CC visualized with FDG PET is shown in Fig. 15.4.

LIVER METASTASES

Virtually all malignant tumors have the potential to disseminate to the liver. The most frequent sources are colorectal,

pancreatic, breast, and lung cancers. Metastases thus represent the most frequent malignant disease of the liver, far ahead of HCC. In addition, the liver is the second most frequent site involved with metastases, following regional lymph nodes. In many cancer patients, the presence of liver involvement is a major prognostic factor, which decisively influences both the treatment options and the long-term survival. This is particularly true in colorectal cancer, as more than 50% of all patients experience metastatic spread to the liver, either at diagnosis or during the course of the disease. Metastases are confined to the liver in about 20% of the cases.[38,39] Long-term survival may be achieved through surgery, especially for colorectal carcinoma. The 5-year survival after resection ranges from 20 to 48%, with low perioperative morbidity and mortality.[40] It should be noted that the most consistent factors of poor prognosis after resection are the presence of extrahepatic disease and tumor-positive resection margins.[41] It is thus of primary importance to obtain an accurate preoperative staging, regarding both intra- and extrahepatic disease. Local tumor ablation, using radiofrequency or cryotherapy is usually performed in unresectable disease or as a complement to resection, possibly in combination with chemotherapy. Given the wide variety of available treatment modalities, and the general trend toward a greater aggressiveness and an increase in the indications for surgical resection, the question of the preoperative staging is, from a clinical perspective, highly relevant.[42] Although most data concern liver metastases from colorectal carcinoma, prolonged survival has also been reported after surgical resection of metastases from genitourinary cancers, breast carcinomas or uveal melanomas.[43]

Several imaging methods are available for intrahepatic staging. The sensitivity ranges from 57 to 100% for US, from 36 to 94% for CT and from 69 to 96% for MRI.[44] Although CT and MRI are considered to be more sensitive than US, most comparative studies failed to demonstrate any statistically significant difference between these techniques.[44] The algorithm for extrahepatic staging varies according to the primary tumor, and usually includes CT of the chest for colorectal cancers, MRI of the brain and bone scintigraphy for noncolorectal tumors.

Evaluation of liver metastases with FDG PET

The first case of liver metastasis depicted with FDG PET was reported in 1982 by Yonekura et al.[45] Since then, numerous publications have established the technique as a highly valuable tool for diagnosing liver metastases from a wide variety of cancers. In 2002 Kinkel et al. published a meta-analysis comparing the diagnostic performances of US, CT, MRI, and FDG PET in the detection of liver metastases from gastrointestinal cancers.[44] The authors analyzed 54 studies out of a total of 111, including nine dealing with US, 24 with CT, 11 with MRI, and nine with PET. Fifty-seven studies were excluded for various reasons, such as the absence of appropriate standard of reference or CT studies performed without contrast agents. The total number of patients was 686 (US), 1747 (CT), 401 (MRI) and 423 (PET). The primary tumor was colorectal in all patients studied with MRI and PET, and in 74% and 78% of the patients studied with US and CT, respectively. Considering the data with a clinically relevant specificity (superior or equal to 85%), the sensitivity (with the 95% CI) was 90% (80–97) for PET, 76% (57–91) for MRI, 72% (63–80) for CT, and 55% (41–68) for US. The difference was statistically significant between PET and CT as well as between PET and US. The authors thus concluded that, at equivalent specificity, FDG PET was the most sensitive noninvasive method for detecting liver metastases from GI tumors (Fig. 15.5). It may be argued that this meta-analysis did not take into account the most recent

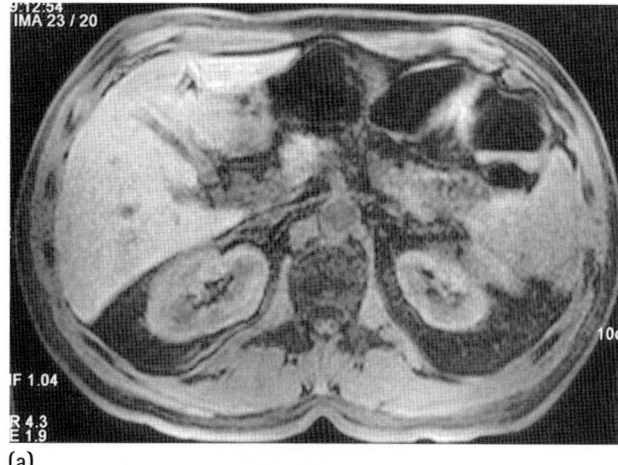

(a)

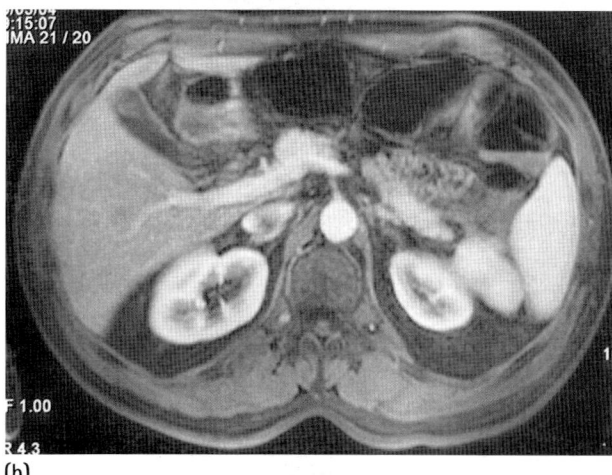

(b)

Figure 15.5 *This patient was initially diagnosed with a carcinoma of the sigmoid colon and synchronous liver metastasis. Both were treated surgically, followed by chemotherapy. Follow-up magnetic resonance imaging (Panel (a), non-enhanced T1-weighted image, and panel (b), Gd-enhanced T1-weighted image) were negative, despite increased blood levels of carcinoembryonic antigen.*

technological developments, as the most recent articles were published in 2000. However, many studies used spiral CT, and the use of superparamagnetic iron oxide enhancement was also described in several MRI articles. In addition, PET technology has also significantly evolved during the past few years, especially with the systematic use of attenuation correction, which has been shown to improve the diagnostic performances, especially in the abdominal region.[46] Interestingly enough, in spite of the wide range of publication (15 years), there was no relationship between the year of publication and the detection rate. It is somewhat surprising that the technological advances obtained during these 15 years did not translate into improved diagnostic accuracy.

Recent articles further demonstrated the excellent performances of PET for diagnosing liver metastases from colorectal cancer. In a series of 47 patients with recurrent colorectal carcinoma, the positive predictive value of PET

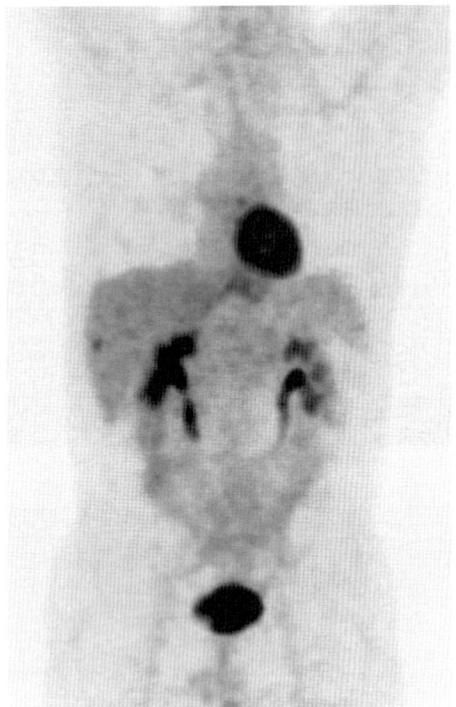

(c)

(d)

Figure 15.5 *(Continued)* *FDG PET reveals a single metastasis in the lateral aspect of the right liver lobe (panel (c), three-dimensional projection image, and panel (d), transaxial view).*

for identifying hepatic lesions was 93%, comparable to intraoperative US (IOUS, 89%) and superior to conventional cross sectional methods (CT and MR, 78%).[47] A direct comparison between PET and conventional methods was biased by the interval of time between the two studies, as CT/MR was performed 37 days on average before PET. Nevertheless, the intrahepatic staging obtained with PET was such that IOUS changed the patient's management in only one case (2%). The sensitivity was 87% for PET, which is very similar to the values reported with the most advanced MRI techniques.[48,49] Interestingly, the comparison between

IOUS and MR with various contrast agents, provided results comparable to those obtained when comparing FDG PET and IOUS. Both techniques had very similar sensitivities (87% for MR, 94% for IOUS), and the patient's management was modified by IOUS in only 4% of the cases.[50] Furthermore, a recent side by side comparison between FDG PET and MRI did not show any statistically significant difference in terms of lesion detection.[51]

The whole-body capability of FDG PET should not be overlooked, as the detection of unsuspected, extrahepatic metastases leads to significant changes in management, with a better patient selection.[52] A preoperative work-up that included PET imaging yielded higher disease-free survival rate and long-term survival after surgical resection of colorectal metastases to the liver than those reported using to conventional methods.[53] Although the test is relatively expensive, including PET in the preoperative algorithm may prove to be cost-effective, as suggested by a decision-tree sensitivity analysis in patients with rising carcino-embryonic antigen and potentially resectable disease limited to the liver.[54] FDG PET is equally effective at detecting hepatic metastases from a wide variety of tumor types, including pancreatic, gastric, and esophageal cancer.[55,56]

The clinical application of PET is not limited to the preoperative staging. Progress has been made in the development of local ablative techniques and new chemotherapy regimens are available in various cancers. Clinicians thus need to assess the response to treatment, either soon after its initiation or after completion. Follow-up is also an issue, as second-line treatments are often proposed for recurrent disease. FDG PET may be decisive in this setting, especially given the well-known limitations of conventional techniques to differentiate active tumor and treatment-related changes.[57,58] In a series of 13 patients with malignant hepatic lesions treated by radio-frequency ablation (RFA), PET correctly identified all recurrent tumors as well as new metastatic sites.[59] MRI was positive in only 43% of the cases. These results are clearly encouraging, in spite of the retrospective design of the study and the long time interval between RFA and PET scanning (9 months on average) (Fig. 15.6). Langenhoff *et al.* evaluated prospectively 56 lesions in 23 patients, treated by RFA (six cases) or cryosurgery ablation (CSA, 17 cases).[60] PET was performed within 3 weeks after treatment. During the follow-up period of 16 months, there was no local recurrence in the 51 lesions that became negative on the post-treatment scan, whereas 4/5 PET-positive lesions developed a local recurrence within 6 months. In these patients, CT became positive much later than PET, in fact months after treatment. The negative predictive value of the early postoperative PET was thus 100%, the positive predictive value 80%. The false positive result was caused by an abscess. Furthermore, PET detected additional intra- and extrahepatic lesions earlier than did CT. PET was found equally effective at evaluating the disease status after hepatic intra-arterial infusion of ^{90}Y glass microspheres[61] and for the surveillance of liver metastases

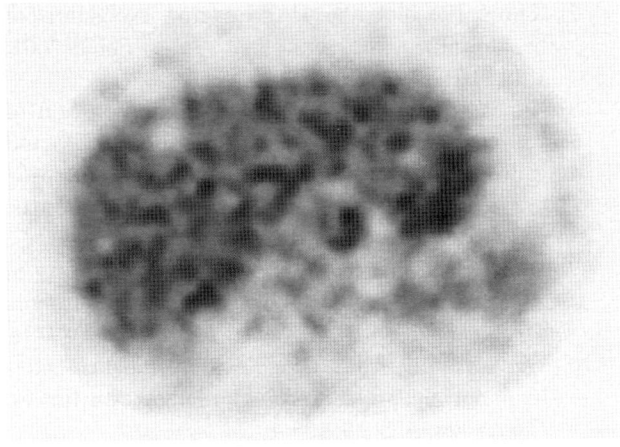

(a)

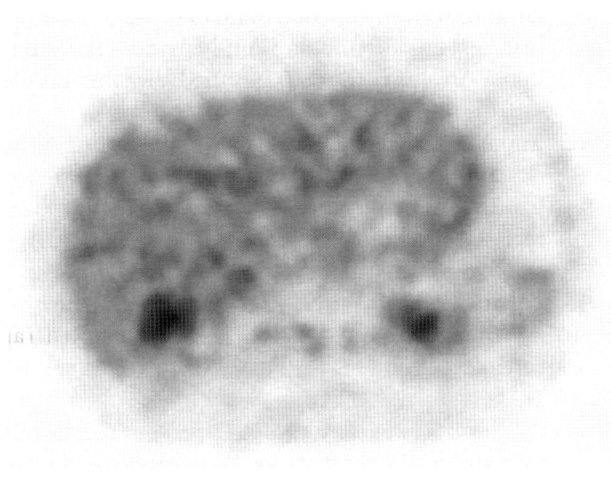

(b)

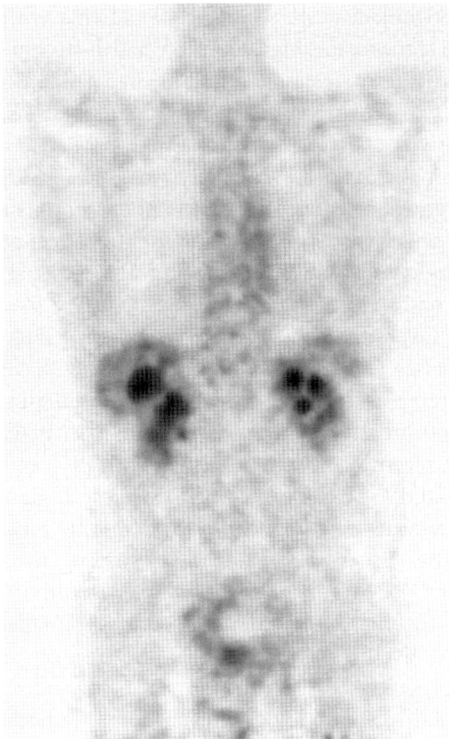

(c)

Figure 15.6 *This patient was treated by radio-frequency ablation and surgery. A follow-up FDG PET study showed the lesion treated by radio-frequency ablation as a defect (a), but a new lesion is visualized in the posterior aspect of the right liver lobe (panel (b), transaxial view, and panel (c), coronal view).*

of various origins, treated by systemic chemotherapy.[62] In a limited series, PET performed as early as 72 h after a single infusion of 5-fluorouracil (5-FU) and folinic acid was able to predict the long-term outcome in liver metastases from colorectal cancer.[63] The available data are therefore very encouraging, even though the patient sample remains very limited and the treatment procedures heterogeneous.

PET imaging with other tracers

5-FU is commonly used in the chemotherapy of gastrointestinal cancers, including for liver metastases from colorectal carcinoma. However, the overall response to such treatment is poor. Therefore, a noninvasive method that could improve patient selection and identify those likely to respond to the treatment would be very helpful. PET with ^{18}F-labeled fluorouracil was largely investigated in this setting, in particular by researchers in Heidelberg. They showed a high variability in the tracer uptake, not only among patients but also among lesions present in a single patient. Most lesions appear as areas of decreased activity, as the normal liver shows a generally high uptake. The most important finding relates to the positive correlation existing between tumor uptake at baseline and the subsequent response to

chemotherapy.[64–66] Eniluracil inactivates the dihydropyrimidine dehydrogenase, thus blocking 5-FU catabolism. Experiments performed in small series of patients showed that pretreatment with this drug increased the tumor uptake, and lowered the uptake by the normal liver.[67]

3′-deoxy-3′-[^{18}F]fluorothymidine (^{18}F-FLT) is a marker for tumor proliferation. It has generated much interest and is increasingly being investigated. The tracer is not appropriate for diagnostic liver imaging, due to the high uptake by the normal liver parenchyma. The sensitivity for detecting liver metastases was only 34% (11/32) in a series of 50 patients with colorectal cancer.[68] Although the assessment of response to treatment is often considered as the most promising clinical application of FLT PET, this issue remains to be fully answered. Indeed, *in vitro* experiments showed an increase in FLT uptake after incubation with 5-FU. These changes reflected activation of salvage pathways of DNA synthesis, rather than inhibition of tumor cell proliferation.[69]

SPECT imaging

The role of SPECT imaging with ^{111}In-pentetreotide (somatostatin receptor scintigraphy, SRS) is limited to a small number of indications, but in those, it is a very important one. Schillaci *et al.* studied 149 patients with neuroendocrine tumors, among whom 65 had histologically confirmed liver metastases.[70] SPECT had a 92.3% (60/65) sensitivity following a patient per patient analysis, and 92.4% sensitivity (171/185) when the analysis was performed based on the lesions. Specificity was 100%. SRS performed better than conventional methods, both in terms of overall sensitivity, specificity and identification of patients with single lesions. SPECT imaging was essential, as planar images had an unacceptably low sensitivity (58.5%, 38/65 patients). Overall, SPECT changed a patient's stage in 19% of the cases (28/149). Comparative studies have shown that SRS remains the method of choice for evaluating neuroendocrine tumors, as it is more sensitive than FDG PET.[71] However, recent data were published with PET and 6-[^{18}F]fluoro-L-DOPA (F-DOPA), which suggest higher diagnostic accuracy using this technique than with SRS, although the difference was not obvious regarding liver involvement: F-DOPA PET had a slightly higher sensitivity but also a lower specificity than SRS (81% and 75%; 86% and 100%, respectively).[72] Larger studies are needed to firmly establish F-DOPA PET in the clinical field, and to define its potential role along with conventional methods and SRS. In addition to its value for diagnosis and staging, SRS is also useful for treatment planning with somatostatin analogs. Repeated measurements of the liver metastases 'functional volume' on the SPECT may also prove useful for evaluating the response to other treatment modalities, with a better predictive value than CT.[73]

REFERENCES

● Seminal primary article
◆ Key review paper

1 Llovet JM, Burroughs A, Bruix J. Hepatocellular carcinoma. *Lancet* 2003; **362**: 1907–17.

2 El-Serag HB, Davila JA, Petersen NJ, McGlynn KA. The continuing increase in the incidence of hepatocellular carcinoma in the United States: an update. *Ann Intern Med* 2003; **139**: 817–23.

3 Befeler AS, Di Bisceglie AM. Hepatocellular carcinoma: diagnosis and treatment. *Gastroenterology* 2002; **122**: 1609–19.

4 Takayama T, Makuuchi M, Hirohashi S, *et al.* Early hepatocellular carcinoma as an entity with a high rate of surgical cure. *Hepatology* 1998; **28**: 1241–6.

5 Llovet JM, Bustamante J, Castells A, *et al.* Natural history of untreated nonsurgical hepatocellular carcinoma: rationale for the design and evaluation of therapeutic trials. *Hepatology* 1999; **29**: 62–7.

6 Valls C, Cos M, Figueras J, *et al.* Pretransplantation diagnosis and staging of hepatocellular carcinoma in patients with cirrhosis: value of dual-phase helical CT. *Am J Roentgenol* 2004; **182**: 1011–17.

7 Kamel IR, Bluemke DA. Imaging evaluation of hepatocellular carcinoma. *J Vasc Interv Radiol* 2002; **13(9 Pt 2)**: S173–84.

8 Kim YK, Kim CS, Lee YH, *et al.* Comparison of superparamagnetic iron oxide-enhanced and gadobenate dimeglumine-enhanced dynamic MRI for detection of small hepatocellular carcinomas. *Am J Roentgenol* 2004; **182**: 1217–23.

9 Weber G, Morris HP. Comparative biochemistry of hepatomas. III. Carbohydrate enzymes in liver tumors of different growth rates. *Cancer Res* 1963; **23**: 987–94.

10 Weber G, Cantero A. Glucose-6-phosphatase activity in normal, pre-cancerous, and neoplastic tissues. *Cancer Res* 1955; **15**: 105–8.

11 Zimmerman RL, Burke M, Young NA, *et al.* Diagnostic utility of Glut-1 and CA 15-3 in discriminating adenocarcinoma from hepatocellular carcinoma in liver tumors biopsied by fine-needle aspiration. *Cancer* 2002; **96**: 53–7.

12 Zimmerman RL, Burke MA, Young NA, *et al.* Diagnostic value of hepatocyte paraffin 1 antibody to discriminate hepatocellular carcinoma from metastatic carcinoma in fine-needle aspiration biopsies of the liver. *Cancer* 2001; **93**: 288–91.

● 13 Torizuka T, Tamaki N, Inokuma T, *et al.* In vivo assessment of glucose metabolism in hepatocellular carcinoma with FDG-PET. *J Nucl Med* 1995; **36**: 1811–17.

● 14 Okazumi S, Isono K, Enomoto K, *et al.* Evaluation of liver tumors using fluorine-18-fluorodeoxyglucose PET: characterization of tumor and assessment of effect of treatment. *J Nucl Med* 1992; **33**: 333–9.

15 Lee JD, Yun M, Lee JM, *et al.* Analysis of gene expression profiles of hepatocellular carcinomas with regard to (18)F-fluorodeoxyglucose uptake pattern on positron emission tomography. *Eur J Nucl Med Mol Imaging* 2004; **31**: 1621–30.

16 Trojan J, Schroeder O, Raedle J, *et al.* Fluorine-18 FDG positron emission tomography for imaging of hepatocellular carcinoma. *Am J Gastroenterol* 1999; **94**: 3314–19.

17 Khan MA, Combs CS, Brunt EM, *et al.* Positron emission tomography scanning in the evaluation of hepatocellular carcinoma. *J Hepatol* 2000; **32**: 792–7.

18 Wudel Jr LJ, Delbeke D, Morris D, *et al.* The role of [18F]fluorodeoxyglucose positron emission tomography imaging in the evaluation of hepatocellular carcinoma. *Am Surg* 2003; **69**: 117–24; discussion 124–6.

19 Jeng LB, Changlai SP, Shen YY, *et al.* Limited value of ^{18}F-2-deoxyglucose positron emission tomography to detect hepatocellular carcinoma in hepatitis B virus carriers. *Hepatogastroenterology* 2003; **50**: 2154–6.

20 Kurtaran A, Becherer A, Pfeffel F, *et al.* ^{18}F-fluorodeoxyglucose (FDG)-PET features of focal

nodular hyperplasia (FNH) of the liver. *Liver* 2000; **20**: 487–90.

21 Shiomi S, Nishiguchi S, Ishizu H, *et al.* Usefulness of positron emission tomography with fluorine-18-fluorodeoxyglucose for predicting outcome in patients with hepatocellular carcinoma. *Am J Gastroenterol* 2001; **96**: 1877–80.

22 Iwata Y, Shiomi S, Sasaki N, *et al.* Clinical usefulness of positron emission tomography with fluorine-18-fluorodeoxyglucose in the diagnosis of liver tumors. *Ann Nucl Med* 2000; **14**: 121–6.

23 Liangpunsakul S, Agarwal D, Horlander JC, *et al.* Positron emission tomography for detecting occult hepatocellular carcinoma in hepatitis C cirrhotics awaiting for liver transplantation. *Transplant Proc* 2003; **35**: 2995–7.

24 Teefey SA, Hildeboldt CC, Dehdashti F, *et al.* Detection of primary hepatic malignancy in liver transplant candidates: prospective comparison of CT, MR imaging, US, and PET. *Radiology* 2003; **226**: 533–42.

25 Dimitrakopoulou-Strauss A, Strauss LG, Gutzler F, *et al.* Pharmacokinetic imaging of ^{11}C ethanol with PET in eight patients with hepatocellular carcinomas who were scheduled for treatment with percutaneous ethanol injection. *Radiology* 1999; **211**: 681–6.

26 Shibata T, Yamamoto K, Hayashi N, *et al.* Dynamic positron emission tomography with ^{13}N-ammonia in liver tumors. *Eur J Nucl Med* 1988; **14**: 607–11.

27 Kempf JS, Hudak R, Abdel-Dayem HM, *et al.* Tl-201 chloride SPECT imaging of hepatocellular carcinoma. *Clin Nucl Med* 1996; **21**: 953–7.

28 Mochizuki T, Takechi T, Murase K, *et al.* Thallium-201/technetium-99m-phytate (colloid) subtraction imaging of hepatocellular carcinoma. *J Nucl Med* 1994; **35**: 1134–7.

29 Fukushima K, Kono M, Ishii K, *et al.* Technetium-99m methoxyisobutylisonitrile single-photon emission tomography in hepatocellular carcinoma. *Eur J Nucl Med* 1997; **24**: 1426–8.

30 Kim YS, Cho SW, Lee KJ, *et al.* Tc-99m MIBI SPECT is useful for noninvasively predicting the presence of MDR1 gene-encoded P-glycoprotein in patients with hepatocellular carcinoma. *Clin Nucl Med* 1999; **24**: 874–9.

31 Ho YJ, Jen LB, Yang MD, *et al.* Usefulness of technetium-99m methoxyisobutylisonitrile liver single photon emission computed tomography to detect hepatocellular carcinoma. *Neoplasma* 2003; **50**: 117–19.

32 Ho YJ, Jeng LB, Yang MD, *et al.* A trial of single photon emission computed tomography of the liver with technetium-99m tetrofosmin to detect hepatocellular carcinoma. *Anticancer Res* 2003; **23**: 1743–6.

33 de Groen PC, Gores GJ, LaRusso NF, *et al.* Biliary tract cancers. *N Engl J Med* 1999; **341**: 1368–78.

● 34 Keiding S, Hansen SB, Rasmussen HH, *et al.* Detection of cholangiocarcinoma in primary sclerosing cholangitis by positron emission tomography. *Hepatology* 1998; **28**: 700–6.

35 Kim YJ, Yun M, Lee WJ, *et al.* Usefulness of (18)F-FDG PET in intrahepatic cholangiocarcinoma. *Eur J Nucl Med Mol Imaging* 2003; **30**: 1467–72.

36 Anderson CD, Rice MH, Pinson CW, *et al.* Fluorodeoxyglucose PET imaging in the evaluation of gallbladder carcinoma and cholangiocarcinoma. *J Gastrointest Surg* 2004; **8**: 90–7.

37 Fritscher-Ravens A, Bohuslavizki KH, Broering DC, *et al.* FDG PET in the diagnosis of hilar cholangiocarcinoma. *Nucl Med Commun* 2001; **22**: 1277–85.

38 Baker ME, Pelley R. Hepatic metastases: basic principles and implications for radiologists. *Radiology* 1995; **197**: 329–37.

39 Weiss L, Grundmann E, Torhorst J, *et al.* Haematogenous metastatic patterns in colonic carcinoma: an analysis of 1541 necropsies. *J Pathol* 1986; **150**: 195–203.

40 Harmon KE, Ryan Jr JA,, Biehl TR, Lee FT. Benefits and safety of hepatic resection for colorectal metastases. *Am J Surg* 1999; **177**: 402–4.

41 Ruers T, Bleichrodt RP. Treatment of liver metastases, an update on the possibilities and results. *Eur J Cancer* 2002; **38**: 1023–33.

42 Nordlinger B, Peschaud F, Malafosse R. Resection of liver metastases from colorectal cancer – how can we improve results? *Colorectal Dis* 2003; **5**: 515–17.

43 Detry O, Warzee F, Polus M, *et al.* Liver resection for noncolorectal, nonneuroendocrine metastases. *Acta Chir Belg* 2003; **103**: 458–62.

◆ 44 Kinkel K, Lu Y, Both M, *et al.* Detection of hepatic metastases from cancers of the gastrointestinal tract by using noninvasive imaging methods (US, CT, MR imaging, PET): a meta-analysis. *Radiology* 2002; **224**: 748–56.

● 45 Yonekura Y, Benua RS, Brill AB, *et al.* Increased accumulation of 2-deoxy-2-[^{18}F]fluoro-D-glucose in liver metastases from colon carcinoma. *J Nucl Med* 1982; **23**: 1133–37.

46 Hustinx R, Dolin RJ, Benard F, *et al.* Impact of attenuation correction on the accuracy of FDG-PET in patients with abdominal tumors: a free-response ROC analysis. *Eur J Nucl Med* 2000; **27**: 1365–71.

47 Rydzewski B, Dehdashti F, Gordon BA, *et al.* Usefulness of intraoperative sonography for revealing hepatic metastases from colorectal cancer in patients selected for surgery after undergoing FDG PET. *Am J Roentgenol* 2002; **178**: 353–8.

48 Bartolozzi C, Donati F, Cioni D, *et al.* Detection of colorectal liver metastases: a prospective multicenter trial comparing unenhanced MRI, MnDPDP-enhanced MRI, and spiral CT. *Eur Radiol* 2004; **14**: 14–20.

49 Vidiri A, Carpanese L, Annibale MD, *et al.* Evaluation of hepatic metastases from colorectal carcinoma with MR-superparamagnetic iron oxide. *J Exp Clin Cancer Res* 2004; **23**: 53–60.

50 Sahani DV, Kalva SP, Tanabe KK, *et al.* Intraoperative US in patients undergoing surgery for liver neoplasms: comparison with MR imaging. *Radiology* 2004; **232**: 810–14.

51 Yang M, Martin DR, Karabulut N, Frick MP. Comparison of MR and PET imaging for the evaluation of liver metastases. *J Magn Reson Imaging* 2003; **17**: 343–9.

52 Ruers TJ, Langenhoff BS, Neeleman N, *et al.* Value of positron emission tomography with [F-18]fluorodeoxyglucose in patients with colorectal liver metastases: a prospective study. *J Clin Oncol* 2002; **20**: 388–395.

● 53 Strasberg SM, Dehdashti F, Siegel BA, *et al.* Survival of patients evaluated by FDG-PET before hepatic resection for metastatic colorectal carcinoma: a prospective database study. *Ann Surg* 2001; **233**: 293–9.

54 Park KC, Schwimmer J, Shepherd JE, *et al.* Decision analysis for the cost-effective management of recurrent colorectal cancer. *Ann Surg* 2001; **233**: 310–19.

55 Delbeke D, Martin WH, Sandler MP, *et al.* Evaluation of benign vs malignant hepatic lesions with positron emission tomography. *Arch Surg* 1998; **133**: 510–15; discussion 515–16.

56 Hustinx R, Paulus P, Jacquet N, *et al.* Clinical evaluation of whole-body 18F-fluorodeoxyglucose positron emission tomography in the detection of liver metastases. *Ann Oncol* 1998; **9**: 397–401.

57 Dromain C, de Baere T, Elias D, *et al.* Hepatic tumors treated with percutaneous radio-frequency ablation: CT and MR imaging follow-up. *Radiology* 2002; **223**: 255–62.

58 Solbiati L, Goldberg SN, Ierace T, *et al.* Radiofrequency ablation of hepatic metastases: postprocedural assessment with a US microbubble contrast agent – early experience. *Radiology* 1999; **211**: 643–9.

59 Anderson GS, Brinkmann F, Soulen MC, *et al.* FDG positron emission tomography in the surveillance of hepatic tumors treated with radiofrequency ablation. *Clin Nucl Med* 2003; **28**: 192–7.

● 60 Langenhoff BS, Oyen WJ, Jager GJ, *et al.* Efficacy of fluorine-18-deoxyglucose positron emission tomography in detecting tumor recurrence after local ablative therapy for liver metastases: a prospective study. *J Clin Oncol* 2002; **20**: 4453–8.

61 Wong CY, Salem R, Raman S, *et al.* Evaluating ^{90}Y-glass microsphere treatment response of unresectable colorectal liver metastases by [^{18}F]FDG PET: a comparison with CT or MRI. *Eur J Nucl Med Mol Imaging* 2002; **29**: 815–20.

62 Mantaka P, Strauss AD, Strauss LG, *et al.* Detection of treated liver metastases using fluorine-18-fluorodeoxyglucose (FDG) and positron emission tomography (PET). *Anticancer Res* 1999; **19**: 4443–50.

63 Bender H, Bangard N, Metten N, *et al.* Possible role of FDG-PET in the early prediction of therapy outcome in liver metastases of colorectal cancer. *Hybridoma* 1999; **18**: 87–91.

64 Dimitrakopoulou A, Strauss LG, Clorius JH, *et al.* Studies with positron emission tomography after systemic administration of fluorine-18-uracil in patients with liver metastases from colorectal carcinoma. *J Nucl Med* 1993; **34**: 1075–81.

65 Kissel J, Brix G, Bellemann ME, *et al.* Pharmacokinetic analysis of 5-[^{18}F]fluorouracil tissue concentrations measured with positron emission tomography in patients with liver metastases from colorectal adenocarcinoma. *Cancer Res* 1997; **57**: 3415–23.

66 Moehler M, Dimitrakopoulou-Strauss A, Gutzler F, *et al.* ^{18}F-labeled fluorouracil positron emission tomography and the prognoses of colorectal carcinoma patients with metastases to the liver treated with 5-fluorouracil. *Cancer* 1998; **83**: 245–53.

67 Aboagye EO, Saleem A, Cunningham VJ, *et al.* Extraction of 5-fluorouracil by tumor and liver: a noninvasive positron emission tomography study of patients with gastrointestinal cancer. *Cancer Res* 2001; **61**: 4937–41.

68 Francis DL, Visvikis D, Costa DC, *et al.* Potential impact of [^{18}F]3′-deoxy-3′-fluorothymidine versus [^{18}F]fluoro-2-deoxy-D-glucose in positron emission tomography for colorectal cancer. *Eur J Nucl Med Mol Imaging* 2003; **30**: 988–94.

69 Dittmann H, Dohmen BM, Kehlbach R, *et al.* Early changes in [^{18}F]FLT uptake after chemotherapy: an experimental study. *Eur J Nucl Med Mol Imaging* 2002; **29**: 1462–9.

70 Schillaci O, Spanu A, Scopinaro F, *et al.* Somatostatin receptor scintigraphy in liver metastasis detection from gastroenteropancreatic neuroendocrine tumors. *J Nucl Med* 2003; **44**: 359–68.

71 Belhocine T, Foidart J, Rigo P, *et al.* Fluorodeoxyglucose positron emission tomography and somatostatin receptor scintigraphy for diagnosing and staging carcinoid tumours: correlations with the pathological indexes p53 and Ki-67. *Nucl Med Commun* 2002; **23**: 727–34.

72 Becherer A, Szabo M, Karanikas G, *et al.* Imaging of advanced neuroendocrine tumors with (18)F-FDOPA PET. *J Nucl Med* 2004; **45**: 1161–7.

73 Gopinath G, Ahmed A, Buscombe JR, *et al.* Prediction of clinical outcome in treated neuroendocrine tumours of carcinoid type using functional volumes on ^{111}In-pentetreotide SPECT imaging. *Nucl Med Commun* 2004; **25**: 253–7.

16

Hematological, reticuloendothelial and lymphatic disorders

16A Anemia and polycythemia

Introduction	675	Studies based on labeled proteins	681
Studies based on radiolabeled red cells	676	Bone marrow imaging	681
Ferrokinetics and metabolic studies	679	References	682

16B Imaging the spleen

Introduction	685	Predicting the response to splenectomy	687
Anatomy and physiology	685	Imaging diseases directly involving the spleen	692
Locating the spleen and assessing its integrity	686	References	693

16C Imaging of lymphomas

Introduction	695	Morphologic imaging modalities	697
Pathological and clinical classification of lymphomas	696	Nuclear medicine imaging modalities	698
Imaging modalities at initial diagnosis and staging of lymphoma	697	Nuclear medicine imaging with fluorodeoxyglucose	702
		References	707

16D Lymphoscintigraphy

Introduction	715	Investigation of a swollen limb	722
Physiological principles	715	References	723
Technique	716		

16A

Anemia and polycythemia

R.W. BARBER, N.G. HARTMAN, AND A.M. PETERS

INTRODUCTION

Nuclear hematology is a broad, wide-ranging discipline based as much on *in vitro* investigations as on imaging. It plays a crucial role in the diagnosis and clinical management of many hematological disorders and, in many institutions, is the responsibility of departments of hematology rather than nuclear medicine. Because nuclear hematology is essentially technique-orientated with a wide range and variety of techniques, this chapter is set out according to techniques rather than diseases. Table 16A.1 lists some of

the commoner procedures with diagnostic reference levels recommended by the Administration of Radioactive Substances Advisory Committee of the United Kingdom (ARSAC).

The investigations can be broadly grouped according to the cell type of interest: red cells (including ferrokinetics and investigation of megaloblastic anemias), platelets, and leukocytes. Whereas labeled leukocytes are important in nuclear medicine for imaging inflammation, they offer little clinical value in the investigation of blood disorders and will not be considered further here. Likewise, platelet

Table 16A.1 *Diagnostic reference levels for hematology studies, as recommended by the Administration of Radioactive Substances Advisory Committee of the United Kingdom (ARSAC)*

Study	Compound	DRL (MBq)	Effective dose (mSv)
Red cell volume	^{51}Cr-normal RBC	0.8	0.3
Red cell survival	^{51}Cr-normal RBC	2	0.6
Sites of sequestration	^{51}Cr-normal RBC	4	1
Spleen imaging	^{99m}Tc-denatured RBC	100	2
Gastrointestinal blood loss	^{51}Cr-normal RBC	4	1
Gastrointestinal protein loss	^{111}In-transferrin	15	3*
Iron metabolism	$^{59}Fe^{2+}$ or $^{59}Fe^{3+}$	0.4	4
Plasma volume	^{125}I-HSA	0.2	0.06
Schilling	^{57}Co-cyanocobalamin	0.04	0.1
White cell imaging	^{111}In-leukocytes	20	9
Platelet kinetics	^{111}In-platelets	20	10
Bone marrow imaging	^{99m}Tc-colloid	400	4

* From ICRP 80. DRL, diagnostic reference level; RBC, red blood cells; HSA, human serum albumin.

disorders are closely related to splenic function and are considered in Chapter 16B. This chapter therefore focuses on polycythemia and anemia.

STUDIES BASED ON RADIOLABELED RED CELLS

In vitro (or more precisely, *ex vivo*) studies based on labeled red cells include measurements of red cell volume (RCV), mean red cell life span (MRCLS), detection, and quantification of gastrointestinal (GI) bleeding and compatibility testing. *In vivo* studies include measurement of splenic function, quantification of splenic red cell pooling, and detection of sites of red cell destruction.[1]

Red cell labeling

CHROMIUM-51

MRCLS and quantification of GI blood loss are based on ^{51}Cr-labeled red cells. A 14-mL sample of venous blood is taken into a syringe containing 2 mL ACD (NIH formula A). The blood is centrifuged at $1000 \times g$ for 5 min, following which the plasma supernatant is removed. Care should be taken not to disturb, and inadvertently remove, the reticulocyte-rich upper surface of the red cell column, which makes an important contribution to MRCLS. Sodium [^{51}Cr]chromate is added to the red cells (approximately 2 MBq for measurement of MRCLS and 0.8 MBq for measurement of RCV) and mixed for 5 min. The unbound ^{51}Cr (usually <10%) is removed by washing the cells in saline. A small aliquot of the labeled cells is retained for the preparation of a counting standard. An anticipated very short MRCLS may be measured using red cells labeled with ^{111}In (see below).

TECHNETIUM-99m

Short-term investigations, such as splenic red cell pooling and tests of splenic function based on blood clearance measurements, should be performed with ^{99m}Tc. The principle of labeling with ^{99m}Tc is to allow the radionuclide to diffuse into the red cells and then to trap it by reduction with stannous ion. The red cells are first 'tinned' by exposure to stannous fluoride and labeled 15 min later by exposure to [^{99m}Tc]pertechnetate. For best results, the cells should be labeled *in vitro* and then washed, although the tinning can be performed *in vivo* by prior intravenous injection of tin. The so-called '*in vivtro*' labeling technique consists of *in vivo* tinning followed by venesection into a syringe containing anticoagulant and pertechnetate. After gentle agitation, the blood in the syringe is then infused back into the patient. Excellent red cell labeling efficiency (>95%) with ^{99m}Tc can nowadays also be obtained by complete *in vivo* labeling for which commercial stannous chloride/citric acid kits are available in various countries.

INDIUM-111

Blood cells can be labeled with ^{111}In by exposure to lipophilic metal chelate complexes, such as ^{111}In-tropolonate or ^{111}In-oxine, which, following penetration of the cell membrane, bind tightly to intracellular proteins. For labeling platelets and neutrophils with ^{111}In or ^{99m}Tc complexes, or with sodium [^{51}Cr]chromate, the cell of interest has first to be isolated from other blood cell types because the labeling is indiscriminate. As far as ^{111}In is concerned, because red cells greatly outnumber other cell types, the ^{111}In complex needs only to be added to whole blood *in vitro* for red cell labeling, followed by washing to remove unbound complex. The labeling efficiency is improved if the complex is added to washed red cells.

Elution of label from red cells is least with ^{51}Cr and greatest with ^{99m}Tc. Red cells are labeled with ^{111}In with a stability almost as high as ^{51}Cr.[2]

Red cell volume

Measurement of RCV is the most frequently performed radionuclide investigation in hematology. A high venous hematocrit in isolation should not be assumed to be due to red cell polycythemia (erthrocytosis). It may equally be the result of a reduced plasma volume (PV), causing relative or pseudo-polycythemia. It is important to identify cases of pseudo-polycythemia as the treatment is venesection rather than myelosuppressive drug therapy. In the occasional patient, usually obese or a smoker, an RCV in the upper normal range and a PV in the lower normal range combine to give a modestly raised venous hematocrit, so-called 'physiological polycythemia'.[3] Cases of pseudoanemia can be identified where the RCV is normal but the PV is expanded, for example in splenomegaly, cirrhosis, and glomerulonephritis. Pseudoanemia is a normal feature of pregnancy and accounts for the reduction in venous hematocrit. When measurement of RCV establishes true polycythemia, the cause should be sought (Table 16A.2).

RCV is most accurately measured with ^{51}Cr-labeled red cells. If it is decided to image splenic red cell pooling, ^{99m}Tc is a satisfactory alternative, although it gives a slight overestimation as a result of radiotracer elution.[2] RCV measurement is based on the dilution principle; a blood sample is taken at about 20 min after injection of a known amount of labeled cells, when complete mixing within the circulation can be assumed. In clinical practice, it is essential to relate the measured RCV to body habitus. Adipose tissue is avascular relative to muscle. In obese patients, RCV expressed in mL/kg may significantly underestimate the degree of polycythemia unless the lean body mass is measured or estimated. Without such correction, true polycythemia may be missed or mis-classified as pseudo-polycythemia. Various formulae based on weight, height, gender, and age have been devised to predict the normal values for RCV

Table 16A.2   *Causes of increased red cell volume*

1. *Primary proliferative polycythemia*

2. *Idiopathic erythrocytosis*

3. *Autonomous high erythropoietin production*

4. *Secondary polycythemia*

   (a) *Hypoxic (with activation of normal erythropoietin mechanism)*

      High altitude

      Hypoxemic lung disease (including intrinsic lung disease, hypoventilation, sleep apnea)

      Cyanotic congenital heart disease

      High oxygen affinity hemoglobins

      Smoking

      Methemoglobinemia

      Red cell metabolic defect

   (b) *With 'inappropriate' secretion of erythropoietin*

      Renal tumor – hypernephroma, nephroblastoma

      Renal ischemia (e.g. cysts, hydronephrosis, renal transplant)

      Hepatoma and liver disease

      Fibroids

      Cerebellar hemangioblastoma

      Bronchial carcinoma

      Pheochromocytoma

   (c) Miscellaneous

      Androgen therapy

      Cushing's disease

      Hypertransfusion

and PV. Pearson *et al.*[4] and the expert panel on radionuclides of the International Council for Standardization in Hematology (ICSH) have proposed predicted normal values and reference ranges based on body surface area, and, for PV for women, age. The recommendations are:

For men

   Mean normal RCV (mL) $= (1486 \times S) - 825$

         98% limits $= \pm 25\%$

   Mean normal PV (mL) $= 1578 \times S$

         99% limits $= \pm 25\%$

For women

   Mean normal RCV (mL) $= (1.06 \times A) + (822 \times S)$

         99% limits $= \pm 25\%$

   Mean normal PV (mL) $= 1395 \times S$

         99% limits $= \pm 25\%$

where A is the subject's age (in years) and S is the surface area (m^2), which is given by

$$W^{0.425} \times h^{0.725} \times 0.007184.$$

W is the subject's weight (in kg) and h is the subject's height (in cm).

Mixing of labeled red cells is prolonged in splenomegaly[5] so the sample should be delayed until 60 min postinjection. PV should be measured (using ^{125}I-labeled albumin) at the same time as RCV in which case at least three samples, usually taken at 10, 20, and 30 min after injection, are obtained. As a result of slow loss of protein into the extra-vascular space, these three samples are used to obtain the appropriate dilution factor for measurement of PV by extrapolation to zero time. The three samples should agree with each other in their estimates of RCV because the limitation here is intra-vascular mixing which should be complete by 10 min unless there is splenomegaly. When the two tests are performed simultaneously, care should be taken to correct for cross-talk from ^{51}Cr into the ^{125}I counting channel: this problem can be avoided by performing the PV study first.

Mean red cell life span

Because of the requirements of intracellular stability and long physical half-life, ^{51}Cr is used for measurement of MRCLS. Blood samples are taken daily after injection of ^{51}Cr-labeled autologous red cells for an appropriate duration judged from the rate of loss of radioactivity from the blood. Because of slow, ongoing elution of ^{51}Cr from the cells, the percentage of ^{51}Cr remaining in blood should be multiplied by a correction factor, increasing with time after injection, that varies from 1.03 at 24 h to 1.6 at 40 days (Table 16A.3).

MRCLS is normally 120 days. It is decreased in hemolytic anemias. It may also be usefully measured in conjunction with GI blood loss studies. In clinical practice, it is usually measured when the cause of an anemia is obscure or multifactorial, for example in patients with known GI blood loss who also have a positive direct anti-globulin (Coombs) test, or in patients with an unexplained transfusion requirement. Blood loss in the stools and sites of red cell destruction can be quantified simultaneously by surface counting (see below).

Gastrointestinal blood loss

GI blood loss is quantified by measuring ^{51}Cr in a 7-day stool collection after the intravenous injection of ^{51}Cr-labeled red cells. The count rate from daily fecal samples is recorded in an *in vitro* counter and compared with the counts from a sample of blood of accurately measured volume (3–5 mL) taken the previous day, placed in a similar carton and diluted to 100 mL. Correction for intravascular ^{51}Cr elution is not usually made; as the elution correction factor at 7 days is only 1.11, the maximal possible error is 10%. Measurement of GI blood loss can also be based on whole-body counting, analogously to the measurements of ^{59}Fe absorption, GI protein loss[6] and granulocyte migration into bowel in inflammatory bowel disease.[7] It should be

Table 16A.3 *Normal range for ^{51}Cr survival curves with correction for elution (from Dacie and Lewis[1])*

Day	Percent ^{51}Cr*	Elution correction factors
1	93–98	1.03
2	89–97	1.05
3	86–95	1.06
4	83–93	1.07
5	80–92	1.08
6	78–90	1.10
7	77–88	1.11
8	76–86	1.12
9	74–84	1.13
10	72–83	1.14
11	70–81	1.16
12	68–79	1.17
13	67–78	1.18
14	65–77	1.19
15	64–75	1.20
16	62–74	1.22
17	59–73	1.23
18	58–71	1.25
19	57–69	1.26
20	56–67	1.27
21	55–66	1.29
22	53–65	1.31
23	52–63	1.32
24	51–60	1.34
25	50–59	1.36
30	44–52	1.47
35	39–47	1.53
40	34–42	1.60

*Corrected for decay; not corrected for elution.

emphasized that ^{51}Cr-labeled red cells are used to prove and quantify GI blood loss, but, as ^{51}Cr is a poor gamma emitter and given in low doses, not to localize GI bleeding in a patient known to be bleeding. Normal daily blood loss is less than 3 mL.

Compatability testing

Compatibility testing takes two forms: a short-term test to confirm that blood for transfusion will survive adequately in the recipient; and a longer-term test to identify a suitable donor for a recipient with multiple antibodies. For the former, a few milliliters of the unit of red cells is removed and labeled with ^{99m}Tc. Following injection into the recipient,

there should be a survival or recovery >90% at 60 min after injection if the blood is compatible. In the longer-term test, red cells from the potential donor are labeled with ^{51}Cr and administered to the recipient. In the absence of antibodies, the cells will show a normal survival, at least initially. If the recipient develops antibodies to the transfused cells, the survival curve abruptly falls at the first appearance of the antibodies several days after injection of the labeled cells. This is called a 'collapsing' survival curve.

Imaging the splenic red cell pool

Abnormal splenic pooling of blood cells may be an important feature of several specific conditions including polycythemia vera (PCV), thrombocytopenia and more rarely granulocytopenia. The term hypersplenism is often used, but it is a misleading term that fails to distinguish between abnormal pooling and abnormally increased cell destruction in the spleen. Pooling is a term which itself requires definition and distinction from the term sequestration. Pooling indicates free exchange of cells between the circulating blood and pool, and as such can be measured as the mean transit time of cells through the pool. Sequestration implies a process whereby cells are temporarily trapped in a vascular bed and are not freely exchangeable with circulating cells. Sequestered cells ultimately re-enter the circulation although they may then be rapidly destroyed elsewhere. Mechanisms, kinetics, and duration of cell sequestration are generally unclear, so the term is best avoided.

Normally, red cell transit time through the spleen is 30–60 s. This is longer than for plasma so the intrasplenic hematocrit is higher than whole-body hematocrit. In contrast, red cells streamline in the hepatic vasculature and consequently the intrahepatic hematocrit is lower than the whole-body hematocrit. In splenomegaly there appears to be an additional red cell pool, with a mean transit time considerably longer than 1 min. This has been inferred from a biphasic uptake of radioactivity in the spleen following bolus injection of labeled red cells.[5] Owing to the presence of this more slowly exchanging pool, equilibration of red cells is longer in the enlarged spleen compared with the normal; this is the reverse to platelets (see Chapter 16B). The markedly enlarged spleen may pool red cells sufficiently to produce pseudo-anemia (reduced venous hematocrit in the presence of normal RCV), although it more readily causes thrombocytopenia. The normal splenic red cell pool is less than 5% of the RCV. It is expanded in PCV to between 5 and 20%, and is even higher in myelofibrosis, typically reaching 30%. The massive splenomegaly of myelofibrosis may cause significant pseudo-anemia as a result of splenic red cell pooling, measurement of which may be helpful for predicting the benefit of splenectomy in patients who are severely transfusion-dependent. In pseudo-polycythemia, the splenic red cell pool is normal. In early

Table 16A.4 *Ferrokinetic patterns in various diseases*

	Plasma clearance half-life	Plasma iron turnover	Red cell utilization
Normal	60–140 min	70–140 mol L^{-1} day^{-1}	70–80%
Iron deficiency	¬	N	↑
Aplastic anemia	↑	N	¬
Secondary anemia	Slightly ¬	N	N
Dyserythropoiesis	Slightly ¬	↑	¬
Myelofibrosis	¬	↑	¬
Hemolytic anemia	¬	↑	↑

¬ = short/decreased, ↑ = prolonged/increased.

PCV, an increased splenic pool is an important diagnostic aid in a patient with a spleen of normal size. In some conditions associated with splenomegaly (e.g. hairy cell leukemia), the splenic red cell volume is increased but not in proportion to the splenomegaly.

Determination of sites of red cell destruction

The importance of identifying sites of blood cell destruction is essentially related to the decision to perform splenectomy in diseases like hemolytic anemias and idiopathic thrombocytopenic purpura in which accelerated cell destruction in the spleen may be pathological. In normal subjects, red cells are destroyed in the reticuloendothelial system.

Because of the relatively long normal life span of red cells, it is usually necessary, even in hemolytic anemias, to label red cells with ^{51}Cr. Sequential surface counting with a scintillation probe over the spleen, liver, precordium, and lumbar spine gives a semiquantitative indication of the major sites of cell destruction. Spleen and liver counts can be corrected for their contained blood pool by normalization to, and comparison with, precordial counts. Thus, assuming that the organ counts immediately after injection of the labeled cells arise only from blood, the 'excess' counts represent the difference between spleen or liver counts and precordial counts. In hereditary spherocytosis, excess counts in the spleen are markedly elevated but not accompanied by an increase in excess hepatic counts. In autoimmune hemolytic anemia, both are increased, although detection of excess counts over the spleen may be helpful in predicting a favorable response to splenectomy. In sickle cell disease, the liver typically shows increased destruction, but, because of autosplenectomy, the spleen does not. ^{111}In-labeled red cells have been used in severe hemolytic anemias associated with a very reduced red cell life span.[8] Nevertheless, although its imaging characteristics are superior, it still has a significant rate of elution.

FERROKINETICS AND METABOLIC STUDIES

Ferrokinetic studies, including erythropoietic bone marrow imaging, are useful in the investigation of suspected aplastic and other dyserythropoietic anemias and diseases associated with myeloid metaplasia, especially myelofibrosis. Iron-59 is administered either orally as the chloride salt for gastrointestinal absorption studies, or intravenously, as citrate for other studies.[9] The interpretation of abnormal findings is summarized in Table 16A.4.

Iron absorption

Iron absorption is measured following an oral dose of ^{59}Fe, given with unlabeled oral ferrous sulfate and ascorbic acid to reduce the radioactive iron to the ferrous form. The unabsorbed iron is then measured by fecal counting. Iron absorption can also be measured by whole-body counting in terms of the percentage difference between counts acquired immediately after ingestion and at 7 and 9 days. The average normal value of iron absorption is about 30%, but the normal range is wide. Values of less than 10% are abnormal. It is increased up to about 90% in iron-deficiency anemia that is not due to iron malabsorption.

Plasma iron clearance

Plasma iron clearance is measured as the rate constant of clearance of intravenously injected, transferrin-bound [^{59}Fe]ferric citrate. If the patient has a reduced transferrin binding capacity, or if transferrin is already saturated (as in aplastic anemia) then ^{59}Fe bound to donor plasma (as diferric transferrin) should be used, otherwise the iron is taken up rapidly by the liver, to form ferritin. If autologous plasma is used, it should be passed through a resin column before injection in order to remove any unbound ^{59}Fe. The plasma disappearance of radioactivity is monoexponential, over a wide range of clearance values, with a normal half-life ranging between 60 and 140 min. The clearance rate is decreased, with a half-life of up to 300 min, in aplastic anemia, and increased in myelofibrosis, polycythemia vera, iron-deficiency anemia and hemolytic anemias, with half-lives typically 20–40 min. Since the disappearance is monoexponential, plasma volume can be measured from the extrapolated zero-time ^{59}Fe plasma concentration.

Plasma iron turnover

Plasma iron turnover, the product of plasma ^{59}Fe clearance and the plasma protein-bound native iron concentration, is an absolute measure of the rate of iron removal from plasma in units of mg mL^{-1} min^{-1}. It clearly reflects plasma iron clearance values, and adds little useful clinical information to iron clearance.

Red cell iron utilization

Red cell utilization (RCU) is the fraction of an injected dose of ^{59}Fe that is incorporated into circulating red cells, and is therefore a measure of effective erythropoiesis. Blood samples are taken on alternate days for 12–14 days following intravenous administration; RCV is then multiplied by the red cell ^{59}Fe concentration in each sample.

RCU can be obtained routinely from PV as determined from the plasma iron clearance, and the whole-body hematocrit (determined as the peripheral venous hematocrit multiplied by 0.9). It is necessary to assume that RCV remains constant over the period of measurement. This can be partially checked by daily venous hematocrit estimations. The daily RCU values rise to a plateau of 70–80% at about 10 days in normal subjects. It is reduced to <10% in aplastic anemia and to between 10 and 50% in myelofibrosis. In iron-deficiency anemia, hemolytic anemia, and true polycythemia, RCU is increased, usually approaching 100%. Where erythropoiesis is ineffective – for example in myelodysplasia or thalassaemias – the red cell utilization is variably reduced, depending on the severity of the disorder.

Iron–59 surface counting

An overall picture of ferrokinetics can be constructed from day-to-day surface counting with a scintillation probe positioned over the liver, spleen, sacrum (for bone marrow) and heart (for blood pool) after an intravenous injection of ^{59}Fe (as ferrous citrate). The counts, corrected for physical decay, give information on sites of erythropoiesis (from early counting), which may be extramedullary, and on sites of red cell destruction (from later counting). Surface counting is rarely performed but does have some clinical value for determining the extent of extramedullary erythropoiesis in the spleen before splenectomy. Positron emission tomography (PET) with ^{52}Fe has demonstrated that active bone marrow may have a patchy distribution, underlining the uncertainty of surface counting.

Iron–52 positron emission tomography

The radionuclides of iron, ^{59}Fe and, in centers with facilities for PET, ^{52}Fe, label the erythron and are used to identify sites of erythropoiesis in aplastic anemia and myelofibrosis. Iron-52 is a positron emitter which, using PET, gives high-resolution images of the distribution of erythropoietic tissue (Fig. 16A.1). The detection of splenic erythropoiesis, absent in uncomplicated PCV and invariably present in myelofibrosis, is helpful in documenting the transition from PCV to a myelofibrotic state. In doubtful cases of essential thrombocythemia, detection of splenic erythropoiesis confirms the presence of a myeloproliferative disorder rather than reactive thrombocytosis. PET can also identify unusual sites of erythropoiesis, for example in retrosternal tissue or lymph nodes.

The indications for ^{52}Fe imaging are the same as for ^{59}Fe surface counting. However, the possibilities with ^{52}Fe extend beyond ^{59}Fe surface counting, such as the demonstration of deep internal sites of erythropoiesis. Although PET imaging maximizes the value of ^{52}Fe, the physical half-life of 8 h is long enough for the radionuclide to be exported from a cyclotron and imaged using a gamma camera fitted with a high-energy collimator suitable for 511 keV photons.

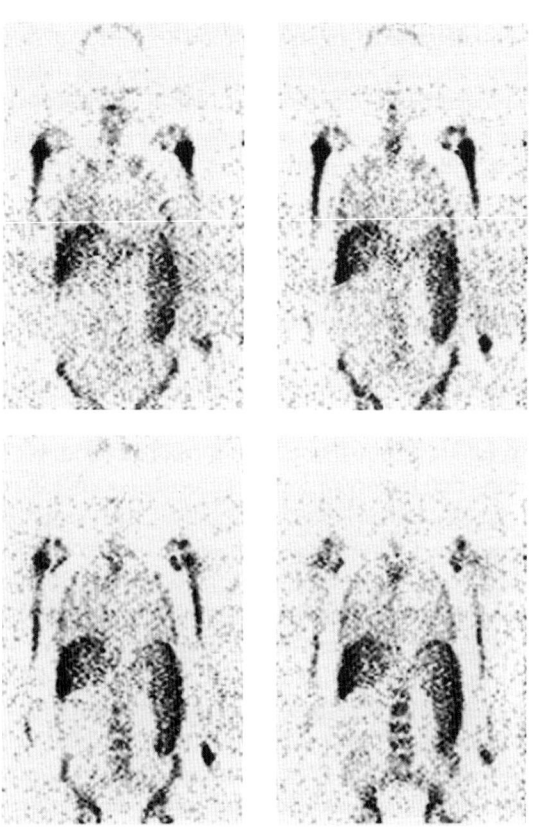

Figure 16A.1 *Coronal whole-body positron emission tomograms in a patient with polycythemia rubra vera following intravenous injection of ^{52}Fe. Although bone marrow uptake is clearly visible, the presence of myeloid metaplasia confirms transition to myelofibrosis.*

Investigation of megaloblastic anemia

Patients with a macrocytic anemia and low serum vitamin B_{12}, or an incidental finding of a consistently low serum vitamin B_{12}, need to be investigated to determine the cause as dietary deficiency, gastric malabsorption or ileal malabsorption. In the classic Schilling test, ^{57}Co-cyanocobalamin (18.5 kBq: GE Healthcare [formally Amersham Healthcare]) is given orally, together with an intramuscular injection of non-radioactive cobalamin to saturate organ pools and stimulate urinary radioactive B_{12} excretion. A 24-h urine collection is made, and aliquots of urine are counted against a known standard. Normal 24-h excretion is 10–40%. If the excretion is 10% or less the test should be repeated with the addition of intrinsic factor (IF) to distinguish between pernicious anemia, and malabsorption from other causes. There should be a 7-day interval between the two parts of the test.

One elegant modification of the test was previously available in dual-labeled kit form (Dicopac test, GE Healthcare) that enabled both parts of the traditional Schilling test to be performed simultaneously. Unfortunately, the kits are no longer marketed, but a description is included here to allow results from this version of the test to be interpreted. The 24-h urinary excretions of 'free' ^{58}Co-labeled cyanocobalamin and ^{57}Co-labeled cyanocobalamin pre-bound to human gastric juices, both administered orally, are compared after a saturating dose of 1 mg intramuscular B_{12}. The normal 24-h urinary excretion of ^{57}Co is >12% and of ^{58}Co, >11%. The ratio of ^{58}Co to ^{57}Co in urine should be > 1.3. An increased ratio suggests gastric malabsorption, while reduced excretion of both agents with a urine ratio of <1.3 suggests ileal malabsorption. The two main causes of error or uncertainty are incomplete 24-h urine collection and subnormal excretion of both isotopes but with a ^{58}Co/^{57}Co ratio of >1.3. The latter is thought to be due to vitamin B_{12} deficiency secondary to ileal malabsorption. The manufacturer recommends that, although ratios of >1.3 are abnormal, only a ratio of >1.7 can be confidently ascribed to low intrinsic factor. This, however, is probably too stringent. The subject is reviewed by Atrah and Davidson,[10] who suggest that a ratio of >1.3 is always suggestive of intrinsic factor deficiency except when the 24-h urine collection is grossly deficient (<500 mL).

STUDIES BASED ON LABELED PROTEINS

Plasma volume

PV can be measured with several radiolabeled proteins, including ^{59}Fe-transferrin, although it is usually measured with ^{125}I-labeled human serum albumin (^{125}I-HSA). As for RCV, the technique is based on the dilution principle. Plasma ^{125}I-HSA concentration, measured in samples taken at 10, 20, and 30 min after injection, is plotted logarithmically

as a function of time in order to establish the fractional rate of loss of albumin from the intravascular compartment. PV is then calculated from the injected dose and the extrapolated zero-time plasma ^{125}I concentration. PV should always be measured independently of RCV in patients with a raised hematocrit to identify patients with pseudo-polycythemia (relative polycythemia). Results should be interpreted using the normal values and reference ranges given by ICSH.[4]

Gastrointestinal protein loss

Protein-losing enteropathy can be diagnosed and quantified by measuring the fecal excretion of intravenously injected ^{51}Cr-labeled albumin,[11] analogously to the measurement of GI bleeding with ^{51}Cr-labeled red cells. Mean loss over 5 days is 0.83 ($\pm$SD 0.32)%.[11] Indium-111-labeled transferrin can also be used and combined with imaging in order to localize the site(s) of loss.[6,12] Fecal collection over 3 days indicated a normal GI loss of 0.48 ($\pm$0.26)%.[12] Whole-body counting for quantification of gastrointestinal protein loss is also possible with ^{111}In-transferrin for the normal whole-body loss is about 1% per day.[6] For localization by imaging without quantification, the best agent may be ^{99m}Tc-labeled human polyclonal immunoglobulin G (^{99m}Tc-HIG), which is more stable than ^{99m}Tc-HSA[13] thereby minimizing pitfalls such as the GI secretion of [^{99m}Tc]pertechnetate.

BONE MARROW IMAGING

Bone marrow sinusoids are lined by fenestrated endothelium with a high permeability to macromolecules. Marrow is partly supplied through what is in effect a portal system via a periosteal network that also supplies bone, explaining why several hematological disorders involving bone marrow, especially granulocytic leukemia and myelofibrosis, give rise to bone scans with superscan features as a result of increased marrow flow. Normal mean bone marrow perfusion measured with H_2^{15}O PET shows wide regional variations. In normal young adults, for instance, Kahn *et al.*[14] obtained values of 14.3 and 11.1 mL min^{-1} (100 mL)$^{-1}$ in two different regions of the pelvis, compared to 17.6 mL min^{-1} (100 mL)$^{-1}$ in the lumbar vertebrae. Martiat *et al.*[15] obtained broadly similar values in normal subjects (10 mL min^{-1} (100 mL)$^{-1}$) but much higher values in hematological disorders, such as PCV (26.9), chronic granulocytic leukemias (25.2) and myelofibrosis (35.1 mL min^{-1} (100 mL)$^{-1}$). Total (i.e. whole-body) skeletal blood flow is difficult to measure but, based on sodium [^{18}F]fluoride blood clearance, has been estimated to be about 300 mL min^{-1}.[16] Given the values above, based on PET, this may be an underestimation.

There are two cellular systems within bone marrow, co-existing throughout red (active) marrow: the reticulo-endothelial system (RES) and the hematopoietic system. The distribution of active marrow throughout the skeleton varies with age. Although usually confined to the central skeleton in the adult, experience with bone marrow imaging has shown that it often extends into the shafts of long bones. Active marrow can be imaged using tracers which target either of the systems, although in disease, aplastic anemia for example, the distribution of the two systems may be divergent.

The indications for bone marrow imaging include: (1) evaluation of a hematological disorder, often as part of a ferrokinetic study; (2) detection of malignant infiltration either from a hematological malignancy such as lymphoma or myeloma or from metastases, which initially infiltrate marrow; and (3) to complement another imaging procedure, for example identification of active bone marrow in the interpretation of a leukocyte scan performed for musculoskeletal infection or of suspected marrow infarction showing increased uptake on a bone scan.

Radiolabeled colloids target the RES, including bone marrow. Small-particle size colloids, such as antimony sulfur colloid, have a relative selectivity for marrow. Radionuclides of iron target the hematopoietic component; high-resolution images of sites of erythropoiesis can be obtained by PET using ^{52}Fe, although the high radiation dose limits the amount that can be given. Indium-111-transferrin is taken up by both components and cannot therefore be used as a surrogate for native iron. Indeed, Chipping et al.[17] observed a distribution of ^{111}In and ^{52}Fe that was concordant in only two of 15 patients with various hematological conditions. Granulocytes pool in bone marrow with kinetics similar to those in the spleen.[18] Radiolabeled leukocytes therefore give clear images of bone marrow within minutes to hours of injection, becoming more prominent over 24 h. Because of its wide distribution, granulocyte pooling in the bone marrow is not as obvious as in the spleen. Nevertheless, the size of the marrow pool is comparable with that of the spleen since the mean granulocyte transit times through, and total blood flows of the two organs are broadly similar.

Labeled anti-granulocyte monoclonal antibodies, recently developed for imaging inflammation, give prominent images of bone marrow because of the large population of myeloid cells expressing the appropriate antigens. As the normal maturation time of myeloid cells in bone marrow is 15 days, compared with a granulocyte life span in the circulation of 10 h, only a small fraction of total antigen within the circulation is available for targeting. Indeed, in blood sampled following the injection of ^{99m}Tc-Leukoscan, an antibody that is commercially available for imaging inflammation, less than 5% of radioactivity is cell-bound.[19] Bone marrow imaging has the potential to demonstrate marrow metastases at a stage before they influence bone remodelling.[20] Technetium-99m-sestamibi, the uptake of which is broadly related to tissue cellularity, is also able to demonstrate bone marrow metastases[21] and hematological malignancies,[22,23] apparently better than [^{18}F]fluorodeoxyglucose PET,[24] although uptake may be influenced by cellular P-glycoprotein expression.[23]

REFERENCES

1 Dacie JV, Lewis SM. *Practical haematology*, 7th edition. Edinburgh: Churchill-Livingstone; 1991.

2 Radia R, Peters AM, Deenmamode M, et al. Measurement of red cell volume and splenic red cell pool using 113m-indium. *Br J Haematol* 1981; **49**: 587–91.

3 Marsh JCW, Liu Yin JA, Lewis SM. Blood volume measurements in polycythaemia: when and why? *Clin Lab Haematol* 1987; **9**: 452–6.

4 Pearson TC, Guthrie DL, Simpson J, et al. Interpretation of measured red cell mass and plasma volume in adults: expert panel on radionuclides of the International Council for Standardization in Haematology. *Br J Haematol* 1994; **89**: 748–56.

5 Tothill P. Red cell pooling in enlarged spleens. *Br J Haematol* 1964; **10**: 347–57.

6 Carpani de Kaski M, Peters AM, Bradley D, Hodgson HJF. Detection and quantification of protein-losing enteropathy with indium-111-transferrin. *Eur J Nucl Med* 1996; **23**: 530–3.

7 Carpani de Kaski M, Peters AM, Knight D, et al. In-111 whole body retention: a new method for quantification of disease activity in inflammatory bowel disease. *J Nucl Med* 1992; **33**: 756–62.

8 Heyns Adu P, Lotter MG, Kotze HF, et al. Kinetics, distribution and sites of destruction of ^{111}In oxine-labelled red cells in haemolytic anaemia. *J Clin Pathol* 1985; **38**: 128–32.

9 Cavill I. Plasma clearance studies. *Methods Haematol* 1986; **14**: 214–44.

10 Atrah HI, Davidson RJL. A survey and critical evaluation of a dual isotope (Dicopac) vitamin B_{12} absorption test. *Eur J Nucl Med* 1989; **15**: 57–60.

11 Rootwelt K. Direct intravenous injection of ^{51}chromic chloride compared with ^{125}I-polyvinylpyrrolidone and ^{131}I-albumin in the detection of gastrointestinal protein loss. *Scand J Clin Lab Invest* 1966; **18**: 405–16.

12 Urita Y. Diagnosis of protein-losing gastroenteropathy by ^{111}In-transferrin scanning and fecal excretion test. *Nippon Shokakibyo Gakkai Zasshi* 1991; **88**: 2644–52.

13 Pain SJ, Barber RW, Purushotham AD, et al. Quantification of lymphatic function for investigation of lymphedema: depot clearance and rate of appearance in blood of soluble macromolecules. *J Nucl Med* 2002; **43**: 318–24.

14 Kahn D, Weiner GJ, Ben-Haim S, et al. Positron emission tomographic measurement of bone marrow

blood flow to the pelvis and lumbar vertebrae in young normal adults. *Blood* 1994; **83**: 958–63.

15 Martiat P, Ferrant A, Cogneau M, *et al.* Assessment of bone marrow blood flow using positron emission tomography: no relationship to bone marrow cellularity. *Br J Haematol* 1987; **66**: 307–10.

16 Wootton R, Reeve J, Veall N. The clinical measurement of skeletal blood flow. *Clin Sci Mol Med* 1976; **50**: 261–8.

17 Chipping P, Klonizakis I, Lewis SM. Indium chloride scanning: a comparison with iron as a tracer for erythropoiesis. *Clin Lab Haematol* 1980; **2**: 255–63.

18 Ussov Y, Aktolun C, Myers MJ, *et al.* Granulocyte margination in bone marrow: comparison with margination in the spleen and liver. *Scand J Clin Lab Invest* 1995; **55**: 87–96.

19 Skehan SJ, White JF, Parry-Jones DR, *et al.* Mechanism of accumulation of ^{99m}Tc-sulesomab in inflammation. *J Nucl Med* 2003; **44**: 11–18.

20 Reske SN. Marrow scintigraphy. In: Murray IPC, Ell PJ. (eds.) *Nuclear medicine in clinical diagnosis and treatment.* Edinburgh: Churchill Livingstone, 1994: 705–9.

21 Wakasugi S, Noguti A, Katuda T, *et al.* Potential of ^{99m}Tc-MIBI for detecting bone marrow metastases. *J Nucl Med* 2002; **43**: 596–602.

22 Fonti R, Del Vecchio S, Zannetti A, *et al.* Bone marrow uptake of ^{99m}Tc-MIBI in patients with multiple myeloma. *Eur J Nucl Med* 2001; **28**: 214–20.

23 Kostakoglu L, Guc D, Campinar H, *et al.* P-glycoprotein expression by technetium-99m scintigraphy in hematological malignancy. *J Nucl Med* 1998; **39**: 1191–7.

24 Mileshkin L, Blum R, Seymour JF, *et al.* A comparison of fluorine-18 fluoro-deoxyglucose PET and technetium-99m sestamibi in assessing patients with multiple myeloma. *Eur J Haematol* 2004; **72**: 32–7.

Imaging the spleen

A.M. PETERS

INTRODUCTION

Radionuclide studies of the spleen make a small contribution to clinical nuclear medicine but they are important because of their general complexity. Clinical imaging of the spleen mostly aims to address its morphology, particularly its size, location and integrity following surgical or accidental trauma. Other important applications concern the intrasplenic kinetics of blood cells, and include the investigation of patients with abnormally low peripheral cell counts, such as idiopathic thrombocytopenic purpura (ITP). Finally, a variety of nuclear investigations complement the cross-sectional imaging modalities of computerized tomography (CT), ultrasound (US) and magnetic resonance imaging (MRI) in evaluating splenic diseases, including focal masses and infiltrative pathologies such as amyloidosis, neoplasia and granulomatous diseases.

ANATOMY AND PHYSIOLOGY

The spleen is located in the upper left quadrant of the abdomen, behind the stomach and above the left kidney. It is shaped like a saucer bent in the middle with the bend running cranio-caudally and the two flat halves located posteriorly and laterally. When viewed from the back or side, its longest dimension is cranio-caudal with a length of 8–13 cm.

Its microanatomy is complex and best summarized from the point of view of functional imaging as consisting mainly of a sinusoidal network called the red pulp served by splenic arterioles and draining into splenic venules (Fig. 16B.1).[1] In the human spleen, about 90% of the incoming blood serving the red pulp is delivered to the interstices of the network, with the remaining 10% being delivered directly to the sinusoidal vessels from where it drains to the splenic veins. The great majority of circulating blood cells on arrival in the spleen are therefore deposited within the interstices. This is a hostile environment containing many macrophages ready to engulf damaged cells. In order to exit the spleen, blood cells have to negotiate clefts between the endothelial cells of the sinusoid, a process requiring them to be deformable because, with the exception of platelets, the diameters of the inter-endothelial clefts are less than their own. Inclusion bodies in red cells, like Heinz bodies, are not deformable and the region of the red cell where they are located becomes trapped in the cleft and pinched off, allowing the cell to subsequently move through. Whilst this is the arrangement in 'couch-potato' species like humans and pigs, more athletic animals, like greyhounds and racehorses, have spleens in which at least 50% of the inflowing blood is delivered directly to the sinusoids, giving the majority of blood cells a fast exit.

Physiology of blood cell pooling in the spleen

The spleen has a remarkable capacity for blood cell storage. In humans, this is not long-term storage but a population of cells in dynamic equilibrium with the corresponding circulating population. The process is appropriately called blood cell pooling; the term sequestration implies prolonged storage of undefined duration and is best avoided. All blood cell types display splenic pooling to some extent.[2] Leukocytes and platelets take on average 10 min to undergo a single splenic transit.[3,4] Interestingly, this includes platelets, which, in view of their small size, is surprising in the context of the sinusoidal arrangement described above. The mechanisms governing blood cell transit time through the spleen are entirely unexplained. Nevertheless, in radiolabeled leukocyte or platelet studies, a prominent splenic image is not only a normal finding but reassuring with respect to cell functional

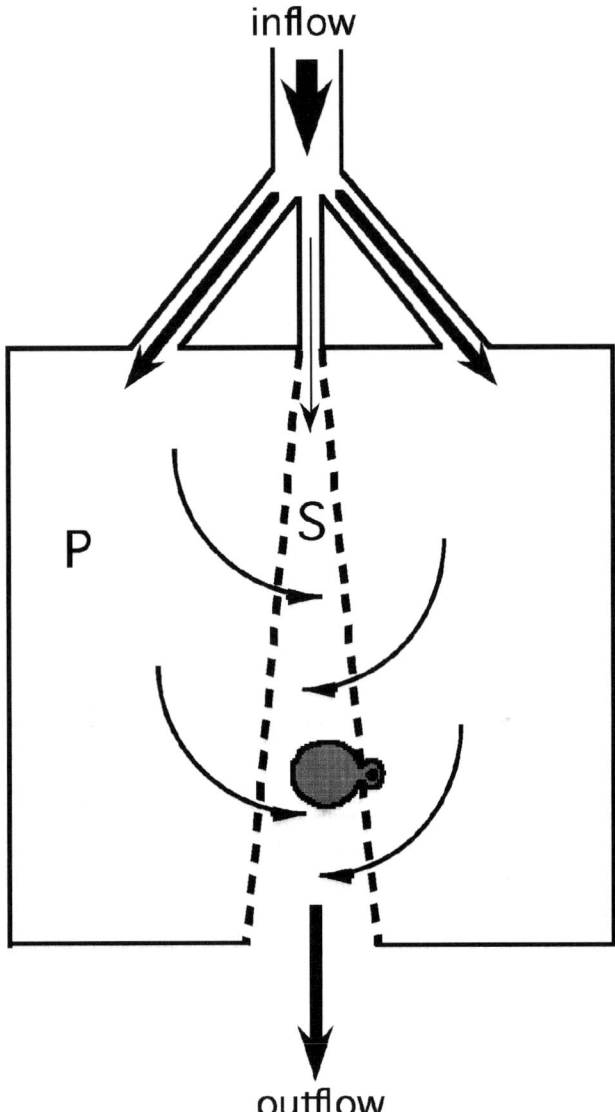

inflow

P

S

outflow

Figure 16B.1 *Diagrammatic illustration of the functional micro-anatomy of the spleen. Most incoming blood (≈90% in humans) enters the pulp meshwork (P) from where the formed elements enter the sinusoidal network (S) by negotiating sinusoidal inter-endothelial clefts that have an aperture smaller than their own diameter. A red cell with a trailing rigid inclusion body is shown. There is a great deal of interspecies variation, with for example more direct inflow to the sinusoids in species such as cat and dog.*

viability. Normal erythrocytes have a much shorter splenic transit time than platelets or leukocytes, but nevertheless still long enough, about 40–60 s, to give the spleen a hematocrit which is significantly higher than whole-body hematocrit, a fact that is evident from a routine multiple-gated cardiac study. The human spleen lacks a significant amount of smooth muscle in its capsule and does not actively contract in response to sympathetic stimulation, in contrast to the feline spleen for example which is able to contract and expel stored red cells. Human spleens do empty themselves of red cells in response, say, to severe short-term exercise but the

process is passive and mediated through a marked reduction in splenic blood flow.[2] The human spleen, in other words, is, in its resting condition, permanently erect.

LOCATING THE SPLEEN AND ASSESSING ITS INTEGRITY

Radiotracers

RADIOCOLLOIDS

About 30% of administered activity accumulates in the spleen about 1 h after injection of labeled leukocytes and platelets.[3,5] This level of selectivity is usually adequate for localizing the spleen or splenunculi with ^{99m}Tc-colloid, although splenic tissue close to the liver is likely to be obscured by hepatic uptake. Single photon emission computed tomography (SPECT) may be helpful in these circumstances. The main advantage of radiocolloids is that they are kit-formulated and therefore convenient.

LABELED RED CELLS

Normal red cells have a relatively long mean transit time through the spleen, which consequently is usually clearly visible on imaging studies for radionuclide ventriculography and localization of gastrointestinal bleeding (Fig. 16B.2). Heat treatment of red cells, traditionally at 49.5°C for 20 min, markedly increases splenic localization. Normal red cells are highly deformable whilst heat-damaged red cells (HDRBCs) are not. As a result, HDRBCs negotiate the spleen very slowly, with a mean time of 10–15 min (in contrast to about 40 s for normal cells), and are ultimately trapped[6] for erythrophagocytosis which occurs some hours later.[7] More than 50% of ^{99m}Tc-labeled HDRBCs localize in the spleen about 1 h after injection, so, compared with radiocolloids, they are more sensitive for localizing small nests of splenic tissue. Coating pre-labeled red cells with immunoglobulin, usually anti-D, is another way of promoting splenic uptake.[8] The rate of splenic accumulation is slower than with HDRBCs but liver uptake is less. The test cannot be used in Rhesus-negative subjects, but this is unimportant because such cells are hardly ever used for clinical imaging.

OTHER LABELED FORMED ELEMENTS

Labeled leukocytes and platelets accumulate in the spleen, about 30%[5] and 60%[3] of administered activity, respectively, at about 1 h post-injection. Apart from marginally less inconvenience, they offer no advantages over ^{99m}Tc-HDRBCs for splenic imaging *per se*.

Normal variants

Splenunculi represent accessory splenic tissue (Fig. 16B.2). They are common, are seen in approximately 10% of the

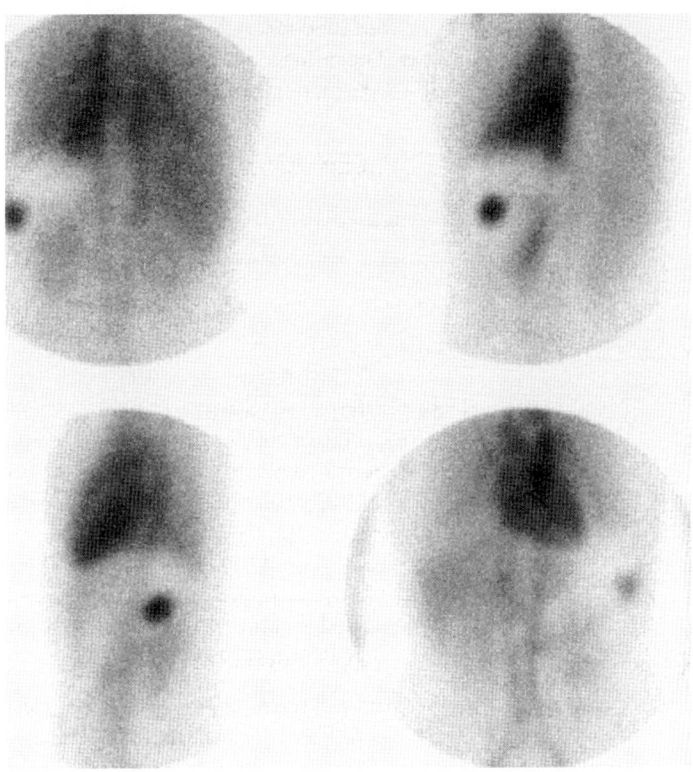

Figure 16B.2   *A splenunculus is visible on this* ^{99m}Tc-*labeled (undamaged) red cell study.*

normal population, may be multiple and occur most frequently around the pancreatic tail and splenic hilum. Splenunculi often enhance after intravenous contrast and therefore may be confused with an adjacent adrenal or lymph node mass. CT or US may suggest accessory splenic tissue but a ^{99m}Tc-colloid scan should be used to confirm this. There may be confusion on CT and US as well as on a colloid scan when the left lobe of the liver occupies the left upper quadrant. SPECT using colloid or the use of ^{99m}Tc-HDRBCs usually delineates the liver from the splenic tissue.

Trauma to the spleen

The integrity of the spleen following prolonged surgical procedures, especially in relation to the pancreas, is often questioned by the surgeon who is concerned about the possibility of intra-operative ischemia and subsequent splenic infarction. Planar imaging with ^{99m}Tc-labeled colloid is usually sufficient, although SPECT may be useful. The spleen is the most frequently injured organ in blunt abdominal trauma. CT can detect contusions, lacerations and splenic fractures and is the primary modality for imaging patients with acute abdominal injuries.

PREDICTING THE RESPONSE TO SPLENECTOMY

Nuclear medicine departments are occasionally called on to predict the response to splenectomy as a treatment for patients with hemolytic anemia or ITP, more often the latter.

The size of the splenic platelet pool is a function of splenic blood flow, which in turn is a function of spleen size. Increased splenic platelet pooling as a result of splenomegaly is a recognized cause of thrombocytopenia, although the spleen must be considerably enlarged to produce a significantly reduced platelet count. Although the size of the splenic platelet pool can be assessed by static quantitative imaging based on any of the cell types mentioned above, a more complete picture of intrasplenic platelet kinetics can be obtained by dynamic gamma camera imaging immediately following intravenous bolus injection of radiolabeled platelets. The blood pool signal in the normal subject falls exponentially over about 30 min asymptotically to a plateau value of about 65% of the maximum (initial) value (Fig. 16B.3). At the same time, the spleen platelet content rises, with a time course that is the mirror image of the blood pool time course, to reach its own plateau representing 30–35% of the labeled cells. Thus the labeled platelets reach dynamic equilibrium between blood and splenic pool after 25–30 min. In splenomegaly, however, increased splenic blood flow promotes earlier equilibration of the labeled platelets between blood and splenic pool and the equilibrium blood level, i.e. recovery, is reduced because of increased delivery of platelets to the spleen with no change in mean transit time (Fig. 16B.4). This is not sequestration but increased splenic pooling. 'Pooling' is a preferable term to 'hypersplenism' which is often used loosely and inappropriately to describe the same process.

Identification of abnormal platelet destruction in the spleen or liver is based on ^{111}In-labeled platelets. Identification of sites of platelet destruction is usually combined with

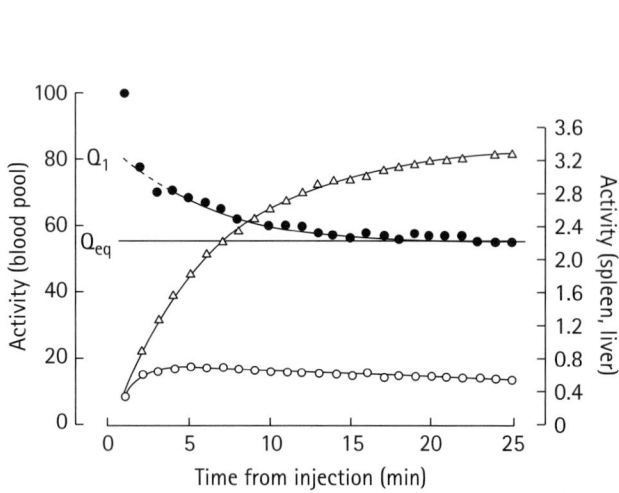

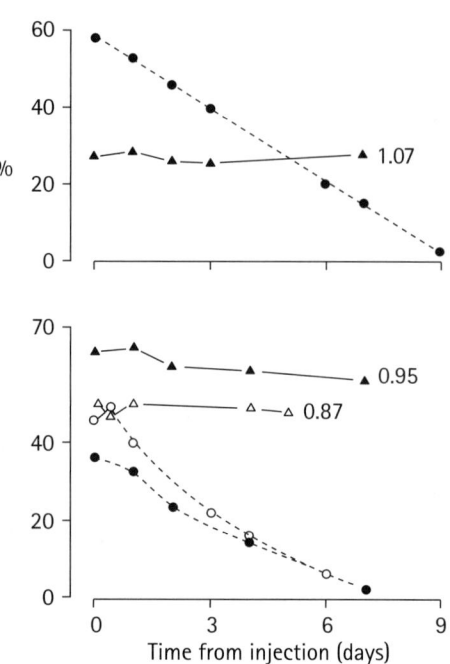

Figure 16B.3   *Time courses over 25 min of blood (filled circles), liver (unfilled circles) and spleen (triangles) activities following intravenous injection of ^{111}In-labeled platelets in a normal subject. The left ordinate refers to blood activity (percent of maximum) and the right ordinate refers to the liver and spleen (counts per frame per pixel). The subject was supine with the gamma camera below. The blood activity approaches a symptote (Q_{eq}) which represents platelet recovery. Extrapolation of the blood activity to 1 min (Q_1) represents the total activity available for equilibration in the model, which summarizes the kinetics. $Q_1 - Q_{eq}$ approximates to the activity in the spleen at equilibrium (reached at about 30 min after injection) and is consistent with a mean intrasplenic platelet transit time of about 10 min. (Reprinted from* Thrombosis and Haemostasis.*)*

Figure 16B.5   *Time courses over several days of blood (circles) and splenic (triangles) activities (per cent of administered activity, corrected for physical decay of the radionuclide, following intravenous injection of ^{111}In-labeled platelets in a normal subject (upper panel) and two patients with splenomegaly and reduced platelet survival (lower panel). The initial splenic activity arises from platelets that are pooling in the spleen while the activity present when the labeled cells have left the blood arises from platelets that have been destroyed in the spleen. In all subjects, initial and final activities (expressed as the destruction-to-pooling ratios) are similar, indicating in each case that the spleen is destroying about the same fraction of the platelet population that it pools. (Reprinted from* British Journal of Haematology.*)*

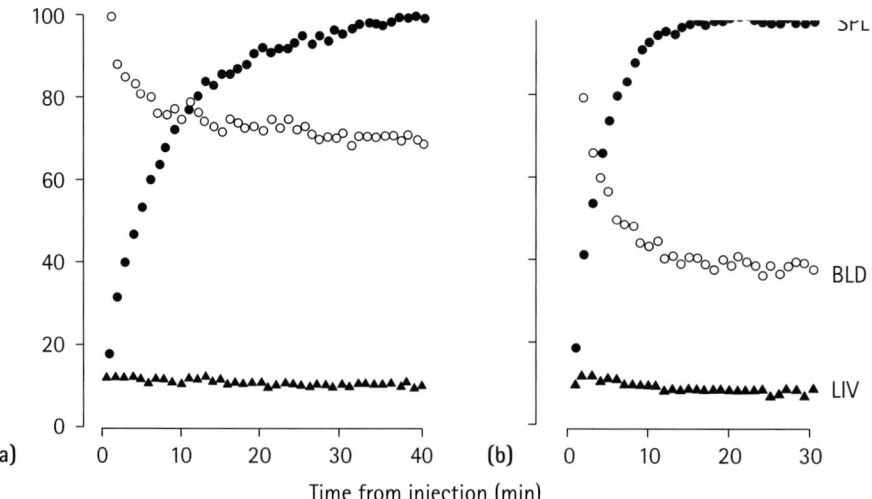

Figure 16B.4   *Time courses over 40 min of blood (unfilled circles), liver (triangles) and spleen (filled circles) activities following intravenous injection of ^{111}In-labeled platelets in a normal subject (a) and a patient with splenomegaly (b). Ordinate: per cent (of initial activity – blood; of maximal splenic activity [counts per pixel per frame] – spleen and liver). There is a lower recovery of platelets and earlier equilibration between blood and spleen in the patient with splenomegaly.*

measurement of the size of the splenic platelet pool and mean platelet life survival in blood (MPLS). Platelets radiolabeled at random (as from a peripheral blood sample) normally leave the blood after re-injection in a linear fashion, consistent with a destruction process based on senescence and a lifespan of 9 days. There are many causes of a reduced MPLS, most of which produce a modest reduction in platelet survival and introduce an element of random destruction, making the survival profile curvilinear. A severe reduction in MPLS gives rise to an exponential disappearance profile, is usually due to ITP and generally results in a platelet count less than about $50 \times 10^9 \, \mathrm{L}^{-1}$. The spleen is not usually enlarged in ITP and splenic platelet pooling is normal.[9] The principal reason for performing platelet kinetic studies with ^{111}In-platelets in these patients is to determine the predominant site of platelet destruction – the liver or spleen – and predict the response of the peripheral platelet count to splenectomy. These studies should be performed with autologous platelets, as labeled homologous platelets may give misleading information.[10]

Indium-111-labeled platelets are almost ideal to address this question as elution of ^{111}In from both platelets and their sites of deposition is very slow.[11] An interesting normal feature

of platelet destruction in the spleen, which forms the basis of the investigation, is that, in the absence of antiplatelet antibodies, its magnitude is matched by the capacity of the splenic platelet pool (Fig. 16B.5). Thus about 30% of circulating platelets are pooled in the spleen and about 30% are destroyed there. As pooling increases in splenomegaly, so does the fraction of platelets destroyed in the spleen. It seems as if, in splenomegaly, the likelihood of a platelet being in the spleen at the moment of its death increases. This means that the fraction of platelets destroyed in the spleen increases appropriately as spleen size increases (Figs 16B.5 and 16B.6).[12]

Several techniques have been used to quantify platelet destruction in the spleen. When ^{51}Cr was used, 'excess' counts were measured in the spleen using a scintillation probe and surface counting, analogously to the excess counts in a ^{51}Cr-labeled red cell study. Excess counts represent the difference between total counts in the spleen and those due to labeled platelets still in the circulation that are pooling in the spleen. The latter fraction is obtainable from the circulating activity. Thus, since the pooled platelets and circulating platelets are in equilibrium, the ratio of the count rates respectively recorded in circulating blood and over the spleen

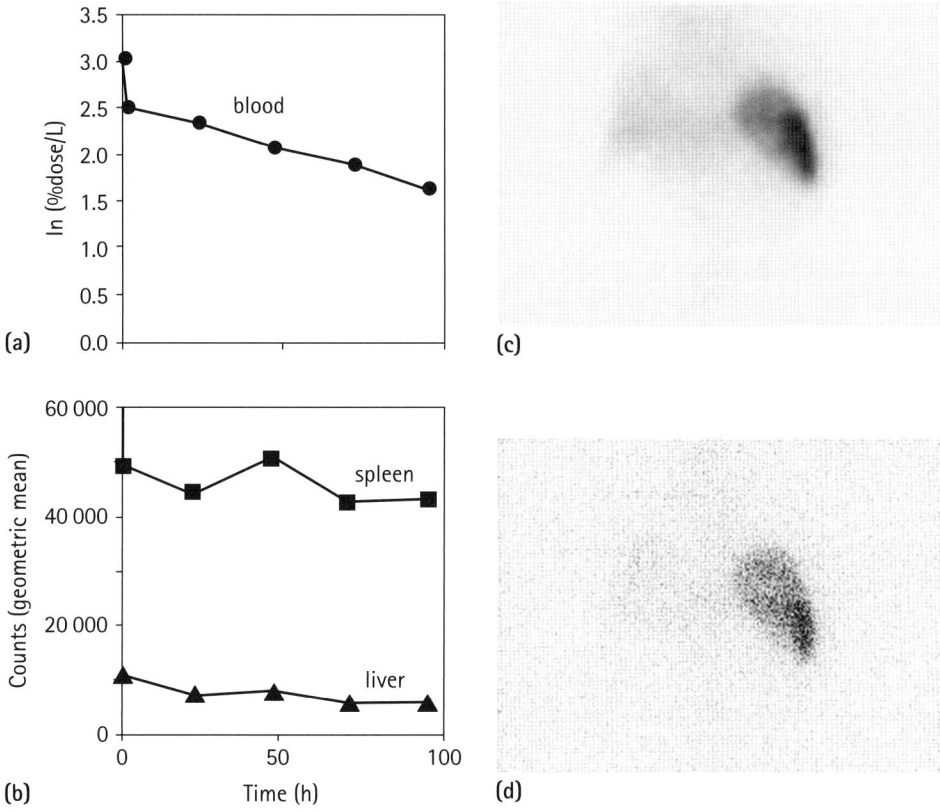

Figure 16B.6   *Time courses of (a) blood and (b) liver and splenic ^{111}In activities in a patient with splenomegaly and a moderately shortened platelet survival following intravenous injection of ^{111}In-labeled platelets (corrected for physical decay of the radionuclide) and corresponding images of liver and spleen obtained at (c) the completion of equilibrium (about 30 min) and (d) completion of blood clearance of labeled platelets (final splenic activity). Final splenic activity is similar to equilibrium activity (ie destruction-to-pooling ratio ≈ 1), indicating that the level of platelet destruction in the spleen is appropriate to splenic size.*

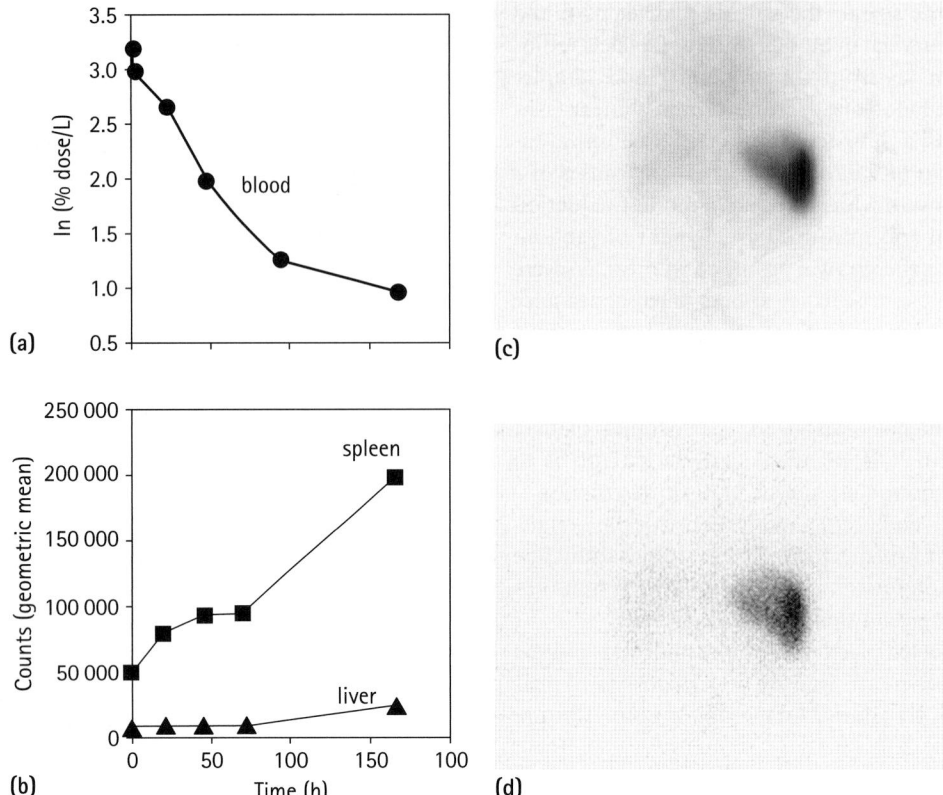

Figure 16B.7 *Time courses of (a) blood and (b) liver and splenic ^{111}In activities in a patient with idiopathic thrombocytopenic purpura following intravenous injection of ^{111}In-labeled platelets (corrected for physical decay of the radionuclide) and corresponding equilibrium and final images (c and d) of liver and spleen. The patient had a significantly shortened platelet survival. The final splenic activity is significantly higher than equilibrium activity, indicating that platelets are undergoing preferential splenic destruction (destruction-to-pooling ratio > 1). The peripheral platelet count would be predicted to increase in response to splenectomy.*

at the time equilibration is achieved (before there has been significant destruction) can be used to calculate the fraction of the splenic signal recorded at later time points that is due to platelet pooling.

Perhaps the most rational approach to quantification of platelet destruction in the spleen is a comparison of the splenic counts at the time when all the labeled platelets have disappeared from the circulation, which reflects destruction, with the counts at the time of equilibrium after the platelets are injected, which reflects pooling. This destruction-to-pooling ratio is then a measure of destruction which takes into account the tendency for destruction in the spleen to be increased (appropriately) in splenomegaly.[12] Re-direction of destruction towards or away from the spleen, as induced by anti-platelet antibodies, for example, will give ratios respectively less than or greater than unity (Figs 16B.7 to 16B.9). The technique becomes less sensitive for detecting abnormal splenic destruction in an enlarged spleen, since there is less scope for destruction to exceed pooling and their ratio tends towards unity. The reverse of this, i.e. detection of abnormal destruction elsewhere, is enhanced, however. An increased destruction-to-pooling ratio is seen in ITP with splenic destruction and in patients who have developed

antibodies to homologous labeled platelets. A decreased destruction-to-pooling ratio is seen in patients in whom hepatic destruction predominates or in patients with thrombocytopenia due to peripheral platelet consumption.

Surface counting of the spleen in anemia

Because of the relatively long normal life span of red cells, it is usually necessary, even in severe hemolytic anemia, to label red cells with ^{51}Cr, which has a physical half-life of 27.8 days. Sequential surface counting with a scintillation probe over the spleen, liver, pre-cordium and lumbar spine gives a semi-quantitative indication of the major sites of cell destruction.[13] Spleen and liver counts can be corrected for their contained blood pool by normalization to, and comparison with, pre-cordial counts. Thus, assuming that the organ counts immediately after injection of the labeled cells arise only from blood, the 'excess' counts represent the difference between spleen or liver counts and pre-cordial counts. In hereditary spherocytosis, excess counts in the spleen are markedly elevated but not accompanied by an increase in excess hepatic counts. In auto-immune hemolytic anemia, both are increased, although detection of excess

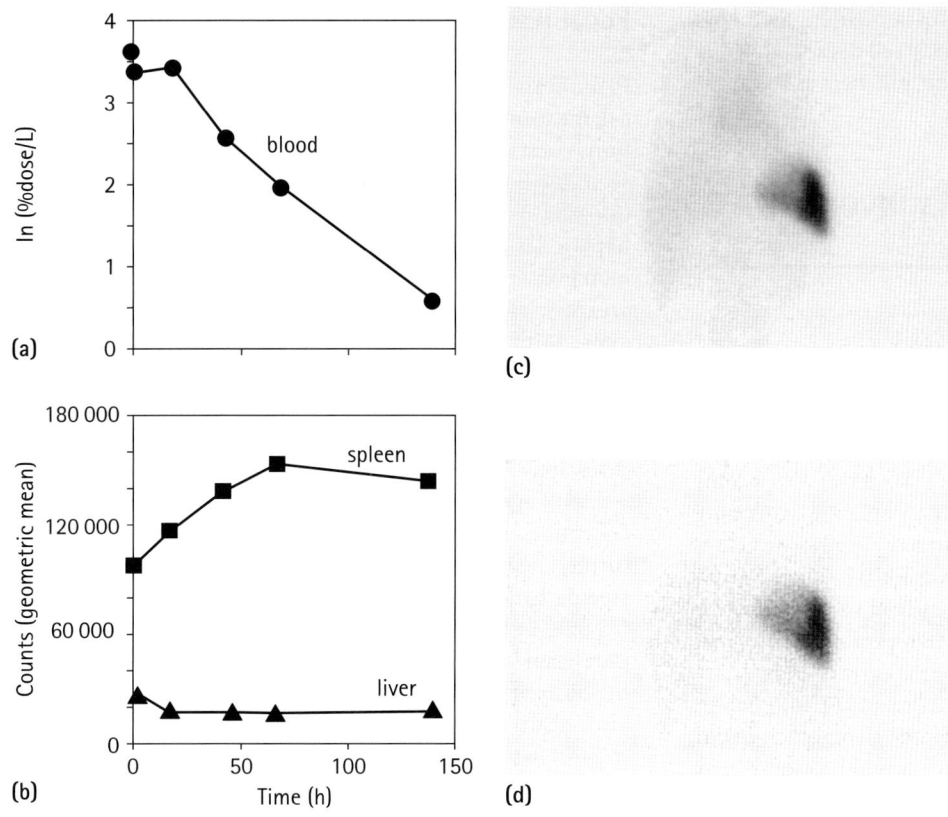

Figure 16B.8 *Time courses of (a) blood and (b) liver and splenic ^{111}In activities in a second patient with idiopathic thrombocytopenic purpura following intravenous injection of ^{111}In-labeled platelets (corrected for physical decay of the radionuclide) and corresponding equilibrium and final images (c and d) of liver and spleen. As with the patient mentioned in Fig. 16B.7, this patient also had a significantly shortened platelet survival. The final splenic activity is significantly higher than equilibrium activity, indicating that platelets are undergoing preferential splenic destruction (destruction-to-pooling ratio > 1). The peripheral platelet count would be predicted to increase in response to splenectomy.*

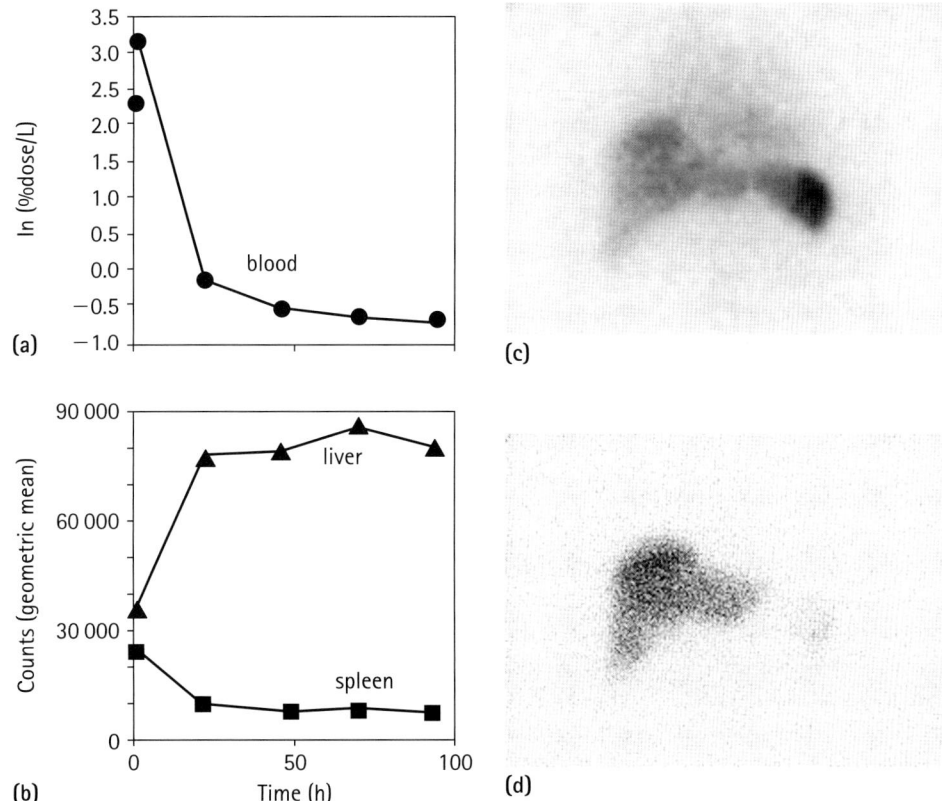

Figure 16B.9 *Time courses of (a) blood and (b) liver and splenic ^{111}In activities in a third patient with idiopathic thrombocytopenic purpura following intravenous injection of ^{111}In-labeled platelets (corrected for physical decay of the radionuclide) and corresponding equilibrium and final images (c and d) of liver and spleen. This patient also had significantly shortened platelet survival. Unlike the patients shown in Figs 16B.7 and 16B.8, the final splenic activity is lower, indicating that platelets are undergoing preferential extrasplenic destruction (destruction-to-pooling ratio < 1), obviously within the liver. The peripheral platelet count would not be predicted to increase in response to splenectomy.*

counts over the spleen may be helpful in predicting a favorable response to splenectomy. In sickle cell disease, the liver typically shows increased destruction, but, because of auto-splenectomy, the spleen does not.

IMAGING DISEASES DIRECTLY INVOLVING THE SPLEEN

Asplenia and polysplenia

In pediatrics, the location of the spleen may be important in the clinical setting of severe congenital heart disease. Splenic congenital anomalies, including asplenia and right-sided spleen, have a high level of association (80–95%) with a complex type of serious cardiovascular malformation, consisting of the following in various combinations: (1) atrial inversion or isomerism, and/or ventricular inversion; (2) single atrium or ventricle, or large atrio-septal or ventriculo-septal defect, or arterio-venous communication; (3) transposition of the great arteries, truncus arteriosus, atresia of the aorta or pulmonary artery, or double outlet of either ventricle; and (4) anomalous drainage of systemic or pulmonary veins or other major anomalies of central veins. Selective splenic imaging may therefore be helpful in the investigation of children suspected of having congenital heart disease, and, conversely, the incidental discovery of asplenia, polysplenia or right-sided spleen should suggest the possibility of co-existent complex cardiovascular malformations. In addition, there is a high incidence of co-existing anomalies of the liver, pancreas and lungs (heterotaxia syndrome). In functional asplenia, there is a morphologically intact organ with no uptake on sulfur colloid scans. This most frequently occurs in sickle cell disease or pathological splenic infiltration.

Ectopic spleen

The presence of splenic tissue in an ectopic location may be congenital or post-traumatic in etiology. It commonly results from seeding of splenic tissue to the peritoneal or pleural surfaces and is difficult to diagnose without utilizing a radiocolloid scan. A 'wandering spleen' is described when the spleen lies ectopically within the abdomen on an abnormally elongated mesentery.

Splenomegaly

In an adult, the upper limit of normal for splenic length is 13 cm.[14] The spleen is also considered to be enlarged if the antero-posterior diameter is greater than two thirds of the abdominal cavity. The degree of splenic enlargement varies with the underlying pathology; hematological malignancies can result in massive splenomegaly. Diffuse enlargement can be demonstrated equally well with ^{99m}Tc-colloid, radiolabeled blood cells, CT or US.

Focal lesions and neoplasms

Plain films frequently demonstrate splenic and parasplenic calcifications, although the location and nature of calcification is best demonstrated on US or CT. The most commonly seen calcifications are vascular and those of granulomatous diseases. Focal masses within the spleen are rarer than hepatic lesions and include benign entities such as cysts, hematomata and abscesses. Pseudocysts, secondary to pancreatitis, are more commonly seen than true congenital cysts. Both appear as a well-defined photopenic area on colloid scanning. Although purulent collections in the spleen are rare, collections close to the spleen are not. Imaging of infected collections with radiolabeled leukocytes, may require an additional image of the spleen with a separate agent, such as radiocolloid, in order to locate the collection. Alternatively, sequential imaging may be performed using a very early splenic image to depict the splenic leukocyte pool as a surrogate for a colloid image. US or CT can differentiate a simple cyst from a more complex lesion such as an abscess, hematoma or hydatid cyst on the basis of calcifications, septae or internal debris. CT will also clearly define changes typical of pancreatic inflammation associated with a pseudocyst. Splenic infarcts are commonly found in patients with hematological diseases and appear as peripherally based wedge shaped areas of decreased uptake on radionuclide images and on CT as non-enhancing low-density defects.

Neoplastic involvement of the spleen is uncommon except in hematological malignancies. The most common benign splenic neoplasm is a hemangioma which is most clearly demonstrated on US as a well-defined echogenic focus. Angiosarcoma is a rare primary tumor of the spleen, lymphoma commonly involves the spleen and metastatic melanoma classically spreads to spleen. Malignancies arising in breast, colon, lung, ovary and prostate may also rarely metastasize to the spleen. Metastatic deposits appear as multiple focal cold areas on ^{99m}Tc-labeled colloid scans and usually appear on CT as multiple hypodense or isodense lesions. Lymphoma is a more common cause of focal splenic deposits than metastases, and in lymphoma, the spleen may be normal in size in a third of cases. Gallium-67 citrate scanning may demonstrate increased uptake in a spleen involved by lymphoma. Granulomatous diseases such as sarcoidosis are also in the differential diagnosis of multifocal defects on ^{99m}Tc-labeled colloid.

Amyloidosis

Amyloid infiltration of the spleen can be readily demonstrated with ^{123}I-labeled serum amyloid P component (SAP) (Fig. 16B.10).[15] In addition to the spleen, the other organs easily seen on SAP scanning when infiltrated with amyloid are the liver, bone marrow, kidneys and adrenals. Other tissues that commonly accumulate amyloid fibrils but are not

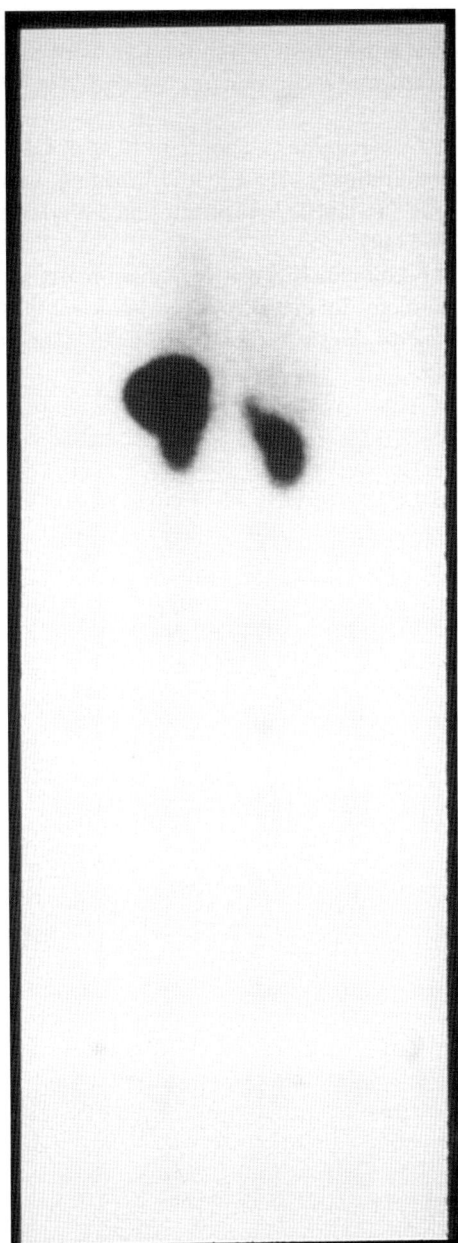

Figure 16B.10 *Whole body (posterior) ^{123}I-serum amyloid component scan in a patient with rheumatoid arthritis who developed AL amyloid. There is intense localization of tracer in the spleen, kidneys and adrenal glands. (With kind permission of Professor Philip Hawkins.)*

easily seen on SAP scanning include the tongue, myocardium, skeletal muscle, skin and gastrointestinal tract. The reason for this organ-based difference is probably related to capillary permeability, which in organs like the spleen and liver is very high, allowing penetration of very large molecules like SAP ($\approx$350 kDa). A much smaller molecule which targets amyloid, the polypeptide aprotenin, has been successfully used to image amyloid in tissues with low endothelial permeability, such as muscle and skin,[16] for which SAP has been unsuccessful.

Extramedullary hematopoiesis

A form of 'physiological' splenic infiltration is myeloid metaplasia, in which the spleen, usually along with the liver and also occasionally with lymph nodes, becomes a site of erythropoiesis. The radionuclides of iron, ^{59}Fe, and, in centers with facilities for PET, ^{52}Fe, label the erythron and are used to identify sites of erythropoiesis in aplastic anemia and myelofibrosis. Iron-52 is a positron emitter which gives high resolution PET images of the distribution of erythropoietic tissue.[17] The detection of splenic erythropoiesis, which is absent in uncomplicated polycythemia vera but invariably present in myelofibrosis, is helpful for documenting the transition from polycythemia to a myelofibrotic state. In doubtful cases of essential thrombocythemia, the detection of splenic erythropoiesis confirms the presence of a myeloproliferative disorder rather than a reactive thrombocytosis.

REFERENCES

1 Weiss L. The spleen. In: Weiss L. (ed.) *Cell and tissue biology*, 6th edition. Baltimore: Urban and Schwarzenberg, 1988: 515–38.

2 Allsop P, Peters AM, Arnot RN, *et al.* Intrasplenic blood cell kinetics in man before and after brief maximal exercise. *Clin Sci* 1992; **83**: 47–54.

3 Peters AM, Klonizakis I, Lavender JP, Lewis SM. Use of indium-111 labelled platelets to measure spleen function. *Br J Haematol* 1980; **46**: 587–93.

4 Peters AM, Saverymuttu SH, Keshavarzian A, *et al.* Splenic pooling of granulocytes. *Clin Sci* 1985; **68**: 283–9.

5 Saverymuttu SH, Peters AM, Keshavarzian A, *et al.* The kinetics of 111-indium distribution following injection of 111-indium labelled autologous granulocytes in man. *Br J Haematol* 1985; **61**: 675–85.

6 Peters AM, Ryan PFJ, Klonizakis I, *et al.* Kinetics of heat damaged autologous red blood cells. Mechanisms of clearance from blood. *Scand J Haematol* 1982; **28**: 5–14.

7 Klausner MA, Hirsch LJ, Leblond PF, *et al.* Contrasting splenic mechanisms in the blood clearance of red blood cells and colloidal particles. *Blood* 1975; **46**: 965–76.

8 Thomson A, Contreras M, Gorick B, *et al.* Clearance of Rh D-positive red cells with monoclonal anti-D. *Lancet* 1990; **336**: 1147–50.

9 Peters AM, Saverymuttu SH, Bell RN, Lavender JP. The kinetics of short-lived indium-111 radiolabelled platelets. *Scand J Haematol* 1985; **34**: 137–45.

10 Peters AM, Porter JB, Saverymuttu SH, *et al.* The kinetics of unmatched and HLA-matched 111-In-labelled homologous platelets in recipients with chronic marrow hypoplasia and anti-platelet immunity. *Br J Haematol* 1985; **60**: 117–27.

11 Peters AM, Klonizakis I, Lavender JP, Lewis SM. Elution of 111-indium from reticuloendothelial cells. *J Clin Pathol* 1982; **35**: 507–9.

12 Peters AM, Saverymuttu SH, Wonke B, *et al.* The interpretation of platelet kinetics studies for the identification of sites of abnormal platelet destruction. *Br J Haematol* 1984; **57**: 637–49.

13 Dacie JV, Lewis SM. *Practical haematology*, 7th edition. Edinburgh: Churchill-Livingstone, 1991.

14 Rosenberg HK, Markowitz RI, Kolbeg H, *et al.* Normal splenic size in infants and children: sonographic measurements. *Am J Roentgenol* 1991; **157**: 119–21.

15 Hawkins PN, Lavender JP, Pepys MB. Evaluation of systemic amyloidosis by scintigraphy with ^{123}I-labeled serum amyloid P component. *N Engl J Med* 1990; **323**: 508–13.

16 Aprile C, Marinone G, Saponaro R, *et al.* Cardiac and pleuropulmonary AL amyloid imaging with technetium-99m labelled aprotinin. *Eur J Nucl Med* 1995; **22**: 1393–401.

17 Jamar F, Lonneux M. Positron emission tomography in haematology. In: Peters AM. (ed.) *Nuclear medicine in radiological diagnosis.* London: Martin Dunitz, 2003: 519–29.

Imaging of lymphomas

L. KOSTAKOGLU, M. COLEMAN, J.P. LEONARD, AND S.J. GOLDSMITH

INTRODUCTION

The prognosis of patients with Hodgkin's disease (HD) and aggressive subtypes of non-Hodgkin's lymphoma (NHL) has significantly improved with the evolution of combination chemotherapy regimens and radiation therapy strategies over the last decade. Accurate staging, restaging and evaluation of therapy response have a significant impact on clinical patient management. Recent technologic advances have enhanced the potential of diagnostic imaging, in the determination of the extent of disease, assessment of prognosis, therapy strategy and subsequent radiotherapy, especially in those patients with bulky lymphomas. The unnecessary use of chemotherapy and external-beam radiation could significantly increase the risk of secondary malignancies and myocardial toxicity. Thus, the early identification of a high-risk population that might benefit from more intensive chemotherapy protocols can potentially improve patient outcome.[1] The magnitude of the risk and poor prognosis associated with some second malignancies warrants more comprehensive screening strategies using more sensitive imaging techniques.[2]

To an extent, there is controversy regarding the exclusive use of anatomic imaging modalities, primarily computed tomography (CT), as the staging and restaging tool in lymphoma. Since the diagnostic sensitivity of these modalities is dependent on size criteria, they fall short in the identification of lymphoma in normal-size lymph nodes. These anatomic modalities cannot also differentiate sterile lymph nodes which are enlarged due to benign or therapy-related causes from malignant ones.[3] Hence, it is not surprising to observe that the failure-free survivals are not significantly different between patients with residual masses and those with complete resolution of lymphoma on post-therapy CT scans. These results may be probably due, in part, to replacement of tumor cells by fibroblasts; as a result no significant volume loss occurs in the original tumor mass.[4–7] Currently, magnetic resonance imaging (MRI) does not yield more specific results than CT for viable tumor and cannot reliably differentiate active lymphoma from infection, hemorrhage or radiation fibrosis.[8,9] Nevertheless, MRI offers advantages over CT in the evaluation of disease process in the central nervous system.

Gallium-67 imaging has been useful for the assessment of therapy response in HD and aggressive NHL (Fig. 16C.1).[6,7,10–12] At initial presentation, however, ^{67}Ga scintigraphy does not contribute significantly to the staging process due to its limited resolution and physiologic uptake in the abdomen. Gallium-67 scintigraphy also lacks specificity in the hilar[13] and abdominal regions. Furthermore, the sensitivity of ^{67}Ga is notoriously low for identifying lesion sites in indolent subtypes compared to HD and aggressive NHL.[14] Thallium-201 or ^{99m}Tc-sestamibi imaging have been proposed as alternative or complementary studies in the assessment of low-grade lymphomas, although similar restrictions apply to both of these radiotracers when imaging infra-diaphragmatic lymphomas.[14,15] While providing complementary information to CT, imaging with these radiotracers lacks accuracy or detection capability to supplant anatomic staging or restaging paradigms.

Positron emission tomography (PET) imaging using [^{18}F]fluorodeoxyglucose (^{18}F-FDG) is a noninvasive functional imaging tool used to characterize rate of glycolysis and high glucose utilization in tumors.[16] FDG PET has been integrated effectively into the staging and restaging algorithm in lymphoma.[17–29] FDG PET has also been a valuable tool to evaluate response to therapy either after

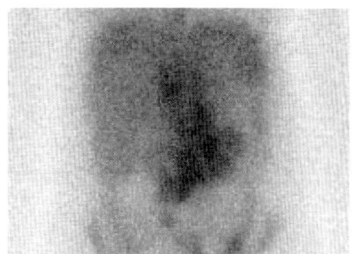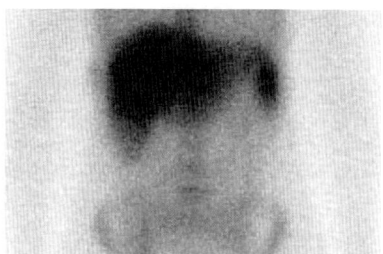

Figure 16C.1   *Patient with a history of stage II abdominal non-Hodgkin's lymphoma underwent a* ^{67}*Ga scintigraphy prior to and after completion of therapy. The pre-therapy study (left panel) demonstrates that there is intense accumulation of the radiotracer in the paraaortic and common iliac lymph node stations consistent with active lymphoma. The post-therapy study (right panel) demonstrates that there is complete resolution of disease. The progression free survival has not been reached for this particular patient after a follow-up period of 36 months.*

completion of or during therapy in lymphoma. With the recent introduction of FDG PET with co-registered CT (PET/CT) scanners, a combined method of metabolic and morphologic imaging has increased the specificity of FDG PET imaging.

This chapter will primarily focus on FDG PET imaging in lymphoma, although applications of traditional radiotracers such as gallium-67 citrate, thallium-201 chloride, and $^{99\,m}$Tc-sestamibi will also be covered briefly.

PATHOLOGICAL AND CLINICAL CLASSIFICATION OF LYMPHOMAS

The development of the revised European–American classification of lymphoid neoplasms (REAL) system in 1994 has incorporated the contributions from immunology, cytogenetics and molecular biology.[30] The World Health Organization (WHO) has also developed a new classification system that encompasses the REAL system with minor modifications.[31] This integrated system is called the WHO/REAL classification used for both HD and NHL.[32] Under this system, although there are more than 30 biologically different lymphoma subtypes, lymphomas are traditionally classified into two broad categories: Hodgkin's disease (HD) and non-Hodgkin's lymphomas (NHLs).

The prevalence of NHLs is higher than that of HD and accounts for 88% of the lymphomas. The overwhelming majority of NHL (~90%) are of B-cell origin and are essentially divided into two main groups: *indolent lymphomas* and *aggressive lymphomas*, based on different therapeutic implications and patient management. Aggressive lymphomas constitute approximately 60% of NHL series[33] while indolent lymphomas account for approximately 40% of new diagnoses.

HD is a relatively rare malignancy accounting for an overall 10–15% of lymphomas. There are two major types of HD according to WHO/REAL system: nodular lymphocyte-predominant HD and classical HD. Classical HD is further classified into nodular sclerosis, mixed cellularity, lymphocyte-rich and lymphocyte-depletion types.

Table 16C.1   *Ann Arbor staging system of lymphomas*

Stage	Features
I	*Involvement of a single lymph node region or involvement of a single extra-lymphatic organ*
II	*Involvement of two or more lymph node regions on the same side of the diaphragm or localized involvement of an extra-lymphatic organ or site plus an involved lymph node region on the same side of the diaphragm*
III	*Involvement of lymph nodes involved on both sides of the diaphragm can be accompanied by extra-lymphatic organ involvement including the spleen*
IV	*Diffuse or disseminated involvement of one or more extra-lymphatic organs with or without associated lymph node involvement*

The presence or absence of the following symptoms should be noted with each stage designation: A = asymptomatic; B = fever, sweats, or weight loss greater than 10% of body weight.

Classical HD usually involves the mediastinum and a late relapse following treatment is uncommon. In patients with nodular lymphocyte-predominant HD, peripheral lymph node involvement is more common; the disease usually progresses slowly, and late relapses are common.

Staging of lymphomas

The Ann Arbor staging system that was primarily formulated for HD and subsequently modified in 1989 remains the most widely used staging system[34] (Table 16C.1). This system is also adapted for the use in NHL where dissemination is more non-contiguous compared to the contiguous spread observed in HD.[35] There are basically four stages of lymphomas as demonstrated in Table 16C.1. Staging can be further modified according to various other risk factors such as the so-called B symptoms (fever higher than 100.5°F, night sweats, and weight loss) and bulky disease (tumor larger than 10 cm) which portend poorer outcomes: stages I and IIA are considered early-stage disease.

Stages IIB (particularly bulky), III and IV are considered advanced-stage disease.

Staging work-up of lymphomas

Lymphomas are typically staged through physical examination, laboratory evaluation (blood counts and chemistries), bone marrow aspirate and biopsy, as well as imaging which usually includes CT scans but may also involve MRI, ^{67}Ga and, lately, FDG PET. Other studies, including organ biopsy and CSF sampling, may be performed in certain clinical situations.

IMAGING MODALITIES AT INITIAL DIAGNOSIS AND STAGING OF LYMPHOMA

From the point of view of a clinician, imaging modalities are of value if they assist in defining prognosis or help to direct a change in management. While stage and extent of disease is important in lymphoma, they are generally subordinate in value to histological assessment. Staging is more clinically relevant in the aggressive NHL than it is in the indolent NHL as 85–90% of patients with indolent lymphomas initially present with advanced stage disease. Thus, imaging has a limited role in the indolent subtypes as treatment is defined more by symptoms than extent of disease. However, one important issue with indolent lymphomas is the common transformation to an aggressive histology which requires more aggressive treatment and generally portends an adverse outcome. Imaging has a role if it has the capability to determine the sites of transformation.

The more aggressive lymphomas, predominantly large cell lymphoma, are potentially curable in approximately 40–50% of patients but, if not, are usually rapidly fatal.[36] Classical HD is potentially curable in over 80% of cases. Staging of extent of disease and determination of response are critical since the stage may determine the treatment and prognosis. Imaging can serve to rule in or rule out disease sites in a way that can direct the appropriate use of radiotherapy in both of these subtypes.

Of greater importance in lymphoma, from the oncologist's perspective, is the possibility that imaging can establish prognosis (if superior or complementary to other information, such as the international prognostic index (IPI) or international prognostic score (IPS)[36,37] in a way that directs a change in management. For this concept to be of practical value, however, simply establishing prognosis is of limited assistance unless this knowledge can be effectively followed up with a treatment change that is necessary and of value in itself to improve outcomes. The second part of this process, improvement of therapy for poor prognosis patients, is not clearly achievable but is under intensive evaluation as part of ongoing clinical trials. Without the added

value of a change in treatment, any added prognostic information through imaging will be limited in its utility.

MORPHOLOGIC IMAGING MODALITIES

Pre-therapy evaluation

The imaging modality of choice for staging HD and NHL has traditionally been whole-body CT scanning. Despite the recent introduction of the fast spin-echo sequences and effective artifact suppression, the overall spatial resolution of MRI is still inferior to that of CT. Nevertheless, MRI offers advantages that include better tissue discrimination, lack of ionizing radiation and use of contrast agents with less risk of systemic effects.[38–41] Imaging characteristics of both CT and MRI can not differentiate between normal findings from malignant changes in normal-size lymph nodes as they both depend on size criteria.

CHEST

While intrathoracic disease is more common with HD (85%) than NHL (40–50%), extranodal involvement of the lung parenchyma, pleura and pericardium is more frequently observed with NHL.[42] For evaluation of chest wall involvement, CT and MRI are equally sensitive and reliable in demonstrating extent of disease.[43] CT plays a significant role for recognizing bulky mediastinal disease which is considered a poor prognostic sign. The additional information from CT, however, is felt to be more useful in early stage disease than in advanced stage disease as treatment strategy may be altered by detection of additional disease sites in the early stage population.[44]

ABDOMEN AND PELVIS

Enlarged lymph nodes (>1 cm), most often retroperitoneal, are generally deemed to harbor lymphoma. In HD, a false-negative rate of 20–80% has been observed in normal-size lymph nodes in the upper abdomen, reflecting the limited sensitivity of CT imaging.[45] MRI with a T2-weighted TSE sequence is considered equivalent to spiral CT and represents an alternative method of examination in abdominal lymphoma. Similar to CT, however, pathological diagnosis using MRI is largely dependent on size criteria.

EXTRANODAL LYMPHOMA

Extranodal NHL encompasses a heterogeneous group of disease presentations of a variety of histologic entities. Bone marrow involvement is more common in NHL than in HD. MRI is more sensitive than biopsy in detecting BM infiltration by lymphoma.[46] It is not practical and cost-effective, however, to routinely assess the entire marrow using MRI. Furthermore, at restaging, therapy-related MRI abnormalities may persist in the BM even in the absence of viable disease.[47] For patients with both bone or BM and adjacent soft tissue involvement, MRI is preferred over CT for better definition of disease for radiotherapy planning.

Primary CNS lymphoma, which is exclusively of the NHL type, is more frequently seen in patients with a history of immunodeficiency or immunosuppression.[48] CT and MRI generally provide findings that are suggestive but not conclusive for CNS lymphoma.[49] Although MR perfusion imaging has been reported to distinguish between AIDS-associated CNS lymphoma and toxoplasmosis, accurate differentiation between these two diseases remains challenging by radiographic criteria.

The detection of hepatic, splenic and small bowel lymphoma is usually achieved by a multimodality approach involving CT, MRI and ultrasound as well as histopathologic assessment.[50]

Post-therapy evaluation

The limitations of current anatomic imaging studies are most evident in the post-therapy setting. As many as 50–80% of patients with HD and 30% of those with NHL have residual masses after treatment. This challenging problem on anatomic imaging has been recognized in the established response criteria classification system for both HD and NHL.[51] Both systems designate residual masses of unclear etiology as CRu, or unconfirmed/uncertain complete responses. Although an aggressive treatment approach is appropriate for residual lymphoma, further treatment in patients with benign post-therapy changes only increases morbidity and risk of second malignancies.[52] Strategies to reduce the risk include limiting the number of CT scans or substituting CT with alternative examinations such as FDG PET studies.[53]

NUCLEAR MEDICINE IMAGING MODALITIES

Imaging with gallium-67 citrate

Gallium-67 imaging has been an effective method of detecting sites of involvement in lymphoma, primarily in the post-therapy setting. However, its role has been declining with the greater availability of FDG PET scanning, both with dedicated PET scanners and combination PET/CT machines.

Gallium-67 is an analog of Fe^{3+} and binds to iron-binding proteins, mainly transferrin in the serum. The accumulation of ^{67}Ga in tumors is mediated by various factors associated with tumor composition and physiology such as tumor-associated transferrin receptors (CD-71), anaerobic tumor metabolism that leads to the dissociation of the Ga–transferrin complex in conditions of low pH, increased tumor perfusion and vascular permeability.[54–57] The biodistribution of ^{67}Ga may be altered in patients with iron overload as ^{67}Ga competes with iron for transferrin binding.

Summaries comparing the imaging techniques are presented in Table 16C.2, while the performance of ^{67}Ga in the evaluation of therapy response and residual disease is

Table 16C.2 *Imaging techniques*

Technique	Dose		Parameters
	MBq	mCi	
FDG PET	370–555	10–15	Fast for 4–6 h fasting. Acquisition starts at 1–2 h after injection. Oral contrast can be given 30 min prior to imaging. Patient's blood glucose level should be $<200\,U\,dL^{-1}$ for an optimal study.
Gallium-67 citrate	296–370	8–10	Acquisition starts at 48–72 h following injection. Whole-body and SPECT images (usually chest) acquired using a medium energy collimator with energy peaks of 93, 185 and 300 keV with setting 20% windows. Additional views can be obtained up to 7 days.
Thallium-201	111–148	3–4	Fast for 4 h. Acquisition starts at 20–30 min following injection. Whole-body and SPECT images acquired using a low-energy collimator with energy peaks of 80 and 167 keV with 20% windows. Additional views can be obtained at 3–4 h.
Technetium-99m sestamibi	740–925	20–25	Fast for 4 h. Acquisition starts at 20–30 min following injection. Whole-body and SPECT images acquired using a low-energy collimator with an energy peak of 140 keV with 15–20% windows. Additional views can be obtained up to 4 h.
Indium-111-octreotide	222	6	Suspend therapy with octreotide acetate during this procedure, if applicable. Whole-body images obtained at 4 and 24 h. SPECT is obtained at 24 h. Whole-body and SPECT images are acquired using a medium energy collimator with energy peaks of 173 and 246 keV with 15–20% windows. Additional views can be obtained at 48–72 h.

presented in Table 16C.3. In the interests of being concise in this text, the reader is referred to the bibliography for additional details.[56–87] Briefly, the highlights of ^{67}Ga imaging are:

- Gallium-67 scintigraphy is more sensitive in the detection of mediastinal disease and at peripheral disease locations than abdominal disease. Clearance of ^{67}Ga through bowels and accumulation in the liver and spleen may pose a diagnostic challenge for evaluation of patients with infradiaphragmatic lymphomas. However, this problem can be avoided to a great extent with the use of SPECT-CT fusion capable gamma cameras (Plate 16C.1).
- Gallium-67 is not specific for malignant lesions as it accumulates in infectious or inflammatory processes. In this regard, therapy-related inflammatory changes may also cause false positive findings on ^{67}Ga studies, especially related to chemo- or radiotherapy induced pneumonia (Fig. 16C.2).
- Gallium-67 scintigraphy is more useful in the post-therapy setting than at initial staging, but a baseline study prior to therapy is necessary to fully assess residual or recurrent disease.
- Gallium-67 imaging after induction chemotherapy has the ability to differentiate chemosensitive patients from those with poor prognosis. A positive post-therapy ^{67}Ga scintigraphy is consistently associated with poor prognosis while a negative result suggests a favorable prognosis. False-negative results, however, may arise due to resolution limitations.
- Gallium-67 scintigraphy can predict therapy outcome as early as after one cycle of therapy.[7,12,88]
- The sensitivity of ^{67}Ga imaging varies among subtypes of lymphoma. It is most sensitive in aggressive NHL (especially diffuse large cell subtype) (Plate 16C.2) and HD and least sensitive in low-grade lymphoma (especially in MALT and small lymphocytic subtype).[65]
- The hilar uptake of ^{67}Ga is often seen only on SPECT, and most likely of benign etiology when symmetric and less intense than the original disease. Asymmetric focal and intense hilar uptake, however, indicates lymphoma (Fig. 16C.3).[13]
- Following chemotherapy, ^{67}Ga uptake in the anterior superior mediastinum is often observed in children and young adults indicating thymic rebound rather than residual disease.[89] If the original disease site is in the superior mediastinum, differentiation of thymic rebound from residual disease may be difficult.
- During or shortly after chemotherapy, ^{67}Ga uptake may be suppressed even if the tumor is viable. There should

Table 16C.3 *Post-therapy ^{67}Ga studies: evaluation of therapy response and residual disease*

Authors	Year	Number of patients	Patient group	ChemoRx cycles	PPV (%)	NPV (%)
Front[7]	*1999*	*31*	*HD*	*1*	*57*	*92*
Front[12]	*2000*	*51*	*NHL*	*1*	*71*	*81*
				3	*74*	*63*
Israel[87]	*2002*	*139*	*NHL*	*1*	*64*	*83*
				3	*77*	*66*
Janicek[6]	*1997*	*30*	*NHL*	*2*	*82*	*94*
Hagemeister[10]	*1994*	*46*	*HD*	*3‡*	*30*	*97*
Ionescu[81]	*2000*	*53*	*HD*	*3–4*	*81*	*86*
Kaplan[86]	*1990*	*37*	*NHL*	*4*	*76*	*70*
Salloum[11]	*1997*	*101*	*HD*	*Completion*	*†*	*83.5*
Front[80]	*1992*	*43*	*HD*	*Completion*	*80*	*84*
		56	*aNHL*	*Completion*	*73*	*84*
Cooper[82]	*1993*	*48*	*HD*	*Completion*	*†*	*73*
Bogart[84]	*1998*	*60*	*HD*	*Completion*	*¶*	*78*
Vose[85]	*1996*	*66*	*aNHL*	*Completion**	*75*	*47*
		77	*LGL*	*Completion**	*76*	*45*

PPV: positive predictive value; NPV: negative predictive value; NHL: non-Hodgkin's lymphoma including low-grade lymphoma; HD: Hodgkin's disease; LGL: low-grade lymphoma; aNHL: aggressive NHL.
*Patients were evaluated after high-dose chemotherapy and bone marrow transplant.
†Inadequate number of patients to determine PPV.
‡Patients were evaluated after three cycles of NOVP (novantrone, vincristine, vinblastine, prednisone) prior to radiotherapy.
¶PPV not given but there was no difference in overall survival between Ga positive or negative patient.

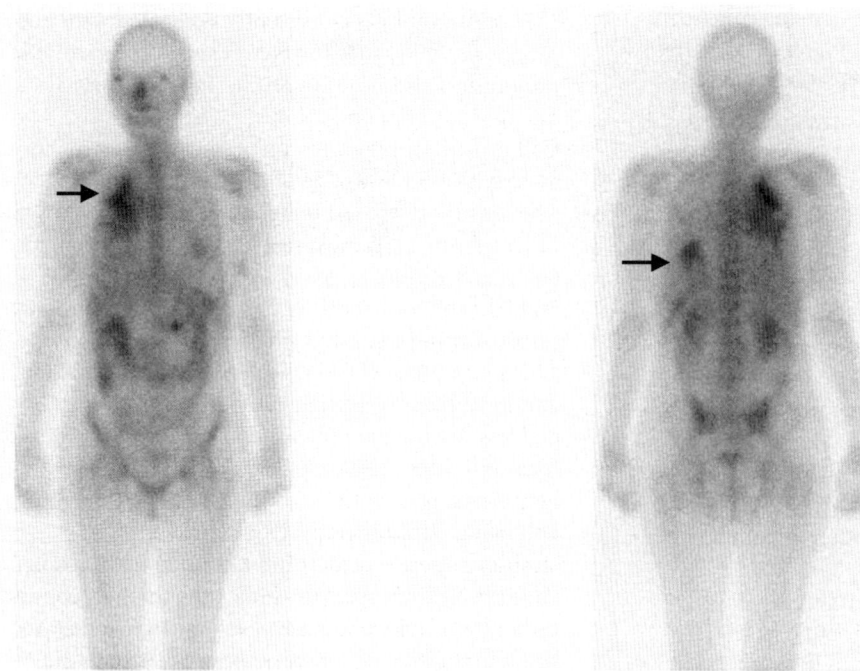

Figure 16C.2 *Patient with a history of abdominal non-Hodgkin's lymphoma underwent ^{67}Ga scintigraphy after completion of therapy. The post-therapy ^{67}Ga whole body scan reveals that there are areas of increased ^{67}Ga uptake in the right upper and left posterior lower lung fields (arrows). These areas demonstrate chemotherapy induced pneumonia which has resolved over time on antibiotic therapy. Note the focal uptake in the left upper quadrant which represents focal physiologic bowel uptake, which resolved at a later imaging time (not shown).*

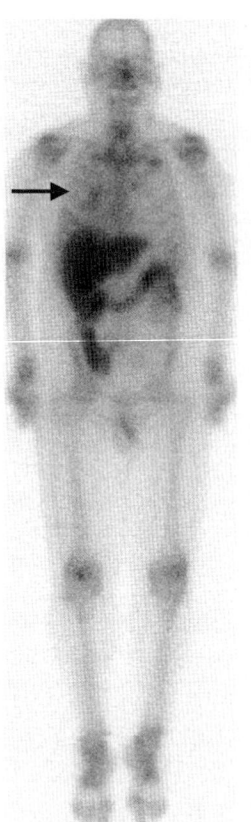
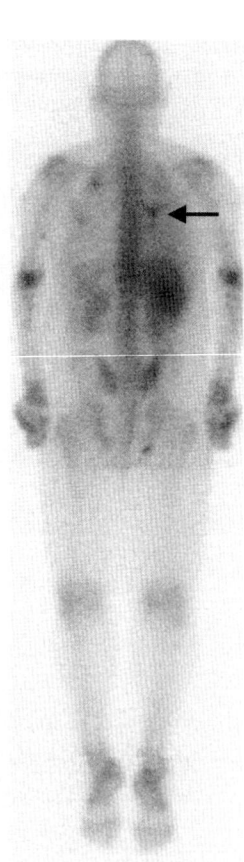

Figure 16C.3 *Patient with a history of mediastinal Hodgkin's lymphoma underwent ^{67}Ga scintigraphy 4 months following therapy completion to evaluate disease status. Anterior and posterior whole body ^{67}Ga images demonstrate asymmetrical hilar uptake, more prominent on the right side (arrows). These findings are consistent with residual lymphoma in the chest. The patient subsequently progressed and received second-line therapy.*

be at least a 3-week interval between last cycle of chemotherapy and ^{67}Ga imaging to avoid false-negative results.[90]

• Biodistribution of ^{67}Ga can be altered to the extent that tumors may not accumulate ^{67}Ga due to conditions resulting in elevated iron levels that compete for transferrin receptors (e.g. recent hemolysis, multiple transfusions, therapeutic iron injections). Additionally, gadolinium used for MRI examinations has been observed to decrease ^{67}Ga localization when given within 24 h of ^{67}Ga injection, probably due to saturation of transferrin by free gadolinium ions.

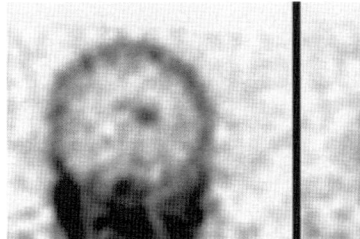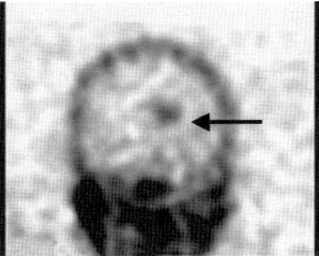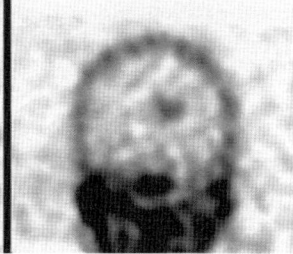

Figure 16C.4 *Patient with HIV+ serology diagnosed with a brain lesion on a recent CT scan, referred for ^{201}Tl imaging to differentiate toxoplasmosis from CNS lymphoma. The ^{201}Tl SPECT coronal images show increased uptake in the left parietal cortex (arrow) corresponding to the lesion on the CT scan, consistent with lymphoma. The patient was subsequently placed on chemotherapy for lymphoma.*

Thallium-201 and ^{99m}Tc-sestamibi imaging in lymphoma

Both ^{201}Tl and ^{99m}Tc-sestamibi (MIBI) are myocardial perfusion agents, although they are also useful radiotracers for tumor imaging as they accumulate mainly within viable tumor tissues.[91]

Cellular uptake of ^{201}Tl within tumors is multifactoral and related to blood flow, tumor viability, the sodium–potassium adenosine triphosphatase (Na–K-ATPase), co-transport system, calcium ion channel mechanisms, and increased cell membrane permeability.[92] Because of the biological similarity of ^{201}Tl to potassium, tumor cells with high Na–K-ATPase activity accumulate ^{201}Tl.[93] Radiotherapy or chemotherapy impacts the activity of Na–K-ATPase on tumor cells, thus decreasing the uptake of thallium-201.[94,95]

Technetium-99 m-sestamibi (MIBI) is a lipophilic monovalent cation that is sequestered into the mitochondria on the basis of transmembrane electrical potentials. MIBI accumulates preferentially in malignant cells, owing to a higher transmembrane electric potential due to higher metabolic rates in malignant cells. The washout of MIBI from the cell is related to the energy dependent transmembrane proteins including the P-glycoprotein pump system (Pgp) and the multidrug resistance protein (MRP).[96–98] Consequently, MIBI tumor washout rate can provide information regarding the presence of multidrug resistance proteins and may impact management. The imaging parameters are shown in Table 16C.2, while the salient points are summarized below. Additional information can be found in the bibliography.[91–105]

The highlights of ^{201}Tl and MIBI imaging in lymphoma are:

- Thallium-201 scintigraphy is primarily used in the diagnosis and follow-up of low-grade lymphomas. Although superior to ^{67}Ga, it still lacks sensitivity in low-grade lymphomas (~70%).[14,100]
- Currently the strength of ^{201}Tl imaging lies in its ability to differentiate CNS lymphoma from toxoplasmosis in immunocompromised patients (Fig. 16C.4).

- The intense uptake in the liver and bowels precludes the use of both ^{201}Tl and MIBI scintigraphy in patients with infra-diaphragmatic lymphoma.
- Because of its close association with multidrug resistance, MIBI scintigraphy can provide information in the prediction of chemotherapy response and could guide the design of the most effective therapy protocols. Nevertheless, evaluation of multidrug resistance is a controversial issue because of the multifaceted problems that stem from nonspecificity of MIBI imaging, tumor heterogeneity, co-existence of various resistance mechanisms, and in clinical practice lack of effective reversal agents.

Indium-111-pentetreotide (octreotide) imaging in lymphoma

Indium-111-octreotide is a somatostatin analog that binds to somatostatin receptors (predominantly receptor subtypes 2 and 5). The uptake of ^{111}In-octreotide is dependent on somatostatin receptor-mediated internalization of the radioligand by the tumor cells. Somatostatin receptor imaging (SRI) is widely used in diagnosing tumors, mainly neuroendocrine tumors with somatostatin receptor expression. However, SRI can also image many other non-neuroendocrine origin tumors expressing somatostatin receptors, including malignant lymphomas.[106] The presence of cellular somatostatin receptors, particularly of subtype 2, has been reported in lymphoma. The imaging parameters are shown in Table 16C.2, while the salient points are summarized below. Additional information can be found in the bibliography.[107–112]

Highlights of SRI are:

- SRI is more sensitive in HD than in NHL.[110,111]
- Generally, SRI has limited detection sensitivity in lymphoma, thus it should not be used as a routine test as part of the initial staging of lymphoma.
- Overall, radiolabeled octreotide scintigraphy is better suited to characterize somatostatin receptor expressing lymphomas than to localize lesion sites. Thus, it may be

useful to determine the patient population that would benefit from therapy with radiolabeled somatostain receptor analogs.

NUCLEAR MEDICINE IMAGING WITH FLUORODEOXYGLUCOSE

FDG PET is a more sensitive staging and a more specific restaging technique compared to traditional modalities including CT and ^{67}Ga scintigraphy in the detection of both nodal and extranodal lymphoma.[24–29] FDG PET has now been incorporated into the existing staging algorithm as well as in the post-therapy evaluation of lymphoma.

Higher FDG uptake in malignant cells is a function of increased glycolysis, overexpression of glucose transporters (GLUT-1), and increase in the levels of the principal enzymes that play a role in glycolysis such as hexokinase.[113–115] FDG enters tumor cells via membrane-located facilitative glucose transporters (GLUTs). It is phosphorylated by hexokinase (HK) as is D-glucose. The FDG-6-phosphate formed, however, cannot undergo further metabolism. Additionally, the dephosphorylating enzyme, glucose-6-phosphatase, is usually expressed at low concentrations in malignant tissues. Thus, FDG is trapped in the cytosol in a time dependent relationship. Recent studies have demonstrated a relationship between GLUT 1 and proliferation rate and tumor grade.[116–119] This issue is not fully clarified, however, as there are conflicting data demonstrating that FDG accumulation correlates with the number of viable cells not with their proliferative rate.[120–122]

Physiologic sites of uptake include cerebral cortex myocardium, distal esophagus, stomach, small intestine, colon, liver, spleen, bone marrow, kidneys, and urinary bladder. Activated skeletal muscles take up FDG, as glycolysis is the main source of energy in the muscle fibers. Delayed imaging (>2 h) should be considered for small lesions and lesions in the liver and spleen.

Clinical applications

HISTOLOGIC SUBTYPES OF LYMPHOMA AND FDG PET IMAGING

Although FDG accumulates in both NHL and HD, the level of uptake measured by standardized uptake values (SUVs) may be considerably lower in low-grade NHLs as compared to high grade NHLs and HD.[17,20,23,29,123,124] Although SUVs depend on various factors including lesion size, patient's weight, glucose levels and the waiting period, low-grade lymphomas usually have an SUV range of 1.5–8.0 while the same range is 3.0–38 for high-grade lymphomas (personal communication) (Plates 16C.3 and 16C.4). In 42 patients with low grade lymphoma, FDG PET was found highly sensitive in follicular lymphoma by detecting 40% more abnormal lymph node areas than conventional staging but in small lymphocytic lymphoma it detected less than 58% of abnormal lymph nodes, mostly in the abdomen.[125] With the evolution of the new generation PET devices, particularly with the integration of CT, the sensitivity of FDG PET imaging may further improve in all subtypes of lymphomas.

One important issue that should be recognized is that low-grade lymphomas may transform to a more aggressive subtype with a rate of 3–5% per year.[65] In such cases, FDG PET can potentially impact management by providing useful information regarding the sites of high-grade transformation for clinicians to obtain tissue confirmation at these particular locations.

The sensitivity of FDG PET is reportedly low in extranodal marginal zone B-cell lymphoma of the mucosa-associated lymphoid tissue (MALT).[126,127] Nodal marginal zone lymphoma appears to be a distinctive lymphoma entity with aggressive characteristics rather than a more advanced stage of MALT. In a restrospective study, none of the patients with MALT showed focal tracer uptake within verified tumor sites, while most patients with nodal marginal zone showed significant FDG uptake within the affected lymph nodes.[126] Generally, FDG PET is positive in both natural killer T-cell lymphomas and mantle cell lymphomas while the uptake is usually lower in peripheral T-cell lymphomas.

STAGING OF LYMPHOMA

Initial staging in lymphoma is crucial for the determination of treatment strategy. Advanced stage disease may be curable with chemotherapy or with a combination therapy with radiotherapy, whereas early stage disease can be cured by local radiotherapy only. FDG PET is an accurate staging technique for lymphoma (Table 16C.4).

The detection sensitivity of FDG PET is superior to CT by revealing additional disease sites in approximately one third of patients with a sensitivity of 83–100%[19–26]) (Table 16C.4) (Plate 16C.5). The sensitivity and specificity of FDG PET is particularly higher in the mediastinal and hilar regions: 96% and 94%, respectively.[26]

Consequently, the greater sensitivity of FDG PET can lead to a stage migration in up to 41% of patients with untreated NHL and HD.[25,128–131] The stage is usually altered within the same risk group (i.e. early stage versus advanced stage) although in some cases, early stage disease can be upstaged to advanced disease or vice versa which results in significant management alterations.[129] Based on the magnitude of stage migration, FDG PET findings may result in major treatment modifications in 10–25% of patients.[128–131]

With respect to extranodal lymphoma, similar to results obtained with nodal lymphoma, FDG PET may provide more information about the extent of disease compared to

Table 16C.4 *Pre-therapy staging with FDG PET: comparison with morphological imaging modalities*

Authors	Year	Study	Number of patients	Patient group	Modality	Sensitivity (%)	Specificity (%)
Hoh[19]	1997	Retrospective	18	NHL+HD	FDG PET	94	NA
					CM*	83	NA
Thill[20]	1997	Retrospective	27	NHL+HD	FDG PET	100	NA
					CT	77	NA
Mainolfi[21]	1998	Prospective	98	NHL+HD	FDG PET	†	†
					CM		
Stumpe[23]	1998	Prospective	50	HD vs NHL	FDG PET	86 vs 89	96 vs 100
				HD vs NHL	CT	81 vs 86	41 vs 67
Bangerter[26]	1999	Retrospective	89	NHL+HD	FDG PET	96	94
					CT	†	†
Wiedmann[27]	1999	Prospective	20	HD	FDG PET	†	†
					CM		
Buchmann[129]	2001	Prospective	52	NHL+HD	FDG PET	99	100
					CT	83	100
Partridge[130]	2000	Retrospective	44	HD	FDG PET	†	†
					CT		
Weihrauch[131]	2002	Prospective	22	HD	FDG PET	88	100
				CT	74	100	

*Conventional modalities: CT, ultrasound, MRI, endoscopy or laparoscopy.

†FDG sensitivity and specificity not given but FDG PET detected more sites than CT or ^{67}Ga scan.

HD: Hodgkin's disease; NHL: non-Hodgkin's lymphoma.

CT.[20,24,27,132] In both NHL and HD splenic involvement is more common than hepatic involvement with an incidence of 22%. Hepatic involvement is more common in NHL than in HD (15% vs 3.2%).[4,24] Conventional imaging is not sufficiently sensitive in the detection of liver, spleen and bone marrow involvement. FDG PET has been shown to be more sensitive, identifying approximately 25% more hepatic and splenic lesions compared to CT.[20]

In HIV positive patients with contrast-enhancing brain tumors, data from the literature suggest that FDG PET may help to discriminate CNS lymphoma from inflammatory. (e.g. toxoplasmosis) lesions with a reported accuracy of 86–89%[133–136]) (Plate 16C.6). Basically, a lesion with an FDG uptake higher than the adjacent gray matter is consistent with a malignant process which prompts biopsy for confirmation rather than treated empirically as infectious. Nonetheless the lesions in the thalamus and basal ganglia may pose challenges due to the intense physiologic FDG uptake. In a recent study, FDG PET was useful for early therapeutic monitoring of CNS lymphoma after chemotherapy.[136]

BM involvement is seen in up to 70% of low-grade, 40% of high-grade NHL and 14% of HD patients.[137] Overall, MRI is more sensitive than BM biopsy due to the high sampling error rate with the latter, but its routine application to evaluate the entire BM is costly and not practical.

Additionally, false negative results can be obtained with MRI in cases with hyperplasia, diffuse lymphoma infiltration as well as with infectious processes. Although physiologic BM uptake is observed on FDG PET images, focal and grossly heterogenous uptake is usually suggestive of pathological BM activity (Plate 16C.7). Diffusely increased FDG uptake is commonly observed in reactive BM, particularly following administration of colony stimulating factors (e.g. G-CSF) (Plate 16C.8).[138,139] The sensitivity and specificity for FDG PET are reported to be 81% and 100%, respectively, in the detection of BM involvement with lymphoma.[93,94] In patients with negative BM biopsy, FDG PET may still reveal focal lymphoma involvement distal from the biopsy site.[140,141] Overall the negative predictive value for FDG PET in the detection of BM involvement is higher than the positive predictive value. Nevertheless, a minimal degree of BM involvement can result in false negative findings due to the resolution limits of FDG PET imaging.[27,140–142]

Primary bone lymphoma accounts for less than 5% of all primary bone tumors. MR imaging is most useful for early identification of this disease entity as well as evaluation of the extent of soft-tissue involvement.[143] Because this is a rare disease, there is no published series using FDG PET, but our experience is that FDG avidly accumulates in bone lesions unlike bone marrow disease.

FDG PET versus ^{67}Ga imaging at initial staging

Multiple studies reported a higher site and patient sensitivity for FDG PET compared to ^{67}Ga imaging[144–148] (Table 16C.4). The patient sensitivity for FDG PET and ^{67}Ga scintigraphy is 87–100% and 63–80%, respectively, in mixed populations of NHL and HD.[144–146] FDG PET is particularly helpful in patients with low grade lymphoma and those with nonspecific hilar uptake on ^{67}Ga scintigraphy.[144] Although there is a paucity of comparative data, the results obtained using dedicated PET cameras also demonstrate that FDG PET has a higher sensitivity and detects more disease sites when compared with ^{67}Ga scintigraphy at initial staging of lymphoma.[147,148] The site sensitivity for FDG PET and ^{67}Ga scintigraphy is reportedly significantly different at 82–96% vs 69–72%.[147,148]

In summary, FDG PET is a highly sensitive and specific staging method that allows for accurate assessment of the extent of nodal and extranodal lymphoma in HD and NHL. Nevertheless, at pre-therapy staging, FDG PET should be either complemented with CT or PET/CT should be used for higher specificity and better assessment of extranodal disease.

Post-therapy evaluation of lymphoma

Following first-line therapy, the identification of recurrent lymphoma during follow-up and insufficient therapy response after completion of chemotherapy prompt initiation of second-line therapy. In early-stage lymphoma, complete response rate is typically high, at 75–90%, irrespective of the histological subtype, but in advanced stage lymphoma, less than 50% of newly diagnosed patients respond to standard treatments.[149,150] Thus, evaluation of response to therapy is more important in the advanced-stage group than that in the early stage. FDG PET performs favorably compared to CT in the discrimination of fibrotic changes from viable residual disease as well as monitoring response to therapy (Table 16C.5).

Compared to CT, FDG PET has a significantly higher specificity (83–92% vs 17–42%) and accuracy (86–96% vs 39–63%) in the differentiation of residual viable disease from post-therapy fibrosis.[21–23,151–153] FDG PET can be used to determine patients who need further treatment after the first-line therapy and also to avoid unwarranted morbidity associated with the ineffective therapy in non-responders (Plates 16C.9 and 16C.10). The negative predictive value for FDG PET, however, may not be reliable due to microscopic residual disease owing to spatial resolution limitations of PET systems.[151]

Incongruent results demonstrating negative FDG PET findings with persistent CT abnormalities, generally indicate post-treatment fibrosis.[21–23,151,152] One should be aware of the false-negative results that originate from lesions that are below the detection limits of PET systems (<0.5 cm) as well as the false-positive findings that can be obtained in infectious or inflammatory processes. However, the positive predictive value of FDG PET is higher than 90% in the detection of residual or recurrent lymphoma (Table 16C.5).

Table 16C.5 *Post-therapy FDG PET in the detection of residual or recurrent lymphoma*

Authors	Year	Study	Number of patients	Patient group	PPV (%)	NPV (%)
Mainolfi[21]	1998	Prospective	32	NHL+HD	†	†
Jerusalem[25]	1999	Prospective	54	NHL+HD	100	90
Cremerius[152]	1999	Retrospective	72	NHL+HD	†	90 vs 67*
Zinzani[158]	1999	Prospective	44	NHL+HD‡	100	96
Mikhaeel[154]	2000	Retrospective	49	NHL	100	83
Hueltenschmidt[150]	2001	Prospective	63	NHL+HD	†	96
Weihrauch[153]	2001	Prospective	28	HD	60	95
Naumann[155]	2001	Prospective	58	NHL+HD	62.5	96
De Wit[156]	2001	Prospective	37	HD	46	96
Spaepen[157]	2001	Prospective	93	NHL	100	83.5
Becherer[165]	2002	Prospective	16	NHL+HD	87.5	100
Spaepen[169]	2002	Prospective	70	NHL+HD	84	100
Kostakoglu[172]	2002	Prospective	27	NHL+HD	90	100
Haioun[170]	2005	Prospective	90	NHL	42	83
Mikhaeel[171]	2005	Prospective	121	NHL	84	89

PPV: positive predictive value; NPV: negative predictive value; NHL: non-Hodgkin's lymphoma; HD: Hodgkin's disease.
*Low-risk vs high-risk patients.
†Either PPV or NPV or both not given.
‡All patients had intra-abdominal lymphoma.

Prediction of therapy outcome after completion of therapy

The IPI for NHL and IPS for HD are the established parameters to predict the risk of disease recurrence and overall survival.[37,38] However, the tumor sensitivity to chemotherapy as evidenced by rapidity of complete response may serve as an indicator for prognosis than IPI. In this regard, sequential FDG PET imaging has a role in the determination of tumor response rates.[25,124,154–161] In this respect, FDG PET may assist in distinguishing patients who are likely to be cured with standard chemotherapy from those who would require a more aggressive treatment approach. Multiple studies have shown that disease relapse occurs in almost all patients with a positive post-therapy FDG PET result while only 25–40% of patients relapse when CT has a positive finding for post-therapy residual masses.[25,154,157]

In a series of 96 patients, Spaepen et al. demonstrated that persistent FDG uptake after first-line chemotherapy was predictive of poor prognosis in aggressive NHL.[157] In the group with negative post-therapy FDG PET, only 20% relapsed and 80% had sustained complete remission with a mean follow-up of 24 months. Conversely, all patients with persistent uptake relapsed with a mean disease-free survival of 3 months.

In HD, similar results were obtained, after the first-line treatment the 1–2 year disease-free survival was rather short for the positive group (0–4%) and significantly longer for the negative group (85–93%).[160,161] In another study, FDG PET was able to predict disease-free survival with better positive and negative predictive values compared to CT and erythrocyte sedimentation rate (ESR), a well-recognized risk factor for HD.[156] Future randomized trials are necessary to determine the optimal therapy for HD using shortened courses of chemotherapy, or chemotherapy combined with lower radiation doses or no radiotherapy in patients with negative post-therapy FDG PET results.

The differentiation of chemosensitive from chemoresistant patients is crucial for the success of high-dose chemotherapy (HDT) followed by autologous stem cell transplantation (SCT).[162,163] Although the reported series are small, FDG PET appears to have a potential in the prediction of relapse after HDT/SCT.[164,165] In patients who had sequential FDG PET before and after HDT, those who had an SUV decrease of less than 25% had progression of disease. Unsurprisingly, 86% of patients with more than 25% of SUV decrease achieved complete remission.[164] These are encouraging results, however, due to the small number of patients, these studies are of preliminary nature.

FDG PET is a powerful tool in the assessment of response after completion of therapy; nonetheless, microscopic disease that accounts for late relapses cannot be excluded with high certainty in cases with negative post-therapy PET results.

Early prediction of response during therapy

Patients with a prompt response to first line therapy are considered to have a better and more durable response than patients who achieve a slow complete remission.[166,167] Anatomic imaging modalities have not yielded successful results in the evaluation of early therapy response as tumor size reduction is usually a late sign of efficacy of treatment. Predictive value of 'early PET' is observed in both the lower-risk and higher-risk groups, indicating prognostic independence from the IPI. Induction chemotherapy may result in a decrease of tumor FDG uptake as early as 7 days after the initiation of treatment.[168] Likewise, persistent FDG uptake after two to four cycles of chemotherapy can accurately predict PFS in patients with aggressive NHL and HD.[160] The relapse rates can be as high as 100% in the PET-positive group compared with 8% for the PET-negative group. Likewise, persistent mid-therapy (after three cycles) FDG uptake usually results in failure to therapy while a negative PET leads to complete response with durable remissions.[169] In one study, at mid-treatment, none of the patients with persistent abnormal FDG uptake achieved a durable complete remission, 84% of patients with negative DG-PET results remained in complete remission with a median follow-up of ~3 years. Furthermore, in a multivariate analysis, FDG PET at mid-treatment was found to be a stronger prognostic factor for PFS than was the IPI.[169]

In a recent study, after completion of induction therapy, 83% of PET-negative patients achieved complete remission compared with only 58% of PET-positive patients. Outcome differed significantly between PET-negative and PET-positive groups; the 2-year estimates of event-free survival reached 82% and 43%, respectively, and the 2-year estimates of overall survival reached 90% and 61%, respectively.[170] Similarly, in a large study of 124 patients with high-grade NHL early interim FDG PET was found to be an accurate and independent predictor of PFS and OS. The estimated 5-year PFS was 89% for the PET-negative group, 59% for the minimal residual group, and 16% for the PET-positive group.[171]

It has also been reported that FDG PET, after one cycle of chemotherapy is predictive of 18-month outcome in patients with aggressive NHL and HD.[159,172] Positive FDG PET images obtained after the first cycle of therapy were associated with a shorter PFS (median: 5 months) compared with negative FDG PET results (PFS medians not reached) with a follow-up period of 36 months. Recently, using a dedicated PET system, in patients with advanced stage or high-risk lymphoma all patients with a negative FDG PET result obtained after first cycle of chemotherapy had sustained complete remission (NPV: 100%) with a follow-up of 12 months whereas nine of ten patients with positive FDG PET results (PPV: 90%) had documented relapse or progressive disease that required further therapy. We can deduce from these data that the chances for relapse are significantly high in patients with persistent FDG uptake after the first cycle of chemotherapy. A negative FDG PET after the first cycle is highly predictive of long-term remission although patients with negative FDG PET studies may still develop tumor progression or relapse.

A recent study reported that compared with International Workshop Criteria (IWC) the IWC+PET-based assessment provided a more accurate response classification in patients with aggressive NHL. In 54 patients with aggressive NHL, PFS was significantly shorter in patients with PR than in those with a CR using IWC while when the two classifications were included in the same multivariate model, only IWC+PET was a statistically significant independent predictor for PFS. In addition, IWC+PET identified a subset of IWC patients with partial response with a more favorable prognosis.[173]

FDG PET versus ^{67}Ga imaging in following therapy

Only limited data are available in terms of direct comparison of ^{67}Ga scintigraphy with FDG PET in lymphoma. Bar-Shalom *et al.* evaluated the performance of ^{67}Ga scintigraphy and FDG PET using a dual-head system in 84 patients.[144] FDG PET had a significantly higher detection rate compared to ^{67}Ga scintigraphy for both nodal and extranodal lymphoma sites. Sensitivity and specificity were 73% and 51%, respectively, for ^{67}Ga scintigraphy, and 93% and 72%, respectively, for camera-based FDG PET. FDG PET was more accurate in the assessment of bone lymphoma compared with ^{67}Ga scintigraphy in (93% vs 29%).

Integrated PET/CT imaging

The principal advantage of PET/CT fusion technology is combining anatomic data with functional/metabolic information in the same imaging session.[174] The metabolic findings that are overlooked due to the subtlety of metabolic changes on FDG PET may result in the detection of residual disease after correlation with the simultaneously acquired CT data. In a recent study, PET/CT performed with non-enhanced CT was found more sensitive and specific than was contrast-enhanced CT for evaluation of lymph node and organ involvement in HD and NHL.[175] For evaluation of lymph node involvement, sensitivity of PET/CT and contrast-enhanced CT was 94% and 88%, and specificity was 100% and 86%, respectively. For evaluation of organ involvement, sensitivity of PET/CT and contrast-enhanced CT was 88% and 50%, and specificity was 100% and 90%, respectively. In addition to the application of fusion technology in the diagnosis and staging and restaging of malignant disease, it is useful in planning radiation therapy and determining the optimum approach for CT-guided biopsy.[174] Consequently, the addition of metabolic imaging can have a great effect on treatment in patients with a residual mass at post-treatment evaluation.

Highlights of FDG PET imaging in lymphoma are:

- FDG PET is an established staging and restaging modality for both nodal and extranodal lymphoma.
- FDG PET is more sensitive than CT and MRI for assessing the nodal or extranodal involvement of lymphoma. As CT and MRI rely on lymph node size tumors in non-enlarged nodes may not be detected.
- FDG PET is more sensitive than ^{67}Ga scintigraphy, in both NHL, including low-grade lymphoma and HD. Although, currently, FDG PET has superseded ^{67}Ga scintigraphy at many centers, ^{67}Ga scintigraphy is still in clinical use at some centers.
- Although FDG accumulates in all types of lymphomas, there may be false-negative findings in patients with MALT.
- Although FDG PET is sensitive in detecting low-grade lymphomas, the degree of FDG uptake (SUV) is often lower than that observed in intermediate- or high-grade lymphomas.
- The sensitivity of FDG PET in detecting bone marrow infiltration has been reported to be low. In addition, FDG PET may yield false-positive as well as negative results. Thus, evaluation of bone marrow should be performed by bone marrow biopsy and MRI when it is indicated. In patients recently administered chemotherapy with colony stimulators, FDG PET should be performed 1 month after discontinuation of colony stimulators.[176]
- Although FDG PET is sensitive to identify disease sites in the chest, false-positive FDG uptake after therapy can be seen at the site of thymic hyperplasia.[89] Thymic hyperplasia is a common phenomenon after treatment, especially in children with an incidence of 16% (Plate 16C.11).
- FDG PET may not differentiate between infectious and malignant processes. In this regard, the specificity of FDG PET is similar to that of ^{67}Ga for the neoplastic tissues versus inflammatory sites which may be more troublesome in the post-therapy setting.
- Reactive lymph nodes in patients with infection or with active granulomatous diseases such as sarcoidosis, tuberculosis and HIV-related lymphoproliferative disorders may also be misinterpreted as malignant processes.
- FDG PET can accurately predict response to therapy after completion of therapy or during therapy, although false-negative findings can arise from microscopic residual disease.
- FDG PET may underestimate the metabolic signals originating from tumors that are smaller than two times the spatial resolution of the scanner (partial volume effect). Detection of a tumor is still possible for low tumor-to-background ratios; objects that measure 5 mm can be recognizable with activity ratios of 3.0.

- The cure rate in patients with early stage lymphoma (stage I–II) is invariably high, therefore the prognostic value of FDG PET in this patient population is questionable.
- With the recent introduction of integrated PET/CT cameras, the specificity of FDG PET has increased by avoidance of false-positive findings that mimic malignant disease process.

REFERENCES

1   Ng AK, Bernardo MV, Weller E, *et al.* Second malignancy after Hodgkin disease treated with radiation therapy with or without chemotherapy: long-term risks and risk factors. *Blood* 2002; **100**: 1989–96.

2   Yasuda S, Ide M, Fujii H, *et al.* Application of positron emission tomography imaging to cancer screening. *Br J Cancer* 2000; **83**: 1607–11

3   Marshall Jr WH, Breiman RS, Harell GS, *et al.* Computed tomography of abdominal para-aortic lymph node disease: preliminary observation with a 6 second scanner. *Am J Roentgenol* 1977; **128**: 759–74.

4   Karimjee S, Brada M, Husband J, McCready VR. A comparison of gallium-67 single photon emission computed tomography and computed tomography in mediastinal Hodgkin's disease. *Eur J Cancer* 1992; **28A**: 1856–7.

5   Castellino RA, Hopper RT, Blank N, *et al.* Computed tomography, lymphography and staging laparotomy: correlations in initial staging of Hodgkin's disease. *Am J Roentgenol* 1984; **143**: 37–41.

6   Janicek M, Kaplan W, Neuberg D, *et al.* Early restaging gallium scans predict outcome in poor-prognosis patients with aggressive non-Hodgkin's lymphoma treated with high-dose CHOP chemotherapy. *J Clin Oncol* 1997; **15**: 1631–7.

7   Front D, Bar-Shalom R, Mor M, *et al.* Hodgkin's disease: prediction of outcome with ^{67}Ga scintigraphy after one cycle of chemotherapy. *Radiology* 1999; **210**: 487–91.

8   Bendini M, Zuiani C, Bazzocchi M, *et al.* Magnetic resonance imaging and ^{67}Ga scan versus computed tomography in the staging and in the monitoring of mediastinal malignant lymphoma: a prospective pilot study. *MAGMA* 1996; **4**: 213–24.

9   Nyman R, Forsgren G, Glimelius B. Long-term follow-up of residual mediastinal masses in treated Hodgkin's disease using MR imaging. *Acta Radiol* 1996; **37**: 323–6.

10 Hagemeister FB, Purugganan R, Podoloff DA, *et al.* The gallium scan predicts relapse in patients with Hodgkin's disease treated with combined modality therapy. *Ann Oncol* 1994; **5**: 59–63.

11 Salloum E, Brandt DS, Caride VJ, *et al.* Gallium scans in the management of patients with Hodgkin's disease: a study of 101 patients. *J Clin Oncol* 1997; **15**: 518–27.

12 Front D, Bar-Shalom R, Mor M, *et al.* Aggressive non-Hodgkin lymphoma: early prediction of outcome with ^{67}Ga scintigraphy. *Radiology* 2000; **214**: 253–7.

13 Frohlich DE, Chen JL, Neuberg D, *et al.* When is hilar uptake of ^{67}Ga-citrate indicative of residual disease after CHOP chemotherapy? *J Nucl Med* 2000; **41**: 269–74.

14 Waxman AD, Eller D, Ashook G, *et al.* Comparison of gallium-67-citrate and thallium-201 scintigraphy in peripheral and intrathoracic lymphoma. *J Nucl Med* 1996; **37**: 46–50.

15 Ohta M, Isobe K, Kuyama J *et al.* Clinical role of Tc-99m-MIBI scintigraphy in non-Hodgkin's lymphoma. *Oncol Rep* 2001; **8**: 841–5.

16 Som P, Atkins HL, Bandophadhyah D. A fluorinated glucose analog, 2-fluoro-2-deoxy-D-glucose (F-18). *J Nucl Med* 1980; **21**: 670–5.

17 Rodriguez M, Rehn S, Ahlstrom H, *et al.* Predicting malignancy grade with PET in non-Hodgkin's lymphoma. *J Nucl Med* 1995; **36**: 1790–6.

18 Jerusalem G, Warland V, Najjar F, *et al.* Whole-body ^{18}F-FDG PET for the evaluation of patients with Hodgkin's disease and non-Hodgkin's lymphoma. *Nucl Med Commun* 1999; **20**: 13–20.

19 Hoh CK, Glaspy J, Rosen P, *et al.* Whole-body FDG-PET imaging for staging of Hodgkin's disease and lymphoma. *J Nucl Med* 1997; **38**: 343–8.

20 Thill R, Neuerburg J, Fabry U, *et al.* Comparison of findings with 18-FDG PET and CT in pretherapeutic staging of malignant lymphoma. *Nuklearmedizin* 1997; **36**: 234–9.

21 Mainolfi C, Maurea S, Varrella P, *et al.* Positron emission tomography with fluorine-18-deoxyglucose in the staging and control of patients with lymphoma. Comparison with clinico-radiologic assessment. *Radiol Med* 1998; **95**: 98–104.

22 Cremerius U, Fabry U, Neuerburg J, *et al.* Positron emission tomography with ^{18}F-FDG to detect residual disease after therapy for malignant lymphoma. *Nucl Med Commun* 1998; **19**: 1055–63.

23 Stumpe KD, Urbinelli M, Steinert HC, *et al.* Whole-body positron emission tomography using fluoro-deoxyglucose for staging of lymphoma: effectiveness and comparison with computed tomography. *Eur J Nucl Med* 1998; **25**: 721–8.

24 Moog F, Bangerter M, Diederichs CG, *et al.* Extranodal malignant lymphoma: detection with FDG PET versus CT. *Radiology* 1998; **206**: 475–81.

25 Jerusalem G, Beguin Y, Fassotte MF, *et al.* Whole-body positron emission tomography using ^{18}F-fluorodeoxyglucose for post-treatment evaluation in Hodgkin's disease and non-Hodgkin's lymphoma has higher diagnostic and prognostic value than classical computed tomography scan imaging. *Blood* 1999; **94**: 429–33.

26 Bangerter M, Kotzerke J, Griesshammer M, *et al.* Positron emission tomography with 18-fluorodeoxyglucose

in the staging and follow-up of lymphoma in the chest. *Acta Oncol* 1999; **38**: 799–804.

27 Wiedmann E, Baican B, Hertel A, *et al*. Positron emission tomography (PET) for staging and evaluation of response to treatment in patients with Hodgkin's disease. *Leuk Lymphoma* 1999; **34**: 545–51.

28 Hany TF, Steinert HC, Goerres GW, *et al*. PET diagnostic accuracy: improvement with in-line PET-CT system: initial results. *Radiology* 2002; **225**: 575–81.

29 Kostakoglu L, Leonard JP, Kuji I, *et al*. Comparison of fluorine-18 fluorodeoxyglucose positron emission tomography and Ga-67 scintigraphy in evaluation of lymphoma. *Cancer* 2002; **94**: 879–88.

30 National Cancer Institute. Sponsored study of classifications of non-Hodgkin's lymphomas: summary and description of a working formulation for clinical usage. The Non-Hodgkin's Lymphoma Pathologic Classification Project. *Cancer* 1982; **49**: 2112–35.

31 Jaffe E, Harris N, Diebold J, Muller-Hermelink H-K. World Health Organization classification of neoplastic diseases of the hematopoietic and lymphoid tissues. A progress report. *Am J Clin Pathol* 1999; **111(suppl 1)**: S8–S12.

32 Harris N, Jaffe E, Diebold J, *et al*. The World Health Organization Classification of Hematological Malignancies Report of the Clinical Advisory Committee Meeting. *Mod Pathol* 2000; **13**: 193–207.

33 Robbins SL, Cotran RS, Kumar V. *Pathological basis of disease*, 2nd edition. Philadelphia: WB Saunders, 1995.

34 Lister TA, Crowther D, Sutcliffe SB, *et al*. Report of a committee convened to discuss the evaluation and staging of patients with Hodgkin's disease: Cotswold meeting. *J Clin Oncol* 1989; **7**: 1630–6.

35 Rosenberg S. Validity of the Ann Arbor staging system classification for the non-Hodgkin's lymphomas. *Cancer Treat Rep* 1977; **61**: 1023–7.

36 Shipp MA. Prognostic factors in aggressive non-Hodgkin's lymphoma: who has 'high-risk' disease? *Blood* 1994; **83**: 1165–73.

37 Hasenclever D, Diehl V. A prognostic score for advanced Hodgkin's disease. International prognostic factors project on advanced Hodgkin's disease. *N Engl J Med* 1998; **339**: 1506–14.

38 Hoane BR, Shields AF, Porter BA, *et al*. Comparison of initial lymphoma staging using computed tomography (CT) and magnetic resonance (MR) imaging. *Am J Hematol* 1994; **47**: 100–5.

39 Skillings JR, Bramwell V, Nicholson RL, *et al*. A prospective study of magnetic resonance imaging in lymphoma staging. *Cancer* 1991; **67**: 1838–43.

40 Jung G, Krahe T, Kugel H, *et al*. Prospective comparison of fast SE and GRASE sequences and echo planar imaging with conventional SE sequences in the detection of focal liver lesions at 1.0 T. *J Comput Assist Tomogr* 1997; **21**: 341–7.

41 Outwater EK, Mitchell DG, Vinitski S. Abdominal MR imaging: evaluation of a fast spin-echo sequence. *Radiology* 1994; **190**: 425–9.

42 Cazals-Hatem D, Lepage E, Brice P, *et al*. Primary mediastinal large B-cell lymphoma: a clinicopathologic study of 141 cases compared with 916 non-mediastinal large B-cell lymphomas – a GELA ('Groupe d'Etude des Lymphomas de l'Adulte') study. *Am J Surg Pathol* 1996; **20**: 877–88.

43 Jeung MY, Gangi A, Gasser B, *et al*. Imaging of chest wall disorders. *Radiographics* 1999; **19**: 617–37.

44 Khoury MD, Godwin JD, Halvorsen R, *et al*. Role of chest CT in non-Hodgkin's lymphoma. *Radiology* 1986; **158**: 659–62.

45 Lee JKT, Stanley RJ, Sagel SS, *et al*. Accuracy of computed tomography in detecting intra-abdominal and pelvic adenopathy in lymphoma. *Am J Roentgenol* 1978; **131**: 675–9.

46 Altehoefer C, Blum U, Bathmann J, *et al*. Comparative diagnostic accuracy of magnetic resonance imaging and immunoscintigraphy for detection of bone marrow involvement in patients with malignant lymphoma. *J Clin Oncol* 1997; **15**: 1754–60.

47 Yuki M, Narabayashi I, Yamamoto K, *et al*. Multifocal primary lymphoma of bone: scintigraphy and MR findings before and after treatment. *Radiat Med* 2000; **18**: 305–10.

48 Lanfermann H, Heindel W, Schaper J, *et al*. CT and MR imaging in primary cerebral non-Hodgkin's lymphoma. *Acta Radiol* 1997; **38**: 259–67.

49 Herrlinger U, Schabet M, Clemens M, *et al*. Clinical presentation and therapeutic outcome in 26 patients with primary CNS lymphoma. *Acta Neurol Scand* 1998; **97**: 257–64.

50 Weissleder R, Elizondo G, Stark DD, *et al*. The diagnosis of splenic lymphoma by MR imaging: value of superparamagnetic iron oxide. *Am J Roentgenol* 1989; **152**: 175–80.

51 Cheson BD, Horning SJ, Coiffier B, *et al*. Report of an international workshop to standardize response criteria for non-Hodgkin's lymphomas. NCI Sponsored International Working Group. *J Clin Oncol* 1999; **17**: 1244–53.

52 Rehani MM, Berry M. Radiation doses in computed tomography. The increasing doses of radiation need to be controlled. *BMJ* 2000; **320**: 593–4.

53 Thomas JL, Barnes PA, Bernadino ME, Hagemeister FB. Limited CT studies in monitoring treatment of lymphoma. *AJR* 1982; **138**: 537–9.

54 Larson SM, Rasey JS, Allen DR, *et al*. Common pathway for tumor cell uptake of gallium-67 and iron-59 via a transferrin receptor. *J Natl Cancer Inst* 1980; **64**: 41–53.

55 Vallabhajosula S, Goldsmith SJ, Lipszyc H, Chahinian AP, Ohnuma T. ^{67}Ga–transferrin and ^{67}Ga–lactoferrin binding to tumor cells: specific versus nonspecific

glycoprotein–cell interaction. *Eur J Nucl Med* 1983; **8**: 354–7.

56 Nejmeddine F, Caillat-Vigneron N, Escaig F, *et al.* Mechanism involved in gallium-67 (Ga-67) uptake by human lymphoid cell lines. *Cell Mol Biol (Noisy-le-grand)* 1998; **44**: 1215–20.

57 Gallamini A, Biggi A, Fruttero A, *et al.* Revisiting the prognostic role of gallium scintigraphy in low-grade non-Hodgkin's lymphoma. *Eur J Nucl Med* 1997; **24**: 1499–506.

58 Kostakoglu L, Yeh SD, Portlock C, *et al.* Validation of gallium-67-citrate single-photon emission computed tomography in biopsy-confirmed residual Hodgkin's disease in the mediastinum. *J Nucl Med* 1992; **33**: 345–50.

59 Front D, Israel O, Epelbaum R, *et al.* Ga-67 SPECT before and after treatment of lymphoma. *Radiology* 1990; **175**: 515–19.

60 Mansberg R, Wadhwa SS, Mansberg V. Tl-201 and Ga-67 scintigraphy in non-Hodgkin's lymphoma. *Clin Nucl Med* 1999; **24**: 239–42.

61 Johnston G, Benua RS, Teates CD, *et al.* ^{67}Ga-citrate imaging in untreated Hodgkin's disease: preliminary report of Cooperative Group. *J Nucl Med* 1974; **15**: 399–403.

62 Cabanillas F, Zornoza J, Haynie TP. Comparison of lymphangiograms and gallium scans in the non-Hodgkin's lymphomas. *Cancer* 1977; **39**: 85–8.

63 Setoin FJ, Pons F, Herranz R, *et al.* Ga-67 scintigraphy for the evaluation of recurrences and residual masses in patients with lymphoma. *Nucl Med Commun* 1997; **18**: 405–11.

64 Ben-Haim S, Bar-Shalom R, Israel O, *et al.* Utility of gallium-67 scintigraphy in low-grade non-Hodgkin's lymphoma. *J Clin Oncol* 1996; **14**: 1936–42.

65 Bastion Y, Berger F, Bryon PA, *et al.* Follicular lymphomas: assessment of prognostic factors in 127 patients followed for 10 years. *Ann Oncol* 1991; **2(suppl 2)**: 123–9.

65 Mclaughlin AF, Southee AE. Gallium scintigraphy in tumor diagnosis and management. In: Murray IPC, Ell PJ. (eds.) *Nuclear medicine in clinical diagnosis and treatment*, vol 1. New York: Churchill Livingstone, 1994: 711–27.

67 Turner DA, Fordham EW, Ali A. Gallium-67 imaging in the management of Hodgkin's disease and other malignant lymphomas. *Semin Nucl Med* 1978; **8**: 205–18.

68 Devizzi L, Maffioli L, Bonfante V, *et al.* Comparison of gallium scan, computed tomography, and magnetic resonance in patients with mediastinal Hodgkin's disease. *Ann Oncol* 1997; **8(suppl 1)**: 53–6.

69 Brascho DJ. Hodgkin's disease and non-Hodgkin's lymphoma. In: *Abdominal ultrasound in the cancer patient.* Brasco DJ, Strawber TH. (eds.) New York: Wiley, 1980.

70 Hussain R, Christie DR, Gebski V, *et al.* The role of the gallium scan in primary extranodal lymphoma. *J Nucl Med* 1998; **39**: 95–8.

71 Zornoza J, Ginaldi S. Computed tomography in hepatic lymphoma. *Radiology* 1981; **138**: 405–10.

72 Israel O, Mekel M, Bar-Shalom R, *et al.* Bone lymphoma: [67]Ga scintigraphy and CT for prediction of outcome after treatment. *J Nucl Med* 2002; **43**: 1295–303.

73 Chajari M, Lacroix J, Peny AM, *et al.* Gallium-67 scintigraphy in lymphoma: is there a benefit of image fusion with computed tomography? *Eur J Nucl Med Mol Imag* 2002; **29**: 380–7.

74 Front D, Bar-Shalom R, Israel O. The continuing clinical role of gallium-67 scintigraphy in the age of receptor imaging. *Semin Nucl Med* 1997; **27**: 68–74.

75 Kostakoglu L, Goldsmith SJ. [F-18] Fluorodeoxyglucose positron emission tomography in staging and follow-up of lymphoma. Is it time to shift gears? *Eur J Nucl Med* 2000; **27**: 564–78.

76 Stroszczynski C, Amthauer H, Hosten N, *et al.* Use of Ga-67 SPECT in patients with malignant lymphoma after primary chemotherapy for further treatment planning: comparison with spiral CT. *Rofo Fortschr Geb Rontgenstr Neuen Bildgeb Verfahr* 1997; **167**: 458–66.

77 Ha CS, Choe JG, Kong JS, *et al.* Agreement rates among single photon emission computed tomography using gallium-67, computed axial tomography and lymphangiography for Hodgkin's disease and correlation of image findings with clinical outcome. *Cancer* 2000; **89**: 1371–9.

78 Even-Sapir E, Bar-Shalom R, Israel O, *et al.* Single-photon emission computed tomography quantitation of gallium citrate uptake for the differentiation of lymphoma from benign hilar uptake. *J Clin Oncol* 1995; **13**: 942–6.

79 Gunay EC, Salanci BV, Barista I, Caner B. Lung hilar Ga-67 uptake in patients with lymphoma following chemotherapy. *Ann Nucl Med* 2004; **18**: 391–7.

80 Front D, Ben-Haim S, Israel O, *et al.* Lymphoma. Predictive value of Ga-67 scintigraphy after treatment. *Radiology* 1992; **182**: 359–63.

81 Ionescu I, Brice P, Simon D, *et al.* Restaging with gallium scan identifies chemosensitive patients and predicts survival of poor-prognosis mediastinal Hodgkin's disease patients. *Med Oncol* 2000; **17**: 127–34.

82 Cooper DL, Caride VJ, Zloty M, *et al.* Gallium scans in patients with mediastinal Hodgkin's disease treated with chemotherapy. *J Clin Oncol* 1993; **11**: 1092–8.

83 Gasparini MD, Balzarini L, Castellani MR, *et al.* Current role of gallium scan and magnetic resonance imaging in the management of mediastinal Hodgkin lymphoma. *Cancer* 1993; **72**: 577–82.

84 Bogart JA, Chung CT, Mariados NF, *et al.* The value of gallium imaging after therapy for Hodgkin's disease. *Cancer* 1998; **82**: 754–9.

85 Vose JM, Bierman PJ, Anderson JR, *et al.* Single-photon emission computed tomography gallium imaging versus computed tomography: predictive value in

patients undergoing high-dose chemotherapy and autologous stem-cell transplantation for non-Hodgkin's lymphoma. *J Clin Oncol* 1996; **14**: 2473–9.

86 Kaplan WD, Jochelson MS, Herman T, *et al.* Gallium-67 imaging: a predictor of residual tumor viability and clinical outcome in patients with diffuse large-cell lymphoma. *J Clin Oncol* 1990; **8**: 1066–70.

87 Israel O, Mor M, Epelbaum R, *et al.* Clinical pretreatment risk factors and Ga-67 scintigraphy early during treatment for prediction of outcome of patients with aggressive non-Hodgkin lymphoma. *Cancer* 2002; **94**: 873–8.

88 Tuli MM, Al-Shemmari SH, Ameen RM. The use of gallium-67 scintigraphy to monitor tumor response rates and predict long-term clinical outcome in patients with lymphoma. *Clin Lymphoma* 2004; **5**: 56–61.

89 Peylan-Ramu N, Haddy TB, Jones E, *et al.* High frequency of benign mediastinal uptake of gallium-67 after completion of chemotherapy in children with high-grade non-Hodgkin's lymphoma. *J Clin Oncol* 1989; **7**: 1800–6.

90 Bekerman C, Hoffer PB, Bitran JD. The role of gallium-67 in the clinical evaluation of cancer. *Semin Nucl Med* 1984; **14**: 296–323.

91 Waxman AD. Thallium 201 in nuclear oncology. In: Freeman LM. (ed.) *Nuclear medicine annual.* New York: Raven, 1991: 193.

92 Abdel-Dayem HM, *et al.* Role of Tl-201 chloride and Tc-99m-sestamibi in tumor imaging. In: *Nuclear medicine annual.* New York: Raven, 1994: 181–234.

93 Sessler MJ, Geck P, Maul FD, *et al.* New aspects of cellular thallium uptake: Tl^+–Na^+–$2Cl(^-)$-cotransport is the central mechanism of ion uptake. *Nuklearmedizin* 1986; **25**: 24–27.

94 Lin J, Leung WT, Ho SKW, *et al.* Quantitative evaluation of thallium-201 uptake in predicting chemotherapeutic response of osteosarcoma. *Eur J Nucl Med* 1995; **22**: 553–5.

95 Elgazzar AH, Fernandes-Ulloa M, Silberstein EB. Tl-201 as a tumour-localizing agent: current status and future considerations. *Nucl Med Commun* 1993; **14**: 96–103.

96 Piwnica-Worms D, Rao VV, Kronauge JF, Croop JM Characterization of multidrug resistance P-glycoprotein transport function with an organotechnetium cation. *Biochemistry* 1995; **34**: 12210–20.

97 Del-Vecchio S, *et al.* Fractional retention of Tc-99m-sestamibi as an index of P-glycoprotein expression in untreated breast cancer patients. *J Nucl Med* 1997; **38**: 1348–51.

98 Kostakoglu L, *et al.* Clinical validation of the influence of P-glycoprotein on Tc-99m-sestamibi uptake in malignant tumors. *J Nucl Med* 1997; **38**: 1003–8.

99 Roach PJ, Cooper RA, Arthur CK, Ravich RB. Comparison of thallium-201 and gallium-67 scintigraphy in the evaluation of non-Hodgkin's lymphoma. *Aust NZ J Med* 1998; **28**: 33–38.

100 Haas RL, Valdes-Olmos RA, Hoefnagel CA, *et al.* Thallium-201-chloride scintigraphy in staging and monitoring radiotherapy response in follicular lymphoma patients. *Radiother Oncol* 2003; **69**: 323–8.

101 Skiest DJ, Erdman W, Chang WE, *et al.* SPECT thallium-201 combined with *Toxoplasma* serology for the presumptive diagnosis of focal central nervous system mass lesions in patients with AIDS. *J Infect* 2000; **40**: 274–81.

102 Lee VW, *et al.* Intracranial mass lesions: Sequential thallium and gallium scintigraphy in patients with AIDS. *Radiology* 1999; **211**: 507–12.

103 Kao CH, Tsai SC, Wang JJ, *et al.* Technetium-99m-sestamethoxyisobutylisonitrile scan as a predictor of chemotherapy response in malignant lymphomas compared with P-glycoprotein expression, multidrug resistance-related protein expression and other prognosis factors. *Br J Haematol* 2001; **113**: 369–74.

104 Liang JA, Shiau YC, Yang SN, *et al.* Prediction of chemotherapy response in untreated malignant lymphomas using technetium-99m methoxyisobutylisonitrile scan: comparison with P-glycoprotein expression and other prognostic factors. A preliminary report. *Jpn J Clin Oncol* 2002; **32**: 140–5.

105 Naddaf SY, Akisik MF, Aziz M, *et al.* Comparison between ^{201}Tl-chloride and ^{99}Tc(m)-sestamibi SPET brain imaging for differentiating intracranial lymphoma from non-malignant lesions in AIDS patients. *Nucl Med Commun* 1998; **19**: 47–53.

106 Ferone D, Semino C, Boschetti M, *et al.* Initial staging of lymphoma with octreotide and other receptor imaging agents. *Semin Nucl Med* 2005; **35**: 176–85.

107 Hanson MW. Scintigraphic evaluation of neuroendocrine tumors. *Appl Radiol* 2001; **30**: 11–17.

108 Leners N, Jamar F, Fiasse R, *et al.* Indium-111-pentetreotide uptake in endocrine tumors and lymphoma. *J Nucl Med* 1996; **37**: 916–22.

109 Van Hagen PM, Krenning EP, Reubi JC, *et al.* Somatostatin analogue scintigraphy of malignant lymphomas. *Br J Haematol* 1993; **83**: 75–9.

110 Lipp RW, Silly H, Ranner G, *et al.* Radiolabeled octreotide for the demonstration of somatostatin receptors in malignant lymphoma and lymphadenopathy. *J Nucl Med* 1995; **36**: 13–18.

111 Lugtenburg PJ, Krenning EP, Valkema R, *et al.* Somatostatin receptor scintigraphy useful in stage I–II Hodgkin's disease: more extended disease identified. *Br J Haematol* 2001; **112**: 936–44.

112 Dalm VA, Hofland LJ, Mooy CM, *et al.* Somatostatin receptors in malignant lymphomas: targets for radiotherapy? *J Nucl Med* 2004; **45**: 8–16.

113 McGowan KM, Long SD, Pekala PH. Glucose transporter gene expression: regulation of transcription and mRNA stability. *Pharmacol Ther* 1995; **66**: 465–505.

114 Wahl RL. Targeting glucose transporters for tumor imaging: 'sweet' idea, 'sour' result. *J Nucl Med* 1996; **37**: 1038–41.

115 Flier JS, Mueckler MM, Usher P, Lodish HF. Elevated levels of glucose transport and transporter messenger RNA are induced by ras or src oncogenes. *Science* 1987; **235**: 1492–5.

116 Ogawa J, Inoue H, Koide S. Glucose transporter type 1 gene amplification correlation with iacyl-Lewis-X-synthesis and proliferation in lung cancer, *Int J Cancer* 1997; **74**: 189–192.

117 Chang S, Lee S, Kim JI, Kim Y. Expression of the human erythrocyte glucose transporter in transitional cell carcinoma of the bladder. *Urology* 2000; **55**: 448–452.

118 Furuido A, Tanaka S, Haruma K, *et al.* Clinical significance of human erythrocyte glucose transporter 1 expression at the deepest invasive site of advanced colorectal carcinoma, *Oncology* 2001; **60**: 162–169.

119 Higashi K, Ueda Y, Sakuma T, *et al.* Comparison of [(18)F]FDG PET and (201)Tl SPECT in evaluation of pulmonary nodules. *J Nucl Med* 2001; **42**: 1489–96.

120 Higashi K, Clavo AC, Wahl RL. *In vitro* assessment of 2-fluoro-2-deoxy-D-glucose, L-methionine and thymidine as agents to monitor the early response of a human adenocarcinoma cell line to radiotherapy. *J Nucl Med* 1993; **34**: 773–9.

121 Buck AC, Schirrmeister HH, Guhlmann CA, *et al.* Ki-67 immunostaining in pancreatic cancer and chronic active pancreatitis: does *in vivo* FDG uptake correlate with proliferative activity? *J Nucl Med* 2001; **42**: 721–5.

122 Brown RS, Leung JY, Kison PV, *et al.* Glucose transporters and FDG uptake in untreated primary human non-small cell lung cancer. *J Nucl Med* 1999; **40**: 556–65.

123 Newman JS, Francis IR, Kaminski MS, *et al.* Imaging of lymphoma with PET with 2-[18F] fluoro-2-deoxy-D-glucose: correlation with CT. *Radiology* 1994; **190**: 111–16.

124 Leskinen-Kallio S, Ruotsalainen U, Nagren K, *et al.* Uptake of carbon-11-methionine and fluorodeoxyglucose in non-Hodgkin's lymphoma: A PET study. *J Nucl Med* 1991; **32**: 1211–18.

125 Jerusalem G, Beguin Y, Najjar F, *et al.* Positron emission tomography (PET) with 18F-fluorodeoxyglucose (18F-FDG) for the staging of low-grade non-Hodgkin's lymphoma (NHL). *Ann Oncol* 2001; **12**: 825–30.

126 Hoffmann M, Kletter K, Becherer A, *et al.* 18F-fluorodeoxyglucose positron emission tomography (18F-FDG-PET) for staging and follow-up of marginal zone B-cell lymphoma. *Oncology* 2003; **64**: 336–40.

127 Najjar F, Hustinx R, Jerusalem G, *et al.* Positron emission tomography (PET) for staging low-grade non-Hodgkin's lymphomas (NHL). *Cancer Biother Radiopharm* 2001; **16**: 297–304.

128 Bangerter M, Moog F, Buchmann I, *et al.* Whole-body 2-[18F]-fluoro-2-deoxy-D-glucose positron emission tomography (FDG-PET) for accurate staging of Hodgkin's disease. *Ann Oncol* 1998; **9**: 1117–22.

129 Buchmann I, Reinhardt M, Elsner K, *et al.* 2-(fluorine-18)fluoro-2-deoxy-D-glucose positron emission tomography in the detection and staging of malignant lymphoma. A bicenter trial. *Cancer* 2001; **91**: 889–99.

130 Partridge S, Timothy A, O'Doherty MJ, *et al.* 2-fluorine-18-fluoro-2-deoxy-D-glucose positron emission tomography in the pretreatment staging of Hodgkin's disease: influence on patients management in a single institution. *Ann Oncol* 2000; **11**: 1273–9.

131 Weihrauch MR, Re D, Bischoff S, *et al.* Whole-body positron emission tomography using 18F-fluorodeoxyglucose for initial staging of patients with Hodgkin's disease. *Ann Hematol* 2002; **81**: 20–5.

132 Rodriguez M, Ahlstrom H, Sundin A, *et al.* 18F FDG PET in gastric non-Hodgkin's lymphoma. *Acta Oncol* 1997; **36**: 577–84.

133 Hoffman JM, Waskin HA, Schifter T, *et al.* FDG-PET in differentiating lymphoma from non-malignant central nervous system lesions in patients with AIDS. *J Nucl Med* 1993; **34**: 567–75.

134 Heald AE, Hoffman JM, Bartlett JA, Waskin HA. Differentiation of central nervous system lesions in AIDS patients using positron emission tomography (PET). *Int J STD AIDS* 1996; **7**: 337–46.

135 Villringer K, Jager H, Dichgans M, *et al.* Differential diagnosis of CNS lesions in AIDS patients by FDG-PET. *J Comput Assist Tomogr* 1995; **19**: 532–6.

136 Palmedo H, Urbach H, Bender H. FDG-PET in immunocompetent patients with primary central nervous system lymphoma: correlation with MRI and clinical follow-up. *Eur J Nucl Med Mol Imaging* 2005; Oct 12: [Epub].

137 Shipp M, Mauch PM, Harris NL. Non-Hodgkin's lymphomas. In: Devita VT, Hellman S, Rosenberg SA. (eds.) *Cancer principles and practice of oncology.* Philadelphia, PA: Lippincott, 1997: 2165–220.

138 Abdel-Dayem HM, Rosen G, El-Zeftawy H, *et al.* Fluorine-18 fluorodeoxyglucose splenic uptake from extramedullary hematopoiesis after granulocyte colony-stimulating factor stimulation. *Clin Nucl Med* 1999; **24**: 319–22.

139 Gundlapalli S, Ojha B, Mountz JM. Granulocyte colony-stimulating factor: confounding F-18 FDG uptake in outpatient positron emission tomographic facilities for patients receiving ongoing treatment of lymphoma. *Clin Nucl Med* 2002; **27**: 140–1.

140 Carr R, Barrington SF, Madan B, *et al.* Detection of lymphoma in bone marrow by whole-body positron emission tomography. *Blood* 1998; **91**: 3340–6.

141 Moog F, Bangerter M, Kotzerke J, *et al.* 18-F-fluorodeoxyglucose-positron emision tomography as a new

approach to detect lymphomatous bone marrow. *J Clin Oncol* 1998; **16**: 603–9.

142 Jerusalem G, Warland V, Najjar F, *et al.* Whole-body ^{18}F-FDG PET for the evaluation of patients with Hodgkin's disease and non-Hodgkin's lymphoma. *Nucl Med Commun* 1999; **20**: 13–20.

143 Krishnan A, Shirkhoda A, Tehranzadeh J, *et al.* Primary bone lymphoma: radiographic–MR imaging correlation. *Radiographics* 2003; **23**: 1371–83.

144 Bar-Shalom R, Yefremov N, Haim N, *et al.* Camera-based FDG PET and ^{67}Ga SPECT in the evaluation of lymphoma: comparative study. *Radiology* 2003; **227**: 353–60.

145 Bar-Shalom R, Mor M, Yefremov N, Goldsmith SJ. The value of Ga-67 scintigraphy and F-18 fluoro-deoxyglucose positron emission tomography in staging and monitoring the response of lymphoma to treatment. *Semin Nucl Med* 2001; **31**: 177–90.

146 Kostakoglu L, Goldsmith SJ. Positron emission tomography in lymphoma: comparison with computed tomography and gallium-67 single photon emission computed tomography. *Clin Lymphoma* 2000; **1**: 67–74.

147 Wirth A, Seymour JF, Hicks RJ, *et al.* Fluorine-18 fluorodeoxyglucose positron emission tomography, gallium-67 scintigraphy, and conventional staging for Hodgkin's disease and non-Hodgkin's lymphoma. *Am J Med* 2002; **112**: 262–8.

148 Shen YY, Kao A, Yen RF. Comparison of ^{18}F-fluoro-2-deoxyglucose positron emission tomography and gallium-67 citrate scintigraphy for detecting malignant lymphoma. *Oncol Rep* 2002; **9**: 321–5.

149 Brandt L, Kimby E, Nygren P, Glimelius B. A systematic overview of chemotherapy effects in Hodgkin's disease. *Acta Oncol* 2001; **40**: 185–97.

150 Coiffier B, Gisselbrecht C, Vose JM, *et al.* Prognostic factors in aggressive malignant lymphomas. Description and validation of prognostic index that could identify patients requiring a more intensive therapy. *J Clin Oncol* 1991; **9**: 211–19.

151 Hueltenschmidt B, Sautter-Bihl ML, Lang O, *et al.* Whole body positron emission tomography in the treatment of Hodgkin disease. *Cancer* 2001; **91**: 302–10.

152 Rigacci L, Castagnoli A, Dini C, *et al.* [18]FDG-positron emission tomography in post treatment evaluation of residual mass in Hodgkin's lymphoma: long-term results. *Oncol Rep* 2005; **14**: 1209–14.

153 Weihrauch MR, Re D, Scheidhauer K, *et al.* Thoracic positron emission tomography using ^{18}F-fluorodeoxyglucose for the evaluation of residual mediastinal Hodgkin disease. *Blood* 2001; **98**: 2930–4.

154 Mikhaeel NG, Timothy AR, O'Doherty MJ, *et al.* 18-FDG-PET as a prognostic indicator in the treatment of aggressive non-Hodgkin's lymphoma – comparison with CT. *Leuk Lymphoma* 2000; **39**: 543–53.

155 Naumann R, Vaic A, Beuthien-Baumann B, *et al.* Prognostic value of positron emission tomography in the evaluation of post-treatment residual mass in patients with Hodgkin's disease and non-Hodgkin's lymphoma. *Br J Haematol* 2001; **115**: 793–800.

156 de Wit M, Bohuslavizki KH, Buchert R, *et al.* [18]FDG-PET following treatment as valid predictor for disease-free survival in Hodgkin's lymphoma. *Ann Oncol* 2001; **12**: 29–37.

157 Spaepen K, Stroobants S, Dupont P, *et al.* Prognostic value of positron emission tomography (PET) with fluorine-18 fluorodeoxyglucose (^{18}F]FDG) after first line chemotherapy in non-Hodgkins lymphoma: is ^{18}F]FDG PET a valid alternative to conventional diagnostic methods? *J Clin Oncol* 2001; **19**: 414–19.

158 Zinzani PL, Magagnoli M, Chierichetti F, *et al.* The role of positron emission tomography (PET) in the management of lymphoma patients. *Ann Oncol* 1999; **10**: 1181–4.

159 Kostakoglu L, Coleman M, Somrov S, *et al.* FDG-PET after one cycle of chemotherapy accurately predicts response to therapy in large cell (aggressive) non-Hodgkin's lymphoma (NHL) and Hodgkin's disease (HD). *J Nucl Med* 2004; **45**: 316P.

160 Mikhaeel NG, Mainwaring P, Nunan T, Timothy AR. Prognostic value of interim and post treatment FDG-PET scanning in Hodgkin lymphoma [abstract]. *Ann Oncol* 2002; **13(suppl 2)**: 21.

161 Spaepen K, Stroobants S, Dupont P, *et al.* Can positron emission tomography with [(18)F]-fluorodeoxyglucose after first-line treatment distinguish Hodgkin's disease patients who need additional therapy from others in whom additional therapy would mean avoidable toxicity? *Br J Haematol* 2001; **115**: 272–8.

162 Stiff PJ, Dahlberg S, Forman SJ, *et al.* Autologous bone marrow transplantation for patients with relapses or refractory diffuse aggressive non-Hodgkin's lymphoma: value of augmented preparative regimes. *J Clin Oncol* 1998; **16**: 48–55.

163 Philip T, Guglielmi C, Hagenbeek A, *et al.* Autologous bone marrow transplantation as compared with salvage chemotherapy in relapses of chemosensitive non-Hodgkin's lymphoma. *N Engl J Med* 1995; **333**: 1540–5.

164 Cremerius U, Fabry U, Wildberger JE, *et al.* Pre-transplant positron emission tomography using fluorine-18-fluoro-deoxyglucose predicts outcome in patients treated with high-dose chemotherapy and autologous stem cell transplantation for non-Hodgkin's lymphoma. *Bone Marrow Transplant* 2002; **30**: 103–11.

165 Becherer A, Mitterbauer M, Jaeger U, *et al.* Positron emission tomography with ^{18}F]2-fluoro-D-2-deoxyglucose (FDG-PET) predicts relapse of malignant lymphoma after high-dose therapy with stem cell transplantation. *Leukemia* 2002; **16**: 260–7.

166 Armitage JO, Weisenburger DD, Hutchins M, *et al.* Chemotherapy for diffuse large-cell lymphoma – rapidly responding patients have more durable remissions. *J Clin Oncol* 1986; **4**: 160–4.

167 Coiffier B, Bryon PA, Berger F, *et al.* Intensive and sequential combination chemotherapy for aggressive malignant lymphomas (protocol LNH-80). *J Clin Oncol* 1986; **4**: 147–53.

168 Romer W, Hanauske A-R, Ziegler S, *et al.* Positron emission tomography in non-Hodgkin's lymphoma: assesment of chemotherapy with fluorodeoxy-glucose. *Blood* 1998; **91**: 4464–71.

169 Spaepen K, Stroobants S, Dupont P, *et al.* Early restaging positron emission tomography with ^{18}F-fluoro-deoxyglucose predicts outcome in patients with aggressive non-Hodgkin's lymphoma. *Ann Oncol* 2002; **13**: 1356–63.

170 Haioun C, Itti E, Rahmouni A, *et al.* [^{18}F]fluoro-2-deoxy-D-glucose positron emission tomography (FDG-PET) in aggressive lymphoma: an early prognostic tool for predicting patient outcome. *Blood* 2005; **106**: 1376–81.

171 Mikhaeel NG, Hutchings M, Fields PA, *et al.* FDG-PET after two to three cycles of chemotherapy predicts progression-free and overall survival in high-grade non-Hodgkin lymphoma. *Ann Oncol* 2005; **16**: 1514–23.

172 Kostakoglu L, Coleman M, Leonard JP, *et al.* Positron emission tomography predicts prognosis after one cycle of chemotherapy in aggressive lymphoma and Hodgkin's disease. *J Nucl Med* 2002; **43**: 1018–27.

173 Juweid ME, Wiseman GA, Vose JM, *et al.* Response assessment of aggressive non-Hodgkin's lymphoma by integrated International Workshop Criteria and fluorine-18-fluorodeoxyglucose positron emission tomography. *J Clin Oncol* 2005; **23**: 4652–61.

174 Townsend DW, Beyer T. A combined PET/CT scanner: the path to true image fusion. *Br J Radiol* 2002; **75**: S24–30.

175 Schaefer NG, Hany TF, Taverna C, *et al.* Non-Hodgkin lymphoma and Hodgkin disease: coregistered FDG PET and CT at staging and restaging – do we need contrast-enhanced CT? *Radiology* 2004; July 23 [Epub ahead of print].

176 Kazama T, Swanston N, Podoloff DA, Macapinlac HA. Effect of colony-stimulating factor and conventional- or high-dose chemotherapy on FDG uptake in bone marrow. *Eur J Nucl Med Mol Imaging* 2005; **32**: 1406–11.

Lymphoscintigraphy

A.M. PETERS AND P.S. MORTIMER

INTRODUCTION

With the increasing importance of sentinel lymph nodes in cancer management, the subject of lymphoscintigraphy has now diverged into two more or less distinct clinical areas: firstly, lymphoscintigraphy for the identification of sentinel nodes and secondly, lymphoscintigraphy in the investigation of the swollen limb and other lymphatic diseases, such as lymph leaks. An increasing level of interest in the first has tended to overshadow interest in the second of these two general clinical applications. This chapter concerns the second, especially lymphoscintigraphy for the investigation of a swollen limb. Lymph leaks are extremely difficult to find using conventional 'extremity lymphoscintigraphy' and will not be considered in this chapter. The interested reader is instead referred to a recent article on the use of an orally administered ^{123}I-labeled medium chain fatty acid, methyl iodophenyl pentadecanoic acid (BMIPP), which, following intestinal re-absorption as the intact molecule, is delivered directly to intestinal lymphatics.[1]

Lymphoscintigraphy (radionuclide lymphography, isotope lymphography, radionuclide lymphangiography, lymphangioscintigraphy) involves the interstitial (usually subcutaneous or intradermal) injection of a radiolabeled tracer that is transported by lymph conducting pathways. The dynamics of tracer movement are usually studied using a large-field-of-view gamma camera although scintillation detectors can also be used.

Lymphoscintigraphy is currently the best method of investigating the lymphatic system in a limb. It can provide functional as well as limited structural information. Its main indication is the investigation of a swollen limb and, in particular, if lymphatic insufficiency is the suspected cause. Unlike conventional direct contrast X-ray lymphography, it does not give good resolution of the lymphatic vessels but can be useful for identifying the direction of lymph draining routes, as in sentinel node mapping, for example. It can be very useful for diagnosing lymphatic obstruction but not the cause of the obstruction. Therefore, additional imaging such as computed tomography (CT), magnetic resonance (MR) or positron emission tomography (PET) may be necessary.

PHYSIOLOGICAL PRINCIPLES

Functions of the lymphatic system

The three main functions of the lymphatic system are as follows.

PRESERVATION OF FLUID BALANCE

Lymph vessels return the capillary ultrafiltrate and escaped plasma proteins to the bloodstream by draining them, ultimately, into the neck veins. This completes the extravascular circulation of fluid and protein and maintains tissue volume homeostasis. If lymphatic function is impaired the tissue develops a severe, protein-rich form of edema called lymphedema.

DEFENSE FUNCTION

Macromolecules, including micro-organisms, are removed from the interstitium by the lymph vessels and transported to the lymph nodes. Lymph drainage is an important component of immunosurveillance as well as 'cleansing' the tissues of unwanted material including malignant cells and inorganic matter such as silica and carbon. The lymph route is the exit route from tissues for immune cells such as lymphocytes, macrophages, and dendritic cells.

NUTRITIONAL FUNCTION

Absorption of fat is conducted from the gut by lacteals.

Transport of macromolecules

Protein and colloids of a certain size are transported exclusively by the lymph. Even fluid drainage from the interstitium proceeds almost exclusively via the lymph routes, contrary to traditional thinking. In most vascular beds, venous capillaries do not continuously reabsorb the filtrate generated in arterial capillaries. Thus, modern evidence demonstrates that well perfused capillaries are normally in a state of filtration along their entire length.[2] The lymph drainage thus bears the responsibility of removing the microvascular filtrate from the tissues. Edema can arise from a high filtration rate that exceeds lymphatic transport capacity or from impaired lymph flow.

Soluble macromolecules, including proteins, are carried across the blood vascular endothelium into the intersitium almost exclusively by convection in contrast to small hydrophilic solutes (such as diethylenetriamine pentaacetic acid) which cross almost exclusively by diffusion. Proteins can therefore only transfer from blood to tissue whereas small solute movement is bi-directional. These rules do not necessarily apply in pathological circumstances. If macromolecules or nanoparticles are radioactively labeled and injected into the body tissue, they can be recorded from the place of injection, along the lymph vessels to the lymph nodes where they are deposited. This is the principle of lymphoscintigraphy.

TECHNIQUE

Agents

The first radiotracers to be applied to lymphoscintigraphy were labeled proteins, especially ^{99m}Tc-human serum albumin.[3–5] These were soon followed by ^{99m}Tc-labeled colloids that were used for imaging the liver. Nowadays, the most widely used agent is ^{99m}Tc-nanocolloid but others have been suggested including ^{99m}Tc-labeled polyclonal human immunoglobulin G (HIG),[6] liposomes labeled with ^{99m}Tc,[7] and dextrans such as ^{99m}Tc-mannosyl dextran.[8] The requirements of the ideal lymphoscintigraphic agent depend on the clinical question being posed, although generally would include a molecular size that favors penetration of lymph vessels from the interstitial space, rather than blood vessels, and a high extraction and retention in loco-regional lymph

nodes. The ideal requirements would, however, vary in some circumstances; for example, to detect a leak in the thoracic duct (a difficult challenge at the best of times), one might choose a small protein, such as albumin to ensure lymphatic entry but a low lymph node extraction fraction, otherwise there will be insufficient tracer made available to the leak. Equally, in breast cancer-related lymphedema, lymph node extraction fraction would be less important because of widespread resection of lymph nodes and the need usually to image lymphatic vessels rather than nodes, although this is more in a clinical research context.

Site of injection

Labeled tracer may be injected into any number of tissue compartments: skin (intradermal), subcutaneous, and intramuscular. The choice of anatomical site for injection depends upon which lymphatic tracts are to be investigated. In the lower limb, imaging anterior epi-fascial lymphatic tracts requires an injection into the web space between first and second toes, the posterior epi-fascial tracts requires an injection behind the external malleolus and for the sub-fascial routes, the injection should be into the calf muscle. In the upper limb, imaging the epi-fascial routes requires a hand injection whereas imaging sub-fascial routes requires a forearm muscle injection.

The most widely used injection depth is the subcutaneous tissues although intradermal routes can be used. Certainty regarding depth of injection is not always straightforward. An intradermal injection should be as superficial as possible thus raising a 'skin bleb'. Injections are usually painful with resistance felt as the plunger is pressed down into the syringe (no resistance felt with subcutaneous injection). Doses of radioactivity are localized and therefore high which is a theoretical disadvantage. Intradermal injections achieve more rapid lymphatic filling and imaging of the drainage routes than subcutaneous injections.[9] Intradermal routes do not appear to be as discriminatory as a subcutaneous injection for determining lymphatic impairment.[10] Therefore intradermal routes appear better for imaging lymph drainage routes, e.g. sentinel node mapping, whereas a subcutaneous injection may be preferable for assessment of lymphatic function, e.g. investigation of swollen limb.

Image acquisition and display

The best method of image acquisition is the use of a dual-headed whole-body gamma camera in whole-body mode at multiple time points starting immediately after injection. For lower limb lymphoscintigraphy the 'sweep', which should start from the feet, takes several minutes and is terminated at upper abdominal level to include the liver. A 5 min or 30 min image, and so on, is the starting point of each individual acquisition. These should be at 5, 30, 60, and about 180 min although it is acceptable to replace the

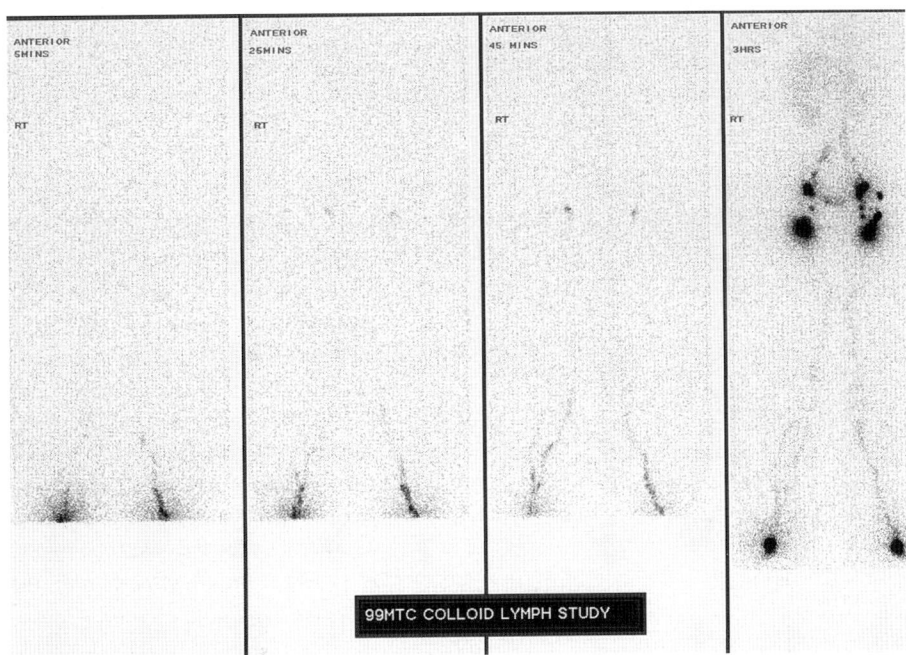

Figure 16D.1 *Normal lymphoscintigraphy. Activity is just visible in inguinal lymph nodes bilaterally at 45 min. There is abundant and symmetrical actvity in inguinal, iliac, and para-aortic nodes at 3 h. The liver is visible only on the delayed image. There is no evidence of re-routing of lymph through the superficial or deep systems.*

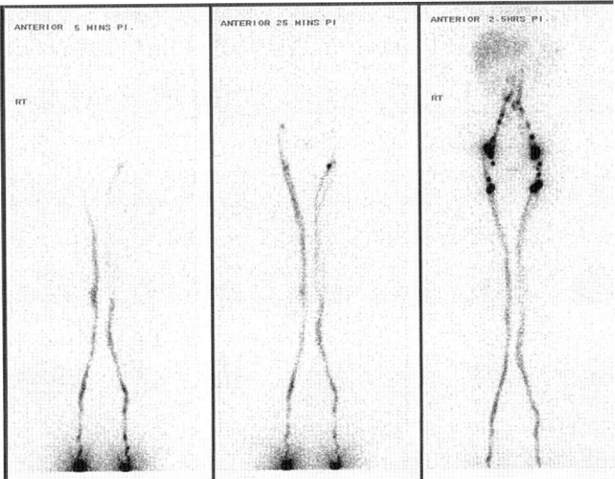

Figure 16D.2 *Another example of a normal study in which lymph transport is somewhat more brisk than in the patient shown in Fig. 16D.1.*

30 min and 60 min images with a 45 min image (Figs 16D.1 and 16D.2). The 3 h image should never be omitted on the grounds that the earlier images appear normal.[11] The reason why the whole-body mode is important is because of the need to view the entire extremity on each acquisition.[12] The four 'half-body' images can then be displayed alongside one another.

Quantification

Even with invasive techniques, it is not possible to measure lymph flow in humans. Nevertheless, serial quantitative measures of lymph transport in a limb are possible.

Following injection, baseline levels of radioactivity are obtained over injection sites. Various protocols for studying lymph transport kinetics have been published but the most commonly used is to draw a region of interest around the imaged regional lymph node chain and then determine the radioactivity as a percentage of that administered.[13] This can be combined with measurement of the rate constant of disappearance of activity in the injection depot. Other analyses may be computerized, e.g. transit time for tracer vanguard. Unfortunately, no standard has been universally agreed and most departments adopt their own protocols. Reproducibility is not that good, making follow-up studies after an intervention unreliable.[14]

Lymph node uptake has proved to be a more reliable measurement than tracer clearance for determining lymphatic impairment within a limb. Nevertheless, the rate at which a radiotracer leaves the injection depot is dependent on local lymph flow. Indeed the rate constant, k, of disappearance represents the local lymph flow per unit volume of tissue in which the tracer is distributed (mL min^{-1} (mL of tissue)$^{-1}$). It has recently been shown with respect to radiolabeled HIG that k correlates strongly with the rate of appearance of radioactivity in central blood (the final destination of lymph after passage through the thoracic duct).[15] There is also strong left to right correlation of k within upper or lower limbs suggesting measurement of fractional removal rate from the injection site may be a more reliable measurement than currently perceived.[16] Clearance studies may be the only way of quantifying lymph transport in circumstances where surgery or radiotherapy has been performed on the regional lymph nodes.

Greater sophistication in the computer analyses of the tracer kinetics has led to the development of the transport index.[17] Five components of the lymphoscintigrams are

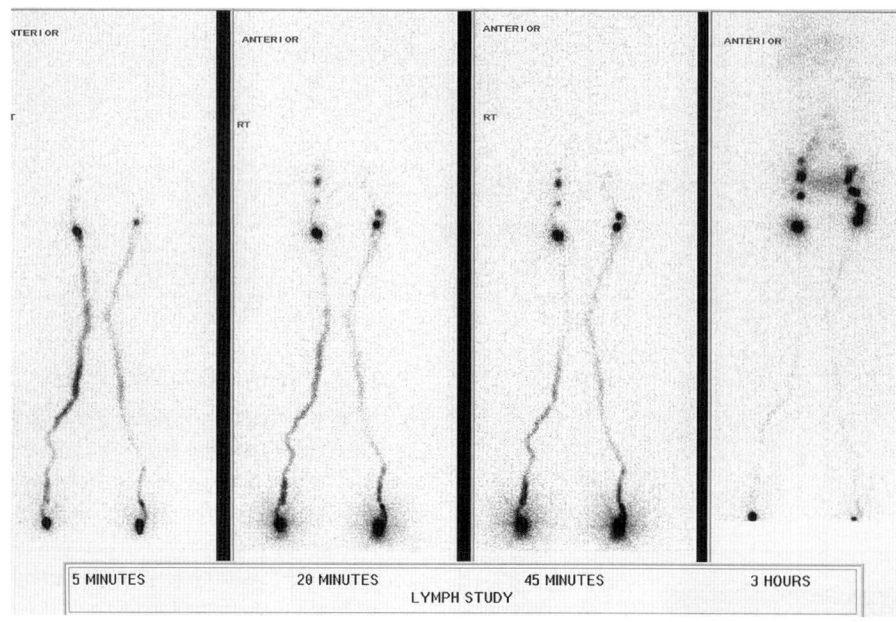

Figure 16D.3 *Lymph transport is rapid bilaterally with abundant inguinal activity present on the image starting at 5 min. These appearances suggest increased capillary filtration, but there is no evidence of lymph re-routing or development of collateral vessels and therefore no evidence that the lymphatic system is having difficulty coping with the increased flow.*

scored: the time for the isotope to reach the lymph nodes, the distribution pattern of the tracer, the transport kinetics, and the appearance of both the lymph vessels and lymph nodes.

Methods that stimulate lymph flow should, in theory, improve the sensitivity for discriminating degrees of lymphatic impairment. Some departments therefore use treadmill walking or running because lymph flow is generally slow at rest.[18] It is important to realize that a standardized exercise protocol is only of use if the subject can reproducibly comply with the requirements. Any infirmity will mean lymph drainage is reduced because of less movement, not because of impaired lymph drainage. Other groups have employed 2 min of massage of hands or feet immediately after the injection.[19]

Qualitative lymphoscintigraphy[19,20]

Following a foot or hand subcutaneous injection, lymph-conducting pathways should start to be visualized within 5 min in a normal study. Inguinal node activity (foot injection) should be detectable within 45 min and perhaps a little earlier for axillary nodes (hand injection). Relatively distinct lymphatic pathways can usually be imaged but from 45 min onwards, the lymphatic vessels tend to fade. In lower limb studies, iliac, and then para-aortic nodes become visible after inguinal nodes in a symmetrical fashion. The liver, the final destination for radiocolloids, becomes visible between 1 and 3 h post-injection.[21]

Increased capillary filtration leads to increased 'washout' of tracer from the interstitium and therefore accelerates tracer transport to and through the lymphatic system (Fig. 16D.3). In the lower limbs, venous disease is

the most common cause. Delayed tracer transport from depot or reduced nodal uptake implies impaired lymph drainage.

Evidence of lymph re-routing (Figs 16D.4 to 16D.6) and the presence of collateral lymph vessels (Fig. 16D.7) both indicate lymphatic dysfunction. If epi-fascial lymph channels are obstructed then lymph finds an alternative route, ascending through dermal lymphatics to give the characteristic appearance of dermal backflow[22] or passing through the connecting vessels to the sub-fascial system and, in the lower limb, entering popliteal nodes. Usually both routes operate so that dermal backflow coexists with popliteal node visualization (Figs 16D.4, 16D.5, and 16D.7). Dermal backflow and popliteal node visualization may not be apparent for some considerable time after injection so it is mandatory to terminate the imaging protocol no sooner than 2.5–3 h after injection, even if everything appears normal at 1 h. Dermal backflow may occur with proximal lymphatic obstruction; for example aplasia of high thigh lymphatic collectors (no inguinal lymph nodes imaged) or ilio-inguinal nodal sclerosis (one or no inguinal nodes imaged) (Fig. 16D.8) or sclerotic metastases within the iliac chain. High levels of superficial radioactivity can also occur with lymph reflux when main lymphatic collector valves are incompetent and consequently lymph refluxes through the skin under the influence of gravity. This is seen in lymphedema – distichiasis syndrome (Fig. 16D.9).

Abnormal collections of radioactivity can be seen at sites of inflammation where lymphatics have presumably been compromised or overloaded as a result of increased capillary fluid filtration. Characteristic images are in the gaiter region following cellulitis or lipodermatosclerosis (Fig. 16D.10). The appearance of multiple lymph collection vessels may be an indication of increased lymph load (and flow)

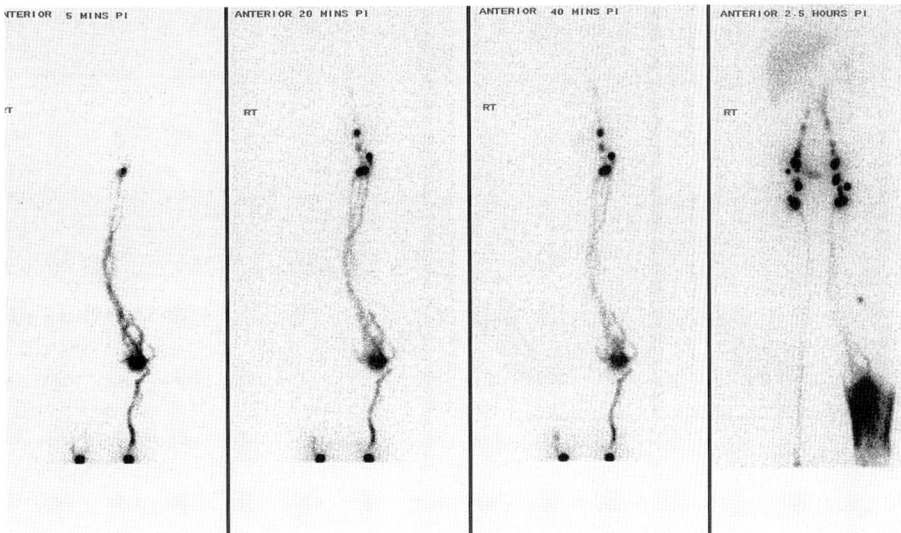

Figure 16D.4 *'Limb in profile' as a result of re-routing of lymph through the skin – so-called dermal backflow – co-existing with popliteal node visualization and indicating re-routing of lymph through the skin and deep system. Transport on the left is rapid, with visualization of inguinal nodes on the image commencing at 5 min post-injection, indicating increased capillary filtration. The re-routing indicates that the lymphatic system is failing to cope with the increased lymph flow. There is what appears to be a grossly dilated lymph vessel, a lymphatic varicosity, just below the knee. Transport on the right is somewhat sluggish but otherwise normal.*

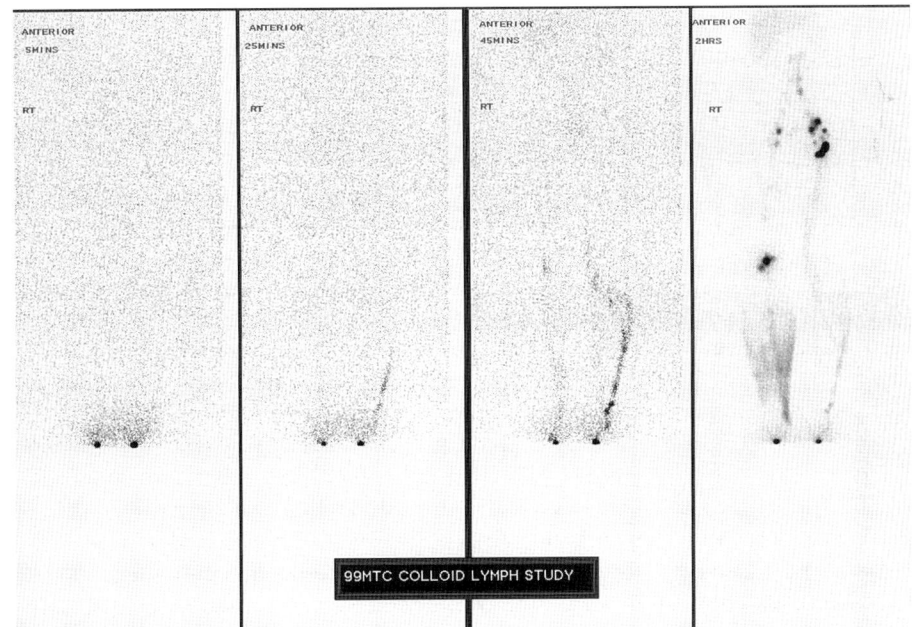

Figure 16D.5 *Another case of dermal backflow co-existing with popliteal node visualization, except in this case, lymph transport on the affected side is reduced.*

(Fig. 16D.7). Occasionally, when using a colloidal radio-tracer, the liver is visualized within minutes of what seemed like a straightforward interstitial injection (Fig. 16D.11, page 722). Whilst this is usually interpreted correctly as inadvertent injection of radiotracer directly into a blood vessel, the possibility should be considered that tracer, having been injected into the intended compartment, subsequently enters the vascular space via a lympho-venous communication. Although the perceived wisdom is that such communications only exist

in the neck, where the major lymphatic trunks return lymph to venous blood, there are several reports in the literature claiming to have demonstrated lympho-venous communications more peripherally, both in humans[23] and experimental animals.[24] The authors recently encountered a patient in whom the study was abandoned because the liver was visualized within 5 min of injection (Fig. 16D.12, page 722). When the study was repeated a few days later exactly the same phenomenon was recorded (Fig. 16D.13, page 723).

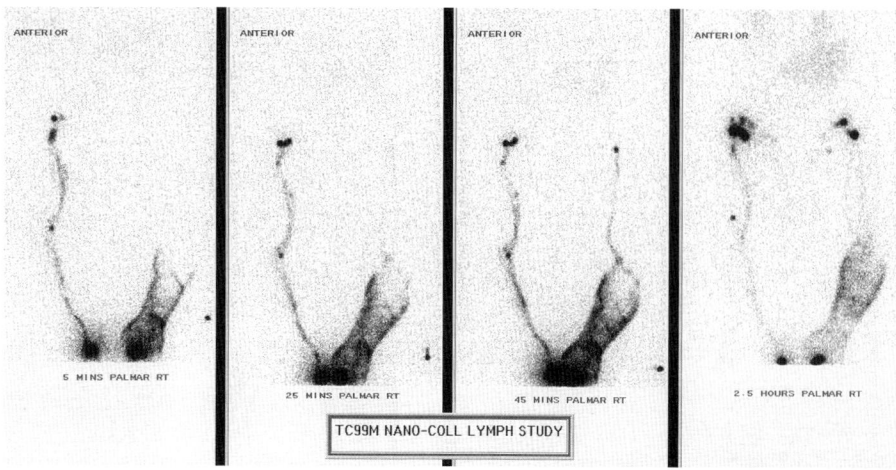

Figure 16D.6 *Dermal backflow in the right lower arm.*

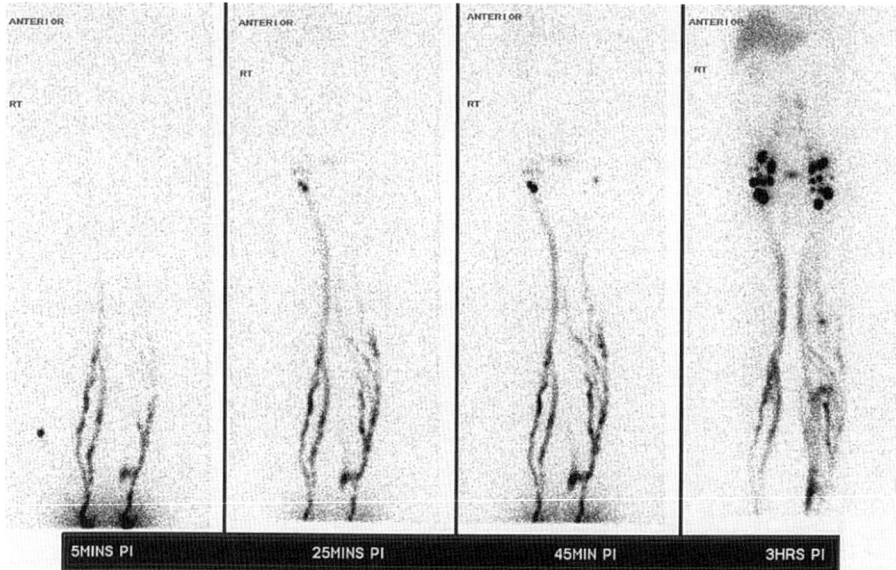

Figure 16D.7 *Marked development of collateral lymph vessels, especially on the left. There is also evident dermal backflow and visualization of a popliteal node.*

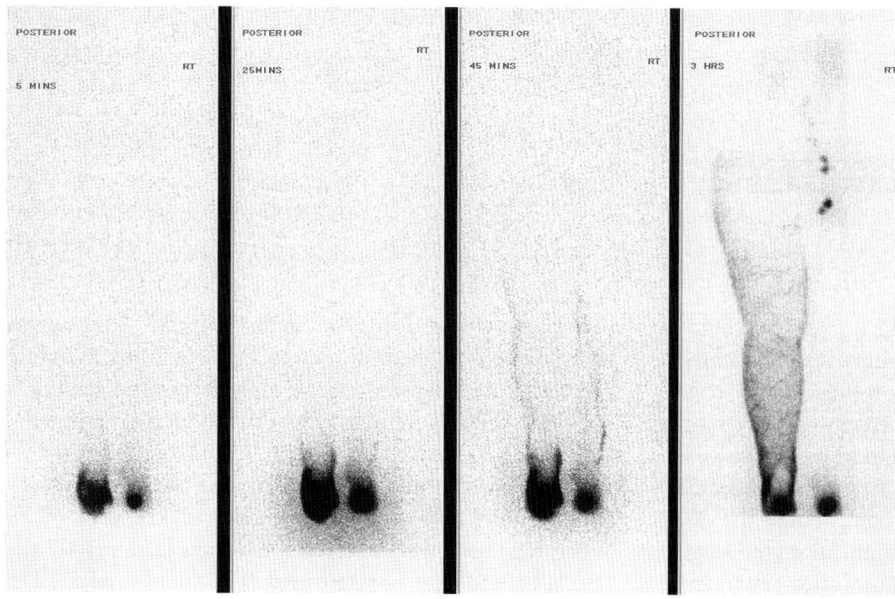

Figure 16D.8 *Proximal unilateral lymphatic obstruction resulting from sclerosis in the ilio-inguinal nodes. There is gross dermal backflow involving the entire limb but only minimal evidence of re-routing through the deep system. Transport up the right lower limb is sluggish but otherwise normal.*

Moreover, it is surprising that the liver is ever visualized at all with radiocolloid injections when one considers the gauntlet run by the radiotracer through the numerous nodes that separate it from its injection site and the proximal end of the thoracic duct. It has recently been shown that nanocolloid, for example, has a nodal extraction efficiency of about 70%.[25] Tracer emerging from the last of a chain of, say, six nodes would therefore be 0.00073 of that entering the first (i.e. $[1 - 0.7]^6$). The quite substantial amounts of tracer eventually accumulating in the liver raise a suspicion of functional lympho-venous communication at some points in the periphery, perhaps within lymph nodes.

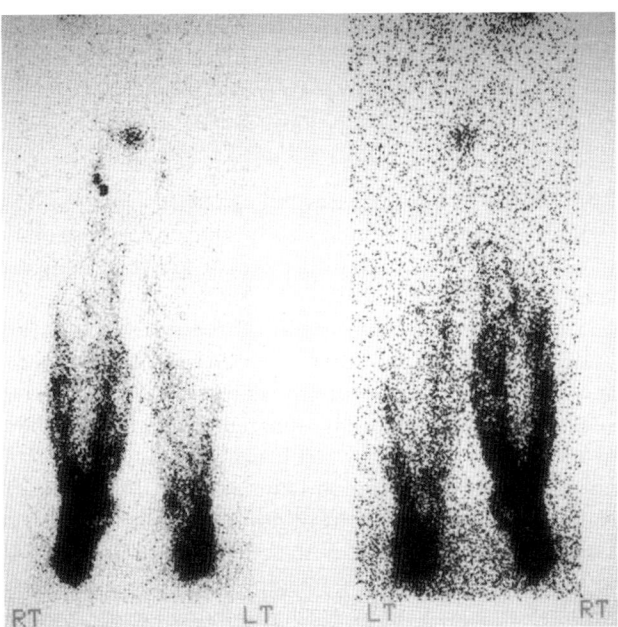

Figure 16D.9 *Lymphedema – distichiasis syndrome.*

Quantitative lymphoscintigraphy

The speed of transit of tracer up the limb is the primary benchmark for increased or decreased lymph transport. Arrival time in minutes and the storage capacity of the regional lymph nodes, i.e. percent uptake of tracer in nodes at 30, 60, and 120 min are the most widely used functional measurements.[18] Lymph drainage declines with age and this has to be taken into consideration when determining normal and abnormal lymphatic transport ranges.[26,27]

Weissleder and Weissleder[18] reported average arrival times in inguinal nodes as 5 min in healthy individuals under standardized physical exercise of running on a treadmill. Nodal uptakes of between 10 and 32% were observed under the same conditions at 120 min. (It should be noted, however, that nodal uptake does not just rely on arrival of tracer in node but also on 'trapping' ability of node and rate of departure of tracer in efferent lymph so it is not an exact measurement.) Differences between right and left legs of up to 20% have no diagnostic significance if the clinical examination is normal.

Using a different protocol, the St Thomas' group in London measured inguinal node uptake following 30 min of rest and then 30 min of walking (total examination time one hour). Good concordance between lymphoscintigraphy and conventional X-ray lymphography was demonstrated.[13,28] The diagnosis of lymphedema was accepted if less than 0.3% of isotope reached the groin nodes by 30 min. An uptake greater than 0.6% was considered normal and greater than 1.5% at 30 min suggested venous disease. The response to exercise between 30 and 60 min appeared to improve sensitivity for diagnosing lymphatic impairment.

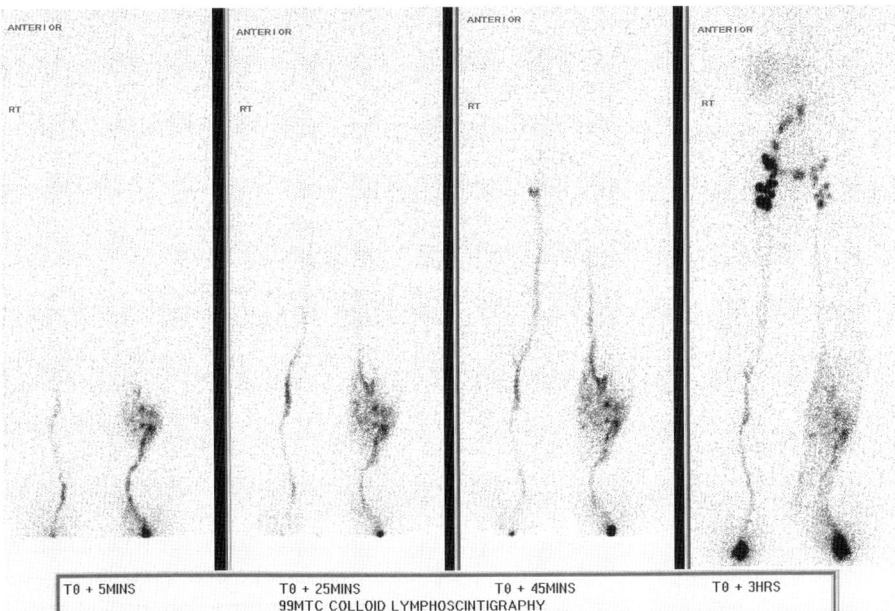

Figure 16D.10 *Cellulitis/lipodermato-sclerosis, with impaired lymph transport on the left and dermal backflow in the gaiter region.*

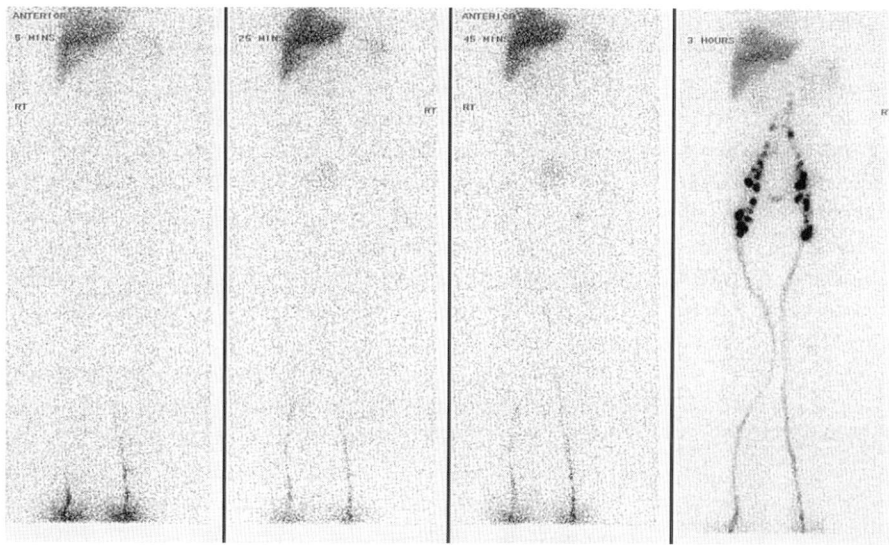

Figure 16D.11 *There is immediate localization of the liver in an otherwise normal study. This was almost certainly the result of inadvertent partial intravascular administration of the tracer.*

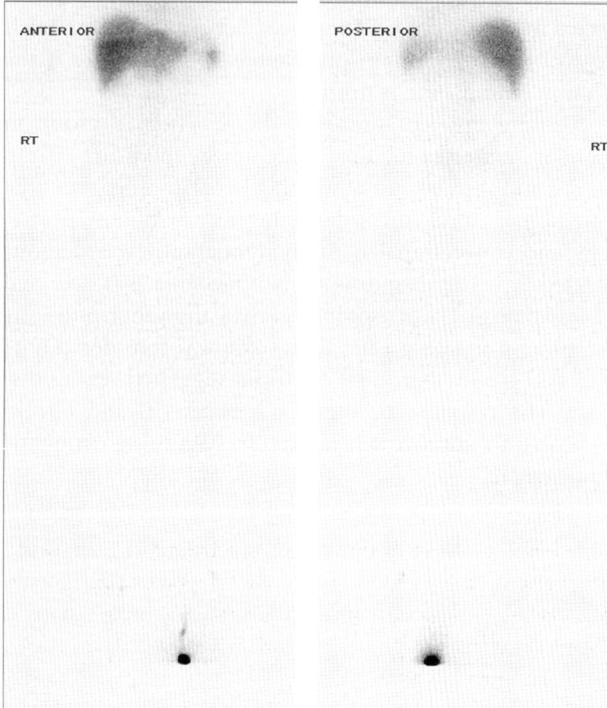

Figure 16D.12 *As in Fig. 16D.11, accidental intravascular administration was assumed and the study therefore abandoned.*

INVESTIGATION OF A SWOLLEN LIMB

A limb may swell for many reasons.[29] Lymphoscintigraphy is the investigation of choice for the diagnosis of lymphatic impairment (lymphedema) but other investigations, e.g. duplex venous Doppler, CT or MRI, may be necessary to determine accurately the cause of swelling. Limb swelling is usually a manifestation of edema but may be the result of an increase in any tissue component, i.e. muscle, fat, blood etc. In Klippel–Trenaunay syndrome, swelling may result from tissue overgrowth, excess filling of the veins as well as (lymph)edema. One should also be alert to the possibility that the limb considered swollen is in fact normal while the contralateral limb has atrophied.

Duplex Doppler venous ultrasound is usually worth undertaking in addition to lymphoscintigraphy. The presence of venous reflux or compression/occlusion of the iliac vein may not be clinically apparent. Indeed correction of the venous lesion may result in improvement or even normalization of the lymphoscintigraphic abnormality.[30] Neither lymphoscintigraphy or duplex Doppler will necessarily identify the cause of obstruction in the case of tumor in which case CT or MR imaging is required. Similarly lymphatic malformations which cause swelling, e.g. lymphangioma, may not be visualized on lymphoscintigraphy because of no communication with normal lymph drainage routes. In these circumstances MR angiography is required to identify the malformation.

Lymphedema

Lymphatics may fail for a number of reasons. First, there may be an intrinsic abnormality of the lymph-conducting pathways, otherwise known as primary lymphedema. In practice, this simply means that no identifiable outside cause can be found. Distal hypoplasia of the leg lymphatics is the commonest form of primary lymphedema. Edema begins in the ankle and extends proximally. The edema is usually bilateral but asymmetrical. A trivial injury may precipitate swelling that in the initial stages is mistaken for soft tissue inflammation or a venous thrombosis. Despite onset at or after puberty, it is assumed that the abnormality represents an underdevelopment of collecting lymphatic vessels (the main limb lymphatics).

Lymphedema of the proximal obstructive type manifests with sudden onset of unilateral whole-limb swelling. After exclusion of causes of proximal obstruction, such as tumor or thrombosis, studies of these cases have demonstrated

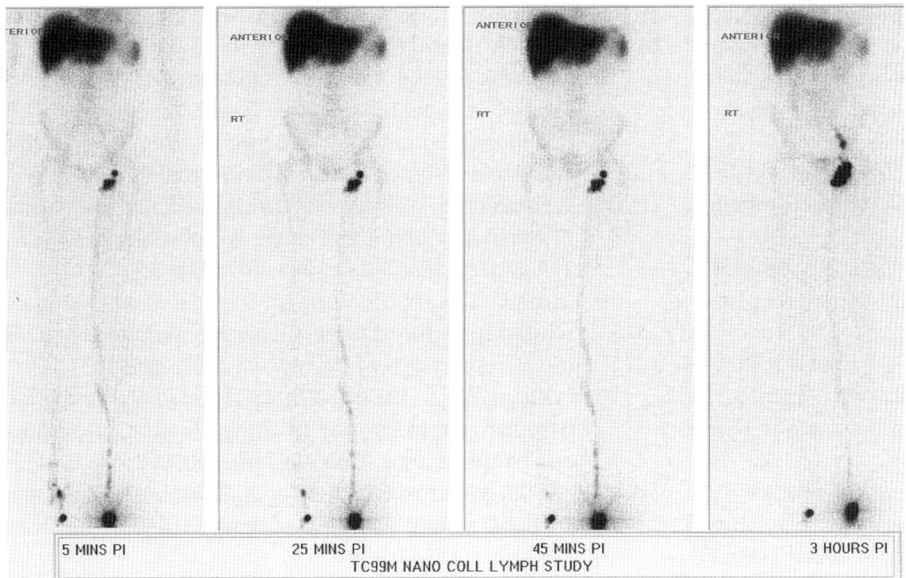

5 MINS PI   25 MINS PI   45 MINS PI   3 HOURS PI
TC99M NANO COLL LYMPH STUDY

Figure 16D.13 *The same administration as for Fig. 16D.11, when it was repeated a few days later. Early hepatic visualization was again evident suggesting the possibility of lymphovenous communications peripherally in the limb. This interpretation is supported by the finding of some interstitial activity at the injection site on the right that decreases over time but is not accompanied by any lymphatic activity more proximally (e.g. no inguinal activity).*

sclerosis and atrophy of draining lymph nodes, but no cause has been identified. Whole-leg swelling, which is sometimes bilateral, can be a manifestation of megalymphatics. Here, grossly dilated (varicose) lymphatics with valvular incompetence give rise to lymph, and sometimes chylous, reflux. An obliterative process, where there is permanent obliteration of the lymphatic lumen and consequently of the vessel itself, probably develops through lymphangiothrombosis or lymphangitis in the same way as for veins. Like blood, lymph will clot, but not so readily. Main (collecting) lymphatic vessels have contractile properties, and under normal circumstances this is the main driving force for limb lymph drainage. Failure of lymphatic contractility will clearly influence lymph drainage. Unfortunately, there is no clinical investigation to confirm lymphangiothrombosis or a failure of contractility.

Secondary lymphedema is swelling arising from a cause extrinsic to the lymph system. In developed countries, surgical removal of lymph nodes or radiation to the lymphatic basin as a necessary part of cancer treatment represents the commonest cause. Lymphedema is rarely the presenting feature of cancer unless the tumor is advanced. Recurrent cancer not uncommonly produces limb swelling because the smaller collateral lymphatics, which have been responsible for preventing lymphedema by acting as the lymph escape route, become blocked with tumor. Trauma to lymphatics either from elective surgery or by accident usually needs to be extensive to induce lymphedema. Filariasis is probably the most common cause of lymphedema worldwide. Progressive and permanent damage to the infested lymphatics causes lymphedema. Recurrent attacks of lymphangitis/cellulitis are associated with lymphedema, and can undermine lymph drainage further.

Venous disease

Raised venous pressure may arise because of venous obstruction (deep vein thrombosis or external compression

of a main vein), valvular failure (post thrombotic syndrome, simple varicose veins), impaired calf muscle pump function (paralysis, arthritis, inactivity) and certain vascular malformations (Klippel–Trenaunay syndrome) or arterio-venous anastomoses (Parkes–Weber syndrome). If increased microvascular fluid filtration exceeds lymphatic transport, edema will develop. In chronic venous disease, sustained filtration may slowly undermine lymphatic transport capacity and lymphedema (lymphatic failure) then ensues. To appreciate fully the contribution of venous and lymphatic failure both duplex venous Doppler and lymphoscintigraphy need to be performed.

Lipedema

Lipedema is a form of lipodystrophy distinct from morbid obesity although the two can co-exist. Lipedema appears to be exclusive to women and manifests with fat, swollen or chunky legs that are out of proportion to the top half of the body. Legs are equally swollen but the feet are spared. Tissue tenderness and easy bruising are accompanying features. There is often a family history suggesting a dominant inheritance through the female line. Fluid accumulation is often present but pitting is initially absent. With time more typical edema develops, so-called lipedema–lymphedema syndrome. Lymphoscintigraphy demonstrates patent lymph drainage pathways with opacification of ilio-inguinal nodes but transit of tracer is sluggish. With time, more typical lymphedema features develop.[31]

REFERENCES

1 Qureshy A, Kubota K, Ono S, *et al.* Thoracic duct scintigraphy by orally administered I-123 BMIPP: normal findings and a case report. *Clin Nucl Med* 2001; **26**: 847–55.

2 Levick JR, Mortimer PS. Fluid balance between microcirculation and intersitium in skin and other tissues; revision of classical filtration – reabsorption scheme. In: Messmer K. (ed.) *Progress in applied microcirculation*. Basle: Karger, 1999; **23**: 42–62.

3 Jepson RP, Simeone FA, Dobyns BM. Removal from skin of plasma protein labelled with radioactive iodine. *Am J Physiol* 1953; **175**: 443–8.

4 Taylor GW, Kinmonth JB, Rollinson E, Rotblat J. Lymphatic circulation studied with radioactive plasma protein. *BMJ* 1957; **i**: 133–7.

5 Hollander W, Reilly P, Burrows BA. Lymphatic flow in human subjects as indicated by the disappearance of ^{131}I labelled albumin from the subcutaneous tissue. *J Clin Invest* 1961; **40**: 222–3.

6 Svensson W, Glass DM, Bradley D, Peters AM. Measurement of lymphatic function with ^{99m}Tc-labelled polyclonal immunoglobulin. *Eur J Nucl Med* 1999; **26**: 504–10.

7 Phillips WT, Andrews T, Liu H-L, *et al.* Evaluation of [^{99m}Tc]liposomes as lymphoscintigraphic agents: comparison with [^{99m}Tc]sulfur colloid and [^{99m}Tc]human serum albumin. *Nucl Med Biol* 2001; **28**: 435–44.

8 Vera DR, Wallace AM, Hoh CK, Mattrey RF. A synthetic macromolecule for sentinel node detection: ^{99m}Tc-DTPA-mannosyl-dextran. *J Nucl Med* 2001; **42**: 951–9.

9 O'Mahony S, Rose SL, Chilvers AJ, *et al.* Finding an optimal method for imaging lymphatic vessels of the upper limb. *Eur J Nucl Med Mol Imaging* 2004; **31**: 555–63.

10 Mostbeck A, Kahn P, Partsch H. Quantitative lymphoscintigraphy in lymphoedema. In: Bollinger A, Partsch H, Wolfe JH. (eds.) *The initial lymphatics*. Stuttgart: George Thieme Verlag, 1985: 123–30.

11 Larcos G, Foster DR. Interpretation of lymphoscintigrams in suspected lymphoedema: contribution of delayed images. *Nucl Med Commun* 1995; **16**: 683–6.

12 McNeill GC, Witte M, Witte CL, *et al.* Whole body lymphangioscintigraphy: preferred method for initial assessment of the peripheral lymphatic system. *Radiology* 1989; **172**: 495–502.

13 Stewart G, Gaunt J, Croft DN, Browse NL. Isotope lymphography: a new method of investigating the role of lymphatics. *Br J Surg* 1985; **72**: 906–9.

14 Kleinhaus E, Baumeister R, Hahn D, *et al.* Evaluation of transport kinetics in lymphoscintigraphy. Follow-up study in patients with transplanted lymphatic vessels. *Eur J Nucl Med* 1985; **10**: 349–52.

15 Pain SJ, Barber RW, Ballinger JR, *et al.* Tissue to blood transport of radiolabelled immunoglobulin injected into the web space of the hands of normal subjects and patients with breast cancer related lymphoedema. *J Vasc Res* 2004; **41**: 183–92.

16 Pain SJ, Barber RW, Ballinger JR, *et al.* Side to side symmetry of radioprotein transfer from tissue space to systemic vasculature following subcutaneous injection

in normal subjects and patients with breast cancer. *Eur J Nucl Med Mol Imaging* 2003; **30**: 657–61.

17 Cambria RA, Gloviczki P, Naessens JM, *et al.* Non-invasive evaluation of the lymphatic system with lymphoscintigraphy: a prospective semiquantitative analysis in 386 extremities. *J Vasc Surg* 1993; **18**: 773–82.

18 Weissleder H, Weissleder R. Lymphoedema: evaluation of qualitative and quantitative lymphoscintigraphy in 238 patients. *Radiology* 1988; **167**: 729–35.

19 Moshiri M, Katz DS, Boris M, Young E. Using lymphoscintigraphy to evaluate suspected lymphoedema of the extremities. *Am J Roentgenol* 2002; **178**: 405–12.

20 Williams WJ, Witte CL, Witte MH, *et al.* Radionuclide lymphangioscintigraphy in the evaluation of peripheral lymphoedema. *Clin Nucl Med* 2000; **25**: 451–64.

21 Ter SE, Alvavi A, Kim CK, *et al.* Lymphoscintigraphy: a reliable test for diagnosis of lymphoedema. *Clin Nucl Med* 1993; **18**: 646–54.

22 Tiedjen KU, Knorz S, Heimann KD. The skin: lymphatic collateral organ? *Scope on Phlebology and Lymphology* 1994; **1**: 7–12.

23 Aboul-Enein A, Eshmawy I, Arafa MS, Abboud A. The role of lymphovenous communication in the development of postmastectomy lymphedema. *Surgery* 1983; **95**: 562–5.

24 Fokin AA, Robicsek F, Masters TN. Transport of viral-size particulate matter after intravenous versus intralymphatic injection. *Microcirculation* 2000; **7**: 357–65.

25 Fowler JC, Solanki CK, Barber RW, *et al.* Measurement of the extraction fractions of nanocolloid and polyclonal immunoglobulin by axillary lymph nodes in patients with breast cancer. *Nucl Med Commun* 2004; **25**: 935–40.

26 Bourgeois P. Effects of age and lateralization on lymphoscintigraphic interpretation. *Nucl Med Commun* 2002; **23**: 257–60.

27 Bull RH, Gane JN, Evans JE, *et al.* Abnormal lymph drainage in patients with chronic venous leg ulcers. *J Am Acad Dermatol* 1993; **28**: 285–290.

28 Burnand KG, McGuinness CL, Lagattolla NR, *et al.* Value of isotope lymphography in the diagnosis of lymphoedema of the leg. *Br J Surg* 2002; **89**: 74–8.

29 Mortimer PS. The swollen limb and lymphatic problems. In: Tibbs DJ, Sabiston DC, Davies MG, *et al.* (eds.) *Varicose veins, venous disorders and lymphatic problems in the lower limbs*. Oxford: Oxford University Press, 1997; 211–33.

30 Raju S, Owen Jr S, Neglen P. Reversal of abnormal lymphoscintigraphy after placement of venous stents for correction of associated venous obstruction. *J Vasc Surg* 2001; **34**: 779–84.

31 Harwood CA, Bull RH, Evans J, Mortimer PS. Lymphatic and venous function in lipoedema. *Br J Dermatol* 1996; **134**: 1–6.

17

Radionuclide therapy

17A Thyroid disease

Introduction   727
Radioiodine therapy for thyrotoxicosis   729
Radioiodine therapy for non-toxic multinodular goiter   733

Radioiodine therapy in malignant thyroid disease   733
Conclusion   739
References   740

17B Endocrine: Peptides

Introduction   745
[^{111}In-DTPA]octreotide   745
[^{90}Y-DOTA,Tyr^3]octreotide and [^{177}Lu-DOTA,Tyr^3]octreotate   747
[^{90}Y-DOTA]lanreotide   750
Patient characteristics   751

[^{90}Y-DTPA-D-GLU]minigastrin   751
Options for improving peptide receptor radionuclide therapy   751
Conclusion   751
References   751

17C Neuroblastoma

The disease   755
Specific targeting of neuroblastoma   755
Indications and contraindications   756
Therapeutic procedure   756
Considerations in radionuclide therapy of children   756

Clinical applications of MIBG therapy in neuroblastoma   757
Possible interventions in ^{131}I-MIBG therapy   759
Conclusion   760
References   762

17D The skeleton

Introduction   765
Available radiopharmaceuticals   765
Patient selection   767
Administration   768
Response assessment   768
Efficacy   768

Toxicity   769
Treatment failure   770
The future   770
Summary   770
References   770

17E The use of ^{32}P

Introduction   773
Relation between polycythemia vera and leukemia   774
Is chemotherapy an alternative to ^{32}P?   774
The role of ^{32}P in the management of polycythemia vera   775

Conclusion   775
References   776
Appendix 1: Dosimetry and practical use of ^{32}P   778
Appendix 2: Mechanism of the risks due to ^{32}P   778

17F The role of dosimetry

Introduction   781
Overview of standard dosimetry   781
Tumor dosimetry   783
Marrow and whole-body dosimetry   784
Cellular and multi-cellular dosimetry   785
Clinical applications of dosimetry   785
Conclusion   785
References   786

Thyroid disease

S.E.M. CLARKE

INTRODUCTION

The role of radioiodine in the management of thyroid disease is well established but exciting new developments are now resulting in improvements in the management of thyroid cancer. Diseases of the thyroid constitute the most common form of endocrine disorders and, over the past 50 years, nuclear medicine has contributed significantly to the management of thyroid patients, both in terms of diagnosis and treatment.[1] Radionuclide therapy for both benign disease (thyrotoxicosis and goiter) and thyroid cancer has served as a model for the development of other radionuclide therapies in recent years.

The first reports of radionuclide therapy for thyrotoxicosis used ^{131}I and this radioisotope rapidly became the favored radionuclide with beta particle and gamma ray emissions and a half-life suitable for therapy.[2] Although thyrotoxicosis was the initial indication for ^{131}I therapy, reports on the treatment of differentiated thyroid cancer soon followed.

Surprisingly, given the length of time for which ^{131}I has been used, significant controversy persists as to which patients are suitable for treatment and what doses of radioiodine should be used. It is only in recent years that prospective studies have been undertaken to clarify some of the unanswered questions in radioiodine treatment. The development of guidelines, both for the treatment of benign and malignant disease, is leading to the standardization of protocols.[3,4]

In this chapter, the theory of radioiodine therapy will be explained, the clinical role explored and the practical aspects of treatment considered. The new developments in clinical practice will also be outlined.

Table 17A.1 *Physical characteristics of ^{131}I and ^{123}I*

Characteristic	Iodine-131	Iodine-123
Half-life	*8.04 days*	*13.3 h*
Principal gamma energies (keV)	*80, 284, 364, 637*	*159*
Beta E$_{max}$	*0.61 MeV*	*N/A*

Iodine-131

The physical properties of ^{131}I are listed in Table 17A.1. Iodine-131 has a physical half-life of 8.04 days, which is well-suited to the biological half-life of iodine in patients with differentiated thyroid cancer. The medium-energy beta-particle emission ($E_{max} = 0.61$ mev) with a path length of about 0.5 mm in tissue, ensures an intracellular radiation dose following the cellular internalization of ^{131}I. The gamma emissions of ^{131}I have both benefits and disadvantages. Gamma-ray emissions facilitate gamma-camera imaging, which enables tracer doses of ^{131}I to be used diagnostically and for dosimetry calculations, and also permits post-therapy imaging to confirm uptake of the therapy dose in all known tumor sites.

The high-energy gamma emissions, however, contribute to the unwanted whole-body radiation burden associated with radionuclide therapy and also to the radiation protection problems for the staff and the patients' relatives.

Synthesis of thyroid hormones

Thyroxine and triiodothyronine are synthesized in the thyroid follicular cells by the iodination of tyrosine (Fig. 17A.1).

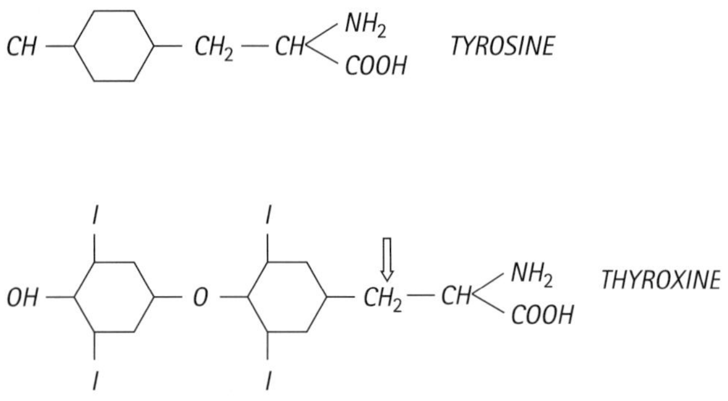

Figure 17A.1 *Synthesis of thyroxine by iodination of tyrosine molecule.*

Iodine is taken up in the follicular cells by an active ATP-dependent transport mechanism through the stimulation of thyroid-stimulating hormone (TSH). In recent years, the thyroid sodium iodide symporter (NIS) has been cloned[5] and *in vitro* and *in vivo* studies have given new insights into iodide transport mechanisms and their defects.[6,7] The iodine pump increases in the presence of iodine deficiency. Peroxidase and hydrogen peroxidase enzymes oxidize the iodine, which is then linked to the tyrosine molecules in the tyrosine-rich thyroglobulin. The iodothyronines are produced, which couple to form triiodothyronine (T3) or tetra-iodothyronine (T4). The process of iodination is inhibited by the presence of excess iodine. The thyroglobulin is then hydrolyzed, liberating T3 and T4, which are secreted into the circulation where they are bound to thyroid-binding globulin, thyroid-binding pre-albumin and albumin. This process of iodination is blocked by perchlorate and by the presence of excess iodine.

The control of thyroid hormone production

The production of TSH occurs in the anterior part of the pituitary. This production is in turn regulated by suppressants and stimulators. Thyroxine, T3, somatostatin and dobutamine all act as suppressors of TSH, and T4 is also believed to have a direct TSH-suppressing action.

The production of TSH is stimulated by thyrotropin-releasing hormone, which is found in various parts of the body including the hypothalamus. The release of TRH is inhibited by T4 and T3. TSH stimulates thyroid hormone production by stimulating cyclic AMP and by activating the incorporation of thyroglobulin in the thyroid follicular cells by a process of endocytosis.

This negative feedback system is utilized in treating patients with Ca thyroid. Discontinuing exogenous thyroxine administration results in the production of high levels of TSH by the pituitary which increases the uptake of radioactive iodine into remnant thyroid tissue or differentiated thyroid cancer cells. A highly purified recombinant source of human thyroid stimulating hormone (rhTSH) has been developed for use in well-differentiated thyroid cancer to stimulate the uptake of radioactive iodine without the necessity of discontinuing thyroxine.[8]

Pathology of the thyroid gland

Like all endocrine organs, the thyroid gland may over- or underproduce hormones or be subject to malignant change. Iodine-131 may be used to treat the various forms of thyroid hormone overproduction, and also for the treatment of differentiated thyroid cancer.

Thyrotoxicosis

The clinical symptoms of thyrotoxicosis are classically those of weight loss, heat intolerance, tremor and palpitations, increased bowel frequency and increased anxiety. The signs include tachycardia and tremor of the outstretched hands. There may be a bruit audible over the thyroid gland, and a systolic flow murmur may be audible over the precordium. In some patients – particularly those with severe disease or a prolonged period before diagnosis – evidence of proximal muscle wasting may be present.

There are two main pathological processes resulting in thyrotoxicosis. The first is a diffuse process affecting the whole gland; the second is a focal process affecting one or several areas of the gland. It is important to differentiate between these two main causes of thyrotoxicosis as the management of these pathologies differs.

TOXIC DIFFUSE GOITER (GRAVES' DISEASE)

Toxic diffuse goiter (Graves' disease) is an autoimmune process caused by the production of a stimulating antibody to the TSH receptor (Fig. 17A.2). The disease may be familial, although the pattern of inheritance is unclear. Various factors have been implicated in the development of Graves' disease and these include pregnancy and stress.[9] The autoimmune process not only affects the thyroid gland but may also affect the eyes in 50% of cases and, more rarely, can be associated with the development of pretibial myxedema and thyroid acropachy. The causative antibody, variously known as thyroid-stimulating immunoglobulin or TSH-receptor antibody, may be assayed and can be demonstrated in 90% of patients with the clinical syndrome of Graves' disease. Although the level of antibody tends to correlate with the severity of clinical symptoms, this is not invariable. The link between TSH-receptor antibody and dysthyroid eye disease remains unclear. It would appear from various studies that the TSH-receptor antibody itself is not the causative factor in dysthyroid eye disease, and recent papers have implicated a 64 kDa protein present in the serum of patients with dysthyroid eye disease which reacts with pig eye muscle.[10]

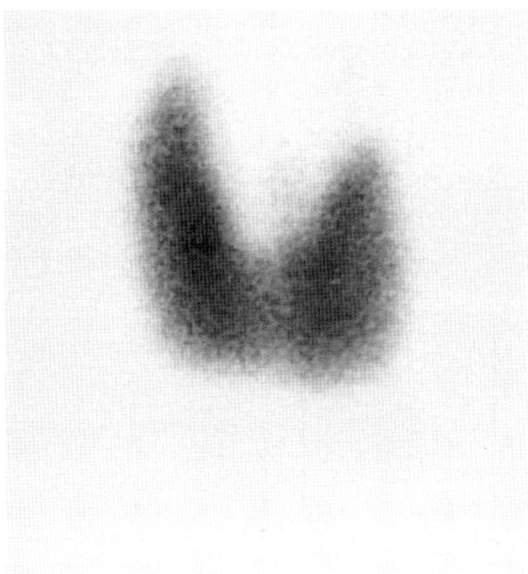

Figure 17A.2 *^{99m}Tc thyroid scan of a patient with toxic diffuse goiter (Graves' disease) showing diffusely increased uptake and visualizing the pyramidal lobe.*

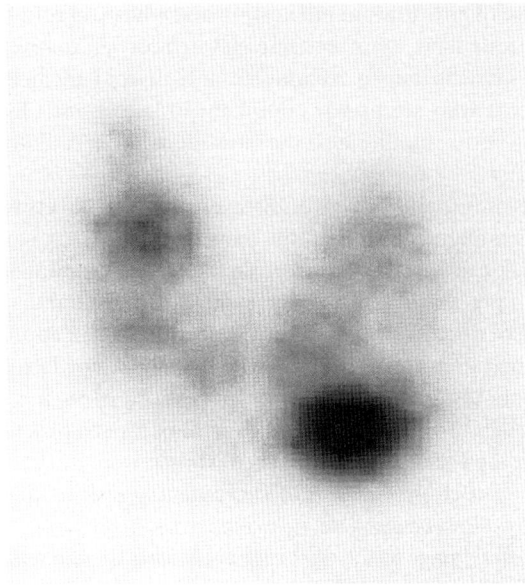

Figure 17A.3 *^{99m}Tc thyroid scan of a patient with a multinodular goiter showing non-homogeneous uptake and developing autonomous nodules at the left lower pole.*

The management of toxic diffuse goiter (Graves' disease) in Europe is generally that of a prolonged course of anti-thyroid medication (carbimazole, methimazole or propylthiouracil). Data show that the continuance of treatment for 12–18 months results in an approximately 50% cure rate on discontinuing anti-thyroid medication.[11] Second-line treatment following failure of anti-thyroid medication, or in patients who are not responding to anti-thyroid treatment, is either ^{131}I or alternatively, surgery.

In the USA, there is a current trend to early ^{131}I treatment with little or no pre-treatment with anti-thyroid medication.[12] The value of pretreatment with anti-thyroid medication, however, is the potential cure rate in half the patients treated, and the rapid control of symptoms that cannot be achieved with ^{131}I, particularly in those patients who are markedly symptomatic.[13] Santos *et al.* have demonstrated in a small series that propylthiouracil reduces the efficacy of radioiodine treatment, however, when compared with no pre-treatment or treatment with methimazole.[14]

TOXIC NODULAR GOITER (PLUMMER'S DISEASE)

In patients with multinodular goiters, there is an increased likelihood of the development of multiple focal areas of thyroid autonomy resulting in elevations of free T4 and free T3 levels. This form of Plummer's disease is particularly common in geographical areas where endemic goiter is prevalent. Germany, Austria and Switzerland are countries with a previous history of dietary iodine deficiency, and there is a higher prevalence of multinodular goiter in these countries compared with the UK (Fig. 17A.3).[15]

Patients may also develop a single nodule, which on isotope imaging is demonstrated to show increased uptake with suppression of the remainder of the gland. Uninodular toxic goiter is diagnosed using conventional biochemical tests and radionuclide imaging with ^{99m}Tc or ^{123}I.

The presenting symptoms of uninodular or multinodular toxic goiter are similar to those of Graves' disease, but with the absence of eye signs, thyroid acropachy or pretibial myxedema. This tends to be a disease of old people and, in the elderly, the clinical presentation may be non-classical with minimal signs and symptoms apart from tachycardia that may progress to atrial fibrillation.

Diagnosis of thyrotoxicosis

The diagnosis of thyrotoxicosis is made on the basis of history, clinical examination and investigations. The investigations include free T4, free T3 and ultra-sensitive TSH investigations. A ^{99m}Tc or an ^{123}I thyroid scan will differentiate toxic diffuse goiter from toxic nodular goiter. Thyroid-stimulating immunoglobulin measurement, if raised, will strongly support a diagnosis of toxic diffuse goiter (Graves' disease), as does the presence of dysthyroid eye disease.

RADIOIODINE THERAPY FOR THYROTOXICOSIS

Selection of patients

TOXIC DIFFUSE GOITER (GRAVES' DISEASE)

As has already been stated, ^{131}I therapy usage is considered in patients who have completed a conventional 12- to 24-month course of anti-thyroid medication and whose thyroid function tests have again become elevated, or alternatively in patients who fail to respond to anti-thyroid medication. Patients who are poorly compliant in taking anti-thyroid medication should also be considered for radioiodine therapy.

As diffuse goiter (Graves' disease) frequently affects young and middle-aged women the issue of using ^{131}I in women of childbearing years has been an issue of discussion. A survey of practice in Europe, Japan and the USA found that one third of doctors in the USA believed ^{131}I to be an appropriate treatment for women of age 19. Only 4% of European doctors thought that ^{131}I was appropriate in such a case, although this does not reflect general European practice.[16]

In the previous decades, such women were not selected for ^{131}I therapy because of the potential risk to the offspring. However, to date, no evidence has been presented to suggest damage to the offspring of patients treated with ^{131}I despite large patient population studies.[17,18]

The use of ^{131}I in young patients remains controversial. In the USA, treatment of patients under the age of 18 with ^{131}I is now taking place routinely. In Europe, however, the concerns about radioiodine treatment in young patients with radiosensitive tissues has led to a general limitation of ^{131}I use to adults. However, it is important to recognize and consider the risks of thyroid surgery in children. It has been estimated that 16–35% of children treated with sub-total thyroidectomy experience acute complications with permanent complications occurring in up to 8% of children.[19,20]

The marked variation in the use of ^{131}I throughout the world, both in terms of the patients who are selected for treatment and the protocols for treatment, is now recognized and surveys of practice undertaken in Europe, Japan, India and the USA confirm this variation.[9,21–23]

The use of surgery as a second-line treatment is less commonly used, although in certain parts of the world it remains the second-line treatment of choice for women of childbearing years. Kuma et al.[24] have shown clearly that there is an increased morbidity associated with surgery compared with ^{131}I therapy. There is also the risk of subsequent recurrence in the residual thyroid. Hypothyroidism is also a post-operative complication of surgery.[20]

TOXIC NODULAR GOITER (PLUMMER'S DISEASE)

Patients with toxic nodular goiter are generally considered to be ideally suited for ^{131}I therapy. A short period of treatment using anti-thyroid medication is recommended in patients who are extremely symptomatic, and in the elderly. It is essential to ensure that the normal thyroid tissue is suppressed at the time of ^{131}I therapy, and this will require an adequate period of discontinuation of anti-thyroid medication before radioiodine treatment (Fig. 17A.4). In patients with mild-to-moderate elevations of thyroid hormone levels and who are relatively asymptomatic, direct treatment with radioiodine may be considered.

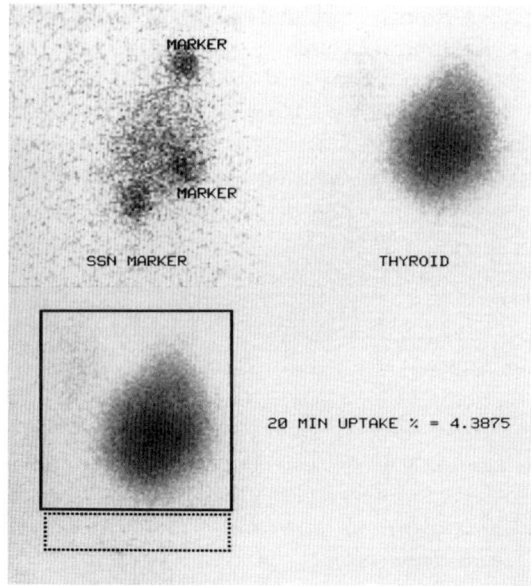

Figure 17A.4 *[99m]Tc thyroid scan showing an autonomously functioning thyroid nodule with complete suppression of the rest of the gland. The radiation dose to the suppressed areas of the gland will be extremely low compared with the dose to the toxic nodule. This explains why hypothyroidism is less common in radioiodine-treated Plummer's disease compared with Graves' disease.*

Practical aspects of therapy

Patients who have been selected for ^{131}I radioiodine treatment should have the implications of therapy explained clearly. It is generally considered good practice to render the patient euthyroid before treatment, as ^{131}I administration will cause a transient elevation in free T4 and free T3 levels approximately 7 days following administration. In the symptomatically well-controlled patient this will have little effect, but in symptomatically toxic patients, this further elevation of thyroid hormone may trigger palpitations, atrial fibrillation and heart failure. This is a particular problem in the elderly. Symptomatic control may be achieved using beta blockade. Since carbimazole blocks the organification of iodine within the thyroid, carbimazole therapy should be discontinued at least 48 h before therapy is undertaken to ensure adequate residence time of ^{131}I within the follicular cells.

There has been controversy as to whether pre-treatment with carbimazole, methimazole or propylthiouracil reduces the subsequent efficacy of radioiodine. Santos et al. have found that pre-treatment with propylthiouracil reduces the effectiveness of radioiodine treatment in patients with Graves' disease. The same effect was not observed with methimazole pre-treatment.[14]

The requirement to admit patients varies considerably across the world. In many countries in Europe, admission is required for doses of 185 MBq and above although in the UK admission is only required for activities above 800 MBq. In the USA, doses up to 1000 MBq may be given as an outpatient. Admission should be considered for the elderly with a risk of heart failure.

Before therapy, patients should be asked to sign a consent form and should be informed of restrictions on working, contact with children and pregnancy before doing so.[4,25,26] The length of time for which restrictions should be observed varies by country, but time should be taken with the patient before treatment to ensure that appropriate restrictions are understood and will be adhered to.

Pregnancy and breast-feeding are absolute contraindications to radioiodine therapy, and it is recommended that a pregnancy test should be undertaken in women of childbearing years who are about to receive radioiodine therapy and in whom pregnancy may be an issue.

The restrictions on work and contact with small children will also depend on national dose limits, and these should be discussed with each patient individually.[4,21] Studies are now being undertaken following radioiodine therapy, and these data confirm that with adequate precautions, the dose to family members is minimal.[27]

In patients in whom thyrotoxicosis is not well controlled before radioiodine therapy, it may be necessary to recommence anti-thyroid medication for a short interval following treatment. All patients should be given written instructions about the precautions to be observed. In addition, the need to avoid pregnancy for 4 months following radioiodine treatment should be emphasized to female patients.

Iodine-131 may be administered in liquid form or as a capsule. The advantages of the capsule are those of radiation protection for staff administering the radioiodine; the disadvantages are those of expense and loss of flexibility in dose. Unusually, ^{131}I may be given intravenously in patients in whom vomiting is a problem. Iodine-131 should be administered in a designated area by trained staff in accordance with the national regulations.

Patients should be encouraged to drink large volumes of fluid for a 24-h period following radioiodine therapy to lower the radiation dose to the bladder. Recommended precautions are included in Table 17A.2.

Dose considerations

The determination of the dose of radioiodine to be administered in patients with thyrotoxicosis remains a topic of controversy. The controversy centers around whether it is possible to avoid hypothyroidism and successfully treat hyperthyroidism by using careful dosimetry calculations. Although much has been written on this subject, there appears to be no consensus as to the optimal protocol for deciding the dose. Current practice therefore ranges from the use of careful dose calculation to a fixed-dose protocol.

DOSIMETRY CALCULATION

Various formulae have been generated which may be used to estimate the administered dose required to deliver an

Table 17A.2 *Precautions following radioiodine therapy*

1. *FOR 24 HOURS AFTER RECEIVING [131]I*

   Drink plenty of fluids and empty bladder regularly

2. *FOR 2–3 WEEKS AFTER RECEIVING [131]I (depending on administered activity)*

   - *Carry this card with you at all times*
   - *Avoid close contact with babies and small children*
   - *Do not breastfeed your child*
   - *Do not spend time with anyone who is pregnant*
   - *Do not share a bed*
   - *Do not go to the cinema or theater or to a restaurant*
   - *Do not travel by public transport if your journey lasts longer than an hour*
   - *Do not return to work unless permission is given by the doctor or physicist*
   - *Keep your own cutlery and crockery separate from the rest of the family*

3. *FOR 4 MONTHS AFTER RECEIVING [131]I*

   Do not become pregnant

effective radiation dose to the gland to render the patient euthyroid and avoid unnecessary radiation being administered.[28] Most formulae require information on ^{131}I uptake and clearance of radioiodine by the gland, and the weight or volume of the gland. The percentage uptake and clearance of radioiodine may be estimated using tracer doses of radioiodine.[29] It is unclear, however, whether tracer doses may have the mild stunning effect on the thyroid follicular cells, thereby altering the uptake and clearance of subsequent therapy doses. In addition, variations in iodine intake in the diet may theoretically affect the reproducibility of radioiodine uptake and clearance.

The volume of the gland may be estimated using ultrasound measurements,[30] but in patients with Plummer's disease or in patients with Graves' disease in a multinodular goiter, the measured volume of the gland does not necessarily correspond to the functioning volume. It is therefore likely that ultrasound estimates of volumes are most accurate in patients with Graves' disease and least accurate in patients with Plummer's disease. Positron emission tomograpy (PET) studies using [124]I have been used by Flower *et al.*[31] to determine more accurately the functioning volume of the thyroid gland.

Results of studies published using these volume estimates to calculate administered dose, however, show that there continues to be an incidence of hypothyroidism and persisting hyperthyroidism in patients treated using these calculations. Other factors such as the duration of pre-treatment with anti-thyroid medication and the issue of varying radiosensitivity may well explain why careful dosimetric measurements fail to predict reliably the dose that will render the patient euthyroid without subsequent hypothyroidism.

Low calculated dose protocols aim to deliver 80 Gy to the thyroid, whereas high calculated dose protocols aim to deliver 300 Gy. Willemsen *et al.*[32] have shown that the administered dose required to deliver a dose of 300 Gy ranged from 240 to 3120 MBq. As might be predicted, Reinhardt *et al.* demonstrated that the frequency of hypothyroidism increased from 27% after 150 Gy to 68% after 300 Gy but that persistent hyperthyroidism decreased from 27% after 150 Gy to 8% after 300 Gy.[33]

FIXED–DOSE PROTOCOL

Fixed-dose protocols range from those that take account of the size of the gland, usually determined clinically by giving smaller doses to small glands on palpation and larger doses to clinically larger glands, and those protocols that attempt electively to ablate the thyroid gland.

As might be predicted, low-dose protocols result in a lower instance of hypothyroidism in the first year, but the long-term outcome shows a significant incidence of hypothyroidism at 15 years (35–40%) compared with 50–70% incidence using high-dose regimes.[34–36]

The administered dose used in an attempt to ablate the thyroid gland varies worldwide, and is usually limited by the maximum permissible dose to be administered as an outpatient. In the USA, 1000 MBq may therefore be administered, whereas in the UK, 500 MBq is the standard upper limit for outpatient administration. Results in the UK published by Kendall-Taylor *et al.*[37] using a fixed dose of 500 MBq show that ablation was achieved in only 64% of patients with a small percentage of patients still remaining hyperthyroid following treatment.

The disadvantage of electively rendering a patient hypothyroid is that, in effect, one pathology is exchanged for another. There is a need to ensure that patients who have been rendered hypothyroid remain on adequate replacement doses of thyroxine for life. The study by Kendall-Taylor *et al.*[37] demonstrated that 2% of patients who had been rendered hypothyroid and started on thyroxine were not taking treatment and a further 3% of patients had been recognized by their physicians to be non-compliant.

Hardisty *et al.*[35] explored the efficacy and cost-effectiveness of varying dose protocols, and concluded that both hypothyroidism and persisting hyperthyroidism were unavoidable whichever dose protocols were used. In addition, they noted that when both cost to the patients and the health service were considered, the use of high fixed-dose attempting to ablate the thyroid gland appeared more cost-effective.[29]

Side–effects and complications

The major complication of radioiodine therapy is hypothyroidism. This may occur in the early post-treatment period, particularly if higher administered doses are given. Alternatively, it may develop gradually in the years following treatment.[29] The later-onset hypothyroidism occurs at a rate of approximately 4% per year, and therefore it has been estimated that follow-up must continue until patient becomes hypothyroid. After 25 years 100% of patients treated with radioiodine will be hypothyroid. It has been postulated that this long-term hypothyroidism relates in part to the natural outcome of Graves' disease.[38] The incidence of post-radioiodine hypothyroidism, however, is markedly lower in patients treated for a solitary toxic nodule compared with those with Graves' disease.[28,39] This is undoubtedly due to the protection of the suppressed area of the gland at the time of treatment and emphasizes the need to ensure that patients have adequate time off antithyroid treatment before radioiodine therapy to ensure good suppression of the normal areas of the gland.

Careful follow-up of patients following radioiodine therapy is therefore mandatory, and should be coordinated by a trained thyroid practitioner. In the early post-therapy period, it is recommended that this follow-up is undertaken within a hospital environment. Subsequently, follow-up may be undertaken in conjunction with a community physician.[10] The management of these patients is greatly facilitated by computer-assisted follow-up programming.

Patients whose hypothyroidism develops rapidly following radioiodine treatment are frequently extremely symptomatic, whereas patients with delayed onset hypothyroidism may not present with classical hypothyroid symptoms. Weight gain and tiredness are key clinical symptoms in diagnosing post-therapy hypothyroidism.

Other side-effects and complications of radioiodine therapy are remarkably few. Patients with large goiters may notice transient swelling of the goiter approximately 1 week following therapy and some discomfort may be associated with this swelling. As has been previously stated, there may be a transient rise in f T4 and f T3 levels 7–10 days following radioiodine treatment, and in patients who have been poorly controlled before radioiodine therapy there may be an exacerbation of palpitations and heart failure. Slight discomfort of the salivary glands may be noted, but this is unusual with the doses used for thyrotoxicosis therapy. Iodine allergy is not a contraindication to radioiodine therapy.

In patients with large goiters in whom tracheal compression is present before therapy, a worsening of pressure symptoms in the immediate post-therapy period may be noticed. This complication is in fact rare. Patients with severe tracheal narrowing should be admitted for therapy with surgical cover. Surgery should be considered as an alternative to radioiodine therapy in this particular group.

DYSTHYROID EYE DISEASE

There has been much discussion as to the effect of radioiodine therapy on dysthyroid eye disease. Reports in the literature yield conflicting information.[40,41]

Catz and Tsao[40] have demonstrated that an improvement in ophthalmopathy can be obtained following ^{131}I ablation of the thyroid, which they believe to be due to the destruction of the antigenic stimulus to antibody formation. Peqqequat *et al.*[42] using non-ablative doses, showed a varying response following therapy with some of the patients improving and a few patients deteriorating. Jones *et al.*[43] observed that while lid retraction improved following ^{131}I treatment in patients with Graves' ophthalmopathy, exophthalmos remained unchanged or deteriorated, and in 50% of the patients periorbital edema was observed following treatment. Bartalena *et al.* in a large prospective study demonstrated that dysthyroid eye disease was exacerbated in 15% of patients after radioiodine and the exacerbation persisted in 8%.[44] It is therefore recommended that patients with severe dysthyroid eye disease should not be treated during an acute exacerbation. A course of high-dose steroids may be considered as a prelude to radioiodine therapy in this small percentage of patients. The prospective study by Bartalena *et al.* also showed that a course of prednisolone given with the radioiodine prevented the exacerbation. Tallstedt *et al.*[45] have studied the effects of thyroxine administered in the early post-radioiodine period, and they conclude that the early administration of thyroxine after radioiodine reduces the occurrence of Graves' ophthalmopathy.

RADIOIODINE THERAPY FOR NON–TOXIC MULTINODULAR GOITER

In recent years, the use of radioiodine in the treatment of non-toxic multinodular goiter has been explored.[46,47] Radioiodine is particularly useful in elderly patients and those with medical contraindications to surgery. Goiter shrinkage is well documented, but multiple doses of radioiodine are frequently required. Varying dose regimes have been described on the basis of dosimetry calculation. High administered doses are required in view of the relatively low overall uptake compared with a toxic goiter. Recently, however, recombinant TSH has been used to increase the uptake of radioiodine in nontoxic goiters by increasing the homogeneity of uptake. The therapeutic dose of radioiodine may be reduced by 50–60% without loss of thyroid volume reduction.[48] Although, historically, patients with evidence of tracheal compression were not deemed suitable for radioiodine therapy, it is now apparent that the theoretical risk of increasing tracheal compression in the immediate post-treatment period does not in fact occur.[40] Nevertheless, in patients with significant stridor, admission is recommended.

Following radioiodine therapy, thyroid function tests should be performed at regular intervals. While hypothyroidism appears an uncommon complication, the development of hyperthyroidism with a picture suggestive of Graves' disease has been reported (Fig. 17A.5).[49] The mechanism for this is unclear, but it is presumed that the release of thyroid antigen may be the trigger for the development of autoimmune thyrotoxicosis. As these patients are frequently elderly and may have cardiovascular disease, careful follow-up is essential as hyperthyroidism may well exacerbate cardiac symptoms in this population.

RADIOIODINE THERAPY IN MALIGNANT THYROID DISEASE

Radioiodine therapy is used both as an adjunct to thyroid surgery in order to completely destroy the normal thyroid tissue and also to treat metastatic disease in patients with recurrent tumor.

Pathology of thyroid cancer

Malignancies of the thyroid may involve the thyroid follicular cells (papillary and follicular thyroid cancers), the parafollicular cells (medullary thyroid cancer) or be lymphoid in origin (primary lymphomas of the thyroid). Rarely, tumors such as breast or renal cancer may metastasize to the thyroid.

Papillary thyroid cancer is the most common form of differentiated cancer, accounting for approximately 65% of all thyroid carcinomas. They occur more commonly in women. Fine-needle aspiration of a papillary thyroid cancer is usually diagnostic as the tumor cells demonstrate typical features of intranuclear grooving and 'orphan Annie' nuclei. Papillary cancers may be found as unexpected asymptomatic lesions in patients undergoing thyroid surgery for benign disease. They are not infrequently multifocal, and spread into cervical lymph nodes is often discovered at the time of presentation. Distant metastases to lung and bone occur less frequently than with follicular tumors. Papillary cancers tend to develop in the third and fourth decades of life. While some pure papillary tumors do not retain the ability to take up iodine, those with follicular elements generally do so and ^{131}I may be used to treat local and distant metastatic spread.

Follicular thyroid cancers are diagnosed when capsular breakthrough of a follicular tumor is demonstrated. They cannot therefore be diagnosed by fine-needle aspiration and lobectomy or total thyroidectomy is required in order to make the diagnosis.

Compared with papillary cancers, follicular thyroid cancers tend to occur in an older population, peaking in the fourth and fifth decades of life. Unlike papillary cancers, they metastasize more commonly to bone and lungs. Liver metastases are rare in both follicular and papillary cancers.

While the majority of follicular cancers take up ^{131}I at the time of presentation, de-differentiation may occur, and as these de-differentiated tumors are more aggressive they frequently lose their ability to take up [131]I. The Hürthle cell variant of follicular cancer is uncommon but is distinguished by the fact that only 10% of these tumors take up [131]I. As medullary thyroid cancers and lymphomas do not

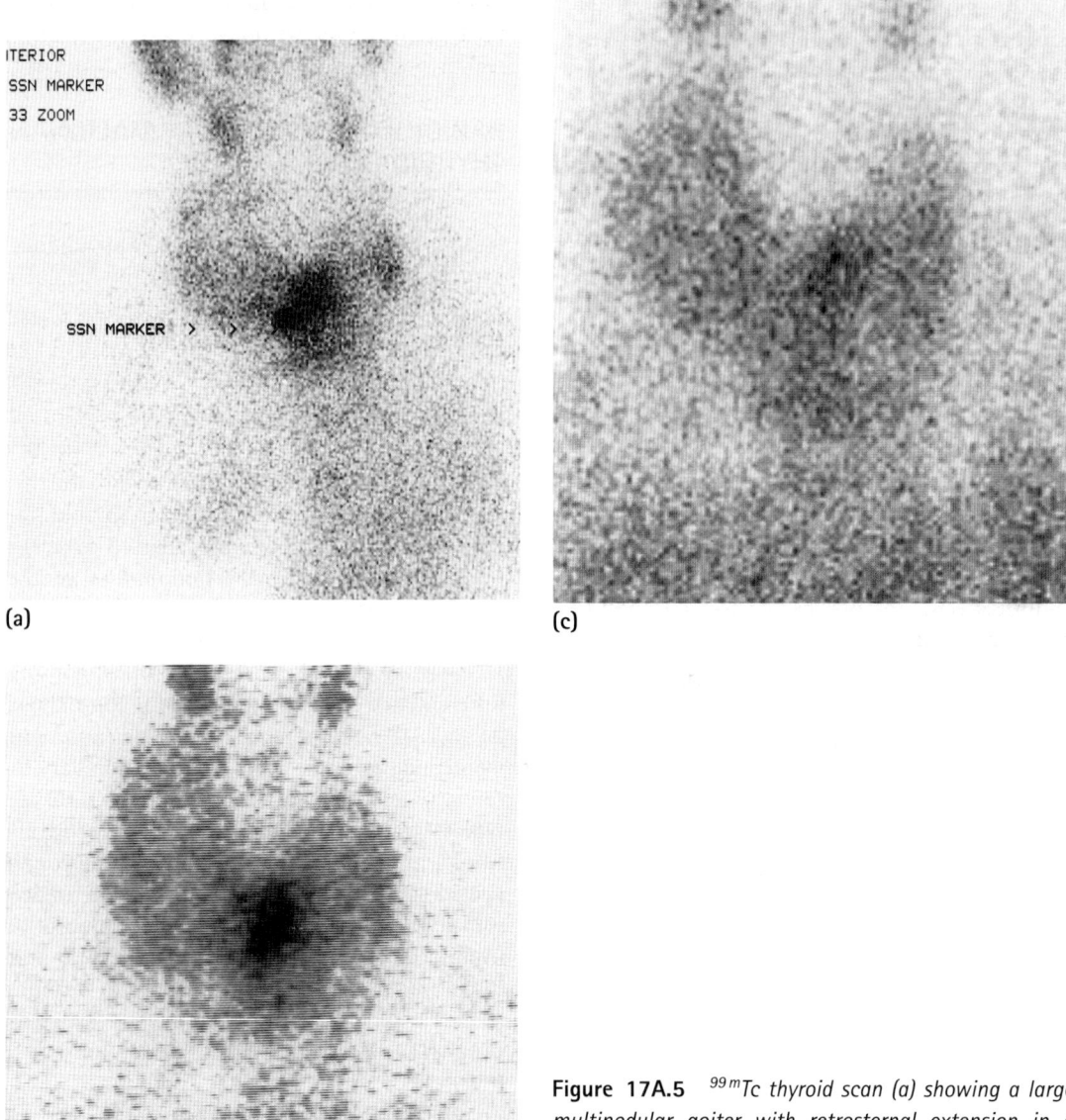

Figure 17A.5 ^{99m}Tc *thyroid scan (a) showing a large multinodular goiter with retrosternal extension in a patient with pressure symptoms and stridor who was unsuitable for surgery. Following treatment with 400 MBq* ^{131}I *the pressure symptoms improved (b), and after a further 400 MBq (c) the goiter was notably smaller.*

take up ^{131}I, its only role is in thyroid remnant ablation (see below). A number of classification systems exist offering prognostic information such as the AMES classification and the MACIS scoring system.[50,51]

Thyroid ablation

The optimal management for patients having thyroid cancer diagnosed either by fine-needle aspiration or at the time of surgery is total thyroidectomy. This may be achieved by a one-stage or a two-stage procedure. Despite careful surgery, however, it is extremely common to demonstrate small residues of normal thyroid tissue on post-operative imaging (Fig. 17A.6).

The data demonstrating an outcome advantage to complete ablation of normal thyroid tissue are unclear. While some series have demonstrated a reduction in relapse rate in patients treated with ^{131}I post-surgery,[52–54] others have failed to show any outcome benefit of radioiodine ablation.[55,56] Sawka *et al.* have conducted a review and meta-analysis of the literature on remnant ablation. They found the data conflicting between studies in low-risk patients which they attributed to the variations in administered activity and the length of follow-up.[57] Tubiana[58] and Mazaferri and Kloos[54] have clearly demonstrated a benefit

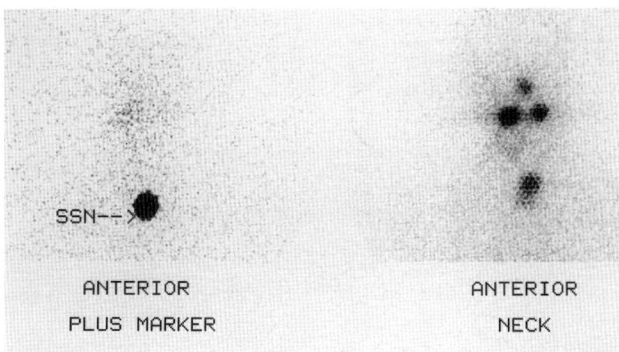

Figure 17A.6 *[131]I scan of the head and neck in a patient following total thyroidectomy for papillary cancer showing residual thyroid tissue in the neck.*

in outcome in patients with poorer prognostic features such as tumors over 1.5 cm.

However, ablation of normal thyroid tissue undoubtedly aids follow-up in the following ways:

- Achieving a negative iodine tracer scan following complete ablation facilitates the interpretation of the subsequent radioiodine tracer scans and the appearance of iodine uptake in the neck subsequent to successful ablation can be reliably interpreted as recurrent tumor.
- As serum thyroglobulin levels play a key role in the follow-up of patients with differentiated thyroid cancer the achievement of undetectable thyroglobulin levels by total thyroid remnant ablation makes subsequent elevations of thyroglobulin levels interpretable as recurrent disease.[59]
- As normal thyroid tissue will trap iodine more efficiently than will tumor cells, ^{131}I therapy will be less immediately effective if recurrences occur as most of the treatment dose will be taken up by the remnant rather than the tumor recurrence.
- Lung metastases may not be visible on a tracer iodine scan if there is persisting normal thyroid tissue.[60]

Ablation doses

One of the main problems of radioiodine thyroid ablation is the stunning effect of the tracer dose before administration of therapy activity. There is now literature evidence confirming that even relatively low tracer doses of radioiodine will significantly reduce the uptake of a subsequent therapy dose.[61,62] It is therefore recommended that doses of 185 MBq or less are used for the tracer scan to minimize the stunning effect of the tracer dose. In an excellent review, Kalinyak and McDougall have reviewed the evidence for and against stunning. They conclude that some of the conflicting data in the literature may be due to a qualitative rather than a quantitative assessment of radioiodine images

in some studies. Stunning appears to be less of a problem if the therapy is given within a week of the tracer scan.[63] New techniques are currently being researched. Park *et al.*[64] are currently exploring the use of high doses of ^{123}I with imaging up to 24 h post-administration to determine the presence of remnant thyroid and to perform uptake measurements for dosimetry calculations. Further data are required to determine whether the substitution of ^{123}I will improve the efficacy of the subsequent therapy dose and reduce the number of ablation doses required, thereby reducing the requirement for admission with both cost savings and improvement in convenience to the patient. Blake *et al.* have demonstrated that a ^{99m}Tc scan instead of a tracer radioiodine scan will allow the assessment of remnant size prior to radioiodine ablation and improve first time ablation rates.[65]

There is now an increasing practice of undertaking ablation therapy without any pre-treatment imaging to avoid the stunning issues. The dose routinely used for ablation varies greatly worldwide. In the USA, 1000 MBq (30 mCi) is commonly used as this dose may be given as an outpatient. de Groot and Reilly[66] have shown that this leads to ablation in only 60% of cases, while Arad *et al.*[67] have reported on the use of fractionated doses using 1.11–1.85 GBq (30–50 mCi) doses at weekly intervals. The success rate is disappointing, however, with only 25% of patients being ablated.[51] Wu *et al.* demonstrated that dividing a 4.4 GBq ablation dose into three weekly fractions led to an overall mean reduction in uptake of 81%.[68] They suggest that intratherapeutic stunning may be occurring. In Europe, larger ablation doses are generally used with 3.7 GBq being the standard dose.[69] Bal *et al.* have prospectively compared the success of using single ablation doses of 925 MBq or 1.85 GBq (25 or 50 mCi) of radioiodine in a large series and found no significant difference in ablation success between the two activies.[70] Post-therapy scans are recommended as, particularly with the higher doses, unsuspected metastatic tumor may also be detected (Fig. 17A.7).

Radioiodine may also be used to ablate remnant thyroid tissue in patients with medullary thyroid cancer while recognizing that these tumors themselves do not take up radioiodine. The rationale for this is the multicentricity of the tumors in patients with familial forms of the disease.

Treatment of differentiated thyroid cancer

Follicular cancers of the thyroid are usually well differentiated and demonstrate a capability of taking up iodine, although the uptake of iodine is significantly less than that of normal thyroid follicular cells. It has also been shown by Mazaferri *et al.*[53] that the majority of papillary carcinomas are also able to take up iodine and the presence of follicular elements on histology is an indicator of iodine uptake capabilities.

TSH levels must be high in order to ensure good uptake of ^{131}I into recurrent sites of differentiated thyroid cancer.

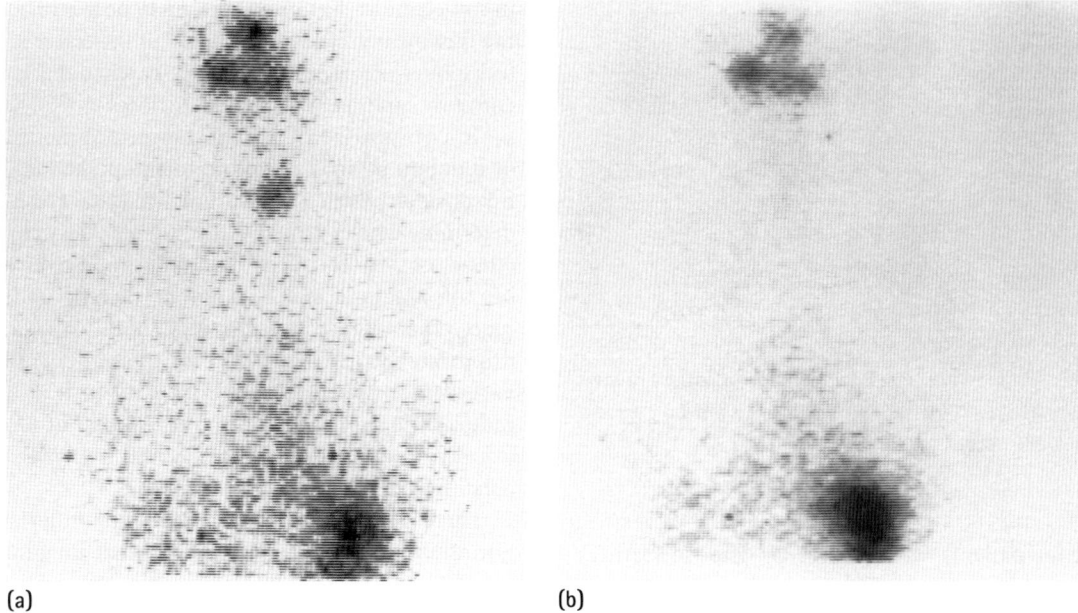

(a)   (b)

Figure 17A.7   *^{131}I scan in patient before (a) and after (b) successful ^{131}I ablation with 3.7 GBq.*

In patients with progressive disease, de-differentiation may occur and poorly differentiated tumor cells lose their ability to take up ^{131}I, although some may continue to secrete thyroglobulin into the circulation. Medullary thyroid cancers, anaplastic carcinomas of the thyroid and lymphomas of the thyroid do not take up ^{131}I which therefore has no role in therapy following ablation of remnant thyroid tissue.

After successful ablation of thyroid tissue with either surgery alone or a combination of surgery and ^{131}I, the subsequent demonstration of focal areas of ^{131}I uptake on whole-body imaging is strongly suggestive of recurrent thyroid tumor. The normal pattern of radioiodine by distribution, however, must be taken into account when interpreting a whole-body scan. Activity is commonly seen in the salivary glands, nasopharynx, stomach, bowel and bladder (Figs 17A.8 and 17A.9). Care should also be taken to ensure that artifacts are not interpreted as focal areas of recurrent tumor. Since ^{131}I is secreted in the saliva, contamination of pocket handkerchiefs is a not uncommon problem and may lead to a false-positive interpretation of a whole-body scan if care is not taken to ensure that no contamination object is imaged. Similarly, urine contamination of underclothes may cause artifacts in the region of the pelvis. Iodine-131 will successfully identify sites of both soft tissue and bone recurrence and may be the first indication of lung metastases.

Before undertaking an ^{131}I tracer scan, the patient should be asked to discontinue thyroid replacement hormone. If the patient is taking thyroxine, a minimum of 4 weeks off treatment is required to ensure adequate TSH levels at the time of imaging. If the patient is taking T3, then a 2-week cessation of therapy is adequate. TSH levels must be measured at the time of undertaking ^{131}I imaging

to ensure the patient's compliance with instructions and to confirm an adequate rise in TSH before a scan is interpreted as negative.

rhTSH administration has been shown to be virtually as effective as thyroid hormone withdrawal in preparing patients for repeat tracer radioiodine imaging with significant improvement in patient quality of life in two large multicenter studies.[71,72] rhTSH is now licensed in Europe and the USA as an alternative to thyroxine withdrawal for preparing patients for tracer imaging. The rhTSH is given as two intramuscular injections on sequential days. The tracer radioiodine dose is given on day 3 and the scan performed, together with a thyroglobulin measurement on day 5.

Many studies have now been reported confirming the successful use of rhTSH prior to ablation therapy and radioiodine therapy of recurrent disease.[73] It has been shown, however, that the effective half-life of radioiodine is shorter with rhTSH preparation compared to thyroxine withdrawal. It is postulated that higher therapy doses may therefore be required.[74] The licensing of rhTSH for therapeutic use is awaiting the results of current multicenter trials.

Recent work at Sloane Kettering has suggested the use of recombinant TSH in patients who have a poor TSH response or in those in whom the time delay necessitated stopping thyroid hormone replacement is clinically unacceptable.[75] Patients with aggressive disease in whom prolonged TSH stimulation may stimulate tumor growth should also be considered for rhTSH rather than thyroxine withdrawal. The use of low iodine diet in the period before tracer imaging will further enhance the avidity of thyroid tumor recurrence for ^{131}I (Table 17A.3).

The amount of ^{131}I to be administered for the tracer scan again varies. The justification for a low tracer dose

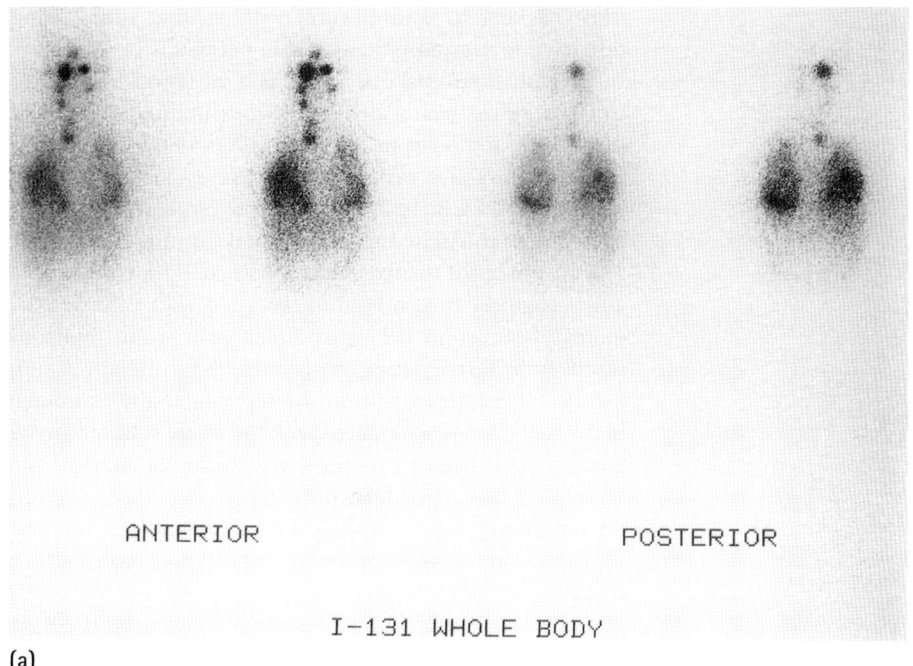

ANTERIOR   POSTERIOR

I-131 WHOLE BODY

(a)

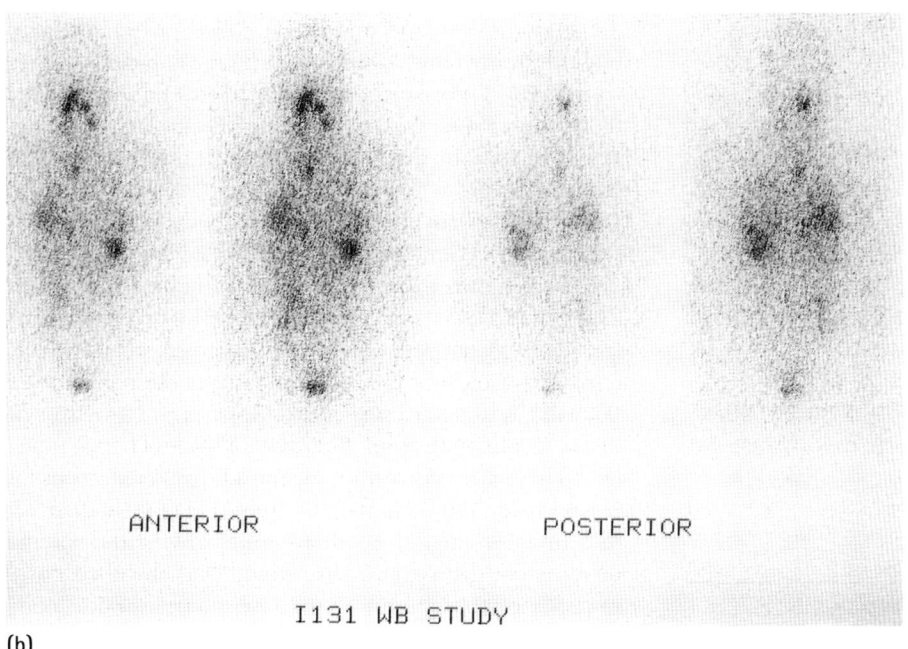

ANTERIOR   POSTERIOR

I131 WB STUDY

(b)

Figure 17A.8 *^{131}I whole-body scans (a) before and (b) 1 week after a 5.5 GBq dose of ^{131}I, showing metastases from a papillary cancer in the neck and lungs which appear more numerous and extensive on the post-therapy scan.*

regime is the avoidance of possible stunning effects of the tracer dose on a subsequent therapy dose. There is little evidence in the literature, however, to suggest that the stunning effects seen in the normal thyroid also occur in thyroid tumor cells and as tumor cells are known to be less radiosensitive than normal cells, it may be postulated that the stunning effect is less important when considering treatment of recurrence compared with ablation of thyroid remnants. The advantage of a high tracer dose (up to 400 MBq) is the higher sensitivity for detecting recurrent disease. The increase in sensitivity with dose is clearly evidenced by the fact that post-therapy scans not uncommonly show lesions

that were not detected on a tracer scan.[76] Siddiqi *et al.* have compared the sensitivity of a whole-body ^{131}I tracer scan with a ^{123}I scan in a small series and showed good concordance between the two methods.[77] This has been extended by Ali *et al.*[78]

Schlumberger[79] recommended a protocol which takes into account the lower sensitivity of the low dose tracer scan regime. He proposes that patients with an elevated thyroglobulin level and a normal tracer scan should receive a therapy dose of ^{131}I. Experience indicated that 50% of patients thus treated show uptake on the post-therapy scan.[55]

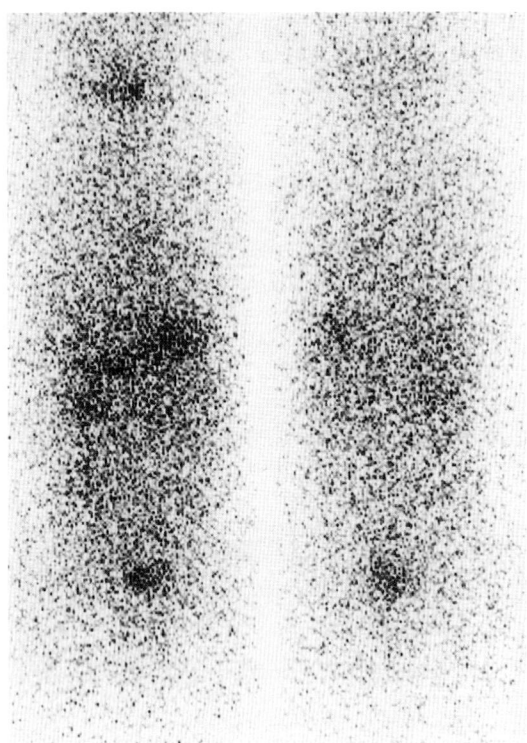

Figure 17A.9 *Normal whole-body ^{131}I scan showing normal biodistribution in the salivary glands, saliva, stomach, bowel and bladder.*

Table 17A.3 *Low iodine diet*

Foods to avoid

- *Sea foods (e.g. shellfish, lobster, crab, prawns, scampi, etc.)*
- *All other types of fish – fresh, frozen, canned, smoked or salted*
- *All fish products (e.g. fish fingers, fish-cakes, fish-paste, etc.)*
- *Vegetables: spinach – fresh or frozen, lettuce, watercress*
- *Iodized salt in cooking*
- *Food colorings*

A patient in whom a tracer scan is performed will be required to observe precautions as for a ^{131}I dose for thyrotoxicosis if they are scanned as an outpatient. Again, extreme care must be taken to ensure that if the patient is a female, they are neither pregnant nor breast-feeding, as both conditions remain absolute contraindications to tracer scanning and subsequent therapy.

In those patients in whom the tracer scan confirms a focal area or areas of recurrence, therapy doses of ^{131}I may be administered. For this, the patient must be admitted into a designated room with en-suite bathroom facilities. Daily monitoring of the patient is required to ensure that the patient is not discharged until the radiation levels fall to those acceptable under national regulations.[80] Visitors

must be kept to a minimum, with visiting times being restricted to not more than 10 min per day.

As with thyrotoxicosis, there is a variation in practice concerning the use of dosimetry measurements obtained from the tracer scan in calculating the therapy dose. The pattern of practice varies between the use of a fixed dose ranging from 5 GBq to 7.4 GBq in some centers to an administered dose calculated from the uptake on the tracer scan. The advantage of the fixed-dose protocol is that it is simple and recognizes the problems associated with volume estimates of recurrent tumor and lack of reproducibility of results from a tracer study compared with the therapy. Again, it must be remembered that the reproducibility of uptake in the therapy dose compared with the tracer scan cannot be guaranteed in view of the potential stunning effect of the tracer scan dose. The dose to the tumor focus is dependent on the uptake of ^{131}I within the tumor and its size, and small foci such as pulmonary metastases may receive doses of up to 300 Gy (30 000 rads).

Centers using dosimetric methods to estimate the dose for individual patients will variably base their dose on uptake and retention measurement obtained from the tracer scan or alternatively blood and urine collections and whole-body counting after tracer dose.[76,80] One approach utilizes so-called BEL dosimetry which calculates the dose to the blood from a tracer study. Doses are selected to give a maximum of 2 Gy to the blood, with no more than 4.4 GBq retained in the whole body at 48 h.[81,82] Doses of up to 16.65 GBq (450 mCi) have been used with no permanent suppression of bone marrow observed. Benua *et al.*[81] however, have shown that average values of radiation delivered to the blood are significantly less than the predicted measurements after tracer doses. This observed fact obviously raises the whole question as to the value of estimating doses following dosimetry calculations. Kosal *et al.*[83] have shown that doses ranging from 4–290 Gy (400–29 000 rads) may be delivered to the tumor using administered doses of 5.5–6.3 GBq (150–170 mCi). O'Connell *et al.* have used ^{124}I PET in an attempt to more accurately define the volume of recurrent disease and have found that absorbed doses in excess of 100 Gy were found to eradicate cervical node metastases. Metastases that did not respond were calculated to have received less than 20 Gy.[84] Sgouros *et al.* have developed three-dimensional imaging-based dosimetry which is patient specific using ^{124}I PET. They have used post-therapy imaging to demonstrate that mean absorbed dose values for individual tumors range from 1.2 to 540 Gy with absorbed doses within tumors ranging from 0.3 to 4000 Gy.[85]

After treatment, the patient should be reinstated on thyroid hormone replacement therapy. The whole process of rescanning and retreatment if required should not be repeated in under 6 months except in patients with rapidly progressive and life-threatening disease. Once a negative radioiodine tracer scan has been obtained, annual follow-up with thyroglobulin measurements is adequate to monitor for disease recurrence. It has been proposed that in high risk patients (patients over 45 years with large tumors and/or local tissue invasion at the time of diagnosis) rhTSH-stimulated thyroglobulin measurements may have increased sensitivity and permit earlier diagnosis of recurrence.

In patients with palpable recurrence localized to the neck, the use of surgery before radioiodine therapy should be considered to debulk the tumor and optimize the efficacy of radioiodine. The combination of surgery and radioiodine has a better outcome compared with the use of surgery alone.[86]

The role of ^{131}I in patients with Hürthle cell tumors is limited and McLeod and Thompson[87] reported that in their experience only 14% of Hürthle cell recurrent tumors take up radioiodine.

De-differentiated tumors

In patients with aggressive disease, the tumor cells may continue to produce thyroglobulin but lose the ability to take up radioiodine as the tumor de-differentiates. Re-differentiation using retinoic acid has proved successful in several series. Prolonged administration of retinoic acid is required and it is unclear from current studies how long re-differentiation will last.[88]

Acute side-effects following ^{131}I therapy for differentiated thyroid cancer

As ^{131}I is taken up and secreted by the salivary glands as well as by recurrent thyroid tumor sites, a significant radiation dose is received by the salivary glands. Becciolini et al.[89] have calculated the absorbed dose to the salivary glands based on external-beam data to range between 0.24 and 2.29 Gy.[64] Patients are commonly aware of swelling and mild discomfort in the region of the salivary gland in the immediate post-therapy period and complain of alteration in taste with a metallic taste frequently noted. While these symptoms generally resolve after the first one or two treatments, subsequent treatments may result in a permanent reduction in salivary flow and a consequent dryness of the mouth and impaired sensation of taste.[90] Attempts to reduce the radiation dose to the salivary glands have been made by suggesting patients chew gum or suck citrus sweets for 24 h following therapy in order to increase salivary flow and thereby increase the rate of excretion of ^{131}I from the salivary gland area. There is little data, however, to confirm the efficacy of this recommendation and Nakada et al. have demonstrated that increasing salivary flow using citrus sweets in the first 24 h after treatment increases salivary gland damage.[91]

Radiation doses to the bladder are minimized by ensuring a high urine output during the admission for therapy. Some patients complain of nausea in the first 48 h after therapy. This appears to be idiosyncratic. It is readily treated with conventional anti-emetics. Transient episodes of marrow

suppression have been observed in patients with widespread bone metastases. This appears to be a greater problem in patients from west Africa and the West Indies.

Transient impairment of testicular function has been demonstrated by Pacini et al.[92] They concluded that approximately 25% of patients treated with ^{131}I suffered no alterations in FSH levels, whereas the remainder had transient rises in FSH levels. Patients treated repeatedly over a prolonged period had a reduced sperm count. Consideration should therefore be given to sperm banking in young men with metastatic thyroid cancer who are likely to require multiple treatments with radioiodine.

Long-term complications of radioiodine therapy for differentiated thyroid cancer

Long-term side effects of ^{131}I therapy – apart from sialadenitis and xerostomia – are remarkably few. In patients with widespread lung metastases – particularly those with miliary metastases – caution must be taken in determining the dose to be administered in view of the risk of radiation fibrosis.[93]

Leukemia has been reported as a complication in patients receiving aggressive therapy with total administered doses exceeding 37 GBq (1 Ci) with intervals of less than 6 months between treatments.[58,66]

Cancer of the bladder is a theoretical long-term complication of ^{131}I therapy given the radiation doses to the bladder in the early phases of treatment. Few reports of cases of cancer of the bladder have been made, although Edmonds and Smith[93] describe patients who have received a cumulative dose of more than 37 GBq (1 Ci). In patients with evidence of lymph node involvement at the time of initial surgery, external-beam radiotherapy may be used in the postoperative period; this is recommended in those who have received more than 37 GBq (1 Ci) of administered radiation. Hall et al.,[94] using the Swedish Cancer Registry, have followed a large cohort of patients with cancer of the thyroid treated with ^{131}I, but have failed to show any long-term increase in incidence of solid tumors (including bladder tumors).

Use of adjunctive external-beam radiotherapy

Patients who are found to have tumor spread to cervical lymph nodes at the time of primary surgery may be considered for external-beam radiotherapy following surgery as an adjunct to ^{131}I therapy. It is optimal to undertake ^{131}I treatment before external-beam therapy to avoid radiation damage to thyroid remnant and residual thyroid tumor cells which may reduce the efficacy of the radioiodine dose.

CONCLUSION

Iodine-131 remains the most frequently used form of radionuclide therapy with its clearly defined role in both benign and malignant disease. With 40 years of experience in its use it has been shown to be safe and effective and the theoretical risks of tumor induction and chromosomal damage have not been demonstrated in practice. The increasing use of recombinant TSH instead of thyroid hormone withdrawal has improved the quality of life of patients undergoing follow-up for thyroid cancer. Many of the lessons learned from the experience with ^{131}I are now proving useful as new radionuclide therapies are developed and integrated into routine management.

Case history

A 56-year-old woman presented with an enlarging goiter and some dysphagia. A [99mTc] thyroid scan demonstrated a multinodular goiter with an normal 20-min uptake value of 2.5% (normal range 0.4–4.0%) (Fig. 17A.10a). Thyroid function tests were normal. As the pressure symptoms were increasing and the patient was reluctant to consider surgery, an 800 MBq dose of ^{131}I was administered as an outpatient. The patient tolerated the treatment well and was clinically and biochemically euthyroid when reviewed 6 and 12 weeks following treatment. Some improvement in pressure symptoms was noted. When seen again 6 months after treatment, the patient felt unwell with weight loss and palpitations. Thyroid function tests confirmed that the patient had become biochemically thyrotoxic and a repeat [99mTc] scan was consistent with Graves' disease in a multinodular goiter (Fig. 17A.10b). The 20-min uptake had increased to 11.1%. The patient was started on carbimazole and was then treated with a further 600 MBq of [131]I. The results of her thyroid function tests fell gradually over the next 6 months until thyroxine treatment was commenced. She is now well 2 years after the second treatment. Her goiter has shrunk significantly and she is asymptomatic.

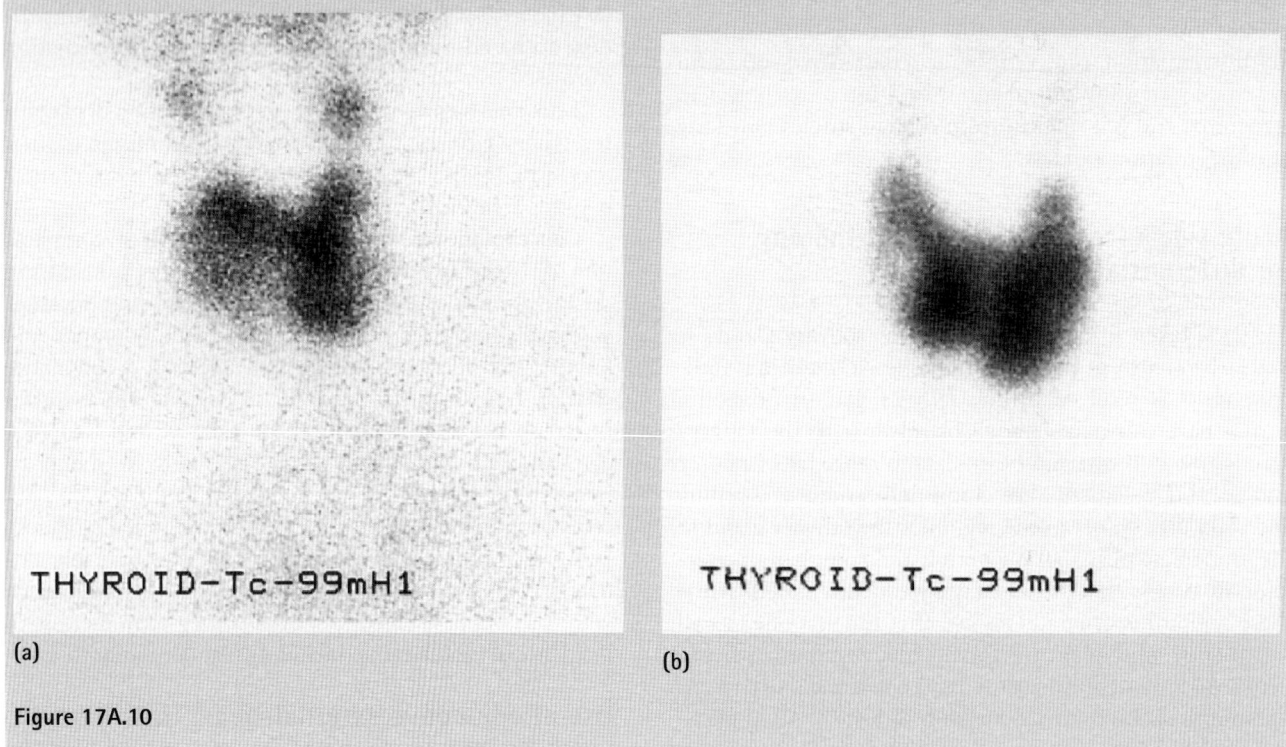

(a)

(b)

Figure 17A.10

REFERENCES

1 Williams RH, Tovery BT, Jaffe H. Radiotherapies. *Am J Med* 1949; **7**: 702–4.

2 Varma VM, Beierwaltes WH, Notal M, *et al.* Treatment of thyroid cancer. *JAMA* 1970; **214**: 1437–42.

3 Meier DA, Brill DA, Becker DV, *et al.* Procedure guidelines for the therapy of thyroid disease with radioiodine. *J Nucl Med* 2202; **43**: 856–61.

4 British Thyroid Association and Royal College of Physicians. *Guidelines for the management of thyroid cancer in adults, 2002.* Available at www.british-thyroid-association.org

5 Dai G, Levy O, Carrasco N. Cloning and characterization of the thyroid iodide transporter. *Nature* 1996; **379**: 458–60.

6 Filetti S, Bidart J-M, Arturi F, *et al.* Sodium/iodide symporter: a key transport system in thyroid cancer cell metabolism. *Eur J Endocrinol* 1999; **141**: 443–57.

7 Dadachova E, Carrasco N. The Na+/I symporter: imaging and therepaeutic applications. *Semin Nucl Med* 2004; **34**: 23–31.

8 Meier CA, Braverman LE, Ebner SA, *et al.* Diagnostic use of recombinant human thyrotropin in patients with thyroid carcinoma (phase I/II study). *J Clin Enocrinol Metab* 1994; **78**: 188–196.

9 Safran M, Paul TL, Roti E, Braverman LE. Environmental factors affecting autoimmune thyroid disease. *Endocrinol Metab Clin North Am* 1987; **16**: 327–42.

10 Boucher CA, Bemard BF, Zhang ZG, *et al.* Nature and significance of orbital autoantigens and their autoantibodies in thyroid associated ophthalmopathy. *Autoimmunity* 1992; **13**: 89–93.

11 Allanic H, Fauchet R, Orgiazzi A. Antithyroid drugs and Graves' disease: a prospective randomised evaluation of the efficacy of treatment duration. *J Clin Endocrinol Metab* 1990; **70**: 675–9.

12 Klein I, Becker DV, Levey GS. Treatment of thyroid disease. *Ann Intern Med* 1994; **121**: 281–8.

13 Lazarus JH, Clarke SEM, Franklyn JA, Harding LK. *Guidelines – the use of radioiodine in the management of hyperthyroidism.* The radioiodine audit subcommittee of the Royal College of Physicians Committee on Diabetes and Endocrinology and the Research Unit of the Royal College of Physicians. London: Chameleon Press Ltd, 1995.

14 Santos RB, Romaldini JH, Ward LS. Propylthiouracil reduces the effectiveness of radioiodine treatment in hyperthyroid patients with Graves' disease. *Thyroid* 2004; **14**: 525–30.

15 Subcommittee for the study of endemic goitre and iodine deficiency of the European Thyroid Association Goitre and iodine deficiency in Europe. *Lancet* 1985; **i**: 1290.

16 Wartofsky L, Glinoer D, Solomon B, *et al.* Differences and similarities in the diagnosis and treatment of Graves' disease in Europe, Japan and the United States. *Thyroid* 1991; **1**: 129–35.

17 Hayek A, Chapman EM, Crawford JD. Long term results of treatment of thyrotoxicosis in children and adolescents with radioactive iodine. *N Engl J Med* 1970; **283**: 949–53.

18 Sarkar SD, Beierwaltes WH, Gill SP, Contey BJ. Subsequent fertility and birth histories of children and adolescents treated with ^{131}iodine for thyroid cancer. *J Nucl Med* 1976; **17**: 460–4.

19 Bacon GE, Laury GH. Experience with surgical treatment of thyrotoxicosis in children. *J Pediatr* 1965; **67**: 1–5.

20 Ching T, Warden MJ, Hefferman RA. Thyroid surgery in children and teenagers. *Arch Otolaryngol* 1977; **103**: 544–6.

21 Schicha H, Scheidhauer K. Radioiodine therapy in Europe – a survey. *Nuklearmedizin* 1993; **32**: 321–4.

22 Kusakabe K, Maki M. Radionuclide therapy of thyroid disease radioactive iodine therapy. *Japn J Nucl Med* 1993; **30**: 813–9.

23 Mithal A, Shah A, Kumar S. The management of Graves' disease by Indian thyroidologists. *Nat Med J India* 1993; **6**: 163–6.

24 Kuma K, Matsuzuka F, Kobayashi A, *et al.* Natural course of Graves' disease after subtotal thyroidectomy and management of patients with postoperative thyroid dysfunction. *Am J Med Sci* 1991; **302**: 8–12.

25 Administration of Radioactive Substances Advisory Committee. *Notes for guidance on the clinical administration of radiopharmaceuticals and the use of sealed radioactive sources.* Didcot, UK: Health Protection Agency, 2006.

26 Singer PA, Cooper DS, Levy EG, *et al.* Treatment guidelines for patients with hyperthyroidism and hypothyroidism. Standards of care committee. American Thyroid Association. *JAMA* 1995; **273**: 808–12.

27 Thompson WH, Harding LK. Radiation protection issues associated with nuclear medicine outpatients. *Nucl Med Commun* 1991; **16**: 879–92.

28 Shapiro B. Optimization of radioiodine therapy: what have we learnt after 50 years. *J Nucl Med* 1993; **34**: 1638–41.

29 Bokisch A, Jamitzy T, Derwantz R, Biersack HJ. Optimized dose planning of radioiodine therapy of benign thyroidal diseases. *J Nucl Med* 1994; **34**: 1632–8.

30 Tsuruta M, Nagayama Y, Izumi M, Nagataki S. Long term follow-up studies on iodine-131 treatment of hyperthyroid Graves' disease based on the measurement of thyroid volume by ultrasonography. *Ann Intern Med* 1993; **7**: 193–7.

31 Flower MA, al-Saadi D, Harmer CL, *et al.* Dose response study on thyrotoxic patients undergoing positron emission tomography and radioiodine therapy. *Eur J Nucl Med* 1994; **21**: 531–6.

32 Willemsen UF, Knesewitsch P, Kreisig T, *et al.* Functional results of radioiodine therapy with a 300 Gy absorbed dose in Graves' disease. *Eur J Nucl Med* 1993; **20**: 1050–5.

33 Reinhardt MJ, Brink I, Alexius Y, *et al.* Radioiodine therapy in Graves' disease based on the tissue absorbed dose calculations: effect of pretreatment thyroid volume on clinical outcome. *Eur J Nucl Med* 2002; **29**: 1118–24.

34 Kinser JA, Roesler H, Furrer T, *et al.* Nonimmunogenic hyperthyroidism: incidence after radioiodine and surgical treatment. *J Nucl Med* 1989; **30**: 1960–5.

35 Hardisty CA, Jones SJ, Hedley AJ, *et al.* Clinical outcome and costs of care in radioiodine treatment of hyperthyroidism. *J R Coll Physicians* 1990; **24**: 36–42.

36 Johnson JK. Outcome of treating thyrotoxic patients with a standard dose of radioactive iodine. *Scottish Med J* 1993; **38**: 142–4.

37 Kendall-Taylor P, Keir M, Ross WM. Ablative radioiodine therapy for hyperthyroidism: long term follow up study. *Br Med J* 1984; **289**: 361–3.

38 Becker DR. Radioactive iodine in the treatment of hyperthyroidism. In: Beckers C. (ed.) *Thyroid disease.* Paris: Pergamon Press, 1982: 145–8.

39 Ng Tang Fui SC, Maisey MN. Standard dose of 131-iodine therapy for hyperthyroidism caused by

autonomously functioning thyroid nodules. *Clin Endocrinol* 1979; **10**: 69–77.

40 Catz B, Tsao J. Total 131-I thyroid remnant ablation for pretibial myxoedema. *Clin Res* 1965; **13**: 130–2.

41 Hamilton R, Mayberry W, McConahey W, Hanson K. Ophthalmopathy of Graves' disease: a comparison between patients treated surgically and patients treated with radioiodine. *Mayo Clin Proc* 1967; **42**: 812–8.

42 Peqquequat E, Mayberry W, McConahey W, Wyse E. Large doses of radioiodine in Graves' disease: effect on ophthalmopathy and long acting thyroid stimulator. *Mayo Clin Proc* 1967; **42**: 802–11.

43 Jones D, Munro D, Wilson G. Observations on the cause of exophthalmos after 131-iodine therapy. *Proc R Soc Med* 1969; **52**: 15–8.

44 Bartalena L, Marocci C, Bogazzi F, *et al.* Relation between therapy for hyperthyroidism and the course of Graves' ophthalmopathy. *N Engl J Med* 1988; **338**: 73–8.

45 Tallstedt L, Lundell G, Blomgren H, Bring J. Does early administration of thyroxine reduce the development of Graves' ophthalmopathy after radioiodine treatment. *Eur J Nucl Med* 1994; **130**: 494–7.

46 Wesche MF, Tie-v-Buul MM, Smits NJ, Wiersinga WM. Reduction in goiter size by ^{131}I therapy in patients with non-toxic multinodular goitre. *Eur J Endocrinol* 1995; **132**: 86–7.

47 Huysmanns DA, Hermus AR, Corstens FH, *et al.* Large compressive goiters treated with radioiodine. *Ann Intern Med* 1994; **121**: 757–62.

48 Nieuwlats WA, Hermus AR, Ross HA, *et al.* Dosimetry of radioiodine therapy in patients with nodular goiter after pretreatment with a single low dose of recombinant human thyroid stimulating hormone. *J Nucl Med* 2004; **45**: 626–33.

49 Nygaards B, Hegedus L, Gervil M, *et al.* Radioiodine treatment of multinodular nontoxic goitre. *Br Med J* 1993; **307**: 828–32.

50 Cat R, Rossi R. A expanded view of risk group definition in differentiated thyroid carcinoma. *Surgery* 1988; **104**: 947–53.

51 Hay ID, Bergstrahl EJ, Goellner JR, *et al.* Predicting outcome in papillary thyroid carcinoma: development of reliable prognostic scoring system in a cohort of 1779 patients surgically treated in one institution during 1940–1989. *Surgery* 1993; **114**: 1050–8.

52 Beierwaltes WH. Carcinoma of the thyroid. Radionuclide diagnosis, therapy and follow-up. *Clin Oncol* 1987; **5**: 23–7.

53 Mazzaferri EL. Papillary thyroid carcinoma: factors influencing prognosis and current therapy. *Semin Oncol* 1987; **14**: 315–32.

54 Mazzaferri EL, Kloos RD. Current approaches to primary therapy for papillary and follicular thyroid cancer. *J Clin Endocrinol Metab* 2001; **86**: 1447–63.

55 Tubiana M. Long term results and prognostic factors with differentiated thyroid carcinoma. *Cancer* 1985; **55**: 794–804.

56 McConahey WM. Papillary thyroid cancer treated at the Mayo Clinic, 1946 through 1970: initial manifestations, pathologic findings, therapy and outcome. *Mayo Clin Proc* 1986; **61**: 978–96.

57 Sawka AM, Thephamongkhol K, Brouwers M, *et al.* A systematic review and meta-analysis of the effectiveness of radioiodine remant ablation for well differentiated thyroid cancer. *J Endocrinol Metab* 2004; **89**: 3662–4.

58 Tubiana M. Thyroid cancer. In: Beckers C. (ed.) *Thyroid diseases.* Paris: Pergamon Press, 1982: 182–227.

59 Pace L, Klain M, Albanese C, *et al.* Short term outcome of differentiated thyroid cancer patients receiving a second iodine-131 therapy on the basis of a detectable serum thyroglobulin level after initial treatment. *Eur J Med Mol Imaging* 2005; **33**: 179–83.

60 Bal CS, Kumar A, Chandra P, *et al.* Is chest X-ray or high resolution CT of the chest sufficient investigation to detect pulmonary metastases in paediatric differentiated thyroid cancer. *Thyroid* 2004; **14**: 217–25.

61 Jeevanram RK, Shah DH, Sharma SM, Ganatra RD. Influence of initial large dose on subsequent uptake of therapeutic radioiodine in thyroid cancer patients. *Nucl Med Biol* 1986; **13**: 277–9.

62 Park JM. Stunned thyroid after high dose 131-I imaging. *Clin Nucl Med* 1992; **17**: 501–2.

63 Kalinyak JE, McDougall IR. Whole-body scanning with radionuclides of iodine, and the controversy of 'thyroid stunning'. *Nucl Med Comm* 2004; **25**: 883–9.

64 Park HM, Perkins OW, Edmonson JW, *et al.* Influence of diagnostic radioiodines on the uptake of ablative doses of iodine-131. *Thyroid* 1994; **4**: 49–54.

65 Blake GM, Patel R, Prescod N, Clarke SEM. Thyroid stunning by a ^{131}I tracer scan prior to radioiodine ablation for thyroid cancer. *Nucl Med Commun* 1998; **19**: 158.

66 de Groot LJ, Reilly M. Comparison of 30 and 50 mCi doses for 131-iodine ablation. *Ann Intern Med* 1982; **96**: 51–2.

67 Arad E, Flannery K, Wilson G, O'Mara R. Fractionated doses of radioiodine ablation of post surgical thyroid tissue remnants. *Clin Nucl Med* 1990; **16**: 676–7.

68 Wu H, Hseu H, Lin W, *et al.* Decreased uptake after fractionated ablative doses of iodine-131. *Eur J Nucl Med Mol Imaging* 2005; **32**: 167–73.

69 Kuni CC, Klingensmith WC. Failure of low doses of ^{131}I to ablate residual thyroid tissue following surgery for thyroid cancer. *Radiology* 1980; **137**: 773–4.

70 Bal CS, Kumar A, Pant GS. Radioiodine dose for remnant ablation in differentiated thyroid carcinoma: a randomized clinical trial in 500 patients. *J Clin Edocrinol Metab* 2004; **89**:1666–73.

71 Haugen BR, Pacini F, Reiners C. A comparison of recombinant human thyrogen and thyroid hormone withdrawal for the detection of thyroid remnant or cancer. *J Clin Endocrinol Metab* 1999; **84**: 3877–85.

72 Ladenson PW, Braverman LE, Mazzaferri EL. Comparison of administration of recombinant human thyrogen with withdrawal of thyroid hormone for radioactive iodine scanning in patients with thyroid carcinoma. *New Engl J Med* 1997; **337**: 888–96.

73 Robbins R. Recombinant human TSH and thyroid cancer management – clinical review. *J Clin Endocrinol Metabol* 2003; **88**: 1933–8.

74 Menzel C, Kranert WT, Dobert N, Diehl M. RhTSH stimulation before radioiodine therapy in thyroid cancer reduces the effective half life of radioiodine. *J Nucl Med* 2003; **44**: 1065–8.

75 Braverman LE, Prat, BM, Ebner S, Longcope C. Recombinant human thyrotropin stimulates thyroid function and radioactive iodine uptake in Rhesus monkeys. *J Clin Endocrinol Metab* 1992; **74**: 1135–9.

76 Maxon HR, Thomas SR, Hertzberg VS. Relation between effective radiation dose and outcome of radioiodine therapy for thyroid cancer. *N Engl J Med* 1983; **309**: 937–41.

77 Siddiqi A, Foley RR, Britton KE, et al. The role of ^{123}I diagnostic imaging in the follow up of patients with differentiated thyroid cancer as compared to ^{131}I scanning: avoidance of negative therapeutic uptake due to stunning. *Clin Endocrinol* 2001; **55**: 515–21.

78 Ali N, Sebastian C, Foley RR, et al. The management of differentiated thyroid cancer using ^{123}I for imaging to assess the need for ^{131}I therapy. *Nucl Med Commun* 2006; **27**: 165–9.

79 Schlumberger M. Detection and treatment of lung metastases of differentiated thyroid cancer in patients with normal chest X-rays. *J Nucl Med* 1988; **29**: 1790–4.

80 Fruhling J. Role of radioactive iodine in the treatment of differentiated thyroid cancer: physiopathological basis, results, considerations from the viewpoint of radioprotection. *Bull Mem Acad R Med Belg* 1994; **149**: 192–206.

81 Benua RS, Cieale NR, Sonenberg M. The relation of radioiodine dose to results and complications in the treatment of metastatic thyroid cancer. *Am J Roentgenol, Radiat Ther Nucl Med* 1962; **87**: 171–82.

82 Leeper RD, Shimaoka K. Treatment of metastatic thyroid cancer. *Clin Endocrinol Metab* 1980; **9**: 383–404.

83 Kosal KF, Adler SF, Carey J, Beierwaltes W. Iodine-131 treatment of thyroid cancer: absorbed dose calculated from post therapy scans. *J Nucl Med* 1986; **27**: 1207–11.

84 O'Connell ME, Flower MA, Hinton PJ, et al. Radiation dose assessment in radioiodine therapy. Dose–response relationships in differentiated thyroid cancer using quantitative scanning and PET. *Radiother Oncol* 1993; **28**: 16–26.

85 Sgouros G, Kolbert MS, Sheikh A, et al. Patient specific dosimetry for ^{131}I thyroid cancer therapy using [124]I PET and 3-dimensional internal dosimetry software. *J Nucl Med* 2004; **45**: 1366–72.

86 Coburn M, Teates D, Wanebo HJ. Recurrent thyroid cancer. Role of surgery versus radioactive iodine. *Ann Surg* 1994; **219**: 587–93.

87 McCleod MK, Thompson WT. Hurthle cell neoplasms of the thyroid. *Otolaryngol Clin North Am* 1990; **23**: 441–52.

88 Simin D, Korber C, Ktrausch M, et al. Clinical impact of retinoids in redifferentiation therapy of advanced thyroid cancer: final results of pilot study. *Eur J Nucl Med Mol Imaging* 2002; **29**: 775–82.

89 Becciolini A, Porciani S, Lanini A, et al. Serum amylase and tissue polypeptide antigen as biochemical indicators of salivary gland injury during iodine-131 therapy. *Eur J Nucl Med* 1994; **21**: 1121–5.

90 Kabra R, Prescod N, Allen S, Clarke SEM. Salivary gland function in patients with Ca thyroid treated with radioiodine. *Nucl Med Commun* 2004; **25**: 402–3.

91 Nakada K, Ishibashi T, Takei T, et al. Does lemon candy decrease salivary gland damage after radioiodine therapy for thyroid cancer. *J Nucl Med* 2005; **46**: 261–6.

92 Pacini F, Gasperi M, Fugazzola L, et al. Testicular function in patients with differentiated thyroid carcinoma treated with radioiodine. *J Nucl Med* 1994; **35**: 1418–22.

93 Edmonds C, Smith T. The long term hazards of treatment of thyroid cancer with radioiodine. *Br J Radiol* 1986; **59**: 45–51.

94 Hall P, Holm LE, Lundell GE. Cancer risks in thyroid cancer patients. *Br J Cancer* 1992; **64**: 159–63.

Endocrine: Peptides

MARION DE JONG, DIK KWEKKEBOOM, ROELF VALKEMA, AND ERIC KRENNING

INTRODUCTION

The 14 amino acid peptide somatostatin plays an important role in the physiologic regulation of hormones and organs in the body. The effects of somatostatin are mediated by high-affinity G-protein coupled membrane receptors, integral membrane glycoproteins. Five different human somatostatin receptor subtypes have been cloned.[1–3] Somatostatin binds to all subtypes with high affinity.

The finding that somatostatin inhibits hormone secretion of various glands led to its use in the treatment of symptoms due to diseases with overproduction of hormones. The native peptide somatostatin is itself unsuitable for treatment, as after intravenous administration it has a very short half-life due to rapid enzymatic degradation. Therefore, somatostatin analogs that are more resistant to enzymatic degradation were synthesized, the molecule was modified in various ways with the preservation of the biological activity of the original molecule, resulting in, for example, the somatostatin analog octreotide, which contains eight amino acids and has a long and therapeutically useful plasma half-life. The affinity of the different somatostatin analogs for these subtypes differs considerably. For example, octreotide binds with high affinity to the somatostatin receptor subtype 2 (sst_2), and with lower affinities to sst_5 and sst_3. It shows no binding to sst_1 and sst_4.[2,4]

Neuroendocrine gastro-entero-pancreatic (GEP) tumors, which comprise pancreatic islet-cell tumors, nonfunctioning neuroendocrine pancreatic tumors and carcinoids, are usually slow growing. When metastasized, the widely used treatment with stable somatostatin analogs results in reduced hormonal overproduction and symptomatic relief in most cases.[5–8] Treatment with somatostatin analogs, whether or

not in combination with interferon-alpha, is seldom successful in terms of CT or MRI assessed tumor size reduction, however.[9]

An interesting application of these peptides in nuclear medicine is the use of radiolabeled analogs for tumor scintigraphy after intravenous injection. The diagnostic peptide [^{111}In-DTPA]octreotide (OctreoScan, ^{111}In-pentetreotide) was approved by the FDA on 2 June 1994 for scintigraphy of patients with these somatostatin receptor-positive tumors. As soon as the success of peptide receptor scintigraphy for tumor visualization became clear, the next logical step was to try to label these peptides with therapeutic radionuclides and to perform peptide receptor radionuclide therapy (PRRT) of receptor-positive GEP tumors.

[^{111}IN–DTPA]OCTREOTIDE

The molecular basis of the use of radiolabeled octreotide in scintigraphy and radionuclide therapy is receptor-mediated internalization and cellular retention of the radionuclide. Internalization of radiolabeled [DTPA]octreotide in somatostatin receptor-positive tumors and tumor cell lines has been investigated;[10–12] it appeared that this process is receptor-specific and temperature dependent. Receptor-mediated internalization of [^{111}In-DTPA]octreotide results in degradation to the final radiolabeled metabolite ^{111}In-DTPA-D-Phe in the lysosomes.[13] This metabolite is not capable of passing the lysosomal and/or other cell membrane(s), and will therefore stay in the lysosomes, causing the long retention time of ^{111}In in sst_2-positive (tumor) cells. Internalization of [^{111}In-DTPA]octreotide is especially important for radionuclide therapy of tumors when radionuclides emitting

Table 17B.1 *Main characteristics of radionuclides presently used in clinical peptide receptor radionuclide therapy studies*

Radionuclide	Half-life (h)	Energy (keV) of main therapeutic particles (type, abundance)	Main gamma energies (keV)	Maximum particle range (mm)
[111]In	67	25 (Auger electrons)	245 (94%), 171 (90%)	0.01
[90]Y	64	2284 (β^-, 100%)	–	12
[177]Lu	161	497 (β^-, 79%), 176 (β^-, 12%), 384 (β^-, 9%)	208 (11%), 113 (7%)	2

Table 17B.2 *Tumor responses in patients with gastro-entero-pancreatic tumors, treated with different radiolabeled somatostatin analogs*

Center (reference)	Ligand	Number of patients	Tumor response					
			CR	PR	MR	SD	PD	CR + PR (%)
Rotterdam[17]	[^{111}In-DTPA]octreotide	26	0	0	5 (19%)	11 (42%)	10 (38%)	0
New Orleans[19]	[^{111}In-DTPA]octreotide	26	0	2 (8%)	NA	21 (81%)	3 (12%)	8
Milan[28]	[^{90}Y-DOTA,Tyr[3]]octreotide	21	0	6 (29%)	NA	11 (52%)	4 (19%)	29
Basel[34,35]	[^{90}Y-DOTA,Tyr[3]]octreotide	74	3 (4%)	15 (20%)	NA	48 (65%)	8 (11%)	24
Basel[7]	[^{90}Y-DOTA,Tyr[3]]octreotide	33	2 (6%)	9 (27%)	NA	19 (57%)	3 (9%)	33
Rotterdam[18]	[^{90}Y-DOTA,Tyr[3]]octreotide	54	0	4 (7%)	7 (13%)	33 (61%)	10 (19%)	7
Rotterdam[43]	[^{177}Lu-DOTA,Tyr[3]]octreotate	76	1 (1%)	22 (29%)	9 (12%)	30 (39%)	14 (18%)	30

CR, complete remission; partial remission; MR, minor remission; SD, stable disease; PD, progressive disease.

therapeutical particles with very short path lengths are used, like those emitting Auger electrons (e.g. [111]In, Table 17B.1). These electrons are only effective in a short distance of only a few nanometers up to millimeters from their target, the nuclear DNA. Recently, Hornick et al.[14] and Wang et al.[15] described *in vitro* cellular internalization, nuclear translocation, and DNA binding of radiolabeled somatostatin analogs, which significantly increased after prolonged exposure. ^{111}In-labeled peptides are therefore suitable for both scintigraphy and radionuclide therapy, all the more so as the decay of Auger electron emitter has recently been shown to lead to a 'bystander effect', an *in vivo*, dose-independent inhibition or retardation of tumor growth in nonradiotargeted cells by a signal produced in cells labeled with an Auger electron emitter.[16]

Clinical studies with [^{111}In-DTPA]octreotide

Initial studies with high dosages of [^{111}In-DTPA]octreotide in patients with metastasized neuroendocrine tumors were encouraging, although partial remissions (PRs) were exceptional.

Fifty patients with somatostatin receptor-positive tumors, of which 26 with GEP tumors, were treated with multiple doses of [^{111}In-DTPA]octreotide in Rotterdam.[17,18] Forty patients were evaluable after cumulative doses of at least 20 GBq up to 160 GBq. Therapeutic effects found in the patients with GEP tumors were: no PRs, minor remissions (MR, i.e. a decrease in tumor size of 25–50%, as measured on CT scans) in five patients, and stabilization of previously progressive tumors in 11 patients (Table 17B.2), underscoring the therapeutic potential of Auger-emitting radiolabeled peptides. The toxicity was generally mild bone marrow toxicity, but three of the six patients who received more than 100 GBq developed a myelodysplastic syndrome (MDS) or leukemia (Table 17B.3). Therefore, 100 GBq was considered the maximum tolerable dose. With a renal radiation dose of 0.45 mGy MBq^{-1} (based on previous studies) a cumulative dose of 100 GBq will lead to 45 Gy on the kidneys, twice the accepted limit for external-beam radiation. However, no development of hypertension, proteinuria or significant changes in serum creatinine or creatinine clearance were observed in the patients, including two patients who received 106 and 113 GBq [^{111}In-DTPA]octreotide without renal protection by infusion with amino acids (see further), over follow-up periods of 3 and 2 years, respectively. These findings show that the radiation of the short-range Auger electrons originating from the cells of the proximal tubules is not harmful for the renal function. The decrease in serum inhibin B and concomitant increase of serum FSH levels in men indicate that spermatogenesis was impaired.

Table 17B.3   *Side-effects in patients with gastro-entero-pancreatic tumors, treated with different radiolabeled somatostatin analogs*

Reference	Ligand	Number of patients	Grade 3–4 hematologic toxicity			Other toxicity
			Platelets (%)	Hemoglobin (%)	White blood cells (%)	
Rotterdam[17]	[^{111}In-DTPA]octreotide	50	10	15	2	3 AML/MDS
New Orleans[19]	[^{111}In-DTPA]octreotide	27	7	11	7	3 Liver, 1 renal
Milan[28]	[^{90}Y-DOTA,Tyr^3]octreotide	40	7	3	7	
Basel[31]	[^{90}Y-DOTA,Tyr^3]octreotide	29	3	7	0	4 Renal*
Basel[35]	[^{90}Y-DOTA,Tyr^3]octreotide	39	0	3	0	1 Renal
Rotterdam[18]	[^{90}Y-DOTA,Tyr^3]octreotide	60	12	8	13	1 MDS, 1 liver, 1 renal
Rotterdam[43]	[^{177}Lu-DOTA,Tyr^3]octreotate	200	3	1	2	1 MDS, 1 renal

Percentages are based on the number of patients. AML, acute myeloid leukemia; MDS, myelodysplastic syndrome. *No amino acid infusion in half of the patients.

At the Louisiana State University Medical Center in New Orleans, a clinical trial was performed to determine the effectiveness and tolerability of therapeutic doses of [^{111}In-DTPA]octreotide in patients with GEP tumors.[19–21] GEP tumor patients who had failed all forms of conventional therapy, with worsening of tumor-related signs and symptoms and/or radiographically documented progressive disease, an expected survival less than 6 months, and somatostatin receptor expression on the tumor as determined by the uptake on a 222 MBq [^{111}In-DTPA]octreotide scan, were treated with at least two monthly 6.6 GBq intravenous injections. Twenty-seven GEP (24 carcinoid neoplasms with carcinoid syndrome and three pancreatic islet cells) patients were accrued. Clinical benefit occurred in 16 (62%) patients. Objective partial responses on CT occurred in two (8%) patients (Table 17B.2). The following transient grades 3/4 side-effects were observed, respectively: leukocytes: 1/1; platelets: 0/2; hemoglobin: 3/0; bilirubin: 1/3; creatinine: 1/0; neurologic: 1/0. The renal insufficiency in one patient was probably not treatment-related, but due to pre-existing retroperitoneal fibrosis. Transient liver toxicity was observed in three patients with widespread liver metastases. Myeloproliferative disease and/or myelodysplastic syndrome had not been observed in the six patients followed-up for 48+ months (Table 17B.3). It was concluded that two doses (6.6 GBq each) of [^{111}In-DTPA]octreotide were safe, well-tolerated, and improved symptoms in 62% of patients, with 8% partial radiographic responses and increased expected survival in GEP cancer patients with somatostatin receptor-expressing tumors.

Both series had relatively high numbers of GEP cancer patients who were in a poor clinical condition upon study entry. Also, many had progressive disease when entering the study. Although in both series favorable effects on symptomatology were reported, CT-assessed tumor regression was observed only in rare cases.

Stokkel *et al.*[22] recently reported on a study that determined the effect of [^{111}In-DTPA]octreotide therapy in patients with progressive radioiodine nonresponsive thyroid cancer. Therapeutic effects were determined in relation to [^{111}In-DTPA]octreotide uptake by tumor localizations assessed on pre-treatment diagnostic [^{111}In-DTPA]octreotide scans. Eleven patients, selected on positive pre-treatment diagnostic scans, were treated with up to four fixed doses of 7400 MBq [^{111}In-DTPA]octreotide with an interval of 2–3 weeks between the doses. In 44% of the patients, stable disease was achieved for up to 6 months after the first treatment. These four patients had relative low pre-treatment thyroglobulin values, representing limited metastasized disease. It was therefore concluded that treatment with high doses [^{111}In-DTPA]octreotide in differentiated thyroid cancer can result in stable disease in a subgroup of patients, whereas low pre-treatment thyroglobulin value, representing a small tumor load, might be a selection criterion for treatment.

It can be concluded that ^{111}In-coupled peptides are not ideal for PRRT because of the small particle range and therefore short tissue penetration. Consequently, various research groups aimed to develop somatostatin analogs that can be linked via a chelator to therapeutic radionuclides. DOTA is a universal chelator capable of formation of stable complexes with metals like ^{111}In, ^{67}Ga, ^{68}Ga, ^{86}Y and ^{64}Cu for imaging as well as with ^{90}Y and with radiolanthanides such as ^{177}Lu for receptor-mediated radionuclide therapy. In addition, new somatostatin analogs were synthesized to improve receptor affinity.

[^{90}Y–DOTA,Tyr^3]OCTREOTIDE AND [^{177}LU–DOTA,Tyr^3]OCTREOTATE

After ^{111}In, the next radionuclide investigated for PRRT was ^{90}Y, which emits beta particles with a high maximum energy (2.27 MeV) and a long maximum particle range (>10 mm, Table 17B.1). The first somatostatin analog radiolabeled with ^{90}Y and applied for PRRT in animals and patients was [^{90}Y-DOTA,Tyr^3]octreotide, in which, in comparison with octreotide, the phenylalanine residue at position 3 has been replaced with tyrosine; this makes the compound more hydrophilic and increases the affinity for sst$_2$, leading to higher uptake in sst$_2$-positive tumors both in preclinical studies and in patients.[23,24]

The next analog investigated in preclinical radionuclide therapy studies was [^{177}Lu-DOTA,Tyr^3]octreotate. ^{177}Lu emits gamma radiation with a suitable energy for imaging and therapeutic beta particles with low to medium energy (maximum 0.50 MeV) (Table 17B.1), so the same compound can be used for both imaging and dosimetry and radionuclide therapy, thus obviating the need for a pretherapeutic dosimetric study. The approximate range of the beta particles is 20 cell diameters, whereas the range of those emitted by ^{90}Y is 150 cell diameters. Less 'cross-fire' induced radiation damage in the radiosensitive renal glomeruli (see also below) can therefore be expected with ^{177}Lu. Also, in comparison with ^{90}Y, a higher percentage of the ^{177}Lu radiation energy will be absorbed in very small tumors and (micro)metastases.

Reduction of renal uptake

A problem during radionuclide therapy may be caused by the uptake and retention of radioactivity in the radiosensitive kidneys; small radiolabeled peptides in the blood plasma are filtered through the glomerular capillaries in the kidneys and subsequently partly reabsorbed by and retained in the proximal tubular cells, thereby reducing the scintigraphic sensitivity for detection of small tumors in the perirenal region and the possibilities for radionuclide therapy. It was shown that the renal uptake of radiolabeled octreotide in rats could be reduced by positively charged amino acids, such as lysine and arginine. About 50% reduction could be obtained by single intravenous administration of 400 mg kg^{-1} L-lysine or D-lysine.[25,26] Therefore, during PRRT an infusion containing the positively charged amino acids L-lysine and L-arginine can be given during and after the infusion of the radiopharmaceutical, in order to reduce the kidney uptake. Various protocols have been described, resulting in up to 55% reduction of renal uptake of radioactivity, thereby allowing a higher administered dose.[27–30] Our preferred protocol comprises a combination of lysine and arginine. Patients receive a 1-L infusion (500 mL of L-lysine HCl 5% plus 250 mL L-arginine HCl 10% plus 250 mL saline, brought to pH 7.4). This infusion lasts 4 h; it starts 30 min prior to the radiopeptide injection, and a constant infusion rate is used throughout the infusion period.[27]

Clinical studies with [^{90}Y-DOTA,Tyr^3] octreotide

Various multicenter phase 1 and phase 2 PRRT trials have been performed using these ^{90}Y- and ^{177}Lu-labeled somatostatin analogs. Otte *et al.* and Waldherr *et al.* (University Hospital Basel, Switzerland) reported different phase 1 and phase 2 studies in patients with neuroendocrine GEP tumors. Otte *et al.*[31–33] described a study in which patients received four or more single doses of [^{90}Y-DOTA,Tyr^3]octreotide with ascending activity at intervals of approximately 6 weeks (cumulative dose 6.12 ± 1.3 GBq m^{-2}) with the aim of performing an intra-patient dose escalation study. In total, 127 single treatments were given. In eight of these 127 single treatments, total doses of ≥3.7 GBq were administered. In an effort to prevent renal toxicity, two patients received Hartmann–Hepa 8% amino acids (including lysine and arginine) solution during all therapy cycles, while 13 patients did so during some but not all therapy cycles; in 14 patients no solution was administered during the therapy cycles. Of the 29 patients, 24 patients showed no severe renal or hematological toxicity (toxicity ≤grade 2 according to the National Cancer Institute grading criteria). These 24 patients received a cumulative dose of ≤7.4 GBq m^{-2}. Five patients developed renal and/or hematological toxicity. All of these five patients received a cumulative dose of >7.4 GBq m^{-2} and had received no Hartmann–Hepa 8% solution during the therapy cycles. Four of the five patients developed renal toxicity; two of these patients showed stable renal insufficiency and two required hemodialysis. Two of the five patients exhibited anemia (both grade 3) and thrombocytopenia (grade 2 and 4, respectively). Twenty of the 29 patients had disease stabilization, two a partial remission, four a reduction of tumor mass <50% and three a progression of tumor growth.

Waldherr *et al.* reported several phase 2 studies in patients with neuroendocrine tumors.[34–36] The patients received four or more single doses of [^{90}Y-DOTA,Tyr^3]octreotide with ascending activity at intervals of approximately 6 weeks. Observed renal or hematological toxicity was ≤grade 2 according to the National Cancer Institute grading criteria. The cumulative dose was ≤7.4 GBq m^{-2}. Complete and partial responses obtained in different studies amounted to 24% (Table 17B.2). In addition, distinct protocols were compared: in the above-mentioned studies, patients received four injections of 1.85 GBq m^{-2} (at intervals of about 6 weeks), while in another study two injections of 3.7 GBq m^{-2} were administered at an interval of 8 weeks. Interestingly, the results from the last study were the most impressive. A higher percentage of complete responses plus partial remissions (24% after four injections versus 33% after two injections) was found, while side-effects were not significantly different.[36] It should be emphasized, however, that this was not a randomized trial comparing two dosing schemes.

Chinol *et al.*[37] from the European Institute of Oncology (Milan, Italy) described dosimetric and dose-finding studies with [^{90}Y-DOTA,Tyr^3]octreotide with and without the administration of kidney protecting agents. No major acute reactions were observed up to an administered dose of 5.6 GBq per cycle. Reversible grade 3 hematological toxicity was found in patients injected with 5.2 GBq, which was defined as the maximum tolerated dose per cycle. None of the patients developed acute or delayed kidney nephropathy, although follow-up was short. Partial and complete remissions were reported by the same group in 28% of 87 patients with neuroendocrine tumors.[38] In more detailed publications from the same group, Bodei *et al.*[28,30] report the results of a phase 1 study in 40 patients with somatostatin receptor-positive tumors, of whom 21 had GEP tumors. Cumulative total treatment doses ranged from 5.9 to 11.1 GBq, given in two treatment cycles. Six of 21 (29%) patients had tumor regression (Table 17B.2). Median duration of the response was 9 months. Bodei *et al.* recently also evaluated the efficacy of [^{90}Y-DOTA,Tyr^3]octreotide therapy in metastatic MTC patients with positive [^{111}In-DTPA]octreotide scintigram, progressing after conventional treatments. Twenty-one patients were retrospectively evaluated after therapy, receiving 7.5–19.2 GBq in 2–8 cycles. Two patients (10%) obtained a CR, while SD was observed in 12 patients (57%); seven patients (33%) did not respond to therapy. The duration of the response ranged between 3 and 40 months.[30]

Another study with [^{90}Y-DOTA,Tyr^3]octreotide (OctreoTher, ^{90}Y-SMT-487) was the phase I Novartis study performed in Rotterdam, Brussels, and Tampa, which aimed to define the maximum tolerated single- and four-cycle doses of [^{90}Y-DOTA,Tyr^3]octreotide and in which patients received escalating doses up to 14.8 GBq m^{-2} in four cycles or up to 9.3 GBq m^{-2} single dose, without reaching the maximum tolerated single dose.[18,39,40] The cumulative radiation dose to kidneys was limited to 27 Gy. All patients received amino acids concomitant with [^{90}Y-DOTA,Tyr^3] octreotide for kidney protection. Three patients had dose-limiting toxicity: one liver toxicity, one thrombocytopenia grade 4 ($<25 \times 10^9$/L), and one MDS. Four out of 54 (7%) patients who had received their maximum allowed dose had PR, and seven (13%) MR (Table 17B.2). The median time to progression in the 44 patients who had either stable disease (SD), MR or PR was 30 months. An important observation in this study was a clear dose–response relationship: the percentage reduction in tumor volume increased with increasing tumor radiation dose (up to about 600 Gy).[41] Prior chemotherapy predisposed to hematological toxicity. Renal toxicity was mild in these patients, with individualized dosimetry and amino acid infusion for kidney protection. Despite the differences in the protocols used, the rate of complete plus partial responses seen in the various aforementioned studies [^{90}Y-DOTA,Tyr^3]octreotide studies consistently exceeds that obtained with [^{111}In-DTPA] octreotide (see above).

Clinical studies with [^{177}Lu-DOTA,Tyr^3]octreotate

Most promising is the use of [^{177}Lu-DOTA,Tyr^3]octreotate. In a comparison in patients, it was found that the uptake of

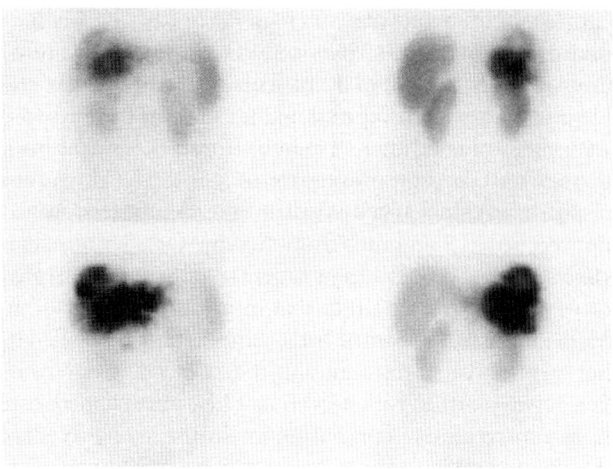

Figure 17B.1   *Abdominal images in a patient with liver metastases from a neuroendocrine pancreatic tumor. Upper row: scintigram, 24 h after injection of 222 MBq [^{111}In-DTPA]octreotide; anterior (left) and posterior abdominal views. Lower row: Post-therapy scan, 1 day after injection of 7.4 GBq [^{177}Lu-DOTA,Tyr^3]octreotate. Note the higher uptake in the metastases after [^{177}Lu-DOTA,Tyr^3]octreotate. Physiologic uptake in the liver, spleen and kidneys is seen on all scans. (Figure reprinted by permission of the Society of Nuclear medicine from: Kwekkeboom DJ, Mueller-Brand J, Paganelli G, et al. An overview of the results of peptide receptor radionuclide therapy with 3 different radiolabeled somatostatin analogs. J Nucl Med 2004; fall supplement, figure 1.)*

radioactivity, expressed as percentage of the injected dose of [^{177}Lu-DOTA,Tyr^3]octreotate, was comparable to that after [^{111}In-DTPA^0]octreotide for kidneys, spleen and liver, but was 3- to 4-fold higher for four of five tumors[29] (Fig. 17B.1). Therefore, [^{177}Lu-DOTA,Tyr^3]octreotate potentially represents an important improvement because of the higher absorbed doses that can be achieved to most tumors with about equal doses to potentially dose-limiting organs and because of the lower tissue penetration range of ^{177}Lu if compared with ^{90}Y, which may be especially important for small tumors.

The first treatment effects of [^{177}Lu-DOTA,Tyr^3]octreotate therapy were described in 35 patients with neuroendocrine GEP tumors, who had a follow-up of 3–6 months after receiving their final dose.[42] Patients were treated with doses of 3.7, 5.6 or 7.4 GBq [^{177}Lu-DOTA,Tyr^3]octreotate, up to a final cumulative dose of 22.2–29.6 GBq, with treatment intervals of 6–9 weeks. The effects of the therapy on tumor size were evaluable in 34 patients. Three months after the final administration a complete remission (CR) was found in one patient (3%), PR in 12 (35%), SD in 14 (41%), and progressive disease (PD) in seven (21%), including three patients who died during the treatment period. The side-effects of treatment with [^{177}Lu-DOTA,Tyr^3]octreotate were few and mostly transient, with mild bone marrow depression as the most common finding. In a more recent update of this treatment in 76 patients with GEP tumors,[43]

CR was found in one patient (1%), PR in 22 (29%), MR in nine (12%), SD in 30 (39%), and PD in 14 patients (18%) (Table 17B.2). Six out of 32 patients who had initially stable disease or tumor regression after the therapy and who were also evaluated after 12 months (mean 18 months from therapy start) became progressive; in the other 26 the tumor response was unchanged. Median time to progression was not reached at 25 months from therapy start. Serious side-effects in the whole group of patients who had been treated or were being treated up to that moment, consisted of an MDS in a patient who had had chemotherapy with alkylating agents 2 years before entering the study, and renal insufficiency in another patient who had had unexplained rises in serum creatinine concentrations in the year preceding the therapy start and who had a urinary creatinine clearance of 41 ml min^{-1} when entering the study. Tumor regression was positively correlated with a high uptake on the [^{111}In-DTPA]octreotide scintigram, limited hepatic tumor mass, and high Karnofsky performance score.

In patients with progressive metastatic (or recurrent) differentiated thyroid carcinoma (DTC), who do not respond to radioiodine therapy or do not show uptake on radioiodine scintigraphy, treatment options are few. As these tumors may express somatostatin receptors, PRRT using somatostatin analogs might be effective, therefore we evaluated the therapeutic efficacy of [^{177}Lu-DOTA,Tyr^3]octreotate in patients with DTC. Furthermore, the uptake of radioactivity in the tumors was studied in relation to treatment outcome. Five patients with DTC were treated with 22.4–30.1 GBq of [^{177}Lu-DOTA,Tyr^3]octreotate. Three patients had Hurthle cell thyroid carcinoma (HCTC), one patient had papillary thyroid carcinoma (PTC) and one had follicular thyroid carcinoma (FTC). The uptake on [^{177}Lu-DOTA,Tyr^3]octreotate scintigraphy was compared with the uptake on the pretherapy [^{111}In-DTPA]octreotide scintigram. After the last treatment with [^{177}Lu-DOTA,Tyr^3]octreotate, one patient had SD as the maximum response, whereas the other two patients had MR and PR, respectively. The response in PTC and FTC was SD and progressive disease, respectively. The patients with MR and PR had the highest [^{177}Lu-DOTA,Tyr^3]octreotate versus [^{111}In-DTPA]octreotide uptake ratios. We concluded that in patients with progressive DTC with no therapeutic option remaining and with sufficient uptake of [^{111}In-DTPA]octreotide in the tumor lesions, [^{177}Lu-DOTA,Tyr^3]octreotate therapy can be effective. This finding is especially important in patients with HCTC, as these patients cannot benefit from radioiodine therapy because of non-iodine avid lesions at diagnosis (*J Nucl Med*, radionuclide therapy supplement, accepted for publication).

Comparison of the different treatments

Treatment with radiolabeled somatostatin analogs is a promising new tool in the management of patients with inoperable or metastasized neuroendocrine tumors. The results that were obtained with [^{90}Y-DOTA,Tyr^3]octreotide and [^{177}Lu-DOTA,Tyr^3]octreotate are very encouraging, although a direct, randomized comparison between the various treatments is lacking. Also, the reported percentages of tumor remission after [^{90}Y-DOTA,Tyr^3]octreotide treatment vary. This may have several causes. Firstly, the administered doses and dosing schemes differ: some studies use dose-escalating schemes, whereas others use fixed doses. Secondly, there are several patient and tumor characteristics that determine treatment outcome, such as amount of uptake on the [^{111}In-DTPA]octreotide scintigram, the estimated total tumor burden, and the extent of liver involvement. Therefore, differences in patient selection may play an important role in determining treatment outcome. Other factors that can have contributed to the different results that were found in the different centers performing trials with the same compounds, may be differences in tumor response criteria, and centralized versus decentralized follow-up CT scoring. Therefore, in order to establish which treatment scheme and which radiolabeled somatostatin analogs or combination of analogs is optimal, randomized trials are needed.

[^{90}Y-DOTA]LANREOTIDE

Virgolini *et al.* developed an ^{111}In- or ^{90}Y-labeled somatostatin analog, [DOTA]lanreotide, for tumor diagnosis and therapy.[44–47] They described that ^{111}In-labeled [DOTA]lanreotide bound with high affinity to hsst$_2$, hsst$_3$, hsst$_4$, and hsst$_5$ and with lower affinity to hsst$_1$ expressed on COS7 cells, making it a universal receptor binder.[48] However, Reubi *et al.*[4] found that [^{90}Y-DOTA]lanreotide had a good affinity for the sst$_5$ in *in vitro* cell lines transfected with the different somatostatin receptor subtypes, whereas it had a low affinity for sst$_3$ (IC$_{50}$ 290 nM) and sst$_4$ (IC$_{50}$ > 10 000 nM). By comparing various compounds, including [DOTA,Tyr^3]octreotide and [DOTA]lanreotide, in rats Froidevaux *et al.*[49] concluded that radiolabeled [DOTA,Tyr^3]octreotide has more potential for clinical application than [DOTA]lanreotide.

Clinical data with [^{90}Y-DOTA]lanreotide

Lanreotide labeled with ^{90}Y was the second analog used for clinical PRRT studies at different centers in the MAURITIUS trial.[46] In this study, cumulative treatment doses of up to 8.58 GBq [^{90}Y-DOTA]lanreotide were given as a short-term intravenous infusion. Treatment results in 154 patients indicated minor responses in 14%. No severe acute or chronic hematological toxicity or changes in renal or liver function parameters due to [^{90}Y-DOTA]lanreotide were reported. In two thirds of patients with neuroendocrine tumor lesions, [^{90}Y-DOTA,Tyr^3]octreotide showed a higher tumor uptake than [^{90}Y-DOTA]lanreotide, which can be explained by the lower affinity of [^{90}Y-DOTA]lanreotide for sst$_2$.

PATIENT CHARACTERISTICS

Despite differences in amounts and types of radioactivity that are administered, there are also shared patient and disease characteristics, as well as similar exclusion and inclusion criteria between the various studies with radiolabeled somatostatin analogs.

Needless to say, all protocols share the feature that the patients' tumors have to show uptake on the diagnostic [^{111}In-DTPA]octreotide scintigram. In some studies, the amount of uptake has at least to equal that of normal liver tissue, in others it is required to be more than that. Most studies also require a patient life expectancy of at least 3–6 months, which makes sense if the administration of the total cumulative dose takes several months and a study objective is to evaluate tumor response. Also, as in all studies with new treatment modalities, other, accepted, treatments have to be exhausted, i.e. in case of neuroendocrine GEP tumors, the tumors have to be inoperable or metastasized. Because of the absorbed radiation doses to especially the kidneys and the bone marrow, most studies require certain minimum kidney function and hematological parameters for study entry and for each new administration. Lastly, the patients have to meet a minimum performance score as they are isolated in a nuclear medicine ward for a variable time, depending on national laws on radiation protection.

[^{90}Y–DTPA–D–GLU]MINIGASTRIN

It has been shown that medullary thyroid carcinoma and other tumors overexpress CCK-B receptors in a high percentage of cases, enabling scintigraphy and radionuclide therapy by targeting of the CCK-B receptors.[50] Radiolabeled CCK analogs have been developed to target these receptors.[51,52] Behr and Behe used a different approach, applying a minigastrin analog with high affinity for the CCK-B receptor and radiolabeled with ^{90}Y via stabilized DTPA (DTPA-D-Glu) as a chelator for PRRT.[53] In eight patients with advanced metastatic disease who received escalating doses of 4×1110 to 4×1850 MBq m^{-2}, a most promising 25% partial response rate was found. Efficacy was associated with the higher dose levels. Hematological and renal toxicities were identified as the dose-limiting toxicities at the 1480 and 1850 MBq m^{-2} levels.

OPTIONS FOR IMPROVING PEPTIDE RECEPTOR RADIONUCLIDE THERAPY

From animal experiments it can be inferred that ^{90}Y-labeled somatostatin analogs may be more effective for larger tumors, whereas ^{177}Lu-labeled somatostatin analogs may be more effective for smaller tumors, but their combination may be the most effective.[54] Therefore, apart from comparisons between radiolabeled octreotate and octreotide, and between somatostatin analogs labeled with ^{90}Y or ^{177}Lu, PRRT with combinations of ^{90}Y- and ^{177}Lu-labeled analogs should also be evaluated. Apart from the combination of analogs labeled with different radionuclides, future directions to improve this therapy will also include efforts to increase the somatostatin receptor number on the tumors, studies on the effects of the use of radiosensitizers as well as development of new peptide analogs. An interesting example is [DOTA, 1-Nal^3]octreotide, which has high affinity for sst$_2$, sst$_3$, and sst$_5$.[55] This compound may allow PRRT of tumors which do not bind octreotide and octreotate with high affinity, i.e. sst$_3$- and sst$_5$-positive tumors.

CONCLUSION

Treatment with radiolabeled somatostatin analogs is a promising new tool in the management of patients with inoperable or metastasized (neuro)endocrine tumors. Symptomatic improvement may occur with all ^{111}In, ^{90}Y or ^{177}Lu-labeled somatostatin analogs that have been used for PRRT. In particular, the results that were obtained with [^{90}Y-DOTA,Tyr^3]octreotide and [^{177}Lu-DOTA,Tyr^3]octreotate are very encouraging in terms of tumor regression. Also, if kidney protective agents are used, the side-effects of this therapy are few and mild, and the duration of the therapy response for both radiopharmaceuticals is more than 2 years. These data compare favorably with the limited number of alternative treatment approaches.

REFERENCES

- ● Seminal primary article
- ◆ Key review paper

- ◆ 1 Patel YC, Greenwood MT, Panetta R, *et al.* The somatostatin receptor family. *Life Sci* 1995; **57**: 1249–65.
- ◆ 2 Patel YC. Somatostatin and its receptor family. *Front Neuroendocrinol* 1999; **20**: 157–98.
- ◆ 3 Schonbrunn A. Somatostatin receptors present knowledge and future directions. *Ann Oncol* 1999; **10**: S17–21.
- ● 4 Reubi JC, Schar JC, Waser B, *et al.* Affinity profiles for human somatostatin receptor subtypes SST1-SST5 of somatostatin radiotracers selected for scintigraphic and radiotherapeutic use. *Eur J Nucl Med* 2000; **27**: 273–82.
- ● 5 Kvols LK, Moertel CG, O'Connell MJ, *et al.* Treatment of the malignant carcinoid syndrome. Evaluation of a long-acting somatostatin analogue. *N Engl J Med* 1986; **315**: 663–6.

◆ 6   Eriksson B, Oberg K. Summing up 15 years of somatostatin analog therapy in neuroendocrine tumors: future outlook. *Ann Oncol* 1999; **10**: S31–8.

◆ 7   Lamberts SW, Krenning EP, Reubi JC. The role of somatostatin and its analogs in the diagnosis and treatment of tumors. *Endocr Rev* 1991; **12**: 450–82.

● 8   Lamberts SW, Reubi JC, Krenning EP. Somatostatin analogs in the treatment of acromegaly. *Endocrinol Metab Clin North Am* 1992; **21**: 737–52.

◆ 9   Janson ET, Oberg K. Long-term management of the carcinoid syndrome. Treatment with octreotide alone and in combination with alpha-interferon. *Acta Oncol* 1993; **32**: 225–9.

● 10 Andersson P, Forssell-Aronsson E, Johanson V, *et al.* Internalization of indium-111 into human neuro-endocrine tumor cells after incubation with indium-111-DTPA-D-Phe1-octreotide. *J Nucl Med* 1996; **37**: 2002–6.

● 11 De Jong M, Bernard BF, De Bruin E, *et al.* Internalization of radiolabelled [DTPA^0]octreotide and [DOTA^0,Tyr^3]octreotide: peptides for somato-statin receptor-targeted scintigraphy and radio-nuclide therapy. *Nucl Med Commun* 1998; **19**: 283–8.

● 12 Hofland LJ, van Koetsveld PM, Waaijers M, Lamberts SW. Internalisation of isotope-coupled somatostatin analogues. *Digestion* 1996; **57**: 2–6.

● 13 Duncan JR, Stephenson MT, Wu HP, Anderson CJ. Indium-111-diethylenetriaminepentaacetic acid-octreotide is delivered in vivo to pancreatic, tumor cell, renal, and hepatocyte lysosomes. *Cancer Res* 1997; **57**: 659–71.

● 14 Hornick CA, Anthony CT, Hughey S, *et al.* Progressive nuclear translocation of somatostatin analogs. *J Nucl Med* 2000; **41**: 1256–63.

● 15 Wang M, Caruano AL, Lewis MR, *et al.* Subcellular localization of radiolabeled somatostatin analogues: implications for targeted radiotherapy of cancer. *Cancer Res* 2003; **63**: 6864–9.

● 16 Xue LY, Butler NJ, Makrigiorgos GM, *et al.* Bystander effect produced by radiolabeled tumor cells in vivo. *Proc Natl Acad Sci USA* 2002; **99**: 13765–70.

● 17 Valkema R, De Jong M, Bakker WH, *et al.* Phase I study of peptide receptor radionuclide therapy with [In- DTPA]octreotide: the Rotterdam experience. *Semin Nucl Med* 2002; **32**: 110–22.

● 18 Valkema R, Pauwels S, Kvols L, *et al.* Long-term follow-up of a phase 1 study of peptide receptor radionuclide therapy (PRRT) with [^{90}Y-DOTA^0, Tyr^3]octreotide in patients with somatostatin receptor positive tumours. *Eur J Nucl Med Mol Imaging* 2003; **30**: S232.

● 19 Anthony LB, Woltering EA, Espenan GD, *et al.* Indium-111-pentetreotide prolongs survival in gastroenteropancreatic malignancies. *Semin Nucl Med* 2002; **32**: 123–32.

◆ 20 McCarthy KE, Woltering EA, Anthony LB. In situ radiotherapy with ^{111}In-pentetreotide. State of the art and perspectives. *Q J Nucl Med* 2000; **44**: 88–95.

◆ 21 McCarthy KE, Woltering EA, Espenan GD, *et al.* In situ radiotherapy with ^{111}In-pentetreotide: initial observations and future directions. *Cancer J Sci Am* 1998; **4**: 94–102.

● 22 Stokkel MP, Verkooijen RB, Bouwsma H, Smit JW. Six month follow-up after ^{111}In-DTPA-octreotide therapy in patients with progressive radioiodine non-responsive thyroid cancer: a pilot study. *Nucl Med Commun* 2004; **25**: 683–90.

● 23 de Jong M, Breeman WA, Bakker WH, *et al.* Comparison of (111)In-labeled somatostatin ana-logues for tumor scintigraphy and radionuclide therapy. *Cancer Res* 1998; **58**: 437–41.

● 24 Kwekkeboom DJ, Kooij PP, Bakker WH, *et al.* Comparison of ^{111}In-DOTA-Tyr^3-octreotide and ^{111}In-DTPA-octreotide in the same patients: bio-distribution, kinetics, organ and tumor uptake. *J Nucl Med* 1999; **40**: 762–7.

● 25 de Jong M, Rolleman EJ, Bernard BF, *et al.* Inhibition of renal uptake of indium-111-DTPA-octreotide in vivo. *J Nucl Med* 1996; **37**: 1388–92.

● 26 Bernard BF, Krenning EP, Breeman WA, *et al.* D-lysine reduction of indium-111 octreotide and yttrium-90 octreotide renal uptake. *J Nucl Med* 1997; **38**: 1929–33.

● 27 Rolleman EJ, Valkema R, de Jong M, *et al.* Safe and effective inhibition of renal uptake of radiolabelled octreotide by a combination of lysine and arginine. *Eur J Nucl Med Mol Imaging* 2003; **30**: 9–15.

● 28 Bodei L, Cremonesi M, Zoboli S, *et al.* Receptor-mediated radionuclide therapy with ^{90}Y-DOTATOC in association with amino acid infusion: a phase I study. *Eur J Nucl Med Mol Imaging* 2003; **30**: 207–16.

● 29 Kwekkeboom DJ, Bakker WH, Kooij PPM, *et al.* [^{177}Lu-DOTA^0,Tyr^3]octreotate: comparison with [^{111}In-DTPA^0]octreotide in patients. *Eur J Nucl Med* 2001; **28**: 1319–25.

◆ 30 Bodei L, Cremonesi M, Grana C, *et al.* Receptor radionuclide therapy with ^{90}Y-[DOTA]^0-Tyr^3-octreotide (^{90}Y-DOTATOC) in neuroendocrine tumours. *Eur J Nucl Med Mol Imaging* 2004; **31**: 1038–46.

● 31 Otte A, Herrmann R, Heppeler A, *et al.* Yttrium-90 DOTATOC: first clinical results. *Eur J Nucl Med* 1999; **26**: 1439–1447.

● 32 Otte A, Herrmann R, Macke HR, Muller-Brand J. [Yttrium 90 DOTATOC: a new somatostatin analog for cancer therapy of neuroendocrine tumors]. *Schweiz Rundsch Med Prax* 1999; **88**: 1263–8.

● 33 Otte A, Mueller-Brand J, Dellas S, *et al.* Yttrium-90-labelled somatostatin-analogue for cancer treatment [Letter]. *Lancet* 1998; **351**: 417–8.

34 Waldherr C, Pless M, Maecke HR, Haldemann A, Mueller-Brand J. The clinical value of [^{90}Y-DOTA]-D-Phe^1-Tyr^3-octreotide (^{90}Y-DOTATOC) in the treatment of neuroendocrine tumours: a clinical phase II study. *Ann Oncol* 2001; **12**: 941–5.

35 Waldherr C, Pless M, Maecke HR, *et al*. Tumor response and clinical benefit in neuroendocrine tumors after 7.4 GBq (90)Y-DOTATOC. *J Nucl Med* 2002; **43**: 610–16.

36 Waldherr C, Schumacher T, Maecke HR, *et al*. Does tumor response depend on the number of treatment sessions at constant injected dose using ^{90}Yttrium-DOTATOC in neuroendocrine tumors? *Eur J Nucl Med* 2002; **29**: S100.

37 Chinol M, Bodei L, Cremonesi M, Paganelli G. Receptor-mediated radiotherapy with Y-DOTA-D-Phe-Tyr-octreotide: the experience of the European Institute of Oncology Group. *Semin Nucl Med* 2002; **32**: 141–7.

38 Paganelli G, Bodei L, Handkiewicz Junak D, *et al*. ^{90}Y-DOTA-D-Phe^1-Try^3-octreotide in therapy of neuroendocrine malignancies. *Biopolymers* 2002; **66**: 393–8.

39 Smith MC, Liu J, Chen T, *et al*. OctreoTher: ongoing early clinical development of a somatostatin-receptor-targeted radionuclide antineoplastic therapy. *Digestion* 2000; **62**: 69–72.

40 Valkema R, Kvols L, Jamar F, *et al*. Phase 1 study of therapy with ^{90}Y-SMT487 (OctreoTher) in patients with somatostatin receptor-positive tumors. *J Nucl Med* 2002; **43**: 33P.

41 Jonard P, Jamar F, Walrand S, *et al*. Tumor dosimetry based on PET ^{86}Y-DOTA-Tyr^3-octreotide (SMT487) and CT-scan predicts tumor response to ^{90}Y-SMT487 (OctreoTher). *J Nucl Med* 2000; **41**: 111P.

42 Kwekkeboom DJ, Bakker WH, Kam BL, *et al*. Treatment of patients with gastro-entero-pancreatic (GEP) tumours with the novel radiolabelled somatostatin analogue [^{177}Lu-DOTA(0),Tyr^3]octreotate. *Eur J Nucl Med Mol Imaging* 2003; **30**: 417–22.

43 Kwekkeboom DJ, Bakker WH, Teunissen JJM, Kooij PPM, Krenning EP. Treatment with Lu-177-DOTA-Tyr3-Octreotate in patients with neuroendocrine tumors: interim results. *Eur J Nucl Med Mol Imaging* 2003; **30**: S231.

44 Virgolini I, Traub T, Novotny C, *et al*. Experience with indium-111 and yttrium-90-labeled somatostatin analogs. *Curr Pharm Des* 2002; **8**: 1781–807.

45 Virgolini I, Szilvasi I, Kurtaran A, *et al*. Indium-111-DOTA-lanreotide: biodistribution, safety and radiation absorbed dose in tumor patients. *J Nucl Med* 1998; **39**: 1928–36.

46 Virgolini I, Britton K, Buscombe J, *et al*. In- and Y-DOTA-lanreotide: results and implications of the MAURITIUS trial. *Semin Nucl Med* 2002; **32**: 148–55.

47 Virgolini I, Kurtaran A, Angelberger P, *et al*. 'MAURITIUS': tumour dose in patients with advanced carcinoma. *Ital J Gastroenterol Hepatol* 1999; **31(Suppl 2)**: S227–30.

48 Smith-Jones PM, Bischof C, Leimer M, *et al*. DOTA-lanreotide: a novel somatostatin analog for tumor diagnosis and therapy. *Endocrinology* 1999; **140**: 5136–48.

49 Froidevaux S, Heppeler A, Eberle AN, *et al*. Preclinical comparison in AR4-2J tumor-bearing mice of four radiolabeled 1,4,7,10-tetraazacyclododecane-1,4,7,10-tetraacetic acid-somatostatin analogs for tumor diagnosis and internal radiotherapy. *Endocrinology* 2000; **141**: 3304–12.

50 Reubi JC, Schaer JC, Waser B. Cholecystokinin (CCK)-A and CCK-B/gastrin receptors in human tumors. *Cancer Res* 1997; **57**: 1377–86.

51 Kwekkeboom DJ, Bakker WH, Kooij PP, *et al*. Cholecystokinin receptor imaging using an octapeptide DTPA-CCK analogue in patients with medullary thyroid carcinoma. *Eur J Nucl Med* 2000; **27**: 1312–17.

52 de Jong M, Bakker WH, Bernard BF, *et al*. Preclinical and initial clinical evaluation of ^{111}In-labeled nonsulfated CCK8 analog: a peptide for CCK-B receptor-targeted scintigraphy and radionuclide therapy. *J Nucl Med* 1999; **40**: 2081–7.

53 Behr TM, Behe MP. Cholecystokinin-B/gastrin receptor-targeting peptides for staging and therapy of medullary thyroid cancer and other cholecystokinin-B receptor-expressing malignancies. *Semin Nucl Med* 2002; **32**: 97–109.

54 De Jong M, Bernard HF, Breeman WAP, *et al*. Combination of ^{90}Y- and ^{177}Lu-labeled somatostatin analogs is superior for radionuclide therapy compared to ^{90}Y- or ^{177}Lu-labeled analogs only. *J Nucl Med* 2002; **43**: 123P–4.

55 Schmitt JS, Wild D, Ginj M, *et al*. DOTA-NOC, a high affinity ligand of the somatostatin receptor subtypes 2, 3 and 5 for radiotherapy. *J Labelled Cpd Radiopharm* 2001; **44**: S697–9.

Neuroblastoma

CORNELIS A. HOEFNAGEL

THE DISEASE

Neuroblastoma is a malignant tumor of the sympathetic nervous system, occurring most frequently in early childhood. The reported incidence is around five children per million population per year. Seventy-five percent of neuroblastoma patients are younger than 4 years and the disease is rare after the age of 14. The symptomatology of this disease is variable and depends on the site and size of the primary tumor and its metastases and the levels of the catecholamines dopamine, norepinephrine, and epinephrine, which more than 90% of neuroblastomas produce in excess.

The prognosis and the choice of treatment depends on the stage of disease: localized disease without distant metastases (TNM stage I and II) is treated by complete surgical excision and has a good prognosis (2-year survival rates of 90%); metastasis to lymph nodes and other organs (TNM stage III–V) is correlated with a poor prognosis and is treated by combination chemotherapy preceding surgery for the primary tumor; this is followed by postoperative chemotherapy, sometimes including high-dose chemotherapy requiring allogenic or autologous bone marrow transplantation. Radiation therapy may be added.[1] Although the initial response rate of this treatment is high (up to 80% complete or partial response[2]), most of these children will relapse. Despite combining chemotherapy, surgery, and conventional radiotherapy, the 5-year survival of stage IV disease remained only 10–20%.[3] This may be due to tumor cells becoming resistant to chemotherapeutic agents.

Prognostic factors are the stage of disease, the patient's age, the site of the primary tumor, the pattern and rate of catecholamine excretion, the serum ferritin level at diagnosis, the tumor histology and genetic parameters, for example the amplification of the *myc*-N oncogene and chromosome 1p36 deletion.[1,4,5] Recently, a new European (ESIOP) clinical trial for high risk neuroblastoma patients was started, aiming to improve the outcome by successive use of intensified chemotherapy, surgery, myeloablative therapy with peripheral stem cell rescue, immuno- and differentiation therapy. New approaches to the diagnosis and therapy of neuroblastoma include targeting of radionuclides via the immunologic (monoclonal antibodies) and metabolic (*meta*-iodobenzylguanidine (MIBG)) route.

SPECIFIC TARGETING OF NEUROBLASTOMA

Targeting of neuroblastoma may be achieved by specific tumor seeking radiopharmaceuticals, interacting with the characteristic features of neuroblastoma, either via the metabolic route (MIBG), via receptor binding (peptides) or via the immunological route (antibodies).

An active uptake-1 mechanism at the cell membrane and neurosecretory storage granules in the cytoplasm of neuroblastoma are responsible for the uptake and retention of ^{131}I-MIBG respectively. Although the radiopharmaceutical may be released from the granules, re-uptake through this specific mechanism maintains prolonged intracellular concentration, in contrast to nonadrenergic tissues which rely on passive diffusion only, resulting in high tumor/nontumor ratios. A number of drugs may interfere with the uptake and/or retention of ^{131}I-MIBG. Cumulative results of ^{131}I-MIBG scintigraphy indicate that more than 90% of neuroblastomas concentrate ^{131}I-MIBG.[6] Moreover, ^{131}I-MIBG uptake in a pediatric tumor is highly specific for neuroblastoma.[7] A good concentration and relatively long retention of ^{131}I-MIBG at tumor sites, as shown by tracer studies, enable therapy with this radiopharmaceutical.

Targeting peptide receptors on the cell surface, the somatostatin analogue ^{111}In-pentetreotide (octreotide) and ^{123}I-labeled vasoactive intestinal peptide (VIP) are currently used for diagnostic scintigraphy of neuroendocrine tumors. By autoradiography somatostatin and VIP receptors have been demonstrated in neuroblastoma in 86% and 57% of cases, respectively.[8] Cumulative results of ^{111}In-pentetreotide scintigraphy show a 77% sensitivity in neuroblastoma.[6] Unlike MIBG and antibodies directed against neuroblastoma, ^{111}In-pentetreotide is not specific for neural crest tumors, and the high uptake of ^{111}In-pentetreotide in the kidneys, liver, and spleen is less favorable for radionuclide therapy. In tumors other than neuroblastoma, however, high doses of ^{111}In-pentetreotide have been applied for therapy and phase I and II studies using [90]Y- or ^{177}Lu-labeled octreotide and lanreotide are being conducted.

Parallel to the introduction of radioiodinated MIBG in the early 1980s, several monoclonal antibodies have been developed to antigens present on the cell surface of neuroendocrine tumors or neural tissue. Goldman et al.[9] reported succesful radioimmunoscintigraphic localization of primary tumors and metastases in eight patients with neuroblastoma, using UJ13A labeled with ^{123}I or ^{131}I and Cheung et al. developed a monoclonal antibody against the oncofetal antigen ganglioside G_{D2}, which, unlike UJ13A, does not react significantly with normal tissues other than the central nervous system. Results of radioimmunoscintigraphy using 111–185 MBq (3–5 mCi) [131]I-3F8 showed T/NT ratios of between 10:1 and 20:1 in neuroblastoma and its radiation dosimetry appeared favorable for therapeutic use.[10] More recently, chimeric antibodies specific for a cell surface glycoprotein of human neuroblastoma (chCE7 and ch14.18) yielded high specific tumor uptakes in neuroblastoma-bearing nude mice.[11] Initial results of scintigraphy in patients are promising.[12]

INDICATIONS AND CONTRAINDICATIONS

The indication for ^{131}I-MIBG therapy is stage III and IV neuroblastoma, showing a high and selective tumor uptake and prolonged retention of MIBG. As a systemic treatment, ^{131}I-MIBG therapy will be directed at both the primary tumor and its distant metastases. Contraindications for ^{131}I-MIBG therapy, as well as for radioimmunotherapy, are severe myelosuppression and renal failure; in addition, any unstable condition of the patient, which does not allow isolation therapy, or lack of understanding of or compliance with radiation protection guidelines by the patient's carer are relative contraindications.

The decision to carry out ^{131}I-MIBG therapy should be based on a tracer study, performed 1, 2, and 3 days after administration of 18.5–37 MBq (0.5–1 mCi) ^{131}I-MIBG

(alternatively scintigraphy using ^{123}I-MIBG), in order to assess the tumor uptake and retention, taking into account the other therapeutic possibilities and the clinical condition of the patient.

THERAPEUTIC PROCEDURE

Before scheduling ^{131}I-MIBG therapy, one must be aware of the medication the patient is using, as many drugs are known or may be expected to interfere with the uptake and/or retention of ^{131}I-MIBG by the tumor cell.[13,14] Patients should be taken off these drugs for at least 1 week prior to diagnostic scintigraphy or therapy using MIBG, and, if necessary, may be put on propanolol and dibenilene (phenoxybenzamide) to control hypertension.

As ^{131}I-MIBG concentrates are usually shipped frozen, upon arrival in the hospital defrosting is achieved by placing the vial within its lead container in a 37°C water bath for 45 min. The total activity is measured using a dose calibrator. Subsequently the concentrate is diluted into an infusion bottle or large syringe containing 0.9% NaCl or 5% glucose solution (dependent on the manufacturer's instructions). A sample is withdrawn for quality control. All these procedures must be carried out in a shielded laminar flow cabinet to reduce the radiation dose to personnel and to ensure sterility of the preparation to be infused.

Before the administration of a therapeutic dose, quality control, checking both the radionuclide and radiochemical purity, may be desirable, as impurities may add to the side-effects of the treatment. High doses of ^{131}I-MIBG with a high specific activity are liable to autoradiolysis, which is dependent on the temperature, the volume, and the presence of stabilizers and scavengers in the formulation.[15]

Generally, a fixed dose of 3.7–7.4 GBq (100–200 mCi) of ^{131}I-MIBG with a high specific activity (up to 1.48 GBq mg^{-1}) is administered intravenously over 1–4 h through a lead-shielded infusion system. An alternative approach is to administer a varying, calculated dose, as assessed by a prior tracer study, aiming for the maximal acceptable 2 Gy bone marrow dose.[16] Several therapeutic doses may be required to attain an objective response, at not less than 4-weekly intervals, depending on the platelet recovery.

Patients must use oral potassium iodide (100 mg daily, starting 1 day before administration of the therapy) to protect the thyroid from free ^{131}I and need to be isolated in a dedicated room suited for radionuclide therapy. The criteria of discharge of patients from the isolation room depend on local legislation.

CONSIDERATIONS IN RADIONUCLIDE THERAPY OF CHILDREN

Isolation may present practical difficulties when treating young children. Problems can be minimized by inviting parents or other relatives to become actively involved in the patient's care. This was found to be both feasible and safe, provided that a number of precautions were taken.[17]

Parents may stay in an adjacent room, linked to the isolation unit by closed circuit television and intercom. When entering the isolation room they must wear a disposable gown, gloves, and shoes which are left in the locker when they leave the room. They need to be instructed to restrict the time of exposure to a minimum, to keep as much distance as possible, not to drink or eat in the isolation room and how to handle radioactive waste. Throughout the isolation period they receive an oral dose of 200 mg potassium iodide daily, starting the day before treatment, to protect the thyroid from inadvertent ^{131}I contamination. Pregnant women and children are to be excluded from patient care and visiting. The external radiation dose to the parent can be measured continuously by a pocket dosemeter and internal contamination may be monitored by measuring a urine sample in a gamma counter. By adding up the measured external radiation dose, the (negligible) internal contamination and the calculated dose received at home assuming a 'mean distance factor', the overall radiation dose these parents theoretically may be exposed to was estimated to vary between 0.4 and 3 mSv.[18] It can therefore be concluded, that the participation of parents in patient care during ^{131}I-MIBG therapy under the conditions mentioned above is safe.

As it is not the treatment but the isolation that will affect children most, they need to be kept busy and amused, e.g. by providing drawing and reading materials, toys, games, and video films. As personal belongings which become contaminated with ^{131}I may have to be stored temporarily, it may not be advisable to bring favorite clothes, toys or other items, the child cannot be without, into the isolation room.

CLINICAL APPLICATIONS OF MIBG THERAPY IN NEUROBLASTOMA

^{131}I–MIBG therapy after conventional treatment

After initial reports in the mid 1980s had indicated the feasibility and therapeutic effect of ^{131}I-MIBG therapy in children with neuroblastoma, small series of patients were reported. In general the following response criteria are used: complete remission (no more evidence of disease), partial remission (>50% reduction of tumor volume), stable disease (<50% reduction of volume or no change). Some groups score a near-total reduction of disease (e.g. by 90%) as a very good partial remission.

Between 1984 and 1991 a phase II study was carried out in 49 children and four adults with progressive recurrent disease after conventional therapy had failed.[19] Using a fixed dose of 3.7–7.4 GBq (100–200 mCi) of ^{131}I-MIBG, infused

in 4 h, the following response was observed: seven complete remissions, 23 partial remissions and arrest of disease (stable disease/no change) in 10 other patients; nine patients had progressive disease and one patient was lost to follow-up. In the majority of patients the duration of objective remissions varied from 2 to 38 months, but in some the response is continuing after up to 14 years. The best results were obtained in patients with bulky soft-tissue disease. Apart from objective response, the palliative effect of the treatment under these conditions was impressive.

Similar results of ^{131}I-MIBG treatment were recorded by Troncone et al.[20] and in a German multicenter study involving 47 patients with stage III or IV neuroblastoma:[21] in the latter study nine children reached a complete or very good partial remission and 13 a partial remission (together giving a 47% objective response). Less favorable results (an objective response rate of 19%) were reported by Garaventa et al.,[22] using lower doses of ^{131}I-MIBG than the studies mentioned above and adjusting the administered dose to the body weight of the child. In a UK multicenter phase I study using dose prescription on the basis of estimated whole body dose, 25 patients with neuroblastoma were treated at whole body dose levels of 1, 2 and 2.5 Gy; the overall response rate was 33% and no correlation between whole body-absorbed dose and tumor response was found.[23]

At international workshops in 1991[24] and 1999 the experience of the major centers in several hundreds of neuroblastoma patients was collected with cumulative results indicating overall objective response rates of 35% and 50%, respectively. This was encouraging, taking into account that most of these patients had stage IV, progressive and intensely pretreated disease, and were only treated with ^{131}I-MIBG after other treatment modalities had failed. In addition, ^{131}I-MIBG therapy provided valuable palliation and improved the quality of life for many children and was well tolerated in comparison with chemotherapy.

^{131}I-MIBG therapy in combination with other treatments

Based upon the observations that oxygen content in tumor cells has a direct influence on the radiosensitivity and hence the effect of radiotherapy, and that a gas enters as a solution into body fluid proportionally to the pressure to which the fluid is exposed (Henry's law), Voûte et al.[25] combined ^{131}I-MIBG therapy with oxygen treatment under hyperbaric conditions, aiming to improve survival in patients with recurrent stage IV neuroblastoma. A number of mechanisms may be active in causing additional damage to the neuroblastoma cells, e.g. the inhibitory effect MIBG has on the mitochondrial respiratory chain, the hyperbaric oxygen inducing the formation of superoxide radicals and the impaired defence mechanism of the neuroblastoma cell to radicals both due to reduced catalase activity and increased ferritin levels. Although it remains difficult to assess the contribution of the individual components, it is postulated that the resulting formation of hydroxyl radicals is toxic to the neuroblastoma cell on top of the ^{131}I-MIBG radiation effect to which it is exposed. Since 1989, 55 patients have been treated with 3.7–7.4 GBq ^{131}I-MIBG, 2–4 days later followed by administration of 5–8 L min^{-1} oxygen at 3 ATA (corresponding to 20 m below sea level) during 1 h in a pressurized chamber once or twice daily for 4 consecutive days. Although this is not a randomized study, the approach proved feasible and encouraging effects on survival were observed. More recently, high dose vitamin C therapy has been added to this regimen to increase the formation of radicals in these ferritin-rich tumors.

Mastrangelo et al.[26] performed pilot studies in 22 patients with advanced neuroblastoma (16 in relapse and six at diagnosis), initially using ^{131}I-MIBG with simultaneous administration of cisplatin. Despite encouraging results long-lasting hematological toxicity occurred; therefore an interval of several days between cisplatin and ^{131}I-MIBG was introduced and subsequently also other chemotherapeutic agents (cyclophosphamide, VP16, vincristine and doxorubicin) were added to this regimen.

Others have chosen to maximize the therapeutic effect of ^{131}I-MIBG by combining it with high-dose chemotherapy followed by autologous bone marrow or stem cell rescue[27,28] or by using ^{131}I-MIBG in a multimodality approach involving high dose melphalan and total-body irradiation with bone marrow rescue.[29] Although complete and partial responses were attained, in such protocols it remains difficult to evaluate to which extent the ^{131}I-MIBG has contributed to the effect and these combinations were associated with severe toxicity.

After a phase I dose-escalating study had established the dose-limiting toxicity of ^{131}I-MIBG at 555 MBq kg^{-1}, Matthay et al.[30] have used myeloablative ^{131}I-MIBG therapy followed by reinfusion of tumor-free, cryopreserved hematopoietic stem cells in 42 patients with refractory neuroblastoma. With administered doses ranging from 3.3 to 31 GBq (median 11.47 GBq) the objective response rate was 38%.

Upfront ^{131}I–MIBG therapy

The observed response to ^{131}I-MIBG therapy in advanced neuroblastoma after conventional therapy, the non-invasiveness of the procedure, and the high metabolic activity which is frequently observed in untreated tumors, led to the concept of substituting ^{131}I-MIBG therapy for combination chemotherapy at diagnosis prior to surgery.[31] The objective of introducing ^{131}I-MIBG therapy as the first therapy in the treatment schedule is to reduce the tumor volume, enabling adequate (>95%) surgical resection of the tumor and to avoid toxicity and the induction of early

drug resistance. The advantages of this approach are that the child's general condition is unaffected or improved before he/she undergoes surgical resection and that chemotherapy is reserved to treat minimal residual disease postoperatively.

Initial results in 31 patients presenting with inoperable stage III or IV neuroblastoma, who were treated according to this protocol, demonstrated the feasibility and effectiveness of this approach.[32] A minimum of two cycles of ^{131}I-MIBG therapy was given to all patients, after which the operability was re-evaluated; patients were then submitted to surgery, or, if still inoperable, received additional ^{131}I-MIBG therapy or were crossed over to combination chemotherapy. After surgery, bone marrow was harvested for high-dose chemotherapy with autologous bone marrow reinfusion at the end of the protocol. The objective response rate of ^{131}I-MIBG therapy at diagnosis was better (>70%) than previously observed after conventional treatment: 19 of 27 evaluable patients had complete or >95% resection of the primary tumor or did not require surgery at all. The case histories on page 760 and the accompanying figures show clinical examples of response to preoperative ^{131}I-MIBG therapy. By 1999, the follow-up of 49 patients showed a survival rate of 38% at 5 years and four of 12 patients with more than 10 years follow-up were alive and well.[33]

Mastrangelo et al.,[34] treating three patients with ^{131}I-MIBG at diagnosis, demonstrated complete dissappearance of the tumor in one patient, persisting for 4 years, and a significant reduction of tumor masses in the other two.

Based upon the results of ^{131}I-MIBG therapy as a single agent in a mixed population of patients, two new protocols have been initiated, integrating upfront ^{131}I-MIBG therapy in two groups of patients, who are divided according to stage and prognostic parameters. The intention is to treat patients with favorable parameters with the least invasive treatment and to intensify the therapy of patients with unfavorable parameters (the so-called high risk group). The first group, patients with unresectable neuroblastoma stage II and III, will receive two cycles of ^{131}I-MIBG therapy only, prior to surgery; only if inoperablity persists, chemotherapy is added. In the second, high risk group (neuroblastoma stage IV, > 1 year of age), upfront ^{131}I-MIBG therapy is combined with topotecan, a topoisomerase I inhibitor enhancing the radiation induced cytotoxicity. Only two therapeutic doses of ^{131}I-MIBG (7.4 and 5.5 GBq, respectively) followed by five daily administrations of 0.7 mg m^{-2} topotecan are administered with an interval of 4 weeks; subsequently four cycles of chemotherapy (VECI) are given prior to surgical resection of the primary tumor. Postoperatively, a single high dose carboplatin and melphalan therapy with peripheral blood stem cells rescue is aimed at treating minimal residual disease, after which 13-cis-retinoic acid is perscribed as a differentiation therapy for 2 years. Initial results of induction therapy with ^{131}I-MIBG and topotecan in 11 patients with high risk neuroblastoma show great effectiveness, but also marrow toxicity.[35]

Therapy using ^{125}I–MIBG

An alternative approach to the management of neuroblastoma is the use of ^{125}I–MIBG for therapy. This may have a role in the treatment of micrometastases and bone marrow infiltration, particularly as the results of ^{131}I-MIBG therapy under these circumstances are poor. Although the range of the [125]I Auger electrons in the storage vesicles would seem to be inadequate to deliver a lethal radiation dose to the nucleus, the finding of a considerable degree of extragranular storage in neuroblastoma[36] may provide a basis for this treatment. After initial experience in five patients with neuroblastoma[37,38] had demonstrated tumor arrest and minor disease regression, results of a phase 1 dose-escalating study showed that higher doses may be administered without causing serious toxicity, as the whole body dose per MBq of ^{125}I-MIBG is about four times lower than that of ^{131}I-MIBG; five of 10 treated patients had over 1 year progression-free survival.[39] The availability of ^{125}I and handling of radioactive waste remain logistical problems of this form of treatment.

Toxicity

In general, both the ^{131}I-MIBG treatment and the isolation are well tolerated by children and the following side-effects may be observed. Hematological effects occur most frequently, predominantly as an isolated thrombocytopenia,[19] which may be partly due to the radiation dose to the bone marrow,[40] but may also be explained by selective uptake of ^{131}I-MIBG into the thrombocytes.[41] Severe bone marrow depression may occur in patients who have bone marrow involvement at the time of MIBG therapy and in patients with delayed renal clearance of ^{131}I-MIBG. In a UK phase I trial, bone marrow suppression was the principal dose-limiting factor: 80% of patients receiving a 2.5 Gy whole-body dose developed grade 3 or 4 thrombocytopenia.[23]

Deterioration of renal function has occasionally been observed in patients whose kidneys have been compromised by intensive pretreatment with cisplatin and ifosfamide.[42] Troncone et al.[20] describe one patient who acquired hypertensive crises shortly after ^{131}I-MIBG therapy requiring alpha-blocking medication. Also hypothyroidism as a consequence of ^{131}I-MIBG therapy in children has been reported.[43,44]

The toxicity of ^{131}I-MIBG therapy at diagnosis is in contrast with the experience of ^{131}I-MIBG therapy after conventional therapy: when used upfront, ^{131}I-MIBG therapy causes isolated thrombocytopenia in fewer patients and bone marrow depression is rare, despite the fact that the bone marrow is invaded in many patients. The relative lack of toxicity of ^{131}I-MIBG therapy at diagnosis indicates that the previously observed more serious side-effects of

^{131}I-MIBG therapy after combination therapy were partly due to the pretreatment, in particular with cisplatin. Both the improvement of the patient's general condition and the minimal toxicity are in contrast with the effects of preoperative combination chemotherapy.

POSSIBLE INTERVENTIONS IN ^{131}I-MIBG THERAPY

Several new applications of MIBG therapy are being investigated, with the aim of improving the therapeutic index. One is the use of other labels for MIBG, for example ^{125}I-MIBG, [211]At-MABG and [76]Br-MBBG.

Tumor targeting may be enhanced by administration of ^{131}I-MIBG by alternative routes, for example the intra-arterial or intraperitoneal route.

By increasing the specific activity and the production of non-carrier-added MIBG it is attempted to improve tumor uptake,[45] but from animal studies and experience with ^{131}I-MIBG therapy in humans, it follows that the optimal specific activity may vary with the tumor type. Excess unlabeled MIBG was found to decrease ^{125}I-MIBG uptake in PC-12 pheochromocytoma xenografts in nude mice, as well as in most normal tissues, but not to influence the uptake in SK-N-SH neuroblastoma.[46]

Pharmacologic interventions may increase the specific uptake and retention of ^{131}I-MIBG, for example by induction of tumor cell differentiation using retinoic acid and interferon,[47] the prolongation of retention by calcium-channel blockers,[48] the blockade of specific normal tissue uptake by unlabeled MIBG[49] or serotonin or by delaying the renal excretion of ^{131}I-MIBG.

The potential contribution of gene therapy to enhancing MIBG uptake by tumors shows promise, particularly in neuroblastoma. The successful introduction of the nor-adrenalin transporter gene (NAT) into NAT negative neuroblastoma cell lines offers the possibility of improving the efficacy of MIBG therapy.[50]

In patients whose neuroblastomas do not or partially concentrate ^{131}I-MIBG, radioimmunotherapy may be an alternative. Although earlier phase I studies, using murine ^{131}I-UJ13A or [131]I-3F8 monoclonal antibodies demonstrated few objective responses, considerable toxicity and limited applicability due to the induction of a human anti-mouse antibody (HAMA) response,[51] new developments include the use of chimeric antibodies, e.g. chCE7 and ch14.18. The therapeutic efficacy of the ^{131}I-labeled anti-L1-CAM antibody chCE7 was demonstrated in nude mice with SK-N-SH neuroblastoma xenograft. In patients, the complementary findings of scintigraphy using ^{123}I-MIBG and ^{131}I-anti-chCE7 underline the heterogeneity of this disease and may have implications for radionuclide therapy of neuroblastoma in the future.[12]

CONCLUSION

In summary, ^{131}I-MIBG therapy is an effective treatment for neuroblastoma, which can be delivered safely, also in children, provided that the bone marrow is free of tumor cells; ^{131}I-MIBG therapy should be used with caution in patients with bone marrow involvement without harvesting stem cells or stored bone marrow support.

^{131}I-MIBG therapy is probably the best palliative treatment for patients with advanced disease, as the invasiveness and toxicity of this therapy compare favorably with that of chemotherapy, immunotherapy, and external beam radiotherapy. The results indicate that ^{131}I-MIBG treatment should be incorporated at an earlier, more favorable moment in the treatment protocol. ^{131}I-MIBG therapy of neuroblastoma at diagnosis may be used instead of combination chemotherapy to attain operability of the primary tumor.

Case history: Case 1

^{131}I-MIBG therapy at diagnosis in a 3-year-old girl with abdominal neuroblastoma metastatic to the bone marrow: three consecutive treatments at 4-week intervals led to significant reduction of metastases and the tumor volume, enabling successful surgical resection.

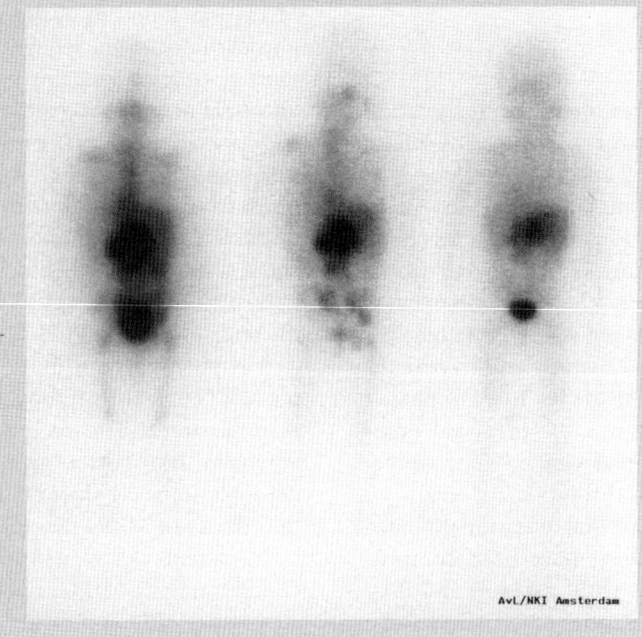

Case history: Case 2

One-year-old boy with a large neuroblastoma in the left upper abdomen and bone marrow involvement, responding well to upfront ^{131}I-MIBG therapy: post-therapy scintigrams (posterior view) show a marked reduction in tumor volume and ^{131}I-MIBG uptake (6.21% dose at second therapy, 1.72% dose at third therapy). Resection of the primary tumor followed.

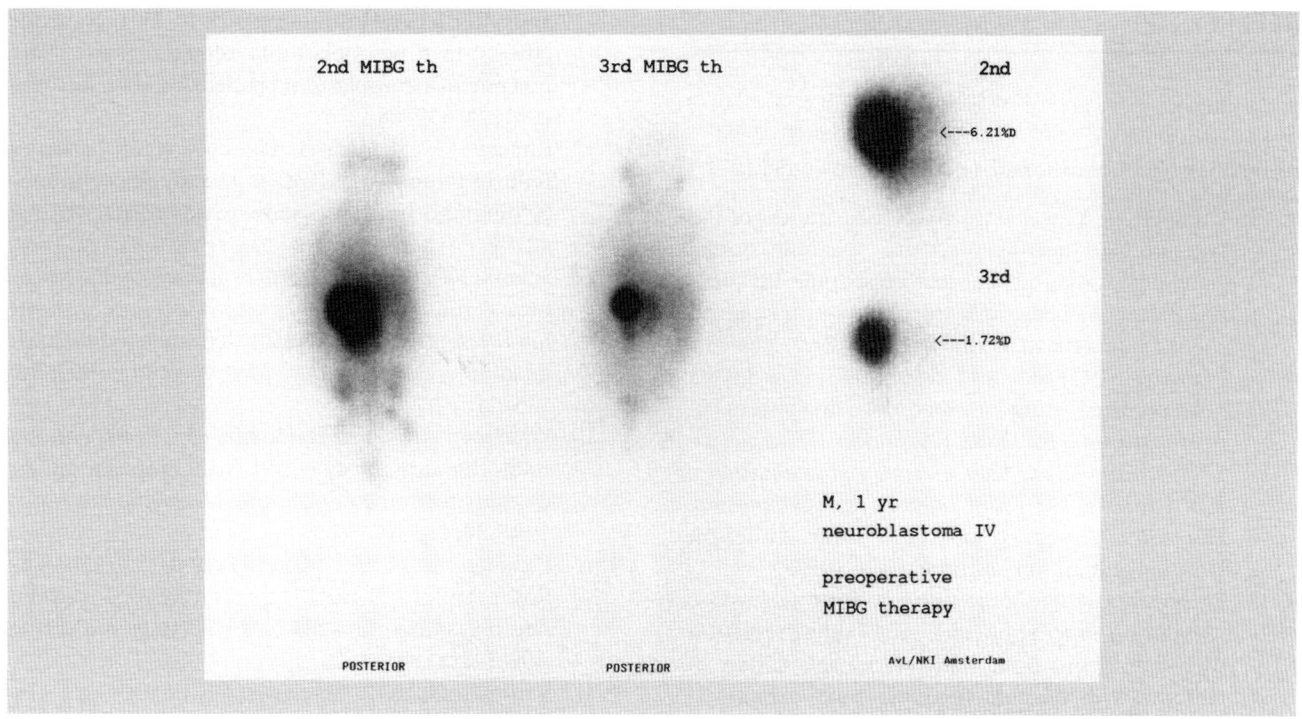

Case history: Case 3

This 2-year-old boy presented with a tumor of the right scapula. It was confirmed to be a neuroblastoma metastasis and ^{131}I-MIBG scintigraphy (left image) demonstrated intense pathological uptake in widespread metastases throughout the bone, bone marrow, and in lymph nodes. However, the location of the primary tumor remained unknown. Upfront treatment with three cycles of ^{131}I-MIBG resulted in a marked regression of disease (middle and right). As there was no primary tumor to be resected, the patient moved on to 'postoperative' chemotherapy directly.

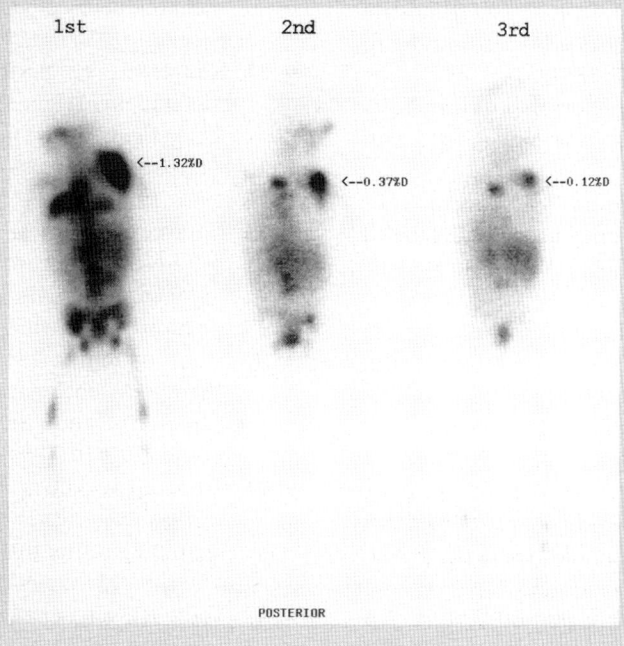

REFERENCES

● Seminal primary article
◆ Key review paper
✱ First formal publication of a management guideline

◆ 1 Voûte PA, de Kraker J, Hoefnagel CA. Tumors of the sympathetic nervous system. Neuroblastoma, ganglioneuroma and phaeochromocytoma. In: Voûte PA, Barrett A, Lemerle J. (eds.) *Cancer in children: clinical management.* Berlin: Springer, 1992: 226–43.

● 2 Pinkerton CR, Pritchard J, de Kraker J, *et al.* ENSG 1-randomized study of high-dose melphalan in neuroblastoma. In: Dicke KA, Spitzer G, Jagannath S. (eds.) *Autologous bone marrow transplantation – Proceedings of the Third International Symposium.* Houston: University of Texas MD Anderson Hospital and Tumor Institute, 1987: 401–5.

● 3 Pinkerton CR, Philip T, Biron P, *et al.* High-dose melphalan, vincristine, and total-body-irradiation with autologous bone marrow transplantation in children with relapsed neuroblastoma: a phase II study. *Med Pediatr Oncol* 1987; **15**: 236–40.

✱ 4 Seeger RC, Brodeur GM, Sather H, *et al.* Association of multiple copies of the N-myc oncogene with rapid progression of neuroblastomas. *N Engl J Med* 1985; **313**: 1111–16.

● 5 Caron H, van Sluis P, van Hoeve M, *et al.* Allelic loss of chromosome 1p36 in neuroblastoma is of preferential maternal origin and correlates with N-myc amplification. *Nature Genetics* 1993; **4**: 187–90.

◆ 6 Hoefnagel CA. Metaiodobenzylguanidine and somatostatin in oncology: role in the management of neural crest tumours. *Eur J Nucl Med* 1994; **21**: 561–81.

● 7 Leung A, Shapiro B, Hattner R, *et al.* The specificity of radioiodinated MIBG for neural crest tumors in childhood. *J Nucl Med* 1997; **38**: 1352–7.

◆ 8 Reubi JC. Neuropeptide receptors in health and disease: the molecular basis for in vivo imaging. *J Nucl Med* 1995; **36**: 1825–35.

✱ 9 Goldman A, Vivian G, Gordon I, *et al.* Immuno-localization of neuroblastoma using radiolabeled monoclonal antibody UJ13A. *J Pediatr* 1984; **105**: 252–6.

● 10 Yeh SDJ, Larson SM, Burch L, *et al.* Radioimmunodetection of neuroblastoma with iodine-131-3F8: correlation with biopsy, iodine-131-metaiodobenzylguanidine and standard diagnostic modalities. *J Nucl Med* 1991; **32**: 769–76.

● 11 Novak-Hofer I, Amstutz HP, Haldemann A, *et al.* Radioimmunolocalization of neuroblastoma xenografts with chimeric antibody chCE7. *J Nucl Med* 1992; **33**: 231–6.

● 12 Hoefnagel CA, Rutgers M, Buitenhuis CKM, *et al.* A comparison of targetting neuroblastoma with mIBG and anti L1-CAM antibody mAB chCE7: therapeutic efficacy in a neuroblastoma xenograft model and imaging of neuroblastoma patients. *Eur J Nucl Med* 2001; **28**: 359–68.

✱ 13 Khafagi FA, Shapiro B, Fig LM, *et al.* Labetalol reduces iodine-131 MIBG uptake by pheochromocytoma and normal tissues. *J Nucl Med* 1989; **30**: 481–9.

◆ 14 Solanki KK, Bomanji J, Moyes J, *et al.* A pharmacological guide to medicines which interfere with the biodistribution of radiolabelled metaiodobenzylguanidine (MIBG). *Nucl Med Commun* 1992; **13**: 513–21.

✱ 15 Wafelman AR, Suchi R, Hoefnagel CA, Beijnen JH. Radiochemical purity of ^{131}I-MIBG infusion fluids; a report from the clinical practice. *Eur J Nucl Med* 1993; **20**: 614–16.

● 16 Fielding SL, Flower MA, Ackery DM, *et al.* The dosimetry of ^{131}I mIBG for treatment of resistant neuroblastoma – results of a UK study. *Eur J Nucl Med* 1991; **18**: 308–16.

● 17 Van der Steen J, Maessen HJM, Hoefnagel CA, Marcuse HR. Radiation protection during treatment of children with ^{131}I-meta-iodobenzylguanidine. *Health Phys* 1986; **50**: 515–22.

◆ 18 Hoefnagel CA. The clinical use of ^{131}I-meta-iodobenzylguanidine (MIBG) for the diagnosis and treatment of neural crest tumors. Thesis, University of Amsterdam, 1989.

● 19 Hoefnagel CA, Voûte PA, de Kraker J, Valdés Olmos RA. ^{131}I-metaiodobenzylguanidine therapy after conventional therapy for neuroblastoma. *J Nucl Biol Med* 1991; **35**: 202–6.

◆ 20 Troncone L, Rufini V, Montemaggi P, *et al.* The diagnostic and therapeutic utility of radioiodinated metaiodobenzylguanidine (MIBG). 5 years experience. *Eur J Nucl Med* 1990; **16**: 325–35.

● 21 Klingebiel T, Berthold F, Treuner J, *et al.* Metaiodobenzylguanidine (MIBG) in treatment of 47 patients with neuroblastoma: results of the German neuroblastoma trial. *Med Pediatr Oncol* 1991; **19**: 84–88.

● 22 Garaventa A, Guerra P, Arrighini A, *et al.* Treatment of advanced neuroblastoma with I-131 meta-iodobenzylguanidine. *Cancer* 1991; **67**: 922–8.

● 23 Lashford LS, Lewis IJ, Fielding SL, *et al.* Phase I/II study of iodine 131 metaiodobenzylguanidine in chemoresistant neuroblastoma: a United Kingdom Children's Cancer Study Group investigation. *J Clin Oncol* 1992; **10**: 1889–96.

◆ 24 Troncone L, Galli G. Proceedings of an international workshop on the role of [^{131}I]metaiodobenzylguanidine in the treatment of neural crest tumors. *J Nucl Biol Med* 1991; **35**: 177–362.

✱ 25 Voûte PA, van der Kleij AJ, de Kraker J, *et al.* Clinical experience with radiation enhancement by hyperbaric oxygen in children with recurrent neuroblastoma stage IV. *Eur J Cancer* 1995; **31A**: 596–600.

26 Mastrangelo R, Tornesello A, Mastrangelo S. Position paper. Role of ^{131}I-metaiodobenzylguanidine in the treatment of neuroblastoma. *Med Pediatr Oncol* 1998; **31**: 22–6.

27 Corbett RP, Pinkerton R, Tait D, Meller S. ^{131}I-metaiodobenzylguanidine and high-dose chemotherapy with bone marrow rescue in advanced neuroblastoma. *J Nucl Biol Med* 1991; **35**: 228–31.

28 Yanik GA, Levine JE, Matthay KK, *et al.* Pilot study of iodine-131-metaiodobenzylguanidine in combination with myeloablative chemotherapy and autologous stem-cell support for the treatment of neuroblastoma. *J Clin Oncol* 2002; **20**: 2142–9.

29 Gaze MN, Wheldon TE, O'Donoghue JA, *et al.* Multi-modality megatherapy with [^{131}I] metaiodobenzylguanidine, high dose melphalan and total body irradiation with bone marrow rescue: feasibility study of a new strategy for advanced neuroblastoma. *Eur J Cancer* 1995; **31A**: 252–6.

30 Matthay KK, Panina C, Huberty J, *et al.* Correlation of tumor and whole-body dosimetry with tumor response and toxicity in refractory neuroblastoma treated with ^{131}I-MIBG. *J Nucl Med* 2001; **42**: 1713–21.

31 Hoefnagel CA, de Kraker J, Voûte PA, Valdés Olmos RA. Preoperative ^{131}I-metaiodobenzylguanidine therapy of neuroblastoma at diagnosis ('MIBG de novo'). *J Nucl Biol Med* 1991; **35**: 248–51.

32 Hoefnagel CA, de Kraker J, Valdés Olmos RA, Voûte PA. ^{131}I-MIBG as first-line treatment in high risk neuroblastoma patients. *Nucl Med Commun* 1994; **15**: 712–17.

33 Hoefnagel CA. Nuclear medicine therapy of neuroblastoma. *Q J Nucl Med* 1999; **43**: 336–43.

34 Mastrangelo R, Lasorella A, Troncone L, *et al.* ^{131}I-metaiodobenzylguanidine in neuroblastoma patients at diagnosis. *J Nucl Biol Med* 1991; **35**: 252–4.

35 Van Noesel MM, de Kraker J, Tytgat GA, *et al.* MIBG and topotecan combined induction therapy for high risk neuroblastomas: a phase I/II pilot study. *Med Pediatr Oncol* 2002; **39**: 257.

36 Smets L, Loesberg L, Janssen M, *et al.* Active uptake and extravesicular storage of metaiodobenzylguanidine in human SK-N-SH cells. *Cancer Res* 1989; **49**: 2941–4.

37 Sisson JC, Hutchinson RJ, Shapiro B, *et al.* Iodine-125-MIBG to treat neuroblastoma: preliminary report. *J Nucl Med* 1990; **31**: 1479–85.

38 Hoefnagel CA, Smets L, Voûte PA, de Kraker J. Iodine-125-MIBG therapy for neuroblastoma. *J Nucl Med* 1991; **31**: 361–2.

39 Sisson JC, Shapiro B, Hutchison RJ, *et al.* Survival of patients with neuroblastoma treated with 125-I MIBG. *Am J Clin Oncol* 1996; **19**: 144–8.

40 Sisson JC, Shapiro B, Hutchinson RJ, *et al.* Predictors of toxicity in treating patients with neuroblastoma by radiolabeled metaiodobenzylguanidine. *Eur J Nucl Med* 1994; **21**: 46–52.

41 Rutgers M, Tytgat GAM, Verwijs-Janssen M, *et al.* Uptake of the neuron-blocking agent meta-iodobenzylguanidine and serotonin by human platelets and neuroadrenergic tumor cells. *Int J Cancer* 1993; **54**: 290–5.

42 Voûte PA, Hoefnagel CA, de Kraker J, Majoor M. Side effects of treatment with ^{131}I-metaiodobenzylguanidine (^{131}I-MIBG) in neuroblastoma patients. In: Evans AE. (ed.) *Advances in neuroblastoma research 2.* New York: Alan R Liss, 1988: 679–87.

43 Picco P, Garaventa A, Claudiani F, *et al.* Primary hypothyroidism as a consequence of 131-I-metaiodobenzylguanidine treatment for children with neuroblastoma. *Cancer* 1995; **76**: 1662–4.

44 Van Santen HM, de Kraker J, van Eck BL, *et al.* High incidence of thyroid dysfunction despite prophylaxis with potassium iodide during ^{131}I-metaiodobenzylguanidine treatment in children with neuroblastoma. *Cancer* 2002; **94**: 2081–9.

45 Mairs RJ, Russell J, Cunningham S, *et al.* Enhanced tumour uptake and in vitro radiotoxicity of no-carrier-added ^{131}I-metaiodobenzylguanidine: implications for the targeted radiotherapy of neuroblastoma. *Eur J Cancer* 1995; **31A**: 576–81.

46 Rutgers M, Buitenhuis C, Smets LA. 'Cold' MIBG pre-treatment: a way to improve the relative neuroblastoma over normal tissue exposure of ^{131}I-MIBG. In: *Proceedings of International Meeting on 'Ten years of experience in neuroblastoma. Quo vadis MIBG? New horizons'.* Westerland: Sylt, 1994.

47 Montaldo PG, Raffaghello L, Guarnaccia F, *et al.* Increase of metaiodobenzylguanidine uptake and intracellular half-life during differentiation of human neuroblastoma cells. *Int J Cancer* 1996; **67**: 95–100.

48 Blake GM, Lewington VJ, Fleming JS, *et al.* Modification by nifedipine of ^{131}I-metaiodobenzylguanidine kinetics in malignant phaeochromocytoma. *Eur J Nucl Med* 1988; **14**: 345–8.

49 Hoefnagel CA, Taal BG, Sivro F, *et al.* Enhancement of ^{131}I-MIBG uptake in carcinoid tumours by administration of unlabelled MIBG. *Nucl Med Commun* 2000; **21**: 755–761.

50 Cunningham S, Boyd M, Brown MM, *et al.* A gene therapy approach to enhance the targeted radiotherapy of neuroblastoma. *Med Pediatr Oncol* 2000; **35**: 708–11.

51 Lashford LS, Clarke J, Kemshead JT. Systemic administration of radionuclides in neuroblastoma as planned radiotherapeutic intervention. *Med Pediatr Oncol* 1990; **18**: 30–6.

The skeleton

V. LEWINGTON

INTRODUCTION

Skeletal pain is common in advancing malignancy. Despite recent advances in radiation oncology, chemotherapy and bisphosphonate treatment, the management of metastatic bone pain remains unsatisfactory for many patients. Practice varies widely, reflecting both the number of different specialties involved in pain management and range of potential treatment options.

Targeted therapy using bone-seeking radiopharmaceuticals has been used successfully for over 30 years. This is an attractive approach for patients with advancing skeletal metastases, being systemic, allowing multiple sites to be treated simultaneously, but reasonably specific, reducing potential toxicity to non-target tissues.

Treatment success depends upon matching the physiological characteristics of the target metastasis to a specific pharmaceutical carrier. Skeletal uptake reflects increased osteoblastic activity and can be predicted from conventional bone scintigraphy. Some therapeutic radionuclides, such as ^{89}Sr and ^{223}Ra have a natural affinity for metabolically active bone. Others, including samarium and rhenium, form stable complexes with the bone-seeking cations phosphate and bisphosphonate.

Several factors influence optimal radionuclide selection. It is essential that the physical half-life ($T_{1/2}$) of the chosen radioisotope matches the biological turnover of the radiopharmaceutical *in vivo*. The half-life dictates dose rate, which in turn governs both the time to symptom benefit and response duration following targeted therapy. Particle range is also important. A long particle range extending across tens of cell diameters increases the risk of normal tissue (i.e. bone marrow) irradiation, and will contribute to myelotoxicity. The gamma photon emission of ^{186}Re and ^{153}Sm allows post-therapy imaging for dosimetry although this is of limited value in routine patient management at present.

AVAILABLE RADIOPHARMACEUTICALS

Licensed products

PHOSPHORUS-32

Initial experience was gained using ^{32}P administered as sodium [^{32}P]orthophosphate. Phosphorus-32 has a physical half-life of 14.3 days and emits a beta particle with a maximum energy (E_{max}) of 1.7 MeV which has a maximum range in tissue of approximately 8.5 mm. Published experience includes a range of fractionated treatment schedules, administering activities of 300–740 MBq (8–20 mCi) over 7–40 days.[1] Efficacy is similar to other therapeutic bone-seeking radiopharmaceuticals[1,2] but most studies report dose-limiting myelosuppression. Despite its significant cost advantage, ^{32}P therapy has been superseded by strontium-89 chloride and by rhenium-186 and samarium-153 bisphosphonates.

STRONTIUM-89

Strontium-89 is a pure beta particle emitter with a physical half-life of 50 days. Following intravenous administration, strontium-89 chloride clears the vascular compartment rapidly and is selectively concentrated at sites of increased osteoblastic activity.[3] Biodistribution studies undertaken using the gamma emitter [85]Sr demonstrated a therapeutic ratio of 10:1 for tumor:normal bone.[4] The biological half-life in normal bone is around 14 days compared with over 50 days in osteoblastic metastases.

SAMARIUM-153

By contrast, [153]Sm has a short physical half-life (approximately 2 days), decaying by the emission of a beta particle with a maximum energy of 0.81 MeV. Bone targeting is achieved via the tetraphosphate, ethylenediamine tetramethylene phosphate (EDTMP). The biological half-life is approximately 12 h with rapid renal excretion. Total skeletal uptake ranges between 55 and 75% depending on the skeletal tumor burden.[5] The short-range beta emission mean path length is in the order of 3.1 mm in soft tissues and 1.7 mm in bone.

RHENIUM-186

Rhenium-186 has a physical half-life of 3 days and is chelated to hydroxyethylidenediphosphonate (HEDP). Peak skeletal uptake occurs 3 h following intravenous administration. Typical biological half-times are in the order of 24 h,[6] whereas the mean biological half-life in bone metastases ranges between 45 ± 6 h (mean $\pm$ SD) and 59 ± 10 h in breast and prostate lesions, respectively.[7]

Products in clinical development

In addition to the licensed products, several alternative radiopharmaceuticals are in clinical development.

RHENIUM-188

Recent interest has focused on the therapeutic potential of [188]Re which has a short physical half-life (16.9 h), decaying by the emission of a high energy, medium range beta particle ($E_{max} = 2.1$ MeV, maximum path length approximately 10 mm in tissue). Rhenium-188 is produced from a [188]W/[188]Re generator, which offers significant advantages in terms of availability and convenience compared with other therapeutic radionuclides. As with [186]Re, targeting is achieved by chelation with HEDP.[8]

TIN-117M

Tin-117m(4+) decays by the emission of low-energy conversion electrons ($E_{max} = 0.13$ and 0.16 MeV) and a low abundance 159 keV gamma photon. The physical half-life is 13.6 days. Optimal blood and soft tissue clearance is achieved by chelation with diethylenetriaminepentaacetic acid (DTPA).[9] Following intravenous administration, peak uptake occurs in normal bone within 24 h but metastatic skeletal uptake occurs slowly over 3–7 days.[10] The short range of conversion electrons reduces the likelihood of normal bone marrow irradiation and no significant myelosuppression has been reported in early clinical trials.[11]

RADIUM-223

Radium-223 has a half-life of 11 days and decays by the emission of four alpha particles via daughter isotopes to [207]Pb, which is a stable isotope. The total decay energy is 28 MeV. As a group II metal, radium has a natural affinity for metabolically active bone. Administered as radium-223 chloride ([223]RaCl$_2$) it is selectively concentrated on bone surfaces relative to soft tissues in murine models. The 30:1 therapeutic ratio (tumor:marrow) is superior to other bone-seeking radiopharmaceuticals. Peak skeletal uptake occurs within 1 h of injection with no subsequent redistribution.[12] Unlike most other bone-seeking radionuclides, excretion is predominantly via the gastro-intestinal tract, with less than 10% renal clearance.[12] Phase II studies are in progress.

The physical characteristics of therapeutic radionuclides used for bone pain palliation are summarized in Table 17D.1.

Table 17D.1 *Physical characteristics of radionuclides used for bone pain palliation*

Radionuclide	Half-life	Maximum beta energy (MeV)	Mean beta energy (MeV)	Maximum beta range	Gamma emission (keV)
[89]Sr	50.5 days	1.4	0.583	7 mm	No
[32]P	14.3 days	1.7	0.695	8.5 mm	No
[117m]Sn	13.6 days	0.13 and 0.16 Mev conversion electrons	$<1 \mu m$	159	
[223]Ra	11.4 days	Alpha particles (average) 5.78 MeV	$<10 \mu m$	154	
[186]Re	3.7 days	1.07	0.362	5 mm	137
[153]Sm	1.9 days	0.81	0.229	4 mm	103
[188]Re	16.9 h	2.1	0.764	10 mm	155

PATIENT SELECTION

The majority of patients are referred for radionuclide therapy having failed other treatment options such as analgesics or external-beam radiotherapy. As there are many causes of chronic pain in this population, it is essential that symptoms be correlated with conventional ^{99m}Tc-methylene diphosphonate (^{99m}Tc-MDP) bone scintigraphy to confirm that individual pain sites are directly attributable to osteoblastic bone metastases (Fig. 17D.1). Nerve root compression, referred pain and vertebral collapse are the most common sources of diagnostic confusion (Fig. 17D.2). Nonfunctional imaging, such as plain radiographs, computed tomography (CT) or magnetic resonance imaging (MRI) do not predict increased bone mineral turnover and are inadequate to plan radionuclide therapy using bone-seeking radiopharmaceuticals.

Patients should be hematologically and biochemically stable prior to treatment. Hemopoietic reserve can be assessed by correlating the peripheral full blood count with tumor extent on radionuclide bone imaging. The platelet or leukocyte trend is more useful than an isolated measurement. Stable platelet and hemoglobin levels at the lower limit of normal ranges suggest reasonable marrow reserve. By comparison, recent, progressive decline in platelet or leukocyte levels suggests advancing marrow compromise and treatment using bone seeking radiopharmaceuticals would be inappropriate in this setting. The absolute threshold for platelets and total white cell count are 100×10^9 L^{-1} and 4.0×10^9 L^{-1}, respectively.[13] As bone-seeking pharmaceuticals are renally excreted, patients should have reasonable renal function – ideally GFR > 30 mL min^{-1}.[13] Renal impairment slows the clearance

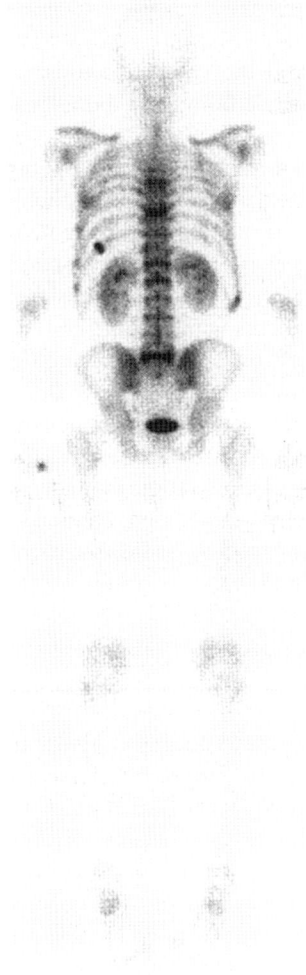

Figure 17D.1 *Hormone refractory prostatic carcinoma. Posterior whole-body ^{99m}Tc-MDP bone image confirming abnormal uptake in multiple osteoblastic bone metastases. Uptake at D12 and L3 corresponded to dominant pain sites on examination.*

Figure 17D.2 *Severe lumbar discomfort in patient with prostatic carcinoma on long-term hormone therapy. Posterior whole-body ^{99m}Tc-MDP bone image. Multiple sites of linear abnormal uptake of activity consistent with osteoporotic vertebral collapse and rib fractures. No evidence of skeletal metastasis.*

Table 17D.2 *Patient selection criteria*

Treatment indications

- *Treatment-refractory bone pain despite analgesics*
- *Positive bone scan – abnormal uptake corresponding to pain sites*
- *Hematology: Hb > 90 g L^{-1}, white cell count > 4.0 × 10^9 L^{-1}, platelets > 100 × 10^9 L^{-1}*
- *Renal function: GFR > 30 mL min^{-1}*

Absolute contraindications

- *Pregnancy*
- *Acute spinal cord compression*
- *Acute/acute on chronic renal failure – glomerular filtration rate < 30 mL min^{-1}*

Precautions

- *Urinary incontinence – catheterize pre-treatment*
- *Vesicoureteric or bladder outflow obstruction – consider ureteric stent or catheterize, as appropriate*

of free drug from the vascular compartment leading to an increased whole-body and bone marrow radiation absorbed dose.

Absolute contraindications to radioisotope therapy include pregnancy and lactation. Radionuclide treatment has no place in the management of acute cord spinal cord compression, which is a neurosurgical or radiotherapy emergency. Isotope therapy can be administered safely to treat bone pain in patients with chronic cord compression but will have no effect on established neurological symptoms. Urinary incontinence carries the risk of radioactive urine contamination and is a relative contraindication to treatment. Bladder catheterization is recommended prior to radiopharmaceutical administration in patients with unmanageable incontinence. Selection criteria for radionuclide therapy using bone seeking radiopharmaceuticals are summarized in Table 17D.2.

ADMINISTRATION

Treatment is given by bolus intravenous injection. In most countries, therapy can be administered on an outpatient basis, depending on local legislation. Patients should be advised to continue their analgesics until the onset of symptom relief and should be given written advice regarding gradual analgesic reduction. It is good practice to monitor the full blood count around 6 weeks post-treatment to exclude significant myelosuppression.

Recommended administered activities are:

^{89}Sr	150 MBq
^{153}Sm-EDTMP	37 MBq kg^{-1}
^{186}Re-HEDP	1.3 GBq

RESPONSE ASSESSMENT

Response is assessed subjectively by monitoring pain severity, analgesic intake, performance status and quality of life. Reductions in tumor markers such as prostatic specific antigen have been observed in activity escalation studies using ^{153}Sm-EDTMP[14] and ^{186}Re-HEDP[15] but this benefit must be weighed against increased toxicity. In routine clinical practice using conventionally approved activities, there is no correlation between tumor marker change and symptom benefit. Significant metastatic regression on follow-up bone imaging is unusual. These observations reflect the different absorbed dose thresholds required to achieve pain palliation as opposed to tumor cell kill.

EFFICACY

Most published series quote symptom benefit in 60–75% of treated patients, irrespective of the radiopharmacuetical administered.[16–18] Up to 25% of patients become pain free.[19] Although patients with very advanced skeletal metastases benefit from radionuclide therapy, the quality of response is generally higher in those treated early in the natural history of their disease.[3] This observation mimics experience using palliative external-beam radiotherapy.

Radionuclide therapy is at least as effective as external-beam irradiation, but offers the advantage of simultaneous multi-site, systemic treatment. Strontium-89 has been shown to delay the development of new bone pain arising from pre-existing clinically silent metastases, underlining the value of early intervention.[20] Optimal responses are reported by patients with predominantly osteoblastic bone metastases, originating from primary tumors such as prostate cancer. Response in breast, lung and gastrointestinal malignancies, which may elicit both osteosclerotic and osteolytic metastases, is less predictable.

If pain recurs, treatment can be repeated safely provided that hematological and biochemical parameters remain stable. Myelotoxicity is cumulative, reflecting both the effects of repeated radionuclide exposure, and more importantly, progressive marrow infiltration in patients with refractory malignancy. The quality of response may decrease with sequential therapies.

The different physical properties of the individual radionuclides influence clinical response. Nuclides with short half-lives, such as ^{153}Sm, ^{186}Re and ^{188}Re, deliver a relatively high dose rate, leading to early symptom relief within 2–7 days of administration. The typical response duration is 2–4 months. The longer physical half-life of ^{89}Sr leads to a lower dose rate and delayed response time from 2 to 4 weeks after administration. Response duration is prolonged at 3 to 6 months. These data are summarized in Table 17D.3.

These differences influence selection of the optimal radiopharmaceutical for individual patients depending on

Table 17D.3 *Characteristics of radiopharmaceuticals used for bone pain palliation*

Radiopharmaceutical	Usual administered activity	Typical response time	Typical response duration	Retreatment interval
$^{89}SrCl_2$	148 MBq	14–28 days	12–26	>3 months
$[^{32}P]orthophosphate\ (Na_2H^{32}PO_4)$	444 MBq (fractionated)	14 days	10 weeks	>3 months
$^{117m}Sn\text{-}DTPA$	2–10 MBq kg^{-1}	5–19 days	12–16 weeks	>2 months
$^{223}RaCl_2$	50–200 kBq kg^{-1}	<10 days	NE	NE
$^{186}Re\text{-}HEDP$	1.3 GBq	2–7 days	8–10 weeks	>2 months
$^{153}Sm\text{-}EDTMP$	37 MBq kg^{-1}	2–7 days	8 weeks	>2 months
$^{188}Re\text{-}HEDP$	1.3–4.4 GBq	2–7 days	8 weeks	NE*

NE, not evaluated.

symptom severity, performance status and life expectancy at the time of treatment. Patients with early metastases, a favorable prognosis (life expectancy > 3 months), reasonable pain control using conventional analgesics and normal marrow function are particularly likely to derive sustained benefit from $^{89}SrCl_2$. By comparison, patients with more advanced metastases, intractable pain and limited marrow reserve would be more appropriately treated using ^{153}Sm-EDTMP or $^{186}Re/^{188}Re$-HEDP.

A temporary increase in pain occurs in up to 50% of patients treated using ^{186}Re-HEDP but is much less frequent following $^{89}SrCl_2$. This may, again, reflect differences in dose rate and the induction of endosseous edema by isotopes with short half-lives.

TOXICITY

The only significant adverse effect of treatment is temporary myelosuppression which typically occurs 4–6 weeks post-administration. Recovery occurs over the next 4–6 weeks. The rate and completeness of recovery reflects the administered activity but, more importantly in routine clinical practice, the underlying bone marrow reserve and effects of previous treatment. Particle range is an important determinant of bone marrow toxicity. Very short range emitters such as ^{117m}Sn-DTPA and $^{223}RaCl_2$ appear significantly less myelosuppressive than the longer range beta particle emitters in preliminary clinical trials.[8,11,21] The longer particle range of ^{89}Sr leads to higher toxicity than ^{153}Sm-EDTMP or ^{186}Re-HEDP, but this is rarely of clinical significance in patients who have been selected appropriately for treatment. Bone marrow recovery may be delayed in patients with diffuse metastases, demonstrated as a superscan appearance on bone scintigraphy (Fig. 17D.3). For this reason, patients with very extensive disease are more appropriately treated using ^{153}Sm-EDTMP or ^{186}Re-HEDP than $^{89}SrCl_2$.

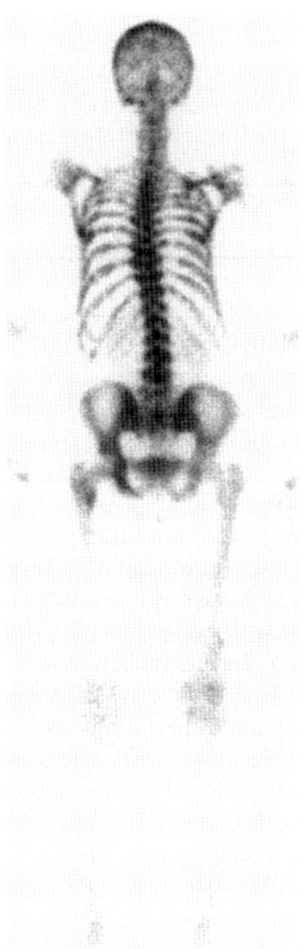

Figure 17D.3 *Posterior whole-body ^{99m}Tc-MDP bone image. Diffuse increased uptake of activity in disseminated breast carcinoma: superscan appearance.*

Prolonged thrombocytopenia has been reported in patients with subclinical disseminated intravascular coagulation (DIC).[22] Pre-treatment clotting studies are recommended in patients with very extensive bone metastases who might be at risk of DIC. Two cases of acute myeloid leukemia following ^{89}SrCl$_2$ therapy have been reported.[23] Both patients had been heavily pre-treated using conventional chemotherapy, external-beam irradiation and investigational drugs, precluding assessment of a causal relationship between hematological malignancy and radionuclide therapy.

TREATMENT FAILURE

Many nonresponders have previously failed to benefit from external-beam radiotherapy suggesting a cohort of patients who have relatively radioresistant bone pain. The commonest reason for treatment failure is incorrect diagnosis, emphasizing the importance of thorough pre-treatment clinical assessment. Response is variable in patients with predominantly osteolytic bone metastases. It is assumed that poor uptake and retention of bone-seeking agents by destructive metastases reduces the absorbed radiation dose delivered below the therapeutic threshold for pain relief.

THE FUTURE

The way forward lies in integrating radionuclide therapy within a multi-modality treatment plan. Several chemotherapy/isotope schedules have been examined. Results consistently suggest superior symptom control and prolonged survival using combined treatment rather than either chemotherapy or radionuclides alone.[24] Evidence supporting the combination of external-beam irradiation with isotope therapy is contradictory.[25,26] Exposure to high dose rate external-beam irradiation might be expected to alter the uptake of bone-seeking radiopharmaceuticals in the irradiated site, depending on the precise sequence of treatment delivery. Further randomized controlled studies will be necessary to clarify the merits of this approach. The potential value of adding bisphosphonates to radionuclide therapy has not been assessed. There is no evidence that the combination is detrimental[27] but randomized controlled trials will be necessary to establish whether this could confer a therapeutic advantage.

The development of alpha particle therapy, using ^{223}Ra for example, appears promising. On the basis of activity escalation trials using beta particle emitters, the high absorbed doses delivered by alpha therapy are predicted to achieve a direct anti-tumor effect in bone. Limited hematological toxicity resulting from the short particle range may allow easier integration with other treatments without incurring additional myelosuppression and offers the opportunity for fractionated therapy to achieve sustained benefit. This has been confirmed by small pre-clinical[12,21] and phase I studies but further large scale trials are required for confirmation.

SUMMARY

Systemic therapy using bone-seeking radioisotopes is a logical approach for patients with refractory, multi-site bone pain. Treatment is well tolerated and delivers sustained symptom relief. The way forward lies in integrating radionuclide therapy within a multi-modality treatment plan and in tailoring treatment, including the choice of radiopharmaceutical, to individual patient circumstances.

The goal of patient-specific activity prescription offers a realistic prospect of enhancing response rates within predictable toxicity limits and of progressing beyond symptom palliation to earlier intervention for survival gain. Future clinical trial design should, therefore, incorporate prospective whole-body and tumor dosimetry to confirm or refute the existence of a dose–response relationship for pain palliation.

REFERENCES

1 Silberstein EB. The treatment of painful osseous metastases with phosphorous-32 labelled phosphates. *Semin Oncol* 1993; **3(suppl)**: 10–21.
2 Fettich J, Paghy A, Nair N, *et al*. Comparative clinical efficacy and safety of phosphorous-32 and strontium-89 in the palliative treatment of metastatic bone pain: results of an IAEA coordinated research project. *World J Nucl Med* 2003; **2**: 226–31.
3 Laing AH, Ackery DM, Bayly RJ, *et al*. Strontium-89 therapy for pain palliation in prostatic skeletal malignancy. *Br J Radiol* 1991; **64**: 816–22.
4 Blake GM, Zivanovic MA, Blacquiere RM, *et al*. Strontium-89 therapy: measurement of absorbed dose to skeletal metastases. *J Nucl Med* 1988; **29**: 549–57.
5 Faranghi M, Holmes RA, Vorhut Q, *et al*. Samarium-153 EDTMP: pharmacokinetics, toxicity and pain response using an escalating dose schedule in treatment of metastatic bone cancer. *J Nucl Med* 1992; **33**: 1451–8.
6 Maxon HR, Thomas SR, Hertzberg VS, *et al*. Rhenium-186 HEDP for the treatment of painful bone metastases. *Semin Nucl Med* 1992; **22**: 33–40.
7 de Klerk JMH, Zonnenberg BA, van het Schip AD, *et al*. Dose escalation study of Re-186 HEDP in patients with metastatic prostate cancer. *Eur J Nucl Med* 1994; **21**: 1113–20.
8 Liepe K, Hliscs R, Kropp J, *et al*. Dosimetry of Re-188 hydroxyethylidenediphosphonate in human prostate cancer skeletal metastases. *J Nucl Med* 2003; **44**: 953–60.
9 Bishayee A, Rao DV, Srivastava SC, *et al*. Marrow sparing effects of Sn-117 m (4+) diethylenetriamine pentaacetic acid for radionuclide therapy of bone cancer. *J Nucl Med* 2000; **41**: 2043–50.
10 Krishnamurthy GT, Swailem FM, Scrivastava SC, *et al*. Tin-117m(4+)DTPA: pharmacokinetics and imaging

characteristics in patients with metastatic bone pain. *J Nucl Med* 1997; **38**: 230–7.

11 Atkins HL, Mausner LF, Scrivastava SC, *et al.* Biodistribution of Sn117m(4+) DTPA for palliative therapy of painful osseous metastases. *Radiology* 1993; **186**: 279–83.

12 Henriksen G, Fisher DR, Roeske JC, *et al.* Targeting of osseous sites with β-emitting [223]Ra: comparison with the β emitter ^{89}Sr in mice. *J Nucl Med* 2003; **44**: 252–9.

13 EANM Guidelines for treatment of metastatic bone pain. Available on www.eanm.org

14 Collins C, Eary JF, Donaldson G, *et al.* Sm-153 EDTMP in bone metastases of hormone refractory prostate carcinoma; a phase I/II trial. *J Nucl Med* 1993; **34**: 1839–44.

15 O'Sullivan JM, McCready VR, Flux G, *et al.* High activity rhenium-186 HEDP with autologous peripheral blood stem cell rescue: a phase I study in progressive hormone refractory prostate cancer metastatic to bone. *Br J Cancer* 2002; **86**: 1715–20.

16 Finlay IG, Mason MD, Shelley M. Radioisotopes for the palliation of metastatic bone cancer: a systematic review. *Lancet Oncol* 2005; **6**: 392–400.

17 Silberstein EB. Teletherapy and radiopharmaceutical therapy of painful bone metastases. *Semin Nucl Med* 2005; **35**: 152–8.

18 Liepe K, Runge R, Kotzerke J. The benefit of bone seeking radiopharmaceuticals in the treatment of metastatic bone pain. *J Cancer Res Clin Oncol* 2005; **1331**: 60–6.

19 Serafini AN. Therapy of metastatic bone pain. *J Nucl Med* 2001; **42**: 895–906.

20 Quilty PM, Kirk D, Bolger JJ, *et al.* A comparison of the palliative effects of strontium-89 and external beam radiotherapy in metastatic prostate cancer. *Radiother Oncol* 1994; **31**: 33–40.

21 Nilsson S, Larsen RH, Fossa SD, *et al.* First clinical experience with alpha-emitting radium-223 in the treatment of skeletal metastases. *Clin Cancer Res* 2005; **11**: 4451–9.

22 Paszkowski AL, Hewitt DJ, Taylor Jr A. Disseminated intravscular coagulation in a patient treated with strontium-89 for metastatic carcinoma of the prostate. *Clin Nucl Med* 1999; **24**: 852–4.

23 Kossman SE, Weiss MA. Acute myelogenous leukaemia after exposure to strontium-89 for the treatment of adenocarcinoma of the prostate. *Cancer* 2000; **88**: 620–4.

24 Tu SM, Millikan RE, Mengistu B, *et al.* Bone targeted therapy for advanced androgen independent carcinoma of the prostate; a randomised phase II trial. *Lancet* 2001; **357**: 336–41.

25 Porter AT, McEwan AJ, Powe JE, *et al.* Results of a randomised phase III trial to evaluate the efficacy of strontium-89 adjuvant to local field external beam irradiation in the management of endocrine resistant metastatic prostate cancer. *Int J Radiat Oncol Biol Phys* 1993; **25**: 805–13.

26 Smeland S, Erikstein B, Aas M, *et al.* Role of strontium-89 as adjuvant to palliative external beam radiotherapy is questionable: results of a double blind randomised study. *Int J Radiat Oncol Biol Phys* 2003; **56**: 1397–404.

27 Marcus CS, Saeed S, Mlikotic, *et al.* Lack of effect of a bisphosphonate (pamidronate disodium) infusion on subsequent skeletal uptake of Sm-153 EDTMP. *Clin Nucl Med* 2002; **27**: 427–30.

FURTHER READING

Lewington VJ. Bone seeking radionuclides for therapy. *J Nucl Med* 2005; **46(suppl 1)**: 38S–47S.

McEwan AJB. Palliation of bone pain. In: Murray IPC, Ell PJ. (eds.) *Nuclear medicine in clinical diagnosis and treatment*, 2nd edition. Edinburgh: Churchill Livingstone, 1998: 1083–99.

17E

The use of ^{32}P

CLAUDE PARMENTIER

INTRODUCTION

The risk of developing cancer, and more specifically acute leukemia, after the use of ^{32}P in patients with polycythemia vera has been recognized for approximately 40 years. As a consequence of this risk, the indications for, and contraindications to, ^{32}P are unclear in the physician's mind. Besides a recent review, this chapter tries to clarify the problem.[1]

Polycythemia vera was first described about a century ago[2,3] and Lawrence introduced the use of ^{32}P for treatment of the disease.[4,5] The incidence of polycythemia vera is between two and three cases per 100 000 persons annually, with a predominance in men.[6] The disease is a clonal malignancy of the pluripotent hematological stem cell, as has been demonstrated in two ways. Firstly, in black women with polycythemia vera, who are simultaneously heterozygotes for two different glucose-6-phosphate dehydrogenase (G6PD) isoenzymes, only a single isoenzyme type is found in the progenitors and the progeny of the three myeloid

hematopoietic series, while equivalent amounts of both inherited isoenzymes are found in nonhematopoietic tissues, which is the signature of a clonal anomaly.[7,8] Secondly, when (in approximately 25% of the cases) a karyotypic anomaly is found, it exists in the three myeloid lines and not in nonhematopoietic tissues.

A karyotypic definition of the disease does not exist, but application of a simple set of diagnostic criteria empirically developed on the basis of clinical experience enables diagnosis of polycythemia vera with high probability. The Polycythemia Vera Study Group, formed in 1966 in the USA by Wasserman and Berlin with the contribution of Italian and French hematologists, defined the diagnostic parameters which are now universally accepted (Table 17E.1). These indicators must be supplemented by the exclusion of secondary polycythemia.

According to present knowledge, polycythemia vera should be treated by bone marrow transplantation. However, the mean age of the patients (60 years) and the lack of matched donors usually preclude this solution. In searching

Table 17E.1 *The Polycythemia Vera Study Group criteria*

Category A	Category B
A1. Increased total red cell volume	B1. Thrombocytosis: platelet count $> 400\,000\,\mu L^{-1}$
Male $> 36\,mL\,kg^{-1}$	B2. Leucocytosis: $12\,000\,\mu L^{-1}$ (no fever or infection)
Female $> 32\,mL\,kg^{-1}$	B3. Increased leukocyte alkaline phosphatase (LAP > 100)
A2. Normal arterial oxygen saturation (92%)	B4. Serum $B_{12} > 900\,pg\,mL^{-1}$ or unbound B_{12} binding
A3. Splenomegaly	capacity $> 0.2200\,pg\,mL^{-1}$

Diagnosis of polycythemia vera is virtually certain in the presence of A1 + A2 + A3 or A1 + A2 + any two from category B.

for an alternative approach and considering the role of ^{32}P, the following questions need to be addressed:

- Can the natural course of polycythemia vera lead to acute leukemia?
- Is ^{32}P responsible for the induction of leukemia as polycythemia vera evolves?
- Is chemotherapy a valuable alternative to ^{32}P?
- What therapeutic role could now be played by ^{32}P?

RELATION BETWEEN POLYCYTHEMIA VERA AND LEUKEMIA

As patients with polycythemia vera must be treated as quickly as possible, precise knowledge of the natural course of the disease is limited. Only two studies may be considered acceptable in this respect. The first dates back to 1950, when Videbaek[9] reported on the natural course of the disease in 125 patients based on data collected from several Danish hospitals between 1920 and 1950. The median survival was 4–5 years for men and 8–9 years for women. The complications were hemorrhage, thrombocytosis, and gastroduodenal ulcer. Eight patients developed malignant tumors leading to death and two died from leukemia. None of the patients were treated with ^{32}P. They were treated by a wide variety of protocols, but most frequently with phlebotomy and X-radiation. The treatment received by the 10 patients who died from malignancy is not known. However, it is generally accepted that the natural history of polycythemia vera leads to leukemia as a terminal event in about 1% of cases. The second acceptable study concerns the phlebotomy arm of the clinical trial initiated by the Polycythemia Vera Study Group; the results from this trial will be reported in the following pages.

In spite of some contradictions,[10] series published before 1965[11,12] showed a clear incidence of acute leukemia in patients treated by ^{32}P. In 1965 a decisive publication by Modan and Lilienfeld[13] definitively established the leukemogenic effect of ^{32}P. In a series of 1222 nonrandomized patients, the incidence of acute leukemia was 11% in the patients treated with ^{32}P but less than 1% in the non-irradiated patients.

Since 1965, many publications have confirmed the excess of leukemia in patients treated by ^{32}P after 10 years of evolution. In these patients at risk, the number of leukemias is 20 times the expected number in a normal population.[14–17]

The Polycythemia Vera Study Group was dissolved in the mid-1980s, but the French team published results until the mid-1990s. The main contribution of the Group lay in the comparison between patients treated by phlebotomy and aspirin only and patients treated by ^{32}P or alkylating agents. Its studies, conducted with great statistical accuracy, (1) clarified the natural history of polycythemia vera (1–2% of natural deaths were found to be caused by leukemia, which corroborated the results reported by Videbaek[9]); (2) showed that alkylating agents (chlorambucil and melphalan) were clearly more dangerous than ^{32}P and than phlebotomy[18]; (3) demonstrated that treatment with phlebotomy only was ethically unacceptable because of the risk of thrombosis, vascular complications, poor patient cooperation, refusal of treatment or intolerance, and early development of myelofibrosis; (4) demonstrated that neither polycythemia nor its treatment predisposes to the development of one particular type of cancer rather than another (the actuarial risk for patients treated with ^{32}P was 15% at the 12th year); and (5) showed that the incidence of myelofibrosis reached 20% after 10 years and 50% after 20 years.[18–20]

Many other publications have clarified further important points. Firstly, the more often ^{32}P activities are used, the earlier leukemia appears. It is commonly accepted that this is due to more rapid evolution of the disease itself. However, in some important studies the increased risk of acute leukemia was proven to be dose dependent.[13,16,17] Secondly, the probability of death due to leukemia increases significantly with time, and represents 16% of patients at risk at the 15th year of follow-up. After the 15th year the number of leukemia cases decreases, but this decrease may be due to statistical fluctuation in the low residual number of patients. Moreover, despite application of the Polycythemia Vera Study Group criteria, some pseudo-polycythemia vera cases could have been included in the cohorts reported in the literature.[16,21,22] Consequently some authors have tried to introduce amendments to the traditional diagnostic criteria.[23]

In some series,[16,17,20,22] prognostic factors (splenomegaly, platelet level) were stressed as possible indicators of leukemia risk after ^{32}P treatment. In fact, it can be stated that these symptoms denote progressing or already advanced disease.[16,22,24,25]

The secondary leukemias that appear in post-polycythemia situations are very aggressive and poorly responsive to chemotherapy.[16,19,22] However, in at least two trials, the life expectancy of ^{32}P-treated patients has been found to be equal to or longer than that of an equivalent control group. This is probably due to a better medical follow-up of these patients than of the population at large.[16,17,26,27]

Finally, it was demonstrated that ^{32}P treatment results in a good life expectancy averaging about 15 years.[16,21]

IS CHEMOTHERAPY AN ALTERNATIVE TO ^{32}P?

Busulfan, an alkylating agent, is still used in the treatment of polycythemia vera. This is probably due to the publication of a randomized trial by the Leukemia and Hematosarcoma Cooperative Group of the European Organisation for Research on Treatment of Cancer.[28] In 293 patients the overall survival was better with busulfan. But, even with too short a follow-up, busulfan appeared more leukemogenic than ^{32}P. Moreover, the leukemogenic effect of busulfan is well established.[29] If busulfan is chosen, the physician in charge must be aware that this drug is rather difficult to guide and is extremely myelosuppressive because of its high level of aggressiveness towards hematopoietic stem cells of the bone marrow.

Hydroxyurea, a nonmutagenic agent used in the treatment of polycythemia vera, which blocks cells in the S phase, has been considered noncarcinogenic.[30] This use of hydroxyurea and its safety were recently revisited. In 1997, Fruchtman et al.,[31] for the Polycythemia Vera Study Group, reported a comparison between 174 patients treated by phlebotomy alone in the 01 group protocol versus 51 patients treated with hydroxyurea. With regard to the leukemogenic effect, a nonsignificant difference was found between the two groups, although the hydroxyurea group showed more leukemias (10% vs. 4%). In another study[32] comparing treatment by hydroxyurea versus treatment by ^{32}P in the Polycythemia Vera Study Group 08 study arm, a lower but non-negligible incidence of leukemia (5.6%) was found in the hydroxyurea group. Overall, it can be accepted that hydroxyurea is less leukemogenic than ^{32}P but more leukemogenic than the natural evolution of the disease. However, the reported studies are rather imprecise, and new statistical trials would be necessary in order to draw more accurate statistical conclusions. Such trials are unrealistic in view of ethical considerations, the long follow-up necessary to reach conclusions and the arrival of new drugs. Moreover progress in cytogenetics and molecular biology can be expected.

Pipobroman is a derivative of piperazine. Its chemical formula is that of an alkylating agent but its essential mechanism of action involves metabolic competition with pyrimidine bases. A randomized trial including 297 polycythemia vera patients treated with hydroxyurea or pipobroman[33] did not report any difference between the two arms in terms of overall survival or incidence of secondary leukemia (5% at the 5th year and 10% at the 13th year).

Anagrelide and interferon-α are under investigation. Some cases respond to imatinib mesylate.[34]

THE ROLE OF ^{32}P IN THE MANAGEMENT OF POLYCYTHEMIA VERA

With the above points in mind, what role might ^{32}P play in the therapeutic management of polycythemia vera? In the USA, ^{32}P is no longer used for the treatment of polycythemia vera.[35] In Europe, studies from Sweden,[36] the United Kingdom,[37] and France[38] recently proposed the following therapeutic indications in polycythemia vera:

- Patients aged over 70 years can benefit from treatment by ^{32}P and supplementation by hydroxyurea does not seem to improve the prognosis.

- Patients who are difficult to survey or who are unable to accept regular intake of drugs must be treated by using ^{32}P.
- Until new drugs have been clearly validated,[35,39,40] patients under 70 years should be treated by using hydroxyurea, given that it is less likely to induce leukemia than other alternatives. However, the treatment must be regularly monitored and adapted as necessary. If major side-effects (painful aphthae, leg ulcers) or resistance develop, the treatment must be interrupted and ^{32}P treatment instituted. (Temporary replacement with pipobroman would not be of any decisive benefit to the patient.) The need for such substitution is generally considered to arise in forms of the disease with a poor prognosis.
- Forms at high thrombotic risk or with progressive thrombocytosis are indications of a myelosuppressive treatment. The almost constant and fast efficiency of ^{32}P can make it useful in such a situation.
- In some young patients, interferon-α or anagrelide should be considered.

In all cases, phlebotomies can avoid vascular accidents. However, the clinician must keep in mind the fact that exclusive use of phlebotomies induces progression towards myelofibrosis and does not represent a baseline treatment for polycythemia vera since it exposes patients to risk of death from vascular complications. Since myelofibrosis may be facilitated by the thrombocythemia caused by phlebotomies, it has been proposed that phlebotomy might be used in combination with low-dose chemotherapy to prevent thrombosis. Such treatment, however, is difficult to guide. With regard to the interest in low-dose aspirin treatment, a large-scale randomized placebo-controlled trial is now under way in 12 European countries. Results of this trial are not yet available. Until that time, it can be considered that aspirin is indicated in those with thrombotic complications, unless they have previously experienced gastrointestinal hemorrhage.[37,38] In cases of granulocytosis, allopurinol is needed to avoid hyperuricemia. A recent paper[41] concludes to the interest of daily low-dose aspirin, but is debated by others.[42]

Recently, a clonal and recurrent mutation in the JH2 pseudo-kinase domain of the Janus kinase 2 (JAK2) gene in more than 80% of polycythemia vera patients was found. This could lead to a new classification of the disease and novel therapeutic approaches.[43]

CONCLUSION

Until better knowledge of the cytogenetic and molecular basis of the disease is obtained, ^{32}P retains a role in the clinical management of polycythemia vera.

Case history

A 65-year-old male patient was diagnosed with polycythemia vera based on the presence of headache, erythrocytosis, and pruritus. The hematological evolution under treatment with ^{32}P is shown in Fig. 17E.1. After the last administration of ^{32}P the blood count normalized. The patient died some years later as a result of coronary thrombosis, without the recurrence of polycythemia but in a state of myelofibrosis.

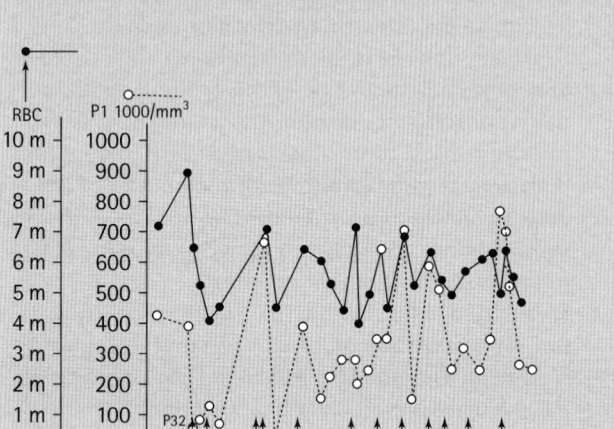

Figure 17E.1   *The hematological evolution of a polycythemia vera patient treated by ^{32}P. After administration of the radioisotope, the blood count was normalized. The patient died as a result of coronary thrombosis some years after the last application of ^{32}P, without recurrence of polycythemia, but with myelofibrosis.*

REFERENCES

● Seminal primary article

◆ Key review paper

★ First formal publication of a management guideline

● 1   Parmentier C. Use and risks of phosphorus-32 in the treatment of polycythaemia vera. *Eur J Nucl Med Mol Imaging* 2003; **30**: 1413–17.

● 2   Vaquez MH. Concerning a special form of cyanosis with accompanying excessive persistent polycythaemia. *Compt Rend Soc Biol* 1892; **44**: 384–8.

● 3   Osler W. Chronic cyanosis with polycythaemia and enlarged spleen: a new clinical entity. *Am J Med Sci* 1903; **126**: 187–201.

★ 4   Lawrence JH. *Polycythaemia physiology, diagnosis and treatment.* New York: Grune and Stratton, 1955.

★ 5   Lawrence JH, Winchell HS, Donald WG. Leukaemia in polycythaemia vera. *Ann Intern Med* 1969; **70**: 763–71.

◆ 6   Berglund S, Zettervall O. Incidence of polycythaemia vera in a defined population. *Eur J Hematol* 1992; **48**: 20–6.

● 7   Adamson JW, Fialkow PJ, Murphy S, *et al.* Polycythaemia vera: stem cell and probable clonal origin of the disease. *N Engl J Med* 1976; **295**: 913–16.

● 8   Fialkow PJ. Clonal and stem cell origin of blood cell neoplams. In: Lobue J, Gordon AS, Silber S. (eds.) *Contemporary hematology oncology*, vol. 1. New York: Plenum, 1980: 1.

◆ 9   Videbaek A. Polycythaemia vera. *Acta Med Scand* 1950; **138**: 179–87.

◆ 10   Halnan KE, Russel MH. Comparison of survival and causes of death in patients managed with and without radiotherapy. *Lancet* 1965; **2**: 760.

◆ 11   Fauvert R, Boivin P, Mallarme J. Conduite et résultats du traitement des polyglobulies par le phosphore 32. *Nouv Rev Fr Hémat* 1961; **1**: 459–67.

◆ 12   Osgood EE. Contrasting incidence of acute monocytic and granulocytic leukaemias in ^{32}P treated patients with polycythemia vera and chronic lymphocytic leukaemia. *J Lab Clin Med* 1964; **64**: 560.

● 13   Modan B, Lilienfeld AM. Polycythaemia vera and leukaemia the role of radiation treatment. A study of 1222 patients. *Medicine* 1965; **44**: 305–44.

◆ 14   Szur L, Lewis SM. Hematological complications of polycythaemia vera and treatment with radioactive phosphorus. *Br J Radiol* 1966; **39**: 122–30.

◆ 15   Harman JB, Ledlie EM. Survival of polycythaemia vera patients treated with radioactive phosphorus. *Br Med J* 1967; **2**: 146.

◆ 16   Tubiana M, Attie E, Parmentier C. Le devenir des polyglobulies essentielles traitées par le phosphore radioactif à propos d'une série de 330 malades suivis pendant 12 à 24 ans. *Nouv Press Med* 1975; **4**: 1781–6.

◆ 17   Landaw SA. Acute leukaemia in polycythaemia vera. *Semin Hematol* 1976; **13**: 33–48.

● 18   Berk PD, Goldberg JD, Donovan PB, *et al.* Therapeutic recommendations in polycythaemia vera based on polycythaemia vera study group protocols. *Semin Hematol* 1986; **23**: 32–143.

● 19   Najean Y, Deschamps A, Dresch C, *et al.* Acute leukaemia and myelodysplasia in polycythaemia vera. A clinical study with long-term follow-up *Cancer* 1988; **61**: 89–95.

● 20 Najean Y, Rain JD, Dresch C, *et al.* Risk of leukaemia, carcinoma, and myelofibrosis in ^{32}P- or chemotherapy-treated patients with polycythaemia vera: a prospective analysis of 682 cases. The French Cooperative Group for the Study of polycythaemias [Review]. *Leuk Lymphoma* 1996; **22(suppl 1)**: 111–19.

● 21 Najean Y, Dresch C, Rain JD. The very-long-term course of polycythaemia: a complement to the previously published data of the polycythaemia vera group. *Br J Haematol* 1994; **86**: 233–5.

● 22 Tubiana M, Flamant R, Attie E, Hayat M. A study of hematological complications occurring in patients with polycythaemia vera treated with ^{32}P (based on a series of 296 patients). *Blood* 1968; **32**: 536–48.

◆ 23 Tefferi A. Polycythaemia vera: a comprehensive review and clinical recommendations [Review]. *Mayo Clin Proc* 2003; **78**: 174–94.

● 24 Charbord P, Caillou B, Lafleur M, Parmentier C. L'érythropoïèse inefficace au cours des splénomégalies myéloïdes: tests au Fer 59, données histologiques et cytologiques médullaires. *Nouv Rev Fr Hématol* 1978; **20**: 443–53.

● 25 Parmentier C, Morardet N, Gardet P, *et al.* Granulocytic progenitor cells (CRC) cultured from patients with polycythaemia vera. *Nouv Rev Fr Hématol* 1980; **22**: 339–55.

● 26 von Heilman E, Köhler T. Polycythaemia vera. *Fortschr Med* 1978; **96**: 941–4.

◆ 27 Parmentier C, Charbord P, Tubiana M. L'avenir lointain de la maladie de Vaquez. *Rev Prat* 1981; **31**: 1533–44.

★ 28 Haanen C, Mathe G, Hayat M. Treatment of polycythaemia vera by radiophosphorus or busulphan: a randomized study. *Br J Cancer* 1981; **44**: 75–80.

● 29 Brodsky I. Busulphan treatment of polycythaemia vera. *J Hematol* 1974; **52**: 1–6.

◆ 30 Nand S, Stock W, Godwin J, Gross-Fisher S. Leukaemogenic risk of hydroxyurea therapy in polycythaemia vera, essential thrombocythemia and myeloid metaplasia with myelofibrosis. *Am J Hemat* 1996; **52**: 42–6.

★ 31 Fruchtman SM, Mack K, Kaplan ME, *et al.* From efficacy to safety: a polycythaemia vera study group report on hydroxyurea in patients with polycythaemia vera. *Semin Hematol* 1997; **34**: 17.

★ 32 Tatarsky I, Sharon R. Management of polycythaemia vera with hydroxyurea. *Semin Hematol* 1997; **34**: 24.

● 33 Najean Y, Rain JD, for the French Polycythaemia Study Group. Treatment of polycythaemia vera: the use of hydroxyurea and piproboman in 292 patients under the age of 65 years. *Blood* 1997; **90**: 33–70.

● 34 Jones CM, Dickinson TM. Polycythaemia vera responds to imatinib mesylate. *Am J Med Sci* 2003; **325**: 149–52.

◆ 35 Streiff MB, Smith B, Spivak JL. The diagnosis and management of polycythemia vera in the era since the polycythaemia vera study group: a survey of American Society of Hematology members practice patterns. *Blood* 2002; **99**: 1144–9.

★ 36 Brandt L, Anderson H. Survival and risk of leukaemia in polycythaemia vera and essential thrombocythaemia treated with oral radiophosphorus: are safer drugs available? *Eur J Hematol* 1995; **54**: 21–6.

★ 37 Pearson TC, Messinezy M, Westwood N, *et al.* A polycythaemia vera up date: diagnosis, pathobiology and treatment. *Hematolgy Am Soc Hematol Educ Program* 2002; 51–67.

★ 38 Conférence de consensus Diagnostic, Pronostic, Traitement et Surveillance des Polyglobulies. Société Française d'Hématologie, 1993.

★ 39 Spivak JL. The optimal management of polycythemia vera. *Br J Hematol* 2002; **116**: 243–54.

★ 40 McMullin MF, Bareford D, Craig J, *et al.* Myeloproliferative Disorders (UK) Study Group. *Br J Haematol* 2003; **120**: 543–4; author reply 544–5. Comment on *Br J Haematol* 2002; **116**: 243–54. The optimal management of polycythaemia vera.

★ 41 Spivak J. Daily aspirin – only half the answer. *N Engl J Med* 2004; **350**: 99–101.

★ 42 Landolfi R, Marchioli R, Kutti J, *et al.* European Collaboration on Low-Dose Aspirin in Polycythemia Vera Investigators. Efficacy and safety of low-dose aspirin in polycythemia vera. *N Engl J Med* 2004; **350**: 114–24.

43 James C, Ugo V, Le Couedic JP, *et al.* A unique clonal JAK2 mutation leading to constitutive signalling causes polycythaemia vera. *Nature* 2005; **434**: 1144–8.

● 44 Silberstein EB. The treatment of painful osseous metastases with phosphorus 32 labeled phosphates. *Semin Oncol* 1993; **20(suppl 2)**: 10–21.

● 45 Spiers FW, Beddoe AH, King SD, *et al.* The absorbed dose to bone marrow in the treatment of polycythaemia by ^{32}P. *Br J Radiol* 1976; **49**: 133–40.

★ 46 Seltzer RA, Kereiakes JG, Saengerpe L. Radiation exposure from radioisotopes on pediatrics. *New Engl J Med* 1964; **271**: 84–90.

◆ 47 Mays CW. Cancer induction in man from internal radioactivity. *Health Phys* 1973; **25**: 585–92.

◆ 48 International Commission on Radiological Protection. *Protection of the patient in radionucleide investigations.* ICPR Publication No 17. Oxford: Pergamon Press, 1971: 64.

● 49 Gilliland DG, Blanchard KL, Levy J, *et al.* Clonality in myeloproliferative disorders: analysis by means of the polymerase chain reaction. *Proc Natl Acad Sci USA* 1991; **88**: 6848–52.

- 50 Jenkins RB, Le Beau MM, Kraker WJ, *et al.* Fluorescence in situ hybridization: a sensitive method for trisomy 8 detection in bone marrow specimens. *Blood* 1992; **79**: 3307–15.
- 51 Bench AJ, Aldred MA, Humphray SJ, *et al.* A detailed physical and transcriptional map of the region of chromosome 20 that is deleted in myeloproliferative disorders and refinement of the common deleted region. *Genomics* 1998; **49**: 351–62.
- 52 Dai CH, Krantz SB, Dessypris EN, *et al.* Polycythemia vera. II. Hypersensitivity of bone marrow erythroid, granulocyte-macrophage, and megakaryocyte progenitor cells to interleukin-3 and granulocyte-macrophage colony-stimulating factor. *Blood* 1992; **80**: 891–9.
- 53 Blomgren H, Petrini B, Wasserman J, *et al.* Changes of the blood lymphocyte population following ^{32}P treatment for polycythemia vera. *Eur J Haematol* 1990; **44**: 302–6.

APPENDIX 1: DOSIMETRY AND PRACTICAL USE OF ^{32}P

^{32}P is produced in a cyclotron and emits pure beta radiation with an average energy of 0.70 MeV and a maximum energy of 1.71 MeV. The beta emission has a range of 3–8 mm in soft tissue. The half-life of this radionuclide is 14.29 days. After administration of ^{32}P, uptake of orthophosphate by the skeleton exceeds that by muscle, fat or skin by a factor of 4–6 at day 1 and 6–10 at day 2. In humans, 5–10% of [^{32}P]orthophosphate is excreted in the urine in the first 24 h, and 20–50% within a week. Less than 2% is excreted in the feces.[44]

Few data are available regarding precise dosimetry in man. Spiers *et al.*[45] measured the dose absorbed by the bone marrow using marrow biopsies taken from the iliac crest and the sternum. For 37 MBq (1 mCi) administered, the doses from activity in trabecular bone, marrow and cortical bone were 10, 13, and 1 cGy, respectively.

Using a compartmental approach, Seltzer *et al.*[46] and Mays[47] found an average skeletal dose of 15 cGy per 37 MBq administered. With some debatable assumptions, the International Commission on Radiological Protection[48] published comparable results.

Practically, ^{32}P is delivered by nuclear facilities in the form of a standardized solution. ^{32}P is administered per os in patients who have fasted for at least 12 h. In nonfasting patients the radionuclide must be administered intravenously through a 0.2 μm membrane to avoid microbial risk.

The activity usually administered is 37×10^6 MBq (1 mCi) per 10 kg of theoretical body weight, i.e. about 185–296 MBq (5–8 mCi).

Phlebotomies are not advisable in the 3 weeks following ^{32}P administration to avoid subtraction of still circulating ^{32}P. If phlebotomies seem useful they must be done before administration of the radionuclide.

The erythrocyte and platelet counts in most of the cases are normalized around 12 weeks after radionuclide administration. At around 10 days the platelet counts can fall to a nadir without any known complication.

^{32}P administrations have to be repeated according to the hematological status of the patient, but a period of time as wide as possible is suitable. Most of the patients are treated once a year.

It is commonly admitted that in patients over 70 years old, the ^{32}P administration must be reduced by 30%. In fact, only the general status and the evolution of the disease have to be taken into account. Many patients over 70 need a complete administration.

APPENDIX 2: MECHANISM OF THE RISKS DUE TO ^{32}P

It is possible that ^{32}P causes leukemia by a genetic process. In a clonal alteration, successive events can lead to cancerization. This explains why acute leukemia exists in the natural evolution of polycythemia vera. Beta emission can be a deleterious event, which could be one of an accumulation of genetic alterations that lead to acute leukemia. There is no specific genetic signature of polycythemia vera although some genetic markers have been described in this disease.

After Fialkow's demonstration with G6PD in women who are G6PD heterozygous, some researchers[49] using restriction enzymes and polymerase chain reaction (PCR) analysis showed an erythroid clonality in erythroid lines in polycythemia vera, as well as in other myeloproliferative diseases. Trisomy 8 has been described in many myeloproliferative syndromes without any specificity. The use of *in situ* hybridization gives accurate sensitivity for detecting this anomaly.[50]

This probably does not provide the clonal alteration which explains polycythemia vera, but can define some molecular alterations found in the emergence of clonal malignancy. Other acquired cytogenetic changes (e.g. del(20q), del(13q), trisomy 9, duplication of segments of 19, and translocations associated with the rare syndrome) have been found. They represent early lesions contributing to the pathogenesis of polycythemia vera and of essential thrombocytosis but do not have a pathognomonic value and can be considered as evolutionary events. The identification of causal gene(s) is an important challenge for both the clinician and fundamental scientist.[51] Hypersensitivity of myeloid progenitors can be considered as consequences of the clonality of the disease.[52] Work on JAK2 gene may constitute an important step in our knowledge of the disease.[53]

The role of immunologic deficit in cancerization

If the lymphocyte counts are within the normal range before treatment, the expression of some membrane antigens detected by monoclonal antibodies (e.g. CD3, CD5, helper/inducer CD4 as well as suppressor/cytotoxic CD8) is slightly reduced. The following observations have also been noted:

- [32]P treatment increases phytohemaglutinin reactivity and the proportion of T cells in the blood.
- After a mean dose of 240 Bq, the peripheral lymphocyte count decreases to 60% at 6 weeks.

- The most reduced lymphocytes are B cells and NK cells, followed by HNK-1 cells and T cells.

Induction of IgM by the *PKW* mitogene was significantly reduced but not that of IgG or IgA. This suggests that, essentially, lymphocytes which mature in bone marrow are affected by ^{32}P treatment.[53] The duration of these anomalies and their possible deleterious effects are unknown.

The role of dosimetry

GLENN FLUX

INTRODUCTION

Radionuclide therapy (RNT) has been carried out for 80 years. As with chemotherapy the treatment is systemic, although in common with external-beam radiotherapy (EBRT) it uses radiation to kill malignant cells. However, in stark contrast to EBRT, for which individual patient treatment planning has become routine practice over the last 30 years, to date neither prospective nor retrospective absorbed-dose calculations have been routinely employed. Typically, administered activities have been fixed or sometimes scaled according to body surface area or weight.

Nevertheless, the principles behind individual treatment planning for EBRT pertain equally to RNT. It is the aim of all therapies to maximize the absorbed dose to target organs whilst minimizing the absorbed dose delivered to normal tissue and there are a number of ways of achieving this with RNT, although the treatment parameters and the problems faced do not entirely coincide with those of EBRT. Whilst concepts such as the number of treatment deliveries ('fractions') and the level of treatment at each fraction are important for both treatment modalities, issues peculiar to RNT include the choice of targeting agent and the radionuclide itself. Of the difficulties specific to RNT, the greatest barrier to accurate dosimetry-based treatment is probably that of image quantification, which is seldom required in routine nuclear medicine practice.

Dosimetry for RNT is complicated by the wide range of target and normal organs that can be irradiated. Whilst normal organs that determine dose-limiting toxicity often include the liver and kidneys, the systemic nature of RNT means that the red marrow is often the most vulnerable organ and treatments are frequently limited by hematological toxicity. A further difficulty is faced by the different scales at which the dosimetry must be considered. The spatial resolution of gamma camera imaging, particularly for ^{131}I, provides a minimum limit to the size of organ in which radionuclide uptake may be accurately quantified, particularly if there is a heterogeneous distribution of activity. However, the therapeutic effect of any given therapy procedure will also be heavily dependent on the uptake pattern at a multi-cellular and cellular scale. These various concerns mean that a comprehensive approach to dosimetry must incorporate a range of techniques and methodologies, each of which must be considered independently as well as part of a global approach.

In recent years, dosimetry for RNT has become an increasingly important field of research, and in conjunction with a new wave of molecular targeting agents and the resurgence of a number of radionuclides, alternative treatments for a range of rare and common cancers are promised. Methodologies have emerged to calculate absorbed-dose distributions arising from heterogeneous uptake of activity at both the microscopic and macroscopic scale and techniques are being further developed to quantify accurately functional image data and absorbed dose depositions. A recent European directive[1] states that for radiotherapeutic procedures, including those pertaining to nuclear medicine for therapeutic purposes, 'exposures of target volumes shall be individually planned; taking into account that doses of non-target volumes and tissues shall be as low as reasonably achievable'. This chapter will cover recent advances in the field of internal dosimetry that can address this directive, and the opportunities subsequently afforded to improve the practice of RNT.

OVERVIEW OF STANDARD DOSIMETRY

In so far as dosimetry has been carried out over the last 30 years for RNT, the most common technique employed has been that devised by the Medical Internal Radiation Dose (MIRD) committee. A series of pamphlets, dose estimate reports, and books have been produced to provide an absolute reference for radiopharmaceutical dosimetry. The basic MIRD schema has found clinical acceptance in part because of its elegant simplicity and the relative ease with which it may be employed in the clinic.

The MIRD schema

To deal with the deposition of absorbed dose from one organ to another, it is convenient to consider separately the organ in which the radionuclide resides, termed the source organ, and the organ for which the dosimetry is to be calculated, termed the target organ. In the case of tumor dosimetry for RNT, the source organ and target organ are the same. In essence, the quantitative determination required to produce absorbed dose estimates can be considered as comprising of just two components, one relating to physical parameters and the other to biological, patient-dependent parameters.

The patient-dependent aspects of internal absorbed dose calculations concern the level of uptake of a radionuclide and its retention within an organ – the greater the uptake and the longer the retention, the greater the absorbed dose to the target organ. This entails calculating the total number of radioactive decays that occur within a source organ, termed the cumulated activity, $\tilde{A}$. This parameter is obtained from the time integral of the activity–time curve for the source organ. For simplicity, if uptake is considered to be instantaneous and a mono-exponential decay is assumed the activity at time t following administration, $A(t)$, is given by

$$A(t) = A_0 e^{-\lambda_{\text{eff}} t}$$

where A_0 is the initial activity (at time $t = 0$) and λ_{eff} is the effective decay constant, related to the effective half-life, T_{eff}, by

$$\lambda_{\text{eff}} = \frac{\ln 2}{T_{\text{eff}}}$$

and to the physical and biological half-lives, λ_{phys} and λ_{biol}, by

$$\lambda_{\text{eff}} = \lambda_{\text{phys}} + \lambda_{\text{biol}}.$$

The cumulated activity is then given by

$$\tilde{A} = A_0 \int_0^\infty e^{-\lambda_{\text{eff}} t} \, dt$$

which under the conditions stated becomes

$$\tilde{A} = \frac{A_0}{\lambda_{\text{eff}}}.$$

The physical parameters are determined by the radionuclide itself and are concerned with the emission energy, Δ, with which the absorbed dose is proportional, the fraction of the emitted energy released in the source organ that is deposited in the target organ, ϕ, with which the absorbed dose is also proportional, and the mass of the target organ itself, m, with which the absorbed dose is inversely proportional. For any standard source–target configuration and for any given radionuclide these parameters are fixed and therefore do not need to be calculated for each treatment. MIRD pamphlets list the combined values of these parameters, called S values, where S is given by

$$S = \frac{\Delta \varphi}{m}$$

and may be defined as the absorbed dose to a target organ from activity in a source organ per unit cumulated activity.

The mean absorbed dose to the target tissue, $\bar{D}$, is then given simply by $\bar{D} = \tilde{A} S$, which is the basic MIRD equation (Fig. 17F.1).

For more detailed exposition of the MIRD methodology and its use, the reader is referred to the many publications and overviews that are available (e.g. Loevinger[2], Siegel et al.[3] and Snyder et al.[4]).

This methodology was initially developed to determine the absorbed doses to normal organs resulting from diagnostic procedures. As such, a number of approximations

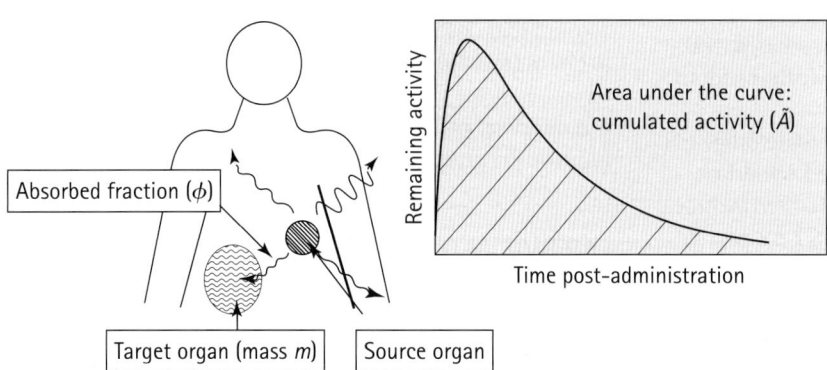

Figure 17F.1 The absorbed dose to a target organ with mass m from a source organ is given by $D = \tilde{A}\Delta\varphi/m$.

and assumptions are made that render it less suitable to therapeutic procedures, including the use of standardized organ sizes and geometries (which of course cannot include abnormal growths such as tumors) and the assumption of a uniform uptake in the source organ. Only a mean absorbed dose to the target organ is calculated. Since its initial exposition, a number of significant advances and alternative methodologies have been made that are more applicable to RNT although the principles and the basic MIRD formalism remain relevant.

TUMOR DOSIMETRY

Accurate tumor dosimetry is difficult to achieve. The approach taken for any specific therapy procedure should be flexible and dependent on the treatment itself and on the scale of uptake. For a relatively small tumor volume, of the order of the spatial resolution of the camera and collimator for the radionuclide imaged, and where a uniform uptake can be assumed, a modification of the MIRD schema can be applied. It is necessary to determine the time-dependent uptake and retention of the radiopharmaceutical which can be attained from a time-sequential series of image data, comprised of either planar or single photon emission computed tomography (SPECT) scans. Regions of interest must be delineated on each of the scans and the counts within the source volume determined for each. The definition of tumor volume itself poses a problem. Anatomical volumes can be determined from computed tomography (CT) or magnetic resonance imaging (MRI) data (which themselves are likely to yield different estimates), and applied to the gamma camera data. Alternatively, a 'functional volume' can be outlined, whereby a threshold of the maximum count can be used, for example. This threshold will vary depending on the radionuclide imaged and on the tumor volume itself. The accuracy with which the time course of activity uptake and retention can be determined is dependent on the number and timing of scans. In the case of a multi-exponential decay a minimum of two scans must be acquired for each phase to characterize the effective half-life, and in order to estimate potential uncertainties in the calculation, three or more scans should be acquired for each phase. This is particularly problematic for the uptake phase. There are practical restrictions to the acquisition of two or more scans over what may be a short period, radiation protection considerations often dictate that the patient should be kept in isolation immediately following administration of a large quantity of radioactivity, and the dead-time characteristics of gamma cameras, particularly of nonparalyzable systems, preclude quantitative imaging at high activities.[5] Hence it is usually convenient to assume instantaneous uptake and to estimate the potential uncertainty involved due to this assumption. In many cases where tumor dosimetry has been performed, the effective decay has been found to be mono-exponential. This minimizes the number of scans required to three, although four or five scans are recommended. An increase in the effective half-life that may occur after the final scan will cause the absorbed dose to be underestimated, which to some extent may counteract the overestimate made from the assumption of instantaneous uptake.

MIRD S values are difficult to ascertain for tumors, since these cannot be standardized and are themselves dependent on both the size and geometry of the tumor. One approach is to use MIRD values derived from similar-sized standard organs (that of a thyroid, kidney or adrenal perhaps), possibly interpolating between values or employing a mass correction factor. Alternatively, if the tumor is assumed to be spherical, S values may be determined according to the diameter or mass of the sphere, an option available within the MIRDOSE and OLINDA software.[6,7] Generation of patient-specific S values necessitates the use of Monte Carlo methodology.[8]

Image quantification

Planar data offer superior spatial resolution to SPECT and are more convenient to acquire and process. However, image contrast is relatively poor, and counts must be corrected for background. In particular, superposition of background and organ counts can be difficult to correct for. SPECT data on the other hand, whilst necessary if the distribution of the uptake is to be visualized, are subject to the reconstruction parameters chosen which will be data dependent and thus are difficult to standardize. Apart from dead-time considerations, the most important parameters affecting image quantification are scatter and attenuation. A number of scatter correction techniques have been proposed, ranging from the application of a single scatter window placed immediately below the peak energy window, to a series of windows and spectral analysis.[9,10] In the case of ^{131}I with its higher energy emissions of 637 keV and 723 keV triple-energy scatter windows are often employed whereby the scatter component in the peak energy window is determined from a linear interpolation between narrow windows placed immediately above and below the peak window. It is worth noting that for ^{131}I imaging 73% of counts within the peak window can be due to septal penetration or scatter within the collimator.[11] There is also a range of options available for applying attenuation corrections. The most simple approach is to assume a uniform attenuation coefficient throughout the phantom or patient and to make corrections accordingly.[12] More complicated approaches are to apply an attenuation map derived from a transmission scan obtained from either an external radionuclide or from a CT scan which may be segmented into regions of varying electron density, notably bone, lung, and soft tissue.[13–16] Quantification of gamma cameras is an increasingly active research area, led by Monte Carlo methodology.[11,17,18] There are a number of methods available to quantify the data. Siegel *et al.*[19] proposed the application of a build-up factor for planar data, whereby the counts are corrected according to their depth in tissue. A common approach is to obtain a calibration factor in counts per megabecquerel from a 'standard' source of known activity imaged along with the patient or in a phantom imaged independently.[20,21] It is worth noting that in many cases where dosimetry calculations are published, no account is taken of either scatter or attenuation correction.

Three-dimensional dosimetry

It is often noted that the difficulties inherent in determining a tumor volume and the non-uniform distribution of activity uptake frequently observed render accurate dosimetry difficult to obtain (EANM group). Both problems may be addressed simultaneously by considering distributions of absorbed dose. For this it is necessary to acquire a series of SPECT scans, register these and then calculate the absorbed dose on a voxel-by-voxel basis.[22,23] As an example, see the case history on page 786. It is then possible to view the dosimetry results as a dose–volume histogram from which maximum, minimum or mean doses may be calculated. Unfortunately, there is no commercially available software package available to perform this patient-specific dosimetry, although a number of in-house packages have been produced.[23–27]

MARROW AND WHOLE-BODY DOSIMETRY

As mentioned, for many radionuclide therapies, the dose-limiting toxicity is hemotological. A number of techniques have been employed to address this issue.

Whole-body dosimetry

If the assumption is made that the absorbed dose to the red marrow is linear with that to the whole body, dosimetry can be performed with relative ease and accuracy. The whole-body absorbed dose may be determined either from total-body imaging[28–30] or from external counts.[31] In the case of imaging the procedure is similar to that of organ dosimetry although in this case a time-sequential series of whole-body scans of the patient must be obtained. The region of interest (ROI) for which the absorbed dose is calculated should encompass the total body and corrections should be made for background activity by placing a suitable ROI outside the body (Fig. 17F.2). Quantification is usually achieved by means of a calibration source, which may be a vial or syringe filled with a known quantity of activity, placed within the field of view (FOV).

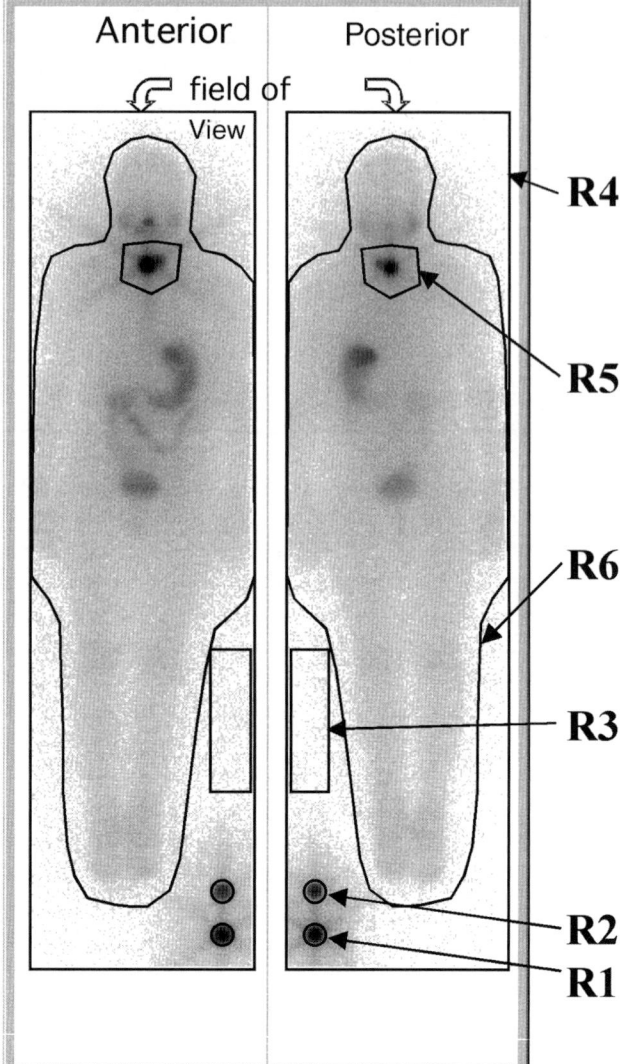

Figure 17F.2 *Outlined regions of interest for multi-center study investigating dosimetry for thyroid cancer. R1: Background source of known activity. R2: A second source of known activity, lower than R1. (To enable dead-time corrections.) R3: Large background region R4: Field of view. R5: ROI incorporating remnant. R6: Whole-body ROI. (Courtesy of M Lassmann)*

A simpler and less resource-intensive approach is to acquire counts from the patient at intervals following administration with a compensated Geiger counter. Quantification in this case is achieved by ensuring that the first reading is obtained immediately after administration of the radiopharmaceutical so that the counts obtained correspond to 100% of the activity. Subsequent readings may then be converted to counts by means of ratios. This method has the advantage of being cost-effective and easy to implement since it does not require the use of imaging, and measurements can be acquired by ward staff or by carers. The accuracy of the method is dependent on the care with which data are acquired, since it is essential that each measurement is obtained in similar conditions; that is, immediately post-void and with the patient lying in the same position relative to the counter. It has been demonstrated in meta-[^{131}I]iodobenzylguanidine (^{131}I-MIBG) treatment for neuroendocrine tumors that the absorbed dose delivered at therapy may be predicted with accuracy from a tracer study.

Marrow dosimetry

In cases of specific uptake and marrow involvement it is possible to use imaging to calculate absorbed marrow dose, using methodology similar to that given above.[32,33] The main problems of this approach are that in the absence of whole-body SPECT, imaging is necessarily limited to either whole-body planar scans or to tomographic scans of selected regions. Conversion of cumulated activity estimates to absorbed dose are complicated by bone–tissue interfaces which will cause backscatter of emitted beta particles and a non-uniform deposition of energy.

Red marrow to blood ratios

Blood samples are usually acquired throughout the course of a therapy procedure and the blood self-absorbed dose can thus be determined directly. Sgouros[34] derived a factor relating the ratio of the absorbed dose to the red marrow from that of the blood by taking into account the relative mass of red and white marrow, bone and blood within the bony matrix. Further development was carried out by Hindorf et al.[35] This technique precludes the need for imaging, although is applicable only in cases where there is no marrow involvement.

At present, although a number of approaches are available,[36,37] marrow dosimetry presents the greatest challenge to dosimetry for RNT. There is no accepted model that is known to predict toxicity reliably, and it is likely that any model to do so will need to take into account previous myelotoxic treatments and bone marrow reserves.

CELLULAR AND MULTI-CELLULAR DOSIMETRY

Whilst macroscopically determined absorbed dose estimates are necessary to implement comprehensive patient-specific treatment planning, it should be noted that treatment efficacy can be largely influenced by the uptake distribution of the radiopharmaceutical at a cellular level. Within any

cluster of cells, either comprising part of a larger tumor or constituting microscopic disease, it is possible that uptake may localize in only a fraction of these cells, or indeed may remain in the extracellular matrix. In this case the critical factor is the energy of emission of the radionuclide and the subsequent degree of crossfire, whereby a cell may be irradiated by activity taken up in a number of adjacent cells. Valimaki et al.[38] developed cellular cluster models to study this effect and others have examined the absorbed dose to the nucleus as a function of the localization of uptake[39–43] showing that the likelihood of inducing double-strand breaks within DNA for any given radionuclide is highly dependent on its localization. The stochastic nature of absorbed dose deposition at a cellular and subcellular level means that average absorbed dose calculations are no longer valid. Instead an approach based on the Monte Carlo method is required. For this purpose a range of Monte Carlo codes are available, including Penelope, MCNP, open gate and EGSnrc.

CLINICAL APPLICATIONS OF DOSIMETRY

Internal dosimetry is being applied to an increasing number of clinical studies and is becoming essential for phase I/II studies.[44–54] A lack of standardized protocols for dosimetry can render quantitative comparisons of results obtained at different centers difficult.[55] In the absence of multi-center protocols it can nevertheless be useful to consider the range of absorbed doses given for any treatment protocol. Many authors have shown that the range of delivered absorbed doses frequently covers one or more orders of magnitude for both tumor and organs at risk. This indicates that many therapies that are administered either as a fixed activity or as a function of patient weight can effectively result in a wide range of treatments.

CONCLUSION

Much of the current research in dosimetry involves model-based techniques and theoretical calculations that are slow to find their way into the clinic. Internal dosimetry for RNT has remained essentially unchanged and largely used only in research applications for several decades. The increasing pressure to demonstrate good clinical practice, the opportunity to evaluate and optimize new (and existing) radiolabeled targeting vectors and the potential for individualized treatment planning will ensure that individual patient dosimetry becomes routine in centers offering radionuclide therapy as a treatment option.

Case history

The patient presented with shoulder metastases from ca thyroid and was treated with 9.0 GBq Na^{131}I. Sequential SPECT scans (Plate 17F.1) were obtained at days 1, 2, and 3 post-administration (a). These scans were spatially registered using mutual information methods (b). A convolution process was used to determine the absorbed dose on a voxel-by-voxel basis. The absorbed dose was first determined for 1 voxel, taking all other source voxels into account, and the process was repeated for all other target voxels (c). The resulting absorbed dose map was displayed both in pseudo-colour and as isodose contours registered to CT to aid visualization (d). In this case a mean absorbed dose of 54 Gy was obtained over an anatomical region outlined by a radiologist. However, the heterogeneous distribution indicated a poor delivery of absorbed dose to the periphery of the large metastasis in the left shoulder and the patient was subsequently treated with external-beam radiotherapy.

REFERENCES

● Seminal primary article
◆ Key review paper
★ First formal publication of a management guideline

★ 1 Nuis A. Health protection of individuals against the dangers of ionising radiation in relation to medical exposure: Council directive 97/43 EURATOM. 30-6-1997.

★ 2 Loevinger R. *MIRD primer for absorbed dose calculations.* New York: Society of Nuclear Medicine, 1988.

★ 3 Siegel JA, Thomas SR, Stubbs JB, *et al.* Techniques for quantitative radiopharmaceutical biodistribution data acquisition and analysis for use in human radiation dose estimates. (MIRD pamphlet no. 16.) *J Nucl Med* 1999; **40**: 37S–61S.

   4 Snyder WS, Ford MR, Warner GG, Watson SB. *Absorbed dose per unit cumulated activity for selected radionuclides and organs,* part 1. Reston, Virginia: Society of Nuclear Medicine, 1975.

   5 Ferrer L, Delpon G, Lisbona A, Bardies M. Dosimetric impact of correcting count losses due to deadtime in clinical radioimmunotherapy trials involving iodine-131 scintigraphy. *Cancer Biother Radiopharm* 2003; **18**: 117–24.

● 6 Stabin MG. MIRDOSE: Personal computer software for internal dose assessment in nuclear medicine. *J Nucl Med* 1996; **37**: 538–46.

   7 Stabin MG, Sparks RB, Crowe E. OLINDA/EXM: the second-generation personal computer software for internal dose assessment in nuclear medicine. *J Nucl Med* 2005; **46**: 1023–7.

   8 Chiavassa S, Bardies M, Guiraud-Vitaux F, *et al.* OEDIPE: a personalized dosimetric tool associating voxel-based models with MCNPX. *Cancer Biother Radiopharm* 2005; **20**: 325–32.

   9 Buvat I, Rodriguezvillafuerte M, Todd-Pokropek A, *et al.* Comparative-assessment of 9 scatter correction methods based on spectral analysis using Monte Carlo simulations. *J Nucl Med* 1995; **36**: 1476–88.

  10 Delpon G, Ferrer L, Lisbona A, Bardies M. Impact of scatter and attenuation corrections for iodine-131 two-dimensional quantitative imaging in patients. *Cancer Biother Radiopharm* 2003; **18**: 191–9.

  11 Dewaraja YK, Ljungberg M, Koral KF. Characterization of scatter and penetration using Monte Carlo simulation in I-131 imaging. *J Nucl Med* 2000; **41**: 123–30.

● 12 Chang LT. A method for attenuation correction in radionuclide computed tomography. *IEEE Trans Nucl Sci* 1978; **25**: 638–43.

  13 Fleming JS. A technique for using CT images in attenuation correction and quantification in SPECT. *Nucl Med Commun* 1989; **10**: 83–97.

  14 Blankespoor SC, Wu X, Kalki K, *et al.* Attenuation correction of SPECT using X-ray CT on an emission–transmission CT system: Myocardial perfusion assessment. *IEEE Trans Nucl Sci* 1996; **43**: 2263–74.

  15 Guy MJ, Castellano-Smith IA, Flower MA, *et al.* DETECT – dual energy transmission estimation CT – for improved attenuation correction in SPECT and PET. *IEEE Trans Nucl Sci* 1998; **45**: 1261–7.

◆ 16 Zaidi H, Hasegawa B. Determination of the attenuation map in emission tomography. *J Nucl Med* 2003; **44**: 291–315.

  17 Ljungberg M, Strand SE, Rajeevan N, King MA. Monte-Carlo simulation of transmission studies using a planar source with a parallel collimator and a line source with a fan-beam collimator. *IEEE Trans Nucl Sci* 1994; **41**: 1577–84.

  18 Autret D, Bitar A, Ferrer L, *et al.* Monte Carlo modeling of gamma cameras for I-131 imaging in targeted radiotherapy. *Cancer Biother Radiopharm* 2005; **20**: 77–84.

  19 Siegel JA, Wu RK, Maurer AH. The buildup factor – effect of scatter on absolute volume determination. *J Nucl Med* 1985; **26**: 390–4.

  20 Koral KF, Dewaraja Y, Li J, *et al.* Update on hybrid conjugate-view SPECT tumor dosimetry and response in I-131-tositumomab therapy of previously untreated lymphoma patients. *J Nucl Med* 2003; **44**: 457–64.

21 Flux GD, Webb S, Ott RJ, *et al.* Three-dimensional dosimetry for intralesional radionuclide therapy using mathematical modeling and multimodality imaging. *J Nucl Med* 1997; **38**: 1059–66.

• 22 Sgouros G, Chiu S, Pentlow KS, *et al.* 3-Dimensional dosimetry for radioimmunotherapy treatment planning. *J Nucl Med* 1993; **34**: 1595–601.

23 Kolbert KS, Sgouros G, Scott AM, *et al.* Implementation and evaluation of patient-specific three-dimensional internal dosimetry. *J Nucl Med* 1997; **38**: 301–8.

24 Guy MJ, Flux GD, Papavasileiou P, *et al.* RMDP: A dedicated package for I-131 SPECT quantification, registration and patient-specific dosimetry. *Cancer Biother Radiopharm* 2003; **18**: 61–9.

25 Mckay E. A software tool for specifying voxel models for dosimetry estimation. *Cancer Biother Radiopharm* 2003; **18**: 379–92.

26 Sjogreen K, Ljungberg M, Wingardh K, *et al.* The LundADose method for planar image activity quantification and absorbed-dose assessment in radionuclide therapy. *Cancer Biother Radiopharm* 2005; **20**: 92–7.

27 Lehmann J, Siantar CH, Wessol DE, *et al.* Monte Carlo treatment planning for molecular targeted radiotherapy within the MINERVA system. *Phys Med Biol* 2005; **50**: 947–58.

28 Monsieurs M, Brans B, Bacher K, *et al.* Patient dosimetry for I-131-MIBG therapy for neuroendocrine tumours based on I-123-MIBG scans. *Eur J Nucl Med Mol Imag* 2002; **29**: 1581–7.

29 Lassmann M, Hanscheid H, Reiners C, Thomas SR. Blood and bone marrow dosimetry in radioiodine therapy of differentiated thyroid cancer after stimulation with rhTSH. *J Nucl Med* 2005; **46**: 900–1.

30 Wahl RL, Kroll S, Zasadny KR. Patient-specific whole-body dosimetry: principles and a simplified method for clinical implementation. *J Nucl Med* 1998; **39**: 14S–20S.

31 Flux GD, Guy MJ, Beddows R, *et al.* Estimation and implications of random errors in whole-body dosimetry for targeted radionuclide therapy. *Phys Med Biol* 2002; **47**: 3211–23.

32 Macey DJ, DeNardo SJ, DeNardo GL, *et al.* Estimation of radiation absorbed doses to the red marrow in radioimmunotherapy. *Clin Nucl Med* 1995; **20**: 117–25.

33 Siegel JA, Lee RE, Pawlyk DA, *et al.* Sacral scintigraphy for bone-marrow dosimetry in radioimmunotherapy. *Nucl Med Biol* 1989; **16**: 553.

34 Sgouros G. Bone-marrow dosimetry for radioimmunotherapy – theoretical derivation of the red marrow to blood activity concentration ratio. *J Nucl Med* 1993; **34**: 160.

35 Hindorf C, Linden O, Tennvall J, *et al.* Time dependence of the activity concentration ratio of red marrow to blood and implications for red marrow dosimetry. *Cancer* 2002; **94**: 1235–9.

36 Siegel JA. Establishing a clinically meaningful predictive model of hematologic toxicity in non-myeloablative targeted radiotherapy: practical aspects and limitations of red marrow dosimetry. *Cancer Biother Radiopharm* 2005; **20**: 126–40.

37 Sgouros G, Stabin M, Erdi Y, *et al.* Red marrow dosimetry for radiolabeled antibodies that bind to marrow, bone, or blood components. *Med Phys* 2000; **27**: 2150–64.

38 Valimaki J, Lampinen JS, Kuronen AA, *et al.* Comparison of different cell-cluster models for cell-level dosimetry. *Acta Oncologica* 2001; **40**: 92–7.

39 Hartman T, Lundqvist H, Westlin JE, Carlsson J. Radiation doses to the cell nucleus in single cells and cells in micrometastases in targeted therapy with I-131 labeled ligands or antibodies. *Intern J Radiat Oncol Biol Phys* 2000; **46**: 1025–36.

40 Malaroda A, Flux GD, Buffa FM, Ott RJ. Multicellular dosimetry in voxel geometry for targeted radionuclide therapy. *Cancer Biother Radiopharm* 2003; **18**: 451–61.

41 Malaroda A, Flux GD, Ott RJ. Integral survival fraction from heterogeneous activity distributions at the multi-cellular scale. *Eur J Nucl Med Mol Imag* 2004; **31**: S476.

42 Gardin I, Faraggi M, Huc E, Bok BD. Absorbed fraction to the cell nucleus for low energy electrons. *Acta Oncologica* 1996; **35**: 953–8.

43 Gardin I, Faraggi M, Huc E, Bok BD. Modeling of the relationship between cell dimensions and mean electron dose delivered to the cell nucleus – application to 5 radionuclides used in nuclear medicine. *Phys Med Biol* 1995; **40**: 1001–14.

44 Gaze MN, Chang YC, Flux GD, *et al.* Feasibility of dosimetry-based high-dose I-131-meta-iodo-benzylguanidine with topotecan as a radiosensitizer in children with metastatic neuroblastoma. *Cancer Biother Radiopharm* 2005; **20**: 195–9.

45 Winter JN, Inwards D, Erwin W, *et al.* Phase I trial combining Y-90 Zevalin and high-dose BEAM chemotherapy with hematopoietic progenitor cell transplant in relapsed or refractory B-cell NHL. *Blood* 2001; **98**: 2835.

46 O'Sullivan JM, McCready VR, Flux G, *et al.* High activity rhenium-186 HEDP with autologous peripheral blood stem cell rescue: a phase I study in progressive hormone refractory prostate cancer metastatic to bone. *Br J Cancer* 2002; **86**: 1715–20.

47 DeNardo SJ, Kramer EL, O'Donnell RT, *et al.* Radioimmunotherapy for breast cancer using indium-111/yttrium-90 BrE-3: results of a phase I clinical trial. *J Nucl Med* 1997; **38**: 1180–5.

48 Breitz HB, Fisher DR, Wessels BW. Marrow toxicity and radiation absorbed dose estimates from

rhenium-186-labeled monoclonal antibody. *J Nucl Med* 1998; **39**: 1746–51.

49 Kraeber-Bodere F, Bardet S, Hoefnagel CA, *et al.* Radioimmunotherapy in medullary thyroid cancer using bispecific antibody and iodine 131-labeled bivalent hapten: preliminary results of a phase I/II clinical trial. *Clin Cancer Res* 1999; **5**: 3190–8S.

50 Murray JL, Macey DJ, Kasi LP, *et al.* Phase-II radioimmunotherapy trial with I-131 CC49 in colorectal cancer. *Cancer* 1994; **73**: 1057–66.

51 Tempero M, Leichner P, Baranowska-Kortylewicz J, *et al.* High-dose therapy with (90)yttrium-labeled monoclonal antibody CC49: a phase I trial. *Clin Cancer Res* 2000; **6**: 3095–102.

52 Vuillez JP, Kraeber-Bodere F, Moro D, *et al.* Radio-immunotherapy of small cell lung carcinoma with the two-step method using a bispecific anti-carcinoembryonic antigen/anti-diethylenetriaminepentaacetic acid (DTPA) antibody and iodine-131 di-DTPA hapten: results of a phase I/II trial. *Clin Cancer Res* 1999; **5**: 3259–67S.

53 Wong JYC, Chu DZJ, Yamauchi D, *et al.* Dose escalation trial of indium-111-labeled anti-carcinoembryonic antigen chimeric monoclonal antibody (chimeric T84.66) in presurgical colorectal cancer patients. *J Nucl Med* 1998; 39: 2097–104.

54 Horning SJ, Younes A, Jain V, *et al.* Efficacy and safety of tositumomab and iodine-131 tositumomab (Bexxar) in B-cell lymphoma, progressive after rituximab. *J Clin Oncol* 2005; **23**: 712–19.

55 Wessels BW, Bolch WE, Bouchet LG, *et al.* Bone marrow dosimetry using blood-based models for radiolabeled antibody therapy: A multi-institutional comparison. *J Nucl Med* 2004; **45**: 1725–33.

18. Pitfalls and artifacts in ^{18}F-FDG PET and PET/CT imaging   791
    G.J.R. Cook

19. Diagnostic accuracy and cost-effectiveness issues   799
    M.N. Maisey

20. Radiopharmaceuticals   813

    20A Introduction   815
    M. Frier

    20B Interactions and reactions   821
    M. Frier

    20C New single-photon radiopharmaceuticals   831
    S.J. Mather

    20D New radiopharmaceuticals for positron emission tomography   839
    E.M. Bednarczyk and A. Amer

21. Technology and instrumentation   847

    21A Solid state and other detectors   849
    R.J. Ott

    21B Image registration   861
    G. Flux and G.J.R. Cook

    21C Attenuation correction in positron emission tomography and single photon emission computed tomography   869
    D.L. Bailey

Pitfalls and artifacts in ^{18}F-FDG PET and PET/CT imaging

GARY J.R. COOK

Introduction	791	False positives and negatives in oncology	794
Normal appearances and variation in		Scanning after therapy	795
^{18}F–FDG PET imaging	791	Specific problems related to PET/CT	795
Patient preparation	794	References	797

INTRODUCTION

As with any diagnostic test there are a number of potential pitfalls, normal variants, and artifacts that may lead to inaccurate interpretation. 2-[^{18}F]Fluoro-2-deoxy-D-glucose (^{18}F-FDG) positron emission tomography (PET) has now become a standard imaging modality, particularly in oncology, and a number of potential pitfalls continue to be described. With careful patient preparation and appropriate imaging protocols, together with adequate experience, many of these may be avoided. Whilst the advent of combined positron emission tomography/computed tomography (PET/CT) has led to a reduction in false positives due to normal variants and an increase in confidence in interpretation of scans, it has also brought some of its own specific artifacts and pitfalls. Already many of these are recognized or overcome by advances in hardware and software and further improvements are anticipated as the combined modality is likely to supersede PET-only scanners in clinical imaging applications.

NORMAL APPEARANCES AND VARIATION IN ^{18}F-FDG PET IMAGING

^{18}F-FDG closely follows the metabolic pathways of glucose and as such can be considered an analog, acting as a tracer of energy substrate metabolism. In oncology, it has been appreciated for many years that malignant cells show a higher glycolytic rate than most normal tissues.[1] On account of this, in addition to the fact that many tumors over-express membrane glucose transporters, malignant tissue shows high uptake of ^{18}F-FDG. Intracellularly, ^{18}F-FDG is converted to ^{18}F-FDG-6-phosphate by hexokinase, but unlike glucose does not undergo significant enzymatic reactions. ^{18}F-FDG-6-phosphate has a negative charge and remains effectively trapped in tissue. Glucose-6-phosphatase mediated dephosphorylation of ^{18}F-FDG-6-phosphate occurs only slowly in most tumors, normal myocardium, and brain, and hence the uptake of ^{18}F-FDG is proportional to glycolytic rate. Rarely, tumors may have higher glucose-6-phosphatase activity resulting in relatively low uptake, a feature that has been described in hepatocellular carcinoma.[2] Some tissues show higher glucose-6-phosphatase activity, including liver, kidney, intestine, and resting skeletal muscle, and show only low uptake.

Although clinical ^{18}F-FDG PET imaging is commonly performed at 60 min following injection, there is evidence in some tumors that uptake as measured by standardized uptake values (SUVs) continues for some hours.[3] Increased glycolysis is not specific to tumor tissue and a number of benign processes, particularly inflammation, may result in uptake of ^{18}F-FDG that is higher than background tissues.[4–6] It would appear that many benign processes do not continue to accumulate ^{18}F-FDG at the same rate as malignant tumors and some groups have exploited this phenomenon by performing imaging at dual time points; for example, at 1 and 2 h.[7,8] Malignant tissue shows an increase in uptake between the time points but benign lesions do not.

In the brain there is high uptake of ^{18}F-FDG into cortical tissue and basal ganglia irrespective of substrate conditions, glucose being the predominant substrate for brain metabolism. The liver, spleen, and bone marrow normally show homogeneous low-grade uptake with bone marrow and spleen appearing less intense than the liver under normal conditions (Fig. 18.1). Some normal lymphatic tissue may show uptake of ^{18}F-FDG and this may be of a moderate intensity in the tonsils in adults as well as the adenoids in children. Thymic activity is commonly seen in children and can also be seen in young adults after chemotherapy, probably as a result of the thymic rebound phenomenon.[9] The typical pattern is of low to moderate uptake in the shape of an inverted 'V' in the anterior mediastinum.

In the chest it has been recognized that there is variation in regional lung activity, this being greater in the inferior and posterior segments, and it has been suggested that this might reduce sensitivity in lesion detection in these regions.[10] Cardiac activity is very variable, ranging from no discernible activity above background blood pool activity, to intense activity throughout the left ventricular myocardium. The degree of uptake depends on substrate availability and in a fasted patient in whom insulin levels are low, the predominant myocardial substrates are fatty acids. For oncology imaging of the thorax it is preferable to minimize cardiac activity by fasting the patient for 4–6 h so that any malignant mediastinal nodes or pericardiac nodules are clearly visualized. It is unusual to see atrial or right ventricular activity unless there is cardiac disease affecting those chambers.[11]

Uptake within the gastrointestinal tract is highly variable. Apart from lymphatic tissues within the oropharynx, salivary glands also often show low to moderate diffuse uptake of ^{18}F-FDG. The esophagus does not usually show significant activity unless inflamed or neoplastic but homogeneous uptake of tracer within the stomach wall is relatively common. Small intestinal uptake is variable and usually of low grade but colonic activity may be quite marked. It is commonest to see diffuse activity at the cecum and in the rectosigmoid region but focal uptake within the colon is unusual unless this is associated with pathology. The cause of intestinal uptake of ^{18}F-FDG is not fully understood and may be multifactorial. In rat studies it appears that only a minority of uptake is associated with intestinal smooth muscle but that the majority is associated either with the intestinal mucosa or with the luminal contents.[12] In order to minimize confounding bowel activity various groups have tried smooth muscle relaxants including glucagon and anticholinergics as well as bowel preparation including laxatives with or without colonic cleansing.[13,14] It is probable that PET/CT imaging will reduce diagnostic uncertainty with respect to physiologic bowel activity by allowing more confident interpretation related to areas of anatomically normal intestine. This may be further enhanced by using bowel contrast agents.[15,16]

Unlike glucose, ^{18}F-FDG is excreted in the urine and activity may therefore be noted in any part of the urinary tract. This explains the limitations of this radiopharmaceutical in imaging primary tumors of renal or urothelial origin. Urinary tract activity also has the potential to cause false positive interpretations for tumor if foci of urinary stasis occur in the ureters. With PET/CT it is easier to correctly differentiate ureteric activity from retroperitoneal lymphadenopathy by direct anatomical correlation. In addition, bladder activity may obscure or mimic pathological activity within the pelvis. Urinary stasis may be minimized

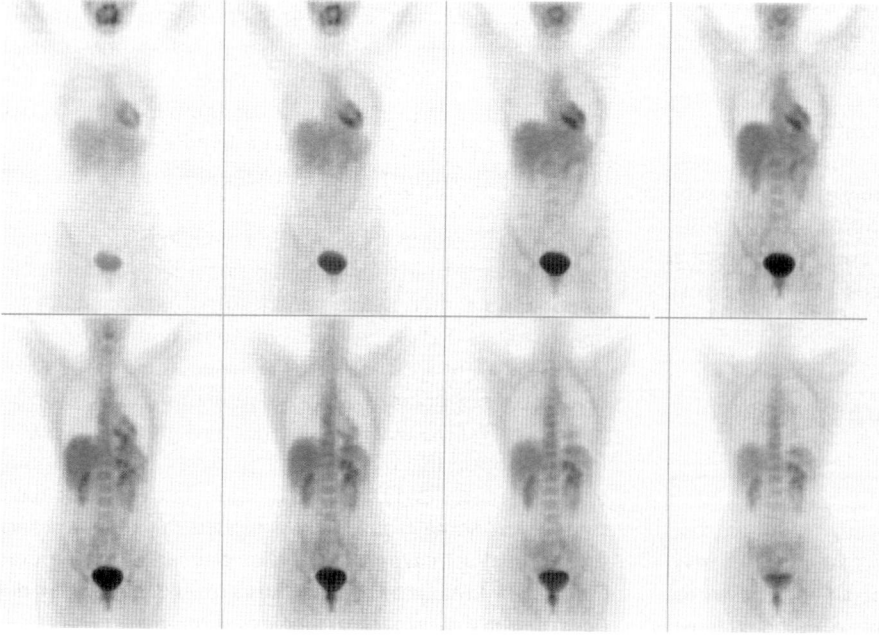

Figure 18.1 *A whole-body attenuation corrected ^{18}F-FDG study demonstrating normal distribution of this radiopharmaceutical on serial coronal slices.*

by good hydration and the use of a diuretic. This can be especially helpful when there is pathology in the pelvis. Rather than trying to empty the bladder by drainage or washout, it is our preference to image the pelvis with a full bladder with dilute ^{18}F-FDG activity. This enables easier differentiation of perivesical lymphadenopathy from small pockets of urinary activity. Some groups catheterize the bladder and perform washouts but we have found this unnecessary in the majority of patients and have found that it can be associated with measurable radiation exposure to technologists. Although excreted ^{18}F-FDG may be seen in any part of the urinary tract, it is important to gain a history of any previous urinary diversion procedures, since these may cause areas of high activity outside the normal renal tract and may result in errors of interpretation unless they are appreciated.

Skeletal muscle uptake is one of the commonest causes of interpretative difficulty. Increased aerobic glycolysis associated with muscle activation leads to increased accumulation of ^{18}F-FDG that may mimic or obscure pathology. Exercise should be prohibited before injection of ^{18}F-FDG and during the uptake period to minimize muscle uptake.

A pattern of symmetrical activity occasionally encountered in the neck, supraclavicular and paraspinal regions (Fig. 18.2) was at one time considered to be due to involuntary muscle tension but with the advent of PET/CT it has become apparent that this activity originates in brown fat, a vestigial organ of thermogenesis that is sympathetically innervated. This appearance, that may mimic or mask pathology, is most commonly seen in children and young adults and is more frequent in winter months and in patients with lower body mass index.[17] It appears that benzodiazepines are able to reduce the incidence of this potentially

confusing appearance, possibly due to a generalized reduction in sympathetic drive.

Even apparently innocent activities such as talking or chewing gum may lead to muscle uptake that simulates malignant tissue. In patients being assessed for head and neck malignancies, it is therefore important that silence is maintained and that patients refrain from chewing during the uptake period. Although vocalization after injection of ^{18}F-FDG may lead to uptake within the laryngeal muscles, in most patients the symmetrical and typical pattern of uptake seen as a result of this (Fig. 18.3) is easily recognized. However, it is prudent to stop the patient from talking during the uptake period if laryngeal pathology is

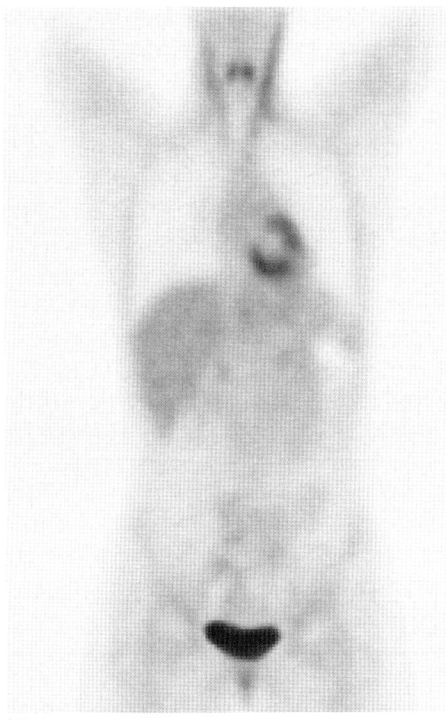

(a)

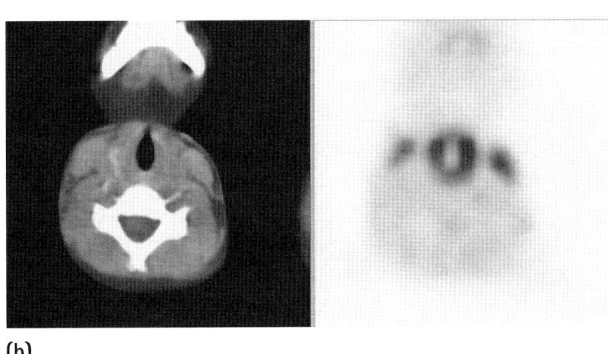

(b)

Figure 18.3 *The typical symmetrical pattern of laryngeal muscle uptake in a patient who talked during the ^{18}F-FDG uptake period on (a) a coronal image and on (b) a transaxial PET/CT image. Symmetrical sternocleidomastoid muscle activity is also seen on the transaxial PET image.*

Figure 18.2 *A whole-body ^{18}F-FDG acquisition in a child showing extensive symmetrical brown fat activation in the neck, supraclavicular, and paraspinal regions.*

suspected. In patients with laryngeal nerve palsies asymmetric uptake may be seen in the larynx.[5]

PATIENT PREPARATION

The key to successful PET imaging is to adequately prepare the patient to minimize the appearance of potential artifactual uptake patterns that make interpretation difficult. For oncology studies it is necessary to starve the patient for 4–6 h prior to injection of ^{18}F-FDG to minimize insulin levels and therefore reduce uptake of ^{18}F-FDG into fat and muscle that may reduce contrast between tumor and normal tissues. This will also reduce cardiac glucose metabolism in favor of fatty acids, reducing left ventricular ^{18}F-FDG activity and improving conspicuity of pathological lesions in the pericardiac region.

To further minimize muscle activity it is important that a patient is relaxed at the time of injection and has not taken vigorous exercise in the hours leading up to the scan. In oncology patients considered at risk of showing activated brown fat or 'muscle tension' then oral benzodiazepines should be considered at least 30 min prior to ^{18}F-FDG injection. Chewing and talking should be forbidden when pathology in the head and neck is suspected.

When malignant disease is suspected close to the urinary tract then good hydration and the use of intravenous diuretics should be considered to minimize urinary stasis and to dilute ^{18}F-FDG activity in the bladder.

FALSE POSITIVES AND NEGATIVES IN ONCOLOGY

A large number of potential false positives with respect to malignancy have been described.[4–6] This reflects the fact that uptake of ^{18}F-FDG is not specific to tumors and that increased glycolysis occurs in a number of physiological and pathological processes. In spite of the large number of reports of potential false positives, in clinical practice with adequate clinical information and an experienced interpreter, real problems are infrequent.

It is well recognized that inflammation may lead to accumulation of ^{18}F-FDG in macrophages and other activated inflammatory cells.[18,19] In oncological imaging, this inflammatory uptake may lead to a decrease in specificity. For example, it may be difficult to differentiate benign postradiotherapy changes from recurrent tumor in the brain, unless the study is optimally timed or unless alternative tracers such as ^{11}C-methionine are used. Apical lung activity may be seen following radiotherapy for breast cancer, and moderate uptake may follow radiotherapy for lung cancer.[20] It may also be difficult to differentiate radiation changes

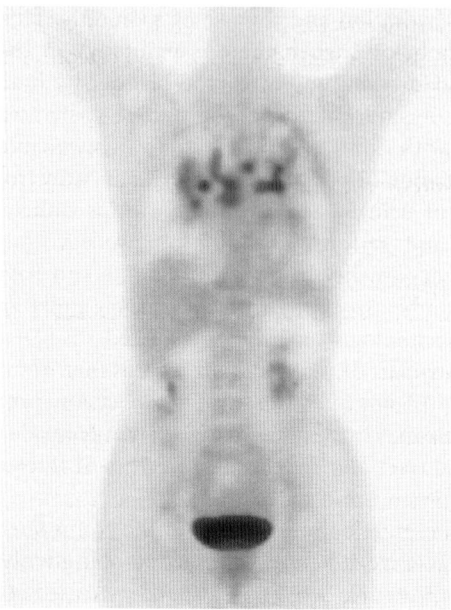

Figure 18.4   *A patient with non-Hodgkin's lymphoma and a previous history of sarcoidosis. The mulifocal activity in the lung hila was due to active sarcoidosis.*

from recurrent tumor in patients who have undergone radiotherapy for rectal cancer within 6 months. A negative scan is helpful but it may be difficult to differentiate residual tumor from inflammatory changes in a positive study.[21]

Pancreatic imaging with ^{18}F-FDG may be problematic. In some cases, uptake into mass-forming pancreatitis may be comparable in degree to uptake in pancreatic cancer. Conversely, false negative results have been described in diabetic patients with pancreatic cancer. However, if diabetic patients and those with raised inflammatory markers are excluded, then ^{18}F-FDG PET may still be an accurate test to differentiate benign from malignant pancreatic masses.[22]

A number of granulomatous disorders have been described as leading to increased uptake of ^{18}F-FDG, including tuberculosis,[23] and sarcoidosis[24] (Fig. 18.4). It is often necessary to be cautious in diagnosing malignancy when ^{18}F-FDG-avid lesions occur in patients who are known to be immunocompromised. It is these patients who often have the unusual infections that may lead to uptake that cannot be differentiated from malignancy. PET remains useful in these patients despite a lower specificity for malignancy, as it is often able to locate areas of disease that have not been identified by other means and which may be more amenable to biopsy.[25]

In the skeleton a diffuse increase in bone marrow activity seen as a result of chemotherapy or colony stimulating factors, is now well recognized.[26] Benign fractures can also lead to false positive uptake of ^{18}F-FDG[27] but it would appear that abnormal uptake is relatively short-lived and usually returns to normal by 3 months, and often considerably sooner, after the fracture.[28] A number of other focal benign skeletal pathologies may result in high ^{18}F-FDG uptake, including Paget's disease,[29] fibrous dysplasia,[30] and osteomyelitis.[31]

A number of benign neoplasms have been described as showing intense ^{18}F-FDG activity including Warthin's tumors of the salivary gland, colonic adenomas, enchondroma, and uterine fibroids,[32–35] amongst many others.

SCANNING AFTER THERAPY

Most oncologic ^{18}F-FDG PET scans are performed at 1 h post-injection but uptake in some tumors may not be maximal until some hours after this.[3] It is likely that a 1-h scan is likely to continue to be the most widely used protocol for practicality, patients' convenience, and because of the relatively short half-life of ^{18}F ($\approx$110 min). To monitor therapy with serial scans it is important to scan patients at exactly the same time after injection of ^{18}F-FDG, as it is possible that differences in timing alone could cause differences in SUVs between studies, independent of any therapy effect. An alternative solution is to scan patients when the uptake curve has reached a plateau, where small differences in timing do not affect measured uptake but as this may be up to 4 h post-injection in some tumors this is a less practical option in most departments.

Controversy exists as to the best time to perform scans following chemotherapy and radiotherapy. To some extent optimal timing may depend on the clinical question being asked. For example, if there is a residual mass following completion of chemotherapy for lymphoma, the timing of the scan after the last course of chemotherapy might be different from when ^{18}F-FDG PET is being used to assess the efficacy of chemotherapy after one or two cycles. It is possible that a 'stunning' phenomenon occurs in some tumors following chemotherapy whereby ^{18}F-FDG uptake is reduced or absent for a period of 2 weeks but subsequently increases again.[36] This phenomenon might explain the apparently poor sensitivity of ^{18}F-FDG PET after neoadjuvant chemotherapy in some cancers with some chemotherapeutic regimes.[37] Alternatively, experiments in mouse tumor models suggest that although early (days 1–3) reduction in ^{18}F-FDG uptake corresponds with reduction in the tumor viable cell fraction, at intermediate time points (days 8–10) uptake may be related to an inflammatory infiltrate.[38]

A flare response has also been described following hormone therapy in breast cancer[39] and in brain tumors[40] following chemotherapy, occurring a few days after therapy and possibly related to an influx of inflammatory cells as a response to tumor cytotoxicity. A number of publications have suggested that it is possible to predict response to chemotherapy at 1–2 weeks following treatment but that scans delayed to 5–6 weeks are more accurate in this regard.[41–44] Further research is required in this area but with the current state of knowledge it would not seem unreasonable to scan patients after one or two cycles of chemotherapy at least 10 days after the last treatment in order to measure whether the therapy is being effective or not. When there is a residual mass at the end of therapy then it would seem better to wait approximately 6 weeks for the most accurate measure of residual viable tumor and prediction of relapse. Allowing for measurement imprecision of approximately 10% and the expected effect of chemotherapy on ^{18}F-FDG uptake after one or more cycles of chemotherapy, the EORTC PET group have suggested guidelines for categorization of treatment response into progressive metabolic disease (PMD), stable metabolic disease (SMD), partial metabolic response (PMR) and complete metabolic response (CMR).[41]

Following radiotherapy there is an inflammatory reaction that may persist for some months and which is associated with uptake of ^{18}F-FDG. It has been suggested that in rectal cancer and head and neck cancers, inflammatory ^{18}F-FDG uptake may persist for 4–6 months after radiotherapy and that accurate diagnosis of residual tumor viability is best made after this time interval.[45,46] A negative scan before this interval is clinically helpful but it may not be possible to differentiate residual tumor activity from inflammatory reaction in positive scans.

SPECIFIC PROBLEMS RELATED TO PET/CT

There is little doubt amongst those with experience of PET/CT that it represents a further advance in imaging although it brings with it its own specific artifacts and pitfalls. This combination modality allows faster patient throughput by the use of the CT data to provide attenuation correction of the emission PET data as well as providing an anatomical and structural background to aid interpretation of the PET images. Acquisition of data within the same scanning gantry minimizes differences in positions of organs and structures between the CT and emission PET scans but any movement between the consecutive acquisitions may lead to misregistration of the two data sets. In most parts of the body misregistration is rare but in the thorax it is relatively common. CT acquisitions are fast enough to ensure that most of the thorax can be acquired either as a breath hold or with minimal respiratory movement but data from the PET scan takes up to 30 min to acquire resulting in the images representing an average position of the respiratory cycle. These differences in breathing patterns between the fast CT and the slower PET acquisitions can lead to misregistration of lung nodules by nearly 15 mm.[47] When the CT data is used for attenuation correction, artifacts may occur particularly at the diaphragm, where differences between the two acquisitions tend to be maximal. A typical appearance of such an artefact is an apparent loss of activity at the diaphragmatic surface (Fig. 18.5). Differences in breathing pattern may also lead to apparent mispositioning of liver metastases into the lung bases when using the CT data to correct for attenuation. It has been shown that differences in breathing patterns may be minimized by performing the CT scan during normal expiration.[48,49]

High-density contrast agents (e.g. oral contrast) or metallic objects can lead to an artifactual overestimation of activity if CT data are used for attenuation correction.[50–56] Such artefacts may be recognized by studying the uncorrected image data. Low-density oral contrast agents can be used without significant artifact[15,16] or the problem may be avoided by using water as a negative bowel contrast agent. Algorithms have been developed to account for the overestimation of activity when using CT-based attenuation correction that may minimize these effects in the future.[56]

The use of intravenous contrast during the CT acquisition may be a more difficult problem. Similarly, the concentrated bolus of contrast in the large vessels may lead to over-correction for attenuation, particularly in view of the fact that the concentrated column of contrast has largely dissipated by the time the PET emission scan is acquired. Artifactual hot spots in the attenuation corrected image[53] or quantitative overestimation of ^{18}F-FDG activity may result. When intravenous contrast is considered essential for a study then the diagnostic aspect of the CT scan is best performed as a third study with the patient in the same position, after first, a low-current CT scan for attenuation correction purposes and second, the PET emission scan.

Whilst many centers have found low-current CT acquisitions to be adequate for attenuation correction and image fusion,[57] it may be necessary to increase CT acquisition settings in larger patients to minimize beam-hardening artifacts on the CT scan that may translate through to incorrect attenuation correction of the PET emission data.[54] This effect can be caused by the patient's arms being in the field of view and may be minimized by placing arms above the head for imaging. Differences in the field of view diameter between the larger PET and smaller CT parts of combined scanners can lead to truncation artifacts at the edge of the CT image but these are generally small and can be minimized by the use of iterative image reconstruction methods.[56]

Despite a number of new artifacts being introduced by combined PET/CT imaging these do not usually have a major negative impact on scan quality or ease of interpretation. New attenuation correction algorithms and the development of respiratory gating techniques may overcome some of the artifacts described above in the future.

It is likely that many pitfalls caused by normal variant uptake may be avoided by the ability to correctly attribute ^{18}F-FDG activity to a structurally normal organ on CT. This may be particularly evident in the abdomen when physiological bowel activity or ureteric activity can otherwise cause interpretative difficulties. PET/CT also has the potential to limit false negative interpretations in tumors that are not very ^{18}F-FDG-avid by recognizing low-grade uptake as being related to structurally abnormal tissue and increasing the diagnostic confidence in tumor recognition by the use of the combined structural and functional data. Similarly, it may be possible to detect small lung metastases on CT lung

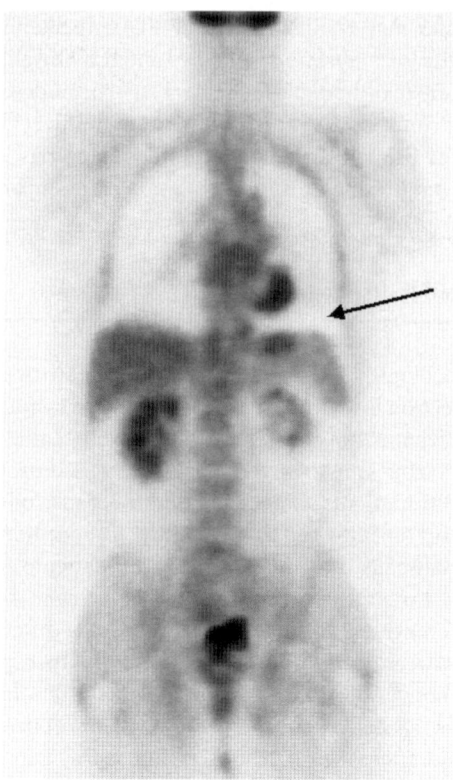

Figure 18.5 *A CT attenuation corrected ^{18}F-FDG PET scan demonstrating artifact at the diaphragm with apparent loss of activity (arrow) due to differences in position of the diaphragm during CT and PET acquisitions.*

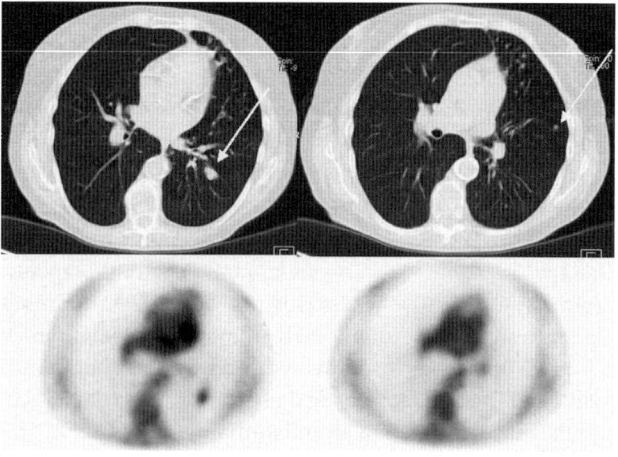

Figure 18.6 *Transaxial ^{18}F-FDG PET and corresponding CT slices from a combined PET/CT acquisition of the thorax. A large left lung metastasis shows clearly on the CT and PET images (left) but a small subcentimeter metastasis on the CT scan (arrow) is not resolved on the PET scan.*

windows that are beyond the resolution of ^{18}F-FDG PET (Fig. 18.6). The full use of the combined data, including the corrected and non-corrected PET emission data, and the inspection of soft-tissue, lung, and bone windows on the CT data, may also allow the description and correct diagnosis of pertinent ^{18}F-FDG negative lesions (e.g. liver cysts) and incidental ^{18}F-FDG negative CT abnormalities (e.g. abdominal aortic aneurysm) to provide an integrated interpretation of all the available data resulting from this technology.

REFERENCES

- ● Seminal primary article
- ◆ Key review paper
- ★ First formal publication of a management guideline

1 Warburg O. On the origin of cancer cells. *Science* 1956; **123**: 309–14.

2 Torizuka T, Tamaki N, Inokuma T, *et al.* In vivo assessment of glucose metabolism in hepatocellular carcinoma with FDG-PET. *J Nucl Med* 1995; **36**: 1811–17.

3 Lodge MA, Lucas JD, Marsden PK, *et al.* A PET study of [18]FDG uptake in soft tissue masses. *Eur J Nucl Med* 1999; **26**: 22–30.

● 4 Cook GJR, Fogelman I, Maisey MN. Normal physiological and benign pathological variants of 18-FDG PET scanning: potential for error in interpretation. *Semin Nucl Med* 1996; **26**: 308–14.

5 Cook GJR, Maisey MN, Fogelman I. Normal variants, artefacts and interpretative pitfalls in PET imaging with 18-fluoro-2-deoxyglucose and carbon-11 methionine. *Eur J Nucl Med* 1999; **26**: 1363–78.

● 6 Shreve PD, Anzai Y, Wahl RL. Pitfalls in oncologic diagnosis with FDG PET imaging: physiologic and benign variants. *Radiographics* 1999; **19**: 61–77.

7 Alavi A, Gupta N, Alberini JL, *et al.* Positron emission tomography imaging in non-malignant thoracic disorders. *Semin Nucl Med* 2002; **32**: 293–321.

8 Hustinx R, Smith RJ, Benard F, *et al.* Dual time point fluorine-18 fluorodeoxyglucose positron emission tomography: a potential method to differentiate malignancy from inflammation and normal tissue in the head and neck. *Eur J Nucl Med* 1999; **26**: 1345–8.

9 Brink I, Reinhardt MJ, Hoegerle S, *et al.* Increased metabolic activity in the thymus gland studied with ^{18}F-FDG PET: age dependency and frequency after chemotherapy. *J Nucl Med* 2001; **42**: 591–5.

10 Miyauchi T, Wahl RL. Regional 2-[^{18}F]fluoro-2-deoxy-D-glucose uptake varies in normal lung. *Eur J Nucl Med* 1996; **23**: 517–23.

11 Fujii H, Ide M, Yasuda S, *et al.* Increased FDG uptake in the wall of the right atrium in people who participated in a cancer screening program with whole-body PET. *Ann Nucl Med* 1999; **13**: 55–9.

12 Qureshy A, Kubota K, Iwata R, *et al.* Localization and reduction of FDG intestinal uptake: tissue distribution and autoradiography study. *Nucl Med Commun* 2002; **23**: 388.

13 Jadvar H, Schambye RB, Segall GM. Effect of atropine and sincalide on the intestinal uptake of F-18 fluorodeoxyglucose. *Clin Nucl Med* 1999; **24**: 965–7.

14 Miraldi F, Vesselle H, Faulhaber PF, *et al.* Elimination of artifactual accumulation of FDG in PET imaging of colorectal cancer. *Clin Nucl Med* 1998; **23**: 3–7.

15 Cohade C, Osman M, Nakamoto Y, *et al.* Initial experience with oral contrast in PET/CT: phantom and clinical studies. *J Nucl Med* 2003; **44**: 412–16.

16 Dizendorf EV, Treyer V, Von Schulthess GK, *et al.* Application of oral contrast media in coregistered positron emission tomography–CT. *AJR* 2002; **179**: 477–81.

● 17 Hany TF, Gharehpapagh E, Kamel EM, *et al.* Brown adipose tissue: a factor to consider in symmetrical tracer uptake in the neck and upper chest region. *Eur J Nucl Med* 2002; **29**: 1393–8.

18 Yamada S, Kubota K, Kubota R, *et al.* High accumulation of fluorine-18-fluorodeoxyglucose in turpentine-induced inflammatory tissue. *J Nucl Med* 1995; **36**: 1301–6.

19 Kubota R, Kubota K, Yamada S, *et al.* Methionine uptake by tumor tissue: a microautoradiographic comparison with FDG. *J Nucl Med* 1995; **36**: 484–92.

20 Nunez RF, Yeung HW, Macapinlac HA, Larson SM. Does post-radiation therapy changes in the lung affect the accuracy of FDG PET in the evaluation of tumour recurrence in lung cancer. *J Nucl Med* 1999; **40**: 234P.

21 Haberkorn U, Strauss LG, Dimitrakopoulou A, *et al.* PET studies of fluorodeoxyglucose metabolism in patients with recurrent colorectal tumors receiving radiotherapy. *J Nucl Med* 1991; **32**: 1485–90.

● 22 Diederichs CG, Staib L, Vogel J, *et al.* Values and limitations of ^{18}F-fluorodeoxyglucose-positron-emission tomography with preoperative evaluation of patients with pancreatic masses. *Pancreas* 2000; **20**: 109–16.

23 Knopp MV, Bischoff HG. Evaluation of pulmonary lesions with positron emission tomography. *Radiologe* 1994; **34**: 588–91.

● 24 Lewis PJ, Salama A. Uptake of fluorine-18-fluorodeoxyglucose in sarcoidosis. *J Nucl Med* 1994; **35**: 1–3.

25 O'Doherty MJ, Barrington SF, Campbell M, *et al.* PET scanning and the human immunodeficiency virus-positive patient. *J Nucl Med* 1997; **38**: 1575–83.

26 Mayer D, Bednarczyk EM. Interaction of colony-stimulating factors and fluorodeoxyglucose positron emission tomography. *Ann Pharmacother* 2002; **36**: 1796–9.

27 Shon IH, Fogelman I. F-18 FDG positron emission tomography and benign fractures. *Clin Nucl Med* 2003; **28**: 171–5.

28 Zhuang HM, Feng Q, Chacho TK, *et al.* Rapid normalization of FDG uptake of skeletal structure following fractures and surgical interventions. *J Nucl Med* 2002; **43**: 38P.

29 Cook GJ, Maisey MN, Fogelman I. Fluorine-18-FDG PET in Paget's disease of bone. *J Nucl Med* 1997; **38**: 1495–7.

30 Dehdashti F, Siegel BA, Griffeth LK, *et al.* Benign versus malignant intraosseous lesions: discrimination by means of PET with 2-[F-18]fluoro-2-deoxy-D-glucose. *Radiology* 1996; **200**: 243–7.

31 Kalicke T, Schmitz A, Risse JH, *et al.* Fluorine-18 fluorodeoxyglucose PET in infectious bone diseases: results of histologically confirmed cases. *Eur J Nucl Med* 2000; **27**: 524–8.

32 Horiuchi M, Yasuda S, Shohtsu A, *et al.* Four cases of Warthin's tumor of the parotid gland detected with FDG PET. *Ann Nucl Med* 1998; **12**: 47–50.

33 Yasuda S, Fujii H, Nakahara T, *et al.* ^{18}F-FDG PET detection of colonic adenomas. *J Nucl Med* 2001; **42**: 989–92.

34 Dobert N, Menzel C, Ludwig R, *et al.* Enchondroma: a benign osseous lesion with high F-18 FDG uptake. *Clin Nuc Med* 2002; **27**: 695–7.

35 Kao CH. FDG uptake in a huge uterine myoma. *Clin Nucl Med* 2003; **28**: 249.

36 Cremerius U, Effert PJ, Adam G, *et al.* FDG PET for detection and therapy control of metastatic germ cell tumour. *J Nucl Med* 1999; **40**: 815–22.

37 Ryu JS, Choi NC, Fischman AJ, *et al.* FDG-PET in staging and restaging non-small cell lung cancer after neoadjuvant chemoradiotherapy: correlation with histopathology. *Lung Cancer* 2002; **35**: 179–87.

● 38 Spaepen K, Stroobants S, Dupont P, *et al.* [(18)F]FDG PET monitoring of tumour response to chemotherapy: does [(18)F]FDG uptake correlate with the viable tumour cell fraction? *Eur J Nucl Med Mol Imaging* 2003; **30**: 682–8.

39 Dehdashti F, Flanagan FL, Mortimer JE, *et al.* Positron emission tomographic assessment of 'metabolic flare' to predict response of metastatic breast cancer to antiestrogen therapy. *Eur J Nucl Med* 1999; **26**: 51–6.

40 De Witte O, Hildebrand J, Luxen A, *et al.* Acute effect of carmustine on glucose metabolism in brain and glioblastoma. *Cancer* 1994; **74**: 2836–42.

★ 41 Young H, Baum R, Cremerius U, *et al.* Measurement of clinical and subclinical tumour response using [^{18}F]-fluorodeoxyglucose and positron emission tomography: review and 1999 EORTC recommendations. European Organization for Research and Treatment of Cancer (EORTC) PET Study Group. *Eur J Cancer* 1999; **35**: 1773–82.

◆ 42 Barrington SF, O'Doherty MJ. Limitations of PET for imaging lymphoma. *Eur J Nucl Med* 2003; **30**: S117–27.

● 43 Romer W, Hanauske AR, Ziegler S, *et al.* Positron emission tomography in non-Hodgkin's lymphoma: assessment of chemotherapy with fluorodeoxyglucose. *Blood* 1998; **91**: 4464–71.

● 44 Findlay M, Young H, Cunningham D, *et al.* Noninvasive monitoring of tumor metabolism using fluorodeoxyglucose and positron emission tomography in colorectal cancer liver metastases: correlation with tumor response to fluorouracil. *J Clin Oncol* 1996; **14**: 700–8.

45 Haberkorn U, Strauss LG, Dimitrakopoulou A, *et al.* PET studies of fluorodeoxyglucose metabolism in patients with recurrent colorectal tumors receiving radiotherapy. *J Nucl Med* 1991; **32**: 1485–90.

46 Greven KM, Williams DW, McGuirt WF, *et al.* Serial positron emission tomography scans following radiation therapy of patients with head and neck cancer. *Head and Neck* 2001; **23**: 942–6.

47 Goerres GW, Kamel E, Seifert B, *et al.* Accuracy of image coregistration of pulmonary lesions in patients with non-small cell lung cancer using an integrated PET/CT system. *J Nucl Med* 2002; **43**: 1469–75.

48 Goerres GW, Kamel E, Heidelberg TN, *et al.* PET-CT image co-registration in the thorax: influence of respiration. *Eur J Nucl Med* 2002; **29**: 351–60.

49 Goerres GW, Burger C, Schwitter MR, *et al.* PET/CT of the abdomen: optimizing the patient breathing pattern. *Eur Radiol* 2003; **13**: 734–9.

50 Dizendorf E, Hany TF, Buck A, *et al.* Cause and magnitude of the error induced by oral CT contrast agent in CT-based attenuation correction of PET emission studies. *J Nucl Med* 2003; **44**: 732–8.

51 Goerres GW, Hany TF, Kamel E, *et al.* Head and neck imaging with PET and PET/CT: artefacts from dental metallic implants. *Eur J Nucl Med* 2002; **29**: 367–70.

52 Kamel EM, Burger C, Buck A, *et al.* Impact of metallic dental implants on CT-based attenuation correction in a combined PET/CT scanner. *Eur Radiol* 2003; **13**: 724–8.

53 Antoch G, Freudenberg LS, Egelhof T, *et al.* Focal tracer uptake: a potential artifact in contrast-enhanced dual-modality PET/CT scans. *J Nucl Med* 2002; **43**: 1339–42.

◆ 54 Cohade C, Wahl RL. Applications of PET/CT image fusion in clinical PET – clinical use, interpretation methods, diagnostic improvements. *Semin Nucl Med* 2003; **33**: 228–37.

55 Goerres GW, Ziegler SI, Burger C, *et al.* Artifacts at PET and PET/CT caused by metallic hip prosthetic material. *Radiology* 2003; **226**: 577–84.

◆ 56 Kinahan PE, Hasegawa BH, Beyer T. X-ray based attenuation correction for PET/CT scanners. *Semin Nucl Med* 2003; **33**: 166–79.

57 Hany TF, Steinert HC, Goerres GW, *et al.* PET diagnostic accuracy: improvement with in-line PET–CT system: initial results. *Radiology* 2002; **225**: 575–81.

19

Diagnostic accuracy and cost-effectiveness issues

M.N. MAISEY

Introduction	799	Receiver operating characteristic curve	804
The goals of diagnostic tests	800	Methodologies	806
The costs and benefits of evaluation	800	References	810
How should new technology be introduced?	800		
Methodology and techniques for evaluating diagnostic performance	800		

INTRODUCTION

New investigations have frequently been introduced with little or no evaluation of either their diagnostic performance or the influence they have on patient management. This deficiency has become particularly important over the past two decades as major new diagnostic technologies, such as positron emission tomography (PET) and magnetic resonance imaging (MRI), have been introduced into clinical medicine, and there has been an increasing pressure to contain costs. The Council on Science and Society report in 1983 noted the haphazard manner in which expensive technologies were introduced, and also that an assessment was considered with very little concern for patient reactions or to the social and psychological consequences. The over-riding reason for an evaluation is to confirm a positive effect on patient management but there are other reasons for increasing effort in this area, which include constraints on the available resources within the health services and a pressure for evidence-based practice. Clinicians and policy makers have the right to know whether the diagnostic services that are offered make a real contribution to patient care at a cost which makes good use of available resources.

This chapter outlines some of the methodologies involved in diagnostic technology performance and cost evaluation, and aims to draw attention to common inadequacies in published studies.

The general methodology for evaluation is common to most diagnostic applications, although the emphasis will depend on the purpose for which the diagnostic method is being used. Diagnostic imaging techniques can be divided into five categories:

1. **Screening of asymptomatic patients for disease**. The prevalence of disease in the referred population will usually be low (e.g. breast or osteoporosis screening). The goal is to detect all patients who have disease, and to accept the need to investigate a proportion of patients without the disease at the cost of not missing any individuals with disease.
2. **The detection and diagnosis of disease in symptomatic patients**. This is the conventional area of diagnostic imaging techniques in hospital. The patients are symptomatic, the prevalence of disease in the investigated population is intermediate and the goal is to detect and characterize disease.
3. **Staging of disease**. The presence of disease will usually have been established by alternative methods. The goal is to identify further sites or the extent of the disease, e.g. staging procedures for the treatment of lung cancer and myocardial perfusion imaging to establish the extent and severity of coronary artery disease (CAD). This will determine optimal management, risk stratification and prognosis.
4. **Monitoring change**. Imaging techniques are being increasingly used to assess the progress of disease and the response to treatment.
5. **Targeting disease**. The use of imaging to target lesions for image-guided biopsy or image-guided therapy (e.g. surgery or radiotherapy).

THE GOALS OF DIAGNOSTIC TESTS

The preceding section classified the applications of imaging procedures. In order for them to be effective, there must be a gain to the individual and to society when they are used. The demonstration of pathology in a patient is not sufficient as a goal in itself. New information should ultimately benefit the patient in one of the following ways:

- Save lives by diagnosis and consequent treatment
- Restore health
- Alleviate suffering (physical and/or psychological) by early detection and treatment
- Prevent occurrence of symptomatic disease by early detection and treatment
- Predict the course of disease (prognosis)

THE COSTS AND BENEFITS OF EVALUATION

Although it appears self-evident that a soundly based evaluation of diagnostic methods in clinical medicine would be beneficial, an argument has to be made for evaluation techniques and it needs to be demonstrated that they are cost-effective.

The benefits of evaluation include:

- Better use of limited resource in patient care within the health service
- Withdrawal of tests which are not shown to be of value and could even do harm
- Prevention of early diffusion of unproven tests into widespread clinical practice
- Earlier adoption of good practice

The direct costs of evaluation may be high and because the methods are often difficult and time-consuming to undertake they may also cause a delay in the introduction of a truly effective test. Similar evaluation costs apply to drug trials and these have undoubtedly been broadly beneficial.

The timing of evaluations is often critical. Early evaluation studies are often like 'trying to hit a moving target' because technology changes so rapidly that the results may be regarded as irrelevant. On the other hand, early evaluation may prevent the widespread application of a test or purchase of equipment and dissemination of a method that is ultimately shown to be useless or at best non-contributory. Early evaluation by a well-designed study may detect an unsuspected morbidity associated with the diagnostic technique, which would have taken much longer to uncover if careful evaluation had not been undertaken. Equally, a too-early evaluation can lead to the premature rejection of a potentially valuable technique; and evaluation that is too late may be unable to prevent the use of a technology that cannot be shown to be useful but is 'believed in' by clinicians and therefore difficult to dislodge. On the other hand, the advantage of late evaluation is that the technology is stable and therefore the results of evaluation more credible.

HOW SHOULD NEW TECHNOLOGY BE INTRODUCED?

There are three ways that new technologies are introduced:

1. **Random diffusion.** New technology is frequently introduced on a random basis depending on a variety of factors such as source of finance, clinical pressures, institutional prestige, commercial interests, and other outside influences.
2. **Evaluation of every new technique.** With the rapid change of technology and the number of established diagnostic methods, this would not be a cost-effective exercise, and is clearly impractical and not realistically achievable.
3. **Selective evaluation.** Both new and old tests can be selectively examined especially if they are expensive, widely used, and applied to disease with a high prevalence. Subsequent resource decisions can then be made on well-established quantifiable data. The choice of what should be evaluated should also be influenced by therapeutic impact and downstream costs.

METHODOLOGY AND TECHNIQUES FOR EVALUATING DIAGNOSTIC PERFORMANCE

The performance of diagnostic tests can be measured at several well-defined hierarchical levels, and form the basis of a classification, which assists in the understanding of the evaluation process. The levels are:

1. Technical capacity
2. Diagnostic accuracy
3. Diagnostic impact
4. Therapeutic impact
5. Patient outcome
6. Cost-effectiveness

Diagnostic tests in the past have usually only been evaluated at the first and second levels, very rarely at the third level, and almost never at the fourth, fifth or sixth levels.

Technical capacity

Evaluation of test performance at this level is essentially a pilot study concerned with questions of safety:

- Are there major hazards?
- Is there morbidity associated with the test?
- What is the patient acceptability?

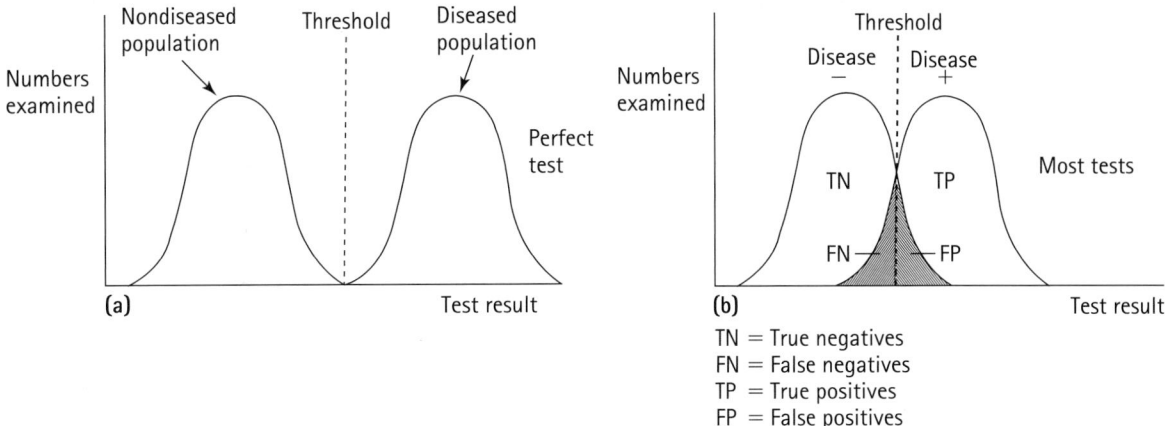

TN = True negatives
FN = False negatives
TP = True positives
FP = False positives

Figure 19.1   *The two graphs show how a threshold may be used to separate normal from diseased populations (a); however, this is almost unknown in medicine; the overlap in (b) is the more usual finding.*

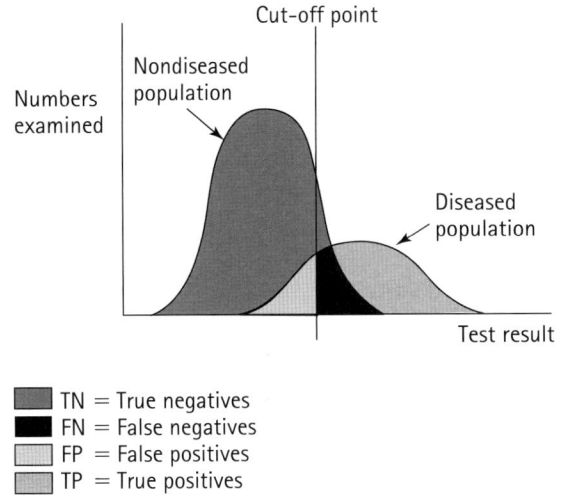

TN = True negatives
FN = False negatives
FP = False positives
TP = True positives

Figure 19.2   *Overlap with false positive and false negative results when the prevalence in the population studied is less than 50%.*

- Does the test perform reliably (i.e. is it repeatable and/or consistent) and does it measure what it claims to measure?
- What is the reproducibility and the precision of the test?

These studies should include an assessment of the engineering reliability of the equipment and the frequency of nondiagnostic tests, test failures and/or patient failures.

Diagnostic accuracy

At this level of evaluation, the purpose is to assess how good the test is at discriminating between patients with the disease from those without the disease. It is very rare for a test in clinical medicine to distinguish completely between a diseased and a nondiseased population; as a consequence of this overlap, a criterion has to be developed for the optimal separation of the two populations with acceptance of

the inevitable false negative (FN) and false positive (FP) diagnoses. Figure 19.1 illustrates this general principle. However, Figure 19.2 is more realistic, because it would be unusual for 50% of the population studied to be diseased and 50% normal. In this case, there are fewer diseased than normal people, i.e. the prevalence of disease in the population is less than 50%.

In nuclear medicine, the diagnostic criterion that is used to separate diseased from nondiseased populations may be quantitative (e.g. thyroid uptake, ejection fraction or SUV), but more often it is qualitative and reported as positive or negative with varying degrees of confidence or probability (e.g. bone and lung scans). Figure 19.3 shows how by changing the criterion or threshold for diagnosing disease alters the numbers of false negatives and false positives.

For any single value of the diagnostic criterion used to separate diseased from nondiseased populations, we can consider the outcome as a 2 × 2 matrix as shown below:

Diagnostic test	Disease Present	Absent	Total
Positive	TP	FP	TP + FP
Negative	FN	TN	FN + TN
Total	TP + FN	FP + TN	TP + FN + FP + TN

Different ways of measuring accuracy of a diagnostic test have been developed, which have both advantages and disadvantages.

ACCURACY

The accuracy of a test is defined as the ratio of true positive results (TP) plus true negative results (TN) to the total number of patients studied.

$$\text{Accuracy} = \frac{\text{TP} + \text{TN}}{\text{TP} + \text{FP} + \text{TN} + \text{FN}} \times 100\%.$$

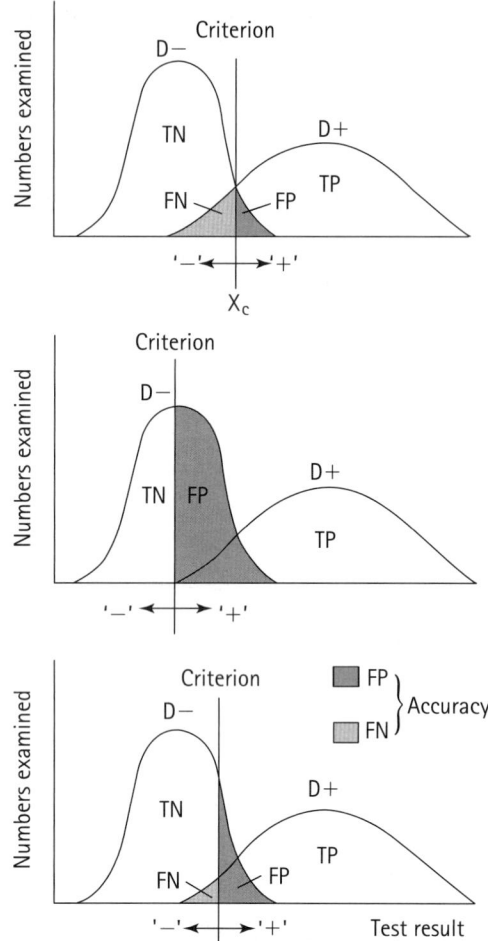

Figure 19.3 *Three graphs showing how when the population prevalence and the test remains constant, the sensitivities and specificities can alter by adjusting the diagnostic criterion.*

This is a global measure of accuracy that does not distinguish between positives and negatives, and is therefore often misleading as a measure of test performance. This problem can be seen graphically from Fig. 19.3 in which the accuracy of the test is the shaded areas divided by the total area under both curves.

The prevalence of the disease in the population studied affects the accuracy of the test, as shown in the following examples.

EXAMPLE 1: PREVALENCE 50%

Test	Disease +	Disease −
+	450	200
−	50	300

$$\text{Accuracy} = \frac{450 + 300}{1000} = 75\%.$$

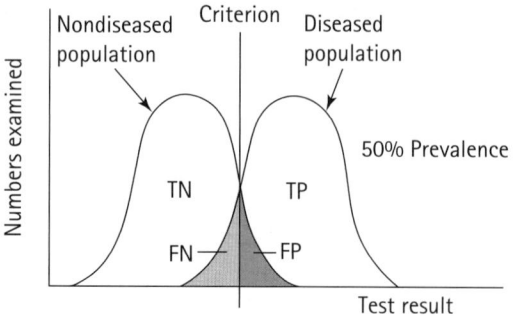

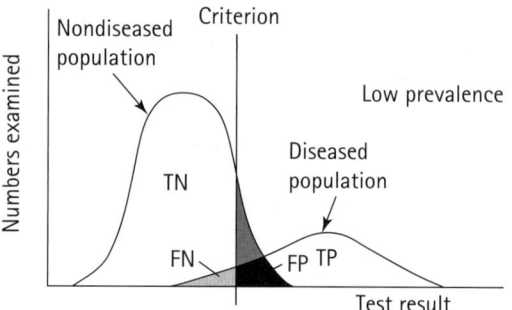

Figure 19.4 *Two graphs showing the effect of changing the disease prevalence in the population on the test performance when the diagnostic criterion remains constant.*

EXAMPLE 2: PREVALENCE 2%

Test	Disease +	Disease −
+	18	392
−	2	588

$$\text{Accuracy} = \frac{18 + 588}{1000} \times 100 = 60.6\%.$$

This effect of prevalence is illustrated in Fig. 19.4 where the disease prevalence is lower but the threshold remains unchanged.

SENSITIVITY AND SPECIFICITY

The information from the matrix can be translated into measurements referred to as the sensitivity and the specificity of the test. **Sensitivity** is defined as the ratio of true positive to true positive plus false negative, or

$$\text{sensitivity} = \frac{\text{TP}}{\text{TP} + \text{FN}} \times 100\%.$$

This can be expressed as 'the proportion of people with the disease that will be detected by the test' (diagnosed by the test set at a particular threshold or criterion). **Specificity** is the ratio of true negative, to true negative plus false positive, or

$$\text{specificity} = \frac{\text{TN}}{\text{TN} + \text{FP}} \times 100\%.$$

This can be expressed as 'the proportion of people without the disease that will be confirmed to be free of the disease'. The closer to 100% each of these measurements approaches the better the test is performing.

It can be seen from Fig. 19.3 that as the criterion or threshold is changed, the number of true positive and false positive cases, and hence the sensitivity and specificity of the test, varies. When the sensitivity and specificity of the test have been measured using a broad enough spectrum of patients with and without the disease, and with a wide range of disease presentations and severity, the prevalence of disease in the test population does not influence the sensitivity and specificity of the test. This can be shown by recalculating the figures in the previous section for sensitivity and specificity, as shown in the following examples.

EXAMPLE 1: PREVALENCE 50%

$$\text{Sensitivity} = \frac{450}{450 + 50} = 90\%.$$

$$\text{Specificity} = \frac{300}{300 + 200} = 60\%.$$

EXAMPLE 2: PREVALENCE 2%

$$\text{Sensitivity} = \frac{18}{18 + 2} = 90\%.$$

$$\text{Specificity} = \frac{588}{588 + 392} = 60\%.$$

This effect can be seen graphically in Fig. 19.4 where these ratios remain constant in spite of much lower disease in the population. Although sensitivity and specificity are good objective measures of the performance of a test, they do not provide any information as to the likelihood of an individual patient whose test is positive or negative being normal or having the disease, and this is the information needed by a clinician for decision making. The measures which provide this information are called the positive and negative predictive accuracies (PPA and NPA) or positive and negative predictive values (PPV and NPV) and are heavily dependent on prevalence of the disease.

POSITIVE AND NEGATIVE PREDICTIVE ACCURACIES

The positive predictive accuracy is the ratio of true positive, to true positive plus false positive results:

$$\text{PPA} = \frac{\text{TP}}{\text{TP} + \text{FP}} \times 100\%$$

or the likelihood of a patient with a positive test actually having the disease.

The negative predictive accuracy is the ratio of true negative, to true negative plus false negative:

$$\text{NPA} = \frac{\text{TN}}{\text{TN} + \text{FN}} \times 100\%$$

or the likelihood of a patient with a negative test being free of the disease. These post-test probabilities are dependent on the prevalence of the disease in the population (pre-test probability of disease), which can be seen by working the same example.

EXAMPLE 1: PREVALENCE 50%

Predictive value of positive test (the PPA) is

$$\frac{450}{450 + 200} \times 100 = 69\%.$$

Predictive value of negative test (the NPA) is

$$\frac{300}{300 + 50} \times 100 = 86\%.$$

EXAMPLE 2: PREVALENCE 2%

Predictive value of positive test (the PPA) is

$$\frac{18}{18 + 392} \times 100 = 4.4\%.$$

Predictive value of negative test (the NPA) is

$$\frac{588}{588 + 2} \times 100 = 99.7\%.$$

The measures so far discussed are sometimes expressed as probabilities: sensitivity (true positive ratio) = P (T+|D+), where

P = the probability of an event occurring
T+ = positive result to a test
| = given
D+ = disease present

that is, the probability of disease being present given a positive test result.

Similarly, specificity (true negative ratio) = P (T−|D−), where

P = the probability of an event occurring
T − = the negative result to a test
| = given
D− = disease absent

and

False positive ratio = P (T+|D+)
False negative ratio = P (T−|D+)
Predictive value of a positive test = P (D+|T+)
Predictive value of a negative test = P (D−|T−)
Prevalence = P (D+).

BAYES' THEOREM

Bayes' theorem provides a general basis for decision theory, from which a mathematical formula can be derived to show how sensitivity and specificity combine with probability of disease to give a predictive value of a positive or negative test; that is, how positive predictive value of a positive or negative test (i.e. how positive predictive value or negative predictive value) can be calculated from sensitivity, specificity, and prevalence.

For example:

$$P(D+ \mid T+) = \frac{P(T+ \mid D+) \times P(D+)}{P(T+)}$$

or

$$= \frac{P(T+ \mid D+) \times P(D+)}{[P(T+ \mid D+) \times P(D+)] + [P(T+ \mid D-) \times P(D-)]}$$

where

P = probability
B = B occurring
D+ = disease present
D− = disease absent
T+ = positive test result
| = given

or

$$PPV = \frac{\text{sensitivity} \times \text{prevalence}}{(\text{sensitivity} \times \text{prevalence}) + [(1 - \text{specificity}) \times (1 - \text{prevalence})]}$$

and

$$NPV = \frac{\text{sensitivity} \times (1 - \text{prevalence})}{[(1 - \text{sensitivity}) \times \text{prevalence}] + [\text{specificity} \times (1 - \text{prevalence})]}.$$

The measures of accuracy, which have been discussed, only apply to disease being present or absent. When the possibility of various different diseases is introduced (i.e. an ordered differential diagnosis), the problem becomes more complex; for example, a chest X-ray may be abnormal because of tuberculosis, cancer or infection.

When two tests (X and Y) are used then the two sensitivities can be combined as shown below:

Test	Sensitivity (%)	Specificity (%)
Ultrasound (test X)	80	60
CT scan (test Y)	90	90
Call positive if X and/or Y is positive*	98	54
Call positive if X and Y are positive**	72	96

*Positive X+ and/or Y+

Sensitivity = {sens. X + [(100 − sens. X) × sens. Y]}/ 100 = 98
Specificity = spec. X × spec. Y/100 = 54

**Positive X+ and Y+

Sensitivity = sens. X × sens. Y/100
Specificity = {spec. X + [(100 − spec. X) × spec. Y]}/100

Thus, it means that insisting that two tests are positive before making a diagnosis will result in a very high specificity (i.e. few false positives) but a low sensitivity (i.e. frequent missed cases).

TEST SELECTION

The choice of which test to use, as well as the threshold for calling a test positive, will depend on the use to which the test is being put. High sensitivity picks up most of the patients who have the disease (few false negatives). It is good for:

- Excluding disease
- Screening especially if there is high morbidity associated with missing the disease

High specificity picks up most of the individuals without the disease (few false positives). It is good for:

- Confirming the presence of disease
- Cases when the risk associated with treating unnecessarily is high

If two or more tests are very sensitive, and the primary purpose of the test is to exclude disease, the gain in sensitivity obtained by using two or more tests may be offset by the decrease in specificity.

RECEIVER OPERATING CHARACTERISTIC CURVE

A further measure of the performance of a diagnostic test is the receiver operating characteristic (ROC) curve, which measures the sensitivities and specificities over a range of criteria. These curves demonstrate graphically how the sensitivities and the specificities change when the diagnostic criterion is altered; that is, the threshold for reporting a test as positive is raised or lowered. If the test has a quantitative measure, the diagnostic criterion for abnormality may be set at different levels; for example, lymph nodes on computed tomography may be called pathological only if they are 5 mm or 10 mm or 20 mm, etc. Although most imaging techniques are reported qualitatively, it is still possible to express the likelihood of their being abnormal semi-quantitatively with different levels of confidence. For example, a chest X-ray may be absolutely normal, or there may be something suspicious, or something almost certainly abnormal, or a gross abnormality. Different levels of likelihood of disease being present are divided into five categories:

- 0: Definitely normal
- 1: Probably normal
- 2: Possibly abnormal
- 3: Probably abnormal
- 4: Definitely abnormal

The evaluation of a test will use these different levels of likelihood and are included in the reporting of the films. From these data, the ROC curves can be constructed and each test, X-ray or imaging method will have its own characteristically shaped curve, which will express the performance of the test quantitatively.

To produce such a curve for an imaging test, a series of scans (using a minimum of 100) are obtained from a representative population with an intermediate prevalence of disease and a wide range of severity of disease. The scans will be read by one individual or a group and put into one of the categories above (i.e. graded 0–4). The positivity of the test is then created five times, i.e. the test is called positive:

1. Only when the definitely abnormals are called positive, i.e. very strict threshold
2. Only when definitely abnormal and probably abnormal, are called positive
3. When definitely abnormal, probably abnormal and possibly abnormal, are called positive (i.e. a lax threshold)
4. Even when cases categorized as probably normal are included, and called positive
5. When cases categorized as definitely normal are also included, i.e. all cases are called abnormal, in which case, no diseased patient will go undetected (100% sensitivity) but all the patients free of disease will be called diseased (0% specificity).

These results are then plotted in the ROC space, the vertical axis being the true positive ratio (the sensitivity correct detection of disease or 'hits') and the horizontal axis being the false positive ratio (1 − specificity) or the 'false alarms' shown in Fig. 19.5.

Typical characteristic curves

These curves can be used to compare the overall performance of tests (Fig. 19.6). Curve A would result from randomly assigning results to one of the categories referred to above and using the outcome to report whether the test was normal or abnormal, and clearly would have no diagnostic value. Curve B describes the shape of a perfect curve when there are no false positive and no false negative results, and as we have already seen, for practical purposes, never occurs clinically. Most tests will have shapes approximating to C and D, where C is a better test than D for detecting a particular condition, because at every threshold or criterion,

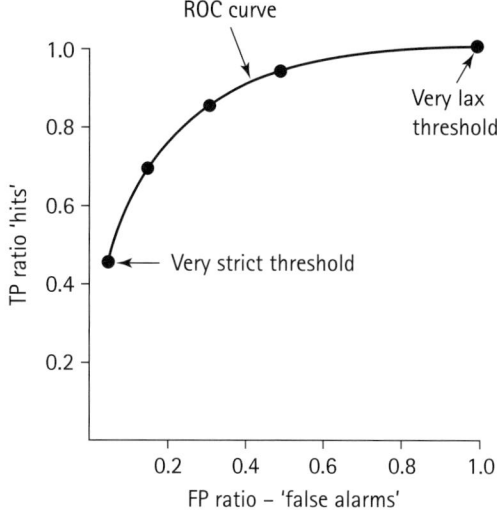

Figure 19.5 *A receiver operating characteristic (ROC) curve from an imaging procedure with five levels of diagnostic probability.*

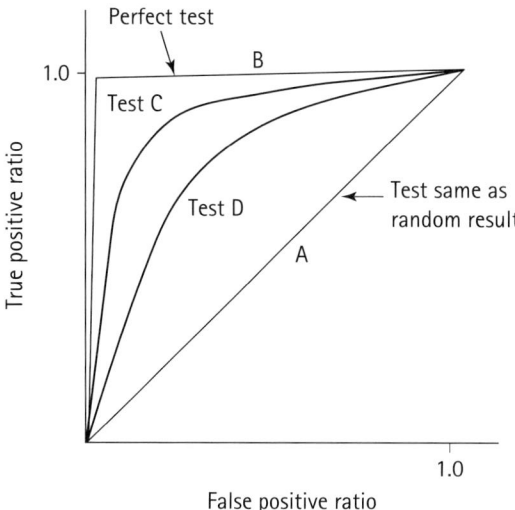

Figure 19.6 *Four theoretical ROC curves showing test performance from perfect (B) to random (A). Curves C and D are typical for many imaging procedures.*

there are more true positives and fewer false positives than for curve D. It can be seen from this that if the result of the scan has to be unequivocally abnormal before it is reported to the clinician as abnormal, then the sensitivity of detection of disease will be low, but the specificity will be high. On the other hand, if we report as positive anything which is possibly abnormal, probably abnormal or definitely abnormal, then the sensitivity for detection of the disease will be much higher but with decreased specificity; that is, there will be more false positives, and will increase the number of patients who are actually free of disease but whom we are diagnosing as having the disease.

The performance of the tests can be assessed by simply inspecting the curves' shapes; however, quantitative values

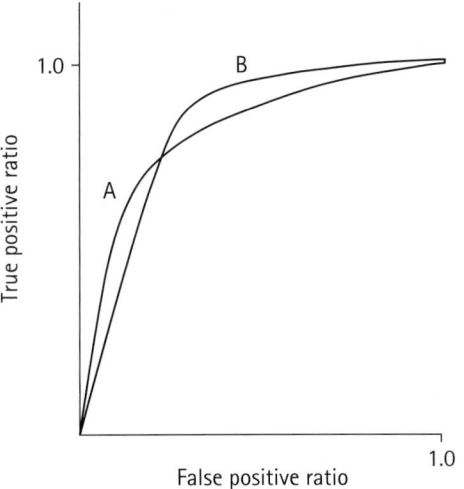

Figure 19.7 *An example of an ROC curve when the total accuracy may be similar but performance differs in different areas of the curve.*

can also be derived from them. The most commonly used method is to integrate the area below the curve and express this as a proportion – the nearer to 1.0, the better the test.

The shape of the ROC curves may be more complex than indicated previously and may cross over as indicated in Fig. 19.7. This illustrates how two tests may be similar in accuracy, because the areas under the curves are identical but the characteristics are different. In this instance, neither of the tests is necessarily better overall, but performance will depend on the use to which it is put. If false positive results are to be avoided, for example when the consequences of a positive diagnosis would be dangerous treatment, test A would be a better test, provided a strict threshold is used; whereas test B may be a better screening test (provided a lax threshold is used) because the sensitivity is higher in this area of the curve.

Showing that a test has a good sensitivity and specificity and performs well using ROC curve measurement does not prove that it is clinically useful. This can be assessed only by measuring the diagnostic and therapeutic impact, and the outcome and cost-effectiveness.

Another way of evaluating a diagnostic test is by determining efficacy; that is, showing whether the test is clinically useful in an ideal clinical and academic environment. The effectiveness of a test also needs to be determined; that is, when it diffuses out to more general health care is efficacy maintained? It is also necessary to determine whether a test is clinically effective when used more widely in the health care system (i.e. is it efficient?) Lastly, is a test worth the extra cost that is incurred by making it generally available (i.e. is it cost-effective?)

It is important to be clear about what the meaning of 'cost-effective'. A useful definition is from Hillman, 'A medical procedure is cost effective if its benefits are sufficiently great to justify its costs and if equal or greater benefits cannot be obtained through less costly means'.[1] Alternatively, the rationale for cost-effectiveness analysis (CEA) is that 'for any given level of resources available society wishes to maximize the total aggregate health benefits conferred' was a definition used by Weinsten and Stason.[2] Cost-effective does not simply mean cheaper it means having an additional benefit which is worth the additional cost. Thus the clinical benefits always have to be considered alongside the costs incurred. A test may be cost-effective if it is less costly and as effective as other procedures. It may be cost-effective if it has a higher cost but is more effective (if the increased costs are worth it) and may be considered cost-effective if it is of lower cost even though it is less effective if the savings are sufficient. From this it can be seen as indicated above that cost-effectiveness is a means to help make a choice and is rarely able to give the answer unequivocally: a judgment is almost always required. In assessing a diagnostic technology it has to be remembered that a procedure may be part of a complex diagnostic strategy or pathway and may have a role in diagnosis, management, detection of disease, risk stratification and prognosis or predicting therapeutic outcome.

Economic analyses of diagnostic technologies or indeed other procedures will therefore never be able to make health care delivery decisions but simply provide a firmer, more robust structure on which these decisions can be taken, based on other issues including clinical, ethical, and political considerations. The information is, in essence, a tool for helping to make these choices by defining the benefits gained from the introduction against the costs involved in doing so. Costs are the opportunity costs, i.e. the next best use of the resources which are involved. The benefits of evaluation include a better utilization of limited health care resources for patient care, the withdrawal of diagnostic procedures which cannot be shown to be of value and which could even do more harm than good, and the prevention of the early diffusion of unproven tests into widespread clinical practice. Possible disadvantages include the cost of evaluation and the potential for delay of the introduction of effective tests into clinical medicine.

METHODOLOGIES

As discussed in the previous section both the costs and the effectiveness need to be measured. Ideally these will be done simultaneously but in practice they are more often undertaken separately and then combined in CEA studies. Clinical benefits or clinical effectiveness may be measured in a number of ways, ranging from case reports to case control studies, management impact studies, and diagnostic randomized prospective control trials but these are rarely performed and may in fact not be the ideal way to evaluate the clinical benefits of diagnostic technologies (Table 19.1). Because cost-effectiveness studies are often not integrated

Table 19.1   *Methods for testing clinical value*

1. *Case reports and case control studies*
2. *Consensus evaluation*
3. *Meta-analysis*
4. *Databases*
5. *Computer modelling and simulation*
6. *Prospective measurement of clinical impact*
7. *Randomized prospective clinical trials*
8. *Epidemiology*

with clinical studies the development and refinement of meta-analysis has become a critical part of the process. A meta-analysis is the integration of the results and outcomes of many studies and trials in such a way that the power of the meta-analysis surpasses the power of individual studies. There are three types of economic methods used for assessing imaging studies: cost-effectiveness analysis, cost utility analysis, and cost-benefit analysis.

Cost-effectiveness analysis

The simplest sub-group of cost-effectiveness analyses is the cost minimalization study which can be employed when it is known or presumed that the clinical effectiveness of two procedures is identical, in which case the only outcome is the total cost of one diagnostic strategy compared with another diagnostic methodology; the lower cost will be selected.

The cost-effectiveness ratio is a comparison of alternative strategies usually comparing the intervention that is under examination with 'usual care'. It may also be used to compare competing interventions or a comparison with no intervention. This ratio is the 'incremental price of obtaining a health unit effect (e.g. dollars or pounds per year gained, or dollars or pounds per quality adjusted life year) from a given health intervention when compared to an alternative. If the intervention is more effective and less costly it is dominating and therefore inappropriate to calculate a cost effectiveness ratio'. The cost-effectiveness ratio is

$$\frac{\text{net increase in cost}}{\text{net increase in health benefit}} = \frac{\text{cost A} - \text{cost B}}{\text{benefit A} - \text{benefit B}}$$

where costs A and B are the costs of strategies A and B, respectively; and benefits A and B are the health benefits of strategies A and B, respectively.

Where the denominator is a clinical outcome measurement (e.g. cases correctly diagnosed) and the denominator is the cost incurred in using the diagnostic method to make the diagnosis this ratio can be expressed as pounds or dollars per case identified and thereby two diagnostic strategies using two different methodologies, for example PET and

CT scanning, can be compared. This method is valuable but limited because it says nothing about the subsequent value of making the diagnosis or the downstream negative effects of misdiagnoses.

Cost utility analysis

Cost utility analysis (CUA) may be considered as a special form of cost-effectiveness analysis where adjustments are made for the 'value attached to the benefits' (i.e. it incorporates patient ultilities). Utilities are a measure of how patients value a health state, usually expressed on a scale of 0–1, where 0 indicates a health state equivalent to death and 1 indicates a health state equivalent to ideal health. Cost utility studies provide a health care outcome in the denominator which can be compared across the whole of a health care system and therefore the 'cost-effectiveness' of, for example, a diagnostic test could theoretically be compared with the introduction of a renal transplant program. In the case of cost utility studies the most widely used health outcome measurement is the quality adjusted life years (QALY). The QALY is a measure of health outcome for a patient which assigns to each period of time a weighting ranging from 1 to zero corresponding to the quality of life during that period and where a weight of 1 corresponds to perfect health and a weight of zero corresponds to a health state judged equivalent to death. This can be expressed as the cost for each quality adjusted life year gained, or saving of resources when a less effective strategy is employed. Conventionally, 'a cost that society is willing to pay' may be used, but this threshold is a societal judgement and although a figure of $50 000 has often been used there is no general consensus and it has been $50 000 for over 10 years and ought to have changed over time. If the introduction of a new technology or procedure costs less than $50 000 for each quality adjusted life year gained it may be regarded as cost-effective. Equally, if you can save more than $50 000 with only one quality adjusted life year forfeited this also may be considered justified as this money, i.e. the opportunity cost, can be applied elsewhere in the health care system more effectively. Although strictly 'willingness to pay' is a method for capital costing of human life.

QALY, as an outcome, has allowed expansion of CEAs to encompass diverse effects of intervention and, more importantly, to compare interventions which have quite different types of outcome.

Cost-benefit analysis

Cost-benefit analysis (CBA) may be regarded as an extension of a cost utility study whereby all the effectiveness measurements, e.g. quality adjusted life years as well as pain and inconvenience, can be given a financial value. This is a classic economic method but uncommonly used in medicine; in spite of the fact that people often object to putting a monetary value on life, you actually have to do this with CEA as well because you have to decide what you are willing to pay for a QALY gained. In medicine, for ethical and other reasons, true CBA is generally not considered to be an appropriate or feasible approach. In attempting to put a monetary value on a life two approaches have been tried. In the human capital approach it is the total contribution usually through earnings that is used to measure the 'value' of a life, and in the second it derives from assessing the 'willingness to pay' for the health care benefit. Both methods have significant limitations and are probably not relevant to diagnostic imaging. Other outcome measures which can be used in CEA instead of QALY across the health care system are lives saved, disability days lost, cases detected, cases correctly staged, disability days avoided, and healthy years equivalent.

Methods adopted for these analyses

In practical terms the methods adopted for these economic analyses described above include:

- Prospective randomized controlled trials of both effectiveness and costs simultaneously
- Retrospective economic evaluation (i.e. attribution of costs) of previously performed clinical trials
- Expert consensus, but this is not regarded as reliable although it may be unavoidable in the absence of data
- Computer modeling methods (usually decision analysis) incorporating meta-analysis and sensitivity analysis

In studies which involve the measurement of cost and the relationship to effectiveness there are a number of important issues and parameters that need to be defined. These have been well summarized by Drummond and Jefferson[3] for example, and are a useful way of understanding and evaluating as well as planning economic studies.

METHODOLOGY ISSUES

When designing a cost-effectiveness study it is necessary to define the parameters listed in Table 19.2 and in order for cost-effectiveness studies to be useful they must be made comparable to one another through agreement on a common set of standards. Time horizons need to be clearly stated; for example, are the costs only incurred during a stay in hospital, for the duration of the disease, for a defined length of time (e.g. 5 years or life-time costs). The issue under study and type of disease will often determine this time frame. The view point or perspective being used, e.g. is that the cost incurred by the provider, the purchaser, the patient or in the best studies the societal perspective which is the optimal one as it takes into account everyone who is affected by the intervention and counts all the significant health outcomes and costs that flow from it irrespective of who experiences the outcomes or costs. Clinical

Table 19.2 *Issues related to cost-effectivness analysis studies*

1. A target audience
2. The type of analysis (e.g. cost-effectiveness analysis, cost utility analysis)
3. The perspective (e.g. societal)
4. Define the intervention program
5. Define the target population for the intervention
6. Define the comparator
7. Compare the comparator in a programme of varying intensity or duration
8. Define the boundaries of the study
9. Define the time horizon

Table 19.3 *Research study designs used for cost-effectiveness analysis*

a. Primary research design
- 'Piggyback studies' (e.g. economic analyses added on to a randomized control trial). These may be either current cost data or retrospective cost data
- A full cost-effectiveness trial where cost-effectiveness is the major element under study.

b. Secondary research design
- Retrospective cohort analysis
- Modeling: usually clinical decision analysis modeling but epidemiology-based models are also used

c. Combination designs
- Retrospective or randomized control trial then using this data to develop a model to extend the conclusions

outcomes need to be clearly stated: quality adjusted life years, lives saved, diagnoses made etc. Are the costs general costs or are they micro-costings where the actual costs incurred are measured in a 'bottom up' fashion. Which type of analysis has been employed – cost-effectiveness, cost minimalization etc. From where have the effectiveness data been obtained must be clear (a single trial, meta-analysis, consensus conference etc.). Is the costing method a prospective micro-costing? Are they marginal or total costs and what type of study is used and is it appropriate, e.g. modeling, prospective controlled trial etc.? Several research designs are used for CEA,[1] as shown in Table 19.3.

ANALYSIS ISSUES

In the analysis of cost-effectiveness data, irrespective of the method employed, it is important that the time horizons for both the costs and the benefits are sufficiently long to capture all costs and benefits of the interventions and are clearly stated. Ideally, this will usually be the full life of the patient group but it may also be, for example, a 5-year or even a shorter time horizon. The discounting rate that has

Table 19.4 *Relationships between costs and benefits*

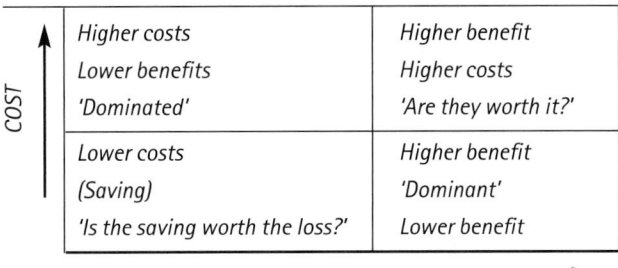

	Higher costs	Higher benefit
	Lower benefits	Higher costs
	'Dominated'	'Are they worth it?'
	Lower costs	Higher benefit
	(Saving)	'Dominant'
	'Is the saving worth the loss?'	Lower benefit

BENEFIT

Table 19.5 *Advantages of modelling*

- Identify key drivers
- Identify key issues for research
- Estimate likely power required
- Test various scenarios rapidly
- Cost-effectiveness
- Generic, used across healthcare systems
- Use for different patient sub-groups
- Interactive for effective dialogue
- Enables the use of appropriate time horizons

Table 19.6 *Examples of data required for a model*

- Population details (age, sex, prevalence etc.)
- Clinical decision variables
- Incidence rates for procedures e.g. angioplasty
- Healthcare costs by procedure
- Diagnostic accuracy
- Diagnostic procedure costs

been used for both costs and benefits needs to be stated (usually 3%) if it has been used, and appropriate allowances must be made for areas where the data is uncertain, which may be by using confidence intervals from meta-analysis or appropriate ranges for a sensitivity analysis in a modeling study.

When the results are presented they will include what other procedures the test under study is compared to – usually an incremental analysis – and what are the major outcomes being presented. A 'dominant' situation exists when the benefits can be shown to be increased at a lower cost or the benefits are less at a higher cost (Table 19.4).

When there is no dominant strategy then the most appropriate presentation is normally by incremental cost-effectiveness per life year lost or life year saved or QALYs saved. Judgement about the cost-effectiveness will usually include a threshold; for example, a medical intervention is worthwhile adopting if it does not cost more than the 'willingness to pay figure' e.g. $50 000 (Table 19.5).

Even if a model is deficient it will, at the very least, provide a guide to studies that need to be undertaken in the field in order to make the model more robust. The starting point in creating a model is a thorough understanding of the clinical process, which is usually much more complex and variable than appears in the first instance. Defining the patients who are eligible to enter the model and the best description of the clinical pathways that a patient may take needs to be produced in collaboration with the relevant clinicians involved in routine management. Where possible a retrospective or prospective cohort sample of actual patients

to validate the model should be obtained and a decision analysis model constructed. The types of data that are required to complete the model include some of those in Table 19.6.

These data will be obtained from published literature, where possible meta-analysis such as that for colorectal cancer which can also incorporate summary receiver operating characteristics [16], cost data that may be in the literature and other sources including small scale micro-costings. Cross-sectional information about a cohort of patients may be the next best way to avoid long-term follow-up of a group of patients. With this type of data collection reasonable estimates of confidence levels can be obtained in some cases and but if the data are weak this must be clearly identified. When patients after initial treatment may at random go through further processes a more complex Markov model may be necessary to provide sufficiently accurate estimates of outcomes. When data are collected and the decision model established it is possible to estimate the cost-effectiveness and incremental cost-effectiveness ratios for the base case. In order to establish the robustness of the conclusions sensitivity analysis is used (e.g. testing over what range of diagnostic accuracy the results still apply and what are these thresholds that can be arrived at). This analysis will identify which are the key drivers to which the model is sensitive and therefore what information needs to be most accurate and, conversely, which parameters do not affect the conclusions over a wide range of possible values. Examples of decision analysis models using PET which illustrate many of these points can be appreciated by working through the papers by Dietlein et al.[4] and Gambhir.[5] A further strength of models is that they may indicate how policy may be changed to make something which is clinically effective more cost-effective and, for example, by concentrating expensive imaging facilities such as FDG PET in one center where the throughput can be extremely high, thus reducing the unit cost and often the quality which may, in turn, improve the accuracy. A further outcome of a good model may be the development of clinical guidelines that have the potential to improve both clinical outcome quality as well as cost-effectiveness. The third outcome may be the identification of a research project to enhance the model with important information allowing the most accurate estimate of the power needed.

In measuring the costs for such a cost-effectiveness model these must be as complete as possible over the appropriate

Table 19.7   *Items in the literature that have been analyzed to date*

Target population	Evaluation method	Reference
Coronary artery disease	Decision analysis model	Garber[6]
		Patterson[7]
		Maddahi[8]
Solitary pulmonary nodule	Decision analysis model	Gambhir[9]
	Decision analysis model	Gould[10]
	Decision analysis model	Dietlein[11]
	Decision analysis	Gould[10]
Staging non-small cell lung cancer	Decision analysis model	Scott[12]
	Decision analysis model	Dietlein[13]
Re-staging colorectal cancer	Decision analysis model	Park[14]
Lymphoma staging	Retrospective costing	Hoh[15]
		Klose[16]
Adenosine vs. dipyridamole	Cost minimalization	Holmberg[17]
General oncology	Retrospective costing	Valk[18]
Neuropsychiatric	–	Small[19]

Table 19.8   *Comparison of costs per year of life saved in different clinical areas*

Procedure	Cost per year of life saved ($)
Liver transplant	43 000–250 000
Mammography (< 50 years)	160 000
Renal dialysis	116 000
Chemotherapy (breast)	46 200
Cardiac transplant	27 200
Coronary artery bypass graft	13 000

time frame and should, for example, incorporate the long-term costs of chemotherapy and palliative care for patients who relapse following therapeutic intervention or those who are misdirected to an inappropriate form of treatment. There are, however, dangers in making models over-complex as well as over-simplified.

Table 19.7 shows the subjects in FDG PET literature which have been analyzed to date with a moderate degree of rigor. Topics include solitary pulmonary nodules, staging non-small cell lung cancer, recurrent colorectal cancer, metastatic melanoma, lymphoma staging, and coronary artery disease.

Cost-effectiveness studies in nuclear medicine including FDG PET studies have been reviewed by Dietlein *et al.*[4] and by Gambhir.[5] These reviews also provide a detailed critique of the individual studies and in the review by Gambhir only six studies in the nuclear medicine literature were found which met all 10 of their quality criteria for cost-effectiveness studies and only one of these (Garber and Solomon[6]) was an FDG PET study. The following is not a comprehensive or detailed analysis of every cost-effectiveness study in the literature but a review of FDG PET related to the more important studies in the literature including some published since the two reviews mentioned above and some that have been completed and will be published shortly. Table 19.8 provides a useful comparison of the PET data with other non-imaging medical interventions.

REFERENCES

1   Hillman BJ, Kahan JP, Neu CR, Hammons GT. Clinical trials to evaluate cost-effectiveness. *Invest Radiol* 1989; **24**: 167–71.

2   Weinstein MC, Stason WB. Foundations of cost-effectiveness analysis for health and medical practices. *N Engl J Med* 1977; **296**: 716–21.

3   Drummond MF, Jefferson TO. Guidelines for authors and peer reviewers of economic submissions to the BMJ. *Br Med J* 1996; **313**: 275–83.

4   Dietlein M, Knapp WH, Lauterbach KW, Schicha H. Economic evaluation studies in nuclear medicine: the need for standardization. *Eur J Nucl Med* 1999; **26**: 663–80.

5   Gambhir SS. Economics of nuclear medicine – introduction. *Q J Nucl Med* 2000; **44**: 103–4.

6   Garber AM, Solomon NA. Cost-effectiveness of alternative test strategies for the diagnosis of coronary artery disease. *Ann Int Med* 1999; **130**: 719.

7   Patterson RE, Eisner RL, Horowitz SF. Comparison of cost-effectiveness and utility of exercise ECG, single-photon emission computed-tomography, positron

emission tomography, and coronary angiography for diagnosis of coronary-artery disease. *Circulation* 1995; **91**: 54–65.

8 Maddahi J, Gambhir SS. Cost-effective selection of patients for coronary angiography. *J Nucl Cardiol* 1997; **4**: S141–51.

9 Gambhir SS, Shepherd JE, Shah BD, *et al.* Analytical decision model for the cost-effective management of solitary pulmonary nodules. *J Clin Oncol* 1998; **16**: 2113–25.

10 Gould MK, Sanders GD, Barnett PG, *et al.* Cost-effectiveness of alternative management strategies for patients with solitary pulmonary nodules. *Ann Int Med* 2003; **138**: 724–35.

11 Dietlein M, Weber K, Gandjour A, *et al.* Cost-effectiveness of FDG-PET for the management of solitary pulmonary nodules: a decision analysis based on cost reimbursement in Germany. *Eur J Nucl Med* 2000; **27**: 1441–56.

12 Scott WJ, Shepherd J, Gambhir SS. Cost-effectiveness of FDG-PET for staging non-small cell lung cancer: a decision analysis. *Ann Thor Surg* 1998; **66**: 1876–83.

13 Dietlein M, Weber K, Gandjour A, *et al.* Cost-effectiveness of FDG-PET for the management of potentially operable non-small cell lung cancer: priority for a PET-based strategy after nodal-negative CT results. *Eur J Nucl Med* 2000; **27**: 1598–609.

14 Park KC, Schwimmer J, Shepherd JE, *et al.* Decision analysis for the cost-effective management of recurrent colorectal cancer. *Ann Surg* 2001; **233**: 310–19.

15 Hoh CK, Glaspy J, Rosen P, *et al.* Whole-body FDG-PET imaging for staging of Hodgkin's disease and lymphoma. *J Nucl Med* 1997; **38**: 343–8.

16 Klose T, Leidl R, Buchmann I, Brambs HJ, Reske SN. Primary staging of lymphomas: cost-effectiveness of FDG-PET versus computed tomography. *Eur J Nucl Med* 2000; **27**: 1457–64.

17 Holmberg MJ, Mohiuddin SM, Hilleman DE, *et al.* Outcomes and costs of positron emission tomography: comparison of intravenous adenosine and intravenous dipyridamole. *Clin Therap* 1997; **19**: 570–81.

18 Valk PE, Abella-Columna E, Haseman MK, *et al.* Whole-body PET imaging with [F-18]fluorodeoxyglucose in management of recurrent colorectal cancer. *Arch Surg* 1999; **134**: 503–11.

19 Small GW. Positron emission tomography scanning for the early diagnosis of dementia – would improve quality of care for patients and save money. *West J Med* 1999; **171**: 293–4.

Glossary

cost-benefit analysis (CBA) An analytical tool for estimating the net social benefit of an intervention as the incremental benefit of the program less the incremental cost, with all benefits and costs measured in currency (euros, pounds sterling, dollars etc.).

cost-effectiveness analysis (CEA) An analytical tool in which costs and effects of a procedure and at least one alternative strategy are calculated and presented as a ratio of incremental cost to incremental effect. Effects are health outcomes, such as cases of a disease diagnosed, years of life gained, or quality adjusted life years, sometimes called cost utility analysis (CUA).

cost-effectiveness ratio The incremental cost of obtaining a unit of health effect (such as dollars per year, or per quality adjusted year, of life expectancy) from a given procedure, when compared with an alternative.

cost-minimization analysis (CMA) An analytic tool used to compare the net costs of procedures that achieve the same clinical outcome.

decision analysis An explicit, quantitative, systematic approach to decision making under conditions of uncertainty in which probabilities of each possible event, along with the consequences of those events, are stated explicitly.

decision tree A graphical representation of a decision, incorporating alternative choices, uncertain events (and their probabilities), and outcomes.

direct costs The value of all goods, services, and other resources that are consumed in the provision of an intervention or in dealing with the side effects or other current and future consequences linked to it.

direct medical costs The value of health resources, (e.g. tests, drugs, supplies, health care personnel, and medical facilities) consumed in the provision of an intervention or in dealing with the side effects or other current and future consequences linked to it.

direct nonmedical costs The value of nonmedical goods, services, and other resources, such as child care or transportation, consumed in the provision of an intervention or in dealing with the side effects or other current and future consequences linked to it.

disability days Days in which activity is restricted due to either a short-term or long-term health problem or condition.

discounting The process of converting future currency and future health outcomes to their present value.

discount rate The interest rate used to compute present value, or the interest rate used in discounting future sums.

dominance The state when an intervention under study is both more effective and less costly than the alternative.

effectiveness The extent to which medical interventions achieve health improvements in real practice settings.

efficacy The extent to which medical interventions achieve health improvements under ideal circumstances.

fixed costs Costs that are held at a constant or fixed level, independent of the level of production and the time frame of the analysis.

health state The health of an individual at any particular point in time. A health state may be modified by the impairments, functional states, perceptions, and social opportunities that are influenced by disease, injury, treatment, or health policy.

incremental cost The cost of one alternative less the cost of another.

incremental cost-effectiveness (ratio) The ratio of the difference in costs between two alternatives to the difference in effectiveness between the same two alternatives.

indirect costs A term used in economics to refer to productivity gains or losses related to illness or death; in accounting it is used to describe overhead or fixed costs of production.

marginal benefit The added benefit generated by the next unit consumed.

marginal cost The added cost of producing one additional unit of output.

marginal cost-effectiveness (ratio) The incremental cost-effectiveness ratio between two alternatives that differ by one unit along some quantitative scale of intensity, dose, or duration. (This term is often used incorrectly as a synonym for incremental cost-effectiveness.)

Markov models A type of mathematical model containing a finite number of mutually exclusive and exhaustive health states, having time periods of uniform length, and in which the probability time of movement from one state to another depends on the current state and remains constant.

meta-analysis A method for combining and integrating the results of independent studies of the effect of a given intervention. Meta-analysis is used broadly to mean the averaging of results across studies. It refers to a defined method for acquiring reports of randomized clinical trials, rating and culling these reports for quality of the research, and statistically combining the results of the remaining studies.

micro-costing A valuation technique which starts with a detailed identification and measurement of all the inputs consumed in a health care intervention and all of its sequelae. Once the resources consumed have been identified and quantified, they are then converted into value terms to produce a cost estimate.

opportunity cost The value of time or any other 'input' in its highest value use. The benefits lost because the next-best alternative was not selected.

perspective The viewpoint from which a cost-effectiveness analysis is conducted.

20

Radiopharmaceuticals

20A Introduction

Introduction	815	Characteristics of selected functional imaging agents	816
The tracer concept	815	References	818
Functional imaging agents	815		

20B Interactions and reactions

Introduction	821	Interactions with PET radiopharmaceuticals	826
Frequency of occurrence	821	Interactions with interventional drugs	826
Reactions	822	Blood labeling	827
Interactions	824	References	827
Interactions with single-photon emitting radiopharmaceuticals	824		

20C New single-photon radiopharmaceuticals

Introduction	831	Neuroreceptor imaging	836
Inflammation imaging	832	Summary	836
Cancer imaging	833	References	836
Cancer therapy	835		

20D New radiopharmaceuticals for positron emission tomography

Introduction	839	Neurodegeneration	841
Bone	841	Neurotransmitters	842
Cardiac imaging agents	841	Oncology	842
Flow	841	References	844

Introduction

MALCOLM FRIER

INTRODUCTION

Radiopharmaceuticals are medicinal products[1] that depend for their action on the presence in their molecule of a radionuclide. The prime requirement of a successful diagnostic radiopharmaceutical is to show selective uptake in or exclusion from an organ or lesion, and for that exclusion or uptake to be of sufficient duration to allow imaging. For a therapeutic material, selective uptake is the prime requirement, with the uptake being of sufficient duration to allow the exertion of a therapeutic effect. The existence of the current armoury of radiopharmaceuticals has derived from the early development of radiotracers.

THE TRACER CONCEPT

The attempts by de Hevesy, early in the 20th century, to separate so-called radium-D from lead were unsuccessful. However, he was quick to suggest that radium-D could be used as a tracer for lead in chemical reactions.[2,3] From the earliest days of working with radionuclides, de Hevesy was very much aware of the limitations imposed by toxicity in using materials such as radium in the investigations of biological systems. It is remarkable that, almost as soon as artificially produced radioactive elements became available,[4] their potential as radiotracers for metabolic pathways, notably those of phosphorus, in biological systems was realized and exploited.[5] The availability of ^{3}H and ^{14}C allowed the synthesis of metabolites and precursors, and it is evident that many of the published reference data relating to the properties of human organs and tissues[6] were obtained through the use of radioactive tracers.[7,8] Many

studies have been focused on the thyroid gland because of the ready availability, following the development of the nuclear reactor, of ^{131}I.

The tracer concept, however, does have serious limitations in that it depends on the availability of ions or molecules that are exact, but radioactive, analogs of the precursor or metabolite they are to mimic. It is true that many relevant biological molecules can be synthesized carrying a ^{14}C or ^{3}H nucleus in their structure, but these do not emit a signal suitable for external imaging given scanners currently available. The introduction of tracers carrying the positron-emitting isotopes of carbon, oxygen, and nitrogen (and fluorine as an analog of hydrogen) has addressed this problem to some extent, but the synthesis and use of such materials will always need to consider the short half-lives of the respective radionuclides. What has developed is a whole range of functional imaging agents based on 'foreign' gamma-emitting radionuclides. These agents demonstrate function through a variety of mechanisms.

FUNCTIONAL IMAGING AGENTS

Functional imaging agents exhibit a wide range of physical and chemical properties. Mechanisms of biodistribution may depend on the physical form, as in the uptake of particulate material by phagocytosis, or may be brought about by the similarity of the radiopharmaceutical agent to a substrate or metabolite, as in the uptake of *meta*-iodobenzylguanidine. Some radiopharmaceuticals are distributed by well-understood mechanisms while the actions of others are poorly defined. The attachment of a radiolabel to a protein or other large biomolecule probably has little effect on the biodistribution of the resulting product. However, many chelates of ^{99m}Tc have very different structures and properties from the starting ligands.

The observed biodistribution of a radiopharmaceutical often cannot be explained in terms of a single mechanism but rather as the result of interaction between many different mechanisms involving initial dilution, passive or active transmembrane transport, protein binding, possible metabolic incorporation and elimination and excretion. The molecule may also undergo degradation and it should be noted that the observed distribution is that of the radiolabel and not necessarily that of the intact molecule.

An important property of a successful functional imaging agent is that it should in itself have no effect on the organ or system it is designed to investigate; in other words, it should be pharmacologically inert. If not inert, then it must be capable of being used at concentrations sufficiently low to exert minimal pharmacological effect. This requirement involves the need for production of materials of very high specific activity; that is, with high levels of radioactivity per unit mass of the radiopharmaceutical.

CHARACTERISTICS OF SELECTED FUNCTIONAL IMAGING AGENTS

Skeletal agents

Technetium-99m diphosphonates are the current agents of choice for the performance of bone scans, demonstrating rapid bone uptake, low background uptake in nonskeletal areas and clearance of nonbound activity by urinary excretion. The half-time for blood clearance of hexamethylene diphosphonate (HDP) has been estimated at 50 min.[9] More than half of the injected dose is taken up by bone, with less than 2% remaining in circulation at 4 h post-injection. Diphosphonates interact with the surface of the hydroxyapatite crystal, and there is crystallographic evidence to suggest a relationship between diphosphonates and the coordination parameters of calcium in hydroxyapatite.[10] The P-C-P link of diphosphonates is very stable, and is not vulnerable to attack by phosphatase enzymes, whereas the P-O-P link found in polyphosphates and pyrophosphates is readily broken (Fig. 20A.1).

Renal agents

Technetium-99m dimercaptosuccinic acid (^{99m}Tc-DMSA) is used for the demonstration of renal morphology. It depends for its function on specific uptake by and long retention within the parenchymal tissue of the kidney. DMSA was introduced into nuclear medicine practice by Lin et al.[11] About 25% of the injected dose is taken up by the kidneys within 1 h, rising to about 40% in 6 h.[12] Less than 10% of the injected activity is excreted in the urine within the first

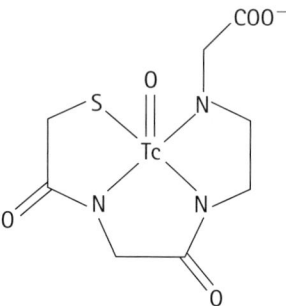

Figure 20A.1 *Comparative structures of medronate (top) and polyphosphate (bottom).*

Figure 20A.2 *Stucture of ^{99m}Tc-mercaptoacetyltriglycine.*

hour. The complex is retained within the cells of the apical part of the proximal convoluted tubules and pars recta, and in the upper part of the loop of Henle. Binding takes place with protein receptors containing sulfhydryl groups.

Stable, water soluble chelates of low molecular weight are generally rapidly excreted by glomerular filtration providing that they do not bind significantly to plasma proteins. Chromium-51 EDTA has a long-established use for this purpose. Technetium-99m diethylenetriaminepentaacetic acid (DTPA)[13] is also excreted exclusively through glomerular filtration. Less than 10% of the activity becomes bound to plasma proteins, leading to a slight underestimation of the glomerular filtration rate.

Technetium-99m mercaptoacetyl triglycine (MAG$_3$)[14] (Fig. 20A.2) is excreted through a combination of glomerular filtration and tubular secretion. Comparative kinetics of MAG$_3$ and hippuran have been evaluated by Pavia et al.[15] who concluded that the mean value of renal excretion constant was equal for the two agents. Clearance values were highly correlated (ratio 0.57). Volumes of distribution differed, being 4.1 L for MAG$_3$ and 7.0 L for hippuran. Between 60 and 70% of the tracers are excreted at 1 h. Protein binding was found to be variable both between and within subjects, more variable for MAG$_3$ and higher for hippuran. Some authors quote a protein binding value of 60–70% for hippuran but the bond is weak and easily broken.

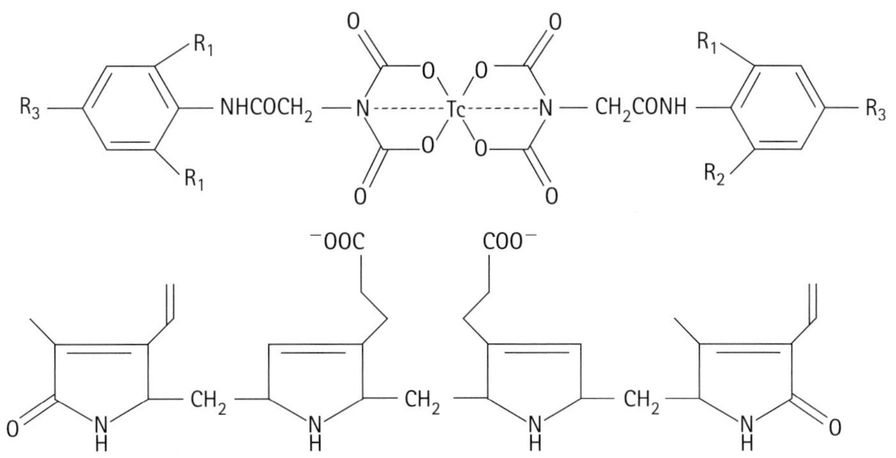

Figure 20A.3 *Comparison between structures of Tc-iminodiacetic acid (top) and bilirubin (bottom).*

Hepatobiliary agents

Many ^{99m}Tc hepatobiliary agents are based on the substituted acetanilide iminodiacetates (the IDAs). These compounds were originally developed during the search for myocardial imaging agents based on lidocaine.[16,17] The free ligand, when labeled with ^{14}C, is excreted predominantly in the urine. The addition of ^{99m}Tc leads to the formation of two or more compounds but only one undergoes rapid biliary excretion.[18] Costello *et al.*[19] have suggested that this is in the form of a bis-dianionic ligand complex of technetium(III). Substitution in the benzene ring increases molecular weight and lipophilicity. Higher molecular weight compounds such as butyl-IDA undergo less competitive inhibition in the presence of elevated serum bilirubin levels, and consequently lower compensatory renal excretion. Comparative structures of IDA and bilirubin are shown on Fig. 20A.3.

Myocardial agents

The most significant advance in studies of the myocardium was made by the introduction of ^{199}Tl as a potassium analog for imaging.[20] The 201 isotope was a later introduction. Although belonging to group III, thallium is thought to be transported into the myocardium by the Na/K/ ATPase system, although the mechanism of facilitated diffusion has been suggested. Its efflux, however, is slower than that of potassium. Within 30 min of injection, 3–4% of the injected dose accumulates in the myocardium. Redistribution occurs within the following 12–18 h, during which time the heart remains clearly visible.

The cationic ^{99m}Tc hexakis-isonitrile complexes (Fig. 20A.4) are not taken up by this mechanism. Experiments with isolated myocytes[21] showed that uptake was not affected by ouabain, indicating no involvement of the Na/K/ATPase system. The lipophilicity of this class of compound certainly contributes to the uptake, and there may be some contribution by assisted diffusion. Sestamibi (MIBI) does show an

MIBI R = — C(CH₃)₂ — CH₂ — O — CH₃

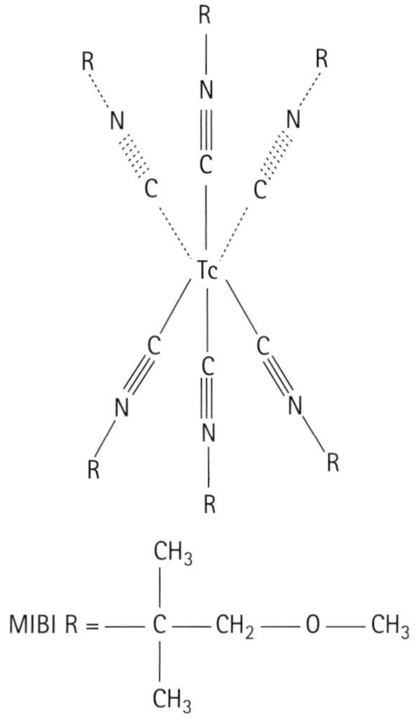

Figure 20A.4 *Structure of ^{99m}Tc-isonitrile.*

affinity for a cytosolic protein of molecular weight 10^4 Da to which it binds[22] with a dissociation constant of 0.77×10^{-5}, and this may serve to explain the slow clearance from the myocardium, activity remaining comparatively stable for some hours at between 2 and 3% of the administered dose. Plasma clearance is rapid with a half-life of 4.3 min.[23]

Tetrofosmin is also a cationic compound of the class (Fig. 20A.5). Uptake is again related to lipophilicity and assisted diffusion, but there is no comparative evidence of intracellular protein binding.

Brain blood–flow agents

Technetium-99m hexamethypropylene amine oxine (HMPAO) is a lipophilic complex of ^{99m}Tc that has found

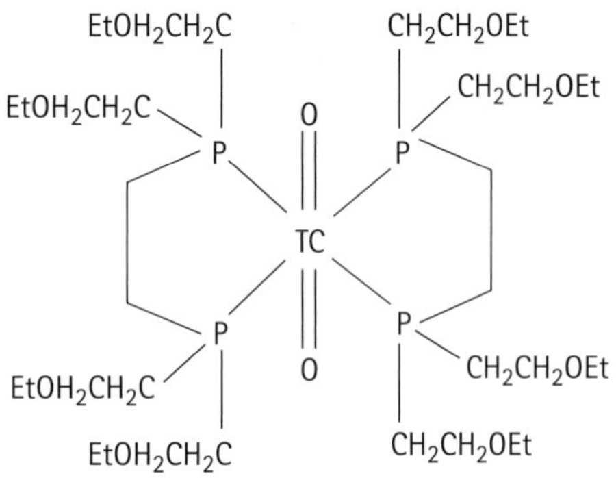

Figure 20A.5 *Structure of ^{99m}Tc-tetrofosmin.*

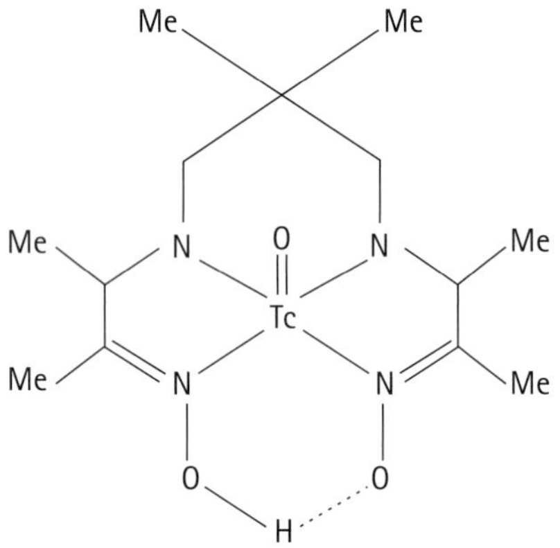

Figure 20A.6 *Structure of ^{99m}Tc-exametazime (hexamethylpropylene amine oxine).*

wide application as a marker for the regional blood flow of the brain. The primary complex (Fig. 20A.6) is highly lipophilic and can cross the blood/brain barrier. It has been proposed[24] that the mechanism of retention is related to the glutathione content of the cell. El Shirbing *et al.*[25] have shown in experimental animals that HMPAO can be found attached mainly to cell organelles. There is also a higher concentration of HMPAO in neuronal nuclei than in glial nuclei for all regions of the brain studied.

Peptide-based radiopharmaceuticals

Products based on peptides exploit the fact that in many pathological conditions, the expression of specific markers can be uprated. Peptides having an affinity for these markers can be used for both diagnostic and therapeutic purposes. The expression of somatostatin receptors is uprated in a number of conditions, including carcinoids, pancreatic endocrine tumours, neuroblastomas, and paragangliomas. The concept of imaging these receptors using small radiolabeled peptides was introduced in 1991.[26] A comparison between the structure of somatostatin and octreotide is shown in Fig. 20A.7. Another peptide, depreotide, with affinity for somatostatin receptors, labeled with ^{99m}Tc, has

Somatostatin

Ala–Gly–Cys–Lys–Asn–Phe–*Phe–Trp–Lys–Thr*–Phe–Thr–Ser–Cys

Octreotide

D–Phe–Cys–*Phe–D–Trp–Lys–Thr*–Cys–Thr(Ol)

Figure 20A.7 *Comparison between the structures of somatostatin and octreotide.*

found application in the imaging of solitary pulmonary nodules. Peptides have also found use in the imaging of apoptosis. A 35 kDa protein, annexin-V, has a nanomolar affinity for the phosphatidylserine and hence ^{99m}Tc-labeled annexin-V has been used for noninvasive detection of apoptosis.[27–29] Annexin imaging has been performed in acute myocardial infarction, myocarditis and acute transplant rejection.[30]

REFERENCES

1 The Medicines (Radioactive Substances) Order 1978, SI No 1004. London: HMSO, 1978.
2 de Hevesy G, Paneth F. RaD als "Indikator" de Bleis Z. *Anorg Chem* 1913; **82**: 323–6.
3 de Hevesy G, Paneth F. Über die Darstellung von Radium D in sichtbaren Mengen und seine chemische Identität mit Blei. *Ber Dt Chem Ges* 1914; **47**: 2784–6.
4 Joliot F, Curie I. Artificial production of a new kind of radioelement. *Nature* 1934; **133**: 201–2.
5 de Hevesey G, Linderstrøm-Lang K, Olsen C. Exchange of phosphorus atoms in plants and seeds. *Nature* 1937; **139**: 149.
6 Lentner C. (ed.) *Geigy scientific tables.* Basel: Ciba-Geigy Ltd, 1981.
7 Moore FD, Olesen KH, McMurrey JD, *et al. The body cell mass and its supporting environment: body composition in health and disease.* Philadelphia: Saunders, 1963.
8 Widdowson FM, Dickerson JWT. Chemical composition of the body. In: Comar CL, Bronner F. (eds.) *The elements, part A.* Mineral metabolism, vol. 11. New York: Academic Press, 1964: 1–247.
9 Weber DA, Makler PT, Watson EE, *et al.* MIRD dose estimate report no. 13. Radiation absorbed dose from technetium-99m labeled bone imaging agents. *J Nucl Med* 1989; **30**: 1117–22.
10 Johanssen B. Principles, problems and trends in radiopharmacology. In: Deckart H, Cox PH. (eds.) *Principles of radiopharmacology.* Dordrecht: Martinus Nijhoff, 1987: 166–82.
11 Lin TH, Khentigan A, Winchell HS. A Tc-99m chelate substitute for organomercurial renal agents. *J Nucl Med* 1979; **15**: 35.

12 McAfee JC. A review of radiopharmaceuticals in nephrourology. In: Joekes AM, Constable AR, Brown NJC, Tauxe WN. (eds.) *Radionuclides in nephrology*. New York: Academic Press, 1982: 3–8.

13 Eckelman WC, Richards P. Instant Tc-99m DTPA. *J Nucl Med* 1979; **1**: 761–2.

14 Fritzberg AR, Kuni CC, Klingensmith III WC, *et al*. Synthesis and biological evaluation of Tc-99m *N,N'*-bis(mercaptoacetyl)-2,3-diaminopropanoate. A potential replacement for (^{131}I)-*o*-iodohippurate. *J Nucl Med* 1982; **23**: 592–8.

15 Pavia J, Ros D, Piera C, *et al*. Comparative study of the kinetics of the renal tracers Tc-99m-MAG-3 and I-131 hippuran. *Nucl Med Commun* 1991; **12**: 529–37.

16 Loberg MD, Cooper M, Harvey H, *et al*. Development of new radiopharmaceuticals based on N-substituted imidodiacetic acid. *J Nucl Med* 1976; **17**: 633–8.

17 Loberg MD, Fields AT. Chemical structure of technetium-99m labelled *N*-(2,6 dimethylphenyl-carbamoylmethyl)imidodiacetic acid (Tc-HIDA). *Int J Appl Radiat Isot* 1978; **29**: 167–73.

18 Fritzberg AR, Lewis D. HPLC analysis of Tc-99m imidodiacetic acid hepatobiliary agents and a question of multiple peaks: concise communication. *J Nucl Med* 1980; **21**: 1180–4.

19 Costello CE, Brodack JW, Jones AG, *et al*. The investigation of radiopharmaceutical components by fast atom bombardment mass spectrometry: the identification of Tc-HIDA and the epimers of Tc-CO2 DADS. *J Nucl Med* 1983; **24**: 353–5.

20 Kawana M, Krizek H, Porte, J, *et al*. Use of Tl-199 as a potassium analogue in scanning [Abstract]. *J Nucl Med* 1970; **11**: 333.

21 Sands H, Delano ML, Gallagher BM. Uptake of hexakis-(*t*-butylisonitrile) technetium(I) and hexakis-(isopropyl-isonitrile) technetium(I) by neonatal rat myocytes and human erythrocytes. *J Nucl Med* 1986; **27**: 404–8.

22 Mousa SA, Williams SJ, Sands H. Characterisation of in-vivo chemistry of cations in the heart. *J Nucl Med* 1987; **28**: 1351–7.

23 Wackers FTJ, Berman DS, Maddahi J, *et al*. Technetium-99m hexakis 2-methoxy isobutyl isonitrile: human biodistribution, dosimetry, safety and preliminary comparison to thallium-201 for myocardial perfusion. *J Nucl Med* 1989; **30**: 301–11.

24 Costa DC, Lui D, Sinha AK, *et al*. Intracellular localisation of ^{99}Tc^m-d,l-HMPAO and ^{201}Tl-DDC in rat brain. *Nucl Med Commun* 1989; **10**: 459–66.

25 El-Shirbiny AM, Sadek S, Owunwanne A, *et al*. Is Tc-99m hexamethyl-propyleneamineoxine uptake in the tissues related to glutathione cellular content? *Nucl Med Commun* 1989; **10**: 905–11.

26 Bakker WH, Albert R, Bruns C, *et al*. (In-111-DTPA-d-Phe)-octreotide, a potential radiopharmaceutical for imaging somatostatin receptor-positive tumours: synthesis, radiolabelling and in-vitro validation. *Life Sci* 1991; **49**: 1593–601.

27 van de Wiele C, Lahorte C, Vermeersch H, *et al*. Quantitative tumor apoptosis imaging using technetium-99m-HYNIC annexin V single photon emission computed tomography. *J Clin Oncol* 2003; **21**: 3483–7.

28 Ohtsuki K, Akashi K, Aoka Y, *et al*. Technetium-99m HYNIC-annexin V: a potential radiopharmaceutical for the in-vivo detection of apoptosis. *Eur J Nucl Med* 1999; **26**: 1251–8.

29 Blankenberg FG, Katsikis PD, Tait JF, *et al*. Imaging of apoptosis (programmed cell death) with ^{99m}Tc annexin V. *J Nucl Med* 1999; **40**: 184–91.

30 Kown MH, Strauss HW, Blankenberg FG, *et al*. In vivo imaging of acute cardiac rejection in human patients using (99m)technetium labeled annexin V. *Am J Transplant* 2001; **3**: 270–7.

Interactions and reactions

MALCOLM FRIER

INTRODUCTION

The diagnostic and therapeutic value of nuclear medicine procedures depends on the predictability of the biodistribution of the radiopharmaceuticals concerned following administration. Assuming that the radiopharmaceutical is intact when administered, and is stable, the observed biodistribution is a true indication of the condition of the patient at the time of receiving the dose. This condition is determined by physiological, pathological, and pharmacological factors including diet, the state of hydration, age-related phenomena, the presence of infection, renal failure, and drug therapy. Any changes in this biodistribution should, ideally, be relatable to a specific pathology and exploited either for diagnostic purposes, or to produce a therapeutic effect. There are circumstances when this pattern is changed in an unexpected way.

Hladik and Norenberg[1] examined problems associated with the clinical use of radiopharmaceuticals and produced a proposed classification system and troubleshooting guide. In it, these authors suggested that problems associated with the clinical use of radiopharmaceuticals could usually be classified into one of four categories comprising modified, unexpected and often unusual diagnostic or therapy outcomes, adverse reactions, unique difficulties encountered in special patient populations, and quality assurance failures. The first of these four categories is further subdivided into altered biodistribution of the radiopharmaceutical, imaging artifacts, and normal anatomical variants. Altered biodistributions may be the result of concomitant drug therapy, other medical procedures such as surgery, dialysis, radiation therapy or biopsy. In addition, there may be the presence of other, undetected pathology,

or there may simply be problems associated with the formulation and stability of the radiopharmaceutical.

Of these factors, the influence of concomitant drug therapy is often the most difficult to predict, because, with few well-documented exceptions, evidence for interaction is scarce, and is often anecdotal. In many circumstances, if an unusual event is seen, patients may be receiving multiple drug therapy, and identifying the specific drug in question may not be straightforward. For similar reasons, linking an observed adverse reaction to the administration of a specific radiopharmaceutical is not always easy, because the response may be to something quite different. In an attempt to overcome some of these problems, Silberstein and Ryan[2] performed a prospective study over a 5-year period commencing in 1989, in which strict criteria were applied to the data collection, specifically excluding vasovagal responses. An algorithm developed to analyze the data categorized the reactions into (1) not related, (2) conditional, unlikely or unrelated, (3) possible, and (4) probable.

FREQUENCY OF OCCURRENCE

Many data concerning both adverse reactions and altered biodistributions are to be found in individual, unrelated publications. Examples include the influence of intravenous etidronate therapy on bone imaging,[3] the possible effects of dipyridamole on erythrocyte labeling efficiency[4] and the benign myocardial uptake of hydroxymethylene diphosphonate.[5] Other, more systematic systems of data collection are operated by some national agencies and professional organizations. In the United States, the reporting route for problems related to all drugs is via the FDA

Table 20B.1 *Summary of adverse event reports received within Europe[7-14]*

Event	Year							
	1993	1994	1995	1996	1997	1998	1999	2000
Adverse event (all)	62	73	64	64	82	68	67	62
Adverse event (high probability)	52			41	52	46	39	38
Altered biodistribution	14	11	6	9	6	2	5	10
Blood labeling						8	8	2
Different radiopharmaceuticals	15	17	13	18	14	18	10	15
Most common product				^{99m}Tc-diphosphonates				

reporting program. Data specific to radiopharmaceuticals have been gathered through the Drug Product Problem Reporting Program for radiopharmaceuticals, jointly supported by the United States Pharmacopoeial Convention, and the Society for Nuclear Medicine.[6] In the United Kingdom, adverse events relating to all drugs are reported to the Medicines and Healthcare Products Regulatory Agency (MHRA). However, within the rest of Europe, the Radiopharmacy Committee of the European Association of Nuclear Medicine operates a reporting scheme specifically for radiopharmaceuticals, and collected data are regularly published. Table 20B.1 includes data from the most recently published reports, showing details of the numbers and nature of reported events, and the numbers of different radiopharmaceuticals implicated.[7-14] In Japan, an annual report appears which relates to reported adverse events.[15-17]

Data gathered from these and other reports can only give a very rough estimate of the frequency of such events, because the reporting process itself is very subjective. Attempts to produce a more objective assessment of the frequency of occurrence of adverse events and altered biodistributions have been undertaken. Silberstein and Ryan[2] gathered data prospectively from 18 nuclear medicine departments in the United States, who each provided monthly returns on the numbers of radiopharmaceutical administrations, and the numbers of adverse events. By analyzing the data according to the algorithm described above, 18 adverse events from 783 525 administrations gave a prevalence of 2.3 (1.2–3.4 at 95% confidence limit) per 10^5 administrations.

In France, where radiopharmaceuticals have been defined as drugs since 1992, few adverse events have been described in the literature. Some authors have reported a rate of 1 to 6 reactions per 100 000 injections. A prospective survey[18] was performed over an 18-month period from November 1993 to May 1995 in the Department of Nuclear Medicine of the University Hospital in Toulouse. Radiopharmaceuticals involved were ^{99m}Tc-phytate, ^{99m}Tc-microspheres of serum albumin, ^{99m}Tc-dimercaptosuccinic acid (DMSA), ^{99m}Tc-hydroxymethyldiphosphonate (HMDP), ^{99m}Tc-colloid, ^{99m}Tc-pyrophosphate, ^{99m}Tc-sestamibi and ^{201}Tl. There were 14 794 injections in total, and three side effects were reported: one case of necrosis at the injection site, one case of vomiting, and one case of dizziness. All the cases occurred with ^{99m}Tc-pyrophosphate. The necrosis was classified as 'serious' by the WHO definition. The causal relationship was unlikely for the first and second case and probable for the third. All patients recovered uneventfully.

Centered in the UK, a prospective survey was performed in 17 nuclear medicine departments during 1996 in an attempt to provide reliable data on the prevalence of adverse reactions to radiopharmaceuticals within Europe.[19] All adverse events following radiopharmaceutical administration were recorded, irrespective of the severity or likelihood of causality, and subsequently analyzed using the same algorithm devised by Silberstein. A prevalence of 11 (3.3–19.2 at the 95% confidence limit) events per 10^5 administrations was obtained with no serious or life-threatening events reported. This rate is slightly higher than that obtained in the United States study of 2.3 events per 10^5 administrations. The difference may be related to the inclusion or exclusion of vasovagal events from the analysis, the way in which the algorithm was used and the comparative size and time scale of the two studies. In any event, the prevalence of adverse reactions is approximately 1000-fold less than that occurring with iodinated contrast media and drugs.

REACTIONS

Single-photon radiopharmaceuticals

Published data from various surveys have identified common features in the recorded adverse events. Some of these are tabulated in Tables 20B.2 and 20B.3. Table 20B.2 is based on data from the USA[2] which are prefaced with the statement that many of the adverse reactions listed are obtained from clinical trials which were not placebo controlled and may have no causative relationship with the radiopharmaceutical. Data in Table 20B.3 are taken from a European study[19] and were classified according to probability of association.

There are numerous case reports in the literature reporting adverse events following administration of

Table 20B.2 *Types of adverse events observed in the United States*

Radiopharmaceutical	Adverse event
[^{99m}Tc]pertechnetate	Chills, nausea, vomiting, diffuse rash, pruritus, hives/urticaria, chest pain, tightness or heaviness, hypertension, dizziness, vertigo, headache, diaphoresis, anaphylaxis
^{99m}Tc-macroaggregated albumin	Chills, nausea, erythema, flushing, diffuse rash, pruritus, hives/urticaria, cardiac arrest, chest pain, tightness or heaviness, hypertension, hypotension, respiratory reaction, tachycardia, syncope or faintness, diaphoresis, cyanosis, anaphylaxis, metallic taste, dyspnea; throat tightness; arm numbness; parosmia.
^{99m}Tc-medronate	Chills, fever, nausea, vomiting, erythema, flushing, diffuse rash, pruritus, hives/urticaria, cardiac arrest, chest pain, tightness or heaviness, hypertension, hypotension, respiratory reaction, tachycardia, seizures, syncope or faintness, dizziness, vertigo, headache, diaphoresis, anaphylaxis, abdominal pain, metallic taste, asthenia, pain/burning in injection site, photophobia, one death secondary to cardiac arrythmia
^{99m}Tc-oxidronate	Nausea, vomiting, erythema, flushing, diffuse rash, pruritus, chest pain, tightness or heaviness, heartburn, seizures, diaphoresis, facial swelling
^{99m}Tc-pentetate	Chills, nausea, erythema, flushing, diffuse rash, pruritus, hives/urticaria, hypertension, hypotension, respiratory reaction, tachycardia, syncope or faintness, headache, cyanosis, anaphylaxis, arthralgia, pain, burning at injection site, cough; wheezing
^{99m}Tc-mertiatide	Nausea, vomiting, erythema, flushing, syncope or faintness, sore, thick throat
^{99m}Tc-mebrofenin	Hives/urticaria
^{111}In-pentetreotide	Fever, nausea, erythema, flushing, hypotension, bradycardia, dizziness, vertigo, headache, diaphoresis, arthralgia and asthenia, one case of anemia
[^{123}I]iodobenguane	Nausea. Erythema, flushing, hypertension, respiratory reaction, syncope or faintness, dizziness and vertigo, tachypnea

Table 20B.3 *Types of adverse events observed in Europe*

Radiopharmaceutical	Adverse event	Likelihood of association
^{99m}Tc-MIBI	Metallic taste on injection	Probable
^{99m}Tc-MIBI	Rash on trunk and extremities 2 days after injection	Possible
^{99m}Tc-oxidronate	Temporary loss of consciousness, profuse sweating	Unlikely
^{99m}Tc-MAG$_3$	Heavy eyes 20 min after injection, followed by eye strain, feeling warm and dizzy	Unlikely
^{99m}Tc-nanocoll	Severe swelling of hands and feet 90 min after local injections	Probable
Sodium [^{131}I]iodide	Sore throat, tender at front of neck 48 h after 406 MBq	Probable
[^{67}Ga]Gallium citrate	Stomach pain and melena 24 h after injection, known cirrhotic, hepatitis, anemia	Unlikely

radiopharmaceuticals. The products appearing most frequently in these reports today are the diphosphonates, which is probably a reflection of the frequency of usage in comparison with other materials. A typical reaction is the delayed appearance, usually within 2–24 h, of an erythematous rash over the trunk and buttocks, accompanied by itching. Less frequent is an urticarial response, an occasional vasomotor reaction, and some complaints of nausea and malaise. Mooser *et al.*[20] reported a delayed-type allergic reaction to ^{99m}Tc-medronate. Balan *et al.*[21] presented a case report showing an unusual severe systemic reaction that occurred in a woman after a ^{99m}Tc-methylene diphosphonate bone scan for which no alternative explanation could be found. The bone scintigram showed diffusely increased uptake in the liver and kidneys accompanied by reversible dysfunction of these organs and dermatological manifestations. The authors speculated that the reaction was the result of an immune-mediated mechanism. Burton and Cashman[22] reported an allergic reaction to nanocolloid during lymphoscintigraphy for sentinel lymph node biopsy. Their comment was in response to an article reporting reaction to the blue dye used in sentinel lymph node imaging. Their patient had not received blue dye, but demonstrated a widespread, non-itchy urticarial skin reaction, being cutaneous symptoms of the grade 1 type. The patient was treated with 10 mg of intravenous chlorpheniramine and recovered uneventfully over the next hour.

Positron emission tomography radiopharmaceuticals

Silberstein[23] has retrospectively reviewed the safety of positron emission tomography (PET) radiopharmaceuticals. In a separate prospective study,[24] he has also examined the prevalence of adverse reactions to positron emitting radiopharmaceuticals in nuclear medicine as well as to non-radioactive drugs used in interventional nuclear medicine during PET studies. The study was conducted over a 4-year period and involved the collaboration of 22 institutions. Information was requested each month during the study about the number of PET procedures performed, the number of adverse reactions to PET radiopharmaceuticals and the number of adverse reactions to interventional non-radioactive pharmaceuticals used. A total of 33 925 radiopharmaceutical doses were recorded in a retrospective examination of records by the 22 participating institutions, and the total prospective number of administered doses recorded by the participants was 47 876, giving a final total of 81 801 administrations. No adverse reactions were found from any PET radiopharmaceutical dose, and there were no deaths or hospitalizations caused by nonradioactive interventional pharmaceuticals used as adjuncts. The study would seem to indicate that PET radiopharmaceuticals have an extraordinary safety record with no adverse reactions reported in over 80 000 administered doses in this study.

INTERACTIONS

In 1982, Hladik[25] reviewed drug-induced changes in the biological distribution of radiopharmaceuticals. The topic was further reviewed in 1994 by Hesslewood and Leung.[26] This review provides information in tabular form on expected interactions between drugs and radiopharmaceuticals on an organ-by-organ basis. There are significant differences between the publications in terms both of the radiopharmaceuticals and the drugs considered. However, the three mechanisms of interaction defined in the scheme proposed by Sampson and Cox[27] remain unchanged.

Direct pharmacological effect of the drug itself

This effect can lead to unusual handling of the radiopharmaceutical. In its simplest form, drugs can have a direct effect upon an organ, which in its turn can handle the radiopharmaceutical in a different way. An example here is that of the narcotic analgesics such as morphine, pethidine, and methadone, which can cause spasm of the biliary tract, and prolong the transit times of hepatobiliary imaging agents.[28] More subtle effects include blocking of receptors or interfering with transport mechanisms. Drug interactions

with *meta*-iodobenzylguanidine (MIBG) have been extensively studied.[29,30]

Direct *in vivo* physicochemical interactions between radiopharmaceutical and drug

This type of interaction has the potential to produce marked changes. Brain imaging with [^{99m}Tc]pertechnetate[31] and liver/spleen imaging with radiocolloids were very susceptible to the presence of aluminum ions,[32] so that even high doses of nonprescription antacid products have been implicated as causing problems. Brain and liver imaging have long been superseded, but the problem highlighted here is that compiling a drug history of prescribed medicines may not always provide the answer if a drug interaction is suspected. Intramuscular iron dextran has produced local accumulation of ^{99m}Tc-medronate at the site of injection.[33] The adverse effect of bisphosphonate therapy for Paget's disease, hypercalcemia of malignancy or osteoporosis on the uptake of bone-seeking radiopharmaceuticals may well be related to the preferential formation of complexes in the circulation, reducing the amounts available for bone uptake, although competition at the skeletal binding site is also a possibility.[34]

Drug-induced, or iatrogenic, disease[35]

Transport of the radiopharmaceutical can be affected, leading to an unexpected biodistribution. Many drugs, including aspirin, paracetamol and some cytotoxic agents can be toxic to the liver, and can affect the clearance of hepatobiliary tracers. Cytotoxic agents can also damage kidney function, bringing about a decrease in glomerular filtration rate, and both doxorubicin and adriamycin are known to be cardiotoxic, possibly related to changes in cell membrane permeability. An example of a possible iatrogenic change has been reported by Hany et al.[36] Focal, intrapulmonary uptake of [^{18}F]fluorodeoxyglucose was observed in three patients, attributed to iatrogenic microembolization.

INTERACTIONS WITH SINGLE-PHOTON EMITTING RADIOPHARMACEUTICALS

Iodobenguane (MIBG)

Many drugs, including labetalol and the tricyclic antidepressants, are known to inhibit the so-called 'uptake-1'[37] mechanism, which is a specific neuronal catecholamine uptake. Some antihypertensive drugs, in particular the adrenergic neuron blockers such as bretylium and guanethidine, can compete with MIBG for transport into storage vesicles.[38] Others, including the angiotensin-converting enzyme inhibitors like captopril and enalapril, and beta

Table 20B.4   *Drugs known to affect the uptake of meta-iodobenzylguanidine (MIBG)*

Drug	Observed effect
Antihypertensives: labetalol,[30] reserpine, adrenergic neuron blockers[29]	*Reduced tumor uptake*
Antidepressants: tricyclics, maprotiline, trazodone[29]	*Reduced tumor uptake*
Antipsychotics: phenothiazines, thioxanthines, butyrophenones[29]	*Reduced tumor uptake*
Sympathomimetics, including OTC preparations containing phenylephedrine, pseudoephedrine, and phenylpropranolamine[29]	*Reduced tumor uptake*
Calcium antagonists[29,39,40]	*Increased tumor retention*

blockers like atenolol, have no significant effect upon MIBG uptake. Table 20B.4 lists some of the drugs that can have an effect on the uptake of MIBG.

[111]In-pentetreotide

Somatostatin analogs such as octreotide are used therapeutically for the treatment of carcinoid syndrome. It might be anticipated that false negative images might be obtained in patients receiving such therapy, because of competition for receptor sites. There is some experience[41] to suggest that detection of liver metastases is enhanced during octreotide therapy. Octreotide therapy also reduced splenic uptake of the radiopharmaceutical, with lesser reductions also being observed in hepatic and renal uptake.

Diphosphonates

The possibility of interaction between etidronate, as used for the treatment of hypercalcemia, and ^{99m}Tc-methylene diphosphonate (MDP), has been investigated by Murphy and colleagues.[34] A review of hospital pharmacy records for a period of 2 years identified 18 patients who had received etidronate. Of this group, six patients (four men and two women, ranging in age from 56 to 76 years) had undergone bone scanning with ^{99m}Tc-MDP while receiving etidronate. Five of the patients had hypercalcemia associated with metastatic disease, and the sixth had hyperparathyroidism. All bone scans demonstrated poor uptake of tracer by bone accompanied by high soft-tissue background. There was loss of bone definition below the mid-thigh, and in five of the six patients there was indistinguishable rib uptake. In one of the patients, there was absence of uptake in two previously defined metastatic lesions. The authors concluded that recent oral or intravenous administration of etidronate is a contraindication to bone scintigraphy,

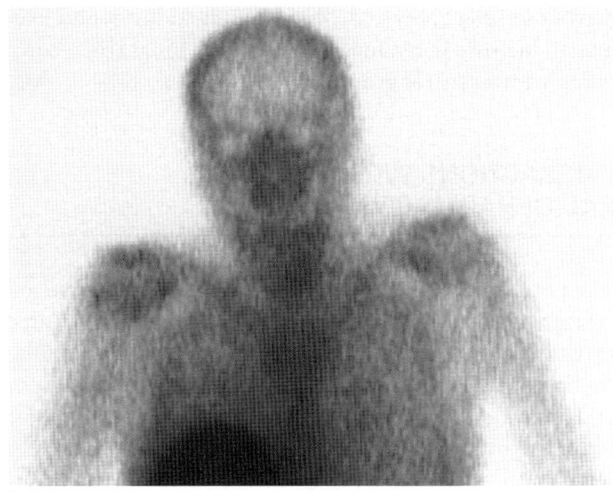

(a)

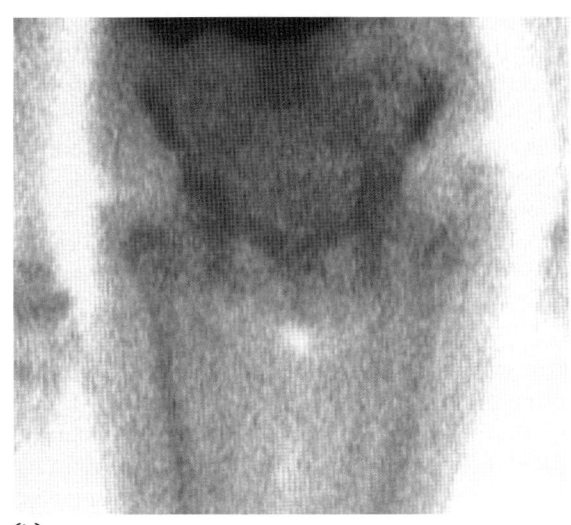

(b)

Figure 20B.1   *Bone scans obtained in a patient known to be taking pamidronate at the time of imaging.*

and markedly decreases sensitivity of detection. Scintigraphy should be delayed for 2–4 weeks from the end of therapy. Figure 20B.1 shows a bone scan obtained in a patient receiving pamidronate therapy.

Other examples

Xavier Holanda[42] examined the effects of the glucantime on the kinetics of biodistribution of ^{99m}Tc-MDP in a rat model. The drug N-methyl meglumine antimoniate (glucantime) is the preferred treatment for leishmaniasis. Glucantime was administered intramuscularly at a dose of 80 mg kg^{-1} day^{-1} for 7 days. ^{99m}Tc-MDP was injected 1 h after the last dose. At sacrifice, organs were isolated and uptake of the radiopharmaceutical assessed in brain, heart, thyroid, lungs, kidneys, testis, stomach, intestines, pancreas, spleen, liver, muscle, bone, and bladder. At 2 h after administration, results indicated a significant reduction of activity in spleen, thyroid, blood, femur, kidneys, and liver and an increase in bladder, pancreas, and lungs when compared with a control group.

INTERACTIONS WITH PET RADIOPHARMACEUTICALS

The potential influence of pharmacological treatments on cerebral uptake of PET radiotracers has been investigated by Cumming et al.[43] It is known that many radiopharmaceuticals for PET are substantially metabolized in peripheral organs, and it is likely that pharmacological treatments intended to alter cerebral metabolism might also alter radiotracer metabolism, and alter cerebral uptake. The application of linear graphical methods to the precursor and metabolite concentrations measured in plasma extracts fractionated by high-performance liquid chromatography allows the calculation of first-order rate constants for the metabolism of PET tracers. Six tracers used for PET studies of neurotransmission were studied: [^{18}F]fluorodopa, a tracer of dopa decarboxylase activity, ^{11}C-deprenyl, a tracer of monoamine oxidase activity, ^{11}C-Sch 23390, a ligand for dopamine D$_1$ receptors, ^{11}C-(S)-nicotine, a ligand for nicotinic receptors, ^{11}C-WIN 35,428, a tropane derivative which labels dopamine uptake sites, and ^{11}C-raclopride, a ligand for dopamine D$_2$ receptors. Amantadine, an antagonist of glutamate receptors, had no effect on the rate of O-methylation of circulating [^{18}F]fluorodopa. ^{11}C-Deprenyl was rapidly metabolized to ^{11}C-methamphetamine and polar metabolites in healthy volunteers. The net rate constant of this metabolism was three times higher in a group of subjects under treatment for epilepsy, consistent with induction of hepatic microsomal enzymes by antiepileptic drugs. The authors suggest that the linear graphic method is useful for estimating the kinetics of the plasma metabolism of many widely used PET tracers, and can reveal drug–drug interactions.

A number of reports[44–46] suggest that interactions can occur between colony-stimulating factors and [^{18}F]fluorodeoxyglucose (^{18}F-FDG) during PET. These reports have been reviewed[47] with the objective of assessing the extent of interference with ^{18}F-FDG imaging and it is suggested that, although this does occur, separating ^{18}F-FDG PET imaging from CSF therapy by 5 days or more may diminish the interference.

INTERACTIONS WITH INTERVENTIONAL DRUGS

Adenosine

Adenosine exerts its action through activation of purine receptors, resulting in vasodilatation in most vascular beds.

Its action is potentiated by dipyridamole, because of the property of this compound to reduce cellular uptake and metabolism of adenosine. Aminophylline, theophylline, and other xanthines, including caffeine, are competitive adenosine antagonists, and therefore markedly reduce the effects. The recommended time for abstention from drinking tea, coffee, and chocolate prior to participating in a cardiac stress test is 12 h. The validity of this requirement has been investigated by Majd-Ardekani and colleagues.[48] Seventy patients undergoing adenosine myocardial perfusion scintigraphy were studied. All patients reported abstention from products containing caffeine in the 12 h prior to the test. Patients were asked about their coffee and tea drinking habits, and serum caffeine levels were determined using high-performance liquid chromatography. Fifty-two patients had measurable serum caffeine levels ranging from 0.1 to 8.8 mg L^{-1}. No significant difference was seen in mean maximum change of pulse rate, systolic and diastolic blood pressure between patients with serum caffeine levels $\geqslant$2.9 mg L^{-1} and those with lower serum caffeine levels. However, significant differences were demonstrated between patients with serum caffeine levels $\geqslant$2.9 mg L^{-1} and those with lower levels, when patients were classified according to the presentation of symptoms. A 12-h abstention from caffeine may be insufficient to be sure of precluding false negative scans.

Dobutamine

The primary action of dobutamine occurs by stimulating the beta-1 receptors of the heart. However, it also possesses some beta-2 and alpha agonistic properties. The presence of beta-adrenergic receptor antagonists can result in peripheral vasoconstriction and hypertension as a result of the alpha agonist properties. Conversely, alpha adrenergic blockade may result in tachycardia and vasodilatation.[49]

Captopril

Captopril-enhanced renography is the noninvasive test of choice for the diagnosis of renovascular hypertension. Bilateral symmetrical changes are associated with many renal conditions, but patients may demonstrate normal renal angiography. In a study of 86 captopril renal scintigraphies (50 using ^{99m}Tc-MAG$_3$ and a 1-day protocol and 36 patients were studied using ^{99m}Tc-DTPA and a 2-day protocol),[50] bilateral symmetrical renal function deterioration was detected in 10 patients. Nine of them were taking calcium antagonists. Control studies performed in five patients without these medications demonstrated normal captopril renograms in four and persistent renal dysfunction in one. It is suggested that calcium antagonists can cause false positive captopril renograms, and that these medications should be stopped before captopril renography.

BLOOD LABELING

Sampson[51] carried out a retrospective study of white cell labeling studies that had been conducted between 1981 and 1997. During that period, some 50 studies were considered abnormal with respect to labeling efficiency, and were subjected to detailed examination. Cells were labeled either with ^{111}In-tropolone or ^{99m}Tc-HMPAO. The subjects of the investigations where labeling efficiencies were deemed unusually low were contacted in an attempt to ascertain what drugs they might have been taking at the time of the test procedure. Those who responded were often taking drugs known to affect white cell function, including cephalosporins, azathioprine, prednisolone, cyclophosphamide, nifedipine, sulfasalazine, iron salts, and heparin. Using Bradford-Hill's criteria to assess whether an association between two variables is also one of causation, it was found that there was a high probability that the taking of these drugs resulted in the observed low labeling efficiencies.

Adverse affects of various drugs on the labeling efficiency of erythrocytes with $[^{99m}$Tc]pertechnetate have been known for several years. Spicer et al.[52] studied the effects of selected antineoplastic agents on the labeling of erythrocytes with ^{99m}Tc using the UltraTag red blood cell kit, which is designed for in vitro labeling. Five different antineoplastic drugs, either alone or in combination, were incubated for 30 min at 37°C with 2-mL samples of whole blood obtained from normal volunteers. Doxorubicin was specifically tested in molar ratios with stannous ion of greater than 1:1 to determine if there was any significant chelation effect that would affect the ability of the kit to label red blood cells. In addition, patients were given a bolus injection of doxorubicin and a blood sample was drawn at 30 min to test whether the metabolites had any effect on labeling. Labeling efficiency using the in vitro method appeared not to be affected in the presence of the drugs studied. However, in a further study using an in vivo method,[53] failures to label red blood cells adequately were observed.

Cyclosporin-A has no effect on labeling efficiencies when using an in vitro technique for labeling erythrocytes with ^{99m}Tc, leukocytes with ^{111}In-oxine, or platelets with ^{111}In-oxine.[54] However, cyclosporin therapy has a definite detrimental effect on labeling efficiency using the in vivo method.[55]

REFERENCES

* First formal publication of a management guideline

* 1   Hladik WB Norenberg JP. Problems associated with the clinical use of radiopharmaceuticals: a proposed classification system and troubleshooting guide. *J Nucl Med* 1996; **23**: 997–1002.

2   Silberstein EB, Ryan J, and the Pharmacopoeia Committee of the Society of Nuclear Medicine. Prevalence of adverse reactions in nuclear medicine. *J Nucl Med* 1996; **37**: 185–92.

3   Hommeyer SH, Varney DM, Eary JF. Skeletal non-visualisation in a bone scan secondary to intravenous etidronate therapy. *J Nucl Med* 1992; **33**: 748–50.

4   Hicks RJ, Eu P, Arkles LB. Efficiency of labelling red blood cells with technetium-99m after dipyridamole infusion for thallium stress testing. *Eur J Nucl Med* 1992; **19**: 1050–3.

5   Jones A, Keeling D. Benign myocardial uptake of hydroxymethylene diphosphonate. *Nucl Med Commun* 1994; **15**: 24–8.

6   Silberstein EB. Adverse reactions to radiopharmaceuticals: the SNM/RSNA USP Drug Product Problem Reporting Program. Society of Nuclear Medicine/ Radiological Society of North America. United States Pharmacopoeial Convention. *J Nucl Med* 1997; **38**: 49N.

7   European System for reporting adverse reactions to and defects in radiopharmaceuticals: annual report 1993. *Eur J Nucl Med* 1994; **21**: BP29–34.

8   European System for reporting adverse reactions to and defects in radiopharmaceuticals: annual report 1994. *Eur J Nucl Med* 1995; **22**: BP29–33.

9   European System for reporting adverse reactions to and defects in radiopharmaceuticals: annual report 1995. *Eur J Nucl Med* 1996; **23**: BP27–31.

10   European System for reporting adverse reactions to and defects in radiopharmaceuticals: annual report 1996. *Eur J Nucl Med* 1997; **24**: BP3–8.

11   European System for reporting adverse reactions to and defects in radiopharmaceuticals: annual report 1997. *Eur J Nucl Med* 1998; **25**: BP45–50.

12   European System for reporting adverse reactions to and defects in radiopharmaceuticals: annual report 1998. *Eur J Nucl Med* 1999; **26**: BP33–8.

13   Hesslewood SR. European System for reporting adverse reactions to and defects in radiopharmaceuticals: annual report 1999. *Eur J Nucl Med* 2001; **28**: BP2–8.

14   Hesslewood SR. European System for reporting adverse reactions to and defects in radiopharmaceuticals: annual report 2000. *Eur J Nucl Med* 2002; **29**: BP13–19.

15   Anonymous. The twenty-first report on survey of the adverse reaction to radiopharmaceuticals (the 24th survey in 1998). Subcommittee of Safety Issue for the Radiopharmaceuticals. Medical and Pharmaceutical Committee. Japan Radioisotope Association. *Jap J Nucl Med* 2000; **37**: 237–48.

16   Kusakabe, Kasaki K, Kosuda S, et al. The twenty-third report on survey of the adverse reaction to radiopharmaceuticals (the 26th survey in 2000). *Jap J Nucl Med* 2002; **39**: 55–65.

17   Anonymous. The 24th report on survey of the adverse reaction to radiopharmaceuticals (the 27th survey in 2001). *Jap J Nucl Med* 2003; **40**: 39–50.

18   Bagheri H, Galian ME, Bastie D, *et al.* Prospective survey on adverse effects of radiopharmaceuticals. *Therapie* 1996; **51**: 550–3.

* 19   Hesslewood SR, Keeling DH. Frequency of adverse reactions to radiopharmaceuticals in Europe. *Eur J Nucl Med* 1997; **24**: 1179–82.

20   Mooser G, Gall H, Peter RU. Delayed-type allergy to technetium-99m. *Contact Dermatitis* 1998; **39**: 269–70.

21   Balan KK, Choudhary AK, Balan A, Wishart G. Severe systemic reaction to (99m)Tc-methylene diphosphonate: a case report. *J Nucl Med Technol* 2003; **31**: 76–8.

22   Burton DA, Cashman JN. Allergic reaction to nanocolloid during lymphoscintigraphy for sentinel lymph node biopsy [Comment]. *Br J Anaesthesia* 2003; **90**: 105.

23   Silberstein EB. Positron-emitting radiopharmaceuticals: how safe are they? *Cancer Biother Radiopharm* 2001; **16**: 13–15.

* 24   Silberstein EB. Prevalence of adverse reactions to positron emitting radiopharmaceuticals in nuclear medicine. Pharmacopeia Committee of the Society of Nuclear Medicine. *J Nucl Med* 1998; **39**: 190–2.

25   Hladik III WB. Drug-induced changes in the biologic distribution of radiopharmaceuticals. *Semin Nucl Med* 1982; **12**: 184–218.

* 26   Hesslewood S, Leung E. Drug interactions with radiopharmaceuticals. *Eur J Nucl Med* 1994; **21**: 348–56.

27   Sampson CB, Cox PH. Effect of patient medication on the biodistribution of radiopharmaceuticals. In: Sampson CB. (ed.) *Textbook of radiopharmacy*, third edition. Amsterdam: Gordon and Breach.

28   Sampson CB. Altered biodistribution of radiopharmaceuticals. In: Theobald AE. (ed.) *Radiopharmacy and radiopharmaceuticals.* London: Taylor and Francis, 1985.

* 29   Solanki KK, Bomanji J, Moyes J, *et al.* A pharmacological guide to medicines which interfere with the biodistribution of radiolabelled metaiodobenzylguanidine (MIBG). *Nucl Med Commun* 1992; **13**: 513–21.

30   Khafagi FA, Shapiro B, Fig LM, *et al.* Labetol reduces I-131 MIBG uptake by phaeochromocytoma and normal tissues. *J Nucl Med* 1989; **30**: 481–9.

31   Bobinet DD, Sevrin R, Zurbriggen MT, *et al.* Lung uptake of ^{99m}Tc-sulfur colloid in patients exhibiting the presence of Al^{3+} in plasma. *J Nucl Med* 1974; **15**: 1220–2.

32   Wang TS, Fawwaz RA, Esser RA, Johnson PM. Altered body distribution of [^{99m}Tc]pertechnetate in iatrogenic hyperaluminemia. *J Nucl Med* 1978; **19**: 391–4.

33   Byun, Rodman SG, Chung KE. Soft-tissue concentration of ^{99m}Tc-phosphates associated with injections of iron dextran complex. *J Nucl Med* 1976; **17**: 374–5.

34   Murphy KJ, Line BR, Malfetano J. Etidronate therapy decreases the sensitivity of bone scanning with methylene diphosphonate labelled with technetium-99m. *Can Ass Radiol J* 1997; **48**: 199–202.

35   Lentle BC, Scott JR. Iatrogenic alterations in radionuclide biodistribution. *Semin Nucl Med* 1979; **9**: 131–41.

36   Hany TF, Heuberger J, von Schulthess GK. Iatrogenic FDG foci in the lungs: a pitfall of PET image interpretation. *Eur Radiol* 2003; **13**: 2122–7.

37   Jaques Jr S, Tobes MC, Sisson JC, *et al.* Comparison of the sodium dependency of uptake of metaiodobenzylguanidine and norepinephrine into cultured bovine adrenomedullary cells. *Mol Pharmacol* 1984; **26**: 539–46.

38   Wieland DM, Brown LE, Tobes MC, *et al.* Imaging the primate adrenal medulla with [^{123}I]- and [^{131}I]-metaiodobenzylguanidine: concise communication. *J Nucl Med* 1981; **22**: 358–64.

39   Blake GM, Lewington VJ, Fleming JS, *et al.* Modification by nifedipine of I-131 metaiodobenzylguanidine kinetics in malignant phaeochromocytoma. *Eur J Nucl Med* 1988; **14**: 345–8.

40   Jaques S, Tobes MC, Sisson JC. Effect of calcium channel blockers on acetylcholine-stimulated and basal release of metaiodobenzyl guanidine and norepinephrine in cultured bovine adrenomedullary cells. *J Nucl Med* 1987; **28**: 639–40.

41   Dorr U, Rath U, Sautter-Bihl ML, *et al.* Improved visualization of carcinoid liver metastases by indium-111 pentetreotide scintigraphy following treatment with cold somatostatin analogue. *Eur J Nucl Med* 1993; **20**: 431–3.

42   Xavier Holanda CM, Cavalcanti Jales RL, Almeida Catanho MT, *et al.* Effects of the glucantime on the kinetic of biodistribution of radiopharmaceuticals in Wistar rats. *Cell Mol Biol* 2002; **48**: 761–5.

43   Cumming P, Yokoi F, Chen A, *et al.* Pharmacokinetics of radiotracers in human plasma during positron emission tomography. *Synapse* 1999; **34**: 124–34.

44   Sugawara Y, Fisher SJ, Zasadny KR, *et al.* Preclinical and clinical studies of bone marrow uptake of fluorine-1-fluorodeoxyglucose with or without granulocyte colony-stimulating factor during chemotherapy. *J Clin Oncol* 1998; **16**: 173–80.

45   Sugawara Y, Zasadny KR, Kison PV, *et al.* Splenic fluorodeoxyglucose uptake increased by granulocyte colony-stimulating factor therapy: PET imaging results. *J Nucl Med* 1999; **40**: 1456–62.

46   Shreve PD, Anzai Y, Wahl RL. Pitfalls in oncologic diagnosis with FDG PET imaging: physiologic and benign variants. *Radiographics* 1999; **19**: 61–77.

47   Mayer D, Bednarczyk EM. Interaction of colony-stimulating factors and fluorodeoxyglucose F^{18} positron emission tomography. *Ann Pharmacotherapy* 2002; **36**: 1796–9.

48   Majd-Ardekani J, Clowes P, Menash-Bonsu V, Nunan TO. Time for abstention from caffeine before an adenosine

myocardial perfusion scan. *Nucl Med Commun* 2000; **21**: 361–4.

49 Association of the British Pharmaceutical Industry. *Compendium of datasheets and summaries of product characteristics*. London: Datapharm Publications Ltd, 2000.

50 Claveau-Tremblay R, Turpin S, De Braekeleer M, *et al*. False-positive captopril renography in patients taking calcium antagonists. *J Nucl Med* 1998; **39**: 1621–6.

51 Sampson CB. Interference of patient medication in the radiolabelling of white blood cells: an update. *Nucl Med Commun* 1998; **19**: 529–33.

52 Spicer JA, Hladik 3rd WB, Mulberry WE. The effects of selected antineoplastic agents on the labeling of erythrocytes with technetium-99m using the UltraTag RBC kit. *J Nucl Med Technol* 1999; **27**: 132–5.

53 Spicer JA, Hladik 3rd WB. Failure to label red blood cells adequately in daily practice using an in vivo method: methodological and clinical considerations. *Eur J Nucl Med* 1998; **25**: 818–19.

54 Owunwanne A, Shihab-Eldeen A. The effect of cyclosporine-A on labeling blood cells with radio-pharmaceuticals. *Nucl Med Biol* 1996; **23**: 1019–21.

55 Spicer JA, Hladik 3rd WB. The effect of cyclosporine concentration on the labeling efficiency of an in vitro technetium-99m red blood cell labeling procedure. *J Nucl Med Technol* 1997; **25**: 70.

New single-photon radiopharmaceuticals

STEPHEN J. MATHER

INTRODUCTION

Any publication with a title that contains the word 'new' is out of date the day after it is submitted to the publisher and this chapter will be no exception. By the time you read this, it is certain that descriptions of several new radiopharmaceuticals, not listed here, will have appeared in the scientific literature. To try to maximize the useful longevity of the information it presents, and due to space restrictions, this chapter will therefore not seek to present a comprehensive list of the very latest radiotracers. Instead it will try to discuss the general trends and areas of application in radiopharmaceutical development over the last decade since it is likely that these trends will continue beyond the date of publication of this book.

In the 50 or so years since the inception of radiopharmaceuticals, their development has proceeded through a number of phases. The early years, the 1950s to mid 1960s, were characterized by the clinical application of naturally occurring radioactive salts such as $[^{131}I]$iodide and $[^{32}P]$phosphate and, following the introduction of ^{99m}Tc, by developments of compounds such as ^{99m}Tc-pyrophosphate for bone scanning. The period up to the early 1980s pursued the aim of developing radiopharmaceuticals that were taken up by the major organs of the body by a variety of different mechanisms: colloids for liver scanning, macroaggregates for lung scanning, ^{99m}Tc-diethylenetriaminepentaacetic acid (DTPA) and dimercaptosuccinic acid (DMSA) for kidney imaging, for example. The 1980s were the years of the application of technetium coordination chemistry and resulted in a number of tracers which measure regional organ perfusion or function: ^{99m}Tc-exametazime[1] for brain perfusion, ^{99m}Tc-sestamibi[2] and tetrofosmin[3] for myocardial perfusion

and ^{99m}Tc-mercaptoacetyl triglycine (MAG$_3$)[4] for renal tubular secretion. In the 1990s a shift occurred towards imaging the characteristics of groups of cells rather than whole organs. Radiolabeled monoclonal antibodies[5] targeting tumor-associated epitopes and neuropeptides such as somatostatin analogs[6] were developed for imaging the overexpression of their receptors on the surface of malignant cells.

This trend has continued in this millennium and is likely to do so for the foreseeable future. The increasing availability of strong competing imaging modalities such as high-field magnetic resonance imaging and spiral computed tomography means that nuclear medicine must concentrate on its unique strengths if it is to continue to prove clinically useful and hence survive into the new century. The two most important attributes of nuclear medicine are (1) the use of very high specific activity tracers which permit the possibility of imaging low capacity mechanisms *in vivo*, and (2) the therapeutic application of targeted radionuclides. The most successful radiopharmaceutical developments in the future will arise from the application of these strengths to the solution of real clinical problems. Thus the directions of radiopharmaceutical research will tend to move from localization of disease to functional assessment of tissues, from targets on the outside of cell membranes to those buried deep within the cytoplasm and cell nucleus, from 'passive' imaging in the nuclear medicine department to interventional applications in the operating theater and from the diagnosis of disease to its treatment.

Many of the radiopharmaceuticals of current interest are based on proteins and peptides which bind to targets on the outside of the cell membrane. Labeling of all of these ligands for single photon emission computed tomography (SPECT) imaging is normally performed using a bifunctional chelate approach.[7] The protein or peptide of interest is first conjugated to a chelator which is suitable for the radionuclide of interest. In the case of trivalent metallic elements such as indium, gallium or yttrium, the chelators of choice are analogs of either DTPA or DOTA since these form strong complexes with these metals.[8] In the case of ^{99m}Tc, different chelators which form strong complexes with technetium must be used. The two most widely used are peptidic chelators (such as MAG$_3$)[9] and hydrazino-nicotinamide (HYNIC).[10] However, in addition to the need for a stable complex that will retain the radionuclide during the process of targeting and localization, the physicochemical nature of the chelator and the radiopharmaceutical as a whole have a profound effect upon disposition of the tracer *in vivo*. Proteins which are larger than about 50–60 kDa are not filtered through the kidneys and so tend to have long circulation times and consequently a high blood background activity for some hours or even days after administration.[11] Proteins and peptides smaller than this are filtered through the glomerus and clear much more rapidly from the blood. Their rate and route of excretion depend upon factors such as charge and lipophilicity. More lipophilic tracers exhibit a higher degree of protein binding and this can slow their clearance.[12] They also tend to be excreted at least in part through the hepatobiliary system with consequent accumulation in the lower gastrointestinal tract. This accumulation can obscure areas of targeted uptake in the pelvis and abdomen and render interpretation of images very difficult in these sites. More hydrophilic tracers show less protein binding and a predominantly renal route of excretion.[12] This provides a clearer background against which sites of abnormal receptor-mediated accumulation can be visualized. However, sometimes a very high retention of radioactivity by the kidney can hinder detection of disease in this region.

The main areas for application of new radiopharmaceuticals are:

- Inflammation imaging
- Cancer imaging
- Cancer therapy
- Neuroreceptor imaging
- Radiopharmaceutical chemistry.

INFLAMMATION IMAGING

The issues in inflammation imaging lie in the complexity of the current 'gold standard' investigation – labeled white cells – and also in its inability to distinguish between inflammation caused by underlying infection and that with other causes. Blood labeling is time consuming, requires special skills and facilities and carries the risk of needle-stick infection from blood-borne infections such as hepatitis and HIV. Attempts to overcome this problem have included the use of tracers which label white cells *in vivo* in whole blood thereby

removing the need for manipulation of the blood *ex vivo*. Perhaps the most widely used example is Leukoscan™ (^{99m}Tc-sulesomab) a radiolabeled antibody fragment which binds to the NCA-90 epitope on white cells.[13] Although developed with the idea that the antibody would bind to circulating white cells which subsequently migrate to the site of infection, it appears that this is not its real mechanism of action.[14] The uptake is due in part to 'nonspecific' extravasation of the labeled antibody at the site of infection followed (perhaps) by binding to local white cells in the vicinity. In order to try to find better, more specific tracers, attention has recently concentrated on the use of smaller ligands which clear much more rapidly from the blood and suffer less from the problem of nonspecific extravasation. These include cytokines and chemotactic peptides which bind to a variety of different receptors on different populations of white cells. The most widely explored cytokines are interleukin-2[15] and interleukin-8.[16] IL-2 has a molecular weight of about 15 kDa and binds to receptors on activated T lymphocytes. Interleukin-8 is a chemotactic cytokine with a molecular weight of about 8.5 kDa which binds to receptors expressed on monocytes and neutrophils, The chemotactic peptides[17] are very small tri- and tetra-peptides that bind with high affinity to receptors on granulocytes and monocytes. All three of these classes of compound have been labeled with technetium using bifunctional chelating approaches and studied in animal models of disease. However, the use of these highly pharmacologically active ligands raises a new question in radiopharmaceutical design – that of toxicity. Some cytokines have a relatively benign toxicological profile. Interleukin-2, for example, is used clinically in repeated doses of a milligram or more. While administration at this level can undoubtedly cause profound pharmacological effects, single doses in the order of tens of micrograms are tolerated very well. On the other hand interleukin-8 in doses of a few micrograms causes profound, if transient, neutropenia in rabbits[18] and a dose of only 10 ng kg^{-1} of the chemotactic peptide f-Met-Leu-Phe caused a drop in white cell count in nonhuman primates.[19] For this reason, IL-8 and chemotactic peptides have not yet been studied in man but ^{99m}Tc-IL2 has been shown to be useful for detection of lymphocytic infiltration in patients with a range of autoimmune diseases.[20]

Although not directly concerned with inflammation a similar approach has been taken to the imaging of thrombosis by the use of peptides which bind to activated platelets.[21] Acutect® or ^{99m}Tc-apcitide (previously known as P280) is a peptide that binds to the GPIIb/IIIa (α_{II}/β_3) integrin receptors which are abundant on newly formed blood clots. Apcitide has the structure shown in Figure 20C.1.[22] It is a dimeric peptide containing a cyclic targeting sequence and a linear labeling sequence. The targeting sequence -Apc-Gly-Asp- is an analog of the common Arg-Gly-Asp (-RGD-) sequence which is found in many integrin binding peptides. Substitution of 'Apc' for 'Arg' provides increased resistance to breakdown by proteolytic enzymes present in the blood while cyclization through the (D)-Tyr residue increases the

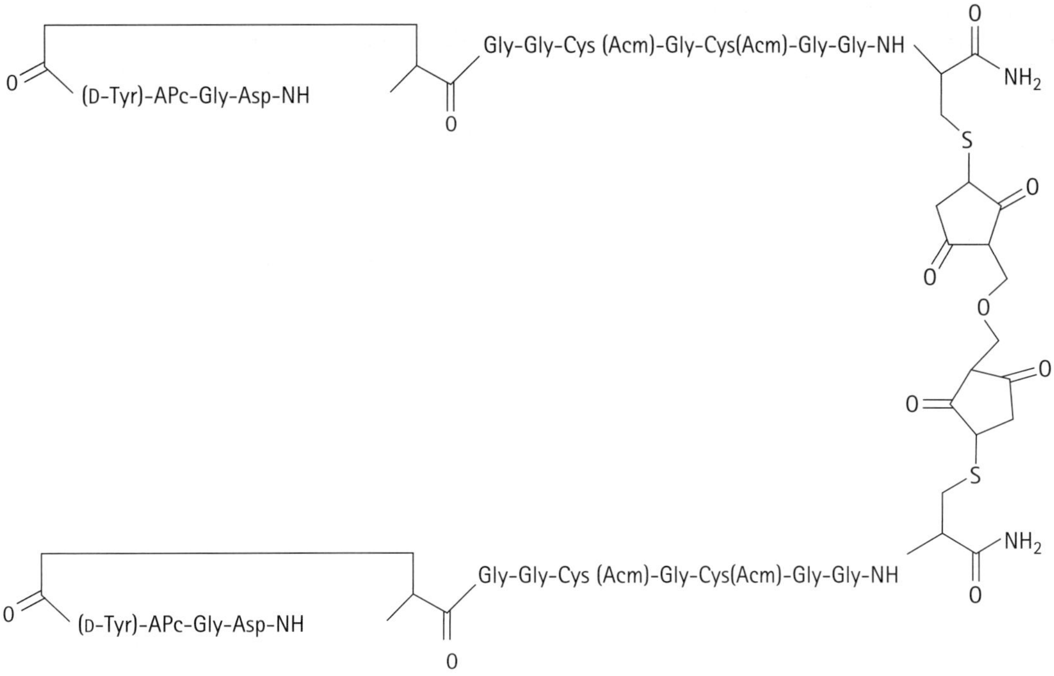

Figure 20C.1 *Amino acid structure of apcitide.*

peptide's affinity for the GPIIb/IIIa receptor. The -Cys-Gly-Cys-Gly- sequence provides a chelating sequence for ^{99m}Tc. Normally the -SH groups present on the cysteine side-chains are protected by the (Acm) blocking group. However, when the peptide is heated during labeling, these Acm groups are released and the ^{99m}Tc binds to the sulfur and nitrogen atoms present in the chelating sequence.

The knowledge that nonspecific mechanisms can contribute to imaging of inflammation has led several research groups to pursue entirely non-white cell mediated solutions to this problem. Among the most successful has been the use of nonspecific immunoglobulins (HIGs)[23] and liposomes.[24] These can be labeled with a variety of radioisotopes, in particular ^{99m}Tc and ^{111}In and therefore have the potential for use in imaging both the same day and for several days after administration. Clinical trials with these agents have demonstrated high sensitivity in the detection of inflammation[25] but neither has achieved widespread use. Perhaps the main reason for this is that, for a variety of reasons, no commercial manufacturer has developed the product, obtained market authorization and made it universally available. Without this commercial development any radiopharmaceutical, however 'good', is likely to remain an item of purely academic interest.

The second important issue in inflammation imaging is identifying the source of the inflammation. The important question is whether to continue the use of antibiotics or not? Thus attempts are being made to develop radiopharmaceuticals which interact not with the body's own defense mechanisms but with the invading micro-organisms themselves. Among the current candidates of interest are the defensins[26] – naturally occurring peptides which bind to a broad spectrum of bacteria. Although these have been shown to have some degree of specificity for infection rather than sterile inflammation, the target-to-background ratios achieved have been relatively modest and their use has not yet been pursued in the clinic. By contrast, the use of ^{99m}Tc-labeled ciprofloxacin, a fluoroquinolone antibiotic, has been studied in almost 1000 patients with encouraging results.[27] In fact, ciprofloxacin is only one of a significant number of antibiotics that have been labeled with the aim of infection imaging and more developments can be expected in this field as antibiotics with more specific bacterial interactions and more favorable patterns of biodistribution are identified. Of particular interest is the use of these drugs for imaging nonbacterial infections. Antibiotics specific for fungal[28] or parasitic infections may be very valuable in the context of adventitious infections in immunocompromised patients or in the developing world.

CANCER IMAGING

The areas of possible application of radiopharmaceuticals in the management of patients with cancer include:

- Population screening
- Primary diagnosis
- Staging of disease
- Measuring response to therapy
- Tailoring and identifying optimal therapies.

In fact, socio-economic issues as well as clinical realities mean that nuclear medicine is unlikely to play a significant role in either screening or primary diagnosis, but it can play in increasingly important part in all four of the subsequent areas of management.

Staging in cancer requires an imaging investigation which provides rapid throughput, whole-body imaging, high sensitivity and high specificity. In recent years it has been recognized that [18F]fluorodeoxyglucose (18F-FDG) can deliver at least the first two of these attributes and the establishment of centers for clinical positron emission tomography (PET) is now the most rapidly evolving application of nuclear medicine in the developed world.[29] At the moment, a SPECT radiopharmaceutical able to compete with FDG in this arena is not on the horizon. New developments are therefore likely to be directed towards producing complementary tracers which can help to overcome the potentially limited specificity of FDG. Among the most widely explored approaches is the use of radiolabeled neuropeptides.[30] Although their application is normally limited to those specific diseases in which expression of the receptors is elevated, these radiopharmaceuticals do have the potential to fill this current deficiency in cancer staging. To date, the most widely explored field of peripheral neuroreceptor imaging remains the family of somatostatin receptors.[31] However, because of its success this application is also encouraging the development of new radiolabeling technology which not only improves the performance of somatostatin receptor imaging, but will have broader utility across the field of neuropeptide receptor targeting. Examples include the development of improved methods for labeling peptides with 99mTc. For example, 99mTc-depreotide (Neospect®) is a new radiopharmaceutical for imaging somatostatin receptors.[22] It applies the same principles followed in the development of Acutect® (above); that is, the combination of a peptide sequence able to bind to the neuropeptide receptor with a sequence able to complex the radionuclide. In this case, the receptor-binding sequence is Tyr-Trp-Lys-Val- while the labeling sequence is a modified Gly-Lys-Cys-, as shown in Figure 20C.2. Although Neospect binds with great affinity to somatostatin receptors (SSTRs) 2, 3, and 5, and does localize specifically in SSTR-expressing tumors, it suffers the disadvantage that it

undergoes significant elimination through the gastrointestinal tract.[32] This means that while it is an excellent tool for imaging SSTR-positive disease above the diaphragm (e.g. lung cancer), it does not perform well in the abdomen and pelvis where sites of disease are obscured by the normal excretory pathway of the radioligand. In attempts to overcome this type of problem, the combination of the use of HYNIC with a variety of co-ligands for technetium coordination has been shown to have a profound influence on the performance of these tracers for imaging[33] and the development of a simple method for producing the tricarbonyl, tri-aqua reactive technetium intermediate[34] provides the opportunity for producing new peptide complexes with novel imaging characteristics. The horizon will see the application of this new chemistry to a range of ligands binding other neuropeptide receptors such as those for neurotensin,[35] gastrin,[36] gastrin-releasing peptide,[37] and vasoactive intestinal peptide.[38]

Many well-established treatments for cancer are highly toxic and one of the major deficiencies in the current management of patients is our inability to identify whether individual patients will benefit from a particular combination of drugs. The classical measure of tumor shrinkage is normally only able to provide information some time after the patient has received a course of often debilitating therapy. An investigation which could provide information on the effectiveness of a particular therapy even after one dose could be very valuable and save not only a large amount of money but also considerable unnecessary toxicity by patients who will not benefit significantly from their treatment. One of the most valuable measures of drug response would be its effect on tumor cell proliferation. In order to try to image this process researchers have labeled a variety of substrates for cell metabolism including a number of different nucleotides and amino acids. One of the most widely studied is 3'-deoxy-3'-[18F]fluorothymidine (FLT), although attempts have also been made to develop SPECT tracers that image proliferation. Perhaps the most well established is 5-iodo-2'-deoxyuridine (IUdR), a thymidine analog which can be incorporated into DNA and which can therefore, as well as imaging proliferation, be potentially used for targeted Auger radiation therapy.[39] Unfortunately, IUdR suffers from the disadvantage that it is rapidly metabolized in vivo with subsequent release of the radioiodine and work is under way to find a more stable analog.[40]

One of the mechanisms by which cancer treatments mediate their effect is by programmed cell death (apoptosis). This arises when cell surveillance systems detect high levels of DNA damage, which, if the cell was allowed to divide normally would lead to a risk of inherited mutations in the genetic code. One of the effects of apoptosis is a refolding of the cell membrane resulting in the exposure on the outside of the cell of elements which are normally on the inner surface. These elements can be used as targets for radiopharmaceuticals which aim to image the apoptotic

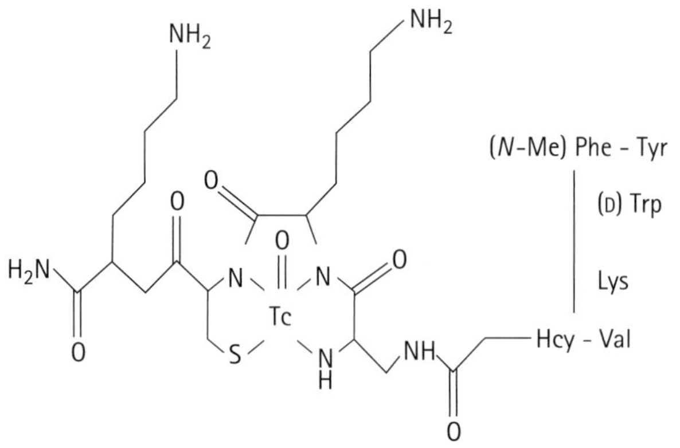

Figure 20C.2 *Structure of 99mTc-depreotide.*

process as a measure of tumor response to therapy. The most well-developed approach is the use of radiolabeled annexin-V.[41] This compound binds to phosphatidylserine which is one of the cell membrane components exposed during the early stages of apoptosis. Annexin-V has been labeled with ^{99m}Tc using HYNIC as a bifunctional complexing agent and studied in a number of clinical trials in which apoptosis is expected to occur. Although originally developed as a marker of tumor response and validated in animal models of such, in fact some of the most impressive images have been acquired in 'natural' apoptosis, such as in myocardial infarction.[42] Although uptake of ^{99m}Tc-annexin-V has been seen in tumors following cytotoxic or radiotherapy,[43] the degree of uptake is very varied and the quality of the images not impressive. There are certainly a number of reasons for this, not least that apoptosis is a transient phenomenon with a variable and unpredictable timing.[44] However, a contributory factor is that annexin-V itself is not an ideal substrate for radiopharmaceutical application. It is a relatively large protein with a molecular weight of about 35 kDa, which clears only slowly from the blood and, like other proteins, diffuses only slowly into tumors. The target-to-background ratios that are achieved are therefore sub-optimal. It seems likely that annexin-V will be a paradigm for a new generation of radiopharmaceuticals for imaging apoptosis which have more ideal pharmacokinetic characteristics.

While these markers of response relate primarily to conventional established cancer therapies, radiopharmaceuticals also have a potential use in defining the role of newly emerging therapies. For example, anti-angiogenic therapies have little immediate effect on tumor size, and their effectiveness cannot be measured using conventional structural imaging. Tracers which target vascular endothelial growth factor (VEGF) and other markers expressed during angiogenesis could be used as surrogate markers of drug efficacy in clinical trials of these compounds.[45]

As well as indicating responses to therapy in cancer, radiopharmaceuticals may also help to identify those patients who will benefit from a particular type of therapy. It has long been known that tumors that are hypoxic are less responsive to external-beam radiation therapy than those with normal oxygen levels. This has prompted a search for radiopharmaceuticals for which the uptake is determined by tissue oxygen levels. The most widely explored class of compounds are the nitroimidazoles. These are preferentially reduced and consequently bound in hypoxic tissues and, if radiolabeled, can potentially be used to image the distribution of oxygen tension in tumors and other important organs such as the heart. Nitroimidazoles have been labeled with a variety of radionuclides including ^{18}F (e.g. ^{18}F-MISO) and ^{123}I (e.g. [^{123}I]iodoazomycin, ^{123}I-IAZA) as well as with ^{99m}Tc.[46] Several of these are in clinical trials although their role and the relationships between uptake and other markers of oxygen tension have yet to be established. A new class of copper-based radiopharmaceuticals which show varying degrees of retention in hypoxic or normoxic tissues has recently emerged. The mechanism of retention of these N4 semi-thiocarbazone tracers is reduction of Cu(II) to Cu(I) followed by loss of the radiometal from the complex. It has been shown that varying the substituents on the periphery of the complex can change the reduction potential of the copper core and by suitable adjustment, a complex which is retained by all normoxic cells (e.g. Cu-ATSM) or only by hypoxic cells (e.g. Cu-PTSM) can therefore be designed.[47]

CANCER THERAPY

As suggested earlier, one of the unique strengths of nuclear medicine is the possibility of targeted radionuclide therapy and recent years have seen a resurgence of interest in this field. The stimulus for this has been the development of two new indications for targeted therapy: radiolabeled anti-CD20 antibodies for therapy of lymphoma[48] and radiolabeled octreotide analogs for treatment of neuro-endocrine cancer.[49] A major difficulty in this area of research is the lack of basic knowledge on what are the important determinants of effective therapy. We employ a variety of different radionuclides with a range of different physical decay properties without a real understanding of what the optimal half-life, type, and energy of particulate emission are. Nor do we know much about the mechanism of action of low-dose targeted radiotherapy. Is it the same as high-dose external beam therapy, i.e. primarily double-stranded DNA cleavage, or do different mechanisms dominate?[50] More basic research is needed to define these parameters. At the same time, it has been argued that irrespective of the underlying mechanisms, the most important type of studies are *in vivo* trials of efficacy either in patients or animal models.[51] For such studies, the most over-riding concern is often the availability of the radioisotope rather than its mode of decay. In recent years the number of commercially available radionuclides has increased with several sources of ^{90}Y and, more recently, ^{177}Lu appearing. Although, to date, the major emphasis has been on targeted radionuclide therapy with beta-emitting radionuclides, there is currently renewed interest in the potential of alpha-particle emitters.[52] Alpha particles have the advantage that they are much more effective since they deposit much greater energy in their target than do beta particles. Since their range is also much shorter they also have the potential for greater selectivity for targeting tumor cells rather than normal adjacent structures. The main difficulty when working with alpha-emitting radionuclides is their complex, often branched schemes of decay through a series of radioactive daughters. A very stable chelation system is needed to cope with the high recoil energies delivered by the radionuclides as they decay, otherwise there is a likelihood that the daughter radionuclides will not remain bound to the targeting vectors.[53]

Irrespective of the radionuclide used for delivering the therapy, there is often a need to undertake a pre-therapy imaging study in order to predict the likely success of the subsequent treatment or to perform dosimetry estimations. For this reason a peptide or protein conjugate that can be labeled with either an imaging or a therapy isotope presents a real advantage. A good example is provided by Zevalin®. This DTPA-anti-CD20 antibody conjugate can be labeled with either ^{111}In for imaging, or ^{90}Y for therapy.[54] Although the biodistribution of the two radiopharmaceuticals may not be completely identical because of differences between the metabolism of the two radionuclide complexes, the sources of error in the dosimetric calculations are likely to outweigh the effects of these differences.

NEURORECEPTOR IMAGING

For many years the development of radiopharmaceuticals for imaging neuroreceptors in the brain has been the preserve of specialist PET chemists. As a consequence of their work a large number of radioligands with affinity for a variety of receptor types and subtypes have been developed[55] but the application of these tracers has been limited to a relatively few specialized centers. If this type of radiopharmaceutical is to become more widely used then either more centers will need to develop access to the technology (a real likelihood with the development of clinical PET) or analogs of these tracers labeled with single-photon emitting radionuclides need to be developed. A significant number of ^{123}I-labeled compounds has now been established and at least one (^{123}I-FP-CIT, [123]I -ioflupane or DatScan™) is now approved for general use. DatScan binds to the dopamine transporter and imaging with this radiopharmaceutical is able to show the loss of transporter function that occurs in diseases such as Parkinson's disease.[56] Since the expense and limited availability of ^{123}I remain a problem attempts have been made to develop ^{99m}Tc-labeled tracers and the most effective to date has been ^{99m}Tc-Trodat-1[57] which shares the same receptor binding structure as DatScan but incorporates a technetium chelating site as shown in Fig. 20C.3. Although the development of ^{99m}Tc-labeled receptor ligands remains the goal of several research groups, its fulfilment remains elusive. A useful neuroreceptor imaging radiopharmaceutical must show high stability (in solution, in serum, and *in vitro*), high *in vitro* binding affinity, good *in vitro* binding selectivity, acceptable brain uptake, and specific receptor uptake *in vivo*. While the first three requirements are achievable, combining these with a sufficient degree of brain uptake presents a real problem.[58] To date, effective tracers have only been developed for one target, the dopamine transporter. It is expected that more lie ahead.

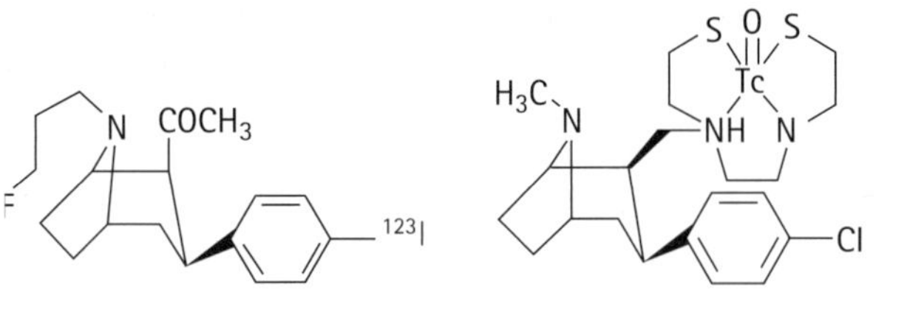

Figure 20C.3 *Chemical structures of ^{123}I-ioflupane and ^{99m}Tc-TRODAT.*

SUMMARY

The underpinning technology which links all of the clinical applications described in this chapter is radiopharmaceutical chemistry. An understanding of the coordination chemistry which allows the preparation of stable complexes and an appreciation of the relationships between this chemistry and the behavior of the radiotracers in biological environments is essential if developments in radiopharmaceutical design are to continue. The ability to manipulate the stability, charge, size, and lipophilicity of bifunctional chelates, in particular, will allow us to generate new complexes with novel physicochemical properties that translate into novel patterns of biodistribution and thus provide a new generation of radiopharmaceuticals beyond the horizon.

REFERENCES

♦ Key review paper

1 Andersen AR, Friberg H, Lassen NA, *et al.* Serial studies of cerebral blood flow using [99]Tc[m]-HMPAO: a comparison with [133]Xe. *Nucl Med Commun* 1987; **8**: 549–57.

2 Jones AG, Abrams MJ, Davison A, *et al.* Biological studies of a new class of technetium complexes: the hexakis (alkylisonitrile) technetium(I) cations. *Int J Nucl Med Biol* 1984; **11**: 225–34.

3 Kelly JD, Forster AM, Higley B, *et al.* Technetium-99m-tetrofosmin as a new radiopharmaceutical for myocardial perfusion imaging. *J Nucl Med* 1993; **34**: 222–7.

4 Fritzberg AR, Kasina S, Eshima D, Johnson DL. Synthesis and biological evaluation of technetium-99m MAG3 as a hippuran replacement. *J Nucl Med* 1986; **27**: 111–16.

♦ 5 Britton KE, Granowska M, Mather SJ. Radiolabelled monoclonal antibodies in oncology I. Technical aspects. *Nucl Med Commun* 1991; **12**: 57–63.

♦ 6 Krenning E, Kwekkeboom D, Pauwels S, *et al.* Somatostatin receptor scintigraphy. *Nuclear medical annual.* New York: Raven Press, 1995: 1–50.

◆ 7 Mather S. Radiolabelling of monoclonal antibodies. In: Shepherd P, Dean C. (eds.) *Monoclonal antibodies, a practical approach*. Oxford: Oxford University Press, 2000: 207–36.

8 Camera L, Kinuya S, Garmestani K, *et al*. Evaluation of the serum stability and in vivo biodistribution of CHX-DTPA and other ligands for yttrium labeling of monoclonal antibodies. *J Nucl Med* 1994; **35**: 882–9.

9 Zamora PO, Gulhke S, Bender H, *et al*. Experimental radiotherapy of receptor-positive human prostate adenocarcinoma with Re-188-RC-160, a directly-radiolabeled somatostatin analogue. *Int J Cancer* 1996; **65**: 214–20.

10 Larsen SK, Abrams MJ, Higgins JD, *et al*. Technetium complex of tricine – useful precursor for the Tc-99m labeling of hydrazino nicotinamide modified human polyclonal IgG. *J Nucl Med* 1994; **35**(5, suppl): 105.

11 Rennen HJ, Makarewicz J, Oyen WJ, *et al*. The effect of molecular weight on nonspecific accumulation of (99m)Tc-labeled proteins in inflammatory foci. *Nucl Med Biol* 2001; **28**: 401–8.

12 Decristoforo C, Mather SJ. 99m-Technetium-labelled peptide-HYNIC conjugates: effects of lipophilicity and stability on biodistribution. *Nucl Med Biol* 1999; **26**: 389–96.

13 Gratz S, Schipper ML, Dorner J, *et al*. LeukoScan for imaging infection in different clinical settings: a retrospective evaluation and extended review of the literature. *Clin Nucl Med* 2003; **28**: 267–76.

14 Skehan SJ, White JF, Evans JW, *et al*. Mechanism of accumulation of ^{99m}Tc-sulesomab in inflammation. *J Nucl Med* 2003; **44**: 11–18.

15 Chianelli M, Sobnack R, Frtizberg AR, *et al*. 99m-Tc-interleukin-2: a new radiopharmaceutical for the in-vivo detection of lymphocytic infiltration. *J Nucl Biol Med* 1994; **38**: 476.

16 van der Laken CJ, Boerman OC, Oyen WJG, *et al*. Imaging of infection in rabbits with radioiodinated interleukin-1 (alpha and beta), its receptor antagonist and a chemotactic peptide: a comparative study. *Eur J Nucl Med* 1998; **25**: 347–52.

17 Babich JW, Fischman AJ. Targeted imaging of infection. *Adv Drug Deliv Rev* 1999; **37**: 237–52.

18 Van der Laken CJ, Boerman OC, Oyen WJ, *et al*. The kinetics of radiolabelled interleukin-8 in infection and sterile inflammation. *Nucl Med Commun* 1998; **19**: 271–81.

19 Fischman AJ, Rauh D, Solomon H, *et al*. In vivo bioactivity and biodistribution of chemotactic peptide analogs in nonhuman primates. *J Nucl Med* 1993; **34**: 2130–4.

20 Signore A, Picarelli A, Annovazzi A, *et al*. ^{123}I-Interleukin-2: biochemical characterization and in vivo use for imaging autoimmune diseases. *Nucl Med Commun* 2003; **24**: 305–16.

21 Bates SM, Lister-James J, Julian JA, *et al*. Imaging characteristics of a novel technetium Tc-99m-labeled platelet glycoprotein IIb/IIIa receptor antagonist in patients with acute deep vein thrombosis or a history of deep vein thrombosis. *Arch Intern Med* 2003; **163**: 452–6.

◆ 22 Lister-James J, Moyer BR, Dean T. Small peptides radiolabeled with ^{99m}Tc. *Q J Nucl Med* 1996; **40**: 221–33.

23 Claessens RA, Boerman OC, Koenders EB, *et al*. Technetium-99m labelled hydrazinonicotinamido human non-specific polyclonal immunoglobulin G for detection of infectious foci: a comparison with two other technetium-labelled immunoglobulin preparations. *Eur J Nucl Med* 1996; **23**: 414–21.

24 Boerman OC, Laverman P, Oyen WJ, *et al*. Radiolabeled liposomes for scintigraphic imaging. *Prog Lipid Res* 2000; **39**: 461–75.

◆ 25 Boerman OC, Rennen H, Oyen WJ, *et al*. Radiopharmaceuticals to image infection and inflammation. *Semin Nucl Med* 2001; **31**: 286–95.

26 Welling MM, Mongera S, Lupetti A, *et al*. Radiochemical and biological characteristics of ^{99m}Tc-UBI 29-41 for imaging of bacterial infections. *Nucl Med Biol* 2002; **29**: 413–422.

27 Britton KE, Wareham DW, Das SS, *et al*. Imaging bacterial infection with (99m)Tc-ciprofloxacin (Infecton). *J Clin Pathol* 2002; **55**: 817–23.

28 Lupetti A, Welling MM, Mazzi U, *et al*. Technetium-99m labelled fluconazole and antimicrobial peptides for imaging of *Candida albicans* and *Aspergillus fumigatus* infections. *Eur J Nucl Med Mol Imaging* 2002; **29**: 674–9.

29 Bomanji JB, Costa DC, Ell PJ. Clinical role of positron emission tomography in oncology. *Lancet Oncol* 2001; **2**: 157–64.

◆ 30 Warner RR, O'Dorisio TM. Radiolabeled peptides in diagnosis and tumor imaging: clinical overview. *Semin Nucl Med* 2002; **32**: 79–83.

31 Breeman WA, de Jong M, Kwekkeboom DJ, *et al*. Somatostatin receptor-mediated imaging and therapy: basic science, current knowledge, limitations and future perspectives. *Eur J Nucl Med* 2001; **28**: 1421–9.

32 Shih WJ, Hirschowitz E, Bensadoun E, *et al*. Biodistribution on Tc-99m labeled somatostatin receptor-binding peptide (depreotide, NeoTec) planar and SPECT studies. *Ann Nucl Med* 2002; **16**: 213–19.

33 Decristoforo C, Mather SJ. Technetium-99m somatostatin analogues: effect of labelling methods and peptide sequence. *Eur J Nucl Med* 1999; **26**: 869–76.

34 Alberto R, Schibli R, Egli A, *et al*. A novel organometallic aqua complex of technetium for the labeling of biomolecules: synthesis of [Tc-99m(OH2)(3)(CO)(3)](+) from [(TcO4)-Tc-99m](-) in

aqueous solution and its reaction with a bifunctional ligand. *J Am Chem Soc* 1998; **120**: 7987–8.

35 Garcia-Garayoa E, Blauenstein P, Bruehlmeier M, *et al*. Preclinical evaluation of a new, stabilized neurotensin (8–13) pseudopeptide radiolabeled with ^{99m}Tc. *J Nucl Med* 2002; **43**: 374–83.

36 Behr TM, Jenner N, Behe M, *et al*. Radiolabeled peptides for targeting cholecystokinin-B/gastrin receptor-expressing tumors. *J Nucl Med* 1999; **40**: 1029–44.

37 Hoffman TJ, Quinn TP, Volkert WA. Radiometallated receptor-avid peptide conjugates for specific in vivo targeting of cancer cells. *Nucl Med Biol* 2001; **28**: 527–39.

38 Virgolini I, Raderer M, Kurtaran A, *et al*. Vasoactive intestinal peptide-receptor imaging for the localization of intestinal adenocarcinomas and endocrine tumors. *N Engl J Med* 1994; **331**: 1116–21.

39 Buchegger F, Vieira JM, Blaeuenstein P, *et al*. Preclinical Auger and gamma radiation dosimetry for fluorodeoxyuridine-enhanced tumour proliferation scintigraphy with [^{123}I]iododeoxyuridine. *Eur J Nucl Med Mol Imaging* 2003; **30**: 239–46.

40 Toyohara J, Hayashi A, Sato M, *et al*. Development of radioiodinated nucleoside analogs for imaging tissue proliferation: comparisons of six 5-iodonucleosides. *Nucl Med Biol* 2003; **30**: 687–96.

41 Blankenberg FG, Tait JF, Strauss HW. Apoptotic cell death: its implications for imaging in the next millennium. *Eur J Nucl Med* 2000; **27**: 359–67.

42 Hofstra L, Liem IH, Dumont EA, *et al*. Visualisation of cell death in vivo in patients with acute myocardial infarction. *Lancet* 2000; **356**: 180–1.

43 Belhocine T, Steinmetz N, Hustinx R, *et al*. Increased uptake of the apoptosis-imaging agent (99m)Tc recombinant human annexin V in human tumors after one course of chemotherapy as a predictor of tumor response and patient prognosis. *Clin Cancer Res* 2002; **8**: 2766–74.

44 Blankenberg F. To scan or not to scan, it is a question of timing: technetium-99m-annexin V radionuclide imaging assessment of treatment efficacy after one course of chemotherapy. *Clin Cancer Res* 2002; **8**: 2757–8.

♦ 45 Weber WA, Haubner R, Vabuliene E, *et al*. Tumor angiogenesis targeting using imaging agents. *Q J Nucl Med* 2001; **45**: 179–82.

♦ 46 Ballinger JR. Imaging hypoxia in tumors. *Semin Nucl Med* 2001; **31**: 321–9.

47 Dearling JL, Lewis JS, Mullen GE, *et al*. Copper bis(thiosemicarbazone) complexes as hypoxia imaging agents: structure–activity relationships. *J Biol Inorg Chem* 2002; **7**: 249–59.

♦ 48 Juweid ME. Radioimmunotherapy of B-cell non-Hodgkin's lymphoma: from clinical trials to clinical practice. *J Nucl Med* 2002; **43**: 1507–29.

49 De Jong M, Valkema R, Jamar F, *et al*. Somatostatin receptor-targeted radionuclide therapy of tumors: preclinical and clinical findings. *Semin Nucl Med* 2002; **32**: 133–140.

♦ 50 Pouget JP, Mather SJ. General aspects of the cellular response to low- and high-LET radiation. *Eur J Nucl Med* 2001; **28**: 541–61.

51 Behr TM. Higher relative biological efficiency of alpha-particles: in vitro veritas, in vivo vanitas? *Eur J Nucl Med* 2001; **28**: 939–40.

♦ 52 McDevitt MR, Sgouros G, Finn RD, *et al*. Radioimmunotherapy with alpha-emitting nuclides. *Eur J Nucl Med* 1998; **25**: 1341–51.

53 McDevitt MR, Ma D, Lai LT, *et al*. Tumor therapy with targeted atomic nanogenerators. *Science* 2001; **294**: 1537–40.

54 Wiseman GA, White CA, Stabin M, *et al*. Phase I/II ^{90}Y-Zevalin (yttrium-90 ibritumomab tiuxetan, IDEC-Y2B8) radioimmunotherapy dosimetry results in relapsed or refractory non-Hodgkin's lymphoma. *Eur J Nucl Med* 2000; **27**: 766–77.

♦ 55 Halldin C, Gulyas B, Langer O, *et al*. Brain radioligands – state of the art and new trends. *Q J Nucl Med* 2001; **45**: 139–52.

56 Seibyl JP, Marek K, Sheff K, *et al*. Iodine-123-beta-CIT and iodine-123-FPCIT SPECT measurement of dopamine transporters in healthy subjects and Parkinson's patients. *J Nucl Med* 1998; **39**: 1500–8.

57 Kung MP, Stevenson DA, Plossl K, *et al*. [^{99m}Tc]TRODAT-1: a novel technetium-99m complex as a dopamine transporter imaging agent. *Eur J Nucl Med* 1997; **24**: 372–80.

♦ 58 Johannsen B, Pietzsch HJ. Development of technetium-99m-based CNS receptor ligands: have there been any advances? *Eur J Nucl Med Mol Imaging* 2002; **29**: 263–75.

New radiopharmaceuticals for positron emission tomography

E.M. BEDNARCZYK AND A. AMER

INTRODUCTION

An extensive library of radiopharmaceuticals labeled with positron emitting isotopes has been developed, many of which have been used in man (Table 20D.1). In spite of this availability, currently only 2-[^{18}F]fluoro-2-deoxy-D-glucose (^{18}F-FDG) has gained widespread clinical acceptance. The result is that ^{18}F-FDG has become almost synonymous with positron emission tomography itself. This does not represent an inherent failure of other molecular probes, but rather represents the natural progression and maturation of radiopharmaceuticals coupled with the adaptation of traditional regulatory pathways. It is beyond the scope of this chapter to exhaustively review all positron emission tomography (PET) tracers that have been used in man; instead, this chapter will focus on radiopharmaceuticals for which there is a growing body of clinical evidence, or that show great potential (although still early in development).

Before presenting data on PET tracers likely to follow ^{18}F-FDG into routine clinical use, we will briefly discuss some of the hurdles that these drugs face. These can be broadly divided into manufacturing and assessment issues. The unique nature of radiopharmaceuticals used in PET (short half-lives, full chemical synthesis versus 'kit' labeling, etc) has created challenges in the standardization and regulation of these drugs. PET tracers saw initial development in research settings (typically universities), where continual optimization and discovery of new synthetic pathways is valued, but which leads to variability in synthetic approaches, and even variability in specific activity between centers or even within centers. While optimization and variability may be acceptable in a research setting, this approach creates problems for existing regulatory mechanisms. Standardization of production methods, and adherence to 'good manufacturing practice' guidelines will be critical for any new PET radiopharmaceutical.

Strategies for labeling a radiopharmaceutical with ^{11}C generally produce a compound that behaves identically to an unlabeled version of the molecule (i.e. distribution and clearance, binding characteristics, etc). This generally means that knowledge gained from work with unlabeled forms of the drug can be applied to the development of the radiopharmaceutical, simplifying the development process. Unfortunately, the nuclear half-life of ^{11}C (approximately 20 min) creates challenges for producing a clinically useful compound, both on standardization of manufacturing technique as well as the extent to which a product can be distributed. Fluorine-18 (or other isotopes with longer half-lives) allow for greater standardization of manufacturing and distribution, but require validation in their own right before use in man, since data from ^{11}C analogs may not be readily applicable to the fluorinated form of the drug.

In order for new tracers to move from research to clinical tools, studies undertaken with the same or greater vigor as those applied to radiopharmaceuticals previously approved for single photon emission computed tomography (SPECT) will have to be conducted. This includes provision of adequate sample size for studies based on realistic estimates of variance. This will have to account for variance from a variety of sources including differences in camera performance characteristics, acquisition and reconstruction protocols, as well as the specific activity of the radiopharmaceutical.

Table 20D.1   *Imaging agents for positron emission tomography*

Agent	Molecular target	Agent	Molecular target
^{18}F-FDG	Metabolism	[^{18}F]fluoroethylketanserin	5HT$_2$
H$_2$^{15}O	Blood flow	^{11}C-methylbromo LSD	5HT$_2$
^{13}NH$_3$	Blood flow	^{18}F-altanserin	5HT$_{2A}$
^{82}Rb	Blood flow	^{11}C-MDL 100907	5HT$_{2A}$ antagonist
C^{15}O	Blood volume	^{11}C-DASB	5HT transporters, D, NE
^{62}Cu-HSA-DTS (human serum albumin-dithiosemicarbazone)	Blood pool	^{11}C-, ^{18}F-McN5652	5HT transporters
		^{11}C-DAPP	5HT transporters, D, NE
^{15}O$_2$	Oxygen extraction	^{11}C-5-hydroxytryptophan (HTP)	Serotonin analog
C^{15}O$_2$	Blood flow	^{11}C-SCH442416	Adenosine 2$_A$
^{15}O-butanol	Blood flow	^{11}C-clorgyline	MAO A
^{11}C-hydroxyephedrine	Presynaptic adrenergic innervation	^{11}C-L-deprenyl	MAO B
		^{11}C-dimethylphenylethylamine	MAO B
^{11}C-metoprolol	β_1-receptors	^{18}F-Ro41-0960	COMT inhibitor
^{11}C-flumazenil (Ro 15-1788)	Benzodiazepine	^{11}C-choline	Choline metabolism
^{11}C-suriclone	Benzodiazepine	^{11}C-pyrrolidinocholine	Choline metabolism
^{18}F-oxoquazepam	Benzodiazepine 1	^{11}C-nicotine	Nicotinic receptor
^{18}F-DOPA	Dopamine	^{11}C-dihydrotetrabenazine (DTBZ)	Monoamine transport
^{11}C-NNC 112	D$_1$	^{11}C-tetrabenazine (TBZ)	Monoamine transport
^{76}Br-SKF 83566	D$_1$	^{11}C-methoxytetrabenazine (MTBZ)	Monoamine transport
[^{76}Br]bromo-SCH 23390	D$_1$	^{18}F-FBT (4-fluorobenzyltrozamicol)	Acetylcholine transport
^{11}C-SCH 23390	D$_1$	^{11}C-N-methyl-4-piperidyl acetate (MP4A)	Acetylcholine analog
^{11}C-raclopride	D$_2$		
^{11}C-FLB457 (also tagged with ^{76}Br)	D$_2$, D$_3$	^{11}C-methylpiperidin propionate	Acetylcholinesterase
^{11}C-fluorophenyl tropane (WIN-35,428)	Dopamine transport	^{11}C-methyl naltrindole (MeNTI)	δ-opioid antagonist
^{11}C-RTI-32	Dopamine transport	^{11}C-carfentanil	μ opioid agonist
^{11}C-D-threo-methylphenidate	Dopamine transport	^{11}C-, ^{18}F-diprenorphine	μ, δ, κ opioid antagonist
^{11}C-cocaine	Dopamine transport	^{11}C-buprenorphine	μ, δ, κ opioid agonist/ antagonist
^{11}C-β-CIT (β-carbomethoxy iodophenyl tropane)	Dopamine transport		
		^{18}F-acetylcyclofoxy	μ, κ opioid antagonist
^{11}C-nomifensine	D, 5HT, piperazine, noradrenergic reuptake	^{11}C-dexetimide	Muscarinic
^{18}F-GBR 13119	D, 5HT, piperazine, noradrenergic reuptake	[^{18}F]fluorodexetimide	Muscarinic
		^{11}C-QNB	Muscarinic
[^{18}F]fluoromethyl-BTCP	D, 5HT, piperazine, noradrenergic reuptake	^{11}C-scopolamine	Muscarinic
		^{11}C-4-MPB (methyl-4-piperidyl benzilate)	Muscarinic cholinergic receptors
^{11}C-, ^{18}F-methylspiperone	D$_2$, 5HT$_2$	^{11}C-3-MPB (methyl-3-piperidyl benzilate)	Muscarinic cholinergic receptors
^{18}F-spiperone	D$_2$, 5HT$_2$		
[^{18}F]fluoroethylspiperone	D$_2$, 5HT$_2$	^{11}C-benztropine	Muscarinic cholinergic receptors
[^{76}Br]bromospiperone	D$_2$, 5HT$_2$		
^{11}C-methylbenperidol	D$_2$, 5HT$_2$	^{11}C-RS 86	Muscarinic
^{11}C-methoxyprogabidic acid	GABA receptors	^{11}C-PK11195	Peripheral benzodiazepine receptors
^{18}F-setoperone	5HT$_{2A}$, D$_2$		
^{11}C-α-methyl-L-tryptophan (α-MTrp)	5HT	^{11}C-PIB	Beta amyloid
^{11}C-WAY-100635	5HT$_{1A}$	^{18}F-FDDNP	Beta amyloid, neurofibrilatory tangles
^{11}C-NAD-299	5HT$_{1A}$		
^{11}C-ketanserin	5HT$_2$	^{11}C-pyrilamine	H1
^{11}C-methylketanserin	5HT$_2$	^{11}C-doxepin	H1

This is in addition to the between and within patient differences introduced by genetically influenced differences in tracer clearance, disease states and concomitant therapeutic agents.

BONE

Given previous clinical use of [^{18}F]fluoride, it would seem inappropriate to include this agent as a 'new' radiopharmaceutical. Early clinical use of [^{18}F]fluoride was limited, in part, by existing camera technology and (at the time) limited tracer availability. The result has been a lack of clinical experience and, for all practical intent, a research-like status for this tracer. In addition to having a well characterized synthesis, with standardized acceptance criteria, [^{18}F]fluoride has the advantage of being readily available and easily shipped. Most of the experience with [^{18}F]fluoride had focused on applications in oncology,[1] but [^{18}F]fluoride has also been shown to be a valid tracer for estimating bone perfusion.[2,3] Briefly, a dynamic scan procedure is used currently requiring an arterial input function (through direct sampling or derived from a region of interest). [^{18}F]Fluoride has also been explored as an agent for the assessment of bone re-mineralization following treatment.[2]

CARDIAC IMAGING AGENTS

Fluorine-18-FDG has matured into a suitable agent for identification of viable myocardial tissue, and ^{13}NH$_3$ and ^{82}Rb have been able to demonstrate advantages over single photon labeled radiopharmaceuticals in some populations. While research with ^{11}C-fatty acids and ^{11}C-acetate continues, a growing body of work probing the sympathetic innervation of the myocardium with ^{11}C-hydroxyephedrine[4–6] is emerging. Carbon-11-hydroxyephedrine is one of the best characterized positron-emitting tracers for pre-synaptic sympathetic nerve terminal assessment. It is a false neurotransmitter with the same neuronal uptake mechanism as norepinephrine, but it is resistant to degradation by monoamine oxidase and catechol-O-methyl-transferase. It accumulates in organs with sympathetic innervation, such as the adrenal medulla and the heart, reflecting uptake-1 capacity; the transporter responsible for re-uptake of norepinephrine from the synaptic cleft into the pre-synaptic nerve ending.

The neuronal function of the heart is compromised in various cardiac disorders, including congestive heart failure, ischemia, cardiac arrhythmias and certain cardiomyopathies. The assessment of neuronal alteration may provide valuable information for disease severity and for appropriate treatments. In this respect, ^{11}C-hydroxyephedrine PET may provide a role for quantitative noninvasive assessment of the re-uptake and storage system in pre-synaptic

terminals. ^{11}C-hydroxyephedrine PET has been used to study the hypothesis that spontaneous sympathetic reinnervation takes place after heart transplantation. Other investigators have utilized this imaging technique to show that cardiac pre-synaptic catecholamine re-uptake is impaired in hypertrophic cardiomyopathy or to evaluate sympathetic nervous system involvement in arrhythmogenesis. Chronic heart failure outcome has been correlated with cardiac uptake of ^{11}C-hydroxyephedrine. Further effort is needed to translate the research results of neuronal function studies into clinical diagnosis and evaluation of various cardiac disorders.[7–10] Because of ^{11}C labeling, it is unlikely that ^{11}C-hydroxyephedrine will emerge into routine clinical use, although it may point to future probes of the adrenergic system. Other drugs (most notably carazolol) have been labeled with fluorine-18,[11] but the value of these drugs in cardiac assessment remains to be seen.

FLOW

The short half-life of ^{15}O (123 s) requires proximity to the production cyclotron and will continue to limit the clinical use of this and related ^{15}O-based flow tracers (such as ^{15}O-butanol). Because of the extent of use, H$_2$^{15}O meets many of the characteristics of established tracers (use in large numbers of subjects, no known pharmacologic effects, validated in a variety of conditions where flow measures are needed). Oxygen-15-based agents will continue to play an important role as a research tool to quantitatively measure blood flow in a variety of tissues.[12]

While ^{13}NH$_3$ and ^{82}Rb are the dominant cardiac PET perfusion agents, a US Food and Drug Administration new drug application (NDA) was filed for a commercially developed ^{62}Zn/^{62}Cu generator eluting ^{62}Cu-PTSM in 2001. ^{62}Cu-PTSM (Cu(II)-pyruvaldehyde bis(N(4)-methylthiosemicarbazone)) was first evaluated in the 1990s and found to have characteristics appropriate for a flow tracer.[13–16] This radiopharmaceutical has been evaluated for cardiac, cerebral,[17] renal[13] and tumor[14,18] perfusion studies. Availability of a commercial ^{62}Cu generator could add an additional useful blood flow radiopharmaceutical.

NEURODEGENERATION

Recently, compounds targeting deposits of beta-amyloid protein and neurofibrilatory tangles, both critical elements in the pathophysiology of Alzheimer's type dementia (AD) have been described. Of these compounds, the one that has generated the greatest degree of clinical interest is N-methyl-[^{11}C]2-(4-methylaminophenyl)-6-hydroxybenzothiazole, (^{11}C-PIB, or 'Pittsburgh compound B').[19,20] Carbon-11-PIB binds to amyloid in the brain, and when used in conjunction with ^{18}F-FDG imaging, is beginning to lend important insight into both the diagnosis and progression of AD. An intriguing application may be for the monitoring of disease-modifying therapies for AD, since amyloid deposition is widely thought to be causative for AD, and is a target of therapeutic agents currently in development. The labeling of this compound with ^{18}F is currently under investigation,[21] and if accomplished and validated, would position PIB as the first clinically relevant amyloid imaging agent. Additional agents specific for binding to neurofibrilatory tangles have been described. 2-(1-{6-[(2-[^{18}F]fluoroethyl)(methyl)amino]-2-naphthyl}ethylidene) malonitrile (^{18}F-FDDNP) binds to both beta amyloid and neurofibrilatory tangles in the brain,[22] and has been administered in man. All of these compounds will add to the understanding of the role of deposition of beta-amyloid in AD as well as to occurrence as part of the normal aging process before a clear diagnostic role is defined.

Another compound, ^{11}C-PK11195 (1-(2-chlorophenyl)-N-methyl-N-(1-methylpropyl)-3-isoquinoline carboxamide), binds to the peripheral benzodiazepine receptor. Within the brain, this receptor is expressed on activated microglia, giving this compound the potential to be applied to the assessment of neuronal damage. Focal binding has been observed in several neurodegenerative disorders including multiple sclerosis,[23] Parkinson's disease,[24] multiple system atrophy,[25] cerebral ischemia,[26] vasculitis and encephalitis.[27,28]

NEUROTRANSMITTERS

L-DOPA is the precursor for the neurotransmitter dopamine. Labeled L-DOPA is taken up by dopaminergic terminals and becomes incorporated into the neurotransmitter. L-^{18}F-DOPA has been used to study pre-synaptic nerve terminals of the nigrostriatal dopaminergic system in Parkinson's disease (PD) and other movement disorders. L-^{18}F-DOPA PET assists in the diagnosis of PD in early disease stages, differentiating clinically unclear cases from other movement disorders, e.g. essential tremor. L-^{18}F-DOPA also permits the follow-up of disease progression and the assessment of medical and surgical PD therapy strategies. A limitation of ^{18}F-DOPA is that some of its peripheral metabolites distribute through the brain and introduce a significant background signal into the PET image.[29–32]

Carbon-11-raclopride became widely used as a PET tracer to study D$_2$ receptors in vivo in both animals and humans shortly after raclopride was investigated as a potential antipsychotic drug in the mid 1980s in Europe. Raclopride, a substituted benzamide, was found to bind with a high selectivity and affinity to D$_2$ dopamine receptors. The drug is highly lipophilic and was shown to penetrate readily into brain tissue. Both in vitro and in vivo studies showed that raclopride binding is saturable and reversible, with a low proportion of nonspecific binding.

A high-affinity ligand with low nonspecific binding and good brain uptake provides a reliable tool to study receptor availability. Investigators have used ^{11}C-raclopride to study changes in D$_2$ receptors in aging, to determine the involvement of D$_2$ receptors in psychiatric disorders such as schizophrenia and substance abuse and in movement disorders such as Parkinson's and Huntington's diseases. In spite of widespread use as a research tool, little clinical use has been proposed. An intriguing possibility for clinical use is suggested by studies assessing of D$_2$ blockade following administration of D$_2$ receptor antagonists (i.e. antipsychotics). In theory, this same approach could be employed on an individualized basis, particularly in refractory patients or those with adverse effects at relatively low doses.[33–36]

Carfentanil is a opiate receptor agonist chemically related to fentanyl. It shows a high degree of specificity for the μ-opioid receptor. Distribution of ^{11}C-carfentanil has been well characterized in the brain, including effects of gender, age and other pathological conditions. ^{11}C-carfentanil has also been used to evaluate the receptor occupancy after administration of opiate antagonists. With renewed interest in the role of endogenous opiates in mediating a variety of addictive behaviours, a new clinical role may emerge for this drug.

Flumazenil is an imidazobenzodiazepine that behaves as a specific benzodiazepine antagonist. Flumazenil binds with high affinity to the benzodiazepine recognition site on the γ-aminobutyric acid (GABA$_A$) receptor, where it competitively antagonizes the binding and allosteric effects of benzodiazepines and other ligands. Carbon-11-flumazenil, administered in tracer amounts, is used for visualization and quantification of benzodiazepine receptors in the brain. Such data are used to localize epileptic foci in patients who are candidates for surgery, particularly when magnetic resonance imaging (MRI) and electroencephalograph (EEG) provide contradictory results. Carbon-11-flumazenil PET has also been used to identify abnormalities of central benzodiazepine receptors and consequently provide information in ischemia or other pathological conditions known to affect neuronal integrity. Its uptake into brain is rapid, and it binds selectively and reversibly to benzodiazepine receptors in the central nervous system, with no pharmacological activity when administered in tracer quantities. Furthermore, although several metabolites are formed, only the parent compound is able to cross the blood–brain barrier.[44–47]

ONCOLOGY

While the role of ^{18}F-FDG in oncology continues to expand, it has certain limitations. Nonspecific uptake is observed with inflammation, muscle use and administration of some drugs such as granulocyte colony stimulating factors (GCSFs). Elimination in urine presents specific challenges when attempting to image malignancies within the pelvis.

To obviate these limitations, and to examine other molecular pathways in cancerous cells, other molecular pathways have been probed. The most widely studied of these agents is ^{11}C-choline. Choline is a component of phospholipids in cellular membranes, with increased uptake observed during cellular proliferation. Carbon-11-choline is rapidly cleared from the blood pool, and has been shown to be taken up by malignant tissue. Because renal elimination accounts for a small fraction of excretion, this has made it an attractive agent for evaluating pelvic malignancies such as prostate cancer.[48,49] In this setting it has shown advantage over ^{18}F-FDG. It has also shown promise in visualizing ovarian and uterine tumors[50] as well as sites outside the pelvis such as the sinuses,[51] brain and musculoskeletal tumors.[52] To date, the published base of patients studied with ^{11}C-choline has been limited, and considerably more data will be needed to understand the limitations of this drug. Localization of ^{11}C-choline in malignant tissue has been promising, but uptake in the gut and pancreas has been observed. Metabolic pathways (in addition to phosphorylation) include oxidation and acetylation. Labeling with ^{11}C limits distribution to centers near production facilities. Fluorine-18-labeled analogs such as [^{18}F]fluoroethylcholine and [^{18}F]fluorocholine have been developed,[53] and appear to have uptake into malignant tissue comparable to ^{11}C-choline. Unfortunately, these analogs undergo significant renal elimination requiring strategies such as early imaging (prior to significant accumulation in the bladder) to be part of the validation process.

Thymidine has long been recognized as a marker of cellular proliferation. This pyrimidine nucleoside is incorporated into DNA, potentially providing higher specificity than FDG by measuring cell proliferation. Initial research focused on ^{11}C-labeled forms, where ^{11}C-thymidine has been used to quantitate uptake into cerebral[54] and abdominal malignancies.[55] It has also been explored as a marker of response to drug treatment,[56] where early response may be a better predictor of outcome than metabolic imaging studies. A recognized limitation of ^{11}C-thymidine is metabolism, with [11]CO_2 as a major breakdown product, requiring some degree of correction in quantitative models.[55] Due to the limitations of ^{11}C and the challenges posed by the metabolite, alternate labeling strategies have been developed.[57] Fluorine-18-thymidine (^{18}F-FLT) is taken up into cells, where, like ^{11}C-thymidine, it is phosphorylated. Unlike ^{11}C-thymidine, FLT becomes trapped intracellularly.[58] FLT has also been evaluated in a variety of tumor types including lung cancer,[59–61] colorectal cancer,[62] and brain tumors,[63,64] including comparative studies with ^{18}F-FDG and ^{11}C-methionine.[61,62,64] Importantly, in comparative studies, FLT did not stand out as a superior agent, rather one that provided complementary information.

Although ^{18}F-DOPA has been used mainly for brain imaging, it also enables detection of neuroendocrine tumors characterized by the capacity to uptake and decarboxylate amine precursors. This focal localization may allow for visualization of tumors missed by conventional anatomic imaging methods, as well as defining the endocrine nature of the tumor. PET radiopharmaceuticals with specific cellular targets offer particular promise in endocrine oncology taking advantage of storage systems and the specific amine precursor uptake and decarboxylation pathways that characterize these tumors. For instance, ^{18}F-DOPA and ^{11}C-5-hydroxytryptophan (^{11}C-5-HTP) are taken up by carcinoid tumor cells. Similarly, 6-[^{18}F]fluorodopamine and ^{11}C-hydroxyephedrine are taken up into pheochromocytoma cells by cell membrane catecholamine transporters and then concentrated in storage vesicles.[65,66]

Carcinoids are tumors of enterochromaffin cells but can also arise in parenchymal organs outside the gastrointestinal tract. Carcinoids characteristically synthesize serotonin; administration of labeled serotonin precursors provides a specific method of tumor visualization. Carbon-11-5-HTP seems well suited for this purpose, especially in the mid-gut, with sensitivity exceeding that of computed tomography (CT). Fluorine-18-DOPA, another amine precursor, was reported to be a useful supplement for diagnostic imaging of carcinoids; its sensitivity exceeds that of ^{18}F-FDG in scanning for primary tumors and lymph node metastases of gastrointestinal carcinoid tumors. False negatives have been reported with undifferentiated carcinoids (poorly differentiated carcinoids with high proliferative activity may be better visualized by ^{18}F-FDG). Other potential limitations of PET using labeled amine precursor are the substantial physiologic uptake in the duodenum and pancreas, which might mask tumors in these sites, and nonspecific accumulations within the intestine or surrounding tissues.[65–68]

Pheochromocytoma is a rare but clinically important tumor of chromaffin cells, characterized by production and secretion of catecholamines. 6-[^{18}F]fluorodopamine is, as suggested by its name, a dopamine analog. In catecholamine-synthesizing cells, 6-[^{18}F]fluorodopamine is transported actively by both the plasma membrane norepinephrine transporter and the intracellular vesicular monoamine transporter. Accumulation of 6-[^{18}F]fluorodopamine in catecholamine storage vesicles enables visualization of sympathetic innervation. Because chromaffin cells express the plasma membrane and vesicular catecholamine transporters, 6-[^{18}F]fluorodopamine was shown to be useful in diagnostic localization of pheochromocytoma when evaluated in clinical studies. Carbon-11-hydroxyephedrine is another agent that has been evaluated in the localization of pheochromocytoma where it was found to be highly sensitive and specific. Rapid and selective tracer accumulation allowed the acquisition of high-quality images within minutes of tracer injection. A potential limitation of this method is the substantial physiologic uptake in other organs.[65,66,69,70]

Numerous PET tracers will continue to emerge as potential clinical tools. These tracers will require vigorous validation of production and utility before they are used as routinely as FDG. If these requirements can be satisfied, they have the potential to provide unique molecular information in the diagnosis and management of a variety of conditions.

REFERENCES

1 Schirrmeister H, Guhlmann A, Elsner K, *et al.* Sensitivity in detecting osseous lesions depends on anatomic localization: planar bone scintigraphy versus ^{18}F PET. *J Nucl Med* 1999; **40**: 1623–9.

2 Frost ML, Cook GJR, Blake GM, *et al.* A prospective study of risedronate on regional bone metabolism and blood flow at the lumbar spine measured by ^{18}F-fluoride positron emission tomography. *J Bone Miner Res* 2003; **18**: 2215–22.

3 Piert M, Zittel T, Machulla H, *et al.* Blood flow measurements with [^{15}O]H$_2$O and [^{18}F]fluoride ion PET in porcine vertebrae. *J Bone Miner Res* 1998; **13**: 1328–36.

4 Rosenspire KC, Haka MS, VanDort ME, *et al.* Synthesis and preliminary evaluation of carbon-11-meta-hydroxyephedrine: a false transmitter agent for heart neuronal imaging. *J Nucl Med* 1990; **31**: 1328–34.

5 Schwaiger M, Kalff V, Rosenspire K, *et al.* Noninvasive evaluation of sympathetic nervous system in human heart by positron emission tomography. *Circulation* 1990; **82**: 457–64.

6 Luisi AJ, Suzuki G, Dekemp R, *et al.* Regional ^{11}C-hydroxyephedrine retention in hibernating myocardium: chronic inhomogeneity of sympathetic innervation in the absence of infarction. *J Nucl Med* 2005; **46**: 1368–74.

7 Carrio I. Cardiac neurotransmission imaging. *J Nucl Med* 2001; **42**: 1062–76.

8 Goldstein D, Holmes C, Cannon R, *et al.* Sympathetic cardioneuropathy in dysautonomias. *N Engl J Med* 1997; **336**: 696–702.

9 Munch G, Nguyen N, Nekolla S, *et al.* Evaluation of sympathetic nerve terminals with [(11)C]epinephrine and [(11)C]hydroxyephedrine and positron emission tomography. *Circulation* 2000; **101**: 516–23.

10 Pietila M, Malminiemi K, Vesalainen R, *et al.* Exercise training in chronic heart failure: beneficial effects on cardiac (11)C-hydroxyephedrine PET, autonomic nervous control and ventricular repolarization. *J Nucl Med* 2002; **43**: 773–9.

11 Salinas C, Muzic RF, Berridge M, Ernsberger P. PET imaging of myocardial b-adrenergic receptors with fluorocarazolol. *J Cardiovas Pharmacol* 2005; **46**: 222–31.

12 Anderson H, Price P. Clinical measurement of blood flow in tumours using positron emission tomography: a review. *Nucl Med Commun* 2002; **23**: 131–8.

13 Barnhart A, Voorhees W, Green M. Correlation of Cu(PTSM) localization with regional blood flow in the heart and kidney. *Intern J Rad Appl Instrum B* 1989; **16**: 747–8.

14 Flower M, Zweit J, Hall A, *et al.* [62]Cu-PTSM and PET used for the assessment of angiotensin II-induced blood flow changes in patients with colorectal liver metastases. *Eur J Nucl Med* 2001; **28**: 99–103.

15 Haynes N, Lacy J, Nayak N, *et al.* Performance of a [62]Zn/[62]Cu generator in clinical trials of PET perfusion agent [62]Cu-PTSM. *J Nucl Med* 2000; **41**: 309–14.

16 Wallhaus T, Lacy J, Stewart R, *et al.* Copper-62-pyruvaldehyde bis(*N*-methyl-thiosemicarbazone) PET imaging in the detection of coronary artery disease in humans. *J Nucl Cardiol* 2001; **8**: 67–74.

17 Mathias CJ, Welch ME, Raichle ME, *et al.* Evaluation of a potential generator produced PET tracer for cerebral perfusion imaging: single-pass cerebral extraction measurements and imaging with radiolabeled Cu-PTSM. *J Nucl Med* 1990; **31**: 351–9.

18 Mathias CJ, Green M, Morrison W, Knapp D. Evaluation of Cu-PTSM as a tracer of tumor perfusion: comparison with labeled microspheres in spontaneous canine neoplasms. *Nucl Med Biol* 1994; **21**: 83–7.

19 Klunk W, Engler H, Nordberg A, *et al.* Imaging brain amyloid in Alzheimer's disease with Pittsburgh compound-B. *Ann Neurol* 2004; **55**: 306–19.

20 Zhang W, Oya S, Kung M, *et al.* F-18 stilbenes as PET imaging agents for detecting beta-amyloid plaques in the brain. *J Med Chem* 2005; **48**: 5980–8.

21 Mathis C, Klunk W, DeKosky S. Imaging technology for neurodegenerative diseases. *Arch Neurol* 2005; **62**: 196–200.

22 Shoghi-Jadid K, Small G, Agdeppa E, *et al.* Localization of neurofibrillary tangles and beta-amyloid plaques in the brains of living patients with Alzheimer disease. *Am J Geriatr Psychiat* 2002; **10**: 24–35.

23 Banati R, Newcombe J, Gunn R, *et al.* The peripheral benzodiazepine binding site in the brain in multiple sclerosis. *Brain* 2000; **123**: 2321–37.

24 Ouchi Y, Yoshikawa E, Sekine Y, *et al.* Microglial activation and dopamine terminal loss in early Parkinson's disease. *Ann Neurol* 2005; **57**: 168–75.

25 Gerhard A, Banati R, Goerres G, *et al.* ^{11}C-R-PK11195 PET imaging of microgial activation in multiple system atrophy. *Neurology* 2003; **61**: 686–9.

26 Pappata S, Levasseur M, Gunn R, *et al.* Thalamic microglial activation is ischemic stroke detected in vivo by PET and [^{11}C]PK11195. *Neurology* 2000; **55**: 1052–4.

27 Cagnin A, Myers R, Gunn R, *et al.* In-vivo visualization of activated glia by [^{11}C](*R*)-PK11195-PET following herpes encephalitis reveals projected neuronal damage beyond the primary focal lesion. *Brain* 2001; **124**: 2014–27.

28 Goerres G, Revesz T, Duncan J, Banati R. Imaging cerebral vasculitis in refractory epilepsy using [^{11}C](*R*)-PK11195 positron emission tomography. *AJR* 2001; **176**: 1016–8.

29 Fischman A. Role of [^{18}F]-DOPA-PET imaging in assessing movement disorders. *Radiol Clin North Am* 2005; **43**: 93–106.

30 Heiss W, Hilker R. The sensitivity of 18-fluorodopa positron emission tomography and magnetic resonance

imaging in Parkinson's disease. *Eur J Neurol* 2004; **11**: 5–12.

31 Seibyl J. Imaging studies in movement disorders. *Semin Nucl Med* 2003; **33**: 105–13.

32 Wahl L, Chirakal R, Firnau G, *et al.* The distribution and kinetics of [18F]6-fluoro-3-*O*-methyl-L-dopa in the human brain. *J Cereb Blood Flow Metab* 1994; **14**: 664–70.

33 Farde L, Von Bahr C, Wahlen A, *et al.* The new selective D2-dopamine receptor antagonist raclopride – pharmacokinetics, safety and tolerability in healthy males. *Int Clin Psychopharmacol* 1989; **4**: 115–26.

34 Farde L, Wiesel F, Halldin C, Sedvall G. Central D2-dopamine receptor occupancy in schizophrenic patients treated with antipsychotic drugs. *Arch Gen Psychiat* 1988; **45**: 71–6.

35 Kohler C, Hall H, Ogren S, Gawell L. Specific *in vitro* and *in vivo* binding of 3H-raclopride. A potent substituted benzamide drug with high affinity for dopamine D-2 receptors in the rat brain. *Biochem Pharmacol* 1985; **34**: 2251–9.

36 Wang G, Volkow ND, Fowler J, *et al.* Age associated decrements in dopamine D2 receptors in thalamus and temporal insula of human subjects. *Life Sci* 1996; **59**: PL31–5.

37 Bencherif B, Wand G, McCaul M, *et al.* Mu-opioid receptor binding measured by [11C]carfentanil positron emission tomography is related to craving and mood in alcohol dependence. *Biol Psychiat* 2004; **55**: 255–62.

38 Frost JJ, Douglas K, Mayberg HS, *et al.* Multicompartment analysis of 11C-carfentanil binding to opiate receptors in humans measured by positron emission tomography. *J Cereb Blood Flow Metab* 1989; **9**: 398–409.

39 Frost JJ, Wagner HN, Dannals RF, *et al.* Imaging opiate receptors in the human brain by positron tomography. *J Comput Ass Tomogr* 1985; **9**: 231–6.

40 Zubieta J, Dannals RF, Frost JJ. Gender and age influences on human brain mu-opioid receptor binding measured by PET. *Am J Psychiat* 1999; **156**: 842–8.

41 Zubieta J, Gorelick D, Stauffer R, *et al.* Increased mu opioid receptor binding detected by PET in cocaine dependent men is associated with increased cocaine craving. *Nat Med* 1996; **2**: 1225–9.

42 Zubieta J, Greenwald M, Lombardi U, *et al.* Buprenorphine-induced changes in mu-opioid receptor availability in male heroin-dependent volunteers: a preliminary study. *Neuropsychopharmacology* 2000; **23**: 326–34.

43 Zubieta J, Smith Y, Bueller J, *et al.* Regional mu opioid receptor regulation of sensory and affective dimensions of pain. *Science* 2001; **293**: 311–15.

44 Asenbaum S, Baumgartner C. Nuclear medicine in the preoperative evaluation of epilepsy. *Nucl Med Commun* 2001; **22**: 835–40.

45 Ihara M, Tomimoto H, Ishizu K, *et al.* Decrease in cortical benzodiazepine receptors in symptomatic patients with leukoaraiosis: a positron emission tomography study. *Stroke* 2004; **35**: 942–7.

46 Maziere M, Hantraye P, Prenant C, *et al.* Synthesis of ethyl 8-fluoro-5,6-dihydro-5-[11C]methyl-6-oxo-4*H*-imidazo[1,5-a][1,4]benzodiazepine-3-carboxylate (RO 15.1788-11C): a specific radioligand for the *in vivo* study of central benzodiazepine receptors by positron emission tomography. *Int J Appl Radiat Isot* 1984; **35**: 973–6.

47 Yamauchi Y, Kudoh T, Kishibe Y, *et al.* Selective neuronal damage and borderzone infarctions in carotid artery acclusive disease: a 11C-flumazenil PET study. *J Nucl Med* 2005; **46**: 1973–9.

48 deJong I, Pruim J, Elsinga PH, *et al.* Preoperative staging of pelvic lymph nodes in prostate cancer by 11C-choline PET. *J Nucl Med* 2003; **44**: 331–5.

49 Hara T, Kosaka N, Kishi H. PET imaging of prostate cancer using carbon-11-choline. *J Nucl Med* 1998; **39**: 990–5.

50 Torizuka T, Kanno T, Futatsubashi M, *et al.* Imaging of gynecologic tumors: comparison of 11C-choline PET with 18F-FDG PET. *J Nucl Med* 2003; **44**: 1051–6.

51 Ninomiya H, Oriuchi N, Kahn N, *et al.* Diagnosis of tumor in the nasal cavity and paranasal sinuses with [11C]choline PET: comparative study with 2-[18F]fluoro-2-deoxy-D-glucose (FDG) PET. *Ann Nucl Med* 2004; **18**: 29–34.

52 Yanagawa T, Watanabe H, Inoue T, *et al.* Carbon-11 choline positron emission tomography in musculoskeletal tumors: comparison with fluorine-18 fluorodeoxyglucose positron emission tomography. *J Comp Ass Tomogr* 2003; **27**: 175–82.

53 Hara T, Kosaka N, Kishi H. Development of 18F-fluoroethylcholine for cancer imaging with PET: synthesis, biochemistry, and prostate cancer imaging. *J Nucl Med* 2001; **43**: 187–99.

54 Eary J, mankoff D, Spence A, *et al.* 2-[C-11]Thymidine imaging of malignant brain tumors. *Cancer Res* 1999; **59**: 615–21.

55 Wells P, Gunn R, Alison M, *et al.* Assessment of proliferation in vivo using 2-[11C]thymidine positron emission tomography in advanced intra-abdominal malignancies. *Cancer Res* 2002; **62**: 5698–702.

56 Wells P, Aboagye E, Gunn R, *et al.* 2-[11C]Thymidine positron emission tomography as an indicator of thymidylate synthetase inhibition in patients treated with AG337. *J Natl Cancer Inst* 2003; **95**: 675–82.

57 Shields A, Briston D, Chandupatla S, *et al.* A simplified analysis of [18F]-3′-deoxy-3′-fluorothymidine metabolism and retention. *Eur J Nucl Med Mol Imaging* 2005; **32**: 1269–75.

58 Wagner M, Seitz U, Buck A, *et al.* 3′-[18F]Fluoro-3′-deoxythymidine ([18F]-FLT) as positron emission tomography tracer for imaging proliferation in a murine B-cell lymphoma model and in human disease. *Cancer Res* 2003; **63**: 2681–7.

59 Buck A, Schirrmeister H, Hetzel M, *et al.* 3-deoxy-3-[^{18}F]fluorothymidine-positron emission tomography for noninvasive assessment of proliferation in pulmonary nodules. *Cancer Res* 2002; **62**: 3331–4.

60 Vesselle H, Grierson J, Muzi M, *et al.* In vivo validation of 3′-deoxy-3′-[^{18}F]fluorothymidine as a proliferation imaging tracer in humans: correlation of [^{18}F]FLT uptake by positron emission tomography with Ki-67 immunohistochemistry and flow cytometry in human lung tumors. *Clin Cancer Res* 2002; **8**: 3315–23.

61 Yap C, Czernin J, Fishbein M, *et al.* Evaluation of thoracic tumors with ^{18}F-fluorothymidine and ^{18}F-fluorodeoxyglucose positron emission tomography. *Chest* 2006; **129**: 393–401.

62 Francis D, Visvikis D, Costa D, *et al.* Potential impact of [^{18}F]-3′-deoxy-3′-fluorothymidine vs [^{18}F]fluoro-2-deoxy-D-glucose in positron emission tomography for colorectal cancer. *Eur J Nucl Med Mol Imaging* 2003; **30**: 988–94.

63 Choi S, Kim J, Kim J, *et al.* [^{18}F]-3′-deoxy-3′-fluorothymidine PET for the diagnosis and grading of brain tumors. *Eur J Nucl Med Mol Imaging* 2005; **32**: 653–9.

64 Jacobs A, Thomas A, Kracht L, *et al.* ^{18}F-Fluoro-L-thymidine and ^{11}C-methylmethionine as markers of increased transport and proliferation in brain tumors. *J Nucl Med* 2005; **46**: 1948–58.

65 Eriksson B, Orlefors H, Oberg K, *et al.* Developments in PET for the detection of endocrine tumors. *Best Pract Res Clin Endocrinol Metab* 2005; **19**: 311–24.

66 Pacak K, Eisenhofer G, Goldstein D. Functional imaging of endocrine tumors: role of positron emission tomography. *Endocr Rev* 2004; **25**: 568–80.

67 Hoegerle A, Altehoefer C, Ghanem N, *et al.* Whole body ^{18}F dopa PET for detection of gastrointestinal carcinoid tumors. *Radiology* 2001; **220**: 373–80.

68 Sundin A, Eriksson B, Bergstrom M, *et al.* Demonstration of [^{11}C]5-hydroxy-L-tryptophan uptake and decarboxylation in carcinoid tumors by specific positioning labeling in positron emission tomography. *Nucl Med Biol* 2000; **27**: 33–41.

69 Pacak K, Eisenhofer G, Carrasquillo J, *et al.* [^{18}F]fluorodopamine positron emission tomographic (PET) scanning for diagnostic localization of pheochromocytoma. *Hypertension* 2001; **38**: 6–8.

70 Trampal C, Engler H, Juhlin C, *et al.* Pheochromocytomas: detection with ^{11}C hydroxyephedrine PET. *Radiology* 2004; **230**: 423–8.

21

Technology and instrumentation

21A Solid state and other detectors

Radiation detectors in nuclear medicine   849
Single-photon imaging   852
Positron cameras   855

Summary   858
References   858

21B Image registration

Introduction   861
Classification   861
Inherent registration   861
Point, line, and surface-based registration   862

Voxel property-based registration   862
Clinical applications of image registration   863
Conclusion   864
References   864

21C Attenuation correction in positron emission tomography and single photon emission computed tomography

Introduction   869
Photon attenuation, scattering and interaction
  with matter   869
Measuring transmission: the key to accurate
  attenuation correction   870

SPECT/CT and PET/CT   872
Correction for attenuation   872
Clinical applications   875
Conclusion   878
References   878

Solid state and other detectors

R.J. OTT

RADIATION DETECTORS IN NUCLEAR MEDICINE

Devices used for nuclear medicine imaging require a high detection efficiency for gamma rays of energy 50–500 keV. At these energies gamma rays interact in material via essentially two mechanisms: the photoelectron effect and Compton scattering (Fig. 21A.1). The electrons produced will ionize or excite the detector material and, if sufficient energy is deposited, the resultant signal used to determine the interaction position and, ideally, the gamma-ray energy. As photoelectron absorption is most efficient for producing energetic electrons, detectors should have a high electron number (Z).

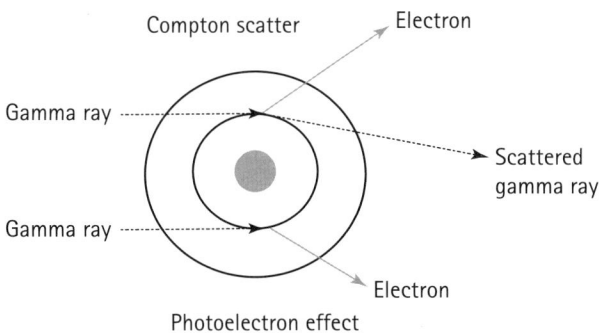

Figure 21A.1 *The two main interaction processes in matter for gamma rays with energies in the range 50–511 keV. The electron energy deposited causes either atomic ionization or excitation.*

Other important detector properties are energy resolution, which determines the ability to reject scattered gamma rays; spatial resolution, which determines the ability to detect small regions of radiotracer uptake; and count-rate performance, which determines the statistical quality of the images. Overall detector efficiency is the ratio of the number of photons detected to the number emitted by the radioactive source and depends on intrinsic gamma-ray detection efficiency (ϵ) and source–detector solid angle ($d\Omega$).

The three main devices used for detecting 50–500 keV gamma rays are scintillation counters, gas-filled detectors, semiconductors, and combinations of the three.

Scintillation detectors

Scintillation detectors[1] are based on coupling a scintillation crystal to a photomultiplier (PMT) or photodiode. Gamma rays interacting in the crystal deposit energy and produce a flash of scintillation light. The properties of some crystals used are shown in Table 21A.1. Thallium-doped sodium iodide, NaI(Tl), is the most commonly used crystal for the detection of gamma rays at energies below 200 keV having a high light output and modest cost. This crystal forms the basis of the gamma camera. For imaging gamma rays with energy above 200 keV a higher Z crystal is desirable. Bismuth germanate (BGO) has been commonly used having 50% higher Z than NaI(Tl). More recently, lutetium oxyorthosilicate (LSO) and gadolinium oxyorthosilicate (GSO) have replaced BGO for high-energy photon imaging having a

Table 21A.1 *The properties of five scintillating crystals used for nuclear medicine imaging*

Crystal	Effective Z	Density (g cm^{-3})	Decay constant ($\times 10^{-9}$ s)	Peak λ (nm)	Relative light output
NaI(Tl)	51	3.67	230	415	1.0
BGO	75	7.13	300	480	0.15
LSO	66	7.4	40	420	0.75
GSO	58	6.7	60	430	0.2
BaF$_2$	54	4.89	0.8/620	~200/310	0.05/0.16

Detection efficiency increases with density and effective atomic weight, Z. High-energy resolution requires high light output whereas count rate depends on the decay constant.
λ, wavelength; BGO, bismuth germanate; LSO, lutetium oxyorthosilicate; GSO, gadolinium oxyorthosilicate.

more intense, faster light output than BGO. Light emitted from a crystal can be detected by a PMT or photodiode and converted to an electronic signal. A PMT (Fig. 21A.2(a)), is a glass vacuum tube with a front surface photosensitive layer (photocathode) which converts optical photons to photo-electrons which are accelerated by high voltage (~1 kV) and collide with a series of electrodes (dynodes) providing electron multiplication. Multiple dynode interactions amplify the signal by ~10^4–10^8 producing a large pulse at the anode. The pulse amplitude/area should be proportional to the energy deposited in the crystal allowing a measurement of the incoming gamma-ray energy. The width of the pulse is determined by the crystal light output decay time and the speed of the PMT. The shorter the pulse the faster the counter will operate. A photodiode (Fig. 21A.2(b)), is a more compact silicon semiconductor device which converts optical photons into many electron–hole pairs, again producing an electronic pulse. A conventional photodiode produces insufficient electron–hole pairs to provide energy measurement but this is overcome by using an avalanche photodiode (APD).

Gaseous detectors

Gaseous detectors are an alternative, low-cost method of detecting gamma rays. A gas-filled proportional counter (Fig. 21A.3) containing planes of wires connected to a high-voltage supply can detect the gas ionization produced by the gamma-ray interactions. The signals produced at the wires determine the position of the ionization and, in principle, the energy deposited in the chamber. Large-area, low-cost gas detectors have a spatial resolution determined by the wire spacing, ~1–2 mm. The gamma-ray detection efficiency depends on the gas pressure and Z value and these detectors are only really viable for detecting gamma rays with energies below 100 keV. For higher energy gamma rays gas detectors require some form of gamma-ray converter such as sheets of lead or high Z scintillation crystals.

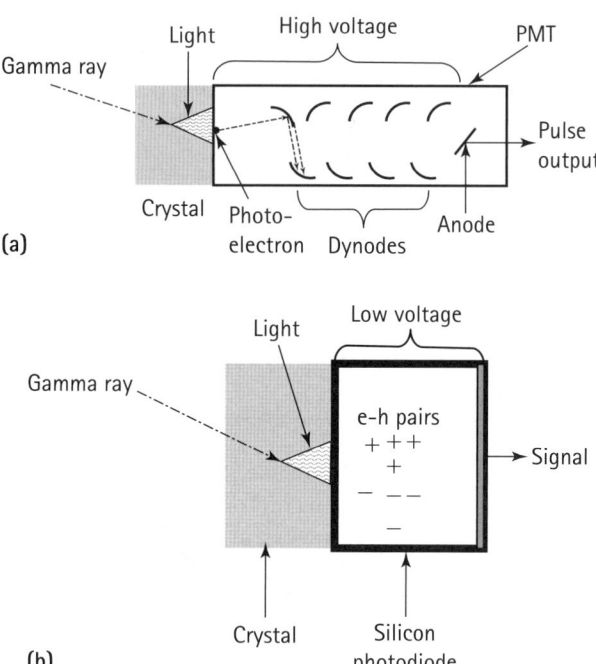

(a)

(b)

Figure 21A.2 *(a) A schematic diagram of a scintillation counter containing a photomultiplier (PMT). Light produced in the crystal is converted to a photoelectron in the photocathode at the front of the PMT. The photoelectron is accelerated via high voltage and multiple dynode collisions produce a substantial pulse at the anode. (b) The same device but using a photodiode. e–h, electron–hole.*

Semiconductor detectors

Semiconductor detectors are the third form of radiation detector in the form of semiconductor diodes which can be considered as a solid-state ionization chamber (Fig. 21A.2(b)) with the production of electron–hole pairs the method of energy transfer. The charge produced is collected by a low applied voltage and can provide an accurate measurement of the gamma-ray energy. A multi-pixel or micro-strip diode

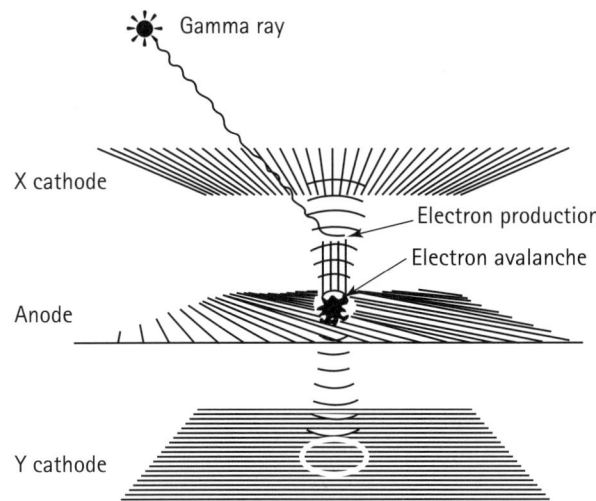

Figure 21A.3 *An example of a multiwire proportional chamber in which the incoming gamma ray induces ionization in the chamber gas. The ionization is amplified by the high voltage between the anode and cathodes and the resultant pulse detected on the cathode wires provides positional signals.*

array can produce images with sub-millimeter spatial resolution. The most common semiconductor material is silicon which has a low Z and poor detection efficiency at energies above 50 keV. Higher Z semiconductors include germanium and cadmium zinc telluride (CZT). Ge detectors have a reasonable detection efficiency above 100 keV but require cooling to reduce thermal noise. CZT is a room temperature semiconductor and can detect 140 keV photons with reasonable efficiency. One major advantage of a semiconductor is the large number of electron–hole pairs giving a high-energy resolution and efficient scatter rejection.

Detector dead-time limits

Detector dead-time limits the detector ability to count individual gamma rays at high count-rates depending upon the time taken to produce and process acceptable signals. Light emission from NaI(Tl) takes more than a microsecond and the amplification/digitization process can take several microseconds. Another gamma ray detected during this time produces a combined signal leading to the production of erroneous spatial and energy information. This effect is called pulse pile-up and at very high count-rates the system may become paralyzed and unable to count individual events (Fig. 21A.4). Electronics can be made insensitive to new events until the previous one has been processed, making the system non-paralyzable although it may saturate. Dead-time is effectively the minimum time required for the detector to count each pulse individually.

Detector performance comparisons are shown in Table 21A.2. Clearly, no one detector system is ideal but the

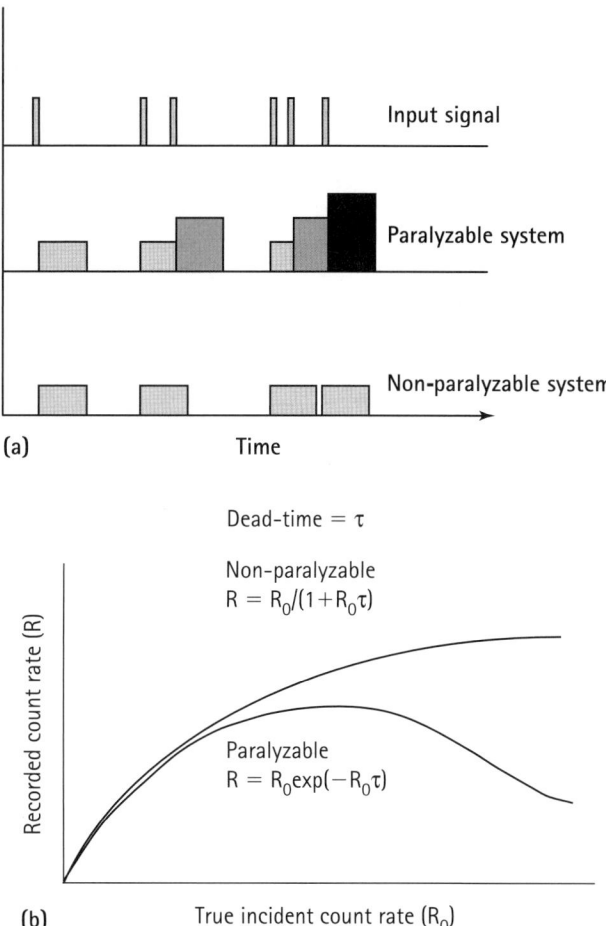

Figure 21A.4 *(a) The output from paralyzable and non-paralyzable detector systems for pulses from the detector. (b) The paralyzable system suffers from pulse pile-up and ultimately becomes incapable of counting whereas the non-paralyzable system loses counts and saturates at high count rates. τ = dead time.*

Table 21A.2 *Comparison of the properties of detector systems used for imaging*

Property	Scintillation counter	Gas detector	Semiconductor
Photon sensitivity	*High*	*Gas only: low Absorber: medium*	*Medium*
Spatial resolution	*~1–10 mm*	*1–2 mm*	*<1 mm*
Count rate limit	*100 kcps*	*100 kcps*	*100 kcps*
Size (one side)	*0.5–50 cm*	*10 cm to several meters*	*0.2–10 cm*
Application	*Gamma camera Positron camera Compton camera*	*Gamma camera Positron camera*	*Gamma camera Compton camera*
Cost	*Medium–high*	*Medium*	*Low–medium*

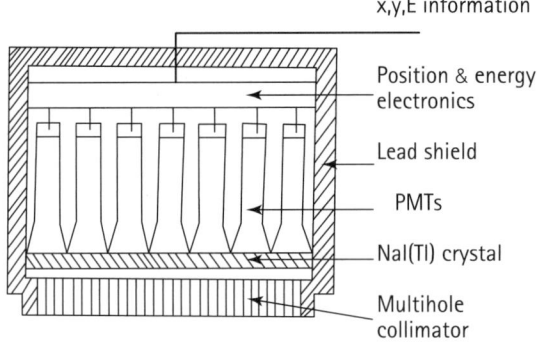

Figure 21A.5 *The main components of a gamma camera. Gamma rays passing through the collimator holes may interact in the crystal which produces light that is detected by photomultipliers (PMTs). The PMT outputs are analyzed by the associated electronics, and the positional and energy pulses are sent to a computer.*

majority of nuclear medicine imaging applications use the scintillation counter.

SINGLE–PHOTON IMAGING

The gamma camera

The workhorse of single-photon imaging is the gamma camera[2–4] which contains a thin, large-area NaI(Tl) crystal coupled on one face to an array of PMTs. The PMTs are connected to electronic circuitry providing positional and energy information used to create an image. The main components of the camera (Fig. 21A.5) are the collimator, the scintillation crystal, the PMTs, the position/energy logic, the camera shield and image display, usually a computer.

The collimator determines the direction of the incident photons allowed to strike the crystal and is, essentially, a thick sheet of lead penetrated by many fine holes. The hole sizes plus the septal and collimator thickness determine the camera sensitivity, spatial resolution and field of view. A parallel-hole collimator has the axes of the holes perpendicular to the camera front face (Fig. 21A.6(a)) allowing only gamma rays incident normal to the collimator surface to reach the crystal. The spatial resolution of several collimators used to image different photon energies is shown in Figure 21A.6(b). A pinhole collimator can be used for imaging small superficial organs and brain imaging is often performed with a fan- or cone-beam collimator to maximize the use of the camera sensitive area.

A parallel-hole collimator of thickness L, hole diameter d and source-to-collimator distance z, has a geometrical spatial resolution (R_c) given by

$$R_c \sim \frac{d(L + z)}{L}. \qquad (21A.1)$$

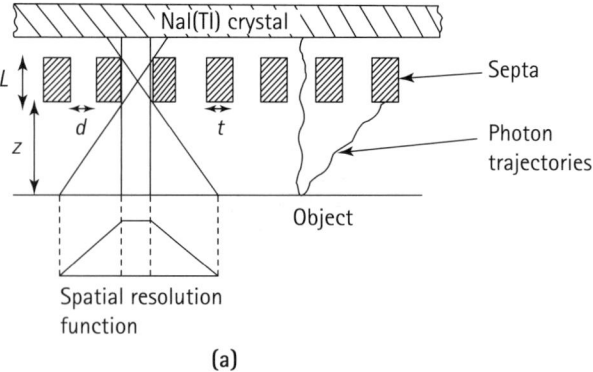

(a)

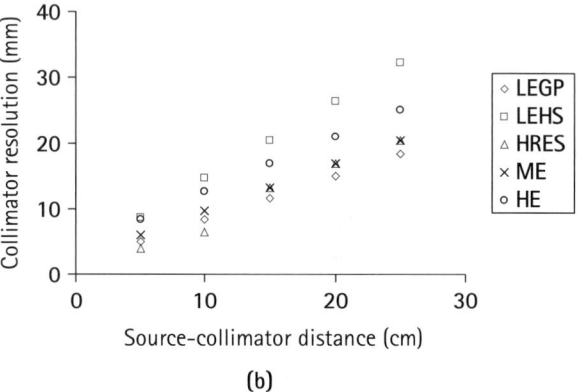

(b)

Figure 21A.6 *(a) How collimator spatial resolution and sensitivity are determined by hole diameter and length, septal thickness and the distance from collimator front surface. The wider the resolution function the worse the resolution but the better the sensitivity determined by the area of this function. (b) The resolution of five different kinds of parallel-hole collimators: (◇) low-energy general purpose; (□) low-energy high sensitivity; (△) high resolution; (×) medium energy; (○) high energy.*

Notice that spatial resolution is improved by increasing the hole length, by reducing the hole diameter and by minimizing the distance z. The intrinsic spatial resolution (R_i) is determined by the PMT information and is typically 3–4 mm. Combined with the R_c, the system spatial resolution (R_s) is

$$R_s = \left(R_i^2 + R_c^2 \right)^{1/2}. \qquad (21A.2)$$

From this it can be seen that R_s is dominated by R_c.

Collimator geometrical efficiency (g) is given by

$$g \propto \left[\frac{Kd^2}{L(d + t)} \right]^2 \qquad (21A.3)$$

where t is septal thickness and K depends upon hole shape. Note that g is not dependent on z. When $z \gg L$ and where $d \gg t$ the relationship becomes

$$g \propto R_c^2. \qquad (21A.4)$$

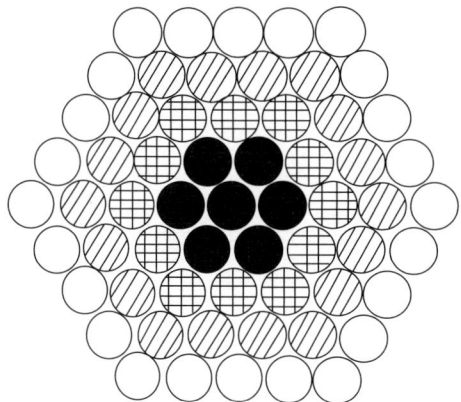

Figure 21A.7 *The hexagonal array of photomultipliers which gives optimal coverage with a circular or hexagonal crystal.*

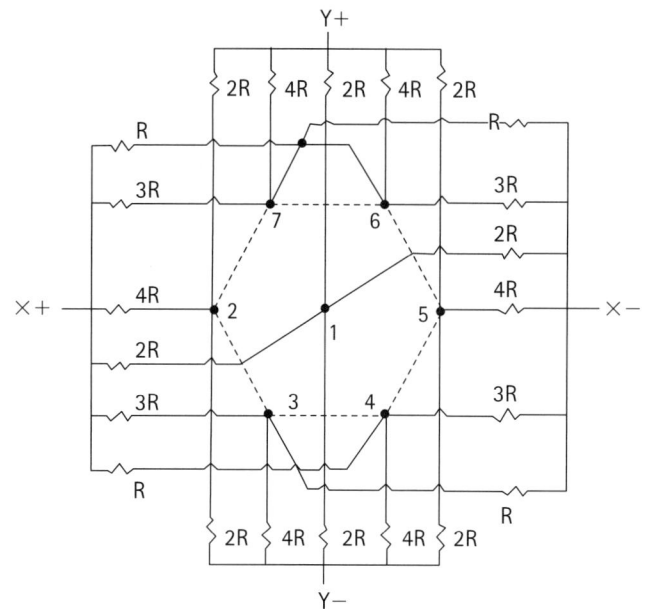

Figure 21A.8 *An example of a resistor network connected to the inner seven photomultipliers (PMTs) showing how X and Y positions are determined from current outputs. Note that the total resistance for each PMT connection is 4R in both X and Y.*

Hence, spatial resolution can only be improved at the expense of reduced sensitivity. Typically only one in a thousand gamma rays hitting the face of the collimator is detected.

Modern cameras usually contain a 50×40 cm^2 rectangular or 40 cm diameter, thin (9–15 mm) single NaI(Tl) crystal which emits 400–500 nm light matching the PMT response characteristics. A 10 mm thick NaI(Tl) crystal has 90% detection efficiency at 140 keV. The light-emission decay constant of 230 ns allows thousands of counts per second (kcps) to be acquired. Although it is hygroscopic and requires hermetic encapsulation, NaI(Tl) is unsurpassed for detecting gamma rays with energies close to 100 keV. The high light output gives an energy resolution of ~9–10% at 140 keV providing good scatter rejection.

The refractive indices of NaI(Tl) and the PMT glass face are 1.85 and 1.5, respectively, producing substantial non-uniform light collection across the face of the crystal. In the past this was minimized by using a light guide with refractive index close to 1.85 shaped to match the PMT to the crystal. Recently, this has been replaced by using microprocessors to correct for sensitivity variations across the field of view.

For cameras with circular crystals a close-packed hexagonal array of PMTs (Fig. 21A.7) is optimal. With 50 mm diameter PMTs the number used on a 40 cm diameter camera was limited to 37. Smaller-diameter (25–30 mm) PMTs enable 61 or 75 tubes to be used, improving spatial resolution. For rectangular crystals, square PMTs can be used. PMTs are chosen to have closely matched gain characteristics so that high-voltage/amplifier adjustments are simplified.

Traditionally, a capacitor or resistor-coupled network (Fig. 21A.8) provides positional and energy information from the PMT analog outputs. The relative PMT outputs determine the X, Y position and the sum gives the event energy (E). This methodology is referred to as 'Anger' or analog logic. Near the edge, one-sided PMT input leads to distortion or 'edge effects'. This part of the camera is usually excluded from the useful field of view reducing the effective size of the camera. E is evaluated using several

energy windows to determine how the signal matches that expected from the detected gamma ray(s).

Recently, low-cost microchip technology has provided a significant improvement in camera uniformity and stability. Although PMTs are 'matched', gain responses are never identical. Additionally, PMT outputs vary with the light intensity and the position where the light hits the photocathode producing spatial non-linearity. PMTs and the associated electronics are also sensitive to changes in temperature, magnetic field and aging and the camera response varies with the energy of the gamma ray detected. PMT gain drift can be minimized by exposure to a fixed light output from a light-emitting diode, for instance. The resultant signals can be stabilized by varying high-voltage or amplifier gain continuously. Stabilized signals can be corrected for spatial and energy response non-linearities. The former is achieved using a distortion map produced by imaging a linearity phantom to correct the measured X, Y positions. The energy response is minimized by using an energy-correction map generated by imaging a range of radionuclides. Further improvements can be achieved to correct for spatial variations in collimator/crystal response using uniform flood source images.

At high count rates, pulse pile-up can mean that the energy signal never returns to baseline causing event mispositioning or complete loss. Accurate signal integration performed with high-speed digitization and digital integration allows shorter integration times at higher count rates, reducing dead time and pulse pile-up.

Position sensitive PMTs (PSPMTs) coupled to crystal arrays can be used for high-resolution single-photon imaging;

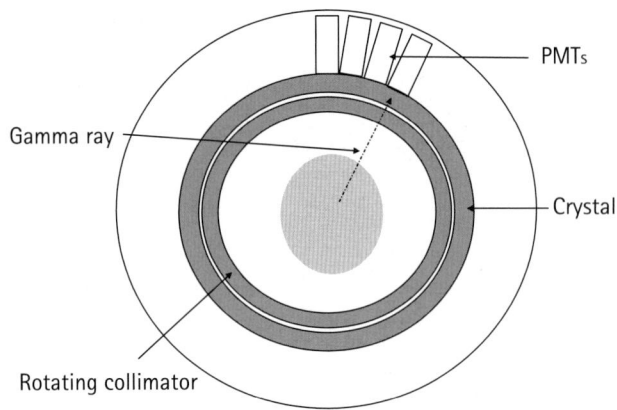

Figure 21A.9 *Outline of the CERASPECT special-purpose brain scanner with the continuous crystal and rotating collimator.*

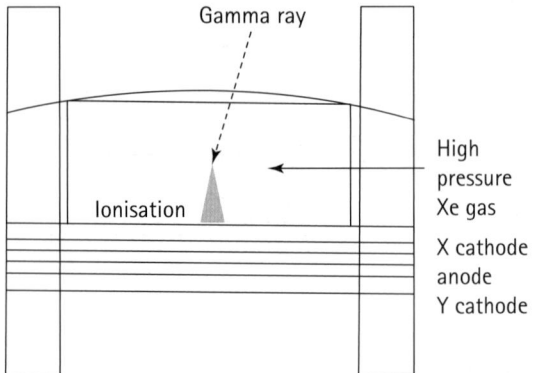

Figure 21A.10 *A multiwire proportional chamber gamma camera in which the gamma ray produces ionization in the high pressure gas which is detected by the wire planes producing positional information.*

for example, for breast imaging or laboratory studies. PSPMTs can localize where light hits the photocathode to a few millimeters allowing spatial resolutions of 1–2 mm to be achieved.[5] Alternatively, a charged coupled device (CCD) coated with 0.5 mm thick Gadox (Gd_2O_2S),[6] has been shown to have sub-millimeter intrinsic spatial resolution and acceptable detection efficiency at 140 keV.

Multi-crystal scanners for single photon emission computed tomography imaging

Dedicated single photon emission computed tomography (SPECT) scanners have been developed using scintillation counters coupled to focused collimators. The Aberdeen Section Scanner Mark II[7] had 24 detectors each attached to a 20 cm focal-length collimator, arranged in a square. The detectors moved tangentially and rotated through 95°. The single-slice spatial resolution was 9 mm within a plane thickness of 14 mm. A recent example designed for brain scanning is the CERASPECT system[8] which contains a single large donut-shaped NaI(Tl) crystal coupled to PMTs via a complex rotating collimator (Fig. 21A.9).

These devices produce either single or a few cross-sectional images with higher sensitivity and spatial resolution than a rotating gamma camera but lack the flexibility to perform planar, dynamic and multiplane SPECT compared to the camera, limiting their development.

Multiwire proportional chamber gamma cameras

Gas-filled detectors have played only a minor role in single-photon imaging. One system of note is the multiwire proportional chamber (MWPC) gamma camera[9] for imaging gamma rays with energy < 100 keV. The camera (Fig. 21A.10) uses high pressure (3–5 Torr) gas (90% xenon, 10% methane) encased in an aluminium pressure vessel with a thin entrance window. Photons ionize the gas and the signal

is detected by parallel wire planes, one anode and two cathodes. The cathode wires are oriented orthogonal to each other providing spatial information. The sensitive area is 25 cm in diameter and the detection efficiency is ~50–60% at 40 keV, falling to 10–15% at 100 keV. The intrinsic energy resolution at 60 keV is 33%, the count rate 850 kcps for a 50% dead-time loss and the intrinsic spatial resolution is ~2.5 mm full width at half maximum (FWHM). The detector can be used to image 50–100 keV gamma rays from ^{133}Xe, ^{201}Tl and ^{178}Ta, for example. A similar system[10] contains ~7.5 × 10^3 Torr (~10 bar) of xenon, has a sensitive area of 25 × 25 cm^2 and a useful sensitivity below 120 keV. The main advantage over crystal-based gamma cameras is the very high count-rate performance and the excellent intrinsic spatial resolution although a collimator will still dominate system resolution.

Semiconductor gamma cameras

The excellent energy resolution of germanium encouraged the development of small-scale semiconductor gamma cameras. The first germanium gamma camera[11] consisted of orthogonal electrical contact strips on a 10 mm thick slice of lithium-drifted germanium to form a detector with a 44 × 44 mm^2 area. The energy resolution was a few keV and the intrinsic spatial resolution 3 mm. A similar camera[12] (Fig. 21A.11) has a 30 × 30 × 5 mm^3 thick crystal giving an energy resolution of 5.5 keV and spatial resolution 1.7 mm. Further development of these devices has been limited by material cost and the need for cryogenics. Recently, CZT at room temperature has been assessed for single-photon imaging. A small CZT camera[13] for breast imaging has a sensitivity ~76% of a NaI(Tl) camera, an energy resolution of 6.5% at 140 keV and a system spatial resolution of <10 mm. The limitations with this material remain the ability to routinely produce large areas with consistent performance. However, semiconductor devices

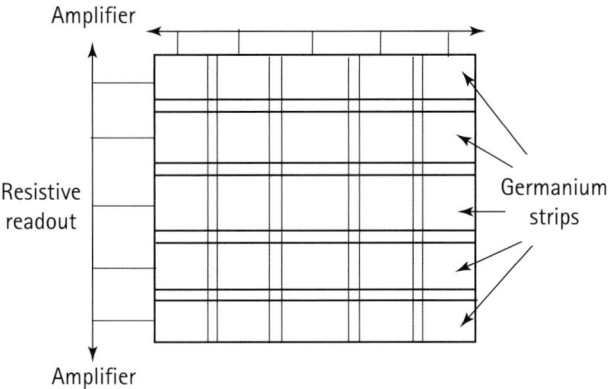

Figure 21A.11 *A schematic of a germanium strip gamma camera using resistive coupling to read out the position of strips hit by the gamma rays.*

have substantial potential for nuclear medicine imaging due to their intrinsic high energy and spatial resolution.

The Compton camera

One device which could overcome the poor sensitivity of a gamma camera/collimator system is the Compton gamma camera. Compton scatter of photons is governed by the relationship

$$\cos\theta = \frac{E - k\delta E}{E - \delta E} \qquad (21A.5)$$

where $k = 1 + m_0 c^2/E$, E is the photon energy, $m_0 c^2$ the electron rest mass, δE the photon energy loss during scatter and θ the photon scatter angle. Two detectors are used, one to scatter the incoming photon and the second to absorb the scattered photon. δE is measured by the first detector and $E - \delta E$ by the second. This information, plus the detection coordinates in the two detectors, allows the incident photon direction to be defined to a conical surface. The radioactive source distribution can, in principle, be obtained using iterative reconstruction techniques. A system[14] containing a 33 × 33 array of 5 × 5 × 6 mm³ thick high-purity germanium (HPGe) elements and an uncollimated gamma camera had a spatial resolution of ≈12 mm at 10 cm from the detector and ~15 times the sensitivity of a conventional collimated gamma camera. As the image reconstruction process introduces image noise, ~10 × events are required to provide similar image quality to a gamma camera. A new design based upon multiple scattering in germanium strip detectors[15] is now being assessed as part of a continued interest in this form of imaging.

POSITRON CAMERAS

Positron emission tomography[16] (PET) requires radionuclides which emit a positive electron (a positron). These

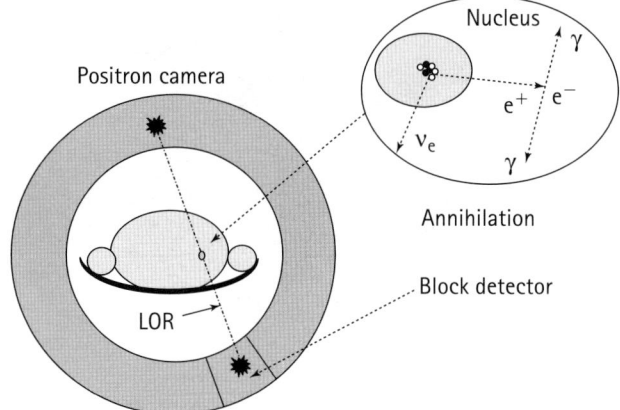

Figure 21A.12 *The annihilation coincidence process. The emitted positron travels a short distance in tissue, slowing down and interacting with an atomic electron. The two annihilation gamma rays, emitted almost back to back, are detected by detectors situated on opposite sides of the patient. If the two detectors give a signal within the resolving time of the camera the event coordinates are recorded in a computer. The event shown is called a 'true coincidence'.*

positrons interact with atomic electrons close to their emission point and, subsequently, annihilate producing two approximately co-linear 511 keV gamma rays. By detecting both gamma rays in fast time coincidence the line through/close to the position of the decaying nucleus can be defined (Fig. 21A.12). This process is annihilation coincidence detection (ACD) and the line is known as a line of response (LOR). Acquisition of millions of LORs allows the production of PET images.

Basic principles of positron emission tomography imaging

The device used for PET imaging is called a positron camera, which usually consists of a large number of scintillation counters surrounding the patient. The counters are made of high-Z, segmented scintillation crystal like BGO (Table 21A.1) connected to several PMTs. Positional information is determined using the PMT analog information. The camera will detect true coincidences where the radionuclide disintegration lies along/close to the LOR (Fig. 21A.13), scattered coincidences, where one or both gamma rays scatter in the patient, and random coincidence events, where the two detected gamma rays come from different radioactive decays – both the latter will produce spurious LORs (Fig. 21A.13). For a positron emitter at the center of the brain, >75% of gamma rays are scattered and for the body this figure is 90–95%. Virtually all first interactions in tissue at this energy are Compton scatters reducing the energy of the gamma rays detected. At 511 keV, a 30° scatter reduces the gamma-ray energy by ~10% and, as BGO has poor energy resolution, the camera cannot discriminate

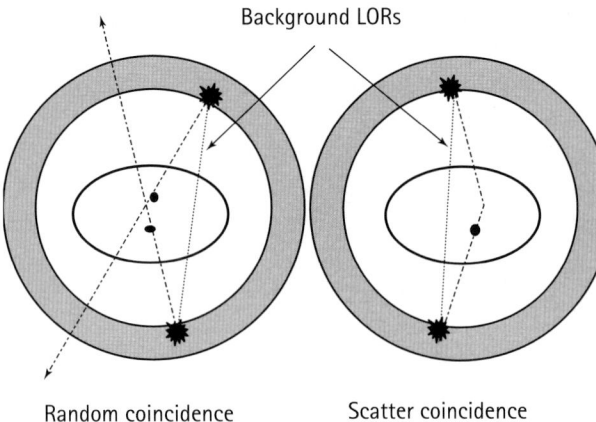

Figure 21A.13   *A random coincidence (left) occurs when single gamma rays from each of two separate radioactive decays are accidentally recorded within the resolving time of the camera. Scatter coincidences (right) occur when one or both of the gamma rays are scattered in the patient.*

against these scattered gamma rays. Additionally, ≈50% of gamma-ray detector interactions are Compton scatters resulting in partial energy deposition in the crystal. These events are detected in the correct position and should be retained. Use of a high-energy threshold will reject these events whereas too low a threshold will accept gamma rays scattered in the patient. In practice a compromise threshold is usually set between 250 and 400 keV. Scatter in PET images can be reduced by using crystals that produce more light than BGO giving a better energy resolution (Table 21A.1, page 850).

Positron camera intrinsic spatial resolution depends on the physics of ACD and on the detector properties. In the brain a resolution of ~4–5 mm FWHM can be obtained but 8–9 mm is more usual in the body. Fundamental limitations on spatial resolution are imposed by the positron range and the annihilation photon acollinearity. A low-energy positron from ^{18}F (E_{max} = 0.94 MeV) contributes a FWHM of 0.13 mm in tissue whilst for ^{82}Rb (E_{max} = 3.35 MeV) the FWHM is 0.42 mm. For body imaging the contribution to the resolution from annihilation photon acollinearity depends on the distance between the detectors and the annihilation point. For 100 cm separation, this contribution is ~2 mm. The main determinant of camera spatial resolution, however, is the size of the crystal elements. Brain imagers use 2 mm crystals and ~1 mm crystals are being used for laboratory imagers. For a whole-body camera crystal blocks are segmented into 4–5 mm elements. The camera spatial resolution is the quadrature combination of the effects of positron range, photon acollinearity and detector size. Note that body tissues other than the brain, move substantially (~5–10 mm) during imaging contributing significantly to the clinical image spatial resolution.

For detector signals of width τ, a coincidence is registered when two signals occur within the resolving time, which is

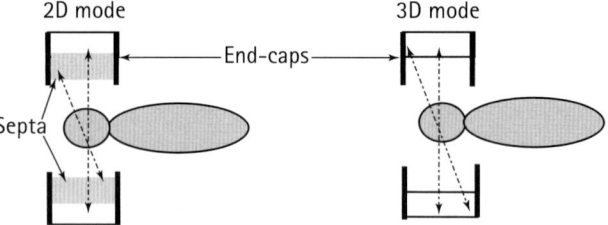

Figure 21A.14   *Two-dimensional positron emission tomography (PET) imaging is performed with interplane septa in place to reduce the number of scattered gamma rays detected. This also reduces the overall efficiency for wide-angle, true events. Three-dimensional imaging is performed with the septa withdrawn increasing the camera efficiency but making it more susceptible to scattered gamma rays and those from radioactivity outside the camera field of view.*

~2τ. The single gamma-ray detection rates (singles rates) are much larger than the coincidence rates due to activity outside the field of view (FoV), one of the gamma rays being undetected or scattered out of the camera or having an energy below the detection threshold. The randoms rate for a given detector pair is

$$R = 2\tau S_1 S_2, \tag{21A.6}$$

where S_1, S_2 are block singles rates. For any pair of blocks, the true coincidence rate (C) is given by

$$C = \varepsilon^2 S, \tag{21A.7}$$

where ϵ is the gamma-ray detection efficiency and S is the mean singles rate. The ratio of random to true events increases in proportion to S:

$$\frac{R}{C} = \frac{2\tau S^2}{\varepsilon^2 S} \sim S. \tag{21A.8}$$

At very high activity levels R/S will be very large. Randoms can be minimized by shielding the detectors from radioactivity outside the FoV and by using crystals with a fast light output so reducing τ.

Positron cameras with $\tau \sim 10^{-9}$s can be made using BaF_2 and CsF which have a fast light decay time. This time difference between two coincidence pulses can give source position uncertainties of ~9 cm. This can improve image quality by reducing background from gamma rays coming from activity outside the FoV. However, the noise reduction achieved is generally outweighed by the lower sensitivity of these crystals.

The sensitivity of a camera depends mainly on the detector sensitive area and on ϵ^2. In two-dimensional (2-D) PET imaging (Fig. 21A.14) detector rings are separated by lead or tungsten septa which absorb out-of-plane gamma rays, reducing scatter and random coincidences. Two-dimensional

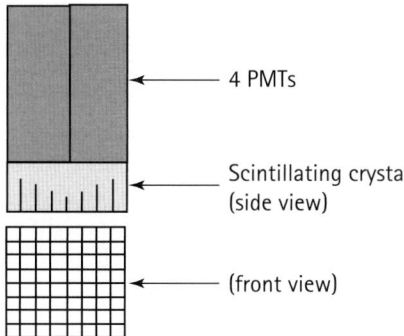

Figure 21A.15 *A 'block detector' consisting of a block of scintillation crystal connected to four photomultipliers (PMTs). The block is segmented so that the light detected by each PMT depends upon the position of the gamma-ray interaction in the crystal. By comparing the size of the PMT signals it is possible to estimate in which segment the gamma ray interacted.*

imaging produces images with a high signal-to-noise ratio (SNR) but at reduced sensitivity to gamma rays emitted at small angles to the patient axis. In the three-dimensional (3-D) mode the camera operates without septa and coincidences are accepted between all detector rings. The number of true coincidences detected is 5–10 times that of the 2-D mode but the camera is far more sensitive to scatter and random coincidences. Three-dimensional brain imaging provides a greater SNR than the 2-D mode but 3-D body imaging requires substantial background correction.

Examples of positron cameras

An example of a modern BGO-based positron camera is the CTI EXACT HR+.[17,18] Here the block detectors (Fig. 21A.15) are made of an 8×8 array of crystal elements, $4.39 \times 4.05 \times 30\,mm^3$ coupled to four PMTs. The elements are produced by cutting the crystal block to different depths allowing light sharing between PMTs. Retractable tungsten septa (0.8 mm thick, 66.5 mm long) separate detector rings and end shields minimize the detection of out-of-field activity gamma rays. The ECAT EXACT HR+ contains four rings of 72 BGO block detectors with a diameter of 82.7 cm and an axial FoV of 15.5 cm. The intrinsic spatial resolution is 4.3 mm FWHM on-axis degrading to 8.3 cm at 20 cm from the axis. This degradation is due to off-axis gamma rays entering the crystal sides. A trues coincidence count rate of ~200–300 kcps can be obtained with this camera.

NaI(Tl)-BASED DETECTORS

NaI(Tl)-based PET detectors have lower detection efficiency than BGO-based cameras but cost less. An example of this type of camera[19] consists of six curved plates of 2.5 cm thick NaI(Tl)/PMT segments in a ring 92 cm in diameter and 25 cm axially. The lower efficiency is partly offset by the long axial FoV. However, each segment must cope with a very high singles rate to produce a modest coincidence rate and the singles/true coincidence ratio may be ~100:1. The good energy resolution allows improved scatter rejection.

DUAL-HEADED GAMMA CAMERAS

Dual-headed gamma cameras operated in coincidence mode[20] have the advantage that the camera can be used for single-photon imaging and PET. Gamma cameras used for ACD have a thick (16–19 mm) NaI(Tl) crystal resulting in increased efficiency for 511 keV gamma rays with acceptable spatial resolution at 140 keV. However, the PET performance is poor due to the very high singles/true count ratio and minimization of dead time and randoms rates requires the use of ~1/3 of the radioactivity used with a BGO-based system.

New positron camera technology

Cerium-doped LSO and GSO are crystals[21,22] with abundant, fast light output as well as high detection efficiency (Table 21A.1). Cameras using these crystals have short resolving times (2τ ~6–8 ns) and low dead time, reducing randoms rates and providing higher true count rates. The high light output can improve detector energy resolution from ~25% with BGO to ~16% with GSO, enhancing scatter rejection.

AVALANCHE PHOTODIODES

PMTs are bulky, expensive and unstable and a reliable semiconductor light detector such as avalanche photodiodes (APDs) could be a replacement. APDs are photodiodes with increased internal gain produced by a larger electric field and provide pulses suitable for energy measurement. APD arrays can be bonded directly onto crystal arrays,[23] but they are still expensive per unit area and require temperature stabilization. Alternatively, PSPMTs can be connected to crystal arrays[24] for small cameras. Both systems provide crystal identification, uniformity of response and lower dead time compared to a block detector.

MULTI-MODALITY SYSTEMS

There is currently much interest in multi-modality systems. The prototype PET–SPECT camera[25] uses block-detector arrays mounted on a rotatable gantry. Each block contains a sandwich of LSO and NaI(Tl) connected to PMTs. The NaI(Tl) is used for SPECT; both crystals are used for PET, providing depth of interaction information. PET–CT systems[26] consisting of BGO/LSO or GSO-based positron cameras mounted co-axially and adjacent to a CT scanner can acquire functional PET images immediately after anatomical CT images. These systems provide excellent image registration

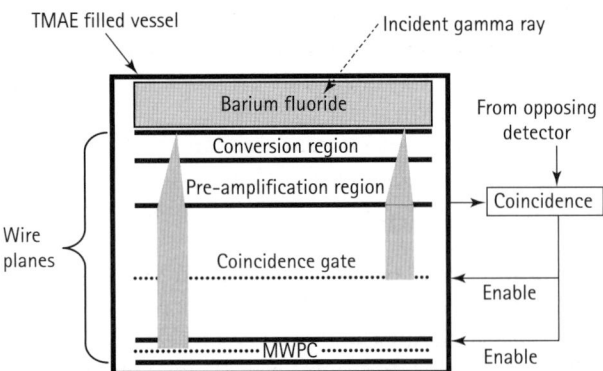

Figure 21A.16   *In the PETRRA camera a gamma-ray interaction in the barium fluoride crystal produces ultraviolet light that enters and ionizes the photosensitive gas, tetrakis methylaminoethylene (TMAE), in the wire chamber. Photoelectrons are produced which are multiplied by the gas to produce a signal. A coincident pulse from the opposing detector 'opens' the coincidence gate allowing the ionization through to the multiwire proportional chamber determining the ionization position.*

with the potential to improve PET quantification and the accuracy of diagnosis.

MULTIWIRE PROPORTION CHAMBER TECHNOLOGY

Several groups have developed positron cameras based on MWPC technology. For example, the PETTRA camera[27] incorporates BaF_2 crystals interfaced to a $60 \times 40\ cm^2$ wire chamber filled with the photosensitive gas, tetrakis dimethyl-amino ethylene (TMAE) (Fig. 21A.16). Ultraviolet light from the crystal photo-ionizes the gas and this ionization is localized by the wire planes. The sensitivity is lower than a BGO system but the camera has excellent timing resolution ($2\tau = 6\ ns$) and spatial resolution $\sim6.5\ mm$. This camera can be produced at lower cost than those with multiple PMTs.

SMALL HIGH-RESOLUTION POSITRON EMISSION TOMOGRAPHY SCANNERS

Small high-resolution PET scanners have been developed for laboratory imaging to help develop and assess new drugs. The CONCORDE microPET system contains units of 8×8 individual LSO crystals ($2 \times 2 \times 10\ mm^3$) read out though fiber optics by a PSPMT. The original camera[28] contained 30 detector units in a 17 cm diameter ring and had a spatial resolution of 2.0 mm. The most recent microPET camera[29] contains smaller crystals and will have a spatial resolution $\sim1\ mm$. The HIDAC MWPC camera[30] has produced images with a spatial resolution less than 1 mm. This camera incorporates a lead channel-plate converting gamma rays to electrons which are then multiplied and detected in an adjacent wire chamber. Similar technology to the PETRRA MWPC system has also been developed in the high-resolution (3 mm), small VUBPET scanner.[31]

SUMMARY

The continued development of new radiation detectors will surely lead to a greater use of semiconductors in nuclear medicine imaging. However, for the present, the scintillation counter remains the detector system of choice. It seems likely that a combination of techniques might be advantageous, combining the strengths of each to overcome present limitations.

REFERENCES

● Seminal primary article
◆ Key review paper

1   Birks JB. *The theory and practice of scintillation counting.* Oxford: Pergamon, 1964.
● 2   Anger HO. Scintillation camera. *Rev Sci Ins* 1958; **29**: 27–33.
◆ 3   Short MD. Gamma-camera systems. *Nucl Instrum Meth Phys Res* 1984; **221**: 142–9.
● 4   Ott RJ, Flower MA, Babich JW, Marsden PK. The physics of radioisotope imaging. In: Webb S. (ed.) *The physics of medical imaging.* Bristol and Philadelphia: Adam Hilger, 1988: 142–318.
5   Pani R, Pellegrini R, Cinti MN, *et al.* A novel compact gamma camera based on flat panel PMT. *Nucl Instrum Meth A* 2003; **513**: 36–41.
6   Lees JE, Fraser GW, Keay A, *et al.* The high resolution gamma imager (HRGI): a CCD based camera for medical imaging. *Nucl Instrum Meth A* 2003; **513**: 23–6.
7   Evans NTS, Keyes WI, Smith D, *et al.* The Aberdeen Mark II single-photon-emission tomographic scanner: specification and some clinical applications. *Phys Med Biol* 1986; **31**: 65–78.
8   Zito F, Savi A, Fazio F. CERASPECT: a brain-dedicated SPECT system. Performance evaluation and comparison with the rotating gamma camera. *Phys Med Biol* 1993; **38**: 1433–42.
9   Lacy JL, Le Blanc AD, Babich JW, *et al.* A gamma camera for medical applications, using a multiwire proportional counter. *J Nucl Med* 1984; **25**: 1003–12.
10   Barr A, Bonaldi L, Carugno G, *et al.* A high-speed, pressurised multi-wire gamma camera for dynamic imaging in nuclear medicine. *Nucl Instrum Meth A* 2002; **477**: 499–504.
11   McCready VR, Parker RP, Gunnerson EM, *et al.* Clinical tests on a prototype semiconductor gamma-camera. *Br J Radiol* 1971; **44**: 58–62.
12   Gerber MS, Miller DW, Schlosser PA, *et al.* Position sensitive gamma-ray detectors using resistive charge division readout. *IEEE Trans Nucl Sci* 1977; **NS-24**: 182–7.

13 Mueller B, O'Connor MK, Blevis I, *et al.* Evaluation of a small cadmium zinc telluride detector for scintimammography. *J Nucl Med* 2003; **44**: 602–9.

14 Sing M, Doria D. An electronically collimated gamma camera for single photon emission computed tomography. Part 1: Theoretical considerations in design criteria. Part 2: Image reconstruction and preliminary experimental measurements. *Med Phys* 1983; **10**: 421–35.

15 Hall CJ, Helsby WI, Lewis RA, *et al.* A nuclear medicine gamma-ray detector based on germanium strip detector technology. *Nucl Instrum Meth A* 2003; **513**: 47–50.

♦ 16 Ott RJ. Positron emission tomography: a view of the body's function. *Contemp Phys* 2003; **44**: 1–15.

17 Casey ME, Nutt R. A multicrystal 2-dimensional BGO detector system for positron emission tomography. *IEEE Trans Nucl Sci* 1986; **33**: 460–3.

18 Dahlbohm M, Hoffman EJ. An evaluation of a two-dimensional array detector for high-resolution PET. *IEEE Trans Med Imag* 1988; **7**: 264–72.

19 Karp JS, Muehllehner G, Geagan MJ, Freifelder R. Whole-body PET scanner using curve-plate (NaI:Tl) detectors. *J Nucl Med* 1998; **39**: 50P, A190.

20 Lewellen TK, Miyaoka RS, Swan WL. PET imaging using dual-headed gamma cameras: an update. *Nucl Med Commun* 1999; **20**: 5–12.

21 Daghighian F, Shenderov P, Pentlow KS, *et al.* Evaluation of cerium-doped lutetium oxyorthosilicate (LSO) scintillation crystal for PET. *IEEE Trans Nucl Sci* 1993; **40**: 1045–7.

● 22 Melcher CL, Schweitzer JS. Cerium-doped lutetium oxyorthosilicate – a fast, efficient new scintillator. *IEEE Trans Nucl Sci* 1992; **39**: 502–5.

23 Pichler B, Boning G, Lorenz E, *et al.* Studies with a prototype high resolution PET scanner based on LSO–APD modules. *IEEE Trans Nucl Sci* 1998; **45**: 1298–302.

24 Nagai S, Watanabe M, Shimoi H, *et al.* A new compact position-sensitive PMT for scintillation detectors. *IEEE Trans Nucl Sci* 1999; **46**: 354–8.

● 25 Schmand M, Dahlbohm M, Eriksson L, *et al.* Performance of a LSO/NaI(Tl) phoswich detector for a combined PET/SPECT imaging system. *J Nucl Med* 1998; **39**(suppl): 24.

● 26 Beyer T, Townsend DW, Brun T, *et al.* A combined PET/CT scanner for clinical oncology. *J Nucl Med* 2000; **41**: 1369–79.

♦ 27 Duxbury DM, Ott RJ, Flower MA, *et al.* Preliminary results from the new large-area PETRRA positron camera. *IEEE Trans Nucl Sci* 1999; **46**: 1050–4.

28 Cherry SR, Shao Y, Silverman W, *et al.* MicroPET: a dedicated PET scanner for small animal imaging. *J Nucl Med* 1996; **37**: 86P, A334.

29 Cherry SR, Shao Y, Slates RB, *et al.* MicroPET II – design of a 1 mm resolution PET scanner for small animal imaging. *J Nucl Med* 1999; **40**: 75P, A303.

30 Jeavons AP, Chandler RA, Dettmar CAR. A 3D HIDAC-PET camera with sub-millimetre resolution for imaging small animals. *IEEE Trans Nucl Sci* 1999; **46**: 468–73.

31 Bruyndonckx P, Liu XA, Tavernier S, Zhang SP. Performance study of a 3D small animal PET scanner based on BaF_2 crystals and a photo sensitive wire chamber. *Nucl Instrum Meth A* 1997; **392**: 407–13.

Image registration

GLENN FLUX AND GARY J.R. COOK

INTRODUCTION

In the course of diagnosis and treatment it is not uncommon for a patient to have a number of scans with various imaging modalities. Image registration (sometimes referred to as 'image co-registration' or 'image fusion') is the practice of aligning two or more image data sets so that a one-to-one spatial correspondence exists between voxel coordinates of each set. Image registration may be applied to image data acquired from different modalities or from the same modality, or may incorporate parametric image data derived from post-acquisition image processing. Although manual registration is employed, automatic or semi-automatic matching of image data relies on the determination of a 'cost function' – a measure of the mis-registration of two image sets that can be quantified and minimized. Image registration is of particular benefit to nuclear medicine as it enables functional image data to be visualized within the context of anatomical information available from computed tomography (CT) and magnetic resonance imaging (MRI). This facilitates localization of focal uptake, identification of normal and pathological regions, and precise volume determination.

CLASSIFICATION

Many methods of image registration have been devised with each having advantages and disadvantages that render them more or less applicable to certain modalities and imaging parameters. Various classification criteria have been devised to categorize registration methods.[1–5] By far the most common transformations used in medical imaging are inelastic (so-called rigid-body registration), whereby all points within one image set are transformed with identical parameters. Elastic registration, which allows deformation of one image set to match another, presents a larger number of problems. However, in principle, this is more suited to medical image data as anatomy is far from rigid, with the exception of isolated segments of bone structure. Registration of image data of the head is usually determined only with rigid techniques[6] although elastic deformations may be used to match brain image data to an atlas, or vice versa.[7] Breast image data are obvious candidates for elastic registration[8,9] although rigid-body techniques have also been applied.[10]

INHERENT REGISTRATION

A simple classification may be made by considering the process of acquiring data that is inherently registered as distinct from manipulating one image set to match the other. Examples of inherent registration include cases of two or more image sets acquired with multiple windows for single photon emission computed tomography (SPECT), emission/transmission imaging for SPECT and positron emission tomography (PET) and two or more image sets acquired simultaneously but with different sequences with MRI. A logical extension of this methodology can be seen with the advent of dual-modality scanners, in particular PET/CT and SPECT/CT[11,12] or by combining MRI and PET.[13] These systems should, in principle, provide the 'gold standard' for multimodality image registration.

In the absence of a dual-modality scanner, inherent image registration of mono- or multimodality image data may be achieved by ensuring that patient set-up and image acquisition parameters are identical for each scan, possibly with the aid of an external mask or frame.[14–20] Ideally, identical slice separations should be obtained for each scan although image re-slicing is possible to overcome this problem. This technique can be difficult to achieve and lacks flexibility, although it has the advantage that little or no post-acquisition data processing is required.

POINT, LINE, AND SURFACE-BASED REGISTRATION

In the absence of precise positional information on the image data at the time of acquisition, one or more common features must be identified in any two image sets to be registered to enable the transformation linking them to be determined post-acquisition. These features may be inherent within the patient data or, where this is not possible or reliable, may be specifically introduced for the purpose of registration. There are a number of possibilities.

An obvious technique for registration is to use corresponding points identified in each image set. A major advantage of this technique is that it is flexible, in that either internal (anatomical) landmarks may be used where these can be identified, or external markers suitable for the relevant modality may be attached to the patient. The solution to the so-called 'Procrustes problem' of determining the optimum transformation spatially linking two sets of points was elegantly solved by Arun et al.[21] using singular value decomposition.

Reliable identification of anatomical landmarks is feasible for high-quality anatomical scans of regions of the body that are relatively immobile. For example Hill et al.[22] used internal landmarks such as the centers of the cochlea for registering magnetic resonance and CT image data of the head for skull base surgery.

In the case of data with poor spatial resolution or lacking in reliably matching points external markers may be affixed to the patient. Whilst this method suffers from the disadvantage of the need for prospective action it benefits from the increased ease of marker localization and provides a method of determining the errors in registration. A number of external markers have been designed for the purpose.[23–28] To increase image contrast markers may contain, for example, ^{99m}Tc for SPECT scans, ^{68}Ge for a PET scan, gadolinium for MRI and barium chloride for CT.

An extreme example of the introduction of an extrinsic feature is the use of a stereotactic head frame, fixed to the patient either with screws into the skull or via a mouthbite.[15,16] The bars of the frame may be filled with a contrast agent suitable for the modality, providing a number of lines to be registered. This can be an extremely accurate method of registration[17,18] although it is, of course, an invasive procedure and thus generally applicable only if the frame is a necessary element of a patient's treatment.

A variety of other frames and masks have also been developed to enable image registration of the head.[19,20]

If the outline of either the patient or of a structure may be delineated on a number of slices in each of the image sets, these obtained surfaces may be used to determine the optimum transformation parameters required for registration.[29] This is a more simple task to carry out on CT or MRI data than on functional data and is more effective for registration of image data of the head. However, functional data of the thorax have also been registered, using, for example, the pleural surfaces of the lungs from PET scans,[30] by wrapping a fiducial band around the patient, filled with a suitable contrast agent,[31] or by using a scatter outline from SPECT data.[32]

In addition to points or surfaces, registration has also been implemented by matching lines. These may be external lines attached to masks or stereotactic frames[33] or principal axes obtained from an imaged organ such as the brain or myocardium.[34,35]

VOXEL PROPERTY-BASED REGISTRATION

A further possibility that has received increasing attention is to use the voxel intensity values themselves to determine the transformation parameters. A number of cost functions have been utilized for this purpose. Transformation parameters are not determined analytically, as in the cases outlined above, but instead an iterative optimization process is performed. Essentially, a cost function of the goodness-of-match of two image sets is computed and the image to be registered is iteratively perturbed either translationally or rotationally with the cost function being recalculated after each iteration until a minimum is attained. Various strategies are employed; for example, re-initializing the search from different starting configurations, to ensure that the final result is not a local minimum. The Powell minimization technique is frequently employed for this purpose.[36]

Variance of intensity ratios

It may be reasoned that in certain cases – time-sequential PET or SPECT scans of radionuclide uptake, for example – the intensity of corresponding voxel values should be identical except for physical decay, so that the ratio of intensity values between corresponding voxels should be constant. Woods et al.[37] introduced a method of registration whereby the cost function to be minimized was the standard deviation of the voxel ratios. This algorithm was extended to deal with registration of PET to MRI image data by assuming that a similar tissue type would result in voxels of similar intensity for either modality. A linear relationship should then exist between the groups of iso-intensity voxels and again the standard deviation between ratios of corresponding groups may be minimized.[38]

Sum of absolute differences

An intuitive measure of the mis-registration of two image sets is the difference between corresponding voxel intensities in each set. Eberl et al.[39] utilized the sum-of-absolute-differences criterion to register SPECT and PET brain phantom scans resulting in accuracy of -0.07 ± 0.46 mm (translation) and $-0.01 \pm 0.20°$ for rotation. The registration accuracy was degraded when SPECT and PET thoracic phantom scans were registered (3.1 ± 1.7 mm).

Image correlation

Image correlation has also been used as a basic criterion to generate cost functions. Bacharach et al.[40] used the correlation coefficient to register PET cardiac scans and achieved registration errors of less than 0.6 mm (translation) and less than 1.5° (rotation). Lin et al.[41] registered dynamic FDOPA PET scans using cross-correlation and achieved errors less than 1 mm. Acton et al.[42] reported a registration accuracy of 2–3 mm to register dynamic SPECT dopamine D_2 receptor brain images by using cross-correlation.

Mutual information

A common and frequently successful technique for registering nuclear medicine data is the use of mutual information. This parameter essentially gives the information held in one image set that is pertinent to another. Entropy-based criteria are highly data-independent and do not make assumptions as to the nature of the relation between the scans to be registered. Maes et al.[43] demonstrated sub-voxel accuracy of the mutual information method compared to stereotactic-frame registration for CT–MRI–PET brain registration. Studholme et al.[44] reported excellent robustness of the mutual information method to the initial starting point in MRI–PET brain registration. Sjogreen et al.[45] developed an automated technique, based on mutual information, to register whole-body emission–emission and emission–transmission scans achieving sub-pixel registration accuracy.

4-D registration

An extrapolation of registration methodology that is particularly relevant to nuclear medicine is its application to 4-D patient studies, as may be acquired for a time-sequential set of scans. In contrast to sequential voxel-based registration methods, 4-D methods compute the similarity criterion by taking into account the entire 4-D dataset simultaneously. Therefore, both the spatial and temporal relationships between the individual scans contribute to the criterion. Acton et al.[42] suggested a 4-D algorithm to register dynamic dopamine-D_2 SPECT series based on principal component analysis. Andersson and Thurfjell[46] described a 4-D mutual information-based method to register dynamic PET brain studies acquired at different time points.

Papvasileiou et al.[47] used the mean sum of squared errors in the least-squares fit algorithm to minimize the variance from a mono-exponential decay within each voxel within a chosen volume over time. This method was applied to 4-D SPECT data to achieve registration errors of less than 3.5 mm and demonstrated that image registration using 4-D can be simpler and more robust than 3-D techniques, particularly when multiple tumor sites with different decay rates are present.

CLINICAL APPLICATIONS OF IMAGE REGISTRATION

The main application of image registration to medical image data is to aid visualization and localization. For example, SPECT data of radionuclide uptake can be particularly difficult for the clinician to localize without the aid of registered anatomical data. Stokking et al.[48] compared observer agreement and confidence in localizing cerebral blood perfusion abnormalities in the peripheral cortex from viewing SPECT images in isolation or registered with MRI data. It was found that both confidence and inter-observer agreement were increased for registered 2-D data, and further increased for registered 3-D data. Mutual information registration has been used to register SPECT and MRI data of the knee to demonstrate that the degree of uptake of [166]Ho-ferric hydroxide macro-aggregates ([166]Ho-FHMA) was associated with the amount of synovitis.[49] Perault et al.[50] registered thoraco-abdominal dual-isotope SPECT data to CT using ^{99m}Tc-hydroxymethylene diphosphonate for bone tomo-scintigraphy and ^{111}In-pentetreotide and ^{131}I or ^{131}I-MIBG for tumor imaging. Overlay of regions of uptake onto the CT image enabled identification of tumor sites that may not have been suspected from CT alone and aided characterization of CT suspicious masses. Further uses have included the measurement of the 3-D distribution of deposition of a radiolabeled aerosol in the lung that could be compared to a computer model.[51] Notably, the uses of registration are not limited to relatively rigid regions but have been extensively applied to mobile regions, in particular the heart.[48–50] However, it should be noted that mis-registration can result in mis-interpretation of image data.[52–55]

Image registration is impacting on the field of radiotherapy planning, where the information from planning CT can be supplemented by functional as well as additional anatomical data.[56–63] The use of registered image data for radiotherapy was explored by Kessler et al.[33] who integrated MRI and PET with CT to alter the delineation of treatment volumes and critical structures in the brain. Adamietz et al.[64] combined SPECT data with CT and found that the therapeutic strategy was changed in seven out of 40 patients.

Image registration is increasingly being applied to the field of radionuclide therapy to aid dosimetry.[47,65] The calculation of absorbed dose to a tumor or critical organ following administration of a radiopharmaceutical is dependent on outlining the relevant volume of interest (VOI) on a series of time-sequential SPECT or planar scans. Consistency in delineation is facilitated by intra-modality registration. Registration also enables calculation of absorbed doses on a voxel-by-voxel basis. Thus a 3-D distribution of absorbed dose can be determined and visualized, eliminating errors due to incorrect outlines and circumventing gross assumptions regarding the heterogeneity of uptake.[66,67] It is then useful to register the resulting 'dose map' with anatomical CT or MRI scans.

An area of image registration having a significant clinical impact is in the relatively recent availability of combined PET/CT and SPECT/CT machines. Although PET/CT scanners have only been commercially available for a few years, current sales far outstrip PET-only scanners. There is mounting evidence that combined anatomical and functional data from these machines improves diagnostic accuracy, particularly in oncology.[68–70] Many authors comment on the increase in diagnostic certainty and fewer equivocal interpretations this combined modality allows. The advantages of each modality (functional sensitivity and specificity of ^{18}F-FDG PET and tissue contrast and high resolution anatomic information from CT) are maximized whilst the relative disadvantages (poor anatomic information of PET, lack of tumor specificity with CT) are minimized. In addition, the use of the low-noise CT data for attenuation correction of the PET data increases patient throughput by as much as 40%. Image registration of PET/CT is by no means perfect and there remain problems with misregistration of tissues near to the diaphragm due to differences in breathing protocols between the CT and PET components of the examination.[71] Work is under way to minimize these artifacts using respiratory gating and other techniques. Potentially, the clinical diagnostic impact from SPECT/CT will be even greater given the poorer resolution and image quality compared to PET. SPECT/CT machines are now also commercially available.

CONCLUSION

Although the use of image registration with clinical image data was initially limited to visualization, further clinical applications continue to emerge. Notable among these at present, and those likely to have a large clinical impact, are the inclusion of various modalities (functional as well as anatomical) for external-beam radiotherapy treatment planning and registration of time-sequential functional data to enable patient-specific 3-D dosimetry for targeted radionuclide therapy.

However, some problems are yet to be fully resolved. The accuracy of image registration, for example, can be difficult to estimate reliably since the parameter judged to provide the most reliable estimate of the error should by definition be that which is used to provide the cost function for registration. The relative accuracy of two methods of registration can therefore be difficult to determine, although in many cases a number of different techniques will produce similar results. It should also be noted that whilst an image registration technique may prove to have a high degree of accuracy in phantom data, the accuracy of the method when applied to patient data is limited by anatomical movement. The brain, for example, can move within the skull by as much as 3 mm.[17] It is recommended that the user visually monitors results, since severe registration errors are always possible.[72] In some cases interactive registration is preferred[73] and it can be argued that in some circumstances this can be quicker and more accurate than using computer-based algorithms.[74] In general, although a large number of registration methods have been devised, the optimum technique for any given case is not well defined and continues to be subject to debate.

Despite the issues concerning registration methodology and verification, image registration and multimodality imaging is a continually expanding field of study that is having a major impact in clinical environments in the course of diagnosis and treatment (see Plate 21B.1).

REFERENCES

● Seminal primary article
◆ Key review paper

◆ 1   Brown LG. A survey of image registration techniques. *Computing Surveys* 1992; **24**: 325–76.

◆ 2   Maurer CR, Fitzpatrick JM. A review of medical image registration. In: Maciunas RJ. (ed.) *Interactive image-guided neurosurgery*. Parkridge, IL: American Association of Neurological Surgeons, 1993: 17–44.

◆ 3   van den Elsen PA, Pol EJD, Viergever MA. Medical image matching – a review with classification. *IEEE Eng Med Biol Magazine* 1993; **12**: 26–39.

◆ 4   Lavallee S. Registration for computer-integrated surgery: methodology, state of the art. In: Taylor RH, Lavallee S, Burdea GC, Mösges R. (eds.) *Computer-integrated surgery*. Cambridge, MA: MIT Press, 1996: 77–97.

◆ 5   Maintz JBA, Viergever MA. A survey of medical image registration. *Medical Image Analysis* 1998; **2**: 1–36.

6   Ge YR, Fitzpatrick JM, Votaw JR, *et al.* Retrospective registration of PET and MR brain images – an algorithm and its stereotaxic validation. *J Comput Assist Tomog* 1994; **18**: 800–10.

7   Rizzo G, Scifo P, Gilardi MC, *et al.* Matching a computerized brain atlas to multimodal medical images. *Neuroimage* 1997; **6**: 59–69.

8   Rueckert D, Sonoda LI, Hayes C, *et al.* Nonrigid registration using free-form deformations: application

to breast MR images. *IEEE Trans Med Imag* 1999; **18**: 712–21.

9   Bruckner T, Lucht R, Brix G. Comparison of rigid and elastic matching of dynamic magnetic resonance mammographic images by mutual information. *Med Phys* 2000; **27**: 2456–61.

10 Meyer CR, Boes JL, Kim B, *et al.* Semiautomatic registration of volumetric ultrasound scans. *Ultrasound Med Biol* 1999; **25**: 339–47.

11 Bocher M, Balan A, Krausz Y, *et al.* Gamma camera-mounted anatomical X-ray tomography: technology, system characteristics and first images. *Eur J Nucl Med* 2000; **27**: 619–27.

12 Beyer T, Townsend DW, Brun T, *et al.* A combined PET/CT scanner for clinical oncology. *J Nucl Med* 2000; **41**: 1369–79.

13 Shao Y, Cherry SR, Farahani K, *et al.* Development of a PET detector system compatible with MRI/NMR systems. *IEEE Trans Nucl Sci* 1997; **44**: 1167–71.

14 Meltzer CC, Bryan RN, Holcomb HH, *et al.* Anatomical localization for PET using MR imaging. *J Comput Assist Tomog* 1990; **14**: 418–26.

● 15 Bergstrom M, Boethius J, Eriksson L, *et al.* Head fixation device for reproducible position alignment in transmission CT and positron emission tomography. *J Comput Assist Tomog* 1981; **5**: 136–41.

16 Mazziotta JC, Phelps ME, Miller J, Kuhl DE. Tomographic mapping of human cerebral metabolism – normal unstimulated state. *Neurology* 1981; **31**: 503–16.

17 Greitz T, Bergstrom M, Boethius J, *et al.* Head fixation system for integration of radiodiagnostic and therapeutic procedures. *Neuroradiology* 1980; **19**: 1–6.

18 Lemieux L, Kitchen ND, Hughes SW, Thomas DGT. Voxel-based localization in frame-based and frameless stereotaxy and its accuracy. *Med Phys* 1994; **21**: 1301–10.

19 Fox PT, Perlmutter JS, Raichle ME. A stereotactic method of anatomical localization for positron emission tomography. *J Comput Assis Tomog* 1985; **9**: 141–53.

20 Miura S, Kanno I, Iida H, *et al.* Anatomical adjustments in brain positron emission tomography using CT images. *J Comput Assist Tomog* 1988; **12**: 363–7.

● 21 Arun KS, Huang TS, Blostein SD. Least-squares fitting of 2 3-D point sets. *IEEE Trans Pattern Analysis and Machine Intelligence* 1987; **9**: 699–700.

22 Hill DLG, Hawkes DJ, Hussain Z, *et al.* Accurate combination of CT and MR data of the head – validation and applications in surgical and therapy planning. *Computerized Medical Imaging and Graphics* 1993; **17**: 357–63.

23 Malison RT, Miller EG, Greene R, *et al.* Computer-assisted coregistration of multislice SPECT and MR brain images by fixed external fiducials. *J Comput Assist Tomog* 1993; **17**: 952–60.

24 van den Elsen PA, Viergever MA. Marker guided registration of electromagnetic dipole data with tomographic images. *Lecture Notes in Computer Science* 1991; **511**: 142–53.

25 Wang MY, Maurer CR, Fitzpatrick JM, Maciunas RJ. An automatic technique for finding and localizing externally attached markers in CT and MR volume images of the head. *IEEE Trans Biomed Eng* 1996; **43**: 627–37.

26 Papavasileiou P, Flux GD, Flower MA, Guy MJ. An automated technique for SPECT marker-based image registration in radionuclide therapy. *Phys Med Biol* 2001; **46**: 2085–97.

27 Papavasileiou P, Flux GD, Flower MA, Guy MJ. A fully-automated image registration method for I-131-MIBG radionuclide therapy using external markers. *J Nucl Med* 2000; **41**: 825.

28 Papavasileiou P, Flux GD, Flower MA, Guy MJ. Automated CT marker segmentation for image registration in radionuclide therapy. *Phys Med Biol* 2001; **46**: N269–79.

29 Pelizzari CA, Chen GTY, Spelbring DR, *et al.* Accurate 3-dimensional registration of CT, PET, and or MR images of the brain. *J Comput Assist Tomog* 1989; **13**: 20–6.

30 Yu JN, Fahey FH, Gage HD, *et al.* Intermodality, retrospective image registration in the thorax. *J Nucl Med* 1995; **36**: 2333–8.

31 Scott AM, Rosa E, Mehta BM, *et al.* In-vivo imaging and specific targeting of p-glycoprotein expression in multidrug-resistant nude-mice xenografts with I-125 MRK-16 monoclonal antibody. *Nucl Med Biol* 1995; **22**: 497–504.

32 Sjogreen K, Ljungberg M, Erlandsson K, *et al.* Registration of abdominal CT and SPECT images using Compton scatter data. *Information Processing in Medical Imaging* 1997; **1230**: 232–44.

● 33 Kessler ML, Pitluck S, Petti P, Castro JR. Integration of multimodality imaging data for radiotherapy treatment planning. *Int J Radiat Oncol Biol Phys* 1991; **21**: 1653–67.

34 He ZX, Maublant JC, Cauvin JC, Veyre A. reorientation of the left-ventricular long-axis on myocardial transaxial tomograms by a linear fitting method. *J Nucl Med* 1991; **32**: 1794–800.

35 Rusinek H, Tsui WH, Levy AV, *et al.* Principal axes and surface fitting methods for 3-dimensional image registration. *J Nucl Med* 1993; **34**: 2019–24.

● 36 Powell MJD. An efficient method for finding the minimum of a function of several variables without calculating derivatives. *Comput J* 1964; **7**: 155–62.

37 Woods RP, Cherry SR, Mazziotta JC. Rapid automated algorithm for aligning and reslicing pet images. *J Comput Assist Tomog* 1992; **16**: 620–33.

38   Woods RP, Mazziotta JC, Cherry SR. MRI–PET registration with automated algorithm. *J Comput Assist Tomog* 1993; **17**: 536–46.

39   Eberl S, Kanno I, Fulton RR, *et al.* Automated interstudy image registration technique for SPECT and PET. *J Nucl Med* 1996; **37**: 137–45.

40   Bacharach SL, Douglas MA, Carson RE, *et al.* 3-dimensional registration of cardiac positron emission tomography attenuation scans. *J Nucl Med* 1993; **34**: 311–21.

41   Lin KP, Huang SC, Yu DC, *et al.* Automated image registration for FDOPA PET studies. *Phys Med Biol* 1996; **41**: 2775–88.

42   Acton PD, Pilowsky LS, Suckling J, *et al.* Registration of dynamic dopamine D-2 receptor images using principal component analysis. *Eur J Nucl Med* 1997; **24**: 1405–12.

43   Maes F, Collignon A, Vandermeulen D, *et al.* Multimodality image registration by maximization of mutual information. *IEEE Trans Med Imag* 1997; **16**: 187–98.

44   Studholme C, Hill DLG, Hawkes DJ. Automated three-dimensional registration of magnetic resonance and positron emission tomography brain images by multiresolution optimization of voxel similarity measures. *Med Phys* 1997; **24**: 25–35.

45   Sjogreen K, Ljungberg M, Wingardh K, *et al.* Registration of emission and transmission whole-body scintillation-camera images. *J Nucl Med* 2001; **42**: 1563–70.

46   Andersson JLR, Thurfjell L. Implementation and validation of a fully automatic system for intra- and interindividual registration of PET brain scans. *J Comput Assist Tomog* 1997; **21**: 136–44.

47   Papavasileiou P, Flux GD, Guy MJ, Flower MA. A novel four-dimensional image registration method for radionuclide therapy dosimetry. *Phys Med Biol* 2004; **49**: 5373–91.

48   Stokking R, Studholme C, Spencer SS, *et al.* Multimodality 3D visualization of SPECT difference and MR images in epilepsy. *J Nucl Med* 1999; **40**: 1270.

49   Vuorela J, Kauppinen T, Sokka T. Distribution of radiation in synovectomy of the knee with Ho-166-FHMA using image fusion. *Cancer Biother Radiopharm* 2005; **20**: 333–7.

50   Perault C, Schvartz C, Wampach H, *et al.* Thoracic and abdominal SPECT–CT image fusion without external markers in endocrine carcinomas. *J Nucl Med* 1997; **38**: 1234–42.

51   Perring S, Summers Q, Fleming JS, *et al.* A new method of quantification of the pulmonary regional distribution of aerosols using combined CT and SPECT and its application to nedocromil sodium administered by metered-dose inhaler. *Br J Radiol* 1994; **67**: 46–53.

52   Makela T, Clarysse P, Sipila O, *et al.* A review of cardiac image registration methods. *IEEE Trans Med Imag* 2002; **21**: 1011–21.

53   Nakajo H, Kumita S, Cho K, Kumazaki T. Three-dimensional registration of myocardial perfusion SPECT and CT coronary angiography. *Ann Nucl Med* 2005; **19**: 207–15.

54   Nishimura Y, Fukuchi K, Katafuchi T, *et al.* Superimposed display of coronary artery on gated myocardial perfusion scintigraphy. *J Nucl Med* 2004; **45**: 1444–9.

55   Loghin C, Sdringola S, Gould KL. Common artifacts in PET myocardial perfusion images due to attenuation–emission misregistration: clinical significance, causes, and solutions. *J Nucl Med* 2004; **45**: 1029–39.

56   Ciernik IF, Huser M, Burger C, *et al.* Automated functional image-guided radiation treatment planning for rectal cancer. *Int J Radiat Oncol Biol Phys* 2005; **62**: 893–900.

57   Fox JL, Rengan R, O'Meara W, *et al.* Does registration of PET and planning CT images decrease interobserver and intraobserver variation in delineating tumor volumes for non-small-cell lung cancer? *Int J Radiat Oncol Biol Phys* 2005; **62**: 70–5.

58   Paulino AC, Koshy M, Howell R, *et al.* Comparison of CT- and FDG-PET-defined gross tumor volume in intensity-modulated radiotherapy for head-and-neck cancer. *Int J Radiat Oncol Biol Phys* 2005; **61**: 1385–92.

59   Van Der Wel A, Nijsten S, Hochstenbag M, *et al.* Increased therapeutic ratio by (18)FDG-PET CT planning in patients with clinical CT stage N2N3M0 non-small-cell lung cancer: a modeling study. *Int J Radiat Oncol Biol Phys* 2005; **61**: 649–55.

60   Gabriele P, Malinverni G, Moroni GL, *et al.* The impact of F-18-deoxyglucose positron emission tomography on tumor staging, treatment strategy and treatment planning for radiotherapy in a department of radiation oncology. *Tumori* 2004; **90**: 579–85.

61   Vrieze O, Haustermans K, De Wever W, *et al.* Is there a role for FGD-PET in radiotherapy planning in esophageal carcinoma? *Radiother Oncol* 2004; **73**: 269–75.

62   Lee YK, Cook G, Flower MA, *et al.* Addition of F-18-FDG-PET scans to radiotherapy planning of thoracic lymphoma. *Radiother Oncol* 2004; **73**: 277–83.

63   Grosu AL, Lachner R, Wiedenmann N, *et al.* Validation of a method for automatic image fusion (BrainLAB System) of CT data and C-11-methionine-PET data for stereotactic radiotherapy using a linac: first clinical experience. *Int J Radiat Oncol Biol Phys* 2003; **56**: 1450–63.

64   Adamietz IA, Baum RP, Schemman F, *et al.* Improvement of radiation treatment planning in squamous-cell head and neck cancer by immuno-SPECT. *J Nucl Med* 1996; **37**: 1942–6.

65   Sjogreen K, Ljungberg M, Wingardh K, *et al.* The LundADose method for planar image activity quantification and absorbed-dose assessment in radionuclide therapy. *Cancer Biother Radiopharm* 2005; **20**: 92–7.

66   Sgouros G, Kolbert KS, Sheikh A, *et al.* Patient-specific dosimetry for I-131 thyroid cancer therapy using I-124 PET and 3-dimensional–internal dosimetry (3D–ID) software. *J Nucl Med* 2004; **45**: 1366–72.

67 Flux GD, Webb S, Ott RJ, *et al.* Three-dimensional dosimetry for intralesional radionuclide therapy using mathematical modeling and multimodality imaging. *J Nucl Med* 1997; **38**: 1059–66.

68 Hany TF, Steinhart H, Goerres G, *et al.* PET diagnostic accuracy: improvement with in-line PET-CT system: initial results. *Radiology* 2002; **225**: 575–81.

69 Lardinois D, Weder W, Hany TF, *et al.* Staging of non-small-cell lung cancer with integrated positron-emission tomography and computed tomography. *N Engl J Med* 2003; **348**: 2500–7.

70 Israel O, Mom M, Guralnik L, *et al.* Is ^{18}F-FDG PET/CT useful for imaging and management of patients with suspected occult recurrence of cancer? *J Nucl Med* 2004; **45**: 2045–51.

71 Cook GJ, Wegner E, Fogleman I. Pitfalls and artefacts in [18]FDG PET and PET/CT oncologic imaging. *Semin Nucl Med* 2004; **34**: 122–33.

72 West J, Fitzpatrick JM, Wang MY, *et al.* Comparison and evaluation of retrospective intermodality brain image registration techniques. *J Comput Assist Tomog* 1997; **21**: 554–66.

73 Habboush IH, Mitchell KD, Mulkern RV, *et al.* Registration and alignment of three-dimensional images: an interactive visual approach. *Radiology* 1996; **199**: 573–8.

74 Pfluger T, Vollmar C, Wismuller A, *et al.* Quantitative comparison of automatic and interactive methods for MRI–SPECT image registration of the brain based on 3-dimensional calculation of error. *J Nucl Med* 2000; **41**: 1823–9.

Attenuation correction in positron emission tomography and single photon emission computed tomography

DALE L. BAILEY

INTRODUCTION

Attenuation correction of emission data in single photon emission computed tomography (SPECT) and positron emission tomography (PET) based on measured transmission data is now accepted as being an improvement over reviewing non-attenuation corrected emission reconstructions. Not only does attenuation correction suppress artifacts in the emission reconstruction but it improves the recovered radio-concentration of tracer from all, and especially deep, regions of the body as well as providing potentially quantitative (kBq mL^{-1}) tomographic emission estimates.

Correction for attenuation can also be applied to planar or conjugate view (e.g. anterior/posterior) data from the gamma camera although this is not very accurate, and of course there is remaining overlying radioactivity. The reader is referred to the following papers by Fleming,[1] Macey and Marshall[2] and Myers et al.[3] for more information on planar corrections. The technology and application of attenuation correction in emission tomography will be the subject of this chapter.

PHOTON ATTENUATION, SCATTERING AND INTERACTION WITH MATTER

Photons with energies in the range 0.1–1.0 MeV predominantly interact with matter via the Compton effect. At energies below this level the photoelectric effect dominates and at energies in the GeV range pair production is the dominant mode of interaction. The physical basis of the Compton effect is utilized in a number of correction schema. The Compton process is shown in Fig. 21C.1. A photon interacts with a loosely bound electron and imparts sufficient energy to it to overcome its binding potential. The atom is ionized and the electron is ejected from the atom.

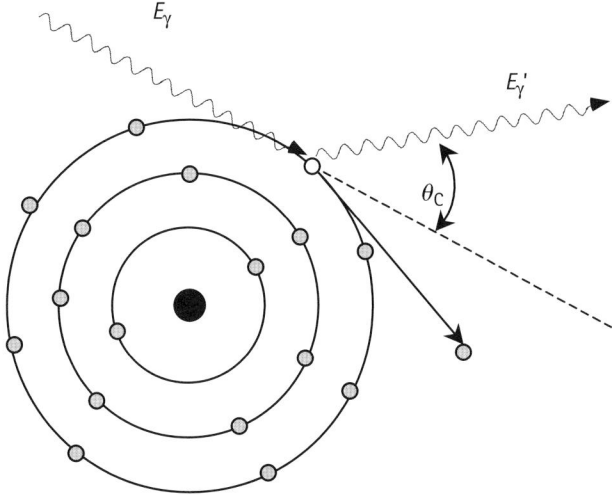

Figure 21C.1 *In the Compton effect an incoming photon interacts with a weakly bound orbital electron and displaces it from the atom (ionization). The photon is deflected through a scattering angle and loses energy in this process.*

The photon undergoes a change of angle and loss of energy, which can be calculated from the Compton equation

$$E'_\gamma = \frac{E_\gamma}{1 + \left(\dfrac{E_\gamma}{m_0 c^2} \right)(1 - \cos \theta_C)} \qquad (21C.1)$$

where E_γ is the incoming photon energy, E'_γ is the resultant photon energy after the interaction, m_0 is the mass of the electron, c is the speed of light and θ_C is the scattering angle. It can be readily calculated from this that a 45° scattering angle for photons with incident energies of 140 and 511 keV results in scattered photons with energies of 130 and 395 keV, respectively. This is often within the energy window set on the gamma camera or PET system due to the limited energy resolution (typically 10–25% full width at half maximum) of the scintillation detectors that are used. In SPECT and three-dimensional PET scatter may constitute 30–50% of the signal recorded and thus correction for scatter as well as attenuation is essential for quantitative measurements.[4]

MEASURING TRANSMISSION: THE KEY TO ACCURATE ATTENUATION CORRECTION

Transmission scanning with nuclear medicine instrumentation has been performed since the mid-1960s.[5–7] Initially, it was done to provide coarse anatomical detail – an early example of multi-modality imaging. In the 1970s and first half of the 1980s it was used to provide data for attenuation correction in the low density lungs based on planar geometric mean emission images[1,2] and for quantification in general.[8,9] In PET, however, it has been used in conjunction with the emission data for attenuation correction from the development of the earliest systems. This is because, as will be seen later in this chapter, correction for attenuation with coincidence annihilation radiation is more straightforward than it is for the single photon case.[10,11] Transmission scanning for the purposes of attenuation correction in SPECT was developed by research groups in the mid-1980s, and introduced into clinical practice by commercial suppliers in the mid-1990s.

There have been numerous attempts to correct for attenuation in SPECT using the emission data alone, i.e. without measuring the photon transmission through the subject. These methods include simple approaches such as the use of elliptical contours to approximate the body outline containing an assumed single 'average' attenuation coefficient throughout, through the more sophisticated iterative methods such as those proposed by Chang,[12] to the more recent attempts to use the inconsistency between the projection data at different angles to estimate the attenuation.[13,14] While interesting and of great potential value, if this can be achieved, the former remain limited to qualitative applications at present and the latter is still work-in-progress.

The problem of attenuation correction in emission tomography can be put very simply: it is comparable to trying to use only one measurement (the attenuated emission data) to solve an equation with two unknowns (emission radionuclide distribution and density/attenuation). By measuring transmission a second measurement is added in an attempt to 'disengage' the effect of attenuation from estimating the unknown radionuclide distribution. For this reason, measuring transmission through the subject for the purposes of attenuation correction, in spite of the added cost and some extra complication, is now the most common method used to provide accurate quantitative reconstructions in both SPECT and PET.

Transmission scanning in SPECT

The first attempts to measure transmission for attenuation correction with rotating gamma cameras all utilized a flood tank or sheet source of radioactivity for the transmission measurement.[15–17] These proved impractical due to the high scatter contamination from the emission nuclide into the transmission measurement, or the need for two separate studies. Two approaches appeared at the end of the 1980s which used a combination of geometrical collimation and pulse height energy discrimination to solve much of the contamination problem. On single- and dual-headed gamma cameras a scanning transmission line source could be used with parallel-hole collimators to reduce scatter contamination and provide good quality transmission measurements.[18] On triple-headed SPECT systems a focusing fan beam collimator could be used on one of the heads with a line source for measuring transmission placed at the focus.[19] The geometry of these systems is shown in Fig. 21C.2.

Table 21C.1 compares the two main SPECT transmission scanning systems. The key to the success of these systems was that they afforded the ability for *simultaneous* measurements of the emission and transmission data.

Gadolinium-153 has been widely used as a transmission source in SPECT. It had previously been used as a transmission source on dual-photon bone mineral densitometry devices in the early 1980s and was introduced for SPECT in the mid-1980s.[17] It emits a pair of photons at 98 and 103 keV which cannot be distinguished by a gamma camera and appear as a single peak at 100 keV. Its half-life is 242 days making it semi-permanent. It is made in a reactor by neutron irradiation of ultra-pure stable ^{152}Gd. The energy of the combined peak was ideal for use in myocardial perfusion scanning with either ^{99m}Tc or ^{201}Tl. A later development in transmission scanning used an array of multiple ^{153}Gd line sources[20] as a stationary 'quasi-flood' source, with collimation, although this suffered from a restricted axial field of view, significant down-scatter contamination, and was not truly simultaneous with nuclides other than ^{99m}Tc. It has proven effective for cardiac scanning, however. Other sources such as ^{133}Ba (302 and 356 keV;

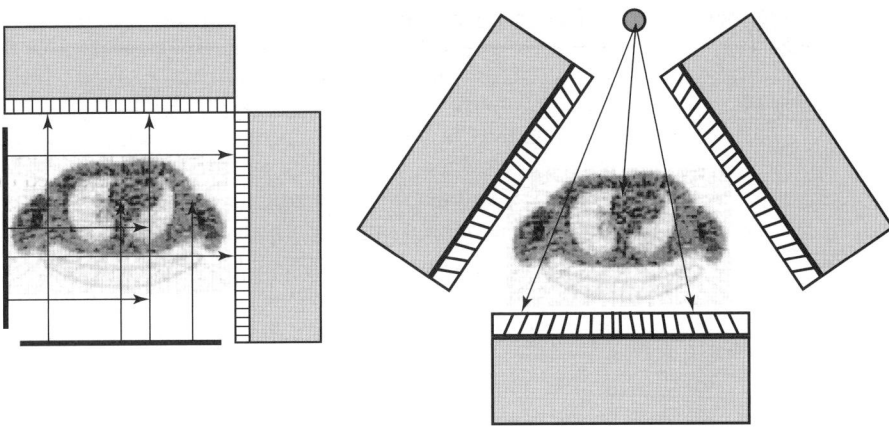

Figure 21C.2 *The most common methods of performing transmission scanning in single photon tomography are to have scanning line sources opposed to dual detector heads in the 90° position (left), or, on a three-headed system, to use fan-beam collimators with a stationary line source at the focus of one of the collimators.*

Table 21C.1 *Comparison of scanning line source and fan-beam stationary line source methods of transmission measurement in SPECT*

Feature	Scanning line source	Fan–beam line source
Radionuclide choice	*Flexible: lower, same as, or higher photon energy than emission nuclide*	*Usually lower photon energy than emission nuclide*
Transverse field-of-view width	*Full field of view*	*Truncated due to fan angle width on central axis of scanner*
Contamination from emission nuclide	*Very small, typically < 5% of emission count rate due to electronic collimation*	*Can be high as the only method of exclusion is pulse height energy separation*
Image separation method(s) employed	*Pulse height energy, electronic source collimation, physical collimation of source*	*Pulse height energy, physical collimation of source*
Emission sensitivity loss in simultaneous emission/transmission mode	*Equal to width of electronic collimation window: 10–15%*	*One third, as one of three heads is dedicated to transmission scanning*
System configuration	*Single or dual head (90°, not 180° opposed); not triple-head systems; mechanical source motion required*	*Implemented on triple-head systems only, but could be used with dual (90° mode) head systems; not single head systems; stationary*
Typical nuclide used	*^{153}Gd, ^{99m}Tc*	*^{153}Gd, ^{241}Am, ^{57}Co*

half-life of 10.7 years) have been used, but ^{153}Gd remains the most commonly used source for transmission scanning. Further information can be found in the paper by Bailey.[21]

Transmission scanning in PET

Attenuation correction of coincidence photons in PET is an analytically straightforward operation and for this reason transmission scanning has been implemented on PET systems from their outset. The most commonly used radionuclide transmission source is ^{68}Ge as it has a half-life of 271 days. It is easily prepared and decays to ^{68}Ga ($t_{1/2}$ = 68.3 min) which emits positrons giving rise to two annihilation photons. PET scanners are usually full-ring devices surrounding the subject. The first and second generation of commercially available PET systems used transmission configurations with a ring of ^{68}Ge which was moved into position between the detector ring and the subject as shown in Fig. 21C.3(a). This configuration did not permit

easy separation of the emission photons from the transmission photons as both have the same energy (511 keV), and therefore simultaneous emission and transmission scanning, or transmission scanning after the injection of the emission radionuclide ('post-injection transmission'), was not possible due to cross-contamination. This approach was modified by replacing the stationary ring source of ^{68}Ge with a rotating rod source. Position encoders on the drive mechanism of the source recorded the instantaneous position of the source, and this allowed the development of electronic collimation, as any recorded event which passed through the known location of the transmission source was considered to be a transmission photon, while the rest were considered emission photons. Configurations with three rotating rod sources have been most commonly used to increase the number of detected events and 'share' the local dead time near the proximal detector over a number of detector modules (Fig. 21C.3(b)).

One disadvantage of this approach was that the half-life for ^{68}Ge is only 271 days, and therefore the sources required

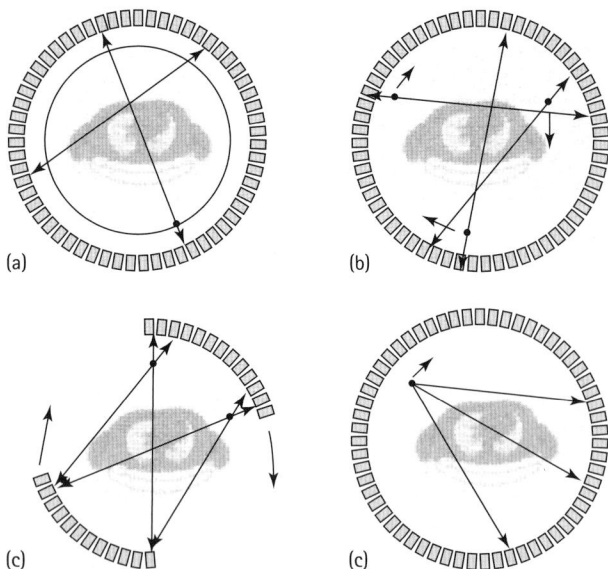

Figure 21C.3 *Configurations that have traditionally been used for transmission scanning in positron tomography include stationary ring sources (a), rotating rod or line sources (b), point sources on a rotating partial ring gantry (c), and a single photon rotating point source (d).*

regular replacement at a significant cost. Another disadvantage of using the rod source approach is that, as a high amount of radioactivity (in the rod source) was close to a single detector module, the dead time on the detector was very high, thus limiting the coincidence count rate for the lines of response incident upon the detector pair. Therefore, alternative methods have been investigated (Fig. 21C.3(c and d)). The high-energy single photon emitting radionuclide ^{137}Cs ($t_{1/2} = 30.2$ years; 663 keV) has been widely used.[22,23] This is a very different acquisition strategy and requires post-processing of the data to remove the large number of scattered photons and for scaling the correction factors from the measured energy of 663 keV to factors appropriate for annihilation radiation at 511 keV.[24] However, count rates and therefore signal quality are extremely high. For more information on the processing strategies the reader is referred to the appropriate chapters in Valk *et al.*[25]

A recent development in PET transmission scanning has been the use of small, dedicated scintillators which serve as one of a pair of coincidence detectors[26] with individual ^{68}Ge/^{68}Ga point sources for high count rate coincidence measurements. The use of a new, fast scintillator (lutetium oxyorthosilicate, LSO) has permitted this development. The sources can be collimated to restrict scatter and can be used with a dedicated, opposed detector to provide simultaneous emission and transmission scans in PET without compromising emission image quality, something which has always remained elusive. This system combines the use of a positron emitter and coincidence detection (thereby reducing scatter) with the high count rates achievable using single photon point sources.

SPECT/CT AND PET/CT

One of the areas of instrumentation development that has grown rapidly in the past few years is combining, in hardware, an emission tomography system (SPECT or PET) with a CT scanner. The aim has been to spatially localize radiopharmaceutical uptake on high-resolution anatomical images. In PET, this has had a significant impact on clinical management.[27] However, the combined datasets have a number of further uses, such as obtaining X-ray electron density maps from which attenuation and scatter correction factors in SPECT and PET can be calculated. For a further discussion of this approach and applications the reader is referred to Townsend *et al.*[28] and Daube-Witherspoon *et al.*[29]

Independent of whether it is PET/CT or SPECT/CT, the X-ray CT data must be converted from the CT values, usually in Hounsfield units (H), to linear attenuation coefficients (μ) for the appropriate photon energy. There are a number of differences between X-ray CT data and transmission of photons in SPECT or PET, namely:

- The polychromatic nature of the X-ray data, as opposed to the mono-energetic nature of the emission photons, and the differences in absorption edges that can affect the conversion to μ values
- The possibility of truncation of the CT field of view compared to the emission tomography field of view
- That the duration of acquisition is usually minutes for SPECT or PET and only seconds for CT, thus introducing the possibility of registration mismatch due to cardiac, respiratory or other physiological movement
- The different attenuation behavior for CT contrast (if given) between X-ray energies and SPECT or PET energies (CT contrast has an attenuation coefficient only 2% higher than water at 511 keV whereas it is extremely radio-opaque to X-rays at energies equivalent to ~70 keV[30])
- Choice of algorithm used to scale the X-ray values to μ values, and whether a distinction is made between soft tissues conversion factors and those for bone

Detailed consideration of these issues is beyond the scope of this chapter but is now well addressed in the usual nuclear medicine literature.

CORRECTION FOR ATTENUATION

SPECT

Prior to the widespread introduction of simultaneous emission and transmission scanning, various approximate corrections were used in SPECT. None attempted to produce

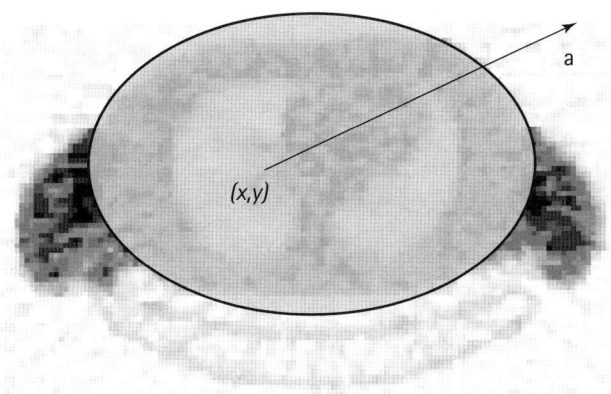

Figure 21C.4 *In the Chang method of calculating attenuation correction factors every point (x, y) in the object has an integral of attenuation coefficients calculated to the detector for each projection over 360°. This provides an approximate mean attenuation correction factor for each pixel.*

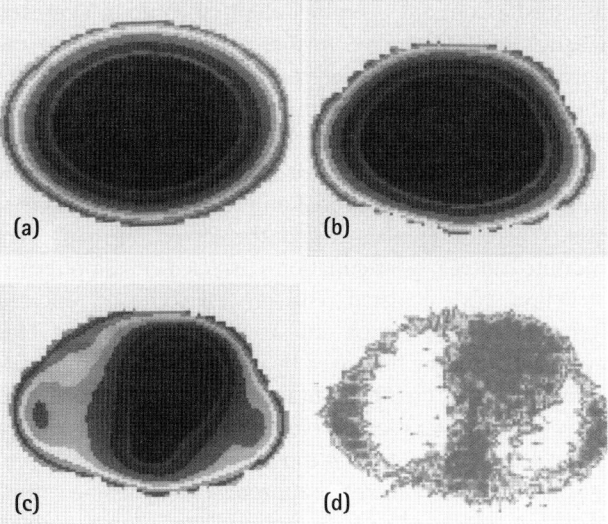

Figure 21C.5 *Attenuation correction factor maps using the Chang method are shown for (a) an ellipse containing a constant attenuation value, (b) an accurate body contour containing a constant attenuation value, and (c) measured values derived from the attenuation map shown in (d).*

quantitatively accurate corrections, but were usually applied to aid qualitative image interpretation. The first step with any correction scheme is to define the boundaries of the subject. The next is to estimate the linear attenuation coefficients within the subject, and, hence, derive a correction factor for each volume element (voxel). The most simple approach was to assume an elliptical boundary within which there was a single, 'average' attenuation coefficient per voxel. Others used an improved approach by obtaining a better estimate of the subject's outline, or the boundary, using either a lower-energy 'scatter' window or, more elaborately, using a low energy radionuclide source, such as ^{133}Xe, to measure it.[31]

Figure 21C.4 shows a measured attenuation reconstruction of the thorax overlaid with an ellipse, as would be done if assuming an elliptical contour for a simple attenuation correction. The crudeness of the approximation can be clearly seen. Usually, no account for the attenuation of the bed is incorporated into such a correction.

To understand the correction applied, the method proposed by Chang is perhaps the most intuitive.[12] A number of variants on this have been developed since the original publication. For the moment, assume that there is an object boundary within which there are discrete linear attenuation coefficients (μ) with units of length^{-1} (i.e. cm^{-1} or pixel^{-1}). The boundary may be an ellipse and the attenuation coefficients may all have the same, assumed value, or the object boundary may be the actual patient outline and the μ values may be measured. Chang's method calculates the integral (or sum) of the μ values along a projection (as illustrated in Fig. 21C.4) for each voxel in the object to the imaginary detector. This is done for many angles, often the same as the acquired number of projection angles. The average of

all of these attenuation factors (A) for each point (x,y) is then determined. Mathematically, this is

$$A(x, y) = \frac{1}{N_p} \sum_{n=1}^{N_p} \exp\left(\sum^{a} \mu_s(i) \Delta i \right)_n \qquad (21C.2)$$

where i represents the direction along the projection to the detector for each projection angle n. Here μ_s signifies that it is the attenuation coefficient for the single photon energy, and N_p is the total number of projections that the correction factor is calculated from. Some examples of attenuation correction maps are shown in Fig. 21C.5.

It can be seen that as more information about the subject is supplied the correction map becomes more contoured and suited to the individual correction. Chang's original method used an ellipse and an average μ value in all voxels. The attenuation correction maps, as seen in Fig. 21C.5, were applied to (multiplied pixel-by-pixel with) the SPECT data reconstructed by filtered back-projection without any empirical attenuation correction. This gives a first-order corrected emission reconstruction. Chang realized that this was only approximate, however. The reason for this is basically that, in SPECT, the count rate recorded is a composite of each individual point's count rate and its attenuation to that point. Therefore, a given count rate seen by the detector from a single emitting source may be the result of a low activity source with little attenuation or a higher activity source at a greater depth, and hence with greater attenuation. This is unlike the case in PET because of the two photons emitted, as attenuation is constant along any projection. In addition, the Chang approach assumed a constant μ and an elliptical contour. However, Chang's method applied further processing to refine the correction. The first-order corrected emission data were then forward projected, with attenuation, to emulate the data acquisition process. The forward projected data were then compared with the measured data, with which they should be identical if the emission reconstruction was correct. Where differences existed, the correction maps were modified and a new attenuation-corrected emission reconstruction was calculated. This process could be repeated iteratively to approach an accurate correction. This approach could be improved by using measured transmission data and therefore accurate attenuation maps. In this case, only one iteration was found to be necessary to provide accurately corrected reconstructions.[17]

More recently, alternative approaches to emission reconstruction by filtered back-projection have become popular. One of the most commonly used approaches is the ordered-subset estimation maximization (OSEM) block-iterative approach.[32] This is one example of a set of methods known as iterative reconstructions. (For further information see Chapter 4 in Valk et al.[25]) A major advantage of these methods is that corrections, such as for attenuation, scatter, and limited spatial resolution, can be built into the reconstruction process, and thus incorporating attenuation maps for correction into the iterative reconstruction becomes a viable proposition. These methods are now widely available on commercial systems. With these approaches accurate attenuation correction can be applied in SPECT.

PET

Attenuation correction in PET is simple to apply. It is physically different to SPECT as the events recorded arise from two photons being detected in coincidence, not just one. Both photons have to traverse the entire body to be recorded and therefore attenuation is constant for the projection; the count rate recorded is independent of the location along the projection of the positron annihilation. Figure 21C.6 illustrates the difference with SPECT. The attenuation correction factors in PET are calculated in the projection space from the equation

$$A(s,\phi) = \exp\left[\sum^{a+b} \mu_{511}(i)\Delta i\right] \quad (21C.3)$$

where μ_{511} indicates that it is an appropriate attenuation coefficient for positron annihilation radiation (511 keV). It can be seen in the equation that the summation is now over the total thickness of the subject for that projection ($a + b$) and therefore this is constant for a point anywhere along the projection. Attenuation correction in PET is applied by multiplying the emission projection data with the calculated attenuation factors on a pixel-by-pixel basis *before* reconstruction. After the attenuation correction is applied,

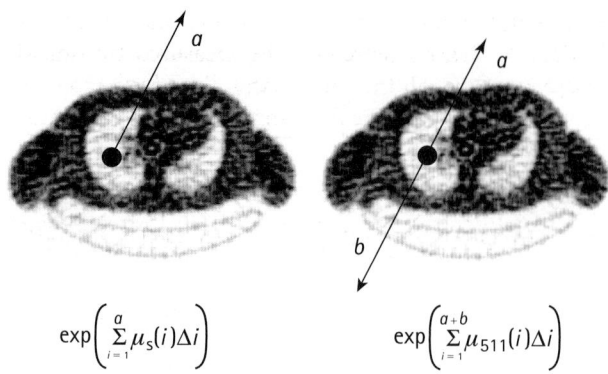

$$\exp\left(\sum_{i=1}^{a} \mu_s(i)\Delta i\right) \qquad \exp\left(\sum_{i=1}^{a+b} \mu_{511}(i)\Delta i\right)$$

Figure 21C.6   *In single photon tomography (left) the attenuation is from the point of interest in the object to the detector in one direction only, while in positron tomography (right) the two photons are both attenuated as they pass through the entire thickness of the subject. This leads to generally higher attenuation factors in PET compared to SPECT in spite of the difference in photon energy and higher linear attenuation coefficient for the lower energy single photons.*

the projection data are fully corrected and no iterating is usually required.[17]

Various processing steps can be applied to the attenuation correction data in PET as they may contain high noise levels because they are calculated on a pixel-by-pixel basis. The data are often spatially smoothed to suppress this noise and if the transmission source was not a positron emitter (such as if ^{137}Cs was used) the data need to be scaled to compensate for the energy difference. Noise can also be suppressed by segmentation of the data and replacing noisy values with an average value for a number of different μ values. (See Bettinardi et al.[33] and Zaidi and Hawegawa[34] for further information on these methods.)

Processing transmission data

While the methods of correcting for attenuation in emission scans differ, the processing of the transmission data for reconstruction of 'attenuation maps' is similar for both SPECT and PET. In PET this is not used in the correction, but merely for anatomical localization, whereas in SPECT it is, in general, used for correcting the emission data. The attenuation factors are calculated by comparing the transmission scan of the subject with a transmission scan acquired without anything in the field of view. This scan is often referred to as a 'reference' or 'blank' scan. This establishes the non-attenuated count rate for each pixel. The transmission equation

$$T(s,\phi) = T_0(s,\phi)\exp\left(-\int \mu(i)\partial i\right) \quad (21C.4)$$

where T is the transmitted count rate and T_0 is the unattenuated count rate (from the reference or blank scan) per pixel in the projection data (s,ϕ). The integral $-\int \mu(i)\partial_i$

represents the sum of attenuation coefficients along the projection. As $T(s, \phi)$ represents the measured transmission count rate through the subject and $T_0(s, \phi)$ the measured unattenuated count rate this can be rearranged to yield the attenuation factors:

$$\frac{T_0(s, \phi)}{T(s, \phi)} = \exp\left(\int \mu(i)\partial i\right) \qquad (21C.5)$$

which are used directly in PET to correct the emission data. In SPECT, a further step is performed. The data are reconstructed after taking the natural logarithm of the equation, i.e.

$$\log_e\left(\frac{T_0(s, \phi)}{T(s, \phi)}\right) = \int \mu(i)\partial i. \qquad (21C.6)$$

This equation is now in the form of a simple summation of the projection and therefore can be reconstructed using the usual algorithms (e.g. filtered back-projection, iterative methods). After reconstruction, the attenuation map (Fig. 21C.5d) can be used in the emission reconstruction for correction, or processed using the Chang approach to produce 'attenuation correction factor' maps (Fig. 21C.5c), and used as described above. If the PET data are to be reconstructed the natural logarithm of the ratio of blank-to-transmission must also be calculated.

The correction factors in PET are, in general, greater than they are in SPECT. This is not always well known. Even though the photon energy of annihilation radiation is higher than the usual gamma energies of single photon emitters, the fact that there are two photons which both must traverse the entire width of the patient, as opposed to a single photon traveling in one direction, means that the attenuation is much greater in PET. In a uniform region of tissue density, such as the abdomen, a 140-keV photon ($\mu = 0.15\,\mathrm{cm}^{-1}$) at the center of the body (assume 35 cm total width, 17.5 cm to the mid-point) will be $\exp(-0.15 \times 17.5) = 7.2\%$ transmission (correction factor of 13.9) whereas for the 511-keV PET equivalent ($\mu = 0.096\,\mathrm{cm}^{-1}$) it is $\exp(-0.096 \times 35) = 3.5\%$ (correction factor of 28.6) – approximately a factor of 2 greater.

CLINICAL APPLICATIONS

Attenuation correction removes distortions in emission reconstructions due to inconsistencies between projections and the spatially varying effect of differential attenuation. The original aim of attenuation correction in SPECT was the same as for PET: to create quantitative, accurate reconstructions of radionuclide distribution. However, it has primarily been used for, and driven by, the desire to remove attenuation artifacts from myocardial perfusion images. We are moving towards a situation where attenuation correction will be routine for all SPECT and PET studies, as this is the only way to ensure distortion-free reconstructions.

SPECT

MYOCARDIAL PERFUSION

By far the most frequent application of attenuation correction in SPECT has been with myocardial perfusion images. The presence of artifacts due to attenuation has been recognized in SPECT for many years. As myocardial perfusion SPECT imaging commenced using ^{201}Tl, with predominantly low-energy photons, the effect was notable and thus attenuation correction produced a profound effect.[35] Artifacts are usually ascribed to different sections of the left ventricle in men and women due to gender differences in muscle bulk in the chest wall, thickness of the diaphragm, and thickness and density of overlying breast tissue. This has necessitated developing separate normal databases for men and women, which is undesirable. Some practitioners advocate re-scanning the subject in the prone (as opposed to supine) position, to dissect out attenuation artifact from true abnormality, i.e. decreased uptake. This is disadvantageous as it greatly lengthens scanning time. Many have just 'learnt to read around the artifact'. Attenuation problems in myocardial perfusion SPECT impact directly on the technique's specificity, which in non-gated SPECT is quoted variably between 70 and 85%. Sensitivity is unaffected and remains in the low 90%s. A typical example is shown in Plate 21C.1.

Radionuclide-based transmission systems are now entering their second generation, with improvements in the quality of the attenuation data produced. The simultaneous acquisition systems allow transmission data to be collected with minimal extension of the scanning time – typically <15% extra – with virtually no loss in image quality for the emission data. Attenuation correction based on measured transmission data has an impact on overall accuracy and specificity. The American Society of Nuclear Cardiology and the Society of Nuclear Medicine have recently released an updated joint statement on attenuation correction of myocardial perfusion data,[36] following their initial position paper of 2002. In that paper, the authors summarized the findings to date for the use of attenuation correction improving sensitivity mildly from 81 to 85%, but more importantly improving specificity from 64 to 81% and normalcy rate from 80 to 89% in over 760 pooled subjects.

OTHER APPLICATIONS: QUALITATIVE

BONE

Not correcting for attenuation can lead to large differences in structures which have relatively uniform uptake but are located in different transverse slices. This was pointed out in a study by Case *et al.* of the differences seen in thoracic and abdominal reconstructions of the spine in a ^{99m}Tc bone scan. An example of this effect is shown in Fig. 21C.7. The uptake in the thoracic vertebra appears greater than that in the abdomen with a clear demarcation at the level of the diaphragm. This is due to the large differences in attenuation between thorax and abdomen, as the thorax has a large component occupied by the air-filled lungs. After applying measured attenuation correction the uptake in the thoracic and abdominal vertebrae are equivalent.

GALLIUM-67

In regions with expected homogeneous radiotracer uptake, lack of correction for attenuation can lead to differences in reconstructed tracer concentration. This is clearly the problem with myocardial perfusion SPECT, but it is particularly well demonstrated in reconstructions of the liver, as it is a larger organ with, in normal cases, homogeneous distribution of many tracers such as ^{67}Ga. The same would apply to other radiotracers with near-homogeneous normal distribution in the liver, e.g. colloid, labelled red blood cells. Figure 21C.8 shows this effect in the liver on a ^{67}Ga scan of a patient with non-Hodgkin's lymphoma.

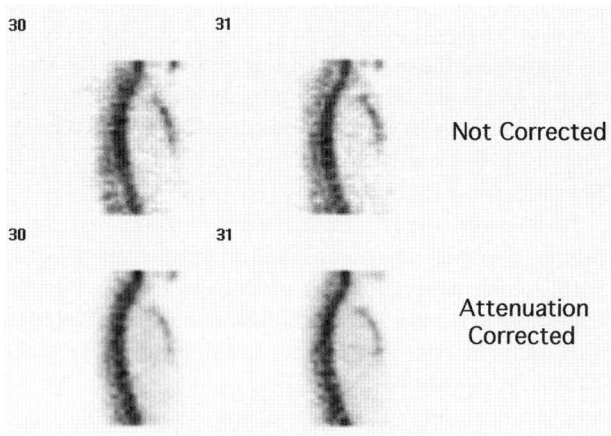

Figure 21C.7 *The qualitative effect of attenuation correction is seen on a ^{99m}Tc bone scan. Before attenuation correction the vertebrae in the thorax appear to have more uptake of the tracer than the vertebrae in the abdomen, while after correction they are seen to all have relatively homogeneous uptake.*

OTHER APPLICATIONS: QUANTITATIVE

Quantification is the ultimate aim for SPECT reconstructions. There are a number of factors which must be addressed to realize this in addition to attenuation correction, such as corrections for scattered photons, partial-volume effects, collimator penetration and distance dependent resolution differences. All of these have been addressed and quantification is certainly achievable in SPECT. (See, for example, Iida *et al.*[37] and Soret *et al.*[38])

Table 21C.2 shows a list of potential applications for quantitative SPECT. Some of these have been achieved already and are indicated by references in the literature while others can be conjectured.

PET

PET studies have traditionally been corrected for attenuation using measured transmission data. The first PET scanners included transmission sources for this purpose.[10,11] There was a tendency to move away from transmission measurements for all but research studies during the 1990s as the transmission scan needed to be acquired prior to injection of the radiopharmaceutical, adding significant time to the entire study. The rotating rod or stationary ring sources of ^{68}Ge/^{68}Ga were not well-suited to post-injection transmission measurements simultaneous with the emission acquisition. As shown by Meikle *et al.*, one reason was that the accidental or 'random' coincidences from the high-activity rod sources were recorded as an emission signal and degraded the quality of the emission scan.[45] Consequently, most centers that perform clinical PET studies did not correct for attenuation on their 'whole-body' scans. Some did acquire transmission data for a single bed position for the purposes of calculating uptake values (e.g. standardized uptake value (SUV)). As can be seen in Fig. 21C.9, though, this introduces significant distortion, enough to spatially 'shift' an abnormal focus. In an even more extreme case, an abnormality that is clearly visible on the PET attenuation reconstruction, can disappear altogether without appropriate attenuation correction (Fig. 21C.10). These studies help to make a compelling case for full attenuation correction in PET. This is now achievable with PET/CT systems that can acquire the transmission (CT) data in a very short

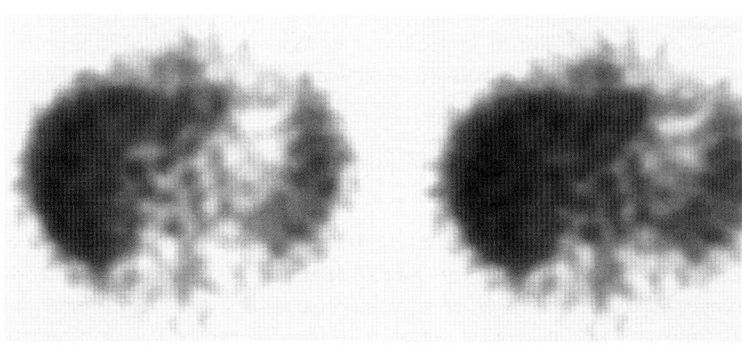

Figure 21C.8 *The effect of attenuation correction on the homogeneous uptake in the liver for a ^{67}Ga scan is shown. Without correction the reconstructed uptake appears to be less towards the center of the body where average attenuation is higher, but after correction the distribution is seen to be far more uniform.*

time. Multi-bed transmission scanning measurements are also possible with rod-based $^{68}Ge/^{68}Ga$ or point-source single-photon ^{137}Cs systems, although the emission and transmission scans must be acquired separately, extending the total acquisition duration. Data acquired with photons of energy other than 511 keV will need to be scaled and pre-treated before they can be applied.

A number of publications have appeared recently which have argued strongly for the need for attenuation correction of all PET data.[46,47] This is to be highly recommended and should be standard practice, within the constraints imposed by the additional time required to collect the transmission data. Hopefully, future tomograph designs will address this issue and there are already promising

Table 21C.2 *Current and future potential applications of quantitative SPECT studies*

Quantitative SPECT study	Radionuclide	Information obtained
Myocardial perfusion	^{99m}Tc	Absolute myocardial uptake; evaluation of triple vessel or left main artery disease (Duvernoy et al.[39])
Gallium scan	^{67}Ga	Quantifying uptake; evaluating response to treatment; derive 'SUV'
Regional cerebral blood flow	^{99m}Tc, ^{123}I	Absolute measure of perfusion in mL $100 g^{-1} min^{-1}$ (Iida et al.[40] and Ito et al.[41])
Cerebral receptors and neurotransmitters	^{99m}Tc, ^{123}I	Absolute uptake measure, reduce need to calculate ratio to reference tissue (Soret et al.[38])
Bone scan	^{99m}Tc	Measure bone uptake, turnover and retention (Bailey et al.[42])
Solitary pulmonary nodules	^{99m}Tc-depreotide	SUV, analogous to PET FDG measurement
Dosimetry planning scan	$^{131}I(^{123}I)$, ^{111}In	Patient-specific dosimetry for radionuclide therapy (Guy et al.[43])
Absolute ventricular volumes; left and right ventricular function	^{99m}Tc	Count-based volume and functional parameters (e.g. LVEF, RVEF) (Bailey et al.[44])

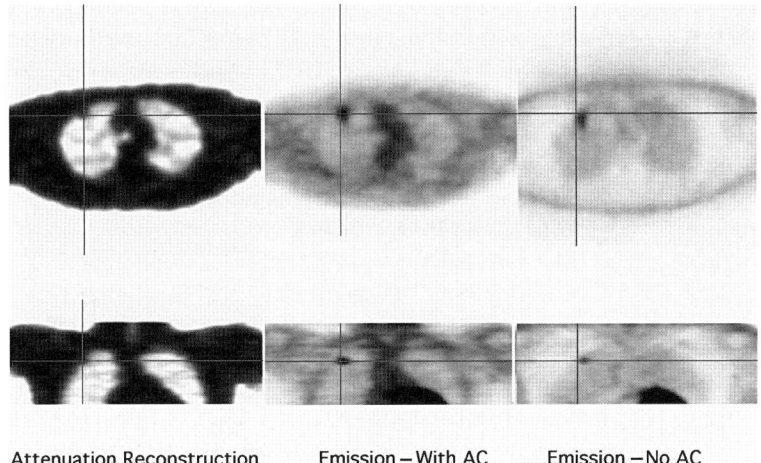

Attenuation Reconstruction   Emission – With AC   Emission – No AC

Figure 21C.9 *Not correcting for attenuation in PET can lead to distortions of the reconstructed data. The example shown here demonstrates a clear displacement of a lesion seen on the attenuation reconstruction (left) and the corrected ^{18}F-FDG emission scan (middle) when no correction is applied (right). AC, attenuation correction.*

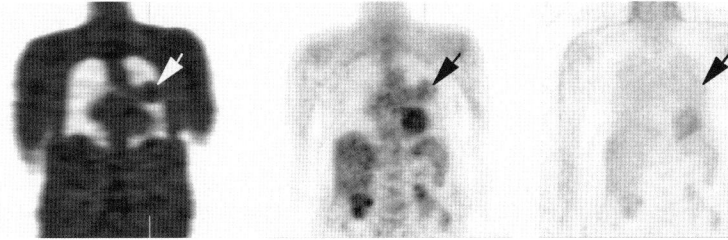

Figure 21C.10 *An extreme example of the need for attenuation correction is shown in this figure. The anatomical lesion seen on the attenuation reconstruction (left) and on the corrected emission scan (middle) virtually disappears without attenuation correction (right). (From: Bai C, Kinahan PE, Brasse D, et al. An analytical study of the effects of attenuation on tumor detection in whole-body PET oncology imaging. J Nucl Med 2003; 44: 1855–86. Image kindly supplied by Dr C. Bai and reproduced with the permission of the Journal of Nuclear Medicine).*

advances such as the dedicated fast detector system mentioned previously.[26]

CONCLUSION

The field of emission tomography is moving towards adopting performing attenuation correction routinely for all investigations. In the past, cost may have been a factor which has restricted the widespread use of attenuation correction in SPECT, there being, in general, no rebate for performing attenuation correction using measured data. In PET it was probably the fact that simultaneous emission/transmission, or rapid post-injection transmission scanning, has not been available that has restricted its use. Both of these issues are being addressed at present and it would appear that the use of attenuation correction will become standard. The measured transmission data are also useful for scatter correction and image co-registration and so will find many uses in current and future routine practice.

REFERENCES

1 Fleming JS. A technique for the absolute measurement of activity using the gamma camera and computer. *Phys Med Biol* 1979; **24**: 176–80.

2 Macey D, Marshall R. Absolute quantitation of radiotracer uptake in lungs using a gamma camera. *J Nucl Med* 1984; **23**: 731–5.

3 Myers MJ, Lavender JP, de Oliviera JB, Maseri A. A simplified method of quantitating organ uptake using a gamma camera. *Br J Radiol* 1981; **54**: 1062–7.

4 Bailey DL, Zito F, Gilardi M-C, *et al.* Performance comparison of a state-of-the-art neuro-SPET scanner and a dedicated neuro-PET scanner. *Eur J Nucl Med* 1994; **21**: 381–7.

5 McRae J, Anger HO. Transmission scintiphotography and its applications. In: *Medical radioisotope scintigraphy*. Salzburg: International Atomic Energy Agency, 1968: 57–69.

6 Kuhl DE, Hale J, Eaton WL. Transmission scanning: a useful adjunct to conventional emission scanning for accurately keying isotope deposition to radiographic anatomy. *Radiology* 1966; **87**: 278.

7 Sorenson JA, Briggs RC, Cameron JR. ^{99m}Tc Point source for transmission scanning. *J Nucl Med* 1969; **10**: 252–3.

8 Tothill P, Galt JM. Quantitative profile scanning for the measurement of organ radioactivity. *Phys Med Biol* 1971; **16**: 625–34.

9 Graham LS, Neil R. *In vivo* quantitation of radioactivity using the Anger camera. *Radiology* 1974; **112**: 441–2.

10 Phelps ME, Hoffman EJ, Mullani NA, Ter-Pogossian MM. Application of annihilation coincidence detection to transaxial reconstruction tomography. *J Nucl Med* 1975; **16**: 210–24.

11 Derenzo SE, Zaklad H, Budinger TF. Analytical study of a high-resolution positron ring detector system for transaxial reconstruction tomography. *J Nucl Med* 1975; **16**: 1166–73.

12 Chang LT. A method for attenuation correction in radionuclide computed tomography. *IEEE Trans Nucl Sci* 1978; **NS-25**: 638–43.

13 Natterer F. Determination of tissue attenuation in emission tomography of optically dense media. *Inverse Problems* 1993; **9**: 731–6.

14 Welch A, Clack R, Natterer F, Gullberg GT. Towards accurate attenuation correction in SPECT without transmission measurements. *IEEE Trans Med Imag* 1997; **MI-15**: 532–41.

15 Morozumi T, Nakajima M, Ogawa K, Yuta S. Attenuation correction methods using the information of attenuation distribution for single photon emission CT. *Med Imag Tech* 1984; **2**: 20–8.

16 Malko JA, Van Heertum RL, Gullberg GT, Kowalsky WP. SPECT liver imaging using an iterative attenuation correction algorithm and an external flood source. *J Nucl Med* 1986; **27**: 701–5.

17 Bailey DL, Hutton BF, Walker PJ. Improved SPECT using simultaneous emission and transmission tomography. *J Nucl Med* 1987; **28**: 844–51.

18 Tan P, Bailey DL, Meikle SR, *et al.* A scanning line source for simultaneous emission and transmission measurements in SPECT. *J Nucl Med* 1993; **34**: 1752–60.

19 Tung C-H, Gullberg GT, Zeng GL, *et al.* Non-uniform attenuation correction using simultaneous transmission and emission converging tomography. *IEEE Trans Nucl Sci* 1992; **39**: 1134–43.

20 Celler A, Sitek A, Stoub E, *et al.* Multiple line source array for SPECT transmission scans: simulation, phantom and patient studies. *J Nucl Med* 1998; **39**: 2183–9.

21 Bailey DL. Transmission scanning in emission tomography. *Eur J Nucl Med* 1998; **25**: 774–87.

22 Karp JS, Muehllehner G, Qu H, Yan X-H. Singles transmission in volume-imaging PET with a ^{137}Cs source. *Phys Med Biol* 1995; **40**: 929–44.

23 Yu SK, Nahmias C. Single-photon transmission measurements in positron emission tomography using ^{137}Cs. *Phys Med Biol* 1995; **40**: 1255–66.

24 Bailey DL, Miller MP, Spinks TJ, *et al.* Experience with fully 3D PET and implications for future high resolution 3D tomographs. *Phys Med Biol* 1998; **43**: 777–86.

25 Valk PE, Bailey DL, Townsend DW, Maisey MN. *Positron emission tomography: basic science & clinical practice.* London: Springer-Verlag, 2003.

26 Jones WF, Moyers JC, Casey ME, *et al.* Fast-channel LSO detectors and fiber-optic encoding for excellent dual photon transmission measurements in PET. *IEEE Trans Nucl Sci* 1999; **NS-46**: 979–84.

27 Lardinois D, Weder W, Hany TF, *et al*. Staging of non-small-cell lung cancer with integrated positron-emission tomography and computed tomography. *N Engl J Med* 2003; **348**: 2500–7.

28 Townsend DW, Beyer T, Blodgett TM. PET/CT scanners: a hardware approach to image fusion. *Semin Nucl Med* 2003; **33**: 193–204.

29 Daube-Witherspoon ME, Zubal IG, Karp JS. Developments in instrumentation for emission computed tomography. *Semin Nucl Med* 2003; **33**: 28–41.

30 Carney J, Beyer T, Brasse D, *et al*. Clinical PET/CT scanning using oral CT contrast agents [Abstract]. *J Nucl Med* 2002; **43(suppl)**: 57P.

31 Jaszczak RJ, Chang LT, Stein NA. Whole body single photon emission computed tomography using large field of view scintillation cameras. *Phys Med Biol* 1979; **24**: 1123–43.

32 Hudson HM, Larkin RS. Accelerated image reconstruction using ordered subsets of projection data. *IEEE Trans Med Imag* 1994; **MI-13**: 601–9.

33 Bettinardi V, Pagani E, Gilardi M, *et al*. An automatic classification technique for attenuation correction in positron emission tomography. *Eur J Nucl Med* 1999; **26**: 447–58.

34 Zaidi H, Hasegawa B. Determination of the attenuation map in emission tomography. *J Nucl Med* 2003; **44**: 291–315.

35 Roach PJ, Hutton BF, Meikle SR, *et al*. Transmission based quantitative SPECT improves the accuracy of Tl-201 myocardial scintigraphy [Abstract]. *Eur J Nucl Med* 1993; **20**: 917.

36 Heller G, Links J, Bateman T, Ziffer J, Ficaro E, Cohen M, *et al*. American Society of Nuclear Cardiology and Society of Nuclear Medicine joint position statement: attenuation correction of myocardial perfusion SPECT scintigraphy. *J Nucl Cardiol* 2004; **11**: 229–30.

37 Iida H, Narita Y, Kado H, *et al*. Effects of scatter and attenuation correction on quantitative assessment of regional cerebral blood flow with SPECT. *J Nucl Med* 1998; **39**: 181–9.

38 Soret M, Koulibaly PM, Darcourt J, *et al*. Quantitative accuracy of dopaminergic neurotransmission imaging with (123)I SPECT. *J Nucl Med* 2003; **44**: 1184–93.

39 Duvernoy CS, Ficaro EP, Karabajakian MZ, *et al*. Improved detection of left main coronary artery disease with attenuation-corrected SPECT. *J Nucl Cardiol* 2001; **7**: 639–48.

40 Iida H, Bloomfield PM, Munaka M, *et al*. A method to quantitate cerebral blood flow using a rotating gamma camera and iodine-123 iodoamphetamine with one blood sample. *Eur J Nucl Med* 1994; **21**: 1072–84.

41 Ito H, Iida H, Bloomfield PM, *et al*. Rapid calculation of regional cerebral blood-flow and distribution volume using iodine-123-iodoamphetamine and dynamic SPECT. *J Nucl Med* 1995; **36**: 531–6.

42 Bailey DL, Hain SF, Adamson KL, *et al*. Quantitative dynamic bone SPECT: a new method to assess skeletal kinetics [Abstract]. *J Nucl Med* 2003; **44(suppl)**: 150P.

43 Guy MJ, Flux GD, Papavasileiou P, *et al*. RMDP: a dedicated package for I-131 SPECT quantification, registration, and patient-specific dosimetry. *Cancer Biother Radiopharm* 2003; **18**: 61–9.

44 Bailey DL, Lewis RE, Clarke GL. Absolute radioactivity quantification using transmission based scatter and attenuation correction [Abstract]. *Eur J Nucl Med* 2001; **28**: 969.

45 Meikle SR, Bailey DL, Hutton BF, Jones WF. Optimisation of simultaneous emission and transmission measurements in PET. In: Klaisner L. (ed.) *IEEE Nuclear Science Symposium and Medical Imaging Conference, 1993*. San Francisco: Institute of Electrical and Electronic Engineers, 1993: 1642–6.

46 Hustinx R, Dolin RJ, Benard F, *et al*. Impact of attenuation correction on the accuracy of FDG-PET in patients with abdominal tumors: a free-response ROC analysis. *Eur J Nucl Med* 2000; **27**: 1365–71.

47 Bai C, Kinahan PE, Brasse D, *et al*. An analytical study of the effects of attenuation on tumour detection in whole-body PET oncology imaging. *J Nucl Med* 2003; **44**: 1855–61.

Index

Figures and tables are comprehensively referred to from the text. Therefore, significant material in figures and tables have in the main been given a page reference only in the *absence* of their concomitant mention in the text referring to that figure.

Entries under the most commonly occurring imaging modalities (positron emission tomography and single photon emission tomography) are for the more significantly mentioned conditions or types of conditions, in addition to technical aspects of the imaging modality or more general aspects of its use in individual organs and tissues. The more minor references of these imaging modalities will be found under the specific (types of) conditions.

Abbreviations used: MAb, monoclonal antibody. Plate numbers are indicated in bold.

abdominal infections 96
abdominal node metastases, testicular cancer 569
Aberdeen Section Scanner Mark II 854
abscess, testicular 598
absolute differences, sum of 863
accuracy of test, measures 801–4
ACE inhibitors 165
acetate, ^{11}C-
    myocardial fatty acid metabolism 150–1
    renal cell carcinoma **Plate 8G.1**
    therapeutic response monitoring 58
        prostate cancer 68–9
acetylcholinergic system imaging 421
Achilles tendoninitis 368
ACTH *see* adrenocorticotrophic hormone
activated protein C resistance 207
activity–time curves *see* time–activity curves
acute coronary syndrome 159–60
acute respiratory distress (adult respiratory distress) syndrome 240, 243
ADAM (2-((2-((dimethylamino) methyl) phenyl) thio)-5-iodophenylamine), ^{123}I- 429
adenocarcinoma, ovarian, radioimmunoscintigraphy 43, 602
adenoma(s)
    adrenal cortical 521, 523, 526, 527, 528, 529
    salivary gland 484
    thyroid, multiple toxic *see* Plummer's disease
adenosine, interactions with xanthines 826
adenosine stress test 153
    post-myocardial infarction risk stratification 162–3
adjuvant chemotherapy, response monitoring in children 409
adjuvant external beam radiotherapy, $_{131}$I-treated thyroid cancer 739
adolescents, hyperthyroidism treatment 500
adrenal gland 521–39
    cortex 522–30
        disorders 523–30
        physiology 522–3
        radiopharmacology 522–3
    incidental mass 526, 528–30
    medulla 530–5
        neuroblastoma 404, 535
        pheochromocytoma *see* pheochromocytoma
        physiology 530–1
    syndromes of excess secretion 521–2

adrenaline *see* epinephrine
adrenocorticotrophic hormone (ACTH; corticotrophin) 521
    excess 523
        ectopic secretion by tumors 33, 523
adult respiratory distress syndrome 240, 243
adverse effects of radiopharmaceuticals 822–4
    frequency of occurrence 821–2
aerosols (lungs) 240
    ^{99m}Tc-DTPA transfer 242
    ^{99m}Tc VQ scans 203–6
affective (mood) disorders 429
age-related occurrence/risk
    fracture 364–5
        bone mineral density and 400
    venous thromboembolism 207
    see also elderly
AIDS *see* HIV disease
airways
    anatomy 197–8
    obstructive disease 201–2
albumin (human)
    ^{51}Cr-, protein-losing enteropathy 681
    macroaggregated *see* MAA
    microspheres (HAM), hysterosalpingoscintigraphy in infertility 588, 589, 591
aldosteronism, primary 526–7
alimentary tract *see* gastrointestinal tract
alkaline phosphatase, placental 602
ALMANAC (Axillary Lymphatic Mapping Against Nodal Axillary Clearance) 133
alpha-fetoprotein 40
alpha particle therapy 79, 835
alveoli 198
Alzheimer's disease 22–4, 416–18, 841–2
    amyloid and *see* amyloid
    early-onset 417–18, **Plate 10A.4**
    late-onset/senile 416–17, **Plates 10A.2–3**
    Lewy body dementia vs 419
    new PET agents 841–2
amine precursor uptake and decarboxylation, tumors capable of (APUDomas) *see* neuroendocrine tumors
amino acid PET neuroimaging, radiolabeled 451
γ -aminobutyric acid and epilepsy 438
amiodarone-induced thyrotoxicosis/hyperthyroidism 498, 502

ammonia, N-^{13}N-
  hepatocellular carcinoma 665
  myocardial perfusion 150, **Plate 6B.2**
amusing children 108–9
amyloid β and Alzheimer's disease 22, 24, 416
  imaging 22, 421
amyloid P component, ^{123}I-serum 692–3
amyloidosis 692–3
anagrelide, polycythemia vera 775
analog logic (Anger) 853
anaplastic/undifferentiated/dedifferentiated thyroid cancer 68, 506
  treatment 739
androgen, excess section in women 527–8
anemia 675–83
  with gastrointestinal blood loss 677–8
    assessment 643
  hemolytic 679, 690
  megaloblastic 681
anesthetic cream, children 109
Anger (analog logic) 853
angina, variant/Prinzmetal's 159
angiogenesis 81
  inhibitors 81
  perfusion restoration to ischemic myocardium by induction of 20
angiography
  coronary 11, 157, 169, **Plate 6A.9**
  CT see computed tomography angiography
  MR, pulmonary embolism 209
  multiplanar gated 183–4
  pelvic and internal pudendal 577
  radionuclide
    shunt quantitation 170–1, **Plates 6A.21–2**
    ventricular function determination 171
  renal artery narrowing 298
angioplasty
  percutaneous coronary 164, **Plate 6A.17**
  renal artery 302
angiosarcoma, spleen 692
angiotensin-converting enzyme inhibitors (angiotensin II synthesis inhibitors) 81, 300
  cortical vs juxtamedullary nephron effects 263–4, 300
animal imaging 12, **Plate 1A.1**
ankle injuries 368–71
ankylosing spondylitis 395–6
Ann Arbor staging system of lymphoma 696
annexin V 69–71, 818
  ^{18}F-, in therapeutic response monitoring 58
  ^{99m}Tc- 818
    in therapeutic response monitoring 58, 69–71, 835
  annihilation coincidence detection 855
  antegrade perfusion of renal pelvis, direct, with pressure measurements 306
  anti-angiogenic drugs 81
  antibacterial drugs (antibiotics), radiolabeled 101, 833
    prosthetic joint infection 388
antibiotics see antibacterial drugs; antifungal drugs; antiparasitic drugs
antibodies (immunoglobulins) 40–1
  biological factors affecting uptake 41–3
  granulocyte see granulocytes
  in HIV disease 246–7
  ^{111}In-labeled polyclonal see indium-111-labeled immunoglobulin
  in inflammation imaging 833
  monoclonal see monoclonal antibodies
  tracer-labeled 6
  see also autoantibodies; Fab' fragment; F(ab')$_2$ fragment; radioimmunoscintigraphy; radioimmunotherapy

anticancer drugs
  cytotoxic see chemotherapy
  discovery, molecular imaging 17–18
  glomerular filtration rate measurement in toxicity prediction 275
anticoagulant therapy, pulmonary embolism 220
antidepressants 429
anti-estrogen therapy, monitoring in breast cancer 66, 553
antifungal drugs 101, 833
antigens 40
  tumor-associated 40
    colorectal cancer 49, 647
    ovarian 601, 602
    prostate cancer 610
antihypertensive actions, captopril 300
antimicrobial drugs see antibacterial drugs; antifungal drugs; antiparasitic drugs
antimicrobial peptides (endogenous) 101–2
antimony sulfide colloid, ^{99m}Tc- 123
antiparasitic drugs 833
antiphospholipid syndrome and venous thromboembolism risk 207
antisense oligonucleotides 7, 9
antithyroid drugs, hyperthyroidism 493, 500, 729
  in block/replacement regime 494, 500
  post-radioiodine therapy 731
  pre-radioiodine therapy 730
anuria, renal transplant 316
anxiety 430
  child 111
  disorders 430
  erection phallography 582
apcitide, ^{99m}Tc- 832–3
aphasia, primary progressive 419
apophyseal injury 364, 365
apoptosis (programmed cell death)
  myocardial 151
  therapy monitoring and 69–71, 834–5
appendages, testicular/gonadal 594
  torsion 594
    imaging 598
aptimers 7, 9
APUDomas see neuroendocrine tumors
arbutamine stress test 154
arcitumomab 42
arm, sports injury 375
arterial supply
  penis 575–6
    angiography 577
    doppler studies 578
    impotence associated with 576, 582, **Plate 13.D1**
    radionuclide studies 578, 579, 580, 581, 582, 583
  testes 594
arteriography see angiography
arthritis
  degenerative (osteoarthritis) 394
  rheumatoid 393
  septic, children 405
arthropathies
  inflammatory 393–6
  seronegative 396
arthroplasty (joint replacement with prosthesis), complications/failure 381–92
  infection 95, 381–92
aseptic loosening of prosthetic joint 381–2
  case history 389
aspirin, polycythemia vera 775
asplenia 692
assessment, child and parent 109–10

association areas, parietotemporal, Alzheimer's disease 416, 417
Association for Eradication of Heart Attack (AEHA) 157
astrocytomas
    histopathological grading/classification 446
    pilocytic 450
    somatostatin receptors 33, 447
asymptomatic patients, screening for disease 799
atherosclerosis 147–8
    coronary 147–8
    plaque 19–20, 147–8
athletic/sports injuries 363, 368–75
atrial septal defect 169, 171
atrial shunts in congenital heart disease 171
atrophy
    Alzheimer's disease 417
    dentatorubral pallidoluysian 460
    multiple system 458–9, **Plates 10E.1–2**
attenuation correction 783, 869–79
    PET 871–2, 874, 874–5
        transmission scanning 871–2, 874–5
    PET, clinical applications
        breast 549
        ^{18}F-FDG whole-body distribution 792
        myocardial perfusion 155, **Plate 6A.2**
    SPECT 870–1, 872–4, 874–5
        clinical applications 876–8
        myocardial perfusion 875, **Plate 21C.1.**
        transmission scanning 870–1, 874–5
attitude, child-centered 110
autoantibodies
    to phospholipids and venous thromboembolism risk 207
    to TSH receptor 728
autoimmune thyroid disease
    Graves' disease 728
    thyroiditis *see* Hashimoto's thyroiditis
autologous transplantation
    bone marrow, following high-dose chemotherapy, neuroblastoma
        758
    stem cells *see* stem cell transplantation
avalanche photodiodes 857
avascular necrosis 396–7
    scaphoid 366, 397
avulsion fractures, pelvis 373
axillary lymph node imaging/biopsy/clearance 127–32, 547–8, 551, 562
    new developments 134
Axillary Lymphatic Mapping Against Nodal Axillary Clearance
        (ALMANAC) 133

B-cell lymphoma
    aggressive vs indolent 696, 697
    extranodal marginal zone 702
B1 (CD20), MAbs to *see* ibritumomab; retuximab; tositumomab
back ache, children 117, 405
bacteria
    antibiotics *see* antibacterial drugs
    antibodies to 94–5
    chemotactic peptides 98
    small bowel, overgrowth 642
    testicular infection 598
Balint's syndrome 23
barium fluoride (BaF$_2$), positron cameras 856
benefit
    clinical 806
    of evaluating diagnostic tests 800
    marginal 812
    see also cost-benefit
benzodiazepine receptor 842

Alzheimer's disease and 421
    antagonist 438–9, 842
    epilepsy and 438–9
beta blockers, hyperthyroidism 493, 500
β -CIT, ^{123}I-, dopaminergic system imaging 420
beta-methyl iodophenyl pentadecanoic acid *see* BMIPP
beta particle therapy 835
    bone metastases 80–1
    gamma imaging for 79, 80
bile acid
    breath test 642
    malabsorption 641
biliary system 643–4
    atresia 115
    carcinoma 648, 665–6
    radiopharmaceuticals used 643–4, 817
biochemical markers of bone turnover 400–1
biodistribution *see* distribution
bioluminescence, optical imaging 12
biomechanics, fracture 363–4
biopsy, sentinel node *see* sentinel lymph nodes
biotherapy, gastrointestinal neuroendocrine tumors 657
bipolar disorder 429
bismuth germanate (BGO) 849, 850, 855, 857
bisphosphonates
    adverse effects 824
    diphosphonate interactions with 825
    osteoporosis 400
    Paget's disease 356–7
bladder
    cancer, ^{131}I therapy-induced 739
    ^{18}F-FDG activity 792–3
    functional assessment 289–92
    radionuclide studies *see* cystography
    urine reflux from *see* vesico-ureteric reflux
bleeding *see* hemorrhage
blood-brain barrier 425
blood cell
    labeling *see* leukocytes; red blood cells
    pooling in spleen *see* spleen
    synthesis *see* hematopoiesis
blood clearance 270
blood dosimetry, related to red marrow 785
blood flow
    cerebral, regional, children 113
    new PET agents 841
    penile
        Doppler studies 577, 578
        flow index (FI) 581–2
        radionuclide methods 578–82
    pulmonary *see* pulmonary vessels
    renal, distribution 263–4
    testicular, Doppler studies 599
blood group compatibility test 678
blood loss *see* hemorrhage
blood pressure
    high *see* hypertension
    reduction by captopril 300
blood supply *see* vascular supply
blood vessel grafts *see* vascular grafts
blue dye (in sentinel node detection) 121–2, 135
    breast cancer 128, 562
    combined with lymphoscintigraphy 125
        breast cancer 130–2
BMIPP (beta-methyl iodophenyl pentadecanoic acid), ^{123}I- 151
    Prinzmetal's angina 159
body outline extraction, prostate cancer imaging 613

body surface area (BSA) as index for physiologic variables
    glomerular filtration rate (GFR) 275
        infants/children 276
    other than GFR 275
bombesin, ^{99m}Tc-, prostate cancer 614
bone
    mass/mineral density measurements 398–401
    metabolic disease 355–62
    PET see positron emission tomography
    radionuclide uptake 332–4, 355
        see also bone scan
    remodelling/turnover 332
        abnormalities 332
        biochemical markers 400–1
        in fracture healing 364
    structure and physiology 331–2
    trauma 363
        fractures see fractures
        pathophysiology 363
bone marrow
    dosimetry 785
    ^{18}F-FDG uptake 792
        false interpretation as malignancy 794–5
    lymphomatous 346, 697–8, 703
    metastases see bone metastases
    suppression (myelosuppression), radioisotope-induced 769
    transplantation
        neuroblastoma, following high-dose chemotherapy 758
        polycythemia vera 773
bone marrow imaging 681–2
    indications 682
    infected joint replacement (±bone scan) 386–8
        disadvantgages 388
bone metastases 337–42
    bone scan see bone scan
    breast cancer 339, 341, 343–4, 552
    case history 349–50
    Ewing's sarcoma 348
    neuroblastoma 535, 760
    pain with see bone pain
    prostate cancer 339, 340, 342, 344, 349–50, 609, 612
    radionuclide therapy 80–1
        gamma imaging for 80
bone pain palliation with radioisotopes 765–71
    administration of radiopharmaceuticals 768
    available radiopharmaceuticals 80, 765–6
    efficacy 768–9
    patient selection 767–8
    response assessment 768
    toxicity of radiopharmaceuticals 769–70
bone scan 332–4
    attenuation correction in SPECT 875–6
    basic principles/background 332–4
        radiopharmaceuticals 332–4, 355, 816
    children 113, 117, 338, 403, 404, 405–8
        injuries 406–8
        reflex sympathetic dystrophy 408
    head and neck cancer 469
    injuries 363–79
        pediatric 406–8
        principles 365
    joint replacement failure 382–3
        combined with gallium scan 383–5
        combined with leukocyte scan 386–8
    metabolic bone disease 355–62
    metastases 80, 338–46
        neuroendocrine tumor 657

radiopharmaceuticals 338
    scintigraphic patterns and correlative imaging 338–42
neuroblastoma 404, 535
osteoarthritis 394
osteomyelitis 95, 117
primary bone tumors 346–9
bone tumors
    primary 346–9
        children 118, 409–11
        lymphoma 703
    secondary see bone metastases
bowel/intestine, ^{18}F-FDG uptake 792
    see also large bowel; small bowel and specific regions
brachial plexopathy, breast cancer 552
brachytherapy (implants)
    brain tumor 449–50
    ovarian cancer 604
brain 413–64
    blood flow see cerebral blood flow; perfusion; perfusion imaging
    CERASPECT scanner 854
    ^{18}F-FDG uptake, normal 448, 792
    functional imaging 20
        in cerebrovascular disease 425–8
        in children, effects of maturation 111
        dementias 416, 418
        psychiatry 428–30
    injury (in head injury) 428
        children 113
    receptor/neurotransmitter imaging
        new PET agents 842
        new SPECT agents 836
    respiratory center 198
brain death 428
    children 113, Plate 4.2
brain registration and analysis of SPECT studies (BRASS) 417
brain tumors 68, 445–55, Plate 21B.1
    epidemiology and etiology 445
    grading 446, 448–9
    histopathological classification 446
    lymphoma 450, 698, 703, Plate 16C.6
    non-radionuclide imaging methods 446–7
    PET 68, 447–52
        false interpretation of 63
    prognostication 449
    somatostatin receptors 33, 447
    SPECT 447
    therapeutic response monitoring 57, 68
BRASS (brain registration and analysis of SPECT studies) 417
breast cancer 65–6, 127–33, 343–4, 541–69
    detection of primaries 544–5, 546–7
    epidemiology 543–67
    guidelines for work-up 543–4
    locally advanced 561–2
    lymph nodes in see axillary lymph node; lymph node metastases;
        mammary nodes
    lymphedema 716
    non-invasive see carcinoma in situ
    occult lesion detection 554
    PET scans 549–54, 564–5, Plate 1D.3
        false interpretation 63, 550, 551, 552
    prognostic factors 543
    radiopharmaceuticals 545
    receptors 564
        somatostatin 33, 545
    recurrence 552, 561
    scintimammography see scintimammography
    screening 128, 544

sentinel node imaging/biopsy 127–33, 551, 562–4
skeletal metastases 339, 341, 343–4, 552
staging and restaging 564–5
therapeutic response monitoring 65–6, 548, 553, 561–2, **Plate 1D.3**
VQ imaging and risk of 218
breast-feeding (lactating) mother, thyroid disease 500
radioiodine contraindicated 500, 731
breath tests 642–3
breathing 198
Breslow thickness 123
busulfan, polycythemia vera 774–5
BW250/183, MAb to 94
bypass grafts, coronary 164–5

CA125 and ovarian cancer 601
cadmium zinc telluride semiconductor detectors 851, 854
caffeine–adenosine interactions 826
calcaneal fracture 369, 370
calcaneonavicular coalition 371
calcification, ectopic, hyperparathyroidism 358
calcium isotopes, skeletal imaging 332
calcium scoring, coronary 157
cameras see gamma cameras
cancellous bone see trabecular bone
cancer see tumors
capacitor-coupled network, SPECT gamma camera 853
capromab pendetide (Prostascint) 42, 610, 612–14, 617–18, **Plates 13H.2–5**
captopril
cortical vs juxtamedullary nephron effects 263–4, 300
drug interactions 826
renal radionuclide studies 300–2, 826
carbimazole, pre-radioiodine therapy 730
carbon dioxide, ^{14}C-
glycolate breath test 642
urea breath test 642
carbon-11-labeled compounds 839, 840
acetate see acetate
adrenaline, pheochromocytoma 534–5
amino acids, brain tumors 451
carfentanil 842
choline see choline
ethanol, hepatocellular carcinoma 665
flumazenil, in epilepsy 438–9, 842
hydroxyephedrine see hydroxyephedrine
5-hydroxytryptophan (HTP), carcinoids 843
molecular targets 840
myocardial fatty acid metabolism 150–1
PIB, Alzheimer's disease 22, 841–2
PK11195 421, 457, 842
raclopride see raclopride
in therapeutic response monitoring 58, 65, 68–9, 843
thymidine see thymidine
carbon-14-labeled compounds
bile acid breath test 642
urease breath test 642
carcinoembryonic antigen (CEA) 40
colorectal cancer 49, 647
^{111}In-labeled MAb to **Plates 1C.2–3**
^{99m}Tc-labeled 50
carcinoid syndrome 654
carcinoid tumors 31, 843
lung **Plate 1D.4**
metastases 7, 10, 30
sites 653
somatostatin receptors 7, 10, 31, 653–4, **Plate 1D.4**
see also neuroendocrine tumors

carcinoma
bile duct 648, 665–6
breast 33
cervical, therapeutic response monitoring 57
colorectal see colorectal cancer
esophageal see esophagus
gastric, therapeutic response monitoring 57, 68
head and neck see head and neck disease, cancer
hepatocellular 648, 661–5
lung see lung cancer
pancreatic 646, **Plate 14D.2**
prostate see prostate cancer
renal cell see renal cell carcinoma
salivary gland 484
skin, trabecular 32
thyroid see thyroid tumors
uterine, skeletal metastases 345
see also adenocarcinoma
carcinoma in situ of breast (in situ carcinoma) 543
PET 550
scintimammography 561
cardiac activity, ^{18}F-FDG 792
cardiac failure 168
cardiology 18–20, 145–82
congenital disease 169–71
ischemic disease see coronary artery disease; ischemic heart disease
PET see positron emission tomography
cardiotoxicity monitoring in chemotherapy 83
carfentanil, ^{11}C 842
carotid artery stenosis 427
carotid body paraganglioma 32
carpal bone fractures 366
CASS (Coronary Artery Surgery Study) 160
catecholamines 530–1
hypersecretion by tumors see paragangliomas
catechol-O-methyltransferase 531
catheterization for direct isotope cystography 287
cavernosography 577
cavernosometry 577
cavernous arteries 575
cavernous body see corpus cavernosum
CD20 (B1), MAbs to see ibritumomab; retuximab; tositumomab
CD66, MAb to 94
CD67, MAb to 94
cell death see apoptosis; necrosis
cell membrane see membrane
cell metabolism, myocardial see metabolism
cell signalling pathways 7
cellular dosimetry 785
cellulitis, children 405
cemented and cementless prosthetic joints 381
central nervous system see brain; spine
CERASPECT brain scanner 854
cerebral blood flow, regional (rCBF) 425
children 113, **Plate 4.1**
imaging 425–8
agents used 425–6, 817–18
epilepsy **Plate 4.4**
subarachnoid imaging **Plate 4.3**
cerebral perfusion see perfusion; perfusion imaging
cerebrovascular disease 425–8
acute 426–7
chronic 427
dementia 418
functional imaging 425–8
parkinsonism 459

cerebrovascular reserve (CVR) 425
  in carotid artery stenosis 427
cervical carcinoma, therapeutic response monitoring 57
cervical node metastases from unknown primary 473
cervical spine, sports injury 374
cesium fluoride (CsF), positron cameras 856
ch14.18 (MAb) 756, 759
Chang method, attenuation correction calculation 873–4
Charnley, Sir John 381
chCE7 (MAb) 756, 759
chemical tumor agents (radioisotopes) 81–2
chemohormonotherapy, breast cancer 553
chemoradiotherapy
  colorectal carcinoma 66–7
  lung cancer (non-small cell) 65
  testicular tumors 570–1
chemotactic peptides, bacterial 98
chemotherapy/cytotoxic drugs (incl. response monitoring) 82
  breast cancer 65–6, 548, 553, 561–2
  children 409
  ^{18}F-FDG imaging after, false interpretation 795
  gastrointestinal tumors
    colorectal carcinoma 66, 67, 647
    esophageal cancer 68, 645–6
    gastric carcinoma 68
    neuroendocrine 657
  glomerular filtration rate measurements in toxicity prediction 275
  liver metastases 668, 669
  lung cancer 60, 63, 64, 65, 230
  lymphoma 699–700, 705–6
    high-dose, followed by stem cell transplantation 705
  neuroblastoma 755
    high-dose, followed by bone marrow or stem cell transplantation 758
  organ toxicity monitoring 82
  polycythemia vera 774–5
  see also chemohormonotherapy; chemoradiotherapy; multidrug-resistant 1 P-glycoprotein
chest/thorax
  disease see lung
  ^{18}F-FDG activity 792
  lymphoma, morphologic imaging pre-therapy 697
  pain, cardiac sources 159
  sports injury 374
  see also mediastinum
children 107–19, 403–12
  cerebral blood flow (regional) 113, **Plate 4.1**
  ^{18}F-FDG whole-body uptake 793
  handling 107–11
  hyperthyroidism treatment 500
  musculoskeletal non-traumatic disorders 403–6, 408–11
  musculoskeletal trauma 365–6, 367, 406–8
    epidemiology 364–5
    non-accidental injury (child abuse) 117, 367, 406–8
  neuroblastoma radionuclide therapy 756
  neurology
    brain death 113, **Plate 4.2**
    brain trauma 113
    epilepsy 113, 439–40
    tumors 445
  renal studies see kidney
chloramine T in radiolabeling technique 46
cholangiocarcinoma 648, 665–6
cholecystitis, acute 644
cholecystokinin 643
  analogs 35, 751
  receptors 35

cholesterol 55
  radiolabeled analogs of 522–3
    adrenal incidentaloma 529–30
    drugs interacting with 522, 526
choline, ^{11}C- 843
  brain tumors 451
  therapeutic response monitoring 58
    prostate cancer 69
  see also fluorocholine
cholinergic system imaging 421
choreatic disorders 460
choriogonadotrophic hormone, MAb 602
chromium-51 chloride test in protein-losing enteropathy 643
chromium-51-labeled compounds and cells
  albumin, protein-losing enteropathy 681
  EDTA 262
  red cells 676
    anemia assessment 643, 680
    blood group compatibility testing 678
    GI blood loss assessment 677–8
    mean red cell life span assessment 677
    red cell destruction site determination 679
chronic regional pain syndrome see reflex sympathetic dystrophy
ciliated fallopian tube cells 586
cine-MRI, myocardial viability assessment 185
cingulate gyrus and Alzheimer's disease 417
ciprofloxacin, ^{99m}Tc- 101, 833
  arthritides 393
  prosthetic joint infection 388
citrate, ^{67}Ga- 93
  adverse reactions 823
  head and neck cancer 467
  joint replacement failure 383–5
  lymphoma 698
  pulmonary infections 96
clearance 269–72, 274
  measurement 270–1
  plasma see plasma clearance
  residence/transit time and 273, 274
  urinary see urine
  ^{131}Xe in phallography 676–7
Clinical Outcomes Utilizing Percutaneous Coronary Revascularization and Aggressive Drug Evaluation (COURAGE) trial 165
CLO test 642
clopidogrel 81
cobalamin see vitamin B$_{12}$
cobalt-57-labeled vitamin B$_{12}$/cyanocobalamin 641, 681
cobalt-57 point or flood source in lymphoscintigraphy 124
  breast cancer 130
  melanoma 125
cobalt-58-labeled vitamin B$_{12}$/cyanocobalamin 681
cocaine derivatives (tropanes), dopaminergic system imaging 420, 458
coincidence detection 855, 872
  annihilation 855
collateral ligaments of knee, injury 373
collecting system in kidney, dilatation in children 116–17
collimators 852
  fan beam 870, 871
  focused, scintillation counters coupled to 854
colloid(s), radiolabeled (^{99m}Tc)
  gastrointestinal tract
    bleeding 623
    esophageal transit 637
  infected joint replacement 386–8
  lymphoscintigraphy 122–3, 125
    breast cancer 128, 132, 562, 563
    injection of see injections

in lymphatic disease/limb swelling 716
  radiation hazard 134
  radiolabeling method 132
reticuloendothelial system 682
splenic imaging 686
  metastases 692
transport in lymphatic system 716
colloid(s), transport in lymph 716
colloid goiter, simple 506–8
colon
  bleeding 623
  ^{18}F-FDG uptake 792
colony-stimulating factor interactions with FDG 826
colorectal cancer (predominantly carcinoma) 49–52, 66–7, 646–7, 648
  case history 648
  false interpretation of PET scans 63
  metastases 13
    liver 7, 13, 51, 646, 647, 667–8, 669
    primary 50–1
  radioimmunoscintigraphy 7, 49–52
  recurrent 51–2, 646–7
  screening 646
  therapeutic response monitoring 57, 66–7, 647, 648
compact bone see cortical bone
compartmental model of kidney 257–8
complement factor 5a 99–100
complementarity determinant region and MAbs 44
Compton camera 855
Compton effect 855, 856, 869
computed tomography (CT)
  adrenal cortical disorders 523
    incidentaloma 529
  brain
    dementia 416
    tumors 446
  breast cancer
    distant metastases 552
    intrathoracic nodal metastases 551
  colorectal carcinoma
    recurrent disease/liver metastases 647
    staging 646
    therapeutic response monitoring 67
  inflammatory bowel disease 633, 634
  liver cancer
    metastatic 667, 668
    primary 661–2
  lung cancer staging 226
  lymphoma
    post-therapy 704
    pre-therapy 697–8
  molecular imaging 11–12
  multichannel/multislice/multidetector, coronary disease 11, 157, 159
  ovarian cancer 602
  positron emission tomography combined with see positron emission tomography/computed tomography
  quantitative, bone mass measurement 399
  radiotherapy planning, combined with image registration in PET or SPECT 863
  single photon emission see single photon emission computed tomography
  single photon emission computed tomography combined with see single photon emission computed tomography/computed tomography
  skeletal metastases 342
  spiral, venous thromboembolism 208
computed tomography angiography 11

coronary 157, 169, **Plate 6A.9**
pulmonary (CTPA), for pulmonary embolism 197, 209, 210, 212, 213, 214, 216, 220
  cancer risk 219
  in pregnancy 217, 218
CONCORDE microPET system 858
congenital anomalies/malformations (developmental abnormalities)
  heart 169–71
  renal tract, infection predisposition 288
  spleen 686–7, 692
  testicular torsion due to 595–6
congenital hypothyroidism (neonatal hypothyroidism) 114, 494–5, 509–10
congenital remnants of thyroid tissue along thyroglossal tract, hypertrophy 509
Conn's syndrome 526–7
contrast agents in PET/CT 796
contrast echocardiography, myocardial 157
  viability assessment 167, 189
contrast-enhanced MR, myocardial viability assessment 167, 185–6
cooperation, child and parent's 111
copper-62 PTSM 841
coronary artery anomalies 171
coronary artery disease 147–69
  diagnosis 156–61
  epidemiology 147
  future prospects for radionuclide imaging 169
  imaging techniques 148–56
    angiography 11, 157, 169, **Plate 6A.9**
  screening 157–8
  therapy 163–5
    revascularization 164–5, 184–5, **Plate 6A.17–19**
  see also ischemic heart disease
Coronary Artery Surgery Study (CASS) 160
coronary spasm 159
corpus cavernosum
  anatomy 575
  blood flow studies in phallography 578, 580
  blood supply/drainage 575, 576
  cavernosometry and cavernosography 577
  dysfunction 582
  injection in phallography 582
    vasoactive drugs 577
    ^{131}Xe 578, 579, 580
  pressure studies 577
corpus spongiosum, anatomy 575
cortex (adrenal) see adrenal gland
cortex (renal)
  nephrons
    captopril effects 263–4, 300
    flow 263–4
  scarring associated with urinary tract infection 289
cortical (compact) bone 331
  remodelling 331
corticobasal degeneration 459, **Plate 10E.3**
  case history 460–1
corticosteroids and fracture risk 400
corticotrophin see adrenocorticotrophic hormone
corticotrophin-releasing hormone-secreting tumors 33
cost
  direct 800, 811
  of evaluating diagnostic tests 800
  fixed 811
  incremental 807, 809, 812
  indirect 812
  marginal 812
  opportunity 806, 807, 812

cost-benefit 807–8, 811
cost-effectiveness 806–7, 808–10
  definition 811
  FDG PET 810
    lung cancer 227–30
  incremental 809, 812
  marginal 812
cost-minimization 811
cost-utility 807
COURAGE (Clinical Outcomes Utilizing Percutaneous Coronary
    Revascularization and Aggressive Drug Evaluation) trial 165
cranium (skull), Paget's disease 356
cremasteric artery 594
Crohn's disease
  case reports 632–4
  diagnosis 630
  follow-up and complications 631
  severity of disease 631
cruciate ligament injury 372–3
crying child 111
crystals, scintillation 849–50
  PET gamma cameras and size of 856
  see also multi-crystal scanners
CTI EXACT HR+ 857
cuboid injury 369
Cushing's syndrome 523–4
  somatostatin receptors 33
cyanocobalamin see vitamin B$_{12}$
cyclosporin A
  blood cell labeling affected by 827
  renal transplant 317
    toxicity problems 318
cyst(s), renal 321, 322
cystography, radionuclide
  direct 286–7
  indirect (IRC) 285–6, 287, 289–90, **Plate 8C.1**
CYT-351, ^{99m}Tc- (Prostatec) 610, **Plate 13H.1**
CYT-356, ^{111}In- (Prostascint) 42, 610, 612–14, 617–18, **Plates 13H.2–5**
CYT-422 610
cytokines
  coronary artery disease and 148
  radiolabeled 98–9, 100–1, 832
cytotoxic anticancer drugs see chemotherapy

D dimer measurement 208, 213
dacryoscintigraphy 485
DaTSCAN see FP-CIT, ^{123}I-
De Quervain's tenosynovitis 375
De Quervain's thyroiditis (subacute thyroiditis)
  diagnosis and clinical features 494, 496, 498–9, 507
  pain 505
  treatment 502
dead-time limits of detectors 851–2
death see apoptosis; brain death; necrosis
decision analysis 809, 811
deconvolution analysis, linear system model of kidney 257–8, 263
dedifferentiation antigens 40
deep vein thrombosis
  clinical presentation 207
  diagnosis 208
  origin 206–7
defecography 640–1
defense role, lymphatic system 715–16
deferential artery 594
dementia 22–4, 419–23, 841–2, **Plates 10A.2–7**
  imaging modalities 416
  types 415

dentatorubral pallidoluysian atrophy 460
depreotide, ^{99m}Tc-labeled 29–30, 834
  lung
    cancer 32–3
    solitary nodule 224–5
  neuroendocrine tumors 657
    pancreatic 31
depression 429
dermis in lymphoscintigraphy
  backflow 718
  injections of radiocolloids see injections
Detection of Ischemia in Asymptomatic Diabetes (DIAD) trial 160–1
detectors (incl. solid-state devices) 849–59
  coincidence see coincidence detection
  dead-time limits 851–2
  performance comparisons 851–2
  scintillation see scintillation detectors
  thallium-doped sodium iodide see thallium-doped sodium iodide
  see also gamma camera
developmental abnormalities see congenital anomalies
dexamethasone suppression scintigraphy 522
  Conn's syndrome 527
  hyperandrogenism 528
diabetes and coronary artery disease 160–1
DIAD (Detection of Ischemia in Asymptomatic Diabetes) trial 160–1
diagnostic imaging 799–812
  categories 799
  economic analysis of 806–10
  evaluation of
    economic 800
    performance evaluation 800–4
  goals 800
  introduction of new technologies 800
dialysis, chronic ambulatory peritoneal, infections 318–19
diaminocyclohexane, ^{99m}Tc- 261
diastolic volume measurement 161
  see also end diastole
diethylenetriamine pentaacetic acid see DTPA
differential renal function, children 116, 283
differentiation status of tumors, degree 42
diffuse goiter
  nontoxic 491
  thyroid scan findings 506
  toxic see Graves' disease
diffuse large B-cell lymphoma 13, **Plate 16C.2**
digestive tract see gastrointestinal tract
dihydroxyphenylalanine see DOPA
di-isopropyl iminodiacetic acid see DISIDA
dimercaptosuccinic acid see DMSA
(2-((2-((dimethylamino) methyl) phenyl) thio)-5-iodophenylamine)
    (ADAM), ^{123}I- 429
diphosphonate compounds, ^{99m}Tc- 333, 355, 816
  adverse events 823
  drug interactions 825
  structure 816
dipyridamole stress testing 153
direct cost 800, 811
discitis (diskitis), children 405
DISIDA (di-isopropyl iminodiacetic acid), ^{99m}Tc-
  biliary atresia 115
  polycystic kidney disease 115
diskitis, children 405
distribution (of agents) 821, 824–6
  functional imaging agents 815–16
  volume of see volume of distribution
diuretic renography (with frusemide) 305, 308–10
  children 116–17

diverticulum, Meckel's 624–5, 626
DMSA (dimercaptosuccinic acid), ^{99m}Tc-
  bone tumors
    primary 347
    secondary (metastases) 338
  head and neck cancer 469
  neuroendocrine tumors 657
  renal studies 261, 269–70, 816
  renal studies in children 113, 117, 283
    abnormal patterns (in general) 284
    in case history 292
    normal kidney incl. variants 283–4
    polycystic kidney disease 117
    renal scarring 285, 288
dobutamine, drug interactions 826
dobutamine stress test 153–4
  contraindications 154
DOPA (dihydroxyphenylalanine) 842
  ^{18}F- see fluorodopa
  metabolism 530
DOPA-responsive dystonia 460
dopamine D_2 receptors
  multiple system atrophy 459
  new PET agents 842
  Parkinson's disease 458
  schizophrenia 429
dopamine transporters (DATs) 457
  Parkinson's disease 458
dopaminergic system 420–1
  Lewy body dementia 420
  movement disorders 457
    Parkinson's disease 20–1, 420, 458
  new PET agents 842
  schizophrenia 429
Doppler sonography
  ovarian cancer 601–2
  penile blood flow 577, 582
    pharmacologically-induced erections 578
  testicular blood flow 599
  venous, swollen limb 722
dose (radiopharmaceutical)
  adrenal scintigraphy 524
  external beam radiotherapy 781
  hysterosalpingoscintigraphy 589–91
  ^{131}I therapy (and its calculation)
    in hyperthyroidism 501, 731
    in thyroid cancer 735, 738, 784
  pediatric, scaling down 108
    musculoskeletal system 403
    renal studies 282
  radionuclide therapy (and its measurement) 90, 781–8
    case history **Plate 17F.1**
    cellular/multicellular dosimetry 785
    clinical applications 785
    image registration 864
    ^{131}I see subheading above
    marrow dosimetry 785
    overview of standard dosimetry 781–2
    ^{32}P in polycythemia vera 778
    tumor dosimetry 783–4
    whole-body dosimetry 784–5
  VQ scan 199, 202
  see also radiation exposure
DOTA compounds
  [DOTA,1-NaI^3]octreotide 751
  ^{68}Ga-DOTA-TOC/NOC, neuroendocrine tumor therapeutic response
    monitoring 69, **Plates 1D.1–2, Plate 1D.4**

^{111}In- see indium-111
^{177}Lu-DOTA-octreotate, neuroendocrine tumor therapy 34, 659, 747–50
double (duplex) kidney 284
DPC11870-11 (LTB$_4$ receptor antagonist) 100
drug-induced conditions 824
  parkinsonism 459–60
  thyrotoxicosis/hyperthyroidism 498, 502
drug interactions (radiopharmaceutical agents) 821–9
  adrenocortical scintigraphic agents 522–3, 533
  with pheochromocytoma 533
drug therapy
  cancer see anticancer drugs
  coronary artery disease 165
  erectile dysfunction 582
  osteoporosis 400
  Paget's disease of bone 356–7
  thyroid disorders
    hyperthyroidism 493, 500, 729
    thyroiditis 502
  see also pharmacological stress test; pharmacologically-induced penile
    erections and specific drugs
DTPA (diethylenetriamine pentaacetic acid)
  dynamic renography, children 112
  Gd-, myocardial viability assessment 166
  ^{111}In- see indium-111
  ^{99m}Tc-
    brain death in children 113
    breast 545
  ^{99m}Tc-, gastrointestinal studies
    gastric emptying 638
    rectal emptying of feces 640
  ^{99m}Tc-, lung
    idiopathic interstitial diseases 243
    immunosuppressed conditions 248
    permeability measurement 240, 241, 242
    VQ scans 203, 205
  ^{99m}Tc-, renal studies 816
    comparisons with other pharmaceuticals 260
    transplant recipients 316, 318, 319
  ^{90}Y-DTPA-minigastrin 751
DTPA-mannosyl-dextran, ^{99m}Tc- 135
dual energy X-ray absorptiometry 398–400
dual-headed gamma cameras
  PET 857
  SPECT 870
dual photon absorptiometry, bone mass measurement 398
ductal carcinoma in situ (DCIS) 543
  PET 550
  scintimammography 561
duplex kidney 284
dynamic stress test 152
dyshormonogenetic goiter 508
dystonia 460

EC (ethylene dicysteine), ^{99m}Tc- 260, 261
ECAT EXACT HR+ 857
ECD (ethyl cysteine dimer), ^{99m}Tc-, cerebral blood flow estimation 425, 426
  epilepsy **Plate 4.4**
ECG see electrocardiography
echocardiography (myocardial)
  acute coronary syndrome 159
  congenital heart disease 170
  contrast see contrast echocardiography, myocardial
  myocardial viability assessment 185, 187–8
  pulmonary embolism 209

economic analysis
    of diagnostic tests 806–10
    in evaluation of diagnostic tests 800
ectopic calcification, hyperparathyroidism 358
ectopic tissue/organ
    kidney 117
    spleen 692
    thyroid 508–9
        pediatric 114–15, 509
        struma ovarii (in ovarian tumor) 498, 503, 604
edema *see* lipedema; lymphedema
EDTA, ^{51}Cr- 262
EDTMP, ^{153}S- 766, 768, 769
education and information, child and parent 108
    renal nuclear medicine 281
EEG, epilepsy 425
effective renal plasma flow (ERPF) 273
effectiveness
    definition 811
    of test 806
        clinical 806
    see also cost-effectiveness
efficacy
    definition 811
    of test 806
egg, fertilization 586–7
ejection fraction, ventricular 18
    left 154, 183, **Plate 6A.1**
        coronary artery disease outcome and 161
        post-myocardial infarction risk stratification and 163
elderly, thyroid dysfunction 500–1
    in sick patients 495
    see also age-related occurrence
electrocardiography (ECG)
    myocardial viability 166
    stress testing *see* stress testing
electroconvulsive therapy 429
electroencephalography, epilepsy 425
embolism, pulmonary
    anticoagulant therapy 220
    clinical presentation 207
    diagnosis 197
        perfusion scan 199–200
    resolution 200
embolization therapy, neuroendocrine tumors hepatic metastases 657–8
embryology, testicular 594
Emergency Room Assessment of Sestamibi for Evaluation of Chest Pain (ERASE) trial 159
emissary veins of penis 576
Emory Cardiac Toolbox 155
end diastole
    surface views **Plate 6B.2**
    volume measurement 161
endarterectomy, carotid 427
endocrine disease 489–539
endocrine pancreatic tumors 31
endocrine therapy *see* chemohormonotherapy; hormone therapy
eniluracil 779
enthesopathy and enthesitis
    in seronegative arthropathy 396
    sport-related 368, 372
environmental risk factors
    brain tumors 445–6
    venous thromboembolism 207
enzymopathies, thyroid hormone metabolism 508

EORTC tumor response criteria 59, 60
epididymitis 593, 598
epilepsy (and epileptic seizures) 435–43, **Plate 4.4, Plates 10C.1–3**
    brain tumors and 449
    case histories 440–1
    children 113, 439–40
    PET 20, 22, 435, 436, 436–9
epinephrine (adrenaline)
    ^{11}C-, pheochromocytoma 534–5
    metabolism 531
epiphysis, slipped capital femoral 364, 406
equilibrium radionuclide ventriculography 183–4
ERASE (Emergency Room Assessment of Sestamibi for Evaluation of Chest Pain) trial 159
ErbB-2 (Her2; neu), MAbs to 604
erection
    dysfunction *see* impotence
    phallography 579, 581–2, 583, **Plate 13.D1**
    pharmacologically-induced *see* pharmacologically-induced penile erections
    physiology 575–6
erythrocytes (red blood cells), ^{99m}Tc- *see* polycythemia; red blood cells
erythropoietin, inappropriate secretion 677
Escherichia coli chemotactic peptides 98
esophagus
    carcinoma 645–6, **Plate 14D.1.**
        therapeutic response monitoring 57, 68, 645–6
    ^{18}F-FDG uptake 792
    transit 637–8
essential tremor 460
estrogens
    ^{18}F-, breast cancer 565
    therapeutic use affecting thyroid function 494
    see also anti-estrogen therapy; oral contraceptives
ethanol, ^{11}C-, hepatocellular carcinoma 665
ethnicity and bone densitometry in fracture risk determination 400
ethyl cysteine dimer *see* ECD
ethylene dicysteine (EC), ^{99m}Tc- 260, 261
ethylenediaminetetraacetic acid, ^{51}Cr- 262
ethylenediaminetetramethylene phosphate (EDTMP), ^{153}S- 766, 768, 769
etidronate–diphosphonate interactions 825
Europe, adverse event reports 822
European American classification of lymphoid neoplasms, revised (REAL) 696
European Organization for Research and Treatment of Cancer, tumor response criteria 59, 60
evaluation, child and parent 109–10
Ewing's sarcoma 348
exametazime *see* HMPAO
excretion, renal *see* output efficiency; urine
exercise stress test 151–2
    indications/contraindications 152
    protocols 152
extracellular fluid volume (ECFV) 273, 274, 275, 278
    infants/children 276
extracellular matrix, skeleton/bone 331
extraction fraction, renal 273, 274
eye disease, dysthyroid 732–3
    TSH receptor antibody and 728

Fab' fragment
    anti-CD66MAb *see* sulesomab
    ^{99m}Tc-labeled, *P. carinii* pneumonia 247

F(ab')$_2$ fragments in radioimmunoscintigraphy 47
factor V Leiden 207
fallopian tubes
    anatomy and physiology 585–6
    imaging *see* hysterosalpingography; hysterosalpingoscintigraphy
fan beam collimation 870, 871
fanolesomab, ^{99m}Tc-, infected joint replacement 388
Fanous technique and index 578, 579
fascitis, plantar 368–9
fatty acid metabolism, cardiac pathology 150–1
    variant/Prinzmetal's angina 159
FDDNP, ^{18}F-, Alzheimer's disease 842
FDG (fluorodeoxyglucose), ^{18}F- 791–8, 839
    adrenal scintigraphy 524
        incidentaloma 530
    bile duct carcinoma 665–6
    breast cancer 549–54, 564–5
        therapeutic response monitoring **Plate 1D.3**
    colony-stimulating factor interactions with 826
    cost-effectiveness *see* cost-effectiveness
    gastrointestinal cancer 68, 645–51
        neuroendocrine tumor staging/restaging 654, 655
    head and neck cancer 471–5
    infection and inflammation 95–8
    prosthetic joint 388
    liver cancer
        metastatic 667–8
        primary 662
    lung
        sarcoidosis 244–5
        solitary nodule 224–5, 225–6
    lung cancer 227–33, 234–5
        distant metastases 227
        impact on management and cost-effectiveness 227–30
        recurrence/relapse 230
        staging 63–4, 226–7
        therapeutic response monitoring 57, 60, 230–2
    lymphoma *see* lymphoma
    metabolism 791–2
    myocardial viability assessment 150, 166, 187–8, 841,
        Plate 6B.2
    neurology
        dementias (incl. Alzheimer's disease) 23, 24, 419
        epilepsy 20, 436–9
        multiple system atrophy **Plate 10E.1**
        Parkinson's disease **Plate 10E.1**
        tumors 68, 447–51, 452, 453
    normal appearances and variations 791–2
    ovarian cancer 604
    patient preparation for imaging with 794
    pitfalls and artifacts 791–8
    pleural disease incl. mesothelioma 233–4
    prostate cancer 611
    skeletal metastases 338, 345–6
    staging 834
        lung cancer 63–4, 226–7
        neuroendocrine tumors 654, 655
    standardized uptake value *see* standardized uptake value
    testicular tumors 570–2
    tumors (in general)
        molecular characterization 12, 13, 14
        residual disease detection 17–18
        therapeutic response 17–18, 57–69
FDG (fluorodeoxyglucose), ^{18}F- 9
feces, rectal emptying 640–1
feet *see* foot

females (women)
    coronary artery disease prognosis 162
    genital tract *see* gynecological disorders
    hyperandrogenism 527–8
femur
    avascular necrosis
        femoral condyles 397
        femoral head 396, 406
    slipped capital epiphysis 364, 406
ferrokinetics 679
fertility problems *see* infertility
fertilization 586–7
fetus, ventilation/perfusion scan risk to 217, 219
fever (pyrexia) of unknown origin (PUO) 96
    HIV-positive patients 246
fibrin D dimer measurement 208, 213
fibrinolytics *see* thrombolytic/fibrinolytic therapy
fibroids, uterine 42
fibrosis
    idiopathic pulmonary 243
    testicular tumors 570
fibular fractures 370, 372
filariasis 723
fine needle aspiration, solitary thyroid nodule 504
first-pass radionuclide angiography, shunt quantitation 170–1,
    Plates 6A.21–2
fixed cost 811
flaccid phallography 579, 580, 582, 583
flare response in cancer
    with bone metastases
        breast cancer 341, 342
        prostate cancer 342
    post-therapy 795
flow, blood *see* blood flow
fluconazole, ^{99m}Tc- 101
fluid
    balance, lymphatic system in 715
    volume, extracellular *see* extracellular fluid volume
flumazenil, ^{11}C-, in epilepsy 438–9, 842
fluorescence, optical imaging 12
fluoride-18, skeletal imaging 332, 333, 841
    Paget's disease of bone 357
    see also barium fluoride
fluorine-18-labeled compounds 839
    DOPA *see* fluorodopa
    dopamine, pheochromocytoma 843
    estrogens, breast cancer 565
    FDDNP, Alzheimer's disease 842
    PIB, Alzheimer's disease 842
    in therapeutic response monitoring 58
    6-thia-hepta-decanoic acid 151
    see also specific fluoro- compounds below
fluorocholine, ^{18}F-
    brain tumors 451
    therapeutic response monitoring 58
fluorodeoxyglucose *see* FDG
fluorodihydroxyphenylalanine, ^{18}F-, therapeutic response monitoring 58
fluorodopa, ^{18}F- 842
    Lewy body dementia 420
    movement disorders 457
        Parkinson's disease 420, **Plate 10E.1**
    multiple system atrophy **Plate 10E.1**
    neuroendocrine tumors 648, 843
fluorodopamine, ^{18}F-, pheochromocytoma 843
fluoro-17-β-estradiol, ^{18}F-, therapeutic response monitoring 58
fluoroethyltyrosine, ^{18}F-, therapeutic response monitoring 58

fluoromisonidazole, ^{18}F- 151
fluoroquinolone antibiotic *see* ciprofloxacin
fluorothymidine, ^{18}F-
  brain tumors 451
  liver metastases 669
  therapeutic response monitoring 58
fluorotyrosine, ^{18}F-, therapeutic response monitoring 58
fluorouracil (5-FU) in colorectal carcinoma 647
  and radiotherapy 66–7
fluorouracil, ^{18}F-, in therapeutic response monitoring 58, 669
  colorectal carcinoma 67
  liver metastases 669
FMISO, ^{18}F- 151
focal seizures *see* partial seizures
focused collimators, scintillation counters coupled to 854
follicular thyroid cancer 733
  radioiodine therapy 735
Fontan procedure 171
foot
  injuries 368–71
  osteoarthritis 394
forearm, sports injury 375
4D image registration 863
4D-MSPECT 155, **Plate 6A.5**
Fourier analysis of image, equilibrium radionuclide ventriculography 184
FP-CIT, ^{123}I- (DaTSCAN; ^{123}I-ioflupane) 836
  corticobasal degeneration **Plate 10E.2**
  Lewy body dementia 420, **Plate 10A.9**
  multiple system atrophy **Plate 10E.2**
  normal appearance **Plate 10A.8**
  parkinsonism
    Parkinson's disease 420, 458, **Plate 10E.2**
    vascular 459
fractional uptake rate (FUR) in kidney 254, 262
fractures 366–7
  biomechanics 363–4
  children 367
  clinical presentation 364
  healing/repair 363–4
    complications 375–6
  insufficiency 367–8
  pathological
    osteomalacia 359
    osteoporosis (or osteopenic) 357–8, 400
    Paget's disease of bone 257
    vertebrae *see* vertebrae
  pathophysiology 363
  sports
    ankle/foot 369, 370
    arm/forearm 375
    rib 374
    spine 374
    thigh/hip/pelvis 373
    tibial region 372
    wrist/hand 375
France, adverse events
  reports 822
  SPECT agents 822
Freiberg's disease 396
frontotemporal dementia 418–19
frusemide *see* furosemide
functional imaging (in general) 815–18
  agents for 815–18
    characteristics of selected agents 816–18
  brain *see* brain
  cardiac disease 145–82

children 111–18
  indications 113–18
  infant maturation and 111–13
  gastrointestinal tract 637–44
  salivary glands *see* salivary glands
  spleen 676, 686–91
  see also specific modalities
functional MRI, brain 20
  epilepsy 425
functional MRS, brain 20
fungal infections, tracers 101, 833
furifosmin, ^{99m}Tc-, myocardial perfusion scan 149
furosemide (frusemide)
  diuresis *see* diuretic renography
  whole body imaging in breast cancer 549–50

G250 (MAb), renal tumor therapy 324–6
GABA and epilepsy 438
gadolinium (Gd/contrast)-enhanced MRI, myocardial viability assessment 167, 185–6
gadolinium orthosilicate (GSO) 849, 850
gadolinium oxisulfide (Gadox) 854
gadolinium-153, SPECT transmission source 870–1
gallbladder function 643
gallium-67 scans
  compounds for 82
    citrate *see* citrate
  head and neck cancer 468
  joint replacement failure 383–5
  lung
    HIV-positive patients 245–6
    infection/inflammation 240
    sarcoidosis 244
  lymphoma 695, 698–700, 876, **Plates 16C.1–2**
    vs PET scans at initial staging 704
    vs PET scans post-therapy 706
  myocardial uptake 246
  renal transplant recipients, for infections 318
gallium-68 somatostatin analogs, neuroendocrine tumor therapeutic response monitoring 69, **Plates 1D.1–2, Plate 1D.4**
gamma-aminobutyric acid (GABA) and epilepsy 438
gamma cameras (and gamma imaging) 852–8
  for beta therapy 79, 80
  breast-specific 547
  myocardial perfusion imaging 149
  new 858
  pediatric imaging 111
  for PET 855–8
  renal imaging, comparison of pharmaceuticals 260
  renal transplant recipients 319
  for SPECT 852–5
  testicular scans 596
  transmission scanning 870
gamma probe, hand-held, sentinel mode imaging 122, 125–6
  new developments 135
gamma rays 849
  detection efficiency (ε) 849
    positron camera 856
  detectors *see* detectors; gamma cameras
  in PET, production/scattering 855
gaseous detectors 850
  performance comparisons with other detectors 851
gastric problems *see* stomach
gastrin, radiolabeled 657, 751
gastrin-releasing peptide receptors and analogs 35
gastrinomas 654
  somatostatin receptors 31

gastroenteropancreatic tumors *see* neuroendocrine tumors
gastrointestinal stromal tumors 69, 648
    drug discovery 17–18, 69
    therapeutic response monitoring 57, 69, 648
gastrointestinal tract 619–72
    bleeding 621–8, 643, 676, 677–8
        anemia *see* anemia
    ^{18}F-FDG uptake 792
    functional studies 637–44
    pediatric 115
    protein loss 643, 681
    tumors 645–60
        neuroendocrine *see* neuroendocrine tumors
        stromal *see* gastrointestinal stromal tumors
gated angiography, multiplanar 183–4
gated myocardial perfusion SPECT 154, 156, **Plates 6A.4–5,**
        Plate 6A.14
    diagnosis of coronary artery disease 156–7
    gated post-myocardial infarction risk stratification 163
    in LV functional assessment 183
gender (sex)
    coronary artery disease prognosis and 162
    fracture risk determination and 400
gene expression, PET studies 71
gene therapy, neuroblastoma 759
generalized seizures
    children 439
    classification 435
genetic causes
    of goiter 508
    of hemostatic disorders predisposing to venous thromboembolism 207
genital/reproductive tract 569–618
    female *see* gynecological disorders
    male 569–83, 609–28
germ cell tumors, non-seminomatous (NSGCT)
    diagnosis and staging 569
    imaging at diagnosis 570
    recurrence and follow-up 570, 571
germanate, bismuth (BGO) 849, 850, 855, 857
germanium semiconductor detectors 851
germanium-68/gallium-67 transmission source 872
germanium-68 transmission source 871–2
Gleason score 344, 611
Gleevec *see* imatinib mesylate
glioblastoma 451
glioma (glial cell tumors)
    etiology 445, **Plate 21B.1**
    grading 448–9
    ^{131}I-monoclonal antibody therapy 449–50
    molecular imaging 14
        somatostatin receptors 33
glomerular filtration flow 254
glomerular filtration rate (GFR) 254, 270–3, 275–8
    filtration marker
        extraction fraction 273
        ideal 270
        volume of distribution 274
    indexation to body size 275–8
    measurement 270–3
        simplified worked example 271–3
glottic cancer, radiotherapy planning **Plate 11A.2**
glucantime–^{99m}Tc-MDP interactions 825–6
glucose (uptake/metabolism)
    myocardial 150
    tumors 61
        lung cancer 64
    see also GLUT-1

glucose-6-phosphatase and ^{18}F-FDG 791
glucose-6-phosphate dehydrogenase isoenzymes and polycythemia vera
        773, 778
GLUT-1 (glucose transporter)
    lymphoma 702
    pancreatic carcinoma 646
glycocholate, ^{14}C-, in bile acid breath test 642
glycolysis, total lesion 61
glycoprotein IIb/IIIa receptor antagonist 832–3
goiter 506–8
    diffuse *see* diffuse goiter
    dyshormonogenetic 508
    intrathoracic/mediastinal 509
    nodular *see* multinodular goiter; nodular goiter
    nontoxic 491, 506–8
    painful 505–6
    thyroid scan in assessment 506
    toxic *see* toxic goiter
grafts and transplants *see* bone marrow; kidney; stem cell
        transplantation; vascular grafts
granulocytes, radiolabeled antibodies 94–5, 682
    HIV disease 247
granulomatous disease/disorders
    ^{18}F-FDG uptake in, false interpretation as malignancy 794
    lungs 240, 243–5
Graves' disease (toxic diffuse goiter) 492, 495, 496, 499–500, 728–9
    diagnosis 496
    somatostatin receptors 34
    treatment 499–500, 729
        radioiodine 499–500, 729–30
gray matter, normal, FDG uptake in tumors relative to 448
growth plates (physis) and their injury 364, 365
    bone scans 113, 405
gut *see* gastrointestinal tract
gynecological disorders
    cancer 601–8
    infertility *see* infertility

hamate fracture 366
hand
    injury 365
    osteoarthritis 395
Hashimoto's (autoimmune) thyroiditis 507–8
    diagnosis 494, 507–8
    pain 505–6
    thyroid lymphoma associated with 507
    treatment 502, 508
Haycock equation 277, 278
HDP (hexamethylpropylene diphosphonate) 816
head and neck disease 465–87
    cancer (predominantly squamous cell carcinoma) 467–82, **Plates**
        11A.1–2
        clinical background 467
        diagnosis and morphologic imaging 467–8
        orbital invasion 487
        prognostication 471
        sentinel node imaging/biopsy 133, 475–7
        types other than squamous carcinoma 467
    salivary glands *see* salivary glands
head frame, stereotactic 862
head injury *see* brain
heart *see entries under* cardio-
heat-damaged red blood cells, splenic imaging 686
HEDP, ^{186}Rh- and ^{188}Rh- 766, 768, 769
helical (spiral) CT, venous thromboembolism 208
helicine arteries of penis 575, 576
Helicobacter pylori infection 642

hematocele 598
hematological disorders 673–724
    ^{131}I-MIBG-induced 759
    malignancy 692
    radioisotope (for bone pain)-induced 769–70
hematological status, radionuclide therapy for bone pain 767
hematoma, renal transplant 316
hematopoiesis 682
    extramedullary 693
hemodynamics, penile 579, 580, 581, 582
hemolytic anemia 679, 690
hemopoiesis see hematopoiesis
hemorrhage/bleeding
    gastrointestinal see gastrointestinal tract
    subarachnoid 427, **Plate 4.3**
hemostatic risk factors for venous thromboembolism 207
hepatic problems see liver
hepatitis, neonatal 115
hepatocellular carcinoma 648, 661–5
Her2, MAbs to 604
hereditary causes see genetic causes
hernia, inguinal 598
heterotopias see entries under ectopic
hexamethylpropylene amine oxime see HMPAO
hexamethylpropylene diphosphonate 816
HIDA (IDA) compounds 643–4, 817
HIDAC MWPC camera 858
high-throughput screening of novel chemical libraries 9
hip
    fractures 366–7, 373
        avascular necrosis 396
    injury 364
        children, and associated pain 406
        sports 373
        see also fractures (subheading above)
    joint replacement failure
        bone scintigraphy 382–3
        bone scintigraphy and gallium scan 383–5
        case histories 389
        leukocyte–marrow imaging 387
    pediatric pathology 117
histo(patho)logy
    Alzheimer's disease 416
    brain tumor classification 446
    sentinel lymph node 126
    breast cancer 132–3
HIV disease/AIDS
    CNS lymphoma 703, **Plate 16C.4**
    lung 245–7
        P. carinii pneumonia (PCP) 240, 241–2, 245, 246, 247
        permeability measurement 241–2
HL91, [99m]Tc- 151
HMFG see human milk fat globule
HMG-CoA reductase inhibitors 165
HMPAO (hexamethylpropylene amine oxime; exametazime), [99m]Tc-
        817–18
    Alzheimer's disease 417, **Plate 10A.2**
    brain death **Plate 4.2**
    brain tumors 447
    cerebrovascular disease 425–6
    depression 429
    frontotemporal dementia 418
    healthy volunteer **Plate 10A.1**
    in leukocyte labeling 629
    Lewy body dementia 419
    occipital seizures **Plate 10C.2**
    subarachnoid hemorrhage **Plate 4.3**

HNP-1 (human neutrophil peptide-1), [99m]Tc- 102
Hodgkin's disease
    somatostatin receptors 33
    staging 696, 702, **Plate 16C.3**
    therapeutic response monitoring 62–3, 698
        children 118
    types/classification 696
hormone therapy monitoring, breast cancer 6, 553
human albumin see albumin
human anti-mouse antibodies (HAMA) 43, 86
human chorionic gonadotrophin (HGC), MAb 602
human milk fat globule (HMFG) 40
    ovarian cancer 43, 602
        in radioimmunotherapy 604
    uterine fibroids 42
human neutrophil peptide-1, [99m]Tc- 102
humanized MAbs 44
Huntington's disease 460
Hürthle cell carcinoma 733
hydrocele 598
hydronephrosis (dilation of collecting/pelvicaliceal system) 306, 308–11
    children 116–17
hydroxyapatite crystals (bone) 331
hydroxyephedrine, [11]C-
    cardiology 841
    pheochromocytoma 843
hydroxyethylidenediphosphonate (HEDP), [186]Rh- and [188]Rh- 766, 768,
        769
5-hydroxytryptamine see serotonin
5-hydroxytryptophan (HTP), [11]C-, carcinoids 843
hydroxyurea, polycythemia vera 775
HYNICTATE see octreotate
hyperandrogenism 527–8
hypercalcemia, SPECT/CT 9
hypermetabolism, brain tumor 449, 450
hyperparathyroidism 358
hyperperfusion, occipital seizures **Plate 10C.3**
hyperplasia
    adrenal 521, 522, 523, 526, 527, 529
    parathyroid 511
hypersplenism 678, 687
hypertension (systemic)
    children 297–303
        renal causes 117, 287–8
    essential/primary, cortical nephron flow and captopril effects in 264
    pheochromocytoma-associated 531
    renovascular see renovascular disorders
hyperthyroidism (thyrotoxicosis) 493–4, 495–503, 728–33
    causes 495
        diagnosis of 496, 499
        excess iodide administration 502
        excess thyroid hormone administration 502
        radioiodine therapy in non-toxic multinodular goiter 733
        in thyroid cancer patients 502–3
    clinical symptoms 728
    diagnosis 729
    diseases associated with 492
    Graves' see Graves disease
    management/treatment 493–4, 496–501, 501–2, 729–33
        radioiodine see iodine-131
    pathophysiology 492–3
hypometabolism
    Alzheimer's disease 417
    epilepsy 436, 437, **Plate 10C.2**
hypoperfusion
    acute ischemic stroke 426
    Alzheimer's disease 417

epilepsy 436, **Plate 10C.1**
head/brain injury 428
subarachnoid hemorrhage 427
transient ischemic attacks 427
hypoplastic lung 115
hypothyroidism 494–5
diagnosis 494
diseases associated with 492
neonatal 114, 494–5, 509–10
pathophysiology 492–3
radioiodine-induced 732
treatment 494–5
hypoxia
myocardial 151
pulmonary vasoconstriction in 198–9
tumor 12–13
head and neck cancer 471
lung cancer 14, 232
hysterosalpingography (HSG) in infertility 587, 588–9, 591
hysterosalpingoscintigraphy (HSS) 588–91
clinical role and indications 591
dosimetry 589–91
findings and interpretation 589
technique 589
hysteroscopy, transcervical, infertility 587

ibritumomab tiuxetan, ^{90}Y- (Zevalin) 42, 85
IBZM (iodobenzamide), ^{123}I-
multiple system atrophy **Plate 10E.2**
Parkinson's disease **Plate 10E.2**
schizophrenia 429
ictal imaging 436
IDA (HIDA) compounds 643–4, 817
image acquisition/processing/display
brain tumors 452–3
cystography (indirect radionuclide) 285–6
lymphoscintigraphy of limbs/lymphatic disease 716–17
lymphoscintigraphy of sentinel nodes 123–4
breast cancer 128
myocardial perfusion SPECT 154–5
renal scintigraphy
dynamic 285
static 282–3
shunts in congenital heart disease 170
testicular scans 596
image correlation 863
image interpretation/analysis
brain tumor FDG PET and MRI 449
cystography (indirect radionuclide) 285
equilibrium radionuclide ventriculography 184
gastrointestinal bleeding 621–2
hysterosalpingoscintigraphy in infertility 589
inflammatory bowel disease 629–30
myocardial perfusion SPECT 155–6
renal imaging 255–6
children 282–4
shunts in congenital heart disease 170
tumor dosimetry and 783–4
VQ scan of pulmonary embolism 209–13, 219
image quality, pediatric 110
image registration (co-registration; fusion) 861–7, **Plate 21B.1.**
clinical applications 863–4
methods 861–3
imatinib mesylate (Glevac) 17–18, 69
polycythemia vera 775
iminodiacetic acid compounds 643–4, 817
immobilization, child 110

immune function, lymphatic system 715–16
immunoglobulins *see* antibodies
immunoscintigraphy *see* radioimmunoscintigraphy
immunosuppression/immunodeficiency
lung infections/inflammation associated with 240
in polycythemia vera 778–9
immunotherapy, radionuclide *see* radioimmunotherapy
impingement syndromes, ankle 368
impotence (erectile dysfunction) 575–83
treatment 582
vasculogenic 576–83, **Plate 13D.1**
etiology and pathogenesis 576–7
non-radionuclide investigations 577–8
radionuclide investigations 578–83
impulse retention function (renal parenchymal) 258
in situ carcinoma *see* carcinoma *in situ*
incidentaloma (incidental mass), adrenal 526, 528–30
incremental cost (incremental price) 807, 809, 812
incremental cost-effectiveness 809, 812
indirect cost 812
indium-111 chloride, protein-losing enteropathy 643
indium-111-labeled blood cells
leukocytes 94
abdominal infections 96
infected joint replacement 387–8
inflammatory bowel disease 629, 630, 631
platelets, predicting response to splenectomy 687, 689
red cells 676
hemolytic anemia 679
indium-111-labeled compounds
DPC11870–11 100
DTPA, lung permeability measurement 241
lanreotide 30
octreotide *see* indium-111-labeled octreotide
transferrin *see* transferrin
indium-111-labeled immunoglobulin/polyclonal antibody
bacterial antigens 94–5
head and neck cancer 469
HIV disease 247
prosthetic joint infection 388
indium-111-labeled monoclonal antibodies (incl. ^{111}In-DTPA) 46
colorectal cancer 49–50, **Plates 1C.2–3**
prostate cancer 42, 610, 612–14, 617–18
renal tumor therapy 325
indium-111-labeled octreotide (incl. ^{111}In-DOTA octreotide and ^{111}In-DTPA-octreotide/^{111}In-pentetreotide) 29, 30, 34, 745–7
adrenal scintigraphy 524
pheochromocytoma 533–4
breast cancer 545
endocrine pancreatic tumors 31
Graves' disease 34
head and neck cancer 469
lymphoma 698, 701–2
meningioma 447
neuroendocrine tumors (incl. carcinoids) 7, 10, 31, 82, 656, 745–7
insulinoma **Plate 14E.1**
staging 654
neuroendocrine tumors (incl. carcinoids), therapeutic use 31, 34, 69, 85, 658, 745–50
neuroblastoma 657
pharmacology
adverse reactions 823
drug interactions 825
sarcoidosis 244
induction therapy *see entries under* neoadjuvant

infants
  functional imaging
    effects of maturation on 111–13
    liver 115
  newborn see neonates
  renal function (GFR etc.) 276
infection 93–106
  bone see osteomyelitis
  prosthetic joint 381–92
  pulmonary 239–40
  radiopharmaceuticals see radiopharmaceuticals
  testicular 598
  thyroid 506
  urinary tract, pediatric 284, 287–94
    acute 289
    case history 292–4
    management, contribution of nuclear medicine 289–92
    rationale for investigation 287–8
    risk factors for renal damage 288
  urinary tract, renal transplant recipient 318–19
  see also septic arthritis and specific diseases and pathogens
infertility 585–92
  anatomy and physiology relevant to 585–7
  causes 585, 587
  male, radioiodine therapy-associated risk 739
  non-radionuclide methods of diagnosis/investigation 585, 587–8
inflammation 93–106
  cells and mediators in 98
  coronary artery disease and 148
  ^{18}F-FDG uptake in, false interpretation as malignancy 794
    post-therapy 795
  prosthetic joint, causing aseptic loosening 381–2
  pulmonary 239–40
  radiopharmaceuticals in see radiopharmaceuticals
  testicular 598
inflammatory arthropathies 393–6
inflammatory bowel disease 629–35
  case reports 632–4
  diagnosis 630–1
  differential diagnosis 631
  follow-up and complications 631–2
  severity of disease 631
information, child and parent see education
inguinal hernia 598
inguinal node visualization 718
inherent image registration 861–2
inherited causes see genetic causes
injections
  intra-/subdermal/peritumoral, radiocolloids for lymphoscintigraphy 124
    breast cancer 128, 132, 563
    melanoma 123
    non-neoplastic lymphatic disease 716
  intravenous
    bone pain-palliating radiopharmaceuticals 768
    contrast agents for PET/CT 796
  intravenous, children 108
    anesthetic cream 109
    renal pharmaceuticals 281–2
  suprapubic, cystoscintigraphy 287
injury (traumatic) 363–79
  children see children
  pathophysiology 363
  prevalence by age and site 364–5
  scrotal 598
  spleen 686
  sports 363, 368–75

inotrope stress testing 153–4
inspiration 198
INSPIRE (AdenosINe 99mTc-Sestamibi SPECT Post-InfaRction Evaluation) trial 162
instrumentation see technology and instrumentation
insufficiency injuries/fractures 367–8
insulin resistance syndrome 158
insulinoma 654, Plate 14E.1
intensity ratios, variance of 862
interferon-α, polycythemia vera 775
interictal imaging 436, 440
interleukin-1 (IL-1) and IL-1 receptor antagonist 98–9
interleukin-2 100, 832
interleukin-8 99, 832
International System for Staging Lung Cancer 223, 224
International Workshop Criteria + PET-based response criteria, lymphoma 62, 706
interosseous membrane fractures 369–70
interstitial lung diseases, idiopathic 242–3
intervertebral diskitis, children 405
intestine see bowel; large bowel; small bowel and specific regions
intradermal injection of radiocolloids for lymphoscintigraphy see injections
intraperitoneal route, ovarian cancer radioimmunotherapy route 604
intrarenal flow distribution 263–4
intrathoracic lymph nodes (incl. internal mammary) imaging 133, 551
intravenous injections see injections
intravenous urography in renovascular hypertension 299
intrinsic factor 641
iodide
  transport into thyroid cell, abnormality 508
  treatment with
    excess, hyperthyroidism due to 502
    in pregnancy, avoidance 500
  see also sodium iodide
iodination of tyrosine see tyrosine
iodine
  diet low, before tracer imaging in ^{131}-treated thyroid cancer 736
  organification defect 508
  radioactive (unspecified isotope), OIH-labeled with, pharmacokinetics 255
iodine-123, thyroid cancer 81–2, 84–5
  recurrent disease 79, 84–5
iodine-123-labeled/iodinated compounds
  ADAM 429
  BMIPP see BMIPP
  dose for children 109
  IBZM see IBZM
  interleukin-2 100
  interleukin-8 99
  MIBG see MIBG
  octreotide 29
  OIH (orthoiodohippurate), comparison with other renal radiopharmaceuticals 260
  in radioimmunoscintigraphy
    neuroblastoma 45–6
    production (radiolabeling) 46
  serum amyloid P component 692–3
  tropanes (cocaine derivatives), dopaminergic system imaging 420, 458
  vasoactive intestinal peptide 756
iodine-125-labeled/iodinated compounds
  MIBG, neuroblastoma therapy 759
  monocyte chemoattractant protein-1 101
iodine-131 (radioiodine) 727–43
  in hyperthyroidism 493, 499
    pre-treatment thyroid scan 501

in hyperthyroidism therapy 729–33
   dose considerations 731–2
   Graves' disease 499–500, 729–30
   Plummer's disease 501–2, 730
   practical aspects of treatment 731–2
   side-effects and complications 732
physical properties 727
sodium iodide *see* sodium iodide
in thyroid cancer scanning 59, 67, 68, 84–5, 736–8
   acute and long-term adverse effects 739
   precautions 738
in thyroid cancer therapy *see* thyroid tumors
iodine-131-labeled monoclonal antibody 85–6
   colorectal cancer scan 7
   neuroblastoma 45–6, 756
   production 46
   therapeutic use 85–6
     brain tumors 449–50
     non-Hodgkin's lymphoma 85–6
     renal tumor 325
iodobenguane *see* MIBG
iodobenzamide *see* IBZM
m-iodobenzylguanidine *see* MIBG
5-iodo-2'-deoxyuridine (IUdR) 834
Iodogen in radiolabeling technique 46
6β-iodomethyl-19-norcholesterol, ^{131}I- *see* NP-59
ionization chamber, solid-state 850–1
iron 679–81
   absorption 679
   plasma
     clearance 679–80
     turnover 680
   red cell utilization 680
iron-52 PET 680
   hematopoiesis 682
     extramedullary 693
iron-59 (^{59}Fe), ferrokinetic studies 679–80
ischemic attacks, transient 427
ischemic heart disease
   algorithm for investigations 189
   definitions of ischemic syndromes 185
   LV dysfunction 184
   see also coronary artery disease
ischemic stroke, acute 426–7, **Plate 10B.1**
isonitriles, ^{99m}TC 817
   2-methoxy isobutyl *see* sestamibi
iterative affine registration, prostate cancer imaging 613
IUdR (5-iodo-2'-deoxyuridine) 834
IWC + PET-based response criteria, lymphoma 62, 706

JAK2 and polycythemia vera 775
jaundice, neonatal/infant 115, 644
joints
   aspiration in children, bone scan prior to 405
   in bone scans of skeletal metastases 341
   false 375–6
   replacement *see* arthroplasty
   see also arthritis; arthropathies
Jones' fracture 369
juxtamedullary nephrons, captopril effects 263–4, 300

Kaposi's sarcoma (KS) 246
Keinbock's disease 396
Khalkhali, Professor Iraj, and scintimammography 559
Ki67 expression, lung cancer 64
kidney 251–327
   adverse effects/toxicity

of chemotherapy, monitoring 83
of ^{131}I-MIBG 759
anatomy 253
   variants 283–4
cancer, molecular characterization 14
chronic failure
   osteodystrophy in 359
   secondary to urinary tract infection 288
damage/scarring
   pediatric *see subheading below*
   transplanted kidney 318
disease (in general), glomerular filtration rate measurements
   275
function 253–5
   activity–time curves *see* renography
   radionuclide measurements, *see subheading below*
   relative 262
models 256–60
obstructive disease *see* obstruction; obstructive nephropathy
output (outflow) efficiency 254, 306–8
pediatric 281–96
   nuclear medicine unit and journey through it 281–2
pediatric, damage (incl. scarring) 285
   cortical scarring 289–90
   tract infection as cause of 288
   vesico-ureteric reflux and 288–9
pediatric, functional studies 116–17, 276
   differential renal function 116, 283
   infant maturation and its effects 112
polycystic disease (PKD), children 115, 117
radionuclide measurements of function 254–64, 269–80
   non-imaging 269–80
   pediatric *see subheading above*
   technique and interpretation 255–6
   see also renography
radiopharmaceuticals *see* radiopharmaceuticals
somatostatin analog uptake, reduction 748
transplants 263, 315–19
   case history 319
   clinical problems 315–19
   donor assessment 315
   rejection 317
   technical aspects of imaging 319
tumors/cancer 321–7, **Plate 8G.1**
   clinical management 321–2
   molecular characterization 14
   mouse **Plate 1A.1**
   PET 322–4
   radionuclide therapy 324–6
   SPECT 321
kinase domains 7
Klippel–Trenaunay syndrome 722, 723
knee
   avascular necrosis 397
   injuries 372–3
   osteoarthritis 394
   replacement, bone scintigraphy 383
Kohler's disease 396
krypton-81m ventilation imaging 202–3

lachrymal studies 485–7
lactation *see* breast-feeding
lanreotide
   ^{111}In-DOTA- 30
   ^{90}Y-DOTA-, therapeutic use 750
laparoscopy (LPC), infertility 587, 588, 591
large B-cell lymphoma, diffuse 13, **Plate 16C.2**

large bowel/intestine
  bleeding 623
  cancer *see* colorectal cancer
  transit 639–40
  see also specific regions
large vessel vascular disease, dementia 418
Larson–Ginsberg index 61
laryngeal muscle, ^{18}F-FDG uptake 793–4
left-to-right shunt in congenital heart disease 170, 171, **Plate 6A.20**
leg *see* lower limb
Legg–Calvé–Perthes' disease 117, 364, 397, 406
leiomyoma (fibroids), uterine 42
Lennox–Gastaut syndrome 439
leukemia
  ^{131}I-induced 739
  polycythemia vera (and its therapy) and 774, 778
  ^{89}SrCl$_2$-induced 739
leukocytes (white blood cells), radiolabeled 94, 827
  abdominal infections 96
  arthritides 393
  bone marrow imaging 682
  drug interactions 827
  inflammatory bowel disease 629, 630, 631
  joint prosthesis infection 95, 388
  osteomyelitis 95
  prosthetic joint infection 385–8
  pulmonary infections 96
  rheumatoid arthritis 393
  splenic imaging 686
  vascular graft infections 97
Leukoscan *see* sulesomab
Leukoscan®, infected joint replacement 95
leukotriene B$_4$ 100
Lewy body dementia 419–20, **Plate 10A.7, Plate 10A.9**
ligamentous injury, ankle/foot 369–71
ligands 8–9
  characteristics 6
  radiolabeled *see* radiopharmaceuticals
limbs
  lower *see* lower limb
  swollen *see* lymphedema; lymphoscintigraphy
  upper, sports injuries 375
line-based image registration 862
line of response (LOR) 855
linear system model of kidney 257–8
  deconvolution analysis 257–8, 263
lingual thyroid 508–9
lipedema 723
liposomes, inflammation imaging 833
liver
  ^{18}F-FDG uptake 792
  pediatric 115
  radiopharmaceuticals used 817
  tumors 661–70
    lymphoma 698, 703, 876
    primary 648, 661–6
    secondary *see* liver metastases
liver metastases 81, 666–70
  breast cancer **Plate 1D.3**
  colorectal cancer 7, 13, 51, 646, 647, 667–8, 669
  neuroendocrine tumors (incl. carcinoids) 7, 10, 30
    embolization therapy 657–8
  radionuclide therapy 81
  vascularity 81
lobes of lung 198
lobular carcinoma *in situ* (DCIS) 543
  PET 550
  scintimammography 561

local anesthetic, children 109
low-density lipoprotein
  cholesterol carriage by 522
  coronary artery disease and 147, 148
  radiolabeled, adrenocortical imaging with 523
lower limb/leg
  sports injury 368–73
  ultrasound, venous thromboembolism deep vein thrombosis 208
lumbar spine
  fusion, complications 375–6
  sports injury 374
lunate
  avascular necrosis 396
  fracture 375
lung 195–250
  adult respiratory distress syndrome 240, 243
  ^{18}F-FDG activity 792
  function 198
  granulomatous diseases 240, 243–5
  idiopathic interstitial diseases 242–3
  infections 96
  nodule (solitary) 223, 224–6
  obstructive disease 201–2
  pediatric imaging 115
    infant maturation and its effects 112
  permeability measurement 240–2
  structure/anatomy 197–8
  VQ imaging *see* ventilation perfusion imaging
lung cancer (predominantly carcinoma) 32–3, 63–5, 223–38
  carcinoid **Plate 1D.4**
  diagnostic tests available 223–4
  distant metastases 227, 324, 450
  hypercalcemia 10
  hypoxic imaging 14, 232
  lymphoma **Plate 16C.1**
  non-small cell *see* non-small cell lung cancer
  PET *see* positron emission tomography
  relapse/recurrence 63, 230
  secondary *see* metastases (distant)
  somatostatin receptors 32–3
  staging 63, 223, 224, 226–7
  therapeutic response monitoring 57, 60, 230–2
lutetium oxyorthosilicate (LSO) 849, 850, 872
lutetium-177-labeling
  MAb, renal tumor therapy 325
  somatostatin analogs (incl. octreotate), neuroendocrine tumor therapy 34, 659, 747–50, 751
lymph node(s), sentinel *see* sentinel lymph nodes
lymph node dissection 121, 122, 125–6
  melanoma 123
  technique and results with sentinel node imaging 125–6
lymph node enlargement, lymphoma 697
lymph node metastases 14–15, 121
  breast cancer 547–8, 551
    intrathoracic (incl. internal mammary) nodes 133, 551
  esophageal cancer 645, **Plate 14D.1**
  head and neck
    from primary head and neck cancer 472
    from unknown primary 473–4
  micrometastatic disease in breast cancer 132–3
  prostate cancer 609, 612, **Plates 13H.5–6**
  renal cell carcinoma 324
  testicular cancer 72, 569
  see also N
lymphatic system/tissue
  ^{18}F-FDG uptake 792
  function 715–16

lymphedema 715, 721, 722–3
  lipedema and (syndrome of) 723
  secondary causes 723
    breast cancer 716
lymphedema–distichiasis syndrome 718
lymphoceles, transplanted kidney 318
lymphography, radionuclide *see* lymphoscintigraphy
lymphoma, Hodgkin's *see* Hodgkin's disease
lymphoma, non-Hodgkin and in general 62–3, 695,
    Plate 16C.1–11
  aggressive vs indolent 696, 697
  classification/types 696, 702
  extranodal 697–8, 702–3
    bone marrow 346, 697–8, 703
    CNS 450, 698, 703, **Plate 16C.6**
    lung **Plate 16C.1**
    thyroid 507, 733, 736
  FDG PET scans 695–6, 698, 702–7, **Plates 16C.3–11**
    false interpretation 63, 703, 704, 706, 707
    summary of important points 706–7
  gallium-67 scans *see* gallium-67 scans
  imaging at initial diagnosis and staging 697, 704
  morphologic imaging modalities 697–8
  pediatric 118, 409
  prognostic indicators 697, 705
  somatostatin receptors 33, 701–2
  staging and restaging 13, 63, 346, 696–7, 702–3
    children 118
  therapy 13
    with radiolabeled MAbs 6, 85–6
    response monitoring 57, 62–3, 64, 65, 698, 699, 704–6, **Plates 16C.9–11**
lymphoscintigraphy 121–39, 715–24
  colloids in *see* colloid; nanocolloid
  physiological principles 715–16
  sentinel node 14–15, 121–39
    alternatives to 134
    breast cancer 128–33, 562, 563
    dynamic lymphoscintigraphy 129
    melanoma 123–5
    standards 134
  swollen limb/other lymphatic diseases 715–24
    qualitative studies 721
    quantitative studies 718–21
    technique 716
lymphovenous communications 719
lysine preventing somatostatin analog renal uptake 748

M (distant metastases in TNM staging)
  breast cancer 564
  head and neck cancer 468
MAA (macroaggregated albumin), ^{99m}Tc-
  adverse reactions 823
  congenital heart disease 171
  hysterosalpingoscintigraphy in infertility 588, 589, 591
  pulmonary perfusion scan 199
macroaggregated albumin *see* MAA
macromolecular transport in lymph 716
MAG$_3$ (mercaptoacetyltriglycine), ^{99m}Tc-, renal imaging 260–1, 262, 307, 816
  adverse reactions 823
  compared with other pharmaceuticals 260
  hypertension 298, 300, 301
    case history 302
  pediatric 112
  structure 816
  transplant recipients 316, 319
magnetic resonance angiography, pulmonary embolism 209

magnetic resonance imaging (MRI) 11
  adrenal incidentaloma 529
  ankylosing spondylitis 396
  brain
    corticobasal degeneration **Plate 10E.3**
    functional *see* functional MRI
    seizures **Plate 10C.1**
    tumors 446, 449, 452
  breast cancer 544–5
    distant metastases 552
  cardiovascular 157
    congenital heart disease 170
    myocardial viability assessment 167, 185
  colorectal carcinoma therapeutic response monitoring 67
  liver cancer
    metastatic 667
    primary 662
  lymphoma, pre-therapy 697–8
  ovarian cancer 602
  skeletal metastases 340
  testicles 599
magnetic resonance spectroscopy (MRS) 11
  brain 20
malabsorption tests 641–2
  vitamin B$_{12}$ 641–2, 681
males (men)
  coronary artery disease prognosis 162
  genital tract disorders 569–83, 609–28
  radioiodine therapy-associated risk of infertility 739
malignant tumors *see* tumors
MALToma 702
mammary nodes, internal (and other intrathoracic nodes), imaging/biopsy/dissection 133, 551
mammography
  radionuclide *see* scintimammography
  standard (X-ray)
    scintimammography added to 560
    screening 544
manic–depressive (bipolar) disorder 429
manubrial metastases 339
marginal cost and benefit 812
marginal zone B-cell lymphoma, extranodal 702
Marine–Lenhart syndrome 497
Markov model 809, 812
masculinization 526, 527
mass/focal lesions
  adrenal, incidental 526, 528–30
  neck, children 114–15
  renal, clinical management 321–2
  splenic 692
  see also tumors
MCP-1 100–1
MDP (methylene diphosphonate), ^{99m}Tc- 333
  adverse reactions 823
  bone tumors
    children 409
    primary 347, 348, 349, 409
    secondary (metastases) 339, 340, 341, 342, 343, 345
  glucantime interactions 825–6
  neuroblastoma 410
  osteomalacia 359
  osteomyelitis 117
  Paget's disease of bone 356
  pediatric musculoskeletal disorders 405
  prostate cancer 611
  renal osteodystrophy 359
MDP (methylene diphosphonate) kit, antibody labeling with ^{99m}Tc 46
MDR1 *see* multidrug-resistant 1 P-glycoprotein

mean parenchymal transit time (MPTT) 254, 259–60, 262–3
    renovascular disorder 299–300
mean platelet life survival 689
mean red cell life span 676, 677
mebrofenin, ^{99m}Tc-, adverse reactions 823
Meckel's diverticulum 624–5, 626
mediastinoscopy, lung cancer staging 226
mediastinum
    in lung cancer, staging 226–7
    mass in upper region in children 114–15
    thyroid gland enlarging downwards into 509
Medical Internal Radiation Dose (MIRD) schema 782–3
medronate
    structure 816
    ^{99m}Tc-, adverse reactions 823
medulla, adrenal see adrenal gland
medulla oblongata, respiratory center 198
medullary thyroid carcinoma 32
    clinical features 503, 507
    somatostatin receptors 32
    treatment 733–4, 736, 751
megaloblastic anemia 681
melanoma 123–5
    radioimmunoscintigraphy 43
    sentinel node imaging (lymphoscintigraphy) 122, 123–5
    somatostatin receptors 33
membrane, cell
    integrity, in myocardial viability assessment 166
    radiopharmaceutical binding to receptors on 81
men see males
meningiomas 450
    somatostatin receptors 33, 447
meniscal injury 372
mercaptoacetyltriglycine see MAG$_3$
Merkel cell tumor 32
mertiatide, ^{99m}Tc-, adverse reactions 823
mesorchium, anomalous 596
mesothelioma 223–4
meta-analysis 807, 809, 812
metabolic bone disease 355–62
metabolic syndrome X 158
metabolic tumor diameter 61
metabolic tumor index (molecular tumor index) 61, 62,
    Plate 1D.2
metabolic tumor volume 61
metabolism
    bone, radionuclide therapy and 80–1
    ^{18}F-FDG 791
    myocardial/myocyte
        in myocardial viability assessment 166–7
        tracers 150–1
    see also hypermetabolism; hypometabolism
meta-iodobenzylguanidine see MIBG
metaphyseal abnormal activity, symmetrical 409
metastases (distant)
    in adrenal 528
    in bone see bone metastases
    in brain 450
    breast cancer 339, 341, 343–4, 552, 564, **Plate 1D.3**
    carcinoid 7, 10, 30
    colorectal cancer 7, 13
    esophageal cancer 645, **Plate 14D.1.**
    head and neck cancer 472, **Plate 11A.1**
        in TNM staging 468
    from kidney (renal cell carcinoma) 323
    in kidney 323
    in liver see liver

    in lung
        renal cell carcinoma 323
        thyroid cancer 736, 737, 739
    lung cancer 227, 324, 450
    from prostate 609, 611–12
        bone pain palliation 767
    in spleen 692
    testicular cancer 569
    thyroid cancer 68, 83–4, 736, 737, 739, 786
metastases (regional =lymph node) see lymph node
    metastases
metatarsals
    second, avascular necrosis 396
    stress fractures 370
metatarsophalangeal joint, osteoarthritis 394
methionine, ^{11}C-
    brain tumors 451
    therapeutic response monitoring 58
2-methoxy isobutyl isonitrile (MIBI) see sestamibi
β-methyl iodophenyl pentadecanoic acid see BMIPP
methylene blue in sentinel node detection see blue dye
methylene diphosphonate see MDP
methylxanthine–adenosine interactions 826
MIBG (meta-iodobenzylguanidine; iodobenguane)
    drug interactions 824–5
    structure and metabolism 531–2, 533
MIBG (meta-iodobenzylguanidine; iodobenguane), ^{123}I 82
    adrenal scintigraphy 524
        pheochromocytoma 532–3, 534
    adverse reactions 823
    cardiac sympathetic innervation 151, 189
    gastrointestinal neuroendocrine tumors 655, 657, 658
    head and neck cancer 469
    neuroblastoma 33, 118, 410, 535
    pheochromocytoma 33
MIBG (meta-iodobenzylguanidine; iodobenguane), ^{125}I-, neuroblastoma
    therapy 759
MIBG (meta-iodobenzylguanidine; iodobenguane), ^{131}I-
    imaging
        adrenal scintigraphy 524
        adrenal scintigraphy, pheochromocytoma 532
        gastrointestinal neuroendocrine tumors 655, 657
        head and neck cancer 469
    therapeutic use, neuroendocrine tumors 34, 69, 82, 95, 535,
        536, 658
        neuroblastoma 755–6, 756–60
    toxicity 759
MIBI see sestamibi
mice see mouse
microchip technology, SPECT gamma camera 853
micrometastatic nodal disease in breast cancer 132–3
microPET camera 858
microspheres, human albumin (HAM), hysterosalpingoscintigraphy in
    infertility 588, 589, 591
milk fat globule, human see human milk fat globule
mineral, bone 331
minigastrin, radiolabeled 751
MIRD (Medical Internal Radiation Dose) schema 782–3
molecular imaging 3–78
    methods and techniques 8–12
    non-oncology applications 11, 18–24
    oncology applications see tumors
    PET agents, targets 840
molecular tumor diameter 61
molecular tumor index 61, 62, **Plate 1D.2**
molecular tumor volume 61
monoamine oxidase 531

monoclonal antibodies (to tumor antigens) 40, 41, 81
 to bacteria 94–5
 biological factors affecting uptake 41–3
 breast cancer, axillary node status 134
 colorectal cancer 49–52, **Plates 1C.2–3**
 ^{131}I-labeled 7
 development 41
 to granulocytes *see* granulocytes
 head and neck cancer 469
 humanized 44
 neuroblastoma 45–6, 756, **Plate 1C.1**
 ovarian cancer 602
 prostate cancer-associated antigens 610–11
 quality control 43–4
 therapeutic use *see* radioimmunotherapy
 see also radioimmunoscintigraphy
monocyte chemoattractant protein-1 100–1
mononuclear cell, infiltrating, tracers 100–2
mood disorders 429
mouse
 antibodies, human antibodies to (HAMA) 43, 86
 renal cell carcinoma **Plate 1A.1**
 transgenic, molecular imaging 12
MoV-18 (MAb) 602, 603
movement disorders 20–1, 457–64
 radiolabeled, ovarian cancer therapy 604
mucin components, MAb to 602
mucosa-associated lymphoid tissue lymphoma 702
MUJ 591 (MAb) 610
mulitiplanar gated angiography 183–4
multicellular dosimetry 785
multicentric breast cancer 547
multichannel/multislice/multidetector CT or CT angiography
 coronary angiography 11, 157, 159
 venous thromboembolism 208
multi-crystal scanners, SPECT 854
multidrug-resistant 1 P-glycoprotein (MDR1)
 breast cancer 66, 546, 561
 head and neck cancer 469
 lymphoma 701
multifocal breast cancer 547
multi-infarct dementia 418, **Plate 10A.5**
multi-modal 3-D change statistical detection, prostate cancer imaging 613
multi-modal imaging *see* positron emission tomography/computed tomography; positron emission tomography/single photon emission computed tomography camera; single photon emission computed tomography/computed tomography
multinodular goiter 504–5, 506–8
 case history 740
 nontoxic 491, 506–8
 radioiodine therapy 733
 toxic 491, 729
multiple-breath steady-state technique 201
multiple endocrine neoplasia
 medullary thyroid carcinoma 507
 type-1 654
multiple system atrophy 458–9, **Plates 10E.1–2**
multi-wire proportional chamber gamma camera 854, 858
muscarinic acetylcholinergic system imaging 421
muscle, skeletal, ^{18}F-FDG uptake 793–4
musculoskeletal system 329–412
 pediatric conditions 403–12
mutual information in image registration 863
myeloid leukemia, ^{89}SrCl$_2$-induced 739
myelosuppression, radioisotope-induced 769

myocardium
 gallium-67 uptake 246
 hibernating 165, 184, **Plate 6A.20**
 detection techniques 166
 infarction 185
 risk stratification following 162–3
 ischemia *see* ischemic heart disease
 molecular imaging 19
 perfusion defects, reversal 155–6
 perfusion scanning 18, 19, 155–69, **Plates 6A.3–15, Plate 6B.2**
 attenuation correction in SPECT 875, **Plate 21C.1.**
 clinical applications 156–69
 in congenital heart disease 171
 post-intervention changes **Plates 6A.17–18**
 radiotracers 149–50
 restoration to ischemic myocardium 20
 radiopharmaceutical imaging agents 149–50, 817
 stunning 165, 185
 repetitive 185
 viability assessment 165–8, 185–9
 FDG 150, 166, 187–8, 188, 841, **Plate 6B.2**
 rationale 184–5
 visual assessment of severity 156, 157
N (nodal involvement in TNM staging)
 breast cancer 564
 head and neck cancer 468, 472
 lung cancer 224, 226, 227
naming memory and semantic dementia 419
nanocolloid, ^{99m}Tc- 123
 adverse reactions 823
 breast cancer 132
NAT (noradrenaline transporter gene) therapy, neuroblastoma 759
navicular–calcaneal coalition 371
NCA-95, MAb to 94
N-DBODC5, ^{99m}Tc- 150
neck
 mass, children 114–15
 nodal metastases from unknown primary 473
 see also head and neck disease
necrosis
 acute tubular (ATN), renal transplant recipients 315, 316, 317
 avascular *see* avascular necrosis
 myocardial 151
 radiation, brain tumor treated areas 449
negative predictive value (NPV) 803, 804
neoadjuvant chemoradiotherapy (preoperative/induction)
 colorectal carcinoma 66–7
 lung cancer (non-small cell) 65
neoadjuvant chemotherapy (preoperative/induction)
 breast cancer 65, 548, 553, 561
 colorectal carcinoma 67
 esophageal carcinoma 68, 645–6
 gastric carcinoma 68
 lymphoma 699
neoadjuvant radiotherapy (preoperative/induction), colorectal carcinoma 67
neonates
 hypothyroidism 114, 494–5, 509–10
 jaundice 115, 644
 osteomyelitis 405
 testicular torsion 594
nephroblastoma (Wilms' tumor) 117
nephrons 253
 cortical *see* cortex
 juxtamedullary, captopril effects 263–4, 300
 in linear system model of kidney 257
nephropathy, obstructive *see* obstructive nephropathy

nephrotoxicity monitoring in chemotherapy 83
nerve supply, penis 576
neu, MAbs to 604
neuroacanthocytosis 460
neuroblastoma 118, 755–63
    adrenal 404, 535
    bone scan 404, 535
    case history 760
    prognostic factors 755
    radioimmunoscintigraphy 45–6
    radionuclide therapy 755–63
    somatostatin receptors 33
neuroendocrine tumors (APUDomas) 69, 653–60
    adrenal gland 531–5
    diagnosis 654
    fluorodopa (^{18}F) 648, 843
    gastroenteropancreatic 31, 648, 653–60
        functionality 653–4
        sites 653, 654
        somatostatin receptors *see subheading below*
    identifying location 654
    liver metastases *see* liver metastases
    non-nuclear therapeutic methods 657–8
        response monitoring 57, 69
    radionuclide therapy 658–9, 745–53
        gamma imaging for beta therapy 80
        somatostatin analogs 31, 34, 69, 85, 658–9, 745–53
    radiopharmaceuticals used for imaging 655–7
    secretory syndromes 654
    somatostatin receptors 31, 653–4, 656–7, **Plates 1D.1–2**
        liver metastases detection 669–70
        as therapeutic targets 31, 34, 69, 85, 658–9, 745–53
    staging and restaging 654–5
    see also carcinoid tumors
neurology 20–4, 413–64
    CERASPECT brain scanner 854
    degenerative disease 841–2
    pediatric 113
    PET *see* positron emission tomography
    tumors *see* brain tumors
neuropeptide receptors, ligands binding to 834
neurotransmission and neurotransmitters 842
    cardiac, tracers 151, 189, 841
    CNS *see* brain
neutrophils
    infiltrating, tracers 98–100
    labeled leukocyte scan accuracy related to presence/absence of 386
    leukocytes (white blood cells), radiolabeled, prosthetic joint infection 385–8
    see also human neutrophil peptide-1
newborns *see* neonates
nicotinic acetylcholinergic system imaging 421
nitrates, myocardial viability assessment 187
nitrogen-13 ammonia *see* ammonia
nitroimidazole, ^{99m}Tc- 151
nocturnal tumescence test 577
nodular goiter
    associated with thyrotoxicosis 497–8
    toxic *see* Plummer's disease
    see also multinodular goiter
nodule(s)
    pulmonary, solitary 223, 224–6
    thyroid
        children 114
        diseases associated with 491, 492
        multiple toxic autonomous *see* Plummer's disease
        see also multinodular goiter; nodular goiter

thyroid, solitary 503–5
    functioning 'hot' nodule 504
    investigation and management 503–4
    and thyrotoxicosis 496–7
    two symmetrical solitary nodules 507
NOET, ^{99m}Tc-, myocardial perfusion scan 149
nofetumomab merpenten 42
non-accidental injury, children 117, 367, 406–8
non-Hodgkin lymphoma *see* lymphoma
non-linear regression analysis, therapeutic response monitoring with PET 60, 62
non-small cell lung cancer (NSCLC) 223, 226–33
    false interpretation of PET scans 63
    relapse/recurrence 63, 230
    staging 226–7
    survival rates 63
    therapeutic response monitoring 60
NORA (normalized residual activity) in kidney 257
noradrenaline (norepinephrine)
    metabolism 531, 532
    transporter gene, neuroblastoma therapy 759
normalized residual activity (NORA) in kidney 257
NP-59 (6β-iodomethyl-19-norcholesterol) 522
    adrenal incidentaloma 529, 530
    technical data on use 524–5

obsessive–compulsive disorder 430
obstruction, urinary outflow tract 305–14
    renal transplant 316
obstructive lung disease 201–2
obstructive nephropathy
    definition 305
    progression, ^{99m}Tc-MAG$_3$ study 311
    transit time 263
obstructive uropathy and obstructing uropathy 308–11
    definitions 305
OC-125 (MAb) 602, 603
occipital lobe epilepsy **Plate 10C.2**
    case histories 440–1
octreotate (HYNICTATE), radiolabeled, neuroendocrine tumor 656–7
    therapy 34, 747–50
octreotide 29, 30
    [DOTA,1-NaI^3]octreotide 751
    ^{111}In- *see* indium-111-labeled octreotide
    structure 818
    ^{99m}Tc-, neuroendocrine tumors 656–7
    ^{90}Y-, neuroendocrine tumors 658, 659, 747–50
ocular disease, dysthyroid *see* eye disease
OIH (orthoiodohippurate), radioiodine-labeled
    comparison with other renal radiopharmaceuticals 260
    pharmacokinetics 255
oligonucleotides, synthetic 7, 9
oncology *see* tumors
oocyte fertilization 586–7
ophthalmopathy disease, dysthyroid *see* eye disease
opiate receptor agonist 842
opportunity cost 806, 807, 812
optical imaging 12
OPTIMA (Oxford Project to Investigate Memory and Ageing) trial 417
oral contraceptives
    interactions with adrenocortical scintigraphic agents 523, 526
    venous thromboembolism and 207
orbital pathology 485–7
ordered subset estimation maximization 874
organ
    clearance 269
    toxicity monitoring in chemotherapy 82

orthoiodohippurate (OIH) *see* OIH
osteitis pubis 364, 373
osteoarthritis 394
osteoblasts 331
osteochondral fractures 363
    ankle 365
osteochondritis dissecans 371, 372
osteoclasts 331–2
osteodystrophy, renal 359
osteoid osteoma 348
osteolytic metastases 338, 341
osteoma, osteoid 348
osteomalacia 358–9
    case history 360
osteomyelitis (bone and marrow infection) 95–6
    in children 117, 405
        chronic non-bacterial/recurrent multifocal 405–6
    fracture-associated 376
osteopenia defined by T score in DEXA scan 400
osteoporosis 357–8
    defined by T score in DEXA scan 400
    drug treatment 400
osteosarcoma 347–8, **Plate 9G.1**
    Paget's disease 357
    pediatric 409, 410
outflow efficiency, renal 254, 306–8
outflow resistance
    chronic 305
    measurement 308–11
outflow tract obstruction, urinary 305–14
    causes 305–6
output (outflow) efficiency, renal 254, 306–8
OV-TL3 (MAb) 602
ovarian tumors 601–8
    adenocarcinoma, radioimmunoscintigraphy 43
    composed of thyroid tissue (struma ovarii) 498, 503, 604
    risk of malignancy index 601
    screening 601
ovum (egg) fertilization 586–7
Oxford Project to Investigate Memory and Ageing (OPTIMA) trial 417
oxidronate, ^{99m}Tc-, adverse reactions 823
oxygen-15 compounds 841
    bone marrow imaging 681
    brain tumors 451
    myocardial perfusion 150

P-glycoprotein *see* multidrug-resistant 1 P-glycoprotein
P280 (^{99m}Tc-apcitide) 832–3
P483H, ^{99m}Tc- 99
Paget's disease (bone) 341, 355–7
pain
    back, children 117, 405
    chronic regional pain syndrome *see* reflex sympathetic dystrophy
    hip, children 406
    thyroid enlargement 505–6
palmitate, ^{11}C- 150
pancreatic tumors
    carcinoma 646, **Plate 14D.2**
    endocrine *see* neuroendocrine tumors, gastroenteropancreatic
    false interpretation with ^{18}F-FDG 794
panic disorders 430
papillary thyroid cancer 733
    radioiodine therapy 735
para-aortic nodes 718
    renal cell carcinoma metastases 324

paragangliomas
    adrenal *see* pheochromocytoma
    extra-adrenal 32, 531
parallel-hole collimator 852
parasitic infections, antibiotics 833
parasympathetic nervous system, penis 576
parathyroid overactivity 358
parenchymal transit time index (PTTI) 254, 259–60, 263
    outflow resistance and 310–11
parents
    assessment 109
    explanations/information *see* education
parietotemporal association areas, Alzheimer's disease 416, 417
Parkes–Weber syndrome 723
Parkinson disease 20–1, 457, 459
    dopaminergic system 20–1, 420, 458
    Lewy body dementia and 419–20, 420
Parkinson disease-dementia complex 420
parkinsonism 458–60
pars interarticularis lesions 374
partial (focal) seizures
    children 439
    classification 435
Patlak–Gjedde analysis, therapeutic response monitoring with PET 60
Patlak–Ratlak plot 262, 307
pediatrics *see* children
Pellegrini–Stieda disease 373
pelvic angiography, impotence 577
pelvic area injuries 364, 367–8
    sports 373–4
pelvic bone (pelvis), insufficiency fractures 367–8
pelvic plexus, penile erection and 576
pelvicaliceal system, dilatation *see* hydronephrosis
pelvis, renal 260
    dilatation *see* hydronephrosis
    direct antegrade perfusion of, with pressure measurements 306
    transit time (PvTT) 259
Pendred's syndrome 508
penile arteries 575
penis
    anatomy 575–6
    blood flow measurements 577
    dynamic scintigraphy *see* phallography
    erection *see* erection
    nocturnal tumescence test 577
pentetate, ^{99m}Tc-, adverse reactions 823
pentetreotide, ^{111}In- *see* indium-111-labeled octreotide
peptides
    antimicrobial (endogenous) 101–2
    bacterial chemotactic 98
    radiolabeled (targeting receptors), as therapeutic agents 745–53, 818
        neuroblastoma 756
        neuroendocrine tumors (in general) 31, 34, 68, 69, 85, 658–9, 745–53
    radiolabeled (targeting receptors), as tracers 6–7, 29–38
        neuroendocrine tumors 656–7
percutaneous coronary interventions 164, **Plates 6A.17–19**
percutaneous suprapubic injections, cystoscintigraphy 287
perfusion
    cerebral/brain, physiology 425
    direct antegrade perfusion of renal pelvis with pressure measurements 306
    testicular 593–600
    see also hyperperfusion; hypoperfusion

perfusion imaging
  cardiac *see* myocardium, perfusion
  cerebral **Plates 10B.1–3**
    cerebrovascular disease 426–8
    psychiatric conditions 428–30
  penile 578
  pulmonary 199–200
  testicular
    non-radionuclide methods 598–9
    radionuclide methods 596–8
pericardial inflammation 246
peripheral vascular disease, impotence associated with *see* impotence
peritoneal cavity as ovarian cancer radioimmunotherapy route 604
peritoneal dialysis, chronic ambulatory, infections 318–19
permeability, lung 240–2
pertechnetate, ^{99m}Tc-
  adverse reactions 823
  lung clearance 241
  Meckel's diverticulum 624–5
  penile blood pool imaging 578
  red cell labeling with ^{99m}Tc using *see* radiolabels
  testicular scans 596
    torsion 597
  thyroid solitary nodule and thyrotoxicosis 497
Perthes' disease 117, 364, 397, 406
PET *see* positron emission tomography
PETTRA camera 858
phage display libraries 9
  antibody (=phage antibodies) 44
phallography 579–83
  erection 579, 581–2, 583, **Plate 13.D1**
  flaccid 579, 580, 582, 583
pharmacodynamics 18
pharmacokinetics of radiopharmaceuticals 821, 824–6
  functional imaging agents 815–16
pharmacological stress test 152–4
  indications 152
    post-myocardial infarction risk stratification 162–3
pharmacologically-induced penile erections 577, 582
  Doppler flow imaging 578
pharmacology, radiotracers in neurology 21
phenylpropanolamine interactions with MIBG 532
pheochromocytoma 531–5, 843
  incidental, prevalence 529
  somatostatin receptors 33, 533–4
phlebotomy, polycythemia vera 775, 778
phobia, social 430
phospholipids, autoantibodies to, and venous thromboembolism risk 207
phosphorus-32 773–9
  adverse effects 778
  bone pain 765
  polycythemia vera 775, 778–9
photodiodes
  avalanche 857
  scintillation detectors 849, 850
photomultiplier (PMT)
  PET gamma camera 857
  scintillation detectors 849, 850
  SPECT gamma camera 852, 853–4
    position-sensitive PMTs 863–4
photon attenuation/scattering/interaction with matter 869–70
physical abuse (non-accidental injury), children 117, 367, 406–8
physical stress test 152
physicochemical interactions, radiopharmaceutical–drug 824

physis *see* growth plates
PIB (Pittsburgh Compound-B)
  ^{11}C-, Alzheimer's disease 22, 841–2
  ^{18}F-, Alzheimer's disease 842
pilocytic astrocytoma 450
pinhole collimator 852
PIOPED *see* prospective investigation of pulmonary embolism diagnosis
pipobroman, polycythemia vera 775
pisiform fracture 366
Pittsburgh Compound-B *see* PIB
pituitary gland
  hypothyroidism due to 494
  tumors 31
    ACTH-secreting 31, 523
PK11195, 421
  ^{11}C- 421, 457, 842
placental alkaline phosphatase 602
plafond fracture, tibial 369–70
plain X-rays/radiography, skeletal metastases 340, 342
planar imaging
  osteoarthritis 394
  somatostatin receptors 30
  tumors
    staging 15
    therapeutic response 17
plantar fasciitis 368–9
plasma clearance 269
  of filtration markers and radiopharmaceuticals 275
  iron 679–80
plasma flow, effective renal (ERPF) 273
plasma volume 681
platelet(s)
  destruction 687–90
  glycoprotein IIb/IIIa receptor antagonist 832–3
  mean life survival 689
  pooling in spleen 685, 687, 689, 690
  radiolabeled, splenic imaging 686
    predicting response to splenectomy 687, 689
  see also thrombocytopenia; thrombocytopenic purpura
platelet factor 4 (PF4) 99
pleural disease 223
  mesothelioma 223–4
plexopathy, brachial, breast cancer 552
plexus, pelvic, penile erection and 576
Plummer's disease (multiple toxic adenomas/autonomous nodules) 496, 501–2
  treatment 501–2, 730
PMMA components in prosthetic joints 381
pneumococcal (*S. pneumoniae*) pneumonia 240, 247
Pneumocystis carinii pneumonia (PCP) 240, 241–2, 245, 246, 247
pneumonia
  Pneumocystis carinii (PCP) 240, 241–2, 245, 246, 247
  Streptococcus pneumonia (pneumococcal) 240, 247
    point-based image registration 862
    polycystic kidney disease (PKD), children 115, 117
    polycythemia (erythrocytosis) 676
    causes 677
      secondary 677
    relative (pseudo-polycythemia) 676, 678–9, 681
    true (polycythemia vera) 678, 680, 773–9
      leukemia and 774, 778
      non-radionuclide therapy 773–4
      radionuclide therapy 775, 778–9
polyethylene, ultrahigh molecular weight, prosthetic joints 381
polymethylmethacrylate components in prosthetic joints 381
polymorphic epithelial mucin antigen 602
polyostotic Paget's disease of bone 356, 357

polyphosphates, structure 816
polysplenia 692
popliteal node visualization 718, 720
position-sensitive photomultipliers 863–4
positive predictive value (PPV) 803, 804
positron, in PET, emission and interactions 855
positron emission tomography (PET) 9–11, 791–8, 839–46, 855–8
    adrenal gland
        incidentaloma 530
        pheochromocytoma 534–5
    attenuation correction see attenuation correction
    basic principles 855–7
    bile duct carcinoma 665–6
    bone marrow imaging 681
    breast see breast cancer
    cardiology/cardiac disease 11, 841
        congenital heart disease 171
        myocardial perfusion 150, 157
    cost-effectiveness see cost-effectiveness
    FDG in see FDG
    ferrokinetics (using ^{52}Fe) see iron-52
    gamma cameras for 855–8
    gastrointestinal cancer 68, 645–51
        neuroendocrine tumor staging/restaging 654, 655
    head and neck cancer 471–5
        follow-up examinations 472–3, **Plate 11A.1**
        lymph node involvement 472
        primary tumor 471–2
        whole-body imaging 472
    infection and inflammation 95–8
        prosthetic joint 388
    liver cancer
        metastatic 667–9, 670
        primary 662–5
    lung cancer 227–33, 234–5
        distant metastases 227
        impact on management and cost-effectiveness 227–30
        recurrence/relapse 230
        staging 63–4, 226–7
        therapeutic response monitoring 57, 60
    lung nodule (solitary) 224–5, 225–6
    lung non-neoplastic disorders 239
        sarcoidosis 244–5
    lymphoma see lymphoma
    molecular imaging (in general) 8, 9–11
    myocardial
        perfusion assessment 19
        viability assessment 166, 185, 187–8
    neurology 11
        cerebrovascular disease 426
        degenerative disease 841–2
        dementias 416, 418, 419
        epilepsy 20, 22, 435, 436–9
        movement disorders 457–64
        tumors see brain tumors
    new agents 839–46
    ovarian cancer 604
    patient preparation for imaging with 794
    pitfalls and artifacts 791–8
    pleural disease incl. mesothelioma 233–4
    prostate cancer 611
    radionuclides used 10
    radiopharmaceuticals used
        adverse reactions 824
        drug interactions 826
    renal tumors 322–4

skeleton 332, 333, 841
    metastases 338, 344–6
    Paget's disease 357
small high-resolution PET scanners 858
technological advances 857–8
testicular tumors 570–2
tumors (in general) 13, 14
    staging 15
    treatment planning 16
    treatment response 17, 57–71
positron emission tomography/computed tomography 795–6, 857–8, 872
    brain tumors 452–3
    breast cancer 552–3
    cardiology 11, 157–8, 169
    head and neck cancer 473, **Plate 11A.2**
    image registration 864
    lung cancer 232–3
    lymphoma 706, 707, **Plates 16C.3–4**, **Plates 16C.8–11**
    molecular imaging 11
        tumor treatment planning 16
    pediatric oncology 118
    problems incl. artifacts 795–6
    skeletal metastases 344–6
    X-ray data and transmission of photons in 872
positron emission tomography/single photon emission computed tomography camera 857
post-synaptic muscarinic imaging 421
post-traumatic stress syndrome 430
PR1A3 and colorectal cancer 49
    ^{99m}Tc-labeled 50
precuneus and Alzheimer's disease 417
predictive value (PV) of tests 803, 804
pregnancy
    pulmonary embolism risk 216–18
    thyroid in
        disease and its management 500, 731
        functional assessment 494
    urinary tract infection in childhood and its impact on 288
    VQ scan risk 199, 216–17
preoperative therapy see entries under neoadjuvant
pressure measurements, antegrade perfusion of renal pelvis with 306
pre-synaptic muscarinic imaging 421
prevalence of disease
    accuracy of test and 802
    predictive value of test and 803
    sensitivity or specificity of test and 803
Prinzmetal's angina 159
processing of data 874–5
prognosis, tumor 13
    see also specific tumors
programmed cell death see apoptosis
progressive aphasia, primary 419
progressive supranuclear palsy 459
proliferation measures, lung cancer 64
propranolol, hyperthyroidism 493, 500
prospective investigation of pulmonary embolism diagnosis (PIOPED) 207, 213, 216
    modified 219
Prostascint (^{111}In-CYT-356; capromab pendetide) 42, 610, 612–14, 617–18, **Plates 13H.2–5**
prostate cancer/carcinoma 68–9, 609–18
    epidemiology 609
    imaging 609–14, **Plates 13H.1–6**
        local recurrence 611
        metastatic disease 611–12

prostate cancer/carcinoma (*contd*)
  imaging (*contd*)
    primary disease 611
    therapeutic response monitoring 57, 68–9, 82, 612
  skeletal metastases 339, 340, 342, 344, 349–50, 609, 612
prostate-specific antigen 82, 344, 610, 612
prostate-specific membrane antigen 82, 610
Prostatec (^{99m}Tc-CYT-351) 610, **Plate 13H.1**
prostheses, joint *see* arthroplasty
protein(s)
  tracer-labeled 6–7
    hematology 681
  transport in lymph 716
protein C, activated, resistance 207
protein-losing enteropathy 643, 681
pseudoarthrosis 375–6
pseudofractures, osteomalacia 359
pseudo-obstruction, renal graft 317
pseudo-polycythemia 676, 678–9, 681
psychiatric disturbances, children 113
psychogenic erection 576
psychogenic parkinsonism 460
PTSN, ^{67}Cu 841
pubic bone, osteitis 364, 373–4
pudendal arteries 594
  internal, angiography in impotence 577
pulmonary non-vascular disorders/problems *see* lung
pulmonary vessels/circulation
  anatomy 198
  blood flow 198
    pediatric 115
  CT angiography *see* computed tomography angiography
  embolism *see* embolism
  hypoxic vasoconstriction 198–9
pulmonary-to-systemic flow ratios (Qp:Qs) in congenital heart disease
    170, 171
pulse pile-up, SPECT gamma camera 853
pyelonephritis, pediatric 284
  case history 292–4
pyrexia *see* fever of unknown origin

QGS (software) 155
qualitative SPECT 875–6
quality-adjusted life years (QALYs) 807, 808
quantitative CT, bone mass measurement 399
quantitative SPECT 876, 877

raclopride, ^{11}C- 842
  multiple system atrophy **Plate 10E.1**
  Parkinson's disease **Plate 10E.1**
radiation detectors *see* detectors
radiation exposure and its burden
  lymphoscintigraphy, protection 134
  pediatric 110
  salivary glands (in thyroid cancer therapy) 483–4
  VQ scan 199, 202, 203, 219
    in pregnancy 199, 217–18
  see also dose
radiation therapy *see* radiotherapy
radiofrequency ablation, liver metastases 668–9
radiography, plain, skeletal metastases 340, 342
radioimmunoscintigraphy (in cancer) 39–55
  clinical protocols and data analysis 47–8
  clinical studies 48–9
    colorectal cancer 7, 49–52, **Plates 1C.2–3**
    neuroblastoma 45–6, 756, **Plate 1C.1**

ovarian cancer 602–3
  prostate cancer 610, 611, 612–14, 617–18, **Plates 13H.2–5**
factors required 39–46
radiolabels 44–7
radioimmunoscintigraphy (in infection and inflammation) 94–5
  P. carinii pneumonia 246–7
radioimmunotherapy 39, 81, 85–6
  neuroblastoma 756, 759
  non-Hodgkin-lymphoma 6, 85–6
  ovarian cancer 604
  renal tumors 324–6
radioiodine *see* iodine-123; iodine-131; thyroid tumors
radiolabel(s) (for tracers)
  labeling with
    antibodies 46
    colloids for lymphoscintigraphy 132
    red blood cells (with pertechnetate) 622
    red blood cells (with pertechnetate), drug interactions affecting
      827
  in radioimmunoscintigraphy 44–7
  see also radiopharmaceuticals
radionecrosis, brain tumor treated areas 449
radionuclide therapy (cancer/proliferative disorders and in general)
    79–91, 725–88, 835–6
  administration 90–1
    personnel for 90
  antibodies in *see* radioimmunotherapy
  bone pain *see* bone pain
  booking method 89
  dose *see* dose
  follow-up 91
  guidelines 89–91
  imaging for 79–82
    intracellular localization 81–2
    principles of localization 80–1
  indications/contraindications 89
  individualization 86
  neuroblastoma 755–63
  neuroendocrine tumors 34, 69, 82, 95, 535, 536
  new agents
    PET 839–46
    SPECT 835–6
  ordering of radiopharmaceutical 89–90
  ovarian cancer 604–5
  patient preparation 90
  polycythemia vera 775, 778–9
  post-therapy scan 91
  preparation and dose measurement 90
  referrers 89
  renal tumors 324–6
  somatostatin analogs *see* somatostatin receptors
  suite decontamination 91
  thyroid cancer 83–5
  waiting time and medication 89
radionuclide therapy (thyroid gland disorders) 727–43
radiopharmaceuticals and radiotracers (incl. radiolabeled ligands)
    813–46
  adrenal cortex 522–3
  atherosclerotic plaque 20
  biliary imaging 643–4, 817
  bone (and bone scans) 332–4, 338, 355, 816
  bone pain palliation 80, 765–6
  breast scintigraphy 545, 559
  cardiology
    myocardial perfusion imaging 149–50, 817
    non-perfusion imaging 150–1

general aspects 5–6, 8–9, 813–46
  concept/principle of (incl. historical perspectives) 5–9, 815
  dose *see* dose
  functional imaging agents *see* functional imaging
  interactions and adverse reactions *see* adverse effects; drug
    interactions
  in PET *see* positron emission tomography
  in SPECT *see* single photon emission computed tomography
  hematology 675
  hepatic imaging 817
  infection and inflammation 93–5, 97–100
    new agents 832–3
  injection *see* injection
  lachrymal gland 485–7
  lymphoscintigraphy 716
    colloids *see* colloids
    newer agents 135
  neuroendocrine tumors 655–7
  neurology
    cerebral blood flow estimation 425–6, 817–18
    neuropharmacologic studies 21
    tumors 450
  renal studies 260–2, 282, 816
    captopril intervention in hypertension 300
    children 282
    outflow resistance measurement 310
    pharmacokinetics 275
    transplant recipients 316
    tumors 321
  splenic imaging 686
  testicular scans 596
  therapeutic use *see* radionuclide therapy
  thyroid scan 492
  ventilation imaging 200–5
  see also radiolabels
radiotherapy (radiation therapy - external beam)
  brain tumor
    hypermetabolic areas 440–50
    testicular tumors 570, 571
  dosimetry 781
  ^{18}F-FDG imaging after, false interpretation 795
  gastrointestinal neuroendocrine tumors 657
  head and neck cancer, planning **Plate 11A.2**
  image registration in planning of 863
  monitoring 82
    breast cancer 65, 66
    colorectal carcinoma 67
    lung cancer 63, 64, 230–2
    parameters for 61
    prostate cancer 612
  neuroblastoma 755
    combined with ^{131}I-MIBG therapy 757–8
  thyroid cancer, adjunct to $_{131}$I therapy 739
  see also brachytherapy; chemoradiotherapy; radionuclide
    therapy
radium-223, bone pain 766, 769
radius
  growth plate injuries 365
  sports injuries 375
rapid urease test 642
Rasmussen's syndrome 439
reabsorption, renal 254
REAL (revised European American classification of lymphoid
    neoplasms) 696
Reaven syndrome 158
receiver operating characteristic curve 804–6

receptors 8–9
  peptide *see* peptides, radiolabeled
  as targets 5–6
    brain *see* brain
    breast cancer *see* breast cancer
    cell membrane 81
    head and neck cancer 469–71
    in infection and inflammation 97–100
    neuroendocrine tumor *see subheading above*
    peptide *see* peptides, radiolabeled
  as targets with neuroendocrine tumors 31, 34, 68, 69, 85, 658–9,
    745–53
    neuroblastoma 756
RECIST (Response Evaluation Criteria in Solid Tumors) criteria 58, 59
rectocele 641
rectum
  cancer *see* colorectal cancer
  fecal emptying 640–1
red blood cells
  ^{51}Cr- *see* chromium-51-labeled red cells
  destruction 679, 690–1
  heat-damaged, splenic imaging 686
  ^{131}In- *see* indium-111-labeled blood cells
  iron utilization 680
  life span, mean (MRCLS) 676, 677
  splenic, pooling 676, 678–9, 686
  ^{99m}Tc- 622–3, 676
    blood group compatibility testing 678
    gastrointestinal bleeding 622–3
    phallography 579, 580
    prostate cancer 611
    technique of production *see* radiolabels
  volume 676–7
  increased *see* polycythemia
red marrow:blood absorbed dose ratio 785
reflex sympathetic dystrophy 365, 397
  children 408
region of interest (ROI) 61
  breast cancer 66
  cystography (indirect radionuclide) 286
  epilepsy, PET 437
  renal scintigraphy
    dynamic 285
    static 283
    transplant recipient 316, 319
  salivary gland functional imaging 483
renal artery narrowing/stenosis
  angiographic 298
  interventions 301–2
  transplanted kidney 318
renal cell carcinoma 322, 323, **Plate 8G.1**
  mouse **Plate 1A.1**
renal problems/disorders *see* kidney
renography/renal scintigraphy (and activity–time curve) 256, 258, 306–7
  characteristics and reporting of abnormal renogram 256
  children 116–17, 282–4, 285
    dynamic 112, 116–17, 285
    static 112, 117, 282–4
  diuretic *see* diuretic renography
  hypertension 298, 299
    captopril intervention 301
renovascular disorders
  functional changes in renovascular disorder 300
  hypertension due to 297–302
    assessment 298
    captopril renal radionuclide study 300–2, 826

reporter genes 7–8, 71
reproductive tract *see* genital/reproductive tract
residence time *see* transit function
resistor-coupled network, SPECT gamma camera 853
resources, sentinel node biopsy 134
respiratory center, medulla oblongata 198
respiratory disease *see* lung
respiratory distress syndrome, adult 240, 243
Response Evaluation Criteria in Solid Tumors criteria (RECIST) 58, 59
reticuloendothelial system 682
retinoic acid therapy, dedifferentiated thyroid cancer 739
retrosternal goiters 509
retuximab (ibritumomab tiuxetan), ^{90}Y- (=Zevalin) 42, 85
revascularization, coronary 164–5, 184–5, **Plates 6A.17–19**
revised European American classification of lymphoid neoplasms (REAL) system 696
rhenium-186, bone pain 80, 766, 768, 769
rhenium-188, bone pain 80, 766, 768, 769
rheumatoid arthritis 393
rheumatology 393–402
ribs
    fractures 374
    metastases 338, 339, 340
right-to-left shunt in congenital heart disease 170, 171
rituximab 42
RP128 (tuftsin receptor ligand) 101
RP517 (LTB$_4$ receptor antagonist) 100
rubidium-81 generator for ^{81m}Kr 202, 203
rubidium-82 (myocardial perfusion) 150
    myocardial viability assessment 166

S value (radiation absorbed dose) 782, 783
sacral fractures 367–8
sacroiliac joint, ankylosing spondylitis 395
salivary glands 483–4, **Plate 11B.1**
    functional imaging 483–4
        infant maturation and its effects on 111–12
    tumors 484
samarium-153, bone pain 766, 769
sarcoidosis 243–5
    pulmonary 243–5
    somatostatin receptors and analogs (incl. octreotide) 34, 243
sarcoma
    Ewing's 348
    Kaposi's (KS) 246
    osteogenic *see* osteosarcoma
    see also angiosarcoma
scaphoid fracture 366
    avascular necrosis associated with 366, 397
    child 365
    sports 375
Schilling test 641, 681
schizophrenia 429–30
scintillation detectors 849–50, 872
    coupled to focused collimators 854
    crystals *see* crystals
    performance comparisons with other detectors 851
scintimammography (mammoscintigraphy) 545–9, 559–62
    indications 560–1
    results of trials 560
    technique 550
screening
    asymptomatic patients for disease 799
    breast cancer 128, 544
    colorectal cancer 646
    coronary artery disease 157–8
    ovarian tumors 601

Screening for Heart Attack Prevention and Education (SHAPE) 157
scrotum, acute
    clinical presentation 593
    etiology/pathogenesis 593
    perfusion imaging *see* perfusion imaging
sedation, child 111
SeHCAT (23-seleno-25-homotaurocholic acid) 641
seizures *see* epilepsy
selenium-75 compounds
    23-seleno-25-homotaurocholic acid (SeHCAT) 641
    6β-selenomethyl-19-norcholesterol *see* SMC
semantic dementia 419
semiconductor detectors 850–1
    gamma cameras with 854–5
    performance comparisons with other detectors 851
seminoma
    residual masses 571
    therapy 570–1
sensitivity of test 802–3, 804
sentinel lymph nodes 121–39
    biopsy 121
        breast cancer 551
        complications 134
        development/procedure 121–2
        resources 134
        standards 134
    definition 122
    imaging 121–39
        breast cancer 127–33, 551, 562–4
        future developments 134–5
        lymphoscintigraphy *see* lymphoscintigraphy
    marking 124
        melanoma 125
septic arthritis, children 405
seronegative arthropathies 396
serotonin (5-HT)
    in carcinoid syndrome/with carcinoid tumors 654, 843
    transporter binding 429
sesamoid injuries 370
sestamibi (MIBI), ^{99m}Tc-
    bone/skeletal tumors
        primary, child 409
        secondary (metastases) 338
    breast cancer 545, 546–7, 559
        locally advanced 561, 562
        lymph nodes 547–8
        non-invasive 561
    head and neck cancer 469
    hepatocellular carcinoma 665
    lymphoma 695, 698, 701
    myocardium
        cell metabolism 166
        hibernation **Plate 6A.20**
        perfusion scan 149–50, **Plate 6A.3**
        viability assessment 185, 186–7
    ovarian cancer 604
    pulmonary nodule (solitary) 224, 225
    therapeutic response monitoring 58
        breast cancer multidrug resistance 66
    see also ERASE; INSPIRE
sex *see* gender
sexual function
    disorders *see* impotence; infertility
    nerves subserving, males 576
SHAPE (Screening for Heart Attack Prevention and Education) 157
shin splints 371

shoulder, sports injuries 375
shunts, congenital heart disease 170–1, **Plate 6A.22**
sickle cell disease 692
siderophore–gallium complex, prosthetic joint infection 383
signalling pathways, cell 7
sildenafil 582
single-breath steady-state technique 201
single-modal 3-D change statistical detection, prostate cancer
    imaging 613
single photon absorptiometry, bone mass measurement 398
single photon emission computed tomography (SPECT) 831–8,
    852–5
  attenuation correction *see* attenuation correction
  bone, thoracic vertebrae 875–6
  bone metastases 341
    radiopharmaceuticals 338
  breast cancer 546
  gamma cameras 852–5
  liver cancer
    metastases 669–70
    primary 665
  lung 239
    solitary nodule 224–5
  lymphoscintigraphy, melanoma 124
  molecular imaging 8
    somatostatin receptors 30
    tumor staging 15
    tumor therapeutic response monitoring 58
  musculoskeletal disorders
    ankylosing spondylitis 395–6
    children 404–5, 411
    femoral head avascular necrosis 396
    knee injuries 372, 373
    metastases *see* skeletal metastases *(subheading below)*
    osteoarthritis 394
    Paget's disease of bone 357
  myocardial perfusion 149, 154–6, 875
    acquisition and processing 154–6
    coronary artery disease prognosis and risk stratification
      161
    gated *see* gated myocardial perfusion SPECT
    hibernating myocardium 168, **Plate 6A.20**
    post-myocardial infarction risk stratification 162
    in syndrome X 158
    viability assessment 185, 186–7
  neuroendocrine tumors 655, 656
  neurology
    Alzheimer's disease 417, **Plates 10A.2–3**
    cerebrovascular disease 426–8
    dopaminergic system imaging 420m 420–1
    epilepsy 435, 436
    frontotemporal dementia 418
    healthy volunteer **Plate 10A.1**
    Lewy body dementia 420
    movement disorders 457–64
    psychiatric conditions 428–30
    tumors 447
  prostate cancer 610, 612
  qualitative 875–6
  quantitative 876, 877
  radioimmunoscintigraphy 47–8
    colorectal cancer 51
  radiopharmaceuticals in 831–8
    adverse effects 822–3
    drug interactions 824–6
    new agents 831–8
  renal tumors 321

single photon emission computed tomography/computed tomography
    872
  image registration 864
  molecular imaging 9, 18–19
  myocardium 18–19, 157, 169
  pediatric musculoskeletal disorders 405
  prostate cancer 612–13
  radioimmunoscintigraphy 47, 48
  X-ray data and transmission of photons in 872
single-headed gamma camera in SPECT 870
size, tumor
  scintimammography and 546–7
  in therapeutic response monitoring 61
  in TNM staging *see* T
  see also volume
skeletal muscle, ^{18}F-FDG uptake 793–4
skeleton
  metastases *see* bone metastases
  radionuclide uptake 332–4, 355
  structure and physiology 332–3
  see also bone
skin
  injection of radiocolloids for lymphoscintigraphy *see* injections
  trabecular carcinoma 32
  see also dermis
skull, Paget's disease 356
SM3 (stripped mucin core antigen) 602, 603
small bowel/intestine
  bacterial overgrowth 642
  bleeding 626
  ^{18}F-FDG uptake 792
  lymphoma 698
  transit 639
small-cell lung cancer 233
  somatostatin receptors 32
small high-resolution PET scanners 858
small vessel vascular disease, dementia 418
SMC (6β-[^{75}S]selenomethyl-19-norcholesterol) 522
  adrenal incidentaloma 529
  technical data on use 524–5
social anxiety disorder 430
sodium iodide
  ^{131}I-
    adverse reactions 823
    thyroid cancer metastatic disease treatment 786
  thallium-doped *see* thallium-doped sodium iodide
soft tissue sports injuries
  ankle/foot 368–9
  knee 372–3
  thigh/hip/pelvis 373–4
  tibial region 371
  wrist/hand 375
software
  myocardial perfusion SPECT 155
  neuroimaging
    Alzheimer's disease 417
    tumors 452
solid-state detectors *see* detectors
somatic nervous system, penis 576
somatostatin, structure 818
somatostatin receptors (and ligands/analogs) 29–34, 745–53
  analogs available 29–30, 34, 745–53
    see also specific analogs
  non-neoplastic disease 34
    sarcoidosis 34, 244
  normal findings and artifacts 30–1
  pulmonary nodule (solitary) 224–5

somatostatin receptors (and ligands/analogs) (contd)
  tumors 31–3
    adrenal pheochromocytoma 33, 533–4
    brain 33, 447
    breast 33, 545
    carcinoid 7, 10, 31, 653–4, **Plate 1D.4**
    head and neck 469
    liver metastases 669–70
    lymphoma 33, 701–2
    neuroendocrine tumors *see* neuroendocrine tumors
    as non-nuclear therapeutic targets 657
    as radionuclide therapeutic targets *see* neuroendocrine tumors
    staging 834
sonography *see* ultrasound
source–detector solid angle (dΩ) 849
spatial resolution
  PET gamma camera 856
  SPECT gamma camera 852–3
specificity of test 802–3, 804
SPECT *see* single photon emission computed tomography
sperm/spermatozoa
  count, and radioiodine therapy 739
  fertilization by 586–7
spermatic cord torsion 594
spermatocele 598
spherocytosis, hereditary 679, 690
spine (vertebral column)
  metastases, uterine carcinoma 345
  sports injury 374
  see also vertebrae
spiral CT, venous thromboembolism 208
spironolactone interactions with adrenocortical scintigraphic agents
    522–3, 526
spleen 685–94
  anatomy 685–6
    normal variants 686–7
  blood cell pooling 685–6
    platelets 685, 687, 689, 690
    red cells 676, 678–9, 686
  diseases directly involving 692–3
  ^{18}F-FDG uptake 792
  function (physiology) 685–6
    assessment 676, 686–91
  integrity assessment 686–7
  localization 686–7
  lymphoma 698, 703
splenectomy, response prediction 679, 687–92
splenomegaly 687, 688, 689, 690, 692
splenunculi 686–7
spondylitis, ankylosing 395–6
spondylodiscitis 95
spondylolysis 374
  pediatric 405
sports injuries 363, 368–75
squamous cell head and neck carcinoma *see* head and neck disease
staging (and restaging), tumors 13–15, 799
  breast cancer 564–5
  colorectal cancer 646
  esophageal cancer 545
  FDG in *see* FDG
  head and neck cancer 467–8
  hepatocellular carcinoma 661
  lung cancer 63, 223, 224, 226–7
  lymphoma *see* lymphoma
  neuroendocrine tumors 654–5
  new SPECT agents 834
  pancreatic cancer 646
  testicular tumors 569–70

standardized uptake value (SUV) of FDG
  adrenal incidentaloma 530
  head and neck cancer 471
  hepatocellular carcinoma 664
  therapeutic response monitoring 60, 62
    breast cancer 66
    lung cancer 64, 230
    sources of error 61
statins 165
statistical change detection, 3D, prostate cancer imaging 612–14
statistical parametric mapping 417
Steele–Richardson–Olszewski syndrome 459
stem cell transplantation following high-dose chemotherapy,
    autologous
  lymphoma 705
  neuroblastoma 758
stents
  coronary 164
    restenosis **Plate 6A.19**
  renal artery 302
stereotactic head frame 862
sternal metastases 339
steroids and fracture risk 400
STICH (Surgical Treatment of Ischemic Congestive Heart Failure) trial
    168
stomach
  carcinoma, therapeutic response monitoring 57, 68
  emptying 638–9
  infant maturation and its effects on functional imaging 111–12
Streptococcus pneumonia (pneumococcal) pneumonia 240, 247
stress fractures
  calcaneus 370
  children 365
  fibula 372
  hip 373
  metatarsals 370
  pars interarticularis 374
  pathophysiology 363
  pelvis 373
  sesamoid 370
  tibia 371, 372
stress testing 151–4, **Plates 6A.6–8, Plates 6A.10–13**
  choice 154
  coronary artery disease prognosis and risk stratification 161
  exercise/treadmill *see* exercise stress test
  image interpretation 155
  pharmacological *see* pharmacological stress test
  post-myocardial infarction risk stratification 162
stripped mucin core antigen (SM3) 602, 603
stroke
  acute ischemic 426–7, **Plate 10B.1**
  rehabilitation and prediction of functional recovery 428
strontium-89, bone pain 80, 765–6, 768, 769
  toxicity 769, 770
struma ovarii (ectopic thyroid tissue in ovarian tumor) 498, 503, 604
Sturge–Weber syndrome, generalized seizures 439
subarachnoid hemorrhage 427, **Plate 4.3**
sublingual thyroid 508–9
substance P receptors and analogs 35
sulesomab, ^{99m}Tc- (Leukoscan) 42, 94, 832
  infected joint replacement 95
sulfur colloid, ^{99m}Tc- 123
  imaging with infected joint replacement 386–8
  lymphoscintigraphy 123
sum of absolute differences 863
supradiaphragmatic node metastases, testicular cancer 569
supranuclear palsy, progressive 459
suprapubic injections, cystoscintigraphy 287

surface-based image registration 862
surface counting
    ^{59}Fe- 680
    spleen in anemia 690–1
surface projection mapping 417
surgery
    renal artery stenosis 301–2
    in thyroid cancer, follow-up after 68
    treatment before/after *see entries under* neoadjuvant; adjuvant
    see also specific procedures
Surgical Treatment of Ischemic Congestive Heart Failure (STICH)
        trial 168
sympathetic nervous system
    cardiac 151, 189, 841
    penis 576
    see also reflex sympathetic dystrophy
symptomatic patients, detection and diagnosis of 799
synapse 6
syndrome X
    cardiac 158
    metabolic 158
systole
    LV function, coronary artery disease outcome and 161
    surface views **Plate 6B.2**

T (primary tumor in TNM staging)
    breast cancer 547
        PET imaging and 550, 551
    head and neck cancer 467–8
    lung cancer 224, 226
T scores/values
    bone densitometry 399–400
    functional MRI in temporal lobe epilepsy 438
talus
    avascular necrosis 396
    sports fractures 369
tamoxifen monitoring, breast cancer 66, 553
targets in molecular imaging 6
    see also receptors
tarsal bones
    coalition 371
    fracture 370
tau protein and Alzheimer's disease 22, 24
teamwork, pediatric imaging 110
teboroxime, ^{99m}Tc-, myocardial perfusion scan 149
technegas generator particles 205
    pulmonary embolism 215
technetium-99m-labeled compounds
    annexin V *see* annexin V
    antimicrobials 101
        prosthetic joint infection 388
    apcitide 832–3
    bombesin, prostate cancer 614
    brain death in children 113
    brain tumors 447
    cardiology
        congenital heart disease 171
        myocardial hypoxia imaging 151
        myocardial perfusion scans 149–50
        myocardial viability assessment 166, 186–7
    cerebral blood flow estimation 425
    colloids *see* colloids
    complement factor 5a 99–100
    CYT-351 (Prostatec) 610, **Plate 13H.1**
    depreotide *see* depreotide
    DISIDA *see* DISIDA
    DMSA *see* DMSA
    dose for children 109

DTPA *see* DTPA
DTPA-mannosyl-dextran 135
ECD *see* ECD
Fab' fragment, *P. carinii* pneumonia 247
head and neck cancer 469
HMPAO *see* HMPAO
human neutrophil peptide-1 102
interleukin-2 100
interleukin-8 99
isonitriles *see* isonitriles
MAG$_3$ *see* MAG$_3$
MDP *see* MDP
mebrofenin, adverse reactions 823
medronate, adverse reactions 823
mertiatide, adverse reactions 823
MIBI *see* sestamibi
monoclonal antibodies 46
    breast cancer axillary node status 134
    colorectal cancer 50
    infected joint replacement 388
monocyte chemoattractant protein-1 101
octreotate (HYNICTATE), neuroendocrine tumors 656–7
octreotide, neuroendocrine tumors 656–7
oxidronate, adverse reactions 823
pentetate, adverse reactions 823
pertechnetate *see* pertechnetate
platelet factor 4 fragment (P483) 99
prostate cancer 610–11
protein-losing enteropathy 681
pulmonary nodule (solitary) 224–5
renal studies 260–1
    captopril intervention in hypertension 300
    case history 302
    outflow resistance measurement 310
RP128 (tuftsin receptor ligand) 101
skeletal imaging 332–3
sulesomab *see* sulesomab
TRODAT 458, 836
ubiquicidin fragment 102
in VQ scan 199
    aerosol ventilation 203–6
    dual imaging with ^{81m}Kr and 202
technetium-99m-labeled leukocytes 94
    infected joint replacement 388
    inflammatory bowel disease 629, 630, 631
    rheumatoid arthritis 393
technology and instrumentation 847–79
    new, introduction 800
temporal lobe
    epilepsy 425, **Plate 10C.1**
        children 439
        perfusion **Plates 10B.1–3**
        PET 22, 436
    medial, Alzheimer's disease and 417
    see also frontotemporal dementia; parietotemporal association areas
tenascin, ^{131}I-labeled MAb, glioma **Plate 21B.1**
    therapeutic use 449–50
tendon injuries/associated pathology
    ankle/foot 368
    hand 366
    wrist/hand 375
teratoma
    ovarian 604
    testicular, mature differentiated (MTD) 570, 571
testicles 569–74, 593–600
    normal scan 596
    perfusion imaging 593–600
    radioiodine therapy-associated dysfunction 739

testicles (*contd*)
  technique and image interpretation in scintigraphy 596–7
  torsion 593–6, 596–8
    anatomy and embryology relevant to 594–6
    clinical features 593–4
    extravaginal 593–4
    intravaginal 594
  tumors 569–74, 598
    diagnosis and staging 569–70
    imaging at diagnosis 570, 598
    residual/recurrent disease 571–2
testicular artery 594
1,4,7,10-tetraazacyclododecane-1,4,7,10-tetraacetic acid *see* DOTA
tetrofosmin, ^{99m}Tc-
  breast cancer 545, 559
  head and neck cancer 469
  myocardial imaging 817
    cell metabolism 166
    perfusion 149, 150
  pulmonary nodule (solitary) 224, 225
thallium-201
  bone tumor
    primary, child 409, 410
    secondary (metastases) 338
  brain tumor 447
  breast cancer 545, 559
  head and neck cancer 468
  Kaposi's sarcoma 246
  lymphoma 695, 698, 701
  myocardial perfusion 149, 817, **Plates 6A.7–8, Plate 6A.10, Plate 6A.12, Plates 6A.18–19**
    myocardial viability assessment 166, 185, 186, 187
thallium-doped sodium iodide (NaI(Tl)) detectors 849, 850
  PET camera 857
  SPECT camera 853
6-thia-hepta-decanoic acid, ^{18}F- 151
thigh injuries 373–4
thoracic spine
  sports injury 374
  vertebrae, attenuation correction in SPECT 875–6
thorax *see* chest
3F8 (MAb), ^{131}I- 756
three-dimensional mode, positron camera 857
three-dimensional statistical change detection, prostate cancer imaging 612–14
three-dimensional tumor dosimetry 784
three-headed gamma camera in SPECT 870
thrombocytopenia 687, 690
  ^{131}I-MIBG-induced 759
  radioisotope (for bone pain)-induced 769–70
thrombocytopenic purpura, idiopathic 685, 690, 691
thromboembolism *see* embolism; venous thromboembolism
thrombolytic/fibrinolytic therapy
  acute ischemic stroke 426
  acute myocardial infarction, prognostication 163
thymidine, ^{11}C- 843
  therapeutic response monitoring 58, 843
    lung cancer 65
  see also fluorothymidine
thymus, ^{18}F-FDG activity 792
thyroglobulin levels in thyroid remnant ablation with ^{131}I 735
  post-treatment monitoring 738–9
thyroid 491–510, 727–43
  classification of diseases 491–2
  dysfunction (non-neoplastic pathology) 728–9
    diagnosis 492–5
    see also hyperthyroidism; hypothyroidism

  ectopic *see* ectopic tissue
  enlargement *see* goiter
  impalpable, and thyrotoxicosis 498
  mass/nodule 114
  pediatric imaging 114–15
  remnant ablation with ^{131}I (in cancer) 734–6
thyroid hormones 727–8
  in hyperthyroidism, administration in block/replacement therapy 494, 500
  in hyperthyroidism, levels 492–3
    post-treatment 493
  in hypothyroidism, levels 493, 494
    neonates 495
  in hypothyroidism, replacement therapy 494
    excess administration causing hyperthyroidism 502–3
    in Hashimoto's thyroiditis 508
    neonates 510
  synthesis and its regulation 727–8
  in thyroid cancer, replacement therapy
    discontinuance for scan following ^{131}I therapy 736
    reinstatement 738
thyroid-stimulating hormone (TSH)
  production and function 728
  receptor, autoantibodies 728
  recombinant, in thyroid cancer patients treated with ^{131}I 736
thyroid tumors (mainly cancer and incl. carcinoma) 32, 67–8, 81–2, 83–4, 733–9
  anaplastic *see* anaplastic thyroid cancer
  distant metastases 68, 83–4, 736, 737, 739, 786
  hyperthyroidism associated with 502–3
  medullary *see* medullary thyroid carcinoma
  nodules and likelihood of
    multiple 505
    solitary 503, 504, 507
  radioiodine (^{131}I) therapy 68, 82, 83, 84, 733–9
    dosimetry 735, 738, 784
    salivary gland pathology following 483–4
    see also iodine-123; iodine-131
  recurrence 79, 80
  therapeutic response monitoring 57, 59, 67–8
thyroidectomy in hyperthyroidism (incl. Graves' disease), subtotal 493, 499
thyroiditis
  acute 491
  acute suppurative 506
  atypical, vs anaplastic thyroid carcinoma 506
  autoimmune/Hashimoto's *see* Hashimoto's thyroiditis
  chronic 491
  subacute/de Quervain's *see* de Quervain's thyroiditis
thyrotoxicosis *see* hypothyroidism
thyroxine (T4)
  in hyperthyroidism, administration in block/replacement therapy 494, 500
  in hyperthyroidism, levels 492–3
    neonates 494
    post-treatment 493
  in hypothyroidism, levels 493, 494
  in hypothyroidism, replacement therapy 494
    in Hashimoto's thyroiditis 508
    neonates 510
  synthesis and its regulation 727–8
thyroxine-binding globulin, abnormal levels 493
tibial injuries 369, 370, 371–2
  children 406
tibialis posterior tendonitis 368
tibiofibular syndesmosis, injury 369, 370
time–activity curves (TACs)

penile 580, 581
rectal emptying 641
renal *see* renography
tin-117m (^{117m}Sn), bone pain 766, 769
TNM staging
    head and neck cancer 467–8
    lung cancer 63, 224, 226
    see also N; T
tositumomab 6, 42, 85–6
toxic goiter
    classification 492
    diffuse *see* Graves' disease
    nodular *see* Plummer's disease
toxicity *see* adverse effects
trabecular (cancellous) bone 331
    remodelling 332
trabecular carcinoma of skin 32
tracer *see* radiopharmaceuticals and radiotracers
transcervical hysteroscopy, infertility 587
transferrin
    ^{67}Ga binding to 93, 383, 698
    ^{111}In- 682
        protein-losing enteropathy 681
transgenic mice, molecular imaging 12
transient ischemic attacks 427
transit function (incl. residence/transit time), gastrointestinal 637–41
transit function (incl. residence/transit time), renal 254, 307
    measurement/analysis 254, 258–60, 262–3, 273–4
        in outflow resistance assessment 305, 310–11
transmission scanning 870–2
    processing of data 874–5
transplants *see* bone marrow; kidney; stem cell transplantation; vascular
        grafts
trapezium fracture 366
trastuzamab (Herceptin) 42
    ovarian cancer 604
trauma *see* injury
treadmill stress test *see* exercise stress test
tremor, essential 460
tri-iodothyronine (T3)
    in hyperthyroidism, administration in block/replacement therapy
        494, 500
    in hyperthyroidism, levels 492–3
        post-treatment 493
    in hypothyroidism, levels 493
    synthesis and its regulation 727–8
trimetazidine 167
triple-headed gamma camera in SPECT 870
TRODAT, ^{99m}Tc- 458, 836
tropanes (cocaine derivatives), dopaminergic system imaging
        420, 458
TSH *see* thyroid-stimulating hormone
tubules, renal
    acute necrosis (ATN) in transplant recipients 315, 316, 317
    captopril effects 300
tuftsin 101
tumor(s) (primarily malignant/cancer) 833–5
    dosimetry 783–4
    drug treatment *see* anticancer drugs
    ^{18}F-FDG imaging, false interpretation 794–5
        post-therapy 795
    ^{131}I therapy-induced 739
    molecular imaging (in general) 12–18
        drug discovery 17–18
        molecular characterization 12–13
        prognostic information 13
        staging and restaging 13–15

therapeutic response *see subheading below*
    treatment planning 15–16
new agents
    PET 842–3
    SPECT 833–5
pediatric 118, 408–11
polycythemia vera-associated risk 774, 778–9
radioimmunoscintigraphy *see* radioimmunoscintigraphy
radionuclide therapy *see* radioimmunotherapy; radionuclide therapy
somatostatin receptors *see* somatostatin receptors
therapeutic optimization 835
therapeutic response monitoring and follow-up 16–17, 57–78, 82–3
    basic principles 58–61
    breast cancer 65–6, 548, 553, 561–2, **Plate 1D.3**
    children 409
    colorectal cancer 57, 66–7, 647, 648
    esophageal cancer 57, 68, 645–6
    gastrointestinal stromal tumors 57, 69, 648
    liver metastases 668–9
    lymphomas 57, 62–3, 64, 65, 698, 699, 704–6, **Plates 16C.9–11**
    new agents 834–5
    in radionuclide therapy 91
    testicular tumors 571–2
venous thromboembolism risk 207
VQ scan-associated risk of induction in pregnant women 217–18,
    219
see also specific sites and types
tumor markers
    antigens as *see* antigen
    ovarian cancer 601, 602
    prostate cancer 610
    testicular tumors, raised 571
tunica vaginalis and testicular torsion 594
two-headed gamma cameras *see* dual-headed gamma cameras
225.28S antimelanoma MAb 43
tyrosine
    ^{11}C-
        brain tumors 451
        therapeutic response monitoring 58
    DOPA synthesis from 530
    iodination 728
        defect 508
tyrosine kinase inhibitor with gastrointestinal stromal tumors 17–18

ubiquicidin fragment 102
UJI3A (MAb), radiolabeled 45, 756, **Plate 1C.1**
    therapeutic use 759
ulcerative colitis
    diagnosis 630
    differential diagnosis 631
    follow-up and complications 631
    severity of disease 631
ultrahigh molecular weight polyethylene, prosthetic joints 381
ultrasound (US; sonography)
    breast cancer 544
    infertility 588
    intravascular coronary 164
    leg, venous thromboembolism deep vein thrombosis 208
    liver cancer
        metastatic 667, 668
        primary 661–2
    renal transplant 316
    in sentinel node detection, guidance using 134
    testicular 598–9
    thyroid solitary nodule 503–4
    see also Doppler sonography; echocardiography
undifferentiated thyroid cancer *see* anaplastic thyroid cancer

United Kingdom, adverse events 823
   reports 822
United States, adverse events
   reports 822
   SPECT agents 822, 823
upper limb, sports injuries 375
uptake function of kidney 254, 306–8
   measurement 254, 257, 262
urea breath test 642
urease test, rapid 642
ureteric complication, renal graft 318
urinary catheterization for direct isotope cystography 287
urinary tract
   disorders
      glomerular filtration rate measurements 275
      infection *see* infection
      outflow tract obstruction *see* obstruction
   ^{18}F-FDG activity 792–3
   see also kidney
urine
   clearance/excretion in (renal excretion) 254, 269, 270
      ^{18}F-FDG 792
   output in renal transplants 316
urography, intravenous, in renovascular hypertension 299
uropathy, obstructive and obstructing *see* obstructive uropathy
uterus
   carcinoma, skeletal metastases 345
   fibroids 42
uveitis 34

variance of intensity ratios 862
vascular dementia 418
vascular grafts
   coronary bypass 164–5
   infection 97
vascular parkinsonism 459
vascular supply
   liver metastases 81
   penis 575–6
      impotence associated with *see* impotence
   testes 594
vasculitis 97
vasoactive intestinal peptide (VIP) 35
   analogs 35
   ^{123}I- 756
   tumors secreting 654
vasoconstriction, hypoxic 198–9
vasodilator stress testing 152–3
venolymphatic communications 719
venotomy (phlebotomy), polycythemia vera 775, 778
venous disease, lymphoscintigraphy 723
   Doppler ultrasound in addition to 722
venous drainage of penis 576
   occlusion/insufficiency 577
      non-radionuclide assessment for 577
      radionuclide assessment for 578, 579, 580, 581, 582
venous thromboembolism 197
   clinical presentation 207
   diagnosis 197, 206–20
      VQ imaging 197, 207, 207–16
   new SPECT agents 832–3
   origins 206–7
   risk factors 207
ventilation imaging 200–6
ventilation perfusion (VQ) imaging 199–206
   pediatric 115
   pulmonary embolism 197, 207, 209–16

   communication of PE risk post-test 216
   formation of post-test diagnosis 213–16
   interpretation 209–13, 219
   role of post-test investigations 218–20
ventilation perfusion (VQ) matching 198–9
ventricular function (and dysfunction) 18, 183–93
   left 183–93, **Plates 6A.15–16**
      algorithm for investigations 189
      in congenital heart disease 171
      coronary artery disease outcome and 161
      image interpretation 155
      post-myocardial infarction risk stratification 162
      reversing dysfunction 184–5
   right, in congenital heart disease 171
   see also specific parameters
ventricular septal defect 169
ventricular shunts in congenital heart disease 171
ventriculography, radionuclide **Plate 6B.1**
   equilibrium 183–4
vertebrae
   fractures (in general) 368
   fractures, pathological 368
      benign vs malignant 340–1
      osteoporosis 357–8
   osteomyelitis 95
   Paget's disease 355–6
   thoracic, attenuation correction in SPECT 875–6
vertebral column *see* spine
vesico-ureteric reflux
   direct radionuclide cystography 286, 287
   indirect radionuclide cystography 285
   renal damage in 288–9
vesicular monoamine transporter genes (*VMAT*) 654, 655
Vidas D dimer measurement 208, 213
VIP *see* vasoactive intestinal peptide
visual assessment of therapy response 61
vitamin B$_{12}$ (cyanocobalamin) 681
   deficiency 681
   malabsorption 641–2, 681
VMAT1/VMAT2 654, 655
volume (tumor) in therapeutic response monitoring 61, 62
   lung cancer radiotherapy 65
   see also size
volume of distribution, renal 273–5
   for filtration markers and renal radiopharmaceuticals 274, 275
voxel property-based image registration 862–3
VQ *see* ventilation perfusion
VUBBET scanner 858

Wada test 440
Warthin's tumor 484
'washout' rate, renal 254
water, ^{15}O- 841
   bone marrow imaging 681
   brain tumors 451
   myocardial perfusion 150
West syndrome 439
white blood cells *see* leukocytes
white matter, normal, FDG uptake in tumors relative to 448
WHO *see* World Health Organization
whole-body clearance 269
whole-body dosimetry 784–5
whole-body imaging
   breast cancer 549–50
   ^{18}F-FDG distribution 792
      child 793
   head and neck cancer 472

lymphoma 698, 700
    prostate cancer, bone pain palliation 767
    radioiodine scan 68
        ^{131}I-treated thyroid cancer patient 737
whole-body transit time for renal radiopharmaceuticals 274
whole kidney transit time (WKTT) 259–60
Wilms' tumor 117
Wilson's disease 460
women see females
World Health Organization (WHO)
    brain tumor grading 446
    lung cancer classification 63
    lymphoma classification 696
    sentinel node biopsy in melanoma 126
    tumor response assessment criteria 58, 59
wrist
    injuries 366
        children 365
        sports 375
    osteoarthritis 395

X-ray absorptiometry, dual energy 398–400
X-ray data in SPECT/CT 872

X-ray radiography, plain, skeletal metastases 340, 342
xanthine–adenosine interactions 826
xenon-127, penile blood pool imaging 578
xenon-133
    cerebral blood flow estimation 425
    penile blood pool imaging 578
    ventilation imaging 200–2

yttrium-90-conjugated to MAb
    chimeric G250 325
    ibritumomab tiuxetan (Zevalin) 42, 85
    ovarian cancer 604
yttrium-90-conjugated minigastrin 751
yttrium-90-conjugated somatostatin analogs, neuroendocrine tumor
        therapy 751
    lanreotide 750
    octreotide 658, 659, 747–50

Z scores (bone densitometry) 400
Zollinger–Ellison syndrome 31, 654